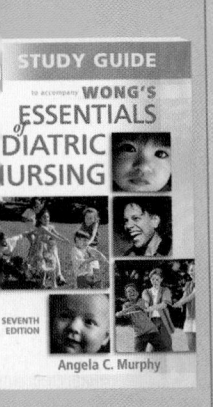
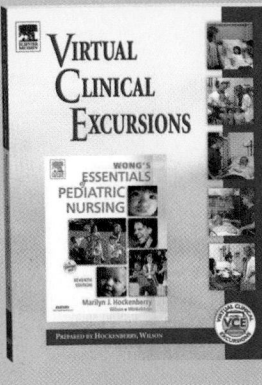

MUST-HAVE PEDIATRIC NURSING RESOURCES!

Get the most out of this text with these essential study tools!

Study Guide
Angela C. Murphy, PhD, RN
This companion **Study Guide** is designed to help you review the essential content in *Wong's Essentials of Pediatric Nursing*. Packed with review questions, case studies, and critical thinking exercises, this guide will enhance your understanding of the theory and applications presented in the text and help you get the most out of your study time.
October 2004 • Approx. 352 pages, • 0-323-03230-3

Virtual Clinical Excursions
Marilyn J. Hockenberry, PhD, RN-CS, PNP, FAAN
This unique teaching-learning system immerses you in a simulated clinical setting where you can work with complex pediatric patients. Each lesson has a core textbook reading assignment with corresponding CD-ROM and workbook activities. The workbook exercises guide you through the process of caring for patients in the virtual hospital, to help you make connections between what you experience on the CD-ROM and what you've read in the textbook.
October 2004 • CD-ROM Software and Workbook
0-323-03282-6

Also available...

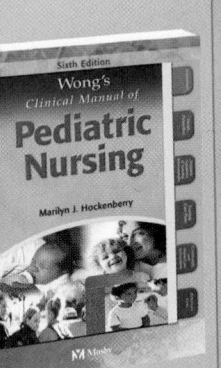
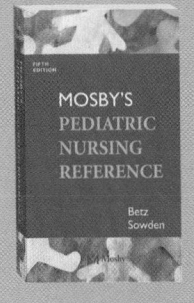

Wong's Clinical Manual of Pediatric Nursing, 6th Edition
Marilyn J. Hockenberry, PhD, RN-CS, PNP, FAAN
This is the only resource of its kind to combine six of the most critical aspects of pediatric nursing — care plans, assessment tools, skills and procedures, patient teaching information, health promotion guidelines, and reference data — into one convenient, portable resource. It's the perfect companion for pediatric clinical rotations!
2004 • 784 pages, 388 illustrations • 0-323-01958-7

Mosby's Pediatric Nursing Reference, 5th Edition
Cecily Lynn Betz, PhD, RN, FAAN; and Linda A. Sowden, MN, RN
This indispensable, compact resource contains the most up-to-date information for nearly 90 common pediatric medical and surgical conditions in a convenient and consistent alphabetical format. Plus, it offers pediatric growth charts, immunization information, laboratory values, abbreviations, psychosocial interventions, and more!
2004 • 832 pages, illustrated • 0-323-01979-X

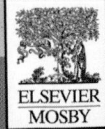

ELSEVIER
MOSBY

GET YOUR COPIES TODAY!
Visit your local bookstore
Call 1-800-545-2522
Order securely at www.elsevierhealth.com

NMX-654

FAMILY HOME CARE BOXES

COMMUNITY FOCUS BOXES

GUIDELINES BOXES

HEALTH AND ... ON

P9-DUQ-060

ESS
of
PED
NU

WONG'S
ESSENTIALS
of
PEDIATRIC
NURSING

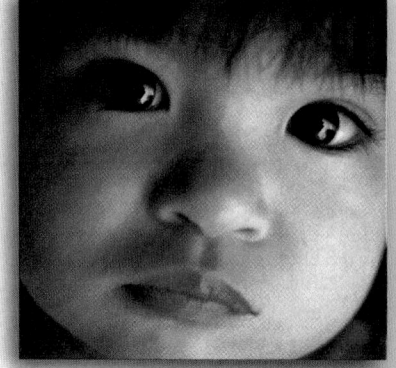

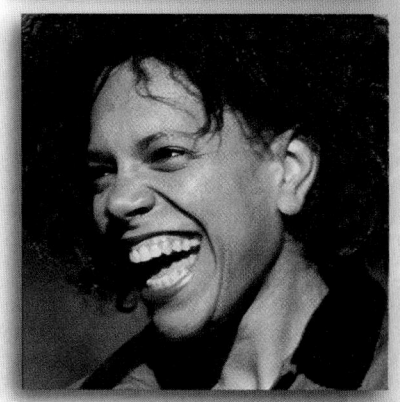

Marilyn J. Hockenberry
PhD, RN-CS, PNP, FAAN

Director, Center for Clinical Research
Nurse Scientist, Texas Children's Hospital;
Director of Nurse Practitioners
Texas Children's Cancer Center;
Professor, Department of Pediatrics
Baylor College of Medicine
Houston, Texas

SEVENTH
EDITION

Section Editors

David Wilson, MS, RNC
Formerly Assistant Professor
Langston University School of Nursing;
Staff Nurse
Children's Hospital Urgent Care Center
Saint Francis Hospital
Tulsa, Oklahoma

Marilyn L. Winkelstein, PhD, RN
Associate Professor
Johns Hopkins University
School of Nursing;
Staff Educator
Johns Hopkins Hospital Children's Center
Baltimore, Maryland

with 645 illustrations

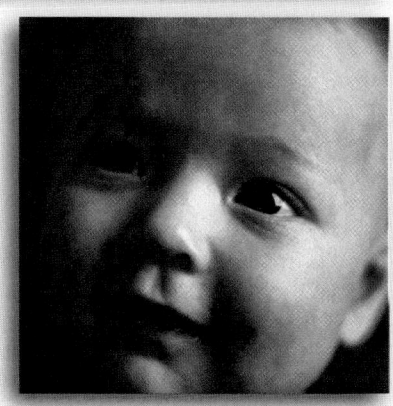

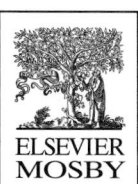

ELSEVIER
MOSBY

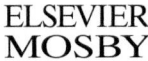

ELSEVIER
MOSBY

11830 Westline Industrial Drive
St. Louis, Missouri 63146

WONG'S ESSENTIALS OF PEDIATRIC NURSING, SEVENTH EDITION   0-323-02593-5

NOTICE

Pediatric Nursing is an ever-changing field. Standard safety precautions must be followed, but as new research and clinical experience broaden our knowledge, changes in treatment and drug therapy may become necessary or appropriate. Readers are advised to check the most current product information provided by the manufacturer of each drug to be administered to verify the recommended dose, the method and duration of administration, and contraindications. It is the responsibility of the licensed prescriber, relying on experience and knowledge of the patient, to determine dosages and the best treatment for each individual patient. Neither the publisher nor the author assumes any liability for any injury and/or damage to persons or property arising from this publication.

Previous editions copyrighted 1982, 1985, 1989, 1993, 1997, 2001.

International Standard Book Number: 0-323-02593-5

Executive Editor: Loren S. Wilson
Senior Developmental Editor: Michele D. Hayden
Publishing Services Manager: Deborah L. Vogel
Senior Project Manager: Ann E. Rogers
Designer: Teresa McBryan

Printed in the United States of America.

Last digit is the print number: 9   8   7   6   5   4   3   2   1

Contributors

CONTRIBUTING EDITOR

PATRICK BARRERA, BS
Research Program Coordinator
Center for Clinical Research
Texas Children's Hospital
Houston, Texas

CONTRIBUTORS

Chris L. Algren, EdD, MSN, RN
Assistant Administrator/Director of Perioperative
    & Procedural Nursing
Vanderbilt Children's Hospital
Nashville, Tennessee

Debra Arnow, MSN, RN, CNA, BC
Assistant Administrator/Director of Nursing
Vanderbilt Children's Hospital
Nashville, Tennessee

Debbie Fraser Askin, MN, RNC
Assistant Professor of Nursing
University of Manitoba;
Neonatal Nurse Practitioner
St. Boniface General Hospital
Winnipeg, Manitoba, Canada

Rose A. Urdiales Baker, MSN, RN, CS
Burn Research Nurse
Clifford R. Boeckman M.D. Regional Burn Trauma Center
Children's Hospital Medical Center of Akron;
Instructor
Kent State University
School of Nursing
Akron, Ohio

Carol C. Bowman, MS, RD, LD
Clinical Dietician
Saint Francis Hospital
Tulsa, Oklahoma

Christine A. Brosnan, DrPH, RN
Assistant Professor
University of Texas
Houston Health Science Center
School of Nursing
Houston, Texas

Rosalind Bryant, MN, RN-CS, PNP
Pediatric Nurse Practitioner
Texas Children's Cancer Center
Texas Children's Hospital;
Clinical Instructor, Department of Pediatrics
Baylor College of Medicine
Houston, Texas

Kimberly Childers, MS, RN, CEN, CPNP
Pediatric Nurse Practitioner
Texas Children's Emergency Center;
Clinical Instructor, Department of Pediatrics
Baylor College of Medicine
Houston, Texas

Christine Chordas, MSN, RN, CPNP
Pediatric Nurse Practitioner
Department of Pediatric Neuro-Oncology
Dana-Farber Cancer Institute
Boston, Massachusetts

Helen Currier, BSN, RN, CNN
Assistant Director, Renal Dialysis and Pheresis Center
Texas Children's Hospital
Houston, Texas

Martha R. Curry, MS, RN, CPNP
Pediatric Nurse Practitioner
Rheumatology Section
Texas Children's Hospital;
Clinical Instructor, Department of Pediatrics
Baylor College of Medicine
Houston, Texas

Carolyn V. Daigneau, MS, RN-CS, PNP
Pediatric Nurse Practitioner
Gastroenterology and Nutrition Section
Texas Children's Hospital;
Clinical Instructor, Department of Pediatrics
Baylor College of Medicine
Houston, Texas

Susan O. Fernbach, BSN, RN
Cardiovascular Genetics Clinic Coordinator
Texas Children's Hospital;
Department of Molecular and Human Genetics
Baylor College of Medicine
Houston, Texas

Melody Brown Hellsten, MSN, RN, APRN-BC, PNP
Coordinator, Pediatric Palliative Care Program
Christus Santa Rosa Children's Hospital;
Pediatric Nurse Practitioner
Department of Pediatrics
University of Texas Health Sciences Center
San Antonio, Texas

Mary C. Hooke, MSN, RN, CPON, CNS
Clinical Nurse Specialist
Pediatric Hematology-Oncology
Children's Hospitals and Clinics
Minneapolis and Saint Paul, Minnesota

Linda M. Kollar, MSN, RN
Director of Clinical Services
Division of Adolescent Medicine
Children's Hospital Medical Center
Cincinnati, Ohio

Kerri Lemance, RN
Instructor
Department of Molecular and Human Genetics
Texas Children's Hospital
Baylor College of Medicine
Genetics Nurse Specialist
Metabolic Clinic at Texas Children's Hospital
Houston, Texas

Shannon Stone McCord, MS, RN, CPNP, CNS, WOCN, CCRN
Pediatric Nurse Practitioner
Wound, Ostomy & Continence Service
Texas Children's Hospital
Houston, Texas

Mary A. Mondozzi, MSN, RN, CPNP
Burn Center Education/Outreach Coordinator
Clifford R. Boeckman M.D. Regional Burn Center
Children's Hospital Medical Center of Akron
Akron, Ohio

Barbara Montagnino, MS, RN, CNS
Clinical Nurse Specialist;
District Sales Manager
Astra Tech, Inc.
Torrance, California

Patricia A. Murray, MN, CPNP, HNC
Pediatric Nurse Practitioner
Grady Health System;
Adjunct Clinical Faculty
Nell Hodgson Woodruff School of Nursing
Emory University
Atlanta, Georgia

Patricia O'Brien, MSN, RN-CS, PNP
Pediatric Nurse Practitioner, Cardiovascular Program
Children's Hospital
Boston, Massachusetts

Amy Nadel Romanczuk, MSN, RN
Formerly Pediatric Ambulatory Care
Medical University of South Carolina
Charleston, South Carolina

Rebecca J. Schultz, MSN, RN, CPNP
Pediatric Nurse Practitioner
Comprehensive Epilepsy Program
Blue Bird Clinic for Pediatric Neurology
Texas Children's Hospital;
Clinical Instructor, Department of Pediatrics
Baylor College of Medicine
Houston, Texas

Sandra Upchurch, PhD, RN, CDE
Assistant Professor
School of Nursing
University of Texas at Houston
Houston, Texas

Reviewers

Jennifer Baxter, MD
Anesthesiologist
Certified Anesthesia Services
Sibley Memorial Hospital
Washington, D.C.

April Catterton, BSN, RN, CPHQ
Director of Clinical Operations
Texas Children's Home Health Services
Texas Children's Hospital
Houston, Texas

Miguel F. da Cunha, PhD
Professor, Department of Nursing for Target Populations;
Director, Office for Teaching Excellence
University of Texas Health Science Center
School of Nursing
Houston, Texas

Scott DeBoer, MSN, RN, CEN, CCRN, CFRN
Founder, Peds-R-Us Medical Education;
Former Flight Nurse Educator
University of Chicago Hospitals Aeromedical Network
Chicago, Illinois

Joseann Helmes DeWitt, MSN, C, RN, CLNC
Assistant Professor
Alcorn State University
School of Nursing
Natchez, Mississippi

Bogdan Dinu
Research Associate
Texas Children's Cancer Center
Texas Children's Hospital
Houston, Texas

Daniel R. Joy, BS, RN, ATC/L
Children's Hospital Urgent Care Center
Saint Francis Hospital
Tulsa, Oklahoma

Mary Lanz
Spanish Translator
Texas Children's Cancer Center
Texas Children's Hospital
Houston, Texas

Cynthia G. Sanders, MS, RN, CPNP
Pediatric Nurse Practitioner
Endocrine Section
Texas Children's Hospital;
Clinical Instructor, Department of Pediatrics
Baylor College of Medicine
Houston, Texas

Susanne N. Suchy, MSN, RN
Instructor, Nursing Division
Henry Ford Community College
Dearborn, Michigan;
Clinical Nurse Specialist
Oncology Patient Services
Karmanos Cancer Institute and Cancer Hospital
Detroit, Michigan

Deborah Jean Throne, MSN, RN
Instructor
Lewis and Clark Community College
Godfrey, Illinois;
Staff Nurse, Emergency Department
Cardinal Glennon Children's Hospital
St. Louis, Missouri

Barbara J. Wheeler, MN, RN, IBCLC
Neonatal Clinical Nurse Specialist
St. Boniface General Hospital;
Lecturer, Faculty of Nursing
University of Manitoba
Winnipeg, Manitoba, Canada

Preface

Essentials of Pediatric Nursing has been a leading book in pediatric nursing since it was first published more than two decades ago. This kind of support places a unique accountability and responsibility on us to earn your future endorsement with each new edition. So, with your encouragement and constructive comments, we offer this extensive revision, the seventh edition of *Essentials of Pediatric Nursing*.

To accomplish this, Marilyn J. Hockenberry, as Editor-in-Chief, along with David Wilson and Marilyn Winkelstein and many expert nurses and multidisciplinary specialists, have revised, rewritten, or authored portions of the text concerning areas that are undergoing rapid and complex change. These areas include community nursing, immunizations, genetics, home care, high-risk newborn care, adolescent health issues, end-of-life care, and numerous diseases. We have carefully preserved aspects of the book that have met with such universal acceptance—its state-of-the-art research-based information; its strong, integrated focus on the family and community; its logical and user-friendly organization; and its easy-to-read style.

We have tried to meet the increasing demands of faculty and students to teach and to learn in an environment characterized by rapid change, enormous amounts of information, fewer traditional clinical facilities, and less time.

This text encourages students to *think critically*. New to this edition are Ethical Case Studies that are designed to reflect complex patient care situations that nurses frequently face in clinical practice. The case studies were established using these principles: Evaluate the issue, Treat all involved with respect, Hear all sides, Initiate action, and Consider the outcome. A complete revision of all Critical Thinking Exercises is included in this edition. The revised Critical Thinking Exercises ask the nurse to examine the evidence, consider the assumptions, establish priorities, and evaluate alternative perspectives regarding each patient situation. The changes in the Critical Thinking Exercises and the addition of Ethical Case Studies support our belief that the science of nursing and related health professions is not black and white. In many instances it includes shades of gray, as in the areas of genetic testing, resuscitation, cultural issues, end-of-life care, and quality of life.

This text also serves as a reference manual for the practicing nurse. The latest recommendations have been included from authoritative organizations such as the American Academy of Pediatrics, the Centers for Disease Control and Prevention, the Institute of Medicine, the Agency for Healthcare Research and Quality, the American Pain Society, the American Nurses Association, and the National Association of Pediatric Nurse Associates and Practitioners. To expand the universe of available information, websites and e-mail addresses have been included for hundreds of organizations and other educational resources.

ORGANIZATION OF THE BOOK

The same general approach to the presentation of content has been preserved from the first edition, although some content has been added, condensed, and rearranged within this framework to improve the flow, minimize duplication, and emphasize health care trends, such as home and community care. The book is divided into two broad parts. The first part of the book, Chapters 1 through 17, sometimes called the "age and stage" approach, considers infancy, childhood, and adolescence from a developmental context. It emphasizes the importance of the nurse's role in health promotion and maintenance and in considering the family as the focus of care. From a developmental perspective, the care of common health problems is presented, giving readers a sense of the normal problems expected in otherwise healthy children and demonstrating when in the course of childhood these problems are most likely to occur. The remainder of the book, Chapters 18 through 32, presents the more serious health problems of infancy, childhood, and adolescence that are not specific to any particular age-group and that frequently require hospitalization, major medical and nursing intervention, and home care.

UNIT ONE (Chapters 1 through 5) provides a longitudinal view of the child as an individual on a continuum of developmental changes from birth through adolescence and as a member of a family unit maturing within a culture and a community. Chapter 1 includes a discussion of morbidity and mortality in infancy and childhood, including Canadian child mortality, and child health care from a historic perspective. Information regarding the Health Insurance Portability and Accountability Act (HIPAA) has been added because of the significant impact this legislation has on daily nursing care. Because of the importance of unintentional injuries as the leading cause of death in children, an overview of this topic is included. The nursing process—with emphasis on nursing diagnoses and outcomes, and the importance of developing critical thinking skills—is presented. The role of the nurse as a care provider, family advocate, health promoter, teacher, counselor, and coordinator of care is discussed.

This book is about families with children, and the philosophy of family-centered care is emphasized. This book is also about providing atraumatic care—care that minimizes the psychologic and physical stress that health promotion and illness treatment can inflict. Features such as Family Focus, Community Focus, and Atraumatic Care boxes bring

Special Features

Much effort has been directed toward making this book easy to teach from and, more important, easy to learn from. In this edition the following features have been included to benefit educators, students, and practitioners.

- A functional and attractive FULL-COLOR DESIGN visually enhances the organization of each chapter, as well as the special features.
- Many of the COLOR PHOTOGRAPHS are new, and anatomic drawings are easy to follow, with color appropriately used to illustrate important aspects, such as saturated and desaturated blood. As an example, the full-color heart illustrations in Chapter 25 clearly depict congenital cardiac defects and associated hemodynamic changes.
- FAMILY HOME CARE boxes help nurses and students teach parents about the special needs of their infants and children.
- ETHICAL CASE STUDIES, new to this edition, have been designed to reflect complex patient care situations that nurses face in clinical practice. The case studies were established using these principles: Evaluate the issue, Treat all involved with respect, Hear all sides, Initiate action, and Consider the outcome.
- EVIDENCE-BASED PRACTICE boxes focus the reader's attention on application of both research and critical thought processes to support and guide the outcomes of nursing care and to provide measurable outcomes that nurses can use to validate their unique role in the health care system.
- COMMUNITY FOCUS boxes address issues that expand to the community, such as increasing immunization rates, preventing lead poisoning, or decreasing smoking among teens.
- CRITICAL THINKING EXERCISES have been completely revised for this edition. The revised exercises ask the nurse to examine the evidence, consider the assumptions, establish priorities, and evaluate alternative perspectives regarding each patient situation.
- CULTURAL AWARENESS boxes integrate concepts of culturally sensitive care throughout the text. The emphasis is on the clinical application of the information, whether it focuses on toilet training or on male or female circumcision.
- ATRAUMATIC CARE boxes emphasize the importance of providing competent care without creating undue physical and psychologic distress. Although many of the boxes provide suggestions for managing pain, atraumatic care also considers approaches to promoting self-esteem and preventing embarrassment.
- NURSING CARE PLANS include RATIONALES for nursing interventions that are not immediately evident to the student. This strengthens the connection between the text and the interventions in the care plans. All care plans include patient and family goals and the most recent NANDA International nursing diagnoses.

Numerous pedagogic devices that enhance student learning have been retained from previous editions:

- CHAPTER OUTLINES with page numbers begin each chapter, which allows readers to quickly locate topics of interest.
- The RELATED TOPICS AND ADDITIONAL RESOURCES box at the beginning of each chapter indicates the chapter or chapters where additional discussion(s) of a given topic can be found. It also highlights additional resources and information included in ancillary products such as the Evolve website, CD Companion, and *Wong's Clinical Manual of Pediatric Nursing*.
- LEARNING OBJECTIVES in each chapter provide the reader with a basic guideline for the major points presented in and learned from the chapter.
- NURSING ALERTS call the reader's attention to considerations that if ignored could lead to a deteriorating or emergency situation. Key assessment data, risk factors, and danger signs are among the kinds of information included.
- NURSING TIPS present handy information of a nonemergency nature that makes patients more comfortable and the nurse's job a little easier.
- GUIDELINES boxes summarize important nursing interventions for a variety of situations and conditions.
- EMERGENCY TREATMENT boxes are flagged by colored thumb tabs, enabling the reader to quickly locate interventions for crisis situations.
- FAMILY FOCUS boxes present issues of special significance to families who have a child with a particular disorder. This feature is another method of highlighting the needs or concerns of families that should be addressed when family-centered care is provided.
- FYI (For Your Information) segments present information of interest that may increase understanding of a concept or spark an interest in reading about a condition. Unlike the Nursing Alerts, which present essential information, the FYIs present information that is optional for the reader and help prioritize what information is most essential for the reader to assimilate.
- KEY TERMS are highlighted throughout each chapter to reinforce student learning.
- Hundreds of TABLES and BOXES highlight key concepts and nursing interventions.
- KEY POINTS, located at the end of each chapter, help the reader summarize major concepts, make connections, and synthesize information.
- A detailed, cross-referenced INDEX allows readers to quickly access discussions.

these philosophies to life throughout the text. Finally, the philosophy of delivering nursing care is addressed. We believe strongly that children and families need consistent caregivers. The establishment of the therapeutic relationship with the child and family is explored as the essential foundation for providing quality nursing care.

The child in the context of family, culture, and community has been broadened to include a separate chapter on community health nursing. Chapter 2 provides important information on community-based nursing care, with em-

phasis on epidemiology as it applies to the detection and identification of causes of morbidity and mortality in pediatrics. A community project presented in this chapter reflects the important components of the nursing process, such as completion of a community needs assessment, planning phase, implementation, and evaluation.

Chapter 3, devoted to the family, further emphasizes the importance of this social group in relation to the health and welfare of children. Family theories establish the tone of the chapter, which includes a variety of parenting situations that reflect contemporary society. An important example is a revised section on nontraditional families. Family strengths and vulnerabilities are addressed, and current findings on adoption, divorce, single-parenting, stepfamilies, and dual-earner families have been incorporated.

Chapter 4 provides the opportunity to expand the discussion of social, cultural, and religious influences on child development and health promotion, including socioeconomic factors, customs, and health beliefs and practices. The content more clearly describes the role of the nurse, with emphasis on cultural sensitivity and culturally competent care. Extensive revisions have been made to the tables detailing cultural and religious factors throughout this chapter to make the information more manageable and user friendly. Cultural Awareness boxes throughout the entire text highlight the influences of culture on children and families. The basic overview of child development in Chapter 5 maintains the same general organization and expands on the theoretic approach to personality development and learning. Biologic systems development is not emphasized in this chapter but is discussed more fully in relation to major systems dysfunction later in the book.

UNIT TWO (Chapters 6 and 7) is concerned with the principles of nursing assessment, including communication and interviewing skills, observation, physical and behavioral assessment, health guidance, and the latest information on preventive care guidelines. Chapter 6 contains guidelines for communicating with children, adolescents, and their families; and a detailed description of a health assessment, including an extensive discussion of family assessment, nutritional assessment, and a sexual history. Content on communication techniques is outlined to provide a concise format for reference. Chapter 7 continues to provide a comprehensive approach to physical examination and developmental assessment, with updated material on temperature measurement, BMI-for-age guidelines, and the latest CDC clinical growth charts.

UNIT THREE (Chapters 8 and 9) stresses the importance of the neonatal period in relation to child survival during the first few months and impact on health in later life. In Chapter 8 several areas have been revised to reflect current issues, especially in terms of the educational needs of the family during short postpartum stays and the recognition of newborn problems in the first few weeks of life. A new intrauterine growth chart is included that reflects a more homogenous sample population than previous growth charts. Other current issues that have been updated include proactive measures to prevent infant abduction, hospital-based baby-friendly breast-feeding initiatives, choices for circumcision analgesia, neonatal hypertension, and newborn screening including universal newborn hearing screening. Newborn skin care guidelines have also been updated, and choices for newborn cord care are discussed. Chapter 9 stresses the nurse's role in caring for the high-risk newborn and the importance of astute observations to the survival of this vulnerable group of infants. Modern advances in neonatal care have mandated extensive revision with a greater sensitivity to the diverse needs of infants, from those with extremely low birth weights to those of normal gestational age who have difficulty making an effective transition to extrauterine life. Updates in Chapter 9 include information on individualized developmental care, preterm infant

nutrition, early discharge of the preterm infant, and neonatal exposure to maternal environmental conditions such as alcohol and tobacco, as well as exposure to viral infections, including HIV. This chapter also includes updates regarding neonatal pain management and detection and management of inborn errors of metabolism.

UNITS FOUR through SIX (Chapters 10 through 17) present the major developmental stages outlined in Unit One, which are expanded to provide a broader concept of these stages and the health problems most often associated with each age-group. Special emphasis is placed on the preventive aspects of care. The chapters on health promotion follow a standard approach that is used consistently for each age-group. New information has been added on Dietary Reference Intakes and vitamin intake and food hypersensitivity, as well as complementary and alternative medicine, motor vehicle child safety restraints, and infant safety. The influence of nutrition in the preschool-age and school-age child (especially decreasing fat intake) in relation to later chronic diseases such as hypertension is also discussed. The sections on childhood immunizations and injury prevention have been updated. The potential negative effects of exposure to violence and terrorism are included as well.

The chapters on health problems in these units primarily reflect more typical and age-related concerns. The information on many disorders has been revised to reflect recent changes. Examples include sudden infant death syndrome, lead poisoning, wound healing, Lyme disease, attention deficit–hyperactivity disorder, contraception, teenage pregnancy, drug abuse, and suicide. The chapters on adolescence include the latest information from the American Medical Association (AMA) guidelines for adolescent prevention services (GAPS), nonsmoking strategies, and current trends in suicide. All psychosocial/physiologic conditions include the latest diagnostic criteria from the *Diagnostic and Statistical Manual of Mental Disorders (DSM-IV-TR)*.

UNIT SEVEN (Chapters 18 through 20) deals with children who have the same developmental needs as growing children but who, because of congenital or acquired physical, cognitive, or sensory impairment, require alternative interventions to facilitate development. Chapter 18 reflects current trends in the care of families and children with chronic illness or disability such as home care, normalizing children's lives, focusing on developmental needs, enabling and empowering families, and providing early intervention. Extensive revisions have been made to reflect increased awareness of the need for quality nursing care at the end of life. This section highlights common fears experienced by the child and family and includes discussion of symptom management and nurses' reactions to caring for dying children.

The content in Chapter 19 on cognitive or sensory impairment includes important updates on the definition and classification of mental retardation. Major updates on hearing impairment include the use of cochlear implants for sensorineural hearing loss. Autism has been added to this chapter to provide a cohesive overview of cognitive and sensory impairments. Chapter 20 provides an overview of home care in light of the current nursing shortage and its impact on the role of the home health care nurse, care provider, and family. This chapter presents updated discussions related to the selection of a home health care agency, the role of the nurse in empowering the family, and case management in home health.

UNIT EIGHT (Chapters 21 and 22) is concerned with the impact of hospitalization on the child and the family and presents a comprehensive overview of the stressors imposed by hospitalization and discusses nursing interventions to prevent or eliminate them. New research on short-stay or outpatient admissions addresses preparing children for these experiences. Chapter 21 provides updated information on the effects of illness and hospitalization on children at specific ages and the effects on their development. There is also an updated section on pain assessment and management, including PCA (patient-controlled analgesia), epidural, and topical analgesia. The increasing role of ambulatory and outpatient settings for surgical procedures is also discussed. Chapter 22 presents information on the safe implementation of procedures with children, including emphasis on the use of therapeutic hugging. We have tried to include as much available research as possible to base the nursing interventions on scientific findings rather than traditional practice. The latest information regarding child pain medications and an expanded table on child and infant pain rating scales have been included in this latest edition. Major revisions include information on intramuscular injections, flushing central venous catheters, maintaining healthy skin, use of patient restraints, and staging of pressure ulcers.

UNITS NINE through TWELVE (Chapters 23 through 32) consider serious health problems of infants and children primarily from the biologic systems orientation, which has the practical organizational value of permitting health problems and nursing considerations to relate to specific pathophysiologic disturbances. Important revisions include discussions of hepatitis, all blood disorders, respiratory syncytial virus, tuberculosis, asthma, effects of passive smoking, seizures, chemotherapy, acquired immunodeficiency syndrome, diabetes mellitus, and burns. The information on orthopedic and muscular injuries in childhood as a result of sports participation or other injuries has been extensively revised to reflect current treatment modalities. Chapter 29 includes focused attention on type 2 diabetes and new information on insulin preparations and types of glucose meters. Once again, major revisions have been made to the discussions on musculoskeletal and articular dysfunction, including newer pharmacologic treatment modalities for spasticity. The sections on idiopathic scoliosis and spinal cord injuries have been extensively revised, and the latest information on myelomeningocele and latex allergy is presented.

Extensive **appendixes** are also included and contain information on family assessment, patterns of inheritance, developmental assessment, growth measurements, pediatric laboratory values, NANDA International–approved nursing diagnoses, and several foreign-language translations of the FACES Pain Rating Scale. New for this edition is an Appendix containing Spanish translations of common terms and phrases used in health care and pediatric nursing. All of the appendix material reflects the most current versions of forms, charts, and measurements. Additional Clinical Growth Charts can be obtained from the Centers for Disease Control and Prevention website: www.cdc.gov/growthcharts.

UNIFYING PRINCIPLES

Several unifying principles have guided the organizational structure of this book since its inception. These principles continue to strengthen the book with each revision in order to produce a text that is consistent in approach throughout each chapter.

The Family as the Unit of Care

The child is an essential member of the family unit. Nursing care is most effective when it is delivered with the belief that *the family is the patient.* This belief permeates the book. When a child is healthy, the child's health is enhanced when the family is a fully functioning, health-promoting system. The family unit can be manifested in a myriad of structures; each has the potential to provide a caring, supportive environment in which the child can grow, mature, and maximize his or her human potential. In addition to the integration of family-centered care into every chapter, an entire chapter is devoted to understanding the family as the core focus in children's lives. Another chapter discusses the social, cultural, and religious influences that impact family beliefs. Separate sections in another chapter deal in depth with family communication and family assessment. The impact of illness, hospitalization, home care, community care, and the death of a child are covered extensively in four additional chapters. The needs of the family are emphasized throughout the text under Nursing Considerations in a separate section on family support. Numerous Family Focus and Family Home Care boxes are included to assist nurses in understanding and providing helpful information to families.

An Integrated Approach to Development

Children are not small adults but special individuals with unique minds, bodies, and needs. No book on pediatric nursing is complete without extensive coverage of communication, nutrition, play, safety, dental care, sexuality, sleep, self-esteem, and, of course, parenting. Nurses promote the healthy expression of all these dimensions of personhood and need to understand how these functions are expressed by different children at different developmental ages and stages. Effective parenting depends on the parent's knowledge of development, and it is often the nurse's responsibility to provide parents with a developmental awareness of their children's needs. For these reasons, coverage of the many dimensions of childhood is integrated within the growth and development chapters, rather than being presented in separate chapters. For example, safety concerns for a toddler are much different from those for an adolescent. Sleep needs change with age, as do nutritional needs. As a result, the units on each stage of childhood contain complete information on all these functions as they relate to the specific age. In the unit on the school-age child, for instance, information is presented on nutritional needs, age-appropriate play and its significance, safety concerns characteristic of the age-group, appropriate dental care, sleep characteristics, and means of promoting self-esteem—a particularly significant concern for school-age children. The challenges of being the parent of a school-age child are presented, and interventions are suggested that nurses can use to promote more healthy parenting. Using the integrated approach, students gain an appreciation for the unique characteristics and needs of children at every age and stage of development.

Focus on Wellness and Illness: Child, Family, and Community

In a pediatric nursing text, a focus on illness is expected. Children become ill, and nurses typically are involved in helping children get well. However, it is not sufficient to prepare nursing students to care primarily for sick children. First, health is more than the absence of disease. Being healthy is being whole in mind, body, and spirit. Therefore the majority of the first half of the book is devoted to discussions that promote physical, emotional, psychosocial, mental, and spiritual wellness. Much emphasis is placed on anticipatory guidance of parents to prevent injury or illness in the child. Second, health care is more than ever prevention focused. The objectives set forth in the "Healthy People 2010" report clearly establish a health care agenda in which solutions to medical and social problems lie in preventive strategies. Third, health care is moving from acute care settings to the community, the home, short-stay centers, and clinics. Nurses must be prepared to function in all settings. To be successful, they must understand the pathophysiology, diagnosis, and treatment of health conditions. Competent nursing care flows from this knowledge and is enhanced by an awareness of childhood development, family dynamics, and communication skills.

Nursing Care

Although the information in this text incorporates information from numerous disciplines (medicine, pathophysiology, pharmacology, nutrition, psychology, sociology), its primary purpose is to provide information on the nursing care of children and families. Discussions of all disorders conclude with a section on Nursing Considerations. In addition, 23 care plans are included. Taken together, they cover the nursing care for virtually every disease, disorder, condition, and crisis of childhood. The purposes of the care plans, like every other feature of the book, are to teach and to convey information. They include all current nursing diagnoses approved by NANDA International that have a potential bearing on the health problem. For every diagnosis, appropriate patient goals, extensive possible interventions with rationales, and outcomes are presented. Thus a complete range of nursing care is presented within the context of a care plan and the nursing process. For every health problem for which a care plan is included in the text, the surrounding narrative text is presented according to the nursing process. In these instances specific headings for assessment, nursing diagnoses, planning, implementation, and evaluation, with unifying logos for the five steps, present appropriate information that is then amplified in the care plan, presented in a standard nursing practice context.

Culturally Competent Care

Increasing cultural diversity in this country requires nurses caring for children and their families to develop expertise in the care of children from numerous backgrounds. Culturally competent nursing care requires more than acquiring knowledge about ethnic and cultural groups. It encompasses not only awareness of the influence of culture on the child and family, but also the ability to intervene appropriately and effectively. The nurse must learn objective skills to focus on the child, family, and community's cultural characteristics. The nurse's self-awareness of unique personal cultural backgrounds must be acknowledged in order to understand how they contribute to cross-cultural communication. The importance of the environment of a cross-cultural care setting is an important consideration when providing clinical nursing care to culturally diverse families. This edition provides numerous learning experiences that examine cross-cultural communication, cultural assessment, cultural interpretation, and appropriate nursing interventions. A revised culture chapter includes major updates and changes in the tables concerning cultural and religious information, the addition of culturally sensitive Critical Thinking Exercises, and the development of new Ethical Case Studies that allow the nurse to evaluate the evidence and formulate assumptions regarding the appropriate priorities for care of children and families from various cultural backgrounds.

The Critical Role of Research and Evidence-Based Practice

This seventh edition is the product of an extensive review of the literature published since the book was last revised. Many readers and researchers have come to rely on the copious references that reflect significant contributions from a broad audience of professionals. To ensure that information is accurate and current, most citations are less than 5 years old, and almost every chapter has entries dated within 1 year of publication. This book reflects the art and science of pediatric nursing. A central goal in every revision is to base care on research, rather than on tradition. Evidence-based practice produces measurable outcomes that nurses can use to validate their unique role in the health care system.

CANADIAN CONTENT

The seventh edition of this text includes updated Canadian statistics regarding infant and child health in Chapter 1 and Canadian immunization schedules in Chapter 10. Numerous Canadian resource organizations are also provided throughout the text. These efforts are intended to make the text as valuable as possible to Canadian readers.

TEACHING/LEARNING PACKAGE

For the seventh edition of this text, extensive ancillary products are offered for instructors and students to use in class and clinical settings.

EVOLVE. Evolve is an innovative website that provides a wealth of continually updated content, resources, and state-of-the-art information on pediatric nursing, including links to related websites, important new content updates, Donna Wong's lectures, and more! Use the web address in the text to access EVOLVE's wide array of information, including course resources for instructors (*Instructor's Manual, Test Bank, Image Collection, PowerPoint slides*) and learning resources for students (WebLinks, interactive case studies, NCLEX-style review questions, pediatric nursing skills).

CD Companion. FREE with every text, this valuable CD-ROM contains a variety of activities to enhance learning through the use of Critical Thinking Exercises, Case Studies, Anatomy Reviews, and Guidelines and Clinical Manifestation boxes. Many Nursing Care Plans are included to build, individualize, and print out. Pediatric nursing skills are included, and 350 NCLEX-style review questions are available for students to practice and hone their studying skills.

Instructor's Electronic Resource.   This innovative electronic resource for the instructor is available online and on CD and contains the following components:

- *Instructor's Manual,* with learning objectives, chapter outlines and accompanying teaching strategies, learning activities, open-book quizzes, and curriculum guides.
- *Electronic Test Bank in ExamView format,* with more than 1,000 NCLEX-style test items, including new alternate format questions. An answer key with page references to the text, rationales, and NCLEX-style coding is included.
- *Electronic Image Collection,* containing more than 400 full-color illustrations and photographs from the text to help instructors develop presentations and explain key concepts. All images on the CD can be printed out as acetates for overhead projection.
- *PowerPoint Slides,* with lecture outlines for each chapter of the book, assist in presenting materials in the classroom.

AVAILABLE FOR PURCHASE:

Study Guide.   This comprehensive and challenging study aid presents a variety of questions to enhance learning of key concepts and content from the text. Multiple-choice, matching, and true-false questions are included, as well as Critical Thinking Case Studies. Answers for all questions are included in the back of the book.

Virtual Clinical Excursions: CD and Workbook Companion.   A CD-ROM and workbook have been developed as a "virtual clinical" experience to expand student opportunities for critical thinking. This package guides the student through a computer-generated virtual clinical environment and helps the user apply textbook content to "virtual patients" in that environment. Case studies are presented that allow students to use this textbook as a reference to assess, diagnose, plan, implement, and evaluate "real" patients using clinical scenarios. The state-of-the-art technologies reflected on this CD-ROM demonstrate *cutting-edge* learning opportunities for students and facilitate knowledge retention of the information found in this textbook. The clinical simulations and workbook represent the next generation of research-based learning tools that promote critical thinking and meaningful learning.

Pediatric Quick Reference.   A handy and invaluable clinical guide for pediatric nursing, the *Pediatric Quick Reference* covers physiologic assessment, pain assessment and management, fluid requirements, intramuscular injections, emergency information, laboratory values, immunization schedules, and references on pain and vaccines.

Wong's Clinical Manual of Pediatric Nursing, sixth edition.   This manual contains a wealth of information for use as a reference for students and in the clinical setting. The manual includes more than 80 Nursing Care Plans, community and home care instructions that can be copied and given to families, detailed descriptions of nursing skills and procedures, and much, much, more!

ACKNOWLEDGMENTS

I am grateful to Donna Wong, whose continued mentorship and support make me a better pediatric nurse. I am also grateful to the many nursing faculty members, practitioners, and students who have offered their comments, recommendations, and suggestions. I am especially grateful to the section editors, **David Wilson** and **Marilyn Winkelstein;** the contributors; and the many reviewers who brought constructive criticism, suggestions, and clinical expertise to this edition. This edition could not have been completed without the dedication of these special people.

I am especially thankful to **Patrick Barrera, Rosalind Bryant,** and **Vanessa Blackstone** for their contributions to this book. Their commitment to excellence and attention to detail are essential to maintaining the quality of this book. Thanks go to **Paul Kuntz** and **Jim Deleon,** photographers at Texas Children's Hospital, for the beautiful color photography; and to the health professionals, children, and parents who generously allowed us to use or take their photographs. Appreciation is also extended to the Library staff at Saint Francis Hospital, Tulsa, Oklahoma—Beth Treasler, Sheryl Roach, and Veronica Stewart.

No book is ever a reality without the dedication and perseverance of the editorial staff. Although it is impossible to list every individual at Mosby who has made exceptional efforts to produce this text, we are especially grateful to **Sally Schrefer, Shelly Hayden, Loren Wilson, and Charlene Ketchum** for their support and commitment to excellence.

Finally, I thank my son **Andrew**—for the unselfish love and endless patience that allow me to devote such a large part of my life to my career. He has given me the opportunity as a mother to directly observe the wonders of childhood.

Marilyn J. Hockenberry

Brief Contents

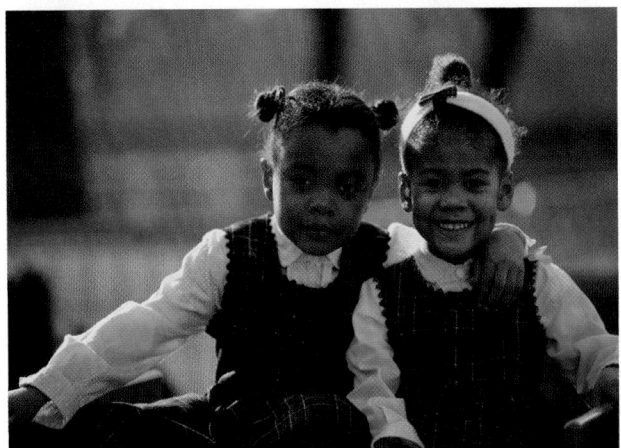

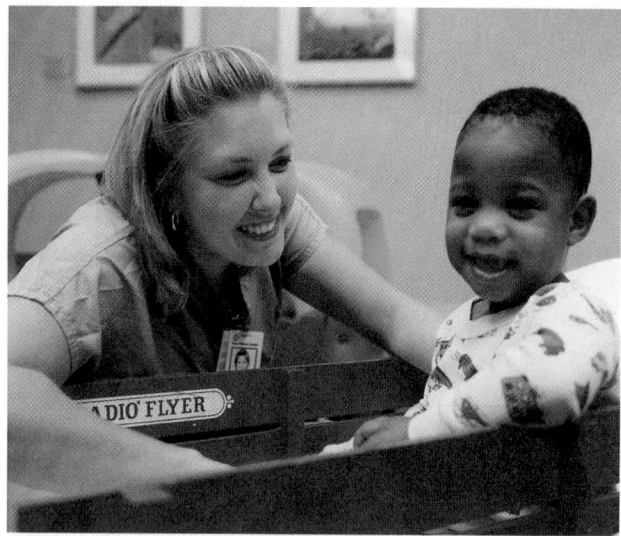

Contents

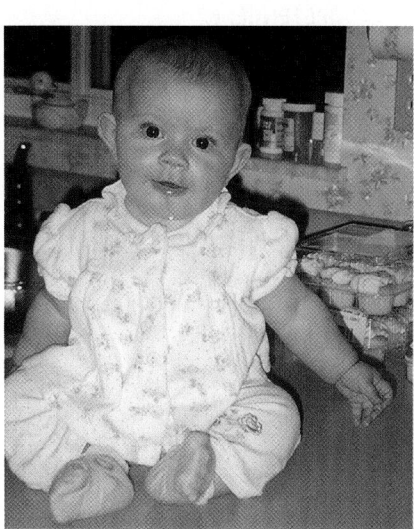

4 Social, Cultural, and Religious Influences on Child Health Promotion, 55

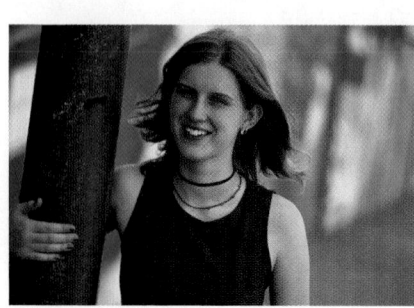

5 Developmental Influences on Child Health Promotion, 79

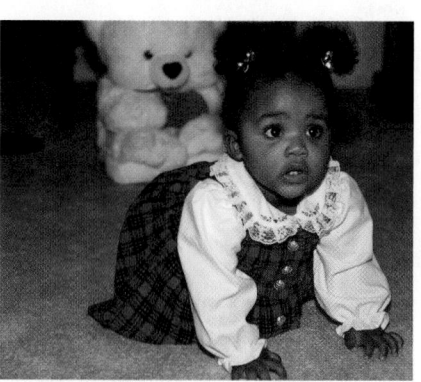

UNIT TWO
Assessment of the Child and Family

UNIT THREE
The Newborn

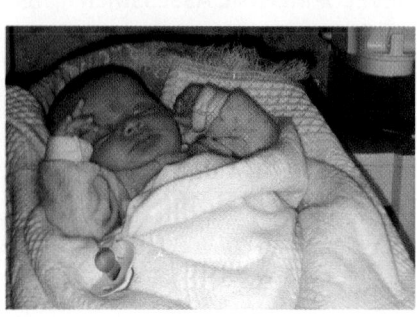

UNIT FOUR
Infancy

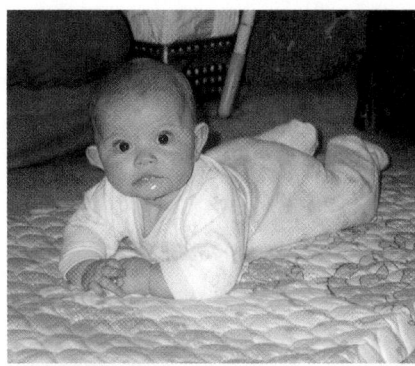

UNIT FIVE
Early Childhood

13 Health Promotion of the Preschooler and Family, 416

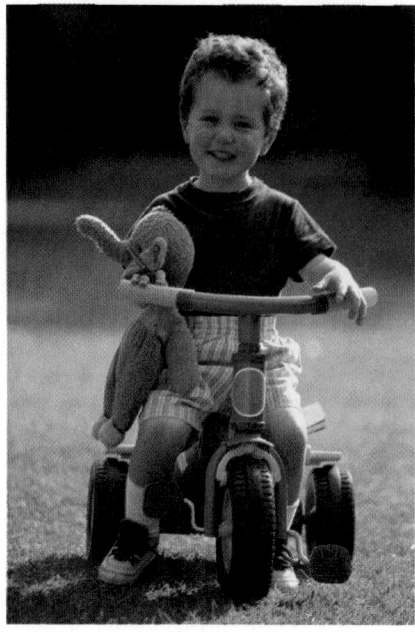

14 Health Problems of Toddlers and Preschoolers, 433

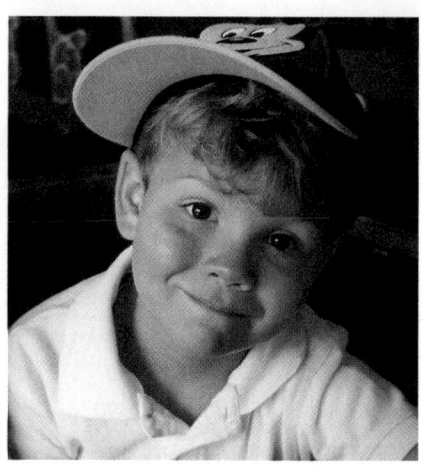

UNIT SIX
Middle Childhood and Adolescence

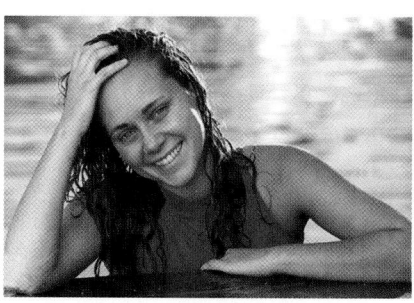

UNIT SEVEN

The Child and Family With Special Needs

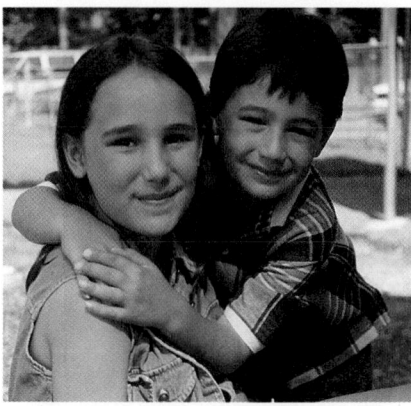

UNIT EIGHT

Impact of Hospitalization on the Child and Family

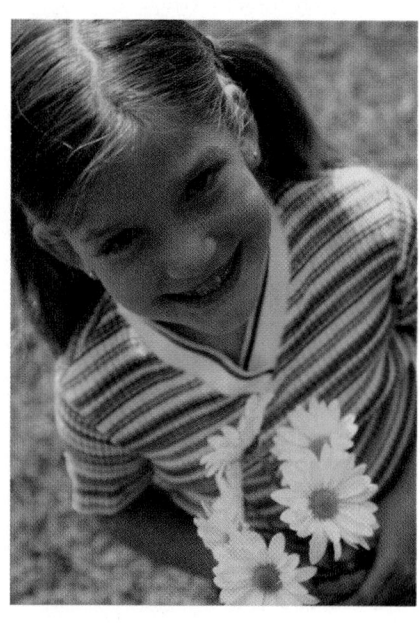

22 Pediatric Variations of Nursing Interventions, 706

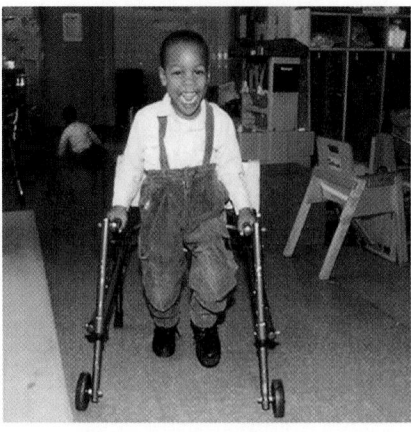

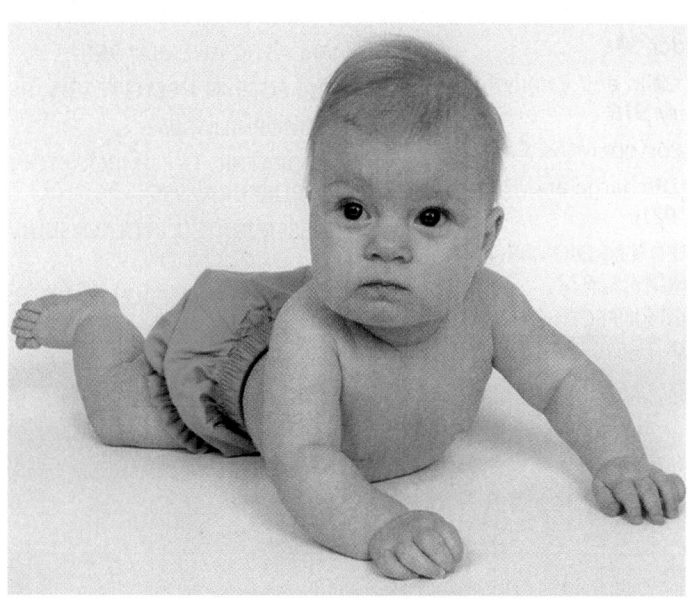

UNIT TEN
The Child With Problems Related to the Production and Circulation of Blood

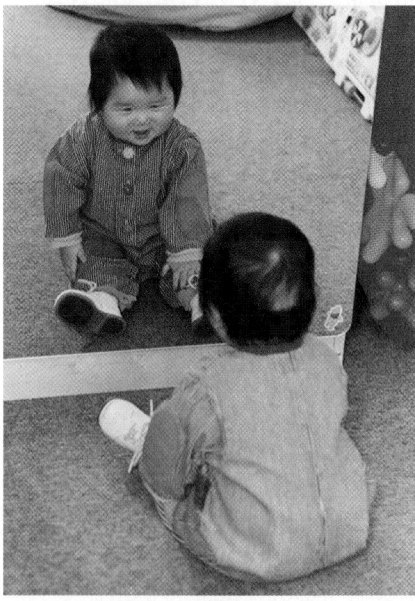

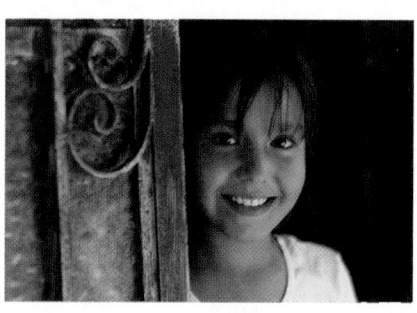

UNIT TWELVE

The Child With a Problem That Interferes With Physical Mobility

31 The Child With Musculoskeletal or Articular Dysfunction, 1147

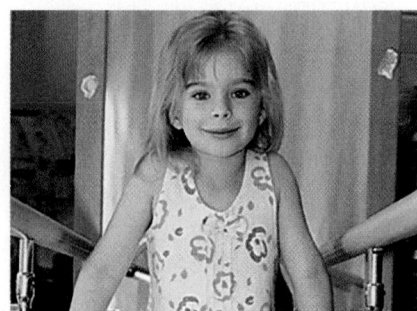

APPENDIXES

Perspectives of Pediatric Nursing

MARILYN L. WINKELSTEIN

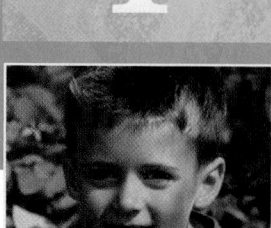

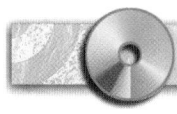 Remember to check out your companion CD-ROM

http://evolve.elsevier.com/Wong/essentials/

CHAPTER OUTLINE

RELATED TOPICS and ADDITIONAL RESOURCES

 IN TEXT

 CD COMPANION

LEARNING OBJECTIVES
On completion of this chapter the reader will be able to:

- Define the terms *mortality* and *morbidity.*
- Identify two ways that knowledge of mortality and morbidity can improve child health.
- List three major causes of death during infancy, early childhood, later childhood, and adolescence.

- List two major causes of illness during childhood.
- Outline four events that were significant in the evolution of child health care in the United States.
- Describe five broad functions of the pediatric nurse in promoting the health of children.

- Define critical thinking.
- Identify the five steps of the nursing process.
- Define nursing diagnosis.
- Differentiate among the three domains of nursing practice: dependent, independent, and interdependent.
- Differentiate a standard care plan from an individualized care plan.

HEALTH DURING CHILDHOOD

The *World Health Organization (WHO)* has defined health as "a state of complete physical, mental, and social well-being and not merely the absence of disease." This is an abstract definition that does not lend itself to concrete specific observations. In reality, information about health is gained by observing *mortality* (death) and *morbidity* (illness) among groups of individuals over specific periods. The balance between physical, mental, and social well-being and the presence of disease is inferred from analysis of data relating to mortality and morbidity.

Mortality and morbidity data also provide information about (1) the causes of death and illness, (2) high-risk age-groups for certain disorders or hazards, (3) advances in treatment and prevention, and (4) specific areas of health counseling. Such information is valuable to nurses because it guides the planning and delivery of nursing care.

"HEALTHY PEOPLE 2000 AND 2010"

Although the health of children in the United States improved dramatically during the twentieth century, several areas of concern remain. Serious domestic problems such as acquired immunodeficiency syndrome (AIDS), drug abuse, violence, and unwanted pregnancies have direct effects on the health of children. Solutions to these problems lie in their *prevention.*

In the last two decades, documents such as *Healthy People 2000* and *Healthy People 2010* established national health objectives and served as the basis for the development of state and community plans. *Healthy People 2010,* released in 2000, contains two overriding goals: (1) to increase the quality and length of healthy life and (2) to eliminate health disparities. The document also contains 10 leading health indicators relating to issues such as substance abuse, injury and violence, and other priority areas for the nation's health. The health indicators serve as focus areas for health improvement efforts. Many states have worked with community coalitions to develop their own versions of *Healthy People 2010.* The *Healthy People Toolkit** found on the Internet provides examples of state and national experiences using the objectives of *Healthy People 2010.*

*www.health.gov/healthypeople/state/toolkit.

MORTALITY

Figures describing rates of occurrence for events such as death in children are referred to as *vital statistics.* In the United States, the **National Center for Health Statistics (NCHS)** is responsible for the collection, analysis, and dissemination of health data. Since 1991, several changes have occurred in the reporting of health statistics. Figures for birth and death are based on the person's state of residence, not the state in which the event occurred. In addition, tabulation of race for live births has changed from the race of the child to the race of the mother. As a result of these changes, figures for births, deaths, and infant mortality rates by race cannot be compared with statistics reported before 1991. *Mortality statistics* describe the incidence or number of individuals who have died over a specific period. These statistics are usually presented as rates per 100,000 and are calculated from a sample of death certificates.

Infant Mortality

The *infant mortality rate* is the number of deaths during the first year of life per 1000 live births. Infant mortality is divided into *neonatal mortality* (<28 days of life) and *postneonatal mortality* (28 days to 11 months). In the United States, there has been a dramatic decrease in infant mortality. At the beginning of the twentieth century the rate was approximately 200 infant deaths per 1000 live births. In 2002, the infant mortality rate was 6.9 per 1000 live births (provisional data; Arias and others, 2003). This decrease resulted primarily from improvements in perinatal care, such as treatment of respiratory distress syndrome and fewer deaths from sudden infant death syndrome (SIDS). The mortality rate in 2001 for white infants was 5.7, and the rate for African-American infants was 14.0 (Arias and others, 2003). The challenge for this century is to reduce the gap between infant mortality for white and African American infants.

From a global perspective, the United States lags behind other developed countries. In 2000, the United States ranked last among nations with the lowest infant death rates. Singapore had the lowest infant death rate (Arias and others, 2003) (Table 1-1). Although the exact reason for the low ranking of the United States is unknown, one explanation may be that many countries with lower infant death rates have national health programs.

TABLE 1-1 ■ Infant Mortality Rate (IMR) for 2000 for Countries of 2,500,000 Population and With IMR Equal to or Less Than the United States Rate for 1999 (rate per 1000 live births)

COUNTRY	INFANT MORTALITY RATE 1999
Singapore	2.9*
Hong Kong	3.0
Japan	3.2*
Sweden	3.2*
Norway	3.8†
Finland	3.8†
Czech Republic	4.1†
Denmark	—
France	4.4*
Spain	4.4*
Germany	4.4*
Italy	4.6
Austria	4.8*
Switzerland	4.9†
Australia	4.9*
Canada	—
Netherlands	5.1†
Greece	5.4†
Belgium	5.2†
Portugal	5.6*
United Kingdom	5.6*
Israel	—
Ireland	5.9*
New Zealand	6.1
Cuba	6.2†
United States	6.9

From Arias E and others: Annual summary of vital statistics 2002, *Pediatrics* 112(6):1225, 2003.
Data from United Nations: *2000 demographic yearbook, Population and Vital Statistics Report*, statistical papers, series A, L111:1, Jan 2001; *Population and Vital Statistics Report*, statistical papers, series A, LIV:1, Jan 2002; *Population and Vital Statistics Report*, statistical papers, series A, LV:1, Jan 2003; OECD health data 2002 on the internet: www.oecd.org/health/.
*Provisional data.
†Organization for Economic Co-operation and Development data source.

Birth weight is considered the major determinant of neonatal death in technologically developed countries. There is a definite relationship between birth weight and mortality (Guyer and others, 2000). The high incidence of ***low birth weight (LBW)*** (<2500 g) in the United States is a key factor in its higher neonatal mortality rates when compared with other countries. Access to and use of high-quality prenatal care is the single most important preventive strategy to decrease early delivery and infant mortality. Other factors that increase the risk of infant mortality include African American race, male gender, short or long gestation, maternal age, and a low level of maternal education (Guyer and others, 2000).

Although there has been a steady and significant decline in infant mortality, the number of deaths in the first year of life is still proportionately high when compared with death

TABLE 1-2 ■ Death Rates by Age and Sex: United States, Preliminary 2001 (rate per 100,000 population)

AGE (years)	ALL RACES		
	BOTH SEXES	MALE	FEMALE
All ages*	848.5	846.4	850.4
<1†	684.8	752.1	614.4
1-4	33.3	37.0	29.5
5-9	15.3	16.7	13.9
10-14	19.2	22.8	15.3
15-19	66.9	93.7	38.5

Modified from Anderson RN, Smith BL: Deaths: leading causes for 2001, *Nat Vital Stat Rep* 52:9, Hyattsville, Md, 2003, National Center for Vital Statistics.
*Figures for ages not stated are included in "All ages" but not distributed among age-groups.
†Death rates for "<1 year" (based on population estimates) differ from infant mortality rates (based on live births).

rates at other ages (Table 1-2). Serious health conditions in preterm LBW infants occur most often during the first 6 months after hospital discharge. In the United States, the death rate for infants younger than 1 year of age is greater than the rate for individuals ages 1 through 54 years. It is not until age 55 and older that the death rate begins to exceed the rate for infants.

In the 1960s, attention was focused on perinatal health care in an effort to decrease the number of neonatal deaths. Neonatal mortality declined from 20.5 per 1000 live births in 1950 to 4.5 per 1000 live births in 2001 (Arias and others, 2003). This decline resulted from advances in neonatal intensive care and better treatment of perinatal illnesses. However, many of the leading causes of death during infancy continue to occur during the perinatal period (Table 1-3). The first four causes—congenital anomalies, disorders related to short gestation and unspecified LBW, SIDS, and newborn affected by maternal complications of pregnancy—account for just over half (50.2%) of all deaths of infants younger than 1 year of age (Minino and others, 2002).

Although a number of perinatal problems have benefited from improved treatment, congenital anomalies continue to be a leading cause of infant mortality. The incidence of the majority of birth defects has remained substantially the same. Heart defects have been rising, but the increase is the result of improved methods of detection, not increased births of affected infants. Anencephaly and spina bifida are expected to decrease with the recommendation of folic acid supplementation for all women of childbearing age (see Spina Bifida [Myelomeningocele], Chapter 32). Reducing LBW will also prevent congenital anomalies. Infant mortality resulting from human immunodeficiency virus (HIV) infection has decreased significantly; in 2000, HIV/AIDS accounted for less than 0.04% of all deaths in children younger than 1 year of age (Minino and others, 2002).

When infant death rates are categorized according to race, infant mortality for whites is lower than for all other races in the United States, and the infant mortality rate for African Americans is twice the rate for whites. The gap between these two racial groups has remained fairly constant. The LBW rate is also higher for African American infants than for any other group. Reasons for these high rates are unknown. One encouraging note is that the gap in mortality rates between white and nonwhite races other than African Americans is narrowing. Infant mortality rates for Hispanics and Asian Pacific Islanders decreased dramatically during the last 20 years (Minino and others, 2002).

Childhood Mortality

Death rates for children older than 1 year of age have always been less than the rate for infants (see Table 1-2). Children ages 5 to 14 years have the lowest rate of death (Table 1-4). However, a sharp rise occurs during later adolescence, primarily from injuries, homicide, and suicide. In 2001, these conditions were responsible for approximately 75% of deaths in teenagers and young adults 15 to 19 years old (Arias and others, 2003). The trend in racial differences that occurs in infant mortality is also seen in childhood deaths for all ages and for both sexes. Whites have fewer deaths for all ages, and male deaths outnumber female deaths.

After 1 year of age, there is a dramatic change in the cause of death. Unintentional injuries (accidents) are the leading cause of death from the youngest ages to the adolescent years. In addition, *violent deaths* are increasing among young people ages 10 through 25 years, especially among African American males. Homicide is the second leading cause of death in the 15- to 19-year age-group (see Table 1-4). Children 12 years of age and older are more likely to be killed by non–family members (acquaintances and gangs, typically of the same race) and most frequently by firearms. Firearm homicide is the leading cause of death among African American males ages 15 to 19 years. *Suicide* is the third leading cause of death among adolescents and young adults 10 to 19 years old (see Table 1-4).

The causes of increased violence against children and self-inflicted violence are not fully understood. In young children, the increase in homicide may represent more accurate identification of child abuse. The problem of child homicides is complex and involves psychologic, social, and economic factors. Nurses need to be aware of young people who are depressed, repeatedly in trouble with the criminal justice system, or associated with groups known to be violent. Prevention requires identification of these individuals and therapeutic intervention by qualified professionals. Pediatric nurses can also assess children and adolescents for risk factors related to violence (such as the presence of a gun in a household) and educate families, teachers, and community leaders about the importance of maintaining safe, nonviolent homes, schools, and neighborhoods.

The major declines in death rates during childhood have occurred in deaths caused by gastrointestinal diseases, infectious diseases, perinatal conditions, neoplasms, and injuries. The absence of infectious diseases as a leading cause of death

---

TABLE 1-3 ■ Mortality Rate and Percentage of Total Deaths for 10 Leading Causes of Infant Death in 2001 (rate per 1000 live births)

RANK	CAUSE OF DEATH*	PERCENT	RATE
—	All races, all causes	100.00	684.8
1	Congenital anomalies	20.0	136.9
2	Disorders relating to short gestation and unspecified low birth weight	16.0	109.5
3	Sudden infant death syndrome	8.1	55.5
4	Newborn affected by maternal complications of pregnancy	5.4	37.2
5	Newborn affected by complications of placenta, cord, and membranes	3.7	25.3
6	Respiratory distress syndrome	3.7	25.1
7	Accidents (unintentional injuries)	3.5	24.2
8	Bacterial sepsis of newborn	2.5	17.3
9	Diseases of the circulatory system	2.3	15.4
10	Intrauterine hypoxia and birth asphyxia	1.9	13.3

Modified from Anderson RN, Smith BL: Deaths: leading causes for 2001, *Nat Vital Stat Rep* 52:9, Hyattsville, Md, 2003, National Center for Vital Statistics.
*Based on World Health Organization: *International statistical classification of diseases and related health problems*, rev 10, Geneva, Switzerland, 1992, WHO.

TABLE 1-4 ■ Five Leading Causes of Death in Children in the United States: Selected Age Intervals—2000—Preliminary Data (rates per 100,000)

RANK	AGES 1-4	RATE	AGES 5-9	RATE	AGES 10-14	RATE	AGES 15-19	RATE
	All causes	33.3	All causes	15.3	All causes	19.2	All causes	66.9
1	Accidents	11.2	Accidents	6.4	Accidents	7.4	Accidents	32.8
2	Congenital anomalies	3.6	Cancer	2.4	Cancer	2.5	Homicide	9.4
3	Cancer	2.7	Congenital anomalies	0.9	Suicide	1.3	Suicide	7.9
4	Homicide	2.7	Homicide	0.7	Congenital anomalies	0.9	Cancer	3.6
5	Heart disease	1.5	Heart disease	0.5	Homicide	0.9	Heart disease	1.7

Modified from Anderson RN, Smith BL: Deaths: leading causes for 2001, *Nat Vital Stat Rep* 52:9, Hyattsville, Md, 2003, National Center for Vital Statistics.

is related to the use of antibacterial agents and immunizations. Deaths caused by infectious diseases have decreased considerably in recent years. In particular, deaths from HIV infection have decreased, and HIV is no longer one of the ten leading causes of death (Anderson and Smith, 2003). Other disorders such as neoplasms have become more prominent causes of death, although childhood deaths from cancer are currently less frequent than ever before (see Leukemias, Chapter 26).

Injuries.   Injuries, the leading cause of death in children older than 1 year of age, are responsible for more childhood deaths and disabilities than all causes of disease combined. As children grow older, the percentage of deaths from injuries increases (Table 1-5). Injuries have not shown the dramatic declines seen in other areas of childhood mortality because injuries have traditionally been regarded as unavoidable accidents or behavioral problems, rather than health problems. The term *accident* suggests a chaotic, random event related to "luck" or "chance." The term *injury* is now preferred because it indicates a sense of responsibility and control.

The pattern of deaths caused by unintentional injuries, especially from motor vehicles, drowning, and burns, is consistent in Western societies. However, the United States exceeds other countries in the number of violent deaths. The leading causes of deaths from injuries for each age-group according to sex are presented in Table 1-5. The majority of deaths from injuries occur in males. It is important to note that accidents account for more teen deaths than any other source (Annie E. Casey Foundation, 2001). Fortunately, prevention strategies such as the use of car restraints, bicycle helmets, and smoke detectors have resulted in a significant decrease in fatalities for younger children. All states have legislation requiring young children to be properly restrained in motor vehicles. Despite safety efforts, however, the overwhelming cause of death in children older than 1 year of age is motor vehicle (MV)–related fatalities, including occupant, pedestrian, bicycle, and motorcycle deaths (Fig. 1-1). Even though the *percentage* of infants dying from MV injuries is small compared with the total number of deaths in infancy, children younger than 1 year of age continue to have a high death rate from MV occupant deaths because they are not properly restrained.

When deaths from injuries are compared according to sex and age, the causes of death differ. The developmental stage of the child determines the type of injury that is most

TABLE 1-5 ■ Mortality From Leading Types of Unintentional Injuries, United States, 1997 (rates per 100,000 population in each age-group)

TYPE OF ACCIDENT	AGE (YEARS)			
	<1	1-4	5-14	15-24
MALES				
All causes	818.0	39.8	24.0	124.4
Unintentional injuries (all types)	22.3	15.2	10.6	52.3
Motor vehicle	4.4 (2)	5.3 (1)	5.8 (1)	38.3 (1)
Drowning	1.8 (4)	3.9 (2)	1.6 (2)	3.2 (2)
Fires and burns	1.5 (5)	2.5 (3)	0.8 (3)	—
Firearms	—	0.5 (4)	1.5 (4)	—
Ingestion of food/object	2.5 (3)	0.5 (5)	—	—
Falls	—	—	—	1.2 (5)
Mechanical suffocation	9.1 (1)	0.6 (4)	0.4 (5)	—
Poisoning	—	—	—	2.8 (3)
All other unintentional injuries	3.1	2.3	1.4	5.3
*Accidents as a percent of all deaths	2.7%	38.2%	44.3%	42.0%
FEMALES				
All causes	662.9	31.8	17.4	46.0
Unintentional injuries (all types)	18.1	10.9	6.7	20.0
Motor vehicle	4.4 (2)	4.7 (1)	4.3 (1)	17.1 (1)
Drowning	1.4 (4)	2.0 (2)	0.6 (3)	0.4 (3)
Fires and burns	1.2 (5)	2.0 (2)	0.7 (2)	—
Firearms	—	—	0.1 (4)	0.1 (5)
Ingestion of food/object	1.5 (3)	0.4 (4)	—	—
Falls	—	—	—	0.2 (4)
Mechanical suffocation	6.9 (1)	0.3 (5)	0.1 (4)	—
Poisoning	—	—	—	0.8 (2)
All other unintentional injuries	2.7	1.5	0.9	1.5
*Accidents as a percent of all deaths	2.7%	34.2%	38.2%	43.4%

Modified from National Safety Council: *Injury facts,* Itaska, Il, 2000, National Safety Council.
Data from National Center for Health Statistics.
*Indicates rank among the leading types of accidents.

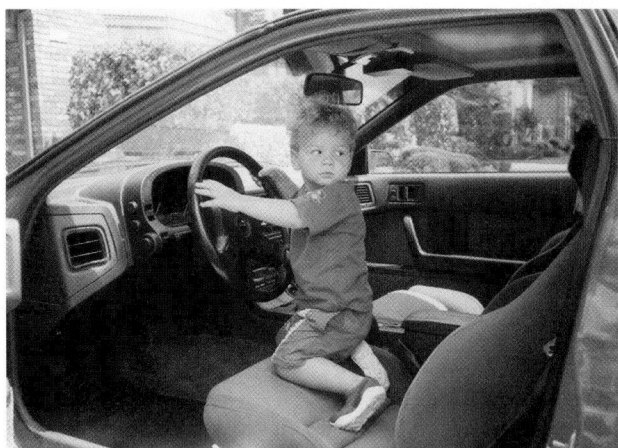

FIG. 1-1 ■ Motor vehicle injuries are the leading cause of death in children older than 1 year of age. The majority of the fatalities involve occupants who are unrestrained.

likely to occur at a specific age. For example, a child between the ages of 1 and 4 years is equally likely to die as an occupant or as a pedestrian in MV injuries. However, children ages 5 to 9 years are more likely to die from pedestrian crashes, and adolescents are more likely to die from occupant crashes. Children ages 5 to 14 are at greatest risk of bicycling fatalities. The majority of bicycling deaths are from head injuries. Helmets reduce the risk of head injury by 85%, but few children wear helmets (National Safety Council, 2000).

Drowning and burns are the second and third leading causes of death in males ages 1 to 14, but the order is reversed in females (Fig. 1-2). Drowning is a significant cause of death in older teenagers. In addition, improper use of firearms is a major cause of death in males (Fig. 1-3). Dur-

ing infancy, more males die from aspiration or suffocation than do females (Fig. 1-4). More than half of all poisonings occur in children younger than 2 years of age (Fig. 1-5). By ages 4 to 5 years, unintentional poisonings are uncommon. Another increase occurs in the 15- to 24-year age-group, in which poisoning is the third leading cause of death in males and the second in females. Poisoning in this age-group is often intentional and represents death from suicide (especially females) or drug abuse.

It is important to remember that not all injuries are unintentional; some may be intentional and represent abuse or suicide. When injuries occur, nurses may need to help determine if they were intentional.

> **!NURSING ALERT**
>
> The history of the injury is essential in assessing intentional injury from abuse or neglect. The following questions are important:
> **When**—Did the parent or guardian seek immediate medical attention or has there been a long delay?
> **Where**—Does the reported location of the accident correlate with the nature of the injury?
> **How**—Are the circumstances surrounding the injury logical?

Injury Prevention. When comparing deaths from injuries with other causes of childhood mortality, it is clear that preventing injuries is the best strategy to improve survival. Nurses play a major role in providing anticipatory guidance to parents and older children regarding hazards during each age period.

Theoretically, all injuries are preventable. Injury prevention is an ongoing part of health promotion for all age-groups. Anticipatory guidance regarding developmental expectations serves to alert parents to the types of injuries most common at any given age. Early in the parent-child re-

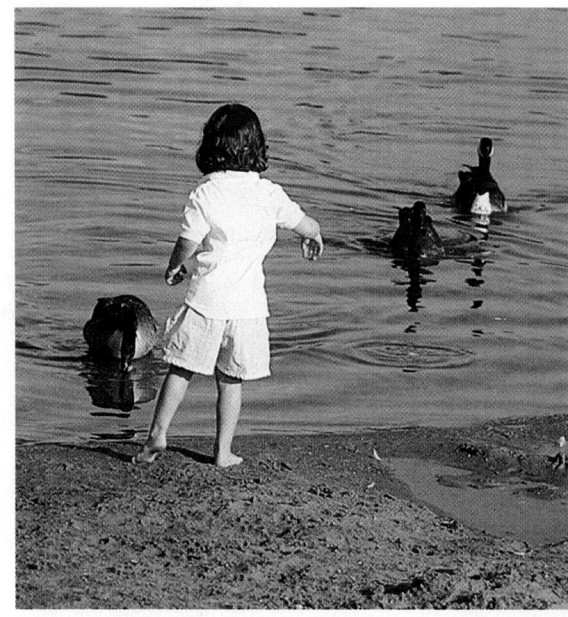

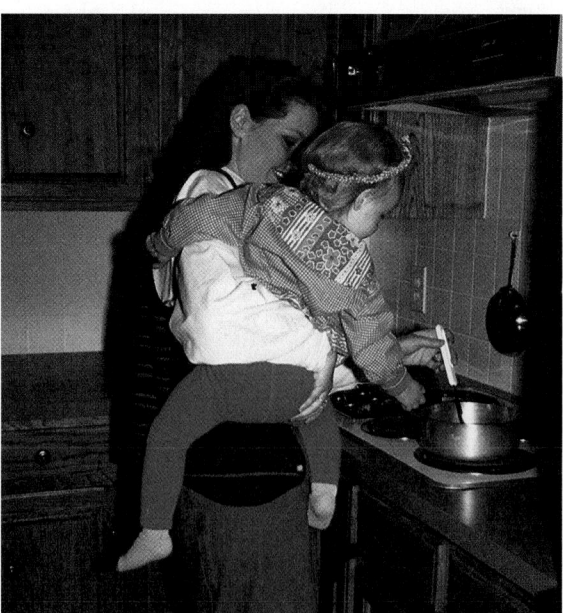

FIG. 1-2 ■ **A,** Drowning is the second leading cause of death from injury in boys and the third in girls ages 5 to 14 years. **B,** Burns are the second leading cause of death from injury in girls and the third in boys ages 1 to 14 years.

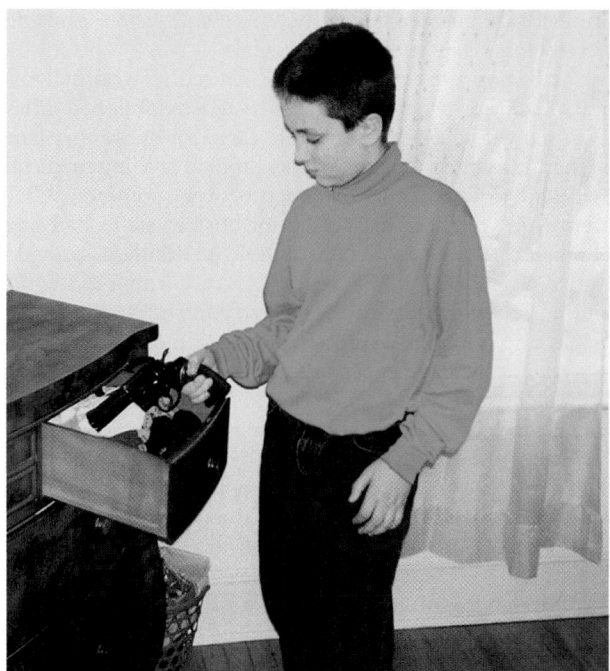

FIG. 1-3 ■ Improper use of firearms is the fourth leading cause of death from injury in boys 5 to 24 years and girls ages 5 to 14 years.

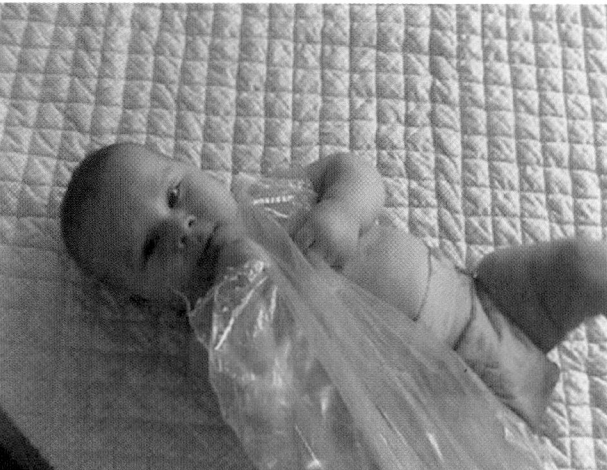

FIG. 1-4 ■ Mechanical suffocation is often the leading cause of death from injury in infants.

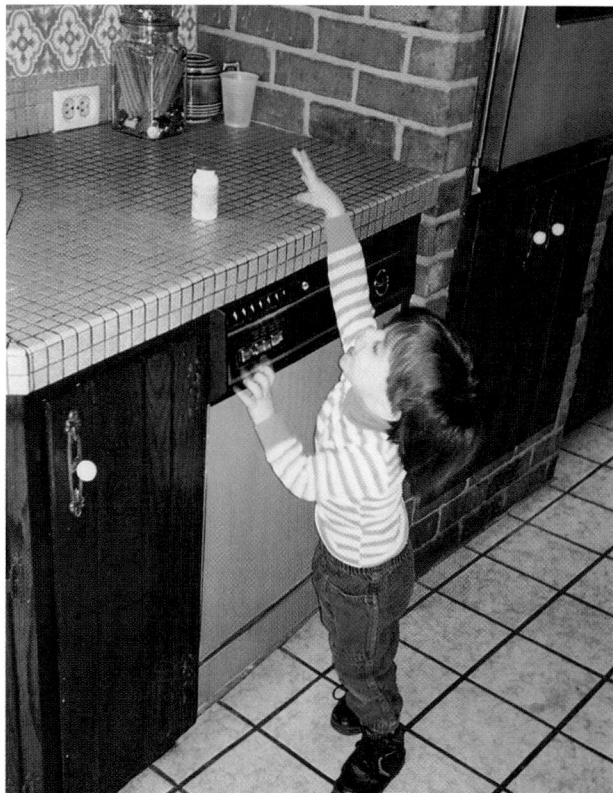

FIG. 1-5 ■ Poisoning causes a considerable number of injuries in children under 4 years of age, but it is the third leading cause of death from injury in males and the second in females (usually from suicide) ages 15 to 24 years.

lationship, parents need advice on how to provide a safe environment. It cannot be assumed that parents of one or more children are familiar with all areas of child safety. The addition of a new infant may cause sibling rivalry, and the new infant may be at risk from a jealous sibling. The American Academy of Pediatrics has developed an injury prevention program *named TIPP: The Injury Prevention Program* that provides useful information and anticipatory guidance on safety issues for parents and health care providers.* Another resource is the **Consumer Product Safety Commission (CPSC)** of the U.S. Government, which provides publications that recommend areas of safety for children.†

MORBIDITY

The prevalence of specific illnesses in the population at a particular time is known as *morbidity statistics.* These are generally presented as rates per 1000 population because of their greater frequency of occurrence. Unlike mortality, morbidity is difficult to define and may denote acute illness, chronic disease, or disability. Sources of data for morbidity statistics include reasons for visits to physicians, diagnoses for hospital admission, and household interviews. Unlike death rates, which are updated annually, morbidity statistics are revised less frequently and may not represent the general population.

Childhood Morbidity

Acute illness is defined as symptoms severe enough to limit activity or require medical attention. Respiratory illness accounts for about 50% of all acute conditions, infections and parasitic disease cause 11%, and injuries cause 15%. The chief illness of childhood is the common cold.

---

*For more information contact the **American Academy of Pediatrics,** 141 Northwest Point Boulevard, Elk Grove Village, IL 60007; (888) 227-1770; fax: (847) 228-1281; www.aap.org.
†For more information call (800) 638-CPSC or (800) 638-2272.

The types of diseases that children contract during child-hood vary according to age. For example, upper respiratory tract infections and diarrhea decrease with age, but other disorders such as acne and headaches increase. Children who have had a particular type of problem are more likely to have that problem again. Morbidity is not distributed randomly in children. Children from poor families tend to have more health problems. This finding suggests a need for heightened efforts to improve access to health care for low-income children.

Recent concern has focused on specific groups of children who have increased morbidity—homeless children, children living in poverty, children of LBW, children with chronic illnesses, foreign-born adopted children, and children in day care centers. Several factors place these groups at risk for poor health. One factor is barriers to health care, especially for the homeless, the poor, and children with chronic health problems. Other factors include improved survival of children with chronic health problems, particularly infants of very LBW. Children living in or exposed to at-risk environments such as the country of origin for adopted children and day care centers may be more likely to have medical problems such as infections (Lears, Guth, and Lewandowski, 1998).

Injuries are an additional factor influencing morbidity. Each year 40,000 to 50,000 children are injured permanently and 1 million children receive medical care because of unintentional injuries.

The most important aspect of morbidity is the degree of disability it produces. *Disability* can be measured in days absent from school or days confined to bed. On average, a child loses 5.3 days per year because of injury or illness. (The incidence of chronic conditions is discussed in Chapter 18.)

For many children childhood is a time of relative health, but it is the rare child who never becomes ill. Education of parents regarding the usual types of childhood illnesses and recognition of symptoms that require treatment is an important part of nursing care. Health promotion and health education are important roles for pediatric nurses.

The New Morbidity

In addition to disease and injury, children face behavioral, social, family, and educational problems that are referred to as the *new morbidity* or *pediatric social illness.* These problems (e.g., poverty, violence, school failure) interfere with children's social and academic development. Estimates of the incidence of these problems vary from 5% to 30%.

Although no conclusive characteristics have been identified for children with new morbidity problems, several findings appear to define at-risk groups. These include (1) children from low socioeconomic status, (2) of the male gender, and (3) with a sibling who has had a previous injury (Altemeier, 2000).

EVOLUTION OF CHILD HEALTH CARE IN THE UNITED STATES

Children in colonial America were born into a world with many hazards to their health and survival. Epidemics were common. Physicians were few, and only a small number had formal training. Midwives were untrained and based their practice on past experiences. Books providing information on childcare and feeding were scarce and, when available, were helpful only to literate parents.

Medical care by physicians was limited to wealthy families who lived in or could travel to more developed cities. Children who lived on farms were cared for by another family member or by a competent neighbor. Traveling medicine men and various forms of quackery were common. Children who were bought as slaves or born to slaves had only as much care as their owner was able or willing to provide. Native American children were treated according to the tradition of their tribe, which was often a mixture of medicine, magic, and religion. With the colonization of America, Native Americans were exposed to new, often fatal, diseases.

Reliable statistics on childhood mortality during the colonial period are unavailable. Epidemic diseases included smallpox, measles, mumps, chickenpox, influenza, diphtheria, yellow fever, cholera, and whooping cough. Dysentery was the most common cause of childhood death. Other diseases that contributed to childhood illness were the "slow epidemics" of tuberculosis, nutritional diseases, and injuries.

Although scientific knowledge was accumulating in the colonial period, there were no organized efforts in the United States to apply this knowledge to the sick until the nineteenth century. At this time, the consequences of childhood illness and injury and the effects of child labor, poverty, and neglect became widely recognized.

The study of pediatrics began in the 1800s, under the influence of a Prussian-born physician, *Abraham Jacobi* (1830-1919), who is referred to as the *Father of Pediatrics.* Jacobi broke new ground in the scientific and clinical investigation of childhood diseases. One outstanding achievement of this time was the establishment of "milk stations," where mothers could bring sick children for treatment and learn the importance of pure milk and its proper preparation.

The crusade for pure milk helped bring the dairy industry under legal control and led to the establishment of infant welfare stations. The remarkable decline in infant mortality since 1900 has been achieved through health-promoting measures such as improved sanitation and pasteurization of milk. Before these regulations existed, unsanitary milk was a source of infantile diarrhea and bovine tuberculosis. Cows were often kept in filthy stables and fed garbage and distillery wastes. Milk from these cows was reported to make infants "tipsy."

At this time, increasing concern developed for the social welfare of children, especially those who were homeless or employed as factory laborers. The work of one reformer, *Lillian Wald* (1867-1940), had far-reaching effects on child health and nursing. Wald founded the Henry Street Settlement in New York City, which eventually provided nursing service, social work, and an organized program of social, cultural, and educational activities. She is regarded as the *founder of public health* or *community nursing,* and was instrumental in establishing the role of the first full-time school nurse, *Lina Rogers.* Soon, other nurses were employed to teach parents and children about the prevention or need for treatment of minor skin conditions, malnutrition, and other illnesses identified in the school. An outgrowth of this nursing involvement in school health was the development of pediatric courses and clinical experience in schools of nursing.

As causes of disease were identified, emphasis on isolation and asepsis occurred. In the early 1900s, children with contagious diseases were isolated from adult patients. Parents were prohibited from visiting because they might transmit disease to and from the home. Even toys and personal articles of clothing were kept from the child. In the 1940s, the investigations of Spitz and Robertson highlighted the effects of isolation and maternal deprivation on institutionalized children. Their research stimulated interest in the psychologic health of children and resulted in changes for hospitalized children, such as rooming-in, sibling visitations, child life programs, prehospitalization preparation, parent education, and hospital schooling.

Influenced by social reformers such as Lillian Wald, national leaders took action to improve children's living conditions. In 1909, President Theodore Roosevelt convened the first *White House Conference on Children,* which focused on the care of dependent children and addressed the deplorable working conditions of youngsters. As a result of this conference, the *U.S. Children's Bureau* was established in 1912. This marked the beginning of a period of studies of economic and social factors related to infant mortality, maternal deaths, and maternal and infant care in rural settings. These studies stimulated the creation of better standards of care for mothers and children and led to the first *Maternity and Infancy Act.* This act provided grants to states to develop a Division of Maternal and Child Health (MCH) as a unit of the health department and influenced the creation of the *American Academy of Pediatrics.*

In 1935, *Title V of the Social Security Act (SSA)* was passed and a federal-state partnership was established under the administration of the Children's Bureau. Title V included federal grants-in-aid to states (matched by state funds) for three types of work: *maternal and child health (MCH), Crippled Children's Services (CCS),* and *child welfare services.* The first programs provided by Title V were prenatal, postnatal, and child health clinics. Another focus of the CCS was orthopedic care. With the recognition that a child's ability to function could be limited by a chronic illness, state CCS programs became involved with children with developmental, behavioral, and educational problems and more recently with home care of children with complex medical conditions. This broadened concept was reflected in the 1985 passage of legislation that changed the name of the CCS to the *Program for Children with Special Health Needs (CSHN).*

Other federal programs that have had a major impact on maternal and child health include the following:

Medicaid. Medicaid was created in 1965 under Title XIX of the Social Security Act to reduce financial barriers to health care for the poor. It is the largest maternal-child health program. A major project under Medicaid is the Child Health Assessment Program (CHAP), which provides services for pregnant women and children. Financial eligibility varies from state to state.

Aid to Families with Dependent Children (AFDC). The SSA of 1935 established AFDC as a cash grant program to enable states to aid needy children without fathers.

MCH Services Block Grant. MCH Services Block Grant provides health services to mothers and children, particularly those with low income or limited access to health services. Its primary purposes are to reduce infant mortality and the incidence of preventable disease and handicapping conditions among children and to increase the availability of prenatal, delivery, and postpartum care to eligible mothers.

Alcohol, Drug Abuse, and Mental Health Block Grant. Established by the Omnibus Budget Reconciliation Act of 1981, this block grant provides funds to states for (1) projects to support prevention, treatment, and rehabilitation related to substance abuse and (2) grants to community mental health centers for the identification, assessment, and treatment of severely mentally disturbed children and adolescents.

Social Services Block Grant. Established under Title XX of the SSA, this grant provides states with funds for child day care, protective and emergency services, counseling, family planning, home-based services, information and referral, and adoption and foster care services.

Women, Infants, and Children (WIC). The WIC Special Supplemental Food Program was started in 1974. It provides nutritious food and nutrition education to low-income, pregnant, postpartum, and lactating women and to infants and children up to age 5 years. Other nutrition programs include Food Stamps, National School Lunch Program, School Breakfast Program, and the Child Care Food Program, which provides financial assistance for nutritious meals to children in day care centers, family and group day care homes, and Head Start centers.

Education for All Handicapped Children Act (P.L. 94-142). P.L. 94-142 was passed in 1975 to provide free public education to all handicapped children ages 3 to 21 years and to provide supportive services (such as speech and counseling) that ensure the benefit of special education.

Education of the Handicapped Act Amendments of 1986 (P.L. 99-457). In 1986, P.L. 99-457 was passed to allow federal funding to states to develop and implement a statewide, comprehensive, coordinated, and multidisciplinary program of early intervention services for handicapped infants and toddlers and their families.

Omnibus Budge Reconciliation Act of 1990. This act required states to extend Medicaid coverage to all children ages 6 to 18 years with family incomes below 133% of the poverty level.

Family and Medical Leave Act (FMLA). FMLA was signed into law in 1993. This act allows eligible employees to take up to 12 weeks of unpaid leave from their jobs every year to care for newborn or newly adopted children; to care for children, parents, or spouses who have serious health conditions; or to recover from their own serious health conditions. After the leave, the law entitles employees to return to their previous jobs or equivalent jobs with the same pay, benefits, and other conditions.

Health Insurance Portability and Accountability Act (HIPAA). The first-ever federal privacy standards to protect patients' medical records and other health information provided to health plans, doctors, hospitals, and other health care providers took effect on April 14, 2003. HIPPA, developed by the Department of Health and Human Services (HHS), contains new standards that provide patients with access to their medical records and more control over how their personal health information is used and disclosed. For further information see the website: http://www.hhs.gov/ocr/hipaa.

Despite federal and state programs available to assist children and families, serious barriers to health care remain. These include (1) *financial barriers,* such as not having insurance, having insurance that does not cover certain services, or being unable to pay for services; (2) *system barriers,* such as having to travel great distances for health care or state-to-state variations in Medicaid benefits; and (3) *knowledge barriers,* such as a lack of understanding of the need for prenatal or child health supervision or an unawareness of the services available. The current thrust in health care is to improve access to health care for all children and their families.

Another major change in health care delivery has been the establishment of a *prospective payment system* based on *diagnosis-related groups (DRGs).* The DRG categories define *pretreatment (prospective) billing* for U.S. hospitals reimbursed by Medicare. When hospitals are held financially responsible if Medicare patients exceed the allotted admission stay, patients are discharged early. Early discharges have created a need for home care and community-based services. Health care cost containment remains a national priority, and currently, many children are enrolled in *managed care companies and health maintenance organizations (HMOs).** In some instances, these companies and organizations have improved access to preventive health care for children, but in other cases, they have reduced access to specialty care for children with chronic conditions (Szilagy, 1998).

PEDIATRIC NURSING

PHILOSOPHY OF CARE

Nursing of infants and children is consistent with the revised *definition of nursing* proposed by the Social Policy Task Force of the American Nurses Association in 2003. This definition states that "nursing is the prevention of illness, the alleviation of suffering, and the protection, promotion, and restoration of health in the care of individuals, families, groups, communities, and populations" (American Nurses Association, 2001; American Nurses Association, 2003). This definition incorporates the four essential features of nursing practice:

1 Attention to the full range of human experiences and responses to health and illness without restriction to a problem-focused orientation
2 Integration of objective data with knowledge gained from an understanding of the patient or group's subjective experience
3 Application of scientific knowledge to the processes of diagnosis and treatment
4 Provision of a caring relationship that facilitates health and healing (American Nurses Association, 2003)

Family-Centered Care†

The philosophy of *family-centered care* recognizes the family as the one constant in a child's life. Three key components of family-centered care are respect, collaboration, and support (Galvin and others, 2000). Families are supported in their caregiving and decision making when health care professionals build on their unique strengths and acknowledge their expertise in caring for their child both within and outside the hospital setting (Newton, 2000). Patterns of liv-

---

*For information on managed care references and resources, contact www.nursingworld.org.
†For additional information, please view "Family-Centered Care" in *Whaley and Wong's Pediatric Nursing Video Series,* St Louis, 1996, Mosby; (800) 426-4545; www.elsevierhealth.com.

BOX 1-1 ■ The Key Elements of Family-Centered Care

Incorporating into policy and practice the recognition that the *family is the constant* in a child's life while the service systems and support personnel within those systems fluctuate
Facilitating *family/professional collaboration* at all levels of hospital, home, and community care:
    Care of an individual child
    Program development, implementation, and evaluation
    Policy formation
Exchanging complete and unbiased information between family members and professionals in a supportive manner at all times
Incorporating into policy and practice the recognition and *honoring of cultural diversity,* strengths, and individuality within and across all families, including *ethnic, racial, spiritual, social, economic, educational,* and *geographic diversity*
Recognizing and respecting *different methods of coping* and implementing comprehensive policies and programs that provide *developmental, educational, emotional, environmental,* and *financial support* to meet the diverse needs of families
Encouraging and facilitating *family-to-family support* and networking
Ensuring that *home, hospital,* and *community service* and *support systems* for children needing specialized health and developmental care and their families are *flexible, accessible,* and *comprehensive* in responding to diverse family-identified needs
Appreciating families as families and children as children, recognizing that they possess a wide range of strengths, concerns, emotions, and aspirations beyond their need for specialized health and developmental services and support

From Shelton TL, Stepanek JS: *Family-centered care for children needing specialized health and developmental services,* Bethesda, Md, 1994, Association for the Care of Children's Health.

ing at home and in the community are promoted, and the needs of all family members, not just the child's, are considered (Box 1-1). The philosophy of family-centered care acknowledges diversity among family structures and backgrounds; family goals, dreams, strategies, and actions; and family support, service, and information needs.

Two basic concepts in family-centered care are enabling and empowerment. Professionals *enable* families by creating opportunities for all family members to display their current abilities and competencies and to acquire new ones that are necessary to meet the needs of the child and family. *Empowerment* describes the interaction of professionals with families in such a way that families maintain or acquire a sense of control over their lives and make positive changes that result from helping behaviors that foster their own strengths, abilities, and actions.

The *parent-professional partnership* is a powerful mechanism for enabling and empowering families.* Parents serve

---

*For information about parent-professional partnerships, a free pamphlet, *Equals in This Partnership,* is available from **The National Center for Infants, Toddlers and Families,** 200 M Street NW, Suite 200, Washington, DC 20036; (202) 638-1144.

as respected equals with professionals and have the right to decide what is important for themselves and their family. The professional supports and strengthens the family's ability to nurture and promote family development. Professionals must also work together as a team to benefit children and their families.

Partnerships imply the belief that partners are capable individuals who become more competent by sharing knowledge, skills, and resources in a manner that benefits all participants. Collaboration is viewed as a continuum. Families have the option of being anywhere along the continuum, depending on their strengths and needs and their relationships with professionals. The nurse can help *every* family, including those with a previous history of serious personal or family problems, to identify their strengths, build on them, and assume a comfortable level of participation. Although caring for the family is strongly emphasized throughout the text, it is highlighted in features such as Cultural Awareness, Family Focus, and Family Home Care boxes.

Atraumatic Care

Although tremendous advances have been made in pediatric care, many changes that have cured illnesses and prolonged life are traumatic, painful, upsetting, and frightening. Unfortunately, minimizing the trauma of medical interventions has not kept pace with technologic advances. Health professionals must be aware of the stresses facing ill children and their families and strive to provide interventions that are safe, effective, and helpful. Health professionals must also attempt to provide atraumatic care.

Atraumatic care is the provision of therapeutic care in settings, by personnel, and through the use of interventions that eliminate or minimize the psychologic and physical distress experienced by children and their families in the health care system. *Therapeutic care* encompasses the prevention, diagnosis, treatment, or palliation of chronic or acute conditions. *Setting* refers to whatever place that care is given—the home, the hospital, or any other health care setting. *Personnel* includes anyone directly involved in providing therapeutic care. *Interventions* range from psychologic approaches, such as preparing children for procedures, to physical interventions, such as providing space for a parent to room in with a child. *Psychologic distress* may include anxiety, fear, anger, disappointment, sadness, shame, or guilt. *Physical distress* may range from sleeplessness and immobilization to the experience of disturbing sensory stimuli such as pain, temperature extremes, loud noises, bright lights, or darkness. Atraumatic care is concerned with the who, what, when, where, why, and how of any procedure performed on a child for the purpose of preventing or minimizing psychologic and physical stress (Wong, 1989).

The overriding goal in providing atraumatic care is *first, do no harm.* Three principles provide the framework for achieving this goal: (1) prevent or minimize the child's separation from the family; (2) promote a sense of control; and (3) prevent or minimize bodily injury and pain. Examples of atraumatic care include fostering the parent-child relationship during hospitalization, preparing the child before any unfamiliar treatment or procedure, controlling pain, allowing the child privacy, providing play activities for expression

BOX 1-2 ■ AHCPR Clinical Practice Guidelines Relevant to Pediatric Practice

Acute pain management: operative or medical procedures and trauma
Urinary incontinence
Pressure ulcers: prediction and intervention
Treatment of pressure ulcers
Diagnosis and treatment of depressed outpatients in primary care settings
Diagnosis and treatment of sickle cell disease
Initial evaluation and early treatment of the HIV-infected individual
Management of cancer-related pain
Diagnosis and treatment of heart failure
Otitis media with effusion

Modified from AHCRP (now known as AHRQ). To order guidelines, contact AHCPR Publications Clearinghouse, PO Box 8547, Silver Spring, MD 20907; (800) 358-9295; website: www.ahcpr.gov.

of fear and aggression, providing choices to children, and respecting cultural differences.

Atraumatic care is an integral part of nursing care discussions in the text. Atraumatic Care boxes highlight selected examples, and several boxes focusing on culture, family teaching, research, and critical thinking incorporate atraumatic care. Chapter 21, Family-Centered Care of the Child During Illness and Hospitalization, is organized according to principles of atraumatic care.

Case Management

Case management developed as an approach to coordinate care and control costs. The benefits of case management include improved patient/family satisfaction, decreased fragmentation of care, and the ability to describe and measure outcomes for a homogeneous group of patients.

Case managers are responsible and accountable for particular groups of patients and often use timelines derived from standards of care. Timelines have a variety of names: critical paths, guidelines for care, case management plans, Caremaps,* coordinated care plans, or other titles agreed on within a specific agency. Regardless of their name, timelines are multidisciplinary plans that include all the components of care for an episode or multiple episodes of illness, as well as the expected outcomes or result of care. Timelines can be confined to inpatient care or the entire continuum of care, including home care (see also Chapter 20).

In addition to providing care in a systematic manner, professional and government organizations often follow *clinical practice guidelines* for the care of an illness, disease, or problem. Care timelines are developed within an institution and reflect local practice patterns, but clinical practice guidelines are developed on a national level and reflect research related to a specific disease or illness. The *Agency for Healthcare Research and Quality (AHRQ)* is a federal agency that has developed several clinical practice guidelines relevant to pediatrics (i.e., acute pain management, the management of otitis media with effusion, and the diagnosis and treatment of sickle-cell disease) (Box 1-2).

---

*Caremap is a registered trademark of the **Center for Case Management, Inc.,** South Natick, MA 01760; (508) 651-2600.

ROLE OF THE PEDIATRIC NURSE
Therapeutic Relationship

A therapeutic relationship is the essential foundation for quality nursing care. Pediatric nurses must relate to children and their families in a meaningful way, and yet remain separate enough to distinguish their own feelings and needs. In a *therapeutic relationship,* caring, well-defined boundaries separate the nurse from the child and family (Peternelj-Taylor, 2002). These boundaries are positive and professional and promote the family's control over the child's health care (Rushton, McEnhill, and Armstrong, 1996). Within a therapeutic relationship, both the nurse and the family are empowered, and open communication is maintained. In a *nontherapeutic relationship,* boundaries are blurred, and many of the nurse's actions may serve personal needs, such as a need to feel wanted and involved, rather than the family's needs. Some settings make the establishment of boundaries more difficult than others. For example, in the home care setting several factors challenge the definition of boundaries. The informal home environment, the casual social conversations among family members, the participation by family members in the care of the child, and the attempt by some families to incorporate the home care nurse into the family all present major challenges to establishing and maintaining clear boundaries.

Exploring whether relationships with patients are therapeutic or nontherapeutic helps nurses identify problem areas early in their interactions with children and families. Although questions for exploring types of involvement can be labeled negative or positive, no one action makes a relationship therapeutic or nontherapeutic. For example, nurses may spend additional time with the family but still recognize their own needs and maintain professional separateness. An important clue to nontherapeutic relationships is the staff's concerns about their peer's actions with the family.

Family Advocacy/Caring

Although nurses are responsible to themselves, the profession, and the institution of employment, their primary responsibility is to the consumer of nursing services—the child and the family. The nurse must work with family members, identify *their* goals and needs, and plan interventions that meet the defined problems. As an advocate, the nurse assists children and their families in making informed choices and acting in the child's best interest. Advocacy involves ensuring that families are aware of all available health services, informed of treatments and procedures, involved in the child's care, and encouraged to change or support existing health care practices. The United Nations Declaration of the Rights of the Child (Box 1-3) provides guidelines for nursing practice to ensure that every child receives optimum care. The nurse uses this knowledge to adapt care for the child and the family.

As nurses care for children and families, they must demonstrate *caring,* compassion, and empathy for others. Aspects of caring include atraumatic care and the development of a therapeutic relationship. Parents perceive caring as a sign of quality nursing care, which is often focused on the nontechnical needs of the child and family. Parents describe "personable" care as nursing actions that include acknowledging the parent's presence, listening, making the

BOX 1-3 ■ United Nations' Declaration of the Rights of the Child

All children need:
To be free from discrimination
To develop physically and mentally in freedom and dignity
To have a name and nationality
To have adequate nutrition, housing, recreation, and medical services
To receive special treatment if handicapped
To receive love, understanding, and material security
To receive an education and develop his or her abilities
To be the first to receive protection in disaster
To be protected from neglect, cruelty, and exploitation
To be brought up in a spirit of friendship among people

parent feel comfortable, involving both the parent and the child in care, showing interest and concern for their welfare, communicating with them, and individualizing the nursing care. Parents perceive "personable" nursing care as an integral of a positive relationship.

The nurse is aware of the needs of children and works with all caregivers to ensure that these needs are met. This often requires the nurse to expand the boundaries of practice to less traditional settings. The nurse may be involved in education, political or legislative change, rehabilitation, screening, administration, and even engineering and architecture. Regardless of how removed from direct patient care nurses become, they must continue to foster health care practices that promote the well-being of children and that incorporate knowledge of child growth and development. For example, as educators, nurses are responsible for helping others learn about and care for children. Their audience may be other nurses, parents, teachers, other members of the health team, or the community at large.

Disease Prevention/Health Promotion

Current health care focuses on prevention of illness and maintenance of health, rather than treatment of disease or disability. Nursing has kept pace with this change. In 1965, *pediatric nurse practitioner (PNP)* programs were developed and led to several specialized ambulatory or primary care roles for nurses. Today, these programs provide education for nurses beyond the basic undergraduate preparation in areas of child health maintenance. Practitioner programs now prepare PNPs in areas such as school health, acute care, and oncology. Although the curriculum varies, the course content includes history taking, physical diagnosis, growth and development, health education, pharmacology, counseling, common childhood problems, and care planning for individuals and groups. These programs are an integral part of graduate nursing education, and graduates from these programs provide high-quality care to children.

The *clinical nurse specialist (CNS)* role was developed in an attempt to provide expert nursing care. Today, the CNS serves as a role model for clinical practice, a researcher to validate nursing observations and interventions, a change agent within the health care system, and a consultant/teacher to the health care team. The CNS is competent in providing nursing care during all stages of illness or wellness and functions in any setting where patients are found—the hospital, home, community, clinic, or long-term facility. The CNS role has developed within each of the traditional specialty areas as well as subspecialties, such as cardiovascular, oncology, and neurology. As with the PNP role, the educational preparation for the CNS includes a graduate degree in nursing. Some graduate programs combine the PNP and CNS roles. Both PNPs and CNSs are commonly called *advanced nurse practitioners* (*ANPs* or *ARNPs*).

Every nurse who is involved with caring for children must practice preventive health. The best approach to prevention is education and anticipatory guidance. In this text, each chapter on health promotion also includes sections on anticipatory guidance. An appreciation of the hazards of each developmental period enables the nurse to guide parents regarding childrearing practices that are aimed at preventing potential problems. One significant example is safety. Because children of every age are at risk for injury, education of the parents is essential to decrease disability and prevent mortality.

Prevention also involves less obvious aspects of care such as promoting mental health. For example, it is not sufficient to administer immunizations without regard for the psychologic trauma associated with administering immunizations.

Health Teaching

Health teaching is inseparable from family advocacy and prevention. Health teaching may be direct as during parenting classes, or indirect as when nurses help parents and children to understand a diagnosis or treatment, encourage children to ask questions about their bodies, refer families to health-related professional or lay groups, supply appropriate literature, and provide anticipatory guidance. To be effective health teachers, nurses need preparation and practice with competent role models. Health education involves transmitting information at the child and family's level of understanding. Effective educators also focus on giving appropriate feedback and evaluation to promote learning.

Support/Counseling

Attention to emotional needs requires support and sometimes counseling. The role of child advocate or health teacher is supportive because this role requires an individualized approach. Support can be offered by listening, touching, and through physical presence. Touching and physical presence are helpful with children because these interventions facilitate nonverbal communication.

Counseling involves a mutual exchange of ideas and opinions that provides the basis for mutual problem solving. It involves support, teaching, fostering expression of feelings or thoughts, and helping families to cope with stress. Optimally, counseling not only helps to resolve a crisis or problem but also enables the family to attain a higher level of functioning, greater self-esteem, and closer relationships. Although advanced practice nurses frequently do most of the formal counseling of parents and children, counseling techniques are discussed in this text to help students and nurses cope with immediate crises and refer families for additional professional assistance.

Restorative Role

The most basic of all nursing roles is the restoration of health through caregiving activities. Nurses are intimately involved

with meeting the physical and emotional needs of children, including feeding, bathing, toileting, dressing, security, and socialization. Although they are responsible for instituting physicians' orders, they are also accountable for their own actions and judgments regardless of written orders.

A significant aspect of restoration of health is continual assessment and evaluation of physical status. The focus throughout this text on physical assessment, pathophysiology, and scientific rationale for therapy assists the nurse in decision making regarding health status. The nurse must be aware of normal findings to identify and document deviations. In addition, the pediatric nurse should never lose sight of the child's individual emotional and developmental needs because these needs influence the course of the disease or illness.

Coordination/Collaboration

The nurse, as a member of the health team, collaborates and coordinates nursing services with the activities of other professionals. Working in isolation does not serve the child's best interest. The concept of "holistic care" can only be realized through a unified interdisciplinary approach. Being aware of individual contributions and limitations to the child's care, the nurse collaborates with other specialists to provide high-quality health services. Failure to recognize limitations can be nontherapeutic and perhaps destructive. For example, the nurse who feels competent in counseling but who is really inadequate in this area may not only prevent the child from dealing with a crisis but also impede future success with a qualified professional.

Even nurses who practice in isolated geographic areas separated from other health professionals are not totally independent. Every nurse works interdependently with the child and family, collaborating on needs and interventions so the final care plan is one that truly meets the child's needs. Unfortunately, collaboration and coordination with the child and the family is sometimes lacking in health care planning. Numerous disciplines often work together to formulate a comprehensive approach without consulting the child and the family. The nurse is in a vital position to include the child and family members in their care, either directly or indirectly, by communicating their thoughts to the health team.

Ethical Decision Making

Ethical dilemmas arise when competing moral considerations underlie various alternatives. Parents, nurses, physicians, and other health care team members may reach different but morally defensible decisions by assigning different weight to the competing moral values. These competing moral values may include *autonomy,* the patient's right to be self-governing; *nonmaleficence,* the obligation to minimize or prevent harm; *beneficence,* the obligation to promote the patient's well-being; and *justice,* the concept of fairness (Cornelison, 1998; Salvatore and Baxter, 1998). Nurses must determine the most beneficial or least harmful action within the framework of societal mores, professional practice standards, the law, institutional rules, religious traditions, the family's value system, and the nurse's personal values.

When ethical conflicts occur, nurses may experience conflicting loyalties to their profession, colleagues, patients and families, institutions, and society. The nurse's role in ethical decision making can be ambiguous. A nurse may be obliged to carry out procedures that are based on physician orders or hospital policy but inconsistent with the patient's best interest. Often, members of the health care team do not seek the nurse's input, leaving the nurse with incomplete information or without a voice in clinical decision making.

The role of nurses as members of the health care team justifies their participation in collaborative ethical decision making. Nurses routinely use a systematic problem-solving method, the *nursing process,* to resolve clinical problems. Using the nursing process, the nurse collects pertinent physiologic and psychosocial data, assesses relevant values held by the patient and family, and incorporates data into a plan of care. Each of these activities is a crucial component of ethical decision making.

Nurses spend most of their time in direct patient care, and are in a unique position to provide insight about the child's condition and response to therapy. They also assist families by interpreting information about the child's condition, prognosis, and treatment options, and by facilitating informed decisions. Because of their relationship to families, nurses represent children and parents' values, beliefs, and preferences. Nurses also serve as the liaison between the family and other health team members.

In their practice, nurses use a professional code of ethics for guidance and professional self-regulation. The Code of Ethics for Nurses with Interpretive Statements (American Nurses Association, 2001) focuses on the nurse's accountability and responsibility to the client and emphasizes the nurse's role as an independent professional one with legal liability (Box 1-4).

Nurses must prepare themselves for collaborative ethical decision making. This is accomplished through formal coursework, continuing education, contemporary literature, and by working in environments that are conducive to ethical discourse. Nurses must be aware of mechanisms for conflict resolution, case review by ethics committees, procedural safeguards, state statutes, and case law.

Nurses frequently face ethical issues regarding patient care, such as the use of lifesaving measures for very LBW newborns or the right of a terminally ill child to refuse treatment. They may struggle with questions regarding truthfulness, their rights and responsibilities in caring for children with AIDS, whistle-blowing, or resource allocation. Throughout the text, ethical dilemmas are addressed in Ethical Case Study boxes. Conflicting arguments are explored and an ethical decision-making model is presented to help nurses clarify all aspects of an ethical dilemma or problem.

Research

Practicing nurses should contribute to research because they are the individuals observing human responses to health and illness. Unfortunately, few nurses systematically analyze their observations. Pediatric nurses often devise innovative methods to encourage children to comply with treatments. When nurses evaluate these clinical interventions and share them with other nurses in research publications, nursing practice becomes based on empiric data or science, not tradition or trial and error.

The emphasis on measurable outcomes to determine the efficacy of interventions (often in relation to the cost) demands that nurses know whether clinical interventions result in positive outcomes for their clients. The current trend toward *evidence-based practice* also necessitates that nurses question *why* an intervention is effective and *if* there is a better approach. The concept of evidence-based practice involves analyzing and translating published clinical research into everyday nursing practice. When nurses base their practice on science and research and document clinical outcomes, they validate their contributions to health not only for clients, third-party payers, and institutions, but also for the nursing profession (Freda, 1998). Evaluation is essential to the nursing process, and research is one of the best ways to accomplish it.

Health Care Planning

Today, the nurse's role has expanded beyond the nucleus of the family to include the community-based health-driven system. Traditionally, nurses were involved in public health either on a continuous or an episodic basis. Nurses were involved in health care planning on a political or legislative level less frequently. Future nurses will need to incorporate a political component into their professional identity and attempt to influence the decision-making body of government.*

As the largest health care profession, nursing has a valuable voice, especially as family/consumer advocate. Nurses must become aware of community needs, interested in the formulation of bills, and supportive of politicians to ensure passage (or rejection) of significant legislation. Nurses also need to become actively involved with groups that are dedicated to the welfare of children (e.g., professional nursing societies, parent-teacher organizations, parent support groups, and volunteer organizations).

Health care planning involves not only providing new services to children and their families but also promoting the highest quality in existing services. In addition to following the Code of Ethics for Nurses, nurses ensure excel-

BOX 1-4 ■ Standard 5. Ethics

THE NURSE INTEGRATES ETHICAL PROVISIONS IN ALL AREAS OF PRACTICE
Measurement Criteria:
The nurse:
1. Delivers care in a manner that preserves/protects patient autonomy, dignity, and rights
2. Maintains patient confidentiality within legal and regulatory parameters
3. Serves as a patient advocate assisting patients in developing skills for self-advocacy
4. Maintains a therapeutic and professional patient-nurse relationship with appropriate professional role boundaries
5. Demonstrates a commitment to practicing self-care, managing stress, and connecting with self and others
6. Contributes to resolving ethical issues of patients, colleagues, or systems
7. Reports illegal, incompetent, or impaired practices.

Modified from *Nursing: Scope and standards of practice,* Washington, DC, 2004, American Nurses Association. Reprinted with permission.

*The following are sources of information on government issues: White House Comment Line: (202) 456-1111, 9 AM to 5 PM EST; White House fax: (202) 456-2461; White House e-mail: president@whitehouse.gov.

lence in their profession by following standards of practice. A *standard of practice* is the level of performance that is expected of a professional. In the past, pediatric nursing has not had national or international standards of care or education. Most pediatric nurses often merged with other specialties within nursing and followed the Standards of Maternal-Child Health Nursing or the standards of several of the pediatric specialties, such as pediatric oncology nursing or school nursing.* However, as the theoretical, practice, and research bases for pediatric nursing mature, the need for standards of practice for all basic pediatric nurses and for advanced practice registered nurses has become more evident. In 2003, the Society of Pediatric Nurses and the American Nurses Association published the *Scope and Standards of Pediatric Nursing*. This document identifies standards of practice that are congruent with current professional policy for both the nurse generalist and the advanced pediatric nurse.†

Throughout the text, the highest standards of nursing practice are reflected in the emphasis on thorough assessment, the focus on scientific rationale as the basis for care, the summary of nursing care goals and responsibilities, and the comprehensive discussion of growth and development.

FUTURE TRENDS

The present shift from treatment of disease to promotion of health has expanded nurses' roles in ambulatory care and highlighted the prevention and health teaching aspects of nursing practice. Prospective payment and the need for home care and community health services require nurses to be more independent and to acquire skills that are useful in settings beyond the hospital. These trends are illustrated throughout the text, with increased emphasis on prevention through anticipatory guidance, child health and family assessment, and discharge planning and care in the home and community. As changing social policy shapes the expanding health care arena, the focus of nursing care is no longer on what we *do for* families, but what we *do in partnership with* them. The philosophy of family-centered care is no longer an option, but a mandate.

Today, technologic advances and the demand for computer knowledge in the work setting are obvious. The current shortage of nurses will persist into the future, and the pressure to create positions in the health care system that do not require a nursing background will become more intense. As new categories of workers enter the health care field, nurses must continue to update their knowledge of technology and prove their unique contribution to health care. Nurses must use technology and learn to work collaboratively with unlicensed assistive personnel. *Unlicensed assistive personnel (UAP)* "are individuals who are trained to function in an assistive role to the registered professional

---

*Available from the **Association of Pediatric Oncology Nurses,** 4700 W. Lake Avenue, Glenview, IL 60025-1485; (847) 375-4724, fax: (877) 734-8755; and the **National Association of School Nurses,** Lamplighter Lane, PO Box 1300, Scarborough, ME 04074; (207) 883-2117; website: www.nasn.org.
†For more information on the Scope and Standards of Pediatric Nursing, contact the Society of Pediatric Nurses, 7794 Grow Drive, Pensacola, FL 32514-7172; (800) 723-2902; fax: (850) 484-8762; website: www.pedsnurses.org

nurse in the provision of [student] care activities as delegated by and under the supervision of the registered professional nurse" (American Nurses Association, 1994).

> ### ! NURSING ALERT
>
> When the registered nurse (RN) determines that someone who is not licensed to practice nursing can safely provide a selected nursing activity or task for a patient and delegates that activity to the individual, the RN remains responsible and legally accountable for the care provided.

Changing demographics will also influence pediatric nursing. Although the actual number of children younger than age 18 years will increase to an estimated 78 million in 2020, their relative importance in terms of the proportion of the total population will decrease from 26% to 24%. In the future, the adult population will grow faster than the pediatric population. The number of younger children will decrease, but the number of older children will increase. Racial composition of the population will also change. The number of whites in the population will decrease, whereas the number of individuals in minority groups will increase. The largest increases will occur in the number of Hispanic and Asian births. The impact of these changes will be an increase in the problems of adolescents and minority groups. Because the elderly will make up a larger percentage of the population, health care dollars will be split between the youngest and oldest groups, with shrinking resources to meet the needs of both. Nurses will need to be aware of developments in adolescent medicine and to continually adapt their care to the cultural milieu in which they practice. Finally, cost containment will present an ever-present challenge to providing quality care.

CRITICAL THINKING AND THE PROCESS OF NURSING CHILDREN AND FAMILIES

CRITICAL THINKING

A systematic thought process is essential to a profession because it helps the professional to meet the needs of the client. *Critical thinking* is purposeful, goal-directed thinking that assists individuals to make judgments based on evidence rather than guesswork (Alfaro-LeFevre, 2004; Sullivan and Decker, 2001). As with the nursing process, critical thinking is based on the scientific method of inquiry.

Critical thinking is a complex developmental process based on rational and deliberate thought. Becoming a critical thinker allows the professional nurse to acquire and apply knowledge that exemplifies disciplined and self-directed thinking. The cognitive skills used in high-quality thinking require intellectual discipline, self-evaluation, counterthinking, opposition, challenge, and support. Critical thinking transforms the ways in which individuals view themselves, understand the world, and make decisions. When thinking is clear, precise, accurate, relevant, consistent, and fair, a logical connection develops between the elements of thought and the problem at hand. Self-evaluation questions that enhance the development of critical thinking are listed in Box 1-5.

Because critical thinking is such an important skill, Critical Thinking Exercises are included throughout this text. These exercises present nursing practice situations that

BOX 1-5 ■ Critical Thinking Process

INTERPRETATION
What is the meaning or significance of the expressed data? How are the evidence/data interpreted?
(includes data categorization or clustering, assigning significance of data, and clarifying meaning of data within the context)

ANALYSIS
What are the intended and actual inferential relationships among the statements or concepts presented? What are some underlying assumptions about the data presented? What priorities of care are appropriate given the data presented?
(includes identifying unstated assumptions, constructing a main conclusion and reasons to support the conclusion)

EVALUATION
Does the evidence presented support the conclusion(s) being drawn? How are the arguments evaluated?
(includes assessing credibility of data or statements expressed, assessing the logical strengths of the actual or intended inferential relationships among statements or descriptions)

INFERENCE
What alternative conclusions or options might be drawn from the expressed data? What alternative perspectives might be presented as options to one's own conclusions? Identifying an underlying cause of an illness/health problem.
(includes process of questioning available evidence, conjecturing alternatives, and drawing conclusions)

EXPLANATION
Justify one's reasoning behind conclusions drawn and arguments (hypotheses) produced based on the evidence or data. Does the contextual evidence support conclusions?
(includes stating results, justifying procedures, and presenting arguments)

SELF-REGULATION
To examine one's own reasoning and validate results. Are biases present that affect one's thinking/conclusions about the data?
(includes self-examination and self-correction)

Modified from Facione P: *Critical thinking: what it is and why it counts,* Millbrae, Calif, 1992, 1998, California Academic Press, retrieved on 4/30/03 from www.insightassessment.com/articles.html; Sullivan EJ, Decker PJ: Problem solving and decision making. In Sullivan EJ, Decker PJ: *Effective leadership and management in nursing,* ed 5, Upper Saddle River, NJ, 2001, Prentice Hall; Alfaro-Lefevre R: *Critical thinking and clinical judgment,* ed 3, Philadelphia, 2004, WB Saunders.

require critical thinking skills. Self-evaluation questions require the student to provide rational and deliberate answers based on self-directed thinking. The aim of these exercises is to enhance sound clinical judgment.

NURSING PROCESS

The nursing process is a method of problem identification and problem solving that describes what the nurse actually does. The nursing process includes assessment, diagnosis, outcome identification, planning, implementation, and evaluation. The second step, nursing diagnosis, is the naming of the child's or family's problem in common nursing language. The American Nurses Association has established Standards of Practice and Professional Performance (Box 1-6) that outline the components included in each step of the nursing process.

● Assessment

Assessment is a continuous process that operates at all phases of problem solving and is the foundation for decision making. It uses multiple nursing skills and consists of purposeful collection, classification, and analysis of data from a variety of sources. To provide an accurate and comprehensive assessment, the nurse must consider information about the patient's biophysical, psychologic, sociocultural, and spiritual background.

● Nursing Diagnosis

The second stage of the nursing process is problem identification and nursing diagnosis. At this point, the nurse must interpret and make decisions about the data gathered. The nurse organizes or clusters data into categories to identify significant areas and makes one of the following decisions:

- **No dysfunctional health problems** are evident; no interventions are indicated.
- **Risk for dysfunctional health problems** exists; interventions are needed to facilitate health promotion.
- **Actual dysfunctional health problems** are evident; interventions are needed to facilitate health promotion.

The nursing diagnosis phase involves the naming of cue clusters that are obtained during the assessment phase. The North American Nursing Diagnosis Association's (NANDA's) accepted definition of *nursing diagnosis* is "a clinical judgment about individual, family, or community responses to actual and potential health problems/life processes." Nursing diagnoses provide the basis for selection of nursing interventions to achieve outcomes for which the nurse is accountable.

At its third national conference, NANDA developed a framework for nursing diagnoses that comprised nine *human response patterns* (Box 1-7). In 2003, NANDA published a nursing diagnosis taxonomy or classification that included 13 domains, 106 classes, and 167 diagnoses (North American Nursing Diagnosis Association, 2003). Marjory Gordon (2000) developed a system for organizing nursing assessment based on 11 *functional health patterns* (Box 1-7). Gordon's system of functional health patterns provides an excellent format for data collection before nursing diagnosis.

BOX 1-6 ■ American Nurses Association Standards of Practice

STANDARDS OF PRACTICE
Standard 1. Assessment: The nurse collects comprehensive data pertinent to the patient's health or the situation.
2. Diagnosis: The nurse analyzes assessment data to determine the diagnoses or issues.
3. Outcomes Identification: The nurse identifies expected outcomes for a plan individualized to the patient or the situation.
4. Planning: The nurse develops a plan of care that prescribes strategies and alternatives to attain expected outcomes.
5. Implementation: The nurse implements the identified plan.
6. Evaluation: The nurse evaluates progress toward attainment of outcomes.

STANDARDS OF PROFESSIONAL PERFORMANCE
Standard 7. Quality of Practice: The nurse systematically enhances the quality and effectiveness of nursing practice.
8. Education: The nurse attains knowledge and competency that reflects current nursing practice.
9. Practice Evaluation: The nurse evaluates one's own nursing practice in relation to professional practice standards and guidelines, relevant statutes, rules, and regulations.
10. Collegiality: The nurse interacts with and contributes to the professional development of peers and colleagues.
11. Collaboration: The nurse collaborates with patient, family, and others in the conduct of nursing practice.
12. Ethics: The nurse integrates ethical provisions in all areas of practice.
13. Research: The nurse integrates research findings into practice.
14. Resource Utilization: The nurse considers factors related to safety, effectiveness, cost and impact on practice in the planning and delivery of nursing services.
15. Leadership: The nurse provides leadership in the professional practice setting and the profession.

Modified from *Nursing: Scope and standards of practice*, Washington, DC, 2004, American Nurses Association. Reprinted with permission.

BOX 1-7 ■ Classification Systems for Nursing Diagnoses

HUMAN RESPONSE PATTERNS*
Exchanging—Mutual giving and receiving
Communicating—Sending messages
Relating—Establishing bonds
Valuing—The assigning of relative worth
Choosing—The selection of alternatives
Moving—Activity
Perceiving—The reception of information
Knowing—The meaning associated with information
Feeling—The subjective awareness of sensation or affect

FUNCTIONAL HEALTH PATTERNS†
Health perception–health management pattern—Perceptions related to general health management and preventive practices
Nutritional-metabolic pattern—Intake of food and fluids related to metabolic requirements
Elimination pattern—Regularity and control of excretory functions, bowel, bladder, skin, and wastes
Activity-exercise pattern—Activity patterns that require energy expenditure and provide for rest
Sleep-rest pattern—Effectiveness of sleep and rest periods
Cognitive-perceptual pattern—Adequacy of language cognitive skills, and perception related to required or desired activities; includes pain perception
Self-perception–Self-concept pattern—Beliefs and evaluation of self-worth
Role-relationship pattern—Family and social roles; especially parent-child relationships
Sexuality reproductive pattern—Problems or potential problems with sexuality or reproduction
Coping-stress tolerance pattern—Stress tolerance level and coping patterns, including support systems
Value-belief pattern—Values, goals, or beliefs that influence health-related decisions and actions

TAXONOMY II DOMAINS‡
Domain 1—Health Promotion
Domain 2—Nutrition
Domain 3—Elimination
Domain 4—Activity/Rest
Domain 5—Perception/Cognition
Domain 6—Self-Perception
Domain 7—Role Relationships
Domain 8—Sexuality
Domain 9—Coping/Stress Tolerance
Domain 10—Life Principles
Domain 11—Safety/Protection
Domain 12—Comfort
Domain 13—Growth/Development

*Modified from the North American Nursing Diagnosis Association: *Nursing diagnoses: definitions and classifications, 1999-2000*, Philadelphia, 1999, The Association.
†Modified from Gordon M: *Manual of nursing diagnosis*, ed 9, St Louis, 2000, Mosby.
‡North American Nursing Diagnosis Association: *Nursing diagnosis: definitions and classification*, 2003-2004, Philadelphia, 2003, The Association.

FAMILY FOCUS

Using Defining Characteristics to Select an Appropriate Nursing Diagnosis

An 18-month-old only child is admitted with respiratory distress and a presumptive diagnosis of epiglottitis. Initial nursing actions focus on the physiologic status of the child. As the condition stabilizes, family assessment data are gathered. The child's immunizations are current, he is clean and well nourished, and his developmental age is appropriate. The parents are both present at admission. The mother is distraught about the sudden onset of respiratory distress. She states that earlier her child had only a "runny nose" and she thought it was just a cold. When the child suddenly began to have difficulty breathing, she felt so helpless and unable to relieve her child's discomfort. She states: "Nothing I did made him any better. If I had known this could happen, I would have brought him to the hospital sooner. I feel like a bad mother." In the hospital, after explanations by the nurses, the mother understands that epiglottitis is a sudden illness that typically follows symptoms of a cold. She is very cooperative and asks what she can do to make her child more comfortable. She implements all the suggestions of the health care team. The father supports both the child and mother, although he assumes a more passive, "listening" role.

Three nursing diagnoses that relate to family/parent situations may be relevant. The first step is to review the diagnoses and the defining characteristics and decide which one is most appropriate:

Parenting, Impaired—inability of the primary caretaker to create, maintain, or regain an environment that nurtures the growth and development of the child

Selected defining characteristics:
Insecure (or lack of) attachment to infant
Poor or inappropriate caretaking skills

Conflict, Parental Role—parent experience of role confusion and conflict in response to crisis

Selected defining characteristics:
Parent expresses concerns about changes in parental role
There is a demonstrated disruption in care or caretaking routines
Parent expresses concerns/feelings of inadequacy to provide for the child's physical and emotional needs during hospitalization or in home
Parent verbalizes or demonstrates feelings of guilt, anger, fear, anxiety, or frustrations about effect of child's illness on family process

Family Processes, Interrupted—a change in family relationships or functioning.

Selected defining characteristics:
Expressions of conflict within the family
Changes in communication patterns among family members

Among these three diagnoses, the most relevant one is *Conflict, Parental Role.* The parents demonstrate attachment behavior to their child and are attentive to his needs. They appear to have appropriate parenting skills and are able to communicate effectively with each other. Neither parent expressed any conflict within the family. The sudden onset of this child's illness has interrupted the mother's usual role and caused her to feel inadequate, anxious, and guilty. However, the mother is able to adapt to this crisis. She demonstrates an ability to cope by learning and implementing new comforting skills for her child. The defining characteristics of the other two diagnoses require maladaptive characteristics that are clearly not demonstrated by these parents.

Actual nursing diagnoses are composed of three components: problem, etiology, and signs and symptoms. The first component—the **problem statement** or diagnostic label—describes the child's response to health pattern deficits in the child, family, or community. This statement represents the child's response to disturbances of life processes, patterns, functions, or development, including those that are secondary to disease.

Not all children, however, have actual health problems. Some may have a potential health problem, which is a risk state requiring nursing intervention to prevent the development of an actual problem. Potential health problems indicate the child or family has the presence of **risk factors** (signs indicating a potential health problem), which predispose the child and family to a dysfunctional health pattern and are limited to individuals at greater risk than the population as a whole. Intervention is directed toward reducing risk factors. To differentiate actual from potential health problems, the word *risk* is included in the nursing diagnosis statement (e.g., *High risk for infection*).

The second component of nursing diagnosis, the **etiology,** describes the physiologic, situational, and maturational factors that cause the problem or influence its development. The etiology is written using NANDA diagnostic categories (e.g., *Noncompliance related to powerlessness*). In formulating nursing diagnoses, it is important that the nurse does not link the problem statement and etiology with words that imply cause and effect. Etiologies are probable causes. Using words that imply cause and effect can result in legal or professional difficulties for the nurse. Although a cause-effect relationship may not be involved, the etiology does influence the problem. Therefore the phrase *related to* is used to indicate a relationship between the problem and its etiology.

Differentiating among various etiologies is important because *interventions to alter the health problem are directed toward the etiology.* This is an important concept in understanding the nursing diagnosis process. For example, a problem statement of *Noncompliance related to dietary restrictions* could have various etiologies, such as (1) knowledge deficit, (2) denial of illness, (3) low economic resources, or (4) cultural conflict. Interventions for a knowledge deficit are very different from interventions for low economic resources.

The third component, **signs and symptoms,** refers to a cluster of cues or defining characteristics that are derived from patient assessment and indicate actual health problems. When a defining characteristic is essential for the nursing diagnosis to be made, it is considered critical. These critical defining characteristics help differentiate between diagnostic categories. For example, in deciding between the diagnostic categories related to family process and parenting, the defining characteristics are important in choosing the most appropriate nursing diagnosis (see Family Focus box).

Nursing diagnoses do *not* describe all the activities of nurses. Nursing practice consists of three dimensions: dependent, interdependent, and independent activities. The differences among these activities reside in the source of authority for the action. **Dependent activities** are areas of nursing practice that hold the nurse accountable for implementing the prescribed treatment. *Interdependent activities* are areas of nursing practice in which nursing responsibility and accountability overlap with other disciplines such as medicine and require collaboration between the two disciplines. *Independent activities* are areas of nursing practice that are the direct responsibility of the nurse.

Throughout the text, Nursing Care Plans incorporate nursing diagnoses that relate to the specific condition or disorder. Because nursing diagnoses prescribe only interventions that nurses can perform independently, or interdependently, an asterisk is used to refer to nursing interventions related to medical management.

Planning

After the nursing diagnosis has been identified, a care plan is developed and *outcomes* or goals are established. The *outcome* is the projected change in the patient's health status, clinical condition, or behavior that occurs after nursing interventions. The ultimate objective of nursing care is to convert the nursing diagnosis into a desired health state. The plan must be established before the interventions can be developed.

The end point of the planning phase is the development of the nursing plan of care. The care plans in this text provide guidelines for the care of children and families with a particular problem and are standard as opposed to individualized care plans (Table 1-6). *Standard care plans* are plans that are sufficiently broad to account for situations that may develop in patients with particular problems. For this reason, the care plans often have numerous nursing diagnoses, both expected and potential. These possible nursing diagnoses guide patient observation and data collection in monitoring the development of adverse reactions. *Individualized care plans* are plans that are concerned with only those diagnoses that apply to a particular patient situation. In actual practice, not all the problems presented in the standard care plan may be relevant. When a standard nursing care plan is used to develop an individualized care plan, problems not pertinent to the situation should be eliminated and the outcomes should be individualized to the specific situation. To help the reader develop an individualized care plan, the nursing diagnoses in the text are listed in order of priority. In general, potential problems are discussed at the end of the plan, except when nursing interventions are essential to prevent a potential problem from becoming an actual problem.

Implementation

The implementation phase begins when the nurse puts the selected intervention into action and accumulates feedback regarding its effects. The feedback returns in observations and communications that provide a database on which to evaluate the outcome of the nursing intervention. Throughout the implementation stage, the patient's safety and psychologic comfort in terms of atraumatic care are the main concerns.

Evaluation

Evaluation is the last step in the decision making involved in the nursing process. The nurse gathers, sorts, and analyzes data to determine if (1) the goal has been met, (2) the plan requires modification, or (3) another alternative should be considered. In the text, observation guidelines are included in the standard care plans to help the reader to identify methods to evaluate whether the goals or outcomes are achieved. The evaluation stage either completes the nursing process or serves as the basis for the selection of other alternatives for intervention in solving the specific problem.

Documentation

Although documentation is not one of the steps of the nursing process, it is essential for evaluation. The nurse can assess and identify problems, plan, and implement without documentation, but evaluation requires written evidence of progress toward outcomes. The documentation elements listed in the Guidelines box should be included in the patient's medical record.

The nursing process has become an integral part of professional practice. The **Joint Commission on Accreditation of Healthcare Organizations (JCAHO)** incorporated the nursing process into the accreditation process. The first JCAHO standard on which nursing service is evaluated states that individualized, goal-directed nursing care is provided to patients through the use of the nursing process. The JCAHO accredits many health care providers such as hospitals, nursing homes, ambulatory services, and home care agencies; organizations that refuse or fail accreditation are unable to receive federal funds, such as Medicare or Medicaid.

TABLE 1-6 ■ Characteristics of Standard and Individualized Nursing Care Plans

	STANDARD CARE PLAN*	INDIVIDUALIZED CARE PLAN
Assessment	Information is specific only to problem	Information is specific to identified problem and to child and family
Nursing diagnosis	All probable nursing diagnoses with general etiologic factors are considered	Only nursing diagnoses specific to child and family are considered; cause of disease directs actual plan of care
Planning	Goals are broad and represent nursing goals and patient goals	Goals are specific and reflect patient outcomes
Implementation	Nursing interventions are broad and applicable to most patients with problem	Nursing interventions are specific and provide direction for nursing care of individual patient
Evaluation	Progress the patient is *expected* to make is identified	Progress the patient has actually made toward outcome is identified

*Describes format used in nursing care plans in the text that may differ from other types of standardized nursing care plans.

GUIDELINES

Documentation of Nursing Care

Initial assessments and reassessments
Nursing diagnoses and/or patient care needs
Interventions identified to meet the patient's nursing care needs
Nursing care provided
Patient's response to, and the outcomes of, the care provided
Abilities of patient and/or, as appropriate, significant other(s) to manage continuing care needs after discharge

Another focus area for JCAHO accreditation is the use of *continuous quality improvement (CQI)*. This process is an ongoing review of systems, problem identification, and resolution that allows institutions to establish and maintain quality care (Sullivan and Decker, 2001). JCAHO standards change over time. For example, in 2000, new standards were added to address the issues of pain assessment and management. In 2003, national patient safety goals were added to address the problem of patient safety in health care organizations.*

Currently, the attention in health care is focused on patient outcomes. Criteria have been established for changes that should occur in the patient as a result of the interaction with the health care team. At discharge, the care is evaluated to ensure that these outcomes were met.

KEY POINTS

- "Healthy People 2010" broadened the health care objectives of the past and focuses on prevention as the method to accomplish health goals.

- The infant mortality rate in the United States is at an all-time low, but the nation continues to lag behind other major countries.

- Low birth weight (LBW), which is closely related to early gestational age, is the leading cause of neonatal death in the United States.

- Injuries are the leading cause of death in children older than age 1 year, with the majority being motor vehicle injuries.

- Childhood morbidity encompasses acute illness, chronic disease, and disability.

- Eighty percent of childhood illness is attributable to infections, with respiratory tract infections occurring two to three times as often as all other illnesses combined.

- The "new morbidity" refers to behavioral, social, and educational problems that can significantly alter a child's health.

- Developmental stage and environment are important factors in the prevalence of injuries at every age and should guide injury preventive measures.

---

*The **Joint Commission on Accreditation of Healthcare Organizations (JCAHO)** has established a toll-free hot line ([800] 994-6610) to encourage patients, their families, caregivers, and others to share concerns regarding quality of care issues at accredited health care organizations. Complaints (may be anonymous) may be sent to the Office of Quality Monitoring, Joint Commission, One Renaissance Boulevard, Oakbrook Terrace, IL 60181; fax: (630) 792-5636; e-mail: complaint@jcaho.org; www.jcaho.org.

- During the early 1900s, public health initiatives such as environmental strategies to control infection and the development of antibiotics were the major advances leading to decreased childhood deaths.

- During the late 1900s, the advancement and application of medical knowledge and technology, specifically in the care of high-risk and LBW newborns, lowered the number of deaths in children, especially the neonatal mortality rate.

- The work of Lillian Wald, a social reformer, had far-reaching effects on child health and nursing. She started visiting nurse services in New York City and was instrumental in establishing the role of the first full-time school nurse.

- The philosophy of family-centered care recognizes the family as the constant in a child's life and that service systems and personnel must support, respect, encourage, and enhance the strength and competence of the family.

- Atraumatic care is the provision of therapeutic care in settings, by personnel, and through the use of interventions that eliminate or minimize the psychologic and physical distress experienced by children and their families in the health care system.

- Managed care is a health care delivery system that attempts to balance cost and quality through a network of health care providers and predetermined prospective payment for services.

- Roles of the pediatric nurse include establishing a therapeutic relationship, family advocacy, disease prevention/health promotion, health teaching, support-counseling, coordination/collaboration of care, ethical decision making, research, and health care planning.

- With the shift in focus from treatment of disease to promotion of health, nurses' roles are expanding beyond traditional health care facilities into ambulatory care centers, schools, the family's home, and the community.

- Changing demographics in the United States will result in greater significance of adolescents' and minority groups' problems and decreasing resources for health care.

- Critical thinking is purposeful, goal-directed thinking based on rational and deliberate thought.

- The process of nursing children and families includes accurate and complete **assessment,** analysis of assessment data to arrive at a **nursing diagnosis, planning** of care, **implementation** of the plan, and **evaluation** of interventions.

References

Alfaro-Lefevre R: *Critical thinking and clinical judgment,* ed 3, Philadelphia, 2004, WB Saunders.

Altemeier WA: Prevention of pediatric injuries: so much to do, so little time, *Pediatr Ann* 29(6):324-325, 2000.

American Nurses Association: *Registered professional nurses and unlicensed assistive personnel,* Washington, DC, 1994, American Nurses Publishing.

American Nurses Association: *Code of ethics for nurses with interpretive statements,* Washington, DC, 2001, American Nurses Publishing.

American Nurses Association, Nursing's Social Policy Statement Revision Task Force: *Nursing's social policy statement, 2003,* Washington, DC, 2003, American Nurses Publishing.

Anderson RN, Smith BL: Deaths: leading causes for 2001, *Nat Vital Stat Rep* 52:9, Hyattsville, Md, 2003, National Center for Health Statistics.

Annie E. Casey Foundation: *Kids count data book: state profiles of child well-being,* Washington, DC, 2001, Center for the Study of Social Policy.

Arias E, MacDorman MF, Strobino DM, Guyer B: Annual summary of vital statistics—2002, *Pediatrics* 112(6):1215-1230, 2003.

Cornelison AH: A profile of ethical principles, *J Pediatr Nurs* 13(6):383-386, 1998.

Freda MC: Toward evidence-based practice, *Maternal Child Nurs* 23:177, 1998.

Galvin E and others: Challenging the precepts of family-centered care: testing a philosophy, *Pediatr Nurs* 26(6):625-632, 2000.

Gordon M: *Manual of nursing diagnosis,* ed 9, St Louis, 2000, Mosby.

Guyer B and others: Annual summary of vital statistics: trends in the health of Americans during the 20th century, *Pediatrics* 106(6): 1307-1317, 2000.

Lears MK, Guth KJ, Lewandowski L: International adoption: a primer for pediatric nurses, *Pediatr Nurs* 24:578-586, 1998.

Minino AM and others: Deaths: final data for 2000, *Nat Vital Stat Rep,* 50:15, Hyattsville, Md, 2002, National Center for Vital Statistics.

National Safety Council: *Injury facts,* 2000 edition, Itaska, Il, 2000, National Safety Council.

Newton MS: Family-centered care: current realities in parent participation, *Pediatr Nurs* 26(2):164-168, 2000.

North American Nursing Diagnosis Association, *Nursing diagnosis: definitions and classification 2003-2004,* Philadelphia, 2003, The Association.

Peternelj-Taylor C: Professional boundaries: a matter of therapeutic integrity, *J Psychosoc Nurs Ment Health Ser* 40(4):22-29, 2002.

Rushton CH, McEnhill M, Armstrong L: Establishing therapeutic boundaries as patient advocates, *Pediatr Nurs* 22(3):185-189, 1996.

Salvatore T, Baxter T: *Administrative ethics: a guide for home care providers,* Springfield, Pa, 1998, HCMA Ltd.

Sullivan EJ, Decker PJ: *Effective leadership and management in nursing,* ed 5, Upper Saddle River, NJ, 2001, Prentice Hall.

Szilagy P: Managed care for children: effect on access to care and utilization of health, *Future Child,* 8(2 summer):39-60, 1998.

Wong D: Principles of atraumatic care. In Feeg V, editor: *Pediatric nursing: forum on the future: looking toward the 21st century,* Pitman, NJ, 1989, Anthony J Jannetti.

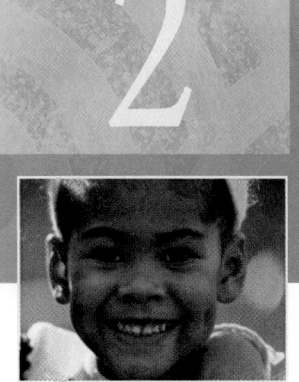

2

Community-Based Nursing Care of the Child and Family

CHRISTINE A. BROSNAN and SANDRA UPCHURCH

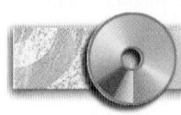
Remember to check out your companion CD-ROM

http://evolve.elsevier.com/Wong/essentials/

CHAPTER OUTLINE

RELATED TOPICS and ADDITIONAL RESOURCES

 IN TEXT

Healthy People 2010: Perspectives of
  Pediatric Nursing, Ch. 1
Nursing Process, Ch. 1
Immunizations, Ch. 1
Family-Centered Home Care, Ch. 20

 CD COMPANION

NCLEX-Style Review Questions

evolve WEBSITE

WebLinks
NCLEX-Style Review Questions

- Define a community.
- Describe community health nursing.
- Identify the roles and functions of the community health nurse.
- Discuss selected aspects of the epidemiologic process.
- Explain the purpose of an economic evaluation.
- Discuss the components of the community nursing process.

NURSING IN THE COMMUNITY

The health of children and their families is greatly influenced by their community, and nurses can make a significant contribution by working with the community to promote children's heath. Nurses working with pediatric populations in the community need an understanding of the concepts and processes critical to address pediatric concerns from a community health perspective. Healthy communities not only provide excellent medical care, but they also provide children a nurturing, safe place to live and grow. Healthy communities address concerns through collaboration between and among citizens, health care providers, businesses, and governmental and private agencies (Flynn and Ivanov, 2000).

In this chapter, community health nursing is discussed as it relates to children. First, it identifies and defines the concepts and principles that serve as the basis of Community Health Nursing. Then, it describes the Community Health Nursing Process, step by step. It concludes by using the process to address a very real child health concern: immunization status.

COMMUNITY CONCEPTS
Community

There are several ways to define a community. A community is a group of individuals with shared characteristics or interests who interact with each other (Allender and Spradley, 2001). A community is a system that includes children and families, the physical environment, educational facilities, safety and transportation resources, political and governmental agencies, health and social services, communication resources, economic resources, and recreational facilities. The community is also the client of the community health nurse (Anderson and McFarlane, 2000). Community health initiatives are directed at either the general health of the community as a whole or at specific populations within the community that have unique needs. In this context, *populations* can be described as groups of people who live in a community, for example, school-age children. *Target populations or subpopulations* are more narrowly defined groups (e.g., nonimmunized preschoolers, obese middle school children) toward whom nurses direct activities to improve the health status of individuals in the group. Common values often guide behaviors of populations and subpopulations in relation to health promotion and disease prevention (Williams, 2000).

Community care involves a collaboration of individuals and groups including health care providers, advocates, government, managed care organizations, businesses, children, and families within a specific community. The goal of the collaborative effort is to provide services that promote the child health initiatives of Healthy People 2010 (Healthy People 2010 website: http://www.healthypeople.gov). Community care is "without walls" in that the services of the health care system are frequently redesigned to meet the changing needs of the community. Those involved in community care partner with the community to identify, plan, intervene, and evaluate activities that improve the health of the community (Anderson and McFarlane, 2000).

Community Health Nursing. *Community health nursing* focuses on promoting and maintaining the health of individuals, families, and groups in the community setting. Community health nursing is a synthesis of nursing and public health. It collaborates with other disciplines to assess, plan, and implement care that emphasizes personal responsibility for health and self-care by community members (Allender and Spradley, 2001; Williams, 2000). Community health nursing, at its best, empowers communities by enabling community members to gain the knowledge and skills needed to fulfill their own needs.

Although community health concepts can be used to address health concerns in any setting, traditional community health settings include the following: home health agencies, schools, doctors' offices, ambulatory health clinics, emergency rooms, triage call centers, insurance agencies, health departments, international relief agencies, health education agencies, juvenile detention facilities, camps, day care centers, foster care facilities, and rehabilitation agencies. The American Nurses Association (1986) has established nine standards for community health nursing to guide practice across settings. They include the following categories: theory, data collection, diagnosis, planning, intervention, evaluation, quality assurance and professional development, interdisciplinary collaboration, and research.

Roles and Functions. The *roles and functions* of the community health nurse continue to evolve. In the future, more pediatric nurses will be working in community settings. The Health Resources and Services Administration (2001) reported that 18.3% of the total registered nurse work force was employed in a community or public health setting and 9.5% in ambulatory care. Only 59% of registered nurses were employed in hospital settings.

Traditionally, the *roles and functions* of community health nurses included caregiver, advocate, case manager, case finder, counselor, educator, epidemiologist, group process leader, health planner, and manager (Clemen-Stone and others, 1998). For example, the nurse, employed in a pediatric outpatient clinic will function in a number of roles to provide care to a child with type 2 diabetes. The nurse provides case management by coordinating care between the disciplines, counsel by supporting the child and family through developmental crisis, and acts as a case finder by identifying risk factors in the child's siblings.

In recent years, the Institute of Medicine developed a list of *core functions* to guide the work of public health professionals, including nurses. The core functions are directed to population-wide services and to personal and home services for people at risk (Institute of Medicine, 1988). The population-wide service is based on assessment of health status monitoring and disease *surveillance, policy development, and assurance* that policies are translated into service. A certain skill set has been identified as important for the nurse in a public health setting. Some of the skills needed include the ability to analyze data, measure health status, connect people to organizations, bring about change in organizations, build strength in diversity, build coalitions, develop interdisciplinary teams, and devise approaches to quality improvement (Gebbie and Hwang, 2000). Consequently, the pediatric nurse employed in a managed care environment may be asked to develop a creative approach to teaching children with asthma about peak flow meters during an emergency room visit. Included in the request may be a mechanism for evaluating the cost of the approach and the occurrence of repeated emergency room visits.

> **!NURSING ALERT**
>
> Nurses must be able to communicate and work with professionals from other disciplines. This includes being able to understand the terms used by demographers, epidemiologists, and economists.

Demography

Demography is the study of population characteristics. *Demographic characteristics* include age, gender, race/ethnicity, socioeconomic status, and education. Individuals, families, and communities may have demographic characteristics that affect their health risks (Anderson and McFarland, 2000). *Risk* is an increased probability of developing a disease, injury, or illness. Age is one of the most important risk factors for disease prevention and certain health conditions. For example, children younger than age 5 are more likely to have respiratory infections than children ages 5 to 17, and those of the older age-group are more likely to suffer fractures and dislocations than children younger than age 5 (Institute of Medicine, 1998). Gender also plays an important role. Males are at much greater risk of hemophilia A and B than females. Race/ethnicity has long been associated with increased risk for disease and disability but it is now thought that, aside from genetic predisposition, there is a complicated relationship between minority status and socioeconomic status that increases the risk for disease and disability (Smith, 2000). Low socioeconomic status predisposes children to a variety of problems. Poor children are more likely to be hospitalized for pneumonia, asthma, dehydration, and gastroenteritis than children from affluent families (Institute of Medicine, 1998). They are less likely to be immunized against childhood illnesses (Ortega and others, 2000)

Epidemiology

Epidemiology is that science of population health applied to the detection of morbidity and mortality in a population. The epidemiologic process identifies the distribution and causes of disease or injury across a population (Anderson and McFarland, 2000). It also serves as an important component in developing health programs. For example, Healthy People 2010 incorporated the process to develop a set of health objectives for the United States. Health professionals in community, state, and national health care organizations use the objectives as a guide to develop programs that have the greatest impact on the health of children.

Distribution of Disease, Injury, or Illness. *Morbidity rates* are used to measure disease and injury and, along with *natality and mortality rates,* present an objective picture of the health status of a community. There are two types of morbidity rates: *incidence* and *prevalence.* Incidence measures the occurrence of *new* events in a population during a period of time. *Prevalence* measures *existing* events in a population during a period of time (Hennekens and Buring, 1987). For example, the incidence of type 1 diabetes in a community is estimated by counting the new cases of type 1 diabetes in a population and dividing that figure by the population at risk. The prevalence of type 1 diabetes is estimated by counting the existing cases of type 1 diabetes in a population and dividing that figure by the population at risk. Both incidence and prevalence are usually given as rates per 1000, 10,000, or 100,000 population depending on their frequency. Box 2-1 presents frequently used mortality and morbidity rates.

BOX 2-1 ■ Frequently Used Mortality and Morbidity Rates

Crude birth rate

$$\frac{\text{Number of births in a population}}{\text{Total population}} \text{ within a time period} \times 1000$$

Crude death rate

$$\frac{\text{Number of deaths in a population}}{\text{Total population}} \text{ within a time period} \times 1000$$

Cause-specific death rate

$$\frac{\text{Number of deaths in a population due to a certain disease}}{\text{Total population}}$$

$$\text{within a time period} \times 1000$$

Age-specific death rate

$$\frac{\text{Number of deaths in a population in a certain age-group}}{\text{Total population in that age-group}}$$

$$\text{within a time period} \times 1000$$

Incidence of disease

$$\frac{\text{Number of new events in a population}}{\text{Total at-risk population}}$$

$$\text{within a time period} \times 1000$$

Prevalence of disease

$$\frac{\text{Number of existing events in a population}}{\text{Total at-risk population}}$$

$$\text{within a time period} \times 1000$$

From National Center for Health Statistics: http://www.cdc.gov/nchs.

Epidemiologic Triangle. Three factors form the epidemiologic triangle, and their interrelationship alters the risk of acquiring a disease or condition (McKeown and Weinrich, 2000). These factors are agent, host, and environment (Fig. 2-1).

An *agent* is responsible for causing a disease and may be an infectious agent such as *Mycobacterium tuberculosis,* a chemical agent such as lead in paint, or a physical agent such as fire. *Host* factors are those that are specific to an individual or group. These may be genetic factors that cannot be controlled, or they can be lifestyle factors; for example, food selections or exercise patterns. *Environmental factors* provide a setting for the host and include the climatic conditions in which the host lives as well as factors related to the home, neighborhood, and school.

Levels of Prevention. Community health programs are based on three classic levels of prevention (Leavell and Clark, 1965). *Primary prevention* focuses on health promotion and prevention of disease or injury. Examples of primary prevention activities include well-child care clinics, immunization programs, safety programs (bike helmets, car seats, seat belts, childproof containers), nutrition programs, environmental efforts (clean air programs), sanitation measures (chlorinated water, garbage removal, sewage treatment), and community parenting classes. *Secondary prevention* focuses on screening and early diagnosis of disease. Examples of secondary interventions include tuberculosis and lead screening programs and mental health counseling for stressful events such as separation, divorce, death, or community natural disasters (e.g., earthquakes, floods, hurricanes). *Tertiary prevention* focuses on optimizing function for children with a disability or chronic disease. Tertiary interventions include rehabilitation and disease management programs for asthma, sickle cell disease, cancer, anorexia, and special education programs for children.

Screening. Community health nurses are frequently involved in *screening,* a secondary prevention activity. The purpose of screening is to detect and treat disease early in the period of pathogenesis to prevent the spread and progression of the disease (Wilson and Jungner, 1968). However, screening is not appropriate for every condition. In a classic article, Wilson and Jungner described 10 principles that will help the nurse determine whether or not a screening program will be useful (Box 2-2). Although screening may bring benefit, there is a certain amount of risk associated with any intervention. In the case of screening, there is the psychologic risk associated with false positive results and the danger that a parent may treat a child differently because of early identification of a disease (Kwon and Farrell, 2000; Clayton, 1999). A great deal of planning is required to ensure that the benefits of screening exceed the risks and cost.

Economics

A basic understanding of the *economics* of health care is essential because it enables the nurse to participate in decision making about the worth of children's health programs. Economists theorize that individuals and societies view health as a basic utility; that is, something that is perceived as valuable (Gold and others, 1996). Other basic utilities are food, shelter, and clothing. People are willing to trade resources, such as money and time, for a program or intervention that will improve their health. Economists measure the amount of resources individuals and communities are willing to pay for good health. They also examine how different groups prioritize health care needs and allocate health care dollars. Methods for defining and estimating cost have been well described, as has the need for a standardized approach to the measurement of cost and effects (Drummond and others, 1997; Brosnan and Swint, 2001).

Economic evaluation provides objective information to establish the value of a program to the community. An example is an evaluation of a school-based hepatitis B vaccination program by Wilson (2000). He concluded that the percentage of vaccinated sixth graders increased from 8%

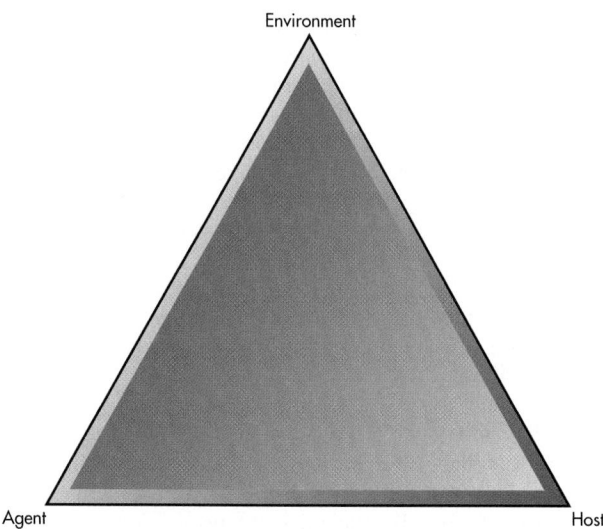

FIG. 2-1 ■ The epidemiologic triangle.

BOX 2-2 ■ Principles of Early Disease Detection

1. The condition sought should be an important health problem.
2. There should be an accepted treatment for patients with recognized disease.
3. Facilities for diagnosis and treatment should be available.
4. There should be a recognizable latent or early symptomatic stage.
5. There should be a suitable test or examination.
6. The test should be acceptable to the population.
7. The natural history of the condition, including development from latent to declared disease, should be adequately understood.
8. There should be an agreed policy on whom to treat as patients.
9. The cost of case-finding (including diagnosis and treatment of patients diagnosed) should be economically balanced in relation to possible expenditures on medical care as a whole.
10. Case-finding should be a continuing process and not a "once and for all" project.

From Wilson JMG, Jungner G: Principles and practice of screening for disease, *Public Health Papers* 34, Geneva, Switzerland, 1968, World Health Organization. Reprinted with permission.

without the program to 82% with the program. The higher vaccination rate potentially saved money that might have eventually been spent to treat these children for hepatitis, cirrhosis, or cancer in the future. The program resulted in potential cost savings of $24 million when compared with the no program alternative.

COMMUNITY NURSING PROCESS

In community nursing, the focus of the nursing process shifts from the individual child and family to the community or target population (Box 2-3). The stages of the process (assessment and diagnosis, planning, intervention, and evaluation) are similar whether the client is one child or a population of children; only the type of interventions and indicators of wellness and illness differ (Anderson and McFarlane, 2000). *Assessment* is focused on collecting subjective and objective information about the target population to *diagnose* problems based on community needs. *Planning* involves the development of community-centered goals. During the *intervention* stage, the nurse works with the community to implement a program that enables members to reach their goals. Finally, the nurse *evaluates* whether or not the goals were met. Community nursing is collaborative, and the nurse is one member of a community team that includes other health professionals, educators, politicians, religious leaders, members of public and voluntary organizations, and consumers. The role of the nurse depends on the scope of the project, the target population, and the expertise of team members. For instance, the school nurse may assume a leadership role in planning for the health needs of elementary school children and serve as a panel member on a city-wide committee assessing environmental pollution.

Community Needs Assessment

The assessment phase of the community nursing process is called a *community needs assessment.* Assessment involves the collection of *subjective and objective information* about a community. Subjective information indicates what community members say are their most important needs and can be determined in a number of ways. One way is to distribute questionnaires to a sample of people living in the community. Another way is to interview community members directly, phoning or meeting with individuals who represent the group or who have a special role in the group. Community leaders are an example of people who have a special role.

Objective information is data that the nurse collects either by direct observation or through written sources. A windshield tour is one method of direct observation. Nurses drive through a neighborhood and take notes about the environment, including the appearance of houses, the presence of sidewalks and gutters, the number of public areas, and so on. Objective information about the health status of the community can also be obtained from such sources as the Chamber of Commerce, Census Bureau, libraries, state health departments, and the internet sites of voluntary health organizations or government agencies. Information about service agencies can be found in resource directories. Resource directories include the local telephone book, community resource directories compiled by such organizations as the United Way, and population-specific books provided by public and voluntary agencies.

BOX 2-3 ■ The Community Nursing Process

Assessment: The nurse collects subjective and objective information about a community and develops a diagnosis based on community needs and problems.
Planning: The nurse develops community-centered goals to address the identified needs and problems.
Intervention: The nurse implements a program that enables community members to reach their goals.
Evaluation: The nurse conducts a systematic evaluation to determine that goals and program objectives were met.

One way to organize an assessment is to use a guide that lists community systems that need to be examined. This process is similar to using a physical assessment guide to examine the different body systems in an individual patient. Anderson and McFarlane (2000) described eight community systems that the nurse should examine: health and social services, communication, recreation, physical environment, education, safety and transportation, politics and government, and economics. During the assessment, the nurse studies how well each component in the community functions and interacts to meet the health needs of children, identifies the strengths of the community, and determines whether any barriers disrupt the components and prevent access to care for children and their families.

After the assessment is completed, the community nurse collaborates with team members to analyze the results of surveys and questionnaires, determine if the needs described by community members can be met by existing community agencies, and identify individuals at highest risk. During the analysis, the demographic characteristics, the morbidity rates, and the mortality rates in the community are compared with a standard. Comparisons can be made on the basis of time or place. In time comparisons, the nurse contrasts the rates in the current year with the rates during an earlier period. In comparisons of place, the nurse contrasts the rates in the community with a standard population. Standard rates may come from another community or from city, state, or national rates. For example, the rate of tuberculosis in a group of preschool children in the *community* in 2002 could be compared with the rate of tuberculosis in preschool children in the *state* in 2002.

A *community health diagnosis* is the reflection of health status, risks, or needs as determined by a causative agent. The format of a community diagnosis is similar to an individual nursing diagnosis with a problem (need) and etiology related to that problem (causative agent). An example of a community nursing diagnosis is "Child abuse related to a violent environment" (Visiting Nurses Association, 1986).

> **NURSING TIP**
>
> All communities have strengths and limitations. The community health nurse draws on the strengths of a community to solve problems.

Community Planning

The nurse collaborates with community members in developing a plan that addresses the needs and problems of the target population. To maximize the use of community resources, problems should first be prioritized on the basis of

BOX 2-4 ■ An Example of Community Assessment and Planning

Meadowlark is an elementary school with 500 children in prekindergarten to sixth grade classes. The school nurse has been asked to conduct a community assessment and develop a plan of care. The children who attend the school and their families are the target population.

COMMUNITY NEEDS ASSESSMENT

The school nurse formed an alliance of community members, including parents, school faculty and staff, health care professionals, local religious leaders, and politicians. The group met at regularly scheduled intervals. Their first task was to complete the community assessment. The alliance members mailed questionnaires to a random sample of families and held focus groups with community members to obtain subjective information about the needs of the community. Alliance members obtained objective data from the local health department, school records, and the US Census Bureau. The nurse also conducted a windshield tour of the neighborhood surrounding the school. The following information was collected:

People: Meadowlark is located in an ethnically diverse community composed of 30% Hispanics, 30% African Americans, 30% non-Hispanic whites, and 10% Asians. It is located in a large southwestern city.

Safety and Transportation: School bus service was rated very good to excellent by a majority of those surveyed. Transportation records indicated that the last school bus accident occurred 10 years ago.

Economics: Although at least one member was fully employed in 94% of the families living in the community, 25% of the families lived below the poverty level. The number below the poverty level had not changed in 10 years.

Education: Of the adult population, 60% had a high school diploma, and 10% had at least 1 year of college. School attendance was higher than overall state attendance rates.

Communication: 95% of homes had telephones compared with 85% 10 years ago. An estimated 10% of the target population did not speak English, and Spanish was the primary language spoken in this group.

Recreation: There were few places where small children were able to play. The focus groups recommended more parks and playgrounds.

Politics and Government: The school system was strongly centralized and headed by a school superintendent. The city had a mayor and city council.

Social: Of families living below the poverty level, 60% received some type of welfare assistance, including food stamps.

Health: Immunization levels for children younger than 2 years of age were 60%, a decrease of 20% in 10 years. Healthy People 2000 recommended that 90% of children in this group be fully immunized. Immunization levels of children younger than 4 years of age were 70%, a decrease of 5% in 10 years. The incidence rate of vaccine-preventable disease was 30/100,000 children younger than 5 years of age compared with the national rate of 24/100,000 children younger than 5 years of age (Teitelbaum and Edmunds, 1999). Responses from questionnaires and focus groups indicated that parents were not always aware of the importance of immunizations, that clinic locations were not well publicized, and that clinic hours were not convenient.

On the basis of these assessments, the following community diagnoses were made:
1. Decreased immunization levels related to knowledge deficit and barriers to access
2. Lack of safe play areas related to an insufficient number of community parks

PLANNING

Alliance members agreed that decreased immunization levels were a priority problem and developed the following goals:
1. Within 2 years immunization levels among children younger than 2 years of age will be 80%.
2. Within 4 years immunization levels of children younger than 4 years of age will be 90%.
3. Within 5 years the incidence of vaccine-preventable disease in the Meadowlark community will be 24/100,000 children younger than 5 years of age.

The alliance members searched the literature for communities that had experienced similar problems, contacted school and health department officials in other areas of the country, examined the results of successful programs, and planned a health program that addressed the unique needs of the target population. Program objectives were:
1. Within 6 months each new mother will receive a pamphlet about the importance of immunizations before hospital discharge. Pamphlets will be available in Spanish and English.
2. Within 1 year auxiliary immunization sites will be established around the community at shopping centers and churches. Clinic hours will be expanded to include evenings and weekends.
3. Each September the nurse will address the school's parent association about the importance of timely immunizations.

The alliance members determined the amount of resources needed to implement the program, including personnel, supplies, and equipment. They estimated the total cost of setting up the program and maintaining it for 5 years and applied for funding to the city and state health departments. The school nurse and other alliance members assumed responsibility for the timely implementation of the health program and the evaluation of program objectives and goals.

their severity, the felt needs of the community, and the ability of the community nurse to bring about change. After the problems are prioritized, the nurse works with community members to develop at least one goal for each problem the members will address. *Goals* are outcomes that give direction to interventions and provide a measure of the change

the interventions produced. Community interventions frequently take the form of *health programs* for improving the health status of the target population. Community health programs are based on the three levels of prevention: primary, secondary, and tertiary. For example, a goal for preventing bicycle injuries is, "Within 1 year all students in the first grade will wear bicycle helmets." The nurse and community members then plan a program that includes a health education program about bicycle safety for students and their parents (primary prevention).

The planning group considers the resources that are already available in the community and resources that will be needed for implementing a health program, including personnel, supplies and equipment, office space, phones, and computers. Decisions are made about the timeline of the program, the budget, and strategies that can be used to obtain funding. The nurse may also contact health professionals who have implemented successful programs in other communities; they can provide valuable, time-saving tips and suggestions. Program descriptions are found through professional contacts, online resources, and by reviewing the literature. An example of a community assessment and planning project is presented in Box 2-4.

Community Intervention

During program implementation, the nurse and community members carry out the intervention. Whether the program is simple or complex, oversight is needed to ensure that everyone involved is communicating with each other, following the guidelines of the plan, keeping within the timeline, and documenting daily activities and expenses. The documentation will prove invaluable during the evaluation phase of the process.

Community Evaluation

Evaluation identifies whether the goals and program objectives were met. There are various models of program evaluation. The structure, process and evaluation method is commonly used by health care organizations. Donabedian (1980) described this approach as:

1 **Structure:** Where and by whom is the care delivered in a program?
2 **Process:** Was the care delivered using operational standards and within the financial guidelines of the program?
3 **Outcomes:** What was the impact to health status? Was there an improvement?

Structure focuses on the qualifications of personnel, the adequacy of buildings and offices, supplies and equipment, and the characteristics of the target population. Process focuses on the interaction of patients and providers. Process indicators include the number of people who attended a health education program, the number of pamphlets distributed, and the efficiency of the program. Outcome focuses on whether program objectives and community goals were met. Program evaluation should be ongoing so that performance improvement initiatives are monitored and so that an improvement in the way health care is delivered will affect the health status of the target population.

KEY POINTS

- Caring for children within a community requires a multidisciplinary approach.
- Healthy communities provide children with not only quality medical care, but also a nurturing, safe place to live and grow.

- Community health nursing focuses on promoting and maintaining the health of individuals, families, and groups in the community setting.
- Individual families and communities may have demographic characteristics that affect their risk for disease or injury.
- Epidemiology is the science of population health applied to the detection of morbidity and mortality in a population.
- Community health programs are based on three levels of intervention: primary, secondary, and tertiary intervention.
- Economic evaluations provide objective information to establish the value of a program to society.
- A community needs assessment involves collection of subjective and objective information about the community.
- A community health diagnosis is a problem with a defined etiology related to a community problem.
- Program planning and implementation in the community require collaboration between the nurse and community members who are in positions to promote change.
- Evaluation of effective community programs includes consideration of the structure, process, and outcomes related to the program.

References

Allender JA, Spradley BW: *Community health nursing: concepts and practice,* Philadelphia, 2001, Lippincott Williams & Wilkins.

American Nurses Association: *Standards of community health nursing practice,* Kansas City, Mo, 1986, American Nurses Association.

Anderson ET, McFarlane J: *Community as partner: theory and practice in nursing,* Philadelphia, 2000, JB Lippincott.

Brosnan CA, Swint JM: Cost analysis: concepts and application, *Public Health Nurs* 18(1):13-18, 2001.

Clayton EW: What should be the role of public health in newborn screening and prenatal diagnosis? *Am J Prev Med* 16(2):111-115, 1999.

Clemen-Stone S, McGuire SL, Eigsti DG: *Comprehensive community health nursing,* St Louis, 1998, Mosby.

Donabedian A: *The definition of quality and approaches to its assessment,* Ann Arbor, 1980, Health Administration Press.

Drummond MF and others: *Methods for the economic evaluation of health care programmes,* ed 2, New York, 1997, Oxford University Press.

Flynn BC, Ivanov LL: Health promotion through healthy cities. In Stanhope M, Lancaster J: *Community & public health nursing,* St Louis, 2000, Mosby.

Gebbie KM, Hwang I: Preparing currently employed public health nurses for changes in the health system, *Am J Public Health* 90(5):716-721, 2000.

Gold MR and others: Identifying and valuing outcomes. In Gold MR and others, editors: *Cost-effectiveness in health and medicine,* New York, 1996, Oxford University Press.

Health Resources and Services Administration: *The registered nurse population,* Rockville, Md, 2001, US Department of Health and Human Services.

Hennekens CH, Buring JE: *Epidemiology in medicine,* Boston, 1987, Little, Brown.

Institute of Medicine: *The future of public health,* Washington, DC, 1988, National Academy Press.

Institute of Medicine: *America's children: health insurance and access to care,* Washington, DC, 1998, National Academy Press.

Kwon C, Farrell PM: The magnitude and challenge of false-positive newborn screening test results, *Arch Pediatr Adolesc Med* 154:714-718, 2000.

Leavell HR, Clark EG: *Preventive medicine for the doctor in his community: an epidemiologic approach,* New York, 1965, McGraw-Hill.

McKeown RE, Weinrich SP: Epidemiologic applications. In Stanhope M, Lancaster J: *Community & public health nursing*, St Louis, 2000, Mosby.

Ortega NA and others: The impact of a pediatric medical home on immunization coverage, *Clin Pediatr* 39:89-96, 2000.

Smith GD: Learning to live with complexity: ethnicity, socioeconomic position, and health in Britain and the United States, *Am J Public Health* 90:1694-1698, 2000.

Teitelbaum M, Edmunds M: Childhood immunization and vaccine-preventable illness, 1992 to 1997, *Stat Bull* 80(2):13-20, 1999.

Visiting Nurse Association of Omaha: *Client management information system for community health nursing agencies*, Rockville, Md, 1986, US Department of Health and Human Services.

Williams CA: In Stanhope M, Lancaster J: *Community & public health nursing*, St Louis, 2000, Mosby.

Wilson JMG, Jungner G: Principles and practice of screening for disease, *Public Health Papers* 34, Geneva, Switzerland, 1968, World Health Organization.

Wilson T: Economic evaluation of a metropolitan-wide, school-based hepatitis B vaccination program, *Public Health Nurs* 17(3):222-227, 2000.

Internet Resources

Children Now. Report Card Guide: http://www.childrennow.org/report_guide.html

Healthy People 2010: http://www.healthypeople.gov

Kids Count Data, Annie E. Casey Foundation: http://www.kidscount.org/

National Center for Health Statistics: http://www.cdc.gov/nchs

National Institute of Environmental Health Sciences: http://www.niehs.nih.gov

National Safe Kids Web Site: www.safekids.org

National Safety Council: http://www.nsc.org

Office of Disease Prevention: http://www.odphp.osophs.dhhs.gov

US Census Bureau, US and state census information: http://www.census.gov/

US Department of Education: http://www.ed.gov/

US Department of Health and Human Services: http://www.os.dhhs.gov/

World Health Organization: http://www.who.int/

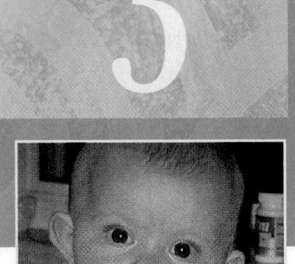

3

Family Influences on Child Health Promotion

PATRICIA MURRAY

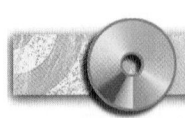
Remember to check out your companion CD-ROM

http://evolve.elsevier.com/Wong/essentials/

CHAPTER OUTLINE

RELATED TOPICS and ADDITIONAL RESOURCES

 IN TEXT

 CD COMPANION

Case Study—Family Functioning
Guidelines—Implementing Discipline
NCLEX-Style Review Questions

evolve WEBSITE

WebLinks
NCLEX-Style Review Questions

GENERAL CONCEPTS

DEFINITION OF FAMILY

The term *family* has been defined in many different ways according to the individual's own frame of reference, value judgment, or discipline. There is no universal definition of family; a family is what an individual considers it to be. Biology describes the family as fulfilling the biologic function of perpetuation of the species. Psychology emphasizes the interpersonal aspects of the family and its responsibility for personality development. Economics views the family as a productive unit providing for material needs. Sociology depicts the family as a social unit interacting with the larger society, creating the context within which cultural values and identity are formed. Others define family in terms of the relationships of the persons who make up the family unit. The most common type of relationships are *consanguineous* (blood relationships), *affinal* (marital relationships), and *family of origin* (family unit a person is born into).

Earlier definitions of family emphasized that family members were related by legal ties or genetic relationships and lived in the same household with specific roles. Later definitions have been broadened to reflect both structural and functional changes. A family can be defined as an institution where individuals, related through biology or enduring commitments, and representing similar or different generations and genders, participate in roles involving mutual socialization, nurturance, and emotional commitment (Lerner, Sparks, and McCubbin, 1999).

Considerable emotion has been generated about the newer concepts of family, such as communal families, single-parent families, and homosexual families. To accommodate these and other varieties of family styles, the descriptive term *household* is used more frequently.

⚠ NURSING ALERT

The knowledge that the nurse has and the sensitivity with which the nurse assesses a household will determine the types of interventions that are appropriate to support family members.

Nursing of infants and children is intimately involved with care of the child *and* the family. Consequently, nurses must be aware of the functions of the family, various types of family structures, and theories that provide a foundation for understanding the changes within a family and for directing family-oriented interventions.

FAMILY THEORIES

A *family theory* can be used to describe families and how the family unit responds to events both within and outside the family. Each family theory makes assumptions about the family and has inherent strengths and limitations. Most nurses use a combination of theories in their work with children and families. Commonly used theories are family systems theory, family stress theory, and developmental theory (Table 3-1).

Family Systems Theory

Family systems theory is derived from general systems theory, a science of "wholeness" that is characterized by interaction among the components of the system and between the system and the environment. *General systems theory* expanded scientific thought from a simplistic view of direct cause and effect (A causes B) to a more complex and interrelated theory (A influences B, but B also affects A). In family systems theory, the family is viewed as a system that continually interacts with its members and the environment. The emphasis is on the interaction between the members; a change in one family member creates a change in other members, which in turn results in a new change in the original member. Consequently, a problem or dysfunction does not lie in any one member but rather in the type of interactions used by the family. Because the interactions, not the individual members, are viewed as the source of the problem, the family becomes the patient and the focus of care. Examples of the application of family systems theory to clinical problems are nonorganic failure to thrive and child abuse. According to family systems theory, the problem does not rest solely with the parent or child but in the type of interactions between the parent and child, and the factors that affect their relationship.

The family is viewed as a whole that is different from the sum of the individual members. For example, in a household of parents and one child there are not only three individuals, but four interactive units. These units include three dyads (the marital relationship, the mother-child relationship, and the father-child relationship) and a triangle (the mother-father-child relationship). The family system functions within a larger system composed of the extended family, the subculture, the culture, and society. This ecologic model of family systems theory places the family dyads in the center of a circle surrounded by the extended family, the subculture, and the culture, with the larger society at the periphery. The concept of *nonsummativity*—"the whole is greater than the sum of its parts"—implies that the nurse

TABLE 3-1 ■ Summary of Family Theories and Applications

ASSUMPTIONS	STRENGTHS	LIMITATIONS	APPLICATIONS
FAMILY SYSTEMS THEORY			
A change in any one part of a family system affects all other parts of the family system (circular causality) Family systems are characterized by periods of rapid growth and change and periods of relative stability Both too little change and too much change are dysfunctional for the family system; therefore, a balance between morphogenesis (change) and morphostasis (no change) is necessary Family system can initiate change, as well as react to it	Applicable for family in normal everyday life, as well as for family dysfunction and pathology Useful for families of varying structure and various stages of life cycle	More difficult to determine cause-and-effect relationships because of circular causality	Mate selection, courtship processes, family communication, boundary maintenance, power and control within family, parent-child relationships, adolescent pregnancy and parenthood
FAMILY STRESS THEORY			
Stress is an inevitable part of family life, and any event, even if positive, can be stressful for family Family encounters both normative expected stressors and unexpected situational stressors over life cycle Stress has a cumulative effect on family Families cope and respond to stressors with a wide range of responses and effectiveness	Potential to explain and predict family behavior in response to stressors and to develop effective interventions to promote family adaptation Focuses on positive contribution of resources, coping, and social support to adaptive outcomes Can be used by many disciplines in health field	Relationships between all variables in framework not yet adequately described Not yet known if certain combinations of resources and coping strategies are applicable to all stressful events	Transition to parenthood and other normative transitions, single-parent families, families experiencing work-related stressors (dual-earner family, unemployment), acute or chronic childhood illness or disability, infertility, death of a child, divorce, teenage pregnancy and parenthood
DEVELOPMENTAL THEORY			
Families develop and change over time in similar and consistent ways Family and its members must perform certain time-specific tasks set by themselves and by persons in the broader society Family role performance at one stage of family life cycle influences family's behavioral options at next stage Family tends to be in stage of disequilibrium, entering a new life-cycle stage, and strives toward homeostasis within stages	Provides a dynamic, rather than static, view of family Addresses both changes within family and changes in family as a social system over its life history Anticipates potential stressors that normally accompany transitions to various stages and when problems may peak because of lack of resources	Traditional model more easily applied to two-parent families with children Use of age of oldest child and marital duration as marker of stage transition may be problematic (e.g., in stepfamilies, single-parent families)	Anticipatory guidance, educational strategies, and developing/strengthening family resources for management of transition to parenthood; family adjustment to children entering school, becoming adolescents, leaving home; management of "empty nest" years and retirement

must consider relationships between family members as well as the family's relationship to their environment. To effect positive change in a family, it is necessary to work with and through the various systems that impact family life.

Another concept, *adaptability,* views the family as a highly adaptable unit. When problems exist within the fam-

ily, change occurs by altering the interaction or feedback messages that perpetuate disruptive behavior. *Feedback* refers to processes in the family that help identify strengths and needs and determine how well goals are accomplished. Positive feedback initiates change; negative feedback resists change. When the family system is disrupted, change can occur at any point in the system. Although family systems theorists pursue the family history to understand current family interaction and problem patterns, the emphasis is on what is occurring *now* and how to change that pattern. This focus allows for sometimes rapid and dramatic changes.

A major factor that influences a family's adaptability is its *boundary,* an imaginary line that exists between the family and its environment. There are varying degrees of openness and closure between these boundaries. The example of one family's capacity to reach out for help, whereas another considers help threatening, demonstrates this concept. Knowledge of boundaries is critical when teaching or counseling families. Families with open boundaries may demonstrate a greater receptivity to interventions, whereas families demonstrating closed boundaries often require increased sensitivity and skill on the part of the nurse to gain their trust and acceptance. The nurse who uses family systems theory should assess the family's ability to accept new ideas, information, resources and opportunities, and plan strategies.

Family Stress Theory

Family stress theory explains how families react to stressful events and suggests factors that promote adaptation to stress. Families encounter *stressors* (events that cause stress and have the potential to effect a change in the family social system), including those that are predictable (e.g., parenthood) and those that are unpredictable (e.g., illness, unemployment). These stressors are cumulative, involving simultaneous demands from work, family, and community life. Too many stressful events occurring within a relatively short period (usually 1 year) can overwhelm the family's ability to cope and place it at risk for breakdown or physical and emotional health problems among its members. When the family experiences too many stressors for it to cope adequately, a state of crisis ensues. For adaptation to occur, a change in family structure or interaction is necessary.

The *resiliency model of family stress, adjustment, and adaptation* emphasizes the stressful situation as not necessarily pathologic or detrimental to the family but demonstrates that the family needs to make fundamental structural or systemic changes to adapt to the situation (McCubbin and McCubbin, 1994). For example, bringing a child with special needs to a treatment facility for therapy might be considered a crisis for a family without a car or money for public transportation, but may be defined as only a minor inconvenience by another family with adequate resources.

Developmental Theory

Developmental theory is an outgrowth of several theories of development. Foremost among the developers is Duvall (1977), who described eight developmental tasks of the family throughout its life span (Box 3-1). The family is described as a small group, a semiclosed system of personalities that interacts with the larger cultural social system. As an interrelated system, changes do not occur in one part without a series of changes in other parts.

Developmental theory addresses family change over time using Duvall's family life cycle stages, based on the predictable changes in the structure, function, and roles of the family, with the age of the oldest child as the marker for stage transition. The arrival of the first child marks the tran-

BOX 3-1 ■ Duvall's Developmental Stages of the Family

STAGE I: MARRIAGE AND AN INDEPENDENT HOME: THE JOINING OF FAMILIES
Reestablish couple identity.
Realign relationships with extended family.
Make decisions regarding parenthood.

STAGE II: FAMILIES WITH INFANTS
Integrate infants into the family unit.
Accommodate to new parenting and grandparenting roles.
Maintain marital bond.

STAGE III: FAMILIES WITH PRESCHOOLERS
Socialize children.
Parents and children adjust to separation.

STAGE IV: FAMILIES WITH SCHOOLCHILDREN
Children develop peer relations.
Parents adjust to their children's peer and school influences.

STAGE V: FAMILIES WITH TEENAGERS
Adolescents develop increasing autonomy.
Parents refocus on midlife marital and career issues.
Parents begin a shift toward concern for the older generation.

STAGE VI: FAMILIES AS LAUNCHING CENTERS
Parents and young adults establish independent identities.
Renegotiate marital relationship.

STAGE VII: MIDDLE-AGED FAMILIES
Reinvest in couple identity with concurrent development of independent interests.
Realign relationships to include in-laws and grandchildren.
Deal with disabilities and death of older generation.

STAGE VIII: AGING FAMILIES
Shift from work role to leisure and semiretirement or full retirement.
Maintain couple and individual functioning while adapting to the aging process.
Prepare for own death and dealing with the loss of spouse and/or siblings and other peers.

Modified from Wright LM, Leahey M: *Nurses and families: a guide to family assessment and intervention,* Philadelphia, 1984, FA Davis.

sition from stage I to stage II. As the first child grows and develops, the family enters subsequent stages. In every stage, the family is faced with certain developmental tasks. At the same time, each member of the family must achieve individual developmental tasks as part of each family life cycle stage.

Developmental theory can be applied to nursing practice. For example, the nurse can assess how well new parents are accomplishing the individual and family developmental tasks associated with transition to parenthood. New applications should emerge as more is learned about developmental stages for nonnuclear and nontraditional families.

FAMILY NURSING INTERVENTIONS

In working with children, the nurse must include family members in their plan of care. To discover family dynamics as well as strengths and weaknesses, a thorough family assessment is necessary (see Chapter 6). When working with families, the nurse's choice of interventions depends on the theoretic family model that is used (Box 3-2) (see also Critical Thinking Exercise). For example, in family systems theory, the focus is on the interaction of family members within the larger environment. In this case, using group dynamics to involve all members in the intervention process and being a skillful communicator are essential. Systems theory also presents excellent opportunities for anticipatory guidance. Because each member of the family reacts to every stress experienced by that system, nurses can intervene to help the family prepare for and cope with changes. At each stress point there is an opportunity for change and learning because families are more open to interventions at this time (Brazelton, 1995). In the family stress theory, crisis intervention strategies are employed to help family members cope with the challenging event. In the developmental theory, the nurse provides anticipatory guidance to prepare members for transition to the next family stage.

FAMILY STRUCTURE AND FUNCTION

FAMILY STRUCTURE

The *family structure,* or *family composition,* consists of individuals, each with a socially recognized status and position, who interact with one another on a regular, recurring basis in socially sanctioned ways. When members are gained or lost through events (e.g., marriage, divorce, birth, death, abandonment, incarceration), the family composition is altered and roles must be redefined or redistributed.

Traditionally, the family structure was either a nuclear or extended family. In recent years, family composition has assumed new configurations, with the single-parent family and blended family becoming prominent forms (Fig. 3-1). The predominant structural pattern in any society depends on the mobility of families as they pursue economic goals and as relationships change. It is not uncommon for children to belong to several different family groups during their lifetime.

BOX 3-2 ■ Family Nursing Interventions

Behavior modification
Case management and coordination
Collaborative strategies
Contracting
Counseling, including support, cognitive reappraisal, and reframing
Empowering families through active participation
Environmental modification
Family advocacy
Family crisis intervention
Networking, including use of self-help groups and social support
Providing information and technical expertise
Role modeling
Role supplementation
Teaching strategies, including stress management, lifestyle modifications, and anticipatory guidance

From Friedman MM: *Family nursing: research theory & practice,* ed 4, Norwalk, Conn, 1998, Appleton & Lange.

Nurses must be able to meet the needs of children from many diverse family structures and home situations. The particular family structure a child participates in affects the direction of nursing care. The US Census Bureau uses four definitions for families: the traditional nuclear family, the

??? CRITICAL THINKING EXERCISE ???

Family Theories

As the school nurse, you are working with a family that consists of a mother, father, and their 10-year-old son and 16-year-old daughter. The daughter, Jenny, has stopped going to school this week.

Although she has had many conflicts with her parents, her relationship with her father is very strained. He recently took away her driving privileges because of curfew violations. Jenny says she is quitting school if she cannot drive. Which family theory would you find most helpful in guiding your nursing care when working with this family?

QUESTIONS

1. Evidence—Is there sufficient evidence to make a decision about which theory to use?
2. Assumptions—Describe an underlying assumption about each of the following theories:
   a. Family systems theory
   b. Family stress theory
   c. Developmental theory
3. What implications for nursing care can be drawn at this time?
4. Does the evidence support your conclusion?
5. What alternative perspectives might you have?

ANSWERS

1. Yes, the nurse has information about a specific situation and the interactions of specific members of a family. The nurse also has information about a specific change that has occurred within this family.
2. **a.** Family systems theory views the family as a system whose members continually interact with each other. An action of one family member affects other members.
   b. Family stress theory is used to explain how a family reacts to stressful events and suggests factors that promote adaptation to stress.
   c. Developmental theory addresses family change over time using family life cycle stages
3. The nurse can help this family by applying family systems theory to examine the interactions that are occurring between the father and the daughter. In this situation, the interactions between the father and daughter are the source of the problem. The first priority is to try to promote better communication between the father and daughter to get the daughter back into school. The nurse might call a family conference at the school in an attempt to get the members of the family—father, mother, and daughter—to communicate. If this approach is unsuccessful, the nurse could refer the family for counseling.
4. There is no evidence to support the use of family stress theory because the family is not experiencing a stress-related problem, and there is no evidence to support crisis intervention. Developmental theory is not appropriate because the family is not entering a new stage. The daughter is in the middle of adolescence, and the conflicts with her parents have been an ongoing problem.
5. The school nurse should perform a thorough assessment of this family to determine whether any other events are influencing the daughter's behavior and interactions. For example, is the daughter experimenting with drugs, or has she recently joined a peer group that is influencing her behavior?

nuclear family, the blended family or household, and the extended family or household.

Traditional Nuclear Family

A traditional nuclear family consists of a married couple and their biologic children. Children in this type of family live with both biologic parents and, if siblings are present, only full brothers and sisters (i.e., siblings who share the same two biologic parents). No other persons are present in the household (i.e., no steprelatives, foster or adopted children, half-siblings, other relatives, or nonrelatives).

Nuclear Family

The nuclear family is composed of two parents and their children. The parent-child relationship may be biologic, step, adoptive, or foster. Sibling ties may be biologic, step, half, or adoptive. The parents are not necessarily married. No other relatives or nonrelatives are present in the household.

Blended Family

A blended family or household includes at least one stepparent, stepsibling, or half-sibling. A stepparent is the spouse of a child's biologic parent but is not the child's biologic parent. Stepsiblings do not share a common biologic parent; the biologic parent of one child is the stepparent of the other. Half-siblings share only one biologic parent. Nurses may have opportunities to interact with blended families in the community (see Family Home Care box).

Extended Family

An extended family or household includes at least one parent, one or more children, and one or more members (related or unrelated) other than a parent or sibling. Parent-child and sibling relationships may be biologic, step-, adoptive, or foster.

In many nations and among many ethnic and cultural groups, the extended family is the norm (Andrews and Boyle, 1995). Within the extended family, grandparents often find themselves rearing their grandchildren (Fig 3-2). Grandparents take over the parental roles for many reasons (e.g. substance abuse, child abuse, neglect, unemployment, divorce). Issues that grandparents face in these situations include financial burdens, lack of involvement with state agencies, and legal and medical dilemmas created by school enrollment and special needs (Woodworth, 1996). In extended families, young parents are often considered too young or too inexperienced to make decisions independently. Often, the older relative holds the authority and makes decisions in consultation with the young parents. Sharing residence with relatives is also beneficial because this arrangement provides assistance with the management

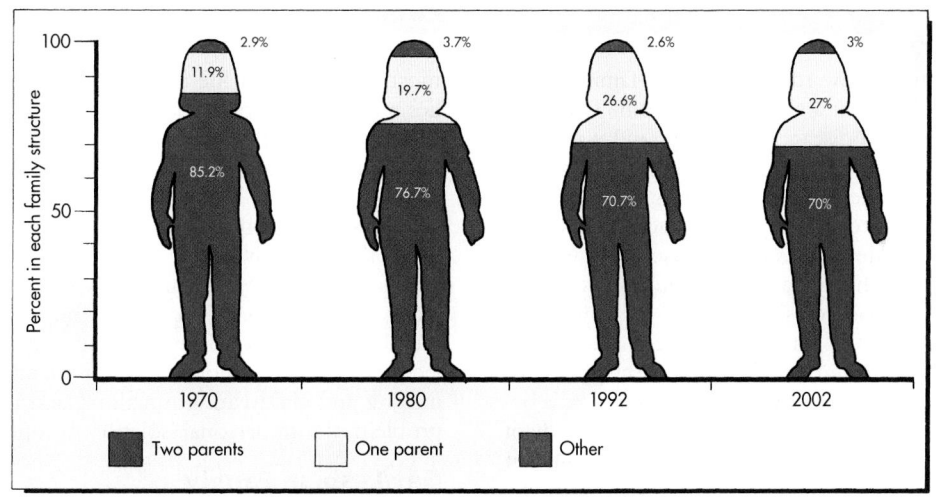

FIG. 3-1 ■ Percentage of children under age 18 living with one or neither parent, 1970, 1980, 1992, and 2002. (Data from the US Census Bureau: *Two married parents the norm,* Washington DC, 2003, Department of Commerce News. Available online: www.census.gov.)

FAMILY HOME CARE

Blended Families and Living "In Step"

Blending families can pose many challenges. If parents bring concerns and questions to health care providers, the following suggestions may be helpful:

Let relationships develop slowly and naturally. Don't expect too much too soon from the children, from your spouse, or from yourself.

Don't criticize or belittle lost (or new) parents or try to erase or replace them. Stepparents are additional parents.

Expect confused feelings, anxieties, competition for attention, bids for loyalty. Decide on standards of discipline and behavior and stick to them.

Communicate. Don't pretend everything is fine if it isn't. Look at problems squarely and deal with them openly.

If you need help, admit it and get it. Read a book, get counseling, join a support group, or call a family meeting.

From Stein B: Yours, mine, and ours: a look at stepfamilies, *Growing Parent* 12(9):1-5, 1984.

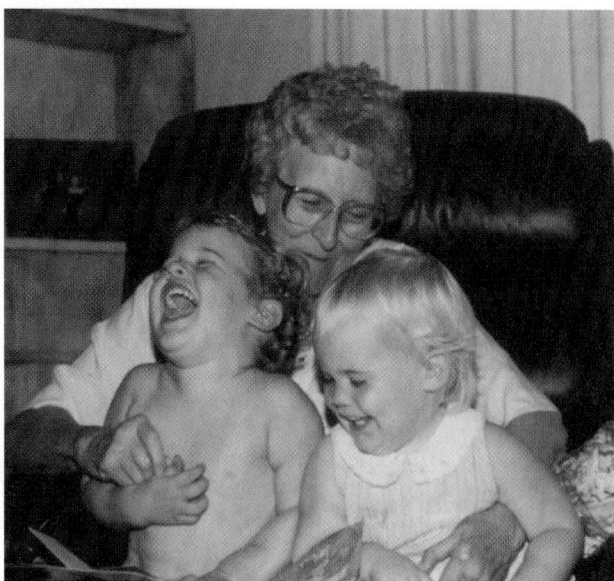

FIG. 3-2 ■ Children benefit from interaction with grandparents, who sometimes assume the parenting role.

of scarce resources and provides childcare for working families. A resource for extended families is the **Grandparent Information Center.** *

Single-Parent Family

Today, there is a trend toward single-parent families. The *single-parent family* is not a new phenomenon. Throughout history, deaths from disease, childbirth, and wars have resulted in many single-parent families, although frequently remarriage occurred. The contemporary single-parent family, however, has emerged partially as a consequence of the women's rights movement and also because more women (and men) have established separate households because of divorce, death, desertion, or illegitimacy. In addition, a more liberal attitude in the courts has made it possible for single people, both male and female, to adopt children. Although mothers usually head single-parent families, it is becoming more common for fathers to be awarded custody of dependent children in divorce settlements. A significant number of single-parent families result when a single woman wishes to have a child but does not choose to have a husband. With the increased psychologic independence of women and the increased acceptability of illegitimacy in society, more unmarried women are deliberately choosing mother-child families. Frequently, these mothers and children are absorbed into the extended family. The challenges of single-parent families are discussed on p. 51.

Binuclear Family

The term *binuclear family* is used to describe the situation that allows parents to continue the parenting role while ter-

minating the spousal unit. The degree of cooperation between households and the time the child spends with each can vary. In *joint custody,* the court assigns divorcing parents equal rights and responsibilities to the minor child or children. These alternate family forms are efforts on the part of those concerned to view divorce as a process of reorganization and redefinition of a family rather than as a family dissolution. Joint custody and co-parenting are discussed further on p. 51.

Polygamous Family

Although it is not legally sanctioned in the United States, the conjugal unit is sometimes extended by the addition of spouses in polygamous matings. *Polygamy* refers to either wives *(polygyny)* or, very rarely, husbands *(polyandry).* Many societies practice polygyny that is further designated as *sororal,* in which the wives are sisters, or *nonsororal,* in which the wives are unrelated. Sororal polygyny is widespread throughout the world. Although plural marriages produce problems of adjustment for the members, co-wives who are sisters are more likely to get along with each other and display less jealousy than co-wives who are unrelated. Most often, mothers and their children share a husband and father, usually with each mother and her children maintaining a separate household, particularly when the wives are unrelated.

Communal Family

The *communal family* emerged from disenchantment with most contemporary life choices. Although communal families may have divergent beliefs, practices, and organization, the basic impetus for formation has been dissatisfaction with the nuclear family structure, social systems, and goals of the larger community. Relatively uncommon today, communal groups share common ownership of property. In cooperatives, there is private ownership of property, but certain goods and services are shared and exchanged without monetary consideration. There is strong reliance on group members and material interdependence. Both provide collective security for nonproductive members, share homemaking and childrearing functions, and help overcome the problem of interpersonal isolation or loneliness.

Gay/Lesbian Family

A *same-sex, homosexual,* or *gay/lesbian family* is one in which there is a common-law tie between two persons of the same sex who have children. Estimates of the number of children of gay or lesbian parents range from 3 to 14 million (Ariel and McPherson, 2000). Although most children in gay/lesbian households are biologic from a former, legal marriage, there are other means by which homosexuals acquire children. They may be foster or adoptive parents; lesbian mothers may conceive through artificial fertilization, or a gay male couple may become parents through use of a surrogate mother.

Disclosure of parental homosexuality ("coming out") to children is a concern for families. There are a number of factors to consider before disclosing this information to children. Parents should be comfortable with their own sexual preference, and it should be discussed with the children before the children know or suspect. The discussion should be

---

*For information, contact the local **American Association of Retired Persons** representative or office; www.aarp.org./confacts/grandparents/grandfacts. Also see www.grandplace.com, a website dedicated to grandparents raising grandchildren.

planned and take place in a quiet setting where interruptions are unlikely. Children should be assured that the parent's relationship with them will not change as a result of the discussion (Lynch and Murray, 2000).

Because this family form is more common than most people may realize, it is important for the nurse to understand that homosexual families are different from the heterosexual family, not necessarily better or worse. The gay or lesbian family environment can be as healthy as any other. Nurses need to be nonjudgmental and to learn to accept differences rather than demonstrate a homophobic prejudice that can have a detrimental effect on the nurse–child-family relationship. Moreover, the more knowledge of the child's family constellation and lifestyle that nurses have, the more help they can provide to the parents and the child (see Critical Thinking Exercise).

FAMILY STRENGTHS AND FUNCTIONING STYLE

Family function refers to the interactions of family members, especially the quality of those relationships and interactions. Researchers are interested in family characteristics that help families to function effectively. Knowledge of these factors guides the nurse throughout the nursing process, and helps the nurse to predict ways in which families may cope and respond to a stressful event, to provide individualized support that builds on family strengths and unique functioning style, and to assist family members in obtaining resources.

Family strengths and unique functioning styles (Box 3-3) are significant resources that nurses can use to meet family needs. Building on qualities that make a family work well and strengthening family resources make the family unit even stronger. All families have strengths as well as vulnerabilities.

FAMILY ROLES AND RELATIONSHIPS

Each individual has a position, or status, in the family structure and plays culturally and socially defined roles in interactions within the family. Each family also has its own traditions and values and sets its own standards for interaction within and outside the group. Each determines the experiences the children should have, those they are to be shielded from, and how each of these experiences meets the needs of family members. When family ties are strong, social control is highly effective, and most members conform to their roles willingly and with commitment. Conflicts arise when people do not fulfill their roles in ways that meet other family members' expectations, either because they are unaware of the expectations or because they choose not to meet them.

PARENTAL ROLES

In all family groups, the socially recognized status of father and mother exists with socially sanctioned roles that prescribe appropriate sexual behavior and childrearing responsibilities. The guides for behavior in these roles serve to control sexual conflict in society and provide for prolonged care of children. The degree to which parents are committed and the way they play their roles are influenced by a number of variables and by the parents' unique socialization experience.

??? CRITICAL THINKING EXERCISE ???

Family Structure

As the nurse, you are interviewing the mother of John, a school-age boy. John's mother states that their family consists of herself, her son, a female friend, and two foster children. John's father lives in another state and has no contact with him. John has one grandparent, who lives in another city in a nursing home. As you plan care for John and his family, what type of family structure do you think John's family represents?

QUESTIONS
1. Evidence—Is there sufficient evidence to draw any conclusions about the structure of this family?
2. Assumptions—Describe the underlying assumption about each of the following types of family structure:
   a. Traditional nuclear family
   b. Single-parent family
   c. Extended family
   d. Gay or lesbian family
3. What implications for nursing care can be drawn from this situation?
4. Does the evidence support your conclusion?
5. What alternatives might you have?

ANSWERS
1. It is very hard to categorize or draw a definite conclusion about the structure of this family. At first glance, the nurse might think that this family is a gay or lesbian family. However, the nurse does not have enough information to draw this conclusion. The nurse needs to gather more data to determine if the mother's female friend is a lesbian and if there is a common-law tie between the mother and this friend. At this point in time, this family does not fit into any of the definitions of typical family structures.
2. a. The traditional nuclear family consists of a married couple and their biologic children.
   b. The single-parent family exists when a single woman has a child, but does not choose to have a husband.
   c. An extended family includes at least one parent, one or more children, and one or more members (related or unrelated) other than a parent or sibling.
   d. A gay or lesbian family is one in which there is a common-law tie between two persons of the same sex who have children.
3. The implication for nursing care is that John's family consists of those people who live in his home at the present time. The nurse needs to recognize that not all families are traditional in their membership or easy to define. Many alternative family structures such as John's occur.
4. The evidence does not support identifying a specific structure for John's family. John's family is whatever John's mother says it is.
5. In the assessment of this family, the nurse should be aware of his or her own thoughts and feelings about family structure. Many alternative family structures such as John's occur, and any preconceived or negative ideas about this family on the part of the nurse could have a negative effect on the nurse's interactions with the family.

Parental role definitions are changing as a result of the changing economy and increased opportunities for women. Women are achieving equality with men in education, more of them are entering the work force, and the number of women who choose to have fewer children or none at all is

BOX 3-3 ■ Qualities of Strong Families

1. A belief and sense of **commitment** toward promoting the well-being and growth of individual family members, as well as that of the family unit
2. **Appreciation** for the small and large things that individual family members do well and **encouragement** to do better
3. Concentrated effort to spend **time** and do things together, no matter how formal or informal the activity or event
4. A sense of **purpose** that permeates the reasons and basis for "going on" in both bad and good times
5. A sense of **congruence** among family members regarding the value and importance of assigning time and energy to meet needs
6. The ability to **communicate** with one another in a way that emphasizes positive interactions
7. A clear set of **family rules, values,** and **beliefs** that establishes expectations about acceptable and desired behavior
8. A varied repertoire of **coping strategies** that promote positive functioning in dealing with both normative and nonnormative life events
9. The ability to engage in **problem-solving** activities designed to evaluate options for meeting needs and procuring resources
10. The ability to be **positive** and see the positive in almost all aspects of their lives, including the ability to see crisis and problems as an opportunity to learn and grow
11. **Flexibility** and **adaptability** in the roles necessary to procure resources to meet needs
12. A **balance** between the use of internal and external family resources for coping and adapting to life events and planning for the future

From Dunst C, Trivette C, Deal A: *Enabling and empowering families: principles and guidelines for practice,* Cambridge, Mass, 1988, Brookline Books.

increasing. As the role of the woman has changed, the complementary role of the man has also changed. Many fathers are taking a more active role in childrearing and household tasks. As the redefinition of sex roles continues in American families, there may be role conflicts in many families because of a cultural lag of the persisting traditional role definitions.

ROLE LEARNING

Roles are learned through the socialization process. During all stages of development children learn and practice, through interaction with others and in their play, a set of social roles and the characteristics of other roles. They behave in patterned and more or less predictable ways because they learn roles that define mutual expectations in typical social relationships. Although role definitions are changing, the basic determinants of parenting remain the same. Three determinants of parenting infants and young children are (1) the parental personality and psychologic well-being, (2) contextual subsystems of support, and (3) child characteristics (Foss, 1996). These determinants have been used as consistent measurements to determine a person's success in fulfilling the parental role.

Parents, peers, authority figures, and other socializing agents who use positive and negative sanctions to ensure conformity to their norms transmit role conceptions. Role behaviors positively reinforced by rewards such as love, af-

fection, friendship, and honors are strengthened. Negative reinforcement takes the form of ridicule, withdrawal of love, expressions of disapproval, or banishment.

In some cultures the role behavior expected of children conflicts with desirable adult behavior. For example, in the United States, children are expected to be submissive in childhood but dominant as adults. This conflict of expectations is known as *role discontinuity.* Other cultures value the same behaviors, such as courage and aggression, both in children and in adults; this provides *role continuity.*

One responsibility of the family is to develop culturally appropriate role behavior in the children. Children learn to perform in expected ways consistent with their position in the family and culture. The observed behavior of each child is a single manifestation—a combination of social influences, as well as individual psychologic processes. In this way the uniting of the child's intrapersonal system (the self) with the interpersonal system (the family) is simultaneously understood as the conduct of the child.

Role structuring initially takes place within the family unit, in which the children fulfill a set of roles and respond to the roles of their parents and other family members. The roles of the children are shaped primarily by the parents, who apply direct or indirect pressures to induce or force children into the desired patterns of behavior or to direct their efforts toward modification of the role responses of the child on a mutually acceptable basis. Parents have their own techniques and determine the course that the process of socialization follows.

Children respond to life situations according to behaviors learned in reciprocal transactions. As they acquire important role-taking skills, their relationships with others change. For instance, when a teenager is also the mother but lives in a household where the grandmother is a co-resident, the adolescent mother may experience more support for the adolescent role than for the parenting role (Black and Nitz, 1996). Children become proficient at understanding others as they acquire the ability to discriminate their own perspectives from those of others. Children who get along well with others and attain status in the peer group have well-developed role-taking skills.

Family Size and Configuration

Parenting practices differ between small and large families. In small families, more emphasis is placed on the individual development of the children. Parenting is intensive rather than extensive, and there is constant pressure to measure up to family expectations. Children's development and achievement are measured against that of other children in the neighborhood and social class. In small families, there is more democratic participation by the children than in larger families. Adolescents in small families identify more strongly with their parents and rely more on their parents for advice. They have well-developed, autonomous inner controls as contrasted with adolescents from larger families, who rely more on adult authority.

Children in a large family are able to adjust to a variety of changes and crises. There is more emphasis on the group and less on the individual (Fig. 3-3). Cooperation is essential, often because of economic necessity. The large number of people sharing a limited amount of space requires a

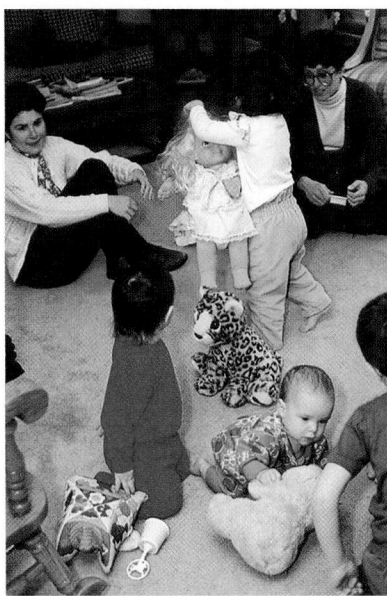

FIG. 3-3 ■ Innumerable relationships and activities are possible in a large family.

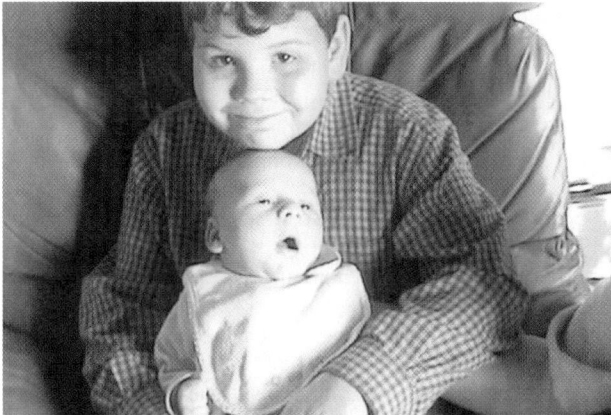

FIG. 3-4 ■ Older school-age children often enjoy taking responsibility for the care of a younger sibling.

greater degree of organization, administration, and authoritarian control. A dominant family member (a parent or older child) wields control. The number of children reduces the intimate, one-to-one contact between the parent and any individual child. Consequently, children turn to each other for what they cannot get from their parents. The reduced parent-child contact encourages individual children to adopt specialized roles to gain recognition in the family.

Older siblings in large families often administer discipline. Siblings are usually attuned to what constitutes misbehavior. Sibling disapproval or ostracism is frequently a more meaningful disciplinary measure than parental interventions. In situations such as death or illness of a parent, an older sibling usually assumes responsibility for the family at considerable personal sacrifice. Large families generate a sense of security in the children that is fostered by sibling support and cooperation. However, adolescents from a large family are more peer-oriented than family-oriented.

Spacing of Children

Age differences between siblings affect the childhood environment, but to a lesser extent than does the sex of the sibling. The arrival of a sibling is difficult for toddlers and preschool children, especially if they are between the ages of 2 and 3 years old. At this age, they are still very attached to their parents and do not understand the concept of sharing. At an older age the child is able to understand the situation and is less likely to see the newcomer as a threat, although the child does feel the loss of the only-child status. Children who are less then 2 years apart have more conflict then children who are spaced further apart (American Academy of Pediatrics, 1996). In general, the narrower the spacing between siblings, the more the children influence one another, especially in emotional characteristics. The wider the spacing, the greater the influence of the parents.

Traditionally, sibling relationships were viewed from a Freudian perspective that emphasized the concept of sibling rivalry. Recently, researchers have viewed siblings through developmental or ecologic frameworks that have focused on interactions within family systems (Friedman, 1998). The results of these broader perspectives provide a picture of rich and varied sibling interactions (Fig. 3-4).

The sibling relationship's most unique feature is its duration. The longest relationship one will share with another human being is the sibling relationship, which lasts through a lifetime (often 50 to 80 years) as compared with the child-parent relationship of approximately 30 to 50 years. Siblings spend long periods together and get to know each other at their best and worst.

Sibling Functions. Siblings exert power, exchange services, and express feelings in reciprocal ways that are often not revealed in the presence of the parents. They see themselves in their brother or sister, experience life vicariously through their sibling's behavior, and begin to expand on their own possibilities. Siblings can also be touchstones for what the other would *not* like to be, and they use each other as yardsticks for comparison. They provide a sounding board for each other, and offer a safe forum for experimenting with new behaviors and roles. Brothers and sisters provide each other with tangible services (e.g., lending money, clothing, toys, sports equipment; teaching a skill), help each other with childhood problems, provide support in dealing with parents or others outside the family, and may provide introductions to new friendship groups. Children learn to negotiate and bargain, and sometimes to manipulate, from their siblings. Their interactions with each other provide opportunities for conflict and conflict resolution. They protect one another from parental-executive abuse of power and can form a coalition to deal with the issues of authority, power, and emotional support. Negotiating with parents is stronger when siblings act together rather than singly.

Siblings interpret the outside world for each other and perform educative functions for the parents. A related function is *pioneering,* in which one sibling initiates a process, thereby giving permission to the others to follow. These patterns include breaking explicit family rules, taking new pathways (such as leaving the family), or adopting different moral or political codes and lifestyles.

Tattling can be an important lever in sibling interactions. On the other hand, there is often a conspiracy of silence among siblings, leaving the parents feeling isolated and excluded. A willingness to maintain each other's privacy often serves as a powerful bond of loyalty that distinguishes the relationship between siblings from that between friends.

More Active Sibling Relationships.   Sibling relationships vary among cultures. Some factors may be giving the sibling relationship greater significance in American families than in the past. Shrinking family size, longer life spans, divorce and remarriage, geographic mobility, maternal employment, alternative sources of child care, competitive pressures, stress, and parental insufficiency may be propelling siblings into greater contact and emotional interdependence than ever before. Siblings often join forces to confront the trauma of divorce, and they frequently rely on each other for support when parents remarry. The large number of working mothers means that young siblings today have significant amounts of time when a personally committed adult does not monitor their relationship. Often an older sibling is required to baby-sit, resulting in children spending more and more time together unsupervised. In a worried, mobile, small-family, high-stress, fast-paced, parent-absent society, children often turn to a brother or sister to meet their needs for contact, constancy, and permanency.

Ordinal Position

It has been observed that the birth position of children affects their personalities. Parents treat children differently, and sibling interactions are different depending on the child's position within the family. Power is unequally distributed among siblings. Older siblings attempt to dominate younger ones. Therefore, younger siblings develop interpersonal skills, the ability to negotiate, and an ability to accept unfavorable outcomes to a greater extent than older siblings. Later-born children are obliged to interact with other siblings from birth and seem to be more outgoing and make friends more easily than firstborns. Children vary tremendously, and generalizations do not always apply to the individual. General characteristics of children in the various ordinal positions are presented in Box 3-4.

The Only Child.   Being the only child in a family has traditionally been considered a disadvantage. Only children have been described as selfish, spoiled, dependent, and lonely. However, a review of 141 research studies indicates that there are no essential personality differences between a child reared alone and one who is reared with one or more siblings (Polit and Falbo, 1987). They do not demonstrate more evidence of maladjustment or self-centeredness than other children and tend to strongly resemble firstborn children in respects such as higher educational goals. Only children perform better on cognitive tests, are more mature, are more socially sensitive, and demonstrate superiority in language facility over other children.

Only children also enjoy the advantage of having parents who can devote more time to them, talk to them, and stimulate them in intellectual activities. However, parents also exert greater pressure for mature behavior at an early age

and for achievement. Relative isolation from peers contributes to intellectual pursuits and encourages a rich fantasy life, independence, and originality.

Multiple Births

A deviation in early development that occurs with variable frequency is multiple births. Twins are not uncommon in the population, but triplets are rare and quadruplets or quintuplets are extremely unusual. In any of these situations, the offspring can be of the like or unlike sex (i.e., derived from a single ovum, from multiple ova, or a combination of the two, which can involve one or more cell divisions). The cause of twinning is unknown, but the increase in the number of larger multiples (quintuplets, sextuplets) during recent years has been associated with fertility-enhancing techniques (ovula-

---

BOX 3-4 ■ Influence of Ordinal Position on Children

FIRSTBORN CHILDREN
Are more achievement-oriented
Are more dominant
Receive more physical punishment
Are allowed to show more aggression to siblings
Have stronger consciences, are more self-disciplined and inner directed
Are more socially anxious
Are prone to feelings of guilt
Identify more with parents than with peers
Are more conservative
Are subject to greater parental expectations
Begin to speak earlier in life
Demonstrate higher intellectual achievement
Plan better and experience fewer frustrations
Are likely to be most wanted

MIDDLE CHILDREN
Have more demands made on them for household help
Are praised less often
Receive less of the parents' time
Learn to compromise and be adaptable
Are less stimulated toward achievement
Are more difficult to characterize because of a variety of positions in the family

YOUNGEST CHILDREN
Are less dependent than firstborn children
Are less tense, more affectionate, and more good-natured
Tend to identify more with peer group than with parents
Are more flexible in their thinking
Are popular with classmates
Have fewer demands placed on them for household help

ONLY CHILDREN
Resemble firstborn children
Are more mature and cultivated
Experience greater parental pressure for mature behavior and achievement
Demonstrate superiority in language facility
Rarely develop into stereotype of spoiled, selfish child
Often enjoy a rich fantasy life as a result of isolation

tion-inducing drugs and assisted reproductive techniques such as in vitro fertilization) (Ventura and others, 1997). Because women in their thirties are almost 2.5 times as likely as women in their twenties to have higher-order plural births, the rise in the multiple-birth ratio has been associated with increased childbearing among older women and the expanded use of fertility drugs (Guyer and others, 1999).

Twins are of two distinct types: *identical,* or *monozygotic (MZ),* and *fraternal* (Fig. 3-5), or *dizygotic (DZ)* (Box 3-5). In the United States the overall twinning rate is approximately 1 in 80 pregnancies; one third are MZ twins and two thirds are DZ twins.

A special kind of sibling relationship is observed in twins, although getting along with each other and quarreling are not much different from these behaviors in any other two siblings, especially if they are different-sex fraternal twins. Twins tend to work out a relationship that is reasonably satisfactory to both and demonstrate early independence from parental attention. They develop a remarkable capacity for cooperative play and considerable loyalty and generosity toward each other. It is not uncommon for them to evolve a private language between themselves that may interfere with the development of the family language.

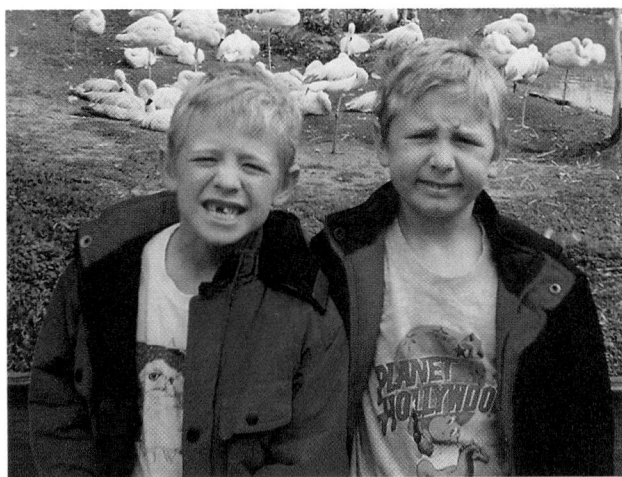

FIG. 3-5 ■ Fraternal twins.

In a twinship, one member of the pair, to a greater or lesser extent, is more dominant, outgoing, and assertive than the other, often to the consternation of their parents. However, the seemingly more passive twin is able to accomplish as much and get his or her way as frequently as the more assertive twin.

It has also been observed that there is a difference in behavior between identical and fraternal twins. There is near-unison in the actions of identical twins (although they alternate in assuming the leadership), but fraternal twins, even of the same sex, do not display this quality. Sibling rivalry can be quite pronounced in fraternal twins, especially in different-sex twins.

Identical twins also differ in their response to the tendency of some parents to treat twins exactly alike. The present philosophy is to determine the degree to which the children demonstrate an inclination toward togetherness. Some twins thrive best when they are constantly in each other's company; others prefer more individuality and separateness. The conservative approach is to allow the children to follow their natural inclinations. Early years of togetherness are often the basis of the children's security, and to separate them too early may produce unnecessary stresses. The tendency is to foster individual differences as they are evidenced to ease the process of separation when it becomes advisable.

Parental Adjustment. The entrance of any new member into a household creates stress, but with multiple births two or more new members must be incorporated into the family at the same time. The problems are obvious. Two infants must be provided with physical care, including feeding, diapering, and all of the purchasing and preparation that accompanies the care of any infant. Scheduling becomes crucial, and advancement in development brings new problems and adjustments (e.g., space and sleeping arrangements, selecting a stroller and other equipment). Care must be observed in selecting toys. As play becomes a serious business, some toys that would be safe and appropriate for a single child become weapons when two infants share a playpen. It is a good idea to select different toys for the children as they grow older and encourage sharing.

It is especially important for parents to maintain relationships with each other and other family members. It is

BOX 3-5 ■ Characteristics of Twins

MONOZYGOTIC (MZ, IDENTICAL TWINS)	DIZYGOTIC (DZ, FRATERNAL TWINS)
Result of one fertilized ovum that became separated early in development	Result of fertilization of two ova
Alike physically and genetically	Differ physically and genetically
Same sex	May be like or opposite sex
Frequency:	Frequency:
Occurs uniformly in all populations	Varies among races (highest—blacks, lowest—Asians, intermediate—whites)
Unaffected by maternal age	More common with advancing maternal age (maximum at age 35-39, then decreases rapidly)
Tendency unaffected by heredity	Marked familial tendency
	Expressed only in the female
	Fathers appear to transmit disposition toward double ovulation to daughters
Similar behavior	Dissimilar behavior; more sibling rivalry

doubly important for parents to arrange time together as often as possible. The **National Organization of Mothers of Twins Clubs, Inc.,*** has local chapters throughout the United States to offer information and support to parents of twins and is highly recommended as a resource for all new parents of twins. *Twins Magazine*† is a place to seek and give advice about parenting multiples.

PARENTING

MOTIVATION FOR PARENTHOOD

A dominant characteristic in all societies is that adults are expected to become parents and to be gratified by the experience. Pressures of tradition, sentiment regarding the state of parenthood, and religious exhortations to fulfill divine commands of fertility profoundly influence decision making because conformity to social-role expectations is a strong influence in family planning.

Factors that influence family size are social class, religion, race, financial stability, type of conjugal-role relationships, and the social-psychologic aspects of sexual relations. How effectively the couple practices contraception may also determine whether the family size remains as planned. In the case of divorce and remarriage, an individual may decide to have more children with the new spouse.

PREPARATION FOR PARENTHOOD

The basic goals of parenting are to promote the physical survival and health of the children, to foster the skills and abilities necessary to be a self-sustaining adult, and to foster behavioral capabilities for maximizing cultural values and beliefs. However, new parents often approach parenthood with limited experience and knowledge. Parents learn by trial and error, committing the same mistakes that have been committed by countless other parents, but they somehow manage to accomplish the task, becoming more skilled with each additional child. Tradition, rather than rational planning, furnishes the chief norms for childrearing. Experience in having been nurtured as a child is an essential component of successful parenting.

Their own parents are probably the only persons who parents observe intimately in the parental role. This results in a *generational continuity*—parents rear their own children in much the same way as they themselves were reared. Other essential skills that parents need to feel comfortable in the parenting role include a basic understanding of childhood growth and development, bathing, feeding, use of play, and interpersonal communication skills.

TRANSITION TO PARENTHOOD

Although there is disagreement as to whether the birth of the first child should be labeled a crisis, the early weeks of an infant's life call for a couple to make drastic adjustments. Although the parents have anticipated and perhaps prepared for the child's arrival, the birth presents the challenge of providing total care 24 hours a day for a new member of the family. A crisis may occur if the event is perceived as disturbing old habits and relationships and eliciting new responses. The birth requires role changes or significantly modifies former relationships. In addition to the roles of husband and wife, the couple must assume the roles of father and mother.

The advent of a new family member requires that the family cope with greater financial responsibilities, a possible loss of income, changes in sleeping habits, and less time for the husband and wife to spend with each other (especially if it is a firstborn) and with other children. If these events are perceived as aversive, it can disrupt the couple's bond and reduce the couple's intimacy and affection. For other couples, the adjustment to parenthood is only mildly stressful.

Parental Factors Affecting Transition to Parenthood

No amount of preparation can fully prepare prospective parents for the constant and immediate needs of an infant. The importance of early parent-infant interactions is addressed in the discussion of the neonate, especially the attachment process (see Chapter 8). Factors affecting parenting are the age of the parents, the quality of the parental relationship, the amount of previous experience with childrearing, parental support systems, and the effects of stress on parental behavior.

Parental Age.   The most satisfactory ages for childbearing are the years between 18 and 35. During this time, parents are considered to be in optimum health, with a predicted life-span that allows sufficient time and vigor to raise a family. However, the age at which parents begin their families has changed over the last few decades in the United States. A substantial increase in the birth rate for women 30 to 44 years of age and a decline for women ages 20 to 29 years have occurred.

Father Involvement.   Current practices that encourage early father-infant interaction indicate that fathers are as intrigued with their newborns as mothers are (see discussion on paternal engrossment under Promote Parent-Infant Bonding [Attachment], Chapter 8). Even fathers who have little initial contact with their neonates become involved with them over the next few months, although the type of interaction is different from that of the mother (Fig. 3-6). For example, mothers are more likely to hold, soothe, care for, or play quietly with their infants, whereas fathers are more boisterous, and engage in more physically stimulating activities. However, fathers are more than just playmates. They are often successful at soothing a distressed infant (Fig. 3-7). A secure attachment to the father can help offset the consequences of an insecure attachment to the mother.

Parenting Education.   First-time parents who have prepared themselves to be parents experience less stress adjusting to the birth of new baby than those who have not. Research suggests that programs designed to take place near the time of birth or soon after are more helpful in easing transitional stress than programs that take place earlier in life (e.g., high school programs).

---

*Executive office, PO Box 438, Thompson's Station, TX 37179-0438; www.nomote.org.
†twinsmagazine.com.

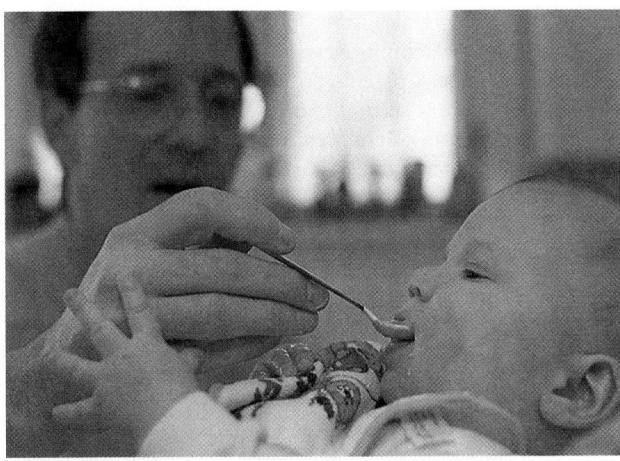

FIG. 3-6 ■ Fathers who assume care of their children may feel more comfortable and successful in their parenting role.

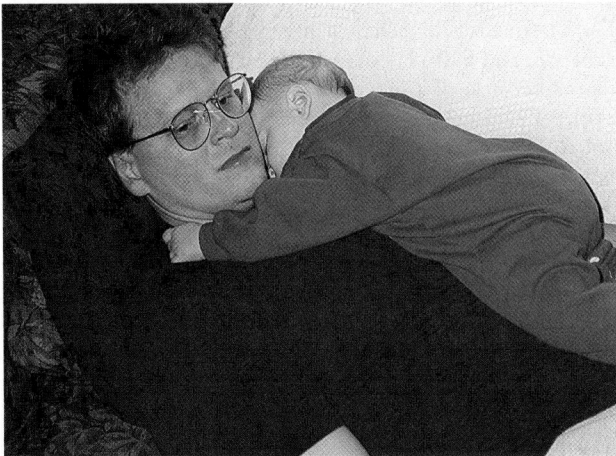

FIG. 3-7 ■ The role of the father is essential to a family's health and well-being.

Many parents are looking for ways to be a better parent. Shifrin (1997) recommends: (1) improving communication by becoming an active listener, (2) being actively involved in the child's education, (3) becoming computer literate, (4) viewing events from the child's point of view, (5) considering the child's temperament, (6) keeping the child healthy with checkups and vaccinations, (7) providing optimal nutrition, (8) maintaining a safe environment, (9) spending time with the child, and (10) evaluating the family's overall functioning.

■ ■ ■

Other factors influencing the transition to the parental role include:

■ Parents with previous experience, such as another child, appear to be more relaxed and have less conflict in disciplinary relationships, and are more aware of normal growth and development.

■ The amount of stress experienced by one or both parents may interfere with their ability to exhibit patience and understanding and to cope with their children's behavior.

■ Special characteristics of the infant, such as being temperamentally difficult, can cause the parents to lose confidence and doubt their abilities. Infants with special care needs (such as those associated with a disability) can be a significant source of added stress.

■ Marital relationships can have a negative effect on parental transition because marital tension can alter caregiving routines and interfere with enjoyment of the infant. Conversely, parents who support and encourage one another serve as a positive influence on establishing a satisfying parental role.

Support Systems.   Successful adaptation to the stress of transition to parenthood involves at least two types of family resources (McCubbin and McCubbin, 1994). *Internal resources* such as adaptability and integration are the first type of resource. Changing from an orderly, predictable life to a relatively disordered, unpredictable one is a universal adaptation that families must make. Rigid schedules are impossible to maintain, and former activities must be curtailed or abandoned. *Adaptation* is reflected in learning to be patient, becoming better organized, and becoming more flexible. *Integration* involves an attempt of the couple to continue some activities they engaged in before they became parents. In this way couples are able to maintain a sense of continuity and appreciate the importance of the husband-wife relationship.

The second resource for coping with stress is the use of *coping strategies* that strengthen the organization and functioning of the family. These include the use of social support systems and community resources and the adoption of a future orientation. Interpersonal supports that provide information, advice, and caretaking are derived from friends, relatives, and neighbors. Relationships with family, friends, and community are essential. For parents, positive, supportive work relationships are important. Equally important is time spent with friends. Arranging for time away from the child or children is also beneficial. One parent can assume care of the family to allow the other parent some time to himself or herself. Adoption of a future orientation provides reassurance to parents that things will get better, that they will cope, and that it is realistic to plan for the time when they will be able to engage in self-fulfilling activities.

It is also reassuring to know that others experience ambivalent feelings toward parenthood and share the same difficulties and frustrations. Exchanging ideas and experiences with other parents provides an opportunity to voice concerns and to learn new ways to cope with multiple childrearing problems.

PARENTING BEHAVIORS
Parental Styles of Control

Parenting styles can be described as authoritarian, permissive, or authoritative. *Authoritarian* or *dictatorial* parents try to control their children's behavior and attitudes through unquestioned mandates. They establish rules and regulations or standards of conduct that they expect to be followed rigidly and unquestioningly. They value and reward absolute obedience, mute acceptance of their word, and unfailing respect for the family's principles and beliefs. They forcefully punish any behavior that is contrary to parental standards. Parental authority is exercised with little explanation and little involvement of the child in decision making. The message is: "Do it because I say so."

Punishment need not be corporal but may be stern withdrawal of love and approval. Careful training often results in rigidly conforming behavior in the children, who tend to be sensitive, shy, self-conscious, retiring, and submissive. They are more apt to be courteous, loyal, honest, and dependable but docile. These behaviors are more typically observed when close supervision and affection accompany parental authority. If not, this style of parenting may be associated with both defiant and antisocial behavior.

Permissive or *laissez-faire* parents exert little or no control over their children's actions. They sometimes confuse permissiveness with license. They avoid imposing their own standards of conduct and allow their children to regulate their own activity as much as possible. These parents consider themselves to be resources for the children, not role models. If rules do exist, the parents explain the underlying reason, encourage the children's opinions, and consult them in decision-making processes. They employ lax, inconsistent discipline, do not set sensible limits, and do not prevent the children from upsetting the home routine. These parents rarely punish the children. Consequently, the children control the parents and are often disobedient, disrespectful, irresponsible, aggressive, and generally defiant of authority.

Authoritative or *democratic* parents combine practices from both of the previously described parenting styles. They direct their children's behavior and attitudes by emphasizing the reason for rules and negatively reinforcing deviations. They respect the individuality of each child and allow the child to voice objections to family standards or regulations. Parental control is firm and consistent but tempered with encouragement, understanding, and security. Control is focused on the issue, not on withdrawal of love or the fear of punishment. These parents foster "inner-directedness," a conscience that regulates behavior based on feelings of guilt or shame for wrongdoing, not on fear of being caught or punished. Parents' realistic standards and reasonable expectations produce children with high self-esteem who are self-reliant, assertive, inquisitive, content, and highly interactive with other children.

There are differing philosophies in regard to parenting. Childrearing is a culturally bound phenomenon, and children are socialized to behave in ways that are important to their family. In the authoritative style, authority is shared and children are included in discussions fostering an independent and assertive style of participation in family life. Other parents value a style that supports family closeness, a more patriarchal style of authority and interpersonal relatedness. When working with individual families, nurses should give these differing styles equal respect.

LIMIT SETTING AND DISCIPLINE

In its broadest sense, *discipline* means to teach or refers to a set of rules governing conduct. In a narrower sense, it refers to the action taken to enforce the rules after noncompliance. *Limit setting* refers to establishing the rules or guidelines for behavior. The clearer the limits that are set and the more consistently they are enforced, the less need there is for disciplinary action. For example, it is often sug-

gested that parents should set limits on the amount of time children spend watching television (Bar-on, 2000).

Nurses can help parents to establish realistic and concrete "rules." Limit setting and discipline are positive, necessary components of childrearing and serve several useful functions as they help children:

- Test their limits of control
- Achieve in areas appropriate for mastery at their level
- Channel undesirable feelings into constructive activity
- Protect themselves from danger
- Learn socially acceptable behavior

Children want and need limits. Unrestricted freedom is a threat to their security and safety. Through testing the limits imposed on them, children learn the extent to which they can manipulate their environment, as well as gain reassurance from knowing that others are there to protect them from potential harm.

Minimizing Misbehavior

The reasons for misbehavior may include attention, power, defiance, and a display of inadequacy (e.g., the child misses classes because of a fear that he or she is unable to do the work). Children may also misbehave because the rules are not clear or consistently applied. Acting out behavior, such as a temper tantrum, may represent uncontrolled frustration, anger, depression, or pain.

The best approach is to structure interactions with children so that unacceptable behavior is prevented or minimized (see Family Home Care box).

General Guidelines for Implementing Discipline

Regardless of the type of discipline used, certain principles are essential to ensure the efficacy of the approach (see Guidelines box). Many strategies, such as behavior modification, can only be implemented effectively when principles of consistency and timing are followed. A pattern of intermittent or occasional enforcement of limits actually prolongs the undesired behavior because children learn that if they are persistent, the behavior is permitted eventually. Delaying punishment weakens its intent, and practices such as telling the child, "Wait until your father comes home," are not only ineffectual, but also convey negative connotations about the other parent.*

Types of Discipline

To deal with misbehavior, parents need to implement appropriate disciplinary action. Many approaches are available. *Reasoning* involves explaining why an act is wrong and is usually appropriate for older children, especially when moral issues are involved. However, young children cannot be expected to "see the other side" because of their egocentrism. Children in the preoperative stage of cognitive development (toddlers and preschoolers) have a limited ability to distinguish between their point of view and those of others. Sometimes children use "reasoning" as a way of gaining at-

---

*For parenting of kindergarten through sixth grade children, see childparenting.about.com and kidshealth.org.

FAMILY HOME CARE

MINIMIZING MISBEHAVIOR

Set realistic goals for acceptable behavior and expected achievements.

Structure opportunities for small successes to lessen feelings of inadequacy.

Praise children for desirable behavior with attention and verbal approval.

Structure the environment to prevent unnecessary difficulties (e.g., place fragile objects in inaccessible area).

Set clear and reasonable rules; expect the same behavior regardless of the circumstances, and if exceptions are made, clarify that the change is for one time only.

Teach desirable behavior through own example, such as using a quiet, calm voice rather than screaming.

Review expected behavior before special or unusual events, such as visiting a relative or having dinner in a restaurant.

Phrase requests for appropriate behavior positively, such as "Put the book down," rather than "Don't touch the book."

Call attention to unacceptable behavior as soon as it begins; use distraction to change the behavior or offer alternatives to annoying actions, such as a quiet toy for one that is excessively noisy.

Give advance notice or "friendly reminders," such as "When the TV program is over, it is time for dinner" or "I'll give you to the count of three and then we have to go."

Be attentive to situations that increase the likelihood of misbehaving, such as overexcitement or fatigue, or decreased personal tolerance to minor infractions.

Offer sympathetic explanations for not granting a request, such as "I am sorry I can't read you a story now, but I have to finish dinner. Then we can spend time together."

Keep any promises made to children.

Avoid outright conflicts; temper discussions with statements such as "Let's talk about it and see what we can decide together" or "I have to think about it first."

Provide children with opportunities for power and control.

 GUIDELINES

Implementing Discipline

Consistency. Implement disciplinary action exactly as agreed on and for each infraction.

Timing. Initiate discipline as soon as child misbehaves; if delays are necessary, such as to avoid embarrassment, verbally disapprove of the behavior and state that disciplinary action will be implemented.

Commitment. Follow through with the details of the discipline, such as timing of minutes; avoid distractions that may interfere with the plan, such as telephone calls.

Unity. Make certain that all caregivers agree on the plan and are familiar with the details to prevent confusion and alliances between child and one parent.

Flexibility. Choose disciplinary strategies that are appropriate to child's age, temperament, and the severity of the misbehavior.

Planning. Plan discipline strategies in advance and prepare child if feasible (e.g., explain use of time-out); for unexpected misbehavior, try to discipline when you are calm.

Behavior-orientation. Always disapprove of the behavior, not the child, with such statements as "That was a wrong thing to do. I am unhappy when I see behavior like that."

Privacy. Administer discipline in private, especially with older children, who may feel ashamed in front of others.

Termination. After the discipline is administered, consider child as having a "clean slate" and avoid bringing up the incident or lecturing.

tention. For example, they may misbehave thinking the parents will give them a lengthy explanation of the wrongdoing and knowing that negative attention is better than no attention. When children use this technique, parents should end the explanation by stating, "This is the rule, and this is how I expect you to behave. I won't explain it any further."

Unfortunately, reasoning is often combined with *scolding,* which sometimes takes the form of shame or criticism.

For example, the parent may state, "You are a bad boy for hitting your brother." Children take such remarks seriously and personally, believing that *they* are bad.

! NURSING ALERT

When reprimanding children, focus only on the misbehavior, not on the child. Use of "I" messages rather than "you" messages expresses personal feelings without accusation or ridicule. For example, an "I" message attacks the behavior—"I am upset when Johnny is punched; I don't like to see him hurt"—not the child.

Positive and negative reinforcement is the basis of *behavior modification* theory—behavior that is rewarded will be repeated; behavior that is not rewarded will be extinguished. Using *rewards* is a positive approach. By encouraging children to behave in specified ways, the tendency to misbehave is lessened. With young children, using paper stars is a very effective method. For older children, the "token system" is appropriate, especially if a certain number of stars or tokens yields a special reward, such as a trip to the movies or a new book. In planning a reward system, the expected behaviors must be explained to the child and the rewards must be reinforcing. A chart should be used to record the stars or tokens, and an earned reward should be given promptly. Verbal approval should always accompany extrinsic rewards.

Consistently *ignoring* behavior will eventually extinguish or minimize the act. Although this approach sounds simple, it is often difficult to implement consistently. Parents frequently "give in" and resort to previous patterns of discipline. Consequently, the behavior is actually reinforced because the child learns that persistence gains parental approval. For ignoring to be effective, parents should (1) understand the process, (2) record the undesired behavior before using ignoring to determine if a problem exists and to compare results after ignoring is begun, (3) determine whether parental attention acts as a reinforcer, and (4) be aware of "response burst." Response burst is a phenomenon that occurs when the undesired behavior increases after ignoring is initiated because the child is "testing" the parents to see if they are serious about the plan.

The strategy of *consequences* involves allowing children to experience the results of their misbehavior. It includes three types:

1 **Natural**—Those that occur without any intervention, such as being late and missing dinner
2 **Logical**—Those that are directly related to the rule, such as not being allowed to play with another toy until the used ones are put away
3 **Unrelated**—Those that are imposed deliberately, such as no playing until homework is completed or the use of time-out

Natural or logical consequences are preferred and effective if they are meaningful to children. For example, the natural consequence of living in a messy room may do little to encourage cleaning up, but allowing no friends over until the room is neat can be motivating! Withdrawing privileges is often an unrelated consequence. After the child experiences the consequence, the parent should refrain from any comment, because the usual tendency is for the child to try to place blame for imposing the rule.

Time-out is actually a refinement of the common practice of "sending the child to his or her room" and is a type of unrelated consequence. It is based on the premise of removing the reinforcer (i.e., the satisfaction or attention the child is receiving from the activity). When placed in an unstimulating and isolated place, children become bored and consequently agree to behave in order to reenter the family group (Fig. 3-8). Time-out avoids many of the problems of other disciplinary approaches. No physical punishment is involved, no reasoning or scolding is given, and the parent does not need to be present for all of the time-out, thus facilitating his or her ability to consistently apply this type of discipline. Time-out offers both the child and the parent a "cooling off" time. To be effective, however, time-out must be planned in advance (see Family Home Care box).

Corporal or *physical punishment* most often takes the form of spanking. Based on the principles of aversive therapy, inflicting pain through spanking causes a dramatic short-term decrease in the behavior. However, there are serious flaws in this approach: (1) it teaches children that violence is acceptable; (2) it may physically harm the child if it is the result of parental rage; and (3) children become "accustomed" to spanking, requiring more severe corporal punishment each time. Spanking can result in severe physical and psychologic injury, and it interferes with effective parent-child interaction. Children who receive corporal punishment are less likely to learn what they should do, because the focus is on what they should not do (American Academy of Pediatrics, 1998). In addition, when the parent is not around, the misbehavior is likely to occur, for children have not learned to behave well for their own sake. Parental use of corporal punishment may also interfere with the child's development of moral reasoning.

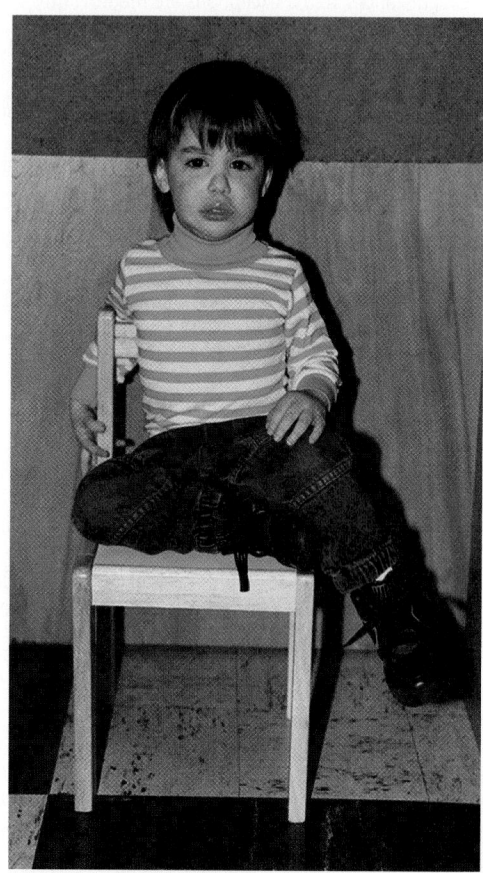

FIG. 3-8 ■ Time-out is an excellent disciplinary strategy for young children.

FAMILY HOME CARE

Using Time-Out

Select an area for time-out that is safe, convenient, and unstimulating, but where the child can be monitored, such as the bathroom, hallway, or laundry room.

Determine what behaviors warrant a time-out.

Make sure children understand the "rules" and how they are expected to behave.

Explain to children the process of time-out:

When they misbehave, they will be given *one* warning.

If they do not obey, they will be sent to the place designated for time-out.

They are to sit there for a specified period of time.

If they cry, refuse, or display any disruptive behavior, the time-out period will begin *after* they quiet down.

When they are quiet for the duration of the time, they can then leave the room.

A rule for the length of time-out is *1 minute per year of age;* use a kitchen timer with an audible bell to record the time rather than a watch.

Implement time-out in a public place by selecting a suitable area or explain to children that time-out will be spent immediately on returning home.

SPECIAL PARENTING SITUATIONS

Parenting is a demanding task under the most ideal circumstances, but when parents and children are faced with situations that deviate from what is considered the norm, the potential for family disruption is increased. Situations that are encountered frequently are divorce, single parenthood, blended families, adoption, and dual-career families. In addition, as cultural diversity increases in our communities, many immigrants are making the transition to parenthood, a new country, culture, and language simultaneously. These families often face isolation, different childrearing customs, and a lack of resources (Foss, 1996). Other situations that create unique parenting challenges are parental alcoholism, homelessness, and incarceration. Although these topics are not addressed here, the reader may wish to investigate them further.

PARENTING THE ADOPTED CHILD

Adoption establishes a legal relationship between a child and parents who are not related by birth, but who have the same rights and obligations that exist between children and their biologic parents. In the past, the biologic mother alone made the decision to relinquish the rights to her child. In recent years, the courts have acknowledged the legal rights of the biologic father regarding this decision. Concerned child advocates have questioned whether decisions that honor the father's rights are in the best interests of the child. As the rights of the child have become recognized, older children have successfully dissolved their legal bond with their biologic parents to pursue adoption by adults of their choice. Furthermore, there is a growing interest and demand within the gay and lesbian community to adopt. Agencies have developed few specific policies in this regard and face questions about the legal and social ramifications of adopting in a relationship not based on marriage, as well as possible consequences of not developing policies (Sullivan, 1995).

Unlike biologic parents who prepare for their child's birth with prenatal classes and the support of friends and relatives, adoptive parents have few sources of support and preparation for the new addition to their family. Nurses can provide the information, support, and reassurance needed to reduce parental anxiety regarding the adoptive process and refer adoptive parents to state parental support groups. Such sources can be contacted through a state or county welfare office. Prospective parents seeking information on international adoptions can contact **Families Adopting Children Everywhere, Inc. (FACE).***

Most problems faced by adoptive parents are not different from those encountered by natural parents, but the desire to be a good parent is often intensified in adoptive parents. Adoptive parents have been portrayed as more apprehensive, insecure, and in need of more assistance than biologic parents. However, some adoptive parents may actually need less assistance than biologic parents. This situation may be related to the adoptive parents' completely voluntary decision to become parents, the relatively long time they have to prepare for parenting, and the maturity associated with adopting.

The sooner infants enter their adoptive home, the better the chances of parent-infant attachment. However, the more caregivers the infant has had before adoption, the greater the risk for attachment problems. The infant must break the bond with the previous caregiver and form a new bond with the adoptive parents. Difficulties in forming an attachment depend on the amount of time the infant has spent with earlier caregivers (e.g., the birth mother, nurse, adoption agency personnel).

Siblings, adopted or biologic, who are old enough to understand should be included in decisions regarding the commitment to adopt, with reassurance that they are not being replaced. Ways that the siblings can interact with the adopted child should be stressed (Fig. 3-9).

Issues of Origin.   The task of telling children that they are adopted is a cause of deep concern and anxiety. There are no clear-cut guidelines for parents to follow in determining when and at what age children are ready for the information. Parents are naturally reluctant to present the children with such unsettling news. However, it is important that parents not withhold the adoption from the child, because it is an essential component of the child's identity (see Critical Thinking Exercise).

The timing arises naturally, as parents become aware of the child's readiness. Most authorities believe that children should be informed at an age young enough so that as they grow older, they do not remember a time when they did not know that they were adopted. The time is highly individual, but must be right for both the parents and the child. It may be when children ask where babies come from, at which time children can also be told the facts of their adoption. If they are told in a way that conveys the idea that they were active participants in the selection process, they will be less likely to feel that they were abandoned victims in a helpless situation. For example, parents can tell children that their personal qualities drew the parents to them. It is wise for parents who have not previously discussed adoption to tell children that they are adopted before the children enter

*PO Box 28058, Northwood Station, Baltimore, MD 21239; (410) 488-2656.

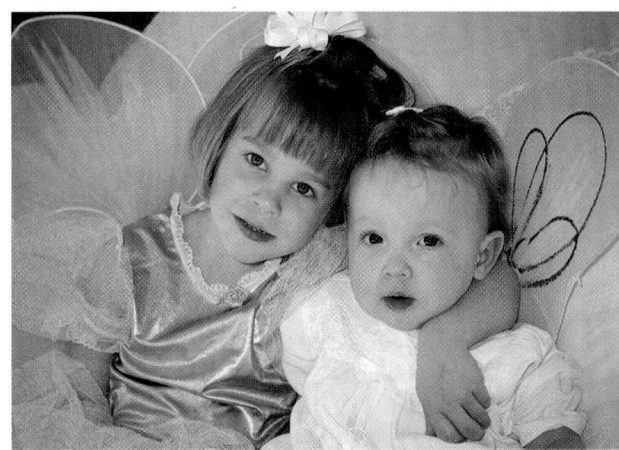

FIG. 3-9 ■ An older sister lovingly embraces her adopted sister.

??? CRITICAL THINKING EXERCISE ???

Parenting the Adopted Child

Twelve-month-old Justin was adopted at birth. His parents tell you that they wonder when they should tell Justin that he is adopted. As the nurse, what counseling and advice should you give Justin's parents?

QUESTIONS

1. Evidence—Is there sufficient information to draw any conclusions about this situation?
2. Assumptions—Describe some underlying assumptions about the following:
   a. The best time to tell children that they are adopted
   b. The manner in which parents should tell their child about adoption
   c. Children's reactions to being told they are adopted
3. What implications for nursing care can be drawn at this time?
4. Does the evidence support your conclusion?
5. Are there alternative perspectives to your conclusion?

ANSWERS

1. Yes. Although there is no one best time to tell children that they are adopted, most authorities believe that children should be informed before they enter school to avoid third parties inadvertently telling them that they are adopted. In addition, authorities agree that children should be told at an age young enough so that, as they grow older, they do not remember a time when they did not know they were adopted.
2. a. The best time is highly individualized and based on the child's readiness. For some children, this time may be when they ask about where babies come from. Children have a more difficult adjustment if disclosure occurs when they are older, and waiting until adolescence is too late to tell the child.
   b. Parents should be completely honest with the child and provide information about the adoption in a matter-of-fact way with complete honesty. Sharing the story of adoption is an important parental responsibility and can be handled much like a parent shares birth experiences with a biologic child.
   c. Parents should anticipate that children may act out after being told that they are adopted. Some children use the fact of their adoption as a weapon to manipulate and threaten their parents. Allowing children to express their feelings and emotions after they have been told about their adoption is very important.
3. Because Justin's parents have requested guidance, it is appropriate for you, as the nurse, to provide information about how and when they should tell Justin that he is adopted. However, the nurse's first priority is to be sure that Justin's parents are comfortable with this information, and that they feel free to ask any further questions and to obtain additional information. Because Justin is only 12 months old, his parents have time to think about how they will present this information to Justin and to prepare for the disclosure. They also have time to discuss how they will react to the feelings, emotions, and behaviors that Justin will demonstrate after he learns that he is adopted.
4. Yes, at the present time, most authorities agree that children should be told about the fact that they are adopted, and that disclosure of this information should occur before the school-age years.
5. The nurse might ask Justin's parents if they would like additional materials such as books and pamphlets. The nurse could also refer Justin's parents to community resources on adoption if they request additional information.

school to avoid third parties inadvertently telling the children before the parents have had the opportunity to do so. Complete honesty between parents and children strengthens the relationship.

Parents should anticipate behavior changes after the disclosure, especially in children who are older. In one study, children who were adopted were two to five times more likely to be referred for psychologic treatment than were nonadopted peers (Grotevant and McRoy, 1996). Children may use the fact of their adoption as a weapon to manipulate and threaten parents. Statements such as "My real mother would not treat me like this" or "You don't love me as much because I'm adopted" hurt parents and increase their feelings of insecurity. Such statements may also cause parents to become overpermissive. Adopted children need the same undemanding love, combined with firm discipline and limit setting, as any other child.

Adolescence. Adolescence may be an especially trying time for parents of adopted children. The normal confrontations of adolescents and parents assume more painful aspects in adoptive families. Adolescents may use their adoption to defy parental authority or as a justification for aberrant behavior. As they attempt to master the task of identity formation, the feeling of abandonment by their biologic parents comes into awareness and may be intensified. Gender differences in reacting to adoption may surface. It has been shown that girls have more difficulty accepting their sexuality, because they may not be able to identify with a nonfertile female parent.

Adopted children fantasize about their biologic parents and may feel the need to discover their parents' identity to define themselves and their own identity. It is important for parents to keep the lines of communication open and to reassure their child that they understand the need to search for their identity. In some states, birth certificates are made legally available to adopted children when they come of age. It is important for parents to be honest with questioning adolescents and to tell them of this possibility (the parents themselves are unable to obtain the birth certificate; it is the children's responsibility if they desire it).

Cross-Racial and International Adoption. Adoption of children from racial backgrounds different from that of the family is commonplace. In addition to the problems faced by adopted children in general, children of a cross-racial adoption must deal with additional differences. It is advised that parents who adopt such children do everything to preserve the adopted children's racial heritage.

> **NURSING ALERT**
>
> As a health care provider, it is important *not* to ask the wrong questions, such as "Is she yours, or is she adopted?" "What do you know about the 'real' mother?" "Are they really brother and sister?" or "How much did she cost?" (Hostetter and Johnson, 1996).

Although the children are full-fledged members of an adopting family and citizens of the adopted country, if they have a strikingly different appearance from other family members or exhibit distinct racial or ethnic characteristics, challenges may be encountered outside the family. Bigotry may appear among relatives and friends. Strangers may make thoughtless comments and talk about the children as though they were not members of the family. It is vital that the family declares to others that this is their child and a cherished member of the family.

In international adoptions,* the medical information the parents receive may be incomplete or sketchy; weight, height, and head circumference are often the only objective information present in the child's medical record (Kronemyer, 2001). Many internationally adopted children were born prematurely, and common health problems such as infant diarrhea and malnutrition delay growth and development. Some children have serious or multiple health problems that can be very stressful for the parents.

PARENTING AND DIVORCE

Since the mid-1960s, a marked change in the stability of families has been reflected in increased rates of divorce, single parenthood, and remarriage. In 1999, the divorce rate for the United States was 4 per 1000 total population (Centers for Disease Control and Prevention, 2002). The divorce rate has changed very little since 1987. In the previous decade, the rate increased yearly, with a peak in 1979. Although almost half of all divorcing couples are childless, more than 1 million children experience divorce each year.

The process of divorce begins with a period of marital conflict of varying length and intensity, followed by a separation, the actual legal divorce, and the reestablishment of different living arrangements (Box 3-6). Because a function of parenthood is to provide for the security and emotional

---

*For more information contact the **International Adoption Clinic,** University of Minnesota, Mailcode 211, 420 Delaware Street SE, Minneapolis, MN 55455; (614) 624-1164; www.peds.umn.edu.

BOX 3-6 ■ Stages of the Divorce Process

ACUTE PHASE
The married couple make the decision to separate. This phase includes the legal steps of filing for dissolution of the marriage and, usually, the departure of the father from the home. The duration of this phase lasts from several months to over a year and is accompanied by familial stress and a chaotic atmosphere.

TRANSITIONAL PHASE
The adults and children assume unfamiliar roles and relationships within a new family structure.
This phase is often accompanied by a change of residence, a reduced standard of living and altered lifestyle, a larger share of the economic responsibility being shouldered by the mother, and radically altered parent-child relationships.

STABILIZING PHASE
The postdivorce family reestablishes a stable, functioning family unit. Remarriage frequently occurs, with concomitant changes in all areas of family life.

Modified from Wallerstein JS: Children of divorce: stress and developmental tasks. In Garmezy N, Rutter M, editors: *Stress, coping, and development in children,* New York, 1983, McGraw-Hill.

---

welfare of children, disruption of the family structure often engenders strong feelings of guilt in the divorcing parents.

During a divorce, parents' coping abilities may be compromised. The parents may be very preoccupied with their own feelings, needs, and life changes and unable to be available and supportive to their children. Newly employed parents, usually mothers, are likely to leave children with new caregivers, in strange settings, or alone after school. The parent may also spend more time away from home, searching for or establishing new relationships. Sometimes, however, the adult feels frightened and alone and begins to depend on the child as a substitute for the absent parent. This dependence places an enormous burden on the child.

Common characteristics in the custodial household after separation and divorce include disorder, coercive types of control, inflammable tempers in both parents and children, reduced parental competence, a greater sense of parental helplessness, poorly enforced discipline, and diminished regularity in enforcing household routines. Noncustodial parents are seldom prepared for the role of visitor, may assume the role of recreational and "fun" parent, and may not have a residence suitable for children's visits. They may also be concerned about maintaining the arrangement over the years to follow.

Impact of Divorce on Children

Numerous studies indicate that divorce has a profound effect on children. Long-term studies indicate that many youngsters suffer for years from psychologic and social difficulties associated with continuing or new stresses in the postdivorce family. One outcome is heightened anxiety about forming enduring relationships as young adults (Thompson, 1998). Even when a divorce is amiable and open, children recall parental separation with the same emotions felt by victims of a natural disaster: loss, grief, and vulnerability to forces beyond their control.

The impact of divorce on children depends on several factors, including the age and sex of the children, the outcome of the divorce, and the quality of the parent-child relationship and parental care during the years following the divorce. Family characteristics are more crucial to the child's well-being than specific child characteristics, such as age or sex. The most important factor is continuing conflict between the divorced parents (Thompson, 1998). High levels of ongoing family conflict are related to problems of social development, emotional stability, and cognitive skills for the child.

Complications associated with divorce include efforts on the part of one parent to subvert the child's loyalties to the other, abandonment to other caregivers, and adjustment to a stepparent. A major problem occurs when children are "caught in the middle" between the divorced parents. They become the message bearer between the parents, are often quizzed about the activities of the other parent, and have to listen to criticisms from one parent about the other. A nurse may be able to intercede by helping the child get out of the middle by stating "I messages" based on the formula of "I feel . . . (state the feeling) when you . . . (state the source). I would like it if you . . ." This approach empowers the child to feel in control. An example of an "I message" is: "I feel uncomfortable when you ask me questions about Mom. I would like it if you would talk to her yourself" (Arbuthnot and Gordon, 1995).

Feelings of children toward divorce vary with age (Box 3-7). Some children feel a sense of shame and embarrassment concerning the family situation. Some feelings cause children to see themselves as different, inferior, or unworthy of love, especially if they feel responsible for the family dissolution. Although the social stigma attached to divorce no longer produces the emotions it did in the past, such feelings may still exist in small towns and can reinforce children's negative self-image. The lasting effects of divorce depend on the children's and the parents' adjustment to the transition from an intact family to a single-parent family and, often, to a reconstituted family.

Although most studies have concentrated on the negative effects of divorce on youngsters, some positive outcomes of divorce have been reported. A successful postdivorce family, either as a single-parent or as a reconstituted family, can improve the quality of life for both adults and children. If conflict is resolved, a better relationship with one or both parents may result, and some children may have less contact with a disturbed parent. Greater maturity, independence, and commitment to sustaining relationships are positive outcomes in some children (Wallerstein and Johnston, 1990).

Age- and Sex-Related Responses to Divorce.   Previously, it was believed that divorce had a greater impact on younger children, but recent observations indicate that divorce constitutes a major disruption for children of all ages. The feelings and behaviors of children may be different for various ages and gender, but all children suffer stress second only to the stress produced by the death of a parent. Although considerable research has looked at sex differences in children's adjustments to divorce, the findings are not conclusive.

Telling the Children.   Parents are understandably hesitant to tell children about their decision to divorce. Most parents neglect to discuss either the divorce or its inevitable changes with their preschool child. Without preparation, even children who remain in the family home are confused by the

BOX 3-7 ■ Feelings and Behaviors of Children Related to Divorce

INFANCY
Effects of reduced mothering or lack of mothering
Increased irritability
Disturbance in eating, sleeping, and elimination
Interference with attachment process

EARLY PRESCHOOL CHILDREN (AGES 2-3 YEARS)
Frightened and confused
Blame themselves for the divorce
Fear of abandonment
Increased irritability, whining, tantrums
Regressive behaviors (e.g., thumb sucking, loss of elimination control)
Separation anxiety

LATER PRESCHOOL CHILDREN (AGES 3-5 YEARS)
Fear of abandonment
Blame themselves for the divorce; decreased self-esteem
Bewilderment regarding all human relationships
Become more aggressive in relationships with others (e.g., siblings, peers)
Engage in fantasy to seek understanding of the divorce

EARLY SCHOOL-AGE CHILDREN (AGES 5-6 YEARS)
Depression and immature behavior
Loss of appetite and sleep disorders
May be able to verbalize some feelings and understand some divorce-related changes
Increased anxiety and aggression
Feel abandoned by departing parent

MIDDLE SCHOOL–AGE CHILDREN (AGES 6-8 YEARS)
Panic reactions
Feelings of deprivation—loss of parent, attention, money, and secure future
Profound sadness, depression, fear, and insecurity

Feelings of abandonment and rejection
Fear regarding the future
Difficulty expressing anger at parents
Intense desire for reconciliation of parents
Impaired capacity to play and enjoy outside activities
Decline in school performance
Altered peer relationships—become bossy, irritable, demanding, and manipulative
Frequent crying, loss of appetite, sleep disorders
Disturbed routine, forgetfulness

LATER SCHOOL-AGE CHILDREN (AGES 9-12 YEARS)
More realistic understanding of divorce
Intense anger directed at one or both parents
Divided loyalties
Able to express feelings of anger
Ashamed of parental behavior
Feel the need for revenge; may wish to punish the parent they hold responsible
Feel lonely, rejected, and abandoned
Altered peer relationships
Decline in school performance
May develop somatic complaints
May engage in aberrant behavior such as lying, stealing
Temper tantrums
Dictatorial attitude

ADOLESCENTS (AGES 12-18 YEARS)
Able to disengage themselves from parental conflict
Feel a profound sense of loss—of family, childhood
Feelings of anxiety
Worry about themselves, parents, siblings
Express anger, sadness, shame, embarrassment
May withdraw from family and friends
Disturbed concept of sexuality
May engage in acting-out behaviors

parental separation. Frequently, children are already experiencing vague, uneasy feelings that are more difficult to cope with than being told the truth about the situation. If possible, the initial disclosure should include both parents and siblings, followed by individual discussions with each child. Sufficient time should be set aside for these discussions, and they should take place during a period of calm, not after an argument. Parents who physically hold or touch their children provide them with a feeling of warmth and reassurance. The discussions should include the reason for the divorce and reassurance that the divorce is not the fault of the children.

Parents should not fear crying in front of the children, because their crying gives the children permission to cry also. Children need to ventilate their feelings. Children may feel guilt, a sense of failure, or that they are being punished for misbehavior. They normally feel anger and resentment and should be allowed to communicate these feelings without punishment. They also have feelings of terror and abandonment. They need consistency and order in their lives. They want to know where they will live, who will take care of them, if they will be with their siblings, and if there will be enough money to live on. Children fear that if their parents stopped loving each other, they could stop loving them. Their need for love and reassurance is tremendous at this time. Children may also wonder what will happen on special days such as birthdays and holidays, whether both parents will come to school events, and whether the child will still have the same friends (Arbuthnot and Gordon, 1995).

Custody and Parenting Partnerships

In the past, when parents separated, the mother was given custody of the children with visitation agreements for the father. Now both parents and the courts are seeking alternatives. Current belief is that neither fathers nor mothers should be awarded custody automatically. Custody should be awarded to the parent who is best able to provide for the children's welfare. In some cases, children experience severe stress when living or spending time with a parent. Many fathers have demonstrated both their competence and their commitment to care for their children.

Often overlooked are the changes that may occur in the children's relationships with other relatives, especially grandparents. Grandparents on the noncustodial side are often kept from their grandchildren, whereas those on the custodial side may be overwhelmed by their adult child's return to the household with grandchildren.*

Two other, less common, custody arrangements are divided custody and joint custody. *Divided,* or *split, custody* means that each parent is awarded custody of one or more of the children, thereby separating siblings. For example, sons might live with the father and daughters with the mother.

Joint custody takes one of two forms. In *joint physical custody,* the parents alternate the physical care and control of the children on a equitable basis while maintaining shared parenting responsibilities legally. This custody arrangement works well for families who live close to each other and whose occupations permit an active role in the care and rearing of the children. In *joint legal custody,* the children reside with one parent but both parents are the children's legal guardians and both participate in childrearing (Arditti, 1992).

Co-parenting offers substantial benefits for the family: children can be close to both parents, and life with each parent can be more normal as opposed to a disciplinarian mother and a recreational father. To be successful, parents in these arrangements must place high value on the commitment to provide normal parenting and to separate their marital conflicts from their parenting roles. No matter what type of custody arrangement is awarded, the primary consideration is the welfare of the children.

SINGLE PARENTING

An individual may acquire single-parent status as a result of divorce, separation, death of a spouse, or through birth or adoption of a child. Although divorce rates have stabilized, the number of single-parent households continues to rise. Approximately 3 of 10 children younger than 18 years of age live in single-parent families, and the majority of single parents are women (US Census Bureau, 2003). It is estimated that at least half of the children born during the 1990s will spend part of their life in a family headed by a divorced, separated, widowed, or never-married mother. Although some women are single parents by choice, most of these women never planned on being single parents, and many feel pressure to marry or remarry.

Managing shortages of money, time, and energy are major concerns for single parents. Studies repeatedly confirm the financial difficulties of single-parent families, particularly in the case of single mothers. Approximately, 41% of female-headed families lived in poverty in 1999. Only 31% of mother-headed households receive any child support or alimony (Annie E. Casey Foundation, 2001). In fact, the stigma of poverty may be more keenly felt than the discrimination associated with being a single parent. These families are often forced by their financial status to live in communities with inadequate housing and personal safety concerns. Single parents often feel guilty about the time spent away from their children. Divorced mothers, from marriages in which the father assumed the role of breadwinner and the mother the household maintenance and parenting roles, have considerable difficulty adjusting to their new role of breadwinner. Many single parents have trouble arranging for adequate child care, and care for a sick child is especially difficult to obtain.

Several authors (Elshtain, 1997; Mackey, 1997; Whitehead, 1997) suggest that the increasing number of single-parent families is harmful to society because children in these families are more likely to be poor, commit crime, and be a source of discipline problems in public education. Zinsmeister (1997) believes the absence of a father in single-parent homes places overwhelming burdens on the mother and deprives the children of a male role model. This situation could lead to poor educational performance, truancy, criminal activity, and psychologic problems for the children. However, Skolnick and Rosencranz (1997) maintain that single-parent families are unfairly stigmatized, and that the harm caused by single or unwed mothers is exaggerated.

Grandparents, a newsletter for grandparents in divided families, is published by Scarsdale Family Counseling Service, 405 Harwood Building, Scarsdale, NY 10583; (914) 723-3281.

Social supports and community resources needed by single-parent families include health care services that are open on evenings and weekends; high-quality child care; respite child care to relieve parental exhaustion and prevent burnout; and parent enhancement centers for advancing education and job skills, providing recreational activities, and offering parenting education. Single parents need social contacts separate from their children for their own emotional growth and that of their children. **Parents Without Partners, Inc.,*** is an organization designed to meet the needs of single parents.

Single Fathers

Fathers who have custody of their children have many of the same problems as divorced mothers. They feel overburdened by the responsibility, depressed, and concerned about their ability to cope with the emotional needs of the children, especially the needs of the girls. The lack of homemaking skills is characteristic of some fathers. They find it difficult at first to coordinate household tasks, school visits, and other activities associated with managing a household alone. Fathers often demand more assistance with household tasks and more independence from their children than custodial mothers do, and they are likely to make use of alternative caregiving and support systems.

PARENTING IN RECONSTITUTED FAMILIES

In the United States, approximately half of all children in homes where parents have divorced will experience another major change in their lives after divorce—a return to a nuclear family and the sudden acquisition of a stepparent when the custodial parent remarries (Dunn, 1995). The entry of a stepparent into a ready-made family requires adjustments for all family members. Some obstacles to the role adjustments and family problem solving include disruption of previous lifestyles and interaction patterns, complexity in the formation of new ones, and lack of social supports. Despite these problems, most children from divorced families want to live in a two-parent home.

Cooperative parenting relationships can allow more time for each set of parents to be alone to establish their own relationship with the children. Under ideal circumstances, power conflicts between the two households can be reduced, and tension and anxiety can be lessened for all family members. In addition, the children's self-esteem can be increased, and there is a greater likelihood of continued contact with grandparents. Flexibility, mutual support, and open communication are critical in successful relationships in stepfamilies and stepparenting situations. Unfortunately, stepfamilies usually do not seek help to prevent problems. Typically, information and counseling are sought only when problems have surfaced and can no longer be ignored. A preventive rather than remedial approach is needed.

PARENTING IN DUAL-EARNER FAMILIES

No change in family lifestyle has had more impact than the large numbers of women entering the workplace. As women moved away from the traditional homemaker pattern, the numbers of dual-earner families increased dramatically. This trend is unlikely to diminish. As a result, the family is subjected to considerable stress as members attempt to meet the challenge of the often competing demands of occupational needs and those regarded as necessary for a rich family life.

Role definitions are frequently altered to arrange an equitable division of time and labor, as well as to resolve conflict, especially conflict related to the traditional norms of the culture. Overload is a common source of stress in a dual-earner family, and social activities are significantly curtailed. Time demands and scheduling are major problems for all individuals who work. When the individuals are parents, the demands can be even more intense. Dual-earner couples may increase the strain on themselves to avoid creating stress for their children. Although there is no evidence to indicate that the dual-earner lifestyle is stressful to children, the stress experienced by the parents may affect the children indirectly.

Working Mothers

Working mothers have become the norm in the United States. However, disapproving attitudes from some health care workers and childcare books, lack of a national policy on childcare, and memories from their own childhood experience with an at-home mother contribute to the sense of stress and guilt that many working mothers experience (Youngblut and others, 2000).

Childcare is critical to the working mother's sense of well-being. The quality of childcare is a persistent concern for all working parents. Determinants of childcare quality are based on health and safety requirements, responsive and warm interaction between staff and children, developmentally appropriate activities and trained staff, limited group size, age-appropriate caregivers, adequate staff to child ratios, and adequate indoor and outdoor space (Scarr, 1998). In general, the quality of childcare is affected by lower ratios, smaller group sizes, and better-qualified teachers. Nurses play an important role in helping families to find suitable sources of childcare and to prepare children for this experience (see Alternate Childcare Arrangements, Chapter 10).

FOSTER PARENTING

The term *foster care* is defined as placement in an approved living situation away from the family of origin. The living situation may be an approved foster home with other relatives or strangers or a preadoptive home (Carlson, 1996). Each state provides a standard for the role of foster parent and a process by which to become one. These "parents" are on contract with the state to provide a "home" for children for a limited duration. Most states require about 27 hours of training before being on contract and at least 12 hours of continuing education a year. Foster parents may be required to attend a foster parent support group that is often separate from a state agency. Each state has guidelines regarding the relative health of the prospective foster parents and their families, background checks regarding legal issues for the adults, personal interviews, and a safety inspection of the residence and surroundings.

Foster homes include both kinship and nonrelative placements. Since 1982, the proportion of children in out-of-home care placed with relatives has increased rapidly and

---

*International Headquarters, 1650 South Dixie Hwy, Suite 510, Boca Raton, FL, 33432; (800) 637-7974; www.parentswithoutpartners.org.

substantially, accompanied by a decrease in the number of foster families (Heger and Scannapieco, 1995). Long-term studies indicate that there is relatively little difference in adult functioning between kinship and nonrelative placements (Benedict and others, 1996). As with their nonfoster counterparts, much of the child's adjustment depends on the stability of the family and available resources (Fein, 1995). Even though foster homes are designed to provide short-term care, it is not unusual for children to stay for many years. In these cases, children consider their foster caregivers "family" and express the feeling that the foster family functions like a normal family (Gardner, 1996; Kufeldt and others, 1995).

Nurses should be aware that nearly 500,000 children will be in foster care at any given time in the United States (American Academy of Pediatrics, 2000). Children in foster care tend to have a higher than normal incidence of acute and chronic health problems (Carlson, 1996). These may include developmental, emotional, medical, and dental problems. Foster children are often at risk because of their previous caretaking environment. Nurses should strive to implement strategies that will improve the health care for this group of children. In particular, assessment and case management skills are required to involve other disciplines to meet their needs.

ACCOMMODATING CONTEMPORARY PARENTING SITUATIONS

During recent years, both the private and government sectors have identified specific problems of contemporary families. Many of these issues involve working parents. One significant stressor for the working single parent or for dual-earner families is when a child becomes ill. The frequency of childhood illness, exclusion practices of most licensed childcare programs, and employer's limited sick-leave policies are other contributing factors. Most authorities agree that a familiar face and place are important components of sick-child care, and some argue that the only place for an ill child is at home with a parent or other relative.

Some employers have become more family focused and provide time off for parents to be with sick children. Increasing numbers are becoming more generous in the amount of time they allow parents (fathers as well as mothers) to remain at home after the birth or adoption of a child. Flexible work schedules and family-oriented legislation can ease the burden of managing family and work responsibilities. The passage of the Family and Medical Leave Act (FMLA) in 1993 set the stage for a greater focus on the issues of contemporary families. The FMLA allows eligible employees to take up to 12 weeks of unpaid leave each year to care for newborn or newly adopted children, parents, or spouses who have serious health conditions, or to recover from their own serious health condition.

KEY POINTS

- Because there is no agreement about the definition of family, a family is what an individual considers it to be.
- Three theories that have significant relevance and application to pediatric nursing are family systems theory, family stress theory, and developmental theory.
- Although the traditional family structure has been nuclear or extended, in recent years other forms, such as the single-parent family, have emerged.
- Family size and positioning within the family structure have a strong impact on a child's development.
- Interpersonal skills and a basic understanding of childhood growth and development are two essential areas of focus for parents.
- Parental control tends to be predominantly one of three types: authoritarian, permissive, or authoritative.
- Three areas of special concern to adoptive families include the initial attachment process, the task of telling the children they are adopted, and identity formation during adolescence.
- Marital factors within the home significantly influence a child's development. The impact of divorce on a child depends on the child's age and sex, the outcome, and the quality of the parent-child relationship and parental care following the divorce.
- Single-parenting and stepparenting create adjustment difficulties and stress to the already-demanding parental role. Significant numbers of children will live in a single-parent or re-constituted family at some point.

References

American Academy of Pediatrics: *Sibling relationships: guidelines for parents*, Elk Grove Village, Il, 1996, AAP Publications.

American Academy of Pediatrics, Committee on Early Childhood, Adoption, and Dependent Care: Development issues for young children in foster care (RE0012), *Pediatrics* 106(5):1145-1150, 2000.

American Academy of Pediatrics, Committee on Psychosocial Aspects of Child and Family Health: Guidance for effective discipline, *Pediatrics* 101(4):723-728, 1998.

Andrews M, Boyle J: *Transcultural concepts in nursing care*, ed 2, Philadelphia, 1995, JB Lippincott.

Annie E. Casey Foundation: *Kids count 2001*, Washington, DC, 2001, Center for the Study of Social Policy.

Arbuthnot J, Gordon D: *Surviving divorce: a student's companion to children in the middle*, Athens, Ohio, 1995, Center for Divorce Education.

Arditti J: Differences between fathers with joint custody and noncustodial fathers, *Am J Orthopsychiatry* 62(2):186-195, 1992.

Ariel J, McPherson DW: Therapy with lesbian and gay parents and their children, *J Marriage Fam Ther* 26(4):421-432, 2000.

Bar-on ME: The effects of television on child health: implications and recommendations, *Arch Dis Child* 83:289-292, 2000.

Benedict M and others: Adult functioning of children who lived in kin versus nonrelative family foster homes, *Child Welfare* 75(5):529-549, 1996.

Black M, Nitz K: Grandmother co-residence, parenting and child development among low income, urban teen mothers, *J Adolesc Health* 18:218-226, 1996.

Brazelton TB: Working with families: opportunities for early intervention, *Pediatr Clin North Am* 42(1):1-10, 1995.

Carlson K: Providing health care for children in foster care: a role for advanced practice nurses, *Pediatr Nurs* 22(5):418-421, 1996.

Centers for Disease Control and Prevention: Births, marriages, divorces, and deaths: provisional data for 2001, *Nat Vital Stat Rep* 50(14):1-2, 2002.

Dunn J: Stepfamilies and children's adjustment, *Arch Dis Child* 73(6):487-489, 1995.

Duvall ER: *Family development*, ed 5, Philadelphia, 1977, JB Lippincott.

Elshtain JB: Single-parent families contribute to the breakdown of society. In Swisher KL, editor: *Single-parent families*, San Diego, 1997, Greenhaven Press.

Fein E: Stability and change: initial findings in a study of treatment foster care placements, *Child Youth Serv Rev* 17(3):379-389, 1995.

Foss G: A conceptual model for studying parenting behaviors in immigrant populations, *Adv Nurs Sci* 19(2):74-87, 1996.

Friedman M: *Family nursing: theory and practice,* ed 4, Norwalk, Conn, 1998, Appleton-Century-Crofts.

Gardner H: The concept of family: perceptions of children in foster care, *Child Welfare* 75:161-182, 1996.

Grotevant H, McRoy R: Emotional disorders in adopted children and youth. In McManus M, editor: Adoption: a lifelong journey for children and families, *Focal Point* 10:1, 1996.

Guyer B and others: Annual summary statistics—1998, *Pediatrics* 104(8):1229-1245, 1999.

Heger R, Scannapieco M: From family duty to family policy: the evolution of kinship care, *Child Welfare* 74(1):200-216, 1995.

Hostetter M, Johnson D; Medical supervision of internationally adopted children, *Pediatr Basics* 77:10-17, 1996.

Kronemyer B: Providing care for internationally adopted children proves rewarding, *Infect Dis Child* 14(1):15, 2001.

Kufeldt K and others: How children in care view their own and their foster families, *Child Welfare* 74(3):695-715, 1995.

Lerner RM, Sparks EE, McCubbin LD: *Family diversity and family policy: strengthening families for America's children,* Boston, 1999, Kluwer Academic Publishers.

Lynch JM, Murray K: For the love of the children: the coming out process for lesbian and gay parents and stepparents, *J Homosex* 39(1):1-24, 2000.

Mackey WC: Single-parent families contribute to violent crime. In Swisher KL, editor: *Single-parent families,* San Diego, 1997, Greenhaven Press.

McCubbin MA, McCubbin HI: Families coping with illness: the resiliency model of family stress, adjustment, and adaptation. In Danielson CB, Bissel BH, Winstead-Fry P, editors: *Families, health, and illness,* St Louis, 1994, Mosby.

Polit D, Falbo T: Only children and personality development, *J Marriage Fam* 49:309-325, 1987.

Scarr S: American child care today, *Am Psychol* 53(2):95-108, 1998.

Shifrin D: Resolved: 10 tips for better parenting in the new year, *AAP News,* January 1997.

Skolnick A, Rosencranz S: The harmful effects of single-parent families are exaggerated. In Sullivan A: Policy issues in gay and lesbian adoption, *Adopt Foster* 19(4):21-25, 1997.

Sullivan A: Policy issues in gay and lesbian adoption, *Adopt Foster* 19(4):21-25, 1995.

Thompson P: Adolescents for families of divorce: vulnerability to physiological and psychological disturbances, *J Psychosoc Nurs* 36(3): 34-39, 1998.

US Census Bureau: *Two married parents the norm,* Washington DC, 2003, Department of Commerce News. Available online: www.census.gov.

Ventura SJ and others: Advance report of final natality statistics, 1995, *Monthly Vital Stat Rep* 44(3 suppl), 1997.

Wallerstein JS, Johnston JR: Children of divorce: recent findings regarding long-term effects and recent studies of joint and sole custody, *Pediatr Rev* 11(7):197-204, 1990.

Whitehead BD: Single-parent families are harmful. In Swisher KL, editor: *Single-parent families,* San Diego, 1997, Greenhaven Press.

Woodworth R: You're not alone . . . you're one in a million, *Child Welfare* 75(5):619-635, 1996.

Youngblut JM and others: Factors influencing single mother's employment status, *Health Care Women Int* 21:125-136, 2000.

Zinsmeister K: Divorce harms children. In Swisher KL, editor: *Single-parent families,* San Diego, 1997, Greenhaven Press.

Social, Cultural, and Religious Influences on Child Health Promotion

CASEY HOOKE

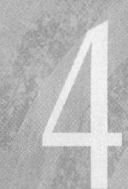

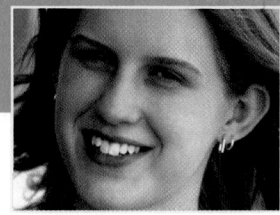

Remember to check out your companion CD-ROM

http://evolve.elsevier.com/Wong/essentials/

CHAPTER OUTLINE

RELATED TOPICS and ADDITIONAL RESOURCES

CULTURE

The future of any society depends on its children; therefore, society must provide for their care, nurture, and socialization. Culture plays a critical role in the socialization agenda of children through particular views of parenting and child development (Yoos and others, 1995). The customs and values of the culture help to organize a society's childrearing system and are transmitted from one generation to the next through the medium of the family.

Culture is the context of the child's experience of health and illness, wellness and sickness (Talabere, 1996). A holistic view of any child requires that nurses develop some understanding of the ways that culture contributes to the development of social and emotional relationships and influences childrearing practices and attitudes toward health.

Transcultural nursing knowledge has become imperative during the past decade because of the increased migration of people worldwide. Professional nurses are providing care to diverse populations from almost every point of the globe (Cooper, 1996). This orientation to transcultural nursing includes an awareness of the nurse's own culture. The nurse who is becoming culturally competent learns about, becomes able to assess from, and shares the culture of others (Dunn, 2002).

Culture is a pattern of assumptions, beliefs, and practices that unconsciously frames or guides the outlook and decisions of a group of people (Buchwald and others, 1994). Culture differs from both race and ethnicity. *Race* is defined as a division of mankind possessing traits that are transmissible by descent and that are sufficient to characterize it as a distinct human type. One classification of race, based on skin color, is Caucasian (white), Negroid (African American), and Mongoloid (yellow). *Ethnicity* is the affiliation of a set of persons who share a unique cultural, social, and linguistic heritage. *Socialization* is the process by which society imparts its competencies, values, and expectations to children (Trawick-Smith, 2000).

Culture is a complex whole in which each part is interrelated. It provides the lens through which all facets of human behavior can be interpreted (Spector, 2000). A culture is composed of individuals who share a set of values, beliefs, practices (language, dress, diet, health care), social relationships, law, politics, economics, and norms of behavior that are learned, integrative, social, and satisfying (Habayeb, 1995). Culture is not a surface veneer that covers a basic outlook shared by all human beings; rather, it is an ingrained orientation to life that serves as a frame of reference for individual perception and judgment. People from one culture differ from those in other cultures in the ways they think, solve problems, and perceive and structure the world. Culture is, essentially, the way of life of a group of people that incorporates experiences of the past, influences thought and action in the present, and transmits these traditions to future group members. Adaptation is necessary, however, for the culture to survive in an ever-changing world. Consciously and unconsciously, the members abandon, modify, or assume new patterns to meet the needs of the group.

The observable components of a culture, such as material objects (dress, art, utensils, and other artifacts) and actions, are sometimes termed the *material overt* or *manifest culture; nonmaterial covert culture* refers to those aspects that cannot be observed directly, such as the ideas, beliefs, customs, and feelings of the culture. Related to the large culture are many *subcultures,* each with an identity of its own. Children are socialized into a particular subculture rather than into the culture as a whole. Subcultural influences, such as ethnicity and social class, are discussed in more detail later in this chapter.

The culture in which children are reared determines the type of food they will eat, the language they will speak, the ideals of behavior they will follow, and the way they will conduct themselves in social roles (Yoos and others, 1995). To be acceptable members of the culture, children must learn how the culture expects them to behave toward others in the group. In turn, they learn how they can expect others to behave toward them.

Cultures and subcultures contribute to the uniqueness of child members in such a subtle way and at such an early age that children grow up to feel that their beliefs, attitudes, values, and practices are the "correct," or "normal" ones. By age 5, children can identify persons who belong to their own race or cultural background. During later primary years, children are able to identify people from different cultures (Trawick-Smith, 2000). A set of values learned in childhood is apt to characterize children's attitudes and behavior for life, guiding their long-range strivings and monitoring their short-range, impulsive inclinations. Thus every ongoing society socializes each succeeding generation to its cultural heritage.

The manner and sequence of the growth and development phenomenon are universal and fundamental features of all children; however, the variations in behavioral responses that children display to similar events are believed to be determined by their culture. Inborn temperament and modes of behavior that prompt children to behave in their own preferred and highly individual manner may be in harmony or in conflict with the culture. Such forces as heredity and maturation impose limits on the influence that parents and other social groups may bring to bear.

The culture fosters and reinforces those behaviors deemed desirable and appropriate; it attempts to depress or extinguish those at conflict with cultural norms. Some cultures encourage aggressive behaviors in their children; others favor amiability and compliance. Some foster individual resourcefulness and competition; others emphasize cooperation and submission to group interest. The child from a culture that values cooperation will not respond to a challenge such as "I'll bet you can get dressed faster than Johnny can," whereas a child from a culture that emphasizes individual achievement will be stimulated by the challenge.

Cultures may also differ in whether status in the group is based on age or on skill. Even children's play and their types of games are culturally determined. In some cultures children play in groups composed of members of the same sex; in others, they play in mixed-sex groups. In some cultures team games predominate; in others, most play is limited to individual games.

Standards and norms vary from culture to culture and from location to location; a practice that is accepted in one area may meet with disapproval or create tension in another. The extent to which cultures tolerate divergence from the established norm varies among cultures and subcultural groups. Although conformity provides a degree of security, it is a decided deterrent to change.

SOCIAL ROLES

Much of children's self-concept is derived from their ideas about their social roles. *Roles* are cultural creations; therefore, the culture prescribes patterns of behavior for persons in a variety of social positions. All persons who hold similar social positions have an obligation to behave in a particular manner. A role prohibits some behaviors and allows others. Because it delineates and clarifies roles, the culture is a significant influence on the development of children's self-concept (i.e., attitudes and beliefs they have about themselves).

A social group consists of a system of roles carried out in both primary and secondary groups. A *primary group* is characterized by intimate, continued, face-to-face contact; mutual support of members; and the ability to order or constrain a considerable proportion of individual members' behavior. Two such groups are the family and the peer group, both of which exert a great deal of influence on the child.

Secondary groups are groups that have limited, intermittent contact and in which there is generally less concern for members' behavior. These groups offer little in terms of support or pressure toward conformity except in rigidly limited areas. Examples of secondary groups are professional associations and church organizations (also considered in relation to subgroups). The childrearing orientation in a secondary-group environment, such as urban communities, differs considerably from that of a primary-group community. An urban community is dynamic and rapidly changing; therefore, many of the traditional behaviors and values do not meet its needs. Consequently, parents are often uncertain about what to teach their children. They may wish to rear their children

with values consistent with their own, but the differences in experience between the generations are too great. As a result, they often grant their children autonomy in some areas of decision making early in the developmental process, and other secondary groups assume a greater influence. The children are exposed to an assortment of social groups with diverse sets of values and expectations. None of the groups is highly dominant in its influence; therefore, the children are exposed to an eclectic set of values, some in agreement and some at conflict with the others. From these they must ultimately select those that they determine to be best for them and adopt them to form a consistent set of roles and behaviors to be incorporated into the self-concept.

Self-Esteem and Culture

A child's sense of self-esteem is influenced by his or her culture (Trawick-Smith, 2000). Some cultures are more collective in thought and action. A child from a collective culture will hold an inclusive view of self. Self-evaluation is related to the accomplishments or competencies of the entire family or community. School experiences that focus on personal achievement may promote positive self-esteem in some children but not in others who are more dependent on the success of a whole family or peer group. A child's sense of control may not come from individual self-reliance but rather from a feeling of worth in one's family or community (Trawick-Smith, 2000).

Families and culture also influence the criteria children use to evaluate their own abilities. Additionally, cultures vary in whether they instill an internal locus of control (a belief in the ability to regulate one's own life). Effects on self-esteem are minimal if these beliefs are directed by parents and are in accordance with cultural customs (Trawick-Smith, 2000). What is damaging to emotional health is helplessness that stems from prejudice. A factor that has helped maintain positive self-image and protect against the damage that prejudice can cause is ethnic pride (Trawick-Smith, 2000).

SUBCULTURAL INFLUENCES

Except in rare situations, children grow and develop in a blend of cultures and subcultures. In a large, complex society such as that of the United States, different groups have their own set of standards, values, and expectations within the collective ways of the large culture. Although many cultural differences are related to geographic boundaries, subcultures are not always restricted by location.

Children's membership in a cultural subgroup is, for the most part, involuntary. They are born into a family with a specific ethnic or racial heritage, socioeconomic level, and religious beliefs. Although in the complex North American society there are countless subcultures and considerable variation in the way of life, those subcultures that seem to exert the greatest influence on childrearing are ethnicity, social class, and occupational role. In addition, schools and peer-group subcultures are strong influences in the socialization of the child.

Ethnicity

Ethnicity is the classification of or affiliation with any of the basic groups or divisions of mankind or any heterogeneous population differentiated by customs, characteristics, language, or similar distinguishing factors. Ethnic differences extend to many areas and include such manifestations as family structure, language, food preferences, moral codes, and expression of emotion. Some standards of behavior result from the cultural heritage of the specific ethnic group. The term ethnic has aroused strong negative feelings and is often rejected by the general population (Spector, 2000).

To establish their place in the group, children learn how to adhere to a mode of behavior that is in accordance with standards distinctive to the group and learn how they can expect others to behave toward them. They take their cues from observing and imitating those to whom they are exposed. For example, children of a racial minority form a perception of their role as a group member by observing the manner in which role models within the subgroup respond to treatment by people outside the subgroup. When they see group members display an attitude of inferiority, they assume this to be the appropriate behavior. These perceptions are then incorporated into their own self-concept.

In the United States the cross-cultural lines are becoming blurred as subcultures are assimilated and blended into the larger culture (Fig. 4-1). It is particularly difficult for persons to attempt to maintain an identity with a subculture while living and conforming to the requirements of the dominant culture. Universal customs and language used in commercial and educational systems are different from those of the minority culture. Consequently, children reared in this environment are confused about roles and values, and they usually adopt those of the more influential or higher status culture. Youths, in particular, are influenced by the locally dominant group.

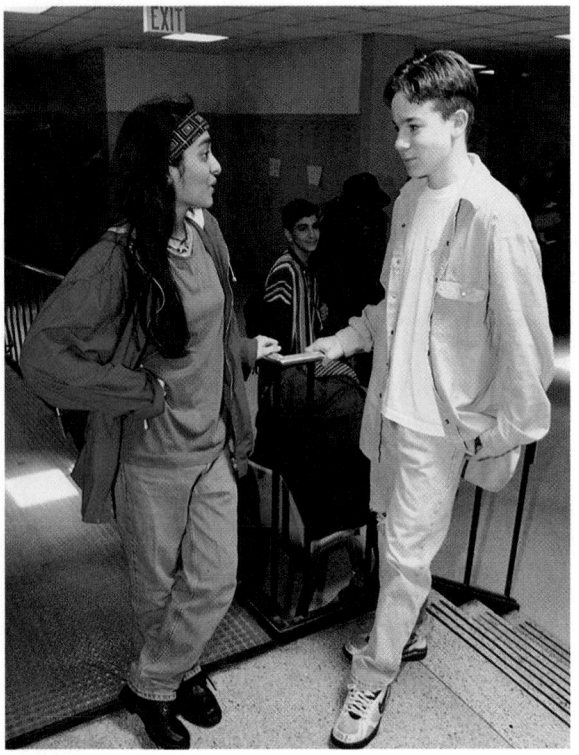

FIG. 4-1 ■ Youngsters from different cultural backgrounds interact within the larger culture.

Ethnocentrism is the emotional attitude that one's own ethnic group is superior to others; that one's values, beliefs, and perceptions are the correct ones; and that the group's ways of living and behaving are the best way (Spector, 2000). *Ethnic stereotyping* or labeling stems from ethnocentric views of people. Ethnocentrism implies that all other groups are inferior and that their ways are not in the best interests of the group. It is a common attitude among a dominant ethnic group and strongly influences the ability of one person to evaluate the beliefs and behaviors of others objectively. This inherent viewpoint of individuals tends to bias their interpretation and understanding of the behavior of others. Sometimes nurses have a tendency to have ethnocentric attitudes when giving care to people from different cultures (Petersen, 1995). The culturally competent nurse, however, has empathy for others, an openness to feeling what the other feels, an attitude of curiosity, a willingness to ask questions to better understand, an attitude of basic respect for self and others, and an acknowledgment of the intrinsic value of all humans (Carillo, Green, and Belancourt, 1999).

Socioeconomic Class

It is important to recognize that family relationships may be stronger among some ethnic or cultural groups than others. However, the influence of socioeconomic class cannot be overlooked.

Socioeconomic class relates to the family's economic and education levels. Strong family relationships exist among those of lower socioeconomic class who have few resources and must rely on the support of a family network to meet physical and emotional needs. Middle- and upper-class people often have resources that reach beyond the extended family. They are able to access physical and emotional support in the community (Giger and Davidhizar, 1999).

The term *socioeconomic class* should not be confused with cultural or ethnic diversity. Children of a specific race are not necessarily of low socioeconomic status. Additionally, children of poverty do not automatically have developmental delays (Trawick-Smith 2000).

Poverty

A subcultural influence closely related to, but different from, social class is the condition known as poverty. It is a relative concept and is usually associated with the general standards of a population. The term *poverty* implies both visible and invisible impoverishment. It is a condition in which families live without adequate resources (Trawick-Smith, 2000). *Visible poverty* refers to lack of money or material resources, which includes insufficient clothing, poor sanitation, and deteriorating housing. *Invisible poverty* refers to social and cultural deprivation, such as limited employment opportunities, inferior educational opportunities, lack of or inferior medical services and health care facilities, and an absence of public services.

An *absolute standard* of poverty attempts to delimit some basic set of resources needed for adequate existence; a *relative standard* reflects the median standard of living in a society and is the term used in referring to childhood poverty in the United States. That is, what appears to be substandard living conditions in one area may be a standard or norm in another.

An important development affecting the American family since the end of World War II is the widening disparity in income status among generations. Research indicates that the safety net (federal financial support) is working less effectively for children than for elderly people and poor adults (Ozawa and Yat-sang, 1996). Growth in the ranking of poor children over the last decade has not been due to an increase in the number of welfare-dependent families. It is because the ranks of the working poor have been growing. Between 1976 and 2000, the number of poor children living in families with income from earnings but no public assistance increased from 4.4 million to 6.9 million. Data on poverty are based on the official poverty measure of $14,494 in 1992 for a family of one adult and two children. These low-income working families are struggling to raise 10.2 million children, or about 15%, of America's children. Forty-two percent of the children are non-Hispanic Caucasian, 22% are non-Hispanic African American, 31% are Hispanic, 4% are non-Hispanic Asian–Pacific Islander, and 1% are non-Hispanic American Indian–Alaskan Native. Two-thirds of these children live with married parents. These low-income working parents also lack crucial benefits such as health insurance and sick leave. Their irregular work schedules, child-care needs, and lack of basic benefits prevent an escape from poverty. Parents who must work during evenings, nights, and weekends may leave children unsupervised and vulnerable (Annie E. Casey Foundation, 2003).

Homelessness

One of the most pressing problems in the United States is the growing number of homeless families. *Homeless individuals* are those who lack resources and community ties necessary to provide for their own adequate shelter. In the past the homeless population traditionally included single adults, mostly men. Currently, 50% of today's homeless are families with children, most of which are headed by single parents (Tropello, 2000).

Homeless children have increased in numbers as poverty has become feminized, minorities have become poorer, and low-income housing has become less accessible. Estimates on the number of homeless children in the United States at any given time range from 68,000 to 100,000. The majority of children are younger than 5 years of age and predominantly from minority groups.

Most homelessness is a direct result of increasing numbers of people in poverty combined with a lack of decent, affordable housing. Government housing subsidies have decreased, whereas the number of working poor has increased (Tropello, 2000). Other reasons include job layoffs, low income, parental mental illness, domestic conflict, and unexpected family or economic crises. Many families move into homelessness gradually after family members and friends are no longer willing to provide housing.

Another group of homeless children are the "runaway" and "throwaway" adolescents. Many runaways are victims of physical and sexual abuse and leave home because of long-term family or school problems. Poor parent-child relationships, extreme family conflict, feelings of alienation from parents, inconsistency in supervision, and unpredictability in discipline are other factors often cited.

Lack of a permanent dwelling deprives children of the most basic necessities for proper growth and development.

Homelessness disrupts a child's friendships and schooling (Strehlow and Amos-Jones, 1999). Homeless children suffer from physical and mental disorders that exceed those found in poor children who have a permanent residence.

Migrant Families

One of the most disadvantaged groups is migrant farm workers and their children. Indications suggest that in the United States there are between 3 and 5 million migrant and seasonal workers and their dependents, whose average yearly income is well below the poverty level. In addition, most of these families have no health care insurance.

The low position of these families on the economic scale and their rootless, mobile existence subject them to inadequate sanitation, substandard housing, social isolation, and lack of educational and medical facilities (Sandhaus, 1998). This lifestyle is especially deleterious to the children. Schooling and health care are inadequate. Children are apt to live in a number of localities and attend a variety of schools in the course of a year, with no continuity in either education or health care. Because both parents work in the fields, children receive little adult supervision; therefore, injury rates are high, and meals are erratic. Except where prohibited and enforced by law, children are even recruited to work in the fields along with the adults.

Some migrants have a home base to which they return at the end of the growing season; others travel continuously, migrating north in summer and south in winter. With most, there is little if any integration into the dominant culture; therefore, migrant groups suffer social isolation. Groups who travel together, especially those with the same ethnic background, develop a cohesiveness and form their own set of values and customs. Sometimes a migrant family will leave the migration stream and became a part of a permanent community. However, this involves adaptation to a new environment and lifestyle that can be stress provoking to these families.

Religion

Probably the most influential factor in shaping the culture of the United States is the Judeo-Christian faith. Many immigrants came to the United States for religious freedom and established a religious and moral atmosphere that persists today. However, there are individual differences that are part of the general culture.

The religious orientation of the family dictates a code of morality and influences the family's attitudes toward education, male and female role identity, and beliefs regarding their ultimate destiny (Fig. 4-2). It may also determine the school that the children attend, the companions with whom they associate, and often their mate selection. In a few instances, such as in the Mennonite and Amish communities, religion is the basis for a common way of life that determines where children are reared and their lifestyle. (See also Religious Beliefs, p. 71.)

Schools

Next to the family, schools exert the major force in providing continuity between generations by conveying a vast amount of culture from the older members to the young. In this way children are prepared to carry out the traditional social roles they are expected to assume as adults in society.

School rules and regulations regarding attendance, authority relationships, and the system of sanctions and rewards based on achievement transmit to the child the behavioral expectations of the adult world of employment and relationships. School is often the only institution in which children systematically learn about the negative consequences of behaviors that deviate from social expectations. Teachers are expected to stimulate and guide the intellectual development of children and their sense of esthetics and to foster their capacity for creative problem solving. Through education, individuals in the lower classes are offered the opportunity for further education and the capacity to move up in the social strata.

Traditionally, the socialization process of school has begun when the child enters kindergarten or first grade. Today, with more than 60% of mothers of preschool children working outside the home, this socialization process begins much earlier for a significant number of children in a variety of childcare settings.

Children of some cultural groups fare less well in school. They come from under-represented groups including African-American, Mexican-American, Puerto Rican, and Native American children (Trawick-Smith, 2000). These cultural variations can be attributed to high rates of poverty as well as different cognitive styles, ineffective schools, and parent viewing of schools as oppressive to cultural and traditional values (Trawick-Smith, 2000).

Communities

Surveys of more than 1 million young persons in the United States grades 6 through 12 have shown that those who experience a higher number of specific assets in their lives are more likely to make healthy choices and avoid high-risk behaviors. These assets offer a framework for positive child and adolescent development. The child's or adolescent's community is made up of the family, school, neighborhood, youth organization, and other members. They all contribute to the young person's experience within any culture (Search Institute, 2003).

Four categories of external assets that youth receive from the community include:

- **Support**—Young people need to feel support, care, and love from their families, neighbors, and others. They also need organizations and institutions that offer positive, supportive environments.
- **Empowerment**—Young people need to feel valued by their community and be able to contribute to others. They need to feel safe and secure.
- **Boundaries and expectations**—Young people need to know what is expected of them and what actions and behaviors are within the community boundaries and what are outside of them.
- **Constructive use of time**—Young people need opportunities for growth through constructive, enriching opportunities and quality time at home.

Internal assets must also be nurtured in the communities young members. These internal qualities guide choices and create a sense of centeredness, purpose, and focus. The four categories of internal assets include:

- **Commitment to learning**—Young people need to development a commitment to education and life-long learning
- **Positive values**—Youth need to have a strong sense of values that direct their choices.
- **Social competencies**—Young people need competencies that help them make positive choices and build relationships.
- **Positive identity**—Young people need a sense of their own power, purpose, worth, and promise (Search Institute, 2003).

Peer Cultures

Peer groups also have an impact on the socialization of children (Fig. 4-3). Peer relationships become increasingly important and influential as children proceed through school. In school, children have what can be regarded as a culture of their own. It is most apparent in the school and in the unsupervised play group. The play group presents this culture in a much purer form than does the school, which is partly produced by adults.

During their lives children are exposed to value systems such as those of the family, ethnic group, and social class. In

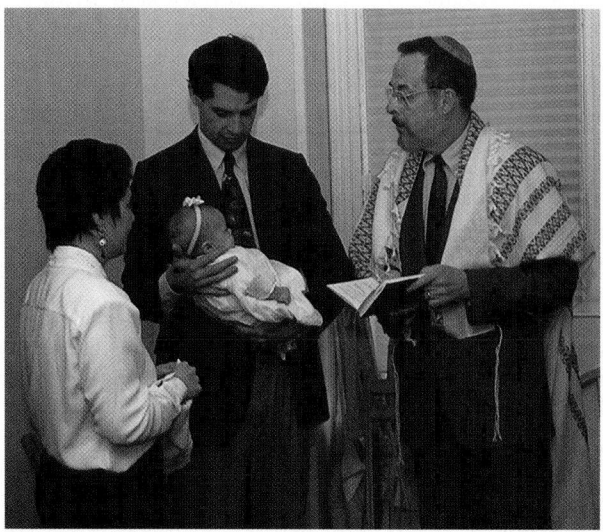

FIG. 4-2 ■ Soon after an infant is born, many families have special religious ceremonies.

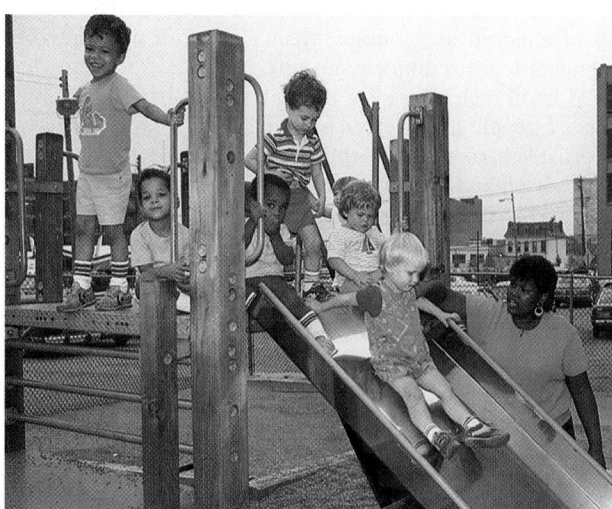

FIG. 4-3 ■ Children from a variety of cultural and ethnic backgrounds begin to socialize in the childcare setting.

peer-group interaction they are confronted with a variety of these sets of values. The values imposed by the peer group are especially compelling because children must accept and conform to them to be accepted as members of the group. When the peer values are not too different from those of family and teachers, the mild conflict created by these small differences serves to separate children from the adults in their lives and to strengthen the feeling of belonging to the peer group.

The kind of socialization provided by the peer group depends on the special subculture that develops from the background, interests, and capabilities of its members. Some groups support school achievement, others focus on athletic prowess, and still others are decidedly antithetic to educative goals. Scholastic achievement is strongly related to the value system of the peer groups. Many conflicts between teachers and students and between parents and students can be attributed to fear of rejection by peers. A conflict between what is expected from parents regarding academic achievement and what is expected from the peer culture is especially pronounced in high school.

Although it has neither the traditional authority of the parents nor the legal authority of the schools for teaching information, the peer group manages to convey a substantial amount of information to its members, especially about taboo subjects such as sex and drugs. Through peer relationships, children learn ways to deal with dominance and hostility and to relate with persons in positions of leadership and authority. The peer subculture relieves boredom and provides recognition that individual members do not receive from teachers and other authority figures.

The peer-group culture has secrets, mores, and codes of ethics with which they promote feelings of group solidarity and detachment from adults. Traditions and folkways are transferred from "generation to generation" of school children and have a great influence over the behavior of all group members. There are age-related games and other activities, and as children move from one level to the next, folkways of the younger group are discarded as those of the older group are adopted. For example, a school-age child rides a bicycle to school; the high school student prefers to drive a car. As they advance, children are forward oriented only—they look forward with anticipation but look backward with contempt.

Biculture

Some children are exposed to the values, role relationships, and lifestyles of two or more cultures. The virtual "straddling" of two cultures is referred to as *biculturation* and involves the ability to efficiently bridge the gap between an individual's culture of origin and the dominant culture (Rogers, 1995). This may occur because the child's parents are from two or more different cultures. In Hawaii, for example, it is common for children to be of four or more cultures. Other children straddle cultures as members of a minority culture within the dominant culture. This biculture is sometimes observed in the play group but usually is not a significant factor until children enter school. Then they must unlearn some of the established practices of one culture in order to become socialized in the other, especially in role relationships. For example, children from Hispanic and Oriental cultures are taught to look away when scolded; in

U.S. schools, the teacher expects direct eye contact—"Look at me when I speak to you." Children learn new roles and social behavior more rapidly than their adult counterparts.

This biculture is particularly marked in language differences. The bilingual child is said to be at a disadvantage in school situations of the dominant culture, in which there is controversy over bilingual education. Those supporting bilingual education adhere to the principle that children will understand more readily and perform more realistically (especially in testing situations) if learning is directed in their own language; others contend that children living in a dominant culture should adopt the ways of that culture, including language. There is less conflict for children when their language and culture are supported by the school, even if the dominant language is used.

THE CHILD AND FAMILY IN NORTH AMERICA

America's orientation toward homogenization—"the great melting pot"—is changing. Increased awareness of the growing proportion of ethnic minorities that make up the U.S. population, coupled with a new positive value and emphasis being placed on ethnic diversity, has resulted in a renewed interest in cultural variation (Patterson and Blum, 1993).

The frontier background of the North American culture has contributed to the overall orientation to life and childrearing. There has always been a basic optimistic view of the world, a belief that things can be better and that the children can and will be better off than the parents. This hopeful outlook and a general future orientation, together with the possibility of upward social mobility, have created a pervasive overall attitude of optimism. Increasing development of self-confidence and autonomy in children is fostered and encouraged. Children in North America are generally permitted a greater degree of freedom than in more tradition-oriented cultures, where individuals remain in one class for life.

Family life in North America is characterized by increasing geographic and economic mobility. There is less reliance on tradition, families are fragmented, and there is limited opportunity to transmit and acquire the traditional and accepted customs of a culture. Consequently, young adults rely to a greater extent on the professed experts, peers, and the mass media for acquisition of acceptable patterns of behavior, including childrearing practices. Conflicting information can be a source of confusion and frustration as parents attempt to determine the comparatively stable, essential components of the culture and transmit these to their children.

Children in North America grow up with a number of adults who differ from one another but who all provide input as role models, teachers, and standards for behavior. Most children live in some form of nuclear family located in sharply differentiated neighborhoods determined by income and ethnic status within a highly technical, largely urban society. Class differences in childrearing persist, but they are becoming less divergent as a result of the increased homogeneity of the culture.

Minority-Group Membership

The United States has more racial, ethnic, and religious minority groups than any other country as a result of high immigration rates and high birth rates among these groups.

Ethnic minority groups are becoming increasingly important because it is anticipated that these groups will produce children at a faster rate than will the majority Caucasian population. Consequently, the minority population is increasing, whereas the majority Caucasian population is decreasing. The term *cultural diversity* refers to the differences that exist among these various groups of people (Habayeb, 1995; Talabere, 1996).

In the Census 2000, there are more than 280 million people in the United States, with 6.8 million reporting more than two races. African Americans alone or in combination with another race comprise more than 35 million, and Hispanic or Latinos of any race comprise more than 35 million. The Hispanic population increased 58%, or 13 million people, from 1990 to 2000 (US Census Bureau, 2000). (See Cultural Awareness Box.)

> **! NURSING ALERT**
>
> Because American cultures and subcultures can be so diverse, it is essential that nurses be aware of and knowledgeable about the predominant groups in their work community and apply the knowledge in their practice.

> **! NURSING ALERT**
>
> Generalizations made about an ethnic group may not apply to certain groups and individuals.

When minority groups emigrate to another country, a certain degree of cultural/ethnic blending occurs through the involuntary process of *acculturation,* those gradual changes produced in a culture by the influence of another culture that cause one or both cultures to be more similar to the other. This process in involuntary in nature; the minority group member is forced to learn the new culture to survive (Spector, 2000). However, the changes occur to various degrees in different families and groups. Many groups continue to identify with their traditional heritage while adapting to the ill-defined concept of the "American way." Acculturation may be referred to as *assimilation,* which is the process of developing a new cultural identity (Spector, 2000).

Evidence indicates that changes in attitudes are slowly taking place in some groups and in some places. *Cultural pluralism* supports the rights of group differences and promotes a mutual respect for the existence of cultural differences (Culley, 1996; Rogers, 1995). With growing awareness, interest, and understanding by increasing numbers of the majority group, which have accompanied the recent emergence of racial and ethnic pride, minority-group children are becoming more secure and confident in their racial or ethnic identity. Individuals vary in their reactions to membership in a minority group, and much of this variation can be attributed to familial factors. As with all children, the most important influences on development of a positive self-image are warm, understanding parents who take an active interest in fostering their children's growth. Parents who accept their children and react positively and constructively rather than in a negative and self-defeating manner will help their children develop feelings of self-worth, self-esteem, and self-acceptance. The more adequate children feel, the more positive will be their attitudes toward both majority and minority children, the greater will be their

CULTURAL AWARENESS

Overview of Race and Hispanic Origin in Census 2000

The federal government defines race and Hispanic origin as two separate and distinct concepts. In the 2000 US Census, responders were first asked if they are of Spanish/Hispanic/Latino origin. The second question asked respondents to report the race or races they considered themselves to be. The definitions of racial groups included the following:

Caucasians are people having "origins in any of the original peoples of Europe, the Middle East, or North Africa."

African Americans are referred to as *blacks* and defined as "any persons whose lineage included ancestors who originated from any of the black racial groups of Africa."

An *Asian* or *Pacific Islander* is any person with "origins in any of the original peoples of the Far East, Southeast Asia, the Indian subcontinent."

Native Hawaiians and *Other Pacific Islanders* are "people having origins in any of the original peoples of Hawaii, Guam, Samoa, or other Pacific Islands."

Native Americans are referred to as *American Indians,* and *Alaska Natives* are defined as "persons having origins in the original peoples of North America, and who maintain cultural identification through tribal affiliations or community attachment."

(US Census Bureau, 2000)

ability to withstand prejudice and intolerance, and the less will be their need for counteraggressive behavior.

CULTURAL SHOCK AND CULTURAL COMPETENCE

The term *cultural shock* describes the "feelings of helplessness and discomfort and a state of disorientation experienced by an outsider attempting to comprehend or effectively adapt to a different cultural group because of differences in cultural practices, values, and beliefs" (Leininger, 1978). This state occurs with both clients and health care providers who move from one cultural setting to another. It can happen to persons who emigrate to a new country (such as Asian refugees) or to those from a subcultural group who must adjust to the ways of an unfamiliar subgroup (such as children entering the school subculture or consumers who enter the hospital subculture). Cultural shock is characterized by the inability to respond to or function in a new or strange situation (see Critical Thinking Exercise).

Numerous factors influence reactions to a new environment. Language barriers, including dialects and jargon (such as medical language) specific to a subcultural group, inhibit effective communication. Habits and customs (such as different role behaviors or etiquette) and differences in attitudes and beliefs are puzzling to the stranger in the new environment. The outsider experiences an intense sense of isolation and feelings of loneliness and nonrelatedness.

Nurses are challenged to overcome cultural shock and develop the dynamics of *cultural sensitivity,* an awareness of cultural similarities and differences. In doing so, the nurse is helped to practice *culturally competent* care. This requires changing the way people think about, understand, and interact within the world around them. Cultural com-

⁇ CRITICAL THINKING EXERCISE ⁇

Reducing Cultural Shock

A woman from the Middle East is visiting her child who is hospitalized for a serious illness. Her husband left for home a short time ago to wash and change clothes. She speaks little English. You need to obtain consent from her for an emergency procedure. She is hesitant and refuses to sign the consent form. What should you do?

QUESTIONS

1. Evidence—are there sufficient data to draw any conclusions about this woman's actions?
2. Assumptions—describe any underlying assumptions about each of the following:
   a. Arab culture
   b. Need for interpreter
   c. Approval for emergency procedures
   d. Documentation of the need for the emergency procedure
3. What priorities for nursing care should be established at this time?
4. Does the evidence support your nursing intervention(s)?
5. What alternative perspectives might you have?

ANSWERS

1. Yes. An understanding of the Arab culture provides insight into the woman's hesitancy to make decisions in her husband's absence.
2. a. Typically in the Arab culture men make the decisions and women are expected to support these decisions.
   b. The need for an interpreter is evident to make sure the mother understands the seriousness of the situation.
   c. Knowledge of the procedures for obtaining approval for emergency procedures without informed consent will facilitate the best care for the child.
   d. Appropriate documentation of how approval was obtained without parent consent is essential.
3. The first priority is to make sure the child is receiving the best care possible and that the necessary procedure is performed as soon as possible. The next priority is to make sure the mother understands the emergency of the situation by using an interpreter.
4. The health status of the child is most important at this time.
5. Attempts should continue to try to reach the father by phone, and continued support of the mother during this stressful time is important.

petence is an ongoing process that is interactive and without end (Dunn, 2002). Six elements included in the process of developing cultural competence are:

- Working on changing one's world view through examining one's own values and behaviors and working to reject racism and institutions that support it.
- Becoming familiar with core cultural issues by recognizing these issues and exploring them with clients.
- Becoming knowledgeable about the cultural groups we work with while learning about each individual client's unique history.
- Becoming familiar with core cultural issues related to health and illness and communicating in a way that encourages clients to explain what an illness means to them.
- Developing a relationship of trust with your client and creating a welcoming atmosphere in the health care setting.
- Negotiating for mutually acceptable and understandable interventions of care (Dunn, 2002).

✏ NURSING ALERT

Because American cultures and subcultures can be so diverse, it is essential that nurses be aware of and knowledgeable about the predominant groups in their work community and apply the knowledge in their practice.

CULTURAL/RELIGIOUS INFLUENCES ON HEALTH CARE

SUSCEPTIBILITY TO HEALTH PROBLEMS

Some groups of people are more susceptible than others to certain illnesses. An innate susceptibility is acquired through generations of evolutionary changes that take place within constrained or segregated populations. The proximity to disease, environmental factors, and the general physical status are significant factors associated with health problems.

Hereditary Factors

Historically, the increased health risks associated with ethnicity have been explained in terms of genetic differences or related factors such as socioeconomic status (Scribner, 1996). The genetic constitution of individuals as groups influences the degree to which they are susceptible to a specific disorder. It may be a result of an inherent lack of resistance to a disease organism, a trait that is an advantage in one environment but places the possessor at a disadvantage in another, or it may be a consequence of intermarriage within a relatively narrow range of geographic, ethnic, or religious restrictions.

A classic example of a geographic constraint is the common communicable disease rubeola (measles). The rubeola virus, or the populations that were continually exposed to it, became altered in such a way that the disease was considered to be a universal disease of childhood from which the majority of children suffered without ill effects. When other populations (e.g., the inhabitants of the Hawaiian Islands) were exposed to the virus by explorers and missionaries, they experienced a violent response that resulted in high mortality.

A number of conditions show ethnic or racial differences. For example, Tay-Sachs disease, characterized by early neurologic deterioration and mental retardation, affects primarily Ashkenazi Jewish families, particularly those of Northeastern European origin, whereas Sephardic Jewish families appear to be no more at risk for the disease than are other populations. The incidence of cystic fibrosis is highest in Caucasians and almost nonexistent in Asians, and the rare affected African Americans are usually in areas where there is apt to be mixed ancestry. A classic disorder of African Americans is sickle cell disease (see Chapter 26); however, the incidence of cardiovascular disease, pneumonia, and diabetes is also high among African Americans. Native Americans are at risk for type 2 diabetes and lactose intolerance. Racial and ethnic differences are further considered in relation to diseases and defects as they are discussed throughout the book.

Common food items and drugs may cause health problems in certain ethnic groups. For example, persons of Mediterranean, African, Near Eastern, and Asian origin frequently have glucose-6-phosphate dehydrogenase deficiency. They may develop acute hemolytic anemia after they ingest fava (horse or broad) beans or certain drugs such as aspirin preparations, sulfonamides, or primaquine. Other groups, especially southern Europeans, Jews, Arabs, African Americans, Asians, and Native Americans, have a deficiency of lactase, the enzyme needed to metabolize lactose. Ingestion of lactose can cause abdominal distention, flatus, and diarrhea. Unknowing but well-meaning health workers may be responsible for these symptoms in their clients when they prescribe foods or food supplements containing lactose as sources of nutrients.

Physical Characteristics.   Among racial groups there are observable differences in physical appearance. The most obvious are skin and hair coloring and texture. Skin color is determined by the amount of melanin pigment present in the skin. Persons from countries located near the equator have darkly pigmented skin, which serves to protect the skin from the year-round exposure to the sun's rays; persons from the northern countries have very light skin, which provides for maximum exposure to the sun's rays (necessary for vitamin D metabolism) during the short daylight hours. There can be wide variations in skin color between these two extremes in terms of geographic origin or from intermixing of dark and light skin color. As a consequence of the dark pigmentation, the detection of skin color changes (e.g., vasomotor alterations, cyanosis, jaundice) can be difficult and requires modification of assessment techniques (see Table 7-8).

Variations in the newborn are often related to racial or ethnic origin. For example, newborn infants of Asian and African-American parents are smaller than infants of Caucasian parentage, and bluish pigmented areas (mongolian spots) on the sacral region are a common observation in Asian, African-American, Native American, and Mexican-American infants. It is important that health care providers be familiar with these birthmarks. They should be documented at newborn exams and subsequent visits so they are not suddenly interpreted as bruises (Garwick and Auger, 2000).

Evaluation of stature and body build reveals some racial tendencies. Children from Asian countries are commonly smaller, falling below the 10th percentile on weight and height charts used for children in the United States (Baze, 1991). This difference in stature can lead to misinterpretation of health status and capabilities. A small child may appear very intelligent for body size but be of average mental ability for age.

Socioeconomic Factors

The most overwhelming adverse influence on health is socioeconomic status. A higher percentage of lower-class individuals are suffering from some health problem at any one time than are those in any other group. The sum of all aspects of their situation contributes to and compounds health problems; this includes crowded living conditions and poor sanitation, which facilitate transfer of disease (e.g., tuberculosis). There is a higher incidence of lead poisoning in children from families from the lower socioeconomic classes because there is more ready access to lead in the environment, especially lead-based paint in old housing (Centers for Disease Control and Prevention, 1997).

In the lower classes children are less likely to be immunized against preventable diseases than are children in the upper and middle classes. Lack of funds or inaccessibility to health services inhibits treatment for any but severe illness or injury. Sometimes health care is inadequate because of lack of information. In some areas a disorder is so commonplace that it is looked on as unavoidable; it is not recognized as something that requires (or is amenable to) treatment. The parents may not have information regarding causes, treatment, outcome of the illness, or preventive measures. The nurse can use the limited opportunities when the family does come into contact with the health care system to inquire about immunizations, screen for vision problems, provide nutritional information, and offer additional prevention and health promotion resources.

Poverty.   A high correlation between poverty and the prevalence of illness has long been observed. Impoverished families suffer from poor nutrition; without medical insurance, they have little if any preventive health care, inadequate health maintenance, and very limited access to medical treatment. One of the most significant health problems related to poverty is a high infant mortality rate. Although the infant mortality rate in the United States is at an all-time low, our nation's infant survival rate remains lower than that of most industrialized nations (Annie E. Casey Foundation, 2003). Day-to-day needs of food, clothing, and lodging take precedence over health care as long as the ailing person feels able to perform activities of daily living.

Poor families are denied access to many health institutions for emergency or other hospital care. Frequently they must travel long distances to service centers that are willing to assume their care. In an emergency they must find money for taxi fare, borrow an automobile, or seek other means of transportation. They must find care for dependents, such as other infants and small children, or have them accompany them when taking the ill child for care. Families tend to delay preventive care indefinitely unless health services are relatively accessible. They are more likely to consult folk practitioners or other persons within their community.

Poor nutrition accounts for many health problems in the lower classes. Lack of funds and knowledge results in a diet that may be seriously lacking in essential food substances, especially protein, vitamins, and iron. This inadequate diet often leads to nutritional deficiency disorders and growth retardation in children. In many the total intake is insufficient to support normal growth. Unstructured eating patterns and irregularly scheduled mealtimes can also contribute to erratic food intake and a proportionately larger consumption of nonnourishing snacks, which can result in excessive weight gain.

Because of deficient preventive care, dental problems are more prevalent. Lack of standard immunizations, together with reduced resistance from poor nutrition, renders the exposed children in poor segments of the population vulnerable to communicable diseases. Poor sanitation and crowded living conditions also contribute to the higher incidence and perpetuation of illness. In general, poor people become ill more frequently and remain ill for longer periods of time than do persons in the general population.

Homelessness.   Research indicates that families are the fastest-growing subgroup of the homeless population. Rural homeless families have been found to be similar to other homeless families in that the majority are headed by women. Unfortunately, rural families are less likely to escape from poverty (Wagner, Menke, and Ciccone, 1995).

Homeless children experience all of the health problems associated with poverty, as well as other types of disorders. Their families have fewer resources with which to control the environment or to promote rehabilitation and prevent disease. Preventive health care, especially immunization and dental care, is seriously lacking. Impaired vision is common among homeless children, perhaps reflecting missed opportunities for vision screening. Homeless children have been found to experience poorer health status and more emergency department visits than low-income housed children (Weinreb and others, 1998).

Children who are homeless have double the health problems, developmental delays, hunger, depression, and behavioral problems (Lewit and Baker, 1996). High rates of iron deficiency among homeless children have also been reported (Fierman and others, 1993; Page, Ainsworth, and Pett, 1993). Lack of adequate food is only part of the problem; homeless families may believe they are meeting nutritional needs when actually the reverse is true. They may also lack knowledge about how to safely prepare and store food.

Estimates of the number of homeless adolescents in the United States range from 500,000 to 2 million (Ensign and Santelli, 1998). Studies indicate that homeless adolescents have poor health compared with the general youth population. Homeless youth have high rates of sexually transmitted diseases, including human immunodeficiency virus (HIV) infection, pregnancy, depression, and injuries (Ensign and Santelli, 1998).

Migrant Families.   Migrants generally suffer more illness, both acute and chronic, than the general population. They are subject to unhealthy environments, poverty, and insufficient medical care; their health-seeking behavior in general is an illness- or injury-oriented recourse to medical care. Affected persons will postpone seeking care for themselves or their children until physical pain or suffering is almost unbearable. The health problems of migrant children appear to be dental caries, upper respiratory tract infections, tuberculosis, otitis media, scabies and lice, intestinal parasites, pesticide exposure, injuries, teenage pregnancy, and growth and development delay.

Tuberculosis rates among migrant families are high. A risk factor for the increased incidence of tuberculosis in children has been the migration of families from high-risk prevalence areas of tuberculosis, such as Asia, Africa, and Latin America (Castiglia, 1997). Also, farm workers are approximately six times more likely to develop the disease than the general population of employed adults. Drug-resistant tuberculosis is an important consideration among this population; it requires altered treatment regimens, and higher rates of resistance have been found in the ethnic and social groups constituting much of the migrant farm workforce (MMWR, 1992).

When medical care is provided to migrant families, follow-up care is usually impossible because of their transient lifestyle. Compliance with medical therapies is primarily related to accessibility and availability. For example, medications provided by health workers are more likely to be taken than those that must be obtained at a pharmacy. In addition, medications are often discontinued following self-perceived recovery.

CUSTOMS AND FOLKWAYS

Nurses must be aware of the need to consider cultural differences in clients when providing health care. An understanding of the various beliefs regarding the causation of illness and disease, as well as traditional health practices, is essential to successful intervention. The more nurses know about the values, beliefs, and customs of other ethnic groups, the better able they are to meet the needs of these families and to gain their cooperation and compliance.

NURSING TIP

Develop a cultural reference manual that includes a brief description of the culture; views on health, illness, diet, and other matters; and how to access interpreters, ethnic community services, or other sources for quick reference (Kuensting and Sanders, 1995).

Cultural Relativity

Although clinical characteristics of a disease or condition are essentially the same across cultures, how a child or family interprets or experiences it varies. Culture as an influence is one obvious explanation for variance. *Cultural relativity* is the concept that any behavior must be judged first in relation to the context of the culture in which it occurs. Nurses must first relate to the family's perceptions and interpretations of experiences from the family's background and cultural belief system before they can effectively intervene.

Some cultures, for example, may view a chronic illness or disability as affecting only particular aspects of a child's life, and the child as a whole is viewed as normal. In contrast, Chinese families frequently describe the illness as having global effects on many aspects of the child's present and future life (Martinson, Armstrong, and Qiao, 1997). These contrasting views may result in a difference in goals and expectations that parents have for their children.

In some cultures the child's gender may influence a family's perception of the implications of an illness or disability. For example, in the Arabic and Asian cultures the male child is held in higher esteem than the female child. This also holds true for some families of Jewish, Italian, Greek, and Indian origin. The male child may receive better health care and more food, because this is the child who will take care of his parents in their old age.

Defining disease or signs and symptoms of illness is also influenced by culture. Some cultures, for example, perceive diarrhea as a cleansing of the body that is essential for health maintenance and illness prevention or cure. Furthermore, signs or symptoms resulting from diarrhea and ensuing dehydration, such as malaise, fever, anorexia, and irritability, may be viewed as separate illness entities.

Nurses can often recognize a family's health-related cultural perceptions and interpretations through discussion and observation. Implications of these perceptions should be explored and considered when planning effective culturally appropriate interventions.

Relationships with Health Care Providers

The manner of relating with health care providers differs considerably among cultural groups. One area of conflict to some nurses is the attitude toward time and waiting that is part of some cultures. For example, African Americans are very flexible in their time orientation; an African-American family may be late for or miss appointments because other issues take precedence over the appointment, and the family may not communicate this to the health agency. Hispanics, too, have a very relaxed view of time. Whereas the dominant culture in the United States says that "time flies," the Hispanic says, "time walks." The Japanese, on the other hand, consider time to be valuable and to be used wisely. They tend to be punctual for medical appointments and persistent in following prescribed regimens. A Vietnamese family will subordinate time to values considered to be more significant, such as propriety. They may be late for an appointment because of an overextended visit by a friend in their home. In general, Asian Americans view the American focus on time as offensive. They spend hours getting to know people and view predetermined, abrupt endings as rude. Introductory small talk is considered good manners.

In many cultural groups the mother assumes the responsibility for health care; in others, both parents are involved equally in relationships with health workers. A somewhat different approach is apparent in some of the Asian cultures. For example, the father in Vietnamese families, as unquestioned head of the family, is traditionally the family member who interacts with persons, including health care providers, outside the family unit (Fig. 4-4).

In the Hispanic family the father, as head of the house, makes decisions regarding illness and treatment of family members, but the grandmother in the extended family is consulted regarding child care. Usually the family confers with other members before reaching a decision regarding treatment or hospitalization of a child. The Arab family also relies on others to give advice and guidance in a time of crisis. A Japanese father may appear to be passive and uninvolved but actually is involved according to his own cultural standards.

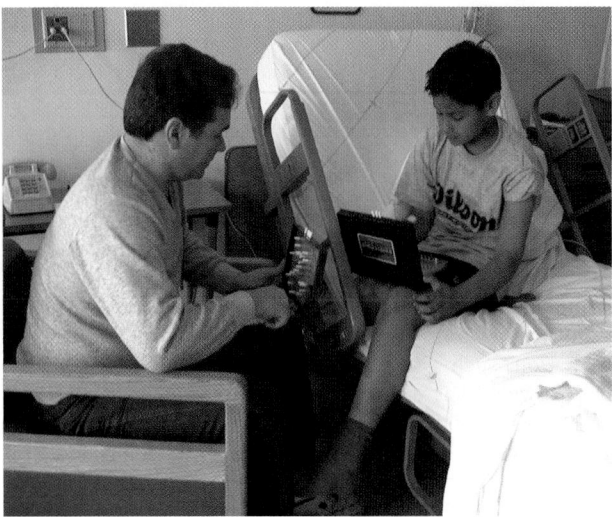

FIG. 4-4 ■ A father with his hospitalized child.

NURSING ALERT

In working with families, it is essential for nurses to identify key members. Failure to include these significant individuals in teaching can seriously hinder adherence to the plan of care.

Nurses should make themselves aware of any specific attitudes regarding the manner of approach to a child in a given culture. Navajo Indians do not like a stranger near their infants. It is feared that the stranger may "witch" the child and cause him or her harm. On the other hand, if a stranger, particularly a woman, lavishes attention on a Latino infant but fails to touch the child, the child will develop symptoms of the "evil eye" (see p. 69). Vietnamese and Korean families may become upset if a newborn is admired at length for fear that the evil spirits will overhear and desire the infant.

Some ethnic groups, such as the Amish, consider a child's admission to the hospital a family affair, with all members gathering to support and console the child and parents. In others, such as the Samoan family, the family is willing to relinquish the care of the child to the hospital authority without interference. Their visits with the child are short, although intense, but this behavior may be misinterpreted by the hospital staff as disinterest or abandonment.

Nurses who are members of a majority culture may encounter tension and distrust in a child from a minority culture as a result of the child's learned perception or relationships with other persons in the majority group. Based on these perceptions, minority children often suspect that nurses may have hostile feelings toward them and fear ill treatment. When such children are hospitalized, this feeling compounds the feelings of loneliness, helplessness, and retribution that accompany fearful happenings and separation from families. The reverse situation may be encountered by a nurse from a minority culture attempting to meet the needs of a child who has been conditioned to view the nurse's cultural or ethnic group as inferior.

Communication. Communication may be a source of distress and misunderstanding between persons from different ethnic groups, especially if the languages are different. Also, prejudice has been found to be one of the biggest barriers to cross cultural communication (Taylor, 1998). The **Office of Minority Health** of the **US Department of Health and Human Services** has established national standards on culturally and linguistically appropriate services in health care. Health care organizations must ensure the competence of language assistance provided to persons with limited English proficiency (LEP) by interpreters and bilingual staff. Family and friends should not be used for interpretation services except on request by the client (Shaw-Taylor, 2002).

Some persons with poor or limited language comprehension may simply smile and nod in agreement if they do not understand the questions or directives. It is vital that the family fully understand all implications of a child's care and management before they sign permits for special procedures or assume responsibility for the child's care. It is not uncommon for a Vietnamese or a Japanese family to indicate "yes" when in fact they mean "no" in order to avoid social disharmony. They tend to use indirectness rather than confrontation and may become evasive when direct questioning makes them feel uncomfortable.

- Have a series of audio and audiovisual recordings in several languages designed to greet and familiarize the family with the hospital.
- In the event that an interpreter is not available, develop a multilingual booklet containing illustrations of commonly used phrases and hospital routines.
- Have legal consent forms and explanations of common diagnostic tests available in several languages.
- Keep cards with common greetings, phrases, and names of body parts in the family's language with the patient's chart, (e.g., *miseries* [pain] and *locked bowels* [constipation] in African Americans and *caida de la mollera* [fallen fontanel from dehydration], *susto* [fright], *dolor, duele,* or *lele* [pain], and *la diarrhea* [diarrhea] in Hispanics).

Nonverbal communication is a practiced art in many Native American tribes, and the members are highly sensitive to body language. They emphasize periods of silence to formulate thoughts in preparation for speech and often remain silent after listening to statements by others to properly assimilate what has been said. Interruption, interjection, or haste to arrive at abrupt conclusions is perceived as immature behavior.

The level of comfort with body space or distance from others varies among cultures. For example, Hispanics tend to get closer, and Asians prefer a greater distance.

Eye contact is viewed differently in cultures. Although Anglos are advised to look people straight in the eye, it is not uncommon for persons in some ethnic groups to avoid eye contact and become uncomfortable when conversing with health workers. A Vietnamese patient may not look directly into the nurse's eyes as a sign of respect. Some Native Americans will make eye contact during the initial greeting, but continued, unwavering eye contact is considered insulting and disrespectful. Asians may consider eye contact a sign of hostility or impoliteness.

Gestures also may have different meanings. For example, some Asians consider finger or foot pointing disrespectful. Native Americans consider vigorous handshaking a sign of aggression, whereas to Anglos the gesture is a sign of good will.

Families may be reluctant to question or otherwise initiate contact with health professionals. In the Asian cultures, for example, it is considered a sign of disrespect to question those who are viewed as persons of authority. A Japanese family may wait silently rather than ask or question. They believe that the health professionals know best and will meet their needs without being asked. It is also important to avoid criticism. Criticism can cause Asians to "lose face," to feel ashamed, which is highly undesirable.

Language has been considered the biggest barrier to the use of health care services by many families, especially Southeast Asians (Mattson, 1995). Often families may have poor language comprehension, so it is necessary to speak slowly and carefully, not loudly, when conversing with them. Many persons are able to read and write English better than they can speak or understand it. Also, the dominant language usually takes over in anxiety-provoking situations, even in those who are able to communicate satisfactorily under ordinary circumstances.

Terms of address and use of first and last names vary among cultures and can create confusion. For example, in Asian cultures the family name is given first in respect for the family and the given name follows. Therefore all siblings in a family have the same first name. Ethiopians have a very complex system whereby women retain their last names after marriage and the paternal grandfather's name becomes the child's last name.

The expression of emotion also varies ethnically. In some cultures (e.g., Hispanic or Jewish) emotions are expressed openly and members are accustomed to sharing their sorrows and joys with family and friends. Conversely, Nordic and Asian groups are more restrained.

Health care providers generally ask questions and use handouts, booklets, and—particularly with children—dolls and pictures as communication aids. This is uncommon in some cultures. For example, Native American healers ask few questions and do not use forms. In some cultures it is inappropriate or considered taboo to look at the inside of the body, even in pictures, or to use dolls or puppets (Malach and Segel, 1990). Nurses need to consider both verbal and nonverbal communication techniques to interact effectively with children and their families from different cultures (see Guidelines box).

Food Customs

Food customs and symbolism are an integral part of various cultural, ethnic, and religious groups. Although in a large country such as the United States most persons have adopted the eclectic food habits that have evolved over countless generations, many ethnic and geographic food traditions and preferences are retained. Special holidays, ceremonies, and life experiences such as births, birthdays, weddings, and death are often marked by special food items or feasts. In many cultures specific food practices are followed during pregnancy in the belief that certain foods damage the developing fetus.

The distinctive food customs of ethnic groups are a product of their native environment, determined by availability. Fish is a staple food of persons living near the ocean, such as people from Japan, Polynesia, southern Europe, and Scandinavia. Fruit and vegetable preferences are directly related to the climate in which they grow naturally or can be cultivated. The types of grain that are ethnically associated are also those that grow best in the native lands. For example, wheat and basmati rice are the staple grains of South Asians, and roti (unleavened bread) is the most commonly eaten bread in the home (Sekhon, 1996). The diet of the Eskimo is predominantly fish and meat, depending on which is the most easily procured in the area. Even in the continental United States there are regional favorites, such as rice, hominy grits, and okra in the Southern states. In some cultures food is highly spiced; in others, foods tend to be bland. Table 4-1 lists the food items common to most cultures and can be used to select foods that most children know and like.

There are a number of restrictions related to food items. Some have a physiologic origin, such as lack of dairy foods in the diets of some persons of African or Asian ancestry in whom a hereditary lactase deficiency prevents digestion of foods containing lactose. Others have religious restrictions, such as kosher foods and food preparation of the Orthodox Jewish faith and the vegetarian diet of Seventh-Day Adventists (see Vegetarian Diets, Chapter 11).

Children in a strange environment, such as the hospital, feel much more comfortable when they are served familiar foods (Fig. 4-5). Hospital food often tastes strange and

bland. The family may be concerned that their child is not receiving foods appropriate to their culture and beliefs. Where possible, it is advisable to provide children's ethnic foods or allow families to bring favorite foods. Concern for differences in food habits and patterns projects an attitude of respect for the family's ethnic or religious heritage.

HEALTH BELIEFS AND PRACTICES
Health Beliefs

Beliefs related to the cause of illness and the maintenance of health are an integral part of the cultural heritage of families. Often inseparable from religious beliefs, they influence the way that families cope with health problems and the way that they respond to health care providers. Predominant among most cultures are beliefs related to natural forces, supernatural forces, and imbalance between forces.

Natural Forces. The most common natural forces held responsible for ill health if the body is not adequately protected include cold air entering the body, impurities in the air, or other natural sources. For example, a Chinese mother may overdress her infant in an effort to keep cold wind from entering the child's body. The Chinese believe that cold weather, rain, and wind are responsible for "cold" conditions.

In the African-American culture, natural phenomena such as phases of the moon, seasons of the year, and planet positions are believed to affect the body and its processes;

GUIDELINES

Culturally Sensitive Interactions

NONVERBAL STRATEGIES

Invite family members to choose where they would like to sit or stand, allowing them to select a comfortable distance.

Observe interactions with others to determine which body gestures (e.g., shaking hands) are acceptable and appropriate. Ask when in doubt.

Avoid appearing rushed.

Be an active listener.

Observe for cues regarding appropriate eye contact.

Learn appropriate use of pauses or interruptions for different cultures.

Ask for clarification if nonverbal meaning is unclear.

VERBAL STRATEGIES

Learn proper terms of address.

Use a positive tone of voice to convey interest.

Speak slowly and carefully, not loudly, when families have poor language comprehension.

Encourage questions.

Learn basic words and sentences of family's language, if possible.

Avoid professional terms.

When asking questions, tell family why the questions are being asked, the way in which the information they provide will be used, and how it might benefit their child.

Repeat important information more than once.

Always give the reason or purpose for a treatment or prescription.

Use information written in family's language.

Offer the services of an interpreter when necessary (see Chapter 6).

Learn from families and representatives of their culture methods of communicating information without creating discomfort.

Address intergenerational needs (e.g., family's need to consult with others).

Be sincere, open, and honest and, when appropriate, share personal experiences, beliefs, and practices to establish rapport and trust.

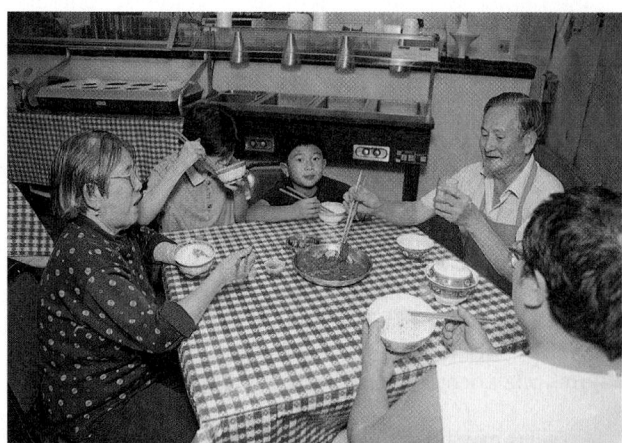

FIG. 4-5 ■ Food customs outside the home can differ significantly from traditional cultural practices.

TABLE 4-1 ■ Foods Common to Most Ethnic Food Patterns

MEAT AND ALTERATIONS	MILK AND MILK PRODUCTS	GRAIN PRODUCTS	VEGETABLES	FRUITS	OTHERS
Pork*	Milk	Rice	Carrots	Apples	Fruit juices
Beef	Ice cream	White bread	Cabbage	Bananas	
Chicken	Yogurt	Noodles, macaroni, spaghetti	Green beans	Oranges	
Eggs		Dry cereal	Greens (especially spinach)	Peaches	
Beans			Sweet potatoes or yams	Pears	
			Tomatoes		

From Endres JB, Rockwell RE: *Food, nutrition, and the young child,* St Louis, 1980, Mosby.
*May be restricted because of religious custom.

therefore, health maintenance is strongly associated with the ability to read "the signs." Most Native Americans consider health to be a state of harmony with nature and the universe.

Supernatural Forces.   High on the list of causes of illness are forces beyond comprehension and logical explanation. Evil influences such as voodoo, witchcraft, or evil spirits are viewed in some cultures as causes of adverse health, especially those illnesses that cannot be explained by other means.

A health belief that is common among people from Latin American, Mediterranean, Near Eastern, some Asian, and some African societies is the concept of the *evil eye* (*malojo* is the Hispanic term) (Leininger, 1995). It is part of the concept of health as a state of balance; illness is a state of imbalance (see Imbalance of Forces). Strength and power are associated with the evil eye. Therefore, as long as an individual's strength and weakness remain in balance, he or she is unlikely to become a victim of the evil eye. Weaknesses are not necessarily physical. For example, an excess of some emotion, such as envy, can create a weakness. Infants and small children, because of immature development of their internal strength-weakness states, are especially vulnerable to the gaze of the evil eye. Consequently, the evil eye concept serves to rationalize an inexplicable onset of illness in children who display such symptoms as restlessness, crying, diarrhea, vomiting, and fever.

Although seldom expressed to health care providers, the belief that a witch can cast a spell over others at the request of someone who wishes them ill is found in Caribbean, African, and Australian aboriginal cultures. The victim is often tortured in effigy by pins driven into a doll at the location where the intended victim is to be hurt. "Voodoo deaths" have occurred from the victim's belief in the curse and may result from dehydration as the victim gives up the will to live and refuses to drink (Chidester, 2001).

Imbalance of Forces.   The concept of balance or equilibrium is widespread throughout the world. One of the most common imbalances supported by the Hispanic, Filipino, Chinese, and Arab cultures is that which exists between "hot" and "cold." This belief is reputedly derived from the Hippocratic theory of humoral pathology, which states that illness is caused by an imbalance of the four humors: phlegm, blood, black bile, and yellow bile. Hot and cold describe certain properties and conditions completely unrelated to temperature. Diseases, areas of the body, foods, and illnesses are classified as either "hot" or "cold." In Chinese health belief the forces are termed *yin (cold)* and *yang (hot).* To maintain health, these hot and cold forces must be kept in balance.

Illness is treated by restoring normal balance through the application of appropriate "hot" or "cold" remedies. A "cold" condition such as a respiratory disease is believed to be caused by exposure to cold weather, rain, or cold wind entering the body; it is treated by administration of "hot" foods, herbs, or drugs. Menstruation is considered to be a "hot" condition; therefore, women are cautioned against ingesting "hot" foods, which might increase menstrual flow or produce cramping. Ingesting too much of either "hot" or "cold" foods can also be interpreted as a cause of illness.

Health care workers who are aware of this belief are better able to understand why some persons refuse to eat certain foods. It is possible to help families devise a diet that contains the necessary balance of basic food groups prescribed by the medical subculture while conforming to the beliefs of the ethnic subculture.

The hot-cold food classification may have adverse effects. For example, newborn infants are often started on evaporated milk formulas. Evaporated milk is considered to be a "hot" food, whereas whole milk is viewed as a "cold" food. Infants tend to develop rashes, which are believed to be caused by "hot" foods; in such cases, parents may decide to switch to whole milk. However, parents fear that it is dangerous to change too rapidly, so they often feed the child some type of neutralizing substance, which may create additional health problems. Such a problem might be averted if the family's preference is determined before discharge from the hospital, with a formula prescribed that is agreeable to both the family and the practitioner.

Health Practices

There are numerous similarities among cultures regarding prevention and treatment of illness. All cultures have some types of home remedies that they apply before seeking help from other persons. Within the ethnic community, folk healers who are endowed with the ability to "cure" maladies are sought for special situations and when home remedies are unsuccessful. There is the *curandero* (male) or *curandera* (female) of the Mexican-American community whose healing powers are believed to be a gift from God. The Asian consults an herbalist, knowledgeable in medicines, or an ethnic practitioner practiced in Asian therapies, including *acupuncture* (insertion of needles), *acupressure* (application of pressure), and *moxibustion* (application of heat). Native Americans consult a variety of healers with specific skills and knowledge. Specialized medicine persons diagnose illness, provide nonsacred treatments (usually by way of massage and herbs), and care for souls. Other specialists perform services or affect cures through spiritual means. Native Hawaiians consult *kahunas* and practice *ho' oponopono* to heal family imbalance or disputes.

The folk healers are very powerful persons in their community. They "speak the language" of the family who seeks help and often combine their rituals and potions with prayer and entreaties to God. They also are able to create an atmosphere conducive to successful management. Furthermore, they exhibit a sincere interest in the family and their problem.

Some folk remedies are compatible with the medical regimen and can be used to reinforce the treatment plan. For example, most of the foods contraindicated for persons with peptic ulcers are "hot" foods and would be avoided because of their belief systems. Also, aspirin (a "hot" medication) is an appropriate therapy for "cold" diseases such as the common cold and arthritis. It is not uncommon to discover that a folk prescription has a scientific basis. However, numerous health remedies or preventive practices have no scientific basis, such as the use of garlic or *asafetida* (a piece of rotten flesh that looks like a dried sponge), which is worn around the neck to prevent contagious diseases. Also, the wearing of copper or silver bracelets to protect the wearer as he or she grows has no scientific basis. Practices that do no harm should be respected.

Overcoming the effect of the evil eye usually requires specialized rituals conducted by the appropriate practitioner. For example, the Chicano *curandera* ascertains that the condition is truly the result of the evil eye by performing an assessment ritual and then, with a confirmed diagnosis, performs a curative ritual. Sometimes the faith in the folk practitioner results in a delay in obtaining needed medical treatment, although the practitioner will usually suggest medical care if his or her ministrations are unsuccessful.

Health practices of different cultures may also present problems in assessment and interpretation. For example, certain cultural practices or remedies can be misdiagnosed as evidence of "child abuse" by uninformed professionals (Box 4-1). It is important to explain why these and other familiar remedies may now be considered harmful. Families need to understand how such practices can place them in jeopardy with child protective services and to explore alternative measures that are more acceptable to the dominant culture (Hayes and Dreher, 1991).

Cultural health remedies that are detrimental to health include eating clay, excessive amounts of salt, or compounds that contain lead or mercury. A careful history can reveal these remedies, but it may require the collaboration of a folk healer to convince a user to stop the practice.

Haitian folk medicine considers it essential to rid the newborn of meconium to ensure neonatal survival. The newborn's first food is a *lok,* or purgative, prepared by cooking a mixture of castor oil, grated nutmeg, sour orange juice, garlic, unrefined sugar, and water. It may be administered several times until the color of the newborn's bowel movement changes from black to yellow. All other oral intake may be restricted until this occurs, which may result in dehydration (DeSantis, 1988).

Faith healing and religious rituals are closely allied with many folk-healing practices. Wearing of amulets, medals, and other religious relics believed by the culture to protect the individual and facilitate healing is a common practice. It is important for health workers to recognize the value of this practice and keep the items where the family has placed them or nearby. It offers comfort and support and rarely impedes medical and nursing care. If an item must be removed during a procedure, it should be replaced, if possible, when the procedure is completed. The reason for its temporary removal is explained to the family, and they are reassured that their wishes will be respected (see Family Focus box).

Nurses can be most effective by operating from a multicultural perspective. Adopting a multicultural perspective means using appropriate aspects of each health cultural orientation under consideration to develop culturally acceptable health care interventions.

BOX 4-1 ■ Cultural Practices Possibly Considered Abusive by the Dominant Culture

Coining—A Vietnamese practice that may produce weltlike lesions on the child's back when a coin, held on edge, is repeatedly rubbed lengthwise on the oiled skin to rid the body of a disease.

Cupping—An Old World practice (also practiced by the Vietnamese) of placing a container (e.g., tumbler, bottle, jar) containing steam against the skin surface to "draw out the poison" or other evil element. When the heated air within the container cools, a vacuum is created that produces a bruiselike blemish on the skin directly beneath the mouth of the container.

Burning—A practice of some Southeast Asian groups whereby small areas of skin are burned to treat enuresis and temper tantrums.

Female genital mutilation (female circumcision)—Removal of or injury to any part of the female genital organ; practiced in Africa, the Middle East, Latin America, India, the Far East, North America, Australia, and Western Europe (Wright, 1996).

Forced kneeling—A child discipline measure of some Caribbean groups in which a child is forced to kneel for a long period of time.

Topical garlic application—A practice of Yemenite Jews in which crushed garlic cloves or garlic–petroleum jelly plaster is applied to the wrists to treat infectious disease; the practice can result in blisters or garlic burns.

Traditional remedies that contain lead—*Greta* and *azarcon* (Mexico; used for digestive problems), *paylooah* (Southeast Asia; used for rash or fever), and *surma* (India; used as a cosmetic to improve eyesight).

FAMILY FOCUS

On Cultural Awareness

I am a pediatric emergency nurse with a high regard for cultural diversities and a respect for healing practices and beliefs. I even made a manual for my emergency department that contains some of the information needed to help us to understand and communicate with subcultures in the urban community that we serve. Although I learned a great deal putting this manual together, it doesn't come close to the lesson I learned with the following experience.

A 15-month-old Bosnian child in status epilepticus was carried in by her parents. They were very frightened and spoke very little English. I learned that the child had received a measles, mumps, and rubella (MMR) immunization the day before. As I proceeded to unwrap her from the blanket she was in, I quickly assessed the ABCs (airway, breathing, and circulation). I noticed that she was very warm (probably a febrile seizure) and that a rag soaked in alcohol was tied around each thigh. Focusing on her potential airway compromise and trying to calm the parents, I proceeded to put an oxygen mask on her, undress her for a full assessment, and remove the alcohol rags. I spoke to the parents all the while in a calm, soothing voice. Once an IV was established and I gave her Ativan, the seizures stopped. So did the communication between her parents and me. I noticed that they would no longer give me eye contact, and the mother would not even speak to me after the seizures stopped. It wasn't until I was returning to the department from admitting her that I realized why they might have stopped communicating with me . . . I had removed the rags! Had I only thought to ask their permission to remove the rags, things may have been different.

Laura L. Kuensting, MSN(R), RN
Cardinal Glennon Children's Hospital
St. Louis, Missouri

Avoid directly criticizing traditional health cultural beliefs and practices as wrong or harmful or implying that biomedical measures are uniformly correct and effective, and the only way to prevent illness or treat sickness. Such criticisms usually result in rejection of both biomedical health care practitioners and their health teaching. When folk practices do not interfere with the welfare of the patient, they need not be discouraged. Often a compromise can be reached that accomplishes the goal of the nurse while maintaining the dignity and self-esteem of the child and family.

Folklore Related to Prenatal Influences

The processes of pregnancy and birth have been surrounded by strongly held beliefs and superstitions that involve taboos and prescriptions for behavior directed toward ensuring the well-being of the unborn child.

It has been a widespread belief that the appearance of the unborn child will be improved if the pregnant woman looks at beautiful people or things. The same concept in reverse has been used to explain birth defects. For example, if a pregnant woman was frightened by a rabbit, it was believed that her child would be born with a cleft lip (harelip); a microcephalic infant was attributed to the mother's seeing a monkey during pregnancy; and the mother's viewing a person with missing limbs would cause the unborn child to be similarly affected. Activities such as a mother reaching her arms above her head, walking in circles, or tying knots were believed to cause the umbilical cord to be knotted or twisted around the neck of the fetus. Even the shape of birthmarks and other skin defects is sometimes believed to reflect maternal impressions. For example, eating strawberries by the mother is associated with nevi. Articles of apparel or adornment, food cravings, emotions such as fright and anger, undesirable thoughts, and the time and manner of announcing the pregnancy are all believed to influence the well-being of the unborn child.

In most instances these customs are relatively harmless and are not in conflict with sound health practices. However, in some situations conformity to cultural or subcultural beliefs may compromise the health and well-being of the mother or fetus (e.g., the practice of eating clay). Nurses and other health care workers must be understanding and take care to explore with the mother all of the ramifications of the practice without creating undue stress and guilt.

Not all of these beliefs are unfounded. There is evidence that maternal emotions may indeed affect the fetus.

RELIGIOUS BELIEFS

Religious and spiritual dimensions of life are among the most important influences in many people's lives. The terms *religion* and *spirituality* are often used interchangeably; however, spirituality subsumes religion. Both religion and spirituality give meaning to life and provide a source of love and relatedness between individuals and their God (Lukoff, Lu, and Turner, 1995). Holistic nursing care is promoted through an integration of spiritual and psychosocial care. The care focuses on activities that support a person's system of beliefs and worship, such as prayer, reading religious materials, and assisting with religious rituals. Meeting the spiritual needs of the child and family can provide strength, whereas unmet spiritual needs can result in spiritual distress and debilitation (Fulton and Moore, 1995). In practice, application of the nursing process for spiritual care (Box 4-2) can provide for the spiritual well-being of the child and family.

Religion affects the way people interpret and respond to illness (Spector, 2000). Among many groups, illness, injury, or death is believed to be sent by God as a punishment for sin. Some may believe that health workers will be unable to help a person whom God is punishing and may express a fatalistic attitude toward treatment, stating it is "the will of God." Others view it as a test of strength, like the testing of Job in the Bible, and strive to remain faithful and overcome the conflicts.

Religious affiliation has implications for many health-related functions and procedures. It is comforting for the family of an ill child to have this need recognized and respected. Nurses need to determine if there are any special considerations, including dietary restrictions, related to spiritual practices that are important to the family. Family members are asked whether they want a clergy member present and whether they prefer hospital staff to call or prefer to do this on their own.

BOX 4-2 ■ Application of the Nursing Process for Spiritual Care

ASSESSMENT

Observe the environment for religious articles.
Observe if the child uses religious rituals, such as prayers or stories, or receives visits from spiritual leaders.
Ask open-ended questions to elicit the importance of religion.
Assess physical and psychosocial behaviors that are indicators of spiritual distress (anger, guilt, fear, alienation, sleeplessness, regression); assess family interactions and relationships.

PLANNING

Be aware of needs related to specific religious beliefs.
Consider the developmental stage of the child, particularly with regard to lack of abstract thinking and the need for a sense of accomplishment and control.
Develop a trusting relationship and include family members in the process.
Teach family interventions to promote spiritual well-being.

IMPLEMENTATION

Offer opportunities for religious rituals and expressions if they are part of the child's spiritual life.
Offer use of self by listening to the concerns of the child and family.
Explore the spiritual dimension through the use of therapeutic play, bibliotherapy, and other forms of artistic expression while involving family members; provide direction and choices to support management of the chronic condition.

OUTCOMES

Use of religious practices, if relevant
Positive statements about meaning and purpose in life
Statements that reflect forgiveness of self and others
Restored relationships with significant others

From Fulton RA, Moore CM: Spiritual care of the school-age child with a chronic condition, *J Pediatr Nurs* 10(4):224-231, 1995.

It is also important to determine the wishes of the family regarding baptism, rites or practices related to death, and other religious rituals (such as circumcision, communion, or use of amulets or icons). Religion, which offers families understanding and spiritual support, is a valuable asset to health care. Characteristics of selected religions with beliefs that affect health care are outlined in Table 4-2.

IMPORTANCE OF CULTURE AND RELIGION TO NURSES

A general agreement exists among nurses to raise the cultural competence of professional nursing practice. To begin to understand and to deal effectively with families in a multicultural community or in a unicultural community that is different from one's own, nurses must be aware of their own attitudes and values regarding a way of life, including health practices (Ahmann, 1994; Phillips and Lobar, 1995). Nurses, too, are a product of their own cultural background. They also need to recognize that they are part of the "nursing culture." Nurses function within the framework of a professional culture with its own values and traditions and, as such, become socialized into their professional culture in their educational program and later in their work environments and professional associations.

Frequently, nurses and other health care workers are not aware of their own cultural values and how those values in-

TABLE 4-2 ■ Religious Beliefs That Affect Nursing Care

BIRTH AND DEATH	DIET AND FOOD PRACTICES	MEDICAL CARE
BUDDHIST		
Birth: No baptism Infant presentation **Death:** Last rite chanting is often practiced at bedside soon after death; the deceased's family or Buddhist priest should be contacted **Organ donation/transplantation:** Believe that organ donation is a matter of individual conscience	No requirements or restrictions Some sects are strictly vegetarian Discourage use of alcohol and drugs	Illness is believed to be a trial to aid development of soul; illness resulting from Karmic causes May be reluctant to have surgery or certain treatments on holy days Cleanliness is believed to be of great importance Family may request Buddhist priest for counseling
CHURCH OF CHRIST SCIENTIST (CHRISTIAN SCIENCE)		
Birth: No baptism **Death:** No last rites; autopsy is not permitted except in cases of sudden death; it is an individual's decision to choose burial or cremation **Organ donation/transplantation:** Church takes no specific position on transplantation or donation as distinct from other medical or surgical procedures	No requirements or restrictions	Oppose human intervention with drugs or other therapies; however, accept legally required immunizations Many adhere to belief that disease is human mental concept that can be dispelled by spiritual truth
CHURCH OF JESUS CHRIST OF LATTER DAY SAINTS (MORMON)		
Birth: No baptism Infant is blessed by church official at first opportunity after birth (in church) Baptism by immersion at 8 years **Death:** Believe that it is proper to bury the dead in the ground; cremation is discouraged **Organ donation/transplantation:** Question of whether one should will his or her organs to be used as transplants is left to the individual	Prohibits tea, coffee, and alcohol Some individuals avoid chocolate and other products that contain caffeine Encourage sparing use of meats Fasting for 24 hours each month	Devout adherents believe in divine healing Medical therapy is not prohibited
HINDU		
Birth: No baptism **Death:** Certain prescribed rites are followed after death; priest may tie thread around neck or wrist to signify blessing; family will wash the body; are particular about who touches their dead; bodies are to be cremated **Organ donation/transplantation:** No religious laws prohibiting donation; individual decision	Many dietary restrictions Beef and veal are not eaten Some are strict vegetarians	Illness or injury is believed to represent sins committed in previous life Accept most modern medical practices

From McQuay JE: Cross cultural customs and beliefs related to health crisis, death, and organ donation/transplantation, *Crit Care Nurs Clin North Am* 7(3):581-594, 1995; Lipson JG, Dibble SL, Minasik PA: *Culture and nursing care: a pocket guide,* San Francisco, 1998, UCSF Nursing Press; Spector RE: *Cultural diversity in health and illness,* ed 5, Upper Saddle River, NJ, 2000, Prentice Hall.

TABLE 4-2 ■ Religious Beliefs That Affect Nursing Care—*cont'd*

BIRTH AND DEATH	DIET AND FOOD PRACTICES	MEDICAL CARE
ISLAM (MUSLIM/MOSLEM)		
Birth: At birth, the first words said to the infant in his or her right ear are Allah-o-Akbar (Allah is great) and the remainder of the Call for Prayer is recited; an Aqeeqa (party) to celebrate the birth of the child is arranged by the parents; circumcision of the male child is practiced **Death:** At the time of death, there are specific rituals (e.g., bathing, wrapping the body in cloth) that must be done; before moving and handling the body, it is preferable to contact someone from the person's mosque or the local Islamic Society to perform these rituals **Organ donation/transplantation:** Permitted; however, there are some stipulations depending on the type of transplant/donation and its effect on the donor and recipient	Prohibit all pork products; fasting is practiced during the ninth month of the Islamic year (Ramadan)	Believers are encouraged in the Qu'ran to seek treatment; it is taught that only Allah cures; however, Muslims are taught not to refuse treatment in the belief that Allah will take care of them because he also chooses at times to work through the efforts of humans
JEHOVAH'S WITNESS		
Birth: No baptism **Death:** No official last rites practiced when death occurs **Organ donation/transplantation:** No definite statement related to this issue		
JUDAISM (ORTHODOX AND CONSERVATIVE)		
Birth: No baptism Ritual circumcision of male infants on eighth day; performed by Mohel (ritual circumciser familiar with Jewish law and aseptic technique) **Death:** According to tradition, during last moments of life, relatives and close friends remain with the deceased **Organ donation/transplantation:** Amputated limbs, or surgically removed tissues should be made available to family for burial; autopsy and organ donation are discouraged but may be permitted if it may save a life or where local law requires it; cremation is not allowed	No ingestion of blood of any kind; can eat animal flesh that has been drained Numerous dietary kosher laws exist Are allowed only meat from animals that are vegetable eaters and are ritually slaughtered; fish that have scales and fins Milk products served first can be followed by meat in a few minutes, but milk may not be consumed for several hours after eating meat Fasting is part of Yom Kippur observance Matzo replaces leavened bread during Passover week	Adherents are generally absolutely opposed to transfusions, including banking of own blood May be opposed to use of albumin, globulin, factor replacement (hemophilia), vaccines Not opposed to non–blood plasma expanders May resist surgical procedures during Sabbath, which extends from sun down Friday until sundown Saturday Seriously ill and pregnant women are exempt from fasting Illness is grounds for violating dietary laws (e.g., patient with congestive heart failure does not have to use kosher meats, which are high in sodium)
ROMAN CATHOLIC		
Birth: Infant baptism; especially urgent if poor prognosis, when it may be performed by anyone **Death:** Sacrament of the Sick is performed if prognosis is poor while patient is alive **Organ donation/transplantation:** Transplantation of organs is viewed by Catholics as ethically and morally acceptable to Vatican; organ donation is viewed as an act of charity	Fasting (eating only one full meal and no eating between meals) and abstaining from meat are practiced on Ash Wednesday and Good Friday; fasting is optional during Lent; no meat on Fridays during Lent as a general rule; children and most hospital patients are exempt from fasting	Encourage anointing of the sick Traditional church teaching does not approve of contraceptives or abortion

TABLE 4-3 ■ Cultural Characteristics Related to Health Care of Children and Families

CULTURAL GROUPS	HEALTH BELIEFS	HEALTH PRACTICES	FAMILY RELATIONSHIPS	COMMUNICATION
African	Illness classified as: **Natural**—affected by forces of nature without adequate protection (e.g., cold air, pollution, food and water) **Unnatural**—God's punishment for improper behavior May see illness as the "will of God"	Self-care and folk medicine very prevalent Folk therapies usually religious in origin Folk therapies often not shared with the medical provider Prayer is common means for prevention and treatment	Strong kinship bonds in extended family; members come to aid of others in crisis Less likely to view illness as a burden Place strong emphasis on work and ambition Elders cared for and respected	Alert to any evidence of discrimination Place importance on nonverbal behavior Affection shown by touching and hugging Silence may indicate lack of trust Eye contact important to establish trust Best to use direct but caring approach
Native American	Believe health is state of harmony with nature and universe Respect of bodies through proper management Depends on individual belief in traditional culture Traditional health beliefs holistic and wellness oriented Health practices include self-sufficiency and harmonious living Participation in religious ceremonies and prayer promotes health	Distinction made between indigenous health problem requiring native healer or practice and Western disease requiring other medical care	Cultures vary in kinship structure Extended family structure—usually includes relatives from both sides of family Elder members assume leadership roles	Most continue to speak their Indian language as well as English Nonverbal communication Individuals usually speak for themselves
Chinese	A healthy body viewed as gift from parents and ancestors and must be cared for Health is one of the results of balance between the forces of *yin* (cold) and *yang* (hot)—energy forces that rule the world Illness caused by imbalance Believe blood is source of life and is not regenerated *Chi* is innate energy	Goal of therapy is to restore balance of yin and yang Acupuncturist applies needles to appropriate meridians identified in terms of yin and yang Acupressure and *tai chi* replacing acupuncture in some areas *Moxibustion* is application of heat to skin over specific meridians Wide use of medicinal herbs procured and applied in prescribed ways Meals may or may not be planned to balance hot and cold	Extended family pattern common Strong concept of loyalty of young to old Respect for elders taught at early age—acceptance without questioning or talking back Children's behavior a reflection on family Family and individual honor and "face" important Self-reliance and self-esteem highly valued; self-expression repressed	Open expression of emotions unacceptable Often smile when they do not comprehend
Vietnamese	Good health considered to be balance between yin and yang Concept of health based on harmony and balance Many use rituals to prevent illness	Family uses all means possible before using outside agencies for health care Regard health as family responsibility; outside aid sought when resources run out Use herbal medicine, spiritual practices, and acupuncture May use cupping, coin rubbing, or pinching skin May use inhaling aromatic oils, herbal teas, or wearing strings tied on body	Family is revered institution Multigenerational families Family is chief social network Children highly valued Individual needs and interests are subordinate to those of a family group Father is main decision maker Women taught submission to men Parents expect respect and obedience from children	Many immigrants are not proficient in speaking and understanding English May hesitate to ask questions Questioning authority is sign of disrespect; asking questions considered impolite May avoid eye contact with health professionals as a sign of respect

Data from Lipson JG, Dibble SL, Minarik PA: *Culture and nursing care: a pocket guide,* San Francisco, 1998, UCSF Nursing Press; Spector RE: *Cultural diversity in health and illness,* ed 5, Upper Saddle River, NJ, 2000, Prentice Hall.

TABLE 4-3 ■ Cultural Characteristics Related to Health Care of Children and Families—cont'd

CULTURAL GROUPS	HEALTH BELIEFS	HEALTH PRACTICES	FAMILY RELATIONSHIPS	COMMUNICATION
Filipino	Health is a result of balance Illness is a result of imbalance To be able to be healthy again is to correct an evil deed	May not respond to illness until it is advanced May use herbal medicine Eating well, not necessarily eating right, promotes good health Physical ailment may be caused by the supernatural	Family is highly valued, with strong family ties Multigenerational family structure common, often including collateral members Members avoid any behavior that would bring shame on the family	Immigrants and older persons may not be able to speak or understand English Sensitive to tone and manner of speaker Limited direct eye contact
Haitian	Illness is a punishment **Natural** cause (*maladi bone die*—disease of the Lord) caused by environmental factors, movement of blood within the body, changes between hot and cold, and bone displacement **Supernatural** (loa—spirits' anger) Good health is the maintenance of equilibrium Prayer and good spiritual habits very important	Health is a personal responsibility Foods have properties of "hot"/"cold" and "light"/"heavy" and must be in harmony with one's life cycle and bodily states Natural illnesses treated by home and folk remedies first May use religious medallions, rosary beads, or figure of saint to pray with	Maintenance of family reputation paramount Lineal authority supreme; children in a subordinate position in family hierarchy Children valued for parental social security in old age and expected to contribute to family welfare at an early age	Recent immigrants and older persons may speak only Haitian Creole Often smile and nod in agreement when do not understand Quiet and gentle communication style and lack of assertiveness lead health care providers to falsely believe they comprehend health teaching and are compliant May not ask questions if health care provider is busy or rushed
Japanese	**Shinto** religious influence Human inherently good Evil caused by outside spirits Illness caused by contact with polluting agents (e.g., blood, corpses, skin diseases) Health achieved through harmony and balance between self and society Disease caused by disharmony with society and not caring for body	Energy restored by means of acupuncture, acupressure, massage, and moxibustion along affected meridians **Kampō** medicine—use of natural herbs Believe in removal of diseased parts Trend is to use both Western and Asian healing methods Care for disabled viewed as family's responsibility Take pride in child's good health Seek preventive care, medical care for illness	Close intergenerational relationships Generational categories: **Issei**—first generation to live in United States **Nisei**—second generation **Sansei**—third generation **Yonsei**—fourth generation Family tends to keep problems to self Value self-control and self-sufficiency Concept of **haji** (shame) imposes strong control; unacceptable behavior of children reflects on family	Issei—born in Japan; usually speak Japanese only Nisei, Sanseri, and Yonsei have few language difficulties Make significant use of non-verbal communication with subtle gestures and facial expression Tend to suppress emotions Will often wait silently
Mexican American	Health controlled by environment, fate, and by will of God Certain illnesses considered hot and cold states and are treated with foods that complement those states Disease based on imbalance between individual and environment	Seek help from **curandero** or **curandera,** especially in rural areas Curandero(a) receives position by birth, apprenticeship, or a "calling" via dream or vision Treatments involve use of herbs, rituals, and religious artifacts Practice for severe illness— make promises, visit shrines, offer medals and candles, offer prayers Adhere to "hot" and "cold" food prescriptions and prohibitions for prevention and treatment of illness	Strong kinship; extended families include *compadres* (godparents) established by ritual kinship Children valued highly and desired, taken everywhere with family Elderly treated with respect	Spanish speaking or bilingual May have a strong preference for native language and revert to it in times of stress May shake hands or engage in introductory embrace Interpret prolonged eye contact as disrespectful Relaxed concept of time— may be late to appointments

continued

TABLE 4-3 ■ Cultural Characteristics Related to Health Care of Children and Families—cont'd

CULTURAL GROUPS	HEALTH BELIEFS	HEALTH PRACTICES	FAMILY RELATIONSHIPS	COMMUNICATION
Puerto Rican	Subscribe to the "hot-cold" theory of causation of illness Believe some illness caused by evil forces Destiny (Si Dios quiere—if God wants) is in control of health	Infrequent use of health care system Seek folk healers (Espiritistas)—use of herbs, rituals Treatment classified as "hot" or "cold" Many varieties of herbal teas used to treat illness and promote healing	Family usually large and home centered—the core of existence Father has authority in family Great respect for elders Children valued—seen as a gift from God Children taught to obey and respect parents	Spanish speaking or bilingual Strong sense of family privacy—may view questions regarding family as impudent

BOX 4-3 ■ Exploring Your Cultural Competence

ASKED Model of Cultural Competence

Awareness: Am I aware of my personal biases and prejudices toward cultural groups different from mine?

Skill: Do I have the skill to conduct a cultural assessment and perform a culturally based physical assessment in a sensitive manner?

Knowledge: Do I have knowledge of the patient's world view and the field of biocultural ecology?

Encounters: How many face-to-face encounters have I had with patients from diverse cultural backgrounds?

Desire: What is my genuine desire to "want to be" culturally competent?

Data from Campinha-Bacote J: Many faces: addressing diversity in health care, *Online J Issues Nurs* 8:1, 2003; available online: http://www.nursingworld.org/ojin/topic20/tpc20_2.htm.

fluence their thoughts and actions. A model for self-examination on cultural competence is the "ASKED" model (Box 4.3). Recognizing that a behavior may be characteristic of a culture rather than an "abnormal" behavior places nurses at an advantage in their relationships with families. When nurses respect the cultural differences of a family, they are better able to determine whether the behavior is distinctive to the individual or a characteristic of the culture.

Cultural standards and values, the family structure and function, and experience with health care influence a family's feelings and attitudes toward health, their children, and health care delivery systems. It is often difficult for nurses to be nonjudgmental and objective in working with families whose behaviors and attitudes differ from or conflict with their own. The nurse needs to understand how one's own cultural background influences the way care is delivered (ANA, 1997). Relying on one's own values and experiences for guidance can result only in frustration and disappointment. It is one thing to know what is needed to deal with a health problem; it is often quite another to implement a fruitful course of action unless nurses work within the cultural and socioeconomic framework of the family.

It is beneficial to adapt ethnic practices to the health needs of the family rather than attempt to change long-standing beliefs. To aid their efforts to understand and respect the cul-

tural beliefs of families, nurses should have a readily available resource file containing pertinent information about the cultural and subcultural characteristics of the community in which they practice (e.g., traditional practices related to infant feeding practices and the time and manner of weaning and toilet training). The nurse needs to develop knowledge on how cultural groups understand life processes, define health and illness, view the causes of illness, and have their healers care for the cultural group's members (ANA, 2003).

Some characteristics of selected cultures are outlined in Table 4-3. Tables 4-2 and 4-3 are presented as beginning frameworks for practicing transcultural nursing. Nurses must assess the cultural and religious practices of families to identify how these practices are similar to and different from those of their own cultural and religious backgrounds. Guidelines for assessing cultural and religious practices of families are described in Box 6-9, pp. 123-124.

!**NURSING ALERT**

These generalizations are presented to help nurses learn the unique beliefs and practices of various groups and are not meant to be stereotypes of any group. It is critical to remember that no cultural group is homogeneous, every racial and ethnic group contains great diversity, and knowledge of a culture may not reflect an individual member's beliefs (Nance, 1995).

KEY POINTS

■ Culture is the sum total of mores, traditions, and beliefs about how people function and encompasses other products of human works and thoughts specific to members of an intergenerational group, community, or population.

■ Nurses have a responsibility to continually develop cultural competence. This includes understanding and respecting the influence of culture, race, and ethnicity on the development of social and emotional relationships, childrearing practices, and attitudes toward health.

■ A child's self-concept evolves from ideas about his or her social roles.

■ Important subcultural influences on children include ethnicity, socioeconomic class, occupation, poverty, religion, schools, community, peers, and biculture.

- A trend that has significantly influenced the American family is increasing geographic and economic mobility.

- Membership in a minority group presents special challenges for children, although changes in societal attitudes are slowly taking place.

- A child's physical characteristics and susceptibility to health problems are strongly related to ethnic and cultural variations of hereditary and socioeconomic forces.

- Hereditary and socioeconomic forces play an important role in a child's susceptibility to health problems.

- Groups of children suffering from greater physical and mental health problems are those living in poverty, those who are homeless, and those who have migrant families.

- Because verbal and nonverbal communication is an important cultural consideration, nurses need to acknowledge and respect their patient's practices for productive interaction to occur.

- Cultural beliefs related to cause of illness and maintenance of health may focus on natural forces, supernatural forces, or imbalance of forces.

- In planning and implementing patient care, nurses need to strive to adapt ethnic practices to the family's health needs rather than attempt to change long-standing beliefs.

- No cultural group is homogeneous; every racial and ethnic group contains great diversity.

References

Ahmann E: "Chunky stew": appreciating cultural diversity while providing health care for children, *Pediatr Nurs* 20:320-324, 1994.

American Nurses Association: *Position statement: cultural diversity in nursing practice, 1997;* available at: http://nursingworld.org/readroom/position/ethics/etcldv.htm.

Annie E. Casey Foundation: *Kids count data book: state profiles of child well-being;* available at: http://www.aecf.org/kidscount/kc2003/pdfs/entire_book.pdf.

Baze S: Measuring physical growth. In Smith D, editor: *Comprehensive child and family nursing skills,* St Louis, 1991, Mosby.

Buchwald D and others: Caring for patients in a multicultural society, *Patient Care* 28(11):105-120, 1994.

Campinha-Bacote J: Many faces: addressing diversity in health care, *Online J Issues Nurs* 8:1, 2003; available at: http://www.nursingworld.org/ojin/topic20/tpc20_2.htm.

Carillo JE, Green AR, Belancourt JR: Cross-cultural primary care: a patient-based approach, *Ann Intern Med* 130:829-834, 1999.

Castiglia PT: Tuberculosis: a pediatric concern, *J Pediatr Health Care* 11(2):75-77, 1997.

Centers for Disease Control and Prevention: *Preventing lead poisoning in young children,* Atlanta, 1997, CDC.

Chidester D: *Patterns of transcendence: religion, death, and dying,* ed 2, Belmont, Calif, 2001, Wadsworth.

Cooper TP: Culturally appropriate care: optional or imperative, *Adv Pract Nurs Q* 2(2):1-6, 1996.

Culley L: A critique of multiculturalism in health care: the challenge for nurse education, *J Adv Nurs* 23:564-570, 1996.

DeSantis L: Cultural factors affecting newborn and infant diarrhea, *J Pediatr Nurs* 3(6):391-398, 1988.

Dunn AM: Culture competence and the primary care provider, *J Pediatr Health Care* 16:105-111, 2002.

Ensign J, Santelli J: Health status and service use: comparison of adolescents at a school-based health clinic with homeless adolescents, *Arch Pediatr Adolesc Med* 152(1):20-24, 1998.

Fierman A and others: Status of immunization and iron nutrition in New York City homeless children, *Clin Pediatr* 32(3):151-155, 1993.

Fulton RA, Moore CM: Spiritual care of the school-age child with a chronic condition, *J Pediatr Nurs* 10(4):224-231, 1995.

Garwick A, Auger S: What do providers need to know about American Indian culture? Recommendations from urban Indian family caregivers, *Fam Systems Health* 18:177-189, 2000.

Giger JN, Davidhizar RE: *Transcultural nursing: assessment and intervention,* ed 3, St Louis, 1999, Mosby.

Habayeb GL: Cultural diversity: a nursing concept not yet reliably defined, *Nurs Outlook* 43(5):224-227, 1995.

Hayes J, Dreher C: Providing culturally sensitive care. In Smith D, editor: *Comprehensive child and family nursing skills,* St Louis, 1991, Mosby.

Kuensting L, Sanders G, editors: *Cultural considerations,* Park Ridge, Il, 1995, Emergency Nurses Association.

Leininger M: *Transcultural nursing,* New York, 1978, John Wiley & Sons.

Leininger M: *Transcultural nursing: concepts, theories, research & practices,* ed 2, New York, 1995, McGraw-Hill.

Lewit EM, Baker LS: Homeless families and children, *Future Children* 6(2):146-158, 1996.

Lukoff D, Lu FG, Turner R: Cultural considerations in the assessment and treatment of religious and spiritual problems, *Psychiatr Clin North Am* 18(3):467-485, 1995.

Malach F, Segel N: Perspectives on health care delivery systems for American Indian families, *Child Health Care* 19(4):219-228, 1990.

Martinson IM, Armstrong V, Qiao J: The experience of the family of children with chronic illness at home in China, *Pediatr Nurs* 23(4):371-375, 1997.

Mattson S: Culturally sensitive perinatal care for Southeast Asians, *J Obstet Gynecol Neonat Nurs* 24(4):335-341, 1995.

Nance TA: Intercultural communications: finding common ground, *J Obstet Gynecol Neonat Nurs* 24(3):249-255, 1995.

Ozawa MN, Yat-sang L: How safe is the safety net for poor children? *Soc Work Res* 20(4):238-254, 1996.

Page A, Ainsworth A, Pett M: Homeless families and their children's health problems: a Utah urban experience, *West J Med* 158(1):30-35, 1993.

Patterson J, Blum R: A conference on culture and chronic illness in childhood: conference summary, *Pediatrics* 91(5):1025-1030, 1993.

Petersen B: Surviving culture shock: lessons learned as a medical missionary in Jamaica, *J Emerg Nurs* 21(6):505-506, 1995.

Phillips S, Lobar S: Performing a culturally competent child health assessment, *Fla Nurse* 43(6):23, 1995.

Prevention and control of tuberculosis in migrant farm workers, *MMWR* 41(RR-10):1-15, 1992.

Rogers G: Educating case managers for culturally competent practice, *J Case Manage* 4(2):60-65, 1995.

Sandhaus S: Migrant health: a harvest of poverty, *Am J Nurs* 98(9):52-54, 1998.

Scribner R: Paradox as paradigm: the health outcomes of Mexican Americans, *Am J Public Health* 86(3):303-304, 1996.

Search Institute: Developmental assets: an overview, 2003; available at: http://www.search-institute.org/assets/.

Sekhon SK: Insights into South Asian culture: food and nutritional values, *Top Clin Nutr* 11(4):47-56, 1996.

Shaw-Taylor Y: Culturally and linguistically appropriate health care for racial or ethnic minorities: analysis of the US Office of Minority Health's recommended standards, *Health Policy* 62:211-221, 2002.

Spector RE: *Cultural diversity in health and illness,* ed 5, Upper Saddle River, NJ, 2000, Prentice Hall.

Strehlow AJ, Amos-Jones T: The homeless as a vulnerable population, *Nurs Clin North Am* 34(2):261-274, 1999.

Talabere LR: Meeting the challenge of cultural care in nursing diversity, sensitivity, competence, and congruence, *J Cult Diversity* 3(2):53-61, 1996.

Taylor R: Check your cultural competence, *Nurs Manage* 29(8):30-32, 1998.

Trawick-Smith J: *Early childhood development: a multicultural perspective,* ed 2, Upper Saddle River, NJ, 2000, Prentice Hall.

Tropello PD: The many faces of homelessness. In Kelley ML, Fitzsimons VM, editors: *Understanding cultural diversity,* Sudbury, Mass, 2000, Jones & Bartlett, pp 199-208.

US Census Bureau: Overview of race and Hispanic origin census 2000 brief, 2000; available at: http://www.census.gov/prod/2001pubs/c2kbr01-1.pdf.

Wagner J, Menke EM, Cicconi MA: What is known about the health of rural homeless families, *Public Health Nurs* 12(6):400-408, 1995.

Weinreb L and others: Determinants of health and service use patterns in homeless and low-income housed children, *Pediatrics* 102(3):554-562, 1998.

Wright J: Female genital mutilation: an overview, *J Adv Nurs* 24:251-259, 1996.

Yoos HL and others: Child rearing beliefs in the African-American community: implications for culturally competent pediatric care, *J Pediatr Nurs* 10(6):343-353, 1995.

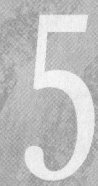

Developmental Influences on Child Health Promotion

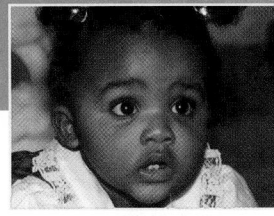

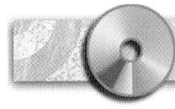 Remember to check out your companion CD-ROM

http://evolve.elsevier.com/Wong/essentials/

CHAPTER OUTLINE

RELATED TOPICS and ADDITIONAL RESOURCES

 IN TEXT

 CD COMPANION

Critical Thinking Exercise—Growth
   Trends During Infancy
NCLEX-Style Review Questions

evolve WEBSITE

WebLinks
NCLEX-Style Review Questions

For additional information, please view "Growth and Development" in *Whaley and Wong's Pediatric Nursing Video Series*, St Louis, 1996, Mosby; (800) 426-4545; website:
www.elsevierhealth.com.

■ Describe major trends in growth and development.
■ Explain the alterations in the major body systems that take place during the process of growth and development.

■ Discuss the development and relationships of personality, cognitive, language, moral, spiritual, and self-concept development.
■ Describe the role of play in the growth and development of children.

■ Demonstrate an understanding of the role of innate and environmental factors in the physical and emotional development of children.

GROWTH AND DEVELOPMENT

FOUNDATIONS OF GROWTH AND DEVELOPMENT

Growth and development, usually referred to as a unit, expresses the sum of the numerous changes that take place during the lifetime of an individual. The entire course is a dynamic process that encompasses several interrelated dimensions:

> **Growth**—an increase in number and size of cells as they divide and synthesize new proteins; results in increased size and weight of the whole or any of its parts
>
> **Development**—a gradual change and expansion; advancement from lower to more advanced stages of complexity; the emerging and expanding of the individual's capacities through growth, maturation, and learning
>
> **Maturation**—an increase in competence and adaptability; aging; usually used to describe a qualitative change; a change in the complexity of a structure that makes it possible for that structure to begin functioning; to function at a higher level
>
> **Differentiation**—processes by which early cells and structures are systematically modified and altered to achieve specific and characteristic physical and chemical properties; sometimes used to describe the trend of mass to specific; development from simple to more complex activities and functions

All of these processes are interrelated, simultaneous, and ongoing; none occurs apart from the others. The processes depend on a sequence of endocrine, genetic, constitutional, environmental, and nutritional influences (Seidel and others, 2003). The child's body becomes larger and more complex; the personality simultaneously expands in scope and complexity. Very simply, growth can be viewed as a *quantitative* change, and development as a *qualitative* change.

Stages of Development

Most authorities in the field of child development conveniently categorize child growth and behavior into approximate age stages or in terms that describe the features of an age-group. The age ranges of these stages are admittedly arbitrary and, because they do not take into account individual differences, cannot be applied to all children with any degree of precision. However, this categorization affords a convenient means to describe the characteristics associated with the majority of children at periods when distinctive developmental changes appear and specific developmental tasks must be accomplished. (A *developmental task* is a set of skills and competencies peculiar to each developmental stage that children must accomplish or master in order to deal effectively with their environment.) It is also significant for nurses to know that there are characteristic health problems peculiar to each major phase of development. The sequence of descriptive age periods and subperiods that are used here and elaborated in subsequent chapters is listed in Box 5-1.

Patterns of Growth and Development

There are definite and predictable patterns in growth and development that are continuous, orderly, and progressive. These patterns, or trends, are universal and basic to all human beings, but each human being accomplishes these in a manner and time unique to that individual.

Directional Trends. Growth and development proceed in regular, related directions or gradients and reflect the physical development and maturation of neuromuscular functions (Fig. 5-1). The first pattern is the *cephalocaudal,* or *head-to-tail,* direction. The head end of the organism develops first and is very large and complex, whereas the lower end is small and simple and takes shape at a later period. The physical evidence of this trend is most apparent during the period before birth, but it also applies to postnatal behavior development. Infants achieve structural control of the head before they have control of the trunk and extremities, hold their back erect before they stand, use their eyes before their hands, and gain control of their hands before they have control of their feet.

Second, the *proximodistal,* or *near-to-far,* trend applies to the midline-to-peripheral concept. A conspicuous illustration is the early embryonic development of limb buds, which is followed by rudimentary fingers and toes. In the infant shoulder control precedes mastery of the hands, the whole hand is used as a unit before the fingers can be manipulated, and the central nervous system develops more rapidly than the peripheral nervous system.

These trends or patterns are bilateral and appear symmetric—each side develops in the same direction and at the same rate as the other. For some of the neurologic functions, this symmetry is only external because of unilateral differentiation of function at an early stage of postnatal development. For example, by the age of approximately 5 years the child has demonstrated a decided preference for the use of one hand over the other, although previously either one had been used.

The third trend, *differentiation,* describes development from simple operations to more complex activities and functions. From very broad, global patterns of behavior, more specific, refined patterns emerge. All areas of development (physical, mental, social, and emotional) proceed in this di-

BOX 5-1 ■ Developmental Age Periods

PRENATAL PERIOD: CONCEPTION TO BIRTH
Germinal: Conception to approximately 2 weeks
Embryonic: 2 to 8 weeks
Fetal: 8 to 40 weeks (birth)
A rapid growth rate and total dependency make this one of the most crucial periods in the developmental process. The relationship between maternal health and certain manifestations in the newborn emphasizes the importance of adequate prenatal care to the health and well-being of the infant.

INFANCY PERIOD: BIRTH TO 12 MONTHS
Neonatal: Birth to 27 or 28 days
Infancy: 1 to approximately 12 months
The infancy period is one of rapid motor, cognitive, and social development. Through mutuality with the caregiver (parent), the infant establishes a basic trust in the world and the foundation for future interpersonal relationships. The critical first month of life, although part of the infancy period, is often differentiated from the remainder because of the major physical adjustments to extrauterine existence and the psychologic adjustment of the parent.

EARLY CHILDHOOD: 1 TO 6 YEARS
Toddler: 1 to 3 years
Preschool: 3 to 6 years
This period, which extends from the time the children attain upright locomotion until they enter school, is characterized by intense activity and discovery. It is a time of marked physical and personality development. Motor development advances steadily. Children at this age acquire language and wider social relationships, learn role standards, gain self-control and mastery, develop increasing awareness of dependence and independence, and begin to develop a self-concept.

MIDDLE CHILDHOOD: 6 TO 11 OR 12 YEARS
Frequently referred to as the "school age," this period of development is one in which the child is directed away from the family group and centered around the wider world of peer relationships. There is steady advancement in physical, mental, and social development, with emphasis on developing skill competencies. Social cooperation and early moral development take on more importance with relevance for later life stages. This is a critical period in the development of a self-concept.

LATER CHILDHOOD: 11 TO 19 YEARS
Prepubertal: 10 to 13 years
Adolescence: 13 to approximately 18 years
The tumultuous period of rapid maturation and change known as adolescence is considered to be a transitional period that begins at the onset of puberty and extends to the point of entry into the adult world—usually high school graduation. Biologic and personality maturation are accompanied by physical and emotional turmoil, and there is redefining of the self-concept. In the late adolescent period the young person begins to internalize all previously learned values and to focus on an individual, rather than a group, identity.

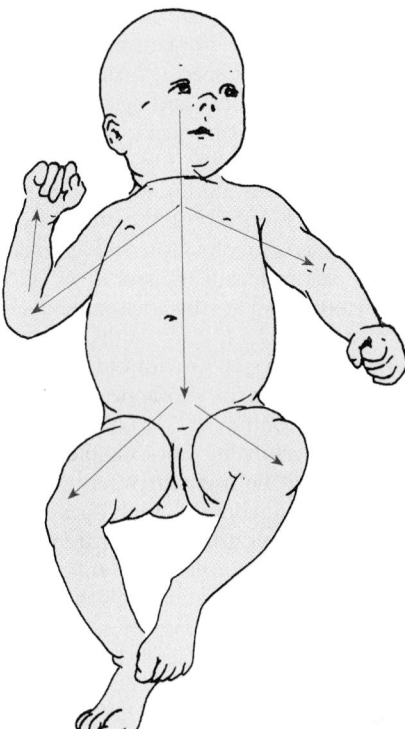

FIG. 5-1 ■ Directional trends in growth.

cialized development; gross, random muscle movements take place before fine muscle control.

Sequential Trends.   In all dimensions of growth and development there is a definite, predictable sequence, with each child normally passing through every stage. Children crawl before they creep, creep before they stand, and stand before they walk. Later facets of the personality are built on the early foundation of trust. The child babbles, then forms words and, finally, sentences; writing emerges from scribbling.

Developmental Pace.   Although there is a fixed, precise order to development, it does not progress at the same rate or pace. There are periods of accelerated growth and periods of decelerated growth in both total body growth and the growth of subsystems. The rapid growth before and after birth gradually levels off throughout early childhood. Growth is relatively slow during middle childhood, markedly increases at the beginning of adolescence, and levels off in early adulthood. Each child grows at his or her own pace. Marked differences are observed between children as they reach developmental milestones.

FYI

Research suggests that normal growth, in particular, height in infants, may occur in brief (possibly even 24-hour) bursts that punctuate long periods in which no measurable growth takes place (Lampl, 1992; Lampl, Johnson, and Frongillo, 2001). Further, findings indicate a stuttering or saltatory pattern of growth that follows no regular cycle and can occur after "quiet" periods that last as long as 4 weeks. Mothers reported that their children were usually fussy and voraciously hungry a day or two before the growth spurt.

rection. Through the process of development and differentiation, early embryonic cells with vague, undifferentiated functions progress to an immensely complex organism composed of highly specialized and diversified cells, tissues, and organs. Generalized development precedes specific or spe-

Sensitive Periods.   There are limited times during the process of growth when the organism will interact with a particular environment in a specific manner. Periods termed *critical, sensitive, vulnerable,* and *optimal* are those times in the lifetime of an organism when it is more susceptible to positive or negative influences.

The quality of interactions during these sensitive periods determines whether the effects on the organism will be beneficial or harmful. For example, physiologic maturation of the central nervous system is influenced by adequacy and timing of contributions from the environment such as stimulation and nutrition. The first 3 months of prenatal life are sensitive periods for physical growth of the fetus.

Psychologic development also appears to have sensitive periods when an environmental event has maximal influence on the developing personality. For example, primary socialization occurs during the first year when the infant makes the initial social attachments and establishes a basic trust in the world. A warm relationship with a parent figure is fundamental to a healthy personality. The same concept might be applied to readiness for learning skills such as toilet training or reading. In these instances there appears to be an opportune time when the skill is best learned.

Individual Differences

Each child grows in his or her own unique and personal way. Great individual variation exists in the age at which developmental milestones are reached. The sequence is predictable; the exact timing is not. Rates of growth vary, and measurements are defined in terms of ranges to allow for individual differences. Some children are fast growers, others are moderate, and some are slower to reach maturity. Periods of fast growth, such as the pubescent growth spurt, may begin earlier or later in some children than in others. Children may grow fast or slowly during the spurt and may finish sooner or later than other children. Gender is an influential factor because girls seem to be more advanced in physiologic growth at all ages.

BIOLOGIC GROWTH AND PHYSICAL DEVELOPMENT

As children grow, their external dimensions change. These changes are accompanied by corresponding alterations in structure and function of internal organs and tissues that reflect the gradual acquisition of physiologic competence. Each part has its own rate of growth, which may be directly related to alterations in the size of the child (e.g., the heart rate). Skeletal muscle growth approximates whole body growth; brain, lymphoid, adrenal, and reproductive tissues follow distinct and individual patterns (Fig. 5-2). When there has been a secondary cause of growth deficiency, such as severe illness or acute malnutrition, recovery from the illness or the establishment of an adequate diet will produce a dramatic acceleration of the growth rate that usually continues until the child's individual growth pattern is resumed.

External Proportions

Variations in the growth rate of different tissues and organ systems produce significant changes in body proportions during childhood. The cephalocaudal trend of development is most evident in total body growth as indicated by these

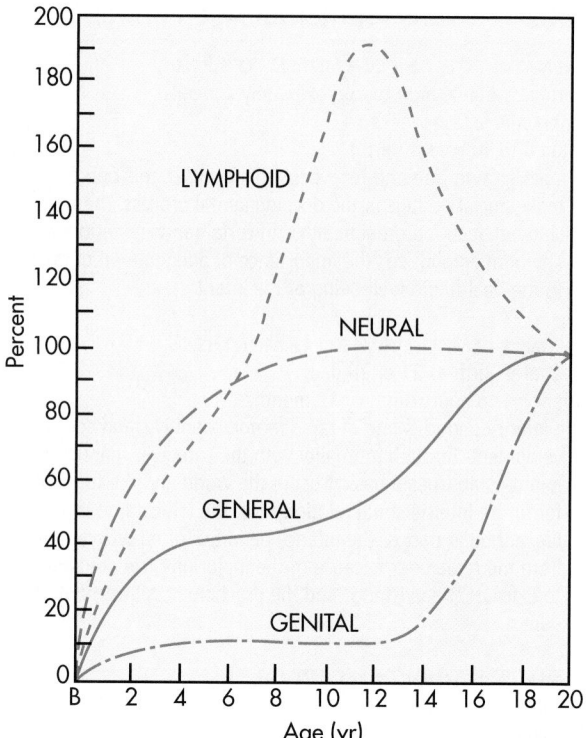

FIG. 5-2 ■ Growth rates for the body as a whole and three types of tissues. *Lymphoid type:* thymus, lymph nodes, and intestinal lymph masses. *Neural type:* brain, dura, spinal cord, optic apparatus, and head dimensions. *General type:* body as a whole; external dimension; and respiratory, digestive, renal, circulatory, and musculoskeletal systems.(From Harris JA and others: *The measurement of man,* Minneapolis, 1930, University of Minnesota Press.)

changes (Fig. 5-3). During fetal development the head is the fastest growing body part, and at 2 months of gestation the head constitutes 50% of total body length. During infancy growth of the trunk predominates; the legs are the most rapidly growing part during childhood; in adolescence, the trunk once again elongates. In the newborn infant the lower limbs are one third the total body length but only 15% of the total body weight; in the adult the lower limbs constitute one half of the total body height and 30% or more of the total body weight. As growth proceeds, the midpoint in head-to-toe measurements gradually descends from a level even with the umbilicus at birth to the level of the symphysis pubis at maturity.

Biologic Determinants of Growth and Development

The most prominent feature of childhood and adolescence is physical growth. Throughout development various tissues in the body undergo changes in growth, composition, and structure. In some tissues the changes are continuous (e.g., bone growth and dentition); in others, significant alterations occur at specific stages (e.g., appearance of secondary sex characteristics). When these measurements are compared with standardized norms, a child's developmental progress can be determined with a high degree of confidence (Table 5-1).

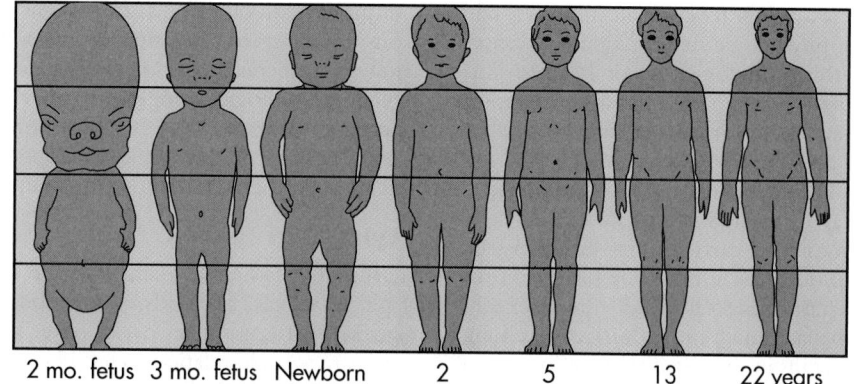

FIG. 5-3 ■ Changes in body proportions from before birth to adulthood. (From Crouch JE, McClintic JR: *Human anatomy and physiology,* ed 2, New York, 1976, John Wiley & Sons.)

TABLE 5-1 ■ General Trends in Height and Weight Gain During Childhood

AGE-GROUP	WEIGHT*	HEIGHT*
INFANTS		
Birth-6 months	Weekly gain: 140-200 g (5-7 oz) Birth weight doubles by end of first 4-7 months†	Monthly gain: 2.5 cm (1 inch)
6-12 months	Weight gain: 85-140 g (3-5 oz) Birth weight triples by end of first year	Monthly gain: 1.25 cm (0.5 inch) Birth length increases by approximately 50% by end of first year
Toddlers	Birth weight quadruples by age 2.5	Height at age 2 is approximately 50% of eventual adult height Gain during second year: about 12 cm (4.75 inches) Gain during third year: about 6-8 cm (2.375-3.25 inches)
Preschoolers	Yearly gain: 2-3 kg (4.5-6.5 lb)	Birth length doubles by age 4 Yearly gain: 5-7.5 cm (2-3 inches)
School-age children	Yearly gain: 2-3 kg (4.5-6.5 lb)	Yearly gain after age 7: 5 cm (2 inches) Birth length triples by about age 13
PUBERTAL GROWTH SPURT		
Females—10-14 years	Weight gain: 7-25 kg (15-55 lb) Mean: 17.5 kg (38.125 lb)	Height gain: 5-25 cm (2-10 inches); approximately 95% of mature height achieved by onset of menarche or skeletal age of 13 Mean: 20.5 cm (8.25 inches)
Males—11-16 years	Weight gain: 7-30 kg (15-65 lb) Mean: 23.7 kg (52.125 lb)	Height gain: 10-30 cm (4-12 inches); approximately 95% of mature height achieved by skeletal age of 15 years Mean: 27.5 cm (11 inches)

*Yearly height and weight gains for each age-group represent averaged estimates from a variety of sources.
†Jung and Czajka-Narins, 1985.

Linear growth, or *height,* occurs almost entirely as a result of skeletal growth and is considered a stable measurement of general growth. Growth in height is not uniform throughout life but ceases when maturation of the skeleton is complete. The maximum growth in length occurs before birth, but the newborn continues to grow at a rapid, though slower, rate.

Double the child's height at the age of 2 years to estimate how tall he or she may be as an adult.

At birth, *weight* is more variable than height and is, to a greater extent, a reflection of the intrauterine environment. The average newborn weighs from 3175 to 3400 g (7 to 7.5 pounds). In general, the birth weight doubles by 4 to 7 months of age and triples by the end of the first year. By the age of 2 to 2.5 the birth weight usually quadruples. After this point the "normal" rate of weight gain, just as the growth in height, assumes a steady annual increase of approximately 2 to 2.75 kg (4.4 to 6 pounds) per year until the adolescent growth spurt.

Both *bone age* determinants and state of *dentition* are used as indicators of development. Because both are discussed elsewhere, neither is elaborated here (see next section for bone age; see also Chapters 10 and 12 for dentition).

Skeletal Growth and Maturation

The most accurate measure of general development is *skeletal* or *bone age,* the radiologic determination of osseous maturation. Skeletal age appears to correlate more closely with other measures of physiologic maturity (such as onset of menarche) than with chronologic age or height. This "bone age" is determined by comparing the mineralization of ossification centers and advancing bony form to age-related standards.

Bone formation begins during the second month of fetal life when calcium salts are deposited in the intercellular substance (matrix) to form calcified cartilage first and then true bone. There are some differences in this bone formation. In small bones the bone continues to form in the center and cartilage continues to be laid down on the surfaces. In long bones the ossification begins in the *diaphysis* (the long central portion of the bone) and continues in the *epiphysis* (the end portions of the bone). Between the diaphysis and the epiphysis, an *epiphyseal cartilage plate* unites with the diaphysis by columns of spongy tissue, the *metaphysis.* Active growth in length takes place in the epiphyseal growth plate. Interference with this growth site by trauma or infection can result in deformity.

The first centers of ossification appear in the 2-month-old embryo, and at birth the number is approximately 400, about half the number at maturity. New centers appear at regular intervals during the growth period and provide the basis for assessment of bone age. Postnatally the earliest centers to appear (at 5 to 6 months of age) are those of the capitate and hamate bones in the wrist. Therefore radiographs of the hand and wrist provide the most useful areas for screening to determine skeletal age, especially before age 6 years. These centers appear earlier in girls than in boys.

Nurses must understand that the growing bones of children possess many unique characteristics. Bone fractures occurring at the growth plate may be difficult to discover and may significantly affect subsequent growth and development (Urbanski and Hanlon, 1996).

Factors that may influence skeletal muscle injury rates and types in children and adolescents include (Kaczander, 1997):

- Less protective sports equipment for children
- Less emphasis on conditioning, especially flexibility
- In adolescents, fractures that are more common than ligamentous ruptures because of the rapid growth rate of the physeal (segment of tubular bone that is concerned mainly with growth) zone of hypertrophy

Neurologic Maturation

In contrast to other body tissues, which grow rapidly after birth, the nervous system grows proportionately more rapidly before birth. Two periods of rapid brain cell growth occur during fetal life: a dramatic increase in the number of neurons between 15 and 20 weeks of gestation and another increase at 30 weeks, which extends to 1 year of age. The rapid growth of infancy continues during early childhood and then slows to a more gradual rate during later childhood and adolescence.

It is believed that no new nerve cells appear after the sixth month of fetal life. Postnatal growth consists of increasing the amount of cytoplasm around the nuclei of existing cells, increasing the number and intricacy of communications with other cells, and advancing their peripheral axons to keep pace with expanding body dimensions. This allows for increasingly complex movement and behavior. Neurophysiologic changes also provide the foundation for language, learning, and behavior development. Neurologic or electroencephalographic development is sometimes used as an indicator of maturational age in the early weeks of life.

Lymphoid Tissues

Lymphoid tissues contained in the lymph nodes, thymus, spleen, tonsils, adenoids, and blood lymphocytes follow a growth pattern unlike that of other body tissues. These tissues are small in relation to total body size, but they are well developed at birth. They increase rapidly to reach adult dimensions by 6 years of age and continue to grow. At about age 10 to 12 years they reach a maximum development that is approximately twice their adult size. This is followed by a rapid decline to stable adult dimensions by the end of adolescence.

Development of Organ Systems

All tissues and organ systems undergo changes during development. Some are striking; others are subtle. Many have implications for assessment and care. Because the major importance of these changes relates to their dysfunction, the developmental characteristics of various systems and organs are discussed throughout the book as they relate to these areas. Physical characteristics and physiologic changes that vary with age are included in age-group descriptions.

PHYSIOLOGIC CHANGES

Physiologic changes that take place in all organs and systems are discussed as they relate to dysfunction. Others such as pulse and respiratory rates and blood pressure are an integral part of physical assessment (see Chapter 7). In addition, there are changes in basic functions, including metabolism, temperature, and patterns of sleep and rest.

Metabolism

The rate of metabolism when the body is at rest (*basal metabolic rate,* or *BMR*) demonstrates a distinctive change throughout childhood. Highest in the newborn infant, the BMR closely relates to the proportion of surface area to body mass, which changes as the body increases in size. In both sexes the proportion decreases progressively to maturity. The BMR is slightly higher in boys at all ages and further increases during pubescence over that in girls.

The rate of metabolism determines the caloric requirements of the child. The basal energy requirement of infants is about 108 kcal/kg of body weight and decreases to 40 to 45 kcal/kg at maturity (Table 5-2). Water requirements remain at approximately 1.5 ml per calorie of energy expended throughout life. Children's energy needs vary considerably at different ages and with changing circumstances. The energy requirement to build tissue steadily decreases with age, following the general growth curve; however, energy needs vary with the individual child and may be considerably higher. For short periods (e.g., during strenuous exercise) and more prolonged periods (e.g., illness), the needs can be very high.

TABLE 5-2 ■ **Recommended Daily Requirements for Calories and Protein Throughout Adolescence***

AGE (years)	ENERGY ALLOWANCE (kCal/kg)	PROTEIN (g)
INFANTS		
0-.5	108	13
0.5-1	98	14
CHILDREN		
1-3	102	16
4-6	90	24
7-10	70	28
MALES		
11-14	55	45
15-18	45	49
FEMALES		
11-14	47	46
15-18	40	44

Data from Food and Nutrition Board: Recommended daily allowances, ed 10, Washington, DC, 1989, National Academy Press.
*See also Dietary Reference Intakes, p. 371.

FYI

Each degree of fever increases the basal metabolism 10% with a corresponding fluid requirement.

Temperature

Body temperature, reflecting metabolism, decreases over the course of development (see inside back cover). Thermoregulation is one of the most important adaptation responses of the infant during the transition from intrauterine to extrauterine life. In the healthy neonate hypothermia can result in several negative metabolic consequences such as hypoglycemia, elevated bilirubin levels, and metabolic acidosis (Bliss-Holtz, 1995). After the unstable regulatory ability in the neonatal period, heat production steadily declines as the infant grows into childhood. Individual differences of 0.5° to 1° F are normal, and occasionally a child normally displays an unusually high or low temperature. Beginning at approximately 12 years of age, girls display a temperature that remains relatively stable, whereas the temperature in boys continues to fall for a few more years. Females maintain a temperature slightly above that of males throughout life.

Even with improved temperature regulation, infants and young children are highly susceptible to temperature fluctuations. Body temperature responds to changes in environmental temperature and is increased with active exercise, crying, and emotional stress. Infections can cause a higher and more rapid temperature increase in infants and young children than in older children. In relation to body weight, an infant produces more heat per unit than children near maturity. Consequently, during active play or when heavily clothed, an infant or small child is likely to become overheated.

Sleep and Rest

Sleep, a protective function in all organisms, allows for repair and recovery of tissues after activity. As in most aspects of development, there is wide variation among individual children in the amount and distribution of sleep at various ages. As children mature, there is a change in the total time they spend in sleep and the amount of time they spend in deep sleep.

Newborn infants sleep much of the time that is not occupied with feeding and other aspects of their care. As infants grow older, the total time spent in sleep gradually decreases, they remain awake for longer periods, and they sleep longer at night. For example, the length of a sleep cycle increases from approximately 50 to 60 minutes in the newborn infant to approximately 90 minutes in adolescence (Anders, Sadeh, and Appareddy, 1995). During the latter part of the first year, most children sleep through the night and take one or two naps during the day. By the time they are 12 to 18 months old, most children have eliminated the second nap. After age 3 years the child has usually given up daytime naps, except in cultures in which an afternoon nap or siesta is customary. During ages 4 to 10 sleep time declines slightly and then increases somewhat during the pubertal growth spurt. The changes in length of sleep at different ages are shown in Fig. 5-4.

There is a change in the quality of sleep as children mature. The time spent in deep, restful sleep increases from 50% in infancy to 80% in the older child.

TEMPERAMENT

Temperament is defined as "the manner of thinking, behaving, or reacting characteristic of an individual" (Chess and Thomas, 1985) and refers to the way in which a person deals with life. From the time of birth, children exhibit marked individual differences in the way that they respond to their environment and the way others, particularly the parents, respond to them and their needs. A generic basis has been suggested for some differences in temperament. Nine characteristics of temperament have been identified through interviews with parents (Box 5-2). Temperament refers to behavioral tendencies, not to discrete behavioral acts. There are no implications of good or bad. Most children can be placed into one of three common categories based on their overall pattern of temperamental attributes:

The easy child. Easy-going children are even-tempered, are regular and predictable in their habits, and have a positive approach to new stimuli. They are open and adaptable to change and display a mild to moderately intense mood that is typically positive. Approximately 40% of children fall into this category.

The difficult child. Difficult children are highly active, irritable, and irregular in their habits. Negative withdrawal responses are typical, and they require a more structured environment. These children adapt slowly to new routines, people, or situations. Mood expressions are usually intense and primarily negative. They exhibit frequent periods of crying, and frustration often produces violent tantrums. This group comprises about 10% of children.

The slow-to-warm-up child. Slow-to-warm-up children typically react negatively and with mild intensity to new stimuli and, unless pressured, adapt slowly with repeated contact. They respond with only mild but passive resistance to nov-

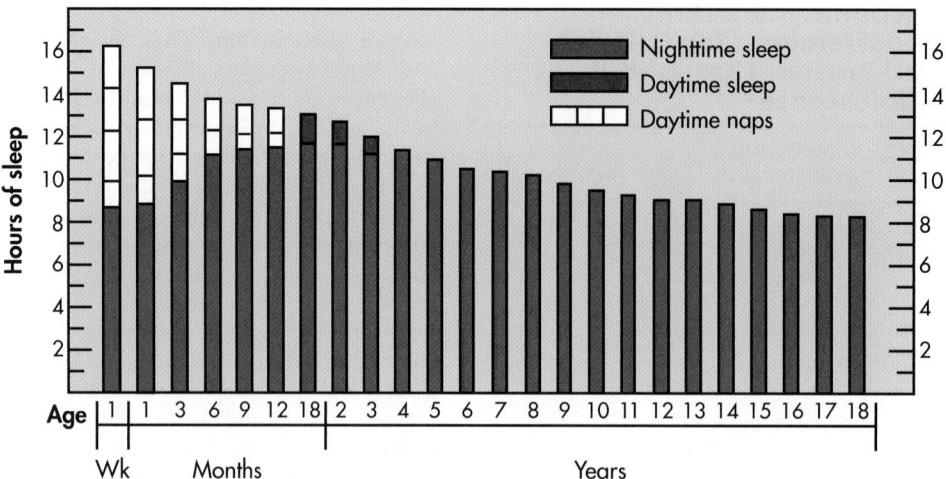

FIG. 5-4 ■ Changes in number of hours of sleep with increasing age. (Modified from Ferber R: *Solve your child's sleep problems,* New York, 1985, Simon & Schuster.)

BOX 5-2 ■ Attributes of Temperament

Activity—level of physical motion during activity such as sleep, eating, play, dressing, and bathing

Rhythmicity—regularity in the timing of physiologic functions such as hunger, sleep, and elimination

Approach-withdrawal—nature of initial responses to a new stimulus such as people, situations, places, foods, toys, and procedures (*Approach* responses are positive and are displayed by activity or expression; *withdrawal* responses are negative expressions or behaviors.)

Adaptability—ease or difficulty with which the child adapts or adjusts to new or altered situations

Threshold of responsiveness (sensory threshold)—amount of stimulation, such as sounds or light, required to evoke a response in the child

Intensity of reaction—energy level of the child's reactions, regardless of quality or direction

Mood—amount of pleasant, happy, friendly behavior compared with unpleasant, unhappy, crying, unfriendly behavior exhibited by the child in various situations

Distractibility—ease with which a child's attention or direction of behavior can be diverted by external stimuli

Attention span and persistence—length of time a child pursues a given activity (*attention*) and the continuation of an activity in spite of obstacles (*persistence*)

elty or changes in routine. They are quite inactive and moody but show only moderate irregularity in functions. Fifteen percent of children demonstrate this temperament pattern.

Thirty-five percent of children either have some, but not all, of the characteristics of one of the categories or are inconsistent in their behavioral responses. Many normal children demonstrate this wide range of behavioral patterns.

Significance of Temperament

Observations indicate that children who display the difficult or slow-to-warm-up patterns of behavior are more vulnerable to the development of behavior problems in early and middle childhood. Any child can develop behavior problems if there is dissonance between the child's temperament and the environment. Demands for change and adaptation that are in conflict with the child's capacities can become excessively stressful. However, authorities emphasize that it is not the temperament patterns of children that place them at risk; it is the *degree of fit* between children and their environment, specifically their parents, that determines the degree of vulnerability. The potential for optimum development exists when environmental expectations and demands fit with the individual's style of behavior and the parents' ability to navigate this period (Gross and Conrad, 1995) (see Failure to Thrive, Chapter 11).

Early identification of temperament provides a useful tool for caregivers in anticipating probable areas of difficulty or risk associated with development. For example, "difficult" children may be prone to colic in infancy, active children require more vigilance to prevent injury, and school entry requires different approaches for children with different temperaments.

Research indicates that irritable and unadaptable infants can raise doubts in mothers about their competence (Beck, 1996). Additional research indicates that a child's temperament can affect parent-child interactions and can influence the parents' self-esteem, marital harmony, mood, and overall satisfaction as parents (Carey, 1998). Studies on the relationship between temperament and the ability to perform a task successfully (mastery motivation) have found that infants with high mastery are more cooperative and less difficult (Morrow and Camp, 1996). Principles that can be used by nurses in direct patient care and in providing anticipatory guidance are listed in Box 5-3.

DEVELOPMENT OF PERSONALITY AND MENTAL FUNCTION

Personality and cognitive skills develop in much the same manner as biologic growth—new accomplishments build on previously mastered skills. Many aspects depend on

BOX 5-3 ■ Activities to Promote Mastery Motivation

Encourage unobtrusive assistance during play.
Share pleasure with infant in accomplishments.
Don't give immediate assistance during tasks.
Don't interrupt infant during tasks.
Let infant initiate activities.
Limit controlling feedback during play.
Provide audio and visually responsive toys.
Provide early kinesthetic stimulation (picking up, rocking).

From Morrow JD, Camp BW: Mastery motivation and temperament of 7-month-old infants, *Pediatr Nurs* 22(3):211-217, 1996.

physical growth and maturation. This is not a comprehensive account of the multiple facets of personality and behavior development. Many aspects are integrated with the child's emotional and social development in later discussion of various age-groups. Table 5-3 summarizes some of the developmental theories.

THEORETIC FOUNDATIONS OF PERSONALITY DEVELOPMENT

According to Freud, all human behavior is energized by psychodynamic forces, and this psychic energy is divided among three components of personality: the id, the ego, and the superego. The *id*, the *unconscious mind,* is the inborn component that is driven by instincts. The id obeys the pleasure principle of immediate gratification of needs, regardless of whether the object or action can actually do so. The *ego,* the *conscious mind,* serves the reality principle. It functions as the conscious or controlling self that is able to find realistic means for gratifying the instincts while blocking the irrational thinking of the id. The *superego,* the *conscience,* functions as the moral arbitrator and represents the ideal. It is the mechanism that prevents individuals from expressing undesirable instincts that might threaten the social order.

Psychosexual Development (Freud)

Freud considered the sexual instincts to be significant in the development of the personality. However, he used the term *psychosexual* to describe any *sensual pleasure.* During childhood certain regions of the body assume a prominent psychologic significance as the source of new pleasures and new conflicts gradually shifts from one part of the body to another at particular stages of development:

Oral stage (birth to 1 year). During infancy the major source of pleasure seeking is centered on oral activities such as sucking, biting, chewing, and vocalizing. Children may prefer one of these over the others, and the preferred method of oral gratification can provide some indication of the personality they develop.

Anal stage (1 to 3 years). Interest during the second year of life centers in the anal region as sphincter muscles develop and children are able to withhold or expel fecal material at will. At this stage the climate surrounding toilet training can have lasting effects on children's personalities.

Phallic stage (3 to 6 years). During the phallic stage the genitals become an interesting and sensitive area of the body. Children recognize differences between the sexes and become curious about the dissimilarities. This is the period around which the controversial issues of the Oedipus and Electra complexes, penis envy, and castration anxiety are centered.

Latency period (6 to 12 years). During the latency period children elaborate on previously acquired traits and skills. Physical and psychic energy are channeled into acquisition of knowledge and vigorous play.

Genital stage (age 12 and older). The last significant stage begins at puberty with maturation of the reproductive system and production of sex hormones. The genital organs become the major source of sexual tensions and pleasures, but energies are also invested in forming friendships and preparation for marriage.

Psychosocial Development (Erikson)

The most widely accepted theory of personality development is that advanced by Erikson (1963). Although built on Freudian theory, it is known as *psychosocial* development and emphasizes a healthy personality as opposed to a pathologic approach. Erikson also uses the biologic concepts of critical periods and epigenesis, describing key conflicts or core problems that the individual strives to master during critical periods in personality development. Successful completion or mastery of each of these core conflicts is built on the satisfactory completion or mastery of the previous core.

Each psychosocial stage has two components—the favorable and the unfavorable aspects of the core conflict—and progress to the next stage depends on resolution of this conflict. No core conflict is ever mastered completely but remains a recurrent problem throughout life. No life situation is ever secure. Each new situation presents the conflict in a new form. For example, when children who have satisfactorily achieved a sense of trust encounter a new experience (e.g., hospitalization), they must again develop a sense of trust in those responsible for their care in order to master the situation. Erikson's life-span approach to personality development consists of eight stages; however, only the first five relating to childhood are included here:

Trust vs mistrust (birth to 1 year). The first and most important attribute to develop for a healthy personality is a basic *trust.* Establishment of basic trust dominates the first year of life and describes all the child's satisfying experiences at this age. Corresponding to Freud's oral stage, it is a time of "getting" and "taking in" through all the senses. It exists only in relation to something or someone; therefore, consistent, loving care by a mothering person is essential to development of trust. *Mistrust* develops when trust-promoting experiences are deficient or lacking or when basic needs are inconsistently or inadequately met. Although shreds of mistrust are sprinkled throughout the personality, from a basic trust in parents stems trust in the world, other people, and oneself. The result is *faith* and *optimism.*

Autonomy vs shame and doubt (1 to 3 years). Corresponding to Freud's anal stage, the problem of *autonomy* can be symbolized by the holding on and letting go of the sphincter muscles. The development of autonomy during the toddler period is centered on children's increasing ability to control their bodies, themselves, and their environment. They want to do things for themselves, using their newly acquired motor skills of walking, climbing, and manipulating and their mental powers of selection and decision mak-

TABLE 5-3 ■ Summary of Personality, Cognitive, and Moral Development Theories

STAGE/AGE	PSYCHOSEXUAL	PSYCHOSOCIAL (ERIKSON)	COGNITIVE STAGES (PIAGET)	MORAL JUDGMENT STAGES (KOHLBERG)
I Infancy *Birth to 1 year*	Oral-sensory	Trust vs mistrust	Sensorimotor (birth to 2 years)	
II Toddlerhood *1-3 years*	Anal-urethral	Autonomy vs shame and doubt	Preoperational thought, pre-conceptual phase (transductive reasoning [e.g., specific to specific]) (2-4 years)	Preconventional (premoral) level Punishment and obedience orientation
III Early childhood *3-6 years*	Phallic-locomotion	Initiative vs guilt	Preoperational thought, intuitive phase (transductive reasoning) (4-7 years)	Preconventional (premoral) level Naive instrumental orientation
IV Middle childhood *6-12 years*	Latency	Industry vs inferiority	Concrete operations (inductive reasoning and beginning logic) (7-11 years)	Conventional level Good-boy, nice-girl orientation Law-and-order orientation
V Adolescence *12-18 years*	Genitality	Identity and repudiation vs identity confusion	Formal operations (deductive and abstract reasoning) (11-15 years)	Postconventional or principled level Social-contract orientation Universal ethical principle orientation (no longer included in revised theory)

*Yearly height and weight gains for each age-group represent averaged estimates from a variety of sources.
†Jung and Czajka-Narins, 1985.

ing. Much of their learning is acquired through imitating the activities and behavior of others. Negative feelings of *doubt* and *shame* arise when children are made to feel small and self-conscious, when their choices are disastrous, when others shame them, or when they are forced to be dependent in areas in which they are capable of assuming control. The favorable outcomes are *self-control* and *willpower.*

Initiative vs guilt (3 to 6 years). The stage of *initiative* corresponds to Freud's phallic stage and is characterized by vigorous, intrusive behavior, enterprise, and a strong imagination. Children explore the physical world with all their senses and powers. They develop a conscience. No longer guided only by outsiders, there is an inner voice that warns and threatens. Children sometimes undertake goals or activities that are in conflict with those of parents or others, and being made to feel that their activities or imaginings are bad produces a sense of *guilt.* Children must learn to retain a sense of initiative without impinging on the rights and privileges of others. The lasting outcomes are *direction* and *purpose.*

Industry vs inferiority (6 to 12 years). The stage of *industry* is the latency period of Freud. Having achieved the more crucial stages in personality development, children are ready to be workers and producers. They want to engage in tasks and activities that they can carry through to completion; they need and want real achievement. Children learn to compete and cooperate with others, and they learn the rules. It is a decisive period in their social relationships with others. Feelings of *inadequacy* and *inferiority* may develop if too much is expected of them or if they believe that they cannot measure up to the standards set for them by others. The ego quality developed from a sense of industry is *competence.*

Identity vs role confusion (12 to 18 years). Corresponding to Freud's genital period, the development of *identity* is characterized by rapid and marked physical changes. Previous trust in their bodies is shaken, and children become overly preoccupied with the way they appear in the eyes of others as compared with their own self-concept. Adolescents struggle to fit the roles they have played and those they hope to play with the current roles and fashions adopted by their peers, to integrate their concepts and values with those of society, and to come to a decision regarding an occupation. Inability to solve the core conflict results in *role confusion.* The outcome of successful mastery is *devotion* and *fidelity* to others and to values and ideologies.

THEORETIC FOUNDATIONS OF MENTAL DEVELOPMENT

The term *cognition* refers to the process by which developing individuals become acquainted with the world and the objects it contains. Children are born with inherited potentials for intellectual growth, but they must develop into that potential through interaction with the environment. By assimilating information through the senses, processing it, and acting on it, they come to understand relationships between objects and between themselves and their world. With cognitive development, children acquire the ability to reason abstractly, to think in a logical manner, and to organize intellectual functions or performances into higher order structures. Language, morals, and spiritual development emerge as cognitive abilities advance.

Cognitive Development (Piaget)

Cognitive development consists of age-related changes that occur in mental activities. The best-known theory regarding children's thinking, and a more comprehensive developmental theory than those already described, was developed by the Swiss psychologist Jean Piaget (1969). According to Piaget, intelligence enables individuals to make adaptations to the environment that increase the probability of survival, and through their behavior individuals establish and maintain equilibrium with the environment.

Piaget proposed three stages of reasoning: (1) intuitive, (2) concrete operational, and (3) formal operational. When they enter the stage of concrete logical thought at about age 7 years, children are able to make logical inferences, classify, and deal with quantitative relationships about concrete things. Not until adolescence are they able to reason abstractly with any degree of competence. Each stage is derived from and builds on the accomplishments of the previous stage in a continuous, orderly process. The course of intellectual development is both maturational and invariant and is divided into the following stages (ages are approximate):

Sensorimotor (birth to 2 years). The sensorimotor stage of intellectual development consists of six substages (see pp. 314 and 392) that are governed by sensations in which simple learning takes place. Children progress from reflex activity through simple repetitive behaviors to imitative behavior. They develop a sense of "cause-and-effect" as they direct behavior toward objects. Problem solving is primarily trial and error. They display a high level of curiosity, experimentation, and enjoyment of novelty and begin to develop a sense of self as they are able to differentiate themselves from their environment. They become aware that objects have *permanence*—that an object exists even though it is no longer visible. Toward the end of the sensorimotor period children begin to use language and representational thought.

Preoperational (2 to 7 years). The predominant characteristic of the preoperational stage of intellectual development is *egocentrism,* which in this sense does not mean selfishness or self-centeredness, but the inability to put oneself in the place of another. Children interpret objects and events, not in terms of general properties, but in terms of their relationships or their use to them. They are unable to see things from any perspective other than their own; they cannot see another's point of view, nor can they see any reason to do so (see Cognitive Development [Piaget], Chapter 13).

Preoperational thinking is concrete and tangible. Children cannot reason beyond the observable, and they lack the ability to make deductions or generalizations. Thought is dominated by what they see, hear, or otherwise experience. However, they are increasingly able to use language and symbols to represent objects in their environment. Through imaginative play, questioning, and other interacting, they begin to elaborate concepts and to make simple associations between ideas. In the latter stage of this period their reasoning is *intuitive* (e.g., the stars have to go to bed just as they do) and they are only beginning to deal with problems of weight, length, size, and time. Reasoning is also *transductive*—because two events occur together, they cause each other, or knowledge of one characteristic is transferred to another (e.g., all women with big bellies have babies).

Concrete operations (7 to 11 years). At this age thought becomes increasingly logical and coherent. Children are able to classify, sort, order, and otherwise organize facts about the world to use in problem solving. They develop a new concept of permanence—*conservation* (see Cognitive Development [Piaget], Chapter 16). That is, they realize that physical factors such as volume, weight, and number remain the same even though outward appearances are changed. They are able to deal with a number of different aspects of a situation simultaneously. They do not have the capacity to deal in abstraction; they solve problems in a concrete, systematic fashion based on what they can perceive. Reasoning is *inductive.* Through progressive changes in thought processes and relationships with others, thought becomes less self-centered. They can consider points of view other than their own. Thinking has become socialized.

Formal operations (11 to 15 years). Formal operational thought is characterized by adaptability and flexibility. Adolescents can think in abstract terms, use abstract symbols, and draw logical conclusions from a set of observations. For example, they can solve the following question: If A is larger than B, and B is larger than C, which symbol is the largest? (The answer is A.) They can make hypotheses and test them; they can consider abstract, theoretic, and philosophic matters. Although they may confuse the ideal with the practical, most contradictions in the world can be dealt with and resolved.

Language Development

Children are born with the mechanism and capacity to develop speech and language skills. However, they will not speak spontaneously. The environment must provide a means for them to acquire these skills. Speech requires intact physiologic structure and function (including respiratory, auditory, and cerebral) plus intelligence, a need to communicate, and stimulation.

The rate of speech development varies from child to child and is directly related to neurologic competence and cognitive development. Gesture precedes speech, and in this way a small child communicates satisfactorily. As speech develops, gesture recedes but never disappears entirely. At all stages of language development, children's comprehension vocabulary (what they understand) is greater than their expressed vocabulary (what they can say), and this development reflects a continuing process of modification that involves both the acquisition of new words and the expanding and refining of word meanings previously learned. By the time they begin to walk, children are able to attach a name to objects and persons.

The first parts of speech used are nouns, sometimes verbs (e.g., "go"), and combination words (such as "bye-bye"). Responses are usually structurally incomplete during the toddler period, although the meaning is clear. Next they begin to use adjectives and adverbs to qualify nouns, followed by adverbs to qualify nouns and verbs. Later, pronouns and gender words are added (such as "he" and "she"). By the time children enter school, they are able to use simple, structurally complete sentences that average five to seven words.

Moral Development (Kohlberg)

Children also acquire moral reasoning in a developmental sequence. Moral development, as described by Kohlberg (1968), is based on cognitive developmental theory and consists of the following three major levels, each of which has two stages:

Preconventional level. The preconventional level of moral development parallels the preoperational level of cognitive development and intuitive thought. Culturally oriented to the labels of good/bad and right/wrong, children integrate these in terms of the physical or pleasurable consequences of their actions. At first children determine the goodness or badness of an action in terms of its consequences. They avoid punishment and obey without question those who have the power to determine and enforce the rules and labels. They have no concept of the basic moral order that supports these consequences. Later, children determine that the right behavior consists of that which satisfies their own needs (and sometimes the needs of others). Although elements of fairness, give and take, and equal sharing are evident, they are interpreted in a very practical, concrete manner without loyalty, gratitude, or justice.

Conventional level. At the conventional stage children are concerned with conformity and loyalty. They value the maintenance of family, group, or national expectations regardless of consequences. Behavior that meets with approval and pleases or helps others is considered to be good. One earns approval by being "nice." Obeying the rules, doing one's duty, showing respect for authority, and maintaining the social order is the correct behavior. This level is correlated with the stage of concrete operations in cognitive development.

Postconventional, autonomous, or principled level. At the postconventional level the individual has reached the cognitive stage of formal operations. Correct behavior tends to be defined in terms of general individual rights and standards that have been examined and agreed on by the entire society. Although procedural rules for reaching consensus become important with emphasis on the legal point of view, there is also emphasis on the possibility for changing law in terms of societal needs and rational considerations.

The most advanced level of moral development is one in which self-chosen ethical principles guide decisions of conscience. These are abstract and ethical but universal principles of justice and human rights with respect for the dignity of persons as individuals. It is believed that few persons reach this stage of moral reasoning.

Spiritual Development

Spiritual beliefs are closely related to the moral and ethical portion of the child's self-concept and, as such, must be considered as part of the child's basic needs assessment. Children need to have meaning, purpose, and hope in their lives. Also, the need for confession and forgiveness is present, even in very young children. Extending beyond religion (an organized set of beliefs and practices), spirituality affects the whole person: mind, body, and spirit. Fowler (1974) has identified seven stages in the development of faith, four of which are closely associated with and parallel cognitive and psychosocial development in childhood:

Stage 0: Undifferentiated. This stage of development encompasses the period of infancy during which children have no concept of right or wrong, no beliefs, and no convictions to guide their behavior. However, the beginnings of a faith are established with the development of basic trust through their relationships with the primary caregiver.

Stage 1: Intuitive-projective. Toddlerhood is primarily a time of imitating the behavior of others. Children imitate the religious gestures and behaviors of others without comprehending any meaning or significance to the activities. During the preschool years children assimilate some of the values and beliefs of their parents. Parental attitudes toward moral codes and religious beliefs convey to children what they consider to be good and bad. Children still imitate behavior at this age and follow parental beliefs as part of their daily lives rather than through an understanding of their basic concepts.

Stage 2: Mythical-literal. Through the school-age years, spiritual development parallels cognitive development and is closely related to children's experiences and social interaction. Most have a strong interest in religion during the school-age years. The existence of a deity is accepted, and petitions to an omnipotent being are important and expected to be answered; good behavior is rewarded, and bad behavior is punished. Their developing conscience bothers them when they disobey. They have a reverence for thoughts and matters and are able to articulate their faith. They may even question its validity.

Stage 3: Synthetic-convention. As children approach adolescence, however, they become increasingly aware of spiritual disappointments. They recognize that prayers are not always answered (at least on their own terms) and may begin to abandon or modify some religious practices. They begin to reason, to question some of the established parental religious standards, and to drop or modify some religious practices.

Stage 4: Individuating-reflexive. Adolescents become more skeptical and begin to compare the religious standards of their parents with those of others. They attempt to determine which to adopt and incorporate into their own set of values. They also begin to compare religious standards with the scientific viewpoint. It is a time of searching rather than reaching. Adolescents are uncertain about many religious ideas but will not achieve profound insights until late adolescence or early adulthood.

DEVELOPMENT OF SELF-CONCEPT

Self-concept is how an individual describes himself or herself (Willoughby, King, and Polatajko, 1996). The term *self-concept* includes all the notions, beliefs, and convictions that constitute an individual's self-knowledge and that influence that individual's relationships with others. It is not present at birth but develops gradually as a result of unique experiences within the self, with significant others, and with the realities of the world. However, an individual's self-concept may or may not reflect reality.

In infancy the self-concept is primarily an awareness of one's independent existence learned in part as a result of social contacts and experiences with others. The process becomes more active during toddlerhood as children explore the limits of their capacities and the nature of their impact on others. School-age children are more aware of differences among people, are more sensitive to social pressures, and become more preoccupied with issues of self-criticism and self-evaluation. During early adolescence children focus more on physical and emotional changes taking place and on peer acceptance. The self-concept is crystallized during later adolescence as young people organize their self-concept around a set of values, goals, and competencies acquired throughout childhood.

Body Image

A vital component of self-concept, *body image* refers to the subjective concepts and attitudes that individuals have toward their own bodies. It consists of the physiologic (the perception of one's physical characteristics), psychologic (values and attitudes toward the body, abilities, and ideals), and social nature of one's image of self (the self in relation to others). All three of the components interrelate with each other. Body image is a complex phenomenon that evolves and changes during the process of growth and development. Any actual or perceived deviation from the "norm" (no matter how this is interpreted) is cause for concern. The extent to which a characteristic, defect, or disease affects children's body image is influenced by the attitudes and behavior of those around them.

The significant others in their lives exert the most important and meaningful impact on children's body image. Labels that are attached to them (such as "skinny," "pretty," or "fat") or body parts (such as "ugly mole," "bug eyes," or "yucky skin") are incorporated into the body image. Because they lack the understanding of deviations from the physical standard or norm, children notice prominent differences in others and unwittingly make "rude" and often cruel remarks about such minor deviations as large or widely spaced front teeth, large or small eyes, moles, or extreme variations in height.

Infants receive input about their bodies through self-exploration and sensory stimulation from others. As they begin to manipulate their environment, they become aware of their bodies as separate from others. Toddlers learn to identify the various parts of their bodies and are able to use symbols to represent objects. Preschoolers become aware of the wholeness of their bodies and discover the genitals. Exploration of the genitals and the discovery of differences between the sexes become important. There is only a vague concept of internal organs and function (Laraia and Stuart, 2000; Selekman, 1983).

School-age children begin to learn about internal body structure and function and become aware of differences in body size and configuration. They are highly influenced by the cultural norms of society and current fads. Children whose bodies deviate from the norm are often criticized or ridiculed.

Adolescence is the age when children become most concerned about the physical self. The unfamiliar body changes and the new physical self must be integrated into the self-concept. Adolescents face conflicts over what they see and what they visualize as the ideal body structure. Body image formation during adolescence is a crucial element in the shaping of identity, the psychosocial crisis of adolescence.

Self-Esteem

Self-esteem is the value that an individual places on oneself and refers to an overall evaluation of oneself (Willoughby, King, and Polatajko, 1996). Self-esteem is described as the affective component of the self, whereas self-concept is the cognitive component; however, the two terms are almost indistinguishable and are often used interchangeably.

The term *self-esteem* refers to a personal, subjective judgment of one's worthiness derived from and influenced by the social groups in the immediate environment and individuals' perceptions of how they are valued by others. Self-esteem changes with development. Highly egocentric toddlers are unaware of any difference between competence and social approval. On the other hand, preschool and early school-age children are increasingly aware of the discrepancy between

their competencies and the abilities of more advanced children. Being accepted by adults and peers outside the family group becomes more important to them. Positive feedback enhances their self-esteem; they are vulnerable to feelings of worthlessness and are anxious about failure.

As children's competencies increase and they develop meaningful relationships, their self-esteem rises. Their self-esteem is again at risk during early adolescence when they are defining an identity and sense of self in the context of their peer group. Unless children are continually made to feel incompetent and of little worth, a decrease in self-esteem during vulnerable times is only temporary. Children assess the following aspects of themselves in forming an overall evaluation of their self-esteem (Sieving and Zirbel-Donisch, 1990):

> **Competence:** How adequate are my cognitive, physical, and social skills?
> **Sense of control:** How well can I complete tasks needed to produce desired actions? Is someone or something specific vs luck or chance responsible for my successes and failures?
> **Moral worth:** How closely do my actions and behaviors meet moral standards that have been set?
> **Worthiness of love and acceptance:** How worthy am I of love and acceptance from parents, other significant adults, siblings, and peers?

Factors that influence the formation of a child's self-esteem include (1) the child's temperament and personality, (2) abilities and opportunities available to accomplish age-appropriate developmental tasks, (3) significant others, and (4) social roles assumed and the expectations of these roles (see also Psychosocial History, Chapter 6).

ROLE OF PLAY IN DEVELOPMENT

Through the universal medium of play children learn what no one can teach them. They learn about their world and how to deal with this environment of objects, time, space, structure, and people. They learn about themselves operating within that environment—what they can do, how to relate to things and situations, and how to adapt themselves to the demands society makes on them. Play is the *work* of the child. In play, children continually practice the complicated, stressful processes of living, communicating, and achieving satisfactory relationships with other people.

CLASSIFICATION OF PLAY

From a developmental point of view, patterns of children's play can be categorized according to content and social character. In both there is an additive effect; each builds on past accomplishments, and some element of each is maintained throughout life. At each stage in development the new predominates.

CONTENT OF PLAY

The content of play involves primarily the physical aspects of play, although social relationships cannot be ignored. The content of play follows the directional trend of the simple to the complex:

> **Social-affective play.** Play begins with social-affective play, wherein infants take pleasure in relationships with people.

As adults talk, touch, nuzzle, and in various ways elicit a response from an infant, the infant soon learns to provoke parental emotions and responses with such behaviors as smiling, cooing, or initiating games and activities. The type and intensity of the adult behavior with children vary among cultures.

Sense-pleasure play. Sense-pleasure play is a nonsocial stimulating experience that originates from without. Objects in the environment—light and color, tastes and odors, textures and consistencies—attract children's attention, stimulate their senses, and give pleasure. Pleasurable experiences are derived from handling raw materials (water, sand, food), from body motion (swinging, bouncing, rocking), and from other uses of senses and abilities (smelling, humming; Fig. 5-5).

Skill play. After infants have developed the ability to grasp and manipulate, they persistently demonstrate and exercise their newly acquired abilities through skill play, repeating an action over and over again. The element of sense-pleasure play is often evident in the practicing of a new ability, but all too frequently the determination to conquer the elusive skill produces pain and frustration (e.g., learning to ride a bicycle).

Unoccupied behavior. In unoccupied behavior children are not playful but focusing their attention momentarily on anything that strikes their interest. Children daydream, fiddle with clothes or other objects, or walk aimlessly. This role differs from that of onlookers, who actively observe the activity of others.

Dramatic, or pretend, play. One of the vital elements in children's process of identification is dramatic play, also known as symbolic or pretend play. It begins in late infancy (11 to 13 months) and is the predominant form of play in the preschool child. After children begin to invest situations and people with meanings and to attribute affective significance to the world, they can pretend and fantasize almost anything. By acting out events of daily life, children learn and practice the roles and identities modeled by the members of their family and society. Children's toys, replicas of the tools of society, provide a medium for learning about adult roles and activities that may be puzzling and frustrating to them. Interacting with the world is one way children get to know it. The simple, imitative, dramatic play of the toddler, such as using the telephone, driving a car, or rocking a doll, evolves into more complex, sustained dramas of the preschooler, which extend beyond common domestic matters to the wider aspects of the world and the society, such as playing police officer, storekeeper, teacher, or nurse. Older children work out elaborate themes, act out stories, and compose plays (Fig. 5-6).

Games. Children in all cultures engage in games alone and with others. Solitary activity involving games begins as very small children participate in repetitive activities and progress to more complicated games that challenge their independent skills such as puzzle solving, solitaire, and computer or video games. Very young children participate in simple, *imitative games* such as pat-a-cake and peekaboo. Preschool children learn and enjoy *formal games* that begin with ritualistic, self-sustaining games such as ring-around-a-rosy and London Bridge. With the exception of some simple board games, preschool children do not engage in *competitive games.* Preschoolers hate to lose and will try to cheat, want to change rules, or demand exceptions and opportunities to change their moves. School-age children and adolescents enjoy competitive games, including cards, checkers, chess, and physically active games such as baseball.

SOCIAL CHARACTER OF PLAY

The play interactions of infancy are between the child and an adult. Children continue to enjoy the company of an adult but are increasingly able to play alone. As age advances, interaction with age-mates increases in importance and becomes an essential part of the socialization process. Through interaction, highly egocentric infants, unable to tolerate delay or interference, ultimately acquire concern for others and the ability to delay gratification or even to reject gratification at the expense of another. A pair of toddlers will engage in considerable combat because their personal needs cannot tolerate delay or compromise. By the time

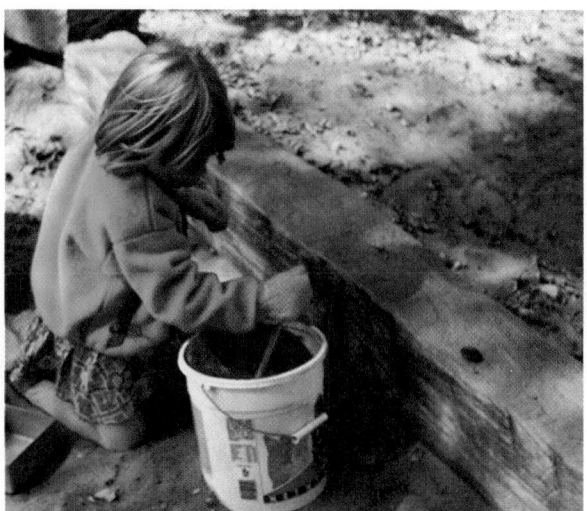

FIG. 5-5 ■ Children derive pleasure from handling raw materials.

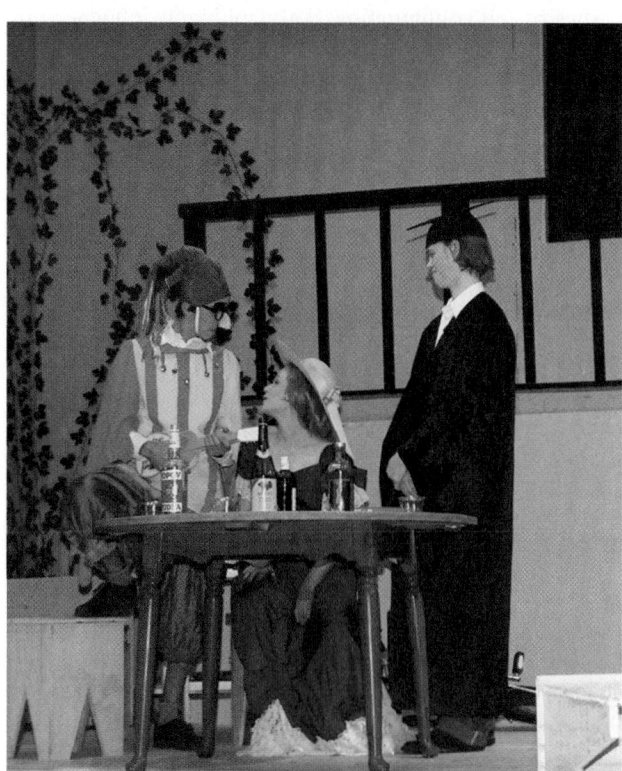

FIG. 5-6 ■ Older children enjoy being in plays.

they reach age 5 or 6 years, children are able to arrive at a compromise or make use of arbitration, usually after they have attempted but failed to gain their own way. Through continued interaction with peers and the growth of conceptual abilities and social skills, children are able to increase participation with others in the following types of play:

Onlooker play. During onlooker play, children watch what other children are doing but make no attempt to enter into the play activity. There is an active interest in observing the interaction of others but no movement toward participating. Watching an older sibling bounce a ball is a common example of the onlooker role.

Solitary play. During solitary play, children play alone with toys different from those used by other children in the same area. They enjoy the presence of other children but make no effort to get close to or speak to them. Their interest is centered on their own activity, which they pursue with no reference to the activities of the others.

Parallel play. During parallel activities children play independently but among other children. They play with toys like those the children around them are using, but as each child sees fit, neither influencing nor being influenced by the other children. Each plays beside, but not with, other children (Fig. 5-7). There is no group association. Parallel play is the characteristic play of toddlers, but it may also occur in other groups of any age. Individuals who are involved in a creative craft with each person separately working on an individual project are engaged in parallel play.

Associative play. In associative play, children play together and are engaged in a similar or even identical activity, but there is no organization, division of labor, leadership assignment, or mutual goal. Children borrow and lend play materials, follow each other with wagons and tricycles, and sometimes attempt to control who may or may not play in the group. Each child acts according to his or her own wishes; there is no group goal (Fig. 5-8). For example, two children play with dolls, borrowing articles of clothing from each other and engaging in similar conversation, but neither directs the other's actions or establishes rules regarding the limits of the play session. There is a great deal of behavioral contagion: when one child initiates an activity, the entire group follows the example.

Cooperative play. Cooperative play is organized, and children play in a group *with* other children (Fig. 5-9). They discuss and plan activities for the purposes of accomplishing an end—to make something, to attain a competitive goal, to dramatize situations of adult or group life, or to play formal games. The group is loosely formed, but there is a marked sense of belonging or not belonging. The goal and its attainment require organization of activities, division of labor, and playing roles. The leader-follower relationship is definitely established, and the activity is controlled by one or two members who assign roles and direct the activity of the others. The activity is organized to allow one child to supplement another's function in order to complete the goal.

FUNCTIONS OF PLAY
Sensorimotor Development

Sensorimotor activity is a major component of play at all ages and is the predominant form of play in infancy. Active play is essential for muscle development and serves a useful

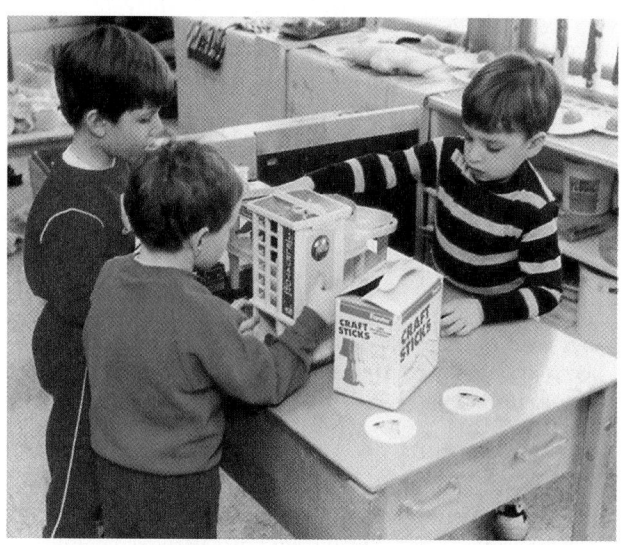

FIG. 5-8 ■ Associative play.

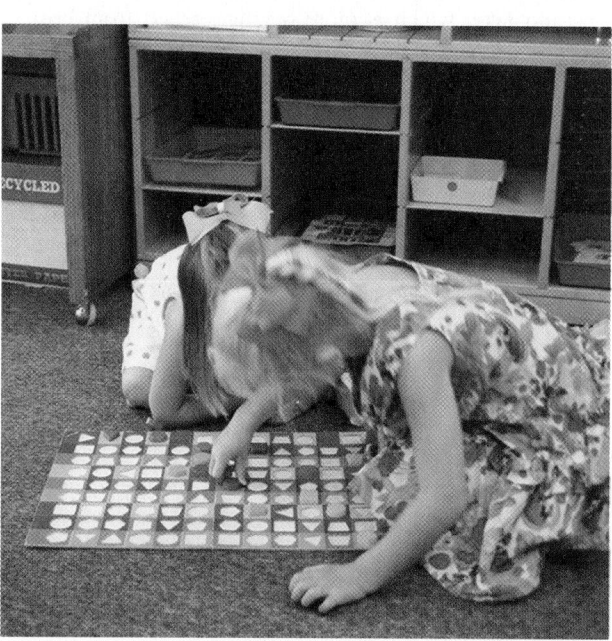

FIG. 5-9 ■ Cooperative play.

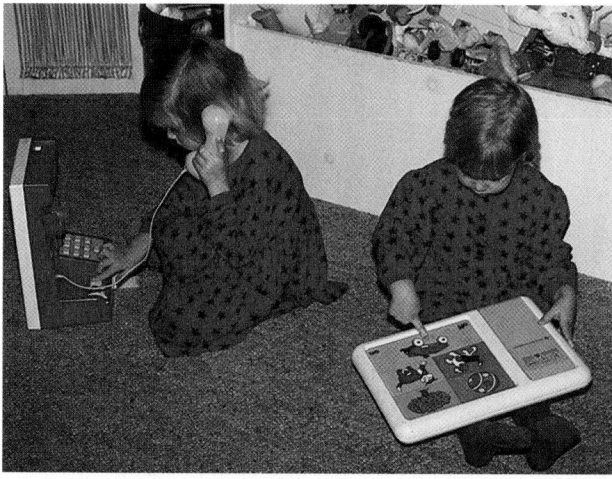

FIG. 5-7 ■ Parallel play.

purpose as a release for surplus energy. Through sensorimotor play, children explore the nature of the physical world. Infants gain impressions of themselves and their world through tactile, auditory, visual, and kinesthetic stimulation. Toddlers and preschoolers revel in body movement and exploration of things in space. With increasing maturity sensorimotor play becomes more differentiated and involved. Whereas very young children run for the sheer joy of body movement, older children incorporate or modify the motions into increasingly complex and coordinated activities such as races, games, roller skating, and bicycle riding.

Intellectual Development

Through exploration and manipulation children learn colors, shapes, sizes, textures, and the significance of objects. They learn the significance of numbers and how to use them; they learn to associate words with objects; and they develop an understanding of abstract concepts and spatial relationships, such as *up, down, under,* and *over.* Activities such as puzzles and games help them develop problem-solving skills. Books, stories, films, and collections expand knowledge and provide enjoyment as well. Play provides a means to practice and expand language skills. Through play, children continually rehearse past experiences to assimilate them into new perceptions and relationships. Play helps children comprehend the world in which they live and distinguish between fantasy and reality.

> **NURSING TIP**
>
> Toys need to have several levels of challenge to keep from becoming obsolete too quickly, such as the Balls in a Bowl (Chase, 1994).

Socialization

From very early infancy children show interest and pleasure in the company of others. Their initial social contact is with the mothering person, but through play with other children they learn to establish social relationships and solve the problems associated with these relationships. They learn to give and take, which is more readily learned from critical peers than from the more tolerant adults. They learn the sex role that society expects them to fulfill, as well as approved patterns of behavior and deportment. Closely associated with socialization is development of moral values and ethics. Children learn right from wrong, the standards of the society, and to assume responsibility for their actions.

Creativity

In no other situation is there more opportunity to be creative than in play. Children can experiment and try out their ideas in play through every medium at their disposal, including raw materials, fantasy, and exploration. Creativity is stifled by pressure toward conformity; therefore, striving for peer approval may inhibit creative endeavors in the school-age or adolescent child. Creativity is primarily a product of solitary activity; yet, creative thinking is often enhanced in group settings where listening to others' ideas stimulates further exploration of one's own ideas. After children feel the satisfaction of creating something new and different, they transfer this creative interest to situations outside the world of play.

Self-Awareness

Beginning with active explorations of their bodies and awareness of themselves as separate from the mother, the process of self-identity is facilitated through play activities. Children learn who they are and their place in the world. They become increasingly able to regulate their own behavior, to learn what their abilities are, and to compare their abilities with those of others. Through play, children are able to test their abilities, to assume and try out various roles, and to learn the effect their behavior has on others.

Therapeutic Value

Play is therapeutic at any age (Fig. 5-10). It provides a means for release from the tension and stress encountered in the environment. In play, children can express emotions and release unacceptable impulses in a socially acceptable fashion. Children are able to experiment and test fearful situations and can assume and vicariously master the roles and positions that they are unable to perform in the world of reality. Children reveal much about themselves in play. Through play, children are able to communicate to the alert observer the needs, fears, and desires that they are unable to express with their limited language skills. Throughout their play, children need the acceptance of adults and their presence to help them control aggression and to channel their destructive tendencies.

Moral Value

Although children learn at home and at school those behaviors considered right and wrong in the culture, the in-

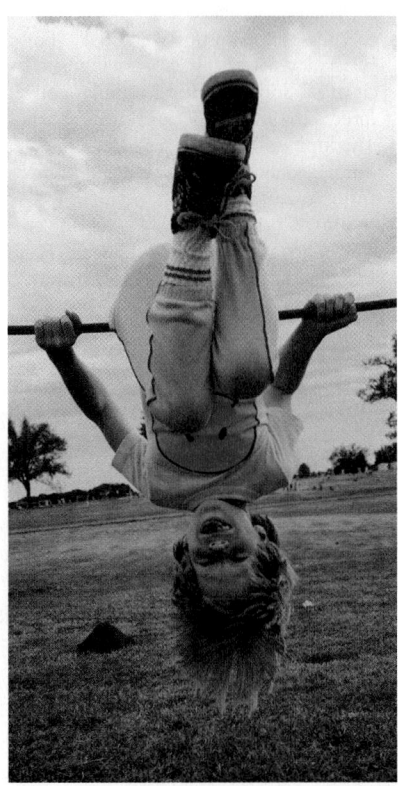

FIG. 5-10 ■ Play is therapeutic at any age and provides a means for release of tension and stress in the environment.

teraction with peers during play contributes significantly to their moral training. Nowhere is the enforcement of moral standards so rigid as in the play situation. If they are to be acceptable members of the group, children must adhere to the accepted codes of behavior of the culture (e.g., fairness, honesty, self-control, consideration for others). Children soon learn that their peers are less tolerant of violations than are adults and that to maintain a place in the play group they must conform to the standards of the group.

TOYS

The type of toys chosen by or provided for children can support and enhance the child's development in the areas just described. Although there is a lack scientific evidence that any toy is necessary for optimal learning, toys offer an opportunity to bring the child and parent together. Research has indicated that a positive parent-child interaction can enhance early childhood brain development (Glassey and others, 2003). Toys that are small replicas of the culture and its tools help children assimilate their culture. Toys that require pushing, pulling, rolling, and manipulating teach them about physical properties of the items and help to develop muscles and coordination. Rules and the basic elements of cooperation and organization are learned through board games.

Because they can be used in a variety of ways, raw materials with which children can exercise their own creativity and imaginations are sometimes superior to ready-made items. For example, building blocks can be used to construct a variety of things, to count, and to learn shapes and sizes.

Toy Safety

Selection of toys and play equipment is a joint effort between parents and children, but evaluation of their safety is the responsibility of the adult. Government agencies do not inspect and police all toys on the market. Therefore, adults who purchase, supervise purchases, or allow children to use play equipment need to evaluate such equipment for its safety, including toys that are gifts or those that are purchased by the children themselves (see Family Home Care box). They should also be alert to notices of toys determined to be defective and recalled by the manufacturers. Parents and health workers can obtain information on a variety of recalled products and can report potentially dangerous toys and child products to the **U.S. Consumer Product Safety Commission (CPSC)*** or, in Canada, the **Canadian Toy Testing Council.**†

SELECTED FACTORS THAT INFLUENCE DEVELOPMENT

HEREDITY

Inherited characteristics have a profound influence on development. The sex of the child, determined by random selection at the time of conception, directs both the pattern of growth and the behavior of others toward the child. In all cultures, attitudes and expectations are different with respect to the sex of the child. Sex and other hereditary determinants strongly affect the end result of growth and the rate of progress toward it. There is a high correlation between parent and child with regard to traits such as height, weight, and rate of growth. Most physical characteristics, including shape and form of features, body build, and physical peculiarities, are inherited and can influence the way in which children grow and interact with their environment. Many dimensions of personality, such as temperament, activity level, responsiveness, and a tendency toward shyness, are believed to be inherited.

Differences in health and vigor of children may be attributed to hereditary traits. An inherited physical or mental disorder will alter or modify a child's physical or emotional growth and interactions. The extent to which disabling conditions interfere with the child's growth and well-being is considered in relation to numerous disabilities throughout the remainder of the book.

NEUROENDOCRINE FACTORS

It has been suggested there may be a growth center in the hypothalamic region responsible for maintaining genetically determined growth patterns. Some functional relationship is believed to exist between the hypothalamus and the endocrine system that influences growth. There is also evidence, based on observations of denervated skeletal muscles, that the peripheral nervous system may influence growth, because muscles deprived of nerve supply degenerate. Many of these effects are not sufficiently explained by disuse or diminished blood supply.

Probably all hormones affect growth in some fashion. Three hormones—growth hormone, thyroid hormone, and androgens—when given to persons deficient in these hormones, stimulate protein anabolism and thereby produce retention of elements essential for building protoplasm and bony tissue. It appears that each of the hormones that has a significant influence on growth manifests its major effect at a different period of growth (see Chapter 29).

NUTRITION

Nutrition is probably the single most important influence on growth. Dietary factors regulate growth at all stages of development, and their effects are exerted in numerous and complex ways. During the rapid prenatal growth period, poor nutrition may influence development from the time of implantation of the ovum until birth. During infancy and childhood the demand for calories is relatively great, as evidenced by the rapid increase in both height and weight. At this time protein and caloric requirements are higher than at almost any period of postnatal development. As the growth rate slows, with its concomitant decrease in metabolism, there is a corresponding reduction in caloric and protein requirements (see Table 5-2).

Growth is uneven during the periods of childhood between infancy and adolescence when there are plateaus and small growth spurts. The child's appetite will fluctuate in response to these variations until the turbulent growth spurt of adolescence, when adequate nutrition is extremely important but may be subjected to numerous emotional influences. Adequate nutrition is closely related to good health

---

*CPSC hotline: (800) 638-CPSC; website: www.cpsc.gov.
†22 Hamilton Avenue North, Ottawa, Ontario, Canada K1Y 1V6; (613) 729-7101.

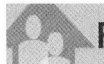 **FAMILY HOME CARE**

Toy Safety*

SELECTION

Select toys that suit the skills, abilities, and interests of children.

Select toys that are safe for the specific child; look for a label that indicates the intended age-group. Toys that are safe for one age may not be safe for another.

For infants, toddlers, and all children who still mouth objects, avoid toys with small parts that may pose a fatal choking or aspiration hazard. Toys in this category are usually labeled, "Not recommended for children under 3 years."

For infants avoid toys with strings or cords that are 7 inches or longer because they may cause strangulation.

For all children younger than 8 years avoid electric toys with heating elements.

For children younger than 5 years avoid arrows or darts.

Check for safety labels such as "flame retardant" or "flame resistant."

Select toys durable enough to survive rough play; look for sturdy construction such as tightly secured eyes, nose, or any small parts.

Select toys light enough that they will not cause harm if one falls on a child.

Look for toys with smooth, rounded edges. Avoid toys with sharp edges that can cut or that have sharp points. Points on the inside of the toy can puncture if the toy is broken.

Avoid toys with any shooting or throwing objects that can injure eyes.

This includes toys with which other missiles such as sticks or pebbles might be used as substitutes for the intended projectiles.

Arrows and darts used by children should have blunt tips and be manufactured from resilient materials; make certain the tips are securely attached.

Make certain that materials in toys are nontoxic.

Avoid toys that make loud noises that might be damaging to a child's hearing.

Even some squeaking toys are too loud when held close to the ear.

If selecting caps for cap guns, look for the label required by federal law to be on boxes or packages of caps, which states: "Warning—Do not fire closer than 1 foot to the ear. Do not use indoors."

If selecting a toy gun, be certain that the barrel or the entire gun is brightly colored to avoid being mistaken for a real gun.

Check toy instructions for clarity. They should be clear to an adult and, when appropriate, to the child.

SUPERVISION

Maintain a safe play environment.

Remove and discard plastic wrappings on toys immediately; they could suffocate a child.

Remove large toys, bumper pads, and boxes from playpens; an adventuresome child can use such items as a means of climbing or falling out.

Set "ground rules" for play.

Supervise young children closely during play.

Teach children how to use toys properly and safely.

Instruct older children to keep their toys away from younger brothers, sisters, and friends.

Keep children who are playing with riding toys away from stairs, hills, traffic, and swimming pools.

Establish and enforce rules regarding protective gear.

Insist that children wear helmets when using bicycles, skateboards, or in-line skates.

Insist that children wear gloves and wrist, elbow, and knee pads when using skateboards or in-line skates.

Instruct children on electrical safety.

Teach children the proper way to unplug an electric toy—pull on the plug, not the cord.

Teach children to beware of electrical appliances and even electrically operated playthings; often children are unfamiliar with the hazards of electricity in association with water.

Teach children the safe use of utensils that under certain circumstances can cause injury—scissors, knives, needles, heating elements, or loops, long string, or cord.

MAINTENANCE

Inspect old and new toys regularly for breakage, loose parts, and other potential hazards.

Look for jagged or sharp edges or broken parts that might constitute a choking hazard.

Check movable parts to make certain they are attached securely to the toys; sometimes pieces that are safe when attached to the toy become a danger when detached.

Examine all outdoor toys regularly for rust and weak or sharp parts that could become a danger to a child.

Check electrical cords and plugs for cracked or fraying parts.

Maintain toys in good repair, without signs of possible hazards such as sharp edges, splinters, weak seams, or rust.

Make repairs immediately, or discard out of reach of children.

Sand sharp wooden toys or splintered surfaces so they are smooth.

Use only paint labeled "nontoxic" to repaint toys, toy boxes, or children's furniture.

STORAGE

Provide a safe place for children to store toys.

Select a toy chest or toy box that is ventilated, is free of self-locking devices that could trap a child inside, and has a lid designed not to pinch a child's fingers or fall on a child's head.

To avoid entrapment and suffocation, containers other than toy chests used for storage purposes should be fitted with spring-loaded support devices if they have a hinged lid.

Teach children to store toys safely to prevent accidental injury from stepping, tripping, or falling on a toy.

Playthings meant for older children and adults should be safely stowed away on high shelves, in locked closets, or in other areas unavailable to younger children.

*Another helpful resource is *Toy safety: guidelines for parents* from American Academy of Pediatrics, Division of Publications, 141 Northwest Point Boulevard, Elk Grove Village, IL 60007; (888) 227-1770; fax (847) 228-1281; website: www.aap.org.

COMMUNITY FOCUS

Healthy Food Choices

Current research indicates that new lower-fat recipes in school lunch programs are well accepted by children (Borja, Bordi, and Lambert, 1996). However, children who were informed about healthier food choices did not consistently select healthier items (Colizza and Colvin, 1995).

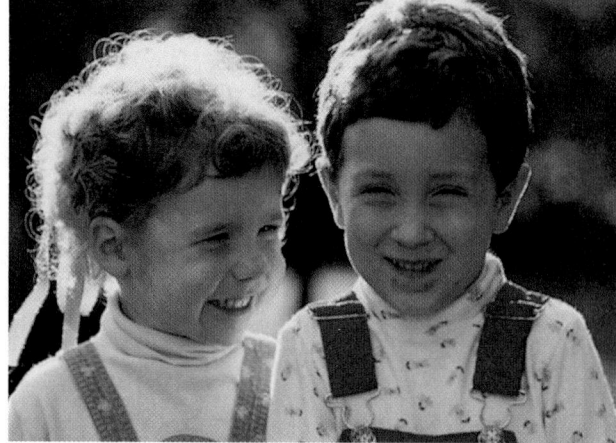

FIG. 5-11 ■ Peers become increasingly important as children develop friendships outside the family group.

throughout life, and an overall improvement in nourishment is evidenced by the gradual increase in size and early maturation of children in this century (see Community Focus box).

INTERPERSONAL RELATIONSHIPS

Relationships with significant others play a critical role in development, particularly in emotional, intellectual, and personality development. Not only do the quality and quantity of contacts with other persons exert an influence on the growing child, but the widening range of contacts is essential to learning and the development of a healthy personality.

The mothering person is unquestionably the single most influential person during early infancy. This person is the one who meets the infant's basic needs of food, warmth, comfort, and love. He or she provides stimulation for the child's senses and facilitates his or her expanding capacities. Through this person the child learns to trust the world and feel secure to venture in increasingly wider relationships.

It is generally the parents who are most influential in helping the child to assume sex-role identification. Parents define and reinforce acceptable sex-role behavior and provide sex-appropriate role models for the child. In the absence of a sex-role model in the family setting, the child may adopt some characteristics of the opposite-sex parent or sibling. Frequently the child identifies with a teacher or other significant person of the same sex.

Siblings are children's first peers, and the way in which they learn to relate to each other affects later interactions with peers outside the family group. The sphere of persons from whom children seek approval widens to include other members of their family, their peers, and, to a lesser extent, other authority figures (e.g., teachers). The increasing importance of the peer group in determining the behavior of school-age children and adolescents is well documented (Fig. 5-11).

When children fail to have quality interpersonal relationships with "mothering" persons, they experience *emotional deprivation.* The most prominent feature of emotional deprivation, particularly during the first year, is developmental delays. Much of the information regarding the adverse effects of interpersonal influences on development has been acquired through retrospective studies of gross deprivation and trauma. The most notable instances involved homeless infants who were placed in institutions for care. Those infants who did not receive consistent mothering care failed to gain weight even with an adequate diet; were pale, listless, and immobile; and were unresponsive to stimuli that usually elicit a response such as smiling or cooing in the normal infant. If emotional deprivation continues for a sufficient length of time, the child may not survive infancy.

Although the most remarkable examples of emotional deprivation were first recognized among infants in institutions, the term *masked deprivation* has been used to describe children reared in homes in which there is a distorted parent-child relationship or otherwise disordered home environment. Infants do not thrive if the caregiving person is hostile, fearful of handling them, or indifferent to them and their needs. Such children exhibit poor growth even though they are apparently free of physical disease. Growth delays in these children are believed to be caused by a psychologically induced endocrine imbalance that interferes with growth. These same infants and children display "catch-up" growth in a changed environment (see Failure to Thrive, Chapter 11).

SOCIOECONOMIC LEVEL

Evidence indicates that the socioeconomic level of children's families has a significant impact on growth and development. At all ages, children from upper- and middle-class families are taller than comparative children of families in the lower socioeconomic strata. The cause of these differences is less definite, although the poorer health and nutrition of lower socioeconomic levels are probably significant factors. Nutritious food sources (especially proteins) are scarce, and other factors (e.g., larger family size and irregularity in eating, sleeping, exercise) may play a role.

Families from lower socioeconomic groups may lack the knowledge or resources needed to provide the safe, stimulating, and enriched environment that fosters optimum development for children. They may be unable to move from unsafe neighborhoods where drug traffic and drive-by shootings are the norm. The effects on the emotional development of children living under these conditions have been compared with those experienced by children living in war zones.

DISEASE

Altered growth and development is one of the clinical manifestations in a number of hereditary disorders. Growth impairment is particularly marked in skeletal disorders, such as the various forms of dwarfism and at least one of the chromosomal anomalies (Turner syndrome). Many of the disorders of metabolism, such as vitamin D–resistant rickets, the mucopolysaccharidoses, and the numerous endocrine disorders, interfere with the normal growth pattern. In other disorders the tendency is toward the upper percentile of height (e.g., Klinefelter and Marfan syndromes).

Many chronic illnesses that are associated with varying degrees of growth failure are congenital cardiac anomalies and respiratory disorders such as cystic fibrosis. Any disorder characterized by the inability to digest and absorb body nutrients will have an adverse effect on growth and development.

ENVIRONMENTAL HAZARDS

Hazards in the environment are a source of concern to health care providers and others interested in health and safety. Physical injuries are the most prevalent consequences of environmental dangers, and these are discussed extensively throughout the book as they apply in relation to age, specific hazards, and selected physical disabilities.

Children are at a high risk for harm resulting from the chemical residues of modern life present in the environment. The hazards of these chemical residues relate to their potential carcinogenicity, enzymatic effects, and accumulation (Baum and Shannon, 1995) (see Community Focus box). The harmful agents most often associated with health risks are chemicals and radiation. Water, air, and food contamination from a variety of origins are well documented. Significant sources of exposure are substances in the immediate environment such as lead and asbestos, chemicals secreted in breast milk (especially prescribed drugs and nicotine), and contamination within well-insulated homes (especially from disinfectants or burning of substances that produce toxic fumes). Passive inhalation of tobacco smoke by infants and children is a hazard at all stages of development. The harmful effects of large doses of radiation are unquestioned, although the effects of low-dose or short-term radiation are debatable, as are the safe versus harmful dosage levels.

STRESS IN CHILDHOOD

Defined from both a physiologic and an emotional point of view, essentially *stress* is "an imbalance between environmental demands and a person's coping resources that . . . disrupts the equilibrium of the person" (Masten and others, 1988).

Although all children experience stress, some youngsters appear to be more vulnerable than others. Children's age, temperament, life situation, and state of health affect their vulnerability, reactions, and ability to handle stress. Also, the responses to a stressor can be behavioral, psychologic, or physiologic. It is impossible, unrealistic, and undesirable to protect children from stress, but providing them with interpersonal security helps them develop coping strategies for dealing with stress. The concept of an *emotional bank,* in which deposits, as well as withdrawals, can be made can help parents and caregivers maintain a proper perspective regarding the effects of stress and coping. Children with a good, positive balance in the account can tolerate significant withdrawal experiences. For children with a low balance, even a minor withdrawal may bankrupt the account, causing it to be overdrawn.

Parents and other caregivers can try to recognize signs of stress to help children deal with stresses before they become overwhelming. Signs of stress take many forms but are typically the same ones seen in children who are abused (see Chapter 14) or depressed (see Chapter 17). If a number of stresses are imposed on children at the same time, the children are more vulnerable. When a succession of stresses produces an excessive stress load, children may experience a serious change in health or behavior.

It is most important that parents and persons working with children understand the nature of childhood stress and ways it can be recognized or anticipated. Caregivers must *listen* to children so they are aware of children's fears and concerns and must let them know that they are important and that what they say matters. Physical contact is comforting and reassuring to children. Simply holding, touching, or hugging children is both relaxing and comforting and facilitates communication. Spending unhurried time with children, family outings, vacations, and exposing children to positive influences help build children's strength and security. Supportive interpersonal relationships are essential to the psychologic well-being of children.

Coping

Coping refers to a special class of individual reactions to stressors—specifically, a reaction to a stressor that resolves, reduces, or replaces the affect state classified as stressful. *Coping strategies* are the specific ways in which children cope with stressors, as distinguished from *coping styles,* which are relatively unchanging personality characteristics or outcomes of coping (Ryan-Wenger, 1992). Research indicates that as children age they tend toward a more internal locus of control and use more vigilant modes of coping

---

COMMUNITY FOCUS

Choosing Children's Sunglasses

Children's sunglasses must absorb at least 99% of ultraviolet radiation (UV). Choose sunglasses with the label "Blocks 99% of UV rays," "UV absorption up to 400 nm," "Special purpose," or "Meets American National Standards Institute (ANSI) requirements." Other guidelines for selecting sunglasses are:

- Allow children to choose their sunglasses.
- A child who wears prescription lenses should also have prescription sunglasses.
- Sunglasses are not a substitute for other protective measures such as wide-brimmed hats and sunscreen.
- The most dangerous time for sun exposure is between 10 AM and 2 PM. High altitude, sand, concrete, snow, and water increase UV exposure.
- Check the predicted index of UV exposure for the following day in the weather section of your local newspaper.
- Teach your child never to look directly at the sun, even when wearing sunglasses.

From Wagner RS: Why children should wear sunglasses, *Patient Care* 29(12):178-184, 1995.

(LaMontagne and others, 1996). Children, as with adults, respond to everyday stress by trying to change the circumstances or trying to adjust to circumstances the way they are. Any strategy that provides relaxation is effective in reducing stress, and most children have their own natural methods such as withdrawal, physical activity, reading, listening to music, working on a project, or taking a nap. Some turn to parents to solve their problems, or they may develop socially unacceptable strategies, such as cheating, stealing, or lying.

Children can be taught stress-reduction techniques to use in coping. First, they must be helped to recognize signs of tension in themselves and then taught any of a variety of appropriate strategies—special exercises, relaxation and breathing, mental imagery, and numerous other simple activities. Also, parents and other caregivers can anticipate possible stress-provoking events and prepare children for coping by role playing a scenario or "talking it through" beforehand. Most of the stress-reducing strategies discussed in Chapter 21 in relation to managing pain are effective for any stress situation.

Probably the most useful tool that children can learn is how to solve problems. When children can view any new situation as a problem to be solved and an opportunity to learn, they are not vulnerable to the control of others. It provides them with a sense of mastery over their own lives and reinforces the fact that they have within themselves the ability and information to handle whatever comes their way. Problem-solving skill gives them the confidence to know where and how to seek help when they need it.

INFLUENCE OF THE MASS MEDIA

Media can have an enormous influence on the developing child. There is no doubt that the media provide children with a means for extending their knowledge about the world in which they live and have contributed to narrowing the differences between classes. However, there is growing concern regarding the enormous influence the media can have on the developing child, because of the large number of hours spent watching television. The images of risky behavior presented by the media may serve to establish or reinforce teenagers' perceptions of their social environment. Children may identify closely with people or characters portrayed in reading materials, movies, video games, and television programs and commercials.

Today, children tend to select media and sports figures as their ideal role models, whereas in the past the majority of children chose their parents or parent surrogates as the people they most wanted to be like (Duck, 1990). This trend can be viewed as a grave concern or a magnificent opportunity to promote positive role models. There is no doubt that the communications media provide children with a means for extending their knowledge about the world in which they live and have contributed to narrowing the differences between classes.

Reading Materials

Books, newspapers, and magazines are the oldest form of mass media. They contribute to children's competence in almost every direction and also provide enjoyment. Recognition of the impact that reading matter used in the schools has on the value system and socialization processes has prompted reevaluation of the content of textbooks in terms of the biased presentation of male and female role models, the sugar-coated view of life situations, and the biased history of minority groups.

Fairy tales, for generations the mainstay of young children's literature, for a time suffered condemnation as being sexist, overly violent in content, and riddled with unfavorable stereotypes, such as the wicked stepmother, dwarfs, and physical unattractiveness associated with evil. They are now believed to provide an excellent medium for explaining puzzling and important topics such as death, stepparents, and inner feelings and turmoils. Although they do not provide solutions, fairy tales confront children with emotional predicaments and offer suggestions for dealing with them.

Comic books and other pulp reading material have been popular in every generation, usually at the expense of literature provided by schools, libraries, and parents. Many children have nothing else to read. The easy reading, quick action, and adventure in brief episodes seem to fulfill a need for children who are striving to understand both aggression in others and their own impulses. Reading ability, intelligence, and school adjustment apparently have no relationship to the number and type of comic books read. Most comic books appear to be relatively harmless to the majority of children and may be beneficial. Comic books seem to have only a minor influence on acquisition of beliefs, values, and behaviors. The popularity of this medium has prompted some educators to encourage translations of literature into comic book form to stimulate students' interest in the classics.

Movies

Movies that are not closely bound to reality and often portray an assortment of socially approved behaviors perhaps make a contribution to children's value systems and do provide opportunities for desirable social learning. On the other hand, children, especially adolescents, flock to the "macho" movies and those whose heroes resort to violent resolution of problems, such as karate and wild automobile chases. The carryover of these influences into daily life and relationships may account in part for the increase in violent behavior of young persons.

Another concern is the plethora of "slasher" and R-rated movies available to children and teenagers in theaters and through cable television and videocassettes. The content of movies has changed markedly during the past few years, with violence and mutilation being major themes. To children who are unable to distinguish between reality and fantasy, these films play on their deepest fears and result in bedtime fears, nightmares, and a fearful view of the world.

Young children can be frightened by some of the movies considered safe for family viewing. For example, *Bambi* can be frightening to young children, and the villainous witches in *Snow White* and the *Wizard of Oz* are terrifying figures. Also, certain classic Disney movies, such as *Snow White* and *Cinderella,* depict stepmothers as evil, destructive persons; such portrayals can have a deleterious effect on children-stepmother relationships or can be confusing to children who have developed a positive relationship with a stepmother.

Children as young as 4 years can recognize that cartoons are "make-believe," but children as old as age 6 continue to assume that noncartoon features are at least roughly analogous to social reality (Downs, 1990). Therefore, young children are especially vulnerable to misinterpreting what they see and need guidance in choosing appropriate programs.

Television

The medium with the most impact on children in North America today is television, which has become one of the most significant socializing agents in the lives of young children. The content of programs and commercials provides multiple sources for acquiring information, modeling behaviors, and observing value orientations. Besides producing a leveling effect on class differences in general information and vocabulary, television exposes children to a wider variety of topics and events than they encounter in day-to-day life. Television always has time to talk to children and is a form of access to the adult world.

FYI

It has been reported that the television is on for more than 6 hours per day in more than half of American homes and that children watch an average of 21 to 28 hours of television per week (Vessey, Yim-Chiplis, and MacKenzie, 1998; Clarke-Pearson, 1997).

Television viewing has a direct impact on child development and behavior. Several studies have found that violence on television and the mass media in general can have a negative influence on the development of unhealthy behaviors

BOX 5-4 ■ Factors That Encourage Learning or Performing Television-Influenced Behaviors

Age. Younger children focus on behaviors rather than on motives or consequences. They view alternatives in a concrete manner, and they are unable to differentiate between central and peripheral plot information. Small children remember various assorted items in the program; for example, they remember the act, not the motive or consequences.

Identification with characters or situations. Children will more often imitate behaviors of persons and situations similar to those in their own lives.

Reward and punishment syndrome. Children will imitate behaviors they see rewarded or not punished when it is expected. They are less likely to repeat an act they see punished; their attention is immediately attracted when they see an act committed that they know should be punished but is not.

Opportunity to reproduce behaviors. Children will imitate behaviors when given the right environment or when violence seems an accepted solution. When children see a situation on television, they will use this information when they encounter a similar situation that requires a solution.

Motivation to reproduce behaviors. Children will imitate behavior when given the appropriate incentives: expectation of reward or lack of punishment. Some children have self-control; others do not.

and violence in children (Earles and others, 2002; Monsen, 2002; Brown and Witherspoon, 2002). Several factors encourage the learning or performing of television-influenced behaviors (Box 5-4).

Most researchers have concluded that protracted television viewing can have detrimental effects on children. Recognizing the negative effects of television viewing, the American Academy of Pediatrics has recommended that children older than age 2 watch less than 2 hours of quality television a day and that children younger than 2 years watch no television (American Academy of Pediatrics, 2001a; Certain and Kahn, 2002).

The passive activity associated with television viewing is frequently accompanied by eating—in many cases, high-calorie snacks. Furthermore, children may expend tremendous mental energy processing the audiovisual messages from television, which may be very exhausting and make them less likely to engage in physical activity later. Andersen and colleagues (1998) found that the incidence of body fat increased in direct proportion to the amount of hours of television watched by children in the United States; as the number of hours of television viewing increased, children were less likely to participate in vigorous physical activities.

In a study to identify children at risk for heart disease, researchers found that more than half of the children with high cholesterol levels watched at least 2 hours of television each day. Using a family history of heart disease or high cholesterol as the screening indicator for cholesterol testing in children, researchers identified three out of four children with high cholesterol levels. When these families were also questioned about the time their children spent watching television, investigators were able to identify 90% of the children with high cholesterol levels by using 2 or more viewing hours as the risk factor (Goldsmith, 1990).

Television programs and commercials, like movies, contain many implicit and explicit messages that promote alcohol consumption, smoking, violence, and promiscuous or unsafe sexual activity. An area of increasing concern is media violence, especially when heavy metal rock groups, whose lyrics and videos sensationalize violent sex, suicide, and satanism, are featured. There is now clear evidence documenting a relationship between television viewing and the use of alcohol or tobacco, violence and aggressive behavior, the use of guns to commit violent acts, and early sexual activity (Strasburger and Donnerstein, 1999). Media advertisement has increasingly been scrutinized out of concern for its effects in encouraging young people to purchase and use alcohol and tobacco.

Parents can help children evaluate television violence by pointing out the subtleties children miss, such as the aggressor's motives and intentions and the unpleasant consequences the perpetrators suffer as a result of their aggressive acts. Often the consequence is separated from the act by a commercial, and therefore children cannot make the correlation. Parents need to point out that conflicts can be resolved without resorting to violent behavior. They can also stress the purpose of the programs—primarily entertainment—and explain why they like or dislike something on television (e.g., "This show is trying to tell you that crime does not pay and that if one does wrong, one will go to jail"). Explanations and discussions can take place between shows (with the volume turned down), and young children can learn from both older children and adults. These discussions can be very effective when begun early and carried out consistently.

It is especially important to identify at-risk children and control their viewing. House rules that specify the type and amount of television help children understand limits, and video-recorded selections of appropriate programs can be substituted for less desirable offerings. Parents need to carefully monitor cable and other pay-television programming because these popular options present more uncensored programming. Locked boxes, V-chips, and blocking devices are available for cable receivers to prevent children from viewing programs when unsupervised. Vessey, Yim-Chiplis, and MacKenzie (1998) suggest that parental role modeling may have a more positive influence on the child's behavior than television programming. They further recommend that parents watch television with children and help children understand the difference between their life and habits and that of persons represented on television.

On the positive side, television has been shown to be a positive influence on children's abilities to deal with a variety of social issues such as divorce, the arrival of a new baby, discrimination, honesty, and helpfulness. Children who view educational programming (such as "Mister Rogers' Neighborhood" and "Sesame Street") for a long period become more affectionate, considerate, cooperative, and helpful toward their playmates. The ways that minority and ethnic characters are portrayed on television can have an impact on the way the majority culture views minority persons and on the self-image of minority children.

Parents need to supervise the amount and type of television programs their children watch and to teach their children how to watch television (see Box 5-5 and Family Home Care box).

NURSING TIP

During an assessment, consider that parents may not be aware of how much time their children spend watching television. Parents may also not understand the child's inability to distinguish between the "fantasy" of television and life events (Vessey, Yim-Chiplis, and MacKenzie, 1998).

Nurses and parents can be powerful forces in influencing the media. They can watch closely for an increase in violence and other undesirable programming and complain to sponsors and television stations if they believe it is not appropriate. Good programming can be both educational and entertaining.

Video Games/Internet

With the growing popularity of home gaming systems, children are spending increased hours playing video games. Unfortunately, many of the video games available are violent in nature with virtual crimes and violence being portrayed, with a significant percentage portraying violence against women. Video games allow the player to be the aggressor, making an ideal environment for a child to learn violent behavior (American Academy of Pediatrics, 2001b). Although video games come with violence and age ratings, many parents are not aware of or choose to ignore the rating appropriate for their child. The American Academy of Pediatrics (2001b) recommend health care providers should encourage parents to adhere to the game ratings and

---

BOX 5-5 ■ Five Important Ideas to Teach Children and Adolescents About Television

1. You are smarter than what you see on your television.
2. Television world is not real.
3. Television teaches that some people are more important than others.
4. Television keeps doing the same things over and over again.
5. Somebody is always trying to make money with television.

Modified from Davis J: Five important ideas to teach your children about TV, *Media Values* 59/60:10-14, 1992. In Strasburger VC, Donnerstein E: Children, adolescents, and the media, *Pediatrics* 103(1):129-139, 1999.

 ## FAMILY HOME CARE

Television Viewing

Provide a positive role model by developing television substitutes such as reading, athletics, physical conditioning, and hobbies.

Construct a time chart of child's activities (homework, television viewing, scheduled outside activities, playing with a friend).

Discuss with child what you both believe to be a balanced set of activities.

At the beginning of each week, select appropriate programs from television schedules.

Allow child to select programs from this approved list.

Limit child's viewing to 2 hours or less per day.

Rule out television at specific times (e.g., before breakfast or on school nights).

Make a list of alternative activities (e.g., riding a bicycle, reading a book, or working on a hobby).

Require that child choose to do something from this list before watching television.

Watch programs with child.

Discuss program and commercial content with child:
  Distinguish between the real and the unreal.
  Correlate consequences with actions.
  Point out subtle messages.
  Explore alternatives to aggressive conflict resolution.
  Stress purpose of program (e.g., entertainment, education).
  Explain likes and dislikes.

Turn the television off after the selected program is over.

Monitor cable and pay television selections; use a lockbox if necessary.

Limit use of television as a safe distraction to potentially stressful times (e.g., keeping the children occupied while the parent gets organized after a difficult day).

limit the amount of time spent playing games and watching television to less than 2 hours a day combined.

The use of computers in both the classroom and household has impacted childhood learning and development. Schools offer a wide variety of computer programs that enable children of all ages to broaden their world views. Computers offer the advantage of interactive learning and hand-eye coordination. Parents have a wide variety of computer software choices for learning and gaming.

Although computer technology has enhanced many forms of learning and recreation, there are potential dangers to children. The Internet and electronic mailing have made correspondence and information available to children from around the world in minutes. Some activities such as "cybersex" and "kiddie porn," as well as some "chat rooms," may expose children to individuals who may attempt to take advantage of the child's naïveté for illicit purposes. Government officials are working to curb illegal activities on the Internet that involve children, yet at the same time maintain freedom of speech. Filtered Internet service providers are available that may serve to protect children from objectionable sites.* Nurses must be involved in encouraging parents to be knowledgeable of their children's Internet activities while providing appropriate learning activities unique to computers. One helpful strategy is to locate the computer in a public area of the home such as the kitchen or family room to enable parents to easily monitor its use.

KEY POINTS

- Growth describes a change in quantity and occurs when cells divide and synthesize new proteins.
- Maturation, a qualitative change, describes the aging process or an increase in competence and adaptability.
- Differentiation refers to a biologic description of the processes by which early cells and structures are modified and altered to achieve specific and characteristic physical and chemical properties.
- Development involves change from a lower to a more advanced stage of complexity.
- The five major developmental periods are prenatal, infancy, early childhood, middle childhood, and later childhood (pubescence and adolescence).
- Growth and development proceed in predictable patterns of direction, sequence, and pace.
- The directional trends in growth and development are cephalocaudal, proximodistal, and mass to specific.
- Physical development includes increase in height and weight and changes in body proportion, dentition, and some body tissues.

- The three broad classifications of child temperament are the easy child, the difficult child, and the slow-to-warm-up child.
- The developmental theories most widely used in explaining child growth and development are Freud's psychosexual stages, Erikson's stages of psychosocial development, Piaget's stages of cognitive development, and Kohlberg's stages of moral development.
- To develop a positive self-concept, children need recognition for their achievements and the approval of others.
- Through play, children learn about their world and how to relate to things, people, and situations.
- Play provides a means of development in the areas of sensorimotor and intellectual progress, socialization, creativity, self-awareness, and moral behavior; it serves as a means for release of tension and expression of emotions.
- Growth and development are affected by a variety of conditions and circumstances, including heredity, physiologic function, gender, disease, physical environment, nutrition, and interpersonal relationships.
- Children's vulnerability and reaction to stress depend to a large extent on their age, coping behaviors, and support systems.
- The mass media can be influential in children's learning and behavior.

References

American Academy of Pediatrics, Committee on Public Education: Children, adolescents, and television, *Pediatrics* 107(2):423-26, 2001a.

American Academy of Pediatrics, Committee on Public Education: Media violence, *Pediatrics* 108(5):1222-26, 2001b.

Anders TF, Sadeh A, Appareddy V: Normal sleep in neonates and children. In Ferber R, Kryger M, editors: *Principles and practice of sleep medicine in the child*, Philadelphia, 1995, WB Saunders.

Andersen RE and others: Relationship of physical activity and television watching with body weight and level of fatness among children, *JAMA* 279(12):938-943, 1998.

Baum C, Shannon M: Environmental toxins: cutting the risks, *Contemp Pediatr* 12(7):20-43, 1995.

Beck CT: A meta-analysis of the relationship between postpartum depression and infant temperament, *Nurs Res* 45(4):225-230, 1996.

Bliss-Holtz J: Methods of newborn infant temperature monitoring: a research review, *Issues Compr Pediatr Nurs* 18(4): 287-298, 1995.

Borja ME, Bordi PL, Lambert CU: New lower fat dessert recipes for the school lunch program are well accepted by children, *J Am Dis Assoc* 96(9):908-910, 1996.

Brown JD, Witherspoon EM: The mass media and American adolescents' health, *J Adolesc Health* 31(6S):153-70, 2002.

Carey WB: Section 5. Communicating with parents and community involvement: teaching parents about infant temperament, *Pediatrics* 102(5):1311-16, 1998.

Certain LK, Kahn RS: Prevalence, correlates, and trajectory of television viewing among infants and toddlers, *Pediatrics* 109(4):634-42, 2002.

Chase RA: Toys, play, and infant development, *J Perinat Educ* 3(2)7-19, 1994.

Chess S, Thomas A: Temperamental differences: a critical concept in child health care, *Pediatr Nurs* 11:167-171, 1985.

Clarke-Pearson KM: Children-media violence-solutions, *NC Med J* 58(4):265-268, 1997.

Colizza DF, Colvin SP: Food choices of healthy school-age children, *J Sch Nurs* 11(4):17-20, 1995.

Downs A: Children's judgments of televised events: the real versus pretend distinction, *Percept Mot Skills* 70:779-782, 1990.

Duck J: Children's ideals: the role of real-life versus media figures, *Austr J Psychol* 42:19-29, 1990.

FamilyConnect, Inc., provides a filtering system that prevents access to pornographic and illegal websites. For further information, call (888) 400-0239; website: www.familyconnect.com. An excellent book that explains the dangers of the Internet and strategies to protect children is *Wicked wild web* by J.R. Robison and C. Ophus (2000), Autumn Sky Publishing, PO Box 702252, Tulsa, OK 74170; (888) 400-0239 (then dial 0 for operator); website: www.wickedwildweb.com.

Earles KA and others: Media influences on children and adolescents: violence and sex, *J Natl Med Assoc* 94(9):797-801, 2002.

Erikson EH: *Childhood and society,* ed 2, New York, 1963, WW Norton.

Fowler JW: Toward a developmental perspective on faith, *Relig Educ* 69:207-219, 1974.

Glassey D, Ramano J, Committee on Early Childhood, Adoption, and Dependent Care–American Academy of Pediatrics: Selecting appropriate toys for young children: the pediatrician's role, *Pediatrics* 111(4):911-13, 2003.

Goldsmith M: Youngsters dialing up cholesterol levels? *JAMA* 264(23):2976, 1990.

Gross D, Conrad B: Temperament in toddlerhood, *J Pediatr Nurs* 10(3):146-151, 1995.

Jung FE, Czajka-Narins DM: Birth weight doubling and tripling times: an updated look at the effects of birth weight, sex, race and type of feeding, *Am J Clin Nutr* 42:182-189, 1985.

Kaczander BI: Pediatric sports medicine: a unique perspective, *Podiatr Manage* 16(2):53-60, 1997.

Kohlberg L: Moral development. In Sills DL, editor: *International encyclopedia of the social sciences,* New York, 1968, Macmillan.

LaMontagne LL and others: Children's preoperative coping and its effects on postoperative anxiety and return to normal activity, *Nurs Res* 45(3):141-147, 1996.

Lampl M: Saltation and stasis: a model of human growth, *Science* 258(5083):801-803, 1992.

Lampl M, Johnson ML, Frongillo, EA Jr: Mixed distribution analysis identifies saltation and stasis growth, *Ann Hum Biol* 28(4):403-411, 2001.

Masten A and others: Competence and stress in school children: moderating effects of individual and family qualities, *J Child Psychol Psychiatry* 29:747-764, 1988.

Monsen RB: Children and the media, *J Pediatr Nurs* 17(4):309-310, 2002.

Morrow JD, Camp BW: Mastery motivation and temperament of 7-month-old infants, *Pediatr Nurs* 22(3):211-217, 1996.

Piaget J: *The theory of stages in cognitive development,* New York, 1969, McGraw-Hill.

Ryan-Wenger N: A taxonomy of children's coping strategies: a step toward theory development, *Am J Orthopsychiatry* 62(2):256-263, 1992.

Seidel HM and others: *Mosby's guide to physical examination,* ed 5, St Louis, 2003, Mosby.

Selekman J: The development of body image in the child: a learned response, *Top Clin Nurs* 5(1):13-21, 1983.

Sieving R, Zirbel-Donisch S: Development and enhancement of self-esteem in children, *J Pediatr Health Care* 4(6):290-296, 1990.

Strasburger VC, Donnerstein E: Children, adolescents, and the media: issues and solution, *Pediatrics* 103(1):129-139, 1999.

Stuart GW, Laraia MT: *Principles and practice of psychiatric nursing,* ed 7, St Louis, 2000, Mosby.

Urbanski LF, Hanlon DP: Pediatric orthopedics, *Top Emerg Med* 18(2):73-90, 1996.

Vessey JA, Yim-Chiplis PK, MacKenzie NR: Effects of television viewing on children's development, *Pediatric Nurs* 23(5):483-486, 1998.

Willoughby C, King G, Polatajko H: A therapist's guide to children's self-esteem, *Am J Occup Ther* 50(2):124-132, 1996.

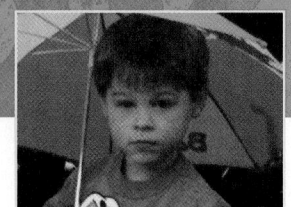

6

Communication and Health Assessment of the Child and Family

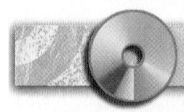
Remember to check out your companion CD-ROM

http://evolve.elsevier.com/Wong/essentials/

CHAPTER OUTLINE

RELATED TOPICS and ADDITIONAL RESOURCES

 IN TEXT

Development of Self-Concept, *Ch. 5*
Developmental Assessment, *Ch. 7*
Family, Structure and Function, *Ch. 3*
Family Theories, *Ch. 3*
Growth Measurements, *Ch. 7*
Immunizations, *Ch. 10*
Nutritional Disturbances, *Ch. 11*
Pain Assessment, *Ch. 21*
Preparation for Procedures, *Ch. 22*
Role of Play in Development, *Ch. 5*
Sex Education: Preschooler, *Ch. 13;* School-Age Child, *Ch. 15;* Adolescent, *Ch. 16*

Sexually Transmitted Diseases, *Ch. 17*
Sleep Problems: Infant, *Ch. 10;* Preschooler, *Ch. 13*
Social, Cultural, and Religious Influences on Child Health Promotion, *Ch. 4*
Spina Bifida, *Ch. 32*
Use of Play in Procedures, *Ch. 22*

 CD COMPANION

Critical Thinking Exercise—The Interview
Case Study—Communicating With Adolescents

Guidelines—Review of Systems; Using an Interpreter; Communicating With Children; Communicating With Adolescents; Analyzing the Symptom: Pain; Initiating a Comprehensive Family Assessment
NCLEX-Style Review Questions

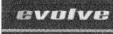 **WEBSITE**

WebLinks
NCLEX-Style Review Questions

For additional information, please view "Communicating With Children and Families" in *Whaley and Wong's Pediatric Nursing Video Series,* St Louis, 1996, Mosby; (800) 426-4545; website: www.elsevierhealth.com.

COMMUNICATION

The forms of communication may be verbal, nonverbal, or abstract. *Verbal communication* may involve language and its expression; vocalizations in the form of laughs, moans, or squalls; or the implications of what is not said in light of what has been said. *Nonverbal communication* is often called body language and includes gestures, movements, facial expressions, postures, and reactions. *Abstract communication* takes the form of play, artistic expression, symbols, photographs, and choice of clothing. Because it is possible to exert greater conscious control over verbal communication, it is a less reliable indicator of true feelings, especially with children.

Many factors influence the communication process. To be successful (gratifying), communication must be appropriate to the situation, properly timed, and clearly delivered. This implies that nurses understand and use techniques of effective communication, including listening. Verbal and nonverbal messages must be congruent; that is, two or more messages sent via different levels must not be contradictory.

VERBAL COMMUNICATION—THE POWER OF WORDS

Words shape reality, and thus they hold tremendous power. A person can change another's perception of reality by the choice of words that are used. For example, if the diagnosis of cancer is always referred to as a tumor, cyst, malignancy, or carcinoma, patients may never really know that they have cancer. Consequently, they may assume less responsibility for their care than if they were aware of the seriousness of the condition. By learning to recognize how patients and health professionals use language to manipulate reality, one can also learn how to change perceptions and communicate more effectively.

Avoidance Language

The most common way that people try to alter reality is by avoiding words that truly describe it. For example, euphemisms such as "passed on" are used instead of "death." Avoidance language indicates that a person wants to hide something, particularly feelings. As a rule, accepting a person's use of euphemisms only serves to perpetuate the fears and never helps the person deal with them. In contrast, use of straightforward, precise, descriptive language lends perspective to the situation and allows the person to discuss the fears. Most often, imagined fears are much worse than reality.

Distancing Language

People may use impersonal words, such as "it" or "others," to shield themselves from the painful reality of a situation. For example, parents may state that they know *someone* with a child who is slow, when they may actually be talking about personal fears regarding *their* child. By realizing that the parents may need to talk about this difficult subject, the nurse can provide sensitive statements that ease them into discussing their situation.

Sometimes distancing is desirable because the topic may be too painful to discuss directly. The use of the third-person technique (see Box 6-4) may be very therapeutic in allowing an individual the opportunity to indirectly approach a subject and receive feedback but still remain in control.

NONVERBAL COMMUNICATION— PARALANGUAGE

In addition to the spoken word, messages are also relayed through nonverbal means, or *paralanguage*—the pitch, pause, intonation, rate, volume, and stress apparent in speech. Young children become very adept at understanding paralanguage; long before they know the meaning of words, they sense anxiety or fear by the rise in pitch or the accelerated rate of the parent's voice. By careful observation of the spoken word, nurses can better understand the meaning of another's verbal message and more accurately control their own paralanguage.

Because most people do not exert conscious control over their paralanguage, it is a valuable clue to feelings and concerns. For example, *pausing* may signify a need to formulate thoughts, recall information, or fabricate a story. Frequent pauses often make the speaker sound unsure. Long pauses may mean that the individual needs more information.

Rate is another characteristic that gives unspoken messages. Talking too fast usually makes the speaker sound glib and insensitive. Talking slowly with a firm tone and appropriate pauses conveys authority. Therefore, a person is much more likely to "hear" instructions if the latter approach is used. Children in particular respond attentively to a slow, even, steady voice.

Confirming and Disconfirming Behaviors

People respond to each other through *confirming behaviors,* such as nodding the head, using direct eye contact, repeating or requesting clarification, and making appropriate comments, or *disconfirming behaviors,* such as tapping fingers or a foot, turning away from the speaker, avoiding eye contact, and interrupting. Because there is a reciprocal relationship between such behaviors, nurses need to use confirming behaviors to receive confirmation in return. This "mirroring" effect is particularly evident in children because of their sensitivity to nonverbal cues.

GUIDELINES FOR COMMUNICATION AND INTERVIEWING

The most widely used method of communicating with parents on a professional basis is the interview process. Unlike social conversation, interviewing is a specific form of goal-directed communication. As nurses converse with children and adults, they focus on the individuals to determine the kind of person they are, their usual mode of handling problems, whether help is needed, and the way in which they react to counseling. Developing interviewing skills requires time and practice, but following some guiding principles can facilitate this process. An organized approach is most effective when using interviewing skills in patient teaching.

ESTABLISHING A SETTING FOR COMMUNICATION
Appropriate Introduction

Introduce yourself to, and ask the name of, each family member who is present. Address parents or other adults by their appropriate titles, such as "Mr." and "Mrs.," unless they specify a preferred name. Record the preferred name on the medical record. Using formal address or their preferred names, rather than using first names or "mother" or "father," conveys respect and regard for the parents or other caregivers (Seidel and others, 2003).

At the beginning of the visit, include children in the interaction by asking them their name, age, and other information. Nurses often direct all questions to adults, even when children are old enough to speak for themselves. This serves to terminate one extremely valuable source of information: the patient. When the child is included, follow the general rules for communicating with children in the Guidelines box on p. 111.

Role Clarification and Explanation of the Interview

During the introduction it is also necessary to clarify the nurse's particular role in the health setting. For example, nurses performing interviews may be pediatric nurse practitioners, inpatient staff nurses, clinic nurses, office nurses, visiting nurses, or school nurses. A parent is much more likely to reveal personal information about the child and family if the relevance and importance of the interview are stressed. If this is not done, parents may refuse to elaborate on certain areas because they feel it has no bearing on the "problem." In addition, because more than one member of the health team may take a history during the course of a hospital admission, it is important to clarify the reason for each interview (Seidel and others, 2003).

Another reason for role clarification is education of the health consumer. With expanded roles in nursing, it is not unusual for families to think that the examiner is a physician rather than a nurse. Role clarification is especially important because some parents may feel deceived if they later are made aware of the nurse's identity. The general consumer acceptance of pediatric nurse practitioners (PNPs) has been very favorable, so it is also important to acknowledge their expertise by emphasizing the PNP's role.

Preliminary Acquaintance

To make the family feel at ease and to develop rapport, begin the interview with some general conversation. The opening statements should be general but still informative. Comments such as "How have things been since your last visit?" "Tell me about Johnny," or (to the child) "What do you think is going to happen today?" allow the parent or child to express the main concern in a casual, relaxed atmosphere.

The preliminary acquaintance conversation also reveals how responsive the informant may be to questions. For example, using open-ended statements, such as "Tell me about the baby," may lead the parent into a lengthy detailed discussion. In this case direct questions toward specific answers to avoid irrelevant remarks. At other times a parent may respond to open-ended questions with only minimal information, in which case continue to use open-ended questions rather than questions with "yes" or "no" answers.

Assurance of Privacy and Confidentiality

The place where the interview is conducted is almost as important as the interview itself. The physical environment should allow for as much privacy as possible, with distractions, such as interruptions, noise, or other visible activity, kept to a minimum. At times it is necessary to turn off a television or radio. The environment should also have some play provision for young children to keep them occupied during the parent-nurse interview (Fig. 6-1). Parents who are constantly interrupted by their children are unable to concentrate fully and tend to give short, brief answers to terminate the interview as quickly as possible.

Confidentiality is also an essential component of the initial phase of the interview. Since the interview is usually shared with other members of the health team or the teacher (as in the case of students), be sure to inform the family of the limits regarding confidentiality. If there is con-

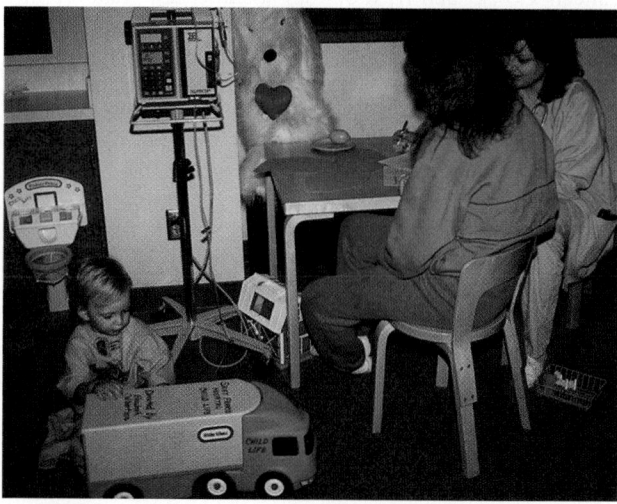

FIG. 6-1 ■ Child plays while nurse interviews parent.

cern regarding confidentiality in a situation, such as talking to a parent suspected of child abuse or a teenager contemplating suicide, deal with this directly and inform the person that in such instances confidentiality cannot be ensured. However, the nurse judiciously protects information of a confidential nature (Sullivan, 1997).

> **!NURSING ALERT**
>
> In 2003, the Health Insurance Portability and Accountability Act was implemented to further ensure patient privacy and limit access to sensitive health information. Nurses and students should become familiar with their institution's policy regarding HIPAA compliance.*

*For more information visit: www.hhs.gov/ocr/hipaa.

COMPUTER PRIVACY AND APPLICATIONS IN NURSING

The use of computer technology to store and retrieve health information has become widespread. The privacy and security of this health information has generated a growing concern throughout the health care community. Any person accessing health information of a confidential nature is charged with managing safeguards for disclosures, because violations might incur civil damages.

In 1994 a committee of the Institute of Medicine recommended a national code of fair health information practices. The suggestion was made that health data organizations (HDOs) should establish data protection units to develop privacy policies and security practices for manual and automated data processing systems. Technologic safeguards, such as encryption and managerial security procedures, can be applied to computer hardware across a network to ensure that individual patient privacy is protected.

Computer and information applications in nursing *(nursing informatics),* such as electronic medical records, are used by many institutions to record care and access information. Two important health care applications are record transmission, including facsimile (fax) and electronic mail (e-mail), and telemedicine. The telemedicine application is capable of two-way video conferencing, transmission of radiographs, and clinical consultation between remote sites and centralized resources.*

TELEPHONE TRIAGE AND COUNSELING

Nurses are increasingly becoming responsible for assessment of children's symptoms and clinical judgment for further medical care *(triage)* via telephone report. Most often, health problems are assessed and prioritized according to urgency, and treatment is judiciously provided via telephone services. Successful outcomes are based on the consistency and accuracy of the information provided, and parents are empowered to participate in their child's medical care. Telephone triage care management has increased access to quality health care services, and patient satisfaction has significantly improved. Unnecessary emergency department and

*Resources: Nicoll LH: *Nurses' guide to the internet,* ed 3, Philadelphia, 2001, JB Lippincott. Also available is a bimonthly publication, *Computers, informatics, nursing.* To order, call (800) 638-3030; fax: (301) 714-2300; e-mail: CustomerService www.cinjournal.com.

clinic visits have decreased, saving medical costs and time (less work absence) for families in need of health care. The most common telephone triage call is for a fever. Approximately 37% of the triage calls related to fever require emergency care, and nearly 50% benefit from home management (Deadrick and Boggess, 1996).

> **!NURSING ALERT**
>
> Legal issues can emerge from errors in telephone triage care management. Always advise that the child should be seen if there is any doubt as to the seriousness of the illness.

A well-designed telephone triage program is essential for safe, prompt, and consistent-quality health care (Rutenberg, 2000). Telephone triage is more than "just a phone call," because a child's life is a high price to pay for poorly managed or incompetent telephone assessment skills. Typically, general guidelines for telephone triage include screening questions; determining when to immediately refer to Emergency Medicine Services (EMS) (dial 911); and determining when to refer to same-day appointments, appointments in 24 to 72 hours, appointments in 4 days or more, or home care (Box 6-1).

COMMUNICATING WITH FAMILIES

COMMUNICATING WITH PARENTS

Although the parent and child are separate and distinct individuals, relationships with the child are frequently mediated via the parent, particularly in the case of younger children. For the most part, information about the child is acquired by direct observation or is communicated to the nurse by

---

BOX 6-1 ■ Telephone Triage Guidelines

Date/time
Background
   Name, age, sex
   Chronic illness
   Allergies, current medications, treatments, or recent
     immunizations
Chief complaint
General symptoms
   Severity
   Duration
   Other symptoms
   Pain
Systems review
Advised to call EMS (911)
Advised to see practitioner
Advice given for home care
Call back if symptoms worsen or fail to improve

RESOURCES FOR TELEPHONE TRIAGE PROTOCOLS
Brown J: *Pediatric telephone medicine: principles, triage and advice,* ed 3, Philadelphia, 1998, JB Lippincott.
Murphy KA: *Pediatric triage guidelines,* St Louis, 1997, Mosby.
Schmitt BD: *Pediatric telephone protocols,* Elk Grove Village, Il, 1998, American Academy of Pediatrics.
Simonsen SM: *Telephone assessment: guidelines for practice,* ed 2, St Louis, 2001, Mosby.

the parents. Usually it can be assumed that because of the close contact with the child, the parent gives reliable information. Making an assessment of the child requires input from the child (verbal and nonverbal), information from the parent, and the nurse's own observations of the child and interpretation of the relationship between the child and the parent. Counseling and guidance must be directed to the caregiver of infants and small children; when children are old enough to be active participants in their own health maintenance, the parent becomes a collaborator in health care.

Encouraging the Parent to Talk

Interviewing parents not only offers the opportunity to determine the health and developmental status of the child, but also offers information about factors that influence the child's life. Whatever the parent sees as a problem should be a concern of the nurse. These problems are not always easy to identify. Nurses need to be alert for clues and signals by which a parent communicates worries and anxieties. Careful phrasing with broad, open-ended questions such as "What is Jimmy eating now?" provides more information than several single-answer questions such as "Is Jimmy eating what the rest of the family eats?"

Sometimes the parent will take the lead without prompting. At other times it may be necessary to direct another question on the basis of an observation, such as "Connie seems unhappy today" or "How do you feel when David cries?" If the parent appears to be tired or distraught, consider asking, "What do you do to relax?" or "What help do you have with the children?" A comment such as "You handle the baby very well. What kinds of experience have you had with babies?" to new parents who appear comfortable with their first child gives positive reinforcement and provides an opening for any questions they might have regarding the care of the infant. Often all that is required to keep parents talking is a nod or saying "yes" or "uh-huh."

When attempting to elicit feelings and covert problem areas, avoid closed-ended questions that begin with "Does . . .," "Did . . .," or "Is . . .," which usually require only a single response. In addition, asking questions such as "Does your son have any problems at school?" subtly implies a lack of parental skills and evokes defensiveness. Instead, say, "What . . .," "How . . .," "Tell me about . . ." and encourage elaboration with "You were saying . . .," "You say that . . .," or reflecting back a key word. Open-ended questions are nonthreatening and encourage description.

Directing the Focus

The ability to direct the focus of the interview while allowing for maximum freedom of expression is one of the most difficult goals in effective communication. One approach is the use of open-ended or broad questions, followed by guiding statements. For example, if the parent proceeds to list the other children by name, say, "Tell me their ages, too." If the parent continues to describe each child in depth, which is not the purpose of the interview, redirect the focus by stating, "Let's talk about the other children later. You were beginning to tell me about Paul's activities at school." This approach conveys interest in the other children but focuses the assessment on the patient.

In the event that the parent has suggested that a problem exists with one of the other children, reintroduce this subject at the end of the interview to assess the need for further family follow-up. Saying to the parent, "Before, you were mentioning that your older son is having trouble in school. Tell me what you see as the problem," reintroduces this subject but only in terms of the possible problem.

Listening and Cultural Awareness

Listening is the most important component of effective communication. When listening is truly aimed at understanding the client, it is an active process that requires concentration and attention to all aspects of the conversation—verbal, nonverbal, and abstract. Major blocks to listening are environmental distraction and premature judgment.

The attitudes and feelings of the nurse are easily injected into an interview. Often nurses' perceptions of a parent's behavior are influenced by their own perceptions, prejudices, and assumptions, which may include racial, religious, and cultural stereotypes. What may be interpreted as passive hostility or disinterest in a parent may be shyness or an expression of anxiety. For example, in Western cultures eye contact and directness are signs of paying attention. However, in many non-Western cultures, including that of Native Americans, directness, such as looking someone in the eye, is considered rude. Children are taught to avert their gaze and to look down when being addressed by an adult, especially one with authority (Seidel and others, 2003). Therefore judgments about "listening," as well as verbal interactions, need to be made with an appreciation of cultural differences (see Guidelines box and Chapter 4).

Although it is necessary to make some preliminary judgments, listen with as much objectivity as possible by clarifying meanings and attempting to see the situation from the parent's point of view. Effective interviewers use conscious control over their reactions, responses, and the techniques they use.

Minimum verbal activity with active listening facilitates parent involvement. It is tempting to spend time explaining, describing, and interpreting health information when the opportunity presents itself. However, it is possible to provide effective health education by timing the information properly and presenting only as much as is necessary at the moment.

Careful listening facilitates the use of clues, verbal leads, or signals from the interviewee to move the interview along. Frequent references to an area of concern, repetition of certain key words, and/or a special emphasis on something or someone serve as cues to the interviewer for the direction of inquiry. Concerns and anxieties are usually mentioned in a casual, offhand manner. Even though they are casual, they are important and deserve careful scrutiny to identify problem areas. For example, a parent who is concerned about a child's habit of bed-wetting may casually mention that the child's bed was "wet this morning."

Because the interview is almost always triangular—between the nurse, parent, and child—the parent may wish to convey information in such a way as to prevent the child from hearing it. This requires active listening on the part of the nurse to hear the unspoken message. The following example illustrates this point:

During a routine health visit, the nurse performed a complete history and physical examination on a 4-year-old girl. The child was accom-

Culturally Sensitive Interactions

NONVERBAL STRATEGIES

Invite family members to choose where they would like to sit or stand, allowing them to select a comfortable distance.

Observe interactions with others to determine which body gestures (e.g., shaking hands) are acceptable and appropriate. Ask when in doubt.

Avoid appearing rushed.

Be an active listener.

Observe for cues regarding appropriate eye contact.

Learn appropriate use of pauses or interruptions for different cultures.

Ask for clarification if nonverbal meaning is unclear.

VERBAL STRATEGIES

Learn proper terms of address.

Use a positive tone of voice to convey interest.

Speak slowly and carefully, not loudly, when families have poor language comprehension.

Encourage questions.

Learn basic words and sentences of family's language, if possible.

Avoid professional terms.

When asking questions, tell family why the questions are being asked, the way in which the information they provide will be used, and how it might benefit their child.

Repeat important information more than once.

Always give the reason or purpose for a treatment or prescription.

Use information written in family's language.

Offer the services of an interpreter when necessary (see Communicating With Families Through an Interpreter, p. 110).

Learn from families and representatives of their culture methods of communicating information without creating discomfort.

Address intergenerational needs (e.g., family's need to consult with others).

Be sincere, open, and honest and, when appropriate, share personal experiences, beliefs, and practices to establish rapport and trust.

panied by her mother, who appeared to be a reliable, well-informed, and talkative informant. During the child's birth history, the mother gave all the information asked. However, during the family history, the mother stated to the nurse, "I had a hysterectomy 6 years ago." Because the nurse gave no indication of acknowledging the significance of this statement, the mother repeated it, only this time she stressed the "6 years." The nurse, who had not been listening as attentively as she should have, realized that the mother was telling her something very important. The mother raised her eyebrows and gently shook her head "no," warning the nurse not to explore this area too openly. The nurse correctly read the cues and stated, "Let's return to your health history later."

At the completion of the physical examination, the nurse took the child to the health center's playroom and took the opportunity to investigate this contradictory information of a "4-year-old child born to a woman with a hysterectomy 6 years ago." The mother revealed that the child was adopted. The mother was greatly concerned about the fact that the child was unaware of this and requested the nurse's advice.

Fortunately, the nurse had "listened" carefully enough to realize the significance of this woman's concern and allowed her the opportunity to discuss it in private.

Listening is also helpful in assessing reliability. For example, the answers elicited at the beginning of the interview may differ from those at the end, when the parent feels more confident in revealing problems. It is important to identify any discrepancies and reintroduce those topics for further investigation.

Using Silence

Silence as a response is often one of the most difficult interviewing techniques to learn. It requires a sense of confidence and comfort on the part of the interviewer to allow the interviewee space in which to think without interruptions. Silence permits the interviewee to sort out thoughts and feelings and search for responses to questions. It also allows for sharing of feelings in which two or more people absorb the emotion to its depth. Silence can also be a clue for the interviewer to go slower, reexamine his or her approach, and not push too hard (Seidel and others, 2003).

Sometimes it is necessary to break the silence and reopen communication. Do this in a way that encourages the person to continue talking about what is considered important. Breaking a silence by introducing a new topic or by prolonged talking essentially terminates the interviewee's opportunity to use the silence. Suggestions for breaking the silence include statements such as "Is there anything else you wish to say?" "I see you find it difficult to continue; how may I help?" or "I don't know what this silence means. Perhaps there is something you would like to put into words but find difficult to say?"

Being Empathic

Empathy is the capacity to understand what another person is experiencing from within that person's frame of reference; it is often described as the ability to put oneself in another's shoes. The essence of empathic interaction is accurately understanding another's feelings (Reynolds, Scott, and Jessiman, 1999; Price and Archbold, 1997; White, 1997). Empathy differs from *sympathy,* which is *having* feelings or emotions in common with another person, rather than *understanding* those feelings. Sympathy is not therapeutic in the helping relationship, because it leads to feeling emotionally overinvolved, and potentially to professional burnout (Yegdich, 1999).

Defining the Problem

To arrive at a solution to a problem, the nurse and the parent must agree that a problem exists. Sometimes the parent may believe that there is a problem that the nurse is unable to see. For example, a mother was overly concerned about every small sniffle, sneeze, or cough in her infant, who had been carefully examined and found to be healthy with no evidence of a respiratory problem. On careful questioning, the nurse discovered that a previous child had died of pneumonia in infancy. Consequently, the nurse was better able to understand the mother's concern and could help the mother deal with her anxieties about her infant; the nurse could also teach her how to recognize any need for concern.

Occasionally, the nurse identifies a problem that the parent denies exists. In this case pursue the situation and either find a way to deal with it or enlist the aid of other health team members. For example, the parents of a child with

Down syndrome may refuse to believe that their child is different from any other child of the same age. They may say, "He is just a little slow," or "All the child needs to do is to try harder." A child with an obvious behavior problem may be described by the parents as "stubborn." Such statements may be clues that the parents have not progressed past the stage of denial in adjusting to the condition.

Solving the Problem

After the problem is identified and agreed on by the parent and the nurse, they can begin to arrive at a solution. A parent who is included in the problem-solving process is more apt to follow through with a course of action. Such questions as "What have you tried so far?" or "What have you thought about doing?" provide leads for exploration and give the parents the feeling that their ideas and solutions are worthwhile. These can be followed by "What prevents you from trying that?" "That sounds like a good plan," or "You seem to be stumped. Have you considered trying this?" Such approaches encourage active participation and reinforce rather than belittle parents' efforts to solve their problems.

Sometimes the parents arrive at a solution that the nurse does not consider the best alternative. If it can be ascertained that it will do no harm and if the parents are convinced of its merits, it is usually best to allow them to continue with the plan. A course of action is more likely to be carried out when parents can reach their own conclusions. However, when parental decisions may be hazardous, nurses are obligated to discuss the risks with the family and try to reach a more beneficial solution. Whenever possible, decisions should be theirs, with the nurse serving as a *facilitator* in problem solving.

Providing Anticipatory Guidance

The ideal way to handle a situation is to deal with it *before* it becomes a problem. The best preventive measure is anticipatory guidance. Traditionally, anticipatory guidance has focused on providing families with information on normal growth and development, as well as nurturing child-rearing practices. For example, one of the most significant areas in pediatrics is injury prevention. Beginning prenatally, parents need specific instructions on home safety. Because of the child's maturing developmental skills, home safety changes must be implemented early to minimize risks to the child.

Many normal developmental changes can disturb unprepared parents, such as a toddler's diminished appetite, negativism, altered sleeping patterns, and anxiety toward strangers. Such topics are discussed in the chapters on health promotion to provide the nurse with knowledge to counsel parents.

However, anticipatory guidance should extend beyond giving information to empowering families to use the information as a means of building competence in their parenting abilities. To achieve this level of anticipatory guidance (Desselle and Pearlmutter, 1997):

- Base interventions on needs identified by the family, not by the professional.
- View the family as competent or as having the ability to be competent.
- Provide opportunities for the family to achieve competence.

Often parents need early guidance with their children (Desselle and Pearlmutter, 1997), and anticipatory guidance builds confidence in their parenting skills.

Avoiding Blocks to Communication

A number of blocks to communication can adversely affect the quality of the helping relationship. Many of these blocks are initiated by the interviewer, such as giving unrestricted advice or forming prejudged conclusions. Another type of block occurs primarily with the interviewees and deals with information overload. When individuals are presented with too much information or information that is overwhelming, they will often demonstrate signals of increasing anxiety or decreasing attention. Such signals should alert the interviewer to give less information or to clarify what has been said. Some of the more common blocks to communication, including signs of information overload, are listed in Box 6-2.

Communication blocks can be corrected by careful analysis of the interview process. One of the best methods for improving interviewing skills is audiotape and/or videotape feedback. With supervision and guidance, the interviewer can recognize the blocks and consciously avoid them.

Communicating With Families Through an Interpreter

Sometimes communication is impossible because two people speak different languages. In this case it is necessary to obtain information through a third party, the interpreter. When an interpreter is used, the same guidelines for interviewing are used. Specific guidelines for using an adult interpreter are presented in the Guidelines box.

BOX 6-2 ■ Blocks to Communication

Socializing
Giving unrestricted and sometimes unasked for advice
Offering premature or inappropriate reassurance
Giving overready encouragement
Defending a situation or opinion
Using stereotyped comments or clichés
Limiting expression of emotion by asking directed, closed-ended questions
Interrupting and finishing the person's sentence
Talking more than the interviewee
Forming prejudged conclusions
Deliberately changing the focus

SIGNS OF INFORMATION OVERLOAD
Long periods of silence
Wide eyes and fixed facial expression
Constant fidgeting or attempting to move away
Nervous habits (e.g., tapping, playing with hair)
Sudden disruptions (e.g., asking to go to the bathroom)
Looking around
Yawning, eyes drooping
Frequently looking at a watch or clock
Attempting to change topic of discussion

Communicating with families through an interpreter requires sensitivity to cultural, legal, and ethical considerations. For example, in some cultures using a child as an interpreter is considered an insult to an adult, because children are expected to show respect by not questioning their elders. In some cultures class differences between the interpreter and the family may cause the family to feel intimidated and less inclined to offer information. Therefore choose the translator carefully, and provide time for the interpreter and family to establish rapport.

Issues of legal and ethical concerns may also arise. For example, in obtaining informed consent through an interpreter, it is important that the family be fully informed of all aspects of the particular procedure that they are consenting to. Issues of confidentiality may arise when family members related to another patient are asked to interpret for the family, thus revealing sensitive information that may be shared with other families on the unit. With increased sensitivity toward patient rights and confidentiality, many institutions are now requiring consent forms to be produced in the primary language of the patient.

When no one else is available to translate, children within the family are often asked to assume this role. In this situation it is important to stress *literal* translation of parent responses. To maximize correct translations, it may be necessary to interrupt the parent and ask the child to translate every few sentences. When using children as interpreters, ask questions directed at specific answers and assess the interpreted translation in terms of nonverbal expressions of communication. It should be noted that some institutions prohibit or discourage the use of children as interpreter; check institutional policy for compliance.*

NURSING ALERT

When using translated materials, such as a health history form, be sure the informant is literate in the foreign language.

COMMUNICATING WITH CHILDREN

Although the greatest amount of verbal communication may usually be carried out with the parent, do not exclude the child during the interview. Pay attention to infants and younger children through play or by occasionally directing questions or remarks to them. Include older children as active participants.

In communication with children of all ages, the nonverbal components of the communication process convey the most significant messages. It is difficult to disguise feelings, attitudes, and anxiety when relating to children. They are very alert to surroundings and attach meaning to every gesture and move that is made; this is particularly true of very young children.

Active attempts to make friends with children before they have had an opportunity to evaluate an unfamiliar person tend to increase their anxiety. It is helpful to continue to talk to the child and parent but go about activities that do not involve the child directly, thus allowing the child to observe from a safe position. If the child has a special toy or doll, "talk" to the doll first. Ask simple questions such as "Does your teddy bear have a name?" to ease the child into conversation. Other guidelines for communicating with children are presented in the Guidelines box. Specific guidelines for preparing children for procedures, a common nursing function, are discussed in Chapter 22.

---

*Interpreting services are also available through American Telephone and Telegraph (AT&T) by calling (800) 628-8486 or (800) 752-6096.

GUIDELINES

Using an Interpreter

Explain to interpreter the reason for the interview and the type of questions that will be asked.

Clarify whether a detailed or brief answer is required and whether the translated response can be general or literal.

Introduce interpreter to family and allow some time before the actual interview so that they can become acquainted.

Communicate directly with family members when asking questions to reinforce interest in them and to observe nonverbal expressions, but do not ignore interpreter.

Pose questions to elicit only one answer at a time, such as "Do you have pain?" rather than "Do you have any pain, tiredness, or loss of appetite?"

Refrain from interrupting family member and interpreter while they are conversing.

Avoid commenting to interpreter about family members, because they may understand some English.

Be aware that some medical words, such as "allergy," may have no similar word in another language; avoid medical jargon whenever possible.

Respect cultural differences; it is often best to pose questions about sex, marriage, or pregnancy indirectly—ask about "child's father" rather than "mother's husband."

Allow time following the interview for interpreter to share something that he or she felt could not be said earlier; ask about interpreter's impression of nonverbal clues to communication and family members' reliability or ease in revealing information.

Arrange for family to speak with same interpreter on subsequent visits whenever possible.

GUIDELINES

Communicating With Children

Allow children time to feel comfortable.

Avoid sudden or rapid advances, broad smiles, extended eye contact, or other gestures that may be seen as threatening.

Talk to the parent if child is initially shy.

Communicate through transition objects such as dolls, puppets, stuffed animals before questioning a young child directly.

Give older children the opportunity to talk without the parents present.

Assume a position that is at eye level with child (Fig. 6-2).

Speak in a quiet, unhurried, and confident voice.

Speak clearly, be specific, use simple words and short sentences.

State directions and suggestions positively.

Offer a choice only when one exists.

Be honest with children.

Allow them to express their concerns and fears.

Use a variety of communication techniques.

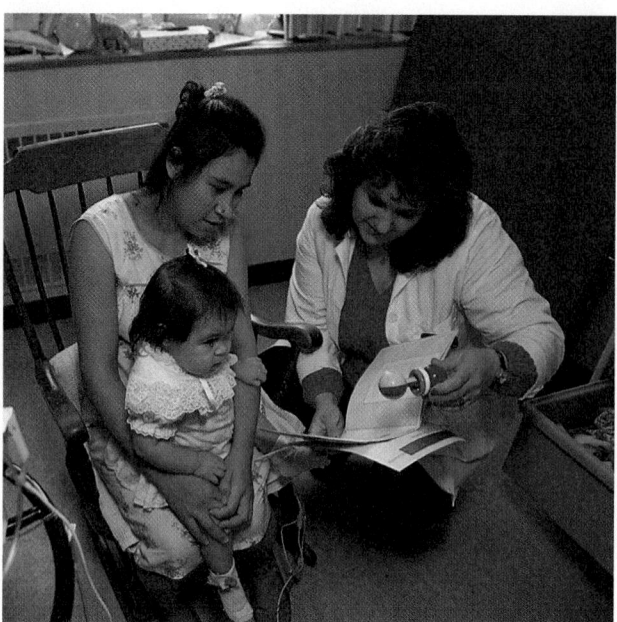

FIG. 6-2 ■ Nurse assumes position at child's level.

Communication Related to Development of Thought Processes

The normal development of language and thought offers a frame of reference in knowing how to communicate with children. Thought processes progress from sensorimotor to perceptual to concrete and finally to abstract, formal operations. The early social communicative development of children has been divided into three stages: (1) *perlocutionary stage*—unintentional communication behavior; (2) *illocutionary stage*—true intent in communication efforts; and (3) *locutionary stage*—intentional communication behaviors and use of symbols (Hoge and Parette, 1995). An understanding of the typical characteristics of these stages provides the nurse with a framework to facilitate social communication (Box 6-3).

Infancy. Because they are unable to use words, infants primarily use and understand nonverbal communication. Infants communicate their needs and feelings through nonverbal behaviors and vocalizations that can be interpreted by someone who is around them for a sufficient amount of time. Infants smile and coo when content and cry when distressed. Crying is provoked by unpleasant stimuli from inside or outside, such as hunger, pain, body restraint, or loneliness. Adults interpret this to mean that an infant needs something and consequently try to alleviate the discomfort and reduce tension. Crying (or the desire to cry) persists as a part of everyone's communication repertoire.

Infants respond to adults' nonverbal behaviors. They become quiet when they are cuddled, patted, or receive other forms of gentle, physical contact. They derive comfort from the sound of a voice, even though they do not understand the words that are spoken. Until infants reach the age at which they experience stranger anxiety, they readily respond to any firm, gentle handling and quiet, calm speech. Loud, harsh sounds and sudden movements are frightening.

BOX 6-3 ■ Stages of Communicative Development in Young Children

PERLOCUTIONARY STAGE (0-8-9 MONTHS)
Characteristics
Child is reflexive to stimuli
Increasing purpose in action

EMERGING ILLOCUTIONARY STAGE (8-9-12-15 MONTHS)
Characteristics
Communicates intentionally with signals and gestures

CONVENTIONAL ILLOCUTIONARY/EMERGING LOCUTIONARY STAGE (12-15-18-24 MONTHS)
Characteristics
Communicates intentionally with gestures, vocalizations, and verbalizations

Modified from Hoge DR, Parette HP: Facilitating communicative development in young children with disabilities, *Transdisciplinary J* 5(2):113-130, 1995.

Older infants' attentions are centered on themselves and their parents; therefore any stranger is a potential threat until proved otherwise. Holding out the hands and asking the child to "come" is seldom successful, especially if the infant is with the parent. If infants must be handled, simply pick them up firmly without gestures. Observe the position in which the parent holds the infant. Most infants have learned to prefer a particular position and manner of handling. In general, infants are more at ease upright than horizontal. Also, hold infants so that they can see their parents. Until they have developed the understanding that an object (in this case the parent) removed from sight can still be present, they have no way of knowing that the object is still there.

Early Childhood. Children younger than 5 years of age are egocentric. They see things only in relation to themselves and from their point of view. Therefore, focus communication on them. Tell them what they can do or how they will feel. Experiences of others are of no interest to them. It is futile to use another child's experience as an attempt to gain the cooperation of very small children. Allow them to touch and examine articles that will come in contact with them. A stethoscope bell will feel cold; palpating a neck might tickle. Although they have not yet acquired sufficient language skills to express their feelings and wants, toddlers are able to communicate effectively with their hands to transmit ideas without words. They push an unwanted object away, pull another person to show them something, point, and cover the mouth that is saying something they do not wish to hear.

Everything is direct and concrete to small children. They are unable to work with abstractions and interpret words literally. Analogies escape them because they are unable to separate fact from fantasy. For example, they attach literal meaning to such common phrases as "two-faced," "sticky fingers," or "coughing your head off." Children who are told they will get "a little stick in the arm" may not be able to envision an injection (Fig. 6-3). Therefore, avoid using a phrase that might be misinterpreted by a small child (see Family Home Care box under Preparation for Procedures, Chapter 22).

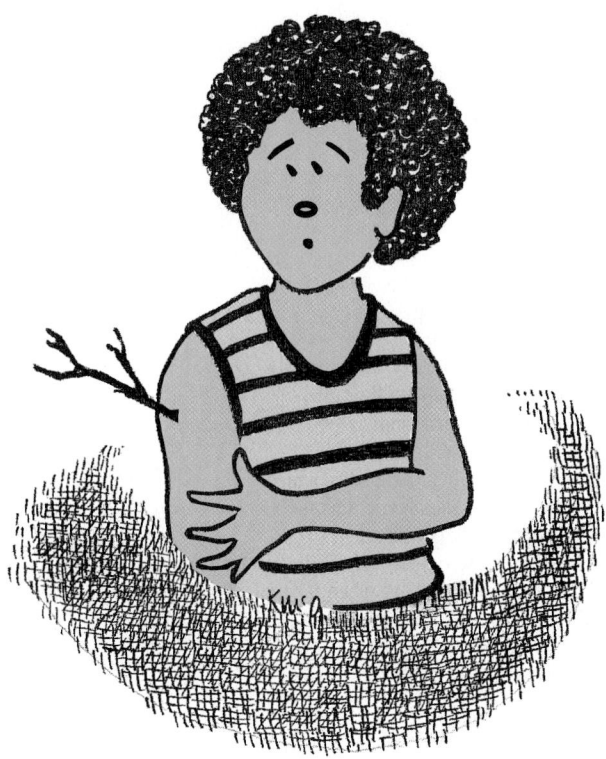

FIG. 6-3 ■ A young child may take the expression "a little stick in the arm" literally.

Use language that is consistent with the child's developmental level. For example, in talking with a toddler, use simple, *short* sentences, repeat words that are *familiar* to the child, and limit descriptions to *concrete* explanations. Be certain that nonverbal messages are consistent with words and actions. For example, do not smile while doing something painful; children may think you enjoy hurting them.

Young children assign human attributes to inanimate objects. Consequently, they fear that objects may jump, bite, cut, or pinch all by themselves. Children do not know that these devices are unable to perform without human direction. To minimize their fear, keep unfamiliar equipment out of view until it is needed.

School-Age Years.   Younger school-age children rely less on what they see and more on what they know when faced with new problems. They want explanations and reasons for everything but require no verification beyond that. They are interested in the functional aspect of all procedures, objects, and activities. They want to know why an object exists, why it is used, how it works, and the intent and purpose of its user. They need to know what is going to take place and why it is being done to them specifically. For example, to explain a procedure such as taking a blood pressure, show the child how squeezing the bulb pushes air into the cuff and makes the "silver" in the tube go up. Let the child operate the bulb. An explanation for the reason might be as simple as "I want to see how far the silver goes up when the cuff squeezes your arm." Consequently, the child becomes an enthusiastic participant.

School-age children have a heightened concern about body integrity. Because of the special importance and value they place on their body, they are overly sensitive to anything that constitutes a threat or suggestion of injury to it. This concern extends to their possessions also, so that they may appear to overreact to loss or threatened loss of treasured objects. Helping children to voice their concerns enables the nurse to provide reassurance and to implement activities that reduce their anxiety. For example, if a shy child dislikes being the center of attention, ignore that particular child by talking and relating to other children in the family or group. When children feel more comfortable, they will usually interject personal ideas, feelings, and interpretations of events.

Older children have an adequate and satisfactory use of language. They still require relatively simple explanations, but their ability to think concretely can facilitate communication and explanation. Commonly, they have sufficient experience with health and health care workers to understand what is transpiring and generally what is expected of them.

Adolescence.   As children move into adolescence, they fluctuate between child and adult thinking and behavior. They are riding a current that is moving them rapidly toward a maturity that may be beyond their coping ability. Therefore, when tensions rise, they may seek the security of the more familiar and comfortable expectations of childhood. Anticipating these shifts in identity allows the nurse to adjust the course of interaction to meet the needs of the moment. No single approach can be relied on consistently, and encountering cooperation, hostility, anger, bravado, and a variety of other behaviors and attitudes can be expected. It is as much a mistake to regard the adolescent as an adult with an adult's wisdom and control as it is to assume that the teenager has the concerns and expectations of a child.

Frequently adolescents are more willing to discuss their concerns with an adult outside the family, and they often welcome the opportunity to interact with a nurse outside of the presence of their parents. They are accepting of anyone who displays a genuine interest in them. However, adolescents are quick to reject persons who attempt to impose their values on them, whose interest is feigned, or who appear to have little respect for who they are and what they think or say.

As with all children, adolescents need to express their feelings. Generally, they talk quite freely when given an opportunity. However, what adolescents say cannot always be taken at face value. When emotional factors are involved, the feelings that are interjected into words are as significant as the words that are used. To give support, be attentive, try not to interrupt, and avoid comments or expressions that convey disapproval or surprise. Avoid prying and asking embarrassing questions, and resist any impulse to give advice. Frequently, adolescents reveal their feelings or a source of concern or ask a question when they are involved in routine matters such as a physical assessment.

Teenagers characteristically have a language and culture all their own that further sets them apart. To avoid misinterpretation, clarify terms frequently. Occasionally, adolescents refuse to answer or answer only in monosyllables. Usually this happens when they are opposed to the contact or do not yet feel safe enough to reveal themselves. In this instance confine discussions to neutral topics to reduce the element of threat until such time as they feel more secure. Be alert for signals indicating that they are ready to talk. The major sources of concern for adolescents are attitudes and feelings toward sex, substance abuse, relationships with parents, peer-group acceptance, and developing a sense of identity.

Interviewing the adolescent presents some special situations. The first may be whether to talk with the adolescent alone, with the adolescent and parents together, or with each person individually. Of course, if the adolescent is alone, there is no question, except whether to suggest to the teenager that the parents may be interviewed at another time. If the parents and teenager are together, talking with the adolescent first has the advantage of immediately identifying with the young person, thus fostering the interpersonal relationship. However, talking with the parents initially may provide insight into the family relationship. In either case, give both parties an opportunity to be included in the interview. If time constraints are important, such as during history taking, clarify these at the onset to avoid appearing to "take sides" by talking more with one person than with the other.

Confidentiality is of great important when interviewing adolescents. Explain to parents and teenagers the limits of confidentiality, specifically that young persons' disclosures will not be shared unless they indicate a need for intervention, as in the case of suicidal behavior.

Another dilemma in interviewing adolescents is that two views of a problem frequently exist—the teenager's and the parents'. Clarification of the problem is a major task. However, providing both parties with an opportunity to discuss their perceptions in an open and unbiased atmosphere can, by itself, be therapeutic. Demonstrating positive communication skills can help families communicate more effectively (see Guidelines box).

NURSING ALERT

Studies have indicated that family communication patterns significantly influence self-esteem in deaf children. Adolescents whose parents used total communication (speech, finger spelling, and sign language) had higher self-esteem scores than those with parents who used speech only (Desselle and Pearlmutter, 1997).

COMMUNICATION TECHNIQUES

In addition to such conventional interviewing methods as reflection and open-ended questions, a number of techniques encourage family members to express their thoughts and feelings in a less directive and confrontational manner. Several approaches are projective—they present nonspecific material that enables individuals to externalize or project inner aspects of themselves to others.

A variety of verbal techniques can be used to encourage communication. Some of these techniques can be used to pose questions or explore concerns in a less threatening manner. Others can be presented as "word games," which are often well received by children. However, for many children and adults, talking about feelings is difficult and verbal communication may be more stressful than supportive. In such instances several nonverbal techniques can be used to encourage communication.

GUIDELINES

Communicating With Adolescents

BUILD A FOUNDATION
Spend time together.
Encourage expression of ideas and feelings.
Respect their views.
Tolerate differences.
Praise good points.
Respect their privacy.
Set a good example.

COMMUNICATE EFFECTIVELY
Give undivided attention.
Listen, listen, listen.
Be courteous, calm, and open-minded.
Try not to overreact. If you do, take a break.
Avoid judging or criticizing.
Avoid the "third degree" of continuous questioning.
Choose important issues when taking a stand.
After taking a stand:
  Think through all options.
  Make expectations clear.

Both verbal and nonverbal techniques are described in Box 6-4. Because of the importance of play in communicating with children, play is discussed more extensively below. Any of the verbal or nonverbal techniques can give rise to strong feelings that surface unexpectedly. Be prepared to handle them or to recognize when issues go beyond your ability to deal with them. At that point, consider an appropriate referral.

Play

Play is a universal language of children. It is one of the most important forms of communication and can be an effective technique in relating to them. Clues about physical, intellectual, and social developmental progress can often be gleaned from the form and complexity of a child's play behaviors. Play requires a minimum of equipment or none at all. Therapeutic play is often used to reduce the trauma of illness and hospitalization (see Chapter 21) and to prepare children for therapeutic procedures (see Chapter 22).

Because their ability to perceive precedes their ability to transmit, infants respond to activities that register on their senses. Patting, stroking, and other skin play convey messages. Repetitive actions, such as stretching infants' arms out to the side while they are lying on their back and then folding them across the chest or raising and revolving the legs in a bicycling motion, will elicit pleasurable sounds. Colorful items to catch the eye or interesting sounds, such as a ticking clock, chimes, bells, or singing, can be used to attract children's attention.

Older infants respond to simple games. The old game of peekaboo is an excellent means of initiating communication with infants while maintaining a "safe," nonthreatening distance. After this intermittent eye-to-eye contact, the nurse is no longer viewed as a stranger but as some-

BOX 6-4 ■ Creative Communication Techniques With Children

VERBAL TECHNIQUES

"I" Messages
Relate a feeling about a behavior in terms of "I."
Describe effect behavior had on the person.
Avoid use of "you."
"You" messages are judgmental and provoke defensiveness.
> *Example:* "You" message—"You are being very uncooperative about doing your treatments."
>
> *Example:* "I" message—"I am concerned about how the treatments are going because I want to see you get better."

Third-Person Technique
Involves expressing a feeling in terms of a third person ("he," "she," "they").
Is less threatening than directly asking children how they feel because it gives them an opportunity to agree or disagree without being defensive.
> *Example:* "Sometimes when a person is sick a lot, he feels angry and sad because he cannot do what others can." Either wait silently for a response or encourage a reply with a statement such as "Did you ever feel that way?"

Approach allows children three choices: (1) to agree and, hopefully, express how they feel; (2) to disagree; or (3) to remain silent, in which case they probably have such feelings but are unable to express them at this time.

Facilitative Responding
Involves careful listening and reflecting back to patients the feelings and content of their statements.
Responses are empathic and nonjudgmental, and legitimize the person's feelings.
Formula for facilitative responses: "You feel _____ because _____."
> *Example:* If child states, "I hate coming to the hospital and getting needles," a facilitative response is, "You feel unhappy because of all the things that are done to you."

Storytelling
Uses the language of children to probe into areas of their thinking while bypassing conscious inhibitions or fears.
Simplest technique is asking children to relate a story about an event, such as "being in the hospital."
Other approaches:
> Show children a picture of a particular event, such as a child in a hospital with other people in the room, and ask them to describe the scene.
> Cut out comic strips, remove words, and have child add statements for scenes.

Mutual Storytelling
Reveals child's thinking and attempts to change child's perceptions or fears by retelling a somewhat different story (more therapeutic approach than storytelling).
Begins by asking child to tell a story about something, followed by another story told by the nurse that is similar to child's tale but with differences that help child in problem areas.
> *Example:* Child's story is about going to the hospital and never seeing his or her parents again. Nurse's story is also about a child (using different names but similar circumstances) in a hospital whose parents visit everyday, but in the evening after work, until the child is better and goes home with them.

Bibliotherapy
Uses books in a therapeutic and supportive process.
Provides children with an opportunity to explore an event that is similar to their own but sufficiently different to allow them to distance themselves from it and remain in control.

General guidelines for using bibliotherapy are:
> Assess child's emotional and cognitive development in terms of readiness to understand the book's message.
> Be familiar with the book's content (intended message or purpose) and the age for which it is written.
> Read the book to the child if child is unable to read.
> Explore the meaning of the book with the child by having child:
> > Retell the story
> > Read a special section with the nurse or parent
> > Draw a picture related to the story and discuss the drawing
> > Talk about the characters
> > Summarize the moral or meaning of the story

Dreams
Often reveal unconscious and repressed thoughts and feelings.
Ask child to talk about a dream or nightmare.
Explore with child what meaning dream could have.

"What If" Questions
Encourage child to explore potential situations and to consider different problem-solving options.
> *Example:* "What if you got sick and had to go the hospital?" Children's responses reveal what they know already and what they are curious about, provide opportunity for helping children learn coping skills, especially in potentially dangerous situations.

Three Wishes
Involves asking, "If you could have any three things in the world, what would they be?"
If child answers, "That all my wishes come true," ask child for specific wishes.

Rating Game
Uses some type of rating scale (numbers, sad to happy faces) to rate an event or feeling.
> *Example:* Instead of asking youngsters how they feel, ask how their day has been "on a scale of 1 to 10, with 10 being the best."

Word Association Game
Involves stating key words and asking children to say the first word they think of when they hear the word.
> Start with neutral words and then introduce more anxiety-producing words, such as "illness," "needles," "hospitals," and "operation."
> Select key words that relate to some event in child's life that is relevant.

Sentence Completion
Involves presenting a partial statement and having child complete it. Some sample statements are:
The thing I like best (least) about school is _____.
The best (worst) age to be is _____.
The most (least) fun thing I ever did was _____.
The thing I like most (least) about my parents is _____.
The one thing I would change about my family is _____.
If I could be anything I wanted, I would be _____.
The thing I like most (least) about myself is _____.

Pros and Cons
Involves selecting a topic, such as "being in the hospital," and having child list "five good things and five bad things" about it.
Is an exceptionally valuable technique when applied to relationships, such as things family members like and dislike about each other.

Continued

BOX 6-4 ■ Creative Communication Techniques With Children—*cont'd*

NONVERBAL TECHNIQUES

Writing

Is an alternative communication approach for older children and adults.

Specific suggestions include:

Keep a journal or diary.

Write down feelings or thoughts that are difficult to express.

Write "letters" that are never mailed (a variation is making up a "pen pal" to write to).

Keep an account of child's progress from both a physical and an emotional viewpoint.

Drawing

Is one of the most valuable forms of communication—both nonverbal (from looking at the drawing) and verbal (from child's story of the picture).

Children's drawings tell a great deal about them because they are projections of their inner selves.

Spontaneous drawing involves giving child a variety of art supplies and providing the opportunity to draw.

Directed drawing involves a more specific direction, such as "draw a person" or the "three themes" approach (state three things about child and ask child to choose one and draw a picture) (Fig. 6-4).

Guidelines for Evaluating Drawings

Use spontaneous drawings and evaluate more than one drawing whenever possible.

Interpret drawings in light of other available information about child and family.

Interpret drawings as a whole rather than on specific details of the drawing.

Consider individual elements of the drawing that may be significant:

Sex of figure drawn first—Usually relates to child's perception of own sex role.

Size of individual figures—Expresses importance, power, or authority.

Order in which figures are drawn—Expresses priority in terms of importance.

Child's position in relation to other family members—Expresses feelings of status or alliance.

Exclusion of a member—May denote feeling of not belonging or desire to eliminate.

Accentuated parts—Usually express concern for areas of special importance (e.g., large hands may be a sign of aggression).

Absence of or rudimentary arms and hands—Suggest timidity, passivity, or intellectual immaturity; tiny, unstable feet may be an expression of insecurity, and hidden hands may mean guilt feelings.

Placement of drawing on the page and type of stroke—Free use of paper and firm, continuous strokes express security, whereas drawings restricted to a small area and lightly drawn in broken or wavering lines may be a sign of insecurity.

Erasures, shading, or cross-hatching—Expresses ambivalence, concern, or anxiety with a particular area.

Magic

Uses simple magic tricks to help establish rapport with child, encourage compliance with health interventions, and provide effective distraction during painful procedures.

Although "magician" talks, no verbal response from child is required.

Play

Is universal language and "work" of children.

Tells a great deal about children because they project their inner selves through the activity.

Spontaneous play involves giving child a variety of play materials and providing the opportunity to play.

Directed play involves a more specific direction, such as providing medical equipment or a dollhouse for focused reasons, such as exploring child's fear of injections or exploring family relationships.

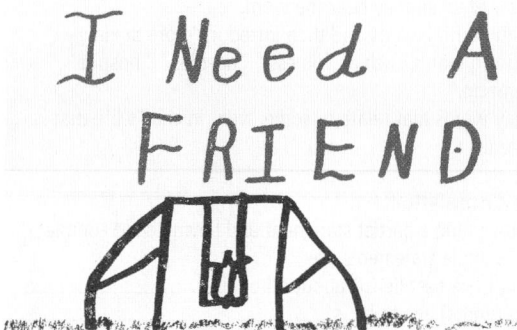

FIG. 6-4 ■ Using the three-themes approach, this child chose the theme, "the first day of school." The drawing and title reveal the child's loneliness and insecurity in a new setting.

one who is a friend. This can be followed by touch games. Clapping an infant's hands together for pat-a-cake or wiggling the toes for "this little piggy" delights an infant or small child. Much of the nursing assessment can be carried out with the use of games and simple play equipment while the infant remains in the safety of the parent's arms or lap. Talking to a foot or other part of the child's body is an effective tactic.

The nurse can capitalize on the natural curiosity of small children by playing games such as "Which hand do you take?" and "Guess what I have in my hand" or by manipulating items such as a flashlight or stethoscope. Finger games are very useful. More elaborate materials, such as puppets and replicas of familiar or unfamiliar items, serve as excellent means of communicating with small children. The variety and extent are limited only by the nurse's imagination.

Through play, children reveal their perceptions of interpersonal relationships with their family, friends, or hospital personnel. Children may also reveal the wide scope of knowledge they have acquired from listening to others around them. For example, through needle play, children may disclose how carefully they have watched each procedure by precisely duplicating the technical skills. They may also reveal how well they remember those who performed procedures. One child who painstakingly reenacted every detail of a tedious medical procedure also played the role of the physician who had repeatedly shouted at her to be still for the long ordeal. Her anger at him was most evident during the play session and revealed the cause for her abrupt withdrawal and passive hostility toward the medical and nursing staff after the test.

Play sessions serve not only as assessment tools for determining children's awareness and perception of their illness, but also as methods of intervention and evaluation. In the previous example, when the child revealed anger toward the physician, the nurse acted the part of the patient but this time did not accept the physician's harsh commands to stay still. Instead, the nurse said to the physician all the things the child had wished she could say.

Subsequent play sessions can also be used to evaluate the child's progress. A change in the type of drawing or the theme of the play may indicate progression toward or away from the ability to deal with anxiety.

HISTORY TAKING

PERFORMING A HEALTH HISTORY

The format used for history taking may be (1) *direct*—the nurse asks for information via direct interview with the informant—or (2) *indirect*—the informant supplies the information by completing some type of questionnaire. The direct method is superior to the indirect approach or a combination of both. However, in view of time constraints, the direct approach is not always practical. If the direct approach cannot be used, review parents' written responses and question them regarding any unusual answers. The categories listed in Box 6-5 encompass children's current and past health status and information about their psychosocial environment.

Identifying Information

Much of the identifying information may already be available from other recorded sources. However, if the parent and youngster seem anxious, use this opportunity to ask about such information to help them feel more comfortable.

Informant.   One of the important elements of identifying information is the informant, the person(s) who furnished the information. Record (1) who the person is (child, parent, or other), (2) an impression of reliability and willingness to communicate, and (3) any special circumstances such as the use of an interpreter or conflicting answers by more than one person.

Chief Complaint

The chief complaint is the specific reason for the child's visit to the clinic, office, or hospital. It may be viewed as the theme with the present illness as the description of the problem. The chief complaint is elicited by asking open-ended neutral questions such as "What seems to be the matter?" "How may I help you?" or "Why did you come here today?" Avoid labeling-type questions such as "How are you sick?" or "What is the problem?" It is possible that the reason for the visit is not an illness or problem.

Occasionally, it is difficult to isolate one symptom or problem as the chief complaint because the parent may identify many. In this situation be as specific as possible when asking questions. For example, asking informants to state which *one* problem or symptom prompted them to seek help now may help them focus on the most immediate concern.

BOX 6-5 ■ Outline of a Pediatric Health History

Identifying information
1. Name	6. Sex
2. Address	7. Religion
3. Telephone	8. Date of interview
4. Birthdate and place	9. Informant
5. Race/ethnic group	

Chief complaint (CC)—To establish the major specific reason for the child's and parents' seeking professional health attention

Present illness (PI)—To obtain all details related to the chief complaint

Past history (PH)—To elicit a profile of the child's previous illnesses, injuries, or operations

1. Birth history (pregnancy, labor, and delivery, perinatal history)	4. Current medications
	5. Immunizations
	6. Growth and development
2. Previous illnesses, injuries, or operations	7. Habits
3. Allergies	

Review of systems (ROS)—To elicit information concerning any potential health problem

1. General	10. Chest
2. Integument	11. Respiratory
3. Head	12. Cardiovascular
4. Eyes	13. Gastrointestinal
5. Ears	14. Genitourinary
6. Nose	15. Gynecologic
7. Mouth	16. Musculoskeletal
8. Throat	17. Neurologic
9. Neck	18. Endocrine

Family medical history—To identify the presence of genetic traits or diseases that have familial tendencies and to assess exposure to a communicable disease in a family member and family habits that may affect the child's health, such as smoking and other chemical use

Psychosocial history—To elicit information about the child's self-concept

Sexual history—To elicit information concerning the child's sexual concerns and/or activities and any pertinent data regarding adults' sexual activity that influence the child

Family history—To develop an understanding of the child as an individual and as a member of a family and a community
1. Family composition
2. Home and community environment
3. Occupation and education of family members
4. Cultural and religious traditions
5. Family function and relationships

Nutritional assessment—To elicit information on the adequacy of the child's nutritional intake and need
1. Dietary intake
2. Clinical examination

Present Illness

The history of the present illness* is a narrative of the chief complaint from its earliest onset through its progression to the present. Its four major components are (1) the details of

---

*The term *illness* is used in its broadest sense to denote any problem of a physical, emotional, or psychosocial nature. It is actually a history of the chief complaint.

onset, (2) a complete *interval* history, (3) the *present* status, and (4) the reason for seeking help *now*. The focus of the present illness is on all factors relevant to the main problem, even if they have disappeared or changed during the onset, interval, and present.

Analyzing a Symptom.   Because pain is often the most characteristic symptom denoting the onset of a physical problem, it is used as an example for analysis of a symptom. Assessment includes (1) type, (2) location, (3) severity, (4) duration, and (5) influencing factors (see Guidelines box; see also Pain Assessment, Chapter 21).

Past History

The past history contains information relating to all previous aspects of the child's health status and concentrates on several areas that are ordinarily deleted in the history of an adult, such as birth history, detailed feeding history, immunizations, and growth and development. Since a great deal of information is included in this section, use a combination of open-ended and fact-finding questions. For example, begin interviewing for each section with an open-ended statement such as "Tell me about your child's birth" to provide the informants with the opportunity to relate what they think is most important. Ask fact-finding questions related to specific details whenever necessary to focus the interview on certain topics.

GUIDELINES

Analyzing the Symptom: Pain

Type. Be as specific as possible. With young children, asking the parents how they know the child is in pain may help describe its type, location, and severity. For example, a parent may state, "My child must have a severe earache because she pulls at her ears, rolls her head on the floor, and screams. Nothing seems to help." Help older children describe the "hurt" by asking them if it is sharp, throbbing, dull, or stabbing. Record whatever words they use in quotes.

Location. Be specific. "Stomach pains" is too general a description. Children can better localize the pain if they are asked to "point with one finger to where it hurts" or to "point to where Mommy or Daddy would put a Band-Aid." Determine if the pain radiates by asking. "Does the pain stay there or move? Show me with your finger where the pain goes."

Severity. Severity is best determined by finding out how it affects the child's usual behavior. Pain that prevents a child from playing, interacting with others, sleeping, or eating is most often severe. Assess pain intensity using a rating scale, such as a numeric scale or faces scale (see Table 21-2).

Duration. Include the duration, onset, and frequency. Describe this in terms of activity and behavior, such as "pain lasted all night, because child refused to sleep and cried intermittently."

Influencing factor. Include anything that causes a change in the type, location, severity, or duration of the pain: (1) precipitating events (those that cause or increase the pain), (2) relieving events (those that lessen the pain, such as medications), (3) temporal events (times when the pain is relieved or increased), (4) positional events (standing, sitting, lying down), and (5) associated events (meals, stress, coughing).

Birth History.   The birth history includes all data concerning (1) the mother's health during pregnancy, (2) the labor and delivery, and (3) the infant's condition immediately after birth. Since prenatal influences have significant effects on a child's physical and emotional development, a thorough investigation of the birth history is essential. Because parents may question what relevance pregnancy and birth have on the child's present condition, particularly if the child is past infancy, explain why such questions are included. An appropriate statement may be, "I will be asking you some questions about your pregnancy and . . . (refer to child by name) birth. Your answers will give me a more complete picture of his (or her) overall health."

Because emotional factors also affect the outcome of pregnancy and the subsequent parent-child relationship, investigate (1) concurrent crises during pregnancy and (2) prenatal attitudes toward the fetus. It is best to approach the topic of parental acceptance of pregnancy through indirect questioning. Asking parents if the pregnancy was planned is a leading statement because they may respond affirmatively for fear of criticism if the pregnancy was unexpected. Rather, encourage parents to disclose their true reactions by referring to specific facts relating to the pregnancy, such as the spacing between offspring, an extended or short interval between marriage and conception, or the concurrent experience of pregnancy and adolescence. The parent can choose to explore such statements with further explanations or, for the moment, may not be able to reveal such feelings. If the parent remains silent, refocus on this topic later in the interview.

Dietary History.   Because parental concerns are common and nursing interventions are important in ensuring optimum nutrition, the dietary history is discussed in detail at the end of this chapter under Nutritional Assessment.

Previous Illnesses, Injuries, and Operations.   When inquiring about past illnesses, begin with a general statement such as "What other illnesses has your child had?" Since parents are most likely to recall serious health problems, ask specifically about colds; earaches; and childhood diseases such as measles, rubella (German measles), chickenpox, mumps, pertussis (whooping cough), diphtheria, tuberculosis, scarlet fever, strep throat, tonsillitis, or allergic manifestations.

In addition to illnesses, ask about injuries that required medical intervention, operations, and any other reason for hospitalization, including the dates of each incident. It is important to focus on injuries such as accidental falls, poisonings, chokings, or burns, because this may be a potential area for parental guidance.

Allergies.   Ask about commonly known allergic disorders such as hay fever and asthma, as well as unusual reactions to drugs, food, or latex products, or other contact agents such as poisonous plants, animals, household products, or fabrics. If asked appropriate questions, most people can give reliable information about drug reactions. (See Guidelines box.)

NURSING ALERT

Information about allergic reactions to drugs or other products is essential. Failure to document a serious reaction places the child at risk if the agent is given.

Current Medications. Inquire about current drug regimens, including vitamins, antipyretics (especially aspirin), antibiotics, antihistamines, decongestants, or antitussives. List all medications, including name, dose, schedule, duration, and reason for administration. Often, parents are unaware of the actual name of the drug. Whenever possible, ask parents to bring the containers with them to the next visit, or ask them for the name of the pharmacy and call for a list of all the child's recent prescription medications. However, this list will not include over-the-counter medications, which are important to know.

Immunizations.   A record of all immunizations is essential. Since many parents are unaware of the exact name and date of each immunization, the most reliable source of information is a hospital, clinic, or private practitioner's record. All immunizations and "boosters" are listed, stating (1) the name of the specific disease, (2) the number of injections, (3) the dosage (sometimes lesser amounts are given if a reaction is anticipated), (4) the ages when administered, and (5) the occurrence of any reaction following the immunization.

> **! NURSING ALERT**
>
> Inquire about previous administration of any horse or other foreign serum, recent administration of gamma globulin or blood transfusion, and anaphylactic reactions to neomycin or chicken eggs.

Growth and Development. The most important previous growth patterns to record are (1) approximate weight at 6 months, 1 year, 2 years, and 5 years of age; (2) approximate length at ages 1 and 4 years; and (3) dentition, including age of onset, number of teeth, and symptoms during teething. Developmental milestones include (1) age of holding up head steadily; (2) age of sitting alone without support; (3) age of walking without assistance; (4) age of saying first words with meaning; (5) present grade in school; (6) scholastic grades; and (7) interaction with other children, peers, and adults.

⟩ GUIDELINES

Taking an Allergy History

Has your child ever taken any drugs or tablets that have disagreed or caused an allergy? If yes, can you remember the name(s) of these drugs?

Can you describe the reaction?

Was the drug by mouth (as a tablet or medicine), or was it an injection?

How soon after starting the drug did the reaction happen?

How long ago did this happen?

Did anyone tell you it was an allergic reaction, or did you decide for yourself?

Has your child ever taken this drug, or a similar one, again? If yes, did your child experience the same problems?

Have you told the doctors or nurses about your child's reaction or allergy?

Modified from Cantrill JA, Cottrell WN: Accuracy of drug allergy documentation, *Am J Health Syst Pharm* 54:1627-1629, 1997.

Use specific and detailed questions when inquiring about each developmental milestone. For example "sitting up" can mean many different activities, such as sitting propped up, sitting in someone's lap, sitting with support, sitting up alone but in a hyperflexed position for assisted balance, or sitting up unsupported with the back slightly rounded. A clue to misunderstanding of the requested activity may be an unusually early age of achievement (see Developmental Assessment, Chapter 7).

Habits.   Habits are an important area to explore (Box 6-6). Parents frequently express concerns during this part of the history. Encourage their input by saying, "Please tell me any concerns you have about your child's habits, activities, or development." Investigate further any concerns that are expressed.

One of the most common concerns relates to sleep. Many children develop a normal sleep pattern, and all that is required during the assessment is a general overview of nighttime sleep and nap schedules. However, a number of children also develop sleep problems (see Sleep Problems, Chapters 10 and 13). When sleep problems occur, a more detailed sleep history is required in order to guide appropriate interventions.*

Habits related to use of chemicals apply primarily to older children and adolescents. If a youngster admits to smoking, drinking, or drug use, ask about the quantity and frequency. Questions such as "Have you ever had a drinking or drug problem?" or "When was the last time you had a drink or took drugs?" may yield more reliable data than questions such as "How much do you drink?" or "How often do you drink or take drugs?" Clarify that "drinking" includes all types of alcohol, such as beer and wine. When quantities such as a "glass" of wine or a "can" of beer are given, ask about the size of the container.

If older children deny use of chemical substances, inquire about past experimentation. Asking, "You mean you never tried to smoke or drink?" implies that the nurse expects some such activity, and the youngster may be more inclined to answer truthfully. Be aware of the confidential nature of such questioning, the adverse effect that the parents' presence may have on the adolescent's willingness to answer,

---

*A sleep history and a sleep chart for the family to record the child's daily sleep and wake activities is available in Hockenberry M: *Wong's clinical manual of pediatric nursing*, ed 6, St Louis, 2004, Mosby.

BOX 6-6 ■ Habits to Explore During the Health Interview

Behavior patterns such as nail biting, thumb sucking, pica (habitual ingestion of nonfood substances), rituals ("security" blanket or toy), and unusual movements (head banging, rocking, overt masturbation, and walking on toes)

Activities of daily living, such as hour of sleep and arising, duration of nighttime sleep and naps, type and duration of exercise, regularity of stools and urination, age of toilet training, and occurrences of daytime or nighttime bed-wetting

Unusual disposition, as well as response to frustration

Use or abuse of alcohol, drugs, coffee, or tobacco

and that self-report may not be an accurate account of chemical abuse.

Review of Systems

The review of systems is a specific review of each body system, similar to the order of the physical examination (Box 6-7). Often the history of the present illness provides a complete review of the system involved in the chief complaint. Since asking questions about other body systems may appear unrelated and irrelevant to the parents or child, precede the questioning with an explanation of why the data are needed (similar to the explanation concerning the relevance of the birth history) and reassure the parents that the child's main problem has not been forgotten.

Begin the review of a specific system with a broad statement such as "How has your child's general health been?" or "Has your child had any problems with his eyes?" If the parent states that there have been past problems with some bodily function, pursue this with an encouraging statement such as "Tell me more about that." If the parent denies any

problems, query for specific symptoms (e.g., "No headaches, bumping into objects, or squinting?"). If the parent reconfirms the absence of such symptoms, record positive statements in the history, such as "Mother denies headaches, bumping into objects, or squinting." In this way, anyone who reviews the health history is aware of exactly what symptoms were investigated.

Family Medical History

The family medical history is used primarily for the purpose of discovering the potential existence of hereditary or familial diseases in the parents and child. In general, it is confined to first-degree relatives (parents, siblings, grandparents, and immediate aunts and uncles). Information for each family member includes age, marital status, state of health if living, cause of death if deceased, and any evidence of the following conditions: heart disease, hypertension, cancer, diabetes mellitus, obesity, congenital anomalies, allergy, asthma, seizures, tuberculosis, sickle cell disease, mental retardation, mental disorders such as depression or psy-

BOX 6-7 ■ Guidelines for Review of Systems

General—Overall state of health, fatigue, recent and/or unexplained weight gain or loss (period of time for either), contributing factors (change of diet, illness, altered appetite), exercise tolerance, fevers (time of day), chills, night sweats (unrelated to climatic conditions), frequent infections, general ability to carry out activities of daily living

Integument—Pruritus, pigment or other color changes, acne, eruptions, rashes (location), tendency for bruising, petechiae, excessive dryness, general texture, disorders or deformities of nails, hair growth or loss, hair color change (for adolescent, use of hair dyes or other potentially toxic substances, such as hair straighteners)

Head—Headaches, dizziness, injury (specific details)

Eyes—Visual problems (ask about behaviors indicative of blurred vision, such as bumping into objects, clumsiness, sitting very close to television, holding a book close to face, writing with head near desk, squinting, rubbing the eyes, bending head in an awkward position), cross-eye (strabismus), eye infections, edema of lids, excessive tearing, use of glasses or contact lenses, date of last optic examination

Nose—Nosebleeds (epistaxis), constant or frequent runny or stuffy nose, nasal obstruction (difficulty in breathing), alteration or loss of sense of smell

Ears—Earaches, discharge, evidence of hearing loss (ask about behaviors, such as need to repeat requests, loud speech, inattentive behavior), results of any previous auditory testing

Mouth—Mouth breathing, gum bleeding, toothaches, toothbrushing, use of fluoride, difficulty with teething (symptoms), last visit to dentist (especially if temporary dentition is complete), response to dentist

Throat—Sore throats, difficulty in swallowing, choking (especially when chewing food—may be from poor chewing habits), hoarseness, or other voice irregularities

Neck—Pain, limitation of movement, stiffness, difficulty in holding head straight (torticollis), thyroid enlargement, enlarged nodes or other masses

Chest—Breast enlargement, discharge, masses, enlarged axillary nodes (for adolescent female, ask about breast self-examination)

Respiratory—Chronic cough, frequent colds (number per year), wheezing, shortness of breath at rest or on exertion, difficulty in breathing, sputum production, infections (pneumonia, tuberculosis), date of last chest x-ray examination, and skin reaction from tuberculin testing

Cardiovascular—Cyanosis or fatigue on exertion, history of heart murmur or rheumatic fever, anemia, date of last blood count, blood type, recent transfusion

Gastrointestinal (much of this in regard to appetite, food tolerance, and elimination habits has been asked elsewhere)—Nausea, vomiting (not associated with eating, may be indicative of brain tumor or increased intracranial pressure), jaundice or yellowing skin or sclera, belching, flatulence, recent change in bowel habits (blood in stools, change of color, diarrhea, or constipation)

Genitourinary—Pain on urination, frequency, hesitancy, urgency, hematuria, nocturia, polyuria, unpleasant odor to urine, force of stream, discharge, change in size of scrotum, date of last urinalysis (for adolescent, sexually transmitted disease, type of treatment; for male adolescent, ask about testicular self-examination)

Gynecologic—Menarche, date of last menstrual period, regularity or problems with menstruation, vaginal discharge, pruritus, date and result of last Pap smear (include obstetric history as discussed under birth history when applicable); if sexually active, type of contraception, sexually transmitted disease and type of treatment

Musculoskeletal—Weakness, clumsiness, lack of coordination, unusual movements, back or joint stiffness, muscle pains or cramps, abnormal gait, deformity, fractures, serious sprains, activity level

Neurologic—Seizures, tremors, dizziness, loss of memory, general affect, fears, nightmares, speech problems, any unusual habits

Endocrine—Intolerance to weather changes, excessive thirst and/or urination, excessive sweating, salty taste to skin, signs of early puberty

chosis, emotional problems, syphilis, or rheumatic fever. Confirm the accuracy of the reported disorders by inquiring about the symptoms, course, treatment, and sequelae of each diagnosis.

Geographic Location.   One of the important areas to explore when assessing the family health history is geographic location, including the birthplace and travel to different areas in or outside of the country, for identification of possible exposure to endemic diseases. Although the primary interest focuses on the child's temporary residence in various localities, also inquire about close family members' travel, especially during tours of military service or business trips. Children are especially susceptible to parasitic infestation in areas of poor sanitary conditions and to vector-borne diseases, such as those from mosquitoes or ticks in warm and humid or heavily wooded regions.

Psychosocial History

The traditional medical history includes a personal and social section that concentrates on children's personal status, such as school adjustment and any unusual habits, and the family and home environment. Since several personal aspects are covered under development and habits, and the social aspects are discussed in detail under Family Assessment, only those issues related to children's ability to cope and their general view of themselves in terms of self-concept are presented here (see Development of Self-Concept, Chapter 5).

Through observation, obtain a general idea of how children handle themselves in terms of confidence in dealing with others, ability to answer questions, and coping with new situations. Observe the parent-child relationship for the types of messages sent to children about their coping skills and self-worth. Do the parents treat the child with respect, focusing on strengths, or is the interaction one of constant reprimands, with emphasis on weaknesses and faults? Do the parents help the child learn new coping strategies or support the ones the child uses?

Messages about body image are also conveyed through the parent-child interaction. Do the parents label the child and body parts, such as "bad boy," "skinny legs," or "ugly scar"? Do the parents handle the child gently, using soothing touch to calm an anxious child, or do they treat the child roughly, using slaps or restraint to force compliance? If the child touches certain parts of the body, such as the genitals, do the parents make comments that suggest a negative connotation?

With older children many of the communication strategies discussed earlier in the chapter are useful in eliciting more definitive information about their coping and self-concept. Children can write down five things they like and dislike about themselves. Sentence completion statements such as "The thing I like best (or worst) about myself is _____," "If I could change one thing about myself, it would be _____," or "When I am scared, I _____," can be used.

Sexual History

The sexual history is an essential component of adolescents' health assessment. The history uncovers areas of concern related to sexual activity, alerts the nurse to circumstances that may indicate screening for sexually transmitted diseases or testing for pregnancy, and provides information related to the need for sexual counseling, such as safe sex practices. Guidelines for anticipatory guidance topics for parents and adolescents are found in Box 6-8.

One approach toward initiating a conversation about sexual concerns is to begin with a history of peer interactions. Open-ended statements such as "Tell me about your social life" or "Who are your closest friends?" generally lead into a discussion of dating and sexual issues. To probe further, include questions about the adolescent's attitudes on such topics as sex education, "going steady," "living together," and premarital sex. Phrase questions to reflect concern rather than judgment or criticism of sexual practices.

In any conversation regarding sexual history, be aware of the language that is used in either eliciting or conveying sexual information. For example, avoid asking if the adolescent is "sexually active," because this term is broadly defined. "Are you having sex with anyone?" is probably the most direct and best understood question. Since homosex-

BOX 6-8 ■ Anticipatory Guidance (Sexuality)

AGES 12 TO 14 YEARS
Have adolescent identify supportive adult to discuss sexuality issues and concerns with.
Discuss delaying sexual activity: advantages.
Discuss making responsible decisions regarding normal sexual feelings.
Discuss role of gender/peer pressure/media in sexual decision making.
Discuss contraceptive options (advantages/disadvantages).
Provide education regarding sexually transmitted diseases (STDs) and human immunodeficiency (HIV) infection; clarify risks and discuss condoms.
Discuss abuse prevention: avoiding dangerous situations, role of drugs and alcohol, and use of self-defense.
Have adolescent clarify values, needs, and ability to be assertive.
If adolescent is sexually active, discuss limiting partners, use of condoms, and contraceptive options.
Have confidential interview with adolescent (including a sexual history).
Discuss the evolution of sexual identity and expression.
Discuss breast examination/testicular examination.

AGES 15 TO 18 YEARS
Support delaying sexual activity.
Discuss alternatives to intercourse.
Discuss "When are you ready for sex?"
Clarify values; encourage responsible decision making.
Discuss consequences of unprotected sex: early pregnancy, STDs, including HIV infection.
Discuss negotiating with partner and barriers to safer sex.
If adolescent is sexually active, discuss limiting partners, use of condoms, and contraceptive options.
Emphasize that sex should be safe and pleasurable for both partners.
Have confidential interview with adolescent.
Discuss concerns about sexual expression and identity.

Modified from Wright K: Anticipatory guidance: developing a healthy sexuality, *Pediatr Ann* 26(2 suppl):S142-S144, C3, 1997.

ual experimentation may occur, refer to all sexual contacts in nongender terms, such as "anyone" or "partners," rather than "girlfriends" or "boyfriends."

A detailed account of sexual partners is needed if the patient has a history of, displays any of the symptoms of, or asks for treatment of a sexually transmitted disease. A difficult but necessary part of the interview is to determine the sites of possible infection. Since sexual diseases can be contracted at any of the body orifices, inform the adolescent that a sexually transmitted disease can be acquired without visible signs of disease at nongenital sites.

FAMILY ASSESSMENT

Assessment of the family, both its structure and function, is an important component of the history-taking process. Because the quality of the functional relationship between the child and family members is a major factor in emotional and physical health, family assessment is discussed separately and in greater detail apart from the more traditional health history.

Family assessment is the collection of data about the composition of the family and the relationships among its members. In its broadest sense, *family* refers to all those individuals who are considered by the family member to be significant to the nuclear unit, including relatives, friends, and other social groups such as the school and church. Although family assessment is not family therapy, it can and frequently is therapeutic. Involving family members in discussing family characteristics and activities often stimulates productive discussion and insight into family dynamics and relationships.

Because of the time involved in performing an in-depth family assessment as presented here, be selective in deciding when knowledge of family function may facilitate nursing care (see Guidelines box). During brief contacts with families, a full assessment is not appropriate, and screening with one or two questions from each category may reflect the health of the family system or the potential need for additional assessment.

ASSESSMENT OF FAMILY STRUCTURE

Family structure refers to the composition of the family—who lives in the home and those social, cultural, religious,

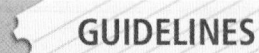

GUIDELINES

Initiating a Comprehensive Family Assessment

Perform a comprehensive assessment on:
  Children receiving comprehensive well-child care
  Children experiencing major stressful life events (e.g., chronic illness, disability, parental divorce, death of a family member)
  Children requiring extensive home care
  Children with developmental delays
  Children with repeated accidental injuries and those with suspected child abuse
  Children with behavioral or physical problems that suggest family dysfunction as the etiology

and economic characteristics that influence the child's and family's overall psychobiologic health (see also Chapters 3 and 4). Since the information elicited in this part of the history is often the most personal and confidential, include it toward the end of the interview when rapport is well established.

The most common method of eliciting information on the family structure is to interview family members. The principal areas of concern (Box 6-9) are (1) family composition, (2) home and community environment, (3) occupation and education of family members, and (4) cultural and religious traditions.

NURSING ALERT

In assessing family composition, it is sometimes difficult to ascertain the status of the adult relationships. If the parent fails to mention the other parent, ask, "Where is the child's father (or mother)?" Avoid saying "husband" or "wife" because this assumes that only marital relationships exist.

Several structural assessment tools can be used to collect and record data about the family composition and environment. Like the interview method, such tools also provide information about relationships, although several additional methods should be used to assess family function.

A *sociogram* is a drawing of circles that indicates the significant persons in an individual's life; its use is appropriate for adults and children as young as 5 years of age. The person is given blank paper and a pencil with the instructions: "Draw a circle to represent you. Around the circle draw circles to represent the most significant persons in your life and label each. Draw the circles in proximity to your circle to represent closeness. For example, the person who is most significant is the circle closest to you." Family members can label the relationships as supportive with a plus sign or negative with a minus sign.

Not only is the sociogram a portrait of the person's significant relationships, it may also uncover unresolved relationships (Fig. 6-5). After completing the sociogram, encourage the family to explore their feelings further with questions such as:

  ▪ How would you change the circles to improve relationships?
  ▪ How do you think you could accomplish these changes?
  ▪ If one person in the circle were to change, what effect do you think that would have on others in the circle?

ASSESSMENT OF FAMILY FUNCTION

Family function is concerned with how the family behaves toward one another and with the quality of the relationships (see also Chapter 3). It is considered the most important component in determining "family health." Assessment of function requires more skill on the part of the interviewer than does assessment of structure and is best approached after structure is assessed. As in assessment of family structure, the more traditional method of eliciting information on family function is by interviewing family members. The principal areas of concern are discussed in Box 6-9.

In addition to observing and interviewing the family to assess family function, several other methods are available and should be used as needed to obtain a comprehensive as-

BOX 6-9 ■ Family Assessment Interview

GENERAL GUIDELINES FOR THE FAMILY INTERVIEW

Schedule the interview with the family at a time that is most convenient for all parties; include as many family members as possible; clearly state the purpose of the interview.

Begin the interview by asking each person's name and their relationship to each other.

Restate the purpose of the interview and the objective.

Keep the initial conversation general to put members at case and to learn the "big picture" of the family.

Identify major concerns and reflect these back to the family to be certain that all parties perceive the same message.

Terminate the interview with a summary of what was discussed and a plan for additional sessions if needed.

STRUCTURAL ASSESSMENT AREAS

Family Composition

Immediate members of the household (names, ages, and relationships)

Significant extended family members

Previous marriages, separations, death of spouses, or divorces

Home and Community Environment

Type of dwelling/number of rooms/occupants

Sleeping arrangements

Number of floors, accessibility of stairs, elevators

Adequacy of utilities

Safety features (fire escape, smoke and carbon monoxide detectors, guardrails on windows, use of car restraint)

Environmental hazards (e.g., chipped paint, poor sanitation, pollution, heavy street traffic)

Availability and location of health facilities, schools, play areas

Relationship with neighbors

Recent crises or changes in home

Child's reaction/adjustment to recent stresses

Occupation and Education of Family Members

Types of employment

Work schedules

Work satisfaction

Exposure to environmental/industrial hazards

Sources of income and adequacy

Effect of illness on financial status

Highest degree or grade level attained

Cultural and Religious Traditions

Religious beliefs and practices

Cultural/ethnic beliefs and practices

Language spoken in home

Assessment questions include:

Does the family identify with a particular religious/ethnic group? Are both parents from that group?

How is religious/ethnic background part of family life?

What special religious/cultural traditions are practiced in the home (e.g., food choices and preparation)?

Where were family members born, and how long have they lived in this country?

What language does the family speak most frequently?

Do they speak/understand English?

What do they believe causes health or illness?

What religious/ethnic beliefs influence the family's perception of illness and its treatment?

What methods are used to prevent/treat illness?

How does the family know when a health problem needs medical attention?

Who is the person the family contacts when a member is ill?

Does the family rely on cultural/religious healers or remedies? If so, ask them to describe the type of healer or remedy.

Who does the family go to for support (clergy, medical healer, relatives)?

Does the family experience discrimination because of their race, beliefs, or practices? Ask them to describe.

FUNCTIONAL ASSESSMENT AREAS

Family Interactions and Roles

Interactions refer to ways family members relate to each other.

Chief concern is amount of intimacy and closeness among the members, especially spouses.

Roles refer to behaviors of people as they assume a different status or position.

Observations include:

Family members' responses to each other (cordial, hostile, cool, loving, patient, short-tempered)

Obvious roles of leadership vs submission

Support and attention shown to various members

Assessment questions include:

What activities do the family perform together?

Whom do family members talk to when something is bothering them?

What are members' household chores?

Who usually oversees what is happening with the children, such as at school or concerning their health?

How easy or difficult is it for the family to change or accept new responsibilities for household tasks?

Power, Decision Making, and Problem Solving

Power refers to individual member's control over others in family; manifested through family decision making and problem solving.

Chief concern is clarity of boundaries of power between parents and children.

One method of assessment involves offering a hypothetical conflict or problem, such as a child failing school, and asking family how they would handle this situation.

Assessment questions include:

Who usually makes the decisions in the family?

If one parent makes a decision, can the child appeal to the other parent to change it?

What input do children have in making decisions or discussing rules?

Who makes and enforces the rules?

What happens when a rule is broken?

Communication

Communication is concerned with clarity and directness of communication patterns.

Further assessment includes periodically asking family members if they understood what was just said and to repeat the message.

Continued

BOX 6-9 ■ Family Assessment Interview—*cont'd*

Observations include:
Who speaks to whom
If one person speaks for another or interrupts
If members appear disinterested when certain individuals speak
If there is agreement between verbal and nonverbal messages
Assessment questions include:
How often do family members wait until others are through talking before "having their say?"
Do parents or older siblings tend to lecture and preach?
Do parents tend to talk "down" to the children?

Expression of Feelings and Individuality
Expressions are concerned with personal space and freedom to grow with limits and structure needed for guidance.

Observing patterns of communication offers clues to how freely feelings are expressed.
Assessment questions include:
Is it OK for family members to get angry or sad?
Who gets angry most of the time? What do they do?
If someone is upset, how do other family members try to comfort this person?
Who comforts specific family members?
When someone wants to do something, such as try out for a new sport or get a job, what is the family's response (offer assistance, discouragement, or no advice)?

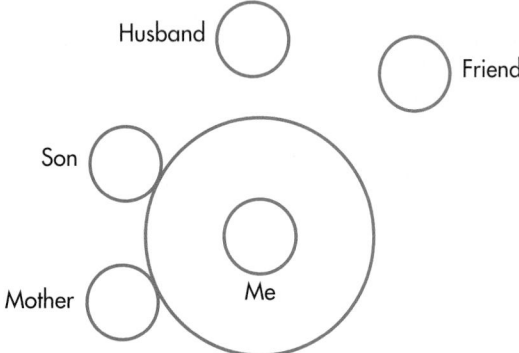

FIG. 6-5 ■ Sociogram of mother with strong, unresolved grief feelings regarding loss of child.

sessment. The following section discusses selected instruments that are reliable and valid but require little or no formal training and minimal time to administer.

The *Family APGAR (FAPGAR)* is a brief screening questionnaire designed to reflect a family member's satisfaction with the functional state of the family (Smilkstein, Ashworth, and Montano, 1982) (see Appendix A). The acronym APGAR stands for *A*daptation, *P*artnership, *G*rowth, *A*ffection, and *R*esolve (commitment). The acronym was chosen because it is familiar to health professionals, but it bears no relationship to the Apgar scoring system for newborns.

The questions in Box 6-10 can be used in the interview without the APGAR ratings to elicit similar types of information. It can be completed in about 5 minutes, can be used by families with traditional and alternative lifestyles and from different cultures, and is appropriate for children 10 years of age or older. Separate forms have been designed to assess relationships with friends and fellow workers, because these groups represent other significant sources of support.

The responses to the five questions are scored as follows: "Almost always"—2; "Some of the time"—1; and "Hardly ever"—0. Each score is totaled. Scores of 7 to 10 suggest a highly functional family; 4 to 6, a moderately dysfunctional family; and 0 to 3, a severely dysfunctional family. Also, a low score in any single item could signal family dysfunction. The family APGAR is not recommended for use with individuals from enmeshed (overly close) or "psychosomatic"

families. Persons with health problems, such as asthma, atopic dermatitis, or irritable bowel syndrome, may report falsely high scores (Smilkstein, 1993).

The *Feetham Family Functioning Survey** provides information about family members' *perception* of relationships that contribute to or are affected by family functioning (Feetham, Perkins, and Carroll, 1993). Although recommended primarily as a research instrument, it can be used clinically without scoring the items to identify areas that may be of concern to the family. The survey consists of 25 ratings of family functioning (household tasks; child care; sexual and marital relationships; interaction with family, children, and friends; community involvement; and sources of emotional support) and two open-ended questions. Each of the questions on family functioning is rated on three 7-point scales of "How much is there now?" "How much should there be?" and "How important is this to me?" (Box 6-11). Discrepancy between the first two ratings, together with the rating of importance, contributes to an assessment of the members' perceptions of family functioning. The survey takes less than 10 minutes to complete and can be used with single-parent and two-parent families (Feetham, Perkins, and Carroll, 1993).

Undoubtedly the richest environment for observing a child's development and interactions with family members is the home. Two tools that can be used to assess the child's home environment are the *Home Observation for Management of the Environment (HOME) Inventory*† (Caldwell and Bradley, 1984) and the *Home Screening Questionnaire (HSQ)*‡ (Frankenburg and Coons, 1986). Both are divided into two age-groups: birth to 3 years of age and 3 to 6 years of age. HOME has an additional inventory for children ages 6 to 10 years. Forms are also available for children with moderate to severe disabilities in each of the three age-groups for visual, auditory, orthopedic, and cognitive impairments.

---

*The survey is available for a fee from **Nursing Systems and Research,** Children's National Medical Center, 111 Michigan Avenue, NW, Washington, DC 20010; (202) 939-4980.
†The forms and an administration manual are available for a fee from the **Center for Research on Teaching and Learning,** College of Education, University of Arkansas at Little Rock, 2801 S. University Avenue, Little Rock, AR 72204; (501) 569-3422.
‡The forms and manual are available for a fee from **Denver Developmental Materials, Inc.,** PO Box 371075, Denver, CO 80237-5075; (303) 355-4729 or (800) 419-4729.

BOX 6-10 ■ Family Apgar

DEFINITION	FUNCTIONS MEASURED BY THE FAMILY APGAR	RELEVANT OPEN-ENDED QUESTIONS
Adaptation is the use of intrafamilial and extrafamilial resources for problem solving when family equilibrium is stressed during a crisis.	How resources are shared, or the degree to which a member is satisfied with the assistance received when family resources are needed	How have family members aided each other in time of need? In what way have family members received help or assistance from friends and community agencies?
Partnership is the sharing of decision-making and nurturing responsibilities by family members.	How decisions are shared, or the member's satisfaction with mutuality in family communication and problem solving	How do family members communicate with each other about such matters as vacations, finances, medical care, large purchases, and personal problems?
Growth is the physical and emotional maturation and self-fulfillment that is achieved by family members through mutual support and guidance.	How nurturing is shared, or the member's satisfaction with the freedom available within the family to change roles and attain physical and emotional growth or maturation	How have family members changed during the past years? How has this change been accepted by family members? In what ways have family members aided each other in growing or developing independent lifestyles?
Affection is the caring or loving relationship that exists among family members.	How emotional experiences are shared, or the member's satisfaction with the intimacy and emotional interaction that exists in the family	How have family members reacted to your desire for change? How have members of your family responded to emotional expressions, such as affection, love, sorrow, or anger?
Resolve is the commitment to devote time to other members of the family for physical and emotional nurturing. It also usually involves a decision to share wealth and space.	How time (and space and money) is shared, or the member's satisfaction with the time commitment that has been made to the family by its members	How do members of your family share time, space, and money?

Modified from Smilkstein G: The Family APGAR: a proposal for a family function test and its use by physicians, *J Fam Pract* 6(6):1231-1239, 1978.

BOX 6-11 ■ Sample Questions From the Feetham Family Functioning Survey

The amount of time you spend with your spouse.
a. How much is there now?

LITTLE   MUCH
1   2   3   4   5   6   7

b. How much should there be?

LITTLE   MUCH
1   2   3   4   5   6   7

c. How important is this to me?

LITTLE   MUCH
1   2   3   4   5   6   7

Reproduced with the permission of Suzanne L. Feetham, PhD, RN, FAAN. Developed from research funded by Division of Nursing, HRA, HHS, NU00632, Detroit, 1977-1980, Wayne State University.

Some of the HOME items require direct observation, whereas others necessitate questioning of the parents. Each item receives a "yes" or "no" response. The number of "yes" responses correlates with the amount of appropriate environmental stimulation. Any "no" responses indicate possible areas for intervention and counseling. Use of HOME requires about a 1-hour home visit with both the child and the major caregiver.

The HSQ was developed using HOME as a guide. The 0- to 3-year form consists of 30 items plus a checklist of toys available to the child in the home. The 3- to 6-year form has 34 items and a similar toy checklist. The questions are written at approximately a third- to sixth-grade reading level and, unlike the HOME, can be completed by the parents in any setting in about 15 to 20 minutes. Scoring directions are detailed in the manual and are based on credits for different answers. For each age-group there is a minimum score for determining suspect or nonsuspect results.

NUTRITIONAL ASSESSMENT

DIETARY INTAKE

Knowledge of the child's dietary intake is a useful and practical component of a nutritional assessment. However, it is also one of the most difficult factors to assess. Individuals' recall of food consumption, especially amounts eaten, is frequently unreliable. In addition, people may be hesitant to reveal their eating patterns if they sense criticism from the nurse. People from different cultures may have difficulty adequately describing the types of food they eat. Despite these obstacles, a food intake record is essential. Several methods are available.

Regardless of the format used in recording food intake, every nutritional assessment should begin with a *dietary history.* The exact questions used to elicit a dietary history vary with the child's age. In general, the younger the child, the more specific and detailed the history should be. Box 6-12 provides a sample dietary history for children and includes additional questions regarding infant feeding.

The overview elicited from the dietary history can be helpful in evaluating food frequency records. It also is concerned with financial and cultural factors that influence food selection and preparation (see Cultural Awareness box.)

The most common and probably easiest method of assessing daily intake is the *24-hour recall.* The child or parent recalls every item eaten in the past 24 hours and the approximate amounts. The 24-hour recall is most beneficial when it represents a typical day's intake. Some of the difficulties with a daily recall are the family's inability to remember exactly what was eaten and inaccurate estimation of portion size. To increase accuracy of reporting portion sizes, the use of food models and additional questioning are recommended. In general, this method is most useful in providing *qualitative* information about the child's diet.

To improve the reliability of the daily recall, the family can complete a *food diary* by recording every food and liquid consumed for a certain number of days. A 3-day record consisting of 2 weekdays and 1 weekend day is representative for most people. Providing specific charts to record intake can improve compliance. The family should record items immediately after eating.

A *food frequency questionnaire* or *record* (Box 6-13) provides information about the number of times in a day, week, or month a child consumes items from the different food groups. In general, it provides a qualitative overview but has the advantage of avoiding recall based on a "typical" day. It can be especially useful when verifying a food history or diary.

CLINICAL EXAMINATION

A significant amount of information regarding nutritional deficiencies is elicited from a clinical examination, especially from assessing the skin, hair, teeth, gums, lips, tongue, and eyes. Hair, skin, and mouth are vulnerable because of the rapid turnover of epithelial and mucosal tissue. Table 6-1 summarizes clinical signs of possible nutritional deficiency or excess. Few are diagnostic for a specific nutrient, and if suspicious signs are found, they must be confirmed with dietary and biochemical data. Generally, the clinical examination does not reveal children *at risk* for a deficiency or excess.

Anthropometry, an essential parameter of nutritional status, is the measurement of height, weight, head circumference, proportions, skinfold thickness, and arm circumference in young children. Height and head circumference reflect past nutrition, whereas weight, skinfold thickness, and arm circumference reflect present nutritional status, especially of protein and fat reserves. Skinfold thickness is a measurement of the body's fat content because approximately half of the body's total fat stores are directly beneath the skin. The upper arm muscle circumference is correlated with measurements of total muscle mass. Since muscle serves as the body's major protein reserve, this measurement is considered an index of the body's protein stores. Ideally, growth measurements are recorded over a period of time, and comparisons are made regarding the *velocity* of growth based on previous and present values. Techniques for anthropomorphic measurement are discussed in Chapter 7.

BOX 6-12 ■ Dietary History

What are the family's usual mealtimes?
Do family members eat together or at separate times?
Who does the family grocery shopping and meal preparation?
How much money is spent to buy food each week?
How are most foods prepared—baked, broiled, fried, other?
How often does the family or your child eat out?
    What kinds of restaurants do you go to?
    What kinds of food does your child typically eat at restaurants?
Does your child eat breakfast regularly?
Where does your child eat lunch?
What are your child's favorite foods, beverages, and snacks?
    What are the average amounts eaten per day?
    What foods are artificially sweetened?
    What are your child's snacking habits?
    When are sweet foods usually eaten?
    What are your child's toothbrushing habits?
What special cultural practices are followed? What ethnic foods are eaten?
What foods and beverages does your child dislike?
How would you describe your child's usual appetite (hearty eater, picky eater)?
What are your child's feeding habits (breast, bottle, cup, spoon, eats by self, needs assistance, any special devices)?
Does your child take vitamins or other supplements? Do they contain iron or fluoride?
Are there any known or suspected food allergies? Is your child on a special diet?
Has your child lost or gained weight recently?
Are there any feeding problems (excessive fussiness, spitting up, colic, difficulty sucking or swallowing)? Are there any dental problems or appliances, such as braces, that affect eating?

What types of exercise does your child do regularly?
Is there a family history of cancer, diabetes, heart disease, high blood pressure, or obesity?

ADDITIONAL QUESTIONS FOR INFANTS
What was the infant's birth weight? When did it double? Triple?
Was the infant premature?
Are you breast-feeding or have you breast-fed your infant? For how long?
If you use a formula, what is the brand?
    How long has the infant been taking it?
    How many ounces does the infant drink a day?
Are you giving the infant cow's milk (whole, low-fat, skim)?
    When did you start?
    How many ounces does the infant drink a day?
Do you give your infant extra fluids (water, juice)?
If the infant takes a bottle to bed at nap or nighttime, what is in the bottle?
At what age did you start cereal, vegetables, meat or other protein sources, fruit/juice, finger food, table food?
Do you make your own baby food or use commercial foods, such as infant cereal?
Does the infant take a vitamin/mineral supplement? If so, what type?
Has the infant shown an allergic reaction to any food(s)? If so, list the foods and describe the reaction.
Does the infant spit up frequently, have unusually loose stools, or have hard, dry stools? If so, how often?
How often do you feed your infant?
How would you describe your infant's appetite?

Numerous *biochemical tests* are available for assessing nutritional status and include analysis of plasma, blood cells, urine, or tissues from liver, bone, hair, and fingernails. Many of these tests are complicated and are not performed routinely. Common laboratory procedures for nutritional status include measurement of hemoglobin, hematocrit, transferrin, albumin, creatinine, and nitrogen. Laboratory values for these tests and more specific nutrient measurements are given in Appendix E.

CULTURAL AWARENESS

Food Practices

Because cultural practices are very prevalent in food preparation, consider carefully the kinds of questions that are asked and the judgments made in regard to counseling. For example, some cultures, such as Hispanic, black, and Native American, include many vegetables, legumes, and starches in their diet that together provide sufficient essential amino acids, even though the actual amount of meat or dairy protein is low. (See Chapter 4 for cultural food practices.)

EVALUATION OF NUTRITIONAL ASSESSMENT

After collecting the data needed for a thorough nutritional assessment, evaluate the findings to plan appropriate counseling. From the data, assess if the child is (1) malnourished, (2) at risk for becoming malnourished, or (3) well nourished with adequate reserves.

Analyze the daily food diary for the variety and amounts of foods suggested in the Food Guide Pyramid (see Fig. 11-1). For example, if the list includes no vegetables, inquire about this rather than assuming that the child dislikes vegetables, because it could be that none were served on that day. Also, evaluate the information in terms of the family's ethnic practices and financial resources. Encouraging increased protein intake with additional meat may be unfeasible for families on a limited budget or in conflict with food practices that use meat sparingly, such as in Asian meal preparation.

Compare findings from clinical examination and anthropometry with the data obtained from the dietary intake. For example, signs of anemia and a dietary record of iron-poor foods suggest laboratory analysis of hemoglobin, hematocrit, and transferrin. Refer any suspicious findings for further evaluation.

BOX 6-13 ■ Food Frequency Record*

FOOD GROUP	NUMBER OF SERVINGS (DAY, WEEK)	SERVING SIZE (IN CUP, TABLESPOON, OR OUNCE PORTIONS)	FOOD GROUP	NUMBER OF SERVINGS (DAY, WEEK)	SERVING SIZE (IN CUP, TABLESPOON, OR OUNCE PORTIONS)
BREADS/CEREALS/RICE/PASTA			**MILK/CHEESE/YOGURT**		
Bread, tortilla			Milk		
Cooked pasta, rice, hot cereal			Cheese		
Dry cereal (not presweetened)			Yogurt		
Crackers			Pudding		
Muffins			Ice cream		
Other			Other		
VEGETABLES			**OTHER PROTEIN FOODS**		
Yellow or orange			Meat		
Green/leafy			Fish		
Other			Poultry		
			Egg		
			Peanut butter		
			Soy legumes (dried beans, peas)		
			Nuts		
			Other		
FRUITS/JUICE			**FATS/OILS/SWEETS**		
Citrus (orange, grapefruit, strawberries, lemon, lime, tangerine)			Butter, oil, margarine, mayonnaise, salad dressing		
Noncitrus			Soda, punch		
Other			Cake/cookie, etc.		
			Candy		
			Presweetened cereal		

*For comparison of actual intake with recommended intake, see Food Guide Pyramid, Fig. 11-1.

TABLE 6-1 ■ Clinical Assessment of Nutritional Status

EVIDENCE OF ADEQUATE NUTRITION	EVIDENCE OF DEFICIENT OR EXCESS NUTRITION	DEFICIENCY/EXCESS*
GENERAL GROWTH		
Within 5th and 95th percentiles for height, weight, and head circumference	Below 5th or above 95th percentiles for growth	Protein, calories, fats, and other essential nutrients, especially vitamin A, pyridoxine, niacin, calcium, iodine, manganese, zinc
Steady gain with expected growth spurts during infancy and adolescence	Absence of or delayed growth spurts; poor weight gain	
Sexual development appropriate for age	Delayed sexual development	Excess vitamin A, D
SKIN		
Smooth, slightly dry to touch	Hardening and scaling	Vitamin A
Elastic and firm	Seborrheic dermatitis	Excess niacin
Absence of lesions	Dry, rough, petechiae	Riboflavin
Color appropriate to genetic background	Delayed wound healing	Vitamin C
	Scaly dermatitis on exposed surfaces	Riboflavin, vitamin C, zinc
	Wrinkled, flabby	Niacin
	Crusted lesions around orifices, especially nares	Protein, calories, zinc
	Pruritus	Excess vitamin A, riboflavin, niacin
	Poor turgor	Water, sodium
	Edema	Protein, thiamine
		Excess sodium
	Yellow tinge (jaundice)	Vitamin B$_{12}$
		Excess vitamin A, niacin
	Depigmentation	Protein, calories
	Pallor (anemia)	Pyridoxine, folic acid, vitamin B$_{12}$, C, E (in premature infants), iron
		Excess vitamin C, zinc
	Paresthesia	Excess riboflavin
HAIR		
Lustrous, silky, strong, elastic	Stringy, friable, dull, dry, thin	Protein, calories
	Alopecia	Protein, calories, zinc
	Depigmentation	Protein, calories, copper
	Raised areas around hair follicles	Vitamin C
HEAD		
Even molding, occipital prominence, symmetric facial features	Softening of cranial bones, prominence of frontal bones, skull flat and depressed toward middle	Vitamin D
Fused sutures after 18 months	Delayed fusion of sutures	Vitamin D
	Hard tender lumps in occiput	Excess vitamin A
	Headache	Excess thiamine
NECK		
Thyroid not visible, palpable in midline	Thyroid enlarged; may be grossly visible	Iodine
EYES		
Clear, bright	Hardening and scaling of cornea and conjunctiva	Vitamin A
Good night vision	Night blindness	Vitamin A
Conjunctiva—Pink, glossy	Burning, itching, photophobia, cataracts, corneal vascularization	Riboflavin
EARS		
Tympanic membrane—Pliable	Calcified (hearing loss)	Excess vitamin D
NOSE		
Smooth, intact nasal angle	Irritation and cracks at nasal angle	Riboflavin
		Excess vitamin A

*Nutrients listed are deficient unless specified as excess.

TABLE 6-1 ■ Clinical Assessment of Nutritional Status—*cont'd*

EVIDENCE OF ADEQUATE NUTRITION	EVIDENCE OF DEFICIENT OR EXCESS NUTRITION	DEFICIENCY/EXCESS*
MOUTH		
Lips—Smooth, moist, darker color than skin	Fissures and inflammation at corners	Riboflavin Excess vitamin A
Gums—Firm, coral pink color, stippled	Spongy, friable, swollen, bluish red or black color, bleed easily	Vitamin C
Mucous membranes—Bright pink, smooth, moist	Stomatitis	Niacin
Tongue—Rough texture, no lesions, taste sensation	Glossitis	Niacin, riboflavin, folic acid
	Diminished taste sensation	Zinc
Teeth—Uniform white color, smooth, intact	Brown mottling, pits, fissures	Excess fluoride
	Defective enamel	Vitamin A, C, D, calcium, phosphorus
	Caries	Excess carbohydrates
CHEST		
In infants, shape is almost circular	Depressed lower portion of rib cage	Vitamin D
In children, lateral diameter increases in proportion to anteroposterior diameter	Sharp protrusion of sternum	Vitamin D
Smooth costochondral junctions	Enlarged costochondral junctions	Vitamin C, D
Breast development—Normal for age	Delayed development	See under General Growth; especially zinc
CARDIOVASCULAR SYSTEM		
Pulse and blood pressure (BP) within normal limits	Palpitations	Thiamine
	Rapid pulse	Potassium Excess thiamine
	Arrhythmias	Magnesium, potassium Excess niacin, potassium
	Increased BP	Excess sodium
	Decreased BP	Thiamine; excess niacin
ABDOMEN		
In young children, cylindric and prominent	Distended, flabby, poor musculature	Protein, calories
	Prominent, large	Excess calories
Older children, flat	Potbelly, constipation	Vitamin D
Normal bowel habits	Diarrhea	Niacin Excess vitamin C
	Constipation	Excess calcium, potassium
MUSCULOSKELETAL SYSTEM		
Muscles—Firm, well-developed, equal strength bilaterally	Flabby, weak, generalized wasting	Protein, calories
	Weakness, pain, cramps	Thiamine, sodium, chloride, potassium, phosphorus, magnesium Excess thiamine
	Muscle twitching, tremors	Magnesium
	Muscular paralysis	Excess potassium
Spine—Cervical and lumbar curves (double S curve)	Kyphosis, lordosis, scoliosis	Vitamin D
Extremities—Symmetric; legs straight with minimum bowing	Bowing of extremities, knock-knees	Vitamin D, calcium, phosphorus
	Epiphyseal enlargement	Vitamin A, D
	Bleeding into joints and muscles, joint swelling, pain	Vitamin C
Joints—Flexible, full range of motion, no pain or stiffness	Thickening of cortex of long bones with pain and fragility, hard tender lumps in extremities	Excess vitamin A
	Osteoporosis of long bones	Calcium; excess vitamin D

Continued

TABLE 6-1 ■ Clinical Assessment of Nutritional Status—cont'd

EVIDENCE OF ADEQUATE NUTRITION	EVIDENCE OF DEFICIENT OR EXCESS NUTRITION	DEFICIENCY/EXCESS*
NEUROLOGIC SYSTEM		
Behavior—Alert, responsive, emotionally stable	Listless, irritable, lethargic, apathetic (sometimes apprehensive, anxious, drowsy, mentally slow, confused)	Thiamine, niacin, pyridoxine, vitamin C, potassium, magnesium, iron, protein, calories
		Excess vitamin A, D, thiamine, folic acid, calcium
Absence of tetany, convulsions	Masklike facial expression, blurred speech, involuntary laughing	Excess manganese
	Convulsions	Thiamine, pyridoxine, vitamin D, calcium, magnesium
		Excess phosphorus (in relation to calcium)
Intact peripheral nervous system	Peripheral nervous system toxicity (unsteady gait, numb feet and hands, fine motor clumsiness)	Excess pyridoxine
Intact reflexes	Diminished or absent tendon reflexes	Thiamine, vitamin E

*Nutrients listed are deficient unless specified as excess.

KEY POINTS

■ Communication, the most important skill nurses must possess in the care of children, has verbal, nonverbal, and abstract components.

■ To effectively establish a setting for communication, nurses must make an appropriate introduction, clarify their role and the purpose of the interview, and ensure privacy and confidentiality.

■ When communicating with parents, nurses need to encourage parental involvement, listen carefully, use silence, and be empathic.

■ Communication with children must reflect their developmental stage.

■ Verbal communication techniques that have proved to be effective include the third-person technique, facilitative responding, storytelling, bibliotherapy, "what if" questions, and other word games.

■ Nonverbal communication with children may take the form of writing, drawing, magic, and play.

■ The objectives of performing a health history are to identify pertinent information, determine the chief complaint, analyze the present illness, secure the patient's health history, review biologic systems, and record a family medical history and child psychosocial and sexual history.

■ Family assessment is the collection of data about family composition and relationships among its members; it also focuses on home and community environment, occupation and education, and cultural and religious traditions.

■ The family function interview examines interaction and roles, power, decision making, problem solving, communication, and expression of feelings and individuality.

■ Nutritional assessment is performed by determination of dietary intake, clinical examination, and biochemical analysis.

References

Bradley RH and others: A reexamination of the association between HOME scores and income, *Nurs Res* 43(5):260-266, 1994.

Caldwell B, Bradley R: *Home observation for measurement of the environment*, rev ed, Little Rock, 1984, University of Arkansas.

Deadrick D, Boggess P: *Pediatrics on telephone line*. Paper presented at the first Annual National Conference for Advanced Practice Nurses, Rutgers University, Nov 6-8, 1996.

Desselle DD, Pearlmutter L: Navigating two cultures: deaf children, self-esteem, and parents' communication patterns, *Soc Work Educ* 19(1):23-30, 1997.

Feetham S, Perkins M, Carroll R: Exploratory analysis: a technique for analysis of dyadic data in research of families. In Feetham S and others, editors: *The nursing of families: theory/research/education/practice*, Newbury Park, Calif, 1993, Sage Publications.

Frankenburg W, Coons C: Home Screening Questionnaire: its validity in assessing home environment, *J Pediatr* 108(4):624-626, 1986.

Hoge DR, Parette HP: Facilitating communicative development in young children with disabilities, *Transdisciplinary J* 5(2):113-130, 1995.

Price V, Archbold J: What's it all about, empathy? *Nurs Educ Today* 17(2):106-110, 1997.

Reynolds WH, Scott B, Jessiman WC: Empathy has not been measured in clients' terms or effectively taught: a review of the literature, *J Adv Nurs* 30(5):1177-1185, 1999.

Rutenberg CD: Telephone triage, *Am J Nurs* 100(3):77-78, 80-81, 2000.

Seidel HM and others: *Mosby's guide to physical examination*, ed 5, St Louis, 2003, Mosby.

Smilkstein G: Family APGAR analyzed, *Fam Med* 25(5):293-294, 1993 (letter).

Smilkstein G, Ashworth C, Montano D: Validity and reliability of the family APGAR as a test of family function, *J Fam Pract* 15(2):303-311, 1982.

Spinetta J and others: The kinetic family drawing in childhood cancer. In Spinetta J, Deasy-Sullivan, GH: Protecting patient's privacy, *RN* 60(6):55-56, 58-59, 1997.

White SJ: Empathy: a literature review and concept analysis, *J Clin Nurs* 6(4):253-257, 1997.

Yegdich T: On the phenomenology of empathy in nursing: empathy or sympathy? *J Adv Nurs* 30(1):83-93, 1999.

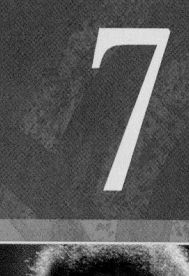

Physical and Developmental Assessment of the Child

7

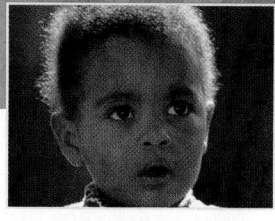
Remember to check out your companion CD-ROM

http://evolve.elsevier.com/Wong/essentials/

CHAPTER OUTLINE

RELATED TOPICS and ADDITIONAL RESOURCES

 IN TEXT

Altered States of Consciousness, *Ch. 28*
Assessment of Cardiac Function, *Ch. 25*
Biologic Development: Adolescent, *Ch. 16*
Dental Problems, *Ch. 15*
Growth and Development, *Ch. 5*
Hearing Impairment; Visual Impairment, *Ch. 19*
History Taking, *Ch. 6*
Neurologic Examination, *Ch. 28*
Physical Assessment (Newborn), *Ch. 8*
Preparation for Procedures, *Ch. 22*
Scoliosis, *Ch. 31*
Sexually Transmitted Diseases, Ch. 17

Skin Lesions, *Ch. 30*
Systemic Hypertension, *Ch. 25*

 CD COMPANION

Critical Thinking Exercise—Cardiovascular Assessment
Case Study—Pediatric Assessment
Anatomy Reviews—Superficial Lymph Nodes; Location of Sinuses; Structures in the Neck; Structures of the Eye; Landmarks of the Pinna; External, Middle, and Inner Ear; External and Internal Structures of the Nose; Interior Structures of the Mouth; Rib Cage; Imaginary Landmarks of the Chest; Percussion Sounds in the

Thorax; Location of Pulses; Direction of Heart Sounds; Location of Hernias
Guidelines—Performing Pediatric Physical Examination; Measuring Triceps Skinfold Thickness; Measuring Blood Pressure; Observing Behavior; Effective Auscultation
NCLEX-Style Review Questions

evolve WEBSITE

WebLinks
NCLEX-Style Review Questions

For additional information, please view "Pediatric Assessment" in *Whaley and Wong's Pediatric Nursing Video Series,* St Louis, 1996, Mosby; (800)426-4545; website: www.elsevierhealth.com.

- Prepare a child for a physical examination based on his or her developmental needs.
- Perform a comprehensive physical examination in a sequence appropriate to the child's age.
- Recognize expected normal findings for children at various ages.
- Record the physical examination according to the head-to-toe format.
- Perform a developmental assessment using a standard screening test.

GENERAL APPROACHES TOWARD EXAMINING THE CHILD

SEQUENCE OF THE EXAMINATION

Ordinarily, the sequence for examining patients follows a head-to-toe direction. The main function of such a systematic approach is to provide a general guideline for assessment of each body area to minimize omitting segments of the examination. The standard recording of data also facilitates exchange of information among different professionals. The typical organization of a physical examination is indicated in the chapter outline. In examining children, this orderly sequence is frequently altered to accommodate the child's developmental needs, although the examination is recorded following the head-to-toe model. Using developmental and chronologic age as the main criteria for assessing each body system accomplishes several goals:

- Minimizes stress and anxiety associated with assessment of various body parts
- Fosters a trusting nurse-child-parent relationship
- Allows for maximum preparation of the child
- Preserves the essential security of the parent-child relationship, especially with young children
- Maximizes the accuracy and reliability of assessment findings

PREPARATION OF THE CHILD

Although the physical examination consists of painless procedures, to a child the use of a tight arm cuff, probes in the ears and mouth, pressing on the abdomen, and listening to the chest with a cold piece of metal can be considerably stressful. Therefore, the same considerations discussed in Chapter 22 for preparing children for procedures are followed here. In addition to that discussion, general guidelines related to the examining process are presented in Box 7-1. The physical examination should be as pleasant as possible, as well as educational. For example, the nurse can use a detailed drawing or anatomically correct doll to help preschoolers and older children learn about their bodies (Vessey, 1995). The paper-doll technique is a useful approach to teaching children about the part of the body that is being examined (Fig. 7-1). At the conclusion of the visit, the child can bring home the paper doll as a memento of the experience.

In most instances children cooperate best when their parents remain with them. There are occasions, however, when older children, particularly adolescents, prefer to be examined alone, such as during the genital examination. Frequently, the child being examined is also accompanied by a sibling, who may be disruptive because of boredom. It is a helpful tactic to involve the sibling in the examination

by allowing the child to hold the stethoscope or a tongue blade and praising the child for the "help" during the assessment.

Table 7-1 summarizes guidelines for positioning, preparing, and examining children at various ages. Because no child fits precisely into one age category, it may be necessary to vary the approach after a preliminary assessment of the child's developmental achievements and needs. Even when the best approach is used, many toddlers are uncooperative and unable to be consoled for much of the physical examination. However, some seem intrigued by the new surroundings and unusual equipment and respond more like preschoolers than toddlers. Likewise, some early preschoolers may require more of the "security measures" employed with younger children, such as continued parent-child contact, and less of the preparatory measures used with preschoolers, such as playing with the equipment before and during the actual examination (Fig. 7-2).

Although the variations in the general approaches are numerous, some of them are elaborated on here because they are more common. For example, the suggested sequence may change considerably when the child is in pain or when obvious physical defects are present. In either situation, examine the affected area last to minimize distress early in the examination and to focus on normal, healthy, or functioning body parts.

Positioning may also be altered because of physical distress. For example, the child who is having difficulty breathing may not be able to lie down; therefore, perform as much of the physical examination as possible with the child in a sitting or slightly reclining position, or complete the examination at another time.

PHYSICAL EXAMINATION

Although the approach to and sequence of the physical examination differ according to the child's age, the following discussion outlines the traditional model for physical assessment. Although the focus includes all pediatric age-groups, the reader is referred to Chapter 8 for a detailed discussion of a newborn assessment. Because the physical examination is a vital part of preventive pediatric care, a schedule for periodic health visits is given in Box 7-2.

GROWTH MEASUREMENTS

Measurement of physical growth in children is a key element in evaluating their health status. Physical growth parameters include weight, height (length), skinfold thickness, arm circumference, and head circumference. Values for these growth parameters are plotted on percentile charts,

BOX 7-1 ■ General Guidelines for Performing Pediatric Physical Examination

Perform examination in appropriate, nonthreatening area.

Have room well lit and decorated with neutral colors.

Have room temperature comfortably warm.

Place all strange and potentially frightening equipment out of sight.

Have some toys, dolls, stuffed animals, and games available for child.

If possible, have rooms decorated and equipped for different-age children.

Provide privacy, especially for school-age children and adolescents.

Provide time for play and becoming acquainted.

Observe behaviors that signal child's readiness to cooperate:

Talking to the nurse

Making eye contact

Accepting the offered equipment

Allowing physical touching

Choosing to sit on examining table rather than parent's lap

If signs of readiness are not observed, use the following techniques:

Talk to parent while essentially "ignoring" child; gradually focus on child or a favorite object, such as a doll.

Make complimentary remarks about child, such as appearance, dress, or a favorite object.

Tell a funny story or play a simple magic trick.

Have a nonthreatening "friend" available, such as a hand puppet to "talk" to child for the nurse (see Fig. 7-22, A).

If child refuses to cooperate, use the following techniques:

Assess reason for uncooperative behavior; consider that a child who is unduly afraid may have had a previous traumatic experience.

Try to involve child and parent in process.

Avoid prolonged explanations about examining procedure.

Use a firm, direct approach regarding expected behavior.

Perform examination as quickly as possible.

Have attendant gently restrain child.

Minimize any disruptions or stimulation.

Limit number of people in room.

Use isolated room.

Use quiet, calm, confident voice.

Begin examination in a nonthreatening manner for young children or children who are fearful:

Use activities that can be presented as games, such as test for cranial nerves (see Table 7-11) or parts of developmental screening tests (p. 169).

Use approaches such as Simon Says to encourage child to make a face, squeeze a hand, stand on one foot, and so on.

Use paper-doll technique.

Lay child supine on an examining table or floor that is covered with a large sheet of paper.

Trace around child's body outline.

Use body outline to demonstrate what will be examined, such as drawing a heart and listening with stethoscope before performing activity on child.

If several children in the family will be examined, begin with most cooperative child to provide modeling of desired behavior.

Involve child in examination process:

Provide choices, such as sitting on table or in parent's lap.

Allow child to handle or hold equipment.

Encourage child to use equipment on a doll, family member, or examiner.

Explain each step of the procedure in simple language.

Examine child in a comfortable and secure position:

Sitting in parent's lap

Sitting upright if in respiratory distress

Proceed to examine the body in an organized sequence (usually head to toe) with the following exceptions:

Alter sequence to accommodate needs of different-age children (see Table 7-1).

Examine painful areas last.

In emergency situation, examine vital functions (airway, breathing, and circulation) and injured area first.

Reassure child throughout examination, especially about bodily concerns that arise during puberty.

Discuss findings with family at end of examination.

Praise child for cooperation during examination; give reward such as a small toy or sticker.

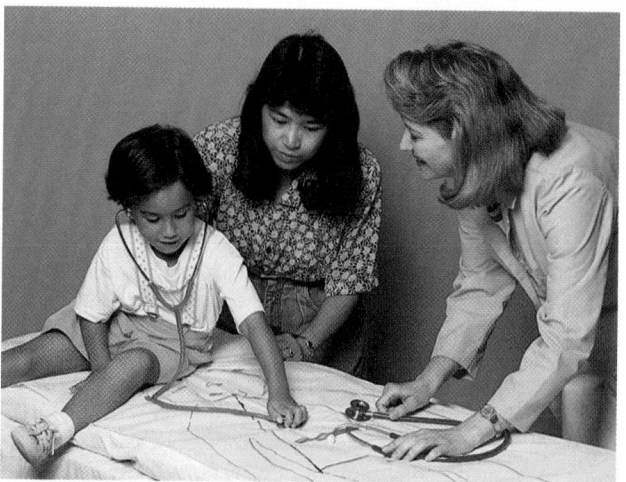

FIG. 7-1 ■ Using paper-doll technique to prepare child.

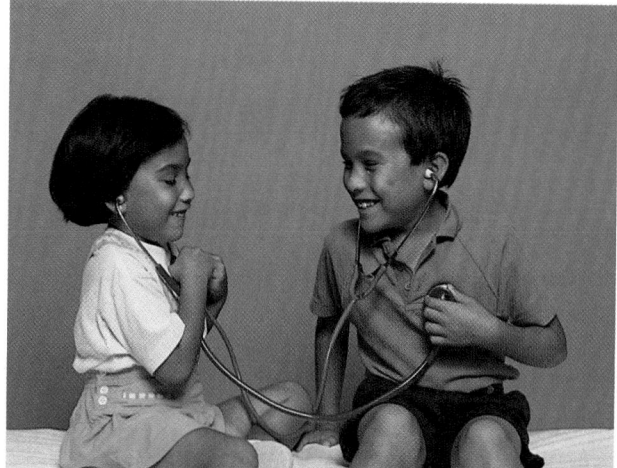

FIG. 7-2 ■ Preparing children for physical examination.

TABLE 7-1 ■ Age-Specific Approaches to Physical Examination During Childhood

POSITION	SEQUENCE	PREPARATION
INFANT		
Before sits alone: supine or prone, preferably in parent's lap; before 4 to 6 months: can place on examining table After sits alone: use sitting in parent's lap whenever possible If on table, place with parent in full view	If quiet, auscultate heart, lungs, abdomen Record heart and respiratory rates Palpate and percuss same areas Proceed in usual head-to-toe direction Perform traumatic procedures last (eyes, ears, mouth [while crying]) Elicit reflexes as body part is examined Elicit Moro reflex last	Completely undress if room temperature permits Leave diaper on male infant Gain cooperation with distraction, bright objects, rattles, talking Smile at infant; use soft, gentle voice Pacify with bottle of sugar water or feeding Enlist parent's aid for restraining to examine ears, mouth Avoid abrupt, jerky movements
TODDLER		
Sitting or standing on or by parent Prone or supine in parent's lap	Inspect body area through play: "count fingers," "tickle toes" Use minimal physical contact initially Introduce equipment slowly Auscultate, percuss, palpate whenever quiet Perform traumatic procedures last (same as for infant)	Have parent remove outer clothing Remove underwear as body part is examined Allow to inspect equipment; demonstrating use of equipment is usually ineffective If uncooperative, perform procedures quickly Use restraint when appropriate; request parent's assistance Talk about examination if cooperative; use short phrases Praise for cooperative behavior
PRESCHOOL CHILD		
Prefer standing or sitting Usually cooperative prone/supine Prefer parent's closeness	If cooperative, proceed in head-to-toe direction If uncooperative, proceed as with toddler	Request self-undressing Allow to wear underpants if shy Offer equipment for inspection; briefly demonstrate use Make up story about procedure: "I'm seeing how strong your muscles are" (blood pressure) Use paper-doll technique Give choices when possible Expect cooperation; use positive statements: "Open your mouth"
SCHOOL-AGE CHILD		
Prefer sitting Cooperative in most positions Younger child prefers parent's presence Older child may prefer privacy	Proceed in head-to-toe direction May examine genitalia last in older child Respect need for privacy	Request self-undressing Allow to wear underpants Give gown to wear Explain purpose of equipment and significance of procedure, such as otoscope to see eardrum, which is necessary for hearing Teach about body functioning and care
ADOLESCENT		
Same as for school-age child Offer option of parent's presence	Same as older school-age child	Allow to undress in private Give gown Expose only area to be examined Respect need for privacy Explain findings during examination: "Your muscles are firm and strong" Matter-of-factly comment about sexual development: "Your breasts are developing as they should be" Emphasize normalcy of development Examine genitalia as any other body part; may leave to end

and the child's measurements in percentiles are compared with those of the general population.

Growth Charts

The most commonly used growth charts in the United States are from the **National Center for Health Statistics (NCHS).** The growth charts have been revised to include the body mass index-for-age (BMI-for-age) charts, 3rd and 97th smoothed percentiles for all charts, and the 85th percentile for the weight-for-stature and BMI-for-age charts (see Appendix D.) The data were collected from five national surveys between 1963 and 1994. The revised charts have eliminated the disjunctions between the curves for infants and other children and have been extended for children

BOX 7-2 ■ Child Preventive Care Timeline

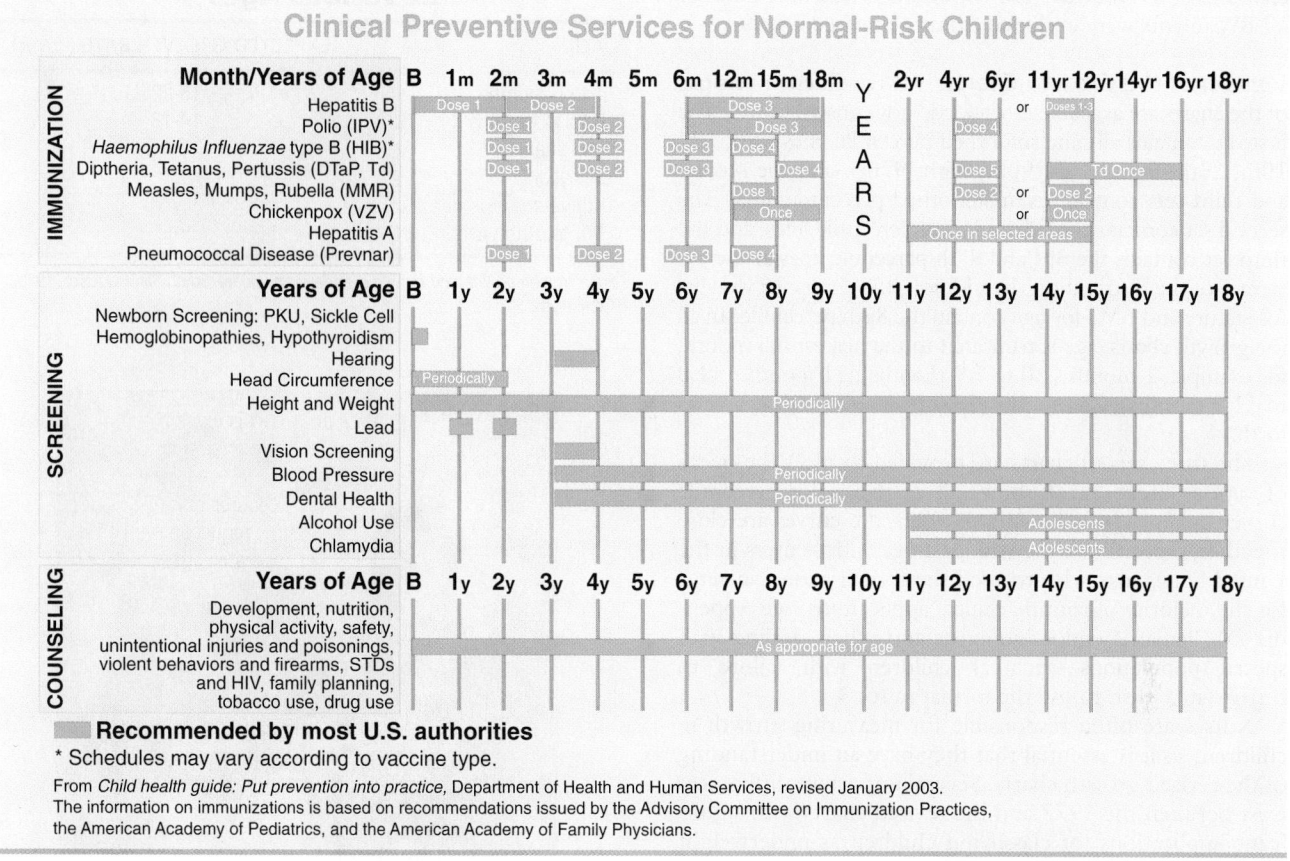

Clinical Preventive Services for Normal-Risk Children

Recommended by most U.S. authorities

* Schedules may vary according to vaccine type.

From *Child health guide: Put prevention into practice,* Department of Health and Human Services, revised January 2003.
The information on immunizations is based on recommendations issued by the Advisory Committee on Immunization Practices,
the American Academy of Pediatrics, and the American Academy of Family Physicians.

and adolescents to 20 years (National Center for Health Statistics, 2000).

The weight-for-age percentile distributions are now continuous between the infant and the older child charts at 24 to 36 months. The length-for-age to stature-for-age and weight-for-length to weight-for-stature curves are parallel in the overlapping ages of 24 to 36 months. The revised weight-for-stature charts provide a smoother transition from the weight-for-length charts for preschool-age children.

The most prominent change to the complement of growth charts for older children and adolescents is the addition of the BMI-for-age growth curves. The BMI-for-age charts were developed with national survey data (1963-1994), excluding data from the 1988-1994 National Health and Nutrition Examination Surveys (NHANES) III for children older than 6 years because an increase in body weight and BMI occurred between NHANES III and previous national surveys. Without this exclusion, the 85th and 95th percentile curves would have been higher, and fewer children and adolescents would have been classified as at risk or overweight. Therefore, the BMI-for-age growth curves do not represent the current population of children older than 6 years of age.

NURSING TIP

The sex-specific BMI-for-age charts for ages 2 to 20 years replace the 1977 NCHS weight-for-stature charts that were limited to prepubescent boys younger than 11.5 years of age and statures less than 145 cm, and to prepubescent girls younger than 19 years of age and statures less than 137 cm.

Breast-fed and Formula-Fed Infants. The national survey data better represent the combined size and growth patterns of the general U.S. population (1971 to 1994). Over the past two decades in the United States, approximately half of all infants were reported ever to have been breast-fed, and approximately one third were breast-fed for 3 months or more. Therefore, compared with the 1977 NCHS growth charts, the nationally representative data on which the revised infant growth charts are based will better represent the combined growth patterns of breast-fed and formula-fed infants in the U.S. population.

With regard to differences in the growth of breast- or formula-fed infants, other research efforts are currently in progress to address this issue. A Working Group of the World Health Organization (WHO) is collecting data at seven international study centers to develop a new set of international growth charts for infants and preschoolers through age 5 years. These charts will be based on the growth of exclusively or predominately breast-fed infants. The basic assumption is that infants from healthy populations, following the current WHO feeding recommendations, are growing optimally.

Special Groups. Although there are differences in size and growth among the major racial and ethnic groups in the United States, these appear to be small and inconsistent. Therefore the revised growth charts include all infants and children whatever their race or ethnicity. Because the growth patterns of preterm, very low-birth-weight (VLBW) (<1500g) infants are considerable different from those of higher-birth-weight term infants and specialized growth charts exist to track the growth of VLBW infants, data for VLBW infants were excluded from the revised charts.

Version of the Growth Charts. Three different versions of the charts are available at www.cdc.gov/growthcharts. The first set contains all nine smoothed percentile lines (3rd, 5th, 10th, 25th, 50th, 75th, 90th, 95th, 97th), and the second and third sets contain seven smoothed percentile lines. The second set contains the 5th and 95th percentile lines, and the third set contains the 3rd and 97th percentile lines at the extremes of the distribution. In addition, the charts for weight-for-stature and BMI-for-age contain the 85th percentile. In all the growth charts, age is truncated to the nearest full month, for example, 1 month (1.0 to 1.9 months), 11 months (11.0 to 11.9 months), 23 months (23.0 to 23.9 months), and so forth.

The three sets of charts are provided to meet the needs of various users. Set 1 shows all of the major percentile curves but may have limitations when the curves are close together, especially at the youngest ages. Most users in the United States may wish to used the format shown in set 2 for the majority of routine clinical applications (see Appendix D). Pediatric endocrinologists and others dealing with special populations—such as children with failure to thrive—may wish to use the format in set 3.

Nurses are often responsible for measuring growth in children, so it is essential that they have an understanding of the revised growth charts. Several important differences exist between the 1977 and the revised charts with significant implications for classifying children as underweight or overweight. Nurses need to become familiar with determining BMI, which only requires information about the child's weight and height.* With the increasing number of overweight children in the United States, the BMI charts will become a critical component of children's physical assessment.

NURSING TIP

BMI-for-age may be used to identify children and adolescents at the upper end of the distribution who are either overweight (≥95th percentile) or at risk for overweight (≥85th and <95th) (Roche and Guo, 2001). Formulas for determining BMI are available at www.cdc.gov/nccdphp/dnpa/bmi/bmi-definiton.htm and in Appendix C.

Children whose growth may be questionable include:

- Children whose height and weight percentiles are widely disparate (e.g., height in the 10th percentile and weight in the 90th percentile, especially with above-average skinfold thickness)
- Children who fail to show the expected growth rates in height and weight, especially during the rapid growth periods of infancy and adolescence (Table 7-2)
- Children who show a sudden increase (except during puberty) or decrease in a previously steady growth pattern

Because growth is a continuous but uneven process, the most reliable evaluation lies in comparing growth measurements

---

*BMI = (Weight in pounds ÷ Height in inches ÷ Height in inches) × 703.

TABLE 7-2 ■ Expected Growth Rates at Various Ages

AGE	EXPECTED GROWTH RATE (cm/yr)
1 to 6 months	18-22
6 to 12 months	14-18
2nd year	11
3rd year	8
4th year	7
5th to 10th years	5-6

From *Human growth and growth disorders: an update,* South San Francisco, 1989, Genentech.

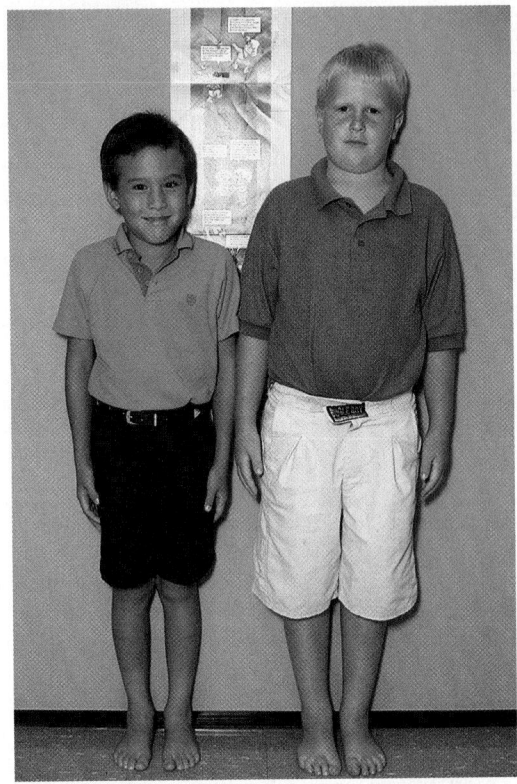

FIG. 7-3 ■ These children of identical age (8 years) are markedly different in size. The child on the left, of Asian descent, is at the 5th percentile for height and weight. The child on the right is above the 95th percentile for height and weight. However, both children demonstrate normal growth patterns.

over time. It is important to remember that normal growth patterns vary among children the same age (Fig. 7-3).

Ethnic Differences in Growth. A potential concern with the U.S. growth charts is their accuracy in evaluating the growth of children from different ethnic and socioeconomic backgrounds. Research findings indicate that these growth charts can serve as a reference guide for all racial or ethnic groups if used from the perspective that different groups of children have varying normal distributions on the growth curves. The NCHS charts are accurate for U.S. African-American children because this group was included

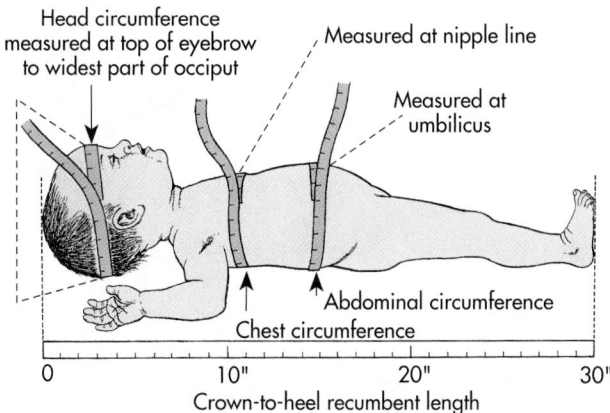

FIG. 7-4 ■ Measurement of head, chest, and abdominal circumference and crown-to-heel (recumbent) length.

in the sample population. Special growth charts for Chinese children are in Appendix D.

Length

The term *length* refers to measurements taken when children are supine (also referred to as *recumbent length*). Until children are 24 months old (36 months if the birth to 36-month chart is used), measure recumbent length. Because of the normally flexed position during infancy, fully extend the body by (1) holding the head in midline, (2) grasping the knees together gently, and (3) pushing down on the knees until the legs are fully extended and flat against the table. If using a measuring board, place the head firmly at the top of the board and the heels of the feet firmly against the footboard.

If such a measuring device is not available, measure length by placing the child on a paper-covered surface, marking the end points of the top of the head and the heels of the feet, and measuring between these two points (Fig. 7-4). For accurate measurement, hold the writing utensil at a right angle to the table when marking the cephalic point; position the feet with the toes pointing directly to the ceiling when marking the heel point. Regardless of the method used, have someone assist in holding the child's head in midline while you extend the legs and take the measurements.

Height

The term *height* (or *stature*) refers to the measurement taken when children are standing upright. Measure height by having the child, with shoes removed, stand as tall and straight as possible, with the head in midline and the line of vision parallel to the ceiling or floor. Be sure the child's back is to the wall or other vertical flat surface, with the heels, buttocks, and back of the shoulders touching the wall and the medial malleoli touching if possible (Fig. 7-5). Check for and correct bending of the knees, slumping of the shoulders, or raising of the heels of the feet.

> **NURSING TIP**
>
> Normally, height is less if measured in the afternoon than in the morning. To minimize this variation, apply modest upward pressure under the jaw or the mastoid processes behind the ears.

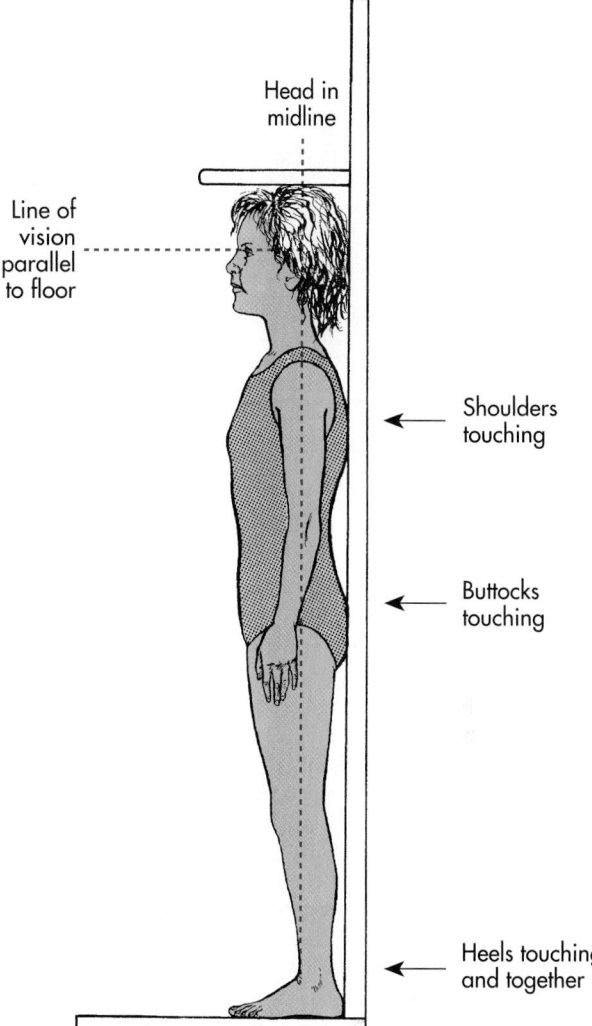

FIG. 7-5 ■ Measurement of height. (Redrawn from *Human growth and growth disorders: an update*, South San Francisco, 1989, Genentech.)

For the most accurate measurement, use a wall-mounted unit (*stadiometer;* see Fig. 7-5). The movable measuring rod of platform scales is accurate only if it maintains a parallel position to the floor and rests securely on the topmost part of the head. To improvise a flat surface for measuring length, attach a paper or metal tape or yardstick to the wall, position the child adjacent to the tape, and place a three-dimensional object, such as a thick book or box, on top of the head. Rest the side of the object firmly against the wall to form a right angle. Measure length or stature to the nearest 1 mm or $\frac{1}{8}$ inch.

Weight

Weight is measured with an appropriately sized beam balance scale, which measures weights to the nearest 10 g or $\frac{1}{2}$ ounce for infants and 100 g or $\frac{1}{4}$ pound for children. Before the child is weighed, the scale is balanced by setting it at zero and noting if the balance registers exactly in the middle of the mark. If the end of the balance beam rises to the top or bottom of the mark, more or less weight, re-

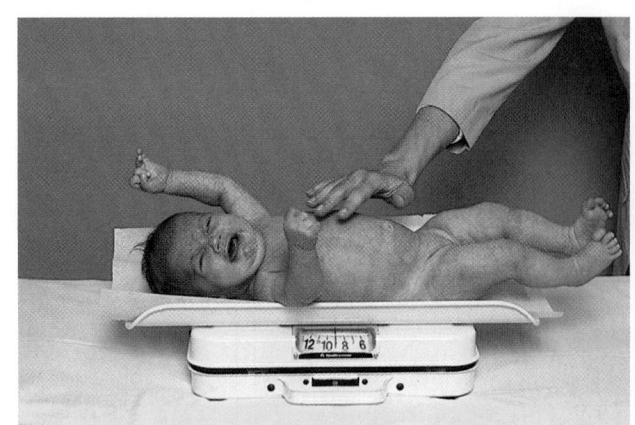

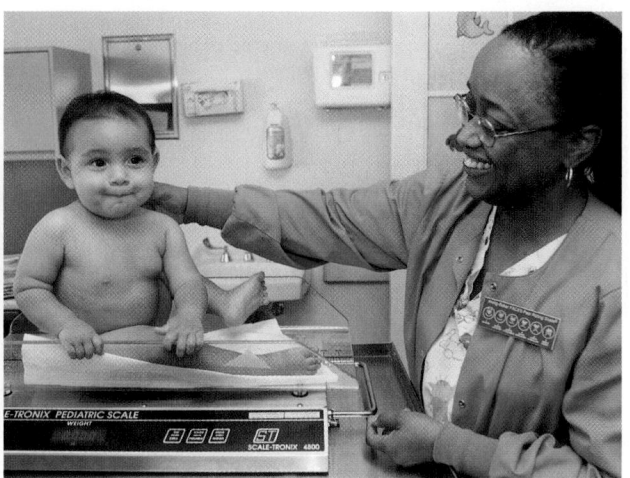

FIG. 7-6 ■ **A,** Infant on scale. **B,** Toddler on scale. Note presence of nurse to prevent falls. (**B,** Courtesy Paul Vincent Kuntz, Texas Children's Hospital.)

spectively, is added. Some scales are designed to allow for self-correction, but others need to be recalibrated by the manufacturer. Scales vary in their accuracy; infant scales tend to be more accurate than adult platform scales, and newer scales tend to be more accurate than older ones, especially at the upper levels of weight measurement. When precise measurements are needed, two nurses should take the weight independently, and if there is a discrepancy, a third reading should be taken.

Take measurements in a comfortably warm room. When the birth to 36-month growth charts are used, children should be weighed nude. Older children are usually weighed while wearing their underpants or a light gown. However, always respect the privacy of all children. If the child must be weighed wearing some article of clothing or some type of special device, such as a prosthesis or an armboard for an intravenous device, note this when recording the weight. Children who are measured for recumbent length are usually weighed on an infant platform scale and placed in a lying-down or sitting position. When weighing children, place your hand lightly above the body of the infant to prevent the child from accidentally falling off the scale (Fig. 7-6, *A*) or stand close to the toddler, ready to prevent a fall (Fig. 7-6, *B*). For maximum asepsis, cover the scale with a clean sheet of paper between each child's measurement.

Skinfold Thickness and Arm Circumference

Measures of relative weight and stature cannot distinguish between adipose (fat) tissue or muscle. One convenient measure of body fat is *skinfold thickness,* which is increasingly recommended as a routine measurement (see also Clinical Examination, Chapter 6). Skinfold thickness is measured with special calipers, such as the Lange calipers. The most common sites for measuring skinfold thickness are the triceps (most practical for routine clinical use), subscapula, suprailiac, abdomen, and upper thigh. For greatest reliability the exact procedure for measurement must be followed and the average of at least two measurements of one site recorded (see Guidelines box).

Arm circumference is an indirect measure of muscle mass. Measurement of arm circumference follows the

GUIDELINES

Measuring Triceps Skinfold Thickness

With child's right arm flexed 90 degrees at elbow, mark mid-point between acromion and olecranon on posterior aspect of arm.

With arm hanging freely, grasp a fold of skin between thumb and forefinger 1 cm above midpoint.

Gently pull fold away from underlying muscle and continue to hold until measurement is completed.

Place caliper jaws over skinfold at midpoint mark and follow directions for using the device.

Estimate reading to nearest 1 mm, 2 to 3 seconds after applying pressure.

Take measurements until duplicates agree within 1 mm.

same procedure for skinfold thickness except measure the midpoint with a paper or steel tape. Place the tape vertically, along the posterior aspect of the upper arm to the acromial process and to the olecranon process; half the measured length is the midpoint. Percentiles for triceps skinfold and arm circumference in children are listed in Appendix D and may be used as reference data. However, the percentiles are not standards or norms, because values between the 5th and 95th percentiles are not ranges of normal.

Head Circumference

Measure head circumference in children up to 36 months of age and in any child whose head size is questionable. Measure the head at its greatest circumference, usually slightly above the eyebrows and pinna of the ears and around the occipital prominence at the back of the skull (see Fig. 7-4). Because head shape can affect the location of the maximum circumference, more than one measurement at points above the eyebrows may need to be taken to obtain the most accurate measure. Use a paper or metal tape because a cloth tape can stretch and give a falsely small measurement. For greatest accuracy, use devices with tenths of a centimeter, because the percentile charts have only 0.5-cm increments.

Plot the head size on the appropriate growth chart under head circumference. Generally, head and chest circumferences are equal at about 1 to 2 years of age. During childhood, chest circumference exceeds head size by about 5 to 7 cm (2 to 3 inches). (For newborns see Physical Assessment, Chapter 8.)

PHYSIOLOGIC MEASUREMENTS

Physiologic measurements, key elements in evaluating physical status of vital functions, include temperature, pulse, respiration, and blood pressure. Compare each physiologic recording with normal values for that age-group (see inside back cover). In addition, compare the values taken on preceding health visits with present recordings. For example, a falsely elevated blood pressure reading may not indicate hypertension if previous recent readings have been within normal limits. The isolated recording may indicate some stressful event in the child's life.

As in most procedures carried out with children, older children and adolescents are treated much the same as are adults. However, special consideration must be given to preschool children (see Atraumatic Care box).

For best results in taking vital signs of infants, count respirations first (before the infant is disturbed), take the pulse next, and measure temperature last. If vital signs cannot be taken without disturbing the child, record the child's behavior (e.g., crying) along with the measurement.

Temperature

Temperature in healthy or ill children can easily be measured at several body sites via oral, rectal, axillary, ear canal, or skin route. Substitutes for the no-longer-used mercury glass thermometer are electronic thermometers, infrared ear-based thermometers, chemical indicator thermometers, skin plastic strips, and digital thermometers, all of which offer advantages (rapid temperature taking, minimal intrusion, and reduced cross contamination) and some disadvantages (see Table 7-3). The accuracy of these instruments may differ, and variations in results may occur if the correct technique is not applied (Fig. 7-7), if the child is febrile, or if the child's age is not appropriately considered (Erickson, 1999; Loveys and others, 1999; Robinson and others, 1998; Romanovsky and others, 1997).

The most frequently used temperature measurement devices (Healthcare Product Comparison System, 1996a, 1996b, and 1996c) in children are:

1 **Electronic continuous thermometers.** Measure the patient's temperature during the administration of general anesthesia, treatment of hypothermia or hyperthermia, and other situations that require continuous monitoring.

2 **Electronic intermittent thermometers.** Measure the patient's temperature at oral, rectal, and axillary sites and are used as primary diagnostic indicators.
3 **Infrared thermometers.** Measure the patient's temperature by collecting emitted thermal radiation from a particular site (e.g., ear canal).

> **NURSING ALERT**
>
> Mercury thermometers should not be used because if broken, inhaled vapors can cause significant toxicity (Goldman and Shannon, 2001).

The routine sites for taking temperature are the sublingual pocket, rectum, axilla, and the ear canal. As a general rule in children, temperature is currently taken in the axilla or rectum in infants and young children, and by mouth after the age of 4 to 5 years when the child understands how to hold the thermometer. Ear-based temperature devices may also be a convenient option (Barone and Rowe, 1999).

The time of the device's placement at the measurement site should be noted. No universal agreement exists regarding the length of time mercury thermometers should be kept in place. Recommendations based on research vary from 8 to 10 minutes for an oral reading, 4 minutes for a rectal reading, and 5 minutes for an axillary reading, but there are researchers who recommend longer placements for oral and axillary routes (Barone and Rowe, 1999). These times may also vary widely within practice settings. Electronic devices considerably lower the measurement time to the range of seconds. However, all efforts should be made to obtain an accurate reading, and devices should be kept in place long enough to achieve this.

Based on the classical literature, the normal core-body temperature is 99° to 100° F (actually assessed for research for surgical and intensive care purposes). The peripheral temperature considered normal in the clinical setting registers as 37.0° C (98.6° F) via the oral route. Temperatures taken at different sites may present small variations from the value of a given reference-criterion site (i.e., oral or rectal) (Childs, Harrison, Hodkinson, 1999; Cretel and others, 1999; Irvin, 1999; Wilshaw and others, 1999). Traditionally it has been assumed that rectal temperatures are around 1° C higher (mean) and axillary temperatures around 1° C lower (mean) than oral temperatures. Recent research reinforces that differences among these sites (rectal, axillary, ear, and oral) may show wide and significant variation across studies (Craig and others, 2000).

> **NURSING TIP**
>
> Because of variations in temperature among rectal, axillary, oral, and ear sites, it is necessary to chart the route along with the recorded temperature reading and to consistently use one route if possible.

Pulse

A satisfactory pulse can be taken radially in children older than 2 years of age. However, in infants and young children, the apical impulse (heard through a stethoscope held to the chest at the apex of the heart) is more reliable (see Fig. 7-29 for location of pulses). Count the pulse for 1 full minute in infants and young children because of possible irregularities in rhythm. However, when frequent apical rates are needed, use shorter counting times (e.g., 15- or 30-second intervals). For greater accuracy, measure the apical rate while the

TABLE 7-3 ■ Comparison of Body Temperature Sites and Techniques*

TEMPERATURE TYPES	COMMENTS
ORAL TEMPERATURE Device to be placed under tongue in right or left posterior sublingual pocket, not in front of tongue. Have child keep mouth closed, without biting on thermometer.	Oral site indicates rapid changes in core body temperature, but accuracy may be an issue when compared to rectal site. (Jensen and others, 2000). Several factors affect mouth temperature: eating/mastication, hot/cold beverages, smoking, open-mouth breathing, ambient temperature (Hooker and Houston, 1996, Rabinowitz and others, 1996).
AXILLARY TEMPERATURE Place tip under arm in center of axilla and keep close to skin, not clothing. Child's arm must be held firmly against side (Fig.7-7, A).	Recommended for children objecting to rectal measurement and for whom oral temperature is not feasible. May be affected by poor peripheral perfusion (results in lower value) or use of radiant warmers or brown fat in cold-stress neonates (results in higher value) (Bliss-Holtz, 1995; Haddock, Merrow, and Swanson, 1996). Advantage: avoids intrusive procedure and eliminates risk of rectal perforation.
RECTAL TEMPERATURE Place well-lubricated tip at maximum 2.5 cm (1 inch) into rectum; securely hold thermometer close to anus. Child may be placed in side-lying, supine, or prone position (i.e., supine with knees flexed toward abdomen); cover penis as procedure may stimulate urination. A small child may be placed prone across parent's lap.	Although very reliable, only recommended when no other route or device can be used (children whose mental age or temperament prevents cooperation, agitated children, and those who have oral/axillary injuries or surgery) (Barone and Rowe, 1999; Jensen and others, 2000). Accuracy is affected by stool in rectum (higher value) (Loveys, 1999). Contraindicated in children with recent rectal surgery, children with diarrhea or anorectal lesions and in those receiving chemotherapy (cancer treatment usually affects mucosa and causes neutropenia) (Hockenberry-Eaton and Kline, 2001). Rectal temperature technique (Fig. 7-7, B).
ELECTRONIC THERMOMETER Senses temperature with an electronic component called thermistor mounted at tip of plastic and stainless steel probe, which is connected to an electronic recorder. Temperature measurement appears on digital display within 60 seconds. Probe can be placed in mouth, axilla, or rectum.	Ideally suited to pediatric use. Devices are safe due to plastic sheath that is unbreakable. Child's mouth can remain open when oral temperature is taken. Accuracy for axillary temperature is supported by some research but not by other studies (Haddock, Merrow, and Swanson, 1996; Wilshaw and others, 1999; Greyling, Viljoen, and Joubert, 2000). Studies recommend that electronic rectal measurements are more accurate than the electronic measurements at axillary, oral, or tympanic sites (Jensen and others, 2000). The penguin electronic thermometer measures rectal temperature in term and near-term infants (Dollberg, Lahav, and Mimouni, 2001).
INFRARED THERMOMETER Infrared thermometers measure thermal radiation from axilla, ear canal, or tympanic membrane. Temperature measurement appears on digital display in approximately 1 second.	Three types of infrared thermometers are available for ear-based use: tympanic, ear-canal, and arterial heat balance via the ear canal (AHBE); often these devices are all inappropriately referred to as "tympanic thermometers." Temperatures measured in this way reflect arterial (bloodstream) temperature (Pompei and Pompei, 1996; Wilshaw and others, 1999).
Ear-Based Temperature Sensor Insert covered tip of probe gently in ear canal, pointing toward midpoint between opposite eyebrow and sideburns (Childs, Harrison and Hodkinson, 1999). For most accurate results: straighten ear canal for sensor to measure heat appropriately (see Fig. 7-7, C), take three measurements, and record highest reading. Most models use "offsets" for internal calculations that transform ear temperature into supposedly equivalent oral or rectal temperatures.	Although frequently used in pediatric settings (especially ambulatory clinics) debate still continues on the reliability of ear-based thermometry in screening of febrile children (Jean-Mary and others, 2002; Lanham and others, 1999; Modell and others, 1998; Saxena and others, 2001). Studies suggest that ear thermometry does not show sufficient agreement with an established method of temperature measurement to be used in situations where body temperature needs to be assessed with precision (Sganga and others, 2000; Craig and others, 2002; Banitelebi and Bangstad, 2002). Although correct probe placement is difficult in infant's ear, accuracy may be affected at this age-group as well (Robinson and others, 1998; Houlder, 2000; Blackburn and others, 2001).

*Revised by Bogdan Dinu.

TABLE 7-3 ■ Comparison of Body Temperature Sites and Techniques—*cont'd*

TEMPERATURE TYPES	COMMENTS
INFRARED THERMOMETER—cont'd	
Ear Sensor (LighTouch LTX)[†]	
Measures the infrared heat energy radiating from canal opening, scans canal for highest temperature reading, and then calculates arterial temperature (correlates highly with core or internal body temperature). Insert hemispheric probe in ear opening; ear tug is not necessary.	Available in two sizes; smaller size of LighTouch Pedi-Q is for infants and toddlers (Wilshaw and others, 1999). Does not calculate offsets; therefore reading is only for arterial temperature (not equivalent to other sites).
Axillary Sensor (LighTouch LTN)[†]	
Measures the infrared heat energy radiating from axilla. Touch covered probe to axilla, depress and release button, remove, and read.	Can be used on wet skin, in incubators, or under radiant heaters, warming pads, or other heat sources. Research suggests that reliability of axillary site may be a general issue when non-mercury thermometers are used (Haddock, Merrow, and Swanson, 1996; Zengeya and Blumenthal, 1996; Craig and others, 2000).
DIGITAL THERMOMETER	
Consists of probe that connects to microprocessor chip, which translates signals into degrees and sends temperature measurement to digital display. Used like an oral electronic thermometer.	More accurate and easier to read, but somewhat more expensive than plastic strip thermometer.
LIQUID CRYSTAL SKIN CONTACT THERMOMETER (CHEMICAL DOT THERMOMETER)	
Single-use, disposable, flexible thermometer with specific chemical mixture in each circle that changes color to measure temperature increments of two tenths of a degree. Two types: Used like mercury thermometer; kept in mouth (1 minute), axilla (3 minutes), or rectum (3 minutes); color change is read 10-15 seconds after removing thermometer. Wearable, continuous-use thermometer, which is placed under axilla; may be read within 2-3 minutes after placement and continuously thereafter; discard and replace every 48 hours.	May underestimate oral temperature and overestimate axillary temperature (Erickson, Meyer, and Woo, 1996). When compared with mercury glass thermometer, they offer less reliable results (Kongpanichkul and Bunjongpak, 2000; Molton, Blacktop, and Hall, 2001). Skin temperature is influenced by clothing, swaddling, and probe placement, especially in neonates and infants (Leick-Rude and Bloom, 1998). Easier to read than plastic strip thermometer (Macqueen, 2001). Tempa.DOT single-use clinical thermometer can be used for routine temperature taking (Macqueen, 2001). Read thermometer away from heat source (e.g., radiant warmer). For older chemical dot thermometers, if unused thermometer changes color from storage in a warm area (above 35° C [95° F]), place in freezer for 1 hour and then at room temperature for 24 hours before using (Py Ma H Corporation, 1994); newer types do not require special storage (Medical Indicators, Inc., 1999). Wearable, continuous-reading thermometer preferred by parents because it requires minimal disturbance to child (i.e., nurse can just lift child's arm to get a temperature reading (Rivera and others, 1997).
PLASTIC STRIP THERMOMETER (THERMOGRAPH)	
Changes color in response to temperature changes. Place strip on forehead until color change occurs; usually takes less than 15 seconds. Some strips are used like oral mercury thermometer.	Accuracy is variable; may be used for screening (Shann and Mackenzie, 1996). Advantages for home and community use include simple instructions and minimal cost (Valadez, Elmore-Meegan, and Morley, 1995).

[†]Manufactured by Exergen Corporation, 51 Water Street, Watertown, MA 02172; (800) 422-3006, (617) 923-9911; website: www.exergen.com.

child is asleep; record the child's behavior along with the rate. Pulses may be graded according to the criteria in Table 7-4. Compare radial and femoral pulses at least once during infancy to detect the presence of circulatory impairment, such as coarctation of the aorta. (See inside back cover for normal rates for pediatric age-groups).

Respiration

Count the respiratory rate in the same manner as for the adult patient. However, in infants observe abdominal movements because respirations are primarily diaphragmatic. Be-

cause the movements are irregular, count them for 1 full minute for accuracy (see also p. 159). (See inside back cover for normal respiratory rates in children.)

Blood Pressure

Blood pressure (BP) measurement by noninvasive methods is part of a routine vital sign determination. BP should be measured annually in children 3 years of age through adolescence and in children with symptoms of hypertension, children in emergency departments and intensive care units, and high-risk infants (Seidel, Rosenstein, and Pathak, 1997;

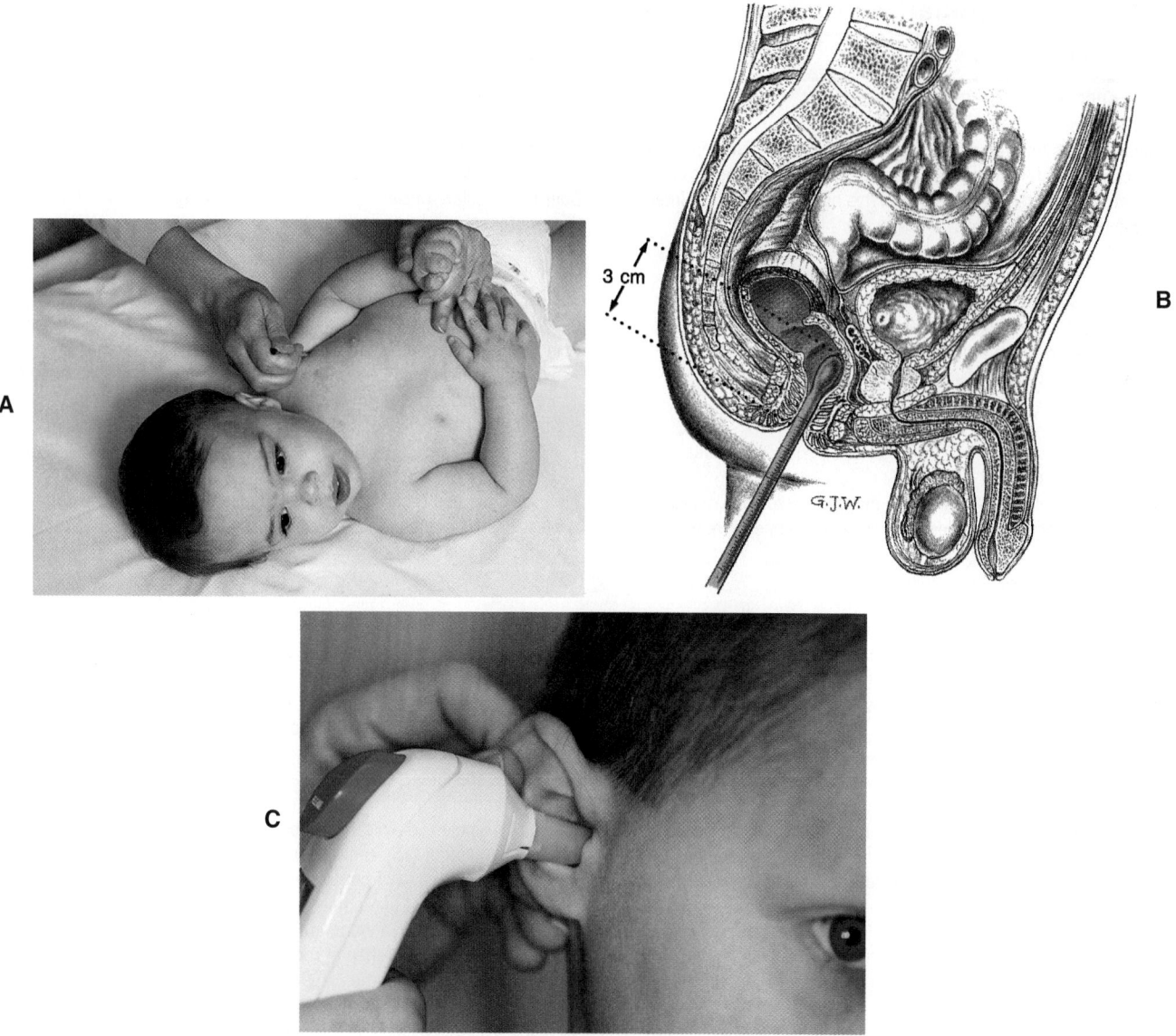

FIG. 7-7 ■ **A,** Position for taking axillary temperature. **B,** Cross-section of rectum illustrates curve approximately 3 cm from anus, where risk of perforation from thermometer is greatest in infants under 3 months of age. **C,** Position for tympanic temperature measurement. Note ear tug to help straighten the canal for the infrared sensor to focus on the eardrum.

National Institutes of Health [NIH], 1996). Ambulatory blood pressure monitoring in children and adolescents is a valuable method for the assessment and management of suspected hypertension (Bald, 2002).

Measurement Devices. BP can also be measured using electronic devices that employ oscillometric or Doppler techniques. In *oscillometry,* pressure changes are transmitted through the arterial wall to the pressure cuff, and the oscillations are detected by a pressure-sensitive indicator. Oscillometers have digital readouts for systolic, diastolic, and *mean arterial pressures (MAP),* and pulse. The MAP is not the same as the mean BP (arithmetic average of systolic and diastolic pressures). Rather, it is a value somewhat lower than the arithmetic mean. BP read-

ings using oscillometry, such as Dinamap, are generally higher and correlate better with direct radial artery values than measurements using auscultation (Amoore, 1998; Wattigney and others, 1996; Gillman and Cook, 1995; Ling and others, 1995) (see Table 7-7). Oscillometry also eliminates common problems found with the auscultation method, such as deflating the cuff too rapidly, not hearing the softest sounds, and rounding numbers for the Korotkoff sounds.

Doppler ultrasound translates changes in ultrasound frequency caused by blood movement within the artery to audible sound by means of a transducer in the cuff. This technique is useful for systolic pressure measurement but is unreliable for diastolic pressure measurement. Oscillometric and Doppler instruments are very useful in measuring BP in

TABLE 7-4 ■ Grading of Pulses

GRADE	DESCRIPTION
0	Not palpable
+1	Difficult to palpate, thready, weak, easily obliterated with pressure
+2	Difficult to palpate, may be obliterated with pressure
+3	Easy to palpate, not easily obliterated with pressure (normal)
+4	Strong, bounding, not obliterated with pressure

infants and have largely replaced the flush method, which reflects only the mean BP, and the auscultatory method.

Selection of Cuff. No matter what type of noninvasive technique is used, the most important factor in accurately measuring BP is the use of an appropriately sized cuff (*cuff size* refers only to the inner inflatable bladder, not the cloth covering). A technique to establish an appropriate cuff size is to choose a cuff having a bladder width that is approximately 40% of the arm circumference midway between the olecranon and the acromion. This will usually be a cuff bladder that covers 80% to 100% of the circumference of the arm (Fig. 7-8) (Beevers, Lip, and O'Brien, 2001; NIH, 1996). Researchers have found that cuff selection of a bladder width to equal forty percent of the upper arm circumference most accurately reflects directly measured radial arterial pressure (Clark and others, 2002).

Using limb circumference for selecting cuff width more accurately reflects direct arterial BP than using limb length, because this method takes into account the variations in thickness of the arm and the amount of pressure required to compress the artery (Gillman and Cook, 1995). For measurement sites other than the upper arms, the limb circumference guidelines can be used, although the shape of the limb (i.e., conical shape of the thigh) may prevent appropriate placement of the cuff and inaccurately reflect intraarterial BP (Table 7-5).

Cuffs that are either too narrow or too wide affect the accuracy of BP measurements. If the cuff size is too small, the reading on the device is falsely high. If the cuff size is too large, the reading is falsely low (Clark and others, 2002).

When another site is used, BP measurements using noninvasive techniques may differ. Generally, systolic pressure in the lower extremities (thigh or calf) is greater than pressure in the upper extremities, and systolic BP in the calf is higher than that in the thigh (Fig. 7-9). These differences are listed in Table 7-6 and apply to oscillometric measurements taken on the right extremities with the child supine and the cuff size based on the circumference method (Park, Lee, and Johnson, 1993).

> **⚠ NURSING ALERT**
>
> In choosing cuff sizes, use an appropriately sized cuff. When the correct size is not available, use an oversized cuff rather than an undersized one or use another site that more appropriately fits the cuff size. Do not choose a cuff based on the name of the cuff (e.g., an "infant" cuff may be too small for some infants).

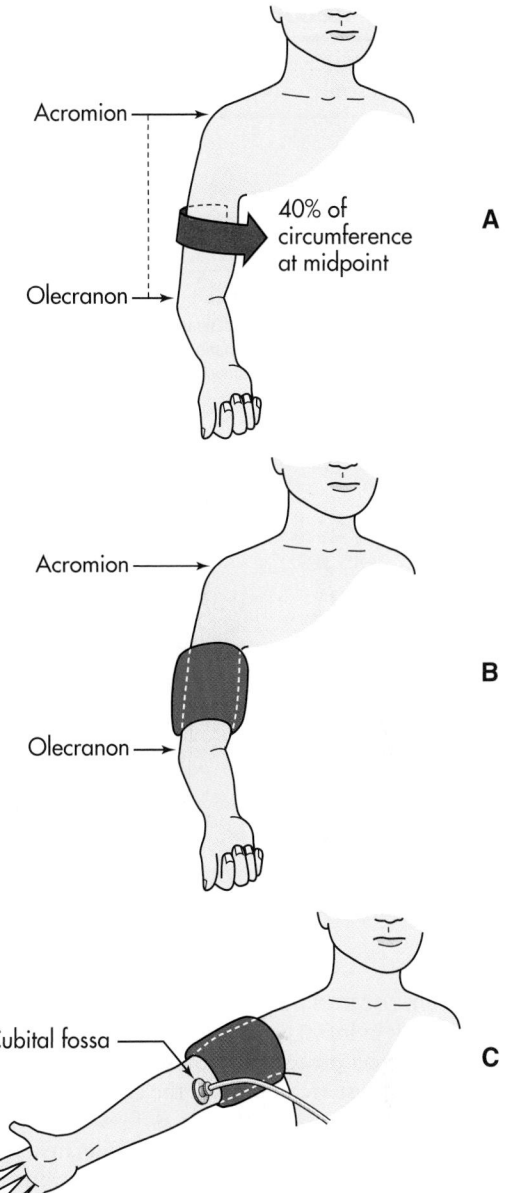

FIG. 7-8 ■ Determination of proper cuff size. **A,** The cuff bladder width should be approximately 40% of the circumference of the arm measured at a point midway between the olecranon and acromion. **B,** The cuff bladder length should cover 80% to 100% of the circumference of the arm. **C,** Blood pressure should be measured with the cubital fossa at heart level. The arm should be supported. The stethoscope bell is placed over the brachial artery pulse, proximal and medial to the cubital fossa and below the bottom edge of the cuff. (From National Institutes of Health, National Heart, Lung, and Blood Institute: *Update on the Task Force Report [1987] on high blood pressure in children and adolescents; a working group report from the National High Blood Pressure Education Program,* Bethesda, Md, NIH pub no 96-3790, Sept 1996.)

> **⚠ NURSING ALERT**
>
> Compare blood pressure in the upper and lower extremities at least once to detect abnormalities, such as coarctation of the aorta, in which the lower extremity pressure is less than the upper extremity pressure.

TABLE 7-5 ■ Recommended Bladder Dimensions for Blood Pressure Cuffs

ARM CIRCUMFERENCE AT MIDPOINT (cm)	CUFF NAME*	BLADDER WIDTH (cm)	BLADDER LENGTH (cm)
5-7.5	Newborn	3	5
7.5-13	Infant	5	8
13-20	Child	8	13
24-32	Adult	13	24
32-42	Wide adult	17	32
42-50	Thigh	20	42

From Frohlich ED and others: Recommendations for human blood pressure determination by sphygmomanometers: report of a special task force appointed by the Steering Committee, American Heart Association, *Circulation* 77:501A, 1988.
*Cuff name does not guarantee that cuff will be appropriate size for a child within that age range.

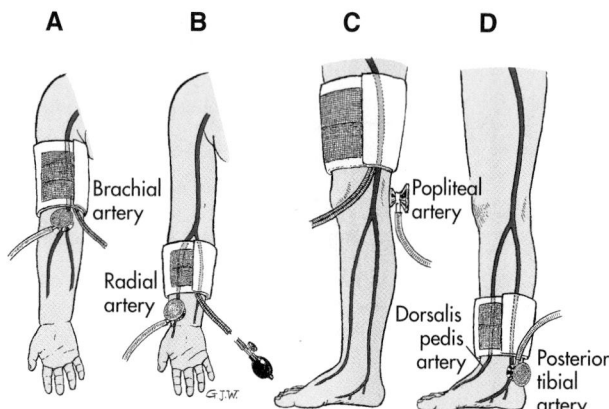

FIG. 7-9 ■ Sites for measuring blood pressure. **A,** Upper arm. **B,** Lower arm or forearm. **C,** Thigh. **D,** Calf or ankle.

TABLE 7-6 ■ Differences in Oscillometric Systolic BP Between Arm and Lower Extremity Sites in Normal Children

	SYSTOLIC BP × (MEAN ± SD)	
AGE-GROUP (years)	ARM-THIGH	ARM-CALF
4-8	−7.1 ± 6.8	−9.3 ± 7.4
9-16	−2.4 ± 7.7	−5.0 ± 26.9

From Park M, Lee D, Johnson GA: Oscillometric blood pressures in the arm, thigh, and calf in healthy children and those with aortic coarctation, *Pediatrics* 91(4): 761-765, 1993.

Measurement and Interpretation. Measuring and interpreting BP in infants and children requires additional attention to correct procedure because (1) limb sizes vary and cuff selection must accommodate the circumference; (2) excessive pressure on the antecubital fossa affects the Korotkoff sounds; (3) children easily become anxious, which can elevate BP; and (4) BP values change with age and growth.

Age, height, weight, and body mass have been shown to be highly correlated with BP (NIH, 1996). Recent studies indicate that height is a more appropriate index of maturation than weight for use with normative BP data and should be considered when evaluating BP in children. Tables are now available that indicate—when height is taken into account—that more short children (10th percentile for age-sex–specific height) and fewer tall children (90th percentile for age-sex–specific height) are likely to be classified as hypertensive (see inside back cover for BP tables).

Although the technique of BP measurement in children is generally the same as that used for adults (see Guidelines box), some aspects of the procedure are especially important. Because children are easily upset by unfamiliar procedures, prepare them for BP measurement. For children of preschool age and above, explain each step of the procedure and tell them how the cuff will feel, such as a tight feeling or an arm hug. Use explanations such as "I want to see how strong your muscle is" or "Let's watch the silver rise in the tube." Because the child should be quiet and relaxed during the procedure, measure BP before performing any anxiety-producing procedures. Infants and small children may be more quiet if the reading is taken while they are sitting in the parent's lap.

Use a pediatric stethoscope and bell for hearing BP sounds in small children and infants. If auscultation is not possible, obtain a systolic reading by palpation; measure the point at which the pulse at the radial or brachial artery reappears as the cuff is deflated. BP should be measured twice, and the average measurement should be recorded (NIH, 1996).

The average BP readings at various ages throughout childhood using sphygmomanometry are listed on the inside back cover, and readings using oscillometry are listed in Table 7-7. A ***normal BP*** is defined as a systolic and diastolic BP less than the 90th percentile for age and sex. (See also Hypertension, Chapter 25.)

> **! NURSING ALERT**
>
> Published norms for BP, such as those on the inside back cover, are valid only if the same method of measurement (auscultation and limb length for cuff size) is used in clinical practice.

GUIDELINES

Measuring Blood Pressure

Use an appropriately sized cuff.

Use same position, preferably sitting, and right arm for brachial artery site (Figs. 7-8 and 7-9, *A*).

Use alternate site as needed to accommodate available cuff sizes.

Use smaller size on forearm: place cuff above wrist and auscultate radial artery (Fig. 7-9, *B*).

Use larger size on thigh: place cuff above knee and auscultate popliteal artery (Fig. 7-9, *C*).

Use larger size on calf: place cuff above malleoli or at mid-calf and auscultate posterior tibial or dorsal pedal artery (Fig. 7-9, *D*).

Position limb at level of heart.

Rapidly inflate cuff to about 20 mm Hg above point at which radial pulse disappears.

Release cuff pressure at a rate of about 2 to 3 mm Hg/sec during auscultation of artery.

Read mercury-gravity manometer at eye level.

Record systolic value as onset of a clear tapping sound (first Korotkoff sound [K1]).

Record diastolic pressure as:

Fourth Korotkoff sound (K4) (low-pitched, muffed sound) for children up to age 12 years

Fifth Korotkoff sound (K5) (disappearance of all sound) for children ages 13 to 18 years

Record also limb, position, cuff size, and method of measurement.

If using electronic monitor, follow manufacturer's instructions and guidelines for correct cuff size.

With oscillometric device (i.e., Dinamap), all four limb sites can be used, but reserve the thigh for last, since it is the most uncomfortable.

Stabilize limb during cuff deflation, since movement interferes with the device's ability to measure blood pressure accurately.

NURSING TIP

Use the following quick formula for average *systolic BP* using auscultation:

1 to 7 years: age in years + 90
8 to 18 years: (2 × age in years) + 83

Use the following formula for average *diastolic BP* using auscultation:

1 to 5 years: 56
6 to 18 years: age in years + 52

GENERAL APPEARANCE

The general appearance of the child is a cumulative, subjective impression of the child's physical appearance, state of nutrition, behavior, personality, interactions with parents and nurse (also siblings if present), posture, development, and speech. Although general appearance is recorded at the beginning of the physical examination, it encompasses all of the observations of the child during the interview and physical assessment.

Note the *facies,* the facial expression and appearance of the child. For example, the facies may give clues to children who are in pain; have difficulty breathing; feel frightened, discontented, or happy; are mentally deficient; or are acutely ill.

Observe the *posture, position,* and types of *body movement.* The child with hearing or vision loss may characteris-

TABLE 7-7 ■ Normative Dinamap BP Values (systolic/diastolic, mean arterial pressure in parentheses)

AGE-GROUP	MEAN	90TH PERCENTILE	95TH PERCENTILE
Newborn (1-3 days)	65/41 (50)	75/49 (59)	78/52 (62)
1 month to 2 years	95/58 (72)	106/68 (83)	110/71 (86)
2-5 years	101/57 (74)	112/66 (82)	115/68 (85)

From Park M, Menard S: Normative oscillometric blood pressure values in the first 5 years in an office setting, *Am J Dis Child* 143(7):860-864, 1989.

tically tilt the head in an awkward position to hear or see better. The child in pain may favor a body part. The child with low self-esteem or a feeling of rejection may assume a slumped, careless, and apathetic pose or posture. Likewise, a child with confidence, a feeling of self-worth, and a sense of security usually demonstrates a tall, straight, well-balanced posture. While observing such "body language," do not interpret too freely but rather record objectively.

Note the child's *hygiene* in terms of cleanliness; unusual body odor; the condition of the hair, neck, nails, teeth, and feet; and the condition of the clothing. Such observations are excellent clues to possible instances of neglect, inadequate financial resources, housing difficulties (e.g., no running water), or lack of knowledge concerning children's needs.

General appearance includes an overall impression of the child's state of *nutrition.* This impression is more than a statement describing body weight or stature, such as "slender and tall." It is an estimation of the quality, as well as the quantity, of nutritional intake. For example, two children can be of the same height and weight, yet one can appear overweight because of flabby, loose skin, whereas the other child appears strong, robust, and well built because of firm, well-defined musculature. Likewise, a small, slender child may be well nourished with no signs of chronic undernutrition, such as bony prominences, a protuberant abdomen, flat buttocks, gaunt facies, and poor muscle tone with evidence of wasting.

Compare your impression of the nutritional state with the parents' history of feeding practices. Discrepancies between the two "impressions" may be a valuable area for nutritional counseling. For example, parents who believe that their child is too thin and eats too little, despite evidence of adequate growth and physical signs of proper nutrition, may find it helpful to keep a daily diary to calculate the child's cumulative food intake. Many parents are surprised at the quantity of food ingested, even though the amounts at each meal or snack are small.

Behavior includes the child's personality, level of activity, reaction to stress, requests, frustration, interactions with others (primarily the parent and nurse), degree of alertness, and response to stimuli. Some mental questions that serve as reminders for observing behavior include: What is the child's overall personality? Does the child have a long attention span or is he or she easily distracted? Can the child follow two or three commands in succession without the need for repetition? What is the youngster's response to delayed gratification or frustration? Is eye-to-eye contact used during conversation? What is the child's reaction to the nurse and family members? Is the child quick or slow to grasp explanations?

Development can be assessed by carefully observing the child, but verify your impressions with screening tests. Various tests for assessing development, speech, vision, and hearing are discussed later in this chapter and in Chapter 19.

Record an overall estimate of the child's speech development, motor skills, degree of coordination, and recent area of achievement under general appearance. For example, the following statement may apply to an 18-month-old child: "Motor development advanced for age; climbs, runs, jumps (most recent motor skill), manipulates small objects with ease; excellent coordination and balance; beginning to name many objects; uses two-word phrases; and enjoys 'talking' to self and others."

SKIN

Skin is assessed for color, texture, temperature, moisture, and turgor. Examination of the skin and its accessory organs primarily involves inspection and palpation. Touch allows the nurse to assess the texture and turgor of the skin as well as the temperature (Turnbull, 2000). The normal *color* in light-skinned children varies from a milky white and rose color to a deeply hued pink color. Dark-skinned children, such as those of Native American, Hispanic, or black descent, have inherited various brown, red, yellow, olive green, and bluish tones in their skin. Asian persons have skin that is normally of a yellow tone.

Several variations in skin color can occur, some of which warrant further investigation. The types of color change and their appearance in children with light or dark skin are summarized in Table 7-8.

Normally the skin *texture* of young children is smooth, slightly dry, and not oily or clammy. Evaluate skin *temperature* by symmetrically feeling each part of the body and comparing upper areas with lower ones. Note any difference in temperature.

Determine *tissue turgor,* or the amount of elasticity in the skin, by grasping the skin on the abdomen between the thumb and index finger, pulling it taut, and quickly releasing it. Elastic tissue immediately assumes its normal position without residual marks or creases. In children with poor skin turgor, the skin remains suspended or tented for a few seconds before slowly falling back on the abdomen. Skin turgor is one of the best estimates of adequate hydration and nutrition.

TABLE 7-8 ■ Differences in Color Changes of Racial Groups

DESCRIPTION	APPEARANCE IN LIGHT SKIN	APPEARANCE IN DARK SKIN
CYANOSIS Bluish tone through skin; reflects reduced (deoxygenated) hemoglobin	Bluish tinge, especially in palpebral conjunctiva (lower eyelid), nail beds, earlobes, lips, oral membranes, soles, and palms	Ashen gray lips and tongue
PALLOR Paleness may be a sign of anemia, chronic disease, edema, or shock	Loss of rosy glow in skin, especially face	Ashen gray appearance in black skin More yellowish brown color in brown skin
ERYTHEMA Redness may be result of increased blood flow from climatic conditions, local inflammation, infection, skin irritation, allergy, or other dermatoses or may be caused by increased numbers of red blood cells as a compensatory response to chronic hypoxia	Redness easily seen anywhere on body	Much more difficult to assess; rely on palpation for warmth or edema
ECCHYMOSIS Large, diffuse areas, usually black and blue in color, caused by hemorrhage of blood into skin; are typically result of injuries	Purplish to yellow-green areas; may be seen anywhere on skin	Very difficult to see unless in mouth or conjunctiva
PETECHIAE Same as ecchymosis except for size: small, distinct pinpoint hemorrhages 2 mm or less in size; can denote some type of blood disorder, such as leukemia	Purplish pinpoints most easily seen on buttocks, abdomen, and inner surfaces of the arms or legs	Usually invisible except in oral mucosa, conjunctiva of eyelids, and conjunctiva covering eyeball
JAUNDICE Yellow staining of the skin usually caused by bile pigments	Yellow staining seen in sclerae of eyes, skin, fingernails, soles, palms, and oral mucosa	Most reliably assessed in sclerae, hard palate, palms, and soles

Accessory Structures

Inspection of the accessory structures of the skin may be performed while the skin is being examined or when the scalp and extremities are being assessed.

Inspect the *hair* for color, texture, quality, distribution, and elasticity. Children's scalp hair is usually lustrous, silky, strong, and elastic. Genetic factors affect the appearance of hair. For example, the hair of black children is usually curlier and coarser than that of white children. Hair that is stringy, dull, brittle, dry, friable, and depigmented may suggest poor nutrition. Record any bald or thinning spots. Loss of hair in infants may indicate lying in the same position and may be a clue for counseling parents concerning the child's stimulation needs.

Inspect the hair and scalp for general cleanliness. Various ethnic groups condition their hair with oils or lubricants,

which, if not thoroughly washed from the scalp, clog the sebaceous glands, causing scalp infections. Also examine the area for lesions; scaliness; evidence of infestation, such as lice or ticks; and signs of trauma, such as ecchymosis, masses, or scars.

In children who are approaching puberty, look for growth of secondary hair as a sign of normally progressing pubertal changes. Note precocious or delayed appearance of hair growth because, although not always suggestive of hormonal dysfunction, it may be of great concern to the early- or late-maturing adolescent.

Inspect the *nails* for color, shape, texture, and quality. Normally the nails are pink, convex, smooth, and hard but flexible (not brittle). The edges, which are usually white, should extend over the fingers. Dark-skinned individuals may have more deeply pigmented nail beds. Short, ragged nails are typical of habitual biting. Uncut, dirty nails are a sign of poor hygiene.

Each individual has a distinct set of handprints and footprints. The patterns, or *dermatoglyphics,* are unique to the individual and vary a great deal in detail and complexity.

The palm normally shows three flexion creases (Fig. 7-10, *A*). In some situations such as Down syndrome, the two distal horizontal creases are fused to form a single horizontal crease (the *single palmar crease,* or *transpalmar crease*) (Fig. 7-10, *B*). If grossly abnormal lines or folds are observed, sketch a picture to describe them and refer the finding to a specialist for further investigation.

LYMPH NODES

Lymph nodes are usually assessed when the part of the body in which they are located is examined. Although the body's lymphatic drainage system is extensive, the usual sites for palpating accessible lymph nodes are shown in Fig. 7-11.

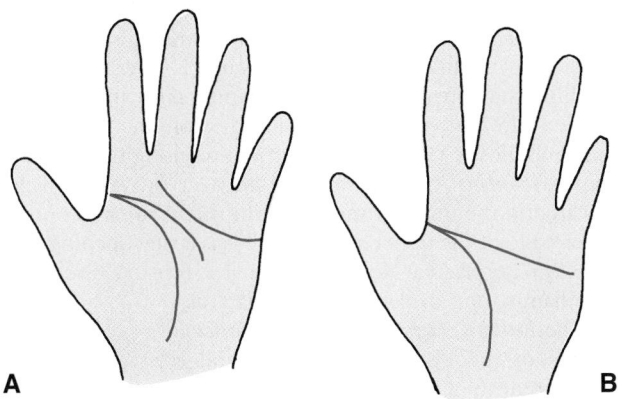

FIG. 7-10 ■ Examples of flexion creases on palm. **A,** Normal. **B,** Transpalmar crease.

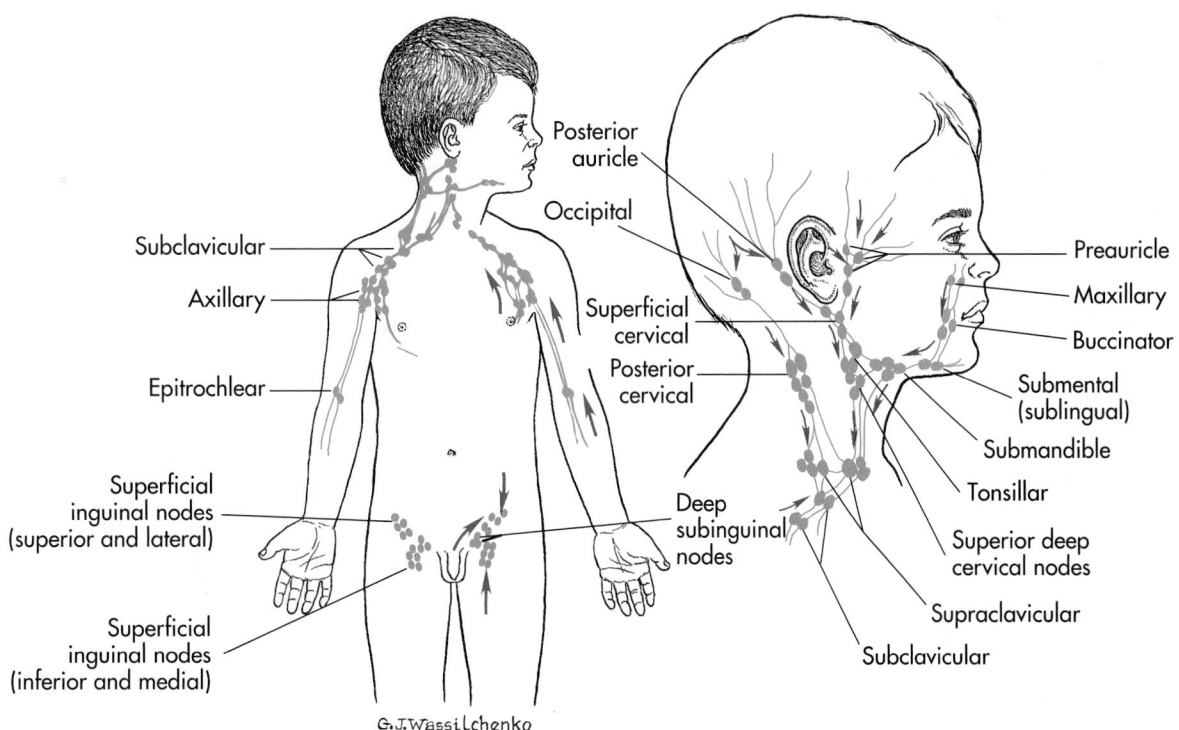

FIG. 7-11 ■ Location of superficial lymph nodes. Arrows indicate directional flow of lymph.

Palpate nodes by using the distal portion of the fingers and gently but firmly pressing in a circular motion along the regions where nodes are normally present. During assessment of the nodes in the head and neck, tilt the child's head upward slightly but without tensing the sternocleidomastoid or trapezius muscles. This position facilitates palpation of the *submental, submaxillary, tonsillar,* and *cervical nodes.* Palpate the *axillary nodes* with the arms relaxed at the sides but slightly abducted. Assess the *inguinal nodes* with the child in the supine position. Note size, mobility, temperature, and tenderness, as well as reports by the parents regarding any visible change of enlarged nodes. In children small, nontender, movable nodes are usually normal. Tender, enlarged, warm lymph nodes generally indicate infection or inflammation close to their location. Report such findings for further investigation.

HEAD AND NECK

Observe the head for general *shape* and *symmetry.* A flattening of one part of the head, such as the occiput, may indicate that the child continually lies in this position. Marked asymmetry is usually abnormal and may indicate premature closure of the sutures (craniosynostosis).

> **! NURSING ALERT**
>
> **Significant head lag after 6 months of age strongly indicates cerebral injury and is referred for further evaluation.**

Note *head control* in infants and *head posture* in older children. Most infants by 4 months of age should be able to hold the head erect and in midline when in a vertical position.

Evaluate range of motion by asking the older child to look in each direction (to either side, up, and down) or manually putting the younger child through each position. Limited range of motion may indicate *wryneck,* or *torticollis,* a result of injury to the sternocleidomastoid muscle in which the child holds the head to one side with the chin pointing toward the opposite side.

> **! NURSING ALERT**
>
> **Hyperextension of the head (opisthotonos) with pain on flexion is a serious indication of meningeal irritation and is referred for immediate medical evaluation.**

Palpate the *skull* for patent sutures, fontanels, fractures, and swellings. Normally the posterior fontanel closes by the second month of life and the anterior fontanel fuses between 12 and 18 months of age. Early or late closure is noted, because either may be a sign of a pathologic condition. (For a more detailed discussion of the cranial bones, see Chapter 8.)

While examining the head, observe the *face* for symmetry, movement, and general appearance. Ask the child to "make a face" to assess symmetric movement and disclose any degree of paralysis. Note any unusual facial proportion, such as an unusually high or low forehead, wide- or close-set eyes, or a small, receding chin.

In addition to assessment of the head and neck for movement, inspect the neck for size and palpate it for associated structures. The neck is normally short, with skinfolds between the head and shoulders during infancy; however, it lengthens during the next 3 to 4 years.

> **! NURSING ALERT**
>
> **If any masses are detected in the neck, report them for further investigation. Large masses can block the airway.**

EYES
Inspection of External Structures

Inspect the *lids* for proper placement on the eye. When the eye is open, the upper lid should fall near the upper iris. When the eyes are closed, the lids should completely cover the cornea and sclera (Fig. 7-12).

Determine the general slant of the *palpebral fissures* or lids by drawing an imaginary line through the two points of the medial canthus and across the outer orbit of the eyes and aligning each eye on the line. Usually the palpebral fissures lie horizontally. However, in Asians, the slant is normally upward.

Also inspect the inside lining of the lids, the *palpebral conjunctiva.* To examine the lower conjunctival sac, pull the lid down while the patient looks up. To evert the upper lid, hold the upper lashes and gently pull *down* and *forward* as the child looks down. Normally the conjunctiva appears pink and glossy. Vertical yellow striations along the edge are the *meibomian* or *sebaceous glands* near the hair follicle. Located in the inner or medial canthus and situated on the inner edge of the upper and lower lids is a tiny opening, the *lacrimal punctum.* Note any excessive tearing, discharge, or inflammation of the lacrimal apparatus.

The *bulbar conjunctiva,* which covers the eye up to the limbus or junction of the cornea and sclera, should be transparent. The *sclera,* or white covering of the eyeball, should be clear. Tiny black marks in the sclera of heavily pigmented individuals are normal.

The *cornea,* or covering of the iris and pupil, should be clear and transparent. Record opacities because they can be signs of scarring or ulceration, which can interfere with vision. The best way to test for opacities is to illuminate the eyeball by shining a light at an angle (obliquely) toward the cornea.

Compare the *pupils* for size, shape, and movement. They should be round, clear, and equal. Test their *reaction to light*

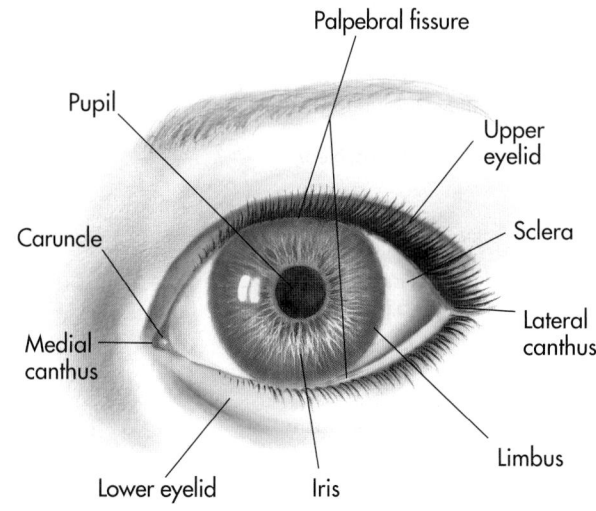

FIG. 7-12 ■ External structures of eye.

by quickly shining a source of light toward the eye and removing it. As the light approaches, the pupils should constrict; as the light fades, the pupils should dilate. Test the pupil/any response of **accommodation** by having the child look at a bright, shiny object at a distance and quickly moving the object toward the face. The pupils should constrict as the object is brought near the eye. Normal findings on examination of the pupils may be recorded as **PERRLA,** which means "*Pupils Equal, Round, React to Light and Accommodation.*"

Inspect the *iris* and pupil for color, size, shape, and clarity. Permanent eye color is usually established by 6 to 12 months of age. As the iris and pupil are inspected, look for the *lens.* Normally the lens is not visible through the pupil.

Inspection of Internal Structures

The ophthalmoscope permits visualization of the interior of the eyeball with a system of lenses and a high-intensity light. The lenses permit clear visualization of eye structures at different distances from the nurse's eye and correct visual acuity differences in the examiner and child. Use of the ophthalmoscope requires practice to know which lens setting produces the clearest image.

The ophthalmic and otic head are usually interchangeable on one "body" or handle, which encloses the power source, either disposable or rechargeable batteries. The nurse should practice changing the heads, which snap on and are secured with a quarter turn, and replacing the batteries and light bulbs. Nurses who are not directly involved in physical assessment are often responsible for ensuring that the equipment functions properly.

Preparing the Child.   The nurse can prepare the child for the ophthalmoscopic examination by showing the child the instrument, demonstrating the light source and how it shines in the eye, and explaining the reason for darkening the room. For infants and young children who do not respond to such explanations, it is best to try to use distraction to encourage them to keep their eyes open. Forcibly parting the lids results in an uncooperative, watery-eyed child and a frustrated nurse. Usually, with some practice, the nurse can elicit a red reflex almost instantly while approaching the child and may also gain a momentary inspection of the blood vessels, macula, or optic disc.

Funduscopic Examination.   Fig. 7-13 shows the structures of the back of the eyeball, or the *fundus.* The fundus is immediately apparent as the *red reflex.* The intensity of the color increases in darkly pigmented individuals.

> **！NURSING ALERT**
>
> A brilliant, uniform red reflex is an important sign because it rules out many serious defects of the cornea, aqueous chamber, lens, and vitreous chamber. Any dark shadows or opacities are recorded because they indicate some abnormality in any of these structures.

As the ophthalmoscope is brought closer to the eye, the most conspicuous feature of the fundus is the *optic disc,* the area where the blood vessels and optic nerve fibers enter and exit from the eye. The color of the disc is creamy pink; it is lighter in color than the surrounding fundus. Normally it is round or vertically oval.

After the optic disc is located, the area is inspected for *blood vessels.* The central retinal artery and vein appear in the depths of the disc and emanate outward with visible branching. The *veins* are darker in color and about one fourth larger in size than the *arteries.* Normally the branches of the arteries and veins cross each other.

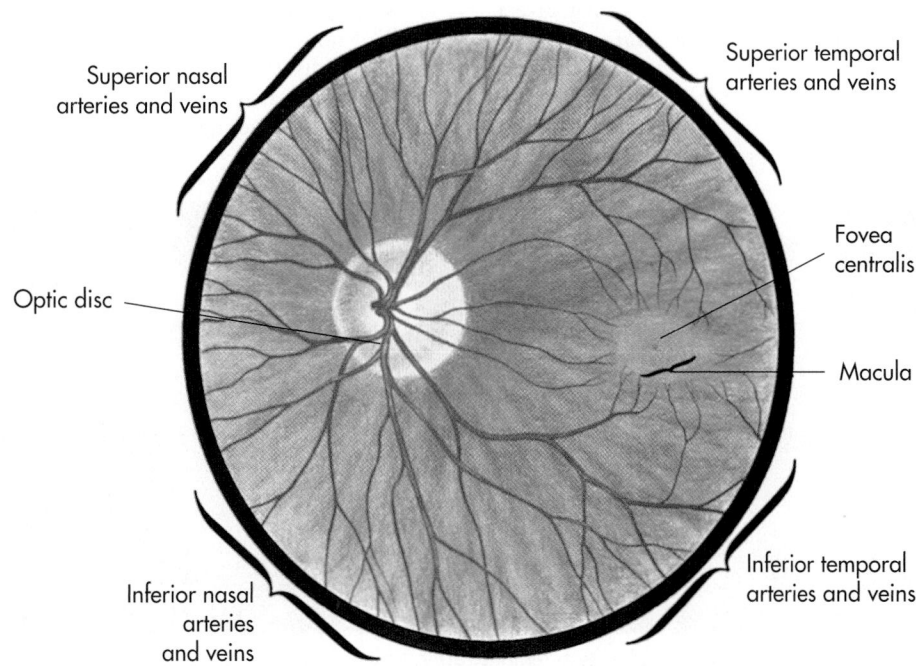

FIG. 7-13 ■ Structures of fundus. (From Seidel HM and others: *Mosby's guide to physical examination,* ed 4, St Louis, 1999, Mosby.)

Other structures that may be seen are the *macula,* the area of the fundus with the greatest concentration of visual receptors, and, in the center of the macula, a minute glistening spot of reflected light called the *fovea centralis;* this is the area of most perfect vision.

Vision Testing

Several tests are available for assessing vision. This discussion focuses on four areas: (1) ocular alignment, (2) visual acuity, (3) peripheral vision, and (4) color vision. Vision screening should be performed at the earliest possible age and at regular intervals (American Academy of Pediatrics [AAP], 2003a; Wall and others, 2002). Behavioral and physical signs that indicate visual impairment are discussed in Chapter 19.

Ocular Alignment. Normally, by the age of 3 to 4 months, children achieve the ability to fixate on one visual field with both eyes simultaneously (binocularity). One of the most important tests for binocularity is alignment of the eyes to detect nonbinocular vision, or *strabismus* (Halle, 2002). In strabismus, or cross-eye, one eye deviates from the point of fixation. If the malalignment is constant, the weak eye becomes "lazy," and the brain eventually suppresses the image produced by that eye. If strabismus is not detected and corrected by age 4 to 6 years, blindness from disuse, known as *amblyopia,* may result.

Tests commonly used to detect malalignment are the corneal light reflex and the cover tests. To perform the *corneal light reflex test,* or *Hirschberg test,* shine a flashlight or the light of the ophthalmoscope directly into the patient's eyes from a distance of about 40.5 cm (16 inches). If the eyes are *orthophoric,* or normal, the light falls symmetrically within each pupil (Fig. 7-14, *A*). If the light falls off center in one eye, the eyes are malaligned. *Epicanthal folds,* excess folds of skin that extend from the roof of the nose to the inner termination of the eyebrow and that partially or completely overlap the inner canthus of the eye, may give a false impression of malalignment (*pseudostrabismus*) (Fig. 7-14, *B*). Epicanthal folds are often found in Asian children.

In the *cover test,* one eye is covered, and the movement of the *uncovered* eye is observed while the child looks at a near (33 cm, or 13 inches) or distant (6 m, or 20 feet) object. If the uncovered eye does not move, it is aligned. If the uncovered eye moves, a malalignment is present because when the stronger eye is temporarily covered, the misaligned eye attempts to fixate on the object.

In the *alternate cover test,* occlusion is shifted back and forth from one eye to the other, and movement of the eye that was *covered* is observed as soon as the occluder is removed while the child focuses on a point in front of him or her. If normal alignment is present, shifting the cover from one eye to the other will not cause the eye to move. If malalignment is present, eye movement will occur when the cover is moved. This test takes more practice than the other cover test because the occluder must be moved back and forth quickly and accurately to see the eye move. Because deviations can occur at different ranges, it is important to perform the cover tests at both close and far distances.

> **❗NURSING ALERT**
>
> The cover test is usually easier to perform if the examiner uses his or her own hand rather than a card-type occluder (Fig. 7-15). Attractive occluders fashioned like an ice cream cone or happy-face lollipop cut from cardboard are also well received by young children.

Photoscreening is a technique used to screen for amblyopia, refractive disorders, and media opacities (AAP, 2003a; Berry and others, 2001). Using a camera, images of the papillary reflexes (reflections) and red reflexes (Bruckner test) are obtained (AAP, 2003a;). Photoscreening offers an effective way to screen infants, preverbal children, and those with developmental delays who are difficult to screen.

Visual Acuity Testing in Children Beyond Infancy. The most common test for measuring visual acuity is the *Snellen letter chart,* which consists of lines of letters of decreasing size (see Appendix C). During testing, the AAP (2003a) now recommends that children stand 10 feet from the chart with their heels at the 10-foot line. When screening for visual acuity in children, the child's right eye is tested first by covering the left. Children who wear glasses

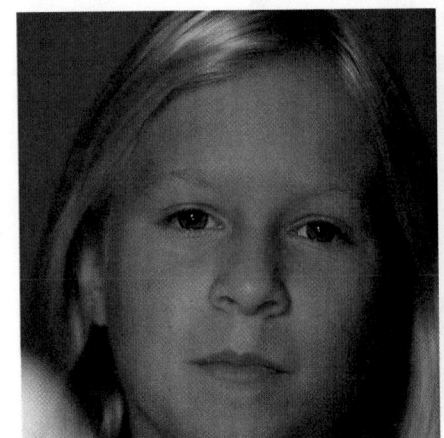
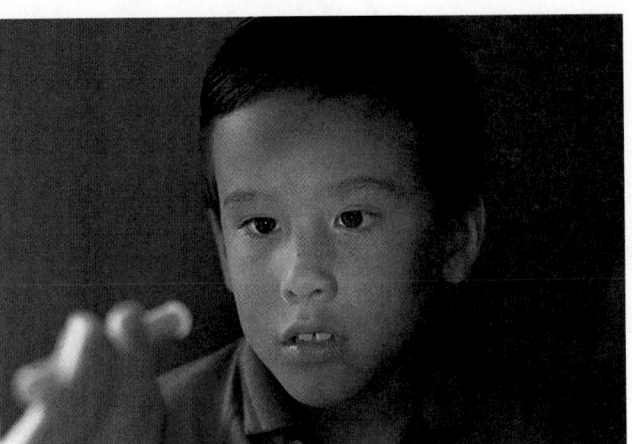

FIG. 7-14 ■ **A,** Corneal light reflex test demonstrating orthophoric eyes. **B,** Pseudostrabismus. Inner epicanthal folds cause eyes to appear malaligned; however, corneal light reflexes fall perfectly symmetrically.

should be screened wearing the lenses. Tell the child to keep both eyes open during the examination. If the child fails the current line, move up the chart to the next larger line. Continue up the chart until a line is found that the child can pass. Then begin moving down the chart again until the child fails to read the line. To pass each line, the child must correctly identify four of six symbols on the line. Repeat the procedure, covering the right eye. Table 7-9 provides a list of visual screening tests for children and guidelines for referral recommended by the AAP (2003a).

For children unable to read letters and numbers, the *tumbling **E*** or ***HOTV test*** is useful (Coats and Jenkins, 1997). The tumbling E test uses the capital letter E to point in four different directions. The child is then asked to point in the direction the E is facing. The HOTV test consists of a wall chart composed of Hs, Os, Ts, and Vs. The child is given a board containing a large H, O, T, and V. The examiner points to a letter on the wall chart, and the child matches the correct letter on the board held in his or her hand. The tumbling E and HOTV are excellent tests for preschool-age children. When a child is unable to perform the tumbling E or HOTV test, the LH symbol or Allen card test may be used. The Allen card test uses common figures to test the child's vision. It is important to assess whether the child is able to identify the pictures before actual vision testing. The examiner walks backward slowly, flipping through the cards and presenting different pictures to the child. The examiner continues to move backward as the child correctly calls out the figures. When the child begins to miss the figure on the cards, the examiner moves forward to confirm that the child is able to identify the figures at that point. All Allen card figures are 20/30 in size. The farthest distance at which the child is able to identify the pictures accurately becomes the numerator, and 30 becomes the denominator. For example, if the child is able to identify the pictures accurately at 15 feet, the visual acuity is recorded as 15/30. This is equivalent to 20/40 or 10/20 visual acuity. The LH symbol test is somewhat different from the Allen card test because it is a spiral-bound set of flash cards. The flash cards contain large pictures of a house, apple, circle, and square. The LH symbol cards contains the symbol size and visual acuity value for a 10-foot testing distance. The visual acuity is determined by the smallest symbols the child is able to identify at 10 feet.

Visual Acuity Testing in Infants and Difficult-to-Test Children. In newborns, vision is tested mainly by checking for *light perception* by shining a light into the eyes and noting responses such as pupillary constriction, blinking, following the light to midline, increased alertness, or refusal to open the eyes after exposure to the light. Although the simple maneuver of checking light perception and eliciting the pupillary light reflex indicates that the anterior half of the visual apparatus is intact, it does not confirm that the infant can see. In other words, this test does not assess whether the brain receives the visual message and interprets the signals.

Another test of visual acuity is the infant's ability to fix on and follow a target. Although any brightly colored or patterned object can be used, the human face is excellent. Hold the infant upright while moving your face slowly from side to side.

> ### NURSING ALERT
> If visual fixation and following are not present by 3 to 4 months of age, further ophthalmologic evaluation is needed.

Other signs that may indicate visual loss or other serious eye problems include fixed pupils, strabismus, constant nystagmus, the setting-sun sign, and slow lateral movements. Unfortunately, it is very difficult to test each eye separately; the presence of such signs in one eye could indicate unilateral blindness.

Special tests are available for testing infants and other difficult-to-test children to assess acuity or confirm blindness. For example, in ***visually evoked potentials,*** the eyes are stimulated with a bright light or pattern, and electrical activity to the visual cortex is recorded through scalp electrodes. Acuity is assessed by using progressively smaller patterns.

Peripheral Vision. In children who are old enough to cooperate, estimate ***peripheral vision,*** or the visual field of each eye, by having children fixate on a specific point di-

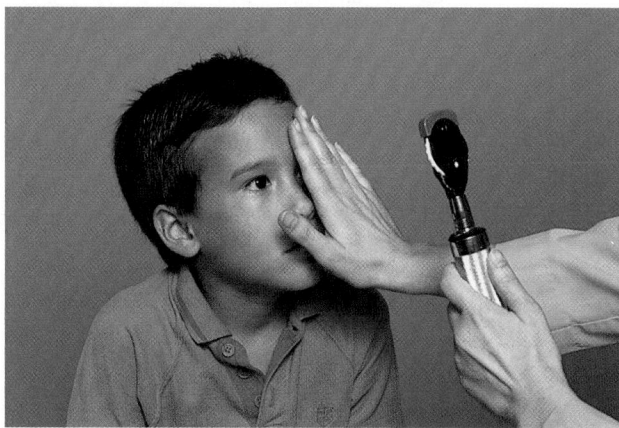
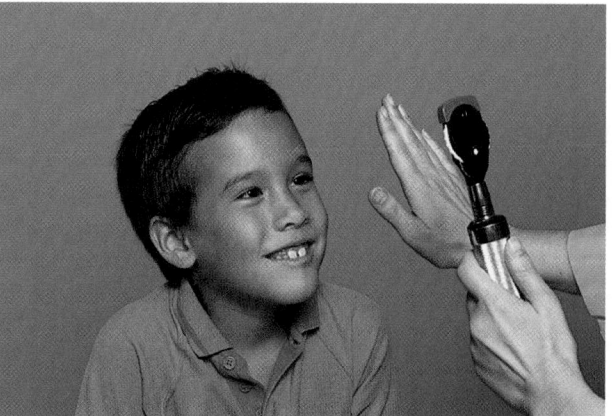

A   **B**

FIG. 7-15 ■ Alternate cover test to detect amblyopia in patients with strabismus. **A,** Eye is occluded, and child is fixating on light source. **B,** If eye does not move when uncovered, eyes are aligned.

TABLE 7-9 ■ Eye Examination Guidelines*

FUNCTION	RECOMMENDED TESTS	REFERRAL CRITERIA	COMMENTS
AGES 3-5 YEARS			

Distance visual acuity	Snellen letters
	Snellen numbers
	Tumbling *E*
	HOTV
	Picture test
	    Allen figures
	    LEA symbols
		1. Fewer than 4 of 6 correct on 20-ft line with either eye tested at 10 ft monocularly (i.e., less than 10/20 or 20/40)
		or
		2. Two-line difference between eyes, even within the passing range (i.e., 10/12.5 and 10/20 or 20/25 and 20/40)
			1. Tests are listed in decreasing order of cognitive difficulty; the highest test that the child is capable of performing should be used; in general, the tumbling *E* or the *HOTV* test should be used for children 3-5 years or age and Snellen letters or numbers for children 6 years and older.
			2. Testing distance of 10 ft is recommended for all visual acuity tests.
			3. A line of figures is preferred over single figures.
			4. The nontested eye should be covered by an occluder held by the examiner or by an adhesive occluder patch applied to eye; the examiner must ensure that it is not possible to peek with the nontested eye.

Ocular alignment	Cross-cover test at 10 ft (3 m) Random dot *E* stereo test at 40 cm Simultaneous red reflex test (Bruckner test)	Any eye movement Fewer than 4 of 6 correct Any asymmetry of pupil color, size, brightness	Child must be fixing on a target while cross-cover test is performed Direct ophthalmoscope used to view both red reflexes simultaneously in a darkened room from 2 to 3 feet away; detects asymmetric refractive errors as well.
Ocular media clarity (cataracts, tumors, etc.)	Red reflex	White pupil, dark spots, absent reflex	Direct ophthalmoscope, darkened room. View eyes separately at 12 to 18 inches; white reflex indicates possible retinoblastoma.
6 YEARS AND OLDER			

Distance visual acuity	Snellen letters
	Snellen numbers
	Tumbling *E*
	HOTV
	Picture test
	    Allen figures
	    LEA symbols
		1. Fewer than 4 of 6 correct on 15-ft line with either eye tested at 10 ft monocularly (i.e., less than 10/15 or 20/30)
		or
		2. Two-line difference between eyes, even within the passing range (i.e., 10/10 and 10/15 or 20/20 and 20/30)
			1. Tests are listed in decreasing order of cognitive difficulty; the highest test that the child is capable of performing should be used; in general, the tumbling *E* or the *HOTV* test should be used for children 3-5 years or age and Snellen letters or numbers for children 6 years and older.
			2. Testing distance of 10 ft is recommended for all visual acuity tests.
			3. A line of figures is preferred over single figures.
			4. The nontested eye should be covered by an occluder held by the examiner or by an adhesive occluder patch applied to eye; the examiner must ensure that it is not possible to peek with the nontested eye.

Ocular alignment	Cross-cover test at 10 ft (3 m) Random dot *E* stereo test at 40 cm Simultaneous red reflex test (Bruckner test)	Any eye movement Fewer than 4 of 6 correct Any asymmetry of pupil color, size, brightness	Child must be fixing on a target while cross-cover test is performed Direct ophthalmoscope used to view both red reflexes simultaneously in a darkened room from 2 to 3 feet away; detects asymmetric refractive errors as well.
Ocular media clarity (cataracts, tumors, etc)	Red reflex	White pupil, dark spots, absent reflex	Direct ophthalmoscope, darkened room. View eyes separately at 12 to 18 inches; white reflex indicates possible retinoblastoma.

From American Academy of Pediatrics, Committee on Practice and Ambulatory Medicine, Section on Ophthalmology: Eye examination in infants, children, and young adults by pediatricians, *Pediatrics* 111(4):902-907, 2003a.

*Assessing visual acuity (vision screening) represents one of the most sensitive techniques for the detection of eye abnormalities in children. The American Academy of Pediatrics, Section on Ophthalmology, in cooperation with the American Association for Pediatric Ophthalmology and Strabismus and the American Academy of Ophthalmology, has developed these guidelines to be used by physicians, nurses, educational institutions, public health departments, and other professionals who perform vision evaluation services.

rectly in front of them as an object, such as a finger or a pencil, is moved from beyond the field of vision into the range of peripheral vision. Check each eye separately and for each quadrant of vision. As soon as children see the object, have them say "stop." At that point measure the angle from the anteroposterior axis of the eye (straight line of vision) to the peripheral axis (point at which the object is first seen). Normally children see about 50 degrees upward, 70 degrees downward, 60 degrees nasalward, and 90 degrees temporally. Limitations in peripheral vision may indicate blindness from damage to structures within the eye or to any of the visual pathways.

Color Vision.   Another important test is for color vision. It is estimated that 8% to 10% of white males and less than half that percentage of black males inherit the X-linked disorder known as *color vision deficit* (less acceptable term, *color blindness*). From 0.5% to 1% of white females are affected. Although the severity of impaired perception of color varies considerably, the two most common types are *protanomaly,* in which the child confuses gray with pink or pale blue with green, and *deuteranomaly,* in which the child confuses gray with pale purple or green. In most of these individuals the color vision deficit causes no major problems. However, some of the difficulties encountered by individuals with more severe deficits may be inability to distinguish amber or red traffic lights, failure to see a red brake light on the rear of a car, difficulty in distinguishing green traffic lights from certain types of incandescent street lamps, and a poor sense of color coordination of clothing. For school-age children the greatest difficulty lies in performance of academic skills that use color as a visual aid. Adolescents may be ineligible for certain vocational opportunities, such as electronics, photography, printing, interior decorating, pharmaceuticals, textiles, police work, and several types of military service.

The tests available for color vision include the *Ishihara test* and the *Hardy-Rand-Rittler (HRR) test.* Each consists of a series of cards (pseudoisochromatic) on which is printed a color field composed of spots of a certain "confusion" color. Against the field is a number or symbol similarly printed in dots but of a color likely to be confused with the field color by the person with a color vision deficit. As a result, the figure or letter is invisible to an affected individual but is clearly seen by a person with normal vision.

EARS
Inspection of External Structures

The entire external earlobe is called the *pinna,* or *auricle,* and is located on each side of the head. Measure the *height* alignment of the pinna by drawing an imaginary line from the outer orbit of the eye to the occiput, or most prominent protuberance of the skull. The top of the pinna should meet or cross this line. Low-set ears are commonly associated with renal anomalies or mental retardation. Measure the *angle* of the pinna by drawing a perpendicular line from the imaginary horizontal line and aligning the pinna next to this mark. Normally the pinna lies within a 10-degree angle of the vertical line (Fig. 7-16). If it falls outside this area, record the deviation and look for other anomalies.

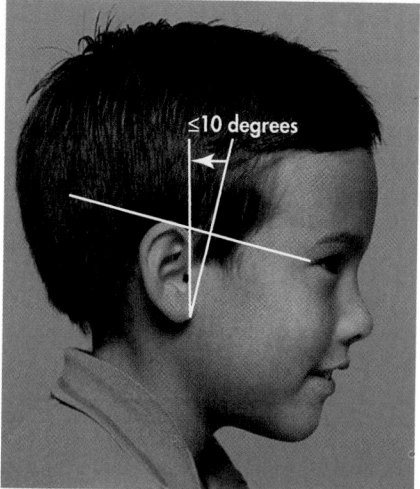

FIG. 7-16 ■ Ear alignment.

Normally the pinna extends slightly outward from the skull. Except in newborn infants, ears that are flat against the head or protruding away from the scalp may indicate problems. Flattened ears in infants may suggest a frequent side-lying position and, just as with isolated areas of hair loss, may be a clue to investigating parents' understanding of the child's stimulation needs.

Inspect the *skin* surface around the ear for small openings, extra tags of skin, or sinuses. If a sinus is found, note this because it may represent a fistula that drains into some area of the neck or ear. Cutaneous tags represent no pathologic process but may cause parents concern in terms of the child's appearance.

Also assess the ear for *hygiene.* An otoscope is not necessary for looking into the external canal to note the presence of *cerumen,* a waxy substance produced by the ceruminous glands in the outer portion of the canal. Cerumen is usually yellow-brown and soft. If an otoscope is used and any discharge is seen, its color and odor are noted. Prevent transmitting potentially infectious material to the other ear or to another child through handwashing and using disposable specula or sterilizing reusable specula between each examination.

Inspection of Internal Structures

The head of the otoscope permits visualization of the tympanic membrane by use of a bright light, a magnifying glass, and a speculum. Some otoscopes have an attachment for a pneumonic device to insert air into the canal to determine membrane compliance (movement). The speculum, which is inserted into the external canal, comes in a variety of sizes to accommodate different canal widths. The largest speculum that fits comfortably into the ear is used to achieve the greatest area of visualization. The lens, or magnifying glass, is movable, allowing the examiner to insert an object, such as a curette, into the ear canal through the speculum while still viewing the structures through the lens.

Positioning the Child.   Before beginning the otoscopic examination, position the child properly and restrain if necessary. Older children usually cooperate and do not need re-

ATRAUMATIC CARE

Reducing Distress From Otoscopy in Young Children

Make examining the ear a game by explaining that you are looking for a "big elephant" in the ear. This kind of make-believe is an absorbing distraction and usually elicits cooperation. After the ear has been examined, clarify that "looking for elephants" was only pretend and thank the child for letting you look in his or her ear. You can also ask the child to put a finger on the opposite ear to keep the light from getting out, which is a great distraction technique.

straint. However, prepare them for the procedure by allowing them to play with the instrument, demonstrating how it works, and stressing the importance of remaining still. A helpful suggestion is to let them observe you examining the parent's ear. Restraint is needed for younger children because the ear examination upsets them (see Atraumatic Care box).

As you insert the speculum into the meatus, move it around the outer rim to accustom the child to the feel of something entering the ear. If examining a painful ear, touch a nonpainful part of the affected ear, then examine the unaffected ear, and finally return to the painful ear. By this time the child is usually less fearful of anything causing discomfort to the ear and will cooperate more.

For their protection and safety, infants and toddlers must be restrained for the otoscopic examination. There are two general positions of restraint. In one the child is seated sideways in the parent's lap with one arm "hugging" the parent and the other arm at the side. The ear to be examined is toward the nurse. With one arm the parent holds the child's head firmly against his or her chest, and with the other arm "hugs" the child, thereby securing the child's free arm. The ear is examined using the same procedure for holding the otoscope as described later (Fig. 7-17, *A*).

The other position involves placing the child on the side, back, or abdomen with the arms at the side and the head turned so that the ear to be examined points toward the ceiling. Lean over the child and use the upper part of the body to restrain the arms and upper trunk movements, and the examining hand to stabilize the head. This position is practical for young infants or for older children who need minimal restraining, but it may not be feasible for other children who protest vigorously. For safety enlist the parent's or an assistant's help in immobilizing the head by firmly placing one hand above the ear and the other on the child's side, abdomen, or back (Fig. 7-17, *B*).

With cooperative children examine the ear with the child in a side-lying, sitting, or standing position. One disadvantage to standing is that the child may "walk away" as the otoscope enters the canal. If the child is standing or sitting, tilt the head slightly toward the child's opposite shoulder to achieve a better view of the drum (Fig. 7-18).

With the thumb and forefinger of the free (usually nondominant) hand, grasp the auricle. For the two positions of restraint, hold the otoscope upside down at the junction of its head and handle with the thumb and index finger. Place the other fingers against the skull to allow the otoscope to move with the child in case of sudden movement. In examining a

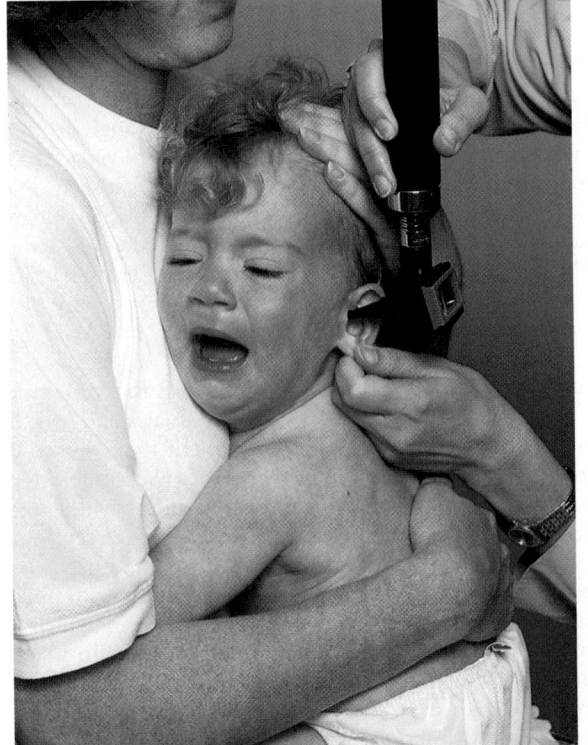

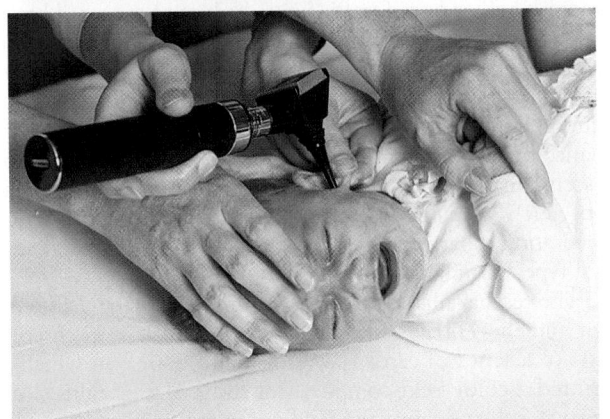

FIG. 7-17 ■ Position for restraining child, **A,** and infant, **B,** during otoscopic examination.

cooperative child, hold the handle with the otic head upright or upside down. Use the dominant hand to examine both ears or reverse hands for each ear, whichever is more comfortable.

Before using the otoscope, visualize the external ear and the tympanic membrane as being superimposed on a clock (Fig. 7-19). The numbers become important geographic landmarks. Introduce the speculum into the meatus between the 3 and 9 o'clock positions in a *downward* and *forward* position. Because the canal is curved, the speculum does not permit a panoramic view of the tympanic membrane unless the canal is straightened. In infants the canal curves upward. Therefore, pull the pinna *down* and *back* to the 6 to 9 o'clock range to straighten the canal (Fig. 7-20, *A*).

With older children, usually those older than 3 years of age, the canal curves downward and forward. Therefore pull the pinna *up* and *back* toward a 10 o'clock position

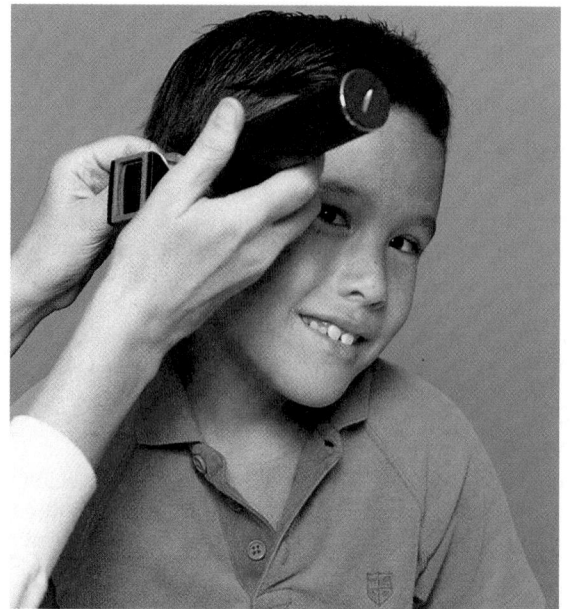

FIG. 7-18 ■ Positioning head by tilting it toward opposite shoulder for full view of tympanic membrane.

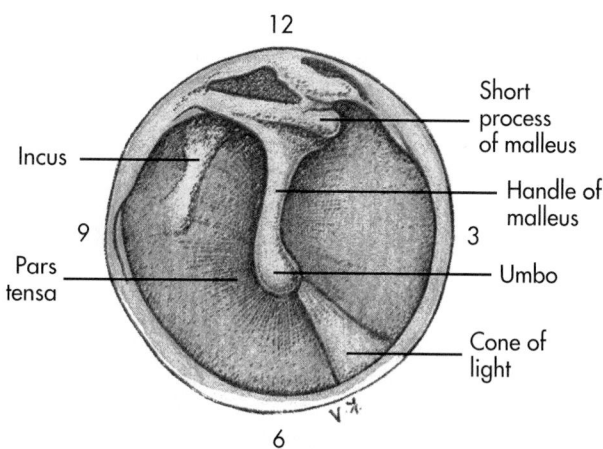

FIG. 7-19 ■ Landmarks of tympanic membrane with "clock" superimposed. (Modified from Potter PA, Perry AG: *Basic nursing: theory and practice,* ed 2, St Louis, 1991, Mosby.)

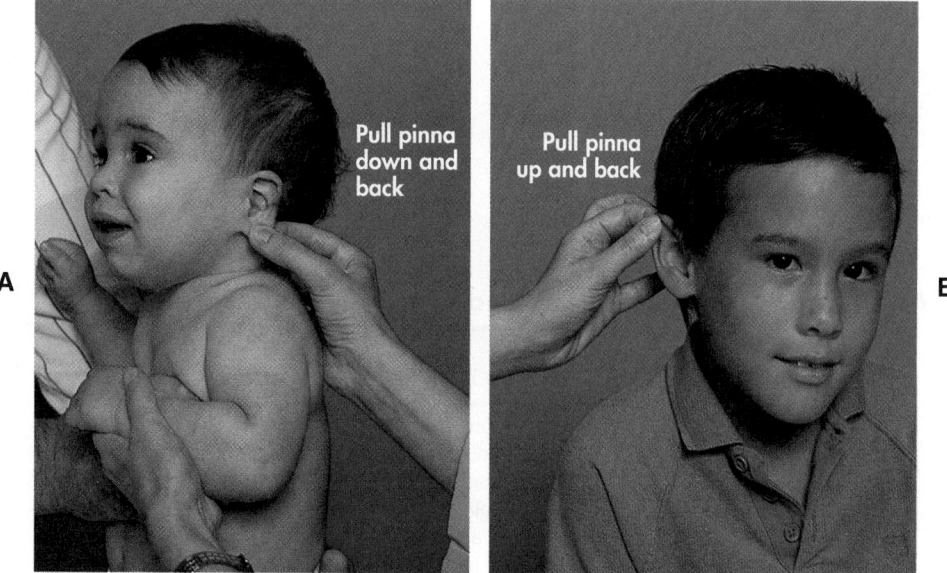

FIG. 7-20 ■ Positioning of eardrum in infant, **A,** and in child older than 3 years of age, **B.**

(Fig. 7-20, *B*). If there is difficulty in visualizing the membrane, try repositioning the head, introducing the speculum at a different angle, and pulling the pinna in a slightly different direction. Do not insert the speculum past the cartilaginous (outermost) portion of the canal, usually a distance of 0.60 to 1.25 cm (¼ to ½ inch) in older children. Insertion of the speculum into the posterior or bony portion of the canal causes pain.

In neonates and young infants the walls of the canal are pliable and floppy because of the underdeveloped cartilaginous and bony structures. Therefore, the very small 2-mm speculum usually needs to be inserted deeper into the canal

than in older children. Great care must be exercised not to damage the walls or drum. For this reason, only an experienced examiner should insert an otoscope into the ears of very young infants.

Otoscopic Examination. As you introduce the speculum into the external canal, inspect the walls of the canal, the color of the tympanic membrane, the light reflex, and the usual landmarks of the bony prominences of the middle ear.

The ***walls*** of the external auditory canal are pink, although they are more pigmented in dark-skinned children. Minute hairs are evident in the outermost portion, where cerumen is produced. Note signs of irritation, foreign bodies, or infection.

Foreign bodies in the ear are not uncommon in children and range from erasers to beans. Symptoms may include pain, discharge, and affected hearing. Soft objects, such as paper or insects, can be removed with forceps. Small, hard objects, such as pebbles, can be removed with a suction tip, a hook, or irrigation. However, irrigation is contraindicated if the object is vegetative matter, such as beans or pasta, which swells when in contact with fluid.

> **! NURSING ALERT**
>
> If there is any doubt about the type of object in the ear and the appropriate method to remove it, refer the child to the appropriate practitioner.

The *color* of the *tympanic membrane* is a translucent, light pearly pink or gray. Note marked erythema (which may indicate suppurative otitis media), a dull nontransparent grayish color (sometimes suggestive of serous otitis media), or ashen gray areas (signs of scarring from a previous perforation). A black area usually suggests a perforation of the membrane that has not healed.

The characteristic tenseness and slope of the tympanic membrane cause the light of the otoscope to reflect at about the 5 or 7 o'clock position. The *light reflex* is a fairly well defined cone-shaped reflection, which normally points away from the face.

The *bony landmarks* of the drum are formed by the *umbo,* or tip of the malleus bone. It appears as a small, round, opaque concave spot near the center of the drum. The *manubrium* (long process or handle) of the malleus appears to be a whitish line extending from the umbo upward to the margin of the membrane. At the upper end of the long process near the 1 o'clock position (in the right ear) is a sharp, knoblike protuberance, representing the *short process* of the malleus. Note the absence of the light reflex or loss or abnormal prominence of any of these landmarks.

Auditory Testing

Several types of hearing tests are available (Table 7-10). The nurse must operate under a high index of suspicion for those children who may have conditions associated with hearing loss and who may have developed behaviors that indicate auditory impairment (Cunningham and Cox, 2003). Types of hearing loss, causes, clinical manifestations, and appropriate treatment are discussed in Chapter 19.

NOSE
Inspection of External Structures

The nose is located in the middle of the face just below the eyes and above the lips. Compare its placement and alignment by drawing an imaginary vertical line from the center point between the eyes down to the notch of the upper lip. The nose should lie exactly vertical to this line, with each side exactly symmetric. Note its location, any deviation to one side, and asymmetry in overall size and in diameter of the nares (nostrils). The *bridge* of the nose is sometimes flat in Asian and black children. Observe the *alae nasi* for any sign of flaring, which indicates respiratory difficulty. Always report any flaring of the alae nasi. Fig. 7-21 illustrates the usual landmarks used in describing the external structures of the nose.

Inspection of Internal Structures

Inspect the *anterior vestibule* of the nose by pushing the tip upward, tilting the head backward, and illuminating the cavity with a flashlight or otoscope without the attached ear speculum.

TABLE 7-10 ■ Audiologic Tests for Infants and Children

AGE OF CHILD	AUDITORY TEST/ AVERAGE TIME	TYPE OF MEASUREMENT	PROCEDURE
All ages	Evoked otoacoustic emissions, 10-min test	Physiologic test specifically measuring cochlear (outer hair cell) response to presentation of a stimulus	Small probe containing a sensitive microphone is placed in the ear canal for stimulus delivery and response detection
Birth to 9 mo	Auditory Brain Stem Response, 15-min test	Electrophysiologic measurement of activity in auditory nerve and brainstem pathways	Placement of electrodes on child's head detects auditory stimuli presented though earphones one ear at a time
9 mo to 2.5 yr	Conditioned oriented responses or visual reinforced audiometry, 30-min test	Behavioral tests measuring responses of the child to speech and frequency-specific stimuli presented through speakers	Both techniques condition the child to associate speech or frequency-specific sound with a reinforcement stimulus, such as a lighted toy
2.5 yr to 4 yr	Play audiometry, 30-min test	Behavioral test measuring auditory thresholds in response to speech and frequency-specific stimuli presented through earphones and/or bone vibrator	Child is conditioned to put a peg in a peg board or drop a block in a box when stimulus tone is heard
4 yr to adolescence	Conventional audiometry, 30-min test	Behavioral test measuring auditory thresholds in response to speech and frequency-specific stimuli presented through earphone and/or bone vibrator	Patient is instructed to raise his or her hand when stimulus is heard

Adapted with permission from Bachmann KR, Arvedson JC: Early identification and intervention for children who are hearing impaired, *Pediatr Rev* 19:155-165, 1998.

Note the *color* of the *mucosal lining,* which is normally redder than the oral membranes, as well as any swelling, discharge, dryness, or bleeding. There should be no discharge from the nose.

On looking deeper into the nose, inspect the *turbinates* or *concha,* plates of bone that jut into the nasal cavity and are enveloped by mucous membrane. The turbinates greatly increase the surface area of the nasal cavity as air is inhaled. The spaces or channels between the turbinates are called *meatus* and correspond to each of the three turbinates. Normally the front end of the inferior and middle turbinate and the middle meatus are seen. They should be the same color as the lining of the vestibule.

Inspect the *septum,* which should divide the vestibules equally. Note any deviation, especially if it causes an occlusion of one side of the nose. A perforation may be evident within the septum. If this is suspected, shine the light of the otoscope into one naris and look for admittance of light. Because olfaction is an important function of the nose, testing for smell may be done at this point or as part of cranial nerve assessment (see Table 7-11).

MOUTH AND THROAT

With a cooperative child, almost the entire examination of the mouth and throat can be accomplished without the use of a tongue blade. Ask the child to open the mouth wide, to move the tongue in different directions for full visualization, and to say "ahh," which depresses the tongue for full view of the back of the mouth (tonsils, uvula, and oropharynx). For a closer look at the buccal mucosa, or lining of the cheeks, ask children to use their fingers to move the outer lip and cheek to one side (see Atraumatic Care box).

Infants and toddlers, however, usually resist attempts to keep the mouth open. Because inspecting the mouth is an upsetting part of the examination, leave it for the end of the physical examination (along with examination of the ears) or do it during episodes of crying. However, the use of a tongue blade (preferably flavored) to depress the tongue is necessary. Place the tongue blade along the *side* of the tongue, not in the center back area where the gag reflex is

elicited. Fig. 7-22, *B,* illustrates proper positioning of the child for the oral examination.

The major structure of the exterior of the mouth is the *lips.* The lips should be moist, soft, smooth, and pink, the color of a deeper hue than the surrounding skin. The lips should be symmetric when relaxed or tensed. Assess symmetry when the child talks or cries.

Inspection of Internal Structures

The major structures that are visible within the oral cavity and oropharynx are the mucosal lining of the lips and cheeks, gums or gingiva, teeth, tongue, palate, uvula, ton-

ATRAUMATIC CARE

Encouraging Opening the Mouth for Examination

Perform the examination in front of a mirror.

Let child first examine someone else's mouth, such as the parent, the nurse, or a puppet (Fig. 7-22, *A*), and then examine child's mouth.

Instruct child to tilt the head back slightly, breathe deeply through the mouth, and hold the breath; this action lowers the tongue to the floor of the mouth without the use of a tongue blade.

Lightly brushing the palate with a cotton swab also may open the mouth for assessment.

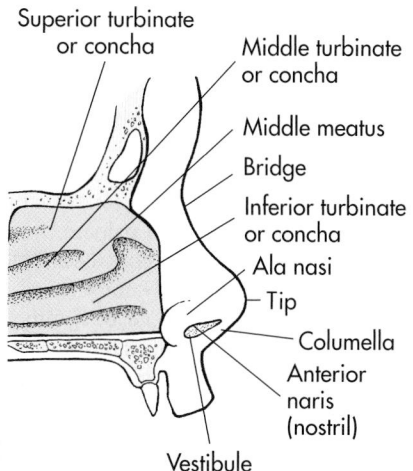

Superior turbinate or concha
Middle turbinate or concha
Middle meatus
Bridge
Inferior turbinate or concha
Ala nasi
Tip
Columella
Anterior naris (nostril)
Vestibule

FIG. 7-21 ■ External landmarks and internal structures of nose.

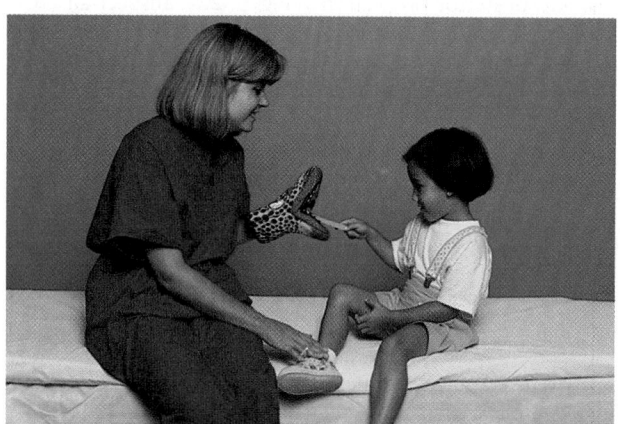

A

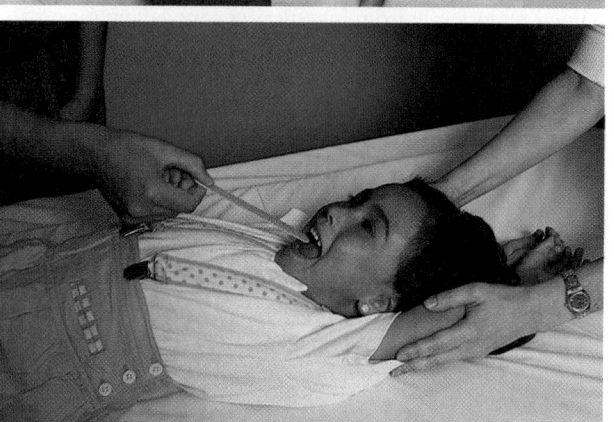

B

FIG. 7-22 ■ **A,** Encouraging child to cooperate. **B,** Positioning child for examination of mouth.

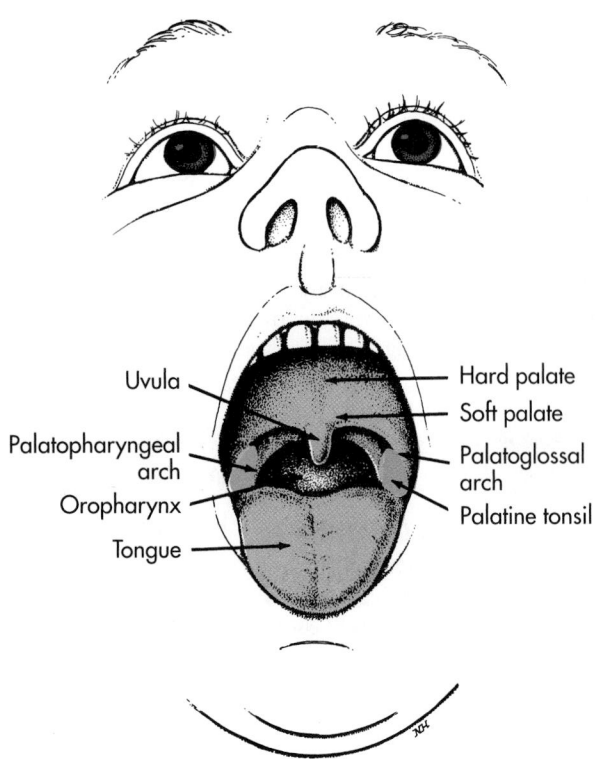

FIG. 7-23 ■ Interior structures of mouth.

Labels: Uvula, Palatopharyngeal arch, Oropharynx, Tongue, Hard palate, Soft palate, Palatoglossal arch, Palatine tonsil

sils, and posterior oropharynx (Fig. 7-23). Inspect all areas lined with *mucous membranes* (inside the lips and cheeks, gingiva, underside of the tongue, palate, and back of the pharynx) for color, any areas of white patches or ulceration, bleeding, sensitivity, and moisture. The membranes should be bright pink, smooth, glistening, uniform, and moist.

Inspect the *teeth* for number in each dental arch, for hygiene, and for occlusion or bite (see also Teething, Chapter 10. Discoloration of tooth enamel with obvious plaque (whitish coating on the surface of the teeth) is a sign of poor dental hygiene and indicates a need for counseling. Brown spots in the crevices of the crown of the tooth or between the teeth may be caries (cavities). Chalky white to yellow or brown areas on the enamel may indicate fluorosis (excessive fluoride ingestion). Teeth that appear greenish black may be stained temporarily from ingestion of supplemental iron.

Examine the *gums (gingiva)* surrounding the teeth. The color is normally coral pink, and the surface texture is stippled, similar to the appearance of orange peel. In dark-skinned children, the gums are more deeply colored, and a brownish area is often observed along the gum line.

Inspect the *tongue* for the presence of papillae, small projections that contain several taste buds and give the tongue its characteristic rough appearance. Note the size and mobility of the tongue. Normally the tip of the tongue should extend to the lips or beyond.

The roof of the mouth consists of the *hard palate,* which is located near the front of the oral cavity, and the *soft palate,* which is located toward the back of the pharynx and which has a small midline protrusion called the *uvula.* Carefully inspect the palates to be sure that they are intact. The arch of the palate should be dome shaped. A narrow, flat roof or a high, arched palate affects the placement of the tongue and

can cause feeding and speech problems. Test movement of the uvula by eliciting a gag reflex. It should move upward to close off the nasopharynx from the oropharynx.

Examine the oropharynx and note the size and color of the *palatine tonsils.* They are normally the same color as the surrounding mucosa; glandular, rather than smooth in appearance; and barely visible over the edge of the palatoglossal arches. The size of the tonsils varies considerably during childhood. However, report any swelling, redness, or white areas on the tonsils.

CHEST

Inspect the *chest* for size, shape, symmetry, movement, breast development, and the presence of the bony landmarks formed by the ribs and sternum. The *rib cage* consists of 12 ribs and the sternum, or breast bone, located in the midline of the trunk (Fig. 7-24). The *sternum* is composed of three main parts. The *manubrium,* the uppermost portion, can be felt at the base of the neck at the *suprasternal notch.* The largest segment of the sternum is the *body,* which forms the *sternal angle (angle of Louis)* as it articulates with the manubrium. At the end of the body is a small, movable process called the *xiphoid.* The angle of the costal margin as it attaches to the sternum is called the *costal angle* and is normally about 45 to 50 degrees. These bony structures are important landmarks in the location of ribs and intercostal spaces.

Intercostal spaces (ICS) are the spaces between the ribs. They are numbered according to the rib directly above the space. For example, the space immediately below the second rib is the second intercostal space.

The *thoracic cavity* is also divided into segments by drawing imaginary lines on the chest and back. Fig. 7-25 illustrates the anterior, lateral, and posterior divisions.

Measure the *size* of the chest by placing the measuring tape around the rib cage at the nipple line (see Fig. 7-4). For greatest accuracy, take two measurements—one during inspiration and the other during expiration, and record the average. Chest size is important, mainly in comparison with its relationship to head circumference, which is discussed on p. 139. Always report marked disproportions because most are caused by abnormal head growth, although some may be a result of altered chest shape, such as *barrel chest* (chest is round) or *pigeon chest* (sternum protrudes outward).

During infancy the *shape* of the chest is almost circular, with the anteroposterior (front-to-back) diameter equaling the transverse, or lateral (side-to-side), diameter. As the child grows, the chest normally increases in the transverse direction, causing the anteroposterior diameter to be less than the lateral diameter. Note the *angle* made by the lower costal margin and the sternum, and palpate the junction of the ribs with the costal cartilage (costochondral junction) and sternum, which should be fairly smooth.

Movement of the chest wall should be symmetric bilaterally and coordinated with breathing. During inspiration the chest rises and expands, the diaphragm descends, and the costal angle increases. During expiration the chest falls and decreases in size, the diaphragm rises, and the costal angle narrows (Fig. 7-26). In children younger than 6 or 7 years of age, respiratory movement is principally abdominal or diaphragmatic. In older children, particularly girls, respirations are chiefly thoracic. In either type, the chest and abdomen

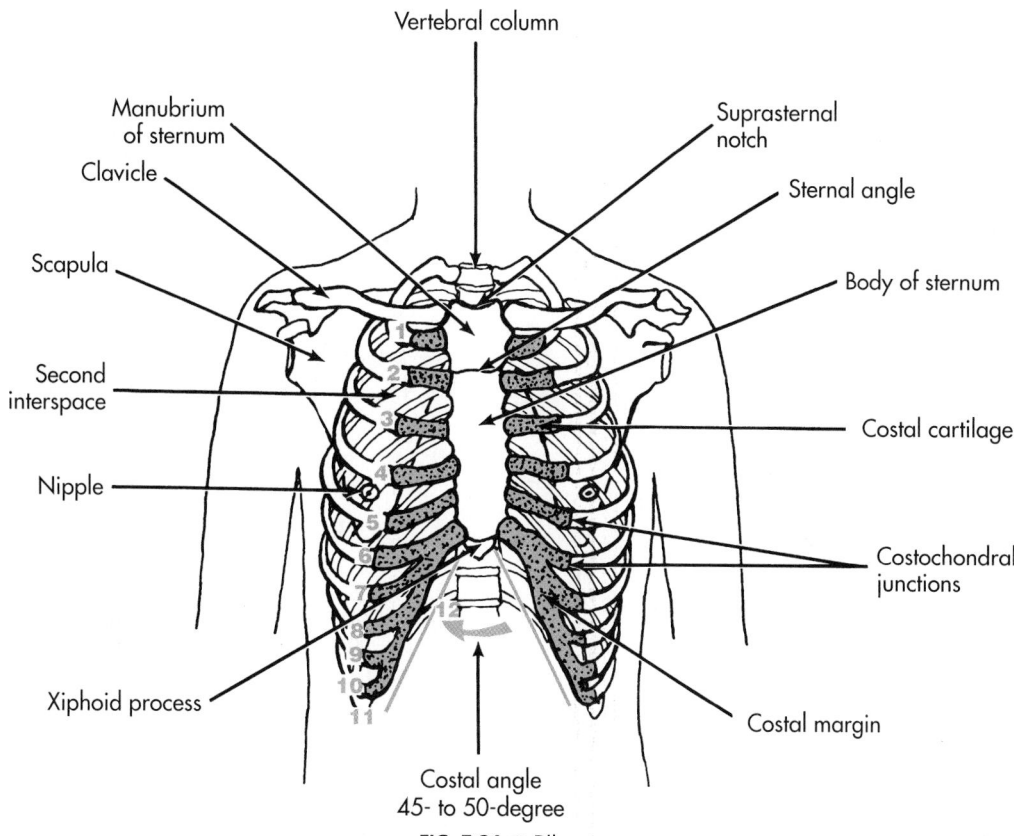

Vertebral column

Manubrium
of sternum

Clavicle

Scapula

Second
interspace

Nipple

Xiphoid process

Suprasternal
notch

Sternal angle

Body of sternum

Costal cartilage

Costochondral
junctions

Costal margin

Costal angle
45- to 50-degree

FIG. 7-24 ■ Rib cage.

should rise and fall together. Always report any asymmetry of movement.

While inspecting the skin surface of the chest, observe the position of the *nipples,* as well as any evidence of *breast development.* Normally the nipples are located slightly lateral to the midclavicular line between the fourth and fifth ribs. Note symmetry of nipple placement and normal configuration of a darker pigmented areola surrounding a flat nipple in the prepubertal child.

Pubertal breast development usually begins in girls between 10 and 14 years of age (see Chapter 16). Record early (precocious) or delayed breast development, as well as evidence of any other secondary sexual characteristics. In males *breast enlargement (gynecomastia)* may be caused by hormonal or systemic disorders, but more commonly it is a result of adipose tissue from obesity or a transitory body change during early puberty. In either situation investigate the child's feelings regarding breast enlargement.

In adolescent females who have achieved sexual maturity, palpate the breasts for evidence of any masses or hard nodules. Use this opportunity to discuss the importance of routine self-breast examination. Emphasize that most palpable masses are benign to decrease any fear or concern that results when a mass is felt.

LUNGS

The *lungs* are situated inside the thoracic cavity, with one lung on each side of the sternum. Each lung is divided into an *apex,* which is slightly pointed and rises above the first rib; a *base,* which is wide and concave and rides on the dome-shaped diaphragm; and a body, which is divided into *lobes.*

The right lung has three lobes: the upper, middle, and lower. The left lung has only two lobes, the upper and lower, because of the space occupied by the heart (Fig. 7-27).

Inspection of the lungs primarily involves observation of respiratory movements, which are discussed previously. Evaluate respirations for rate (number per minute), rhythm (regular, irregular, or periodic), depth (deep or shallow), and quality (effortless, automatic, difficult, or labored). Note the character of breath sounds, such as noisy, grunting, snoring, or heavy.

Evaluate respiratory movements by placing each hand flat against the back or chest with the thumbs in midline along the lower costal margin of the lungs. The child should be sitting during this procedure and, if cooperative, should take several deep breaths. During respiration your hands will move with the chest wall. Assess the amount and speed of respiratory excursion and note any asymmetry of movement.

Experienced examiners may percuss the lungs. The anterior lung is percussed from apex to base, usually with the child in the supine or sitting position. Each side of the chest is percussed in sequence to compare the sounds. When the posterior lung is percussed, the procedure and sequence are the same, although the child should be sitting. Resonance is heard over all the lobes of the lungs that are not adjacent to other organs. Any deviation from the expected sound is recorded and reported.

Auscultation

Auscultation involves using the stethoscope to evaluate breath sounds (see Guidelines box). Breath sounds are best heard if the child inspires deeply (see Atraumatic Care box).

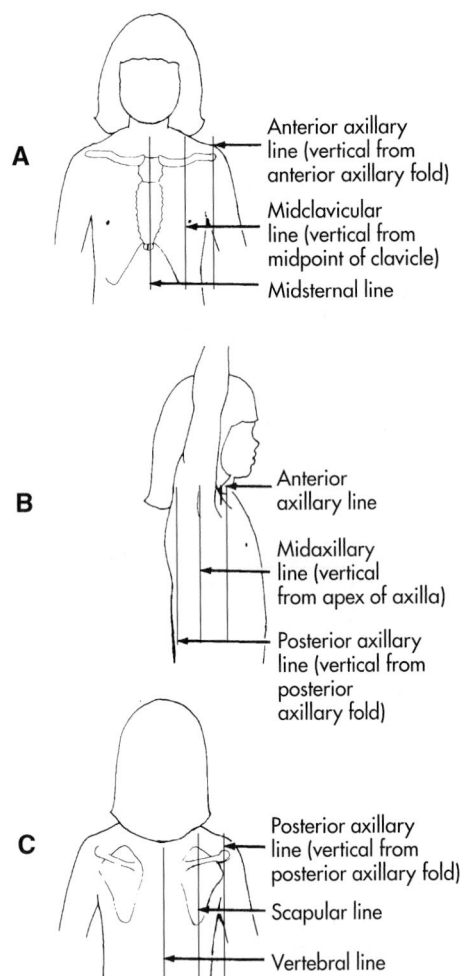

FIG. 7-25 ■ Imaginary landmarks of chest. **A,** Anterior. **B,** Right lateral. **C,** Posterior.

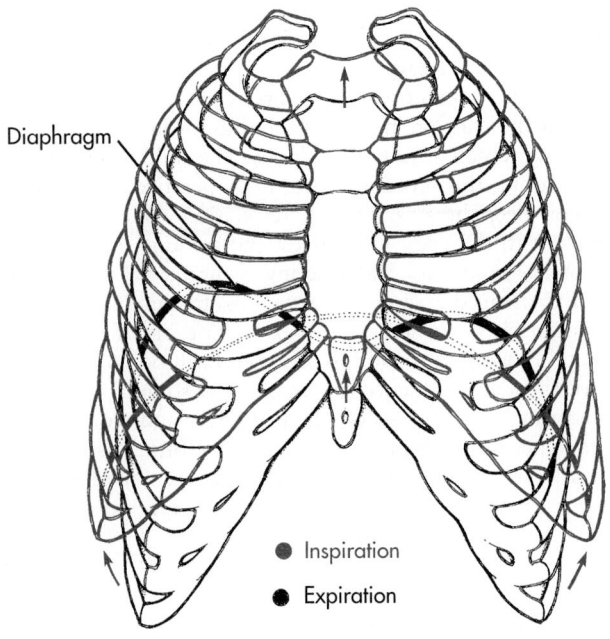

FIG. 7-26 ■ Movement of chest during respiration.

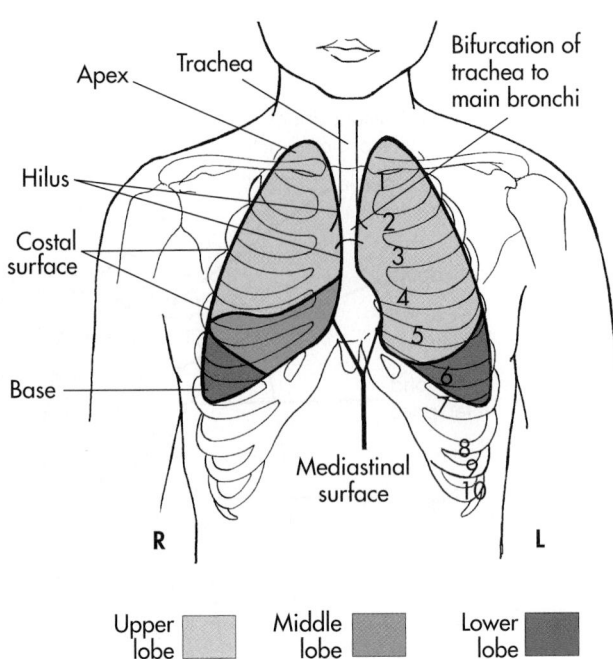

FIG. 7-27 ■ Location of lobes of lungs within thoracic cavity.

In the lungs breath sounds are classified as vesicular, bronchovesicular, or bronchial (Box 7-3).

Absent or *diminished breath sounds* are always an abnormal finding warranting investigation. Fluid, air, or solid masses in the pleural space all interfere with the conduction of breath sounds. Diminished breath sounds in certain segments of the lung can alert the nurse to pulmonary areas that may benefit from chest physiotherapy. Increased breath sounds following pulmonary therapy indicate improved passage of air through the respiratory tract. Terms used to describe various respiration patterns are found in Box 7-4.

Various pulmonary abnormalities produce *adventitious sounds* that are not normally heard over the chest. These sounds occur in addition to normal or abnormal breath sounds. They are classified into two main groups: *crackles,* which result from the passage of air through fluid or moisture, and *wheezes,* which are produced as air passes through narrowed passageways, regardless of the cause, such as exudate, inflammation, spasm, or tumor. Considerable practice with an experienced tutor is necessary to differentiate the various types of lung sounds. Often it is best to describe the type of sound heard in the lungs rather than trying to label it. Always report any abnormal sounds for further medical evaluation.

HEART

The heart is situated in the thoracic cavity between the lungs in the mediastinum and above the diaphragm (Fig. 7-28). About two thirds of the heart lies within the left side of the rib cage, with the other third on the right side as it crosses the sternum. The heart is positioned in the thorax like a trapezoid:

Vertically along the right sternal border (RSB) from the second to the fifth rib
Horizontally (long side) from the lower right sternum to the fifth rib at the left midclavicular line (LMCL)

GUIDELINES

Effective Auscultation

Make sure child is relaxed and not crying, talking, or laughing. Record if child is crying.

Check that room is comfortable and quiet.

Warm stethoscope before placing it against skin.

Apply firm pressure on chestpiece but not enough to prevent vibrations and transmission of sound.

Avoid placing stethoscope over hair or clothing, moving it against skin, breathing on tubing, or sliding fingers over chestpiece, which may cause sounds that falsely resemble pathologic findings.

Use a symmetric and orderly approach to compare sounds.

ATRAUMATIC CARE

Encouraging Deep Breaths

Ask child to "blow out" the light on an otoscope or pocket flashlight; discreetly turn off the light on the last try so that the child feels successful.

Place a cotton ball in child's palm; ask child to blow the ball into the air and have parent catch it.

Place a small tissue on the top of a pencil and ask child to blow the tissue off.

Have child blow a pinwheel, a party horn, or bubbles.

BOX 7-3 ■ Classification of Normal Breath Sounds

VESICULAR BREATH SOUNDS
Heard over entire surface of lungs, with exception of upper intrascapular area and area beneath manubrium.
Inspiration is louder, longer, and higher pitched than expiration.
Sound is soft, swishing noise.

BRONCHOVESICULAR BREATH SOUNDS
Heard over manubrium and in upper intrascapular regions where trachea and bronchi bifurcate.
Inspiration is louder and higher in pitch than in vesicular breathing.

BRONCHIAL BREATH SOUNDS
Heard only over trachea near suprasternal notch.
Inspiratory phase is short, and expiratory phase is long.

BOX 7-4 ■ Various Patterns of Respiration

Tachypnea—Increased rate
Bradypnea—Decreased rate
Dyspnea—Distress during breathing
Apnea—Cessation of breathing
Hyperpnea—Increased depth
Hypoventilation—Decreased depth (shallow) and irregular rhythm
Hyperventilation—Increased rate and depth
Kussmaul breathing—Hyperventilation, grasping and labored respiration, usually seen in diabetic coma or other states of respiratory acidosis
Cheyne-Stokes respirations—Gradually increasing rate and depth with periods of apnea
Biot breathing—Periods of hyperpnea alternating with apnea (similar to Cheyne-Stokes except that depth remains constant)
Seesaw (paradoxic) respirations—Chest falls on inspiration and rises on expiration
Agonal—Last gasping breaths before death

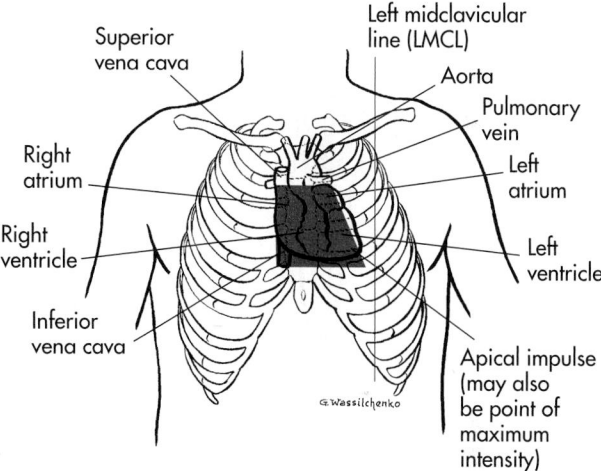

FIG. 7-28 ■ Position of heart within thorax.

Diagonally from the left sternal border (LSB) at the second rib to the LMCL at the fifth rib
Horizontally (short side) from the RSB and LSB at the second ICS—base of the heart

Inspection is best done with the child sitting in a semi-Fowler position. Look at the anterior chest wall from an angle, comparing both sides of the rib cage with each other. Normally they should be symmetric. In children with thin chest walls, a pulsation may be visible. Because comprehensive evaluation of cardiac function is not limited to the heart, also consider other findings such as the presence of all pulses (especially the femoral pulses) (Fig. 7-29), distended neck

veins, clubbing of the fingers, peripheral cyanosis, edema, blood pressure, and respiratory status.

Use palpation to determine the location of the *apical impulse (AI)*, the most lateral cardiac impulse that may correspond to the apex. The AI is found:

- Just lateral to the left MCL and fourth ICS in children >7 years of age
- At the left MCL and fifth ICS in children <7 years of age

Although the AI gives a general idea of the size of the heart (with enlargement, the apex is lower and more lateral), its normal location is quite variable, making it a rather unreliable indicator of heart size.

The *point of maximum intensity (PMI),* as the name implies, is the area of most intense pulsation. Usually the PMI is located at the same site as the AI, but it can occur elsewhere. For this reason, the two terms should not be used synonymously.

Assess *capillary filling time,* an important test for peripheral circulation, by pressing the skin lightly on a central

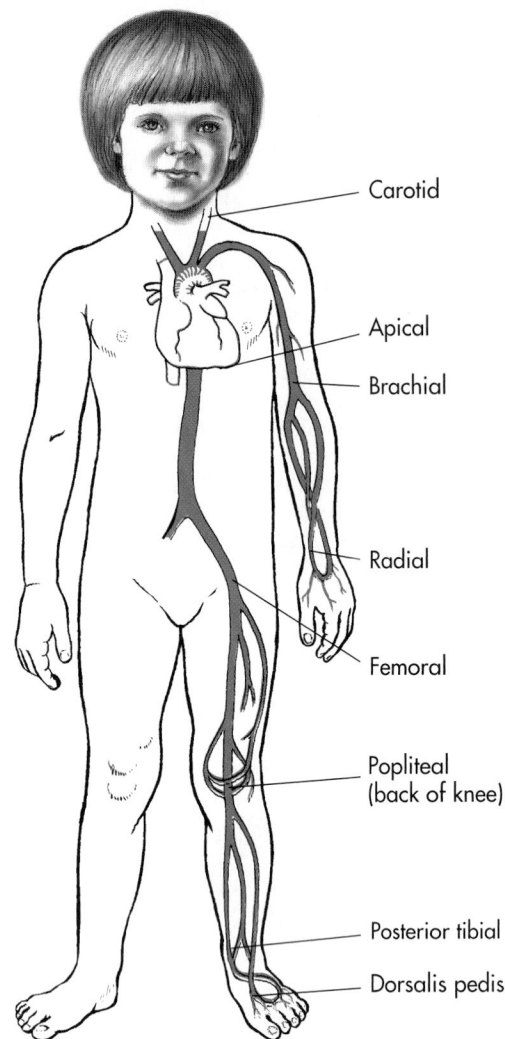

FIG. 7-29 ■ Location of pulses.

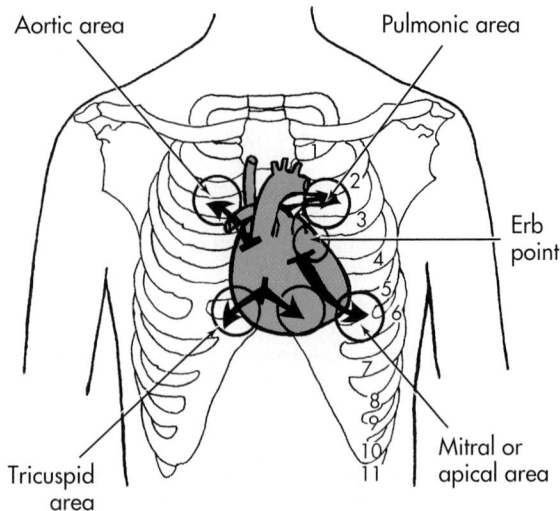

FIG. 7-30 ■ Direction of heart sounds for anatomic valve sites and areas (circled) for auscultation.

site, such as the forehead, or a peripheral site, such as the top of the hand, to produce a slight blanching. The time it takes for the blanched area to return to its original color is the *capillary refill time.*

> **⚠ NURSING ALERT**
>
> Capillary refill should be brisk—in less than 2 seconds; prolonged refill may be associated with poor systemic perfusion, as well as a cool ambient temperature.

Auscultation

Origin of Heart Sounds. The heart sounds are produced by the opening and closing of the valves and the vibration of blood against the walls of the heart and vessels. Normally two sounds—S_1 and S_2—are heard, which correspond respectively to the familiar "lub dub" often used to describe the sounds. S_1 is caused by closure of the *tricuspid* and *mitral valves* (sometimes called the *atrioventricular valves*). S_2 is the result of closure of the *pulmonic* and *aortic valves* (sometimes called *semilunar valves*). Normally the split of the two sounds in S_2 is distinguishable and widens during inspiration. *Physiologic splitting* is a significant normal finding.

> **⚠ NURSING ALERT**
>
> "Fixed splitting," in which the split in S_2 does not change during inspiration, is an important diagnostic sign of atrial septal defect.

Two other heart sounds—S_3 and S_4—may be produced. S_3 is normally heard in some children; S_4 is rarely heard as a normal heart sound; if heard, it usually indicates the need for further cardiac evaluation.

Another important category of heart sounds is *murmurs,* sounds that are produced by vibrations within the heart chambers or in the major arteries from the back-and-forth flow of blood. The description and classification of murmurs are skills that require considerable practice and training. Consult with an experienced practitioner whenever a murmur is identified or suspected.

Differentiating normal heart sounds. Fig. 7-30 illustrates the approximate anatomic position of the valves within the heart chambers. Note that the anatomic location of valves does not correspond to the area where the sounds are heard best. The auscultatory sites are located in the direction of the blood flow through the valves.

Normally S_1 is louder at the apex of the heart in the mitral and tricuspid area, and S_2 is louder near the base of the heart in the pulmonic and aortic area. Listen to each sound by inching down the chest. The following areas should also be auscultated for sounds, such as murmurs, which may radiate to these sites: sternoclavicular area above the clavicles and manubrium, area along the sternal border, area along the left midaxillary line, and area below the scapulae.

> **NURSING TIP**
>
> To distinguish between S_1 or S_2 heart sounds, simultaneously palpate the carotid pulse with the index and middle finger and listen to the heart sounds; S_1 is synchronous with the carotid pulse.

Auscultate the heart with the child in at least two positions: sitting and reclining. If adventitious sounds are de-

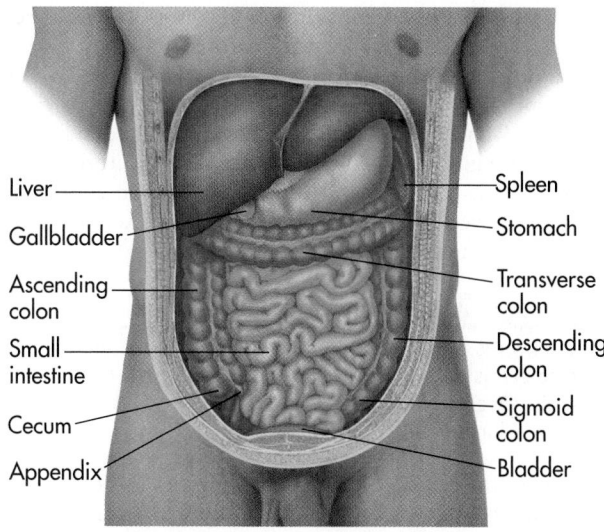

FIG. 7-31 ■ Location of structures in abdomen. (From Seidel HM, Ball JW, Dains JE, Benedict GW: *Mosby's guide to physical examination,* ed 5, St Louis, 2003, Mosby.)

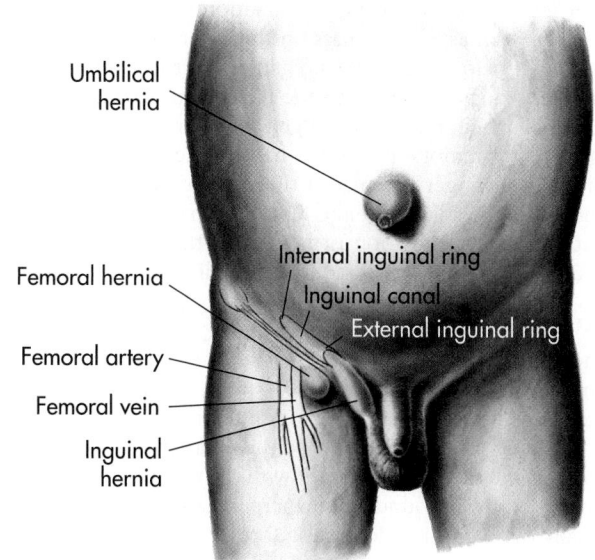

FIG. 7-32 ■ Location of hernias.

tected, further evaluate them with the child standing, sitting and leaning forward, and lying on the left side. For example, atrial sounds such as S_4 are heard best with the person in a recumbent position and usually fade if the person sits or stands.

Evaluate heart sounds for (1) *quality* (should be clear and distinct, not muffled, diffuse, or distant); (2) *intensity,* especially in relation to the location or auscultatory site (should not be weak or pounding); (3) *rate* (should be the same as the radial pulse); and (4) *rhythm* (should be regular and even). A particular arrhythmia that occurs normally in many children is *sinus arrhythmia,* in which the heart rate increases with inspiration and decreases with expiration. Differentiate this rhythm from a truly abnormal arrhythmia by having children hold their breath. In sinus arrhythmia, cessation of breathing causes the heart rate to remain steady.

ABDOMEN

Examination of the abdomen involves inspection, followed by auscultation and then palpation. Perform palpation last because it may distort the normal abdominal sounds. Knowledge of the anatomic placement of the abdominal organs is essential to differentiate normal, expected findings from abnormal ones (Fig. 7-31).

For descriptive purposes the abdominal cavity is divided into four quadrants by drawing a vertical line midway from the sternum to the pubic symphysis and a horizontal line across the abdomen through the umbilicus. Each section is named as follows:

■ Left upper quadrant
■ Left lower quadrant
■ Right upper quadrant
■ Right lower quadrant

Inspection

Inspect the *contour* of the abdomen with the child erect and supine. Normally the abdomen of infants and young children is quite cylindric and, in the erect position, fairly prominent because of the physiologic lordosis of the spine. In the supine position the abdomen appears flat. A midline protrusion

from the xiphoid to the umbilicus or pubic symphysis is usually *diastasis recti,* or failure of the rectus abdominis muscles to join in utero. In a healthy child a midline protrusion is usually a variation of normal muscular development.

> **❗ NURSING ALERT**
>
> A tense, boardlike abdomen is a serious sign of paralytic ileus and intestinal obstruction.

The *skin* covering the abdomen should be uniformly taut, without wrinkles or creases. Sometimes silvery, whitish striae ("stretch marks") are seen, especially if the skin has been stretched as in obesity. Superficial veins are usually visible in light-skinned, thin infants, but distended veins are an abnormal finding.

Observe *movement* of the abdomen. Normally chest and abdominal movements are synchronous. In infants and thin children *peristaltic waves* may be visible through the abdominal wall; they are best observed by standing at eye level to and across from the abdomen. Always report this finding.

Examine the *umbilicus* for size, hygiene, and evidence of any abnormalities, such as hernias. The umbilicus should be flat or only slightly protruding. If a herniation is present, palpate the sac for abdominal contents and estimate the approximate size of the opening. *Umbilical hernias* are common in infants, especially in black children.

Hernias may exist elsewhere on the abdominal wall (Fig. 7-32). An *inguinal hernia* is a protrusion of peritoneum through the abdominal wall in the inguinal canal. It occurs mostly in males, is frequently bilateral, and may be visible as a mass in the scrotum. To locate a hernia, slide the little finger into the external inguinal ring at the base of the scrotum and ask the child to cough. If a hernia is present, it will hit the tip of the finger.

> **NURSING TIP**
>
> If the child is too young to cough, have the child blow up a balloon or laugh to raise the intraabdominal pressure sufficiently to demonstrate the presence of an inguinal hernia.

A *femoral hernia,* which occurs more frequently in girls, is felt or seen as a small mass on the anterior surface of the thigh just below the inguinal ligament in the femoral canal (a potential space medial to the femoral artery). Feel for a hernia by placing the index finger of your right hand on the child's right femoral pulse (left hand for left pulse) and the middle ring finger flat against the skin toward the midline. The ring finger lies over the femoral canal, where the herniation occurs. Palpation of hernias in the pelvic region is often part of the examination of genitalia.

Auscultation

The most important finding to listen for is *peristalsis,* or *bowel sounds,* which sound like short metallic clicks and gurgles. Their frequency per minute should be recorded (e.g., 5 sounds/min). Bowel sounds may be stimulated by stroking the abdominal surface with a fingernail. Report absence of bowel sounds or hyperperistalsis because either usually denotes an abdominal disorder.

Palpation

Two types of palpation are performed: superficial and deep. In *superficial palpation,* lightly place your hand against the skin and feel each quadrant, noting any areas of tenderness, muscle tone, and superficial lesions, such as cysts. Because superficial palpation is often perceived as tickling, several techniques can be used to minimize this sensation and provide relaxation (see Atraumatic Care box). Admonishing the child to stop laughing only draws attention to the sensation and decreases cooperation.

Deep palpation is used for palpating organs and large blood vessels and for detecting masses and tenderness that were not discovered during superficial palpation. Palpation usually begins in the lower quadrants and proceeds upward to avoid missing the edge of an enlarged liver or spleen. Except for palpating the liver, successful identification of other organs, such as the spleen, kidney, and part of the colon, requires considerable practice with tutored supervision. Report any questionable mass. The lower edge of the *liver* is sometimes felt in infants and young children as a superficial mass 1 to 2 cm (0.4 to 0.8 inch) below the right costal margin (the distance is sometimes measured in fingerbreadths). Normally, the liver descends during inspiration as the diaphragm moves downward. Do not mistake this downward displacement as a sign of liver enlargement.

> ! **NURSING ALERT**
>
> If the liver is palpable 3 cm below the right costal margin or the spleen is palpable more than 2 cm below the left costal margin, these organs are enlarged—a finding that is always reported for further medical investigation.

Palpate the *femoral pulses* by placing the tips of two or three fingers (index, middle, or ring) along the inguinal ligament about midway between the iliac crest and pubic symphysis. Feel both pulses simultaneously to make certain that they are equal and strong (Fig. 7-33).

> ! **NURSING ALERT**
>
> Absence of femoral pulses is a significant sign of coarctation of the aorta and is referred for medical evaluation.

GENITALIA

Examination of genitalia conveniently follows assessment of the abdomen while the child is still supine. In adolescents inspection of the genitalia may be left to the end of the examination. The best approach is to examine the genitalia matter-of-factly, placing no more emphasis on this part of the assessment than on any other segment. It helps to relieve children's and parents' anxiety by telling them the results of the findings; for example, the nurse might say, "Everything looks fine here."

If it is necessary to ask questions, such as about discharge or difficulty in urinating, respect the child's privacy by covering the lower abdomen with the gown or underpants. To prevent embarrassing interruptions, keep the door or curtain closed and post a "do not disturb" sign. Have a drape ready to cover the genitalia if someone enters the room.

🖐 ATRAUMATIC CARE

Promoting Relaxation During Abdominal Palpation

Position child comfortably, such as in a semireclining position in the parent's lap, with knees flexed.

Warm the hands before touching the skin.

Use distraction, such as telling stories or talking to child.

Teach child to use deep breathing and to concentrate on an object.

Give infant a bottle or pacifier.

Begin with light, superficial palpation and gradually progress to deeper palpation.

Palpate any tender or painful areas last.

Have child hold the parent's hand and squeeze it if palpation is uncomfortable.

Use the nonpalpating hand to comfort child, such as placing the free hand on the child's shoulder while palpating the abdomen.

To minimize sensation of tickling during palpation:

Have children "help" with palpation by placing their hand over the palpating hand.

Have them place their hand on the abdomen with the fingers spread wide apart, and palpate between their fingers.

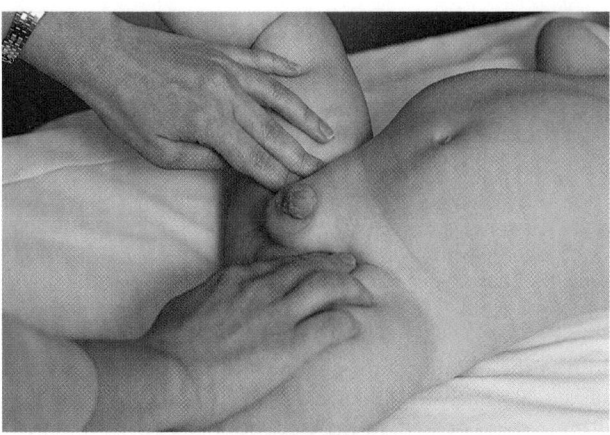

FIG. 7-33 ■ Palpating for femoral pulses.

In examining the genitalia, wear gloves whenever touching body substances. It might be helpful for the adolescent to know that wearing gloves also prevents skin-to-skin contact.

The genital examination is an excellent time for eliciting questions of concern about body functioning or sexual activity. Also use this opportunity to increase or reinforce the child's knowledge of reproductive anatomy by naming each body part and explaining its function. This part of the health assessment is an opportune time to teach self-testicular examination to boys.*

Male Genitalia

Note the external appearance of the glans and shaft of the penis, the prepuce, the urethral meatus, and the scrotum (Fig. 7-34). The *penis* is generally small in infants and young boys until puberty, when it begins to increase in both length and width. In an obese child the penis often looks abnormally small because of the folds of skin partially covering it at the base. Be familiar with normal pubertal growth of the external male genitalia to compare the findings with the expected sequence of maturation (see Chapter 16).

Examine the *glans* (head of the penis) and *shaft* (portion between the perineum and prepuce) for signs of swelling, skin lesions, inflammation, or other irregularities. Any of these signs may indicate underlying disorders, especially sexually transmitted diseases.

The *urethral meatus* is carefully inspected for location and evidence of discharge. Normally it is centered at the tip of the glans.

Hair distribution is also noted. Normally, before puberty, no pubic hair is present. Soft, downy hair at the base of the penis is an early sign of pubertal maturation. In older adolescents hair distribution is diamond-shaped from the umbilicus to the anus.

The location and size of the *scrotum* are noted. The scrota hang freely from the perineum behind the penis, and the left scrotum normally hangs lower than the right. In infants the scrota appear large in relation to the rest of the genitalia. The skin of the scrotum is loose and highly rugated (wrinkled). During early adolescence the skin normally becomes redder and coarser. In dark-skinned children the scrota are usually more deeply pigmented.

Palpation of the scrotum includes identification of the testes, epididymis, and, if present, inguinal hernias. The two *testes* are felt as small ovoid bodies about 1.5 to 2 cm (0.6 to 0.8 inch) long—one in each scrotal sac. They do not enlarge until puberty, when they approximately double in size.

When palpating for the presence of the testes, avoid stimulating the *cremasteric reflex,* which is stimulated by cold, touch, emotional excitement, or exercise. This reflex pulls the testes higher into the pelvic cavity. Several measures are useful in preventing the cremasteric reflex during palpation of the scrotum. First, warm the hands. Second, if the child is old enough, examine him in a tailor or "Indian" position, which stretches the muscle, preventing its contraction (Fig. 7-35, *A*). Third, block the normal pathway of ascent of the testes by placing the thumb and index finger over the upper part of the scrotal sac along the inguinal canal (Fig. 7-35, *B*). If there is any question concerning the existence of two testes, place the index and middle fingers in a scissors fashion to separate the right and left scrotum. If after using these techniques the testes have not been palpated, feel along the inguinal canal and perineum to locate masses that may be undescended testes. Although undescended testes may descend at any time during childhood and are checked at each visit, failure to palpate testes is reported.

*For free information on testicular cancer, contact **Jason A. Struble Memorial Cancer Fund, Inc.,** 624 Kehrs Mill Road, Ballwin, MO 63011.

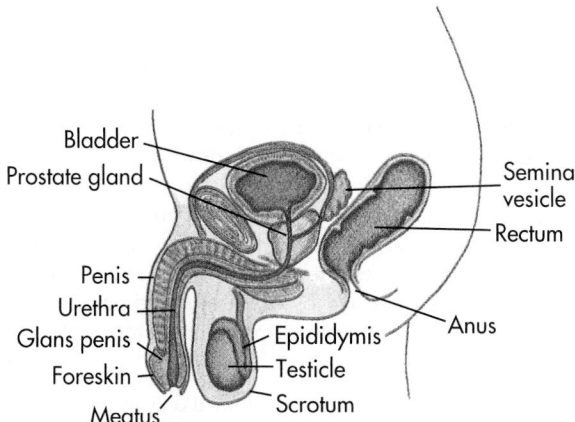

FIG. 7-34 ■ Major structures of genitalia in uncircumcised postpubertal male. (From Potter PA, Perry AG: *Basic nursing: theory and practice,* ed 3, St Louis, 1995, Mosby.)

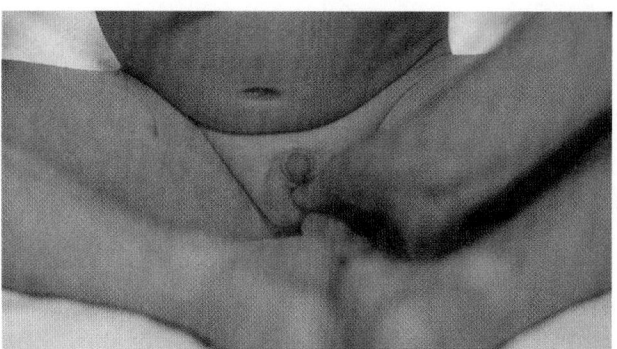

A

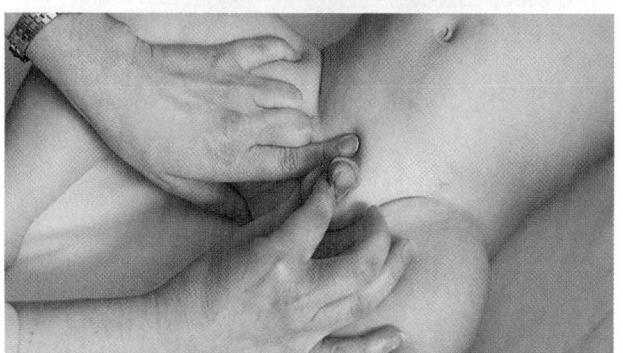

B

FIG. 7-35 ■ **A,** Preventing cremasteric reflex by having child sit in "tailor" position. **B,** Blocking inguinal canal during palpation of scrotum for descended testes.

Female Genitalia

The examination of female genitalia is limited to inspection and palpation of external structures. If a vaginal examination is required, an appropriate referral is made unless the nurse is qualified to perform the procedure. A convenient position for examination of the genitalia involves placing the young child supine on the examining table or in a semireclining position on the parent's lap with the feet supported on your knees as you sit facing the child. Divert the child's attention from the examination by instructing her to try to keep the soles of her feet pressed against each other. Separate the labia majora with the thumb and index finger and retract outward to expose the labia minora, urethral meatus, and vaginal orifice.

Examine the female genitalia for size and location of the structures of the *vulva* or *pudendum* (Fig. 7-36). The *mons pubis* is a pad of adipose tissue over the symphysis pubis. At puberty the mons is covered with hair, which extends along the labia. The usual pattern of female *hair distribution* is an inverted triangle. The appearance of soft, downy hair along the labia majora is an early sign of sexual maturation. Note the size and location of the *clitoris.* It is a small erectile organ located at the anterior end of the labia minora. It is covered by a small flap of skin, the *prepuce.*

The *labia majora* are two thick folds of skin running posteriorly from the mons to the posterior commissure of the vagina. Internal to the labia majora are two folds of skin called the *labia minora.* Although the labia minora are usually prominent in the newborn, they gradually atrophy, which makes them almost invisible until their enlargement during puberty.

The inner surface of the labia should be pink and moist. Note the size of the labia and any evidence of fusion, which may suggest male scrota. Normally no masses are palpable within the labia.

The *urethral meatus* is located posterior to the clitoris and is surrounded by Skene glands and ducts. Although not a prominent structure, the meatus appears as a small V-shaped slit. Note its location, especially if it opens from the clitoris or inside the vagina. Gently palpate the glands, which are common sites of cysts and sexually transmitted lesions.

The *vaginal orifice* is located posterior to the urethral meatus. Its appearance varies depending on individual anatomy and sexual activity. Ordinarily, examination of the vagina is limited to inspection. In virgins a thin crescent-shaped or circular membrane, called the *hymen,* may cover part of the vaginal opening. In some instances it completely occludes the orifice. After rupture, small rounded pieces of tissue called *caruncles* remain. Although an imperforate hymen denotes lack of penile intercourse, a perforate one does not necessarily indicate sexual activity (see also Sexual Abuse, Chapter 14).

> **! NURSING ALERT**
>
> In females who have been circumcised, the genitalia will appear different. Do not show surprise or disgust, but note the appearance and discuss the procedure with the young woman.

Surrounding the vaginal opening are *Bartholin glands,* which secrete a clear, mucoid fluid into the vagina for lubrication during intercourse. Palpate the ducts for cysts. Also note the discharge from the vagina, which is usually clear or white.

ANUS

After examination of the genitalia, the anal area is easily examined, although the child should be placed on the abdomen. Note the general firmness of the *buttocks* and symmetry of the *gluteal folds.* Assess the tone of the anal sphincter by eliciting the *anal reflex.* Gently scratching the anal area results in an obvious quick contraction of the external anal sphincter.

BACK AND EXTREMITIES
Spine

The general *curvature* of the spine is noted. Normally the back of a newborn is rounded or C shaped from the thoracic and pelvic curves. The development of the cervical and lumbar curves approximates development of various motor skills, such as cervical curvature with head control, and gives the older child the typical double S curve.

Marked curvatures in posture are abnormal (see Fig. 31-18). *Scoliosis,* lateral curvature of the spine, is an important childhood problem, especially in girls. Although scoliosis may be identified by observing and palpating the spine and noting a sideways displacement, more objective tests include:

■ With the child standing erect, clothed only in underpants (and bra if older girl), observe from behind, noting asymmetry of the shoulders and hips.
■ With the child bending forward so that the back is parallel to the floor, observe from the side, noting asymmetry or prominence of the rib cage.

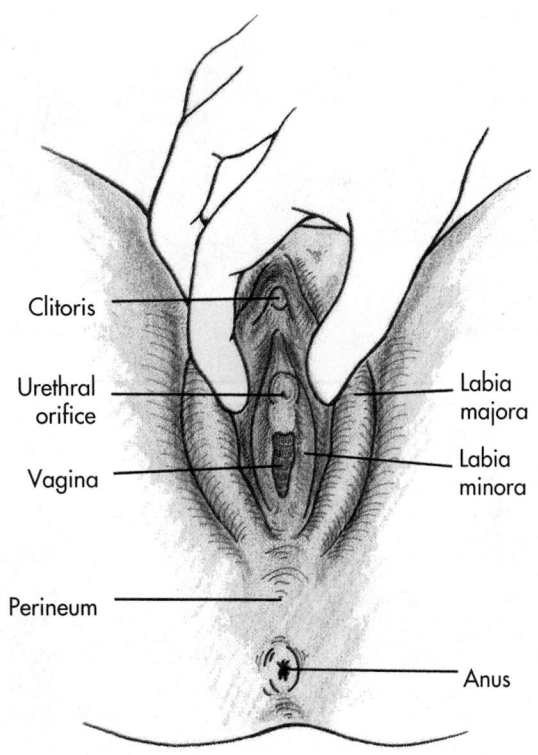

Clitoris
Urethral orifice
Vagina
Perineum
Labia majora
Labia minora
Anus

FIG. 7-36 ■ External structures of genitalia in postpubertal female. Labia are spread to reveal deeper structures. (From Potter PA, Perry AG: *Basic nursing: theory and practice,* ed 4, St Louis, 1999, Mosby.)

A slight limp, a crooked hemline, or complaints of a sore back are other signs and symptoms of scoliosis.

Inspect the *back,* especially along the spine, for any tufts of hair, dimples, or discoloration. *Mobility* of the vertebral column is easily assessed in most children because of their propensity for constant motion during the examination. However, mobility can be tested by asking the child to sit up from a prone position or to do a modified sit-up exercise.

Movement of the cervical spine is an important diagnostic sign of neurologic problems, such as meningitis. Normally movement of the head in all directions is effortless.

> **! NURSING ALERT**
>
> Hyperextension of the neck and spine, or *opisthotonos,* which is accompanied by pain when the head is flexed, is always referred for immediate medical evaluation.

Extremities

Inspect each extremity for symmetry of length and size; refer any deviation for orthopedic evaluation. Count the fingers and toes to be certain of the normal number. This is so often taken for granted that an extra digit (*polydactyly*) or fusion of digits (*syndactyly*) may go unnoticed.

Inspect the arms and legs for *temperature* and *color,* which should be equal in each extremity, although the feet may normally be colder than the hands.

Assess the *shape* of bones. Several variations of bone shape may be observed in children. Although many of them cause parents concern, most are benign and require no treatment. *Bowleg,* or *genu varum,* is lateral bowing of the tibia. It is clinically present when the child stands with the medial malleoli (rounded prominence on either side of the ankle) opposite each other and the space between the knees is greater than approximately 5 cm (2 inches) (Fig. 7-37). Toddlers are usually bowlegged after beginning to walk until all of their lower back and leg muscles are well developed. Unilateral or asymmetric bowlegs that are present beyond the age of 2 to 3 years, particularly in black children, may represent pathologic conditions requiring further investigation.

Knock-knee, or *genu valgum,* appears as the opposite of bowleg, in that the knees are close together but the feet are spread apart. It is determined clinically by using the same method as for genu varum but by measuring the distance between the malleoli, which normally should be less than 7.5 cm (3 inches) (Fig. 7-38). Knock-knee is normally present in children from about 2 to 7 years of age. Knock-knee that is excessive, asymmetric, accompanied by shortened stature, or evident in a child nearing puberty requires further evaluation.

Next inspect the *feet.* Infants' and toddlers' feet appear flat because the foot is normally wide and the arch is covered by a fat pad. Development of the arch occurs naturally from the action of walking. Normally, at birth the feet are held in a valgus (outward) or varus (inward) position. To determine whether a foot deformity at birth is a result of intrauterine position or development, scratch the outer, then inner, side of the sole. If the foot position is self-correctable, it will assume a right angle to the leg. As the child begins to walk, the feet turn outward less than 30 degrees and inward less than 10 degrees.

Toddlers have a "toddling" or broad-based gait, which facilitates walking by lowering the center of gravity. As the child reaches preschool age, the legs are brought closer together. By school age the walking posture is much more graceful and balanced.

The most common gait problem in young children is *pigeon toe,* or *toeing in,* which usually results from torsional deformities, such as internal tibial torsion (abnormal rotation or bowing of the tibia). Tests for tibial torsion include measuring the thigh-foot angle, which requires considerable practice for accuracy.

Elicit the *plantar* or *grasp reflex* by exerting firm but gentle pressure with the tip of the thumb against the lateral sole of the foot from the heel upward to the little toe and then across to the big toe. The normal response in children who are walking is flexion of the toes. *Babinski sign,* dorsiflexion of the big toe and fanning of the other toes, is nor-

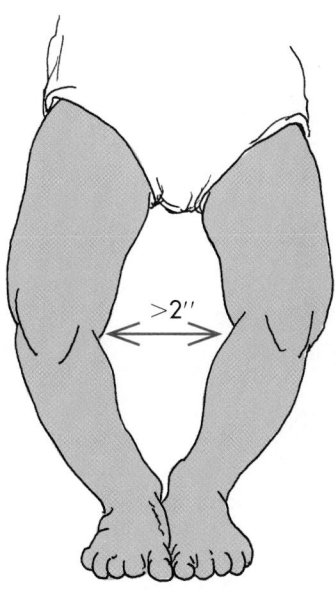

FIG. 7-37 ■ Bowleg.

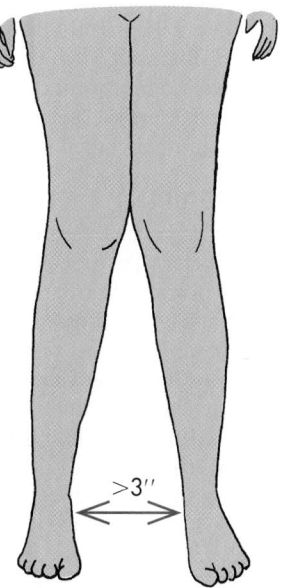

FIG. 7-38 ■ Knock-knee.

mal during infancy but abnormal after about 1 year of age or when locomotion begins (see Fig. 8-9).

Joints

Evaluate the joints for *range of motion.* Normally this requires no specific testing if the nurse has been observant of the child's movements during the examination. However, the hips should be routinely investigated in infants for congenital dislocation. Signs of congenital hip dislocation are discussed in Chapter 31. Report any evidence of joint immobility or hyperflexibility.

Palpate the joints for *heat, tenderness,* and *swelling.* These signs, as well as redness over the joint, warrant further investigation.

Muscles

Note symmetry and quality of muscle development, tone, and strength. Observe *development* by looking at the shape and contour of the body in both a relaxed and a tensed state. Estimate *tone* by grasping the muscle and feeling its firmness when it is relaxed and contracted. A common site for testing tone is the biceps muscle of the arm. Children are usually willing to "make a muscle" by clenching their fist.

Estimate *strength* by having the child use an extremity to push or pull against resistance, as in the following examples:

Arm strength. Child holds the arms outstretched in front of the body and tries to raise the arms while downward pressure is applied.
Hand strength. Child shakes hands with nurse and squeezes one or two fingers of the nurse's hand.
Leg strength. Child sits on a table or chair with the legs dangling and tries to raise the legs while downward pressure is applied.

Note symmetry of strength in the extremities, hands, and fingers, and report evidence of paresis or weakness.

NEUROLOGIC ASSESSMENT

The assessment of the nervous system is the broadest and most diverse part of the examining process, because every human function, both physical and emotional, is controlled by neurologic impulses. Much of the neurologic examination has already been discussed, such as assessment of behavior, sensory testing, and motor functioning. The following focuses on a general appraisal of cerebellar functioning, deep tendon reflexes, and the cranial nerves.

Cerebellar Functioning

The cerebellum controls balance and coordination. Much of the assessment of cerebellar functioning is included in observing the child's posture, body movements, gait, and development of fine and gross motor skills. Tests such as balancing on one foot and the heel-to-toe walk assess balance. Test *coordination* by asking the child to reach for a toy, button clothes, tie shoes, or draw a straight line on a piece of paper, provided that the child is old enough to do these activities. Coordination can also be tested by any sequence of rapid successive movements, such as quickly touching each finger with the thumb of the same hand.

Several tests for cerebellar function are described in Box 7-5 and can be performed as games. When the Romberg test is done, stay beside the child if there is a possibility that the child may fall. School-age children should be able to perform these tests, although, in the finger-to-nose test, preschoolers normally can only bring the finger within 5 to 7.5 cm (2 to 3 inches) of the nose. Difficulty in performing these exercises indicates poor sense of position (especially with the eyes closed) and incoordination (especially with the eyes opened).

Reflexes

Testing reflexes is an important part of the neurologic examination. Persistence of primitive reflexes (see Chapter 8), loss of reflexes, or hyperactivity of deep tendon reflexes is usually a result of a cerebral insult.

Elicit reflexes by using the rubber head of the reflex hammer, flat of the finger, or side of the hand. If the child is easily frightened by equipment, use your hand or finger. Although testing reflexes is a simple procedure to perform, the child may inhibit the reflex by unconsciously tensing the muscle. To avoid tensing, distract younger children with toys or talk to them. Older children can concentrate on the exercise of grasping their two hands in front of them and trying to pull them apart. This diverts their attention away from the testing and causes involuntary relaxation of the muscles.

Deep tendon reflexes are stretch reflexes of a muscle. The most common deep tendon reflex is the *knee jerk,* or *patellar reflex* (this is sometimes called the *quadriceps reflex*). The reflexes normally elicited are described in Figs. 7-39 to 7-42. Report any diminished or hyperreflexic response for further evaluation.

BOX 7-5 ■ Tests for Cerebellar Function

Finger-to-nose test. With child's arm extended, ask child to touch the nose with the index finger with eyes open and then closed.
Heel-to-shin test. While standing, have child run the heel of one foot down the shin or anterior aspect of the tibia of the other leg, both with eyes opened and then closed.
Romberg test. With eyes closed, have child stand with heels together; falling or leaning to one side is abnormal and is called *Romberg sign.*

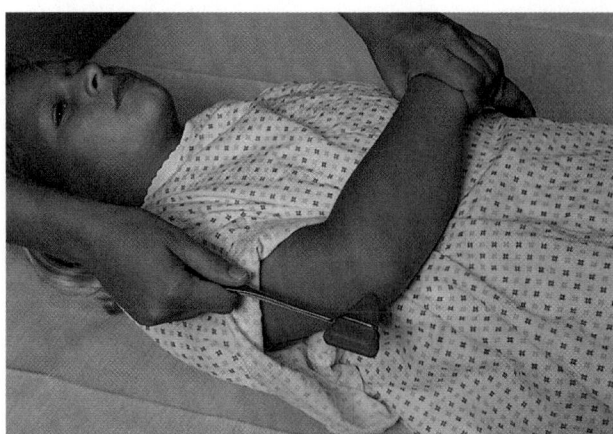

FIG. 7-39 ■ Testing for triceps reflex. Child is placed supine, with forearm resting over chest, and triceps tendon is struck. Alternate procedure: child's arm is abducted, with upper arm supported and forearm allowed to hang freely. Triceps tendon is struck. Normal response is partial extension of forearm.

Cranial Nerves

Assessment of the cranial nerves is an important area of neurologic assessment (Table 7-11). With young children, present the tests as games to encourage trust and security at the beginning of the examination. Or include the cranial nerve test when each "system" is examined, such as tongue movement and strength, gag reflex, swallowing, cardinal positions of gaze (Fig. 7-43), and position of the uvula during examination of the mouth.

DEVELOPMENTAL ASSESSMENT

One of the most essential components of a complete health appraisal is assessment of developmental functioning. *Screening* procedures are designed to identify quickly and reliably those children whose developmental level is below normal for their age and who therefore require further investigation. They also provide a means of recording objective measurements of present developmental functioning for future reference. Since the passage of P.L. 99-457, the Education of the Handicapped Act Amendments of 1986, much greater emphasis is placed on developmental assessment of children with disabilities, and nurses can play a vital role in providing this service. All of the procedures discussed in this section can be administered in a variety of settings—home, school, day care center, hospital, practitioner's office, or clinic.

DENVER II

The most widely used developmental screening tests for young children has been the series of tests developed by Dr. William Frankenburg and his colleagues in Denver, Colorado.

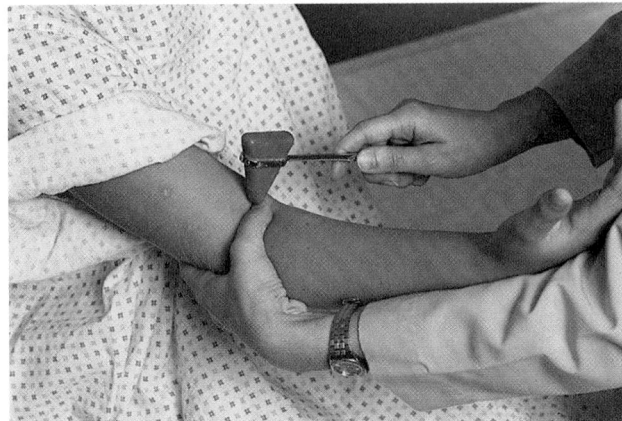

FIG. 7-40 ■ Testing for biceps reflex. Child's arm is held by placing partially flexed elbow in examiner's hand with thumb over antecubital space. Examiner's thumbnail is struck with hammer. Normal response is partial flexion of forearm.

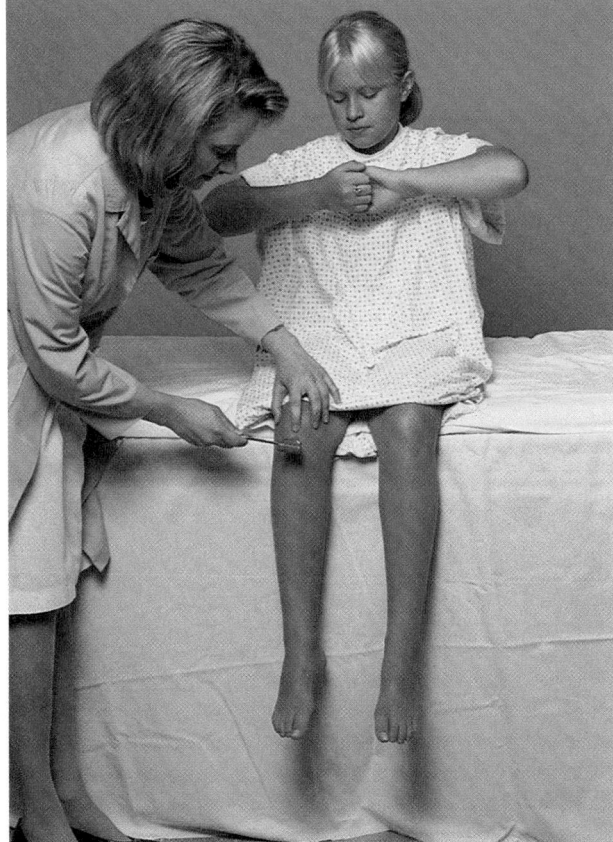

FIG. 7-41 ■ Testing for patellar, or knee jerk, reflex, using distraction. Child sits on edge of examining table (or on parent's lap) with lower legs flexed at knee and dangling freely. Patellar tendon is tapped just below kneecap. Normal response is partial extension of lower leg.

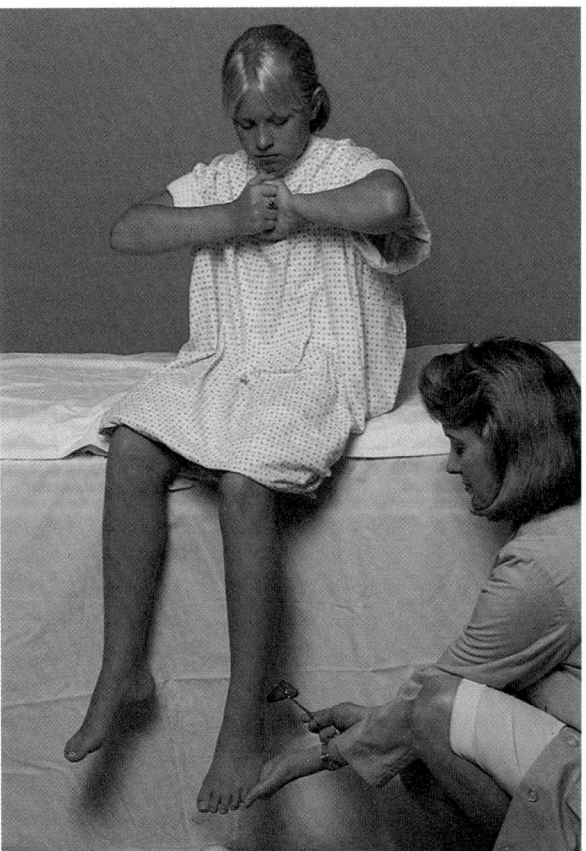

FIG. 7-42 ■ Testing for Achilles reflex. Child should be in same position as for knee jerk reflex. Foot is supported lightly in examiner's hand, and Achilles tendon is struck. Normal response is plantar flexion of foot (foot pointing downward).

TABLE 7-11 ■ Assessment of Cranial Nerves

DESCRIPTION/FUNCTION	TESTS
I—OLFACTORY NERVE Olfactory mucosa of nasal cavity Smell	With eyes closed, have child identify odors such as coffee, alcohol from a swab, or other smells; test each nostril separately
II—OPTIC NERVE Rods and cones of retina, optic nerve Vision	Check for perception of light, visual acuity, peripheral vision, color vision, and normal optic disc

III—OCULOMOTOR NERVE
Extraocular muscles (EOM) of eye:
    Superior rectus (SR)—moves eyeball up and in
    Inferior rectus (IR)—moves eyeball down and in
    Medial rectus (MR)—moves eyeball nasally
    Inferior oblique (IO)—moves eyeball up and out
Pupil constriction and accommodation
Eyelid closing
	Have child follow an object (toy) or light in the six cardinal positions of gaze (see Fig. 7-43)
	
	Perform PERRLA
	Check for proper placement of lid

IV—TROCHLEAR NERVE Superior oblique muscle (SO) Moves eye down and out	Have child look down and in (see Fig. 7-43)
V—TRIGEMINAL NERVE Muscles of mastication Sensory: face, scalp, nasal and buccal mucosa	Have child bite down hard and open jaw; test symmetry and strength With child's eyes closed, see if child can detect light touch in mandibular and maxillary regions Test corneal and blink reflex by touching cornea lightly (approach from side so that child does not blink before cornea is touched)
VI—ABDUCENS NERVE Lateral rectus (LR) muscle Moves eye temporally	Have child look toward temporal side (see Fig. 7-43)
VII—FACIAL NERVE Muscles for facial expression Anterior two thirds of tongue (sensory)	Have child smile, make funny face, or show teeth to see symmetry of expression Have child identify a sweet or salty solution; place each taste on anterior section and sides of protruding tongue; if child retracts tongue, solution will dissolve toward posterior part of tongue
VIII—AUDITORY, ACOUSTIC, OR VESTIBULOCOCHLEAR NERVE Internal ear Hearing/balance	Test hearing; note any loss of equilibrium or presence of vertigo
IX—GLOSSOPHARYNGEAL NERVE Pharynx, tongue Posterior one third of tongue (sensory)	Stimulate posterior pharynx with a tongue blade; child should gag Test sense of sour or bitter taste on posterior segment of tongue
X—VAGUS NERVE Muscles of larynx, pharynx, some organs of gastrointestinal system, sensory fibers of root of tongue, heart, lung, and some organs of gastrointestinal system	Note hoarseness of voice, gag reflex, and ability to swallow Check that uvula is in midline; when stimulated with a tongue blade, should deviate upward and to stimulated side
XI—ACCESSORY NERVE Sternocleidomastoid and trapezius muscles of shoulder	Have child shrug shoulders while applying mild pressure; with examiner's hands placed on shoulders, have child turn head against opposing pressure on either side; note symmetry and strength
XII—HYPOGLOSSAL NERVE Muscles of tongue	Have child move tongue in all directions; have child protrude tongue as far as possible; note any midline deviation Test strength by placing tongue blade on one side of tongue and having child move it away

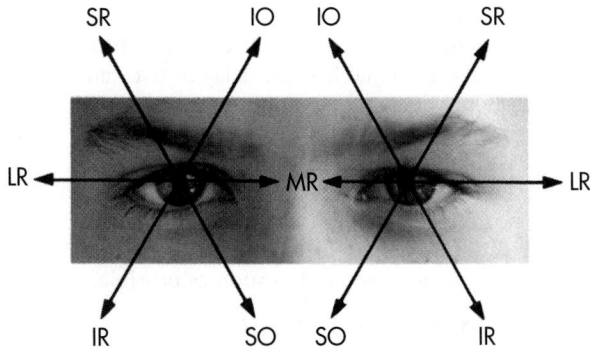

FIG. 7-43 ■ Testing cardinal positions of gaze.

The oldest and best known, the ***Denver Developmental Screening Test (DDST)*** and its revision, the ***DDST-R,*** have been revised, restandardized, and renamed the ***Denver II.*** Before administering the Denver II, the examiner should be trained by, and receive a certificate from, a master instructor who has been trained by the Denver faculty.* The Denver II differs from the DDST in items, test form, interpretation, and referral (see Appendix C). The previous total of 105 items has been increased to 125, including an increase from 21 DDST to 39 Denver II language items. Previous items that were difficult to administer or interpret have been either modified or eliminated. Many items that were previously tested by parental report now require observation by the examiner.

Each item was evaluated to determine if significant differences exist on the basis of sex, ethnic group, maternal education, and place of residence. Items for which clinically significant differences exist were replaced or, if retained, are discussed in the Denver II's Technical Manual. When evaluating children delayed on one of these items, the examiner can look up norms for the subpopulations to consider if the delay may be caused by sociocultural or environmental differences.

The items on the test form are arranged in the same format as the DDST-R. The norms for the distribution bars were updated with the new standardization data but retain the 25th, 50th, 75th, and 90th percentile divisions. The test form contains a place to rate the child's behavioral characteristics (compliance, interest in surroundings, fearfulness, and attention span).

To determine relative areas of advancement and areas of delay, sufficient items should be administered to establish the basal and ceiling levels in each sector. By scoring appropriate items as "pass," "fail," "refusal," or "no opportunity," and relating such scores to the age of the child, each item can be interpreted as described in the accompanying box. To identify cautions, all items intersected by the age line are administered. To screen solely for developmental delays, only the items located totally to the *left* of the child's age line are administered. Criteria for referral are based on the availability of resources in the community (Box 7-6).

Research on the Denver II's validity and accuracy continues. One study found that most children with even sub-

tle developmental problems were identified. However, almost half of the children without developmental problems received suspect scores, resulting in a high rate of overreferrals (Glascoe and others, 1992). To minimize overreferrals, a decision for referral depends not only on the results of the Denver II, but also on the practitioner's clinical judgment after considering the child's developmental history; general health status; social, cultural, and emotional environment; and the availability of local resources for diagnosis and treatment (Frankenburg, 1994a; 1994b).

Although it is not the purpose of this discussion to detail the instruction manual, some points concerning preparation, administration, and interpretation of the Denver II are important to stress. Before beginning the screen, ask if the child was born prematurely and correctly calculate the adjusted age. Up to 24 months of age, allowances are made for infants born prematurely by subtracting the number of weeks of missed gestation from their present age and testing them at the adjusted age. For example, a 16-week-old infant who was born 4 weeks early is tested at a 12-week adjusted age level. Explain to the parents and child, if appropriate, that the screenings are *not* intelligence tests but rather are a method of showing what the child can do at a particular age. Emphasize that the child is *not* expected to perform each item on the test.

Tell the parent before the screening begins that the results of the child's performance will be explained after all of the items have been concluded. It is the nurse's responsibility to properly inform parents of any testing or screening procedure before its administration so that they are fully aware of its purpose and intent.

---

*Forms and complete instructions are available from Denver Developmental Materials, Inc., PO Box 6919, Denver, CO 80206-9019; (303) 355-4729. The DDST and DDST-R are no longer available because they have been replaced by the Denver II.

Prepare toddlers and preschoolers for the procedure by presenting it as a game. Frequently, the Denver II is an excellent way to begin a health appraisal because it is nonthreatening, requires no painful or unfamiliar procedures, and capitalizes on the child's natural activity of play. Because children are easily distracted, perform each item quickly and present only one toy from the kit at a time. After that toy's purpose is concluded, such as building a tower of blocks or identifying its color, replace the toy in the bag and take out another one. Other temporary factors that may interfere with the child's performance include fatigue, illness, fear, hospitalization, separation from the parent, or general unwillingness to perform the activities. In addition, undiagnosed mental retardation, hearing loss, vision loss, neurologic impairment, or a familial pattern of slow development greatly influences the child's performance.

After completion of the Denver II, ask the parent if the child's performance was typical of behavior at other times. If the parent replies affirmatively and the child's cooperation was satisfactory, explain the results, emphasizing all successful items first, then those items failed but that the child was not expected to pass, and finally those items that were delays. If the parent replies that the child's performance was not typical of usual behavior, it is best to defer any scoring or discussion of results, especially if the refusals yield a suspect score. In this situation reschedule testing for a time when the child is more likely to cooperate.

In explaining a normal score, focus on how well the child performed and reinforce the parents' efforts in satisfactorily stimulating their child. In addition to assessing the child's present developmental level, the Denver II can be used to guide parents toward those activities that are appropriate, although not necessarily expected, for the child's age. By testing for items to the right of the age line (ones the child is not expected to perform), children with advanced development, who may be gifted, can be identified.

In explaining delays, carefully note the parent's response, especially casual acceptance such as "He'll catch up" or questions such as "Does this mean my child is retarded?" Be aware of personal anxieties during these situations and refrain from giving glib reassurances such as "I'm sure he will do better next time." Rather, respond honestly to parents' questions, yet with appropriate flexibility and concern, stressing the need for further developmental testing.

DENVER II PRESCREENING DEVELOPMENTAL QUESTIONNAIRE

The Denver II Prescreening Developmental Questionnaire (PDQ-II) is a further revision of the PDQ and the R-PDQ. This version uses the norms (90th and 75th percentiles) from the Denver II. The PDQ-II is a parent-answered prescreen consisting of 91 questions from the Denver II, although only a subset of questions are asked for each age-group. The form may need to be read to parents and caregivers who are less educated.

Four different forms are available and are selected based on age: orange (0 to 9 months), purple (9 to 24 months), cream (2 to 4 years), and white (4 to 6 years). The caregiver answers questions until (1) three "nos" are circled (they do not have to be consecutive) or (2) all the questions on both sides of the form have been answered. Scoring is based on the number of delays or cautions (see Box 7-6). Children who have no delays or cautions are considered to be developing normally. If a child has one delay or two cautions, the caregiver is provided with age-appropriate developmental activities to pursue with the child, and a rescreen with the PDQ-II is done 1 month later. If on rescreening the child has one or more delays, the Denver II is administered as soon as possible. If a child has two or more delays or three or more cautions on the first screening with the PDQ-II, the Denver II is administered as soon as possible.

DEVELOPMENTAL SCREENING AND INTERPRETATION

Although screening tests are an effective method of applying the knowledge of children's expected rate of development to a large segment of the population, they are only as successful as the individual's expertise in administering them. Because many of the screening tests are devised to be used by paraprofessionals, there are inherent risks in screening if such individuals are not properly trained or supervised. For example, false-positive findings can label the child as developmentally delayed and cause problems that otherwise might not have existed. False-negative findings can prevent children with problems from receiving the help they need.

Nurses administering developmental screening or supervising paraprofessionals' testing need to assess the child's "whole picture" and not rely solely on any screening procedure. Development, like growth and health, is a dynamic process. Tests such as the Denver II should be used as part of *developmental surveillance,* a continuous comprehensive primary health care approach that includes the parents as partners with professionals (Frankenburg, 1994b). Evaluation of the child's total well-being is the result of evaluating data from a comprehensive health and family history, physical examination, and developmental screening.

KEY POINTS

■ The most common approach to examining children follows a head-to-toe sequence.

■ Growth measurements during the physical examination focus on length, height, weight, skinfold thickness, and arm and head circumference. Assessment of growth is measured against standard growth charts to determine a child's status in comparison with other children of the same age.

■ Measurements of temperature, pulse, respiration, and blood pressure constitute the physiologic approach to assessment.

■ The general appearance of a child is a cumulative, subjective impression of physical appearance, state of nutrition, behavior, personality, interactions with parents and nurse, posture, development, and speech.

■ Assessment of the skin, which primarily involves inspection and palpation, focuses on color, texture, temperature, moisture, and turgor. The nurse needs to be aware of both physiologic and ethnic factors that may affect these areas.

■ In assessment of the lymph nodes, the nurse examines, by palpation, the part of the body in which the glands are located.

■ The head is inspected for shape, symmetry, mobility, and muscle control.

- Examination of the eyes includes placement and alignment, inspection of external and internal structures, and vision testing.

- The ears are examined for placement and alignment, inspection of external and internal structures, and auditory testing.

- The lungs are examined by methods of inspection, palpation, percussion, and auscultation.

- Auscultation is the most important procedure for examining the heart.

- Abdominal assessment follows an orderly sequence of inspection, auscultation, and palpation, since palpation may distort normal abdominal sounds.

- Examination of the genitalia may provoke anxiety in the child, and the nurse must avoid any transference of anxiety.

- Neurologic assessment addresses behavior; motor, sensory, and cerebellar functioning; reflexes; and cranial nerves.

- The Denver II, a major revision and a restandardization of the DDST, differs from the DDST in items included in the test, the test form, and the interpretation of scoring.

References

American Academy of Pediatrics, Committee on Practice and Ambulatory Medicine, Section on Ophthalmology: Eye examination in infants, children, and young adults by pediatricians, *Pediatrics* 111(4): 902-907, 2003a.

American Academy of Pediatrics, Committee on Practice and Ambulatory Medicine, Section on Otolaryngology and Bronchoesophagology: Hearing assessment in infants and children: recommendations beyond neonatal screening, *Pediatrics* 111(2):436-440, 2003b.

Amoore JN: A comparative evaluation of the DINAMAP 8100 and DINAMAP Compact TS using a non-invasive blood pressure simulator, *Blood Press Monit* 3(5):309-314, 1998.

Androkites AL, Werger AM, Young ML: Comparison of axillary and infrared tympanic membrane thermometry in a pediatric oncology outpatient setting, *J Pediatr Oncol Nurs* 15(4):216-222, 1998.

Bald M: Ambulatory blood pressure monitoring in children and adolescents, *Minerva Pediatr* 54(1):13-24, 2002.

Banitalebi H and Bangstad HJ: Measurement of fever in children—is infrared tympanic thermometry reliable? *Tidsskr Nor Laegeforen* 122(28):2700-2701, 2002.

Barone MA, Rowe PC: Pediatric procedures. In McMillan JA, DeAngelis CD, Feigin RD, editors: *Oski's pediatrics—principles and practice,* ed 3, Philadelphia, 1999, Lippincott Williams & Wilkins.

Beevers G, Lip GYH, O'Brien E: ABC of hypertension blood pressure measurement, part I: Sphygmomanometry: factors common to all techniques, *BMJ* 322(7292):981-985, 2001.

Berry BE and others: Preschool vision screening using the MTI-Photoscreener, *Pediatr Nurs* 27(1):27-34, 2001.

Blackburn S and others: Neonatal thermal care, part III: the effect of infant position and temperature probe placement, *Neonatal Netw* 20(3):25-30, 2001.

Bliss-Holtz J: Methods of newborn infant temperature monitoring: a research review, *Issues Compr Pediatr Nurs* 18(4):287-298, 1995.

Childs C, Harrison R, Hodkinson C: Tympanic membrane temperature as a measure of core temperature, *Arch Dis Child* 80(3):262-266, 1999.

Clark JA and others: Discrepancies between direct and indirect blood pressure measurements using various recommendations for arm cuff selection, *Pediatrics* 110(5):920-923, 2002.

Coats DK, Jenkins RH: Vision assessment of the pediatric patient: refinements, *Am Acad Ophthalmol* 1(1):1-12, 1997.

Craig JV and others: Infrared ear thermometry compared with rectal thermometry in children: a systematic review, *Lancet* 360:603-609, 2002.

Craig JV and others: Temperature measured at the axilla compared with rectum in children and young people: systematic review, *BMJ* 320(7243):1174-1178, 2000.

Cretel E and others: A comparative study of body temperature using rectal and tympanic measurement, *Rev Med Intern* 20(11):981-984, 1999.

Cunningham M, Cox, EO: Hearing assessment in infants and children: Recommendations beyond neonatal screening, *Pediatrics* 111(2): 436-440, 2003.

Dollberg S, Lahav S, Mimouni FB: Precision of a new thermometer for rapid rectal temperature measurement in neonates, *Am J Perinatol* 18(2):103-105, 2001.

Erickson RS: The continuing question of how best to measure body temperature, *Crit Care Med* 27(10):2307-2310, 1999.

Erickson RS, Meyer LT, Woo TM: Accuracy of chemical dot thermometers in critically ill adults and children, *Image J Nurs Sch* 28(1): 23-28, 1996.

Frankenburg WK: Preventing developmental delays: is developmental screening sufficient? part I: Developmental screening and the Denver II, *Pediatrics* 93(4):586-589, 1994a.

Frankenburg WK: Preventing developmental delays: is developmental screening sufficient? part II: Partners in health care, *Pediatrics* 93(4): 589-593, 1994b.

Gillman MW, Cook NR: Blood pressure measurement in childhood epidemiological studies, *Circulation* 92(4):1049-1057, 1995.

Glascoe FP and others: Accuracy of the Denver-II in developmental screening, *Pediatrics* 89:1221-1225, 1992.

Goldman LR, Shannon MW: Technical report: mercury in the environment: implications for pediatricians, *Pediatrics* 108(1):197-205, 2001.

Greyling G, Viljoen MJ, Joubert G: Axillary temperature compared to tympanic membrane temperature in children, *Curationis* 23(3):54-61, 2000.

Haddock BJ, Merrow DL, Swanson MS: The falling grace of axillary temperatures, *Pediatr Nurs* 22(2):121-125, 1996.

Halle C: Achieve new vision screening objectives, *Nurse Practitioner* 27(3):15-35, 2002.

Healthcare Product Comparison System: *Thermometers, electronic, continuous,* Plymouth Meeting, Pa, 1996a, ECRI.

Healthcare Product Comparison System: *Thermometers, electronic, intermittent,* Plymouth Meeting, Pa, 1996b, ECRI.

Healthcare Product Comparison System: *Thermometers, infrared, ear,* Plymouth Meeting, Pa, 1996c, ECRI.

Hockenberry-Eaton M, Kline NE: Nursing support of the child with cancer. In Pizzo PA, Poplack DP, editors: *Principles and practices of pediatric oncology,* vol 4, Philadelphia, 2001, JB Lippincott.

Hooker EA, Houston H: Screening for fever in an adult emergency department: oral vs tympanic thermometry, *South Med J* 89(2): 230-234, 1996.

Houlder LC: The accuracy and reliability of tympanic thermometry compared to rectal and axillary sites in young children, *Pediatr Nurs* 26(3):311-314, 2000.

Irvin SM: Comparison of the oral thermometer versus the tympanic thermometer, *Clin Nurs Spec* 13(2):85-89, 1999.

Jean-Mary MB, Dicanzio J, Shaw J, Bernstein HH: Limited accuracy and reliability of infrared axillary and aural thermometers in a pediatric outpatient population, *J Pediatr* 141(5):671-676, 2002.

Jensen BN and others: Accuracy of digital tympanic, oral, axillary, and rectal thermometers compared with standard rectal mercury thermometers, *Eur J Surg* 166(11):848-851, 2000.

Kongpanichkul A, Bunjongpak S: A comparative study on accuracy of liquid crystal forehead, digital electronic axillary, infrared tympanic with glass-mercury rectal thermometer in infants and young children, *J Med Assoc Thai* 83(9):1068-1076, 2000.

Lanham DM and others: Accuracy of tympanic temperature readings in children under 6 years of age, *Pediatr Nurs* 25(1):39-42, 1999.

Leick-Rude MK, Bloom LF: A comparison of temperature-taking methods in neonates, *Neonatal Netw* 17(5):21-37, 1998.

Ling J and others: Clinical evaluation of the oscillometric blood pressure monitor in adults and children based on the 1992 AAMI SP-10 standards, *J Clin Monit* 11(2):123-130, 1995.

Loveys AA and others: Comparison of ear to rectal temperature measurements in infants and toddlers, *Clin Pediatr* 38(8):463-466, 1999.

Macqueen S: Clinical benefits of 3M Tempa.DOT thermometer in paediatric settings, *Br J Nurs* 10(1):55-58, 2001.

Medical Indicators, Inc: *NexTemp single-use clinical thermometers: the quick, accurate, "no-hassle" way to take a temp,* Pennington, NJ, Jan 1999, NCFI.

Modell JG and others: Unreliability of the infrared tympanic thermometer in clinical practice: a comparative study with oral mercury and oral electronic thermometers, *South Med J* 91(7):649-654, 1998.

Molton AH, Blacktop J, Hall CM: Temperature taking in children, *J Child Health Care* 5(1):5-10, 2001.

National Center for Health Statistics: CDC growth charts: United States, *Adv Data* 314, 2000.

National Institutes of Health, National Heart, Lung, and Blood Institute: *Update on the Task Force Report (1987) on high blood pressure in children and adolescents: a working group report from the National High Blood Pressure Education Program,* Bethesda, Md, NIH pub no 96-3790, Sept 1996.

Park M, Lee D, Johnson CA: Oscillometric blood pressures in the arm, thigh and calf in healthy children and those with aortic coarctation, *Pediatrics* 92(4):761-765, 1993.

Pompei F, Pompei M: *Physicians reference handbook on temperature,* Watertown, Mass, 1996, Exergen.

Py Ma H Corporation: *Tempa Dot single use thermometer: technical information,* Flemington, NJ, 1994, The Corporation.

Rabinowitz RP and others: Effects of anatomic site, oral stimulation, and body position on estimates of body temperature, *Arch Intern Med* 156(7):777-780, 1996.

Rivera AY and others: Evaluation of a liquid crystal contact thermometer in children with fever, *J Investig Med* 45:1, 1997.

Robinson JL and others: Comparison of esophageal, rectal, axillary, bladder, tympanic, and pulmonary artery temperatures in children, *J Pediatr* 133:553-556, 1998.

Roche AF, Guo S: The new growth charts, *Pediatr Basics* 94:2-13, 2001.

Romanovsky AA and others: A difference of 5 degrees C between ear and rectal temperatures in a febrile patient, *Am J Emerg Med* 15(4):383-385, 1997.

Saxena AK, Topp SS, Heinecke A, Willital GH: Application criteria for infrared ear thermometers in pediatric surgery, *Technol Health Care* 9(3):281-285, 2001.

Seidel HM, Rosenstein BJ, Pathak A: *Primary care of the newborn,* ed 2, St Louis, 1997, Mosby.

Sganga A, Wallace R, Kiehl E, Irving T, Witter L: A comparison of four methods of normal newborn temperature measurement, *MCN* 25(2): 76-79, 2000.

Shann F, Mackenzie A: Comparison of rectal, axillary and forehead temperatures, *Arch Pediatr Adolesc Med* 150:74-78, 1996.

Turnbull R: Skin assessment in children: a methodical approach, *Nurs Times* 96(41):33-34, 2000.

Valadez JJ, Elmore-Meegan M, Morley D: Comparing liquid crystal thermometer readings and mercury thermometer readings of infants and children in a traditional African setting, *Trop Geogr Med* 47(3):130-133, 1995.

Vessey JA: Developmental approaches to examining young children, *Pediatr Nurs* 21(1):53-56, 1995.

Wall TC and others: Compliance with vision-screening guidelines among a national sample of pediatricians, *Ambulatory Pediatr* 2(6):449-455, 2002.

Wattigney WA and others: Utility of an automatic instrument for blood pressure measurement in children: the Bogalusa Heart Study, *Am J Hypertens* 9(3):256-262, 1996.

Wilshaw R and others: A comparison of the use of tympanic, axillary, and rectal thermometers in infants, *J Pediatr Nurs* 14(2):88-93, 1999.

Zengeya ST, Blumenthal I: Modern electronic and chemical thermometers used in the axilla are inaccurate, *Eur J Pediatr* 155(12): 1005-1008, 1996.

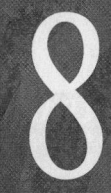

Health Promotion of the Newborn and Family

DAVID WILSON

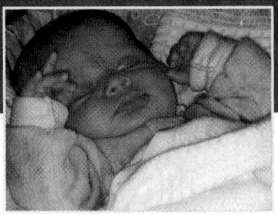

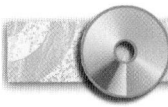 Remember to check out your companion CD-ROM

http://evolve.elsevier.com/Wong/essentials/

CHAPTER OUTLINE

RELATED TOPICS and ADDITIONAL RESOURCES

 IN TEXT

 CD COMPANION

Critical Thinking Exercises—Circumcision, Formula Preparation
Case Studies—Breast-Feeding, The Normal Newborn
Anatomy Review—Location of Sutures and Fontanels
Guidelines—Assessing Attachment Behaviors, Physical Examination of the Newborn, Ophthalmia Neonatorum Prophylaxis
Nursing Care Plan
NCLEX-Style Review Questions

 WEBSITE

WebLinks
NCLEX-Style Review Questions

WONG'S CLINICAL MANUAL OF PEDIATRIC NURSING, ED 6

Community and Home Care Instructions: Using a Bulb Syringe
Guidelines for Car Seat Safety

*For additional information, please view "Pediatric Assessment" in *Whaley and Wong's pediatric nursing video series*, St Louis, 1996, Mosby; (800) 426-4545; website: www.elsevierhealth.com.

- Identify the principal cardiorespiratory changes that occur during transition to extrauterine life.
- Identify the immature physiologic functioning of each body system and its significance to nursing care of the newborn.
- Perform an initial and transitional assessment of the newborn including the Apgar score and gestational age assessment.
- Perform a newborn physical assessment based on recognition of expected normal findings.
- Outline a nursing care plan for the newborn.
- Assess and promote parent-infant attachment behaviors.

ADJUSTMENT TO EXTRAUTERINE LIFE

The most profound physiologic change required of the neonate is transition from fetal or placental circulation to independent respiration. The loss of the placental connection means the loss of complete metabolic support, especially the supply of oxygen and the removal of carbon dioxide. The normal stresses of labor and delivery produce alterations of placental gas exchange patterns, acid-base balance in the blood, and cardiovascular activity in the infant. Factors that interfere with this normal transition or that increase fetal *asphyxia* (a condition of hypoxemia, hypercapnia, and acidosis) will affect the fetus's adjustment to extrauterine life.

IMMEDIATE ADJUSTMENTS
Respiratory System

The most critical and immediate physiologic change required of the newborn is the onset of breathing. The stimuli that help initiate the first respiration are primarily chemical and thermal. *Chemical factors* in the blood (low oxygen, high carbon dioxide, and low pH) initiate impulses that excite the respiratory center in the medulla. The primary *thermal stimulus* is the sudden chilling of the infant who leaves a warm environment and enters a relatively cooler atmosphere. This abrupt change in temperature excites sensory impulses in the skin that are transmitted to the respiratory center.

The significance of *tactile stimulation* is questionable. Descent through the birth canal and normal handling during delivery may have some effect on initiation of respiration. Recent evidence suggests that the establishment of adequate *pulmonary perfusion* through the pulmonary vasculature may have a more significant role in the establishment of respirations than previously believed. After the capillary network surrounding the alveoli expands (capillary erection) with increasing blood flow and pressure, the alveoli begin to open partially. As air enters the partially deflated alveoli, lung fluid diffuses across the alveolar-capillary membrane, further enhancing alveolar expansion. Mercer and Skovgaard (2002) assert that delaying cord clamping and allowing more blood volume into the newborn's circulation may have an important role in the establishment of adequate blood volume, adequate pulmonary perfusion, and subsequent onset of respirations in the newborn.

The initial entry of air into the lungs is opposed by the surface tension of the fluid that filled the fetal lungs and the alveoli. Some lung fluid may also be removed during the normal forces of labor and delivery. As the chest emerges from the birth canal, fluid is squeezed from the lungs through the nose and mouth. After complete delivery of the chest, a brisk recoil of the thorax occurs.

In the alveoli the surface tension of the fluid is reduced by *surfactant,* a substance produced by the alveolar epithelium that coats the alveolar surface. The effect of surfactant in facilitating breathing is discussed in relation to respiratory distress syndrome (see Chapter 9).

Circulatory System

Equally important as the initiation of respiration are the circulatory changes that allow blood to flow through the lungs. These changes, which occur more gradually, are the result of pressure changes in the lungs, heart, and major vessels. The transition from fetal to postnatal circulation involves the functional closure of the fetal shunts: the foramen ovale, the ductus arteriosus, and eventually the ductus venosus. (For a review of fetal circulation, see Chapter 25.) Increased blood flow dilates the pulmonary vessels, pulmonary vascular resistance decreases, and systemic resistance increases, thus maintaining blood pressure. As the lungs receive blood, the pressure in the right atrium, right ventricle, and pulmonary arteries decreases. Left atrial pressure increases above right atrial pressure with subsequent foramen ovale closure. With the increase in pulmonary blood flow and dramatic reduction of pulmonary vascular resistance, the ductus arteriosus begins to close.

The most important factors controlling ductal closure are the increased oxygen concentration of the blood and the fall in endogenous prostaglandins. The foramen ovale closes functionally at or soon after birth. The ductus arteriosus is closed functionally by the fourth day. Anatomic closure takes considerably longer. Failure of the ductus arteriosus or foramen ovale to close results in persistence of fetal shunting of blood away from the lungs (see Chapter 25).

Because of the reversible flow of blood through the ductus during the early neonatal period, a functional murmur occasionally may be heard. In conditions such as crying or straining, the increased pressure shunts unoxygenated blood from the right side of the heart across the ductal opening, causing transient cyanosis.

PHYSIOLOGIC STATUS OF OTHER SYSTEMS
Thermoregulation

Next to establishing respiration, heat regulation is most critical to the newborn's survival. Although the newborn's capacity for heat production is adequate, several factors predispose the newborn to excessive heat loss:

1 The newborn's large surface area facilitates heat loss to the environment, although this is partially compensated for by

the newborn's usual position of flexion, which decreases the amount of surface area exposed to the environment.

2 The newborn's thin layer of subcutaneous fat provides poor insulation for conservation of heat.

3 The newborn's mechanism for producing heat is different from that of the adult, who can increase heat production through shivering. The chilled neonate cannot shiver but produces heat through *nonshivering thermogenesis,* which involves increased metabolism and oxygen consumption.

The principal thermogenic sources are the heart, liver, and brain. However, there is an additional source unique to the newborn known as *brown adipose tissue,* or *brown fat.* Brown fat, which owes its name to its larger content of mitochondrial cytochromes, has a greater capacity for heat production through intensified metabolic activity than does ordinary adipose tissue. Heat generated in brown fat is distributed to other parts of the body by the blood, which is warmed as it flows through the layers of this tissue. Superficial deposits of brown fat are located between the scapulae, around the neck, in the axillae, and behind the sternum. Deeper layers surround the kidneys, trachea, esophagus, some major arteries, and adrenals. The location of brown fat may explain why the nape of the neck often feels warmer than the rest of the infant's body.

Although newborns' ability to conserve heat is usually a matter of concern, they also can have difficulty dissipating heat in an overheated environment, which increases the risk of hyperthermia.

Hemopoietic System

The *blood volume* of the newborn depends on the amount of placental transfer of blood. The blood volume of the full-term infant is about 80 to 85 mL/kg of body weight. Immediately after birth the total blood volume averages 300 mL, but depending on how long cord clamping is delayed, as much as 100 mL can be added to the blood volume. Blood values for the newborn are listed in Appendix E.

Fluid and Electrolyte Balance

Changes occur in the *total body water volume,* extracellular fluid volume, and intracellular fluid volume during the transition from fetal to postnatal life. At birth the total weight of the infant is 73% fluid, compared with 58% in the adult. The infant has a proportionately higher ratio of extracellular fluid than the adult and consequently has a higher level of total body sodium and chloride and a lower level of potassium, magnesium, and phosphate.

A very important aspect of fluid balance is its relationship to other systems. Besides the rate of fluid exchange being seven times greater in the infant than in the adult, the infant's *rate of metabolism* is twice as great in relation to body weight. As a result, twice as much acid is formed, leading to more rapid development of acidosis. In addition, the immature kidneys cannot sufficiently concentrate urine to conserve body water. These three factors make the infant more prone to problems of dehydration, acidosis, and possible overhydration or water intoxication.

Gastrointestinal System

The ability of the newborn to digest, absorb, and metabolize foodstuff is adequate but limited in certain functions. Enzymes are adequate to handle the proteins and simple carbohydrates (monosaccharides and disaccharides), but deficient production of pancreatic amylase impairs use of complex carbohydrates (polysaccharides). Deficiency of pancreatic lipase limits absorption of fats, especially with ingestion of foods with high saturated fatty acid content such as cow's milk.

The liver is the most immature of the gastrointestinal organs. The activity of the enzyme *glucuronyl transferase* is reduced, which affects the conjugation of bilirubin with glucuronic acid and contributes to the physiologic jaundice of the newborn. The liver is also deficient in forming plasma proteins. The decreased plasma protein concentration probably plays a role in the edema usually seen at birth. Prothrombin and other coagulation factors are also low. The liver stores less glycogen at birth than later in life. Consequently, the newborn is prone to hypoglycemia, which may be prevented by early and effective feeding, especially breast-feeding.

Some salivary glands are functioning at birth, but the majority do not begin to secrete saliva until about the age of 2 to 3 months, when drooling is frequent. Stomach capacity is limited to about 90 mL; thus, the infant requires frequent small feedings. The colon also has a small volume; the newborn may have a bowel movement after each feeding. Newborns who breast-feed usually have more frequent feedings and more frequent stools than infants who receive formula. However, the pattern may change after the first few weeks.

The infant's *intestine* is longer in relation to body size than that of the adult. Therefore, there are a larger number of secretory glands and a larger surface area for absorption as compared with the adult's intestine. There are rapid peristaltic waves and simultaneous nonperistaltic waves along the entire esophagus. These waves, called the migrating motor complex (MMC), propel nutrients forward. The relative immaturity of the MMC, combined with decreased lower esophageal sphincter (LES) pressure, inappropriate relaxation of the LES, and delayed gastric emptying, make regurgitation a common occurrence. Progressive changes in the stooling pattern indicate a properly functioning gastrointestinal tract (Box 8-1).

BOX 8-1 ■ Change in Stooling Patterns of Newborns

MECONIUM
Infant's first stool; composed of amniotic fluid and its constituents, intestinal secretions, shed mucosal cells, and possibly blood (ingested maternal blood or minor bleeding of alimentary tract vessels).
Passage of meconium should occur within the first 24 to 48 hours, although it may be delayed up to 7 days in very-low-birth-weight infants.

TRANSITIONAL STOOLS
Usually appear by third day after initiation of feeding; greenish brown to yellowish brown, thin, and less sticky than meconium; may contain some milk curds.

MILK STOOL
Usually appears by fourth day.
In *breast-fed infants* stools are yellow to golden, are pasty in consistency, and have an odor similar to that of sour milk.
In *formula-fed infants* stools are pale yellow to light brown, are firmer in consistency, and have a more offensive odor.

Renal System

All structural components are present in the renal system, but there is a functional deficiency in the kidney's ability to concentrate urine and to cope with conditions of fluid and electrolyte stress such as dehydration or a concentrated solute load.

Total volume of urine per 24 hours is about 200 to 300 mL by the end of the first week. However, the bladder voluntarily empties when stretched by a volume of 15 mL, resulting in as many as 20 voidings per day. The first voiding should occur within 24 hours. The urine is colorless and odorless and has a specific gravity of about 1.020.

Integumentary System

At birth all the structures within the skin are present, but many of the functions of the integument are immature. The two layers of the skin, the epidermis and dermis, are loosely bound to each other and very thin. *Rete pegs,* which later in life anchor the epidermis to the dermis, are not developed. Slight friction across the epidermis, such as from rapid removal of adhesive tape, can cause separation of these layers and blister formation. The transitional zone between the cornified and living layers of the epidermis is effective in preventing fluid from reaching the skin surface.

The *sebaceous glands* are very active late in fetal life and in early infancy because of the high levels of maternal androgens. They are most densely located on the scalp, face, and genitalia and produce the greasy vernix caseosa that covers the infant at birth. Plugging of the sebaceous glands causes *milia.*

The *eccrine glands,* which produce sweat in response to heat or emotional stimuli, are functional at birth, and palmar sweating on crying reaches levels equivalent to those of anxious adults by 3 weeks of age. The eccrine glands produce sweat in response to higher temperatures than those required in adults, and the retention of sweat may result in miliaria. The *apocrine glands* remain small and nonfunctional until puberty.

The growth phases of *hair follicles* usually occur simultaneously at birth. During the first few months the synchrony between hair loss and regrowth is disrupted, and there may be overgrowth of hair or temporary alopecia. Boys' hair grows faster than girls' hair, and in both sexes scalp hair growth is slower at the crown.

Because the amount of *melanin* is low at birth, newborns are lighter skinned than they will be as children. Consequently, they are more susceptible to the harmful effects of the sun.

Musculoskeletal System

At birth the *skeletal system* contains larger amounts of cartilage than of ossified bone, although the process of ossification is fairly rapid during the first year. The nose, for example, is predominantly cartilage at birth and may be temporarily flattened or asymmetric by the force of delivery. The six skull bones are relatively soft and are separated only by membranous seams. The sinuses are incompletely formed in the newborn.

Unlike the skeletal system, the *muscular system* is almost completely formed at birth. Growth in size of muscular tissue is caused by hypertrophy, rather than hyperplasia, of cells.

Defenses Against Infection

The infant is born with several defenses against infection. The first line of defense is the *skin* and *mucous membranes,* which protect the body from invading organisms. The second line of defense is the *cellular elements* of the immunologic system, which produce several types of cells capable of attacking a pathogen. The *neutrophils* and *monocytes* are phagocytes, which means they can engulf, ingest, and destroy foreign agents. *Eosinophils* also probably have a phagocytic property, because they increase in number in the presence of foreign protein. The *lymphocytes* (T cells and B cells) are capable of being converted to other cell types, such as monocytes and antibodies. Although the phagocytic properties of the blood are present in the infant, the inflammatory response of the tissues to localize an infection is immature.

The third line of defense is the formation of specific *antibodies* to an antigen. Exposure to various foreign agents is necessary for antibody production to occur. Infants are generally not capable of producing their own immunoglobulins (Ig) until the beginning of the second month of life, but they receive considerable passive immunity in the form of IgG from the maternal circulation and from human milk (see p. 205). They are protected against most major childhood diseases, including diphtheria, measles, poliomyelitis, and rubella for about 3 months, provided the mother has developed antibodies to these illnesses.

Endocrine System

Ordinarily the endocrine system of the newborn is adequately developed, but its functions are immature. For example, the posterior lobe of the pituitary gland produces limited quantities of *antidiuretic hormone,* or *vasopressin,* which inhibits diuresis. This renders the young infant highly susceptible to dehydration.

The effect of maternal *sex hormones* is particularly evident in the newborn. The labia are hypertrophied, and the breasts may be engorged and secrete milk (witch's milk) from the first few days of life to as long as 2 months of age. Female newborns may have *pseudomenstruation* (more often seen as a milky secretion than actual blood) from a sudden drop in progesterone and estrogen levels.

Neurologic System

At birth the nervous system is incompletely integrated but sufficiently developed to sustain extrauterine life. Most neurologic functions are *primitive reflexes.* The *autonomic nervous system* is crucial during transition, because it stimulates initial respirations, helps maintain acid-base balance, and partially regulates temperature control.

Myelination of the nervous system follows the cephalocaudal-proximodistal (head-to-toe—center-to-periphery) laws of development and is closely related to observed mastery of fine and gross motor skills. *Myelin* is necessary for rapid and efficient transmission of some, but not all, nerve impulses along the neural pathway. The tracts that develop myelin earliest are the sensory, cerebellar, and extrapyramidal tracts. This accounts for the acute senses of taste, smell, and hearing in the newborn, as well as the perception of pain. All *cranial nerves* are present and myelinated except for the optic and olfactory nerves.

Sensory Functions

The newborn's sensory functions are remarkably well developed and have a significant effect on growth and development, including the attachment process.

Vision.   At birth the eye is structurally incomplete. The *fovea centralis* is not yet completely differentiated from the macula. The *ciliary muscles* are also immature, limiting the ability of the eyes to accommodate and focus on an object for any length of time. The infant can track and follow objects. The *pupils* react to light, the blink reflex is responsive to a minimal stimulus, and the corneal reflex is activated by a light touch. *Tear glands* usually do not begin to function until 2 to 4 weeks of age.

The newborn has the ability to focus momentarily on a bright or moving object that is within 20 cm (8 inches) and in the midline of the visual field. In fact, the infant's ability to fixate on coordinated movement is greater during the first hour of life than during the succeeding several days. *Visual acuity* is reported to be between 20/100 and 20/400, depending on the vision measurement techniques.

The infant also demonstrates visual preferences: medium colors (yellow, green, pink) over bright (red, orange, blue) or dim colors; black-and-white contrasting patterns, especially geometric shapes and checkerboards; large objects with medium complexity rather than small, complex objects; and reflecting objects over dull ones.

Hearing.   After the amniotic fluid has drained from the ears, the infant probably has *auditory acuity* similar to that of an adult. The neonate reacts to a loud sound of about 90 decibels with a startle reflex. The newborn's response to sounds of low frequency versus those of high frequency differs; the former, such as the sound of a heartbeat, metronome, or lullaby, tends to decrease an infant's motor activity and crying, whereas the latter elicits an alerting reaction. There is also an early sensitivity to the sound of human voices, although not specifically speech sounds. For example, infants younger than 3 days of age can discriminate the mother's voice from that of other females. As early as age 5 days, newborns can differentiate between stories repeated to them during the last trimester of pregnancy by their mother and the same stories recited after birth by a different woman.

The internal and middle *ear* are large at birth, but the external canal is small. The mastoid process and the bony part of the external canal have not yet developed. Consequently the tympanic membrane and facial nerve are very close to the surface and can be easily damaged.

Smell.   Newborns react to strong odors such as alcohol or vinegar by turning their heads away. Breast-fed infants are able to smell breast milk and will cry for their mothers when the breasts are engorged and leaking. Infants are also able to differentiate the breast milk of their mother from the breast milk of other women by smell. Maternal odors are believed to influence the attachment process and successful breast-feeding. Unnecessary routine washing of the breast may interfere with establishment of early breast-feeding.

Taste.   The newborn has the ability to distinguish between tastes. Various types of solutions elicit differing gusto-facial reflexes. A tasteless solution elicits no facial expression; a sweet solution elicits an eager suck and a look of satisfaction; a sour solution causes the usual puckering of the lips; and a bitter liquid produces an angry, upset expression. Newborns demonstrate preferential taste for glucose water to sterile water. During early childhood the taste buds are distributed mostly on the tip of the tongue.

Touch.   At birth the infant is able to perceive tactile sensation in any part of the body, although the face (especially the mouth), hands, and soles of the feet seem to be most sensitive. There is increasing documentation that touch and motion are essential to normal growth and development. Gentle patting of the back or rubbing of the abdomen usually elicits a calming response from the infant. However, painful stimuli, such as a pinprick, will elicit an upsetting response.

NURSING CARE OF THE NEWBORN AND FAMILY

● Assessment

The newborn requires thorough, skilled observation to ensure a satisfactory adjustment to extrauterine life. Physical assessment following delivery can be divided into four phases:

1 The initial assessment using the Apgar scoring system
2 Transitional assessment during the periods of reactivity
3 Assessment of gestational age
4 Systematic physical examination.

In addition, the nurse must be aware of behaviors that signal successful attachment between the infant and parents. Awareness of the expected normal findings during each assessment process helps the nurse recognize any deviation that may prevent the infant from progressing uneventfully through the early postnatal period. With increasingly shorter hospitalizations, the accomplishment of thorough newborn assessment and parent teaching has become a challenge.

Initial Assessment: Apgar Scoring

The most frequently used method to assess the newborn's immediate adjustment to extrauterine life is the *Apgar* scoring system (Papile, 2001). The score is based on observation of heart rate, respiratory effort, muscle tone, reflex irritability, and color (Table 8-1). Each item is given a score of 0, 1, or 2. Evaluations of all five categories are made at 1 and 5 minutes after birth and repeated until the infant's condition stabilizes. Total scores of 0 to 3 represent severe distress, scores of 4 to 6 signify moderate difficulty, and scores of 7 to 10 indicate absence of difficulty in adjusting to extrauterine life. The Apgar score is affected by the degree of physiologic immaturity, infection, congenital malformations, maternal sedation or analgesia, and neuromuscular disorders.

The Apgar score reflects the general condition of the infant at 1 and 5 minutes based on the five parameters described previously. The Apgar score is not a tool, however, that stands on its own to either interpret past events or predict future events linked to the infant's eventual neurologic or physical status. There has been a considerable amount of discussion and controversy in the past about Apgar scoring because of its misuse as an indicator for the presence or absence of perinatal asphyxia in the medicolegal field (American Academy of Pediatrics and American College of Obstetricians and Gynecologists, 1996, 2002). In addition, the Apgar score is not used to determine the newborn's need for resuscitation at birth.

TABLE 8-1 ■ Infant Evaluation at Birth—Apgar Scoring System

SIGN	0	1	2
Heart rate	Absent	Slow, <100	>100
Respiratory effort	Absent	Irregular, slow, weak cry	Good, strong cry
Muscle tone	Limp	Some flexion of extremities	Well flexed
Reflex irritability	No response	Grimace	Cry, sneeze
Color	Blue, pale	Body pink, extremities blue	Completely pink

ESTIMATION OF GESTATIONAL AGE BY MATURITY RATING

NEUROMUSCULAR MATURITY

A PHYSICAL MATURITY   MATURITY RATING

FIG. 8-1 ■ A, New Ballard Scale for newborn maturity rating. Expanded scale includes extremely premature infants and has been refined to improve accuracy in more mature infants. (A, From Ballard JL and others: New Ballard Score, expanded to include extremely premature infants, *J Pediatr* 119:418, 1991.)

Clinical Assessment of Gestational Age

Assessment of gestational age is an important criterion because perinatal morbidity and mortality are related to gestational age and birth weight. A frequently used method of determining gestational age is the simplified *Assessment of Gestational Age* by Ballard, Novack, and Driver (1979) (Fig. 8-1). This scale, an abbreviated version of the *Dubowitz scale,* can be used to measure gestational ages of infants between 35 and 42 weeks. It assesses six external physical and six neuromuscular signs. Each sign has a number score, and the cumulative score correlates with a maturity rating of from 26 to 44 weeks of gestation.

The "new" *Ballard Scale,* a revision of the original scale, can be used with newborns as young as 20 weeks of gestation. The tool has the same physical and neuromuscular sections but includes −1 and −2 scores that reflect signs of extremely premature infants, such as fused eyelids; imperceptible breast tissue; sticky, friable, transparent skin; no lanugo; and square-window (flexion of wrist) angle of greater than 90 degrees (see Fig. 8-1, *A,* and the description of the tests in Box 8-2). The examination of infants with a gestational age of 26 weeks or less should be performed at a postnatal age of less than 12 hours. For infants with a gestational age of at least 26 weeks, the examination can be performed up to 96 hours after birth. To ensure accuracy, it is recommended that the initial examination be performed within the first 48 hours of life. Neuromuscular adjustments after birth in extremely immature neonates require that a follow-up examination be performed to further validate neuromuscular criteria. The scale overestimates gestational age by 2 to 4 days in infants younger than 37 weeks of gestation, especially at gestational ages of 32 to 37 weeks (Ballard and others, 1991). In one study the Ballard scale was shown to overestimate gestational age of infants less that 28 weeks' gestation by as much as 1.2 to 3.3 weeks; therefore, other indices should be used as well (Donovan and others, 1999).

Weight Related to Gestational Age. The weight of the infant at birth also correlates with the incidence of perinatal morbidity and mortality. However, birth weight alone is a poor indicator of gestational age and fetal maturity. Maturity implies functional capacity—the degree to which the neonate's organ systems are able to adapt to the requirements of extrauterine life. Therefore, gestational age is more

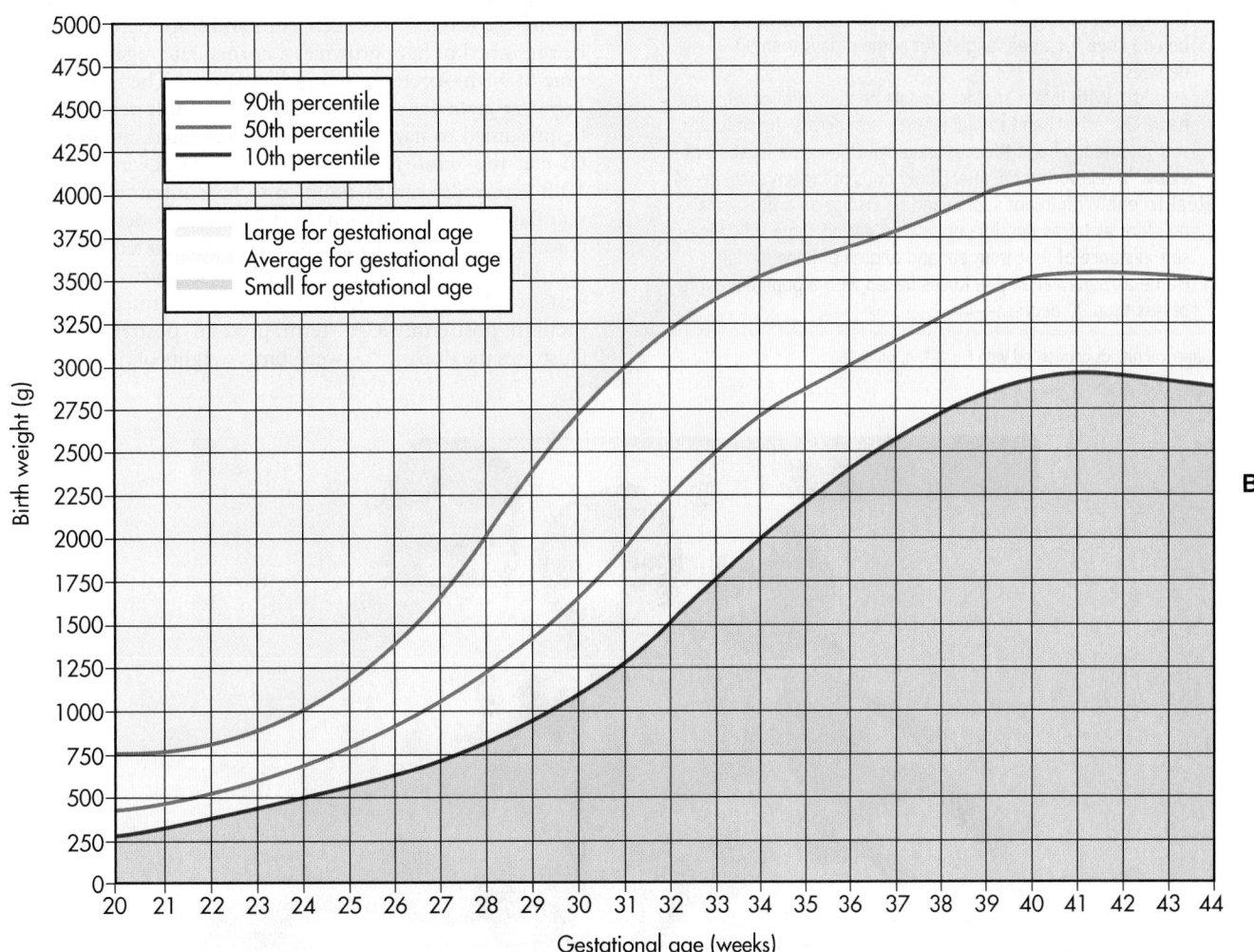

B

FIG. 8-1—*cont'd* ■ **B,** Intrauterine growth: birth weight percentiles based on live single births at gestational ages 20 to 44 weeks. (**B,** Data from Alexander GR and others: A United States national reference for fetal growth, *Obstet Gynecol* 87(2):163-168, 1996.)

closely related to fetal maturity than is birth weight. Because heredity influences a newborn's size, noting the size of other family members is part of the assessment process.

Intrauterine growth curves developed by Battaglia and Lubchenco (1967) have been used to classify infants according to birth weight and gestational age. Since that time, other

BOX 8-2 ■ Tests Used in Assessing Gestational Age

Posture. With infant quiet and in a supine position, observe degree of flexion in arms and legs. Muscle tone and degree of flexion increase with maturity. Full flexion of the arms and legs—4.*

Square window. With thumb supporting back of arm below wrist, apply gentle pressure with index and third fingers on dorsum of hand without rotating infant's wrist. Measure angle between base of thumb and forearm. Full flexion (hand lies flat on ventral surface of forearm)—4.

Arm recoil. With infant supine, fully flex both forearms on upper arms, hold for 5 seconds; pull down on hands to fully extend and rapidly release arms. Observe rapidity and intensity of recoil to a state of flexion. A brisk return to full flexion—4.

Popliteal angle. With infant supine and pelvis flat on a firm surface, flex lower leg on thigh and then flex thigh on abdomen. While holding knee with thumb and index finger, extend lower leg with index finger of other hand. Measure degree of angle behind knee (popliteal angle). An angle of less than 90 degrees—5.

Scarf sign. With infant supine, support head in midline with one hand; use other hand to pull infant's arm across the shoulder so that infant's hand touches shoulder. Determine location of elbow in relation to midline. Elbow does not reach midline—4.

Heel to ear. With infant supine and pelvis flat on a firm surface, pull foot as far as possible up toward ear on same side. Measure distance of foot from ear and degree of knee flexion (same as popliteal angle). Knees flexed with a popliteal angle of less than 90 degrees—4.

*Numerical ratings correspond with Fig. 8-1, *A*, on p. 180.

intrauterine growth charts have emerged to reflect a more heterogenous sample population than previously described (Cunningham and others, 2001). The primary intrauterine growth charts that provide national reference data include the work of Alexander and colleagues (1996), which is representative of more than 3.1 million live births in the United States and Thomas and colleagues (2000); and that of Arbuckle, Wilkins, and Sherman (1993), and Kramer and colleagues (2001), are representative of intrauterine growth among the Canadian population. Thomas and colleagues (2000) concluded that intrauterine growth measured by head circumference, birth weight, and length varies according to race and gender. These researchers also found that altitude did not seem to significantly affect birth weight as has been suggested by other authors. It is recommended that the reader access and use the most current intrauterine growth chart specific to the referent population being evaluated.

Classification of infants at birth by both ***birthweight*** and ***gestational age*** provides a more satisfactory method for predicting mortality risks and providing guidelines for management of the neonate than estimating gestational age or birth weight alone. The infant's birth weight, length, and head circumference are plotted on standardized graphs that identify normal values for gestational age (for birth weight see Fig. 8-1, *B*). The infant whose weight is ***appropriate for gestational age (AGA)*** (between 10th and 90th percentiles) can be presumed to have grown at a normal rate regardless of the time of birth—preterm, term, or postterm. The infant who is ***large for gestational age (LGA)*** (above 90th percentile) can be presumed to have grown at an accelerated rate during fetal life; the ***small-for-gestational-age (SGA)*** infant (below 10th percentile) can be assumed to have intrauterine growth retardation or delay. When gestational age is determined according to the Ballard scale, the newborn will fall into one of the following nine possible categories for birth weight and gestational age: AGA—term, preterm, postterm; SGA—term, preterm, postterm; LGA—term, preterm, postterm. Fig. 8-2 illustrates the disparity between birth weights of three preterm

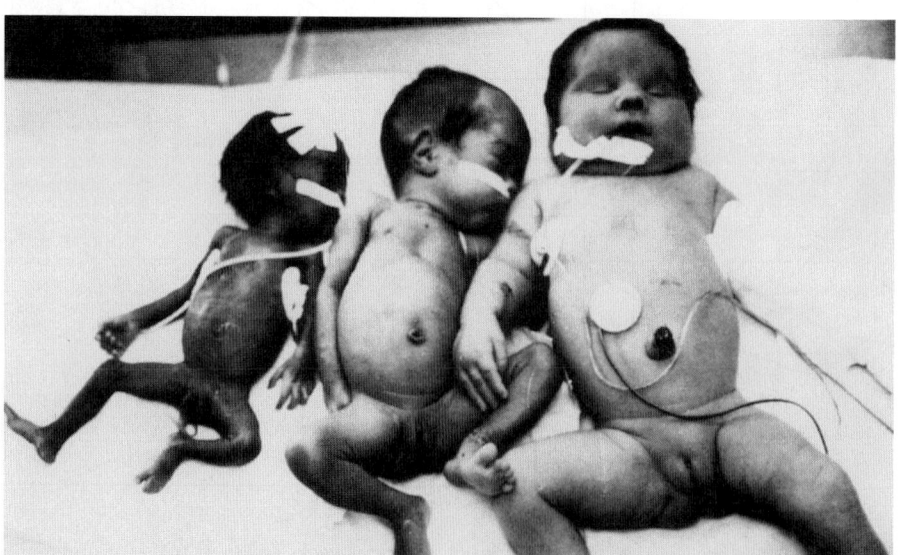

FIG. 8-2 ■ Three infants, same gestational age, weight 600, 1400, and 2750 g, respectively, from left to right. (From Korones SB: *High-risk newborn infants: the basis for intensive nursing care,* ed 4, St Louis, 1986, Mosby.)

infants of the same gestational age of 32 weeks. The infant with a birth weight of 600 g has more than a 50% mortality, the infant weighing 1400 g has a 25% to 50% mortality, and the infant weighing 2750 g has less than a 4% mortality. Therefore, birth weight influences mortality—the lower the birth weight and gestational age, the higher the mortality.

General Measurements. Several important measurements of the newborn have significance when compared with each other as well as when recorded over time on a graph. For the full-term infant, average *head circumference* is between 33 and 35.5 cm (13 to 14 inches). Head circumference may be somewhat less, immediately after birth, because of the molding process that occurs during a vaginal delivery. Usually by the second or third day the skull is normal in size and contour.

Chest circumference is 30.5 to 33 cm (12 to 13 inches). Head circumference is usually about 2 to 3 cm (about 1 inch) greater than chest circumference. Because of the molding of the head during delivery, these measurements may initially appear equal.

Head circumference may also be compared with crown-to-rump length, or sitting height. *Crown-to-rump* measurements are usually 31 to 35 cm (12.5 to 14 inches) and are approximately equal to head circumference. The relationship of the head and crown-to-rump measurements is more reliable than that of the head and chest.

Neonatal head circumference and crown-to-rump length may provide a more accurate means for identifying infants at risk; head circumference has been shown to be equal to or up to 1 cm more than crown-to-rump length in 62% of the infants examined and determined to be normocephalic.

Abdominal circumference in the newborn may be measured just above the level of the umbilicus, because the umbilical cord is still attached, making measurements across the umbilicus too variable in newborns. Measuring the abdominal circumference below the umbilical region is unsuitable because bladder status may affect the reading. In the event of abdominal distention, serial measurements are taken to determine changes in girth.

Head-to-heel length is also measured. Because of the usual flexed position of the infant, it is important to extend the leg completely when measuring total body length. The average length of the newborn is 48 to 53 cm (19 to 21 inches) (Fig. 8-3).

Measure *body weight* soon after birth because weight loss occurs fairly rapidly. Normally the neonate loses about 10% of the birth weight by 3 to 4 days of age because of loss of excessive extracellular fluid and meconium, as well as limited food intake, especially in breast-fed infants. The birth weight is usually regained by the tenth day of life. Most newborns weigh 2700 to 4000 g (6 to 9 pounds), the average weight being about 3400 g (7.5 pounds). Accurate birth weights and lengths are important because they provide a baseline for assessment of future growth.

Another category of measurements is vital signs. *Axillary temperatures* are taken because insertion of a thermometer into the rectum can potentially cause perforation of the mucosa if performed incorrectly (see Fig. 7-7, B). Core body temperature varies according to the periods of reactivity but is usually 36.5° to 37.6° C (97.7° to 99.7° F). Skin temperature is slightly lower than core body temperature. There-

fore, axillary temperature may be less than rectal temperature, although the difference is small (as little as 0.2° F) between axillary and rectal sites. Because brown adipose tissue is located in the axillary pocket, axillary readings may be elevated whenever nonshivering thermogenesis (NST) occurs. However, axillary readings may be normal in cold-stressed infants when NST is not triggered or is overwhelmed.

The single best method for determining the newborn infant's temperature in any given situation remains elusive when considering the available studies. There is controversy regarding the accuracy of tympanic membrane sensors for measuring neonatal temperature. Studies have found tympanic membrane temperatures to have high variability according to neonatal environment (bassinet or open crib, radiant warmer, and incubator) (Leick-Rude and Bloom, 1998) and limited usefulness for use in critically ill neonates (Weiss, Poeltler, and Gocka, 1993), and at least one study concluded that tympanic membrane temperatures were unacceptable for detecting fever in children younger than 6 years of age (Lanham and others, 1999). Infrared axillary and digital thermometers are used in many neonatal units because they give rapid readings and are easy to clean; studies demonstrate their usefulness in well term newborns (Sganga and others, 2000), whereas accuracy with critically ill neonates is less predictable (Seguin and Terry, 1999; Wilshaw and others, 1999). Skin temperature readings have also been found to vary with probe site placement, bed type, and environmental temperature, and the use of blankets, clothing, and nesting devices (Leick-Rude and Bloom, 1998). Thomas (2003) found considerable variation between axillary and abdominal temperature measurements in a small sample of term newborns and suggests that trends of temperature measurements be evaluated over time. Temporal artery thermometers do not appear to provide an adequate measurement of body temperature in infants when compared with rectal thermometer readings (Greenes and Fleischer, 2001).

In most studies regarding newborn temperature, the glass mercury thermometer is the gold standard against which other methods are compared. There is no universal agreement on placement times for glass thermometers, although 3 minutes for rectal temperature and 5 minutes for axillary temperature are considered to be adequate.

Nurses must be cognizant of the many variables involved (site—axillary, rectal, tympanic, skin; skin blood flow at site of measurement; environment—radiant warmer, open crib,

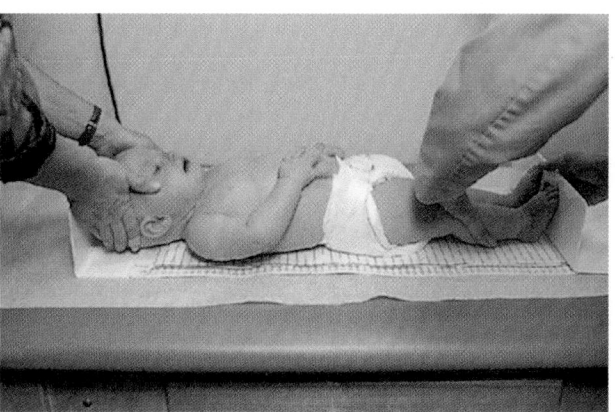

FIG. 8-3 ■ Measurement of infant length.

incubator, clothing, or nesting; purpose—fever, possible sepsis, in which case the temperature may be lower than normal in newborns, and thermoregulation in the transition phase; instrument—electronic, digital, infrared) and able to make clear clinical decisions based on accurate and objective data. Further research is needed to perfect thermometers that accurately reflect the infant's core temperature in order to effectively plan nursing care and maintain a stable temperature.

Pulse and *respirations* also vary according to the periods of reactivity and the infant's behaviors but are usually in the range of 120 to 140 beats/min and 30 to 60 breaths/min, respectively. Both are counted for a full 60 seconds to detect irregularities in rate or rhythm. The heart rate is taken apically with a stethoscope, and the femoral arteries are palpated for equality of strength or fullness.

Measurement of *blood pressure* is recommended; it provides useful baseline data and may indicate cardiac problems. Blood pressure is most easily and accurately assessed using oscillometry (Dinamap), although the device is less reliable when mean arterial pressure is below 40 mm Hg (Chia and others, 1990) (Fig. 8-4). The average oscillometric systolic/diastolic pressure is 65/41 at 1 to 3 days of age. Compare blood pressure in the upper and lower extremities, which should be equal.

A suggested schedule for monitoring heart, respiratory rate, and temperature is on admission to the nursery, once every 30 minutes until the newborn has been stable for 2 hours (American Academy of Pediatrics and American College of Obstetricians and Gynecologists, 2002), then once every 8 hours until discharge. However, this schedule may vary according to institutional policy. Any change in the infant, such as in color, breathing, muscle tone, or behavior, necessitates more frequent monitoring.

! NURSING ALERT

Although uncommon, the presence of neonatal hypertension may be a sign of a significant underlying problem such as renal, cardiac or thromboembolic pathology, or associated with a medication treatment regimen. Neonatal hypertension is brought to the primary practitioner's attention for further evaluation.

General Appearance.   Before each body system is assessed, it is important to describe the general *posture* and behavior of the newborn. The overall appearance yields valuable clues to the physical status of the infant.

In the full-term neonate the posture is one of complete *flexion* as a result of in utero position. Most infants are born in a vertex presentation with the head flexed and the chin resting on the upper chest, the arms flexed with the hands clenched, the legs flexed at the knees and hips, and the feet dorsiflexed. The vertebral column is also flexed. It is important to recognize any deviation from this very characteristic fetal position.

The infant's *behavior* is carefully noted, especially the degree of alertness, drowsiness, and irritability, which are common signs of neurologic problems. Some questions to mentally ask when assessing behavior include the following:

- Is the infant awakened easily by a loud noise?
- Is the infant comforted by rocking, sucking, or cuddling?

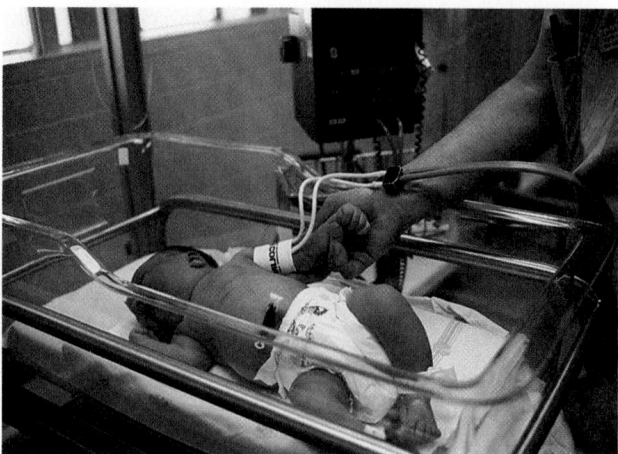

FIG. 8-4 ■ Measurement of blood pressure using oscillometry.

- Do there seem to be periods of deep and light sleep?
- When awake, does the infant seem satisfied after a feeding?
- What stimuli elicit responses from the infant?
- When disturbed, how much does the infant protest?

Skin.   The *texture* of the newborn's skin is velvety smooth and puffy, especially about the eyes, the legs, the dorsal aspect of the hands and the feet, and the scrotum or labia. Skin *color* depends on racial and familial background and varies greatly among newborns. In general, the Caucasian infant is usually pink to red; the African-American newborn may appear a pinkish or yellowish brown. Infants of Hispanic descent may have an olive tint or a slight yellow cast to the skin. Infants of Asian descent may be a rosy or yellowish tan. The color of Native American newborns depends on the tribe and can vary from a light pink to a dark, reddish brown. By the second or third day the skin turns to its more natural tone and is drier and flakier. Several other color changes that may be noted on the skin are described later in this chapter (see Table 8-4).

Head.   General observation of the *contour* of the head is important, because molding occurs in almost all vaginal deliveries. In a vertex delivery the head is usually flattened at the forehead, with the apex rising and forming a point at the end of the parietal bones and the posterior skull or occiput dropping abruptly. The usual, more oval contour of the head is apparent by 1 to 2 days after birth. The change in shape occurs because the bones of the cranium are not fused, allowing for overlapping of the edges of these bones to accommodate to the size of the birth canal during delivery. Such molding usually does not occur in infants born by cesarean section.

Six bones—the frontal, occipital, two parietals, and two temporals—make up the cranium. Between the junction of these bones are bands of connective tissue called *sutures.* At the junction of the sutures are wider spaces of unossified membranous tissue called *fontanels.* The two most prominent fontanels in infants are the *anterior fontanel,* formed by the junction of the sagittal, coronal, and frontal sutures, and the *posterior fontanel,* formed by the junction of the sagittal and lambdoid sutures (Fig. 8-5, *A*).

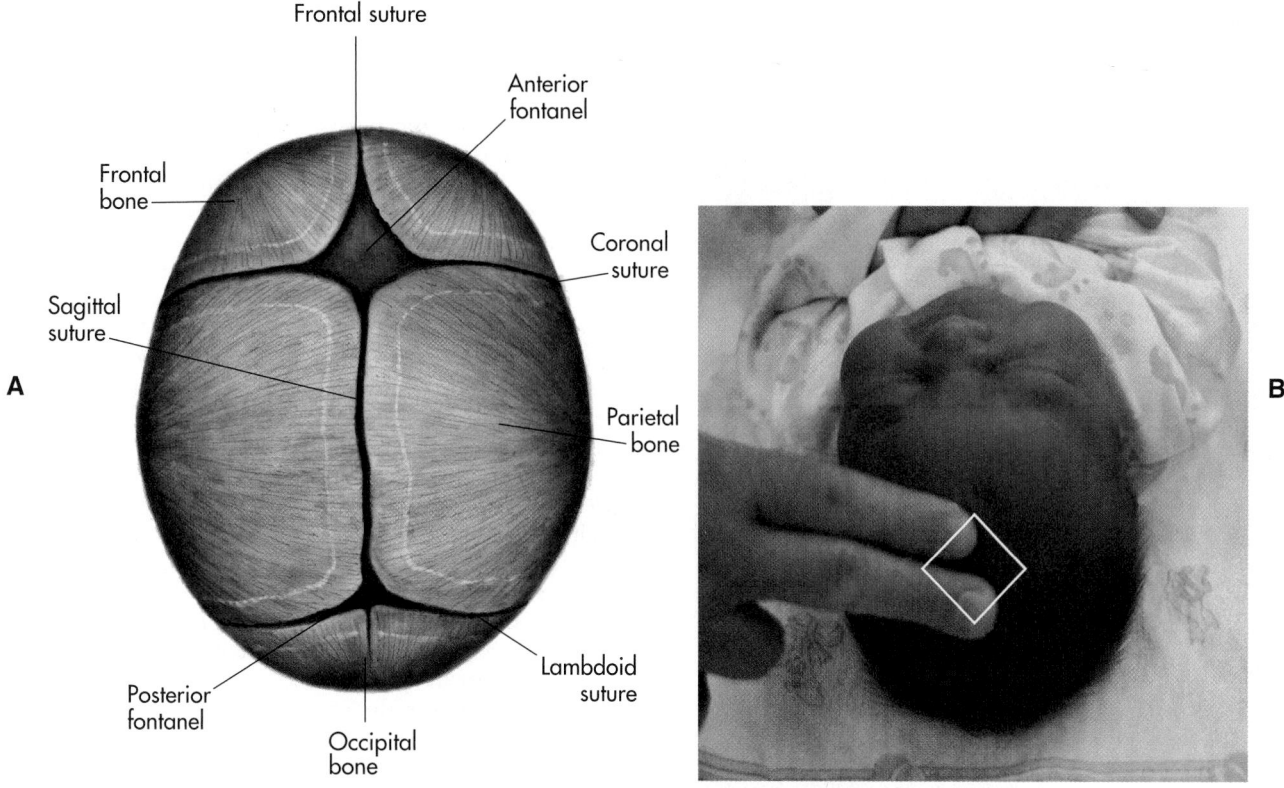

FIG. 8-5 ■ **A,** Location of sutures and fontanels. **B,** Palpating anterior fontanel.

The location of the suture is easily remembered because the coronal suture "crowns" the head and the sagittal suture "separates" the head.

The skull is palpated for all patent sutures and fontanels, noting size, shape, molding, or abnormal closure. The sutures feel like cracks between the skull bones, and the fontanels feel like wider *soft spots* at the junction of the sutures. These are palpated by using the tip of the index finger and running it along the ends of the bones (Fig. 8-5, *B*).

The anterior fontanel is diamond shaped and measures anywhere from barely palpable to 4 to 5 cm (about 2 inches) at its widest point (from bone to bone, rather than from suture to suture). The posterior fontanel is easily located by following the sagittal suture toward the occiput. The posterior fontanel is triangular, usually measuring between 0.5 and 1 cm (less than ½ inch) at its widest part. The fontanels should feel flat, firm, and well demarcated against the bony edges of the skull. Frequently pulsations are visible at the anterior fontanel. Coughing, crying, or lying down may temporarily cause the fontanels to bulge and become more taut.

Palpate the skull for any unusual masses or prominences, particularly those resulting from birth trauma, such as caput succedaneum or cephalhematoma (see Chapter 9). Because of the pliability of the skull, exerting pressure at the margin of the parietal and occipital bones along the lambdoid suture may produce a snapping sensation similar to the indentation of a Ping-Pong ball. This phenomenon, known as

physiologic craniotabes, may be found normally, especially in newborns of breech birth, but also may indicate hydrocephalus, congenital syphilis, or rickets.

Assess the degree of *head control.* Although *head lag* is normal in the newborn, the degree of ability to control the head in certain positions should be recognized. If the supine infant is pulled from the arms into a semi-Fowler position, marked head lag and hyperextension are noted (Fig. 8-6, *A*). However, as the infant is brought forward into a sitting position, the infant will attempt to control the head in an upright position. As the head falls forward onto the chest, many infants will attempt to right it into the erect position. Also, if the infant is held in ventral suspension (i.e., held prone above and parallel to the examining surface), the infant will hold the head in a straight line with the spinal column (Fig. 8-6, *B*). When lying on the abdomen, the newborn has the ability to lift the head slightly, turning it from side to side. Marked head lag is seen in neonates with Down syndrome, prematurity, hypoxia, and brain damage.

Eyes.   Because newborns tend to have their eyes tightly closed, it is best to begin the examination of the eyes by observing the lids for edema, which is normally present for the first 2 days after delivery. The eyes are observed for symmetry. *Tears* may be present at birth, but purulent discharge from the eyes shortly after birth is abnormal. To visualize the surface structures of the eye, the infant is held supine, and the head is gently lowered. The eyes will usually open, similar to the mechanism of a doll's eyes. The *sclera* should be white and clear.

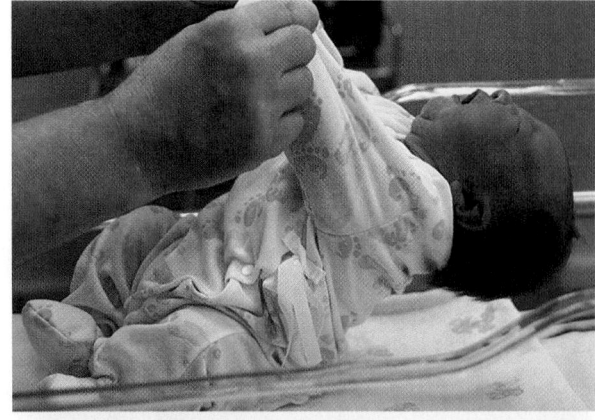

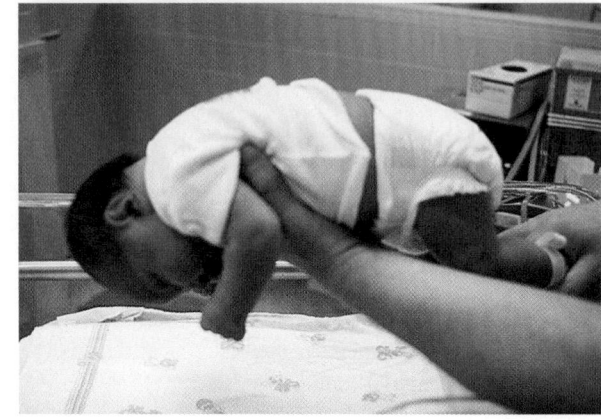

FIG. 8-6 ■ Head control in infant. **A,** Inability to hold head erect when pulled to sitting position. **B,** Ability to hold head erect when placed in ventral suspension.

The cornea is examined for the presence of any opacities or haziness. The *corneal reflex* is normally present at birth but is generally not elicited unless brain or eye damage is suspected. The pupil will usually respond to light by constricting. The pupils are normally malaligned. A searching *nystagmus* is common. *Strabismus* is a normal finding because of the lack of binocularity. The color of the iris is noted. Most light-skinned newborns have slate gray or dark blue eyes, whereas dark-skinned infants have brown eyes.

A funduscopic examination is quite difficult to perform because of the infant's tendency to keep the eyes tightly closed. However, a *red reflex* should be elicited (see Chapter 7).

> **NURSING TIP**
>
> To elicit a red reflex place, the infant in a dark room. In an alert state many newborns will open the eyes in a supported sitting position.

Ears.   The ears are examined for position, structure, and auditory function. The top of the pinna should lie in a horizontal plane to the outer canthus of the eye (see Fig. 7-16). The pinna is often flattened against the side of the head from pressure in utero. An otoscopic examination is ordinarily not performed because the *canals* are filled with vernix caseosa and amniotic fluid, making visualization of the *tympanic membrane* difficult.

Auditory ability is tested by a number of objective hearing tests (see p. 156). Making a loud noise close to the infant's head may or may not elicit a response; the lack of a response, however, is not a definite indication of hearing loss. The *startle reflex* (see Table 8-2) may be observed when there is a sudden loud noise near the infant or the bassinet is accidentally bumped suddenly, but this will often depend on the infant's state at the time.

Nose.   The nose is usually flattened after birth, and bruises are common. Patency of the *nasal canals* can be assessed by holding the hand over the infant's mouth and one canal and noting the passage of air through the unobstructed opening. If nasal patency is questionable, it is reported, because most newborns are obligatory nose breathers. Sneezing and thin white mucus are common.

Mouth and Throat.   An external defect of the mouth such as cleft lip is readily apparent; however, the internal structures require careful inspection. The *palate* is normally highly arched and somewhat narrow. Rarely teeth may be present. A common finding is *Epstein pearls,* small, white, epithelial cysts along both sides of the midline of the hard palate. They are insignificant and disappear in several weeks.

The *frenulum* of the upper lip is a band of thick, pink tissue that lies under the inner surface of the upper lip and extends to the maxillary alveolar ridge. It is particularly evident when the infant yawns or smiles. It disappears as the maxilla grows.

The *lingual frenulum* attaches the underside of the tongue to the lower palate midway between the ventral surface of the tongue and the tip. In some cases a tight lingual frenulum, formerly referred to as tongue-tie, may restrict adequate sucking. Further evaluation may be required to ascertain adequate sucking, particularly in breast-fed infants. A frenuloplasty may be required if the lingual frenulum is tight enough to impair successful breastfeeding (Barclay, 2002; Ballard, Auer, and Khoury, 2002).

Elicit the *sucking reflex* by placing a nipple or non-latex gloved finger in the infant's mouth. The infant should exhibit a strong, vigorous suck. The *rooting reflex* is elicited by stroking the cheek and noting the infant's response of turning toward the stimulated side and sucking (Fig. 8-7).

The *uvula* can be inspected while the infant is crying and the chin is depressed. However, it may be retracted upward and backward during crying. Tonsillar tissue is generally not seen in the newborn. *Natal teeth,* teeth present at birth, as opposed to *neonatal teeth,* which erupt during the first month of life), are seen infrequently and erupt chiefly at the position of the lower incisors. Teeth are reported because they are frequently found with developmental abnormalities and syndromes, including cleft lip and palate. Most natal teeth are loosely attached. However, current thinking suggests preserving them until they exfoliate naturally (McDonald and Avery, 2000), unless the tooth is attached loosely or breast-feeding is impaired from the neonate biting the breast.

Neck.   Because the newborn's neck is short and covered with folds of tissue, adequate assessment of the neck requires allowing the head to fall gently backward in hyperextension

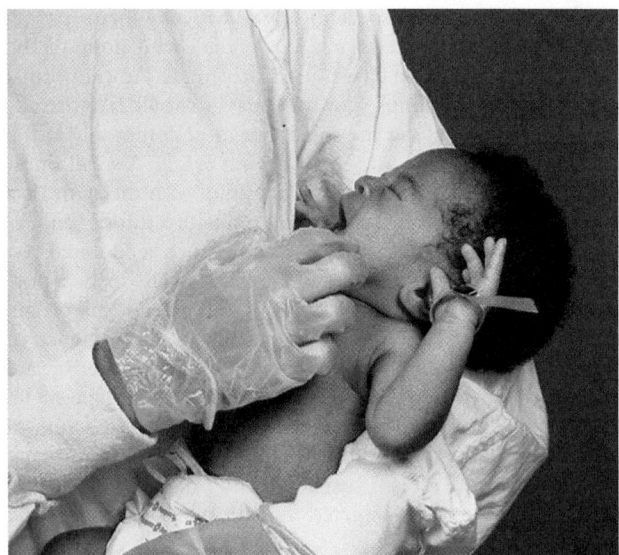

FIG. 8-7 ■ Eliciting rooting reflex. (From Seidel HM and others: *Mosby's guide to physical examination*, ed 3, St Louis, 1995, Mosby.)

while the back is supported in a slightly raised position. Observe for range of motion, shape, and any abnormal masses, and palpate and compare each clavicle for possible fractures.

Chest.   The *shape* of the newborn's chest is almost circular because the anteroposterior and lateral diameters are equal. The ribs are very flexible, and slight intercostal retractions are normally seen on inspiration. The xiphoid process is commonly visible as a small protrusion at the end of the sternum. The sternum is generally raised and slightly curved.

Inspect the *breasts* for size, shape, and nipple formation, location, and number. Breast enlargement appears in many newborns of either sex by the second or third day and is caused by maternal hormones. Occasionally a milky substance, sometimes called *"witch's milk,"* is secreted by the infant's breasts by the end of the first week. *Supernumerary nipples* may be found on the chest or even in the axilla.

Lungs.   The normal *respirations* of the newborn are irregular and abdominal, and the rate is between 30 and 60 breaths/min. Pauses in respiration less than 20 seconds in duration are considered normal. After the initial forceful breaths required to initiate respiration, subsequent breaths should be easy and fairly regular in rhythm. Occasional irregularities occur in relation to crying, sleeping, and feeding.

Perform auscultation when the infant is quiet. Bronchial breath sounds should be equal bilaterally. Any differences in auscultatory findings between symmetric sites is reported. *Crackles* soon after birth indicate the presence of fluid, which represent the normal transition of the lungs to extrauterine life. However, wheezes, persistence of medium or coarse crackles after the first few hours of life, and stridor should be reported for further investigation.

Heart.   *Heart rate* is auscultated and may range from 100 to 180 beats/min shortly after birth and, when the infant's condition has stabilized, from 120 to 140 beats/min. The

point of maximum intensity (PMI) may be palpated and is usually found in the fourth to fifth intercostal space, medial to the left midclavicular line. The PMI gives some indication of the location of the heart, which may be displaced in conditions such as congenital diaphragmatic hernia or pneumothorax. *Dextrocardia,* an anomaly wherein the heart is on the right side of the body, is reported, because the abdominal organs may also be reversed, with associated circulatory abnormalities.

NURSING TIP

Because auscultation of neonatal breath sounds and heart tones is often difficult for the untrained ear, practice auscultating one parameter at a time. Close your eyes and mentally block out the extraneous sounds heard, such as room noise or neonatal movement; offer the newborn a pacifier or a nonlatex gloved finger. Auscultation of a murmur and decreased air movement in specific lung fields requires patience and practice; it may require auscultating the heart tones or breath sounds for 1 to 3 minutes each.

Auscultation of the specific components of the *heart sounds* is difficult because of the rapid rate and effective transmission of respiratory sounds. However, the *first (S1)* and *second (S2)* sounds should be clear and well-defined; the second sound is somewhat higher in pitch and sharper than the first. A *murmur* is frequently heard in the newborn, especially over the base of the heart or at the left sternal border in the third or fourth interspace. Ordinarily a murmur is not associated with specific cardiac defects, but frequently represents the incomplete functional closure of fetal shunts. However, always record and report any murmur or other unusual sounds.

Abdomen.   The normal *contour* of the abdomen is cylindric and usually prominent with few visible veins. Bowel sounds are heard within the first 15 to 20 minutes after birth. Visible peristaltic waves may be observed in some newborns.

Inspect the *umbilical cord* to determine the presence of two arteries, which look like papular structures, and one vein, which has a larger lumen than the arteries and a thinner vessel wall. At birth the cord appears bluish white and moist. After clamping, it begins to dry and appears a dull, yellowish brown. It progressively shrivels in size and turns greenish black.

If the umbilical cord appears unusually large in diameter at the base, inspect for the presence of a hematoma or small omphalocele. If the cord is clamped over an existing omphalocele, part of the intestine will be clamped, causing tissue necrosis. One practical rule of thumb is to cut the cord distally 4 to 5 inches from a questionable enlargement until further examination is carried out by a practitioner. The extra length can later be cut once no pathology has been identified.

NURSING ALERT

A cord that is draining and erythematous at the base should be investigated by the primary practitioner. The cord undergoes a process of dry gangrene decay, which has an odor; therefore, odor alone may not be a reliable index of suspicion for omphalitis.

Palpate after inspecting the abdomen. The *liver* is normally palpable 1 to 3 cm (about ½ to 1 inch) below the right costal margin. The tip of the *spleen* can sometimes be felt, but a palpable spleen more than 1 cm below the left costal margin suggests enlargement and warrants further investigation. Although both *kidneys* should be palpated, this maneuver requires considerable practice. When felt, the lower half of the right kidney and the tip of the left kidney are 1 to 2 cm above the umbilicus.

During examination of the lower abdomen, it is particularly important to palpate for *femoral pulses,* which should be strong and equal bilaterally.

Female Genitalia.

Normally, the *labia minora, labia majora,* and *clitoris* are edematous, especially after a breech delivery. However, the labia and clitoris must be carefully inspected to identify any evidence of ambiguous genitalia or other abnormalities. Normally, in a female, the urethral opening is located behind the clitoris.

Virtually all female newborns have hymens, and this fact should be noted on the chart for future reference in case of concern regarding sexual abuse. A *hymenal tag* is occasionally visible from the posterior opening of the vagina. It is composed of tissue from the hymen and the labia minora. It usually disappears in several weeks. Generally, the vaginal vault is not inspected.

Vaginal discharge may be noted during the first week of life. This *pseudomenstruation* is a manifestation of the abrupt decrease of maternal hormones and usually disappears by 2 to 4 weeks. Fecal discharge from the vaginal opening indicates a rectovaginal fistula and is always reported. Vernix caseosa may be present in large amounts between the labia.

Male Genitalia.

The *penis* is inspected for the location of the urethral opening, which is located at the tip. However, the opening may be totally covered by the prepuce, or foreskin, which covers the glans penis. A tight prepuce is a very common finding in the newborn. It should not be forcefully retracted; locating the urinary meatus is usually possible without retracting the foreskin. *Smegma,* a white cheesy substance, is commonly found around the glans penis, under the foreskin. Small, white, firm lesions called *epithelial pearls* may be seen at the tip of the prepuce. An erection is common in the newborn.

The *scrotum* may be large, edematous, and pendulous in the full-term neonate, especially in the infant born in breech position. It is more deeply pigmented in dark-skinned races. A noncommunicating *hydrocele* commonly occurs unilaterally and disappears within a few months. Always palpate the scrotum for the presence of *testes* (see Chapter 7). In small newborns, particularly preterm infants, the undescended testes may be palpable within the inguinal canal. Absence of the testes may also be a sign of ambiguous genitalia, especially when accompanied by a small scrotum and penis. *Inguinal hernias* may or may not be manifested immediately after birth. A hernia is more easily detected when the infant is crying. Palpable *lymph nodes* are most commonly found in the inguinal area.

Back and Anus.

Inspect the *spine* with the infant prone. The shape of the spine is gently rounded, with none of the characteristic S-shaped curves seen later in life. Any abnormal openings, masses, dimples, or soft areas are noted. A protruding sac anywhere along the spine, but most commonly in the sacral area, indicates some type of *spina bifida.* A small sinus, which may or may not be communicating with the spine, is a *pilonidal sinus.* It is frequently covered with a tuft of hair. Although it may have no pathologic significance, a pilonidal cyst may indicate the existence of spina bifida occulta or be a portal of entry into the spinal column. With the infant still prone, note symmetry of the gluteal folds. Report any evidence of asymmetry; tests for developmental dysplasia of the hip are performed by trained (or skilled) examiners (see Chapter 31).

The presence of an anal orifice and passage of meconium during the first 24 to 48 hours of life indicates *anal patency.* If an imperforate anus is suspected and not readily visible, a small catheter may be inserted into the anal opening by the practitioner.

> **! NURSING ALERT**
>
> The presence of meconium or stool in the rectal area is not an indication of rectal patency; a fistula may exist wherein stool is evacuated via the vagina, scrotum, or raphe. Therefore, it is imperative that anal patency be checked with a small rubber catheter should any doubt regarding patency exist.

Extremities.

Examine the extremities for symmetry, range of motion, and reflexes. Count the fingers and toes, and note supernumerary digits *(polydactyly)* or fusion of digits *(syndactyly).* A partial syndactyly between the second and third toes is a common variation seen in otherwise normal infants. The nail beds should be pink, although slight blueness is evident in acrocyanosis.

The palms of the hands should have the usual creases (see Fig. 7-10). The full-term newborn usually has creases covering the entire sole of the foot. The soles of the feet are flat with prominent fat pads.

Observe *range of motion* of the extremities throughout the entire examination. The newborn will demonstrate full range of motion in the elbow, hip, shoulder, and knee joints. Movements should be symmetric, smooth, and unrestricted. The absence of arm movement signals a potential birth injury paralysis such as Klumpke or Erb-Duchenne palsy. An asymmetric or partial Moro reflex should alert the practitioner to further evaluate upper extremity mobility. Examine the lower extremities for limb length, symmetry, and hip abduction and flexion.

Also assess *muscle tone.* By attempting to extend a flexed extremity, determine if tone is equal bilaterally. Extension of any extremity is usually met with resistance, and when released, the extremity returns to its previous flexed position. *Hypotonia* suggests some degree of hypoxia or neurologic disorder and is common in Down syndrome. *Asymmetry* of muscle tone may indicate a degree of paralysis from brain damage or nerve damage. Failure to move the lower limbs suggests a spinal cord lesion or injury. *Tremors, twitches,* and *myoclonic jerks* characterize neonatal seizures or may indicate neonatal narcotic withdrawal syndrome. Quivering or momentary tremors are usually normal.

Two reflexes are elicited. The first is the *grasp reflex.* Touching the palms of the hands or soles of the feet near the base of the digits causes flexion or grasping (Fig. 8-8, *A*). The other is the *Babinski reflex.* Stroking the outer sole of the foot upward from the heel across the ball of the foot causes the big toe to dorsiflex and the other toes to hyperextend (Fig. 8-8, *B*).

Neurologic System.   Assessing neurologic status is a critical part of the physical examination of the newborn. Much of the neurologic testing takes place during evaluation of body systems, such as eliciting localized reflexes and observing posture, muscle tone, head control, and movement. However, several important mass (total body) reflexes also need to be elicited. Test these at the end of the examination, because they may disturb the infant and interfere with auscultation. These reflexes, as well as several local reflexes, are described in Table 8-2. Record and report the absence, asymmetry, persistence, or weakness of a reflex.

Transitional Assessment: Periods of Reactivity

The newborn exhibits behavioral and physiologic characteristics that may at first appear to be signs of stress. However, during the initial 24 hours, changes in heart rate, respiration, motor activity, color, mucus production, and bowel activity occur in an orderly, predictable sequence that is normal and indicates lack of stress.

For 6 to 8 hours after birth, the newborn is in the *first period of reactivity.* During the first 30 minutes the infant is very alert, cries vigorously, may suck the fist greedily, and appears very interested in the environment. At this time the neonate's eyes are usually open, suggesting that this is an excellent opportunity for mother, father, and child to see each other. Because the newborn has a vigorous suck, this

is also an opportune time to begin breast-feeding. The infant will usually grasp the nipple quickly, satisfying both mother and infant. This is particularly important for nurses to remember, because after this initially highly active state the infant may be quite sleepy and uninterested in sucking. Physiologically, the respiratory rate during this period is as high as 80 breaths/min, crackles may be heard, heart rate reaches 180 beats/min, bowel sounds are active, mucus secretions are increased, and temperature may decrease.

After this initial stage of alertness and activity, the infant enters the *second stage* of the first reactive period, which generally lasts 2 to 4 hours. Heart and respiratory rates decrease, temperature continues to fall, mucus production decreases, and urine or stool is usually not passed. The infant is in a state of sleep and relative calm. Any attempt at stimulation usually elicits a minimal response. Because of the continued decrease in body temperature, undressing or bathing is avoided during this time.

The *second period of reactivity* begins when the infant awakes from this deep sleep; it lasts about 2 to 5 hours and provides another excellent opportunity for child and parents to interact. The infant is again alert and responsive, heart and respiratory rates increase, the gag reflex is active, gastric and respiratory secretions are increased, and passage of meconium frequently occurs. This period is usually over when the amount of respiratory mucus has decreased. After this stage is a period of stabilization of physiologic systems and a vacillating pattern of sleep and activity.

Behavioral Assessment

Another important area of assessment is observation of behavior. Infants' behavior helps shape their environment, and their ability to react to various stimuli affects how others relate to them. The principal areas of behavior for newborns are sleep, wakefulness, and activity, such as crying.

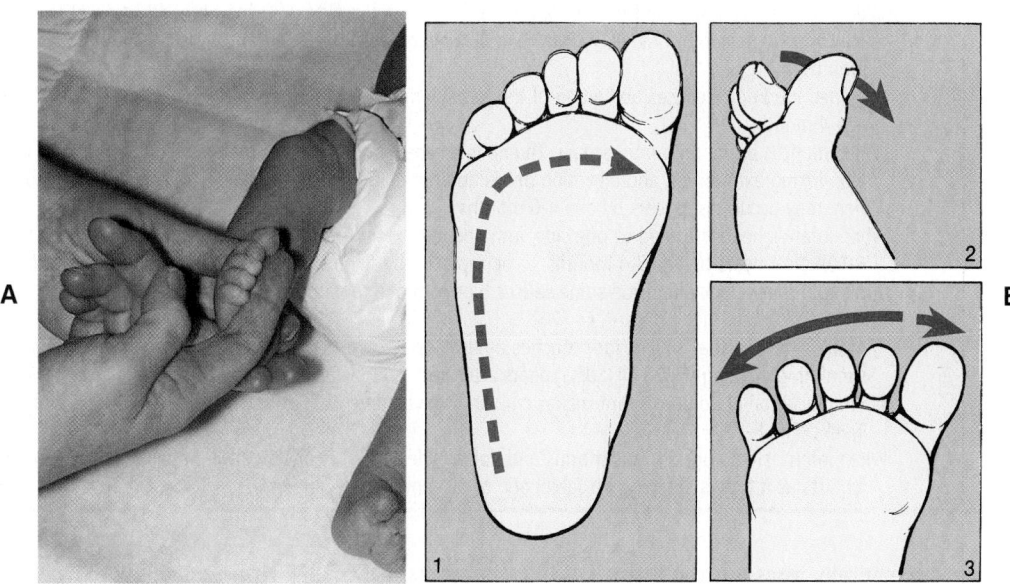

FIG. 8-8 ■ **A,** Plantar or grasp reflex. **B,** Babinski reflex. 1, Direction of stroke. 2, Dorsiflexion of big toe. 3, Fanning of toes. (**A,** From Zitelli BJ, Davis HW: *Atlas of pediatric physical diagnosis,* ed 4, St Louis 2002, Mosby.)

TABLE 8-2 ■ Assessment of Reflexes in the Newborn

REFLEXES	EXPECTED BEHAVIORAL RESPONSES
LOCALIZED	
Eyes	
Blinking or corneal reflex	Infant blinks at sudden appearance of a bright light or at approach of an object toward cornea; persists throughout life
Pupillary	Pupil constricts when a bright light shines toward it; persists throughout life
Doll's eye	As head is moved slowly to right or left, eyes lag behind and do not immediately adjust to new position of head; disappears as fixation develops; if persists, indicates neurologic damage
Nose	
Sneeze	Spontaneous response of nasal passages to irritation or obstruction; persists throughout life
Glabellar	Tapping briskly on glabella (bridge of nose) causes eyes to close tightly
Mouth and Throat	
Sucking	Infant begins strong sucking movements of circumoral area in response to stimulation; persists throughout infancy, even without stimulation, such as during sleep
Gag	Stimulation of posterior pharynx by food, suction, or passage of a tube causes infant to gag; persists throughout life
Rooting	Touching or stroking the cheek along side of mouth causes infant to turn head toward that side and begin to suck; should disappear at about age 3-4 months, but may persist for up to 12 months (see Fig. 8-7)
Extrusion	When tongue is touched or depressed, infant responds by forcing it outward; disappears by age 4 months
Yawn	Spontaneous response to decreased oxygen by increasing amount of inspired air; persists throughout life
Cough	Irritation of mucous membranes of larynx or tracheobronchial tree causes coughing; persists throughout life; usually present after first day of birth
EXTREMITIES	
Grasp	Touching palms of hands or soles of feet near base of digits causes flexion of hands and toes (see Fig. 8-8, *A*): palmar grasp lessens after age 3 months, to be replaced by voluntary movement; plantar grasp lessens by 8 months of age
Babinski	Stroking outer sole of foot upward from heel and across ball of foot causes toes to hyperextend and hallux to dorsiflex (see Fig. 8-8, *B*); disappears after age 1 year
Ankle clonus	Briskly dorsiflexing foot while supporting knee in partially flexed position results in one to two oscillating movements ("beats"); eventually no beats should be felt
MASS	
Moro	Sudden jarring or change in equilibrium causes sudden extension and abduction of extremities and fanning of fingers, with index finger and thumb forming a C shape, followed by flexion and adduction of extremities; legs may weakly flex; infant may cry (Fig. 8-9); disappears after age 3-4 months, usually strongest during first 2 months
Startle	A sudden loud noise causes abduction of the arms with flexion of elbows; hands remain clenched; disappears by age 4 months
Perez	While infant is prone on a firm surface, thumb is pressed along spine from sacrum to neck; infant responds by crying, flexing extremities, and elevating pelvis and head; lordosis of the spine, as well as defecation and urination, may occur; disappears by age 4-6 months
Asymmetric tonic neck	When infant's head is turned to one side, arm and leg extend on that side, and opposite arm and leg flex (Fig. 8-10); disappears by age 3-4 months, to be replaced by symmetric positioning of both sides of body
Trunk incurvation (Galant) reflex	Stroking infant's back alongside spine causes hips to move toward stimulated side; disappears by age 4 weeks
Dance or step	If infant is held so that sole of foot touches a hard surface, there is a reciprocal flexion and extension of the leg, simulating walking (Fig. 8-11); disappears after age 3-4 weeks, to be replaced by deliberate movement
Crawl	When placed on abdomen, infant makes crawling movements with arms and legs; disappears at about age 6 weeks (Fig. 8-12)
Placing	When infant is held upright under arms and dorsal side of foot is briskly placed against hard object, such as table, leg lifts as if foot is stepping on table; age of disappearance varies

One method of systematically assessing the infant's behavior is the use of the ***Brazelton Neonatal Behavioral Assessment Scale (BNBAS)*** (Brazelton and Nugent, 1996). The BNBAS is an interactive examination that assesses the infant's response to 28 items organized according to the clusters in Box 8-3. It is generally used as a research or diagnostic tool and requires special training.

In addition to its use as an initial and ongoing tool to assess neurologic and behavioral responses, the scale can be used as an assessor of initial parent-child relationships, as a

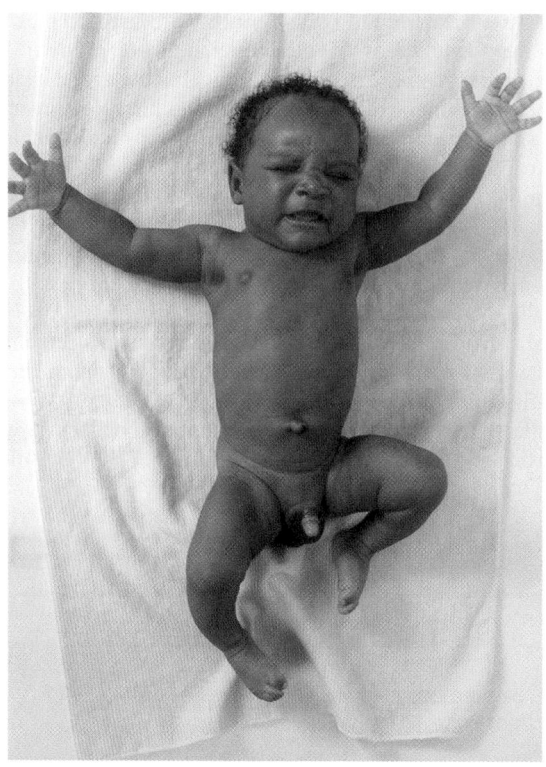

FIG. 8-9 ■ Moro reflex. (Photo by Paul Vincent Kuntz, Texas Children's Hospital.)

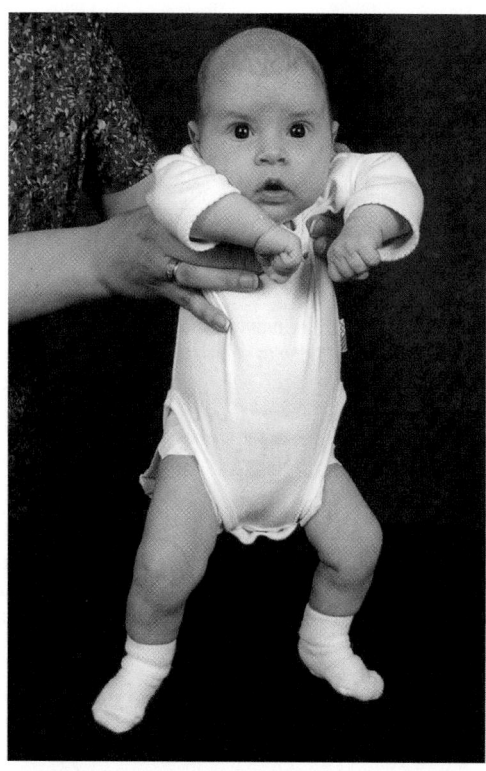

FIG. 8-11 ■ Dance reflex. (Photo by Paul Vincent Kuntz, Texas Children's Hospital.)

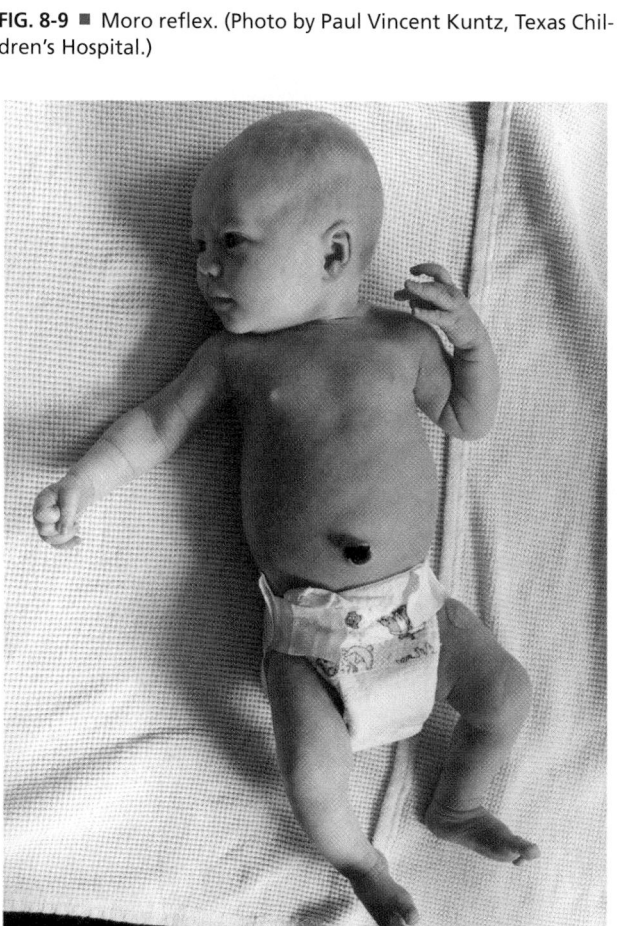

FIG. 8-10 ■ Tonic neck reflex. (Photo by Paul Vincent Kuntz, Texas Children's Hospital.)

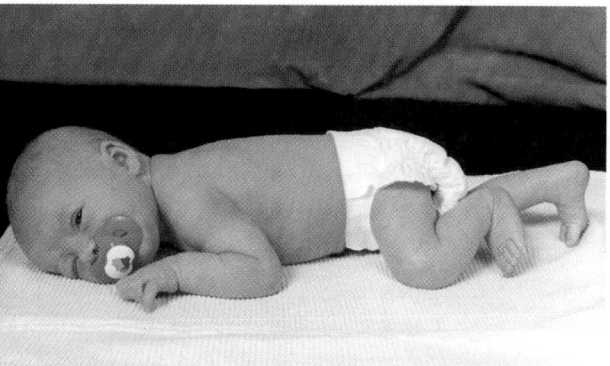

FIG. 8-12 ■ Crawl reflex. (Photo by Paul Vincent Kuntz, Texas Children's Hospital.)

BOX 8-3 ■ Clusters of Neonatal Behaviors in Brazelton Neonatal Behavioral Assessment Scale

Habituation—Ability to respond to and then inhibit responding to discrete stimulus (light, rattle, bell, pinprick) while asleep
Orientation—Quality of alert states and ability to attend to visual and auditory stimuli while alert
Motor performance—Quality of movement and tone
Range of state—Measure of general arousal level or arousability of infant
Regulation of state—How infant responds when aroused
Autonomic stability—Signs of stress (tremors, startles, skin color) related to homeostatic (self-regulating) adjustment of the nervous system
Reflexes—Assessment of several neonatal reflexes

preventive instrument that identifies the caregiver as one who may benefit from a role model, and as a guide to help parents focus on their infant's individuality and develop a deeper attachment to their child. Studies have demonstrated that showing parents the unique characteristics of their infant causes a more positive perception of the infant to develop, with increased interaction between infant and parent.

Patterns of Sleep and Activity. Newborns begin life with a systematic schedule of sleep and wakefulness that is initially evident during the periods of reactivity. After this initial period, it is not unusual for the infant to sleep almost constantly for the next 2 to 3 days to recover from the exhausting birth process.

Infants have six distinct sleep-wake states, which represent a particular form of neural control (Table 8-3). As gestational

TABLE 8-3 ■ States of Sleep and Activity

STATE/BEHAVIOR	IMPLICATIONS FOR PARENTING
DEEP SLEEP (QUIET)	
Closed eyes	Continue usual house noises because external stimuli do not arouse infant
Regular breathing	Leave infant alone if sudden loud noise awakens infant and child cries
No movement except for occasional sudden bodily twitch	Do not attempt to feed
No eye movement	
LIGHT SLEEP (ACTIVE)	
Closed eyes	External stimuli that did not arouse infant during regular sleep may minimally arouse child
Irregular breathing	Periodic groaning or crying is usual; do not interpret as an indication of pain or discomfort
Slight muscular twitching of body	
Rapid eye movement (REM) under closed eyelids	
May smile	
DROWSY	
Eyes may be open	Most stimuli arouse infant but may return to sleep state
Irregular breathing	Pick infant up during this time rather than leaving in crib
Active body movement variable, with occasional mild startles	Provide mild stimulus to awaken
	May enjoy nonnutritive sucking
QUIET ALERT	
Eyes wide open and bright	Satisfy infant's needs such as hunger or nonnutritive sucking
Responds to environment by active body movement and staring at close-range objects	Place infant in area of home where activity is continuous
Minimal body activity	Place toys in crib or playpen
Regular breathing	Place objects within 17.5-20 cm (7-8 inches) of infant's view
Focuses attention on stimuli	Intervene to console
ACTIVE ALERT	
May begin with whimpering and slight body movement	Remove intense internal or external stimuli because has increased sensitivity to stimuli
Eyes open	
Irregular breathing	
CRYING	
Progresses to strong, angry crying and uncoordinated thrashing of extremities	Comforting measures that were effective during alert state are usually ineffective
Eyes open or tightly closed	Rock and swaddle to decrease crying
Grimaces	Intervene to reduce fatigue, hunger, or discomfort
Irregular breathing	

Portions adapted from Blackburn S, Loper DL: *Maternal, fetal, and neonatal physiology: a clinical perspective*, Philadelphia, 1992, WB Saunders.

and postconceptional maturity increases, each state becomes more precisely defined according to the behaviors observed. *State* is defined as a "group of characteristics that regularly occur together" (Blackburn, 2003) and comprise body activity, eye and facial movements, respiratory pattern, and response to internal and external stimuli. The six sleep-wake states are: quiet (deep) sleep, active (light) sleep, drowsy, awake (quiet), active alert, and crying. Infants respond to internal and external environmental factors by controlling sensory input and regulating the sleep-wake states; the ability to make smooth transitions between states is called *state modulation.* The ability to regulate sleep-wake states is essential in the neurobehavioral development of the infant. The more immature the infant, the less able he or she is able to cope with external/internal factors that affect the sleep-wake patterns.

Recognition and knowledge of sleep-wake states is important in the planning of nursing care. It is also important for nurses to help parents and caregivers understand the significance of the infant's behavioral responses to daily caregiving and how these states can be altered. A classic example is the newborn who feeds vigorously in the active alert state rather than the deep sleep state. The neurologic assessment of a newborn in the active alert state will differ significantly from the deep sleep state. Newborns typically spend as much as 16 to 18 hours sleeping and do not necessarily follow a pattern of light-dark diurnal rhythm. With increasing age, sleep-wake states will change, with increasing amounts of time spent in awake alert states and decreasing amounts of sleep time. Approximately 50% of total sleep time is spent in irregular or rapid eye movement sleep.

Cry.   The newborn should begin extrauterine life with a strong, lusty cry. The sounds produced by crying can be described as hunger, anger, pain, and "bid for attention" cries.

Discomfort (pain) sounds initially consist of gasps and cries in which the consonant *H* is clearly distinguishable. The duration of crying is as highly variable in each infant as is the duration of sleep patterns. Some newborns may cry as little as 5 minutes or as much as 2 hours or more per day. Feeding usually terminates the state of crying when hunger is the cause. Swaddling or wrapping an infant snugly in a blanket promotes sleep and maintains body temperature. Rocking the infant reduces crying and induces quiet alertness or sleep. Variations in the initial cry can indicate abnormalities. A weak, groaning cry or grunting during expiration usually indicates respiratory disturbance. Absent, weak, or constant crying requires further investigation for possible drug withdrawal or a neurologic problem.

Assessment of Attachment Behaviors

One of the most important areas of assessment is careful observation of behaviors that are thought to indicate the formation of emotional bonds between the newborn and family, especially the mother. Such behaviors include the *en face position;* undressing and touching the infant; smiling, kissing, and talking to the infant; and holding, rocking, and cradling the child close to the body (see Guidelines box). However, because assessment is closely related to interventions that promote attachment (e.g., encouraging these behaviors in parents), the major portion of assessing attachment behaviors is discussed on pp. 211-212.

Physical Assessment

An essential aspect of the care of the newborn is a thorough physical assessment that includes estimation of gestational age and physical examination to identify normal characteristics and existing abnormalities. These initial and ongoing assessments are critical to establishing baseline data for planning, implementing, and evaluating care and are a nursing

---

GUIDELINES

Assessing Attachment Behavior

When the infant is brought to the parents, do they reach out for the child and call the child by name?

Do the parents speak about the child in terms of identification—whom the infant looks like; what appears special about their child over other infants?

When parents are holding the infant, what kind of body contact is there—do they feel at ease in changing the infant's position; are fingertips or whole hands used; are there parts of the body they avoid touching or parts of the body they investigate and scrutinize?

When the infant is awake, what kinds of stimulation do the parents provide—do they talk to the infant, to each other, or to no one; how do they look at the infant—direct visual contact, avoidance of eye contact, or looking at other people or objects?

How comfortable do the parents appear in terms of caring for the infant? Do they express any concern regarding their ability or disgust for certain activities, such as changing diapers?

What type of affection do they demonstrate to the newborn, such as smiling, stroking, kissing, or rocking?

If the infant is fussy, what kinds of comforting techniques do the parents use, such as rocking, swaddling, talking, or stroking?

GUIDELINES

Physical Examination of the Newborn

Provide a normothermic and nonstimulating examination area.

Undress only body area examined to prevent heat loss.

Proceed in an orderly sequence (usually head to toe) with the following exceptions:

Observe infant's attitude and position of flexion first to avoid disturbing him or her.

Perform all procedures that require quiet next, such as auscultating the lungs, heart, and abdomen.

Perform disturbing procedures, such as testing reflexes, last.

Measure head, chest, and length at same time to compare results.

Proceed quickly to avoid stressing infant.

Check that equipment and supplies are working properly and are accessible.

Comfort infant during and after the examination.

Talk softly.

Hold infant's hands against chest.

Swaddle and hold.

Offer pacifier or nonlatex gloved finger to suck.

Use containment and positioning to maximize developmental state regulation.

priority in caring for the newborn. The discussion of physical examination focuses on normal findings and variations from the norm that require little or no intervention. The reader is encouraged to review the material in Chapter 7 for further discussions of examination techniques. General guidelines for conducting a physical examination are presented in the Guidelines box. Table 8-4 summarizes physical examination of the newborn.

● *Nursing Diagnosis*

A number of nursing diagnoses are prominent in the nursing care of the newborn and family, and others spe-

cific to individual cases become evident. The most common nursing diagnoses are outlined in the Nursing Care Plan on pp. 216-218.

● *Planning*

The goals for the newborn and family are as follows:

1 Infant will maintain a patent airway.
2 Infant will maintain a stable body temperature.
3 Infant will experience no infections or injuries.
4 Infant will receive optimum nutrition.
5 Family will exhibit attachment behavior.
6 Family will be prepared for discharge and home care.

TABLE 8-4 ■ Summary of Physical Assessment of the Newborn

USUAL FINDINGS	COMMON VARIATIONS/ MINOR ABNORMALITIES	POTENTIAL SIGNS OF DISTRESS/MAJOR ABNORMALITIES
GENERAL MEASUREMENTS		
Head circumference—33-33.5 cm (13-14 inches); about 2-3 cm (1 inch) larger than chest circumference	Molding after birth may alter head circumference Head and chest circumferences may be equal for first 1-2 days after birth	Head circumference <10th or >90th percentile
Chest circumference—30.5-33 cm (12-13 inches) *Crown-to-rump length*—31-35 cm (12.5-14 inches); approximately equal to head circumference *Head-to-heel length*—48-53 cm (19-21 inches)		
Birth weight—2700-4000 g (6-9 pounds)	Loss of 10% of birth weight in first week; regained in 10-14 days, depending on feeding method	Birth weight <10th or >90th percentile
VITAL SIGNS **Temperature** Axillary—36.5°-37° C (97.9°-98° F)	Crying may increase body temperature slightly Radiant warmer will falsely increase axillary temperature	Hypothermia Hyperthermia
Heart Rate Apical—120-140 beats/min	Crying will increase heart rate; sleep will decrease heart rate During first period of reactivity (6 to 8 hours), rate can reach 180 beats/min	Bradycardia—Resting rate below 80-100 beats/min Tachycardia—Rate above 160-180 beats/min Irregular rhythm
Respirations 30-60 breaths/min	Crying will increase respiratory rate; sleep will decrease respiratory rate During first period of reactivity (6 to 8 hours), rate can reach 80 breaths/min	Tachypnea—Rate above 60 breaths/min Apnea—20 seconds or more
Blood Pressure Oscillometric—65/41 mm Hg in arm and calf	Crying and activity will increase blood pressure (BP) Placing cuff on thigh may agitate infant; thigh BP may be higher than arm or calf BP by 4-8 mm Hg	Oscillometric systolic pressure in calf 6-9 mm Hg less than in upper extremity (sign of coarctation of aorta)
GENERAL APPEARANCE *Posture*—Flexion of head and extremities, which rest on chest and abdomen	Frank breech—Extended legs, abducted and fully rotated thighs, flattened occiput, extended neck	Limp posture, extension of extremities

TABLE 8-4 ■ Summary of Physical Assessment of the Newborn—*cont'd*

USUAL FINDINGS	COMMON VARIATIONS/ MINOR ABNORMALITIES	POTENTIAL SIGNS OF DISTRESS/MAJOR ABNORMALITIES
Skin		
At birth, bright red, puffy, smooth Second to third day, pink, flaky, dry Vernix caseosa Lanugo Edema around eyes, face, legs, dorsa of hands, feet, and scrotum or labia *Acrocyanosis*—Cyanosis of hands and feet *Cutis marmorata*—Transient mottling when infant is exposed to decreased temperature	Neonatal jaundice after first 24 hours Ecchymoses or petechiae caused by birth trauma *Milia*—Distended sebaceous glands that appear as tiny white papules on cheeks, chin, and nose *Miliaria or sudamina*—Distended sweat (eccrine) glands that appear as minute vesicles, especially on face *Erythema toxicum*—Pink papular rash with vesicles superimposed on thorax, back, buttocks, and abdomen; may appear in 24 to 48 hours and resolve after several days *Harlequin color change*—Clearly outlined color change as infant lies on side; lower half of body becomes pink, and upper half is pale *Mongolian spots*—Irregular areas of deep blue pigmentation, usually in sacral and gluteal regions; seen predominantly in newborns of African, Native American, Asian, or Hispanic descent *Telangiectatic nevi ("stork bites")*—Flat, deep pink localized areas usually seen in back of neck	Progressive jaundice, especially in first 24 hours Generalized cyanosis Pallor Mottling Grayness Plethora Hemorrhage, ecchymoses, or petechiae that persist *Sclerema*—Hard and stiff skin Poor skin turgor Rashes, pustules, or blisters *Café-au-lait spots*—Light brown spots *Nevus flammeus*—Port-wine stain
Head		
Anterior fontanel—Diamond shaped; size varies from barely palpable to 4-5 cm (0.5 to 2 inches) (see Fig. 8-5) *Posterior fontanel*—Triangular, 0.5-1 cm (0.2-0.4 inch) Fontanels should be flat, soft, and firm Widest part of fontanel measured from bone to bone, not suture to suture	Molding following vaginal delivery Third sagittal (parietal) fontanel Bulging fontanel because of crying or coughing *Caput succedaneum*—Edema of soft scalp tissue *Cephalhematoma* (uncomplicated)—Hematoma between periosteum and skull bone	Fused sutures Bulging or depressed fontanels when quiet Widened sutures and fontanels *Craniotabes*—Snapping sensation along lambdoid suture that resembles indentation of Ping-Pong ball
Eyes		
Lids usually edematous Color—Slate gray, dark blue, brown Absence of tears Presence of red reflex Corneal reflex in response to touch Pupillary reflex in response to light Blink reflex in response to light or touch Rudimentary fixation on objects and ability to follow to midline	Epicanthal folds in Asian infants Searching nystagmus or strabismus *Subconjunctival (scleral) hemorrhages*—Ruptured capillaries, usually at limbus	Pink color of iris Purulent discharge Upward slant in non-Asians Hypertelorism (3 cm or greater) Hypotelorism Congenital cataracts Constricted or dilated fixed pupil Absence of red reflex Absence of pupillary or corneal reflex Inability to follow object or bright light to midline Yellow sclera
Ears		
Position—Top of pinna on horizontal line with outer canthus of eye Startle reflex elicited by a loud, sudden noise Pinna flexible, cartilage present	Inability to visualize tympanic membrane because of filled aural canals Pinna flat against head Irregular shape or size Pits or skin tags	Low placement of ears Absence of startle reflex in response to loud noise Minor abnormalities may be signs of various syndromes, especially renal

continued

TABLE 8-4 ■ Summary of Physical Assessment of the Newborn—cont'd

USUAL FINDINGS	COMMON VARIATIONS/ MINOR ABNORMALITIES	POTENTIAL SIGNS OF DISTRESS/MAJOR ABNORMALITIES
Nose Nasal patency Nasal discharge—Thin white mucus Sneezing	Flattened and bruised	Nonpatent canals Thick, bloody nasal discharge Flaring of nares (alae nasi) Copious nasal secretions or stuffiness (may be minor)
Mouth and Throat Intact, high-arched palate Uvula in midline Frenulum of tongue Frenum of upper lip Sucking reflex—Strong and coordinated Rooting reflex Gag reflex Extrusion reflex Absent or minimal salivation Vigorous cry	*Natal teeth*—Teeth present at birth; benign but may be associated with congenital defects *Epstein pearls*—Small, white epithelial cysts along midline of hard palate	Cleft lip Cleft palate Large, protruding tongue or posterior displacement of tongue Profuse salivation or drooling *Candidiasis (thrush)*—White, adherent patches on tongue, palate, and buccal surfaces Inability to pass nasogastric tube Hoarse, high-pitched, weak, absent, or other abnormal cry
Neck Short, thick, usually surrounded by skinfolds Tonic neck reflex	*Torticollis (wry neck)*—Head held to one side with chin pointing to opposite side	Excessive skinfolds Resistance to flexion Absence of tonic neck reflex Fractured clavicle
Chest Anteroposterior and lateral diameters equal Slight sternal retractions evident during inspiration Xiphoid process evident Breast enlargement	Funnel chest (pectus excavatum) Pigeon chest (pectus carinatum) Supernumerary nipples Secretion of milky substance from breasts ("witch's milk")	Depressed sternum Marked retractions of chest and intercostal spaces during respiration Asymmetric chest expansion Redness and firmness around nipples Wide-spaced nipples
Lungs Respirations chiefly abdominal Cough reflex absent at birth, present by 1-2 days Bilateral equal bronchial breath sounds	Rate and depth of respirations may be irregular, periodic breathing Crackles shortly after birth	Inspiratory stridor Expiratory grunt Retractions Persistent irregular breathing Periodic breathing with repeated apneic spells Seesaw respirations (paradoxical) Unequal breath sounds Persistent fine, medium or coarse crackles Wheezing Diminished breath sounds Peristaltic bowel sounds on one side, with diminished breath sounds on same side
Heart *Apex*—Fourth to fifth intercostal space, lateral to left sternal border S₂ slightly sharper and higher in pitch than S₁	*Sinus arrhythmia*—Heart rate increases with inspiration and decreases with expiration Transient cyanosis on crying or straining	Dextrocardia—Heart on right side Displacement of apex, muffled Cardiomegaly Abdominal shunts Murmur Thrill Persistent central cyanosis Hyperactive precordium

TABLE 8-4 ■ Summary of Physical Assessment of the Newborn—*cont'd*

USUAL FINDINGS	COMMON VARIATIONS/ MINOR ABNORMALITIES	POTENTIAL SIGNS OF DISTRESS/MAJOR ABNORMALITIES
Abdomen		
Cylindric in shape	Umbilical hernia	Abdominal distention
Liver—Palpable 2-3 cm below right costal margin	*Diastasis recti*—Midline gap between recti muscles	Localized bulging
Spleen—Tip palpable at end of first week of age	*Wharton's jelly*—unusually thick umbilical cord	Distended veins
Kidneys—Palpable 1-2 cm above umbilicus		Absent bowel sounds
Umbilical cord—Bluish white at birth with two arteries and one vein		Enlarged liver and spleen
Femoral pulses—Equal bilaterally		Ascites
		Visible peristaltic waves
		Scaphoid or concave abdomen
		Moist umbilical cord
		Presence of only one artery in cord
		Urine, stool, or pus leaking from cord or cord insertion site
		Periumbilical erythema
		Palpable bladder distention following scanty voiding
		Absent femoral pulses
		Cord bleeding or hematoma
Female Genitalia		
Labia and clitoris usually edematous	*Pseudomenstruation*—Blood-tinged or mucoid discharge	Enlarged clitoris with urethral meatus at tip
Urethral meatus behind clitoris	Hymenal tag	Fused labia
Vernix caseosa between labia		Absence of vaginal opening
Urination within 24 hours		Meconium from vaginal opening
		No urination within 24 hours
		Masses in labia
		Ambiguous genitalia
Male Genitalia		
Urethral opening at tip of glans penis	Urethral opening covered by prepuce	*Hypospadias*—Urethral opening on ventral surface of penis
Testes palpable in each scrotum	Inability to retract foreskin	*Epispadias*—Urethral opening on dorsal surface of penis
Scrotum usually large, edematous, pendulous, and covered with rugae; usually deeply pigmented in dark-skinned ethnic groups	*Epithelial pearls*—Small, firm, white lesions at tip of prepuce	*Chordee*—Ventral curvature of penis
Smegma	Erection or priapism	Testes not palpable in scrotum or inguinal canal
Urination within 24 hours	Testes palpable in inguinal canal	No urination within 24 hours
	Scrotum small	Inguinal hernia
		Hypoplastic scrotum
		Hydrocele—Fluid in scrotum
		Masses in scrotum
		Meconium from scrotum
		Discoloration of testes
		Ambiguous genitalia
Back and Rectum		
Spine intact, no openings, masses, or prominent curves	Green liquid stools in infant under phototherapy	Anal fissures or fistulas
Trunk incurvation reflex	Delayed passage of meconium in very-low-birth-weight neonates	Imperforate anus
Anal reflex		Absence of anal reflex
Patent anal opening		No meconium within 36-48 hours
Passage of meconium within 48 hours		Pilonidal cyst or sinus
		Tuft of hair along spine
		Spina bifida (any degree)

continued

TABLE 8-4 ■ Summary of Physical Assessment of the Newborn—cont'd

USUAL FINDINGS	COMMON VARIATIONS/ MINOR ABNORMALITIES	POTENTIAL SIGNS OF DISTRESS/MAJOR ABNORMALITIES
Extremities		
Ten fingers and toes	Partial syndactyly between second and third toes	*Polydactyly*—Extra digits
Full range of motion	Second toe overlapping into third toe	*Syndactyly*—Fused or webbed digits
Nail beds pink, with transient cyanosis immediately after birth	Wide gap between first (hallux) and second toes	*Phocomelia*—Hands or feet attached close to trunk
Creases on anterior two thirds of sole	Deep crease on plantar surface of foot between first and second toes	*Hemimelia*—Absence of distal part of extremity
Sole usually flat	Asymmetric length of toes	Hyperflexibility of joints
Symmetry of extremities	Dorsiflexion and shortness of hallux	Persistent cyanosis of nail beds
Equal muscle tone bilaterally, especially resistance to opposing flexion		Yellowing of nail beds
Equal bilateral brachial pulses		Sole covered with creases
		Transverse palmar (simian) crease
		Fractures
		Decreased or absent ROM
		Dislocated or subluxated hip
		Limitation in hip abduction
		Unequal gluteal or leg folds
		Unequal knee height (Allis or Galeazzi sign)
		Audible clunk on abduction (Ortolani sign)
		Asymmetry of extremities
		Unequal muscle tone or range of motion
NEUROMUSCULAR SYSTEM		
Extremities usually maintain some degree of flexion	Quivering or momentary tremors	*Hypotonia*—Floppy, poor head control, extremities limp
Extension of an extremity followed by previous position of flexion		*Hypertonia*—Jittery, arms and hands tightly flexed, legs stiffly extended, startles easily
Head lag while sitting, but momentary ability to hold head erect		Asymmetric posturing (except tonic neck reflex)
Able to turn head from side to side when prone		*Opisthotonic posturing*—Arched back
Able to hold head in horizontal line with back when held prone		Signs of paralysis
		Tremors, twitches, and myoclonic jerks
		Marked head lag in all positions

● *Implentation*

Maintain a Patent Airway

Establishing a patent airway is a primary objective in the delivery room and is the responsibility of the attending nurses and practitioners. However, maintaining a patent airway continues to be a priority goal in the nursery, with attention to proper positioning of the infant to facilitate drainage of secretions, especially after feeding. The American Academy of Pediatrics (2000a) recommends the supine position during sleep for healthy newborns. This recommendation is based on the possible association between sleeping prone and sudden infant death syndrome (see Chapter 11). A bulb syringe is kept near the infant and is used if suctioning is required. Used bulb syringes should probably be replaced every 24 hours in the hospital and boiled for 10 minutes before reuse in the home to eliminate bacterial contamination.

If more forceful removal of secretions is required, mechanical suction is used. The use of the proper-size catheter and correct suctioning technique is essential to prevent mucosal damage and edema. Gentle suctioning is necessary to prevent reflex bradycardia, laryngospasm, and cardiac arrhythmias from vagal stimulation. Oropharyngeal suctioning is performed for 5 seconds, with sufficient time between suctioning to allow the infant to reoxygenate.

▌NURSING ALERT

To avoid aspiration of amniotic fluid or mucus, clear the pharynx first, then the nasal passages using a bulb syringe. In some nurseries the stomach is routinely emptied with a feeding tube to remove amniotic fluid, blood, and mucus, which may cause abdominal distention and interfere with the establishment of respiration. Passing a catheter to the stomach also rules out esophageal atresia. Vital signs are closely monitored, and any indication of respiratory distress is immediately reported.

▌NURSING ALERT

The cardinal signs of respiratory distress in the newborn include tachypnea, nasal flaring, grunting, intercostal retractions, and cyanosis.

Maintain Stable Body Temperature

Conserving the newborn's body heat is an essential nursing goal. At birth a major cause of heat loss is *evaporation,* the loss of heat through moisture. The amniotic fluid that bathes the infant's skin favors evaporation, especially when combined with the cool atmosphere of the delivery room. Heat loss through evaporation is minimized by rapidly drying the skin and hair with a warmed towel and placing the infant in a heated environment.

Another major cause of heat loss is *radiation,* the loss of heat to cooler solid objects in the environment that are not in direct contact with the infant. Loss of heat through radiation increases as these solid objects become colder and closer to the infant. The temperature of ambient or surrounding air in the incubator essentially has no effect on loss of heat through radiation. This is a critical point to remember when attempting to maintain a constant temperature for the infant, because even though the temperature of the ambient air is optimal, the infant can become hypothermic.

The use of radiant heating devices such as heat lamps or phototherapy lights with an incubator may cause overheating of the infant, because infants cannot effectively dissipate radiant heat through the Plexiglas wall of the incubator. For this same reason, an incubator should not be exposed to direct sunlight.

An example of radiant heat loss is the placement of the incubator close to a cold window, drafty doorway, or air-conditioning unit. The cold from either source will cool the walls of the incubator and, subsequently, the body of the neonate. To prevent this, the infant is placed as far away as possible from walls, windows, and ventilating units. If heat loss continues to be a problem, a radiant warmer may be placed over the infant or infant and mother.

Heat loss can also occur through conduction and convection. *Conduction* involves loss of heat from the body because of direct contact of skin with a cooler solid object. This can be minimized by placing the infant on a padded, covered surface and providing insulation through clothes and blankets rather than by placing the infant directly on a hard table. Placing the newborn close to the mother, such as in her arms or on her abdomen immediately after delivery, is physically beneficial in terms of conserving heat, as well as fostering maternal attachment.

Convection is similar to conduction, except that heat loss is aided by surrounding air currents. For example, placing the infant in the direct flow of air from a fan or air-conditioner vent will cause rapid heat loss through convection. Transporting the neonate in a crib with solid sides reduces airflow around the infant.

Protect from Infection and Injury

The most important practice for preventing cross-infection is thorough handwashing of all individuals involved in the infant's care. A common practice in many newborn nurseries is the use of cover gowns and "scrub" clothes to prevent infection. Studies have shown that this practice is ineffective and costly. Donning a long-sleeved cover gown over regular clothing is recommended when the neonate is held outside the bassinet (American Academy of Pediatrics and American College of Obstetricians and Gynecologists, 2002). Several other procedures to prevent infection include eye care, umbilical care, bathing, and care of the circumcision. Vitamin K is administered to protect against hemorrhage. In addition, several safety measures are practiced, particularly in terms of proper identification, and screening tests are used to detect various disorders.

Identification.   Proper identification of the newborn is absolutely essential. The nurse must verify that identifying bands are securely fastened and verify the information (name, sex, mother's admission number, date, and time of birth) against the birth records and the child's actual gender. This identification process should take place optimally in the delivery room. Some institutions use methods of infant identification such as a color photograph kept in the medical record, storage of blood for DNA genotyping, or electronic surveillance systems for infant security. Footprinting or fingerprinting alone is *not* currently recommended for newborn identification (American Academy of Pediatrics and American College of Obstetricians and Gynecologists, 2002); however, the National Center for Missing and Exploited Children (NCMEC) does recommend the use of footprints as a form of identification in addition to a cord blood sample, which is stored until the day after discharge. Electronic tags that give off a radio frequency may also be used to prevent newborn abductions.

A proactive hospital emergency plan should be implemented to prevent infant abduction and to respond promptly and effectively in the event of such an event. A mock newborn abduction drill is an effective method that can be used to evaluate staff competence and response to the incident (Shogan, 2002). *All* hospital personnel should be educated regarding newborn abduction, preventive aspects, and methods to identify the potential risk of such an occurrence.

The nurse needs to discuss safety issues with the mother the first time the infant is brought to her. It has been reported by the **National Center for Missing and Exploited Children (NCMEC)*** that 55% of infant abductions occur in the mother's room (Rabun, 2000). A written copy of the safety instructions should also be given to the parent. Parents are instructed to look at identification badges of nurses and hospital personnel who come to take infants and not to relinquish their infants to anyone without proper identification. Mothers are also advised not to leave the infant alone in the crib while they shower or use the bathroom; rather, they should ask to have the infant observed by a health care worker if a family member is not present in the room. Parents and staff are encouraged to use a password system when the newborn is taken from the room as a routine security measure (Carroll, 2000). The nurse should document in the chart that these instructions were given and that appropriate identification band checks are routinely made throughout each shift. Nursing staff are also educated regarding the "typical" abductor profile and to be constantly aware of visitors with unusual behavior.

---

*(800)THE LOST; website: www.missingkids.com. *Safeguard Their Tomorrows* is a printed resource available through NCMEC's website (courtesy Mead Johnson) for expectant and new parents and health care workers. Parents and health care workers will find a number of useful educational resources available at this website, including information on selecting safe day care and babysitters. Another resource is *Creating a Secure Workplace: Effective Policies and Practices in Health Care,* available from American Hospital Publishing; (800) 621-6902; website: www.amphi.com.

The typical profile of an abductor is a female between the ages of 15 and 44 who is often overweight and has low self-esteem; she may be emotionally disturbed because of the loss of her own child or inability to conceive and may have a strained relationship with her husband or partner. The typical abductor may also be seen visiting the newborn nursery or neonatal intensive care unit area before the abduction and may ask questions about the care of or the health of a specific newborn. The abductor may familiarize herself with the hospital routine and may also impersonate a health care worker. Parents are made aware of the fact that infant safety measures must be implemented in the home as well. Measures to prevent and decrease infant abduction after discharge to the home include discontinuing the publication of birth announcements in the local newspaper and avoiding using yard decorations to announce a newborn's arrival (Shogan, 2002).

Eye Care.   Prophylactic eye treatment against *ophthalmia neonatorum,* infectious conjunctivitis of the newborn, includes the use of (1) silver nitrate (1%) solution, (2) erythromycin (0.5%) ophthalmic ointment or drops, or (3) tetracycline (1%) ophthalmic ointment or drops (preferably in single-dose ampules or tubes) (see Guidelines box). *Chlamydia trachomatis* is the major cause of ophthalmia neonatorum in the United States. Silver nitrate is effective against gonococcal conjunctivitis.

Topical antibiotics such as tetracycline and erythromycin, silver nitrate, and a 2.5% povidone-iodine solution (currently unavailable in commercial form in the United States) have not proved to be effective in the treatment of chlamydial conjunctivitis.

A 14-day course of oral erythromycin or an oral sulfonamide may be given for chlamydial conjunctivitis (American Academy of Pediatrics and American College of Obstetrician and Gynecologists, 2002). Administration of oral erythromycin in infants younger than 6 weeks old has been associated with infantile hypertrophic pyloric stenosis. It is also recommended that eye prophylaxis be administered for newborns born by cesarean section in the event of an ascending intrauterine infection. Herpes simplex virus may also cause neonatal conjunctivitis; treatment in such cases involves the use of topical and systemic antiviral medications.

Because studies on maternal attachment emphasize that in the first hour of life a newborn has a greater ability to focus on coordinated movement than at any other time during the next several days and because eye contact is very important in the development of maternal-infant bonding, the routine administration of silver nitrate or topical ophthalmic

antibiotics can be postponed for up to 1 hour in the United States and up to 2 hours in Canada. However, there must be some kind of checklist to ensure that the drug is given.

NURSING TIP

A chemical conjunctivitis may occur within 24 hours of instillation of ophthalmic prophylaxis—the clinical features include mild lid edema and a sterile, nonpurulent eye discharge (Fuloria and Kreiter, 2002). Purulent eye discharge should be reported to the primary practitioner for further investigation.

Vitamin K Administration.   Shortly after birth, vitamin K is administered as a single intramuscular dose of 0.5 to 1 mg to prevent hemorrhagic disease of the newborn, also called *vitamin K deficiency bleeding.* Normally, vitamin K is synthesized by the intestinal flora. However, because the infant's intestine is sterile at birth and because breast milk contains low levels of vitamin K, the supply is inadequate for at least the first 3 to 4 days. The major function of vitamin K is to catalyze the synthesis of prothrombin in the liver, which is needed for blood clotting and coagulation. The vastus lateralis muscle is the traditionally recommended injection site, but the ventrogluteal (not dorsogluteal) muscle can be used. Oral vitamin K preparations are commercially unavailable in the United States but may be given in other countries. A single oral dose of vitamin K may be inadequate to raise serum vitamin K levels; therefore, it is recommended that oral doses of vitamin K be given shortly after birth, at 1 to 2 weeks of age, and a third dose at 1 month to prevent hemorrhagic disease (Puckett and Offringa, 2000).

Hepatitis B (HBV) Vaccine Administration.   To decrease the incidence of HBV in children and its serious consequences, cirrhosis and liver cancer, in adulthood, the first of three doses of HBV vaccine is recommended soon after birth and before hospital discharge for all newborns; this first dose may also be given by age 2 months if the mother is HB surface antigen (HBsAg) negative. The injection is given in the vastus lateralis muscle. This muscle is used because this site is associated with a better immune response than is the dorsogluteal area (a muscle typically not used in infants in the United States) (see also Immunizations, Chapter 10). Giving the infant oral sucrose can reduce the pain of the injection.

Premature infants born to HBsAg-negative women should be vaccinated just before hospital discharge, provided that the infant weighs 2000 g or more; the vaccination should be delayed until 2 months of age if the infant weighs less than 2000 g. Infants born to HBsAg-positive mothers should be immunized within 12 hours after birth with HBV vaccine and hepatitis B immune globulin at separate sites, regardless of gestational age or birth weight (American Academy of Pediatrics, 2003c). In Canada, HBV vaccine is given to the newborn only if the mother is HBsAg-positive at birth (see Immunizations, Chapter 10).

Newborn Screening for Disease.   A number of genetic disorders can be detected in the newborn period. There is no national policy for such detection in the United States; therefore, the extent of neonatal screening is deter-

---

GUIDELINES

Ophthalmia Neonatorum Prophylaxis

Clean the eyelids with sterile cotton and sterile water if needed.
Separate lids and apply 2 drops or a 1- to 2-cm (½ inch) ribbon of ointment in each conjunctival sac.
Massage lids to ensure spread of the medication.
Wipe excess medication from eye with sterile cotton 1 minute after application.
Do not rinse eyes with sterile normal saline.

mined by state laws and voluntary guidelines. Most states require screening for phenylketonuria (PKU), hypothyroidism, galactosemia, and sickle cell disease (see Chapters 9 and 26). Because concern has been voiced regarding the inconsistency among states in screening for such conditions based on cost, population demographics, resource availability, and political environment, the Task Force on Newborn Screening was formed by the American Academy of Pediatrics and other federal health care agencies to address this issue. A number of resolutions and policies have been developed to better address the issue of newborn screening (see American Academy of Pediatrics, 2000b).

The nurse's responsibility is to educate parents regarding the importance of screening and to collect appropriate specimens at the recommended time (after 24 hours of age). With early newborn discharge before 24 hours, adequate screening for PKU requires a follow-up test within 2 weeks (American Academy of Pediatrics and American College of Obstetricians and Gynecologists, 2002). Accurate screening depends on good-quality blood spots on approved filter paper forms. The blood should completely saturate the filter paper spot on one side only. The paper should not be handled, placed on wet surfaces, or contaminated with any substance, such as coffee or tea. (See Atraumatic Care box.)

The American Academy of Pediatrics and American College of Obstetricians and Gynecologists (2002) also recommend routine prenatal and perinatal human immunodeficiency virus (HIV) counseling and testing for all pregnant women and their newborns. Benefits of early identification of HIV-infected infants are early antiretroviral therapy and aggressive nutritional supplementation; appropriate changes in their immunization schedule; monitoring and evaluating immunologic, neurologic, and neuropsychologic functions for possible changes caused by antiretroviral therapy; initiation of special educational needs; evaluation for the need of other therapies, such as immunoglobulin for the prevention of bacterial infections; tuberculosis screening and treatment; and management of communicable disease exposures. In addition, vertical transmission of HIV from mother to newborn may be reduced to 2% with a cesarean section before the rupture of membranes and onset of labor (American Academy of Pediatrics and American College of Obstetri-

ATRAUMATIC CARE

Heel Punctures

Repeated heel lancing may be necessary to obtain sufficient blood for a number of newborn blood tests, including newborn screening. It has been anecdotally observed that newborns appear to withdraw the heel when touched for subsequent heel punctures. In fact, Taddio and colleagues (2002) found that infants of diabetic mothers exposed to multiple heel punctures in the first 24 to 36 hours of life learned to anticipate pain and exhibited more intense pain responses. The use of automated lancet devices such as Tenderfoot* has been found to cause less pain and require fewer punctures than using manual lance blades (Blain-Lewis, 1992; Paes and others, 1993). Additional studies have shown that venipuncture performed by an experienced phlebotomist elicited fewer pain responses (as measured by the Premature Infant Pain Profile) from term newborns than did heel punctures (Shah and Ohlsson, 2001). In addition, the need for additional skin punctures was reduced with venipuncture. Although maternal anxiety was initially higher in the venipuncture group, mothers who observed the venipuncture reported observing less pain response than mothers who observed heel punctures. Oral sucrose and nonnutritive sucking has proved effective in decreasing the pain associated with heel punctures in preterm and term infants during the first week of life (Stevens, Yamada, and Ohlsson, 2001; Gibbins and others, 2002), however the exact dose range that proves effective varies among several studies (Stevens, Yamada, and Ohlsson, 2001). In one study, infants experiencing venipuncture were given either oral sucrose (30%) and a skin placebo or the eutectic mixture of local anesthetic (EMLA). Pain scores were measured with the Premature Infant Pain Profile (PIPP), and infants receiving the oral sucrose solution exhibited fewer pain symptoms than those in the EMLA group (Gradin and others, 2002). Giving newborns 2 mL of oral sucrose solution (25% and 50%) significantly demonstrated a reduction in crying time and heart rate after 3 minutes in comparison with controls (given sterile water) during heel stick sampling for serum bilirubin concentrations (Haouari and others, 1995).

Evidence indicates that as little as 2 mL of a 24% oral sucrose solution is effective in decreasing pain in term and preterm infants. In addition, the best analgesic effect is achieved when sucrose is administered 2 minutes before the painful procedure with a pacifier or syringe. In one study protocol wherein oral sucrose was effective, 0.5 mL of 24% oral sucrose solution was administered 2 minutes before the heel puncture, during, and 5 minutes following the heel puncture (Gibbins and others, 2002). Monitoring for adverse effects must accompany each administration (Noerr, 2001).

The mother's holding the infant in skin-to-skin contact has also been shown to significantly reduce the child's distress during the procedure (Blass and Watt, 1999; Gray, Watt, and Blass, 2000). Breast-feeding during heel puncture in term newborns has been shown to be effective in decreasing pain scores when compared to placebo or a 30% oral sucrose solution (Carbajal and others, 2003).

The benefit of applying the topical anesthetic EMLA to reduce the pain of heel lance has produced mixed results in term and preterm infants (Fitzgerald, Millard, and McIntosh, 1989; Taddio and others, 1998; Stevens and others, 1999).

From these studies it is evident that there are a number of effective ways to decrease the pain associated with heel puncture in term and preterm newborns. It is essential that nurses use all available resources to advocate for the prevention and management of neonatal pain during such procedures as heel puncture.

A number of commercially available oral sucrose solutions now exist and include, but are not limited to, the following: Ora-Sweet (54% solution), Paddock Labs, Inc., which can be diluted 1:1 to produce a 27% solution; Sweet-Ease, a 24% sucrose solution, Childrens Medical Ventures, Norwell, MA. When these are not available the pharmacy may mix an oral sucrose solution to ensure a clean product. An approximate 25% sucrose solution is made by mixing 1 teaspoon of granulated (table) sugar with 4 teaspoons of sterile water; however, this method is the least desirable to prevent contamination of the solution and subsequent problems.

*Manufactured by International Technidyne, Inc., Edison, NJ.

cians and Gynecologists, 2002). As a result of virologic diagnostic techniques such as HIV culture, polymerase chain reaction, and immune complex–dissociated p24 antigen, diagnosis of HIV infection can be made in 30% to 50% of infants at birth and in 100% of infants by 4 to 6 months of age. For information on several diseases that may be included in newborn screening, see Newborn Screening Fact Sheets (American Academy of Pediatrics, 1996a).

Universal Newborn Hearing Screening. Approximately 1 to 6 per 1000 newborns may have significant hearing loss, which may go undetected until later in life. Such deficits may lead to subsequent speech and language delays which could be treated with early detection. The Joint Committee on Infant Hearing, American Academy of Pediatrics (2000c), recommends that all birthing hospitals establish programs to screen all newborn infants before discharge for hearing loss by auditory brainstem response or evoked otoacoustic emissions. It is estimated that screening by high-risk factors alone fails to identify approximately 50% of all newborns with a congenital hearing loss. Newborns who fail the initial screening require documentation and referral for further testing by 1 month of age; newborns who do not receive initial screening before discharge should also be tested by 1 month. The Academy also recommends adequate training of nursery staff to perform the hearing screening and reimbursement by third-party providers. Guidelines for screening infants and older children for hearing loss have recently been published (American Academy of Pediatrics, 2003a).

Bathing. Bath time is an opportunity for the nurse to accomplish much more than general hygiene. It is an excellent time for observations of the infant's behavior, state of arousal, alertness, and muscular activity. Bathing is usually performed after the vital signs have stabilized, especially the temperature.

With the possibility of transmission of viruses such as HBV and HIV via maternal blood and blood-stained amniotic fluid, the traditional timing of the newborn's bath has been questioned. The newborn must be considered a potential contamination source until proved otherwise. As part of *standard precautions,* nurses should wear gloves when handling the newborn until blood and amniotic fluid are removed by bathing.

In a study of 97 healthy full-term newborns bathed at age 1 hour (experimental group) and 4 hours (control group), there were no significant differences in rectal temperatures at 1 and 2 hours after the bath among the two groups. The researcher concluded that healthy full-term newborns with a rectal temperature greater than 36.5° C (97.7° F) can be bathed after the initial assessment to decrease the chance of contamination (Penny-MacGillivray, 1996). This study has been recently replicated by another group of nurse researchers who also found that the timing of the initial bath in the term newborn does not negatively affect temperature stability. Newborns bathed within 1 hour of birth did not experience thermoregulation difficulties as a result of the timing of the bath (Behring, Vezeau, and Fink, 2003). Nurses are cautioned, however, to avoid instituting routine newborn bathing according to a rigid sched-

ule; nursing interventions such as bathing should be based on individualized assessment and family interaction needs rather than a schedule.

The bath time provides an opportunity for the nurse to involve the parents in the care of their child, to teach correct hygiene procedures, and to learn about their infant's individual characteristics (Fig. 8-13). The appropriate types of bathing supplies and the need for safety in terms of water temperature and supervision of the infant at all times during the bath are stressed. For example, if sponges are used, they need to dry thoroughly between each use (may require a clothes dryer) to prevent growth of organisms.

Parents are encouraged to examine their infant closely during bathing. Frequently, normal variations such as Epstein pearls, mongolian spots, or "stork bites" cause parents much worry because they are unaware of the significance of such findings. Minor birth injuries may appear as major defects to them. Explaining how these occurred and when they will disappear reassures parents of their infant's normalcy. Common variations are discussed further in Chapter 9.

One of the most important considerations in skin cleansing is preservation of the skin's "acid mantle," which is formed from the uppermost horny layer of the epidermis, sweat, superficial fat, metabolic products, and external substances such as amniotic fluid, microorganisms, and chemicals. The infant's skin surface has a pH of about 5 soon after birth, and the bacteriostatic effects of this pH are significant. Consequently, only plain warm water should be used for the bath. Alkaline soaps, oils, powder, and lotions are not used because they alter the acid mantle, thus providing a medium for bacterial growth. Talcum powder has the added risk of aspiration if it is applied too close to the infant's face. A safer alternative is a cornstarch-based powder (see also Diaper Dermatitis, Chapter 30).

Parents should be involved in a discussion regarding the newborn's bath at home. It is recommended that for the first 2 weeks the infant be bathed no more than two or three times per week with a plain warm sponge bath. This practice will help maintain the integrity of the newborn's skin and allow time for the umbilical cord to completely dry. Routine

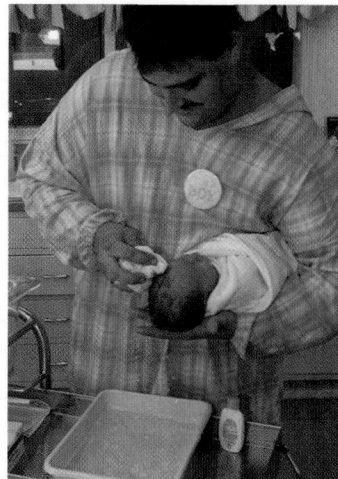

FIG. 8-13 ■ Bath time is an excellent opportunity for parents to learn about their newborn.

daily soap bathing for newborns is no longer recommended (AWHONN, 2001; Darmstadt and Dinulos, 2000).

Cleansing proceeds in the cephalocaudal (head-to-toe) direction. The eyes are carefully wiped from the inner to the outer aspect of the lid. The face is cleansed next. The scalp is usually wiped, although it is sometimes necessary to shampoo the hair. Shampooing is best accomplished by positioning the infant's head over a small basin, lathering the scalp with a mild soap, and rinsing by pouring water from a small vessel over the head into the basin. The rest of the body is kept covered during this procedure. The head is dried quickly to prevent heat loss from evaporation. The ears are cleaned with the twisted end of a washcloth, not with a cotton-tipped swab, which, if inserted into the canal, can damage the ear.

The rest of the body is washed in a similar manner. Although the infant's skin requires little rubbing for adequate cleansing, certain areas (e.g., folds of neck, axillae, creases at joints) need special attention. The genitalia of both sexes require careful cleansing. Cleansing of the vulva is done in a front-to-back direction. The bath is a perfect opportunity to stress this part of hygiene to the mother, for both the infant's and her protection against urinary tract infection.

Cleansing the male genitalia involves washing the penis and scrotum. Sometimes smegma needs to be removed by wiping around the glans. The foreskin is not retracted, because it is normally tight in newborns. It remains adhered to the glans for approximately 3 to 14 years.

After the foreskin can be easily retracted, the boy should be taught to gently wash the glans with soap, rinsing well afterward. During the act of urination, retraction of the foreskin will help avoid irritation of the glans with urine. Parents are also instructed to be aware of the signs of urinary tract infections, which may be more common in uncircumcised infant males. Symptoms include irritability or fussiness on urination (from discomfort), voiding in small amounts and frequently, and unusual voiding urgency.

The buttocks and anal area are thoroughly cleansed of any fecal material. As with the rest of the body, the area is dried to prevent a warm, moist environment that fosters growth of bacteria.

! NURSING ALERT

If the male infant is not circumcised, the parents are taught how to cleanse under and around the foreskin by retracting it gently only as far as it will go, then returning it to its normal position after cleansing. Leaving the foreskin retracted may cause edema and discomfort of the glans penis.

A diaper is applied after the bath. It should fit snugly around the thighs and abdomen to prevent urine from leaking. In males cloth diapers are folded with extra thickness in the front to provide greater absorbency. In females the placement of the extra fold depends on whether the infant is prone or supine. Diapers are fastened with the back side overlapping the front side to allow full flexion of the hips.

The nurse should discuss the choice of cloth or disposable diapers with parents. In the United States the most commonly used diapers are disposable paper diapers. Other choices are home-laundered or commercially laundered cloth diapers. A number of factors—cost, convenience, skin care benefits, in-fection control, and environmental concerns—influence the relative merits of these three diaper types. In general, home-laundered diapers are the least expensive when human labor cost is not included. When human labor cost is included, the price difference between disposable diapers, diaper service reusable diapers, and home-laundered diapers is quite small, although paper diapers tend to cost the most. Disposable diapers are the most convenient, although a diaper service eliminates the need to shop for replacement diapers.

Disposable diapers with absorbent gelling material have benefits related to preserving healthy skin, preventing diaper dermatitis, especially beyond the neonatal period (see Chapter 30), and controlling contamination of the environment because of their better containment of urine and feces.

Care of the Umbilicus.   Because the umbilical stump is an excellent medium for bacterial growth, various methods of cord care are practiced. Common methods used include the use of an antimicrobial agent such as bacitracin or triple dye, whereas others advocate the use of alcohol alone, soap and water, or sterile water alone. The use of antiseptic agents has been shown to prolong cord drying and separation (Zupan and Garner, 2000). Studies regarding bacterial growth and colonization according to the cleansing method used have produced varied results (Janssen and others, 2003; Golombek, Brill, and Salice, 2002; Zupan and Garner, 2000; Dore and others, 1998). Current recommendations for cord care by AWHONN include cleaning the cord with sterile water or a neutral pH cleanser; subsequent care entails cleansing the cord with water (AWHONN, 2001). Nurses working in neonatal care must carefully evaluate the available studies and compare the risks and benefits regarding the method of cord care within their own population of newborns and families. Regardless of the method used, nurses must include cord care teaching in the discharge planning because it has been demonstrated to be a concern for parents following discharge to the home.

The diaper is folded in front below the cord to avoid irritation and wetness on the site. The area is kept free of urine and stool and cleansed daily with the cleanser of choice. Parents are instructed regarding stump deterioration and proper umbilical care. The stump deteriorates through the process of dry gangrene. Cord separation time is influenced by a number of factors, including type of cord care, type of delivery, and other perinatal events. The average cord separation time is 10 to 14 days.

It takes a few more weeks for the cord base to heal completely following cord separation. During this time care consists of keeping the cord clean and dry and may include wiping the base with alcohol.

! NURSING ALERT

With early hospital discharge newborns may be discharged before it is safe to remove the cord clamp. Teach the parent how to safely remove the clamp once the newborn is at least 24 hours old and no oozing from the cord is noted.

Circumcision.   Circumcision, the surgical removal of the foreskin on the glans penis, is usually done in the hospital, although it is not a common practice in most countries. Despite the frequency of the procedure in the United States, there is still much controversy regarding the benefits and risks (Box 8-4). The American Academy of Pediatrics (1999a) issued a circumcision policy statement stating that the medical benefits of male newborn circumcision are not sufficiently significant to recommend it as a routine procedure. The American Academy of Pediatrics statement emphasizes parental autonomy to determine what is in the best interest of their male newborn infant. The policy encourages the physician to ensure that parents have been given accurate and unbiased information about the risks, benefits, and alternatives before making an informed choice and that they understand that circumcision is an elective procedure. In addition to examining the medical benefits of male newborn circumcision, the Academy recommended that if parents decide to have their male infant circumcised, procedural analgesia should be provided.

This policy statement has direct implications for nurses caring for newborns and their families. First, because nurses are in a unique position to help educate parents regarding the care of their newborns, they must take responsibility for ensuring that each parent has accurate and unbiased information by which to make an informed decision regarding the appropriateness of the circumcision procedure for their newborn. Parents need to know the options for pain control, especially the choice of topical or injected anesthesia, and their option of observing the procedure.* Nurses should also be proactive in advocating for circumcision analgesia.

Second, in the event that anesthesia is not used, the nurse should use every nonpharmacologic intervention that can reduce the pain of this operative procedure (see Atrau-

---

Circumcision: Information for Parents is available from the American Academy of Pediatrics, 141 Northwest Point Boulevard., Elk Grove Village, IL 60009-1098; (888) 227-1770; Fax: (847) 228-1281; www.aap.org.

BOX 8-4 ■ Risks and Benefits of Neonatal Circumcision

RISKS	BENEFITS
Complications:	Prevention of penile cancer
Hemorrhage	and posthitis (inflammation
Infection	of prepuce)
Dehiscence (separation of approximated edges of skin)	Decreased incidence of balanitis (inflammation of glans) and, possibly, urinary
Meatitis (from loss of protective foreskin)	tract infection in infant males, as well as some sexually transmitted diseases
Adhesions	later in life
Concealed penis	Prevention of complications
Urethral fistula	associated with later cir-
Meatal stenosis	cumcision
Pain in unanesthetized infants (long-term consequences unknown, but short-term stresses include increased heart rate, behavior changes, prolonged crying, increased cortisol levels, and decreased blood oxygenation)	Preservation of male's body image that is consistent with peers (in countries where procedure is common)

matic Care box). Despite adequate scientific evidence that newborns feel and respond to pain, circumcisions are still being performed in the United States with either insufficient analgesia or no analgesia at all. Nurses can use the Academy's policy statement to advocate more effectively for the use of optimal pain relief for circumcision. The American College of Obstetricians and Gynecologists (2001) has also issued a statement in support of administering analgesia during neonatal circumcision.

Circumcision is usually performed in the nursery. It should not be performed immediately after delivery because of the neonate's unstabilized physiologic status and increased susceptibility to stress. Preoperative nursing care usually includes allowing the infant nothing by mouth before the procedure to prevent aspiration of vomitus (about 2 hours); however, the necessity of this practice has recently been questioned (Kraft, 2003). Additional measures include checking for a signed consent form and adequately restraining the infant, usually on a special board (Fig. 8-14) or physiologic circumcision restraint chair. The circumcision chair is padded and allows free movement of the newborn's extremities without compromising the surgical field. In addition, the chair allows the infant to sit at a 30- to 45-degree angle, and it is adjustable to accommodate smaller newborns (Stang and others, 1997). All of the equipment used for the procedure, such as gloves, instruments, dressings, and draping towels, must be sterile.

The procedure involves freeing the foreskin from the glans penis by using a scalpel, Gomco or Mogen (see Cultural Awareness box) clamp, or Plastibell. In the *Gomco technique* the foreskin is clamped, cut with a scalpel, and removed; the clamp crushes the nerve endings and blood vessels, promoting hemostasis. In the *Plastibell procedure* the foreskin is removed using a plastic ring and a string tied around the foreskin like a tourniquet. The excess foreskin is trimmed. In about 5 to 8 days the plastic ring separates and falls off.

After the procedure is completed, the infant is released from the restraints and comforted. If the parents were not present during the procedure, they are informed of the infant's status and reunited with their son.

Care of the circumcision depends on the type of procedure. If a clamp (Gomco or Mogen) was used, a petrolatum

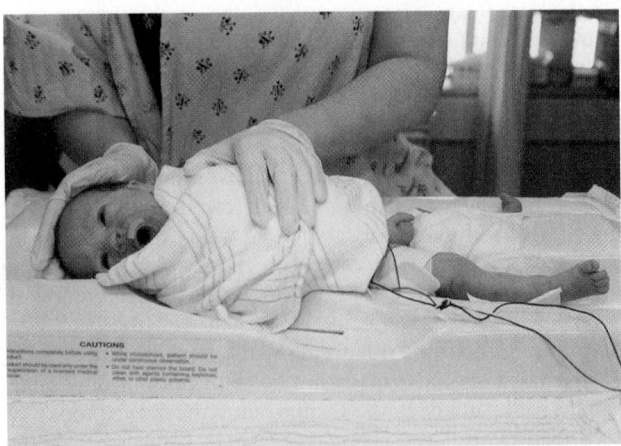

FIG. 8-14 ■ Proper positioning of infant in Circumstraint. (Photo by Paul Vincent Kuntz, Texas Children's Hospital.)

gauze dressing may be applied loosely to prevent adherence to the diaper. If the Plastibell was applied, no special dressing is required. Because the area is tender, the diaper is applied loosely to prevent friction against the penis. The circumcision is evaluated for excessive bleeding in the first few hours after the procedure, and the first void is recorded. A recommended standard is to evaluate the site every 30 minutes for at least 2 hours and then at least every 2 hours thereafter (Williamson, 1997).

> ### NURSING TIP
>
> To check for the first void in disposable diapers made of absorbent gelling material, pinch the crotch of the diaper for a "clumpy, doughy" feeling, because these diapers will feel dry despite voiding.

Normally, on the second day a yellowish white exudate forms as part of the granulation process. This is not a sign of infection and is not forcibly removed. As healing progresses, the exudate disappears. Parents are educated to report any evidence of bleeding, unusual swelling, or absence of voiding to the practitioner.

Provide Optimal Nutrition

Selection of a feeding method is one of the major decisions faced by parents. In general, there are three acceptable choices: human milk, commercially prepared whole cow's milk formula, and modified evaporated cow's milk. There are significant nutritional, economic, and psychologic advantages and differences among these methods. Nurses should be at the forefront in providing the parent(s) with accurate and unbiased information needed to make a conscientious informed decision regarding the feeding method. In general, there are two primary choices: human milk and commercially prepared cow's milk–based formula. There are significant nutritional, economic, and psychologic advantages and differences between these two methods.

Human Milk.   Human milk is the best option for infant nutrition up to 1 year of age. Breast milk consists of a number of micronutrients that are called bioavailable, meaning these nutrients are available in quantities and qualities that make them easily digestible by the newborn's intestine and absorbed for energy and growth. Breast milk offers a variety of immunologic properties that are found exclusively in human milk. Human milk has been shown to be effective in protecting the newborn against respiratory infections, gastrointestinal infections caused by enterococci, otitis media, numerous allergies, and atopy. The fat content of human milk is composed of lipids, triglycerides, and cholesterol; cholesterol is an essential element for brain growth. The function of these lipids is to allow optimal intestinal absorption of essential fatty acids and polyunsaturated fatty acids (PUFAs). Furthermore, lipids contribute approximately 50% of the total calories in human milk (Lawrence and Lawrence, 1999). Although the overall fat content in human milk is higher than in cow's milk, it is used more efficiently by the infant.

The primary source of carbohydrate in human milk is lactose, which is present in higher concentrations (6.8 g/dL) than in cow's milk–based formula (4.9 g/dL). The carbohydrates not only serve as a large portion of total calories in human milk but they also have protective functions; the oligosaccharides in human milk stimulate the growth of *Lactobacillus bifidus* and prevent bacteria from adhering to epithelial surfaces. Additional carbohydrates found in human milk include glucose, galactose, and glucosamine.

Human milk also contains two proteins, whey (lactalbumin) and casein (curd), in a ratio of approximately 60:40 (80:20 in most cow-milk based formula). This ratio in human milk makes it more digestible and produces the soft stools seen in breast-fed infants. Thus human milk has a laxative effect and constipation is uncommon. The whey protein, lactoferrin, in human milk has iron-binding characteristics with bacteriostatic capabilities, particularly against gram-positive and gram-negative aerobes, anaerobes, and yeasts (Lawrence and Lawrence, 1999).

Lysozyme is found in large quantities in human milk with bacteriostatic functions against gram-positive bacteria and Enterobacteriaceae. Human milk also contains numerous other host defense factors such as macrophages, granulocytes, and T- and B-lymphocytes. Casein in human milk greatly enhances the absorption of iron, thus preventing iron-dependent bacteria from proliferating in the gastrointestinal tract (Biancuzzo, 1999). Secretory IgA is found in high levels in colostrum, but levels gradually decline over the first 14 days of life. Secretory IgA prevents bacteria and viruses from invading the intestinal mucosa in breast-fed newborns, thus protecting from infection (Hanson and Korotkova, 2002). The whey protein is also believed to play an important role in preventing the development of certain allergies.

Several digestive enzymes also present in human milk include amylases, lipases, proteases, and ribonucleases, which enhance the digestion and absorption of various nutrients. The amounts of lipid and water-soluble vitamins as well as electrolytes, minerals, and trace elements in human milk are

---

CULTURAL AWARENESS

Circumcision

In the Jewish culture circumcision is performed during a ceremony called a **berith**, or **brit**, which takes place on the eighth day of life. A specially trained professional known as a **mohel** stretches the prepuce over the glans, pulling it though a slit in a shield (usually a Mogen clamp) and cutting it with a knife. The traditional technique is not sterile, and bleeding is controlled by tight bandaging around the penis (Cohen and others, 1992). The infant may be given some sweet wine before the procedure. Blankets instead of straps are usually used to restrain the infant to a board, and the parents are present (Trochtenberg, 1990).

Female circumcision (mutilation) is also practiced, particularly in Africa, the Middle East, and Southeast Asia—and in immigrants from these countries to the United States, Australia, Canada, and Europe. In the most extensive operation (excision or infibulation) the clitoris, labia minora, and medial aspects of the labia majora are removed. The remaining labia majora are sewn closed, except for a small opening for urine and menses (American Academy of Pediatrics, 1998a; McCleary, 1994). Anesthesia is used very rarely. In African and Asian cultures, female circumcision is used to prove virginity and to reduce sexual pleasure, thus promoting fidelity. The World Health Organization condemns all forms of female genital mutilation (Female genital mutilation, 1994).

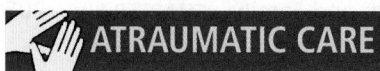

Guidelines for Pain Management During Neonatal Circumcision

PHARMACOLOGIC INTERVENTIONS

Use of Topical Anesthetic

One hour before the procedure, administer acetaminophen.

Place a thick layer (1 g) of EMLA* cream around the penis where the prepuce (foreskin) attaches to the glans. Avoid placing cream on the tip of the penis where EMLA may come in contact with urethral opening.

Cover the penis with a "finger cot" that is cut from a vinyl or latex glove, or a piece of plastic wrap and secure bottom of covering with tape. Avoid using Tegaderm or large amounts of tape on the skin because removing the adhesive causes pain and can irritate or remove the fragile skin.

If the infant urinates during the time EMLA is applied (1 hour) and a significant amount of EMLA is removed, reapply the cream and covering. The total application of EMLA should not exceed a surface area of 10 cm² (1.25 × 1.25 inches).

Remove cream with clean cloth or tissue. Blanching of skin is an expected reaction to EMLA's application under an occlusive dressing; erythema and some edema may occur also.

During procedure, give the infant a concentrated sucrose solution (24%). Use this solution to coat the pacifier (recoat several times before and during the procedure) or administer 2 mL to the tongue 2 minutes before the procedure.

Following procedure, apply petrolatum or A&D ointment on a 4×4 dressing before diapering infant to prevent the wound from adhering to the dressing or diaper. Topical anesthetic alone is not recommended for pain management of circumcision.

Use of Dorsal Penile Nerve Block (DPNB) or Ring Block

One hour before procedure administer acetaminophen.

One hour before procedure, apply EMLA. For the DPNB apply EMLA to the prepuce as described previously and at the penile base. For the ring block apply EMLA to the prepuce as described previously and to the shaft of the penis. A topical anesthetic should be used in conjunction with the dorsal penile nerve block or ring block to avoid the pain of injecting the anesthetic.

Use a 30-gauge needle to administer the lidocaine.[†] For the DPNB, 0.4 mL of the lidocaine is infiltrated at the 10:30 o'clock and 1:30 o'clock positions in Buck's fascia at the penile base. For the ring block, 0.4 mL of lidocaine is infiltrated subcutaneously on each side of the shaft of the penis below the prepuce. Using buffered lidocaine (with sodium bicarbonate) and warming the solution may further decrease pain. (Lidocaine with epinephrine is not used in neonates).

For maximum anesthesia, wait 5 minutes following the injection of lidocaine. An alternative anesthesia is chloroprocaine, which is as effective as lidocaine after 3 minutes.

During the circumcision, administer sucrose as described previously.

Apply A&D ointment or petrolatum as described previously.

Acetaminophen

Administer acetaminophen as ordered by the practitioner (10-15 mg/kg) every 4 to 6 hours for 24 hours not to exceed five doses in 24 hours or a maximum dose of 75 mg/kg/day

Oral Sucrose

Administer 2 mL of a concentrated solution (12%-25%) of oral sucrose 2 min before procedure

Allow infant to suck on pacifier dipped in oral sucrose during procedure.

NONPHARMACOLOGIC INTERVENTIONS (TO ACCOMPANY PRECEDING PHARMACOLOGIC INTERVENTIONS)

If Circumstraint board is used, pad with blankets or other thick, soft material such as "lamb's wool." A more comfortable, padded, and physiologic restraint that places the infant semi-reclining can also decrease distress (Stang and others, 1997).[‡]

Provide the parents, caregiver, or another staff member with the option to hold the infant during the procedure or to be present during the circumcision.

Swaddle the upper body and legs during the procedure to provide warmth and containment and to reduce movement.

If the patient is not swaddled and is unclothed, use a radiant warmer to prevent hypothermia. Shield infant's eyes from overhead lights as needed.

Prewarm any topical solutions to be used in sterile preparation of the surgical site by placing in a warm blanket or towel.

Play infant relaxation music§ before, during, and after procedure; allow parents or other caregiver the option to provide the music of choice.

Following the procedure, remove restraints and swaddle. Immediately have the parent, other caregiver, or nursing staff hold the infant. Continue to have the infant suck on pacifier or offer feeding.

Recommend use of combination analgesia: or oral sucrose, acetaminophen and topical anesthetic; oral sucrose, acetaminophen, topical anesthesia, and DPNB or Ring Block, in addition to nonpharmacologic comfort measures.

Data from Broadman LM and others: Post-circumcision analgesia: a prospective evaluation of subcutaneous ring block of the penis, *Anesthesiology* 67:339-402, 1987; Howard CR, Howard FM, Weitzman ML: Acetaminophen analgesia in neonatal circumcision: the effect on pain, *Pediatrics* 93(4):641-646, 1994; Lander J and others: Comparison of ring block, dorsal penile nerve block, and topical anesthesia for neonatal circumcision, *JAMA* 278:2157-2162, 1997; Mintz MR, Grillo R: Dorsal penile nerve block for circumcision, *Clin Pediatr* 28:590-591, 1989; Serour F, Mandelberg A, Mori J: Slow injection of local anesthetic will decrease pain during dorsal penile nerve block, *Acta Anesthesiol Scand* 42:926-928, 1998; Spencer DM and others: Dorsal penile nerve block in neonatal circumcision: chloroprocaine versus lidocaine, *Am J Perinatol* 9(3):214-218, 1992; Stang H and others: Beyond dorsal penile nerve block: a more humane circumcision, *Pediatrics* 100(2):E3, 1997 (www.pediatrics.org/cgi/content/full/100/2/e3); Stevens B and others: The efficacy of sucrose for relieving procedural pain in neonates—a systematic review and meta-analysis, *Acta Pediatr* 86:837-842, 1997; Taddio A and others: Efficacy and safety of lidocaine-prilocaine cream (EMLA) for pain during circumcision, *N Engl J Med* 336(17):1197-1201, 1997; Taddio A: Pain management for neonatal circumcision, *Paediatr Drugs* 3(2):101-111, 2001; Taddio A, Ohlsson K, Ohlsson A: Lidocaine-prilocaine cream for analgesia during circumcision in newborn boys, *Cochrane Syst Rev* 2003(1):CD000496; Geyer and others: An evidence-based multidisciplinary protocol for neonatal circumcision pain management, *J Obstet Gynecol Neonatal Nurs* 31(4):403-410, 2002; Taddio A and others: Combined analgesia and local anesthesia to minimize pain during circumcision, *Arch Pediatr Adol Med* 154(6): 620-623, 2000; Kraft NL: A pictorial and video guide to circumcision without pain, *Adv Neonatal Care* 3(2): 50-64, 2003.

*Note: In March, 1999, the FDA approved the use of EMLA in infants age 37 weeks of gestation. Although the package insert lists under "Warnings" that patients taking drugs associated with drug-induced methemoglobinemia, such as acetaminophen, are at greater risk for developing methemoglobinemia, there have been no reported cases of this complication occurring in children taking acetaminophen and using EMLA. In fact, there is no evidence that acetaminophen is a methemoglobin-inducing drug in humans. (Prescott LF: *Paracetamol (acetaminophen): a critical bibliographic review*, Bristol, 1996, Taylor & Francis.) The only reported cases of methemoglobinemia from acetaminophen have been in cats and dogs (Hjelle JJ, Grauer GF: Acetaminophen-induced toxicosis in dogs and cats, *J Am Vet Med Assoc* 188(7):742-749, 1986.)

†Note: In one study, the use of buffered lidocaine, which normally reduces the stinging sensation of lidocaine, did not provide effective anesthesia for DPNB (Stang and others, 1997). The study on slow injection of the anesthetics lidocaine and bupivacaine compared 40 vs 80 seconds in patients ages 15-53 years (Serour F, Mandelberg A, Mori J: Slow injection of local anesthetic will decrease pain during dorsal penile nerve block, *Acta Anesthesiol Scand* 42:926-928, 1998).

‡For information on the Stang Circ Chair, contact Pedicraft, 4134 Augustine Rd., Jacksonville, FL 32207; (800) 223-7649; e-mail: info www.pedicraft.com.

§Suggested infant relaxation music: *Heartbeat Lullabies* by Terry Woodford. Available from Baby-Go-To-Sleep Center, Audio Therapy Innovations, Inc., PO Box 550, Colorado Springs, CO 80901; (800) 537-7748.

sufficient for growth, development, and energy needs during the first 6 months of life. The one possible exception to the vitamin content is vitamin D, which is found in varying amounts depending on the mother's intake of vitamin D–fortified food and exposure to ultraviolet light. Therefore, to prevent vitamin-D–deficiency rickets, the American Academy of Pediatrics (2003b) now recommends that infants who are exclusively breast-fed, and consuming less than 500 mL vitamin D–fortified formula or milk per day, or who are ingesting less than 500 mL per day of vitamin-D–fortified formula or milk, be supplemented with 200 IU vitamin D (oral) per day. In addition, older children who are not regularly exposed to sunlight, do not take a multivitamin supplement containing at least 200 IU vitamin-D–or do not consume at least 500 mL of vitamin-D–fortified milk, should receive a supplement of 200 IU vitamin D daily.

Additional beneficial components of human milk include prostaglandins, epidermal growth factor, desoxyhexanoic acid (DHA), arachidonic acid, taurine, cystine, carnitine, cytokine, interleukins, and natural hormones such as thyroid-releasing hormone, gonadotrophin-releasing hormone, and prolactin. Studies have demonstrated that breast-feeding is associated with a decrease in the incidence of type 2 diabetes (Kue Young and others, 2002), a decrease in the incidence of hospital admissions for respiratory tract illnesses in generally healthy infants (Bachrach, Schwarz, and Bachrach, 2003), and higher intelligence scores than cow's-milk–based formula-fed infants (Anderson, Johnstone, and Remley, 1999).

Some studies have demonstrated that breast-feeding has an analgesic effect on newborns during painful procedures such as heel puncture (Carbajal and others, 2003; Gray and others, 2002).

Breast-Feeding. Human milk is the preferred form of nutrition for all infants. The incidence of breast-feeding in the United States declined in the 1980s, but data from 1990 to 2001 show an overall increase of more than 26% in the number of mothers initiating breast-feeding in the hospital; in addition, there was an increase (32.5%) in the number of mothers breast-feeding at 6 months (Ryan, Wenjun, and Acosta, 2002). There has been concern voiced that the increasingly early discharge of new mothers from hospitals, more aggressive marketing of infant formulas to the public, and more employed mothers have contributed to the decline of breast-feeding in the 1980s. There is evidence that hospital practices intended to provide optimal maternal-newborn health may instead undermine breast-feeding. Early separation of mother and newborn, delays in initiating breast-feeding, provision of formula in the hospital and in discharge packs, conflicting information by health care workers, and formula coupons given at discharge have been implicated in the decline of breast-feeding following discharge. Rooming-in has correlated positively with successful breast-feeding, whereas the use of a pacifier has sometimes been associated with earlier weaning from breast to bottle. Changing hospital practices that were perceived as detrimental to breast-feeding significantly improved the overall duration of breast-feeding in one study (Wright, Rice, and Wells, 1996). Although some studies have shown that the availability of commercial formula from hospital "discharge packs" may influence mothers to bottle-feed,

other studies have found no such effect (Donnelly and others, 2000; Dungy and others, 1997).

A survey of breast-feeding mothers indicated that the determining factors for changing to bottle-feeding included the mother's perception of the father's attitude toward breast-feeding and the mother's uncertainty regarding the amount of milk the infant would receive (Arora and others, 2000). These findings have important implications for involving fathers in education and discussion regarding breast-feeding before and during the pregnancy. Fathers may express concerns of feeling left out during the newborn period if they have little involvement other than diapering and holding the infant. Encouraging fathers regarding their positive role in supporting the mother to breast-feed may help decrease feelings of isolation, benefit mother-infant interaction, and decrease a sense of helplessness and isolation.

The American Academy of Pediatrics (2004) has reaffirmed its position exclusively recommending breastfeeding until at least 1 year of age as the best form of infant nutrition. The Academy also supports programs that enable women to continue breast-feeding after returning to work. In its support of breast-feeding practices, the Academy further discourages the advertisement of infant formula to breast-feeding mothers and distribution of formula discharge packs without the advice of a health care provider.

The *Baby-Friendly Hospital Initiative (BFHI)* is a joint effort of the World Health Organization and the United Nations Children's Fund to encourage, promote, and support breast-feeding as the model for optimum infant nutrition. Ten research-supported practices were developed by BFHI as a guideline for maternity facilities worldwide to promote breast-feeding (Wright, Rice, and Wells, 1996; Kyenkya-Isabirye, 1992) (Box 8-5).

BOX 8-5 ■ Ten Steps to Successful Breast-Feeding

Every facility providing maternity services and care for newborn infants should:

1. Have a written breast-feeding policy that is routinely communicated to all health care staff.
2. Train all health care staff in skills necessary to implement this policy.
3. Inform all pregnant women about the benefits and management of breast-feeding.
4. Help mothers initiate breast-feeding within a half-hour of birth.
5. Show mothers how to breast-feed and how to maintain lactation, even if they should be separated from their infants.
6. Give newborn infants no food or drink other than breast milk, unless medically indicated.
7. Practice rooming-in—allow mothers and infants to remain together—24 hours a day.
8. Encourage breast-feeding on demand.
9. Give no artificial teats or pacifiers (also called dummies or soothers) to breast-feeding infants.
10. Foster the establishment of breast-feeding support groups and refer mothers to them on discharge from the hospital or clinic.

From Kyenkya-Isabirye M: UNICEF launches the Baby-Friendly Hospital Initiative, *MCN* 17(4):177-179, 1992; Wright A, Rice S, Wells S: Changing hospital practices to increase the duration of breastfeeding, *Pediatrics* 97(5):669-676, 1996.

In addition to the physiologic qualities of human milk, the most outstanding psychologic benefit of breast-feeding is the close maternal-child relationship. The infant is nestled very close to the mother's skin, can hear the rhythm of her heartbeat, can feel the warmth of her body, and has a sense of peaceful security. The mother has a very close feeling of union with her child and feels a sense of accomplishment and satisfaction as the infant sucks milk from her.

Human milk is the most economical form of feeding. It is always available, ready to serve at room temperature, and free of contamination. Although human milk is not sterile, healthy full-term infants can tolerate varying amounts of nonpathogenic and pathogenic organisms. The protection against infection can provide additional cost savings in terms of fewer medical visits and less time lost from work for the employed mother.

Breast-fed infants, especially beyond 2 to 3 months of age, tend to grow at a satisfactory but slower rate than bottle-fed infants.

Contraindications to breast-feeding include (Lawrence and Lawrence, 2001):

- Maternal cancer therapy
- Active tuberculosis not under treatment in mother
- HIV in mother
- Galactosemia in infant
- Cytomegalovirus (CMV)—primary risk is to premature infants receiving CMV-infected donor milk, not to infected mother's infant, who already has CMV
- Maternal substance abuse (e.g., cocaine and marijuana)
- Human T-cell leukemia virus type 1

Mastitis is usually not a contraindication if the discomfort is tolerable. The Centers for Disease Control and Prevention currently does not consider maternal hepatitis C to be a contraindication for breast-feeding (Lawrence and Lawrence, 2001).

Breast-feeding can also be done with twin births. If both twins are full term, they can begin feedings immediately after birth (Fig. 8-15). Simultaneous feeding promotes the rapid production of milk needed for both infants and makes the milk that would normally be lost in the letdown reflex available to one of the twins. When only one infant is hun-

gry, the mother should feed singly. She should also alternate breasts when feeding each infant and avoid favoring one breast for one infant. The suckling patterns of infants vary, and each infant needs the visual stimulation and exercise that alternating breasts provides.

A disadvantage of breast-feeding to many mothers is the perceived inconvenience of loss of freedom and independence. Being committed to feeding the infant every 2 to 3 hours can be overwhelming, especially to women with multiple responsibilities. Many women resume their careers shortly after their pregnancy and prefer to use bottle-feeding. However, breast-feeding and employment are possible, and suggestions for the mother are discussed in Chapter 10. Although breast-feeding is the preferred form of infant feeding, mothers' decisions regarding their preferences must be supported and respected.

Successful breast-feeding probably depends more on the mother's desire to breast-feed, satisfaction with breast-feeding, and available support systems than on any other factors. Contrary to popular belief, breast-feeding is not instinctive. Mothers need support, encouragement, and assistance during their postpartum hospital stay and at home to enhance their opportunities for success and satisfaction.

Three main criteria have been proposed as essential in promoting positive breast-feeding: correct sucking technique, absence of a rigid feeding time schedule, and correct positioning of the infant at the breast to achieve latch-on. Correct suckling for breast-feeding is defined as a wide-open mouth, tongue under the areola, and expression of milk by slow, deep suckling (Fig. 8-16).

The following interventions promote breast-feeding:

- Frequent and early breast-feeding, especially during the first hour of life; immediate skin-to-skin contact; rooming-in; feeding on demand; and careful control of drugs that may decrease maternal milk supply or affect the mother's ability to breast-feed
- Direct modeling of the importance of breast-feeding by health care providers, such as implementing demand nurs-

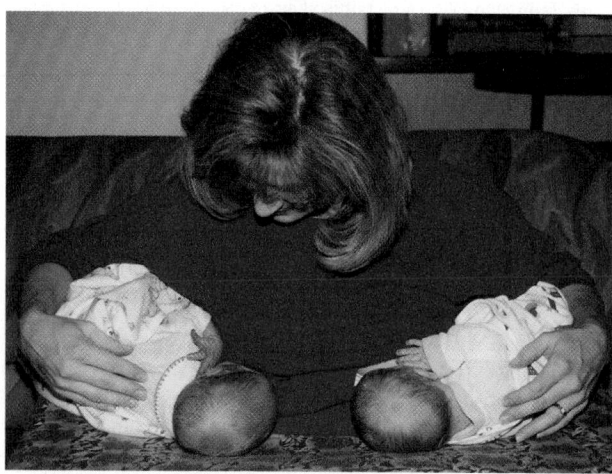

FIG. 8-15 ■ Simultaneous breast-feeding of twins.

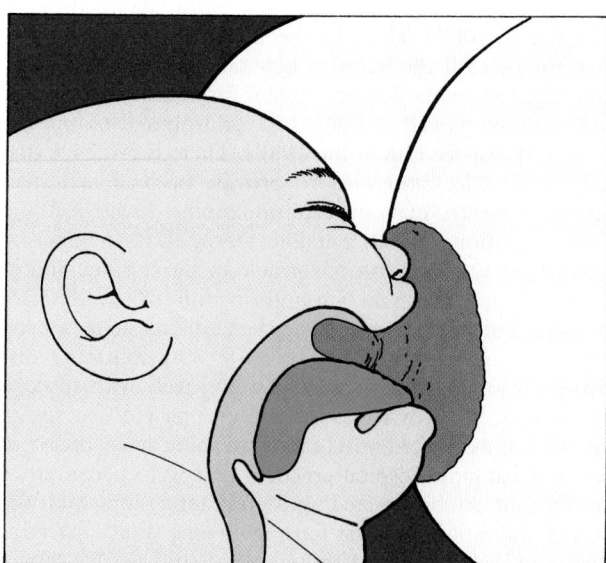

FIG. 8-16 ■ The tongue is under the areola, with the tip of the nipple at the back of the wide-open mouth.

ing with no formula supplementation and decreased emphasis on infant formula products

- Increased information and support to mothers following discharge, especially phone follow-up
- Early breast pumping every 2 to 3 hours for 10 to 15 minutes bilaterally if the newborn is unable to nurse immediately (increases oxytocin production and thus milk production)

Nurses play a very significant role in the breast-feeding decision and must make themselves available to families for guidance and support. Several excellent books and organizations, such as **LaLeche League,** * are available as resources for professionals and breast-feeding mothers.

!**NURSING ALERT**

Do not use microwaving to defrost frozen human milk. High-temperature microwaving (72° to 98° C [162° to 208° F]) significantly destroys the antiinfective factors and vitamin C content. The safety of low-temperature microwaving (20° to 53° C [68° to 127° F]) remains questionable. One of the best ways to thaw frozen human milk is to place the bottle under a warm flow of tap water until the milk is thawed. Another option is to let the frozen milk thaw overnight in the refrigerator to maintain high levels of secretory IgA (Biancuzzo, 1999). Test the temperature of the milk before feeding.

Bottle-Feeding.   Bottle-feeding generally refers to the use of bottles for feeding commercial or evaporated milk formula rather than using the breast, although human milk may be expressed and fed with a bottle when necessary. Bottle-feeding is an acceptable method of feeding. However, nurses should not assume that new parents automatically know how to bottle-feed their infant. Parents who choose bottle feeding also need support and assistance in meeting their infant's needs.

Providing newborns with nutrition is only one aspect of the feeding. Holding them close to the body while rocking or cuddling them helps to ensure the emotional component of feeding. Like breast-fed infants, bottle-fed infants need to be held on alternate sides of the lap to expose them to different stimuli. The feeding should not be hurried. Even though they may suck vigorously for the first 5 minutes and seem to be satisfied, they should be allowed to continue sucking. Infants need at least 2 hours of sucking a day. If there are six feedings per day, then about 20 minutes of sucking at each feeding provides for oral gratification.

NURSING TIP

An angled bottle is preferable to a straight bottle, because it encourages more physiologic positioning of the infant, improves the infant's comfort level, and decreases the need for burping (Farber, Van Fossen, and Koontz, 1995).

Propping the bottle is discouraged for the following reasons:

- It denies the infant the important component of close human contact.
- The infant may aspirate formula while sleeping.

---

*1400 N. Meacham, Schaumburg, IL 60173; (800) LA-LECHE, (800) 525-3243; website: www.lalecheleague.org. In Canada: PO Box 29, 18C Industrial Drive, Chesterville, Ontario, KOC 1HO; (613) 448-1842, (800) 665-4324; website: www.lalecheleaguecanada.org.

- It may facilitate the development of middle ear infections. As the infant lies flat and sucks, milk that has pooled in the pharynx becomes a suitable medium for bacterial growth. Bacteria then enters the eustachian tube, which leads to the middle ear, causing acute otitis media.
- It encourages continuous pooling of formula in the mouth, which can lead to nursing caries when the teeth erupt (see Chapter 12).

!**NURSING ALERT**

Warming bottles in the microwave oven is not recommended because of the risk of burns from bottles exploding or the hot temperature of the fluid. When milk is warmed in the microwave it is not warmed evenly and some may be too hot, causing mouth burns.

Preparation of Formula.   The two traditional ways of preparing formula are the terminal heat method (all of the utensils and formula are boiled together for 25 minutes) and the aseptic method (the equipment is boiled separately, after which the formula is poured into the bottles). Because of improved sanitary conditions in developed countries, neither of these methods is essential. The clean technique is satisfactory, including using a dishwasher. Persons preparing the formula wash their hands well and then wash all of the equipment used to prepare the formula, including the cans of formula or evaporated milk. The formula is prepared and bottled immediately before each feeding. Warming the formula is optional, although many parents prefer to warm it before feeding. Any milk remaining in the bottle after the feeding is discarded, because it is an excellent medium for bacterial growth. Opened cans of formula are covered and refrigerated until the next feeding. The recent incident involving contamination of powdered formula with *Enterobacter sakazakii* and subsequent infant death in a neonatal unit has brought attention to formula preparation in the hospital; formula preparation for in-hospital use is further discussed in Chapter 9.

Recommendations for labeling infant formulas require that the directions for preparation and use of the formula include pictures and symbols for nonreading individuals. In addition, manufacturers are translating the directions into foreign languages, such as Spanish and Vietnamese, to prevent misunderstanding and errors in formula preparation.

!**NURSING ALERT**

Impress on families that the proportions of powdered and concentrated formulas must not be altered or diluted to extend the amount of formula, nor concentrated to provide more calories (except under medical supervision).

Commercially Prepared Formulas.   The analysis of human and whole cow's milk indicates that the latter is unsuitable for infant nutrition. Whole cow's milk has a high protein content, low fat and lipid content, and there has been evidence that it may cause intestinal bleeding and lead to iron-deficiency anemia in infants. There has also been some question regarding the unmodified protein content of whole cow's milk, which may trigger an undesired immune response and thus increase the incidence of allergies in children at an early age.

Commercially prepared formulas are cow's milk–based and have been modified to closely resemble the nutritional content of human milk. These formulas are altered from cow's milk by removing butterfat, decreasing the protein content, and adding vegetable oil and carbohydrate. Some cow's milk–based formulas have demineralized whey added to yield a whey:casein ratio of 60:40. The standard cow's milk–based formulas, regardless of the commercial brand, have essentially the same compositions of vitamins, minerals, protein, carbohydrates, and essential amino acids, with minor variations such as the source of carbohydrate (Akers and Groh-Wargo, 1999), nucleotides to enhance immune function, and long-chain polyunsaturated fatty acids (LCPUFAs) DHA and arachidonic acid, which are thought to improve brain function (Georgieff, 2001). Furthermore, the Food and Drug Administration (FDA) regulates the manufacture of infant formula in the United States to ensure product safety. Standard cow's milk–based formulas are sold as low-iron and iron-fortified; however, only the iron-fortified formulas meet the requirements of infants (Akers and Groh-Wargo, 1999).

There are four main categories of commercially prepared infant formulas: (1) *cow's milk–based formulas,* available in 20 kcal/fl oz as liquid (ready to feed), as powder (requires dilution with water), or as a concentrated liquid (requires dilution with water); (2) *soy-based formulas,* available commercially in ready-to-feed 20 kcal/fl oz powder and concentrated liquid forms, commonly used for children who are lactose- or cow's milk protein- intolerant; (3) *casein- or whey-hydrolysate formulas,* commercially available in ready-to-feed and powder forms and used primarily for children who cannot tolerate or digest cow's milk or soy-based formulas (Wilson and Bowman, 2000); and (4) *amino acid formulas.*

The American Academy of Pediatrics (2004) recommends the use of soy protein–based formulas for infants with galactosemia, hereditary lactase deficiency, documented IgE allergies caused by cow's milk, and documented evidence of lactose intolerance. Soy protein–based formulas, however, have not been proved to be effective against colic or in the prevention of allergy in healthy or high-risk infants (American Academy of Pediatrics, 1998b).

The casein- or whey-hydrolysate formulas are considered to be less antigenic than either cow's milk–based or soy-based formulas. The protein hydrolysate formulas (casein and whey) are derived from cow's milk–based formulas by a process of heat, filtration, and enzyme treatment designed to break the peptide chains into more digestible and nonallergic proteins. The hydrolysate formulas have the disadvantage of tasting bad; however, these may be made more palatable by adding a hypoallergenic flavoring such as Vari-Flavor (Christie, 1999).

Neocate and Elecare (Ross Labs) are extensively hydrolyzed amino acid formulas, designed for infants who are sensitive to cow's milk–based, soy-based, and partially hydrolyzed casein- and whey-based formulas. Both products are available in powder form. A wide variety of formulas are manufactured for infants and children with special needs; it is not within the scope of this text to discuss each one, but a formula company representative can provide product books that describe the purpose and content of each formula.

Follow-up formulas are marketed as a transitional formula for infants older than 6 months who are also eating solid foods. These generally contain a higher percentage of calories from protein and carbohydrate sources, a higher amount of iron and vitamins, and a lower amount of fat than standard cow's milk–based formulas. Many nutrition experts and the Academy of Pediatrics (2004), however, discount the necessity of follow-up formulas if the infant is receiving an adequate amount of solid foods containing sufficient iron, vitamins, and minerals.

Alternate Milk Products. In the United States few infants are fed *evaporated milk formula,* and its use is not recommended by the American Academy of Pediatrics. However, it has many advantages over whole milk. It is readily available in cans, needs no refrigeration if unopened, is less expensive than commercial formula, provides a softer, more digestible curd, and contains more lactalbumin and a higher calcium:phosphorus ratio. Disadvantages of evaporated milk for infant nutrition include low iron and vitamin C concentrations, excessive sodium and phosphorus, decreased vitamin A and D (except in fortified forms), and poorly digested fat (Akers and Groh-Wargo, 1999). A common rule for preparing evaporated milk formula is diluting the 13-ounce can of milk with 19½ ounces of water and adding 3 tablespoons of sugar or commercially processed corn syrup.

Evaporated milk must not be confused with condensed milk, which is a form of evaporated milk with 45% more sugar. Because of its high carbohydrate concentration and disproportionately low fat and protein content, condensed milk is not used for infant feeding. Likewise, skim and low-fat milk must not be used for infant milk because they are deficient in caloric concentration, significantly increase the renal solute load and water demands, and deprive the body of essential fatty acids.

Goat's milk is a poor source of iron and folic acid. It has an excessively high renal solute load as a result of its high protein content, making it unsuitable for infant nutrition. Some parents believe that goat's milk is less allergenic than other available milk sources and may feed it to their infant to reduce allergic milk reactions. However, infants who indeed have a reaction to foreign proteins in cow's milk will likewise react to the foreign proteins in goat's milk (Fomon, 1993). Raw, unpasteurized milk from any animal source is unacceptable for infant nutrition.

Feeding Schedules. Ideally, feeding schedules should be determined by the infant's hunger. *Demand feedings* involve feeding infants when they signal readiness. *Scheduled feedings* are arranged at predetermined intervals. Some hospital routines involve a 4-hour feeding schedule for healthy term newborns. Although this may be satisfactory for bottle-fed infants, it hinders the breast-feeding process. Breast-fed infants tend to be hungry every 2 to 3 hours because of the easy digestibility of the milk; therefore, they should be fed on demand.

Supplemental feedings should *not* be offered to breast-fed infants before lactation is well established, because they may satiate the infant and may cause nipple preference. Supplemental water is not needed in breast-fed infants, even in hot climates. Furthermore, giving infants electrolyte-free water may result in water intoxication, hyponatremia, and subsequent seizures. Satiated infants suck less vigorously at the breast, and milk production depends on the breast being emptied at each feeding. If milk is allowed to accumulate in the ducts, causing breast engorgement, ischemia results, suppressing the activity of the acini or milk-secreting cells. Consequently, milk production is reduced. In addition, the process of sucking from a bottle is different from breast nipple compression. The relatively inflexible rubber nipple prevents the tongue from its usual rhythmic action. Infants learn to put the tongue against the nipple holes to slow down the more rapid flow of fluid. When infants use these same tongue movements during breast-feeding, they may push the human nipple out of the mouth and may not grasp the areola properly.

Usually by 3 weeks of age lactation and a predictable feeding pattern are established. Bottle-fed infants retain about 2 to 3 ounces of formula at each feeding and are fed approximately six times a day. The quantity of formula consumed is based on the caloric need of 108 kcal/kg/day; therefore, a newborn who weighs 3 kg requires 324 kcal/day. Because commercial formula has 20 kcal/oz, approximately 16 ounces (480 mL) will provide the daily caloric requirement. Breast-fed infants may feed as frequently as 10 to 12 times a day. Larger infants are able to retain increased amounts because of greater stomach capacity; as a result, they generally sleep through the night sooner than smaller infants or breast-fed infants.

Feeding Behavior.   Five behavioral stages occur during successful feeding. Recognizing these steps can assist nurses in identifying potential feeding problems caused by improper feeding techniques. *Prefeeding behavior,* such as crying or fussing, demonstrates the infant's level of arousal and degree of hunger. To encourage the infant to grasp the breast properly, it is preferable to begin feeding during the quiet alert state, before the infant becomes upset. *Approach behavior* is indicated by sucking movements or the rooting reflex. *Attachment behavior* includes activities that occur from the time the infant receives the nipple and sucks (sometimes more pronounced during initial attempts at breast-feeding). *Consummatory behavior* consists of coordinated sucking and swallowing. Persistent gagging might indicate unsuccessful consummatory behavior. *Satiety behavior* is observed when infants let the parent know that they are satisfied, usually by falling asleep.

Promote Parent-Infant Bonding (Attachment)

The process of parenting is based on a mutual relationship between parent and infant. As more is learned of the complexity of neonates and of their potential for influencing and shaping their environments, particularly their interaction with significant others, it is apparent that promoting positive parent-child relationships necessitates an understanding of factors involved in identifying behavioral steps in attachment, variables that enhance or hinder this process, and methods of teaching parents ways to develop a stronger relationship with their children, especially by recognizing potential problems. (See also Assessment of Attachment Behaviors, p. 193.)

Infant Behavior.   Nurses must appreciate the individuality and uniqueness of each infant. According to the individual temperament, the infant will change and shape the environment, which will undoubtedly influence future development. (See Patterns of Sleep and Activity, p. 192.) Obviously, an infant who sleeps 20 hours a day will be exposed to fewer stimuli than one who sleeps 16 hours a day. In turn, each infant will likely elicit a different response from parents. The infant who is quiet, undemanding, and passive may receive much less attention than the infant who is responsive, alert, and active. Behavioral characteristics such as irritability and consolability can influence the ease of transition to parenthood and the parent's perception of the infant.

Nurses can positively influence the attachment of parent and child. The first step is recognizing individual differences and explaining to parents that such characteristics are normal. For example, some people believe that infants sleep throughout the day, except for feedings. For some newborns this may be true, but for many it is not. Understanding that the infant's wakefulness is part of biologic rhythm and not a reflection of inadequate parenting can be crucial in promoting healthy parent-child relationships. Another aspect of helping parents concerns supplying guidelines on how to enhance the infant's development during awake periods. Placing the child in a crib to stare at the same mobile every day is not exciting, but carrying the infant into each room as one does daily chores can be fascinating. A few suggestions can make life more stimulating for the infant and gratifying for the parents (Box 8-6).

Maternal Attachment.   Research has suggested that there is a *maternal sensitive period* immediately and for a short time after birth when parents have a unique ability to attach to their infants (Klaus, Kennell, and Klaus, 1995). Mothers demonstrate a predictable and orderly pattern of behavior during the development of the attachment process. When mothers are presented with their nude infants, they begin to examine the infant with their fingertips, concentrating on touching the extremities, and then proceed to massage and encompass the trunk with their entire hands. Assuming the *en face position,* in which the mother's and infant's eyes meet in visual contact in the same vertical plane, is significant in the formation of affectional ties (Fig. 8-17). Although similar patterns of touching have been

---

BOX 8-6 ■ How to Make the Infant's World More Exciting*

Infants prefer animated and auditory objects.
Infants enjoy novelty, quickly tire of seeing same objects; mobile should be changed frequently.
Infants prefer to look at medium-intensity colors and contrasting colors, such as black and white.
Infants like geometric shapes and checkerboards; prefer patterns over straight lines.
Contrasting lights and reflective surfaces such as mirrors are especially interesting.
But most of all, nothing is as fascinating as the human face and voice!

*Objects should be placed about 20 cm (8 inches) away from infant.

observed, additional studies demonstrate different patterns for mothers, as well as the same pattern for nonmaternal persons, such as male and female nurses. Consequently, nurses must exercise caution in interpreting behaviors such as touching.

Several studies have attempted to substantiate the long-term benefits of providing parents with opportunities to optimally bond with their infant during the initial postpartum period. Although there has been some evidence that increased parent-child contact encourages prolonged breast-feeding and may minimize the risks of parenting disorders, conclusions about the long-term effects of such early intervention on parenting and child development must be viewed cautiously. In addition, some authorities claim that the emphasis on bonding has been unjustified and may lead to guilt and fear in parents who did not have early contact with their infant. There is also concern over the literal interpretation of "sensitive" or "critical" to imply that without early contact, optimum bonding cannot occur or, conversely, that early contact alone is sufficient to ensure competent parenting. Examples of cases where a strong maternal-infant attachment develops in less than ideal situations include adoption and the birth of a child with a congenital defect (Billings, 1995).

Certainly it should be stressed to parents that, although early parent-infant is valuable, it does not represent an "all or none" phenomenon. Throughout the child's life there will be multiple opportunities for the development of parent-child attachment. Bonding is a complex process that develops gradually and is influenced by numerous factors, only one of which is the type of initial contact between the newborn and parent.

In a concept analysis of parent-infant attachment, Goulet and colleagues (1998) describe attributes of parent-infant attachment as proximity, reciprocity, and commitment. Within these attributes are further dimensions, which include contact, emotional state, individualization, complementarity, sensitivity, centrality, and parent role exploration. The researchers describe the parent-infant attachment process as one that is complex and therefore cannot be evaluated simply by the observations of attitudes and behaviors of parents toward their infants (Goulet and others, 1998). Further research into the reciprocal relationships between infant and parent and the situational factors that influence such relationships are recommended.

Another component of successful maternal attachment is the concept of *reciprocity* (Brazelton, 1974). As the mother responds to the infant, the infant must respond to the mother by some signal, such as sucking, cooing, eye contact, grasping, or molding (conforming to other's body during close physical contact). The first step is *initiation,* in which interaction between infant and parent begins. Next is *orientation,* which establishes the partners' expectations of each other during the interaction. Following orientation is *acceleration* of the attention cycle to a peak of excitement. The infant reaches out and coos, both arms jerk forward, the head moves backward, the eyes dilate, and the face brightens. After a short time, *deceleration* of the excitement and *turning away* occur, in which the infant's eyes shift away from mother's and the child grasps his or her shirt. During this cycle of nonattention, repeated verbal or visual attempts to reinitiate the infant's attention are ineffective. This deceleration and turning away probably prevent the infant from being overwhelmed by excessive stimuli. In a good interaction both partners have synchronized their attention-nonattention cycles. Parents or other caregivers who do not allow the infant to turn away and who continually attempt to maintain visual contact encourage the infant to turn off the attention cycle and thus prolong the nonattention phase.

Although this description of reciprocal interacting behavior is usually observed in the infant by 2 to 3 weeks of age, nurses can use this information to teach parents how to interact with their infant. Recognizing the attention versus nonattention cycles and understanding that the latter is not a rejection of the parent helps parents develop competence in parenting.

Paternal Engrossment.   Fathers also show specific attachment behaviors to the newborn. This process of *paternal engrossment,* forming a sense of absorption, preoccupation, and interest in the infant, includes (1) visual awareness of the newborn, especially focusing on the beauty of the child; (2) tactile awareness, often expressed in a desire to hold the infant; (3) awareness of distinct characteristics with emphasis on those features of the infant that resemble the father; (4) perception of the infant as perfect; (5) development of a strong feeling of attraction to the child that leads to intense focusing of attention on the infant; (6) experiencing a feeling of extreme elation; and (7) feeling a sense of deep self-esteem and satisfaction. These responses are greatest during the early contacts with the infant and are intensified by the neonate's normal reflex activity, especially the grasp reflex and visual alertness. In addition to behavioral reactions, fathers also demonstrate physiologic responses such as increased heart rate and blood pressure during interactions with their newborns.

The process of engrossment has significant implications for nurses. It is imperative to recognize the importance of early father-infant contact in releasing these behaviors. Fathers need to be encouraged to express their positive feelings, especially if such emotions are contrary to any popular

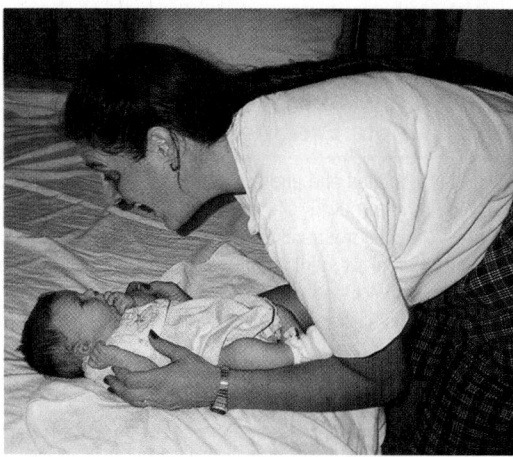

FIG. 8-17 ■ *En face* position between parent and infant can be significant in attachment process.

belief that fathers should remain stoic. If this is not clarified, fathers may feel confused and attempt to suppress the natural sensations of absorption, preoccupation, and interest in order to conform with societal expectations.

Mothers also need to be aware of the responses of the father toward the newborn, especially because one of the consequences of paternal preoccupation with the infant is less overt attention toward the mother. If both parents are able to share their feelings, each can appreciate the process of attachment toward their child and will avoid the unfortunate conflict of being insensitive and unaware of the other's needs. In addition, a father who is encouraged to form a relationship with his newborn is less likely to feel excluded and abandoned after the family returns home and the mother directs her attention toward caring for the infant.

Ideally, the process of engrossment should be discussed with parents before the delivery, such as in prenatal classes, to reinforce the father's awareness of his natural feelings toward the expected child. Focusing on the future experience of seeing, touching, and holding one's newborn may also help expectant fathers become more comfortable in accepting their paternal feelings toward the unborn child. This in turn can assist them in being more supportive toward the mother, especially as the labor and delivery event draws near.

At the infant's birth, the nurse can play a vital role in helping the father express engrossment by assessing the neonate in front of the couple; pointing out normal characteristics; encouraging identification through consistent referral to the child by name; encouraging the father to cuddle, hold, talk to, or feed the infant; and demonstrating whenever necessary the soothing powers of caressing, stroking, and rocking the child (Fig. 8-18). Fathers are encouraged to be with the mother during labor and delivery, to spend time alone with the mother and newborn after delivery, and to "room in" with the mother and infant. Many birthing centers have adopted a family-centered focus including sleeping accommodations that more closely resemble the home environment for the new mother and father.

Fathers, like mothers, may demonstrate attachment not only after the infant's birth but during fetal life as well. Paternal attachment may proceed at a different pace than maternal attachment. Paternal preoccupation with events of labor and delivery and the spouse's health may detract from paternal attachment (Anderson, 1996). Preliminary research indicates that genetic factors may also play an important role in the development of parent-infant attachment (Kendler, 1996).

The nurse observes for the same indications of affection from the father as those expected in the mother, such as visual contact in the en face position and embracing the infant close to the body. When present, such behaviors are reinforced. If such responses are not obvious, the nurse needs to assess the father's feelings regarding this birth, cultural beliefs that may affect his expression of emotions, and other factors that influence his perception of the infant and the mother in order to help him facilitate a positive attachment during this critical period.

Siblings. Although the attachment process has been discussed almost exclusively in terms of the parents and infants, it is essential that nurses be aware of other family members, such as siblings and members of the extended family, who need preparation for the acceptance of this new child. Young children in particular need sensitive preparation for the birth to minimize sibling jealousy.

In support of *family-centered care,* there is an increasing trend to allow siblings to visit the mother on the postpartum unit, hold the newborn, and participate in the care of the new sibling according to the child's age (Fig. 8-19). Another trend has been the presence of siblings at childbirth. Unlike sibling visitation, the evidence supporting this practice has been controversial, yet the nature of truly providing family-centered care encompasses siblings, grandparents, and other significant persons who comprise the extended family unit (Tomlinson, Bryan, and Esau, 1996). The American Academy of Pediatrics and the American College of Obstetricians and Gynecologists (2002) support the presence of siblings at childbirth and visitation of the newborn and mother; basic guidelines for infection control and adult supervision are also recommended.

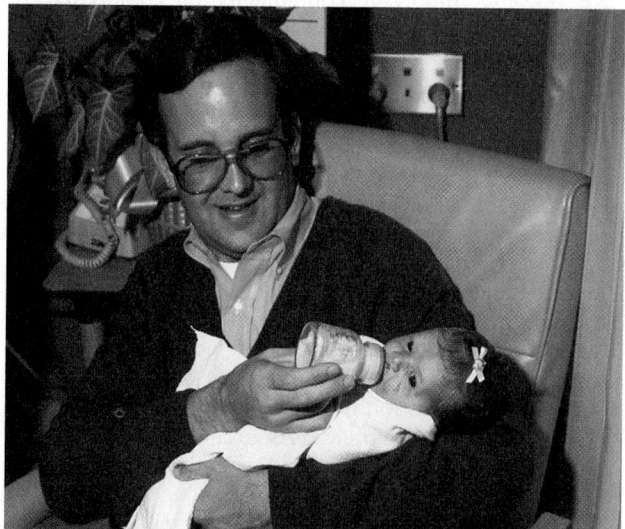

FIG. 8-18 ■ A desire to hold the infant and participate in caregiving activities is an indication of paternal engrossment.

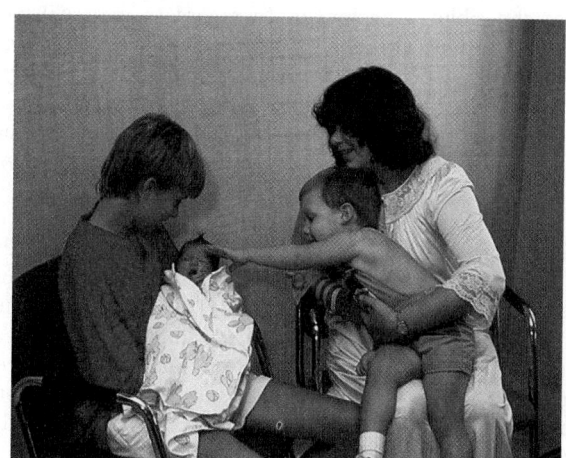

FIG. 8-19 ■ Sibling visitation shortly after birth can be significant in the attachment process.

Children exhibit different degrees of involvement in the birth process. Some reported benefits include children's increased knowledge of the birth process, less regressive behavior after the birth, and more mothering and caregiving behavior toward the infant. Some practitioners add facilitated family bonding and assimilation of the newborn into the family as positive outcomes. Parents whose children attended the birth have echoed these same benefits and have expressed their desire to repeat the experience should another pregnancy occur. Despite these positive findings, opponents believe that allowing children to observe a delivery could lead to emotional difficulties, although there is no research to support this contention. As research mounts, birthing centers that allow siblings at the birth are developing more definitive guidelines, such as an age requirement of at least 4 to 5 years, the presence of a supportive person for the sibling only, and an adequate sequence of preparation in which parents explore all options for preparing their other children.

From observations during sibling visitation, there is evidence that sibling attachment occurs. However, the en face position is assumed much less often among the newborn and siblings than between mother and newborn, and when this position is used, it is brief. Siblings focus more on the head or face than on touching or talking to the infant. The siblings' verbalizations are focused less on attracting the infant's attention and more on addressing the mother about the newborn. Children who have established a prenatal relationship with the fetus have demonstrated more attachment behaviors, supporting the suggestion of encouraging prenatal acquaintance. Additional research is needed to establish theories on sibling bonding as have been constructed for parental bonding.

Multiple Births and Subsequent Children.
A component of attachment that has special meaning for families with multiple births, *monotropy* refers to the principle that a person can become optimally attached to only one individual at a time. If a parent can form only one attachment at a time, how can all the siblings of a multiple birth receive optimum emotional care? Research on bonding and multiple births is still lacking despite the recent increase in multiple births, and even less is known about paternal engrossment and sibling attachment. In regard to maternal-twin bonding, the conclusions of different authors vary. Some report that mothers bond equally to each twin at the time of birth, even if one twin is ill. Others suggest that mothers of twins may take months or even years to form individual attachments to each child and even longer if the twins are identical.

Nurses can be instrumental in promoting bonding of multiple births. The most important principle is to assist the parents in recognizing the individuality of the children, especially in monozygotic (identical) twins. The mother should visit with each newborn, including a sick infant, as much as possible after birth. Rooming-in and breast-feeding are encouraged. Any characteristics that are unique to each child are emphasized, and each infant is called by name, rather than calling them "the twins." Asking the family questions such as "How do you tell Sally and Amy apart?" and "In what ways are Sally and Amy different and similar?" helps point out their individual characteristics. Behaviors on the Brazelton Neonatal Behavioral Assessment Scale can be used to illustrate these differences and to stress effective strategies for dealing with multiple personalities at the same time. Co-bedding of twins or other multiples may also be encouraged in the hospital and home to maintain the bond between siblings that was formed in utero (Della Porta, Aforismo, and Butler-O'Hara, 1998) (see also Sudden Infant Death Syndrome, Chapter 11). Other strategies for promoting individualism are discussed under Multiple Births in Chapter 3.

Another area of attachment that has received minimal attention is maternal bonding of multiparous mothers. Research suggests that there are several additional tasks to "taking on" a second child. These include:

- Promoting acceptance and approval of the second child
- Grieving and resolving the loss of an exclusive dyadic relationship with the first child
- Planning and coordinating family life to include a second child
- Reformulating a relationship with the first child
- Identifying with the second child by comparing this child with the first child in terms of physical and psychologic characteristics
- Assessing one's affective capabilities in providing sufficient emotional support and nurturance simultaneously to two children

Employed mothers who have a second child report fewer concerns regarding general aspects of separation from their child and the effect of separation on the child, but they have similar concerns regarding separation due to employment as they had with the first child. It appears that although experience may decrease some concerns, it may not minimize others.

Prepare for Discharge and Home Care

With increasingly shorter maternity admissions, as well as a trend toward *mother-infant care,* also called *dyad* or *couplet care,* discharge planning, referral, and home visiting have become important components of comprehensive newborn care. First-time, as well as "experienced," parents benefit from guidance and assistance with the infant's care, such as breast- or bottle-feeding, and with the family's integration of a new member, particularly sibling adjustment.

To assess and meet these needs, teaching must begin early, ideally *before the birth.* Not only is the postpartum stay short (12 to 24 hours), but also mothers are in the *taking-in phase,* where they demonstrate passive and dependent behaviors. Therefore, on the first postpartum day mothers may not be able to absorb large amounts of information. This time may need to be spent highlighting essential aspects of care, such as infant safety and feeding. Parents may also be given a list of mother and infant care topics as part of the nursing admission history to choose issues they wish to review. Concerns before discharge should focus on newborn feeding patterns, stool cycles, jaundice, and excessive crying.

Many concerns have been voiced regarding early discharge and newborn hospitalizations for dehydration, jaundice, breast-feeding failure, congenital heart disease, and certain congenital metabolic diseases such as PKU. Legislation has passed in many states mandating that third-party insurers provide coverage for postpartum stays of at least 48 hours after vaginal delivery and 96 hours after cesarean delivery. The federal government passed the Newborns' and Mothers' Health Protection Act in 1996 mandating that health plans could not restrict benefits for hospitalized infants and mothers to less than 48 hours for vaginal delivery and less than 96 hours for cesarean delivery. Studies in various parts of the United States continue to show varied results with respect to newborn rehospitalizations, emergency room visits, and infant morbidities (Brown and others, 2002; Gries, Phyall, Barfield, 2000; Malkin and others, 2000). The American Academy of Pediatrics (1995) recommended that newborns discharged early receive follow-up care within 48 hours of a short stay either in the primary practitioner's office or in the home. In a study of newborn discharge and follow-up care in California, 67.5% of the newborns discharged early did not receive appropriate follow-up according to the Academy's guidelines. Inadequate follow-up care was especially high among newborns receiving Medicaid and low-income Latino and non–English-speaking homes (Galbraith and others, 2003).

To better meet the needs of mothers being discharged soon after delivery, many institutions have implemented programs to provide early follow-up postpartum care at no additional cost to the mother (Locklin and Jansson, 1999; Brown and Johnson, 1998). (See Community Focus boxes.)

Although many mothers and newborns may be safely discharged within 12 to 24 hours without detriment to their health, others may require a longer stay. Follow-up home care within days (or even hours after discharge when minor problems are anticipated) appears to be the emerging trend in an effort to curtail hospital costs and provide adequate maternal-newborn care with minimal complications. Despite the changing spectrum of well newborn health care, the nurse's role continues to be that of providing ongoing assessments of each mother-newborn dyad to ensure a safe transition to home and a successful adaptation into the family unit (Weekly and Neumann, 1997; Brown, Towne, and York, 1996).

With family structures changing, it is essential that nurses identify the primary caregiver, which may not always be the mother but may be a father, grandparent, or baby-sitter. Depending on the family composition, the mother's primary support system in the care of the newborn may not always be the traditional husband or male companion.

Nurses should not assume that terminology associated with mother-infant care is understood. Words relating to the anatomy (e.g., "meconium," "labia," "edema," and "genitalia") and to breast-feeding (e.g., "areola," "colostrum," and "let-down reflex") may be unfamiliar to mothers. Mothers with other children do not necessarily understand more words, and young age and less education decrease comprehension.

An essential area of discharge counseling is the safe transportation of the newborn home from the hospital. Ideally this information should also be provided *before* delivery to allow parents an opportunity to purchase a suitable infant car safety seat restraint.

When purchasing a car safety seat restraint, parents should consider cost and convenience. The convertible-type

---

COMMUNITY FOCUS

Early Newborn Discharge Checklist

Feeding—Adequate latch-on demonstrated for breast-feeding newborn; successfully feeding at least 1 to 2 ounces of formula every 3 to 4 hours with minimal spitting up or absence of vomiting

Elimination—Voiding every 4 to 6 hours or more often; stool—one stool passed in first 24 to 48 hours

Circumcision—Evidence of voiding; nonbleeding circumcision (does not require pressure)

Color—Pink centrally and buccal mucosa moist; no evidence of jaundice in first 24 hours

Cord—Cleansing/antibacterial agent applied per unit protocol

Newborn screening—Completed PKU and others per state law—follow-up scheduled as necessary

Vital signs—Stable heart rate, respiratory rate, and temperature for at least 8 to 12 hours; no apnea

Activity—Wakeful periods before feedings; moves all extremities

Home visit/primary practitioner visit—Appointment made within 2 to 3 days after discharge

---

COMMUNITY FOCUS

Newborn Home Care After Early Discharge*

Wet diapers—6 to 10 per day

Breast-feeding—Successful latch-on and feeding every 1.5 to 3 hours daily

Formula feeding—Successfully, voiding as above, taking at least 1 to 2 ounces every 3 to 4 hours

Circumcision—Wash with warm water only; yellow exudate forming nonbleeding; Plastibell intact 48 hours

Stools—At least one every 48-72 hours (bottle-feeding), or two to three per day (breast-feeding)

Color—Pink to ruddy when crying; pink centrally when at rest or asleep

Activity—Has four to five wakeful periods per day and alerts to environmental sounds and voices

Jaundice—Physiologic jaundice (not appearing in first 24 hours); feeding, voiding, and stooling as noted above or practitioner notification for suspicion of pathologic jaundice (appears within 24 hours of birth, ABO/Rh problem suspected), decreased activity, poor feeding, dark orange skin color persisting fifth day in light-skinned newborn

Cord—Kept above diaper line; drying, no drainage; periumbilical area nonerythematous

Vital signs—Heart rate 120 to 140 beats/min at rest; respiratory rate 30 to 55 at rest without evidence of sternal retractions, grunting, or nasal flaring; temperature 36.3° to 37° C (97.3° to 98.6° F) axillary

Position of sleep—Back

*Any deviation from the above or suspicion of poor newborn adaptation should be reported to the practitioner at once.

NURSING CARE PLAN   The Normal Newborn and Family

NURSING DIAGNOSIS ■ **Ineffective airway clearance related to excess mucus, improper positioning**

PATIENT GOAL 1: Will maintain a patent airway

NURSING INTERVENTIONS/*RATIONALES*

Suction mouth and nasopharynx with bulb syringe as needed
  Compress bulb before insertion and aspirate pharynx, then nose, *to prevent aspiration of fluid*
With mechanical suction, limit each suctioning attempt to 5 seconds, with sufficient time between attempts *to allow reoxygenation*
Position infant on right side after feeding *to prevent aspiration*
Position infant on back during sleep *to decrease risk of sudden infant death syndrome*
Perform as few procedures as possible on infant during first hour and have oxygen ready for use if respiratory distress should develop
Take vital signs according to institutional policy and more frequently if necessary
Observe for signs of respiratory distress and report any of the following immediately:
  Apnea
  Tachypnea
  Grunting, stridor
  Abnormal breath sounds
  Nasal flaring
  Cyanosis or pallor
  Retractions
Keep diapers, clothing, and blankets loose enough *to allow maximum lung (abdominal) expansion and to avoid overheating*
Clean nares of any crusted secretions during bath or when necessary
Check for patent nares

EXPECTED OUTCOMES
Airway remains patent
Breathing is regular and unlabored
Respiratory rate is within normal limits (see inside back cover for normal limits)

NURSING DIAGNOSIS ■ **Risk for altered body temperature related to immature temperature control, change in environmental temperature**

PATIENT GOAL 1: Will maintain stable body temperature

NURSING INTERVENTIONS/*RATIONALES*

Dry thoroughly and remove wet linen immediately after birth
Wrap infant snugly in a warmed blanket
Place infant in a preheated environment (under radiant warmer or next to mother)
Place infant on a padded, covered surface
Take infant's temperature on arrival at nursery or mother's room; proceed according to hospital policy regarding method and frequency of monitoring
Maintain room temperature between 24° and 25.5° C (75° to 78° F) and humidity about 40% to 50%
Give initial bath according to hospital policy
  Prevent chilling of infant during bath
  Postpone bath if there is any question regarding stabilization of body temperature

Dress infant in a shirt and diaper and swaddle in a blanket or cover with blanket
Provide infant with a head covering if heat loss is a problem, *because large surface area of head favors heat loss*
Keep infant away from drafts, air conditioning vents, or fans
Place infant in a recessed cubicle with high-enough walls to *shield from cross-ventilation*
Warm all objects used to examine or cover infant (e.g., place them under radiant warmer)
Uncover only one area of body for examination or procedures
Postpone circumcision until after temperature stabilizes, or use radiant warmer during procedure
Be alert to signs of hypothermia or hyperthermia

EXPECTED OUTCOME
Infant's temperature remains at optimum level (36.5° to 37.5° C [97.7° to 99.5° F])

NURSING DIAGNOSIS ■ **Risk for infection or inflammation related to deficient immunologic defenses, environmental factors, maternal disease**

PATIENT GOAL 1: Will exhibit no evidence of infection

NURSING INTERVENTIONS/*RATIONALES*

Wash hands before and after caring for each infant
Wear gloves when in contact with body secretions
Use of cover gowns is controversial *because studies show they do not decrease infection rates but do increase costs*
Make certain appropriate eye prophylaxis has been carried out
Check eyes daily for evidence of inflammation or discharge
Keep infant from potential sources of infection (e.g., persons with respiratory or skin infections, improperly prepared food sources, other unclean items)
Clean vulva in posterior direction *to prevent fecal contamination of vagina or urethra;* stress this to parents
While cleaning penis, do not retract foreskin; gently wipe away smegma
Maintain asepsis during circumcision
*If infant has been circumcised, cover area with a petrolatum jelly gauze dressing (except when Plastibell is used)
Check for voiding and bleeding after circumcision; disposable diaper may feel dry when wet, but crotch area will feel "clumpy" or "doughy" and heavy
Keep umbilical stump clean and dry
  Place diapers below umbilical stump
  Assess cord daily for odor, color, and drainage
*Apply antibacterial/ cleansing agent to cord per hospital protocol
*Administer hepatitis B vaccine (HBV) in vastus lateralis muscle (in Canada, only if mother is HBsAg- positive)

EXPECTED OUTCOMES
Infant exhibits no evidence of infection or inflammation
Eyes remain clear with no evidence of irritation
Genital area is free of irritation
Cord appears dry, surrounding area free of infection
Infant receives HBV vaccine

*Dependent nursing action.

NURSING DIAGNOSIS ■ **Risk for trauma related to physical helplessness**

PATIENT GOAL 1: Will be clearly and correctly identified

NURSING INTERVENTIONS/*RATIONALES*

Make certain infant is properly identified *for placement with correct mother*
  Ensure that identification (ID) band(s) are properly and securely placed
  Check infant's ID band frequently *to ensure correct infant identity*
Discuss safety issues with parents, especially mother, *to prevent possible kidnapping*
Observe staff's ID badge and give infant only to properly identified personnel
Never leave infant unobserved alone in crib or room

EXPECTED OUTCOMES

Infant is clearly and correctly identified at all times
Parents observe safety practices
ID bands remain in place

PATIENT GOAL 2: Will have no physical injury

NURSING INTERVENTIONS/*RATIONALES*

Avoid using rectal thermometer *because of risk of rectal perforation*
Never leave infant unsupervised on a raised surface without sides
Always close diaper pins (if used) and place them away from infant's body
Keep pointed or sharp objects away from infant
Keep own fingernails short and trimmed; avoid jewelry that can scratch infant
Use appropriate methods of handling and transporting infant

EXPECTED OUTCOME

Infant remains free of physical injury

PATIENT GOAL 3: Will exhibit no evidence of bleeding

NURSING INTERVENTIONS/*RATIONALES*

*Administer vitamin K intramuscularly (per hospital protocol), using vastus lateralis muscle as site of injection
Check circumcision site; assess for any oozing *that may indicate bleeding tendencies*

EXPECTED OUTCOME

Infant exhibits no evidence of bleeding

NURSING DIAGNOSIS ■ **Altered nutrition: less than body requirements (risk) related to immaturity, parental knowledge deficit**

PATIENT GOAL 1: Will receive optimal nutrition

NURSING INTERVENTIONS/*RATIONALES*

Assess strength of suck and coordination with swallowing *to identify possible problem affecting feeding*
Offer initial intake according to parent's preference, hospital policy, and practitioner's protocol
Prepare for demand feeding of breast-fed infants; night feedings determined by condition and preferences of mother
Offer bottle-fed infants 2 to 3 ounces of formula every 3 to 4 hours or on demand

Support and assist breast-feeding mothers during initial feedings and more frequently if necessary
Avoid routine water or supplemental feedings for breast-feeding infants because they may *decrease the desire to suck and cause nipple preference*
Encourage father or other support person to remain with mother to help her and infant with positioning, relaxation, and reinforcement
Encourage father or other support person to participate in bottle-feeding
Place infant on right side after feeding *to prevent aspiration*
Observe stool pattern

EXPECTED OUTCOMES

Infant demonstrates strong suck
Infant retains feedings
Infant receives an adequate amount of nutrients (specify amount and frequency of feedings)
Infant loses less than 10% of birth weight

NURSING DIAGNOSIS ■ **Altered family processes related to maturational crisis, birth of term infant, change in family unit**

PATIENT (FAMILY) GOAL 1: Will exhibit parent-infant interaction behaviors that are consistent with enhancing bonding

NURSING INTERVENTIONS/*RATIONALES*

As soon after delivery as possible, encourage parents to see and hold infant; place newborn close to face of parents *to establish visual contact*
Ideally, perform eye care after initial meeting of infant and parents, within 1 hour after birth *when infant is alert and most likely to visually relate to parent*
Identify for parents specific behaviors manifested by infant (e.g., alertness, ability to see, vigorous suck, rooting behavior, and attention to human voice)
Discuss with parents their expectations of fantasy child vs real child if indicated
Encourage parents to "talk out" their labor and delivery experience; identify any events that signify loss of control to either parent, especially mother
Identify behavioral steps in attachment process, and evaluate aspects that could be considered positive and those that may represent inadequate or delayed parenting
Encourage family to room-in or to call for infant frequently if not rooming-in
Observe and assess reciprocity of cues between infant and parent *to identify behaviors that may need strengthening*
Assist parents in recognizing attention-nonattention cycles and in understanding their significance
Assess variables affecting development of attachment through observing infant and parent and interviewing each parent or other significant caregiver

EXPECTED OUTCOMES

Parents establish contact with infant immediately or soon after birth
Parents demonstrate attachment behaviors, such as touch, eye contact, naming and calling infant by name, talking to infant, participating in caregiving activities
Parents recognize attention-nonattention cycles

*Dependent nursing action.

continued

NURSING CARE PLAN   The Normal Newborn and Family—*cont'd*

PATIENT (SIBLING) GOAL 2: Will demonstrate adjustment/attachment behaviors toward newborn

NURSING INTERVENTIONS/*RATIONALES*

Allow to visit and touch newborn when feasible

Explain physical differences in newborn, such as bald head, umbilical stump and clamp, circumcision, *to lessen any fear siblings might have*

Explain to siblings realistic expectations regarding newborn's abilities and needs
    Requires complete care
    Is not a playmate

Encourage siblings to participate in care at home *to make them feel part of the experience*

Encourage parents to spend individual time with other children at home *to reduce feelings of jealousy toward new sibling*

EXPECTED OUTCOME

Siblings express interest in newborn and realistic expectations for their age

PATIENT (FAMILY) GOAL 3: Will be prepared for discharge and home care

NURSING INTERVENTIONS/*RATIONALES*

Discuss with parents correct preparation of formula
    Stress that proportions must not be altered to dilute or concentrate the formula

Discourage microwaving of bottles *to avoid burns*

Encourage use of support persons, such as lactation specialist or members of La Leche League, for assistance with breast-feeding

Instruct in other aspects of newborn care
    Bathing
    Umbilical cord and circumcision care
    Recognize states of activity for optimum interaction (see Table 8-3)

Encourage participation in parenting classes, if offered

Discuss importance and proper use of federally approved car seat restraints
    If infant is small, advise parents to use rolled blankets and towels in crotch area to *prevent slouch* and along sides *to minimize lateral movement* (or place seat at a 45-degree reclining angle), but never use padding underneath or behind infant, *because it creates slackness in harness, leading to possible ejection from seat in a crash*
    Refer to organizations that may rent appropriately equipped car seat restraints

If parent-infant attachment is at risk, refer to appropriate agencies (social services, family and child services, at-risk programs)

EXPECTED OUTCOMES

Family demonstrates ability to provide care for infant

Family keeps appointments for follow-up care

Infant rides home in federally approved car seat restraint

Family members avail themselves of needed services

---

seats are more expensive initially but cost less than two separate systems. Convenience is a major factor, because a cumbersome restraint may be used less and improperly. Before buying a car safety seat restraint, it is best to try out different models. For example, some types are too large for subcompact cars. Asking friends about the advantages and disadvantages of their restraints is helpful, but borrowing their car seat or purchasing a used one can be dangerous. Parents should use only a restraint that has directions for use and a certification label stating that it complies with federal motor vehicle safety standards (both should be on the seat). They should not use a restraint that has been involved in a crash. Some service clubs and hospitals have loan programs for restraints. Information about approved models and other aspects of car safety seat restraints is available from several organizations and sources.*

Parents are cautioned against placing an infant in the front seat of a car with a passenger-side air bag. Infants weighing less than 9.07 kg (20 pounds) or younger than 1 year should always be placed in a rear-facing child safety seat in the back seat of the car (American Academy of Pediatrics, 2002).

---

*American Academy of Pediatrics, 141 Northwest Point Boulevard, Elk Grove Village, IL 60007; (888) 227-1770, fax: (847) 228-1281; website: www.aap.org; and local division of traffic safety; or **National Highway Traffic Safety Administration Auto Safety Hotline,** (800) 424-9393.

! NURSING ALERT

Padding is never placed underneath or behind the infant, because it creates slackness in the harness, leading to the possibility of the child's ejection from the seat in the event of a crash. In vehicles with front passenger-side air bags, the rear-facing safety seat must be placed in the back seat to avoid injury to the infant from the released air bag forcing the safety seat against the vehicle seat or passenger door.

Although federal safety standards do not specify the *minimum* weight of an infant and the appropriate type of restraint, newborns weighing 2 kg (4 pounds, 8 ounces) receive relatively good support in convertible seats with a seat back–to-crotch strap height of 14 cm ($5\frac{1}{2}$ inches) or less. Rolled blankets and towels may be needed between the crotch and legs to prevent slouching and can be placed along the sides to minimize lateral movements. Placing the infant in a safety seat at a 45-degree angle will prevent slumping and airway obstruction (American Academy of Pediatrics, 2002). Seats with shields (large padded surfaces in front of the child) and armrests (found on some other models) are unacceptable because of their proximity to the infant's face and neck. (For a discussion of appropriate car restraints for preterm infants, see p. 252, and for infants, see Motor Vehicle Injuries in Chapter 10 and 12.)

In the United States and Canada all states and provinces have mandated the use of child restraints. Therefore, hospitals and birthing centers should have policies regarding the safe discharge of a newborn in a car safety seat and provisions for parents to learn to use the device correctly. In addition, hospital personnel should ensure that infants born before 37 weeks' gestation have a period of observation in the selected car seat to monitor for possible apnea, bradycardia, and oxygen desaturation (American Academy of Pediatrics, 1999b). Parents are more likely to use a restraint correctly and consistently if the proper use of one is demonstrated and its necessity is stressed. Infants and children continue to be hurt and killed because car seat restraints are not installed properly.

● *Evaluation*

The effectiveness of nursing interventions is determined by continual reassessment and evaluation of care based on the following observational guidelines:

1. Observe infant's color and respiratory patterns.
2. Monitor axillary temperature regularly; observe for signs of temperature instability, such as respiratory distress.
3. Observe for any evidence of infection, especially at the umbilicus or site of circumcision; check identification bands; check medical record for documentation of prophylactic eye treatment, vitamin K injection, HBV vaccine, and metabolic screening tests.
4. Monitor daily weight.
5. Observe interactions between infant and family members; interview family regarding their feelings about the newborn.
6. Observe parents' ability to provide care for infant; interview parents regarding any concerns about infant's care at home.
7. Observe parents' correct use of car safety seat restraint on discharge.

The *expected outcomes* are described in the Nursing Care Plan on pp. 216-218.

KEY POINTS

- Transition from fetal or placental circulation to independent respiration is the most important physiologic change required of the newborn.
- Chemical and thermal factors help initiate the neonate's first respiration.
- Circulatory changes in the neonate result from shifts in pressure in the heart and major vessels and from functional closures of the fetal shunts.
- The newborn's large surface area, thin layer of subcutaneous fat, and unique mechanism for producing heat predispose the newborn to excessive heat loss.
- The infant's high rate of metabolism is closely correlated with the rate of fluid exchange, which is seven times greater in the infant than in the adult.
- The skin and mucous membranes, the reticuloendothelial system, and antibodies are the first, second, and third lines of defense against infection.
- Apgar scoring, the initial assessment of the newborn, focuses on heart rate, respiratory effort, muscle tone, reflex irritability, and color.
- Physical assessment of the newborn includes clinical assessment of gestational age, general measurements, general appearance, head-to-toe assessment, and parent-infant attachment or bonding.

- Neurologic assessment focuses on localized reflexes and posture, muscle tone, head control, and movement and is best accomplished during the general physical examination.
- Behavioral assessment of newborns with the Brazelton Neonatal Behavioral Assessment Scale examines responses to seven categories: habituation, orientation, motor performance, range of state, regulation of state, autonomic regulation, and reflexes.
- An instrument for assessing the reciprocal interchange between parent and infant is the Nursing Child Assessment Feeding Scale.
- Physical care for the newborn includes maintaining a patent airway, maintaining a stable body temperature, protecting from infection and injury, and providing optimal nutrition.
- Although the attachment, or bonding, process primarily affects infants and parents, siblings also play an important role.
- With short maternity admissions, teaching needs to begin before birth and continue after discharge with telephone or home follow-up.
- An essential aspect of discharge teaching is ensuring the newborn's safe transportation home in a federally approved, backward-facing car safety seat restraint.

References

Akers SM, Groh-Wargo SL: Normal nutrition during infancy. In Samour PQ, Helm KK, Lang CE, editors: *Family handbook of pediatric nutrition*, ed 2, Gaithersburg, Md, 1999, Aspen.

Alexander GR and others: A United States national reference for fetal growth, *Obstet Gynecol* 87(2):163-168, 1996.

American Academy of Pediatrics, Clinical Report: Prevention of rickets and vitamin D deficiency: new guidelines for vitamin D intake, *Pediatrics* 111(4):908-910, 2003b.

American Academy of Pediatrics, Committee on Bioethics: Female genital mutilation, *Pediatrics* 102(1):153-156, 1998a.

American Academy of Pediatrics, Committee on Fetus and Newborn, and American College of Obstetricians and Gynecologists, Committee on Obstetric Practice: Use and abuse of the Apgar Score, *Pediatrics* 98(1):141-142, 1996.

American Academy of Pediatrics, Committee on Fetus and Newborn: Hospital stay for healthy term newborns, *Pediatrics* 96(4):788-790, 1995.

American Academy of Pediatrics, Committee on Genetics: Newborn screening facts sheet, *Pediatrics* 98(3):473-490, 1996a.

American Academy of Pediatrics, Committee on Infectious Diseases, *Red book: 2003 report of the Committee on Infectious Diseases,* ed 26, Elk Grove Village, Il, 2003c, The Academy.

American Academy of Pediatrics, Committee on Injury and Poison Prevention: Safe transportation of newborns at hospital discharge, *Pediatrics* 104(4):986-988, 1999b.

American Academy of Pediatrics, Committee on Injury and Poison Prevention: Selecting and using the most appropriate car safety seats for growing children: guidelines for counseling parents, *Pediatrics* 109(3):550-553, 2002.

American Academy of Pediatrics, Committee on Nutrition: *Pediatric nutrition handbook,* ed 5, Elk Grove Village, Il, 2004, The Academy.

American Academy of Pediatrics: Hearing assessments in infants and children: recommendations beyond neonatal screening, *Pediatrics* 111(2):436-440, 2003a.

American Academy of Pediatrics, Joint Committee on Infant Hearing: Year 2000 Position Statement: principle and guidelines for early hearing detection and intervention. *Pediatrics* 106(4):798-824, 2000c.

American Academy of Pediatrics, Task Force on Circumcision: Circumcision policy statement, *Pediatrics* 103(3):686-693, 1999a.

American Academy of Pediatrics, Task Force on Infant Sleep Position and Sudden Infant Death Syndrome: Changing concepts of sudden infant death syndrome: implications for infant sleeping environment and sleep position, *Pediatrics* 105(3):650-656, 2000a.

American Academy of Pediatrics: Serving the family from birth to the medical home: newborn screening: a blueprint for the future, Pediatrics 106(2 pt.2):389-427, suppl., 2000b.

American Academy of Pediatrics and American College of Obstetricians and Gynecologists: *Guidelines for perinatal care,* ed 5, Elk Grove Village, Il, 2002, The Academy.

American College of Obstetricians and Gynecologists, Committee on Obstetric Practice: ACOG committee opinion: circumcision, *Obstet Gynecol* 98(4):707-708, 2001.

Anderson AM: The father-infant relationship: becoming connected, *J Soc Pediatr Nurs* 1(2):83-92, 1996.

Anderson JW, Johnstone BM, Remley DT: Breastfeeding and cognitive development: a meta-analysis, *Am J Clin Nutr* 70(4):525-535, 1999.

Arbuckle T, Wilkins R, Sherman G: Birth weight percentiles by gestational age in Canada, *Obstet Gynecol* 81(1):39-48, 1993.

Arora S and others: Major factors influencing breastfeeding rates: mother's perception of father's attitude and milk supply, *Pediatrics* 106(5):e67, 2000.

Association of Women's Health, Obstetric and Neonatal Nursing (AWHONN): *Evidence-based clinical practice guideline: neonatal skin care,* Washington, DC, 2001, The Association.

Bachrach VR, Schwarz E, Bachrach LR: Breastfeeding and the risk of hospitalization for respiratory disease in infancy, *Arch Pediatr Adolesc Med* 157(3):237-243, 2003.

Ballard JL, Auer CE, Khoury JC: Ankyloglossia: assessment, incidence, and effect of frenuloplasty on the breastfeeding dyad, *Pediatrics* 110(5):e63, 1001, 2002.

Ballard JL, Novak KK, Driver M: A simplified score for assessment of fetal maturation of newly born infants, *J Pediatr* 95(5):769-774, 1979.

Ballard JL and others: New Ballard score, expanded to include extremely premature infants, *J Pediatr* 119:417-423, 1991.

Barclay L: Frenuloplasty corrects ankyloglossia disrupting breastfeeding, *Pediatrics* 110:63, 2002.

Battaglia FC, Lubchenco LO: A practical classification of newborn infants by weight and gestational age, *J Pediatr* 71(2):159-161, 1967.

Behring A, Vezeau TM, Fink, R: Timing of the newborn first bath: a replication, *Neonat Netw* 22(1):39-46, 2003.

Biancuzzo M: *Breastfeeding the newborn: clinical strategies for nurses,* St Louis, 1999, Mosby.

Billings JR: Bonding theory—tying mothers in knots? a critical review of the application of a theory to nursing, *J Clin Nurs* 4(4):207-211, 1995.

Blackburn ST: *Maternal, fetal, and neonatal physiology: a clinical perspective,* Philadelphia, ed 2, 2003, WB Saunders.

Blain-Lewis N: Comparative studies of bruising and healing after heelstick, *Neonat Intensive Care* 5(5):18-21, 1992.

Blass EM, Watt LB: Suckling- and sucrose-induced analgesia in human newborns, *Pain* 83(3):611-623, 1999.

Brazelton TB: Mother-infant reciprocity. In Klaus M and others, editors: *Maternal attachment and mothering disorders,* New Brunswick, NJ, 1974, Johnson & Johnson Baby Products.

Brazelton TB, Nugent JK: *Neonatal behavioural assessment scale,* London, 1996, MacKeith Press.

Brown S and others: Early postnatal discharge from hospital for healthy mothers and term infants, *Cochrane Database Syst Rev* 2002(3): CD002958, 2002.

Brown SG, Johnson BT: Enhancing early discharge with home follow-up: a pilot project, *JOGNN* 27(1):33-38, 1998.

Brown LP, Towne SA, York R: Controversial issues surrounding early postpartum discharge, *Nurs Clin North Am* 31(2):333-339, 1996.

Carbajal R and others: Analgesic effect of breast feeding in term neonates: randomized controlled trial, *BMJ* 326(7379):13, 2003.

Carroll V: Infant abduction: lowering the risk, *AWHONN Lifelines* 3(6):25-27, 2000.

Chia F and others: Reliability of the Dinamap noninvasive monitor in the measurement of blood pressure of ill Asian newborns, *Clin Pediatr* 29(5):262-267, 1990.

Christie L: Food hypersensitivities. In Samour PQ, Helm KK, Lang CE, editors: *Handbook of pediatric nutrition,* ed 2, Gaithersburg, Md, 1999, Aspen.

Cohen HA and others: Postcircumcision urinary tract infection, *Clin Pediatr* 31(6):322-324, 1992.

Cunningham FG and others, editors: *Williams obstetrics,* ed 21, New York, 2001, McGraw Hill.

Darmstadt GL, Dinulos JG: Neonatal skin care, *Pediatr Clin North Am* 47(4):757-782, 2000.

Della Porta K, Aforismo D, Butler-O'Hara M: Co-bedding of twins in the neonatal intensive care, *Pediatr Nurs* 24(6):529-531, 1998.

Donnelly A and others: Commercial hospital discharge packs for breastfeeding women, *Cochrane Database Syst Rev* 2000(2):CD002075, 2000.

Donovan EF and others: Inaccuracy of Ballard scores before 28 weeks' gestation, *J Pediatr* 135(2 pt 1):147-152, 1999.

Dore S and others: Alcohol versus natural drying for newborn cord care, *JOGNN* 27(6):621-627, 1998.

Dungy CI and others: Hospital infant formula discharge packages: do they affect the duration of breast-feeding? *Arch Pediatr Adolesc Med* 151(7):724-729, 1997.

Farber SD, Van Fossen RL, Koontz SW: Quantitative and qualitative video analysis of infants feeding: angled- and straight-bottle feeding systems, *J Pediatr* 126(6):S118-S124, 1995.

Female genital mutilation, *AAP News* 10(2):3, 1994.

Fitzgerald M, Millard C, McIntosh N: Cutaneous hypersensitivity following peripheral tissue damage in newborn infants and its reversal with topical anaesthesia, *Pain* 39:31-36, 1989.

Fomon SJ: *Infant nutrition,* St Louis, 1993, Mosby.

Fuloria M, Kreiter S: The newborn examination: Part I. Emergencies and common abnormalities involving the skin, head, neck, chest, and respiratory and cardiovascular systems, *Am Fam Physician* 65(1):61-68, 2002.

Galbraith AA and others: Newborn early discharge revisited: are California newborns receiving recommended postnatal visits? *Pediatrics* 111(2):364-371, 2003.

Georgieff MK: Taking a rational approach to the choice of formula, *Contemp Pediatr* 18(8):112-130, 2001.

Geyer J and others: An evidence-based multidisciplinary protocol for neonatal circumcision pain management, *JOGNN* 31(4):403-410, 2002.

Gibbins S and others: Efficacy and safety of sucrose for procedural pain relief in preterm and term neonates, *Nurs Res* 51(6):375-382, 2002.

Golombek SG, Brill PE, Salice AL: Randomized trial of alcohol versus triple dye for umbilical cord care, *Clin Pediatr* 41(6):419-423, 2002.

Goulet C and others: A concept analysis of parent-infant attachment, *J Adv Nurs* 28(5):1071-1081, 1998.

Gradin M and others: Pain reduction at venipuncture in newborns: oral glucose compared with local anesthetic cream, *Pediatrics* 110(6): 1053-1057, 2002.

Gray L, Watt L, Blass EM: Skin-to-skin contact is analgesic in healthy newborns, *Pediatrics* 105(1):110-111, 2000; available at www.pediatrics.org/cgi/content/full/105/1/e14.

Gray L and others: Breastfeeding is analgesic in healthy newborns, *Pediatrics* 109(4):590-593, 2002.

Greenes DS, Fleischer GR: Accuracy of a noninvasive temporal artery thermometer for use in infants, *Arch Pediatr Adolesc Med* 155(3): 376-381, 2001.

Gries DM, Phyall G, Barfield WD: Evaluation of early discharge program for infants after childbirth in a military population, *Mil Med* 165(8):616-621, 2000.

Hanson LA, Korotkova M: The role of breastfeeding in prevention of neonatal infection, *Semin Neonatol* 7(4):275-281, 2002.

Haouari N and others: The analgesic effect of sucrose in full-term infants: a randomised controlled trial, *BMJ* 310:1498-1500, 1995.

Hicks MA: A comparison of the tympanic and axillary temperatures of the preterm and term infant, *J Perinatol* 16(4):261-267, 1996.

Janssen PA and others: To dye or not to dye: a randomized, clinical trial of a triple dye/alcohol regime versus dry cord care, *Pediatrics* 111(1):15-20, 2003.

Kendler KS: Parenting: a geneti-epidemiologic perspective, *Am J Psychiatry* 153(1):11-20, 1996.

Klaus MH, Kennell JH, Klaus PH: *Bonding: building the foundations of secure attachment and independence,* Menlo Park, Calif, 1995, Addison-Wesley.

Kraft NL: A pictorial and video guide to circumcision without pain, *Adv Neonatal Care* 3(2):50-64, 2003.

Kramer MS and others: A new and improved population-based Canadian reference for birth weight for gestational age, *Pediatrics* 108(2):e35, 462, 2001.

Kue YT and others: Type 2 diabetes mellitus in children: prenatal and early infancy risk factors among native Canadians, *Arch Pediatr Adolesc Med* 156(7):651-655, 2002.

Kyenkya-Isabirye M: UNICEF launches the Baby-Friendly Hospital Initiative, *MCN* 17(4):177-179, 1992.

Lanham DM and others: Accuracy of tympanic temperature readings in children under 6 years of age, *Pediatr Nurs* 25(1):39-42, 1999.

Lawrence RA, Lawrence RM: *Breastfeeding: a guide for the medical profession,* ed 5, St Louis, 1999, Mosby.

Lawrence RA, Lawrence RM: The evidence for breastfeeding: given the benefits of breastfeeding, what contraindications exist?, *Pediatr Clin N Am* 48(1): 235-251, 2001.

Leick-Rude MK, Bloom LF: A comparison of temperature-taking methods in neonates, *Neonat Netw* 17(5):21-37, 1998.

Locklin MP, Jansson MJ: Home visits: strategies to protect the breastfeeding newborn at risk, *J Obstet Gynecol Neonatal Nurs* 28(1): 33-40, 1999.

Malkin JD and others: Infant mortality and early postpartum discharge, *Obstetr Gynecol* 96(2): 183-188, 2000.

McCleary PH: Female genital mutilation and childbirth: a case report, *Birth* 21(4):221-223, 1994.

McDonald RE, Avery DR: *Dentistry for the child and adolescent,* ed 7, St Louis, 2000, Mosby.

Mercer JS, Skovgaard RL. Neonatal transition physiology: A new paradigm, *J Perinat Neonat Nurs* 15(4):56-75, 2002.

Noerr B: Sucrose for neonatal procedural pain, *Neonat Netw* 20(7): 63-67, 2001.

Paes B and others: A comparative study of heel-stick devices for infant blood collection, *Am J Dis Child* 147(3):346-348, 1993.

Papile LA: The Apgar score in the 21st century, *N Engl J Med* 344(7):519-520, 2001.

Penny-MacGillivray T: A newborn's first bath: when? *J Obstet Gynecol Neonatal Nurs* 25(6):481-487, 1996.

Puckett RM, Offringa M: Prophylactic vitamin K for vitamin K deficiency bleeding in neonates, *Cochrane Database Syst Review* 2000(4): CD002776.

Rabun J: For healthcare professionals: guidelines on prevention of and response to infant abductions, ed 6, Alexandria, Va, 2000, National Center for Missing and Exploited Children.

Ryan AS, Wenjun Z, Acosta A: Breastfeeding continues to increase in the new millennium, *Pediatrics* 110(6): 1103-1109, 2002.

Seguin J, Terry K: Neonatal infrared axillary thermometry, *Clin Pediatr* 38(1):35-40, 1999.

Sganga A and others: A comparison of four methods of normal newborn temperature measurement, *MCN* 25(2): 76-79, 2000.

Shah V, Ohlsson A: Venepuncture versus heel lance for blood sampling in term neonates, *Cochrane Database Syst Rev* 2001(2):CD001452.

Shogan MG: Emergency management plan for newborn abduction, *J Obstet Gynecol Neonatal Nurs* 31(3): 340-346, 2002.

Stang HJ and others: Beyond dorsal penile nerve block: a more humane circumcision, *Pediatrics* 100(2):e3, 1997; available at www.pediatrics.org/cgi/content/full/100/2/e3.

Stevens B, Yamada J, Ohlsson A: Sucrose for analgesia in newborn infants undergoing procedures, *Cochrane Database Syst Rev* 2001(4): CD001069.

Stevens B and others: Management of pain from heel lance with lidocaine-prilocaine (EMLA) cream: is it safe and efficacious in preterm infants? *J Dev Behav Pediatr* 20 (4): 216-221, 1999.

Taddio A and others: A systematic review of lidocaine-prilocaine cream (EMLA) in the treatment of acute pain in neonates, *Pediatrics* 101(2):e1, 1998; available at www.pediatrics.org/cgi/content/full/101/2/e1.

Taddio A and others: Conditioning and hyperalgesia in newborns exposed to repeated heel lances. *JAMA* 288(7):857-861, 2002.

Thomas KA. Comparability of infant abdominal skin and axillary temperatures: newborn infant, *Nurs Rev* 3(4):173-178, 2003.

Thomas P and others: A new look at intrauterine growth and the impact of race, altitude, and gender, *Pediatrics* 106(2):e21, 2000.

Tomlinson PS, Bryan AA, Esau AL: Family centered intrapartum care: revisiting an old concept, *JOGNN* 25(4):331-337, 1996.

Trochtenberg DS: Neonatal circumcision, *N Engl J Med* 323(17): 1206, 1990 (letter to the editor).

Weekly SJ, Neumann ML: Speaking up for baby: the case for individualized neonatal discharge plans, *AWHONN Lifelines* 1(1):24-29, 1997.

Weiss ME, Poeltler D, Gocka I: Infrared tympanic thermometry for neonatal temperature assessment, *J Obstet Gynecol Neonatal Nurs* 23(9):798-803, 1993.

Williamson ML: Circumcision anesthesia: a study of nursing implications for dorsal penile nerve block, *Pediatr Nurs* 23(10):59-63, 1997.

Wilshaw R and others: A comparison of the use of tympanic, axillary, and rectal thermometers in infants, *J Pediatr Nurs* 14(2):88-93, 1999.

Wilson D, Bowman C: Infant nutrition: building blocks for the future, *Mother Baby J* 5(4):17-22, 2000.

Wright A, Rice S, Wells S: Changing hospital practices to increase the duration of breast-feeding, *Pediatrics* 97(5):669-676, 1996.

Zupan J, Garner P: Topical umbilical cord care at birth, *Cochrane Database Syst Rev* 2000(2):CD001057, 2000.

9

Health Problems of Newborns

DEBBIE FRASER ASKIN and DAVID WILSON

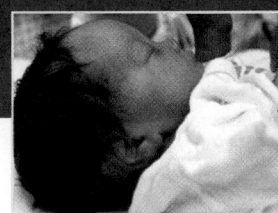

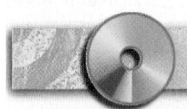

Remember to check out your companion CD-ROM

http://evolve.elsevier.com/Wong/essentials/

CHAPTER OUTLINE

RELATED TOPICS and ADDITIONAL RESOURCES

 IN TEXT

Administration of Medications, *Ch. 22*
Assessment (Newborn), *Ch. 8*
Cognitive Impairment, *Ch. 19*
Collection of Specimens, *Ch. 22*
Congenital Adrenogenital Hyperplasia, *Ch. 29*
Diaper Dermatitis, *Ch. 30*
Family-Centered Home Care, *Ch. 20*
Impact of Chronic Illness, Disability, or Death on the Child and Family, *Ch. 18*
Infant Mortality, *Ch. 1*
Infection Control, *Ch. 22*
Pain Assessment; Pain Management, *Ch. 21*
Preparing for Discharge and Home Care, *Ch. 21*
Procedures for Maintaining Respiratory Function, *Ch. 22*

Procedures Related to Alternative Feeding Techniques, *Ch. 22*
Promotion of Parent-Infant Bonding (Attachment), *Ch. 8*

 CD COMPANION

Critical Thinking Exercises—Jaundice, The High-Risk Newborn, Infant of a Diabetic Mother, Patent Ductus Arteriosus, Fetal Alcohol Syndrome/Effects
Case Study—Health Problems of the Newborn
Guidelines—Physical Assessment, Neonatal Skin Care, Developmental Interventions, Referral Regarding Genetic Counseling
Manifestations of Acute Pain in the Neonate
Clinical Manifestations of Respiratory Distress Syndrome

Manifestations Observed in Neonatal Sepsis
Nursing Care Plans
NCLEX-Style Review Questions

 WEBSITE

WebLinks
NCLEX-Style Review Questions
WONG'S CLINICAL MANUAL OF PEDIATRIC NURSING, 6/E

Nursing Care Plans
Community and Home Care Instructions—The Child With an Ostomy, Measuring a Child's Temperature

For additional information on physical assessment, please view "Pediatric Nursing: Newborn Assessment" in *Whaley and Wong's Pediatric Nursing Video Series,* St Louis, 1996, Mosby; (800) 426-4545; website: www.elsevierhealth.com.

LEARNING OBJECTIVES
On completion of this chapter the reader will be able to:

- Recognize common deviations from normal characteristics in the newborn.
- Perform a systematic assessment of a high-risk newborn.
- Outline a general plan of care for a high-risk infant.
- Recognize physiologic factors that compromise the preterm infant's health status.

- Discuss the role of the nurse in facilitating positive parent-infant relationships.
- Contrast physical characteristics of preterm and full-term infants.
- Discuss the basis for screening newborns for health problems.

- Discuss the rationale for performing newborn screening and genetic counseling when a newborn has a hereditary condition.
- Modify a general plan of care to meet the needs of an infant with specific high-risk health needs.

BIRTH INJURIES

Several factors predispose an infant to birth injuries (Mangurten, 2002; Paige and Carney, 2002). Maternal factors include uterine dysfunction that leads to prolonged or precipitous labor, preterm or postterm labor, and cephalopelvic disproportion. Injury may result from dystocia caused by fetal macrosomia, multifetal gestation, abnormal or difficult presentation (not caused by maternal uterine or pelvic conditions), and congenital anomalies. Intrapartum events that can result in scalp injury include the use of intrapartum monitoring of fetal heart rate (FHR) and collection of fetal scalp blood for acid-base assessment. Obstetric birth techniques can cause injury. Forceps birth, vacuum extraction, version and extraction, and cesarean birth are potential contributory factors. Often more than one factor is present, and multiple predisposing factors may be related to a single maternal condition.

SOFT-TISSUE INJURY

Various types of soft-tissue injury may be sustained during the process of birth, primarily in the form of bruises or abrasions secondary to dystocia. Soft-tissue injury usually occurs when there is some degree of disproportion between the presenting part and the maternal pelvis (cephalopelvic disproportion). The use of forceps to facilitate a difficult vertex delivery may produce discoloration or abrasion on the sides of the neonate's face. Petechiae or ecchymoses may be observed on the presenting part after a breech or brow delivery. After a difficult or precipitous delivery, the sudden release of pressure on the head can produce scleral hemorrhages or generalized petechiae over the face and head. Petechiae and ecchymoses may also appear on the head, neck, and face of an infant born with a nuchal cord, giving the infant's face a cyanotic appearance. A well-defined circle of petechiae and ecchymoses or abrasions may also be seen on the occipital region of the newborn's head when a vacuum suction cup is applied during delivery. Rarely, lacerations occur during cesarean section.

These traumatic lesions generally fade spontaneously within a few days, without treatment. However, petechiae may be a manifestation of an underlying bleeding disorder or a systemic illness such as an infection and should be further evaluated as to their origin. Nursing care is primarily directed toward assessing the injury and providing an explanation and reassurance to the parents.

HEAD TRAUMA

Trauma to the head and scalp that occurs during the birth process is usually benign but occasionally results in more serious injury. The injuries that produce serious trauma, such as intracranial hemorrhage and subdural hematoma, are discussed in relation to neurologic disorders in the newborn (see Table 9-11). Skull fractures are discussed in association with other fractures sustained during the birth process. The three most common types of extracranial hemorrhagic injury are caput succedaneum, subgaleal hemorrhage, and cephalhematoma.

Caput Succedaneum

The most commonly observed scalp lesion is ***caput succedaneum,*** a vaguely outlined area of edematous tissue situated over the portion of the scalp that presents in a vertex delivery (Fig. 9-1). The swelling consists of serum or blood, or both, accumulated in the tissues *above* the bone, and it often extends beyond the bone margins. The swelling may be associated with overlying petechiae or ecchymoses. No specific treatment is needed, and the swelling subsides within a few days.

Cephalhematoma

Infrequently, a cephalhematoma is formed when blood vessels rupture during labor or delivery to produce bleeding into the area between the bone and its periosteum. The injury occurs most often with primiparous delivery and is often associated with forceps delivery and vacuum extraction. Unlike caput succedaneum, the boundaries of the cephalhematoma are sharply demarcated and do not extend beyond the limits of the bone (suture lines) (Fig. 9-1, C). The cephalhematoma may involve one or both parietal bones. The occipital bones are less commonly affected, and the frontal bones are rarely affected. The swelling is usually minimal or absent at birth and increases in size on the second or third day. Blood loss is usually not significant.

No treatment is indicated for uncomplicated cephalhematoma. Most lesions are absorbed within 2 weeks to 3 months. Lesions that result in severe blood loss to the area or that involve an underlying fracture require further evaluation. Hyperbilirubinemia may result during resolution of the hematoma. A local infection can develop and is sus-

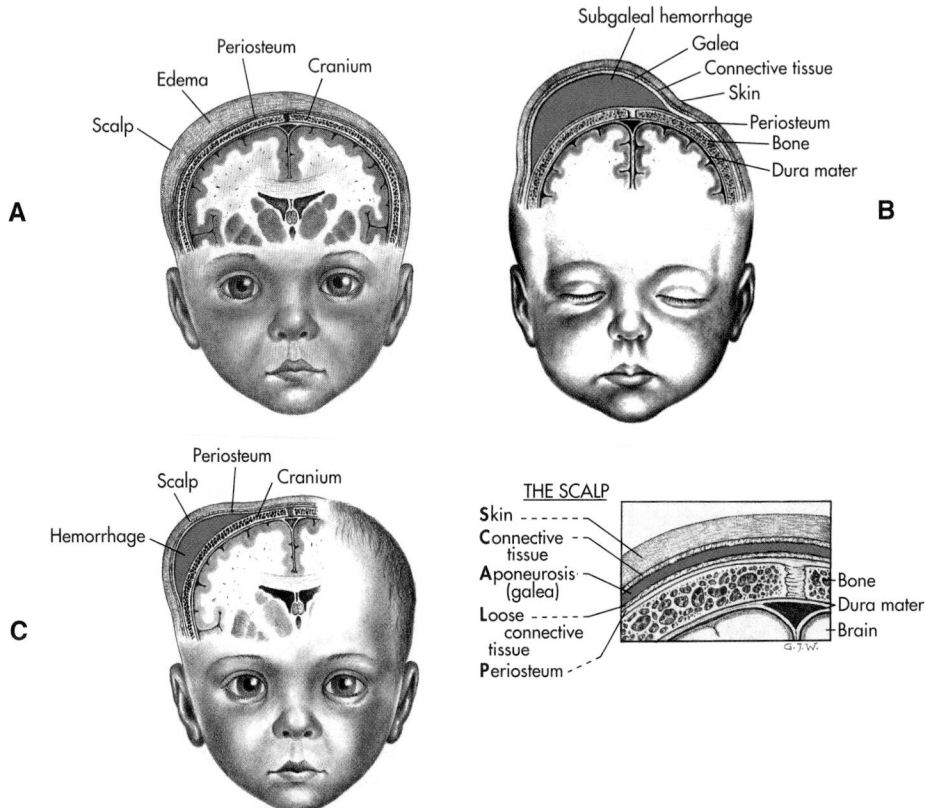

FIG. 9-1 ■ **A,** Caput succedaneum. **B,** Subgaleal hemorrhage. **C,** Cephalhematoma. (**A** and **C** from Seidel HM and others: *Mosby's guide to physical examination,* ed 5, St Louis, 2003, Mosby.)

pected when a sudden increase in swelling occurs. Parents should be counseled that, in some cases, a small area of calcification may develop and persist.

Subgaleal Hemorrhage

Subgaleal hemorrhage is bleeding into the subgaleal compartment (Fig. 9-1, *B*). The *subgaleal compartment* is a potential space that contains loosely arranged connective tissue; it is located beneath the galea aponeurosis, the tendinous sheath that connects the frontal and occipital muscles and forms the inner surface of the scalp. The injury occurs as a result of forces that compress and then drag the head through the pelvic outlet (Paige and Carney, 2002). There have been reports of concern regarding the increased use of the vacuum extractor at birth and an association with cases of subgaleal hemorrhage, neonatal morbidity, and deaths (Garas and others, 2001; Ross, Fresquez, and El-Haddad, 2001); however, the rates of such outcomes are reportedly declining (Putta and Spencer, 2000). The bleeding extends beyond bone, often posteriorly into the neck, and continues after birth, with the potential for serious complications such as anemia or hypovolemic shock.

Early detection of the hemorrhage is vital; serial head circumference measurements and inspection of the back of the neck for increasing edema and a firm mass are essential. A boggy scalp, pallor, tachycardia, and increasing head circumference may also be early signs of a subgaleal hemorrhage (Putta and Spencer, 2000). Computed tomography or magnetic resonance imaging is useful in confirming the diagnosis. Replacement of lost blood and clotting factors is required in acute cases of hemorrhage. Another possible early sign of subgaleal hemorrhage is a forward and lateral positioning of the newborn's ears because the hematoma extends posteriorly. Monitoring the infant for changes in level of consciousness and a decrease in the hematocrit are also key to early recognition and management. An increase in serum bilirubin levels may be seen as a result of the degradating blood cells within the hematoma.

Nursing Considerations

Nursing care is directed toward assessment and observation of the common scalp injuries and vigilance in observing for possible associated complications such as infection or, rarely, acute blood loss and hypovolemia. Because these visible injuries resolve spontaneously, parents need reassurance of their usual benign nature.

FRACTURES

The *clavicle,* or *collarbone,* is the bone most frequently fractured during the birth process. It is often associated with shoulder dystocia or a difficult vertex or breech delivery of infants who are large for gestational age. *Crepitus* (the coarse crackling sensation produced by the rubbing together of fractured bone fragments) may be felt or heard on examination. A palpable, spongy mass, representing localized edema and hematoma, may also be a sign of a fractured clavicle. The infant may be reluctant to move the arm on the affected side, and the Moro reflex may be asymmetric. Radiographs usually reveal a complete fracture with overriding of the fragments.

Fractures of *long bones,* such as the femur or the humerus, are difficult to detect by radiographic examination. Although osteogenesis imperfecta is a rare finding, a newborn infant with a fracture should be assessed for other evidence of this congenital disorder.

Fractures of the neonatal *skull* are uncommon. The bones, which are less mineralized and more compressible than bones in older infants and children, are separated by membranous seams that allow sufficient alteration in the head contour so that it adjusts to the birth canal during delivery. Skull fractures usually follow a prolonged, difficult delivery or forceps extraction. Most fractures are linear, but some may be visible as depressed indentations that compress or decompress like a Ping-Pong ball. A similar finding in neonates is *craniotabes,* which is usually benign or may be associated with prematurity, or hydrocephalus (Johnson, 2003). In this condition the cranial bone(s) move freely on palpation and may easily compress.

> **! NURSING ALERT**
>
> The newborn with a fractured clavicle may have no symptoms, but suspect a fracture if an infant has limited use of the affected arm, malpositioning of the arm, asymmetric Moro reflex, focal swelling or tenderness, or cries in pain when the arm is moved. Eliciting the scarf sign (extending arm across chest toward opposite shoulder) for assessment of gestational age is contraindicated if a fractured clavicle is suspected.

> **! NURSING ALERT**
>
> Any newborn who is large for gestational age or weighs more than 8.5 pounds and is delivered vaginally should be evaluated for a fractured clavicle.

Nursing Considerations

Often, no intervention may be prescribed other than maintaining proper body alignment, careful dressing and undressing of the infant, and handling and carrying that support the affected bone. For example, if the infant has a fractured clavicle, it is important to support the upper and lower back rather than pull the infant up from under the arms. Positioning the infant side-lying with the affected side down is also avoided. Linear skull fractures usually require no treatment. A Ping-Pong ball–type skull fracture may require decompression by surgical intervention. The infant is carefully observed for signs of neurologic complications. The parents of infants with a fracture of any bone should be involved in caring for the infant during hospitalization as part of discharge planning for care at home.

PARALYSES
Facial Paralysis

Pressure on the facial nerve during delivery may result in injury to cranial nerve VII. The primary clinical manifestations are loss of movement on the affected side, such as an inability to completely close the eye, drooping of the corner of the mouth, and absence of wrinkling of the forehead and nasolabial fold (Fig. 9-2). The paralysis is most noticeable when the infant cries. The mouth is drawn to the unaffected side, the wrinkles are deeper on the normal side, and the eye on the involved side remains open.

No medical intervention is necessary. The paralysis usually disappears spontaneously in a few days but may take as long as several months.

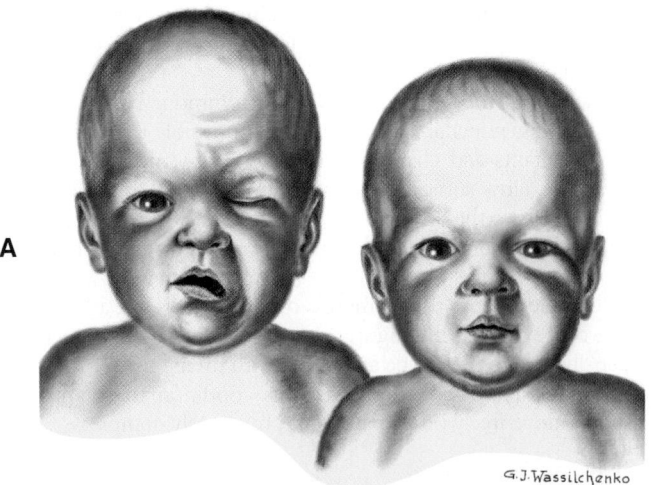

FIG. 9-2 ■ **A,** Paralysis of right side of face 15 minutes after forceps delivery. Absence of movement on affected side is especially noticeable when infant cries. **B,** The same infant 24 hours later.

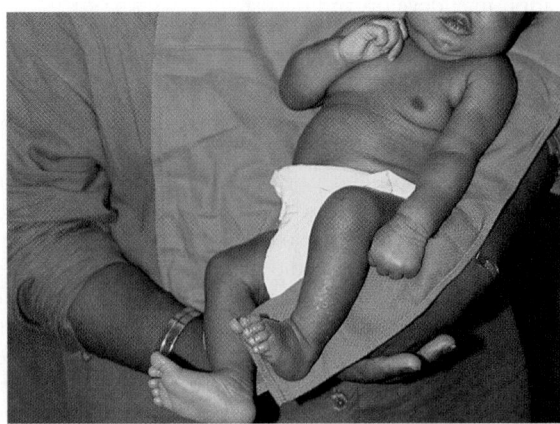

FIG. 9-3 ■ Left-sided brachial plexus (Erb) palsy. Note extended, internally rotated arm and pronated wrist on affected side.

Brachial Palsy

Plexus injury results from forces that alter the normal position and relationship of the arm, shoulder, and neck. *Erb palsy (Erb-Duchenne paralysis)* is caused by damage to the upper plexus and usually results from a stretching or pulling away of the shoulder from the head such as might occur with shoulder dystocia or with a difficult vertex or breech delivery. The less common lower plexus palsy, or *Klumpke palsy,* results from severe stretching of the upper extremity while the trunk is relatively less mobile.

The clinical manifestations of Erb palsy are related to the paralysis of the affected extremity and muscles. The arm hangs limp alongside the body. The shoulder and arm are adducted and internally rotated. The elbow is extended, and the forearm is pronated, with the wrist and fingers flexed; a grasp reflex may be present because finger and wrist movement remain normal (Tappero, 2003) (Fig. 9-3). In lower plexus palsy the muscles of the hand are paralyzed, with consequent wrist drop and relaxed fingers. In a third and more severe form of brachial palsy, the entire arm is paralyzed and hangs limp and motionless at the side. The Moro reflex is absent on the affected side for all of the forms of brachial palsy.

Treatment of the affected arm is aimed at preventing contractures of the paralyzed muscles and maintaining correct placement of the humeral head within the glenoid fossa of the scapula. Complete recovery from stretched nerves usually takes 3 to 6 months. However, avulsion of the nerves (complete disconnection of the ganglia from the spinal cord that involves both anterior and posterior roots) results in permanent damage. For those injuries that do not improve spontaneously by 3 months, surgical intervention may be needed to relieve pressure on the nerves or to repair the nerves with grafting (Volpe, 2001). In some cases injection of botulinum toxin A into the triceps muscle may be effective in reducing muscle contractures after birth-related brachial plexus injuries (Rollnik and others, 2000).

Phrenic Nerve Paralysis

Phrenic nerve paralysis results in diaphragmatic paralysis as demonstrated by ultrasonography, which shows paradoxic chest movement and an elevated diaphragm. Initially, radiography may not demonstrate an elevated diaphragm if the neonate is receiving positive pressure ventilation (Volpe, 2001). The injury sometimes occurs in conjunction with brachial palsy. Respiratory distress is the most common and important sign of injury. Because injury to the phrenic nerve is usually unilateral, the lung on the affected side does not expand, and respiratory efforts are ineffectual. The infant is positioned on the affected side to facilitate maximum expansion of the uninvolved lung. Breathing is primarily thoracic, and cyanosis, tachypnea, or complete respiratory failure may be seen. Pneumonia and atelectasis on the affected side may also occur.

Nursing Considerations

Nursing care of the infant with facial nerve paralysis involves aiding the infant in sucking and helping the mother with feeding techniques. Because part of the mouth cannot close tightly around the nipple, the use of a soft rubber nipple with a large hole may be helpful. The infant may require gavage feeding to prevent aspiration. Breast-feeding is not contraindicated, but the mother will need additional assistance in helping the infant grasp and compress the areolar area.

If the lid of the eye on the affected side does not close completely, artificial tears can be instilled daily to prevent drying of the conjunctiva, sclera, and cornea. The lid is often taped shut to prevent accidental injury. If eye care is needed at home, the parents are taught the procedure for administering eye drops before the infant is discharged from the nursery (see Chapter 22).

Nursing care of the newborn with brachial palsy is concerned primarily with proper positioning of the affected arm. The affected arm should be gently immobilized on the upper abdomen; passive range-of-motion exercises of the shoulder, wrist, elbow, and fingers are initiated in the latter part of the first week (Volpe, 2001). Wrist flexion contractures may be prevented with the use of supportive splints. In dressing the infant, preference is given to the affected arm. Undressing begins with the unaffected arm, and redressing begins with the affected arm to prevent unnecessary manipulation and stress on the paralyzed muscles. Parents are taught to use the "football" position when holding the infant and to avoid picking the child up from under the axillae or by pulling on the arms.

The infant with phrenic nerve paralysis requires the same nursing care as any infant with respiratory distress. As with other birth injuries, the emotional needs of the family are similar to those discussed for soft-tissue injury (p. 223). Follow-up is also essential because of the extended length of recovery. Parents may wish to contact the **Brachial Plexus Foundation** and visit the website for further information.*

COMMON PROBLEMS IN THE NEWBORN

ERYTHEMA TOXICUM NEONATORUM

Erythema toxicum neonatorum, also known as *flea-bite dermatitis* or *newborn rash,* is a benign, self-limiting eruption of unknown cause that usually appears within the first 2 days of life. The lesions are firm, 1- to 3-mm, pale yellow or white papules or pustules on an erythematous base; they resemble flea bites. The rash appears most commonly on the face, proximal extremities, trunk, and buttocks, but it may be located anywhere on the body except the palms and soles. The rash is more obvious during crying episodes. There are no systemic manifestations, and successive crops of lesions heal without pigmentation. The rash usually lasts about 5 to 7 days. The etiology is unknown. However, a smear of the pustule will show numerous eosinophils and a relative absence of neutrophils. When the diagnosis is questionable, bacterial, fungal, or viral cultures should be obtained. Although no treatment is necessary, parents are usually concerned about the rash and need to be reassured of its benign and transient nature.

CANDIDIASIS

Candidiasis, also known as *moniliasis,* is not uncommon in the newborn. *Candida albicans,* the usual organism responsible, may cause disease in any organ system. It is a yeastlike fungus (it produces yeast cells and spores) that can be acquired from a maternal vaginal infection during delivery, by person-to-person transmission (especially poor handwashing technique), or from contaminated hands, bottles, nipples, or other articles. Mucocutaneous, cutaneous, and disseminated candidal infections are all observed in this age-group. It is usually a benign disorder in the neonate, often confined to the oral and diaper regions. Diaper dermatitis caused by *Candida* presents as a moist, erythematous eruption with small white or yellow pebbly pustules. Small areas of skin erosion may also be seen.

Oral Candidiasis

Oral candidiasis *(thrush)* is characterized by white, adherent patches on the tongue, palate, and inner aspects of the cheeks (Fig. 9-4). It is often difficult to distinguish from coagulated milk. The infant may refuse to suck because of pain in the mouth, but this is uncommon.

This condition tends to be acute in the newborn and chronic in infants and young children. Thrush appears

*210 Spring Haven Circle, Royersford, PA 19468; website: www.membrane.com/bpp/index.html.

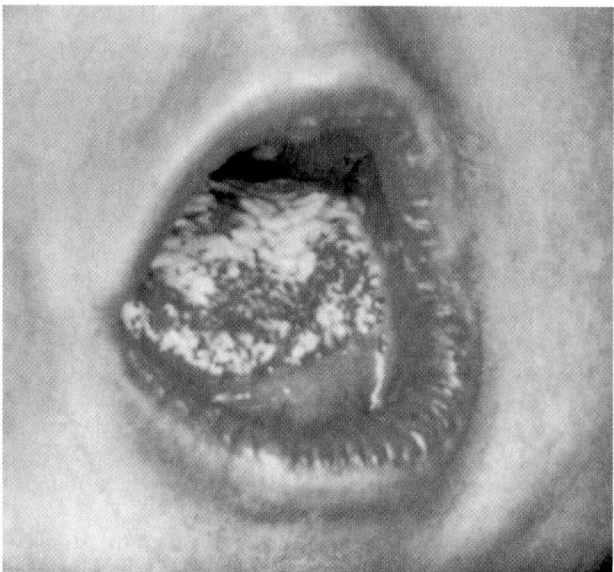

FIG. 9-4 ■ Oral candidiasis (thrush). (From *Variations and minor departures in infants,* Evansville, Ind, 1978, Mead Johnson & Co.)

when the oral flora is altered as a result of antibiotic therapy or poor handwashing by the infant's caregiver. Although the disorder is usually self-limiting, spontaneous resolution may take as long as 2 months, during which time lesions may spread to the larynx, trachea, bronchi, lungs, and along the gastrointestinal tract. The disease is treated with good hygiene, application of a fungicide, and correction of any underlying disturbance. The source of infection, usually the mother, should be treated to prevent reinfection.

Topical application of 1 mL nystatin (Mycostatin) over the surfaces of the oral cavity four times a day, or every 6 hours, is usually sufficient to prevent spread of the disease or prolongation of its course. Several other drugs may be used, including amphotericin B (Fungizone), clotrimazole (Lotrimin, Mycelex), fluconazole (Diflucan), or miconazole (Monistat, Micatin) given intravenously, orally, or topically. To prevent relapse, therapy should be continued for at least 2 days after the lesions disappear (Zenk, 2000). Gentian violet solution may be used in addition to one of the antifungal drugs in chronic cases of oral thrush; however, the former does not treat gastrointestinal *Candida* and may be irritating to the oral mucosa.

> ### ❗ NURSING ALERT
>
> Oral candidiasis can be distinguished from coagulated milk when attempts to remove the patches with a tongue blade are unsuccessful. The primary caregiver may also report that the infant does not nurse well or bottle-feed as previously.

HERPES

Neonatal herpes is one of the most serious viral infections in the newborn, with a mortality rate of up to 60% in those infants with disseminated disease. The rash appears as vesicles or pustules on an erythematous base. Clusters of lesions are common. The lesions ulcerate and crust over rapidly. 50% to 70% of infants with neonatal herpes eventually develop this characteristic rash, but not always before they exhibit other signs and symptoms (Margileth, 1999). Neonatal herpes may also present ophthalmologic clinical findings such as chorioretinitis and microphthalmia and neurologic involvement such as microcephaly and encephalomalacia (Kimberlin, 2002).

Nursing Considerations

Nursing care is directed toward preventing spread of the infection and correct application of the prescribed topical medication. For candidiasis in the diaper area, the caregiver is taught to keep the diaper area clean and to apply the medication to affected areas as prescribed (see also Diaper Dermatitis, Chapter 30).

Oral nystatin is applied after feedings. The medication is distributed over the surface of the oral mucosa and tongue with an applicator or syringe; the remainder of the dose is deposited in the mouth to be swallowed by the infant to treat any gastrointestinal lesions. The intravenous (IV) administration of amphotericin B must be closely monitored to prevent tissue damage and phlebitis.

In addition to good hygienic care, other measures to control thrush include rinsing the infant's mouth with plain water after each feeding before applying the medication and boiling reusable nipples and bottles for at least 20 minutes after a thorough washing (spores are heat-resistant). If used, pacifiers should be boiled for at least 20 minutes once daily, and the nipples of breast-feeding mothers should be treated to prevent reinfection. Infants with candidal diaper dermatitis can introduce the yeast into the mouth from contaminated hands. Placing clothes over the diaper can prevent this cycle of self-infection.

Neonates with herpes virus or suspected infection should be carefully evaluated for clinical manifestations and contact precautions (in addition to standard precautions) instituted according to American Academy of Pediatrics/American College of Obstetricians and Gynecologists' guidelines or hospital protocol. Herpes cultures are obtained, and antiviral therapy with acyclovir is initiated after positive cultures are obtained or if there is strong suspicion of herpes infection (American Academy of Pediatrics and American College of Obstetricians and Gynecologists, 2002).

BIRTHMARKS

Discolorations of the skin are very common findings in the newborn infant (see discussion on skin assessment of the newborn, Chapter 8). Most, such as mongolian spots or telangiectatic nevi, involve no therapy other than reassurance to parents of the benign nature of these discolorations. However, some can be a manifestation of a disease that suggests further examination of the child and other family members (e.g., the multiple light brown *café-au-lait spots* that often characterize the autosomal-dominant hereditary disorder neurofibromatosis and are common findings in Albright syndrome).

Darker or more extensive lesions demand further scrutiny, and excision of the lesion is recommended when feasible or when excisional biopsy is performed. Such lesions include the reddish brown solitary nodule that appears on the face or upper arm and usually represents a spindle and epithelioid cell nevus *(juvenile melanoma);* a *giant pigmented nevus* (or *bathing trunk nevus*), a dark brown to black, irregular plaque that is at risk of transformation to malignant melanoma; and the dark brown or black macules

that become more numerous with age *(junctional* or *compound nevi).*

Vascular birthmarks may be divided into the following categories: vascular malformations, capillary hemangiomas, and mixed hemangiomas. *Vascular stains (malformations)* are permanent lesions that are present at birth and are initially flat and erythematous. Any vascular structure, capillary, vein, artery, or lymphatic may be involved. The two most common vascular stains are the *port-wine stain* and *nevus flammeus.* The port-wine lesions are pink, red, or, rarely, purple stains of the skin that thicken, darken, and proportionally enlarge as the child grows (Fig. 9-5, *A*). The nevus flammeus ("stork bite or "salmon patch") is usually located on the glabella or nape of the neck (Dohil, Baugh, and Eichenfield, 2000).

Port-wine stains may also be associated with structural malformations, such as glaucoma or leptomeningeal angiomatosis (tumor of blood or lymph vessels in the pia-arachnoid) *(Sturge-Weber syndrome)* or bony or muscular overgrowth *(Klippel-Trenaunay-Weber syndrome).* Children with port-

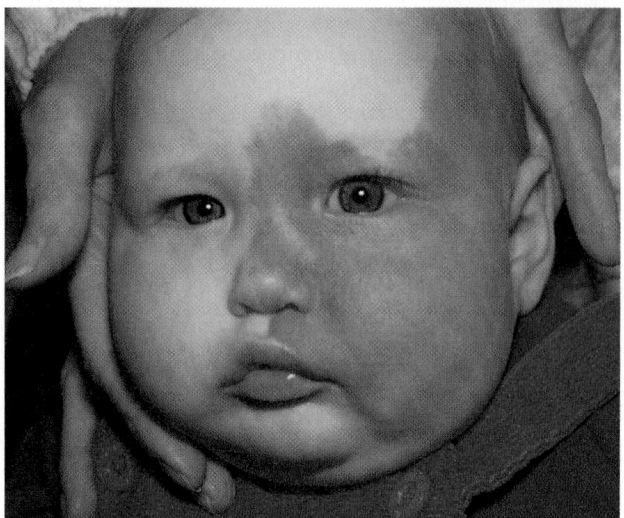

A

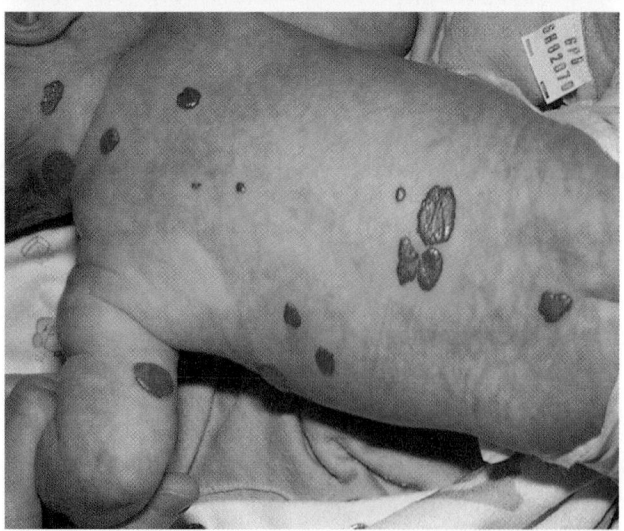

B

FIG. 9-5 ■ **A,** Port-wine stain. **B,** Strawberry hemangioma. (From Zitelli BJ, Davis HW: *Atlas of pediatric physical diagnosis,* ed 4, St Louis, 2002, Mosby.)

wine stains on the eyelids, forehead, cheeks, or extremities should be monitored for these syndromes with periodic ophthalmologic examination, neurologic imaging, and measurement of extremities.

The treatment of choice for port-wine stains is the use of the flashlamp-pumped pulsed dye laser. A series of treatments are usually needed. The treatments can significantly lighten or completely clear the lesions with almost no scarring or pigment change.

Capillary hemangiomas, also sometimes referred to as *strawberry hemangiomas,* are benign cutaneous tumors that involve only capillaries. These are often not apparent at birth but may appear within a few weeks and enlarge considerably during the first year of life and tend to resolve spontaneously by 2 to 3 years of age. These hemangiomas are bright red, rubbery nodules with a rough surface and a well-defined margin (Fig. 9-5, *B*).

Cavernous venous hemangiomas involve deeper vessels in the dermis and have a bluish red color and poorly defined margins. These latter forms may be associated with the trapping of platelets *(Kasabach-Merritt syndrome)* and subsequent thrombocytopenia (Witt, 2003; Szlachetka, 1998).

Although most hemangiomas usually require no treatment because of their high rate of spontaneous involution, some vision and airway obstruction may necessitate therapy. The pulsed dye laser can effectively reduce some hemangiomas; systemic prednisone administered for 2 to 3 weeks or longer may also deter further growth. Subcutaneous injections of interferon alfa-2a or interferon alfa-2b may be required if prednisone therapy and the pulsed dye laser fail to control a problematic hemangioma; however, associated side effects may outweigh the benefits of therapy in some cases (Dohil, Baugh, and Eichenfield, 2000).

Nursing Considerations

Birthmarks, especially those on the face, are upsetting to parents. Families need an explanation of the type of lesion, its significance, and possible treatment.* They can benefit from seeing photographs of other infants before and after treatment for port-wine stains or after the passage of time for hemangiomas. Pictures taken to follow the involution process may further help parents gain confidence that progress is taking place.

If laser therapy is performed, the lesion will have a purplish black appearance for 7 to 10 days, after which the blackness will fade and give way to redness with an eventual lightening of the treated area. During the treatment phase parents are cautioned to avoid any trauma to the lesion or picking at the scab. The child's fingernails are trimmed as an added precaution. Washing the area gently with water and dabbing it dry is adequate, although in some cases a topical antibiotic ointment may be used. No salicylates should be taken during the treatment phase because they decrease the effects of the therapy. The child should be kept out of the sun for several weeks and then protected with a sunscreen of

at least SPF 25. Complications associated with laser treatment include possible secondary infection, keloid or pyogenic granuloma formation, localized dermatitis, and hyperpigmentation or hypopigmentation (Vanderhoof, Doidge, and Maughan, 1998).

NURSING CARE OF THE HIGH-RISK NEWBORN AND FAMILY

IDENTIFICATION OF HIGH-RISK NEWBORNS

The *high-risk neonate* can be defined as a newborn, regardless of gestational age or birth weight, who has a greater-than-average chance of morbidity or mortality because of conditions or circumstances superimposed on the normal course of events associated with birth and the adjustment to extrauterine existence. The high-risk period encompasses human growth and development from the time of *viability* (the gestational age at which survival outside the uterus is believed to be possible, or as early as 23 weeks of gestation) up to 28 days following birth and includes threats to life and health that occur during the prenatal, perinatal, and postnatal periods.

Classification of High-Risk Newborns

High-risk infants are most often classified according to birth weight, gestational age, and predominant pathophysiologic problems. The more common problems related to physiologic status are closely associated with the state of maturity of the infant and usually involve chemical disturbances (e.g., hypoglycemia, hypocalcemia) and consequences of immature organs and systems (e.g., hyperbilirubinemia, respiratory distress, hypothermia). Because high-risk factors are common to several specialty areas—particularly obstetrics, pediatrics, and neonatology—specific terminology is needed to describe the developmental status of the newborn (Box 9-1).

Formerly, weight at birth was considered to reflect a reasonably accurate estimation of gestational age. That is, if an infant's birth weight exceeded 2500 g (5.5 pounds), the infant was considered to be mature. However, accumulated data have shown that intrauterine growth rates are not the same for all infants and that other factors (e.g., heredity, placental insufficiency, maternal disease) influence intrauterine growth and the birth weight of the infant. From these data a more definitive and meaningful classification system that encompasses birth weight, gestational age, and neonatal outcome has been developed. It has also been determined that the lowest perinatal mortality is found in the infant who weighs between 3000 and 4000 g and whose gestational age is more than 36 weeks (Behrman and Shiono, 2002). (See Fig. 8-2 for size comparison of newborn infants.)

ASSESSMENT

At birth the newborn is given a rapid, yet thorough, assessment to determine any apparent problems and identify those that demand immediate attention. This examination is primarily concerned with the evaluation of cardiopulmonary and neurologic functions. The assessment includes the assignment of an Apgar score (see Chapter 8) and an evaluation for any obvious congenital anomalies or evidence of neonatal distress. Delivery rooms are equipped with a

*Information is available from **Birthmarks and Hemangiomas InterNET Support;** website: http://members.tripod.com/Michelle_G/indexH.htm/ and go to Support Group; and **Vascular Birthmarks Foundation,** (877) VBF LOOK, days; (877) VBF 4646, evenings and weekends; website: www.birthmark.org/.

BOX 9-1 ■ Classification of High-Risk Infants

CLASSIFICATION ACCORDING TO SIZE

Low-birth-weight (LBW) infant—An infant whose birth weight is less than 2500 g, regardless of gestational age

Very-low-birth-weight (VLBW) infant—An infant whose birth weight is less than 1500 g

Extremely-low-birth-weight (ELBW) infant—An infant whose birth-weight is less than 1000 g

Appropriate-for-gestational-age (AGA) infant—An infant whose weight falls between the 10th and 90th percentiles on intrauterine growth curves

Small-for-date (SFD) or small-for-gestational-age (SGA) infant—An infant whose rate of intrauterine growth was slowed and whose birth weight falls below the 10th percentile on intrauterine growth curves (see also Fig. 8-1, *B*)

Intrauterine growth restriction (IUGR)—Found in infants whose intrauterine growth is restricted (sometimes used as a more descriptive term for the SGA infant)

Symmetric IUGR: Growth restriction in which the weight, length, and head circumference are all affected

Asymmetric IUGR: Growth restriction in which the head circumference remains within normal parameters while the birth weight falls below the 10th percentile

Large-for-gestational-age (LGA) infant—An infant whose birth weight falls above the 90th percentile on intrauterine growth charts

CLASSIFICATION ACCORDING TO GESTATIONAL AGE

Premature (preterm) infant—An infant born before completion of 37 weeks of gestation, regardless of birth weight

Full-term infant—An infant born between the beginning of the 38 weeks and the completion of the 42 weeks of gestation, regardless of birth weight

Postmature (postterm) infant—An infant born after 42 weeks of gestational age, regardless of birth weight

CLASSIFICATION ACCORDING TO MORTALITY

Live birth—Birth in which the neonate manifests any heartbeat, breathes, or displays voluntary movement, regardless of gestational age

Fetal death—Death of the fetus after 20 weeks of gestation and before delivery, with absence of any signs of life after birth

Neonatal death—Death that occurs in the first 27 days of life; early neonatal death occurs in the first week of life; late neonatal death occurs at 7 to 27 days

Perinatal mortality—Total number of fetal and early neonatal deaths per 1000 live births

special resuscitation area where infants with evidence of distress are stabilized and evaluated before being transported to the neonatal intensive care unit (NICU) for therapy and more extensive assessment (see Clinical Assessment of Gestational Age, Chapter 8).

Systematic Assessment

A thorough systematic physical assessment (see Guidelines box) is an essential component in the care of the high-risk infant. Subtle changes in feeding behavior, activity, color, oxygen saturation (SaO₂), or vital signs often indicate an underlying problem. The low-birth-weight (LBW) preterm infant, especially the very-low-birth-weight (VLBW), or

extremely-low-birth-weight (ELBW) infant, is ill-equipped to withstand prolonged physiologic stress and may die within minutes of exhibiting abnormal symptoms if the underlying pathologic process is not corrected. The alert nurse is aware of subtle changes and reacts promptly to implement interventions that promote optimum functioning in the high-risk neonate. Changes in the infant's status are noted through ongoing observations of the infant's adaptation to the extrauterine environment.

Observational assessments of the high-risk infant are made according to the infant's acuity; the critically ill infant requires close observation and assessment of respiratory function, including continuous pulse oximetry, electrolytes, and evaluation of blood gases. Accurate documentation of the infant's status is an integral component of nursing care. With the aid of continuous, sophisticated cardiopulmonary monitoring, nursing assessments and daily care may be coordinated to allow for minimal handling of the infant (especially the VLBW or ELBW infant) to decrease the effects of environmental stress.

Monitoring Physiologic Data

Most neonates under intensive observation are placed in a controlled thermal environment and monitored for heart rate, respiratory activity, and temperature. The monitoring devices are equipped with an alarm system that indicates when the vital signs are above or below preset limits. However, it is essential to check the apical heart rate and compare it with the monitor reading.

Blood pressure (BP) is monitored routinely in the sick neonate by either internal or external means. Direct recording with arterial catheters is often used but carries the risks inherent in any procedure in which a catheter is introduced into an artery. An umbilical venous catheter may also be used to monitor the neonate's central venous pressure. Oscillometry (Dinamap) or Doppler transcutaneous apparatus are simple, effective means for detecting alterations in systemic BP (hypotension or hypertension). Normal BP ranges for healthy premature infants are listed in Table 9-1. Infants who have birth asphyxia, have low Apgar scores, or are mechanically ventilated have lower systolic and diastolic pressures. In the NICU, frequent laboratory examinations and their interpretation are integral parts of the ongoing assessment of infants' progress. Accurate intake and output records are kept on all acutely ill infants. An accurate output can be obtained by collecting urine in a plastic urine collection bag specifically made for premature infants (see Urine Specimens, Chapter 22) or by weighing the diapers, which is the simplest and least traumatic means of measuring urinary output. The preweighed wet diaper is weighed on a gram scale, and the gram weight of the urine is converted directly to milliliters (e.g., 25 g = 25 mL).

One study has shown that urine obtained from disposable diapers containing absorbent gelling material yields inaccurate results for urine specific gravity, pH, and protein. Urine samples obtained from cotton balls of 100% cotton that were strategically placed in the diaper proved to be the most accurate, whereas samples from absorbent gelling material liners and cloth diapers yielded inaccurate results for specific gravity, pH, and protein (Kirkpatrick, Alexander, and Cain, 1997).

⚡ GUIDELINES

Physical Assessment

GENERAL ASSESSMENT

Using electronic scale, weigh daily, or more often if ordered.

Measure length and head circumference periodically.

Describe general body shape and size, posture at rest, ease of breathing, presence and location of edema.

Describe any apparent deformities.

Describe any signs of distress: poor color, hypotonia, lethargy, apnea.

RESPIRATORY ASSESSMENT

Describe shape of chest (barrel, concave), symmetry, presence of incisions, chest tubes, or other deviations.

Describe use of accessory muscles: nasal flaring or substernal, intercostal, or subclavicular retractions.

Determine respiratory rate and regularity.

Auscultate and describe breath sounds: stridor, crackles, wheezing, wet or diminished sounds, grunting, diminished air entry, equality of breath sounds.

Describe cry if not intubated.

Describe ambient oxygen and method of delivery; if intubated, describe size of tube, type of ventilator and settings, and method of securing tube.

Determine oxygen saturation by pulse oximetry and partial pressure of oxygen and carbon dioxide by transcutaneous oxygen ($tcPo_2$) and transcutaneous carbon dioxide ($tcPco_2$).

CARDIOVASCULAR ASSESSMENT

Determine heart rate and rhythm.

Describe heart sounds, including any murmurs.

Determine the point of maximum intensity (PMI), the point at which the heartbeat sounds and palpates loudest (a change in the PMI may indicate a mediastinal shift).

Describe infant's color (may be of cardiac, respiratory, or hematopoietic origin): cyanosis, pallor, plethora, jaundice, mottling.

Assess color of mucous membranes, lips.

Determine blood pressure. Indicate extremity used and cuff size; check each extremity at least once.

Describe peripheral pulses, capillary refill (<2 to 3 seconds), peripheral perfusion (mottling).

Describe monitors, their parameters, and whether alarms are in "on" position.

GASTROINTESTINAL ASSESSMENT

Determine presence of abdominal distention: increase in circumference, shiny skin, evidence of abdominal wall erythema, visible peristalsis, visible loops of bowel, status of umbilicus.

Determine any signs of regurgitation, and time related to feeding; character and amount of residual if gavage fed; if nasogastric tube is in place, describe type of suction, drainage (color, consistency, pH, guaiac).

Describe amount, color, consistency, and odor of any emesis.

Palpate liver margin (1-3 cm below right costal margin)

Describe amount, color, and consistency of stools; check for occult blood or reducing substances if ordered or indicated by appearance of stool.

Describe bowel sounds: presence or absence (must be present if feeding).

GENITOURINARY ASSESSMENT

Describe any abnormalities of genitalia.

Describe amount (as determined by weight), color, pH, labstick findings, and specific gravity of urine (to screen for adequacy of hydration).

Check weight (the most accurate measure for assessment of hydration).

NEUROLOGIC-MUSCULOSKELETAL ASSESSMENT

Describe infant's movements: random, purposeful, jittery, twitching, spontaneous, elicited; level of activity with stimulation; evaluate based on gestational age.

Describe infant's position or attitude: flexed, extended.

Describe reflexes observed: Moro, sucking, Babinski, plantar reflex, and other expected reflexes.

Determine level of response and consolability.

Determine changes in head circumference (if indicated); size and tension of fontanels, suture lines.

Determine pupillary responses in infant >32 weeks of gestation.

Check hip alignment (only experienced practitioner should perform).

TEMPERTATURE

Determine skin and axillary temperature.

Determine relationship to environmental temperature.

SKIN ASSESSMENT

Describe any discoloration, reddened area, signs of irritation, blisters, abrasions, or denuded areas, especially where monitoring equipment, infusions, or other apparatus come in contact with skin; also check and note any skin preparation used (e.g., povidone-iodine tape).

Determine texture and turgor of skin: dry, smooth, flaky, peeling, etc.

Describe any rash, skin lesion, or birthmarks.

Determine whether IV infusion catheter or needle is in place, and observe for signs of infiltration.

Describe parenteral infusion lines: location, type (arterial, venous, peripheral, umbilical, central, peripheral central venous); type of infusion (medication, saline, dextrose, electrolyte, lipids, total parenteral nutrition); type of infusion pump and rate of flow; type of catheter or needle; and appearance of insertion site.

Blood examinations are a necessary part of the ongoing assessment and monitoring of the high-risk newborn's progress. The tests most often performed are blood glucose, bilirubin, calcium, hematocrit, serum electrolytes, and blood gases. Samples may be obtained from the heel; by venipuncture; by arterial puncture; or by an indwelling catheter in an umbilical vein, umbilical artery, or peripheral artery (see Atraumatic Care box, p. 201, and Chapter 22, Collection of Specimens).

When numerous blood samples must be drawn, it is important to maintain an accurate record of the amount of blood being removed, especially in ELBW and VLBW infants, who can ill afford to have their blood supply depleted

TABLE 9-1 ■ Blood Pressure Ranges in Different Weight Groups of Healthy Premature Infants*

BIRTH WEIGHT (g)	SYSTOLIC (mm Hg)	DIASTOLIC (mm Hg)
501-750	50-62	26-36
751-1000	48-59	23-36
1001-1250	49-61	26-35
1251-1500	46-56	23-33
1501-1750	46-58	23-33
1751-2000	48-61	24-35

Modified from Hegyi T and others: Blood pressure ranges in premature infants. I. The first hours of life, *J Pediatr* 124(4):630, 1994.
*Defined as infants without a history of maternal hypertension, Apgar scores of less than 3 at 1 minute and less than 6 at 5 minutes, pneumothorax, hematocrit 32, serum pH 7.1, use of dopamine, infusion of erythrocytes or colloid, mechanical ventilation, or cardiopulmonary resuscitation.

during the acute phase of their illness. There is an increased emphasis upon drawing as little blood as possible from high-risk neonates to minimize the depletion of blood volume and avoid blood transfusions and associated complications. To obtain frequent samples for monitoring arterial blood gas levels without repeated arterial punctures, pulse oximetry, which measures the saturation or percent of oxygen in the hemoglobin, is typically used. An in-line arterial blood gas monitor also decreases the need for blood waste and peripheral punctures. Although used less frequently than pulse oximetry, some situations warrant the monitoring of transcutaneous oxygen ($tcPo_2$) and carbon dioxide ($tcPco_2$). The nurse notes changes in oxygenation (or other aspects being monitored) associated with handling and adjusts the infant's care accordingly. The frequency of vital signs is determined by the infant's acuity level (seriousness of condition) and response to handling.

● Nursing Diagnoses

Many nursing diagnoses may be evident after a careful assessment of the infant at risk. Some apply to all infants; others vary according to the needs and characteristics of individual infants and their families. The nursing diagnoses that represent general guides for nursing intervention are found in the Nursing Care Plan on pp. 255 to 259. Because a number of health problems accompany the high-risk infant, the nurse is also alert to other conditions and complications discussed later in this chapter and elsewhere in the book.

● Planning

The nursing care plan for the high-risk infant depends to a large extent on the diagnosis of the health problem that places the infant at risk. However, the following are basic goals for all high-risk infants and their families:

1 Infant will exhibit adequate oxygenation.
2 Infant will maintain stable body temperature.
3 Infant will exhibit no evidence of nosocomial infection.
4 Infant will receive adequate hydration and nutrition.
5 Infant will maintain skin integrity.
6 Infant will exhibit normal intracranial pressure and no evidence of intraventricular hemorrhage (unless preexisting condition).

7 Infant will experience no pain or a reduction of pain.
8 Infant receives appropriate developmental support and care.
9 Family receives appropriate support, including preparation for home care or for infant's death.

● Implementation

Respiratory Support

The primary objective in the care of high-risk infants is to establish and maintain respiration. Many infants require supplemental oxygen and assisted ventilation. All infants require appropriate positioning in order to maximize oxygenation and ventilation. Oxygen therapy is provided on the basis of the infant's requirements and illness (see Respiratory Distress Syndrome, p. 271).

Thermoregulation

After or concurrent with the establishment of respiration, the most crucial need of the LBW infant is application of external warmth. Prevention of heat loss in the distressed infant is absolutely essential for survival, and maintaining a neutral thermal environment is a challenging aspect of neonatal intensive nursing care. Heat production is a complicated process that involves the cardiovascular, neurologic, and metabolic systems, and the immature neonate has all of the problems related to heat production that are faced by the full-term infant (see Thermoregulation, Chapter 8). However, LBW infants are placed at further disadvantage by a number of additional problems. They have an even smaller muscle mass and fewer deposits of brown fat for producing heat, lack insulating subcutaneous fat, and have poor reflex control of skin capillaries.

To delay or prevent the effects of cold stress, at-risk newborns are placed in a heated environment immediately after birth, where they remain until they are able to maintain **thermal stability**—the capacity to balance heat production and conservation and heat dissipation. Because overheating produces an increase in oxygen and calorie consumption, the infant is also jeopardized in a hyperthermic environment. A **neutral thermal environment** is one that permits the infant to maintain a normal core temperature with minimum oxygen consumption and calorie expenditure. Studies indicate that optimum thermoneutrality cannot be predicted for every high-risk infant's needs. Guidelines for providing an optimum thermal environment for the VLBW infant suggest maintaining the infant's core temperature at rest within a range of 36.7° to 37.3° C (98.1° to 99.1° F) with core and mean temperatures changing less than 0.2° C and 0.3° C an hour (Sauer, Dane, and Visser, 1984).

VLBW and ELBW infants, with thin skin and almost no subcutaneous fat, can control body heat loss or gain only within a very limited range of environmental temperatures. In these infants heat loss from radiation, evaporation, and transepidermal water loss is three to five times greater than in larger infants, and a decrease in body temperature is associated with an increase in mortality. Further research is needed to define a neutral thermal environment for the ELBW infant.

The consequences of cold stress that produce additional hazards to the neonate are (1) hypoxia, (2) metabolic acidosis, and (3) hypoglycemia. Increased metabolism in response to chilling creates a compensatory increase in oxygen and calorie consumption. If available oxygen is not increased to accommodate this need, arterial oxygen ten-

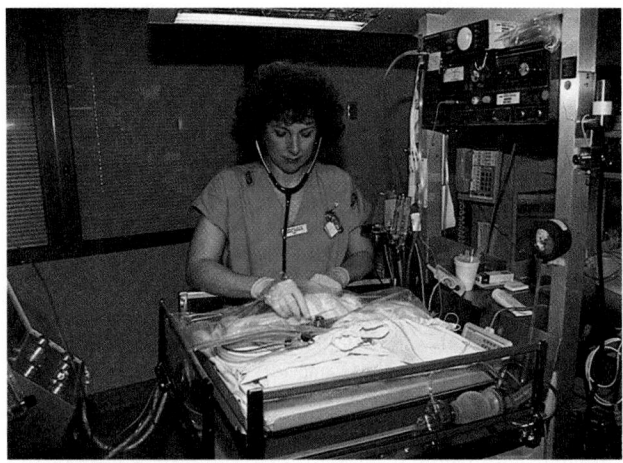

FIG. 9-6 ■ Nurse caring for infant under overhead warming unit. Note use of nesting with blankets.

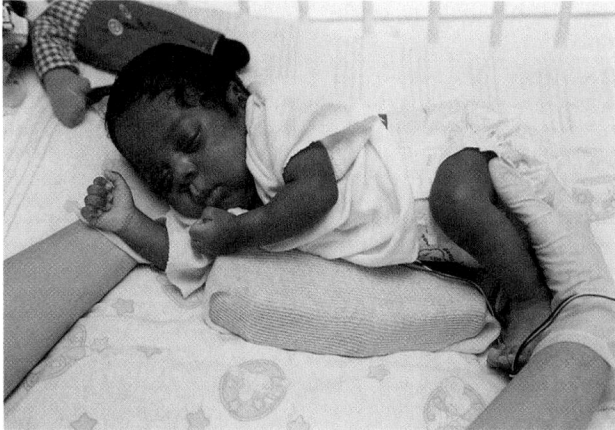

A

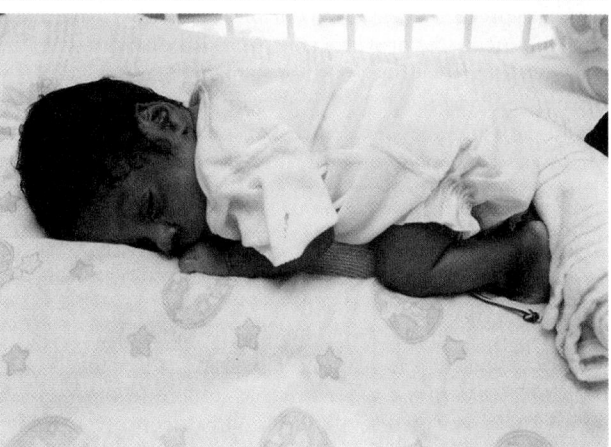

B

FIG. 9-7 ■ **A,** Preterm infant slowly and gently transitioned to prone position on prone roll designed with stockinette-covered foam cut to individual specification to prevent flattening of shoulders and pelvis against the mattress and to support a stable breathing base for the infant. **B,** Preterm infant positioned on prone roll. (Courtesy Texas Children's Hospital, Houston, Tex; photo by Paul Vincent Kuntz.)

sion is decreased. This is further complicated by a smaller lung volume in relation to the metabolic rate, which creates diminished oxygen in the blood and concurrent pulmonary disorders. A small advantage is gained by the presence of fetal hemoglobin because its increased capacity to carry oxygen allows the infant to exist for longer periods in conditions of lowered oxygen tension.

The three primary methods for maintaining a neutral thermal environment are the use of an incubator, a radiant warming panel (Figs. 9-6 and 9-7), and an open bassinet with cotton blankets. The dressed infant under blankets can maintain a certain temperature within a wider range of environmental temperatures; however, the close observations required with a high-risk infant are best accomplished if the infant remains partially unclothed. The incubator should always be prewarmed before placing an infant in it. The use of *double-walled incubators* significantly improves the infant's ability to maintain a desirable temperature and reduce energy expenditure related to heat regulation. The infant is clothed and warmly wrapped in blankets when removed from the warm environment of the incubator for feeding or cuddling. Inside or outside the incubator, head coverings are effective in preventing heat loss. A fabric-insulated or wool cap is more effective than one fashioned from stockinette (Blackburn, 2003). The use of a heated gel mattress with radiant heat has been shown to significantly decrease the incidence of radiation heat loss and preserve an adequate neutral thermal environment for the VLBW neonate (Vogtman, Mockel, and Tillig, 1996).

An effective means for maintaining the desired range of temperature in the infant is the use of a *manually adjusted* or *automatically controlled (servo-controlled) incubator.* The latter mechanism, when set at the upper and lower limits of the desired circulating air temperature range, adjusts automatically in response to signals from a thermal sensor attached to the abdominal skin. If the infant's temperature drops, the warming device is triggered to increase heat output. The servo control is usually set to a desired skin temperature between 36° and 36.5° C (96.8° to 97.7° F) (Blake and Murray, 2002).

Disadvantages are always inherent in any mechanical device; therefore, an important part of nursing assessment is

to compare the infant's temperature with the temperature in the incubator. For example, if the infant's temperature fluctuates in response to sepsis, the servo-controlled mechanism would respond by decreasing or increasing the ambient air temperature. Therefore a critical observation could be easily overlooked.

A high-humidity atmosphere contributes to body temperature maintenance by reducing *evaporative heat loss.* A number of "microenvironments" may be used with the VLBW and ELBW infant to minimize evaporative and *insensible water losses.* These include items such as thermal blankets or plastic wrap, humidified reservoirs for incubators, and humidified plastic heat shields covered with plastic wrap. When such environments are used, special care must be taken to avoid bacterial contamination of the warm and humid environment by such "water bugs" as *Pseudomonas* and *Serratia;* postnatally acquired pneumonia from such organisms may be fatal, particularly in VLBW infants. In one study, ELBW and VLBW infants were placed in a polyethylene wrap from the neck down immediately after delivery. There was a significant decrease in heat loss in infants born at 23 to 27 weeks of gestation (Vohra and others, 1999).

The use of emollient creams (Aquaphor) and semiocclusive dressings (Tegaderm, Op-Site) have been used to reduce evaporative heat loss in VLBW infants. Again, care must be taken to avoid disrupting the integrity of the skin and to guard against the use of products that have additives that can be absorbed through the skin.

Skin-to-skin (kangaroo) contact between the stable preterm infant and parent is also a viable option for interaction because of the maintenance of appropriate body temperature by the infant. Other benefits of skin-to-skin contact are discussed later in this chapter.

Protection From Infection

Protection from infection is an integral part of all newborn care, but preterm and sick neonates are particularly susceptible. The protective environment of a regularly cleaned and changed incubator provides effective isolation from airborne infective agents. However, thorough, meticulous, and frequent handwashing is the foundation of a preventive program. This includes *all* persons who come in contact with infants and their equipment. After handling another infant or equipment, no one ever touches an infant without first washing hands.

Personnel with infectious disorders are either barred from the unit until they are no longer infectious or are required to wear suitable shields, such as masks or gloves, to reduce the likelihood of contamination. In some areas an annual influenza vaccination is recommended for NICU personnel. *Standard precautions* as a method of infection control are instituted in all nursery areas to protect the infants and staff (see Chapter 22). The benefit of "gowning" by visitors and hospital staff to control infection is not supported by research. Sibling visitation in the NICU has not been shown to increase nosocomial infections (Polak, Ringler, and Daugherty, 2004).

The sources of infection rise in direct relationship to the number of persons and pieces of equipment coming in contact with the infants. Equipment used in the care of infants is cleaned on a regular basis in accordance with the manufacturer's recommendations or institutional protocol; this includes cleaning of cribs, mattresses, incubators, radiant warmers, cardiorespiratory monitors, pulse oximeters, and vital sign–monitoring equipment after usage with one infant and before usage with another. Because organisms thrive best in water, plumbing fixtures and humidifying equipment are particularly hazardous. Disposable equipment used for water-related therapies, such as nebulizers and plastic tubing, is changed regularly.

Hydration

High-risk infants often receive supplemental parenteral fluids to supply additional calories, electrolytes, or water. Adequate hydration is particularly important in preterm infants because their extracellular water content is higher (70% in full-term infants and up to 90% in preterm infants), their body surface is larger, and the capacity for osmotic diuresis is limited in preterm infants' underdeveloped kidneys. Therefore these infants are highly vulnerable to fluid depletion.

Parenteral fluids may be given to the high-risk neonate via several routes depending on the nature of the illness, the duration and type of fluid therapy, and unit preference.

Common routes of fluid infusion include peripheral, peripherally inserted central venous (or percutaneous central venous), surgically inserted central venous and, at times, umbilical venous. The preferred sites for peripheral IV infusions in neonates are the peripheral veins on the dorsal surfaces of the hands or feet. Alternative sites are scalp veins and antecubital veins. Special precautions and frequent observations must accompany the use of peripheral lines with hypertonic solutions (dextrose 10%) and total parenteral nutrition (Wilson, 2000). In many neonatal centers the percutaneous central venous catheter, also commonly called the peripherally inserted central venous catheter, is used for parenteral therapy and medication administration because of less expense and decreased neonatal trauma.

In most facilities NICU nurses insert peripheral IV catheters and maintain the infusions. IVs must always be delivered by continuous infusion pumps that deliver minute volumes at a preset flow rate. The catheter is secured to the skin with a minimum amount of tape (see Skin Care, p. 238), with care taken not to cause undue pressure from the catheter hub and tubing. Because all infants, especially those who are ELBW and VLBW, are highly vulnerable to any fluid shifts, infusion rates are very carefully regulated and are checked hourly to prevent tissue damage from extravasation, fluid overload, or dehydration. Pulmonary edema, congestive heart failure, patent ductus arteriosus, and intraventricular hemorrhage may occur with fluid overload. Dehydration may cause electrolyte disturbances (particularly Na^-), with potentially serious central nervous system (CNS) effects.

Infants who are ELBW, tachypneic, receiving phototherapy, or in a radiant warmer have increased insensible water losses that require appropriate fluid adjustments. Nurses must monitor fluid status by daily (or more frequent) weights and accurate intake and output of all fluids, including medications and blood products. Urine-specific gravity and dipstick measurements are monitored per unit protocol, and serum electrolytes are obtained as warranted by the infant's condition. ELBW infants often require more frequent monitoring of these parameters because of their inordinate transepidermal fluid loss, immature renal function, and propensity to dehydration or overhydration. Intolerance of even dextrose 5% is not uncommon in the ELBW infant, with subsequent glycosuria and osmotic diuresis. Alterations in behavior, alertness, or activity level in these infants receiving IV fluids may signal an electrolyte imbalance, hypoglycemia, or hyperglycemia. The nurse is also observant for tremors or seizures in the VLBW or ELBW infant, because these may be a sign of hyponatremia or hypernatremia.

> ### ⚠ NURSING ALERT
>
> Nurses should be constantly alert for signs of IV infiltration (e.g., erythema, edema, color change of tissue, blanching at site) and for signs of overhydration (weight gain of more than 30 g in 24 hours, periorbital edema, tachypnea, and crackles on lung auscultation).

A common problem observed in infants who have an umbilical artery catheter in place is vasoconstriction of peripheral vessels, which can seriously impair circulation. The response is triggered by arterial vasospasm caused by the presence of the catheter, the infusion of fluids, or injection of medication. Blanching of the buttocks, genitalia, or legs or feet is an indication of vasospasm. The problem is recognized promptly and reported to the practitioner. The nurse must also observe for signs of thrombi in infants with umbilical venous or arterial lines. The precipitation of microthrombi in the vascular bed with the use of such catheters is commonly manifested by a sudden bluish discoloration seen in the toes, called "cath toes." The problem is promptly reported to the practitioner because failure to alleviate the existing pathology may result in the loss of toes or even a foot or leg.

NURSING ALERT

Circulatory effects are observed first in the toes but may extend to include the legs and buttocks. The toes first flush and then turn a mulberry color, and, if the condition is not corrected, there may be serious complications involving the loss of a limb. The infant with an umbilical venous or arterial catheter should also be observed closely for catheter dislodging and subsequent bleeding or hemorrhage; urinary output, renal function, and gastrointestinal function are also evaluated in these infants. Although the intent of such catheters is to effectively deliver IV fluids (and sometimes medications) and to obtain arterial blood gas samples, they are not without inherent complications.

Nutrition

Optimum nutrition is critical in the management of LBW and preterm infants, but there are difficulties in providing for their nutritional needs. The various mechanisms for ingestion and digestion of foods are not fully developed; the more immature the infant, the greater the problem. In addition, the nutritional requirements for this group of infants are not known with certainty. It is known that all preterm infants are at risk because of poor nutritional stores and several physical and developmental characteristics.

An infant's need for rapid growth and daily maintenance must be met in the presence of several anatomic and physiologic disabilities. Although some sucking and swallowing activities are demonstrated before birth and in premature infants, coordination of these mechanisms does not occur until approximately 32 to 34 weeks of gestation, and they are not fully synchronized until 36 to 37 weeks. Initial sucking is not accompanied by swallowing, and esophageal contractions are uncoordinated. The gag reflex may not be developed until 36 weeks of gestation. Consequently, infants are highly prone to aspiration and its attendant dangers. As infants mature, the suck-swallow pattern develops but is slow and ineffectual, and these reflexes may also become easily exhausted.

The amount and method of feeding are determined by the size and condition of the infant. Nutrition can be provided by either the parenteral or enteral route or by a combination of the two. Infants who are ELBW, VLBW, or critically ill have often been fed exclusively by the parenteral route because of their inability to digest and absorb enteral nutrition. Illness factors resulting in hypoxia and major organ immaturity further preclude the use of enteral feeding until the infant's condition has stabilized; necrotizing enterocolitis has previously been associated with enteral feedings in acutely ill or distressed infants (see Necrotizing Enterocolitis, p. 284). Total parenteral nutritional support of acutely ill infants may be accomplished quite successfully with commercially available IV solutions specifically designed to meet the infant's nutritional needs, including protein, amino acids, trace minerals, vitamins, carbohydrates (dextrose), and fat (lipid emulsion).

Studies have shown that there are benefits to the early introduction of small amounts of enteral feedings in metabolically stable preterm infants. These *minimal enteral* or *trophic feedings* have been shown to stimulate the infant's gastrointestinal tract, preventing mucosal atrophy and subsequent enteral feeding difficulties. Minimal enteral feedings with as little as 0.1 to 4 mL/kg preterm formula or breast milk may be given by gavage as early as the second or third postnatal day. Parenteral hydration and nutrition is continued until the infant is able to tolerate an amount of enteral feeding sufficient to sustain growth. An increased incidence of necrotizing enterocolitis in those VLBW infants fed enterally has not been substantiated (Evans and Thureen, 2001). In fact, minimal enteral feedings have been proved to increase mineral absorption, increase serum calcium and alkaline phosphatase activity, and substantially decrease the incidence of bilious gastric residuals and feeding intolerance in preterm infants (Schanler and others, 1999). Minimal enteral feedings have been recommended as the standard of care for feeding VLBW infants (Kliegman, 1999).

Although the timing of the first feeding has been a matter of controversy, most authorities now believe that early feeding (provided that the infant is medically stable) reduces the incidence of complicating factors such as hypoglycemia, dehydration, and the degree of hyperbilirubinemia. The feeding regimen used varies in different units. The initial enteral feeding is usually not attempted until infants have adapted to extrauterine existence as evidenced by adequate oxygenation; evidence of gastrointestinal motility, including passage of meconium; and stable cardiopulmonary status.

Breast-Feeding.   There is now sufficient evidence indicating that human milk is the best source of nutrition for term and preterm infants. Studies indicate that even small preterm infants are able to breast-feed if they have adequate sucking and swallowing reflexes and there are no other contraindications, such as respiratory complications, or concurrent illness (Morton, 2002). Mothers who wish to breast-feed their preterm infants are encouraged to pump their breasts until their infants are sufficiently stable to tolerate breast-feeding.

Appropriate guidelines for the storage of *expressed mother's milk (EMM)* should be followed to decrease the risk of milk contamination and destruction of its beneficial properties.

Preterm infants may be able to successfully breast-feed earlier than previously believed (28 to 36 weeks); in addition, preterm infants who are breast-fed rather than bottle-fed demonstrate fewer oxygen desaturations, absence of bradycardia, warmer skin temperature, and better coordination of breathing, sucking, and swallowing (Gardner, Snell, and Lawrence, 2002). The preterm infant should be carefully evaluated for readiness to breast-feed, including assessment of behavioral state, ability to maintain body temperature outside an artificial heat source, respiratory status, and readiness to suckle at the mother's breast. The latter may be accomplished with nonnutritive suckling at the breast during skin-to-skin (kangaroo) contact so that the mother and new-born may become accustomed to each other (Gardner, Snell, and Lawrence, 2002). Nasal cannula oxygen may also be provided during preterm breast-feeding on the basis of the infant's assessed requirements.

Time, patience, and dedication on the part of the mother and the nursing staff are needed to help infants with breast-feeding. The process is begun slowly—beginning with one feeding daily and gradually increasing the feedings as the infant tolerates them. Supplementary bottle-feeding is inefficient because the infant expends energy and calories to feed twice. Supplementing by gavage feeding or using a training nipple is more energy and calorie efficient. Breast-feeding the preterm infant often requires additional guidance by a lactation consultant; continued support and encouragement by the nursing staff is essential to breast-feeding preterm infants. In addition, postdischarge breast-feeding often requires further guidance, counseling, and support by nursing staff (Morton, 2002).

Nipple Feeding.   Vigorous infants can be fed from a nipple with little difficulty, whereas compromised preterm infants will require alternative methods. The amount to be fed is determined largely by the infant's weight gain and tolerance of previous feeding and is increased by small increments until a satisfactory caloric intake is ensured.

The rate of increase that is well tolerated varies from one infant to another, and determining this rate is often a nursing responsibility. Preterm infants require more time and patience to feed as compared with full-term infants, and the oral-pharyngeal mechanism may be stressed by an attempt to feed too rapidly. It is important not to tire the infants or overtax their capacity to retain the feedings. When infants require a prolonged time (arbitrarily, more than 30 minutes) to complete a feeding, gavage feeding may be considered for the next time.

A developmental approach to feeding considers the individual infant's readiness rather than initiated feedings based on weight and age, or a predetermined time schedule. Feeding readiness is determined by each infant's medical status, energy level, ability to sustain a brief quiet alert state, gag reflex (demonstrated with a gavage tube insertion), spontaneous rooting and sucking behaviors, and functional sucking reflex (Hunter, 2001). The preterm infant may experience difficulty coordinating sucking, swallowing, and breathing, with resultant apnea, bradycardia, and decreased oxygen saturation. The infant's ability to suck on a pacifier does not indicate complete readiness for nipple feeding or ability to coordinate the above-mentioned activities without some degree of stress; a gradual introduction of nippling in preterm infants is based on careful evaluation of their ability to maintain adequate cardiopulmonary functions while feeding. When infants are unable to tolerate bottle-feedings, intermittent feedings by gavage are instituted until they gain enough strength and coordination to use the nipple.

The nipple used should be relatively firm and stable. Although a high-flow, pliable nipple requires less energy to use, it may provide a flow rate that is too rapid for some preterm infants to manage without risk of aspiration. A firmer nipple facilitates a more "cupped" tongue configuration and allows for a more controlled, manageable flow rate.

The infant is positioned in the feeder's arms or placed semiupright in the lap (Fig. 9-8) and is held with the back curved slightly to simulate the position assumed naturally by most full-term newborns. The use of gentle cheek and jaw support for preterm infants has been shown to facilitate feedings. Stroking the infant's lips, cheeks, and tongue be-

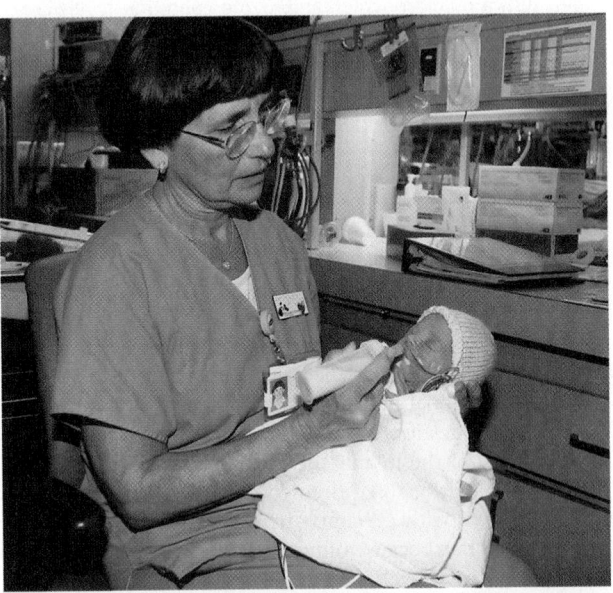

A

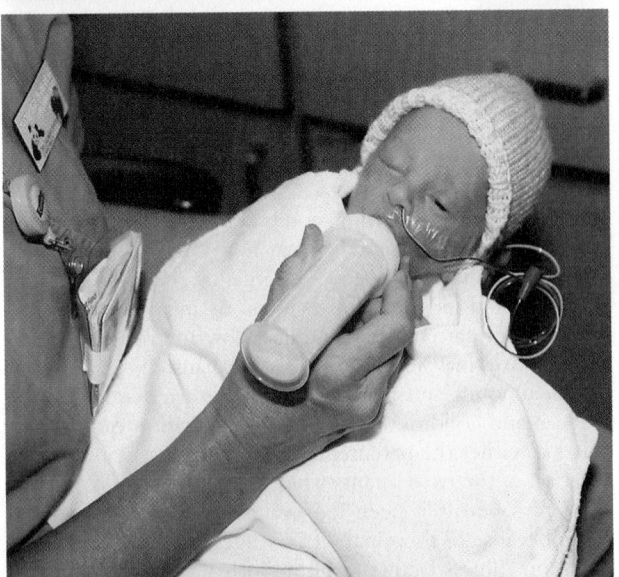

B

FIG. 9-8 ■ Nipple feeding the preterm infant. **A,** Infant is first brought to a quiet alert state in preparation for feeding. **B,** After readiness is demonstrated, infant is nipple fed. (Courtesy Jeff Barnes, Education and Eastern Oklahoma Perinatal Center, St. Francis Hospital, Tulsa, Okla.)

fore feeding helps promote oral sensitivity. Inward and upward support to the infant's cheeks and a slightly upward lift to the chin are provided by the fingers to assist nipple compression during feeding.

Bottle-feedings are continued if infants are able to tolerate the feedings and take the required amount. Some premature infants respond more slowly than full-term infants; therefore, the feeding interval, as well as the amount of the feeding, is individualized. Preterm infants are often slow feeders and require patience, frequent rest periods, and burping (or bubbling).

Gavage Feeding. Gavage feeding is a safe means of meeting the nutritional requirements of infants who are younger than 32 weeks of gestation or weigh less than 1500 g. These infants are usually too weak to suck effectively, are unable to coordinate swallowing, and lack a gag reflex. Gavage feedings may be provided by continuous drip regulated via infusion pump or by intermittent bolus feedings. Studies have demonstrated an overall decrease in total milk fat concentration delivery when continuous gavage infusions are administered, which suggests that intermittent or bolus gavage of expressed mother's milk be administered when possible (Premji and others, 2002). Intermittent gavage feeding is used as an energy-conserving technique for infants learning to nipple feed who become excessively tired, listless, or cyanotic.

A size 5, 6, or 8 French feeding tube is used to instill the formula, and the usual methods for determining correct placement are used (see Chapter 22 for technique). Although the more relaxed lower esophageal sphincter makes passage of the tube easier, there may be changes in heart rate and blood pressure in response to vagal stimulation. The procedure is best accomplished when an infant is in a prone or a right side-lying position with the head slightly elevated. It is preferable to insert the tube through the mouth rather than the nares. Nasal insertion obstructs nose breathing and may irritate the delicate nasal mucosa. Passage through the mouth also provides an opportunity to observe the sucking response. However, because of less stimulation of the gag reflex, nasal tube gavage may be used in certain situations, such as when continuous or frequent feedings (every 2 hours) are required or in older preterm infants who need supplementation after nipple feeding but who fight, gag, and vomit with oral tube management.

The stomach is aspirated, the contents measured, and the aspirate returned as part of the feeding. However, this practice may vary depending on circumstances and individual unit protocol. The amount of aspirate depends on the length of time since the previous feeding or concurrent illness. Whether or not the amount of the aspirate is deducted from the total feeding varies among units. Some advocate deducting the amount aspirated to avoid overdistending the stomach.

The milk or formula is allowed to flow by gravity, and the length of time varies. This procedure is not used as a timesaving method for the nurse. Complications of indwelling tubes include obstructed nares, mucous plugs, purulent rhinitis, epistaxis, infection, and possible stomach perforation.

> **! NURSING ALERT**
>
> Contamination of powdered infant formula in hospitals by *Enterobacter sakazakii* has been associated with serious neonatal infections, necrotizing enterocolitis, and mortality (MMWR, 2002; Van Acker and others, 2001). When possible, alternatives to powdered formula should be chosen; otherwise, such formula should be carefully mixed in a designated preparation room using aseptic technique, and continuous infusion of powdered formula should not exceed 4 hours (MMWR, 2002).

The nurse must observe preterm infants closely for behaviors that indicate readiness for oral feedings. These include (1) a strong, vigorous suck; (2) coordination of sucking and swallowing; (3) a gag reflex; (4) sucking on the gavage tube, hands, or a pacifier; and (5) rooting and wakefulness before and sleeping after feedings. When these behaviors are noted, infants can be challenged with nipple feedings that are introduced slowly.

The infant may be held during gavage feedings by the caregiver or parent. Oxygen may be supplied via nasal cannula to facilitate handling. It is not recommended that the infant be removed from a primary source of oxygen (e.g., a hood or tent) for feedings, because doing so decreases oxygen availability. Flow-by oxygen may be given for brief episodes of desaturation, but this is inadequate for the duration of feedings, either by gavage or nipple. Nonnutritive sucking on a pacifier may help bring the infant to a quiet alert state in preparation for feeding. When compared with other LBW infants, those who are allowed nonnutritive sucking are ready for oral feeding earlier, require fewer tube feedings, demonstrate better weight gain, are discharged earlier, and have fewer complications. Nonnutritive sucking also increases oxygenation during tube feeding.

> **! NURSING ALERT**
>
> An increase in gastric residuals, abdominal distention, bilious vomiting, temperature instability, apneic episodes, and bradycardia may be indicative of early necrotizing enterocolitis (NEC) and should be reported to the practitioner.

Feeding Resistance

Any feeding technique that bypasses the mouth precludes the opportunity for the child to practice sucking and swallowing, or the opportunity to experience normal hunger and satiation cycles. Infants may demonstrate aversion to oral feedings by such behaviors as averting the head to the presentation of the nipple, extruding the nipple by tongue thrust, gagging, or even vomiting.

Developmental delays have been noted in the areas of perceptual-motor performance as measured by standard tests, although the area of intellectual function measured remains within normal limits. Other observations include disinterest in or active resistance to oral play, diminished spontaneity and motivation, and shallow interpersonal relationships, probably related to the absence of some early incorporative patterns of normal oral experiences. The longer the period of nonoral feeding, the more severe the feeding problems, especially if this period occurs during a time when the infant progresses from reflexive to learned and voluntary feeding actions. Infancy is the period during which the mouth is the primary instrument for reception of stimulation and pleasure.

Infants identified as being at risk for feeding resistance should be provided with regular oral stimulation such as stroking the oral area from cheeks to lips, touching the tongue, placing some of the feeding on the lips and tongue, and associating feeding with pleasurable activities (holding, talking, making eye contact) based on the child's developmental level. Those who exhibit feeding aversion should begin a stimulation program to overcome resistance and acquire the ability to take nourishment by the oral route. Because management requires long-term commitment, successful implementation of a plan for oral stimulation depends on maximum parental involvement and promotion of primary nursing (see Family Focus box).

Energy Conservation

One of the major goals of care for the high-risk infant is conservation of energy. Much of the care described in this section is toward this end (e.g., disturbing the infant as little as possible, maintaining a neutral thermal environment, gavage feeding as appropriate, promoting oxygenation, judiciously implementing any caregiving activities that increase oxygen and caloric consumption). The infant who is not required to expend energy to cope with efforts to breathe, eat, or alter body temperature can use this energy for growth and development. Diminishing environmental noise levels and shading the infant from bright lights also promote rest (see Developmental Care, p. 240).

Early in hospitalization, the prone position is best for most preterm infants and results in improved oxygenation, better-tolerated feedings, and more organized sleep-rest patterns. Infants exhibit less physical activity and energy expenditure when placed in the prone position. However, others appear to prefer a flexed side-lying posture. Prolonged supine positioning for preterm infants is not desirable, because they appear to lose their sense of equilibrium when supine and use vital energy in attempts to recover balance by postural changes. In addition, prolonged supine positioning is associated with long-term problems such as decreased flexion of the limbs, pelvis, and trunk; widely abducted hips (frog-leg position); retracted and abducted shoulders; ankle and foot eversion; increased neck extension; and increased trunk extension with neck and back arching (Holditch-Davis, Blackburn, and VandenBerg, 2003). The American Academy of Pediatrics (1996c) continues to affirm its position that *healthy* infants be placed to sleep in a nonprone position. When medically stable, preterm infants should be placed in a nonprone position to sleep unless conditions such as gastroesophageal reflux or upper airway anomalies make this impractical (see also Sudden Infant Death Syndrome, Chapter 11). Prone positioning for play should be provided in the nursery and encouraged following discharge.

Skin Care

The skin of premature infants is characteristically immature relative to that of full-term infants. In most preterm infants the skin barrier properties resemble those of the term infant by 2 to 4 weeks' postnatal age, regardless of gestational age at birth. Because of its increased sensitivity and fragility, no alkaline-based soap that might destroy the "acid mantle" of the skin is used. The increased permeability of the skin facilitates absorption of ingredients. All skin products (e.g., alcohol or povidone-iodine) should be used with caution; the skin is rinsed with water afterward because these substances may cause severe irritation and chemical burns in VLBW and ELBW infants.

The skin is easily excoriated and denuded; therefore, care must be taken to avoid damage to the delicate structure. The total skin is thinner than that of full-term infants and lacks "rete pegs," appendages that anchor the epidermis to the dermis. Therefore there is less cohesion between the thinner skin layers. Adhesives used after heel sticks or to secure monitoring equipment or IV infusions may excoriate the skin or adhere to the skin surface so well that the epidermis can be separated from the dermis and pulled away with the tape. The use of pectin barriers and hydrocolloid adhesives may be useful as these products mold well to skin contours and adhere in moist conditions. Recommendations for protecting the integrity of premature skin include using minimal adhesive tape, backing the tape with cotton, and delaying adhesive and pectin barrier removal until adherence is reduced (Lund and Kuller, 2003). An emollient such as Eucerin or Aquaphor may also be used to promote skin integrity and prevent dry, cracking, and peeling skin in infants at risk for skin breakdown (Horii and Lane, 2001; Polak, Ringler, and Daugherty, 2004). It is unsafe to use scissors to remove dressings or tape from the extremities of very small and immature infants, because it is easy to snip off tiny extremities or nick loosely attached skin. Solvents used to remove tape are avoided because they tend to dry and burn the delicate skin. Guidelines for skin care are listed in the Guidelines box.

During skin assessment of preterm infants, nurses are alert to the subtle signs that indicate zinc deficiency, a problem sometimes seen in infants who have inadequate intake or abnormal losses of zinc. Breakdown usually occurs in the areas around the mouth, buttocks, fingers, and toes. In preterm and VLBW infants it may also occur in the creases of the neck, wrists, and ankles, and around wounds. Zinc deficiency is most likely to appear in preterm infants with inadequate zinc intake, an ileostomy, short bowel syndrome, or chronic diarrhea. Suspicious lesions are reported to the practitioner so that zinc supplements can be prescribed.

Skin injuries have been reported during the use of phototherapy blankets. Caution is warranted in using these products in ELBW infants or infants who are at risk for skin breakdown.

FAMILY FOCUS

Feeding Resistance

Our son was in the NICU for several months. Now at 6 years of age he is normal in every way except one—he refuses almost all food. He lives on a diet of mashed bananas, mashed potatoes, fruit juice, milk, and a daily multivitamin/mineral pill. Getting him to eat has been a 6-year battle that we have lost. Now I know that simple oral stimulation techniques could have prevented or lessened this problem. Please tell nurses the importance of these interventions when any infant is NPO for a prolonged time.

A mother and a nurse

Neonatal Skin Care

GENERAL SKIN CARE

Assessment

Assess skin every day or once a shift for redness, dryness, flaking, scaling, rashes, lesions, excoriation, or breakdown.

Evaluate and report abnormal skin findings and analyze for possible causes.

Intervene according to interpretation of findings or physician order.

BATHING

Initial bath

Assess for stable temperature a minimum of 2 to 4 hours before first bath.

Use cleansing agents with neutral pH or minimal dyes or perfume, in water

Do not completely remove vernix.

Bathe preterm infant <32 weeks in sterile water only.

Routine

Decrease frequency of baths to every second or third day by daily cleansing of eye, oral, and diaper areas and pressure points.

Use cleanser or soaps no more than 2-3 times a week.

Avoid rubbing skin during bathing or drying.

Immerse stable infants fully (except head) in an appropriate-size tub.

Use swaddled immersion bathing technique: slow unwrapping after gently lowering into water for sensitive, but stable, infants needing assistance with motor system reactivity.

Emollients

Follow hospital protocol or consider the following:

Apply petroleum-based ointment without preservative sparingly to body (avoid face, head) every 6 to 12 hours during the first 2 to 4 weeks for infants <32 weeks (except when neonate is in radiant heat source).

Apply emollient as needed to infants >32 weeks for dry, flaking skin.

Adhesives

Decrease use as much as possible.

Use transparent adhesive dressings to secure IVs, catheters, and central lines.

Use hydrogel or limb electrodes.

Consider pectin barriers (Hollihesive,* Duoderm†) beneath adhesives to protect skin.

Secure pulse oximeter probe or electrodes with elasticized dressing material (carefully avoid restricting blood flow).

Do not use adhesive remover, solvents, or bonding agents.

Avoid removing adhesives for at least 24 hours after application.

Adhesive removal can be facilitated using water, mineral oil, or petrolatum.

Remove adhesives or skin barriers slowly, supporting the skin underneath with one hand and gently peeling away the product from the skin with the other hand.‡

Antiseptic Agents

Apply before invasive procedures.

Apply povidone-iodine two times, air dry for 30 seconds; remove completely with sterile water or sterile saline solution following procedure.

Avoid use of alcohol.

Transepidermal Water Loss (TEWL)

Minimize TEWL and heat loss in small premature infants <30 weeks by:

Measuring ambient humidity during first weeks of life.

Considering an increase in humidity to >70% by using one or more of the following options or hospital guidelines:

Transparent dressings

Emollient application every 6 to 8 hours or according to hospital protocol

Servo-controlled humidifying incubator

SKIN BREAKDOWN

Prevention

Decrease pressure from externally applied forces using water, air, or gel mattresses, sheepskin, or cotton bedding.

Provide adequate nutrition, including protein, fat, and zinc.

Apply transparent adhesive dressings to protect arms, elbows, and knees from friction injury.

Use tracheostomy and gastrostomy dressings for drainage and relief of pressure from trach or G tube (Hydrasorb or Lyofoam).†

Use emollient in the diaper area (groin and thighs) to reduce urine irritation.

Treating Skin Breakdown

Irrigate wound every 4 to 8 hours with warm half-strength normal saline (NS) using a 30-mL or larger syringe and 20-gauge Teflon catheter.

Culture wound and treat if signs of infection are present (excessive redness, swelling, pain on touch, heat, or resistance to healing).

Use transparent adhesive dressing for uninfected wounds.

Apply hydrogel with or without antibacterial or antifungal ointments (as ordered) for infected wounds (may need to moisten before removal).

Use hydrocolloid for deep, uninfected wounds (leave in place for 5 to 7 days) or as an ostomy barrier and to improve appliance adhesion; warm barrier in hand for several minutes to soften before applying to skin.

Avoid use of antiseptic solutions for wound cleansing (used for intact skin only).

Treating Diaper Dermatitis

Maintain clean, dry skin; use absorbent diapers and change often.

If mild irritation occurs, use petrolatum barrier.

For developing dermatitis, apply a generous quantity of zinc-oxide barrier.

For severe dermatitis, identify cause and treat (frequent stooling from spina bifida, severe opiate withdrawal, or malabsorption syndrome).

Modified from Kuller JM: Skin breakdown: risk factors, prevention, and treatment, *NINR* 1(1):33-42, 2001; Johnson FE, Maikler VE: Nurses' adoption of the AWHONN/NANN Neonatal Skin Care Project, *NINR* 1(1):59-67, 2001; Lund CH, Kuller J, Lott JW: Neonatal skin care: clinical outcomes of the AWHONN/NANN evidence-based clinical practice guideline, *J Obstet Gynecol Neonat Nurs* 30(1):41-51, 2001; Taquino LT: Promoting wound healing in the neonatal setting: process versus protocol, *J Perinat Neonat Nurs* 14(1):108-118, 2000; Lund C, Lane A, Raines DA: Neonatal skin care: the scientific basis for practice, *J Obstet Gynecol Neonat Nurs* 28(3):241-254, 1999; Malloy MB, Perez-Woods R: Neonatal skin care: prevention of skin breakdown, *Pediatr Nurs* 17(1):41-48, 1991.

*Hollister, Libertyville, Il.

†ConvaTec/Bristol-Myers Squibb Co, Princeton, NJ.

‡**Caution:** Scissors are not to be used for tape or dressing removal because of hazard of cutting skin or amputating tiny digits.

Continued

GUIDELINES

Treating Diaper Dermatitis—*cont'd*

Treat *Candida albicans* with antifungal ointment or cream.
Avoid powders and antibiotic ointments (not recommended). (See Cord and Circumcision Care, Chapter 8.)

OTHER SKIN CARE CONCERNS
Use of Substances on Skin
Evaluate all substances that come in contact with infant's skin.
Before using any topical agent, analyze components of preparation and:
   Use sparingly and only when necessary.
   Confine use to smallest possible area.
   Whenever possible and appropriate, wash off with water.
   Monitor infant carefully for signs of toxicity and systemic effects.

Use of Thermal Devices
Avoid heat lamps because of increased potential for burns. If needed, measure actual temperature of exposed skin every 15 minutes.
When using heating pads (Aqua-K pads):
   Change infant's position every 15 minutes initially and then every 1 to 2 hours.
   Preset temperature of heating pads <40° C (104° F)

When using preheated transcutaneous electrodes:
   Avoid use on infants
   Set at lowest possible temperature
   Use pulse oximetry rather than transcutaneous monitoring whenever possible.
When prewarming heels before phlebotomy, avoid temperatures >40° C
Provide warm ambient humidity, direct away from infant; use aerosolized sterile water and maintain ambient temperature so as not to exceed 40° C.
Document use of all heating devices.

Use of Fluid Therapy/Hemodynamic Monitoring
Be certain fingers or toes are visible whenever extremity is used for IV or arterial line.
Secure catheter or needle with transparent dressing/tape to promote easy visualization of site.
Assess site hourly for signs of ischemia, infiltration, and inadequate perfusion (check capillary refill).
Avoid use of restraints (e.g., arm boards); if used, check that they are secured safely and not restricting circulation or movement (check for pressure areas).
Use commercial IV protector (i.e., I.V. House) with minimal tape.

Administration of Medications

Administration of therapeutic agents such as drugs, ointments, IV infusions, and oxygen requires judicious handling and meticulous attention to detail. The computation, preparation, and administration of drugs in minute amounts often require collaboration between nurses, physicians, and pharmacists to reduce the chance for error. In addition, the immaturity of an infant's detoxification mechanisms and inability to demonstrate symptoms of toxicity (e.g., signs of auditory nerve involvement from ototoxic drugs such as gentamicin) complicate drug therapy and require that nurses be particularly alert for signs of adverse reaction. (See Administration of Medication, Chapter 22.)

Nurses should be aware of the hazards of administering bacteriostatic and hyperosmolar solutions to infants. Benzyl alcohol, a common preservative in bacteriostatic water and saline, has been shown to be toxic to newborns and should not be used to flush IV catheters, to dilute or reconstitute medications, or as an anesthetic to start IVs. It is recommended that medications with preservative such as benzyl alcohol be avoided whenever possible. *Nurses must read labels carefully to detect the presence of preservatives in any medication to be administered to an infant.*

Hyperosmolar solutions present a potential danger to preterm infants. Hyperosmolar solutions given orally to infants can produce clinical, physiologic, and morphologic alterations, the most serious of which is necrotizing enterocolitis. Oral and parenteral medications should be sufficiently diluted to prevent complications related to hyperosmolality.

Developmental Care

Much attention has been focused on the effects of early developmental intervention on both normal and preterm infants. Infants respond to a great variety of stimuli, and the atmosphere and activities of the NICU are overstimulating. Consequently, infants in the NICU are subjected to *inappropriate* stimulation that can be harmful. For example, the noise level that results from monitoring equipment, alarms, and general unit activity has been correlated with the incidence of intracranial hemorrhage, especially in the ELBW or VLBW infant. Personnel should reduce noise-generating activities, such as closing doors (including incubator portholes), listening to loud radios, talking loudly, and handling equipment (e.g., trash containers). Gray and Philbin (2000) suggest monitoring sound levels in the nursery in order to address problem areas. Nursing care activities, such as taking vital signs, changing the infant's position, weighing, and changing diapers, are associated with frequent periods of hypoxia, oxygen desaturation, and elevated intracranial pressure. The more immature the infant, the less able the neonate is to habituate to a single procedure, such as taking an oscillometric BP, without becoming overstimulated.

Twenty-four-hour surveillance of sick infants implies maximum visibility and often bright lights. Units should establish a night-day sleep pattern by either darkening the room, covering cribs with blankets, or placing eye patches over the infant's eyes at night. Infants need scheduled rest periods during which the lights are dimmed, the incubators are covered with blankets, and the infants are not disturbed for handling of any kind (Holditch-Davis, Blackburn, and VandenBerg, 2003). Sleep periods should be undisturbed for at least 50 minutes to allow complete sleep cycles.

Infants' eyes should shielded from bright procedure lights to prevent potential harm. Glass (1994) questions the need for prolonged, intense patterned visual stimulation, suggesting that just because the infant is able to respond to the stimulus does not necessarily mean the level of stimulation is beneficial. Many experts suggest that the human face, especially the parent's, is the best visual stimulus and that visual stimuli be kept to a minimum early in development. Developmental care, accentuating the infant's unique ability to achieve behavioral state organization, is tailored to the developmental level and tolerance of each infant based on a comprehensive behavioral assessment. During the early stages of development (especially before 33 weeks of gestation), external stimulation produces uncoordinated, random activity, such as jerky limb extension, hyperflexion, and irregular vital signs. At this stage infants need to have *minimum* environmental stimulation. Using the developmental model of supportive care, the nurse closely monitors physiologic and behavioral signs to promote organization and well-being of the high-risk infant during handling. As much as possible, attempts are made to avoid disrupting infant sleep cycles for care or nurturing. Softly calling the infant by name and then gently placing a hand on the body signals care is beginning and alleviates the abrupt interruption that precedes caregiving. They are handled with slow, controlled movements (some infants are unstable if moved abruptly), and their random movements are controlled with limbs held flexed close to their bodies during turning or other position changes. This containment or facilitated tucking may also be used before invasive procedures such as heel stick to alleviate distress. Blanket swaddling and nesting or containment has been shown to decrease physiologic and behavioral stress during routine care procedures such as bathing, weighing, and heel stick. A nest constructed by placing blanket rolls underneath the bedsheet helps infants in maintaining an attitude of flexion when prone or side lying.

Although it must be individually adjusted, ***skin-to-skin (STS)*** contact (***kangaroo care***) and short periods of gentle massage can help to reduce stress in preterm infants. Regular passive skin-to-skin contact between parents (mother or father) and LBW infants has been shown to alleviate stress. The parent wears a loose-fitting, open-front top that provides a modified marsupial-like pocket carrier for the infant. The undressed (except for diaper) infant is placed in a vertical position on the parent's bare chest, which permits direct eye contact, skin-to-skin sensations, and close proximity (Fig. 9-9). Skin-to-skin contact between parent and infant, in addition to being a safe and effective method for VLBW infant-parent acquaintance, can have a positive healing effect for the mother with a high-risk pregnancy. Mothers may experience psychologic healing related to preterm delivery and regain the mothering role through early skin-to-skin contact with their VLBW infants. Additional benefits of skin-to-skin care include earlier contact with mechanically ventilated infants, maintenance of neonatal thermal stability and oxygen saturation, increased feeding vigor, maintenance of organized state, and minimal untoward effects of being held (Conde-Agudelo, Diaz-Rossello, and Belizan, 2000; Anderson, 1999; Moran and others, 1999). In full-term newborns, skin-to-skin contact has a strong analgesic effect during procedures such as heel lance (Gray, Watt, and Blass, 2000). LBW infants receiving skin-to-skin contact with breast-feeding mothers maintained a higher oxygen saturation and were less likely to have desaturations below 90%, and their mothers were more likely to continue breast-feeding both in the hospital and for 1 month after discharge. Kangaroo care of preterm infants fosters appropriate neu-

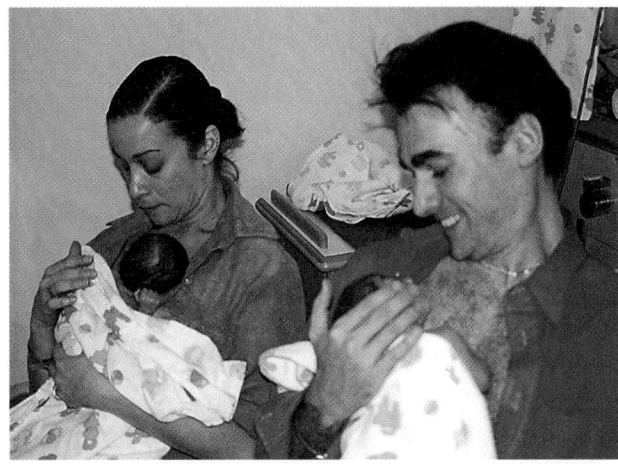

FIG. 9-9 ■ Kangaroo care. Each parent has the opportunity to place one twin against the body. Note: The blanket has been lowered for photographic purposes. (Courtesy Kathy Connor, RN, Hillcrest Medical Center, Tulsa, Okla.)

robehavioral development by promoting stability of heart and respiratory function, minimizes purposeless movements, offers maternal proximity for attention, improves the infant's behavioral state, and permits self-regulating behaviors (Ludington-Hoe and Swinth, 1996).

Co-bedding of twins (or *multiples*) is another developmental intervention that has recently been implemented in several institutions in the United States to provide a better environment for neonatal growth and development (Altimier and Lutes, 2001; DellaPorta, Aforismo, and Butler-O'Hara, 1998). Co-bedding involves placing twins or other multiples together in the same crib or incubator. Preliminary data from a multicenter study indicate that twins who are co-bedded have improved thermoregulation, have significantly fewer apnea and bradycardia episodes, gain weight more quickly than their single counterparts, and have decreased length of stay. Parental satisfaction is also significantly greater with co-bedded newborns (Lutes, 1998). One major concern with co-bedding is cross-transmission of infection between the neonates, but increased infection rates have not occurred with co-bedding (Altimier and Lutes, 2001). Some manufacturers are developing incubators to accommodate the size and needs of two infants.

Additional research studies have confirmed the beneficial effects of developmental care with preterm infants. In addition to requiring fewer days of mechanical ventilation, preterm infants who received individualized developmental care had shorter hospital stays; a significant decrease in complications such as intraventricular hemorrhage and bronchopulmonary dysplasia; less need for sedation when critically ill; improved neurodevelopmental scores at 9, 18, and 36 months of life; and a decrease in feeding intolerance (Symington and Pinelli, 2003; Buehler and others, 1995; Als and others, 1994).

The arena of developmental care for preterm infants has expanded to include a wide variety of interventions such as infant massage, soothing soft music, recordings of parents reading stories, positioning to enhance self-regulatory abilities, enhancement of hand-to-mouth activities, uninterrupted sleep periods, decreased environmental light and

BOX 9-2 ■ Signs of Stress or Fatigue in Neonates

SUBSYSTEM	SIGNS OF STRESS
AUTONOMIC	**PHYSIOLOGIC INSTABILITY**
Respiratory	Tachypnea, pauses, gasping, sighing
Color	Mottled, flushed, dusky, pale or gray
Visceral	Hiccups, gagging, choking, spitting up, grunting and straining as if having a bowel movement; coughing, sneezing, yawning
Autonomic	Tremors, startles, twitches
MOTOR	**FLUCTUATING TONE, LACK OF CONTROL OVER MOVEMENT, ACTIVITY, AND POSTURE**
Flaccidity	Low tone in trunk; limp, floppy upper and lower extremities; limp, drooping jaw (gape face)
Hypertonicity	Arm or leg extensions, arm(s) outstretched with fingers splayed in salute gesture, fingers stiffly outstretched, trunk arching, neck hyperextended
Hyperflexion	Trunk, extremities, fisting
Activity	Squirming; frantic diffuse activity or little or no activity or responsiveness
STATE	**DISORGANIZED QUALITY TO STATE BEHAVIORS, INCLUDING AVALABLE STATES, MAINTENANCE OF STATE CONTROL, AND TRANSITION FROM ONE STATE TO ANOTHER**
Sleep	Whimpering sounds, facial twitching, irregular respirations, fussing, grimacing, restless appearance
Awake	Glazed, unfocused look, staring, worried or pained expression, hyperalert or panicked appearance, eye roving, crying, cry-face, actively averting gaze or closing eyes, irritability, prolonged awake periods, inconsolability, frenzy
	Abrupt or rapid state changes
OTHER STATE-RELATED BEHAVIORS AND ATTENTION-INTERACTION	**EFFORTS TO ATTEND TO AND INTERACT WITH ENVIRONMENTAL STIMULATION ELICITS SIGNS OF STRESS AND DISORGANIZED SUBSYSTEM FUNCTIONING**
Autonomic	Physiologic instability of varying degrees with autonomic, respiratory, color, and visceral responses
Motor	Fluctuating tone, increased motor activity, progressively frantic diffuse activity if stimulation continues
State	Roving eyes, gaze averting, glazed-unfocused look or worried, panicked expression, weak cry, cry-face, irritability
	Closed eyes and sleeplike withdrawal
	Abrupt state changes
	Signs of stress when presented with more than one type of stimulus at a time

Modified from Als H: Toward a synactive theory of development: promise for the assessment and support of infant individuality, *Infant Mental Health J* 3(4):229-243, 1982; Als H: A synactive model of neonatal behavior organization: framework for the assessment of neurobehavioral development in the premature infant and for support of infants and parents in the neonatal intensive care environment, *Phys Occup Ther Pediatr* 6:3-55, 1986; Hunter JG: The neonatal intensive care unit. In Case-Smith J, Allen AS, Pratt PN, editors: *Occupational therapy for children,* ed 4, St Louis, 2001, Mosby.

noise, and even the use of stuffed animals to facilitate infant positioning. As a result of such interventions, parents may perceive the NICU environment as less threatening. Active participation in providing such an environment for their special infant also involves the parents in the provision of daily care when the newborn is critically ill and cannot be fed or held.*

When infants have reached sufficient developmental organization and stability (especially between 34 and 36 weeks of gestation), interventions are designed and implemented to support their growing abilities. Nurses and parents become adept at learning to read infants' behavioral cues and supplying appropriate interventions (Box 9-2). Clues include both approach and avoidance behaviors. Approach behaviors that are supported and enhanced include tongue extension, hand clasp, hand-to-mouth movements, sucking, looking, and coo-

ing. Signs of stress or fatigue that signal the infant's need for "time-out" are described in Box 9-2.

An intervention program for convalescing infants must be individualized and include parents and siblings early in the infant's hospitalization; teaching parents to be responsive to the infant's individual cues is an important function of the NICU nurse. When infants are recovering and are free of support systems, medically stable, and on room air or smaller amounts of oxygen, they are assessed to document behavioral state organization and ability to self-regulate. An effective program may be designed to provide limited sensory stimulation involving one or two senses or multisensory experiences that include tactile, visual, auditory, vestibular, olfactory, and gustatory stimuli as appropriate for each infant. Parents and siblings, as well as health care providers, are encouraged to adhere to the established developmental care plan to avoid disruption in sleep/wake cycles and minimize inappropriate stimuli.

When the condition of an infant is sufficiently advanced to begin developmental intervention, some activities are individualized according to each infant's cues, temperament,

*A resource for parents interested in developmental care products is Children's Medical Ventures, Inc., 275 Longwater Drive, Norwell, MA 02190; (800) 377-3449; (781) 871-6226; website: www.childmed.com/.

GUIDELINES

Developmental Interventions

GENERAL GUIDELINES

Individualize interventions for each infant.
Offer stimulus only during periods of alertness.
Begin one type of stimulus at a time.
Provide intervention for short periods.
Space periods according to infant's tolerance.
Continually assess infant's response to developmental interventions.
Titrate interventions according to infant's cues.
Terminate stimulation if infant displays evidence of overstimulation (see Box 9-2).
Provide 50-minute uninterrupted sleep periods.
Handle to promote/maintain behavioral organization providing for flexion, containment, firm pressure, grasp, and nonnutritive sucking.

TACTILE

Stroke skin slowly and gently in head-to-toe direction (assess tolerance first); begin with trunk and move to more sensitive areas, such as face.
Provide alternate textures (e.g., satin, velvet).
Provide firm boundaries, foot bracing, blankets, "nesting."
Encourage skin-to-skin (kangaroo) holding by parents and siblings as tolerated.
Containment holding in cupped palms of hand provides nesting and comfort.

AUDITORY

Reduce noise levels.
Mother's voice is the best.
Maintain 50 dB with maximum 55 dB for only 10 minutes per hour.
Play tape of parents' and siblings' voices.
Softly play simple, soothing music, recording of womb sounds, or music box for short periods only.*
Call infant by name at each interaction.

VESTIBULAR

Position with limbs and trunk in flexion, with hands to face at midline.
Slowly change position during handling; avoid quick position changes.
Side-to-side slow movement is preferred over rocking.
Place in sling (hammock) and rock.
Close infant's fist around cloth toy.
Lift head to upright position, tip to right and then to left, stopping at midline (only with stable, more mature infants).
Avoid rapid horizontal to vertical movements in ill infant to minimize intracranial pressure and autonomic consequences—desaturations, apnea, bradycardia.

OLFACTORY

Pass open container or a cotton gauze dipped in breast milk or formula under nose.
Cloth doll that has been in close contact with mother' skin—avoid perfumes, scented soaps, powders.
Use a pacifier dipped in mother's breast milk during gavage feeding for nonnutritive sucking.

GUSTATORY

Place infant's hand or a pacifier in mouth when sucking movements are observed or during gavage feeding.
Place 1 or 2 drops of milk in infant's mouth with each tube feeding.
Provide nonnutritive suckling at mother's breast.

VISUAL

Reduce light levels and protect eyes from direct lights such as examination or procedure lights.
Place photographs of parents and siblings in visual range (19 to 22 cm) in *en face* position (maintain for short periods when awake and alert; constant picture in close proximity may be too much stimulus).
Initiate eye contact, repeat as tolerated once the infant reaches 30 weeks' gestation. Monitor carefully for stress responses.

*Suggested infant relaxation music: "Heartbeat Lullabies" by Terry Woodford. Available from Baby-Go-To-Sleep Center, Audio Therapy Innovations, Inc., PO Box 550, Colorado Springs, Colo 80901; (800) 537-7748; website: www.babygotosleep.com.

---

state, behavioral organization, and particular needs. Intervention periods are short (e.g., 2 to 3 minutes of voices, 5 minutes of quiet music). Interventions are initiated according to the maturational development of the infant. Hearing and vestibular interventions are initiated earlier than visual stimulation. One type of intervention at a time is applied to document the infant's tolerance and response (see Guidelines box). The types and duration of any stimuli are adjusted on an individual basis, and the parents are involved as early as possible in learning about their infant's particular developmental needs.

Developmental care of the preterm neonate is an ongoing process in the NICU and is incorporated into the daily care given to each infant. The nurse is cognizant of the preterm infant's developmental needs, temperament, and newborn state, as well as environmental conditions that adversely affect the infant; nursing care is planned accordingly to enhance optimum physical, psychosocial, and neurologic development. This task is often difficult to accomplish when

invasive treatments or interventions are required to stabilize the critically ill neonate.

Neonatal Pain

Until fairly recently it was believed that the nerve pathways of newborn infants were not sufficiently myelinated to transmit painful stimuli, that the infant did not possess sufficiently integrated cortical function to interpret or recall pain experiences, and that the risk of anesthesia was too great to justify any possible benefit of pain relief (Hadjistavropoulos and others, 1997; McLaughlin and others, 1993; Shapiro, 1989; Anand and Hickey, 1987). Nurses have been found to hold similar beliefs and to give significantly higher pain intensity ratings to full-term as opposed to preterm neonates (Shapiro, 1993; Franck, 1987). Consequently, invasive procedures (including some types of surgery) have been performed on infants without an anesthetic (Johnston and others, 1997).

This traditional view has been refuted by a number of research studies that indicate that both preterm and full-term infants perceive and react to pain in much the same manner as children and adults. Evidence indicates that pain pathways, cortical and subcortical centers needed for pain perception, and neurochemical systems associated with pain transmission and modulation are intact and functional in the neonate. Pain perception has both physiologic and psychologic components, and it is accepted that newborns recognize and respond to painful stimuli. However, pain is a sensation with strong emotional associations, and the relationship of the consciousness of the newborn to the perception of pain has not been agreed on by researchers. Therefore the term *nociception* (the perception by the *nerves* of injurious influences or painful stimuli) is often used to discuss pain in the neonate (Anand and Hickey, 1987).

Physiologic responses in neonates to painful stimuli have been well documented by numerous studies. The summary of these observations indicates that painful stimuli cause a global stress response in infants undergoing surgery with minimal or no analgesia. This response is evidenced by cardiorespiratory changes (marked increases in heart rate and blood pressure, and decreased $tcPO_2$ or oxygen saturation), palmar sweating, increased intracranial pressure, and hormonal (release of catecholamines, growth hormone, glucagon, cortisol, other corticosteroids, and aldosterone and by hyperglycemia) and metabolic changes (increased plasma lactate, pyruvate, ketone bodies, and some fatty acids) (Evans, 2001). With adequate analgesia and anesthesia, infants experience less of a stress response and less postoperative mortality and morbidity (Anand, 1998). Pain control during procedures can shorten periods of oxygen desaturation (Pokela, 1994). The use of *preemptive analgesia* (prevention of pain) in premature infants may also decrease the incidence of intraventricular hemorrhage and periventricular leukomalacia (Anand and others, 1999).

All infants, regardless of gestational age, should receive appropriate analgesia or anesthesia for potentially painful procedures (Anand and International Evidence-Based Group for Neonatal Pain, 2001; American Academy of Pediatrics, 2000). Local or systemic pharmacologic agents are available to permit anesthesia or analgesia to neonates and are indicated for those undergoing surgical procedures (American Academy of Pediatrics, 2000).

Other effects of pain may include increased wakefulness and irritability, as well as alterations in feeding, vomiting, loss of appetite, and loss of interest in or energy for sucking. Interruptions in sleep-wake patterns, behavioral states, and parent-infant interactions also occur and may interfere with recovery from surgery.

Assessment of pain in the preverbal child is difficult, especially in the neonate, because the most reliable indicator of pain, self-report, is not possible. Evaluation must be based on physiologic changes and behavioral observations (Box 9-3). Although behaviors such as vocalizations, facial expressions, body movements, and general state are common to all infants, they vary with different situations. Crying associated with pain is more intense and sustained. Facial expression is the most consistent and specific characteristic; scales are available to systematically evaluate facial features, such as eye squeeze, brow bulge, and open mouth and taut tongue (see Fig. 21-3) (Gibbins and Stevens, 2001; Hadjistavropoulos and others, 1997). Most infants respond with

BOX 9-3 ■ Manifestations of Acute Pain in the Neonate

PHYSIOLOGIC RESPONSES
Vital signs: observe for variations
  Increased heart rate
  Increased blood pressure
  Rapid, shallow respirations
Oxygenation
  Decreased arterial oxygen saturation (SaO_2)
Skin: observe color and character
  Pallor or flushing
  Diaphoresis
  Palmar sweating
Other observations
  Increased muscle tone
  Dilated pupils
  Decreased vagal nerve tone
  Increased intracranial pressure
  Laboratory evidence of metabolic or endocrine changes
    Hyperglycemia
    Decreased pH
    Elevated corticosteroids

BEHAVIORAL RESPONSES
Vocalizations: observe quality, timing, and duration
  Crying
  Whimpering
  Groaning
Facial expression: observe characteristics, timing, orientation of eyes and mouth (see Fig. 21-3)
  Grimaces
  Brow furrowed
  Chin quivering
  Eyes tightly closed
  Mouth open and squarish
Body movements and posture: observe type, quality, and amount of movement or lack of movement; relationship to other factors
  Limb withdrawal
  Thrashing
  Rigidity
  Flaccidity
  Fist clenching
Changes in state: observe sleep, appetite, activity level
  Changes in sleep/wake cycles
  Changes in feeding behavior
  Changes in activity level
  Fussiness, irritability
  Listlessness

increased body movements, but the infant may be experiencing pain even when lying quietly with eyes closed (Shapiro, 1989). The preterm infant's response to pain may be behaviorally blunted or absent. An infant who receives a muscle-paralyzing agent such as vecuronium will also be incapable of mounting a behavioral or visible pain response.

Several pain assessment tools have been developed for the assessment of pain in the neonate (Table 9-2). One pain assessment tool used by nurses in the neonatal intensive care setting is called **CRIES** (Table 9-3). This tool has been developed for use by nurses who work with premature and full-term infants. CRIES is an acronym for the physiologic and

TABLE 9-2 ■ Summary of Pain Assessment Scales for Infants

AGES OF USE	AUTHORS	RELIABILITY AND VALIDITY	SCORING VARIABLES	RANGE
POSTOPERATIVE PAIN SCORE (POPS)				
1-7 months	Attia J and others: Measurement of postoperative pain and narcotic administration in infants using a new clinical scoring system, *Anesthesiology* 67(3A):A532, 1987.	Not tested by original authors. Later tested by Joyce BA and others (1994); high interrater agreement (reliability); discriminant validity ($P < 0.0001$); reliability with high Cronbach alpha ranging from 0.79-0.88	Sleep (0-2) Flexion fingers/toes (0-2) Facial expression (0-2) Sucking (0-2) Quality of cry (0-2) Tone (0-2) Spontaneous motor activity (0-2) Consolability (0-2) Spontaneous excitability (0-2) Sociability (0-2)	0 = worst pain 20 = no pain
NEONATAL INFANT PAIN SCALE (NIPS)				
Average gestational age 33.5 weeks	Lawrence J and others: The development of a tool to assess neonatal pain, *Neonat Netw* 12(6):59-66, 1993.	Interrater reliability = 0.92 and 0.97. Construct validity using analysis of variance between before, during, and after procedure scores: $F = 18.97$, $df = 2.42$, $P < 0.001$. Concurrent validity between NIPS and VAS using Pearson correlations = 0.53-0.84. Internal consistency using Cronbach alpha = 0.95, 0.87, and 0.88 for before, during, and after procedure scores	Facial expression (0-1) Arms (0-1) Cry (0-2) Legs (0-1) Breathing patterns (0-1) State of arousal (0-1)	0 = no pain 7 = worst pain
PAIN ASSESSMENT TOOL (PAT)				
27 weeks' gestational age—full term	Hodgkinson K and others: Measuring pain in neonates: evaluating an instrument and developing a common language, *Aust J Adv Nurs* 12(1): 17-22, 1994.	No reliability or validity discussed by original authors	Posture/tone (1-2) Respirations (1-2) Sleep pattern (0-2) Heart rate (1-2) Expression (1-2) Saturations (0-2) Color (0-2) Blood pressure (0-2) Cry (0-2) Nurse's perception (0-2)	4 = no pain 20 = worst pain
PAIN RATING SCALE (PRS)				
1-36 months	Joyce BA and others: Reliability and validity of preverbal pain assessment tools, *Issues Comp Pediatr Nurs* 17:121-135, 1994.	Interrater agreement: $r = .65$-0.84, $P < 0.0001$. Discriminant validity: statistically significant t-tests ($P < 0.0001$)	0—smiling, sleeping, no change when moved/touched 1—takes small amount orally, restless, moving, cries 2—not drinking/eating, short periods of cries, distracted with rocking or pacifier 3—change in behavior, irritable, arms/legs shake/jerk, facial grimace 4—flailing, high-pitched wailing, parents request pain medication, unable to distract 5—sleeping prolonged periods interrupted by jerking, continuous crying, rapid and shallow respirations	0 = no pain; 5 = worst pain

Continued

TABLE 9-2 ■ Summary of Pain Assessment Scales for Infants—*cont'd*

AGES OF USE	AUTHORS	RELIABILITY AND VALIDITY	SCORING VARIABLES	RANGE
CRIES				
32-60 weeks' gestational age	Krechel SW, Bildner J: CRIES: a new neonatal postoperative pain measurement score: initial testing of validity and reliability, *Pediatr Anaesth* 5:53-61, 1995.	Concurrent validity between CRIES and POPS = 0.73 ($P < 0.0001$, n = 1382); Spearman correlation between subjective report and POPS and CRIES = 0.49 ($P < 0.0001$, n > 1300) Discriminant validity using before and after analgesia scores: Wilcoxon Sign rank test = mean decline of 3.0 units ($P < 0.0001$, n = 74) Interrater reliability using Spearman correlation coefficient: $r = 0.72$ ($P < 0.0001$, n = 680)	Crying (0-2) Requires increased oxygen (0-2) Increased vital signs (0-2) Expression (0-2) Sleepless (0-2)	0 = no pain; 10 = worst pain
PREMATURE INFANT PAIN PROFILE (PIPP)				
28-40 weeks' gestational age	Stevens B and others: Premature Infant Pain Profile: development and initial validation, *Clin J Pain* 12:13-22, 1996. See also Ballantyne and others, 1999.	Internal consistency using Cronbach alpha = 0.75-0.59; standardized item alpha for 6 items = 0.71 Construct validity using handling vs. painful situations: statistically significant differences (paired $t = 12.24$, two-tailed $P < 0.0001$, and Mann-Whitney $U = 765.5$, $P < 0.00001$) and using real vs. sham heel stick procedures with infants ages 28-30 weeks' gestational age ($t = 2.4$, two-tailed $P < 0.02$, and Mann-Whitney $U = 132$, $P < 0.016$) and with full-term males undergoing circumcision with topical anesthetic vs. placebo ($t = 2.6$, two-tailed $P < 0.02$, or nonparametric equivalent Mann-Whitney U test, $U = 145.7$, two-tailed $P < 0.02$)	Gestational age (0-3) Eye squeeze (0-3) Behavioral state (0-3) Nasolabial furrow (0-3) Heart rate (0-3) Oxygen saturation (0-3)	0 = no pain 21 = worst pain
SCALE FOR USE IN NEWBORNS (SUN)				
0-28 days	Blauer T, Gerstmann D: A simultaneous comparison of three neonatal pain scales during common NICU procedures, *Clin J Pain* 14(1):39-47, 1998.	No reliability; face validity, content validity, construct validity using extreme groups	Brow bulge (0-3) CNS state (0-4) Movement (0-4) Breathing (0-4) Tone (0-4) Heart rate (0-4) Face (0-4) Mean BP (0-4)	0 = no pain 28 = worst pain Average baseline score 10-14 A 2 represents normal or baseline value
NEONATAL PAIN, AGITATION, AND SEDATION SCALE (NPASS)				
Birth (23 weeks' gestational age) and term newborns up to 100 days	Puchalski M, Hummel P: Loyola University Chicago, Loyola University Medical Center.	Interrater reliability using ICC: 95% CI for pre- and postintervention pain scale; 95% CI for pre- and postintervention sedation scale Internal consistency (Cronbach alpha): Preintervention pain scale, 0.75 and 0.71 raters 1 and 2 Postintervention pain scale, 0.25 and 0.27 raters 1 and 2 Preintervention sedation scale, 0.88 and 0.81 raters 1 and 2 Postintervention sedation scale, 0.86 and 0.89 raters 1 and 2	Cry/irritability (0-2) Behavior/state (0-2) Facial expression (0-2) Extremities/tone (0-2) Vital signs—HR, RR, BP, Sao_2 (0-2)	Pain score: 0-10 (0 = no pain; 10 = intense pain) Sedation score: 0-10 (0 = no sedation; 10 = deep sedation)

TABLE 9-3 ■ CRIES Neonatal Postoperative Pain Scale

	0	1	2
Crying	No	High pitched	Inconsolable
Requires O₂ for sat >95%	No	<30%	>30%
Increased vital signs	Heart rate and blood pressure = preoperative state	Heart rate and blood pressure increase <20% of preoperative state	Heart rate and blood pressure increase >20% of preoperative state
Expression	None	Grimace	Grimace/grunt
Sleepless	No	Wakes at frequent intervals	Constantly awake

Neonatal pain assessment tool developed at the University of Missouri–Columbia. Copyright S. Krechel, MD, and J. Bildner, RNC, CNS, 1995.

behavioral indicators of pain used in the tool. The indicators include Crying, Requiring increased oxygen, Increased vital signs, Expression, and Sleeplessness. Each indicator is scored from 0 to 2—similar to the Apgar score for neonates. The total possible pain score, which represents the worst pain, is 10. A pain score greater than 4 should be considered significant. This tool has been tested for reliability and validity for postoperative pain in infants between the ages of 32 weeks of gestation and 20 weeks postterm (Bildner and Krechel, 1996; Krechel and Bildner, 1995).

The *Premature Infant Pain Profile (PIPP)* is unique because it has been developed specifically for preterm infants (Stevens and others, 1996). The category "gestational age at time of observation" gives a higher pain score to infants with lower gestational age.

The **Neonatal Pain and Sedation Scale (NPASS)** was originally developed to measure pain/sedation in preterm infants after surgery. It measures five criteria (cry/irritability, behavior/state, facial expression, extremities/tone, and vital signs) in two dimensions (pain and sedation) and may be used in neonates as young as 23 weeks' gestation up to infants 100 days old. Extra points are added in the pain dimension for preterm infants based on gestational age. The other observational categories are listed in Table 9-2.

Preterm infants are subjected to a variety of repeated noxious stimuli, including multiple heel sticks, venipuncture, endotracheal intubation and suctioning, arterial sticks, chest tube placement, and lumbar puncture. The effects of pain caused by such procedures are not fully known, but researchers have begun to investigate the potential consequences. Fitzgerald, Millard, and McIntosh (1989) supported this statement with evidence of hypersensitivity to repeated heel stick procedures in preterm infants born at 27 to 32 weeks of gestational age.

The memory of pain has been a well-investigated phenomenon. Neither adults nor infants have the capacity to remember the sensation of pain. Only the experiences associated with pain can be remembered (Anand and Hickey, 1987). Grunau and others (1994) demonstrated the phenomenon of memory in toddlers with a history of ELBW and long stays in the NICU. These toddlers had higher somatic complaints of unknown origin than children who had been full-term healthy infants. Others have found that full-term newborns undergoing circumcision without an anesthetic reacted more intensely to immunization injections at 4 to 6 months of age than newborns who had an anesthetic (Taddio and others, 1997).

Nurses' anecdotal reports suggest that infants show memory by exhibiting defensive behaviors when painful procedures are repeated. Nurses often describe infants who stiffen and withdraw when touched because human touch has repeatedly been associated with pain. Such infants often become hypervigilant and gaze intently at the hands rather than at the eyes of people who approach them. These reports not only indicate that infants remember painful events, but also show that continual exposure to pain affects development, especially in response to human contact. Taddio and others (2002) described hypervigilance in infants of diabetic mother who received multiple heel punctures during the first 24 hours of life.

The immediate and long-term consequences of infant pain are still being investigated by researchers. However, the limited amount of available knowledge suggests serious potential deleterious effects of untreated pain (Box 9-4). The early experience of untreated pain may permanently alter peripheral and central pain mechanisms. For example, peripheral tissue injury such as repeated heel lance can produce a hyperalgesic state (skin tenderness) for weeks to months (Dickenson and Rahman, 1999). Nurses who care for infants and children should consider the potential acute and long-term effects of pain on their young patients and be active advocates in treating and preventing pain.

Despite current research on the neonate's experience of pain, infant pain remains inadequately managed. The mismanagement of infant pain is partially the result of misconceptions regarding the effects of pain on the neonate, as well as a lack of knowledge of the consequences of untreated pain.

Nonpharmacologic measures used to alleviate pain are discussed in Chapter 21. Those used to reduce discomfort in the NICU include repositioning, swaddling, containment, cuddling, rocking, soft music, reducing environmental stimulation, tactile comfort measures, skin-to-skin contact with the mother, and nonnutritive sucking. However, nonpharmacologic measures may not be sufficient to decrease physiologic distress, even if behavioral responses such as crying are lessened. In premature infants, additional stimulation such as stroking may increase physiologic distress. Breast-feeding has recently been reported to be an effective analgesic to alleviate newborn pain during procedures such as heel puncture.

Available pharmacologic options for managing neonatal pain include the use of the topical anesthetic EMLA, concentrated oral sucrose solution, localized nerve block for

BOX 9-4 ■ Consequences of Untreated Pain in Infants

ACUTE CONSEQUENCES

Periventricular intraventricular hemorrhage
Increased chemical and hormone release
Breakdown of fat and carbohydrate stores
Prolonged hyperglycemia
Higher morbidity for NICU patients
Memory of painful events
Hypersensitivity to pain
Prolonged response to pain
Inappropriate innervation of the spinal cord
Inappropriate response to nonnoxious stimuli
Lower pain threshold

POTENTIAL LONG-TERM CONSEQUENCES

Higher somatic complaints of unknown origin
Greater physiologic and behavioral responses to pain
Increased prevalence of neurologic deficits
Psychosocial problems
Neurobehavioral disorders
Cognitive deficits
Learning disorders
Poor motor performance
Behavioral problems
Attention deficits
Poor adaptive behavior
Inability to cope with novel situations
Problems with impulsivity and social control
Learning deficits
Emotional temperament changes in infancy or childhood
Accentuated hormonal stress responses in adult life

Data from Anand, Grunau, and Oberlander, 1997; Anand and Hickey, 1987; Barba and others, 1991; Fitzgerald, 1995; Fitzgerald, Millard, and McIntosh, 1989; Grunau and others, 1994; Langland and Langland, 1988; Penticuff 1987; Perry and others, 1990; Sexon and others, 1986; Wong, 1992.

ATRAUMATIC CARE

Use of Opioids and Extubation Practice

Traditional belief holds that the continued use of opioids for neonates in the postoperative period results in prolonged intubation. Consequently, traditional practice is to discontinue all opioids several hours before and after extubation, preventing pain relief. Furdon and others (1998) found that continuous opioid infusion in infants without an underlying pulmonary or neurologic pathologic condition actually shortened the time to extubation and caused no problems of respiratory depression that required reintubation. There is preliminary evidence that the use of preemptive analgesia with a continuous infusion of low-dose morphine reduces the incidence of poor neurologic outcomes in preterm neonates who require ventilatory support.

---

circumcision (dorsal penile nerve block and ring block), and opioid analgesics.

Morphine and fentanyl are the most widely used opioid analgesics for pharmacologic management of neonatal pain. Continuous or bolus IV infusion of opioids provides effective and safe pain control (American Academy of Pediatrics, 2000a) (see Atraumatic Care box, above right). Ketorolac (Toradol) has been shown to be effective in the management of postoperative neonatal pain (Burd and Tobias, 2002). Postoperative neonatal pain should be managed with around-the-clock dosing or use of a continual drip; dosing as needed is not considered to be an effective management of chronic or postoperative pain (Hummel and Puchalski, 2001). Other methods for managing neonatal pain are epidural infusion, local and regional nerve blocks, and intradermal or topical anesthetics (Anand and International Evidence-Based Group for Neonatal Pain, 2001; American Academy of Pediatrics, 2000a; Taddio and others, 1998). (See Pain Management, Chapter 21, for more information on pharmacologic management of pain in the infant.)

Study results vary when EMLA is used in newborns for heel punctures; some find the topical anesthetic to be beneficial in managing heel stick pain while others do not.

However, EMLA does reduce the pain of circumcision, venous or arterial puncture, and percutaneous venous catheter placement (Taddio and others, 1998). A concentrated sucrose solution, especially administered with a pacifier, can decrease pain associated with heel lance and venipuncture (Gradin and others, 2002; Stevens, Yamada, and Ohlsson, 2001; Blass and Watt, 1999; Ramenghi and others, 1999) (see also Atraumatic Care, Heel Punctures box, Ch. 8, p. 201).

Parents are universally concerned that their infants are suffering pain during procedures. Nurses need to address these concerns and encourage the parents to speak with the health care professionals involved. Parents have the right to withhold consent for invasive procedures and are entitled to honest answers from those responsible for the infant's care. When permissible, they can also help provide comfort measures for the infant. It is important that parents are aware that nurses are sensitive to the infant's pain and are reassured that the infant will not suffer unduly.

Family Support and Involvement

Professional health workers often are so absorbed in the life-saving physical aspects of care that the emotional needs of infants and their families are ignored. The significance of early parent-child interaction and infant stimulation has been documented by reliable research. Nurses, aware of these infant and family needs, must incorporate activities that facilitate family interaction into the nursing care plan.

The birth of a preterm infant is an unexpected and stressful event for which families are emotionally unprepared. They find themselves simultaneously coping with their own needs, the needs of their infant, and the needs of their families (especially when there are other children). To compound the situation, the precarious nature of their infant's condition engenders an atmosphere of apprehension and uncertainty. They are faced with multiple crises and overwhelming feelings of responsibility, helplessness, and frustration.

All parents have some anxieties about the outcome of a pregnancy, but after a premature birth the concern is heightened regarding both the viability and the normalcy of their infant. Mothers may see their infant only briefly before the newborn is removed to the intensive care unit or even to another hospital, leaving them with just the recollection of the infant's very small size and unusual appearance. They usually feel alone or lost on the mother-baby unit, belonging neither with mothers who have lost their infants nor with those who have delivered healthy, full-term infants. The staff and physicians are often guarded in discussing the infant's condition; mothers are continually expecting to hear that their infant has died, and they are sensitive to the anxieties of other mothers and staff members. Going home without their infant only serves to compound their feelings of disappointment, failure, and deprivation.

When an infant is to be transported from the hospital, the parents need a description of the facility where the infant is going. They need to know the location, reputation, and nature of the facility and the care that the infant is expected to receive. The name of the infant's physician and the telephone number of the nursery should be given to them, and unfamiliar terms such as "neonatologist," "ventilator," "infusion," and "incubator" should be explained. Explanations are kept simple, and parents are given the opportunity to ask questions. If booklets are available that describe the facility, they are given to the family.

Perhaps most important of all, the parents should have some contact with the infant before the transport. To be able to see, touch, and (if possible) hold their infant may help decrease the parents' anxiety. Often a photograph, or even a videotape, of their infant can serve as tangible evidence of the newborn's existence until the parents are able to travel to the regional facility. When possible, it is often advisable to transfer the mother to the same institution as her infant.

Parents need to be informed of their infant's progress and reassured that the infant is receiving proper care. They need to understand the smallest aspects of the infant's condition and treatment. Parents need a realistic, honest, and direct assessment of the situation. Using nonmedical terminology, moving at a pace that is comfortable for parents to assimilate the information, and avoiding lengthy technical explanations facilitate communication with family members. Psychologic tasks that must be accomplished by parents during their infant's care are presented in Box 9-5.

Facilitating Parent-Infant Relationships

Because of their physiologic instability, infants are separated from their mothers immediately and surrounded by a complex, impenetrable barrier of glass windows, mechanical equipment, and special caregivers. There is some evidence indicating that the emotional separation that accompanies the physical separation of mothers and infants may interfere with the normal maternal-infant attachment process discussed in Chapter 8. Maternal attachment is a cumulative process that begins before conception, strengthens by significant events during pregnancy, and matures through maternal-infant contact during the neonatal period and infancy.

When an infant is sick, the necessary physical separation appears to be accompanied by an emotional estrangement by the parents, which may seriously damage the capacity for parenting their infant. This detachment is further hampered by the tenuous nature of the infant's condition. When survival is in doubt, parents may be reluctant to establish a relationship with their infant. They prepare themselves for the

BOX 9-5 ■ Psychologic Tasks of Parents of a High-Risk Infant

Work through the events surrounding labor and delivery.
Acknowledge that the infant's life is endangered and begin the anticipatory grieving process.
Confront and recognize feelings of inadequacy and guilt in not delivering a healthy child.
Adapt to the neonatal intensive care environment.
Resume parental relationships with the sick infant and initiate the caregiving role.
Prepare to take the infant home.

Modified from Siegel R, Gardner SL, Merenstein GB: Families in crisis: theoretical and practical considerations. In Merenstein GB, Gardner SL, editors: *Handbook of neonatal intensive care*, ed 5, St Louis, 2002, Mosby.

death of the infant while continuing to hope for recovery. This anticipatory grief (see Chapter 18) and hesitancy to embark on a relationship are evidenced by behaviors such as delay in giving the infant a name, reluctance in visiting the nursery (or when they do visit, focusing on equipment and treatments rather than on their infant), and hesitancy to touch or handle the infant when given the opportunity.

Family-centered care of high-risk newborns includes encouraging and facilitating parental involvement rather than isolating parents from their infant and associated care. This is particularly important in relation to mothers; to reduce the effects of physical separation, mothers are united with their newborn at the earliest opportunity. Preparing the parents to see their infant for the first time is a nursing responsibility.

Before the first visit, the parents are prepared for their infant's appearance, the equipment attached to the child, and some indication of the general atmosphere of the unit. The initial encounter with the intensive care unit is a stressful experience, and the frightening array of people, equipment, and activity is likely to be overwhelming. A book of photographs or pamphlets describing the NICU environment (infants in incubators or under radiant warmers, monitors, mechanical ventilators, and IV equipment) provides a useful and nonthreatening introduction to the NICU.

Parents are encouraged to visit their infant as soon as possible. Even if they saw the infant at the time of transport or shortly after birth, the infant may have changed considerably, especially if there are a number of medical and equipment requirements associated with the infant's hospitalization. At the bedside the nurse should explain the function of each piece of equipment and the role it plays in facilitating recovery. Explanations may often need to be patiently repeated because parents' anxiety over the infant's condition and the surroundings may prevent them from really "hearing" what is being said. When possible, some items related to therapy can be removed; for example, phototherapy can be temporarily discontinued and eye patches removed to permit eye-to-eye contact.

Parents appreciate the support of a nurse during the initial visit with their infant, but they may also appreciate some time alone with the infant for a short while. It is important during the early visits to emphasize the positive aspects of their infant's behavior and development so that parents can focus on their infant as an individual rather than on the equipment that surrounds the child. For example, the nurse may describe the infant's spontaneous behaviors during care, such as the grasp reflex, Moro reflex, and spontaneous movement, or make comments about the infant's biologic functions. Most institutions have open visiting policies so that parents and siblings may visit their infant as often as they wish.

Parents vary greatly in the degree to which they are able to interact with their infant. Some may wish to touch or hold their infant during the first visit, whereas others may not feel comfortable enough even to enter the nursery. These reactions depend on a variety of prenatal and postnatal factors, such as the parity of the mother and her preparation before birth; the size, condition, and physical appearance of the infant; and the type of treatment the infant is receiving. It is essential to recognize that the individualized pacing and quality of the interactions are more important than an early onset of these interactions. Parents may not be receptive to early and extended infant contact because they need time to adjust to the impact of an infant with birth problems and must be helped to grieve before acceptance of their infant can occur.

The parents' inability to focus on their infant is a clue for the nurse to assist the parents in expressing feelings of guilt, anxiety, helplessness, inadequacy, anger, and ambivalence. Nurses can help parents deal with these distressing feelings and recognize that they are normal responses shared by other parents. It is important to point out and reinforce the positive aspects of parents' behavior and interactions with their infant.

Most parents feel shaky and insecure about initiating interaction with their infant. Nurses can sense parents' level of readiness and offer encouragement in these initial efforts. Parents of preterm infants follow the same acquaintance process as do parents of term infants. They may quickly proceed through the process or may require several days, or even weeks, to complete the process. Parents begin by touching their infant's extremities with their fingertips and poking the infant tenderly, and then proceed to caresses and fondling (Fig. 9-10). Touching is the first act of communication between parents and child. Parents need to be prepared for their infant's exaggerated and generalized startle responses to touch so that they will not interpret these as negative reactions to their overtures. It may be necessary to limit tactile stimuli when the infant is critically ill and labile, but the nurse can offer other options such as speaking softly or sitting at the bedside.

Parents of acutely ill preterm infants may express feelings of helplessness and lack of control. Involving the parent in some type of caregiving activity, no matter how minor it may seem to the nurse, enables the parent to "take on" a more active role. Examples of such caregiving for the acutely ill infant who cannot be held and is seemingly not responding positively include moistening the infant's lips with a small amount of sterile water on a cotton-tipped swab or slipping the diaper from under the infant when it is wet or soiled.

Eventually, parents begin to endow their infant with an identity—as part of the family. When an infant no longer appears as a foreign object and begins to take on aspects of

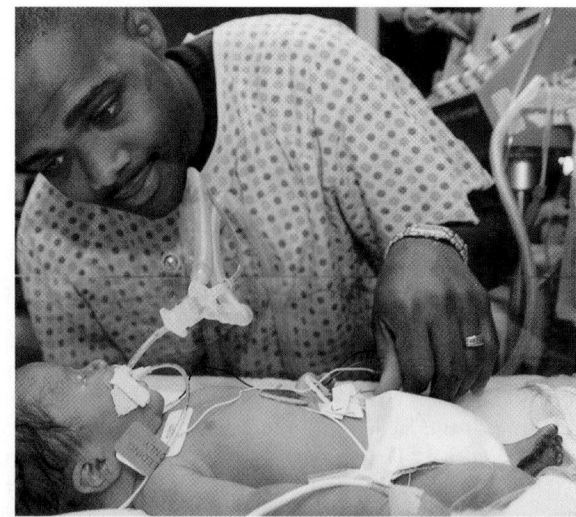

A

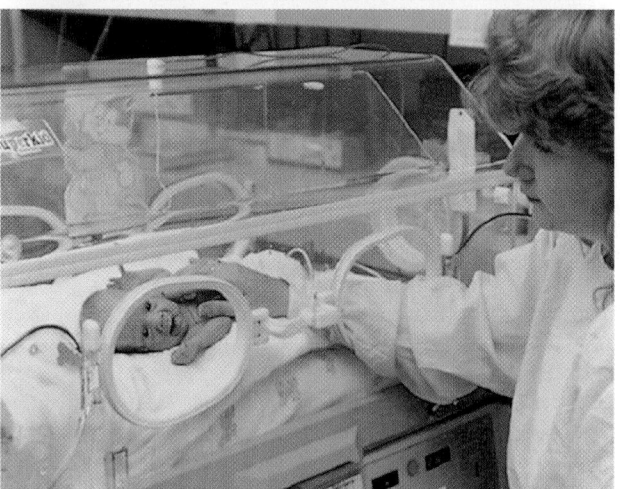

B

FIG. 9-10 ■ **A,** Father interacting with newborn receiving intensive care. **B,** Encouraging interaction of mother and her preterm infant in intensive care unit facilitates mother-infant attachment process.

family members, such as the father's chin or the sister's nose, nurses can facilitate this incorporation. Parents are encouraged to bring in clothes, a toy, a stuffed animal, or a family snapshot for their infant, and the nurse can help parents set goals for themselves and for the infant. Parents may become involved by reading a children's storybook or nursery rhymes in a soft, soothing voice. Some families tape record the parents' voices telling or reading stories and play the tapes when the infant is able to cope with such stimuli. Feeding schedules are discussed, and parents are encouraged to visit at times when they can become involved in the care of their infant (Fig. 9-11).

Throughout the parent-infant acquaintance process, the nurse listens carefully to what the parents say to assess their concerns and their progress toward incorporating their infant into their lives. The manner in which parents refer to their infant and the questions they ask reveal their worries and feelings and can serve as valuable clues to future relationships with the infant. The alert nurse is attuned to these subtle indications of parents' needs, which provide guide-

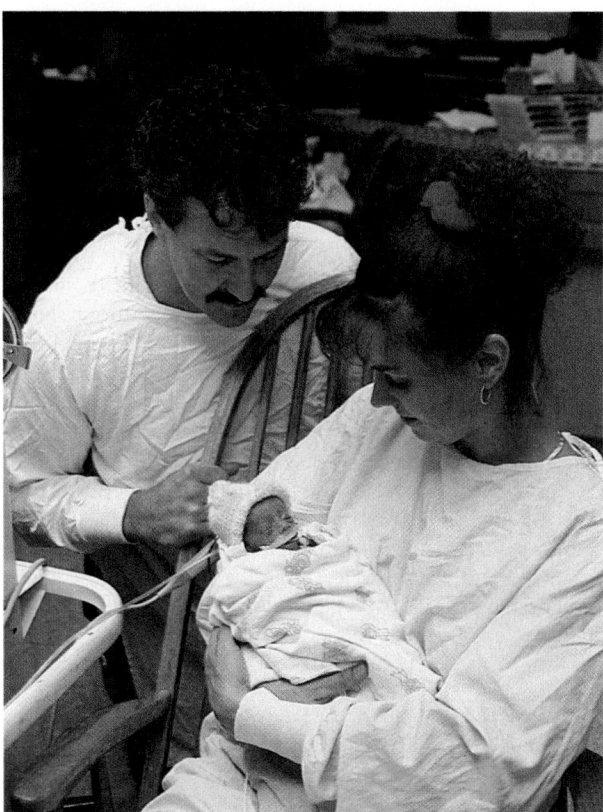

FIG. 9-11 ■ Mother and father visit their newborn infant.

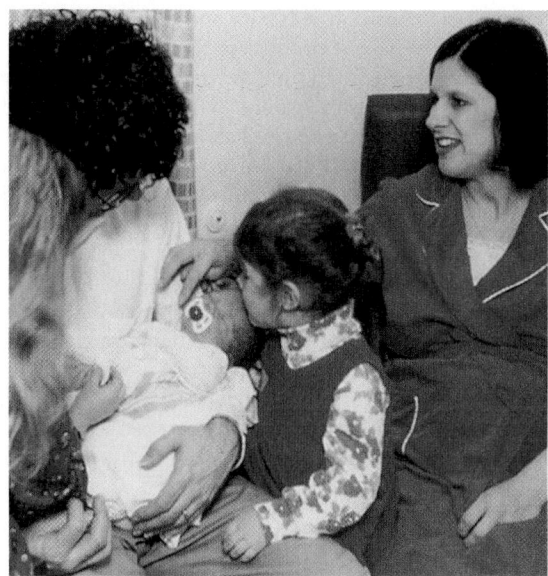

FIG. 9-12 ■ Big sister gets acquainted with the new baby.

lines for nursing intervention. Often all that the parents need is reassurance that they will have the support of the nurse during caregiving activities and that the behaviors about which they are concerned are normal reactions and will disappear as the infant matures (e.g., an exaggerated Moro reflex or inability to coordinate swallowing, breathing, and taking milk orally).

Parents need guidance in their relationships with their infant and assistance in their efforts to meet their infant's physical and developmental needs. The nursing staff must help parents understand that their preterm infant offers few behavioral rewards and show them how to accept small rewards from their infant. The infant's reactions and behaviors are explained to parents, who take their infant's jerky, rejective behavior personally. They need reassurance that these behaviors are not a reflection on their parenting skills. Parents are taught to recognize their infant's cues regarding stimulation, handling, and other interaction, especially aversive behaviors that indicate a need for rest. Nurses need to include parents in planning their infant's care and sensory stimulation materials, such as a music box or recording.

Above all, nurses must encourage and reinforce parents during their caregiving activities and interactions with their infant to promote healthy parent-child relationships. It is also helpful for the parents to have contact and communication with a consistent group of nurses. This decreases the amount of different information given to parents and often instills confidence that although the parents cannot be at their infant's bedside 24 hours a day, there are competent and caring nurses whom they may call to inquire about the infant's status. Periodic parent conferences involving the staff caring for the child serve to clarify misunderstandings or problems related to the infant's condition.

Siblings. In the past, concerns about sibling visitation in the NICU focused on fears of infection and disruption of nursing routines. These fears have not been substantiated, and sibling visits should be a part of the normal operation of NICUs (Fig. 9-12). Clearly defined policies and procedures should be developed to facilitate sibling visitation (American Academy of Pediatrics and American College of Obstetricians and Gynecologists, 2002).

The birth of a preterm infant is a difficult time for siblings, who rely on the support of understanding parents. When the happy anticipation is changed to sadness, worry, and altered routines, siblings are bewildered and deprived of their parents' attention. They know something is wrong, but they have only a dim understanding of what it is. Concern about the negative effects on visiting siblings of seeing the ill newborn has not been confirmed. Children have not hesitated to approach or touch the infant, and children younger than 5 years of age have been less reluctant than older children; in addition, there have been no measurable differences between previsit and postvisit behaviors.

The potential benefits of sibling visits must be weighed against exposure of the child to the environment of the NICU. Children must be prepared for the unfamiliar NICU atmosphere, but contact with the infant appears to have a positive effect on siblings by helping them to deal with the reality rather than the bizarre fantasies that are characteristic of young children. Such visits also help to bond the family as a unit.

Support Groups. Parents need to feel that they are not alone. Parent support groups have been of immeasurable value to families of infants in the NICU. Some groups consist of parents who have infants in the hospital and share the same anxieties and concerns. Other groups include parents who have had infants in the NICU and who have dealt with the crisis effectively. The groups are usually under the leadership of a staff person and involve physicians, nurses, and social workers, but it is the parents who can offer other parents something that no one else can provide.

The **Family Resource Coalition*** is a North American network of family support programs designed to help families of preterm infants.

An excellent resource for parents of preterm infants is the book by J. Zaichkin, *Newborn Intensive Care: What Every Parent Needs to Know* (2002).† This resource has technical and anecdotal information regarding different problems facing preterm infants, common treatments and therapies, preparation for home discharge, and home care for the preterm infant. Another resource for parents wanting more information about kangaroo care is by S.M. Ludington-Hoe, *Kangaroo Care: The Best You Can Do to Help Your Preterm Infant* (1993).‡

Discharge Planning and Home Care

Parents become very apprehensive and excited as the time for discharge approaches. They have many concerns and insecurities regarding the care of their infant. They fear that the child may still be in danger, that they will be unable to recognize signs of distress or illness in their infant, and that the infant may not yet be ready for discharge. Nurses need to begin early to assist parents in acquiring or increasing their skills in the care of their infant. Appropriate instruction must be provided and sufficient time allowed for the family to assimilate the information and learn the continuing special care requirements. Where rooming-in or other live-in arrangements are available, parents can stay for a few days and nights and assume the care of their infant under the supervision and support of the nursery staff.

There should be appropriate medical and nursing follow-up and referrals to services that can benefit the family, including developmental follow-up. Parents of preterm infants should also be given adequate information about immunizations with other discharge planning information. Home health agencies provide nursing supervision, counseling, and referrals for nursing visits. With the trend toward early discharge, many hospital-based home health care agencies become involved in the follow-up and care of the NICU "graduate" in the home. For the parents of an infant being discharged with equipment such as an oxygen tank, apnea monitor, or even a ventilator, discharge planning requires interdisciplinary collaborative practice to ensure that the family has not only the appropriate resources, but also the available assistance for dealing with the infant's needs. Organized support groups are a part of many communities, including those discussed previously, those designed for parents of infants who require special care because of specific defects or disabilities, and those for parents of multiple

births. Some manufacturers provide for the special needs of such infants. For example, premature-size disposable diapers are available from the manufacturers of Pampers.*

Car seat safety is an essential aspect of discharge planning, and infants younger than 37 weeks of gestation should have a period of observation in an appropriate car seat to monitor for possible apnea, bradycardia, and decreased SaO$_2$ (American Academy of Pediatrics, 1999). Several models can be adapted for small infants with the placement of blanket rolls on each side of the infant to support the head and trunk. For adequate support without slumping, the seat back–to-crotch strap distance must be 14 cm (5.5 inches) or less; a small rolled blanket may be placed between the crotch strap and the infant to reduce slouching. The distance from the lower harness strap to the seat bottom should be 10 inches or less to decrease the potential for the harness straps to cross the infant's ears (American Academy of Pediatrics, 1996b). The Centers for Disease Control and Prevention also recommends that infants younger than 1 year old and weighing less than 20 pounds not be placed in rear-facing car seats on the passenger side of cars with an air bag because of the increased risk of injury when the air bag is inflated (Update: fatal air bag, 1997). Additional guidelines are available from the American Academy of Pediatrics (1996b, 2002), including a video tape for the safe transportation of preterm and LBW infants. (See Chapter 10 for a discussion of infant car restraints and AAP website: www.aap.org for a complete list of appropriate car seats for infants.)

Knowing that members of the staff are available for telephone or personal contact when the parents take the infant home provides a measure of security to anxious parents. Many NICU facilities maintain a policy of open communication between staff and parents both during the infant's hospitalization and after discharge. It is the responsibility of the NICU staff to make certain that parents are prepared to care for their infant, both emotionally and physically. At the same time, it is important that parents establish a trusting relationship with the infant's primary care provider in the community before discharge from the acute care facility.

Neonatal Loss

The precarious nature of many high-risk infants makes death a very real and ever-present possibility. (See Ethical Case Study.) Although infant mortality has been reduced sharply with improved technology, the mortality rate is still greatest during the neonatal period. Nurses in the NICU are the persons who must prepare the parents for an inevitable death, provide end-of-life care for the infant and family, and facilitate a family's grieving process after an expected or unexpected death.

The loss of an infant has special meaning for the grieving parents. It represents a loss of a part of themselves (especially for mothers), a loss of the potential for immortality that offspring represent, and the loss of the dream child that has been fantasized throughout the pregnancy. There is a sense of emptiness and failure. In addition, when an infant

---

*20 N. Whacker Drive, Suite 1100, Chicago, IL 60606; (312) 338-0900; website: www.familysupportamerica.org.
†Available from NICU Ink, Petaluma, CA; (707) 762-2646 or (888) 642-8465; website: www.neonatalnetwork.com/nicuink/.
‡Available from Bantam/Random House, New York; website: www.randomhouse.com.

---

*Procter & Gamble; to place order, phone toll free (800) 543-4932; in Ohio (800) 582-2623.

ETHICAL CASE STUDY

Ethical Decision Making Model	Britt is a 6.5-month-old infant in the neonatal intensive care unit. He was born at 28 weeks' gestation and as a result of prematurity he has numerous health problems including postnecrotizing enterocolitis, short bowel syndrome and subsequent ileostomy, chronic lung disease, and is ventilator-dependent with a tracheostomy, grade III periventricular hemorrhage, and partial blindness from retinopathy of prematurity, and bilateral hearing deficit that will eventually require hearing aids. Britt is dependent on intravenous total parenteral nutrition for nutrition and fluids. Britt's parents are Josh and Debi; they are 22 and 23 years old, respectively, and have another child, Darlene, who is 22 months old. Darlene was also a preemie and has various health care needs including tube feedings through a skin-level feeding tube, atopy, and recurrent urinary tract infections due to reflux. The parents are only able to visit the neonatal intensive care unit every other week because they live 120 miles from the hospital and they cannot take off work because of financial problems. The extended family has no relationship with the parents because of a recent squabble over money loaned by the grandparents, which the parents have been unable to repay.
Evaluate the issue	Britt has had 19 cardiac arrests, 3 of which occurred within the last 48 hours, and he has responded to drugs and higher ventilator and oxygen settings but shows signs of gradual decline in mental alertness and ability to maintain adequate cardiorespiratory and metabolic function. The nursing staff are concerned about Britt's quality of life and have suggested that the next time he "codes," the physician allow him to die a natural death. Britt's parents are unable to visit at this time but have requested by telephone conference that all available means be employed to keep Britt alive; they want to bring him home soon to be with the rest of the family. They further indicate that they have a lot of faith in a Higher Being and that Britt will soon be healed. Several nurses have refused to care for Britt because they "cannot stand to see him suffer."
Treat all involved with respect	The parents' concerns regarding Britt's condition and resuscitation efforts should be objectively addressed in person with a conference of nursing, medical, social worker, and perhaps clergy or spiritual advisors close to the family. Britt's mother has expressed strong guilt feelings regarding his illness and their inability to care for him as they care for Darlene. The extended family has instilled additional guilt over the financial situation and the parents' inability to visit Britt on a regular basis. The nurses must realize the parents' guilt over not being able to completely care for Britt as they have cared for Darlene.
Hear all sides	The nurses must first consider the parents' views on Britt's health status. It is important to evaluate the parents' perception of Britt's health status and that of the daughter, Darlene. Are there parallels that may be drawn between the two children's course of illness? What considerations have the parents given to home care of Britt and Darlene? Does the family have religious beliefs that preclude allowing the child to die without further intervention? Do the parents fully understand the essence of Britt's health status?
Initiate action	Which of the following actions is most appropriate for the nursing staff to take at this time? ■ Tell the parents that Britt is going to die regardless of resuscitation efforts and that his death is the best solution to prevent further suffering. ■ Enlist the assistance of the parents' pastor (spiritual advisor) to help the family see the reality of Britt's suffering and eventual death. ■ Persuade the primary care practitioner to request a Do Not Resuscitate order from the parents. ■ Contact the local hospice facility for end-of-life care for Britt and the family.
Consider the outcome	A number of ethical issues must be considered in this case. One dilemma the parents are facing is the deteriorating health and possible death of a child they have formed a bond with and have loved for 6.5 months. The second ethical dilemma facing the parents is their religious belief about Britt's healing. The lack of support from extended family further complicates the situation. An ethical dilemma the nurses face is the issue of whether Britt has what would be considered a positive quality of life or experiences pain and suffering as a result of his deteriorating physical status.

has lived for such a short time, there may be few, if any, pleasant memories to serve as a basis for the identification and idealization that are part of the resolution of a loss.

To help parents understand that the death is a reality, it is important that they be encouraged to hold their infant before death and, if possible, be present at the time of death so that their infant can die in their arms if they choose. Many who deny the need to hold the infant later regret the decision.

Parents are given the opportunity to actually "parent" the infant in any manner they wish or are able to do before and after the death. This may include seeing, touching, holding, caressing, and talking to their infant privately; the parents may also wish to bathe and dress the infant. If parents are hesitant about seeing their dead infant, it is advisable to keep the body in the unit for a few hours, because many parents change their minds after the initial shock of the death.

Parents may need to see and hold the infant more than once—the first time to say "hello" and the last time to say "good-bye." If parents wish to see the infant after the body has been taken to the morgue, the infant should be retrieved, wrapped in a blanket, rewarmed in a radiant warmer, and taken to the mother's room or other private place. The nurse should stay with the parents and provide them an opportunity for private time alone with their dead infant. Individual grief responses of the mother and father should be recognized and handled appropriately; gender differences and cultural and religious beliefs will affect the parents' grief responses.

Some units have implemented a hospice approach for families with infants for whom the decision has been made not to prolong life and who are receiving only palliative care. A special "family" room is set aside and contains all supportive equipment needed for the care of the infant. It also provides a homelike atmosphere for the family. All hospice services are available to the family, and the infant remains under the care and supervision of a primary nurse on the NICU staff. (See Chapter 18 for further discussion of hospice care.)

A photograph of the infant taken before or after death is highly desirable. Parents may wish to have a special family portrait taken with the infant and other family members; this often helps personalize and make the experience more tangible. The parents may not wish to see the photograph at the time of death, but the chance to refer to it later will help to make their infant seem more real, which is a part of the normal grief process. A photograph of their infant being held by the hand or touched by an adult offers a more positive image than a morgue type of photograph. Many NICUs have a bereavement or memory packet made up for the grieving parents, which may include the infant's handprints and footprints, a lock of hair, the bedside name card and, as appropriate to the family's religious beliefs, a certificate of baptism. In some units special knitted clothing is made by hospital volunteer groups and donated for dressing the infant postmortem. Other tangible remembrances or mementos of the child can be provided, such as name tags, armbands, and locks of hair shaved for IV insertion or other procedures. Naming the deceased infant is an important step in the grieving process. Some parents may hesitate to give the newborn a name that had been chosen during the pregnancy for their special "baby." However, having a tangible person for whom to grieve is an important component of the grieving process.

A primary nurse who is familiar to the family should be present during the discussion about the dead or dying infant. An **RTS (Resolve Through Sharing)** counselor or bereavement counselor is often involved in helping the family through this difficult period. The nurse should talk with parents openly and honestly about funeral arrangements, because few of them have had experience with this aspect of death. Many funeral homes now offer inexpensive arrangements for these special cases. Someone from the NICU should take the responsibility for acquiring this type of information. It is often helpful to parents for the NICU to have a list of local funeral homes, services offered, and a price for the service offered. Families need to be informed of the options available, but it is preferable to encourage a funeral because the ritual provides an opportunity for parents to feel the support of friends and relatives. A member of the clergy of the appropriate faith may be notified if the

parents wish. Issues regarding an autopsy or organ donation (when appropriate) are approached in a multidisciplinary fashion (primary practitioner and primary nurse) with respect, sensitivity to cultural and religious beliefs, tact, and consideration of the family's wishes. (See also Grief and Perinatal Loss in Merenstein and Gardner, 2002, and Jansen, 2003, for additional suggestions for helping families who experience neonatal loss).

Before the parents leave the hospital, they are given the telephone number of the unit (if they do not have it) and invited to call any time they have any further questions. Many intensive care units make it a point to contact the parents several weeks after a neonatal death to assess the parents' coping mechanisms, evaluate the grieving process, and provide support as needed. Several organizations are available to offer support and understanding to families who have lost a newborn, including **The Compassionate Friends,* Aiding Mothers and Fathers Experiencing Neo-Natal Death (AMEND),†** and **SHARE Pregnancy & Infant Loss Support, Inc.‡** (See also Chapter 18 for further discussion of the family and the grief process.)

Nurses who care for critically ill infants also experience grief; NICU nurses may feel helpless and sorrowful. It is important that such grief be allowed and that nurses attend the funeral or memorial service as a part of working through the grief process. Nurses may fear that showing emotion is unprofessional and that the expression of grief indicates "loss of control." These fears are unfounded. Studies have demonstrated that to continue to be effective managers and providers of care, nurses must be allowed to grieve and support each other through the process (Gardner, Hauser, and Merenstein, 2002).

Baptism.   Because many Christian parents wish to have their child baptized if death is anticipated or is a decided possibility, this becomes a nursing responsibility. Whenever possible, it is most desirable that a representative of the parents' faith (e.g., a Roman Catholic priest or a Protestant minister) perform such a ritual. When death is imminent, a nurse or a physician can perform the baptism by simply pouring water on the infant's forehead (a medicine dropper is a convenient means) while repeating the words, "I baptize you in the name of the Father and of the Son and of the Holy Spirit." This includes a birth of any gestational age, particularly when the parents are of the Roman Catholic faith.

When the faith of the parents is uncertain, a conditional baptism can be carried out by saying, "If you are capable of receiving baptism, I baptize you in the name of the Father and of the Son and of the Holy Spirit." The baptism is recorded in the infant's chart, and a notice is placed on the

---

*PO Box 3696, Oakbrook, IL 60522; (630) 990-0010, (877) 969-0010; website: www.compassionatefriends.org.

†Information available at www.amendinc.com, PO Box 20260, Wichita, KS 67208-1260; (316) 268-8441.

‡SHARE Pregnancy & Infant Loss, Inc., (800) 821-6819, (636) 947-6164; website: www.nationalshareoffice.com/helpfromshare.asp; offers a variety of services for grieving parents and family members.

crib or incubator. Parents are informed at the first opportunity.

● Evaluation

The effectiveness of nursing interventions is determined by continual reassessment and evaluation of care based on the following observational guidelines.

1 Take vital signs and perform respiratory assessments at time intervals based on infant's condition and needs; observe infant's respiratory efforts and response to therapy; check functioning of equipment; review laboratory test results.

2 Measure abdominal skin and axillary temperatures at specified intervals.

3 Observe infant's behavior and appearance for evidence of sepsis.

4 Assess for hydration; assess and measure fluid intake; observe infant during feeding; measure amount of formula or parenteral intake; weigh daily.

5 Observe infant's skin for signs of irritation and breakdown.

6 Observe infant for evidence of increased intracranial pressure or signs of intraventricular hemorrhage.

7 Observe infant's physiologic and behavioral response to pain and pain control interventions.

8 Observe infant's response to developmental care.

9 Observe parental interaction with infant; interview family regarding their feelings, concerns, and readiness for home care.

10 Assess family and observe their behaviors during and after the death of their infant.

The *expected outcomes* are described in the Nursing Care Plan on pp. 255 to 259.

HIGH RISK RELATED TO DYSMATURITY

PRETERM INFANTS

Prematurity accounts for the largest number of admissions to an NICU. Immaturity of most organ systems places infants at risk for a variety of neonatal complications (e.g., hyperbilirubinemia, respiratory distress syndrome). The actual cause of prematurity is not known in most instances (Box 9-6). The incidence of prematurity is lowest in the middle to high socioeconomic classes, in which pregnant women are generally in good health, are well nourished, and receive prompt and comprehensive prenatal care. The incidence is highest in the lower socioeconomic class, in which a combination of deleterious circumstances is present. Other factors, such as multiple pregnancies, pregnancy-induced hypertension, and placental

---

NURSING CARE PLAN   The High-Risk Infant*

NURSING DIAGNOSIS ■ Ineffective breathing pattern related to pulmonary and neuromuscular immaturity, decreased energy, and fatigue

PATIENT GOAL 1: Will exhibit adequate oxygenation parameters (specify)

NURSING INTERVENTIONS/*RATIONALES*

Position for optimal air exchange (note: prone positioning is associated with optimal oxygenation; however, the supine position for sleeping is still recommended) *to maximize oxygenation.*

Avoid neck hyperextension *because it reduces diameter of trachea*

Observe for signs of respiratory distress—nasal flaring, retractions, tachypnea, apnea, grunting, cyanosis, low oxygenation saturation (SaO_2)

Suction *to remove accumulated mucus from nasopharynx, trachea, and endotracheal tube*

Suction only as necessary based on assessment (e.g., auscultation of chest, evidence of decreased oxygenation, increased infant irritability)

Avoid routine suctioning, *because it may cause bronchospasm, bradycardia due to vagal nerve stimulation, hypoxia, and increased intracranial pressure (ICP), predisposing infant to intraventricular hemorrhage (IVH)*

Use proper suctioning technique *because improper suctioning can cause infection, airway damage, pneumothoraces, and IVH*

Use two-person suction technique *because assistant can provide immediate hyperoxygenation before and after catheter insertion*

Avoid using Trendelenburg position, *because it can contribute to increased ICP and reduced lung capacity from gravity pushing organs against diaphragm*

During diaper changes, raise infant slightly under hips and not by raising feet and legs

Use semiprone or side-lying position *to prevent aspiration in infant with excessive mucus or who is being fed*

Carry out regimen prescribed for supplemental oxygen therapy (maintain ambient O_2 concentration at minimum FiO_2 level based on arterial blood gases and SaO_2)

Maintain neutral thermal environment *to conserve utilization of O_2*

Closely monitor blood gas measurements and SaO_2 readings

Apply and manage monitoring equipment correctly (i.e., cardiac or oxygen)

Demonstrate understanding of function of respiratory support apparatus

    Mechanical ventilation apparatus

    Insufflation bags with masks or endotracheal tube adaptor

    Oxygen hood

    Humidifier warmers

    Nasal cannula

    CPAP delivery modality

Observe and assess infant's response to ventilation and oxygenation therapy

EXPECTED OUTCOMES

Airway remains patent

Breathing provides adequate oxygenation and CO_2 removal

Respiratory rate and pattern are within appropriate limits for age and weight (specify)

Arterial blood gases and acid-base balance are within normal limits for gestational age

Tissue oxygenation is adequate

---

*Relates primarily to very-low-birth-weight (VLBW) and low-birth-weight (LBW) infants.

Continued

NURSING DIAGNOSIS ▦ **Ineffective thermoregulation related to immature temperature control and decreased subcutaneous body fat**

PATIENT GOAL 1: Will maintain stable body temperature

NURSING INTERVENTIONS/*RATIONALES*

Place infant in incubator, radiant warmer, or warmly clothed in open crib *to maintain stable body temperature*

Monitor axillary temperature in unstable infants (use skin probe or air temperature control; check function of servocontrolled mechanism when used)

Regulate servocontrolled unit or air temperature control as needed *to maintain skin temperature within accepted thermal range*

Use plastic heat shield as appropriate *to decrease body heat and water losses*

Monitor for signs of hyperthermia—redness, flushing, diaphoresis (rarely)

Check temperature of infant in relation to ambient temperature and temperature of heating unit *to decrease radiant heat loss*

Avoid situations that might predispose infant to heat loss, such as exposure to cool air, drafts, bathing, cold scales, or cold mattress

Monitor serum glucose values *to ensure euglycemia*

EXPECTED OUTCOME

Infant's axillary temperature remains within normal range for post-conceptional age (specify)

NURSING DIAGNOSIS ▦ **Risk for infection related to deficient immunologic defenses**

PATIENT GOAL 1: Will exhibit no evidence of nosocomial infection

NURSING INTERVENTIONS/*RATIONALES*

Ensure that all caregivers wash hands before and after handling infant *to minimize exposure to infective organisms*

Ensure that all equipment in contact with infant is clean

Prevent personnel with upper respiratory tract or communicable infections from coming into direct contact with infant

Isolate other infants who have infections according to institutional policy

Instruct health care workers and parents in infection control procedures

*Administer antibiotics as ordered (specify)

Ensure strict asepsis or sterility with invasive procedures and equipment such as peripheral IV therapy, lumbar puncture, and arterial/venous catheter insertion

EXPECTED OUTCOME

Infant exhibits no evidence of nosocomial infection

NURSING DIAGNOSIS ▦ **Imbalanced nutrition: less than body requirements related to inability to ingest nutrients because of immaturity or illness**

PATIENT GOAL 1: Will receive adequate nourishment, with caloric intake to maintain positive nitrogen balance and exhibit appropriate weight gain

NURSING INTERVENTIONS/*RATIONALES*

*Maintain parenteral fluid or total parenteral nutrition therapy as ordered (specify)

Monitor for signs of intolerance to total parenteral therapy, especially protein and glucose

Assess readiness to nipple-feed: ability to maintain quiet alert state and ability to coordinate swallowing and breathing

Provide opportunities for the medically stable infant to "practice breast-feeding"

Provide nonnutritive sucking before bottle- or breast-feeding and during gavage feeding *to enhance digestion of nutrients, bring to quiet alert state for feeding, and promote neurobehavioral regulation*

Nipple feed infant if strong sucking, swallowing, and gag reflexes are present (usually at gestational age of 34 to 35 weeks) *to minimize risk of aspiration*

Follow unit protocol for advancing volume and concentration of formula *to avoid feeding intolerance*

Use orogastric feeding if infant tires easily or has weak sucking, gag, or swallowing reflexes, *because prolonged or stressful nipple feeding may result in weight loss*

Assist mother with expressing breast milk *to establish and maintain lactation until infant can breast-feed*

Assist mother with breast-feeding when feasible and desirable

EXPECTED OUTCOMES

Infant receives an adequate amount of calories and essential nutrients

Infant demonstrates a steady weight gain (approximately 20 to 30 g/day) after acute phase of illness

NURSING DIAGNOSIS ▦ **Risk for imbalanced fluid volume related to immature physiologic characteristics of preterm infant or immaturity or illness**

PATIENT GOAL 1: Will exhibit adequate hydration status

NURSING INTERVENTIONS/*RATIONALES*

Monitor fluid and electrolytes closely when therapies that increase insensible water loss (IWL) (e.g., phototherapy, radiant warmer) are used

Implement strategies to minimize IWL, such as plastic covering, increased ambient humidity

Ensure adequate parenteral/oral fluid intake

Assess state of hydration (e.g., skin turgor, blood pressure, edema, weight, mucous membranes, urine specific gravity, electrolytes, fontanel)

Regulate parenteral fluids closely *to avoid dehydration, overhydration, or extravasation into surrounding tissues*

Avoid administering hypertonic fluids (e.g., undiluted medications, concentrated glucose infusions) *to prevent excess solute load on immature kidneys and fragile veins*

Monitor urinary output and laboratory values *for evidence of dehydration or overhydration* (adequate urinary output 1-2 mL/kg/hr)

Minimize use of adhesives *to preserve intact skin barrier*

EXPECTED OUTCOME

Infant exhibits evidence of fluid homeostasis

NURSING DIAGNOSIS ▦ **Risk for impaired skin integrity related to immature skin structure, physical immobility, decreased nutritional state, and invasive procedures**

PATIENT GOAL 1: Will maintain skin integrity

NURSING INTERVENTIONS/*RATIONALES*

See Guidelines box, Neonatal Skin Care, pp. 239-240

EXPECTED OUTCOME

Skin remains clean and intact with no evidence of irritation, injury or breakdown

*Dependent nursing action

NURSING DIAGNOSIS ▪ **Risk for injury from variable cerebral blood flow, systemic hypertension or hypotension, and decreased cellular nutrients (glucose and oxygen) related to immature central nervous system and physiologic stress response**

PATIENT GOAL 1: Will receive care to prevent injury and maintain appropriate systemic and cerebral blood flow, as well as adequate cerebral glucose and oxygen; will not exhibit evidence of intraventricular hemorrhage (unless preexisting condition)

NURSING INTERVENTIONS/*RATIONALES*

Avoid sudden position changes and transferring from horizontal to vertical position *to minimize autonomic stress and increased intracranial pressure*

Speak softly to infant and call by name before initiating handling for care and procedures

Decrease environmental stimulation: noise, visual, tactile, and vestibular *because stress responses, especially increased blood pressure, increase risk of elevated ICP*

Establish a routine that provides for undisturbed sleep/rest periods *to eliminate or minimize times of stress and to promote adequate sleep/wake cycle*

Use minimal handling, and handle or disturb infant only when absolutely necessary

Keep extra diapers under buttocks to facilitate changing soiled diapers; raise infant's hips, not feet and legs

Organize (cluster) care during normal waking hours as much as possible *to minimize sleep disruption and frequent intermittent noise*

Close and open drapes or dim lights *to allow for day/night schedule*

Cover incubator with cloth and place "do not disturb" sign nearby *to decrease light and alert others to infant's rest period*

Use diffuse lighting; avoid bright examination or procedure lights— shield infant's eyes from same

Refrain from loud talking or laughing

Limit number of visitors and staff near infant

Explain meaning of unfamiliar sounds to family

Keep equipment and other noise to minimum (<50 dB)

  Turn alarms as low as safely possible

  Attend to alarms and telephones immediately

  Place bedside equipment, such as ventilator or IV pump, away from head of bed

  Turn outflow valve from ventilator away from infant's ear

  Turn off bedside equipment that is not in use, such as suction and oxygen

  Avoid loud, abrupt noises, such as discarding items in trash can, dropping items, placing items on top of incubator, closing doors and drawers, heavy traffic

  Avoid use of noisy radios or televisions

Assess and manage pain using pharmacologic and nonpharmacologic methods, *since pain increases blood pressure*

Recognize signs of physical stress and overstimulation *to institute appropriate interventions promptly*

Avoid hypertonic medications and solutions *because they increase cerebral blood flow*

Elevate head of bed or mattress between 15 and 20 degrees *to decrease ICP*

Maintain adequate oxygenation *because hypoxia increases cerebral blood flow and ICP* (see interventions under nursing diagnosis of ineffective breathing pattern on p. 255)

Avoid any sudden turning of head to side, *which restricts carotid artery blood flow and adequate oxygenation to brain*

EXPECTED OUTCOME

Infant exhibits no evidence of increased ICP or IVH

NURSING DIAGNOSIS ▪ **Pain, acute or chronic, related to procedures, diagnosis, treatment**

PATIENT GOAL 1: Will experience no pain or a reduction of pain

NURSING INTERVENTIONS/*RATIONALES*

Recognize that infants, regardless of gestational age, feel pain

Differentiate between clinical manifestations of pain and stress/fatigue (see Boxes 9-2 and 9-4)

*Administer analgesics or topical agents as prescribed and advocate for more effective pain control (specify)

Use nonpharmacologic pain control measures appropriate to infant's age and condition: repositioning, flexion, swaddling, containment, cuddling, rocking (as appropriate), music, reducing environmental stimulation, tactile comfort measures such as firm touching, nesting and nonnutritive sucking (pacifier or breast as appropriate)

Assess effectiveness of nonpharmacologic pain control measures *because some measures (e.g., stroking) may increase premature infant's distress*

Encourage parents to provide comfort measures when possible

Convey an attitude of sensitivity and compassion for infant's discomfort

Discuss with family their concerns about infant's pain

Encourage family to speak with health practitioner about their concerns

EXPECTED OUTCOME

Infant exhibits no or minimal signs of pain

NURSING DIAGNOSIS ▪ **Delayed growth and development related to preterm birth, NICU environment, separation from parents, physiologic immaturity, and effects of concomitant illnesses**

PATIENT GOAL 1: Will attain normal growth and development potential

NURSING INTERVENTIONS/*RATIONALES*

Provide optimum nutrition *to ensure steady weight gain and brain growth*

Provide regular periods of undisturbed rest *to decrease unnecessary O_2 use and caloric expenditure*

Provide age-appropriate developmental intervention, including positioning

Recognize signs of overstimulation (flaccidity, yawning, staring, active averting, irritability, crying) *so that infant is allowed to rest*

Promote parent-infant interaction, *because it is essential for normal growth and development*

Promote self-regulating behaviors (e.g., midline, flexed extremities, hands to mouth, "nesting")

EXPECTED OUTCOMES

Infant exhibits a steady weight gain once past the acute phase of illness

Infant is exposed only to appropriate auditory, vestibular, olfactory, and visual stimuli

Infant demonstrates quiet alert state interspersed with uninterrupted sleep periods of 50 to 60 minutes

*Dependent nursing action

Continued

NURSING CARE PLAN The High-Risk Infant—*cont'd*

NURSING DIAGNOSIS ■ **Interrupted family processes related to preterm birth, situational/maturational crisis, knowledge deficit (birth of a preterm or ill infant), interruption of adequate and appropriate parental interaction**

PATIENT (FAMILY) GOAL 1: Will be informed of infant's progress

NURSING INTERVENTIONS/*RATIONALES*

Prioritize information *to help parents understand most important aspects of care, signs of improvement, or deterioration in infant's condition*

Encourage parents to ask questions about child's status

Answer questions, facilitate expression of concern regarding care and prognosis

Be honest; respond to questions with correct answers *to establish trust*

Encourage mother and father to visit and/or call unit often *so they are informed of infant's progress*

Encourage parents to be involved in aspects of infant's care (as appropriate) *to foster parents' sense of hope, caring and decrease sense of helplessness*

Emphasize positive aspects of infant's status *to encourage sense of hope*

EXPECTED OUTCOME

Parents express feelings and concerns regarding infant and prognosis and demonstrate understanding and involvement in care

PATIENT (FAMILY) GOAL 2: Will exhibit positive parent-infant interaction and attachment behaviors

NURSING INTERVENTIONS/*RATIONALES*

Encourage parents to visit as soon as possible *so that attachment process is initiated*

Encourage parents to:

Visit infant frequently

Touch, hold, and caress infant as appropriate for infant's physical condition

Help parents establish a routine for visiting, handling and touching *to allow uninterrupted periods of infant sleep*

Become actively involved in infant's care

Bring clothing to dress infant as soon as condition permits

Reinforce parents' endeavors *to increase their self-confidence*

Be alert to signs of tension and stress in parents

Enable parents to spend time alone with infant

Help parents interpret infant's responses; comment regarding any positive response and signs of overstimulation, stress or fatigue

Help parents by demonstrating infant care techniques and offer support

Identify resources (e.g., transportation, baby-sitting) *to enable parents to visit*

EXPECTED OUTCOMES

Parents visit infant soon after birth and at frequent intervals

Parents relate positively with infant (e.g., call infant by name, look at and touch infant)

Parents provide care for infant and demonstrate an attitude of comfort in relationships with infant

Parents identify signs of stress or fatigue in infant

PATIENT (SIBLINGS) GOAL 3: Will exhibit positive sibling-infant interaction and attachment behaviors

NURSING INTERVENTIONS/*RATIONALES*

Encourage siblings to visit infants when feasible

Explain environment, events, appearance of infant, and why infant cannot come home *to prepare them for* visiting

Provide photos of infant or other items if siblings are unable to visit

Encourage siblings to make pictures or bring other small items, such as a letter or drawing, for infant and place in incubator or crib

EXPECTED OUTCOMES

Siblings visit infant in NICU or nursery

Siblings exhibit an understanding of explanations (specify)

Siblings receive infant-related items (specify)

PATIENT (FAMILY) GOAL 4: Will be prepared for home care

NURSING INTERVENTIONS/*RATIONALES*

Assess readiness of family (especially mother or other primary caregiver) to care for infant in home setting *to facilitate parents' transition to home with infant*

Teach necessary infant care techniques and observations

Encourage parent(s), when possible, to spend one or two nights in a hospital predischarge room before discharge with infant *to foster confidence in caring for infant at home*

Reinforce follow-up medical care

Refer to appropriate agencies or services *so that needed assistance is provided*

Encourage and facilitate involvement with parent support group or refer to appropriate support group(s) *for ongoing support*

Offer family opportunity to learn infant cardiopulmonary resuscitation and response to choking incident

EXPECTED OUTCOMES

Family demonstrates ability to provide care for infant

Family members state how and when to contact available services

Family members recognize importance of follow-up medical care

NURSING DIAGNOSIS ■ **Anticipatory grieving related to unexpected birth of high-risk infant, grave prognosis, or death of infant**

PATIENT (FAMILY) GOAL 1: Will acknowledge possibility of child's death and demonstrate healthy grieving behaviors

NURSING INTERVENTIONS/*RATIONALES*

Provide family with the opportunity to hold their infant before death and, if possible, to be present at the time of death

Support family's decision for terminating life support and end-of-life care

Arrange for or perform appropriate baptism rite for infant

Provide family with the opportunity to see, touch, hold, bathe, caress, examine, and talk to their infant privately before and after death

Keep infant's body available for a few hours *to give family members who are hesitant an opportunity to see deceased infant if they change their minds; rewarm as necessary*

Provide photographs taken before and after infant's death for family *to refer to at a later time to make infant real*

NURSING CARE PLAN The High-Risk Infant—*cont'd*

Take photograph of infant being held or touched by an adult; avoid morgue-type photograph *because it depersonalizes child*

Dress infant in an appropriate dress or suit *to personalize child*

Provide other tangible remembrances of child's death (e.g., name card, identification band, lock of hair, footprints, blanket, clothing, toy)

Encourage family to name infant if they have not done so

Identify resources to assist with funeral arrangements *to facilitate parental grieving*

EXPECTED OUTCOME

Family discusses the reality of the death and conveys an attitude of realization

---

PATIENT (FAMILY) GOAL 2: Will receive adequate emotional and physical support

NURSING INTERVENTIONS/*RATIONALES*

Be available to family *to provide support*

Provide appropriate religious support (e.g., clergy)

Discuss infant's illness and end-of-life care with family (as appropriate)

Talk with family openly and honestly about funeral arrangements

Have information available regarding inexpensive services in the community

Inform family of all options available *so that they can make informed decisions*

Provide opportunity for family to call or visit the unit if they have any questions regarding infant's illness and death

May contact family after the death *to assess coping and status of grieving process*

Refer family to appropriate support group(s) *for ongoing support*

EXPECTED OUTCOMES

Family grieves for infant's death appropriately

Family demonstrates appropriate (influenced by cultural, religious, and social factors) grieving behaviors over infant's death

---

BOX 9-6 ■ Etiology of Preterm Birth

Unknown
  Maternal Factors
    Malnutrition
    Chronic diseases
      Heart disease
      Renal disease
      Diabetes
  Factors Related to Pregnancy
    Hypertension
    Abruptio placenta or placenta previa
    Incompetent cervix
    Premature rupture of membranes or chorioamnionitis
    Polyhydramnios
  Fetal Factors
    Chromosomal abnormalities
    Intrauterine infection
    Anatomic abnormalities

---

problems that interrupt the normal course of gestation before completion of fetal development, are responsible for a large number of preterm births.

The outlook for preterm infants is largely, but not entirely, related to the state of physiologic and anatomic immaturity of the various organs and systems at the time of birth. Infants at term have advanced to a state of maturity sufficient to allow a successful transition to the extrauterine environment. Infants born prematurely must make the same adjustments but with functional immaturity proportional to the stage of development reached at the time of birth. The degree to which infants are prepared for extrauterine life can be predicted to some extent by birth weight and estimated gestational age (see Clinical Assessment of Gestational Age, Chapter 8).

Diagnostic Evaluation

Preterm infants have a number of distinct characteristics at various stages of development. Identification of these characteristics provides valuable clues to the gestational age and hence to the physiologic capabilities of infants. The general, outward physical appearance changes as the fetus progresses to maturity. Characteristics of skin, general attitude (or posture) when supine, appearance of hair, and amount of subcutaneous fat provide cues to a newborn's physical development. Observation of spontaneous, active movements and response to stimulation and passive movement contribute to the assessment of neurologic status. The appraisal is made as soon as possible after admission to the nursery, because much of the observation and management of infants depends on this information.

On inspection, preterm infants are very small and appear scrawny because they lack or have only minimal subcutaneous fat deposits (or none in some cases) and have a proportionately large head in relation to the body, which reflects the cephalocaudal direction of growth. The skin is bright pink (often translucent, depending on the degree of immaturity), smooth, and shiny (may be edematous), with small blood vessels clearly visible underneath the thin epidermis. The fine lanugo hair is abundant over the body (depending on gestational age) but is sparse, fine, and fuzzy on the head. The ear cartilage is soft and pliable, and the soles and palms have minimal creases, resulting in a smooth appearance. The bones of the skull and the ribs feel soft, and the eyes may be closed. Male infants have few scrotal rugae, and the testes are undescended; the labia and clitoris are prominent in females. Figure 9-13 compares the features of full-term and preterm infants.

In contrast to full-term infants' overall attitude of flexion and continuous activity, preterm infants may be inactive and listless. The extremities maintain an attitude of extension

CLINICAL EVALUATION

PRETERM   TERM

Posture—The preterm infant lies in a "relaxed attitude," limbs more extended; the body size is small, and the head may appear somewhat larger in proportion to the body size. The term infant has more subcutaneous fat tissue and rests in a more flexed attitude.

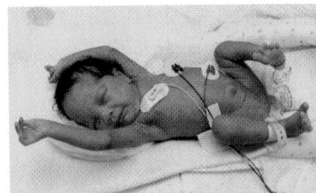 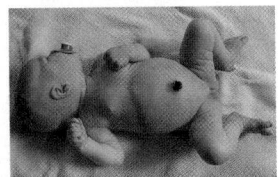

Ear—The preterm infant's ear cartilages are poorly developed, and the ear may fold easily; the hair is fine and feathery, and lanugo may cover the back and face. The mature infant's ear cartilages are well formed, and the hair is more likely to form firm, separate strands.

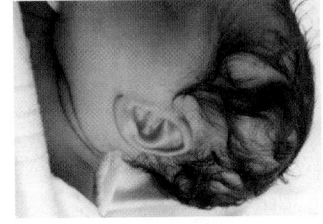 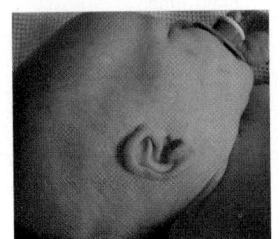

Sole—The sole of the foot of the preterm infant appears more turgid and may have only fine wrinkles. The mature infant's sole (foot) is well and deeply creased.

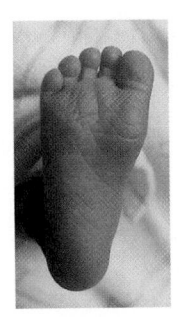 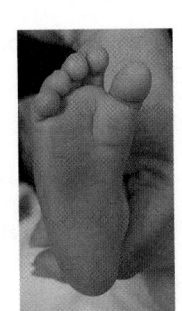

Female genitalia—The preterm female infant's clitoris is prominent, and labia majora are poorly developed and gaping. The mature female infant's labia majora are fully developed, and the clitoris is not as prominent.

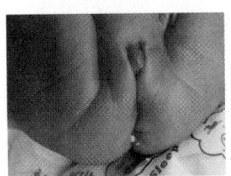 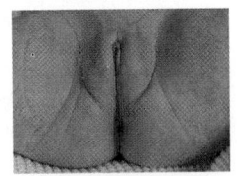

Male genitalia—The preterm male infant's scrotum is undeveloped and not pendulous; minimal rugae are present, and the testes may be in the inguinal canals or in the abdominal cavity. The term male infant's scrotum is well developed, pendulous, and rugated, and the testes are well down in the scrotal sac.

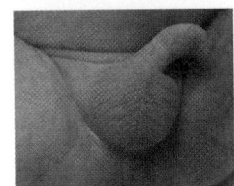 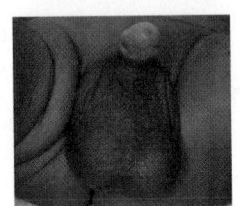

Scarf sign—The preterm infant's elbow may be easily brought across the chest with little or no resistance. The mature infant's elbow may be brought to the midline of the chest, resisting attempts to bring the elbow past the midline.

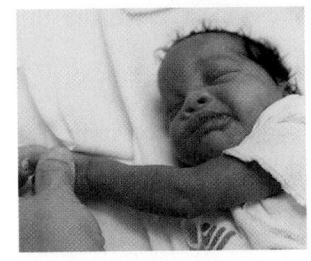 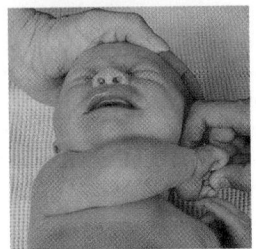

FIG. 9-13 ■ Clinical and neurologic examinations comparing preterm and full-term infants. (Photos by Paul Vincent Kuntz, Texas Children's Hospital, Houston, Tex.)

NEUROLOGIC EVALUATION

PRETERM   TERM

Grasp reflex—The preterm infant's grasp is weak; the term infant's grasp is strong, allowing the infant to be lifted up from the mattress.

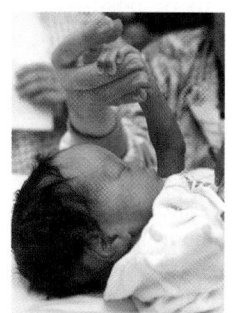
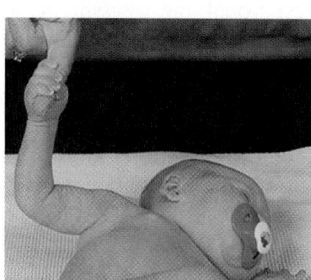

Heel-to-ear maneuver—The preterm infant's heel is easily brought to the ear, meeting with no resistance. This maneuver is not possible in the term infant, since there is considerable resistance at the knee.

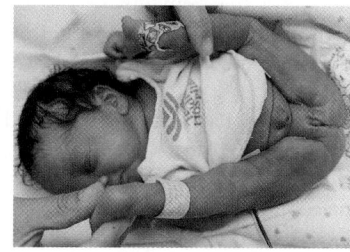
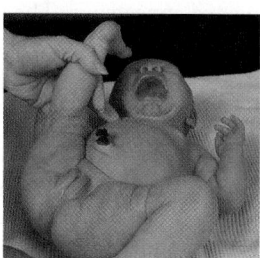

FIG. 9-13—cont'd ■ Clinical and neurologic examinations comparing preterm and full-term infants. (Photos by Paul Vincent Kuntz, Texas Children's Hospital, Houston, Tex.)

and remain in any position in which they are placed. Reflex activity is only partially developed—sucking is absent, weak, or ineffectual; swallow, gag, and cough reflexes are absent or weak; and other neurologic signs are absent or diminished. Physiologically immature, preterm infants are unable to maintain body temperature, have limited ability to excrete solutes in the urine, and have increased susceptibility to infection. A pliable thorax, immature lung tissue, and an immature regulatory center lead to periodic breathing, hypoventilation, and frequent periods of apnea. They are more susceptible to biochemical alterations such as hyperbilirubinemia and hypoglycemia, and they have a higher extracellular water content that renders them more vulnerable to fluid and electrolyte derangements. Preterm infants exchange fully half of their extracellular fluid volume every 24 hours as compared with one seventh of the volume in adults.

The soft cranium is subject to characteristic nonintentional deformation, or "preemie head," caused by positioning from one side to the other on a mattress. The head looks disproportionately longer from front to back, is flattened on both sides, and lacks the usual convexity seen at the temporal and parietal areas. This positional molding is often a concern to parents and may influence the parents' perception of the infant's attractiveness and their responsiveness to the infant. Positioning the infant on a waterbed or gel mattress can reduce or minimize cranial molding.

Neurologic impairment (such as intraventricular hemorrhage) and serious sequelae correlate with the size and gestational age of infants at birth and with the severity of neonatal complications. The greater the degree of immaturity, the greater the degree of potential disability. A greater incidence of cerebral palsy, attention deficit hyperactivity disorder, visual-motor deficits, and altered intellectual functioning is observed in preterm than in full-term infants. However, behavioral development can be enhanced when families are provided with support and infants are referred to appropriate services for neurologic and developmental interventions. Parental interest and involvement are very important variables in the developmental progress of infants.

Therapeutic Management

When delivery of a preterm infant is anticipated, the intensive care nursery is alerted and a team approach implemented. Ideally, a neonatologist, an advanced practice nurse, a staff nurse, and a respiratory therapist are present for the delivery. Infants who do not require resuscitation are immediately transferred in a heated incubator to the NICU, where they are weighed and where IV lines, oxygen therapy, and other therapeutic interventions are initiated as needed. Resuscitation is conducted in the delivery area until infants can be safely transported to the NICU.

Subsequent care is determined by the status of the infant. The general care of the preterm infant differs from that of the full-term infant primarily in the areas of respiratory support, temperature regulation, nutrition, susceptibility to infection, activity intolerance, and other consequences of physical immaturity.

Nursing Considerations

The nursing care, like the therapeutic management, is individualized for each infant. See appropriate discussions under Nursing Care of the High-Risk Newborn and Family for additional details of care.

POSTMATURE INFANTS

Infants born of a gestation that extends beyond 42 weeks as calculated from the mother's last menstrual period (or by gestational age assessment) are considered to be postmature, or postterm, regardless of birth weight. This constitutes 3.5% to 15% of all pregnancies. The cause of delayed birth is unknown. Some infants are appropriate for gestational age but show the characteristics of progressive placental dysfunction. These infants, often called postmature infants, display characteristics such as absence of lanugo, little if any vernix caseosa, abundant scalp hair, and long fingernails. The skin is often cracked, parchment-like, and desquamating. A common finding in postmature infants is a wasted physical appearance that reflects intrauterine deprivation. Depletion of subcutaneous fat gives them a thin, elongated appearance. The little vernix caseosa that remains in the skinfolds may be stained a deep yellow or green, which is usually an indication of meconium in the amniotic fluid.

There is a significant increase in fetal and neonatal mortality in postterm infants as compared with those born at term. They are especially prone to fetal distress associated with the decreasing efficiency of the placenta, macrosomia, and meconium aspiration syndrome. The greatest risk occurs during the stresses of labor and delivery, particularly in infants of *primigravidas*, or women delivering their first child. Close surveillance with fetal assessment and induction of labor is usually recommended when infants are significantly overdue.

HIGH RISK RELATED TO PHYSIOLOGIC FACTORS

HYPERBILIRUBINEMIA

The term *hyperbilirubinemia* refers to an excessive level of accumulated bilirubin in the blood and is characterized by *jaundice,* or *icterus,* a yellowish discoloration of the skin, sclerae, and nails. Hyperbilirubinemia is a common finding in the newborn and in most instances is relatively benign. However, in extreme cases, it can indicate a pathologic state.

Hyperbilirubinemia may result from increased unconjugated or conjugated bilirubin. The unconjugated form or indirect hyperbilirubinemia (Table 9-4) is the type most commonly seen in newborns. The following discussion of hyperbilirubinemia is limited to unconjugated hyperbilirubinemia.

TABLE 9-4 ■ Comparison of Major Types of Unconjugated Hyperbilirubinemia*

PHYSIOLOGIC JAUNDICE	BREAST-FEEDING–ASSOCIATED JAUNDICE (EARLY ONSET)	BREAST MILK JAUNDICE (LATE ONSET)	HEMOLYTIC DISEASE
CAUSE			
Immature hepatic function plus increased bilirubin load from red blood cell (RBC) hemolysis	Decreased milk intake related to fewer calories consumed by infant before mother's milk is well established; enterohepatic shunting	Possible factors in breast milk that prevent bilirubin conjugation Less frequent stooling	Blood antigen incompatibility causes hemolysis of large numbers of RBCs Liver unable to conjugate and excrete excess bilirubin from hemolysis
ONSET			
After 24 hours (preterm infants, prolonged)	Second to fourth day	Fifth to seventh day	During first 24 hours (levels increase faster than 5 mg/dL/day)
PEAK			
72-90 hours	Third to fifth day	Tenth to fifteenth day	Variable
DURATION			
Declines on fifth to seventh day	Variable	May remain jaundiced for 3-12 weeks or more	Dependent on severity and treatment
THERAPY			
Phototherapy if bilirubin levels increase significantly (rise in bilirubin greater than 5 mg/dL/day)	Frequent (10-12 times/day) breast-feeding Phototherapy for bilirubin 17-22 mg/dL in healthy term infants (Maisels, 1994) and continue breast-feeding; possibly alternate formula feedings; avoid glucose water and water supplements	Increase frequency of breast-feeding; use no supplementation such as glucose water; cessation of breast-feeding no longer recommended If bilirubin levels reach 16 mg/dL, may discontinue breast-feeding for 12 hours; if bilirubin levels decrease, breast-feeding can resume May include home phototherapy without discontinuing breast-feeding	*Postnatal*—Phototherapy; if severe, exchange transfusion *Prenatal*—Transfusion (fetus) Prevent sensitization (Rh incompatibility) of Rh-negative mother with RHIG (RhoGAM)

*Table depicts patterns of jaundice in term infants; patterns in preterm infants will vary according to factors such as gestational age, birth weight, and illness.

Pathophysiology

Bilirubin is one of the breakdown products of the hemoglobin that results from red blood cell (RBC) destruction. When RBCs are destroyed, the breakdown products are released into the circulation, where the hemoglobin splits into two fractions: heme and globin. The globin (protein) portion is used by the body, and the heme portion is converted to *unconjugated bilirubin,* an insoluble substance bound to albumin.

In the liver the bilirubin is detached from the albumin molecule and, in the presence of the enzyme *glucuronyl transferase,* is conjugated with glucuronic acid to produce a highly soluble substance, *conjugated bilirubin,* which is then excreted into the bile. In the intestine, bacterial action reduces the conjugated bilirubin to urobilinogen, the pigment that gives stool its characteristic color. Most of the reduced bilirubin is excreted through the feces; a small amount is eliminated in the urine.

Normally the body is able to maintain a balance between the destruction of RBCs and the use or excretion of byproducts. However, when developmental limitations or a pathologic process interferes with this balance, bilirubin accumulates in the tissues to produce jaundice. Possible causes of hyperbilirubinemia in the newborn are:

- Physiologic (developmental) factors (prematurity)
- An association with breast-feeding or breast milk
- Excess production of bilirubin (e.g., hemolytic disease, biochemical defects, bruises)
- Disturbed capacity of the liver to secrete conjugated bilirubin (e.g., enzyme deficiency, bile duct obstruction)
- Combined overproduction and undersecretion (e.g., sepsis)
- Some disease states (e.g., hypothyroidism, galactosemia, infant of a diabetic mother)
- Genetic predisposition to increased production (Native Americans, Asians)

The most common cause of hyperbilirubinemia is the relatively mild and self-limited *physiologic jaundice,* or *icterus neonatorum.* Unlike hemolytic disease of the newborn (see p. 268), physiologic jaundice is not associated with any pathologic process. Although almost all newborns experience elevated bilirubin levels, only about half demonstrate observable signs of jaundice.

Two phases of physiologic jaundice have been identified in term infants. In the first phase, bilirubin levels gradually increase to approximately 6 mg/dL on the third day of life, then decrease to a plateau of 2 to 3 mg/dL by the fifth day. Bilirubin levels maintain a steady plateau state in the second phase without increasing or decreasing until approximately 12 to 14 days, at which time levels decrease to the normal value of 1 mg/dL (Volpe, 2001; Maisels, 1999). This pattern varies according to racial group, method of feeding (breast versus bottle), and gestational age (Maisels, 1999). In preterm infants serum bilirubin levels may peak as high as 10 to 12 mg/dL at 4 to 5 days and decrease slowly over a period of 2 to 4 weeks (Blackburn, 1995; Gartner, 1994).

On average, newborns produce twice as much bilirubin as do adults because of higher concentrations of circulating erythrocytes and a shorter life span of RBCs (only 70 to 90 days, in contrast to 120 days in older children and adults). In addition, the ability of the liver to conjugate bilirubin is reduced because of limited production of glucuronyl transferase. Newborns also have a lower plasma-binding capacity for bilirubin because of reduced albumin concentrations as compared with older children. Normal changes in hepatic circulation after birth may contribute to excess demands on liver function.

Normally, conjugated bilirubin is reduced to *urobilinogen* by the intestinal flora and excreted in feces. However, the sterile and less motile newborn bowel is initially less effective in excreting urobilinogen. In the newborn intestine the enzyme β-glucuronidase is able to convert conjugated bilirubin into the unconjugated form, which is subsequently reabsorbed by the intestinal mucosa and transported to the liver. This process, known as *enterohepatic circulation,* or *shunting,* is accentuated in the newborn and is thought to be a primary mechanism in physiologic jaundice (Maisels, 1999). Feeding (1) stimulates peristalsis and produces more rapid passage of meconium, thus diminishing the amount of reabsorption of unconjugated bilirubin, and (2) introduces bacteria to aid in the reduction of bilirubin to urobilinogen. Colostrum, a natural cathartic, facilitates meconium evacuation.

Breast-feeding is associated with an increased incidence of jaundice. Two types have been identified. *Breast-feeding–associated jaundice (early-onset jaundice)* begins at 2 to 4 days of age and occurs in approximately 10% to 25% of breast-fed newborns. The jaundice is related to the process of breast-feeding and probably results from decreased caloric and fluid intake by breast-fed infants before the milk supply is well established, because fasting is associated with decreased hepatic clearance of bilirubin (Porter and Dennis, 2002).

Breast milk jaundice (late-onset jaundice) begins at age 5 to 7 days and occurs in 2% to 3% of breast-fed infants. Rising levels of bilirubin peak during the second week and gradually diminish. Despite high levels of bilirubin that may persist for 3 to 12 weeks, these infants are well. The jaundice may be caused by factors in the breast milk (pregnanediol, fatty acids, and β-glucuronidase) that either inhibit the conjugation or decrease the excretion of bilirubin. Less frequent stooling by breast-fed infants may allow for extended time for reabsorption of bilirubin from stools.

Diagnostic Evaluation

The degree of jaundice is determined by serum bilirubin measurements. Normal values of unconjugated bilirubin are 0.2 to 1.4 mg/dL. In the newborn, levels must exceed 5 mg/dL before jaundice (icterus) is observable (see Table 9-5). It is important to note, however, that the evaluation of jaundice is not based solely on serum bilirubin levels, but also on the timing of the appearance of clinical jaundice, gestational age at birth, age in days since birth, family history including maternal Rh factor, evidence of hemolysis, feeding method, infant's physiologic status, and the progression of serial serum bilirubin levels. The following criteria are indicators of pathologic jaundice that, when present, warrant further investigation as to the cause of the jaundice.

- Appearance of jaundice within 24 hours of birth
- Persistent jaundice after 1 (term neonate) or 2 (preterm) weeks
- Total serum bilirubin levels 12 to 13 mg/dL
- Increase in serum bilirubin 5 mg/dL/day
- Direct bilirubin 1.5 to 2 mg/dL

Noninvasive monitoring of bilirubin via cutaneous reflectance measurements (*transcutaneous bilirubinometry*) allows for repetitive estimations of bilirubin. These devices work well on dark- and light-skinned infants and correlate fairly well with serum determinations of bilirubin levels in full-term infants. With shorter maternity stays, the value of transcutaneous bilirubin measurements as an assessment tool in follow-up home care has been demonstrated in a homogenous population (Ruchala, Seibold, and Stemsterfer, 1996). However, because transcutaneous bilirubin measurements are affected by race, gestational age, and birth weight, their use in heterogenous populations remains limited for diagnostic purposes (Engle and others, 2002; Maisels, 1999). Also, the intensity of jaundice is not always related to the degree of hyperbilirubinemia. Transcutaneous bilirubin measurements may reduce the need for blood sampling in full-term neonates (Briscoe, Clark, and Yoxall, 2002). After phototherapy has been initiated, transcutaneous bilirubinometry is no longer useful as a screening tool.

The use of hour-specific serum bilirubin levels to predict newborns at risk for rapidly rising levels has now become an official recommendation by the American Academy of Pediatrics (2004) for the monitoring of healthy neonates ≥ 35 weeks' gestation before discharge from the hospital. The use of a nomogram with three levels (high, intermediate, or low risk) of rising total serum bilirubin values assists in the determination of which newborns might need further evaluation after discharge (Bhutani, Johnson, and Sivieri, 1999). It is now recommended that healthy infants receive follow-up care and assessment of bilirubin within 3 days of discharge if discharged at less than 24 hours and a risk assessment with transcutaneous bilirubin or the hour-specific nomogram. Newborns discharged at 24 to 47.9 hours should receive follow-up evaluation within 4 days (96 hours), and those discharged between 48 and 72 hours should receive follow-up within 5 days (American Academy of Pediatrics, 2004). The serum bilirubin may be obtained at the time of the metabolic screening, thus precluding the need for additional blood sampling.

Newer technologies that are currently being evaluated for noninvasive monitoring of neonatal serum bilirubin values include carbon monoxide indices in exhaled breath (carbon monoxide is produced when RBCs are broken down) and the use of a transcutaneous bilirubin meter (BiliCheck) that measures the total serum bilirubin and provides a prediction of risk for hyperbilirubinemia in newborns before discharge (Stevens and others, 2001; Bhuttani and others, 2000).

Complications. Unconjugated bilirubin is highly toxic to neurons; therefore, an infant with severe jaundice is at risk of developing *bilirubin encephalopathy* (interchangeably referred to as kernicterus), a syndrome of severe brain damage resulting from the deposition of unconjugated bilirubin in brain cells. *Kernicterus* describes the yellow staining of the brain cells that may result in bilirubin encephalopathy (Canadian Pediatric Society, 1999). The damage occurs when the serum concentration reaches toxic levels, regardless of cause. There is evidence that a fraction of unconjugated bilirubin crosses the blood-brain barrier in neonates with physiologic hyperbilirubinemia. When certain pathologic conditions exist in addition to elevated bilirubin levels, there is an increase in the permeability of the blood-brain barrier to unconjugated bilirubin and, thus,

potential irreversible damage. The exact level of serum bilirubin required to cause damage is not yet known.

Multiple factors contribute to bilirubin neurotoxicity; therefore, *serum bilirubin levels alone do not predict the risk of brain injury.* Factors that enhance the development of bilirubin encephalopathy include metabolic acidosis, lowered serum albumin levels, intracranial infections such as meningitis, and abrupt increases in blood pressure. In addition, any condition that increases the metabolic demands for oxygen or glucose (e.g., fetal distress, hypoxia, hypothermia, hypoglycemia) also increases the risk of brain damage despite lower serum levels of bilirubin.

The signs of bilirubin encephalopathy are those of central nervous system depression or excitation. Prodromal symptoms consist of decreased activity, lethargy, irritability, hypotonia and seizures. Later these subtle findings are followed by development of athetoid cerebral palsy, mental retardation, and deafness (Canadian Pediatric Society, 1999). Those who survive may eventually show evidence of neurologic damage, such as mental retardation, attention deficit hyperactivity disorder, delayed or abnormal motor movement (especially ataxia or athetosis), behavior disorders, perceptual problems, or sensorineural hearing loss.

Therapeutic Management

The primary goals in the treatment of hyperbilirubinemia are to prevent bilirubin encephalopathy and, as in any blood group incompatibility, to reverse the hemolytic process (p. 268). The main form of treatment involves the use of phototherapy. Exchange transfusion is generally used for reducing dangerously high bilirubin levels that occur with hemolytic disease.

The pharmacologic management of hyperbilirubinemia with phenobarbital has centered primarily on the infant with hemolytic disease, and phenobarbital is most effective when given to the mother several days before delivery. Phenobarbital promotes (1) hepatic glucuronyl transferase synthesis, which increases bilirubin conjugation and hepatic clearance of the pigment in bile, and (2) protein synthesis, which may increase albumin for more bilirubin binding sites. However, the use of phenobarbital in either the antenatal or the postnatal period has not proved to be as effective as other treatments in reducing bilirubin. Bilirubin production in the newborn can be decreased by inhibiting heme oxygenase—an enzyme needed for heme breakdown (to biliverdin)—with *metalloporphyrins,* especially tin-protoporphyrin and tin-mesoporphyrin. The use of heme-oxygenase inhibitors provides a preventive approach to hyperbilirubinemia (Martinez and others, 1999).

Full-term infants with jaundice may also benefit from early initiation of feedings and frequent breast-feeding. These preventive measures are aimed at promoting increased intestinal motility, decreasing enterohepatic shunting, and establishing normal bacterial flora in the bowel to effectively enhance the excretion of unconjugated bilirubin.

Phototherapy consists of the application of fluorescent light to the infant's exposed skin. Light promotes bilirubin excretion by *photoisomerization,* which alters the structure of bilirubin to a soluble form *(lumirubin)* for easier excretion. Studies indicate that blue fluorescent light is more effective in reducing bilirubin. However, because blue light alters the coloration of the infant, the normal light of fluorescent bulbs

TABLE 9-5 ■ Management of Hyperbilirubinemia in the Healthy Term Newborn

AGE (hours)	TSB LEVEL (mg/dL μmol/L)*			
	CONSIDER PHOTOTHERAPY	PHOTOTHERAPY	EXCHANGE TRANSFUSION IF INTENSIVE PHOTOTHERAPY FAILS	EXCHANGE TRANSFUSION AND INTENSIVE PHOTOTHERAPY
24†	—	—	—	—
25-48	≥ 12 (170)	≥ 15 (260)	≥ 20 (340)	≥ 25 (430)
49-72	≥ 15 (260)	≥ 18 (310)	≥ 25 (430)	≥ 30 (510)
>72	≥ 17 (290)	≥ 20 (340)	≥ 25 (430)	≥ 30 (510)

From American Academy of Pediatrics, Provisional Committee for Quality Improvement and Subcommittee on Hyperbilirubinemia: Practice parameter: management of hyperbilirubinemia in the healthy term newborn, *Pediatrics* 94(4):558-562, 1994.
*TSB indicates total serum bilirubin.
†Term infants who are clinically jaundiced at 24 hours old are not considered healthy and require further evaluation.

in the spectrum of 420 to 460 nm is often preferred so that the infant's skin can be better observed for color (jaundice, pallor, cyanosis) or other conditions. For phototherapy to be effective, the infant's skin must be fully exposed to an adequate amount of the light source. When serum bilirubin levels are rapidly increasing or approximating critical levels, double or intensive phototherapy is recommended; this technique involves the application of conventional overhead lamps while the infant is lying on a fiberoptic blanket. The color of the infant's skin does not influence the efficacy of phototherapy. Best results occur within the first 24 to 48 hours of treatment.

An alternative to traditional phototherapy "bililights" is the *fiberoptic blanket* or *panel* (Wallaby,* Biliblanket†), which consists of a light-generating illuminator, a bundle of plastic fibers affixed to a panel that distributes the energy, and a soft, disposable, light-permeable cover to protect the infant. The blanket delivers therapeutic light consistently and continuously to the infant and achieves the same photoisomerization as conventional phototherapy. The fiberoptic blanket is especially suited for home phototherapy. The portable blanket permits more infant-parent interaction, as well as better temperature control because the infant can be covered. It also eliminates the need for using eye patches *(if eyes are not exposed to a direct light source)* in some cases and placing the lights at the correct distance. However, special caution should be taken to ensure that the plastic pad is completely covered and to prevent exposing the fragile skin of extremely immature or compromised infants to the fiberoptic blanket, because dermal injury has been reported in at least two instances (Woo, 1998; Hussain and Sharief, 1996).

The American Academy of Pediatrics (1994) practice parameter provides suggestions for initiating phototherapy in healthy, term infants (Table 9-5). The authors emphasize that the initiation of phototherapy should always be based on individual clinical judgment rather than serum bilirubin levels alone.

Some clinicians believe that preterm infants have a higher risk of developing pathologic jaundice at lower serum bilirubin levels than do healthy, term infants because of associated illness factors that may increase the entry of bilirubin into the brain; however, research has failed to confirm this belief (Maisels, 1999; Yeo, Perlman, and Hao, 1998). Until further research is completed, the recommen-

dations for starting phototherapy in infants weighing 1500 g is at levels of 5 to 8 mg/dL; for those weighing 1500 to 1999 g, levels of 8 to 12 mg/dL; and for those weighing 2000 to 2499 g, levels of 11 to 14 mg/dL (Maisels, 1999). However, each infant should be carefully evaluated with other illness and risk factors in mind, rather than depending on absolute values for all infants in a specific group.

Recommendations for prevention and management of early-onset jaundice in breast-fed infants include encouraging frequent breast-feeding, preferably every 2 hours, and avoiding glucose water, formula, or water supplementation. Bilirubin levels are monitored in late-onset jaundice, and treatment options vary. Breast-feeding may be discontinued for up to 12 hours when bilirubin levels reach 16 mg/dL. Breast-feeding is resumed after bilirubin levels decrease (Lawrence and Lawrence, 1999). Parents should be offered the option of continuing breast-feeding, because no harmful effects have been found in healthy, term infants with bilirubin levels less than 20 mg/dL who continue to consume human milk (Frank and others, 2002). Based on these findings, Maisels (1999) suggests that when feasible, phototherapy be implemented without the interruption of breast-feeding. Home phototherapy and continued breast-feeding are another option. Phototherapy as a treatment for hyperbilirubinemia is discussed on p. 264.

Prognosis. Early recognition and treatment of hyperbilirubinemia prevents severe brain damage (bilirubin encephalopathy). The characteristic impaired neurologic functions associated with bilirubin encephalopathy include athetosis (involuntary writhing movements), sensorineural hearing loss, paralytic gaze palsy, and other gaze abnormalities. Motor skills are delayed, and dental enamel hypoplasia may also occur.

Nursing Considerations
● Assessment

Part of the routine physical assessment includes observing for evidence of jaundice at regular intervals. Jaundice is most reliably assessed by observing the infant's skin color from head to toe and the color of the sclerae and mucous membranes. Applying direct pressure to the skin, especially over bony prominences such as the tip of the nose or the sternum, causes blanching and allows the yellow stain to be more pronounced. For dark-skinned infants, the color of the sclera, conjunctiva, and oral mucosa is the most reliable

---

*Fiberoptic Medical Products, Inc., Allentown, Pa.
†Ohmeda, Columbia, Mo.

indicator. Also, bilirubin (especially at high levels) is not uniformly distributed in skin. The nurse observes the infant in natural daylight for a true assessment of color.

The transcutaneous bilirubin meter is a useful screening device and is used to detect neonatal jaundice in full-term infants. Because phototherapy reduces the accuracy of the instrument, its value is limited to assessments made before the initiation of phototherapy. Institutions in which the device is used set up their own criteria based on their experience with their particular instrument. Blood samples are also taken for the measurement of bilirubin in the laboratory.

With short hospital stays, jaundice may appear after discharge. A careful history from the parents may reveal significant familial patterns of hyperbilirubinemia (older siblings of the infant). Other considerations in assessment include the ethnic origin of the family (e.g., higher incidence in Asian infants), type of delivery (e.g., induction of labor), and infant characteristics such as weight loss after birth, gestational age, sex, and the presence of any bruising. The method and frequency of feeding are assessed.

NURSING ALERT

Evidence of jaundice that appears before the infant is 24 hours of age is an indication for assessing bilirubin levels.

NURSING ALERT

While blood is drawn, phototherapy lights are turned off and the blood is transported in a covered tube to avoid a false reading as a result of bilirubin destruction in the test tube.

Nursing Diagnoses

Based on the nursing assessment, a number of nursing diagnoses may be evident (Box 9-7). Some are the same as for any high-risk infant; others may be related to concomitant health problems, such as prematurity or sepsis.

Planning

The goals for the infant with hyperbilirubinemia and the family are as follows:

1 Infant will receive appropriate therapy if needed to reduce serum bilirubin levels.
2 Infant will experience no complications from therapy.
3 Family will receive emotional support.
4 Family will be prepared for home phototherapy (if prescribed).

Implementation

Basic nursing care of the child with hyperbilirubinemia differs from that of any newborn infant only in management of specific therapy (see Nursing Care of the Newborn and

BOX 9-7 ■ Nursing Diagnoses: Infant With Hyperbilirubinemia

Body temperature, risk for imbalanced related to use of phototherapy
Fluid volume, risk for deficient related to phototherapy
Family processes, interrupted, related to situational crisis, prolonged hospitalization of infant, or rehospitalization for therapy
Injury, risk for, related to phototherapy

Family, Chapter 8, and Nursing Care of the High-Risk Newborn and Family, p. 229).

Prevention of physiologic and breast-feeding jaundice may be possible with early introduction of feedings and frequent nursing without supplementation. Every effort is made to provide an optimum thermal environment to reduce metabolic needs.

Phototherapy. The infant who receives phototherapy is placed nude under the light source and repositioned frequently to expose all body surface areas to the light. After phototherapy has been initiated, frequent serum bilirubin levels (every 4 to 12 hours) are necessary because visual assessment of jaundice is no longer considered valid.

Several precautions are instituted to protect the infant during phototherapy. The infant's eyes are shielded by an opaque mask to prevent exposure to the light (Fig. 9-14). The eye shield should be properly sized and correctly positioned to cover the eyes completely but prevent any occlusion of the nares. The infant's eyelids are closed before the mask is applied, because the corneas may become excoriated if they come in contact with the dressing. On each nursing shift the eyes are checked for evidence of discharge, excessive pressure on the lids, or corneal irritation. Eye shields are removed during feedings, which provide the opportunity to provide visual and sensory stimulation.

Infants who are in an open crib must have a protective Plexiglas shield between them and the fluorescent lights to minimize the amount of undesirable ultraviolet light reaching their skin and to protect them from accidental bulb breakage. Their temperature is closely monitored to prevent hyperthermia or hypothermia. Maintaining the infant in a flexed position with rolled blankets along the sides of the body helps maintain heat and provides comfort.

Accurate charting is another important nursing responsibility and includes (1) times that phototherapy is started and stopped, (2) proper shielding of the eyes, (3) type of fluorescent lamp (by manufacturer), (4) number of lamps, (5) distance between surface of lamps and infant (should be no less than 18 inches), (6) use of phototherapy in combination with an incubator or open bassinet, (7) photometer measurement of light intensity, and (8) occurrence of side effects.

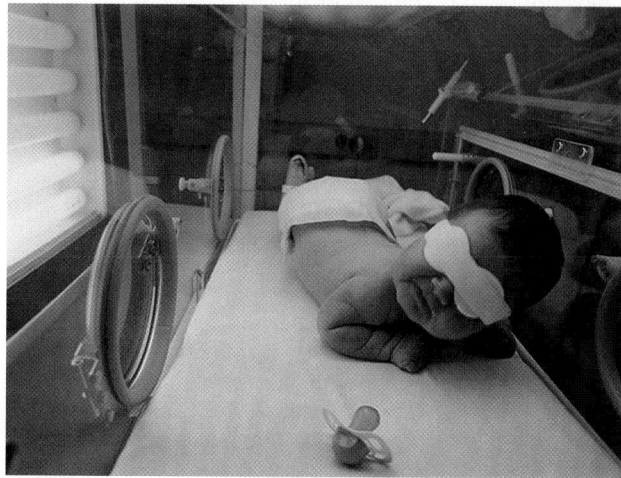

FIG. 9-14 ■ Infant under phototherapy unit. Note that the eyes are shielded and a diaper is used to contain the diarrheal stools.

Minor side effects for which the nurse should be alert include loose, greenish stools; transient skin rashes; hyperthermia; increased metabolic rate; dehydration; electrolyte disturbances, such as hypocalcemia; and priapism. To prevent or minimize these effects, the temperature is monitored to detect early signs of hypothermia or hyperthermia, and the skin is observed for evidence of dehydration and drying, which can lead to excoriation and breakdown. Oily lubricants or lotions are not used on the skin in order to prevent increased tanning or a "frying" effect. Full-term infants receiving phototherapy may require additional fluid volume to compensate for insensible and intestinal fluid loss. Because phototherapy enhances the excretion of unconjugated bilirubin through the bowel, loose stools may indicate accelerated bilirubin removal. Frequent stooling can cause perianal irritation; therefore, meticulous skin care, especially keeping the skin clean and dry, is essential.

After phototherapy is permanently discontinued, there is often a subsequent increase in the serum bilirubin level, often called the "rebound effect"; this is usually transient and resolves without resuming therapy.

Family Support.   Parents need reassurance concerning their infant's progress. All of the procedures are explained to familiarize them with the benefits and risks. Parents need to be reassured that the naked infant under the bilirubin light is warm and comfortable. Parents may be concerned about the eye shields, because "blindness" is a frightening experience. Eye shields are removed when the parents are visiting to facilitate the attachment process. The parents can be reassured that the neonate is accustomed to darkness after months of intrauterine existence and benefits a great deal from auditory and tactile stimulation (see Family Focus box).

The initiation of any treatment requires ***informed consent*** by the parents for the therapy prescribed; however, in the case of phototherapy considerable anxiety may rightfully occur when such words as "kernicterus" and "brain damage" are used to describe possible effects of nontreatment. It is imperative that nurses remain sensitive to parents' feelings and information needs during this process; an important nursing intervention is the assessment of the parents' understanding of the treatment involved and clarification of the nature of the therapy. One of the most important nursing interventions is recognition of breast-feeding jaundice. Lack of familiarity among health professionals has caused many newborns prolonged hospitalization, termination of breast-feeding, and unnecessary phototherapy. Care of the new mother may include supporting successful and frequent breast-feeding. Parents also need reassurance of the benign nature of the jaundice and encouragement to resume breast-feeding if temporary cessation is prescribed. In some situations jaundice may increase the risk of breast-feeding being discontinued and development of the vulnerable child syndrome—the belief of parents that their child has suffered a "close call" and is vulnerable to serious injury (see Critical Thinking Exercise).

Discharge Planning and Home Care.   With short hospital stays, mothers and infants may be discharged before evidence of jaundice is present. It is very important for the nurse to discuss signs of jaundice with the mother, because any clinical symptoms will probably appear at home. Home visits within 2 to 3 days after discharge to evaluate feeding and elimination patterns and jaundice are becoming routine for many health care organizations.

If home phototherapy is instituted, the hospital or home health care nurse is usually responsible for teaching family members and assessing their abilities to implement the treatment safely. General guidelines for home care preparation and education are discussed in Chapter 20. Written instructions and supervision of care—especially the application of eye shields, if needed—are essential. The minor side effects of phototherapy are reviewed, and parents may need instruction in taking axillary temperatures and recording times and amounts of feedings and the number of wet diapers and stools. Regardless of how benign the disorder or the therapy, these parents need support and understanding. Siblings also benefit from an explanation of the therapy to allay fears or misconceptions.

In jaundice associated with breast-feeding, follow-up blood studies are usually required to assess the progress of the jaundice. If temporary cessation of breast-feeding is prescribed, mothers should be taught to pump the breasts every 3 to 4 hours to maintain lactation; the expressed milk is frozen for use after breast-feeding is resumed.

● *Evaluation*

The effectiveness of nursing interventions is determined by continual reassessment and evaluation of care based on the following observational guidelines:

1 Observe skin color; review bilirubinometric or laboratory findings.
2 Observe for signs of neurologic impairment.
3 Check placement of eye shields; observe skin for signs of dehydration; monitor core temperature.
4 Interview family members and observe parent-infant interactions.

Expected outcomes:

1 Healthy newborn begins feeding soon after birth.
2 Parents receive instructions about clinical jaundice before discharge.

FAMILY FOCUS

Phototherapy and Parent-Infant Interaction

The traditional use of phototherapy has evoked concerns regarding a number of psychobehavioral issues, including parent-infant separation, potential social isolation, decreased sensorineural stimulation, altered biologic rhythms, altered feeding patterns, and activity changes. Parental anxiety is greatly increased, particularly at the sight of the newborn blindfolded and under special lights. The interruption of breast-feeding for phototherapy is a potential deterrent to successful maternal-infant attachment and interaction. Because research has demonstrated that bilirubin catabolism occurs primarily within the first few hours of the initiation of phototherapy, there is increased support for the removal of the infant from treatment for feeding and holding. Intermittent phototherapy may be just as effective as continuous therapy when used correctly. The benefits of stopping phototherapy for parental feeding and holding outweigh concerns related to the clearance of bilirubin (Blackburn, 2003). Home phototherapy offers an additional opportunity to foster parent-infant attachment.

??? CRITICAL THINKING EXERCISE ???

Jaundice

A full-term, 5-day-old newborn is brought to the minor emergency department late in the evening for evaluation of newborn jaundice. A home health nurse visited earlier in the day and a serum bilirubin was drawn by heel stick with the results of a total bilirubin 14.6, direct bilirubin 0.9. The father is very concerned because a home health care worker mentioned that the newborn might develop brain damage if the bilirubin levels were to increase to high levels. The mother is breastfeeding every 2-3 hours and the newborn has had four wet diapers and three semiliquid stools over the past 18 hours. The newborn's birth weight was 6 lb, 4 oz, and her current weight (nude) is 6 lb. On examination the infant is active and alert, with visibly jaundiced skin and sclerae, intact reflexes, and strong suck reflex. By history there were no prenatal or delivery complications. Apgar scores at 1 and 5 minutes were 8 and 9, and the initial assessment did not reveal any problems. The mother's blood type is A positive, and the direct Coombs test (DAT) is negative. The newborn was discharged from the birth hospital on the second day of life in apparent good health.

QUESTIONS

1. Evidence—Is there sufficient evidence to draw any conclusions about the newborn's condition at this time?
2. Assumptions—Describe some underlying assumptions about the following:
   a. Newborn jaundice in healthy term infant
   b. Serum bilirubin levels and the newborn's age in days—other pertinent laboratory values—may refer to Table 9-5
   c. Nutritional and excretory function and relation to bilirubin metabolism
   d. The physical status of the infant per assessment data
3. What implications and priorities for nursing care can be drawn at this time?
4. Does the evidence objectively support your argument (conclusion)?
5. Are there alternative perspectives to your argument? What are they?

ANSWERS

1. Yes, there are sufficient data to arrive at some possible conclusions.
2. a. See text pages 263-266
   b. Levels are in acceptable limits based on available data; based on available data, ABO incompatibility–related hemolysis is not evident but may warrant further investigation
   c. Oral intake is adequate; urine and stool output is appropriate
   d. The assessment of behavior and reflexes indicates no particular concerns; the newborn seems to be healthy
3. No immediate intervention to reduce bilirubin is warranted at this time although the treatment is a medical decision. Nursing care should focus on alleviating parents' concerns regarding condition of infant, who appears to be healthy, and address their concerns about the misinformation concerning the potential for brain damage (which is a nonexistent problem at this point). Encourage the mother to continue breastfeeding on demand and observe the infant's activity levels, intake, and urine and stool output. Emphasize that jaundice and hyperbilirubinemia are transient conditions of the newborn. At this point a follow-up appointment should be scheduled with the primary practitioner in 24 hours to monitor the bilirubin level, address the parents' concerns, and monitor the infant's weight.
4. Yes—the infant's laboratory data and physical assessment data support these conclusions. Additionally, knowledge about physiologic hyperbilirubinemia of the newborn supports these conclusions. Phototherapy does not seem warranted at this time based on the available data.
5. One might question the need to interrupt breastfeeding; however, this does not seem necessary at this point. The available data do not point to a pathologic process; however, some may elect to obtain further laboratory data (CBC, reticulocyte count).

---

3 Newborn is exposed to prescribed light source (if phototherapy is indicated).
4 Infant exhibits no signs of adverse effects of phototherapy: eyes remain free of irritation, infant remains well hydrated, and temperature remains below 38° C (100.4° F).
5 Family members demonstrate an understanding of the condition and its therapy; they interact with infant appropriately.
6 Infant displays no evidence of neurologic complications.

HEMOLYTIC DISEASE OF THE NEWBORN

Hyperbilirubinemia in the first 24 hours of life is most often the result of hemolytic disease of the newborn (HDN) (erythroblastosis fetalis), an abnormally rapid rate of RBC destruction. Anemia caused by this destruction stimulates the production of RBCs, which in turn provides increasing numbers of cells for hemolysis. Major causes of increased erythrocyte destruction are isoimmunization (primarily Rh) and ABO incompatibility.

Blood Incompatibility

The membranes of human blood cells contain a variety of *antigens,* also known as *agglutinogens,* substances capable of producing an immune response if recognized by the body as foreign. The reciprocal relationship between antigens on RBCs and antibodies in the plasma causes *aggluti-nation* (clumping). In other words, antibodies in the plasma of one blood group (except the AB group, which contains no antibodies) produce agglutination when mixed with antigens of a different blood group. In the *ABO blood group system* the antibodies occur naturally. In the *Rh system* the person must be exposed to the Rh antigen before significant antibody formation takes place and causes a sensitivity response known as *isoimmunization.*

Rh Incompatibility (Isoimmunization). The Rh blood group consists of several antigens (with D being the most prevalent). For simplicity, only the terms *Rh positive* (presence of antigen) and *Rh negative* (absence of antigen) are used in this discussion. The presence or absence of the naturally occurring Rh factor determines the blood type.

Ordinarily, no problems are anticipated when the Rh blood types are the same in both mother and fetus or if the mother is Rh positive and the infant is Rh negative. Difficulty may arise when the mother is Rh negative and the infant is Rh positive. Although the maternal and fetal circulations are separate, fetal RBCs (with antigens foreign to the mother) sometimes gain access to the maternal circulation through minute breaks in the placental vessels. The mother's

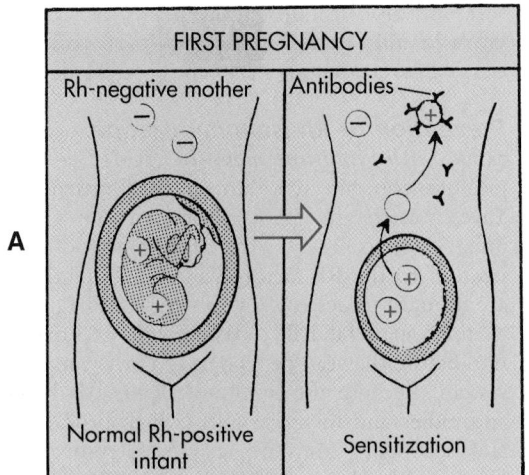 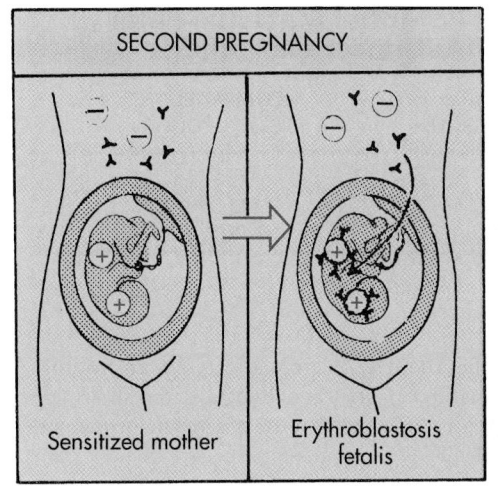

FIG. 9-15 ■ Development of maternal sensitization to Rh antigens. **A,** Fetal Rh-positive erythrocytes enter maternal system. Maternal anti-Rh antibodies are formed. **B,** Anti-Rh antibodies cross placenta and attack fetal erythrocytes.

natural defense mechanism responds to these alien cells by producing anti-Rh antibodies.

Under normal circumstances, this process of isoimmunization has no effect on the fetus during the first pregnancy with an Rh-positive fetus because the initial sensitization to Rh antigens rarely occurs before the onset of labor. However, with the increased risk of fetal blood being transferred to the maternal circulation during placental separation, maternal antibody production is stimulated. During a subsequent pregnancy with an Rh-positive fetus, these previously formed maternal antibodies to Rh-positive blood cells enter the fetal circulation, where they attack and destroy fetal erythrocytes (Fig. 9-15). Multiple gestation, abruption placenta, placenta previa, manual removal of the placenta, and cesarean delivery increase the incidence of transplacental hemorrhage and subsequent isoimmunization (Moise, 2002).

Because the condition begins in utero, the fetus attempts to compensate for the progressive hemolysis and anemia by accelerating the rate of erythropoiesis. As a result, immature RBCs *(erythroblasts)* appear in the fetal circulation, hence the term *erythroblastosis fetalis.*

There is wide variability in the development of maternal sensitization to Rh-positive antigens. Sensitization may occur during the first pregnancy if the woman had previously received an Rh-positive blood transfusion. No sensitization may occur in situations in which a strong placental barrier prevents transfer of fetal blood into the maternal circulation. In approximately 10% to 15% of sensitized mothers, there is no hemolytic reaction in the newborn. In addition, some Rh-negative women, even though exposed to Rh-positive fetal blood, are immunologically unable to produce antibodies to the foreign antigen (Neal, 2001).

In the most severe form of erythroblastosis fetalis *(hydrops fetalis),* the progressive hemolysis causes fetal hypoxia, cardiac failure, generalized edema (anasarca), and effusions into the pericardial, pleural, and peritoneal spaces. The fetus may be delivered stillborn or in severe respiratory distress. Early intrauterine detection of isoimmunization by ultrasonography, amniocentesis, fetal blood sampling, and subsequent

treatment by fetal blood transfusions have dramatically improved the outcome of affected fetuses (Moise, 2002).

ABO Incompatibility. Hemolytic disease can also occur when the major blood group antigens of the fetus are different from those of the mother. The major blood groups are A, B, AB, and O. In the North American white population, 46% have type O blood, 42% have type A blood, 9% have type B blood, and 3% have type AB blood.

The presence or absence of antibodies and antigens determines whether agglutination will occur. Antibodies in the plasma of one blood group (except the AB group, which contains no antibodies) will produce agglutination (clumping) when mixed with antigens of a different blood group. Naturally occurring antibodies in the recipient's blood cause agglutination of a donor's RBCs. The agglutinated donor cells become trapped in peripheral blood vessels, where they hemolyze, releasing large amounts of bilirubin into the circulation.

The most common blood group incompatibility in the neonate is between a mother with O blood group and an infant with A or B blood group (see Table 9-6 for possible ABO incompatibilities). Naturally occurring anti-A or anti-B antibodies already present in the maternal circulation cross the placenta and attack the fetal RBCs, causing hemolysis. Usually the hemolytic reaction is less severe than in Rh incompatibility. Unlike the Rh reaction, ABO incompatibility may occur in the first pregnancy. The risk of significant hemolysis in subsequent pregnancies is thought to be unchanged from that of the first (Luchtman-Jones, Schwartz, and Wilson, 1997).

Clinical Manifestations

Jaundice may appear shortly after birth (during the first 24 hours) in the newborn affected by HDN, and serum levels of unconjugated bilirubin rise rapidly. Anemia results from the hemolysis of large numbers of erythrocytes, and hyperbilirubinemia and jaundice result from the liver's inability to conjugate and excrete the excess bilirubin. Most newborns with HDN are not jaundiced at birth. However, hepatosplenomegaly and varying degrees of hydrops may

TABLE 9-6 ■ Potential Maternal-Fetal ABO Incompatibilities

MATERNAL BLOOD GROUP	INCOMPATIBLE FETAL BLOOD GROUP
O	A or B
B	A or AB
A	B or AB

be evident. If the infant is severely affected, signs of anemia (notably, marked pallor) and hypovolemic shock are apparent. Hypoglycemia may occur as a result of pancreatic cell hyperplasia.

Diagnostic Evaluation

Early identification and diagnosis of RhD sensitization is important in the management and prevention of fetal complications. A maternal antibody titer *(indirect Coombs test)* should be drawn at the first prenatal visit. Genetic testing allows early identification of paternal zygosity at the RhD gene locus, thus allowing earlier detection of the potential for isoimmunization and precluding further maternal or fetal testing (Moise, 2002). Amniocentesis can be used to test the fetal blood type of a woman whose antibody screen is positive. Chorionic villus sampling has drawbacks that preclude its use, including possible spontaneous abortion of the fetus and fetomaternal hemorrhage, which would essentially make the situation worse. An additional diagnostic method to determine isoimmunization is an amniocentesis using polymerase chain reaction to determine the fetal blood type. With either method the determination of an Rh-negative fetus requires no further treatment. Ultrasonography is considered an important adjunct in the detection of isoimmunization; alterations in the placenta, umbilical cord, and amniotic fluid volume, as well as the presence of fetal hydrops, can be detected with high-resolution ultrasonography and allow early treatment before the development of erythroblastosis. Doppler ultrasonography of fetal middle cerebral artery peak velocity has been used to detect and measure fetal hemoglobin and, subsequently, fetal anemia (Moise, 2002). Erythroblastosis fetalis caused by Rh incompatibility can also be monitored by evaluating rising anti-Rh antibody titers in the maternal circulation or by testing the optical density of amniotic fluid (delta OD_{450} test), because bilirubin discolors the fluid (Doyle and others, 1999).

The disease in the newborn is suspected on the basis of the timing and appearance of jaundice (see Table 9-4) and can be confirmed postnatally by detecting antibodies attached to the circulating erythrocytes of affected infants *(direct Coombs test or direct antiglobulin test).* The Coombs test may be performed on cord blood samples from infants born to Rh-negative mothers if there is a history of incompatibility or further investigation is warranted.

Therapeutic Management

The primary aim of therapeutic management of isoimmunization is prevention. Postnatal therapy is usually phototherapy for mild cases and exchange transfusion for more severe forms. Although phototherapy may control bilirubin levels in mild cases, the hemolytic process may continue, causing severe anemia between 7 and 21 days of life.

Prevention of Rh Isoimmunization. The administration of ***Rho immune globulin (RhIg),*** a human gamma globulin concentrate of anti-D, to all unsensitized Rh-negative mothers after delivery or abortion of an Rh-positive infant or fetus prevents the development of maternal sensitization to the Rh factor. The injected anti-Rh antibodies are thought to destroy (by subsequent phagocytosis and agglutination) fetal RBCs passing into the maternal circulation before they can be recognized by the mother's immune system. Because the immune response is blocked, anti-D antibodies and memory cells (which produce the primary and secondary immune responses, respectively) are not formed (Blackburn, 2003; Shaw, 2003). The inhibition of memory cell formation is especially important because memory cells provide long-term immunity by initiating a rapid immune response after the antigen is reintroduced (McCance and Huether, 1998).

To be effective, RhIG (such as RhoGAM) must be administered to unsensitized mothers within 72 hours (but possibly as long as 3 to 4 weeks) after the first delivery or abortion and repeated after subsequent ones. The administration of RhIG at 26 to 28 weeks of gestation further reduces the risk of Rh isoimmunization. RhIG is not effective against existing Rh-positive antibodies in the maternal circulation.

Intrauterine Transfusion. Infants of mothers already sensitized may be treated by intrauterine transfusion, which consists of infusing blood into the umbilical vein of the fetus. The need for therapy is based on the antenatal diagnosis of isoimmunization by determining the optical density of amniotic fluid (by amniocentesis) as an index of fetal hemolysis or by serial ultrasonography, which may detect the presence of fetal hydrops as early as 16 weeks of gestation. With the advance of ultrasound technology, fetal transfusion may be accomplished directly via the umbilical vein, infusing Rh O-negative packed RBCs to raise the fetal hematocrit to 40% to 50%; fetal movement and transfusion risks are minimized by administering vecuronium bromide for temporary fetal paralysis. The frequency of intrauterine transfusions may vary according to institution and fetal hydropic status yet may be as often as every 2 weeks until the fetus reaches pulmonary maturity at approximately 37 to 38 weeks of gestation (Moise, 2002). The use of intraperitoneal blood transfusions is employed less commonly for isoimmunization because of higher associated fetal risks; however, it may be used for cases in which intravascular access is impossible.

Exchange Transfusion. Exchange transfusion, in which the infant's blood is removed in small amounts (usually 5 to 10 mL at a time) and replaced with compatible blood (such as Rh-negative blood), is a standard mode of therapy for treatment of severe hyperbilirubinemia and is the treatment of choice for hyperbilirubinemia and hydrops caused by Rh incompatibility. Exchange transfusion removes the sensitized erythrocytes, lowers the serum bilirubin level to prevent bilirubin encephalopathy, corrects the anemia, and prevents cardiac failure. Indications for exchange transfusion in full-term infants may include a rapidly increasing serum bilirubin level and hemolysis despite intensive phototherapy (as noted in Table 9-5). An infant born with hydrops fetalis or signs of cardiac failure is a candidate for immediate exchange transfusion with fresh whole blood.

For exchange transfusion, fresh whole blood is typed and crossmatched to the mother's serum. The amount of donor blood used is usually double the blood volume of the infant, which is approximately 85 mL/kg body weight, but is limited to no more than 500 mL. The two-volume exchange transfusion replaces approximately 85% of the neonate's blood.

An exchange transfusion is a sterile surgical procedure. A catheter is inserted into the umbilical vein and threaded into the inferior vena cava. Depending on the infant's weight, 5 to 10 mL of blood is withdrawn within 15 to 20 seconds, and the same volume of donor blood is infused over 60 to 90 seconds. If the blood has been citrated (addition of citrate phosphate dextrose adenine to prevent coagulation), calcium gluconate may be given after the infusion of each 100 mL of donor's blood to prevent hypocalcemia.

> **NURSING ALERT**
>
> RhIG is administered intramuscularly only to Rh-sensitized women—*never* to the newborn or father.

Prognosis. The severe anemia of isoimmunization may result in stillbirth, shock, congestive heart failure, or pulmonary or cerebral complications such as cerebral palsy. As a result of early detection and intrauterine treatment, erythroblastotic newborns are rare and exchange transfusions for the condition are less common. Despite the availability of effective preventive measures, Rh HDN continues to cause significant fetal morbidity and mortality in the United States.

Nursing Considerations

The initial nursing responsibility is recognizing jaundice. The possibility of hemolytic disease can be anticipated from the prenatal and perinatal history. Prenatal evidence of incompatibility and a positive Coombs test result are cause for increased vigilance for early signs of jaundice in an infant.

If an exchange transfusion is required, the nurse prepares the infant and the family and assists the practitioner with the procedure. Documentation of blood volume exchanged, including the amount of blood withdrawn and infused, the time of each procedure, and the cumulative record of the total volume exchanged, is kept. Vital signs, monitored electronically, are evaluated frequently and correlated with the removal and infusion of blood. If signs of cardiac or respiratory problems occur, the procedure is stopped temporarily and resumed after the infant's cardiorespiratory function stabilizes. The nurse also observes for signs of blood transfusion reaction.

Throughout the procedure attention must be given to the infant's thermoregulation. Hypothermia increases oxygen and glucose consumption, causing metabolic acidosis. Not only do these consequences hinder the infant's overall physical ability to withstand the long procedure, but they also inhibit the binding capacity of albumin and bilirubin and the hepatic enzymatic reactions, thus increasing the risk of kernicterus. Conversely, hyperthermia damages the

donor erythrocytes, elevating the free potassium content and predisposing the infant to cardiac arrest.

The exchange transfusion is performed with the infant under a radiant warmer. However, the infant is usually covered with sterile drapes that may prevent the radiant heat from sufficiently warming the skin. The blood is also warmed (using specially designed devices, *never* a microwave oven) before infusion.

After the procedure is completed, the nurse inspects the umbilical site for evidence of bleeding. The catheter may remain in place in case repeated exchanges are required.

> **NURSING ALERT**
>
> Signs of blood exchange transfusion reaction include tachycardia or bradycardia, respiratory distress, dramatic change in blood pressure, temperature instability, and generalized rash.

Family Support. Parents often feel guilty because they think they have caused the blood incompatibility. Parents should never be made to feel responsible or negligent. They are encouraged to verbalize and express their thoughts. Actions that were taken to prevent any problems, such as frequent antepartum examinations and blood tests, should be referred to and praised.

METABOLIC COMPLICATIONS

The high-risk infant is subject to a variety of complications related to physiologic function and the transition to extrauterine life. Prominent among these are fluid and electrolyte derangements, hypoglycemia, and hypocalcemia. These complications often occur concurrently with or as a secondary result of other neonatal disorders and may therefore be difficult to differentiate from other conditions. The major characteristics of hypoglycemia and hypocalcemia are outlined in Table 9-7.

RESPIRATORY DISTRESS SYNDROME

Respiratory distress is a name applied to respiratory dysfunction in neonates and is primarily a disease related to developmental delay in lung maturation. The terms *respiratory distress syndrome (RDS)* and *hyaline membrane disease* are most often applied to this severe lung disorder, which is not only responsible for more infant deaths than any other disease, but also carries the highest risk in terms of long-term respiratory and neurologic complications (see Chapter 23 for a discussion of adult RDS). It is seen almost exclusively in preterm infants. The disorder is rare in drug-exposed infants or infants who have been subjected to chronic intrauterine stress (e.g., maternal preeclampsia or hypertension). Respiratory distress of a nonpulmonary origin in neonates may also be caused by sepsis, cardiac defects (structural or functional), exposure to cold, airway obstruction (atresia), intraventricular hemorrhage, hypoglycemia, metabolic acidosis, acute blood loss, and drugs. Pneumonia in the neonatal period is respiratory distress caused by bacterial or viral agents and may occur alone or as a complication of RDS.

Pathophysiology

Preterm infants are born before the lungs are fully prepared to serve as efficient organs for gas exchange. This appears to be a critical factor in the development of RDS. Although

TABLE 9-7 ■ Metabolic Abnormalities

HYPOGLYCEMIA	HYPOCALCEMIA
DEFINITION	
Blood glucose concentration significantly lower than that in the majority of infants of the same age and weight (usually <45 mg/dL)	Abnormally low levels of calcium in circulating blood
TYPE	
Increased or impaired glucose utilization—Large- or normal-size infants who appear to suffer from hyperinsulinism; infants born to women with diabetes; infants with increased metabolic demands such as those with cold stress, sepsis, or after resuscitation; infants with enzymatic or metabolic endocrine defects *Decreased glucose stores*—Small or growth-restricted infants, premature infants	*Early onset*—Appears in first 48 hours, appears in preterm infants who experienced perinatal hypoxia; sometimes in infant of diabetic mother *Late onset*—Cow's milk–induced hypocalcemia (neonatal tetany); apparent after first 3-4 days (high phosphorus/calcium ratio of cow's milk depresses parathyroid activity, reducing serum calcium levels); infants with intestinal malabsorption, hypoparathyroidism, or hypomagnesemia
CLINICAL MANIFESTATIONS	
Vague, often indistinguishable from other newborn conditions *Cerebral signs*—Jitteriness, tremors, twitching, weak or high-pitched cry, lethargy, limpness, apathy, convulsions, and coma *Other*—Cyanosis, apnea, rapid irregular respirations, sweating, eye rolling, poor feeding Signs often transient but recurrent	*Early onset*—Jitteriness, apnea, cyanotic episodes, edema, high-pitched cry, abdominal distention *Late onset*—Twitching, tremors, seizures
SCREENING	
Bedside monitoring or serum blood glucose should be done for all infants at risk	
LABORATORY DIAGNOSIS	
Plasma glucose concentrations less than 47 mg/dL (2.6 mmol/L) to 50 mg/dL (2.8 mmol/L) in any newborn regardless of gestational age at birth	Serum calcium less than 7.8-8 mg/dL (1.95-2.0 mmol/L) in full-term infant *or* Ionized calcium less than 4.4 mg/dL (1.1 mmol/L)
TREATMENT	
Early feeding in normoglycemic infants (preventive); IV glucose administration if feedings not tolerated or glucose level extremely low	*Early onset*—Increased formula feedings, administration of calcium supplements (sometimes) *Late onset*—Administration of calcium gluconate orally or intravenously (slowly); vitamin D Correct hypoparathyroidism
NURSING	
See Nursing Care of the High-Risk Newborn and Family, p. 229 Identify infants at risk or with hypoglycemia Reduce environmental factors that predispose to hypoglycemia (e.g., cold stress, respiratory distress) Administer IV glucose as prescribed Initiate early feedings in healthy infant Ensure adequate intake of carbohydrate (breast milk or formula)	See Nursing Care of the High-Risk Newborn and Family, p. 229 Identify infants at risk or with hypocalcemia Administer calcium as prescribed* Observe for signs of acute hypercalcemia (e.g., vomiting, bradycardia) Manipulate environment to reduce stimuli that might precipitate a seizure or tremors (e.g., picking up infant suddenly, sudden jarring of crib)

***Nursing Alert:** Calcium preparations should *never* be administered by bolus rapid infusion in infants.

the precise cause is still undetermined, several features in the development of the disorder have been established, and there are a number of interdependent relationships that complicate the situation.

There is evidence of fetal respiratory activity before birth. The lungs make feeble respiratory movements, and fluid is excreted through the alveoli. Because the final un-folding of the alveolar septa, which increases the surface area of the lungs, occurs during the last trimester of pregnancy, preterm infants are born with numerous underdeveloped and many uninflatable alveoli. There is limited pulmonary blood flow, which results from the collapsed state of the fetal lungs—from poor vascular development in general and an immature capillary network in particular. Because of increased pulmonary vascular resistance, the major portion of fetal blood is shunted from the lungs by way of the ductus arteriosus and foramen ovale.

At birth, infants must initiate breathing and keep the previously fluid-filled lungs inflated with air. At the same time, the pulmonary capillary blood flow must be increased approximately tenfold to provide for adequate lung perfusion and to alter the intracardiac pressure that closes the fetal cardiac structures. Most full-term infants successfully accomplish these adjustments, but preterm infants with respiratory distress are unable to do so. Although numerous factors are involved, most authorities believe that the central factor responsible for this adaptation is normal development of the surfactant system.

Surfactant is a surface-active phospholipid secreted by the alveolar epithelium. Acting much like a detergent, this substance reduces the surface tension of fluids that line the alveoli and respiratory passages, resulting in uniform expansion and maintenance of lung expansion at low intraalveolar pressure. Immature development of these functions produces consequences that seriously compromise respiratory efficiency. Deficient surfactant production causes unequal inflation of alveoli on inspiration and the collapse of alveoli on end expiration. Without surfactant, infants are unable to keep their lungs inflated and therefore exert a great deal of effort to reexpand the alveoli with each breath. With increasing exhaustion, infants are able to open fewer and fewer alveoli. This inability to maintain lung expansion produces widespread atelectasis.

In the absence of alveolar stability (normal functional residual capacity) and with progressive atelectasis, pulmonary vascular resistance (PVR) increases, whereas with normal lung expansion it would decrease. Consequently, there is hypoperfusion to the lung tissue, with a decrease in effective pulmonary blood flow. The increase in PVR causes partial reversion to the fetal circulation, with a right-to-left shunting of blood through the persisting fetal communications—the ductus arteriosus and foramen ovale.

Inadequate pulmonary perfusion and ventilation produce hypoxemia and hypercapnia. Pulmonary arterioles, with their thick muscular layer, are markedly reactive to diminished oxygen concentration. Thus a decrease in oxygen tension causes vasoconstriction in the pulmonary arterioles that is further enhanced by a decrease in blood pH. This vasoconstriction contributes to a marked increase in PVR. In normal ventilation with increased oxygen concentration, the ductus arteriosus constricts and the pulmonary vessels dilate to decrease PVR.

Prolonged hypoxemia activates anaerobic glycolysis, which produces increased amounts of lactic acid. An increase in lactic acid causes metabolic acidosis; inability of the atelectatic lungs to blow off excess carbon dioxide produces respiratory acidosis. Acidosis causes further vasoconstriction. With deficient pulmonary circulation and alveolar perfusion, partial pressure of oxygen in arterial blood continues to fall, pH falls, and the materials needed for surfactant production are not circulated to the alveoli.

Pulmonary interstitial emphysema develops in preterm infants with RDS and immature lungs as a result of overdistention of distal airways; this condition further complicates adequate oxygenation in the immature airways.

BOX 9-8 ■ Clinical Manifestations of Respiratory Distress Syndrome

RESPIRATORY SIGNS AND SYMPTOMS
Tachypnea (up to 80 to 120 breaths/min) initially*
Dyspnea
Pronounced intercostal and/or substernal retractions (Fig. 9-16)
Fine inspiratory crackles
Audible expiratory grunt
Flaring of the external nares
Cyanosis or pallor

MANIFESTATIONS AS THE DISEASE PROGRESSES
Apnea
Flaccidity
Absent spontaneous movement
Unresponsiveness
Diminished breath sounds
Mottling

MANIFESTATIONS ASSOCIATED WITH SEVERE DISEASE
Shocklike state
Decreased cardiac output and bradycardia
Low systemic blood pressure

*Not all infants born with RDS will manifest these characteristics; the VLBW and ELBW infant may have respiratory failure and shock at birth because of physiologic immaturity.

Diagnostic Evaluation

The diagnosis of RDS is made on the basis of clinical manifestations (Box 9-8) and radiographic studies. Radiographic findings characteristic of RDS include (1) a diffuse granular pattern over both lung fields that closely resembles ground glass and represents alveolar atelectasis and (2) dark streaks, or bronchograms, within the ground glass areas that represent dilated, air-filled bronchioles. It is important to distinguish between RDS and pneumonia in infants with respiratory distress. The extent of respiratory function and acid-base balance is determined by blood gas analysis. Criteria for visually evaluating the degree of respiratory distress are illustrated in Fig. 9-16. Pulse oximetry and carbon dioxide monitoring, as well as pulmonary function studies, assist in differentiating pulmonary and extrapulmonary illness and are used in the management of RDS.

Therapeutic Management

The treatment of RDS involves immediate establishment of adequate oxygenation and ventilation and supportive care and measures required for any preterm infant, as well as those instituted to prevent further complications associated with preterm birth. The supportive measures most crucial to a favorable outcome are to (1) maintain adequate ventilation and oxygenation, (2) maintain acid-base balance, (3) maintain a neutral thermal environment, (4) maintain adequate tissue perfusion and oxygenation, (5) prevent hypotension, and (6) maintain adequate hydration and electrolyte status. Nipple and gavage feedings are contraindicated in any situation that creates a marked increase in respiratory rate because of the greater hazards of aspiration. In addition, administering enteral substrate to the infant with transient

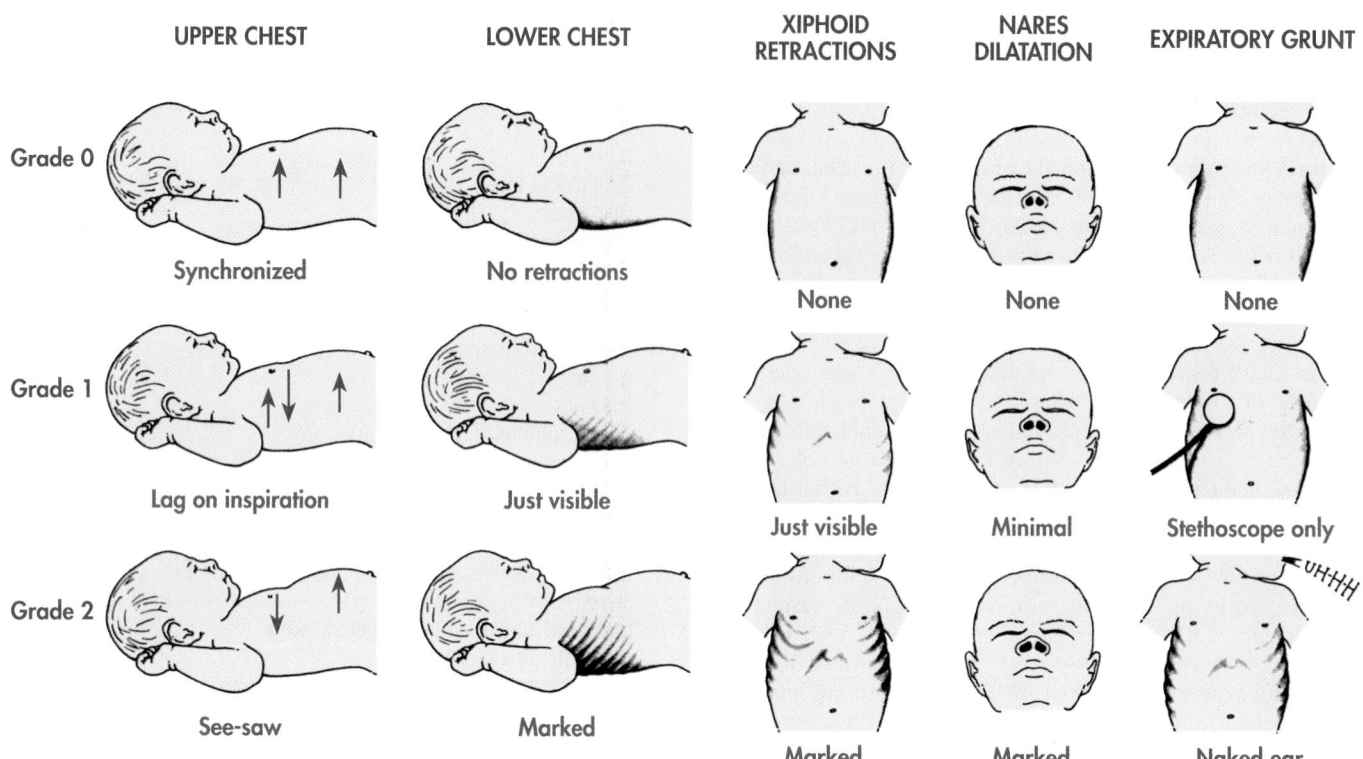

UPPER CHEST	LOWER CHEST	XIPHOID RETRACTIONS	NARES DILATATION	EXPIRATORY GRUNT
Grade 0 Synchronized	No retractions	None	None	None
Grade 1 Lag on inspiration	Just visible	Just visible	Minimal	Stethoscope only
Grade 2 See-saw	Marked	Marked	Marked	Naked ear

FIG. 9-16 ■ Criteria for evaluating respiratory distress. (Modified from Silvermann WA, Anderson DH: *Pediatrics* 17:1, 1956.)

hypoxia places the infant at risk for necrotizing enterocolitis. Nutrition is provided by parenteral therapy during the acute stage of the disease.

The administration of *exogenous surfactant* to preterm neonates with RDS has become an accepted and common therapy in most neonatal centers worldwide. Numerous clinical trials involving the administration of exogenous surfactant to infants with or at high risk for RDS demonstrate improvements in blood gas values and ventilator settings, decreased incidence of pulmonary air leaks, decreased deaths from RDS, and an overall decreased infant mortality rate (Merrill and Ballard, 2003). The overall rates of some associated comorbidities (chronic lung disease, necrotizing enterocolitis, patent ductus arteriosus, intraventricular hemorrhage) have not decreased with surfactant replacement. Exogenous surfactant is derived from a natural source (e.g., porcine, bovine) or from the production of artificial surfactant.

Complications seen with surfactant administration include pulmonary hemorrhage and mucous plugging. Additional studies are under investigation for the potential benefits of surfactant in infants with meconium aspiration, infectious pneumonia, sepsis, persistent pulmonary hypertension, and lung hypoplasia concomitant with congenital diaphragmatic hernia. Surfactant may be administered at birth as a preventive or prophylactic treatment of RDS or later on in the course of RDS as a rescue treatment. Surfactant is administered via an endotracheal (ET) tube directly into the infant's trachea; the exact number of doses (single versus multiple) that is most effective has yet to be determined. Nursing responsibilities with surfactant administration include assistance in the delivery of the product, collection and monitoring of arterial blood gases, scrupulous monitoring of oxygenation with pulse oximetry, and assessment of the infant's tolerance of the procedure. After surfactant is absorbed, there is usually an increase in respiratory compliance that requires adjustment of ventilator settings to decrease mean airway pressure and prevent overinflation or hyperoxemia. Suctioning is usually delayed for an hour or so (depending on the type of surfactant and unit protocol) to allow maximum effects to occur. Current research is in progress to investigate the possibility of delivering an aerosolized surfactant. This method would decrease the problems associated with current delivery systems (contamination of the airway, interruption of mechanical ventilation, and loss of the drug in the endotracheal tubing from reflux).

The goals of oxygen therapy are to provide adequate oxygen to the tissues, prevent lactic acid accumulation resulting from hypoxia, and at the same time avoid the potentially negative effects of oxygen barotrauma. Numerous methods have been devised to improve oxygenation (Table 9-8). All require that the gas be warmed and humidified before entering the respiratory tract. If the infant does not require mechanical ventilation, oxygen can be supplied to a plastic hood placed over the infant's head to supply variable concentrations of humidified oxygen (see Oxygen Therapy, Chapter 22). If oxygen saturation of the blood cannot be maintained at a satisfactory level and the carbon dioxide level ($Paco_2$) rises, infants will require ventilatory assistance.

TABLE 9-8 ■ Common Methods for Assisted Ventilation in Neonatal Respiratory Distress

METHOD	DESCRIPTION	HOW PROVIDED
CONVENTIONAL METHODS		
Continuous positive airway pressure (CPAP)	Provides constant distending pressure to airway in spontaneously breathing infant	Nasal prongs Endotracheal tube Face mask Nasal cannula
Positive end-expiratory pressure (PEEP)*	Provides increased end-expiratory pressure during expiration and between mandatory breaths, which prevents alveolar collapse; maintains residual airway pressure	Endotracheal intubation and either volume-limited or pressure-limited ventilator
Intermittent mandatory ventilation (IMV)*	Allows infant to breathe spontaneously at own rate but provides mechanical cycled respirations and pressure at regular preset intervals	Endotracheal intubation and ventilator
Synchronized intermittent mandatory ventilation (SIMV)	Mechanically delivered breaths are synchronized to the onset of spontaneous patient breaths; assist/control mode facilitates full inspiratory synchrony; involves signal detection of onset of spontaneous respiration from abdominal movement, thoracic impedance, and airway pressure or flow changes	Patient-triggered infant ventilator with signal detector and assist/control mode; endotracheal tube
Volume guarantee ventilation	Delivers a predetermined volume of gas using an inspiratory pressure that varies according to the infant's lung compliance (often used in conjunction with SIMV)	Volume guarantee ventilator with flow sensor; endotracheal tube
ALTERNATIVE METHODS		
High-frequency oscillation (HFO)	Application of high-frequency, low-volume, sine-wave flow oscillations to airway at rates between 480 and 1200 breaths/min	Variable-speed piston pump (or loudspeaker, fluidic oscillator); endotracheal tube
High-frequency jet ventilation (HFJV)	Uses a separate, parallel, low-compliant circuit and injector port to deliver small pulses or jets of fresh gas deep into airway at rates between 250 and 900 breaths/min	May be used alone or with low-rate IMV; endotracheal tube

*Also referred to as conventional ventilation (vs HFV).

Prevention. The most successful approach to prevention of RDS is prevention of premature delivery, especially in elective early delivery and cesarean section. Improved methods for assessing the maturity of the fetal lung by amniocentesis, although not a routine procedure, allow a reasonable prediction of adequate surfactant formation. Because estimation of a delivery date can be miscalculated by as much as 1 month, such tests are particularly valuable when scheduling an elective cesarean section. The combination of maternal steroid administration before delivery and surfactant administration postnatally seems to have a synergistic effect on neonatal lungs, with the net result being a decrease in infant mortality, decreased incidence of intraventricular hemorrhage, fewer pulmonary air leaks, and fewer problems with pulmonary interstitial emphysema and RDS.

Prognosis

RDS is a self-limiting disease. After a period of deterioration (approximately 48 hours) and in the absence of complications, affected infants begin to improve by 72 hours. Often heralded by the onset of diuresis, this improvement has been attributed primarily to increased production and greater availability of surface-active material.

Infants with RDS who survive the first 96 hours have a reasonable chance of recovery. However, complications of RDS include associated respiratory conditions and problems associated with prematurity: patent ductus arteriosus and congestive heart failure, intraventricular hemorrhage, bronchopulmonary dysplasia, retinopathy of prematurity, pneumonia, air leak syndrome, sepsis, necrotizing enterocolitis, and neurologic sequelae.

Nursing Considerations

● *Assessment*

Care of infants with RDS involves all of the observations and interventions previously described for high-risk infants. In addition, the nurse is concerned with the complex problems related to respiratory therapy and the constant threat of hypoxemia and acidosis that complicates the care of patients in respiratory difficulty.

The respiratory therapist, an important member of the neonatal intensive care team, is often responsible for the maintenance of respiratory equipment. Although it may be the responsibility of the respiratory therapist to regulate the apparatus, nurses should understand the equipment and be able to recognize when it is not functioning correctly. The most essential nursing function is to observe and assess the infant's response to therapy. Continuous monitoring and close observation are mandatory because an infant's status can change rapidly and because oxygen concentration and ventilation parameters are prescribed according to the infant's blood gas measurements and pulse oximetry readings.

Changes in oxygen concentration are based on these observations. The amount of oxygen administered, expressed as the fraction of inspired air (FiO_2), is determined on an individual basis according to pulse oximetry or direct or indirect measurement of arterial oxygen concentration. Capillary samples collected from the heel (see Chapter 22 for procedure) are useful for pH and $PaCO_2$ determinations but *not* for oxygenation status. Continuous transcutaneous or pulse oximetry readings are recorded at least hourly. Blood sampling is performed after ventilator changes for the acutely ill infant and thereafter when clinically indicated.

● Nursing Diagnoses

Many of the diagnoses associated with any high-risk infant are appropriate for the infant with RDS. Diagnoses that are more specifically related to respiratory distress are listed in Box 9-9.

● Planning

The major goals for the infant with respiratory distress are the same as for any high-risk infant (such as infant and family support), with special emphasis on respiratory needs:

1 Infant will exhibit optimum air exchange and oxygenation.
2 Infant will exhibit desired respiratory, cardiac, thermoregulatory, neurologic, and metabolic function (unless preexisting conditions are present).

❗ NURSING ALERT

Suctioning is not an innocuous procedure (it may cause bronchospasm, bradycardia resulting from vagal nerve stimulation, hypoxia, or increased intracranial pressure [ICP], predisposing the infant to intraventricular hemorrhage) and should *never* be carried out on a routine basis. Improper suctioning technique can also cause infection, airway damage, or even pneumothoraces.

● Implementation

Mucus may collect in the respiratory tract as a result of the infant's pulmonary condition. Secretions interfere with gas flow and predispose the infant to obstruction of the passages, including the ET tube. Suctioning should be performed only when necessary and should be based on individual infant assessment, which includes auscultation of the chest, evidence of decreased oxygenation, excess moisture in the ET tube, or increased infant irritability. During suctioning a variety of techniques can be used to minimize complications including hyperventilation or hyperoxygenation and the use of a closed suctioning system (Cifuentes, Segars, and Carlo, 2003).

When nasopharyngeal passages, the trachea, or the ET tube is being suctioned, the catheter should be inserted gently but quickly; intermittent suction is applied as the catheter is withdrawn. It is imperative that the time the airway is obstructed by the catheter be limited to no more than 5 seconds, because continuous suction removes air from the lungs along with the mucus. It is recommended that the "two-person" suctioning procedure be used on infants who are acutely ill and who do not tolerate any procedure without profound decreases in oxygen saturation, BP, and heart rate. However, this procedure may not be necessary with an in-line suction device. The object of suctioning an artificial airway is to maintain patency of that airway, not the bronchi. Suction applied beyond the ET tube can cause traumatic lesions of the trachea. Some recommend that the FiO_2 be increased by 10% before suctioning to compensate for a decrease in FiO_2 during the procedure (see Chapter 22). The use of in-line suction catheters may decrease airway contamination and hypoxia.

The most advantageous positions for facilitating an infant's open airway are on the side with the head supported in alignment by a small folded blanket or, when on the back, positioned to keep the neck slightly extended. With the head in the "sniffing" position, the trachea is opened at its maximum; hyperextension reduces the tracheal diameter in neonates. The supported side-lying position can also be used effectively.

Inspection of the skin is part of routine infant assessment. Position changes and the use of water pillows are helpful in guarding against skin breakdown.

Mouth care is especially important when infants are receiving nothing by mouth, and the problem is often aggravated by the drying effect of oxygen therapy. Drying and cracking can be prevented by good oral hygiene using sterile water. Irritation to the nares or mouth that occurs from appliances used to administer oxygen may be reduced by the use of a water-soluble ointment. (See also Nursing Care Plan: The High-Risk Infant, pp. 255-259.)

The nursing care of an infant with RDS is a demanding role; meticulous attention must be given to subtle changes in the infant's oxygenation status. The importance of attention to detail cannot be overemphasized, particularly in regard to medication administration.

● Evaluation

The effectiveness of nursing interventions is determined by continual reassessment and evaluation of care based on the following observational guidelines:

1 Perform frequent respiratory assessment (see assessment guidelines, p. 275).
2 Observe infant's behavior; weigh daily or as prescribed, take vital signs, and observe for signs of sepsis and respiratory complications (atelectasis, pneumothorax, pneumonia).

BOX 9-9 ■ Nursing Diagnoses: Infant With Respiratory Distress Syndrome

Ineffective breathing pattern related to surfactant deficiency, alveolar instability, and pulmonary immaturity
Ineffective breathing pattern related to decreased energy
Impaired gas exchange related to immature alveolar structure
Impaired gas exchange related to inability to maintain lung expansion
Risk for trauma (brain tissue) related to hypoxemia and hypercapnia

Expected Outcomes

1 Respiratory rate and pattern are within appropriate limits for age and weight.
2 Tissue oxygenation is adequate; arterial blood gases and acid-base balance are within appropriate limits for postconceptional age.

RESPIRATORY COMPLICATIONS

The newborn infant is vulnerable to a variety of pulmonary complications, some requiring oxygen therapy (Table 9-9). For example, the preterm infant is subject to periods of apnea, and in term, near-term, and postterm infants, intrauterine stress often causes the fetus to pass meconium, which may be aspirated before or during birth. Oxygen therapy, although life-saving, is not without its hazards. Positive pressure introduced by mechanical apparatus has created an increase in the incidence of ruptured alveoli and subsequent *pneumothorax* and *bronchopulmonary dysplasia (chronic lung disease).* The use of nasal CPAP (continuous positive airway pressure) decreases the incidence of adverse effects associated with intubation and positive pressure ventilation in preterm infants with RDS (Davis and Henderson-Smart, 2003). *Retinopathy of prematurity* is observed almost exclusively in preterm infants and is related primarily to prematurity and oxygen therapy (see Table 9-9; Table 9-11). There has been increased interest in the resuscitation of asphyxiated newborns with 21% oxygen rather than 100% oxygen; preliminary studies demonstrate no significant neurologic morbidities at 18 to 24 months in newborns resuscitated with 21% oxygen (Saugstad and others, 2003). Proponents for room air resuscitation suggest there are fewer complications associated with oxidative stress and hyperoxemia when room air is administered (Vento and others, 2003). Large multicenter studies are currently in progress to determine the optimum concentration of oxygen for resuscitation.

Inhaled nitric oxide (INO), extracorporeal membrane oxygenation (ECMO), and *liquid ventilation* are additional therapies used in the treatment of respiratory distress and respiratory failure in neonates. INO is used in term and near-term infants with conditions such as persistent pulmonary hypertension, meconium aspiration syndrome (see Table 9-9), pneumonia, sepsis, and congenital diaphragmatic hernia to decrease or reverse pulmonary hypertension, pulmonary vasoconstriction, acidosis, and hypoxemia. Nitric oxide is a colorless, highly diffusable gas that can be administered through the ventilator circuit blended with oxygen. INO therapy may be used in conjunction with surfactant replacement therapy, high-frequency ventilation, or ECMO. INO has not proved to be significantly effective in decreasing RDS or in improved survival rates in preterm infants, although clinical trials are still ongoing (Kinsella and others, 1999; Kinsella and Abman, 1999). Clinical trials have demonstrated that the use

TABLE 9-9 ■ Respiratory Complications

DESCRIPTION	CLINICAL MANIFESTATIONS	TREATMENT	NURSING CONSIDERATIONS
MECONIUM ASPIRATION SYNDROME (MAS)			
Aspiration of amniotic fluid containing meconium into fetal or newborn trachea in utero or at first breath	Meconium stained at birth Tachypnea Hypoxia Hyperventilation (early) Hypoventilation (later)	Suction hypopharynx at birth Intubate and suction trachea Treat for respiratory distress Prevent acidosis and hypoxemia May use exogenous surfactant, INO, or ECMO	See Nursing Care of Infant With Respiratory Distress Syndrome, p. 275
APNEA OF PREMATURITY			
Lapse of spontaneous breathing for 20 seconds or longer, that may or may not be followed by bradycardia, oxygen desaturation, and color change	Persistent apneic spells	Observe for apnea Check for thermal stability Administer theophylline or caffeine as ordered Administer nasal continuous positive airway pressure (NCPAP) as ordered	Provide continuous electronic monitoring (respiratory and heart rates) Observe for presence of respirations Observe color Provide gentle tactile stimulation Suction nose and oropharynx if still apneic Apply artificial ventilation with bag-valve-mask and with sufficient pressure to lift rib cage Assess for and manage any precipitating factors (e.g., temperature instability, abdominal distention, ambient oxygen) Observe for signs of theophylline or caffeine toxicity: tachycardia (rate 180 to 190 beats/min) and (later) vomiting, restlessness, irritability Assess skin (with NCPAP) for breakdown, irritation at nasal septum

Continued

TABLE 9-9 ■ Respiratory Complications—*cont'd*

DESCRIPTION	CLINICAL MANIFESTATIONS	TREATMENT	NURSING CONSIDERATIONS
PNEUMOTHORAX			
Presence of extraneous air in pleural space as a result of alveolar rupture	Tachypnea or apnea Systemic hypotension Sudden or persistent oxygen desaturation Grunting, nasal flaring Retractions Absent or diminished breath sounds Shift in point of maximum intensity of heart sounds Bradycardia/cyanosis	Evacuate trapped air in pleural space through needle aspiration or insertion of chest tube	Maintain close vigilance of infants with respiratory distress or those on assisted ventilation Provide appropriate care of chest drainage apparatus Keep emergency needle aspiration setup at bedside
CHRONIC LUNG DISEASE (BRONCHOPULMONARY DYSPLASIA [BPD])			
Pathologic process related to alveolar damage from lung disease, prolonged exposure to high peak inspiratory pressures and oxygen, and immature alveoli and respiratory tract	Dyspnea Barrel chest Inability to wean from mechanical ventilation after course of RDS (surfactant deficiency) Wheezing	Prevention: Administer maternal steroids, exogenous surfactant postnatally Provide early detection with pulmonary function tests Use synchronized or volume guarantee ventilation, decreased inspiratory pressures, or nasal CPAP Prevent air leaks Use high-frequency ventilation Prevent or control respiratory or systemic infections Diagnosis established: Support respiratory efforts Maintain adequate oxygenation and avoid hyperoxemia Administer steroids, diuretics, bronchodilators Provide supplemental oxygen in hospital/home	Provide developmental care and enhancement Provide opportunities for additional rest during feedings Observe for signs of fluid overload or pulmonary edema Assist with home oxygen therapy as needed Assess susceptibility to upper respiratory tract infections and need for frequent hospitalization for respiratory dysfunction Provide increased caloric density (feedings) with medium-chain triglycerides and glucose polymers

of INO improved ventilatory status in infants with pulmonary hypertension, decreased requirements for ventilatory support (Sadiq and others, 2003), and decreased the need for ECMO (Kinsella and Abman, 2000).

ECMO may be used in the management of term infants with acute severe respiratory failure for the same conditions as those mentioned for INO. This therapy involves a modified heart-lung machine, although in ECMO the heart is not stopped and blood does not entirely bypass the lungs. Blood is shunted from a catheter in the right atrium or right internal jugular vein by gravity to a servo-regulated roller pump, pumped through a membrane lung where it is oxygenated and through a small heat exchanger, then returned to the systematic circulation via a major artery such as the carotid artery to the aortic arch. ECMO provides oxygen to the circulation and allows the lungs to "rest," and decreases pulmonary hypertension and hypoxemia in such conditions as persistent pulmonary hypertension of the newborn, congenital diaphragmatic hernia, sepsis, meconium aspiration, and severe pneumonia.

Liquid ventilation has been used experimentally in various neonatal clinical trials to increase pulmonary compliance, decrease lung surface tension, and decrease inflating pressures and subsequent barotrauma in newborn respiratory failure. This therapy involves the use of *perfluorocarbons,* which are inert liquids derived by replacing all the carbon-bound hydrogen atoms on organic compounds with fluorine. Oxygen delivery in the compromised neonate is significantly improved with perfluorocarbons; antibiotics and surfactant may be administered directly into the lungs with liquid ventilation, and removal of debris such as meconium is facilitated.

CARDIOVASCULAR COMPLICATIONS

The most serious cardiovascular disorders of the newborn are the congenital heart defects. Other conditions that oc-

TABLE 9-10 ■ Cardiovascular and Hematologic Complications

DESCRIPTION	CLINICAL MANIFESTATIONS	THERAPEUTIC MANAGEMENT	NURSING CONSIDERATIONS
PATENT DUCTUS ARTERIOSUS (PDA)			
See Chapter 25	Decreased Po_2 Increased Pco_2 Recurrent apnea Bounding peripheral pulses Systolic or continuous murmur	Regulate parenteral fluids Provide respiratory support Administer indomethacin or perform surgical ductal ligation	See Nursing Care of the High-Risk Infant, p. 229
PERSISTENT PULMONARY HYPERTENSION OF THE NEWBORN (PPHN)			
Severe pulmonary hypertension and large right-to-left shunt through foramen ovale and ductus arteriosus	Hypoxia Marked cyanosis Tachypnea with grunting and retractions Decreased peripheral pulses and prolonged capillary refill (poor perfusion) Shock	Regulate IV fluids Provide supplemental oxygen and assisted ventilation Administer vasodilators Maintain acid-base balance Prevent hypoxemia and hypercarbia Administer inhaled nitric oxide or extracorporeal membrane oxygenation (ECMO)	See Nursing Care of the High-Risk Infant, p. 229; Respiratory Distress Syndrome, p. 271 Provide nursing care to reduce stress to infant, especially noxious stimuli that cause increased oxygen demands Decrease physical manipulation and disturbance
ANEMIA			
Loss of blood from hemorrhage during delivery or due to frequent blood specimen withdrawal and inadequate erythropoiesis (in acutely ill infant)	Pallor Apnea Tachycardia Diminished activity Poor feeder Poor weight gain Respiratory distress: grunting, nasal flaring, intercostal retractions Respiratory difficulty	Administer volume expanders for hypovolemia at birth (5% albumin) Transfuse with packed RBCs or administer recombinant human erythropoietin	Use microsamples for blood tests Monitor amount of blood drawn for tests Administer recombinant human erythropoietin as prescribed Administer iron supplements as prescribed
POLYCYTHEMIA/HYPERVISCOSITY SYNDROME			
Venous hematocrit 65% or greater as a result of twin-to-twin, mother-to-fetus transfusion, increased RBC production, or possibly lengthy delay in clamping cord at birth	High incidence of: Cardiovascular symptoms (PPHN, cyanosis, apnea) Seizures Hyperbilirubinemia Gastrointestinal abnormalities	Implement partial exchange transfusion with blood product or appropriate volume expander Provide appropriate therapy for associated problems	See Nursing Care of the High-Risk Infant, p. 229; Hyperbilirubinemia, p. 262
VITAMIN K DEFICIENCY BLEEDING (FORMERLY HEMORRHAGIC DISEASE OF THE NEWBORN)			
Bleeding disorder resulting from transient deficiency of vitamin K–dependent blood factors	Oozing blood from umbilicus or circumcision Bloody or black stools Hematuria Ecchymoses	Administer prophylactic vitamin K	Administer vitamin K via intramuscular route

cur in the newborn period are usually related to prematurity (e.g., anemia, patent ductus arteriosus) or other diseases (e.g., respiratory distress). Some of these disorders are outlined in Table 9-10.

CEREBRAL COMPLICATIONS

Cerebral injury in newborn infants is not an uncommon observation. Newborn infants are particularly vulnerable to ischemic injury caused by variable (both increased and decreased) cerebral blood flow subsequent to asphyxia, and preterm infants, with a fragile cerebrovascular network, are highly prone to periventricular or intraventricular hemorrhage. Fragility and increased permeability of capillaries and prolonged prothrombin time predispose the preterm infant to trauma when delicate structures are subjected to the forces of labor. The more common cerebral complications are outlined in Table 9-11.

The highest incidence of abnormal neurologic findings occurs in infants with intracranial hemorrhage and VLBW. Major neurologic problems, such as cerebral palsy, seizures,

TABLE 9-11 ■ Neurologic Complications

DESCRIPTION	CLINICAL MANIFESTATIONS	THERAPEUTIC MANAGEMENT	NURSING CONSIDERATIONS
RETINOPATHY OF PREMATURITY (ROP)			
Gradual replacement of retina by fibrous tissue and blood vessels Multifactorial etiology	Progressive vascular growth of retina Eventual blindness if not treated Diagnosed by ophthalmologic examination	Prevent preterm birth Provide early screening and detection in infants born at <28 weeks' gestation and weight <1500 g Decrease exposure to bright direct lighting; although exposure to bright light has not proven to contribute to ROP, such exposure is nevertheless undesirable from a neurobehavioral developmental perspective Use supplemental oxygen judiciously and monitor oxygen blood levels carefully; prevent wide fluctuations in oxygen blood levels (hyperoxia and hypoxia) Arrest vascular proliferation process—cryotherapy and laser photocoagulation; surgical repair of detached retina	See Nursing Care of the High-Risk Infant, p. 229 Provide preventive care by closely monitoring blood oxygen levels, responding promptly to saturation alarms, and preventing fluctuations in blood oxygen levels Provide postoperative pain management when surgery is indicated Provide parental education and support Provide nursing care using principles of individualized developmental care
HYPOXIC-ISCHEMIC BRAIN INJURY			
Nonprogressive neurologic (brain) impairment caused by intrauterine or postnatal asphyxia resulting in hypoxemia or cerebral ischemia Hypoxic-ischemic encephalopathy (HIE) is the resultant cellular damage causing the clinical manifestations	Appears within first 6-12 hours after hypoxic episode Seizures Abnormal muscle tone (usually hypotonia) Disturbance of sucking and swallowing Apneic episodes Stupor or coma Muscular weakness in hips and shoulders (full term), lower limb weakness (preterm)	Prevent hypoxia Provide supportive care Provide adequate ventilation Maintain cerebral perfusion Prevent cerebral edema Treat underlying cause Administer antiseizure drugs	See Nursing Care of the High-Risk Infant, p. 229 Observe for signs that indicate cerebral hypoxia Monitor ventilatory and IV therapy Observe for and manage seizures Support family Provide guidelines for family management of mild to severe neurologic damage
GERMINAL MATRIX/INTRAVENTRICULAR HEMORRHAGE (GM/IVH)			
Hemorrhage into and around ventricles caused by ruptured vessels as a result of an event that increases cerebral blood flow to area	Sudden deterioration in condition if bleed is large Most bleeds are initially asymptomatic Tense, bulging anterior fontanel Neurologic signs: 　Twitching 　Stupor 　Apnea 　Seizures 　Evident on cranial ultrasonography or tomography	Supportive care: 　Provide ventilatory support 　Maintain oxygenation 　Regulate fluid and electrolytes, acid-base balance 　Suppress or prevent seizures 　Ventricular shunting or drainage	See Nursing Care of the High-Risk Infant, p. 229 Prevent increased cerebral blood pressure Avoid events that may increase/decrease cerebral blood flow (e.g., pain, unnecessary stimulation, endotracheal suctioning, hypoxia, hyperosmolar drugs, rapid volume expansion) Elevate head of bed 20 to 30 degrees; keep head in midline Support family Monitor for posthemorrhagic hydrocephalus after diagnosis Provide developmental care and enhancement
INTRACRANIAL HEMORRHAGE			
Subdural Subarachnoid Intracerebellar	Sudden decrease in hematocrit Change in sensorium Poor feeding See Chapter 28	See Chapter 28	Same as for PVH/IVH

and hydrocephalus, are usually diagnosed in the first 2 years of life. Less severe deficits, such as learning disorders, hyperactivity, and fine and gross motor incoordination, may not be diagnosed until preschool or even school age. Cerebral palsy is one of the most common neurologic deficits in survivors of prematurity (see Chapter 32).

NEONATAL SEIZURES

Seizures in the neonatal period are usually the clinical manifestation of a serious underlying disease. The most common cause of seizures in the neonatal period (for term and preterm) is hypoxic ischemic encephalopathy secondary to perinatal asphyxia (Volpe, 2001). Although not life threatening as an isolated entity, seizures constitute a medical emergency because they signal a disease process that may produce irreversible brain damage. Consequently, it is imperative to recognize a seizure and its significance so that the cause, as well as the seizure, can be treated (Box 9-10).

The features of neonatal seizures are different from those observed in the older infant or child. For example, the well-organized, generalized tonic-clonic seizures seen in older children are rare in infants, especially preterm infants. The newborn brain, with its immature anatomic and physiologic status and less cortical organization, is insufficient to allow ready development and maintenance of a generalized seizure. Instead, signs of seizures in newborns, especially preterm neonates, are subtle and include findings such as lip smacking, tongue thrusting, eye rolling, and arching (Volpe, 2001)

Jitteriness or tremulousness in the newborn is a repetitive shaking of an extremity or extremities that may be observed with crying, occur with changes in sleeping state, or are elicited with stimulation. Jitteriness is relatively common in newborns, and in a mild degree may be considered normal during the first 4 days of life. Jitteriness can be distinguished from seizures by several characteristics: jitteriness is not accompanied by ocular movement as are seizures; the dominant movement in jitteriness is tremor, whereas seizure movement is clonic jerking that cannot be stopped by flexion of the affected limb; and jitteriness is highly sensitive to stimulation, whereas seizures are not.

A *tremor* is defined as repetitive movements of both hands (with or without movement of legs or jaws) at a frequency of 2 to 5 per second and lasting more than 10 minutes. It is common in newborn infants and has a variety of causes, including neurologic damage, hypoglycemia, and hypocalcemia. In most instances tremors are of no pathologic significance.

Neonatal seizures can be divided into four major types. These classifications are outlined in order of frequency in Table 9-12 and consist of clonic, tonic, myoclonic, and subtle seizures (Volpe, 2001). Clonic, multifocal clonic, and migratory clonic seizures are more common in term infants.

Diagnostic Evaluation

Early evaluation and diagnosis of seizures is urgent. In addition to a careful physical examination, the pregnancy and family histories are investigated for familial and prenatal causes. Blood is drawn for glucose and electrolyte examination, and cerebrospinal fluid is obtained for examination for gross blood, cell count, protein, glucose, and culture. Electroencephalography may help identify subtle seizures but is less helpful in establishing a diagnosis. Other diagnostic procedures, such as computed tomography, magnetic resonance imaging, and echoencephalography, may be indicated. A video electroencephalogram may be used to identify seizure activity in some newborns.

Therapeutic Management

Treatment is directed toward prevention of cerebral damage and involves correction of metabolic derangements, respiratory and cardiovascular support, and suppression of the seizure activity. The underlying cause is treated (e.g., glucose infusion for hypoglycemia, calcium for hypocalcemia, antibiotics for infection). If needed, respiratory support is provided for hypoxia, and anticonvulsants may be administered, especially when the other measures fail to control the seizures. Phenobarbital, given intravenously or orally, has

---

BOX 9-10 ■ Causes of Neonatal Seizures

METABOLIC
Hypoglycemia; hyperglycemia
Hypocalcemia
Hypernatremia; hyponatremia
Hypomagnesemia
Pyridoxine deficiency
Aminoacidurias (e.g., phenylketonuria, maple syrup urine disease)
Hyperammonemia

TOXIC
Uremia
Bilirubin encephalopathy (kernicterus)

PRENATAL INFECTIONS
Toxoplasmosis
Syphilis
Cytomegalovirus
Herpes simplex
Hepatitis

POSTNATAL INFECTIONS
Bacterial meningitis
Viral meningoencephalitis
Sepsis
Brain abscess

TRAUMA AT BIRTH
Hypoxic brain injury
Intracranial hemorrhage
Subarachnoid, subdural hemorrhage
Intraventricular hemorrhage

MALFORMATIONS
Central nervous system agenesis
Hydroencephalopathy
Parencephalopathy
Tuberous sclerosis

MISCELLANEOUS
Narcotic withdrawal
Degenerative disease
Benign familial neonatal seizures

TABLE 9-12 ■ Classifications of Neonatal Seizures

TYPE	CHARACTERISTICS
Clonic	Slow rhythmic jerking movements
	Approximately 1 to 3 per second
Focal	Involves face, upper or lower extremities on one side of body
	May involve neck or trunk
	Infant is conscious during event
Multifocal	May migrate randomly from one part of the body to another
	Movements may start at different times
Tonic	Extension/stiffening movements
Generalized	Extensions of all four limbs (similar to decerebrate rigidity)
	Upper limbs are maintained in a stiffly flexed position (resembles decorticate rigidity)
Focal	Sustained posturing of a limb
	Asymmetric posturing of trunk or neck
Subtle	May develop in either full-term or preterm infants but are more common in preterm
	Often overlooked by inexperienced observers
	Signs:
	Horizontal eye deviation
	Repetitive blinking or fluttering of the eyelids, staring
	Sucking or other oral-buccal-lingual movements
	Arm movements that resemble rowing or swimming
	Leg movements described as pedaling or bicycling
	Apnea (common)
	Signs may appear alone or in combination
Myoclonic	Rapid jerks that involve flexor muscle groups
Focal	Involves upper extremity flexor muscle group
	No electroencephalogram (EEG) discharges observed
Multifocal	Asynchronous twitching of several parts of the body
	No associated EEG discharges observed
Generalized	Bilateral jerks of upper and lower limbs
	Associated with EEG discharges

Modified from Volpe J: Neonatal seizures. In Volpe J: *Neurology of the newborn*, ed 4, Philadelphia, 2001, WB Saunders.

been the drug of choice and is used if seizures are severe and persistent. Other drugs that may be used are phenytoin (Dilantin), lorazepam, and diazepam (Valium).

A newer drug, fosphenytoin sodium, is a water-soluble prodrug and has been designed to replace phenytoin. Fosphenytoin metabolizes to form phenytoin in the body yet can easily be diluted or mixed in dextrose and normal saline and may be given via IV or intramuscular routes. In addition, fosphenytoin does not cause pain during IV administration.

Nursing Considerations

The major nursing responsibilities in the care of infants with seizures are to recognize when the infant is having a seizure so that therapy can be instituted, to carry out the therapeutic regimen, and to observe the response to the therapy and

any further evidence of seizures or other symptomatology. Assessment and other aspects of care are the same as for all high-risk infants. Parents need to be informed of their infant's status, and the nurse should reinforce and clarify the explanations of the practitioner. The infant's behaviors need to be interpreted for the parents, and the infant's responses to the treatment must be anticipated and their significance explained. Parents are encouraged to visit their infant and perform the parenting activities consistent with the plan of care. Seizures are a frightening phenomenon and generate a great deal of anxiety and fear, which is easily compounded by the justifiable concern of the staff. Providing support and guidance is an important nursing function.

HIGH RISK RELATED TO INFECTIOUS PROCESSES

SEPSIS

Sepsis, or *septicemia*, refers to a generalized bacterial infection in the bloodstream. Neonates are highly susceptible to infection as a result of diminished nonspecific (inflammatory) and specific (humoral) immunity, such as impaired phagocytosis, delayed chemotactic response, minimal or absent immunoglobulin-A and immunoglobulin-M (IgA and IgM), and decreased complement levels. Because of the infant's poor response to pathogenic agents, there is usually no local inflammatory reaction at the portal of entry to signal an infection, and the resulting symptoms tend to be vague and nonspecific. Consequently, diagnosis and treatment may be delayed.

Sepsis in the neonatal period can be acquired prenatally across the placenta from the maternal bloodstream or during labor from ingestion or aspiration of infected amniotic fluid. Prolonged rupture of the membranes always presents a risk for this type from maternal-fetal transfer of pathogenic organisms. In utero transplacental transfer can occur with organisms and viruses such as cytomegalovirus, toxoplasmosis, and *Treponema pallidum* (syphilis), which cross the placental barrier during the latter half of pregnancy.

Early sepsis (less than 3 days) is acquired in the perinatal period; infection can occur from direct contact with organisms from the maternal gastrointestinal and genitourinary tracts. The most common infecting organisms are group B streptococcus (GBS) and *Escherichia coli*, which may be present in the vagina. GBS has emerged as an extremely virulent organism in neonates, with a high (50%) death rate in affected infants. *Haemophilus influenzae* and coagulase-negative staphylococci are also commonly seen in early-onset sepsis in VLBW infants. Other pathogens that are harbored in the vagina and that may infect the infant include gonococci, *Candida albicans*, herpes simplex virus (type II), *Listeria* organisms, and chlamydia.

Late sepsis (1 to 3 weeks after birth) is primarily nosocomial, and the offending organisms are usually staphylococci, *Klebsiella*, enterococci, and *Pseudomonas*. Coagulase-negative staphylococcus is commonly found to be the cause of septicemia in ELBW and VLBW infants. Bacterial invasion can occur through sites such as the umbilical stump; the skin; mucous membranes of the eye, nose, pharynx, and ear; and internal systems such as the respiratory, nervous, urinary, and gastrointestinal systems.

Postnatal infection is acquired by cross-contamination from other infants, personnel, or objects in the environment. Bacteria that are commonly called "water bugs" (because they are able to grow in water) are found in water supplies, humidifying apparatus, sink drains, suction machines, and most respiratory equipment. Organisms such as coagulase-negative staphylococcus, which usually colonize the skin, may infect indwelling venous and arterial catheters used for infusions, blood sampling, and monitoring of vital signs. Neonatal sepsis is most common in the infant at risk, particularly the preterm infant or the infant born after a difficult or traumatic labor and delivery, who is least capable of resisting such bacterial invasion. These organisms are often transmitted by the personnel from person to person or object to person by poor handwashing and inadequate housecleaning.

Diagnostic Evaluation

Diagnosis of sepsis is often based on suspicion of presenting clinical signs and symptoms. Because sepsis is so easily confused with other neonatal disorders, the definitive diagnosis is established by laboratory and radiographic examination. Isolation of the specific organism is always attempted through cultures of blood, urine, and cerebrospinal fluid. Blood studies may show signs of anemia, leukocytosis, or leukopenia. Leukopenia is usually an ominous sign because of its frequent association with high mortality. An elevated number of immature neutrophils, decreased or increased total neutrophils, and changes in neutrophil morphology also suggest an infectious process in the neonate. There is some evidence that C-reactive protein serial measurements may have a significant role in establishing or excluding the diagnosis of sepsis in suspected infants and minimizing exposure to antibiotic treatment (Hengst, 2003).

Prevention. Several measures are important in the prevention of both early- and late-onset infection. Programs to screen pregnant women for GBS colonization (culture-based) and treatment of those women in labor have dramatically reduced the incidence of GBS infection in the neonate (Centers for Disease Control and Prevention, 2002). Screening programs for other maternal infections including hepatitis B and human immunodeficiency virus (HIV) have also been recommended.

Nursery procedures aimed at minimizing the risk of nosocomial infections include the practice of good handwashing techniques, appropriate isolation precautions where indicated, and the adoption of recommended standards for spacing of infant beds (see American Academy of Pediatrics and American College of Obstetricians and Gynecologists, 2002).

Therapeutic Management

In addition to the institution of vigorous therapeutic measures, early recognition (Box 9-11) and diagnosis are essential to increase the infant's chance for survival and reduce the likelihood of permanent neurologic damage. Antibiotic therapy is initiated before laboratory results are available for confirmation and identification of the exact organism. Treatment consists of circulatory support, respiratory sup-

---

BOX 9-11 ■ Manifestations Observed in Neonatal Sepsis

GENERAL SIGNS
Infant generally "not doing well"
Poor temperature control—hypothermia, hyperthermia (rare)

CIRCULATORY SYSTEM
Pallor, cyanosis, or mottling
Cold, clammy skin
Hypotension
Edema
Irregular heartbeat—bradycardia, tachycardia

RESPIRATORY SYSTEM
Irregular respirations, apnea, or tachypnea
Cyanosis
Grunting
Dyspnea
Retractions

CENTRAL NERVOUS SYSTEM
Diminished activity—lethargy, hyporeflexia, coma
Increased activity—irritability, tremors, seizures
Full fontanel
Increased or decreased tone
Abnormal eye movements

GASTROINTESTINAL SYSTEM
Poor feeding
Vomiting
Diarrhea or decreased stooling
Abdominal distention
Hepatomegaly
Hemoccult-positive stools

HEMATOPOIETIC SYSTEM
Jaundice
Pallor
Petechiae, ecchymosis
Splenomegaly

---

port, aggressive administration of antibiotics, and immunotherapy.

Supportive therapy usually involves administration of oxygen (if respiratory distress or hypoxia is evident), careful regulation of fluids, correction of electrolyte or acid-base imbalance, and temporary discontinuation of oral feedings. Blood transfusions may be needed to correct anemia and shock, and electronic monitoring of vital signs and regulation of the thermal environment are mandatory.

Antibiotic therapy is continued for 7 to 10 days if cultures are positive, discontinued in 3 days if cultures are negative and the infant is asymptomatic, and most often administered via IV infusion. Antifungal and/or antiviral therapies are implemented as appropriate, depending on causative agents.

Prognosis. The prognosis for neonatal sepsis is variable. Severe neurologic and respiratory sequelae may occur in ELBW and VLBW infants as a result of early-onset sepsis. Late-onset sepsis and meningitis may also result in poor outcomes for immunocompromised neonates. The trend in antenatal diagnosis of maternal GBS and subsequent maternal and neonatal treatment with antibiotic therapy has decreased the incidence of early-onset GBS disease by 70% (0.5 cases per 1000 live births in 1999), although rates of late-onset perinatal GBS disease remained constant (Centers for Disease Control and Prevention, 2002). New rapid tests for identification of maternal GBS at delivery are being developed and will soon be implemented to facilitate detection and treatment; a vaccine to prevent perinatal GBS is still some years away from being implemented. There has been a recent increase in the incidence of gram-negative organisms seen in early-onset sepsis, with *Escherichia coli* being the predominant isolated organism.

Nursing Considerations

Nursing care of the infant with sepsis involves observation and assessment as outlined for any high-risk infant. Recognition of the existing problem is of paramount importance; it is usually the nurse who observes and assesses infants and identifies that "something is wrong" with them. Awareness of the potential modes of infection transmission also helps the nurse identify those at risk for developing sepsis. Much of the care of infants with sepsis involves the medical treatment of the illness. Knowledge of the side effects of the specific antibiotic and proper regulation and administration of the drug are vital.

Prolonged antibiotic therapy poses additional hazards for affected infants. Antibiotics predispose the infant to growth of resistant organisms and superinfection from fungal or mycotic agents, such as *Candida albicans*. Nurses must be alert for evidence of such complications. Nystatin oral suspension is swabbed on the buccal mucosa for prophylaxis against oral candidiasis.

A number of specimens may be needed to help identify the cause and source of the infection. It is recommended that the fully flexed position be avoided for obtaining spinal fluid and that the side-lying position (modified with neck extension) or sitting position be used for obtaining spinal fluid specimens. Continual cardiorespiratory and pulse oximetry monitoring provides an ongoing assessment of the infant's condition during the procedure.

Part of the total care of infants with sepsis is to decrease any additional physiologic or environmental stress. This includes providing an optimum thermoregulated environment and anticipating potential problems such as dehydration or hypoxia. Precautions are implemented to prevent the spread of infection to other newborns, but to be effective, activities must be carried out by all caregivers. Proper handwashing, the use of disposable equipment (e.g., linens, catheters, feeding supplies, IV equipment), disposing of excretions (e.g., vomitus, stool), and adequate housekeeping of the environment and equipment are essential. Because nurses are the most consistent caregivers involved with sick infants, it is usually their responsibility to oversee that standard precautions are maintained by everyone.

Another aspect of caring for infants with sepsis involves observation for signs of complications, including meningitis and septic shock, a severe complication caused by toxins in the bloodstream.

✐NURSING ALERT

Artificial and long natural fingernails worn by nurses have been associated with serious neonatal infection and morbidity from *Pseudomonas aeruginosa* in the NICU (Moolenaar and others, 2000).

NECROTIZING ENTEROCOLITIS

NEC is an acute inflammatory disease of the bowel with increased incidence in preterm infants. Three factors appear to play an important role in the development of NEC: intestinal ischemia, colonization by pathogenic bacteria, and substrate (formula feeding) in the intestinal lumen. The precise cause of NEC is still uncertain, but it appears to occur in infants whose gastrointestinal tract has suffered vascular compromise. Intestinal ischemia of unknown etiology, immature gastrointestinal host defenses, bacterial proliferation, and feeding substrate are now believed to have a multifactorial role in the etiology of NEC. Prematurity remains the most prominent risk factor in the development of NEC.

The damage to mucosal cells lining the bowel wall is great. Diminished blood supply to these cells causes their death in large numbers; they stop secreting protective, lubricating mucus; and the thin, unprotected bowel wall is attacked by proteolytic enzymes. Thus the bowel wall continues to swell and break down; it is unable to synthesize protective immunoglobulin-M, and the mucosa is permeable to macromolecules (e.g., exotoxins), which further hampers intestinal defenses. Gas-forming bacteria invade the damaged areas to produce *pneumatosis intestinalis,* the presence of air in the submucosal or subserosal surfaces of the bowel.

A consistent relationship has been observed between the development of NEC and enteric feeding of hypertonic substances (e.g., formula, hyperosmolar medications). It is unclear whether this connection is a result of the formula imposing a stress on an ischemic bowel, serving as a substrate for bacterial growth, or both.

Diagnostic Evaluation

Radiographic studies show a sausage-shaped dilation of the intestine that progresses to marked distention and the characteristic pneumatosis intestinalis—"soapsuds," or the bubbly appearance of thickened bowel wall and ultralumina. There may be air in the portal circulation or free air observed in the abdomen, indicating perforation. Laboratory findings may include anemia, leukopenia, leukocytosis, metabolic acidosis, and electrolyte imbalance. In severe cases coagulopathy (disseminated intravascular coagulation) or thrombocytopenia may be evident. Organisms are often cultured from blood, although bacteremia or septicemia may not be prominent early in the course of the disease.

Therapeutic Management

Treatment of NEC begins with prevention. Oral feedings may be withheld for at least 24 to 48 hours from infants who are believed to have suffered birth asphyxia and as long as deemed necessary from ELBW and VLBW infants. Breast milk is the preferred enteral nutrient because it confers some passive immunity (immunoglobulin-A), macrophages, and lysozymes.

Minimal enteral feedings (trophic feeding, gastrointestinal priming) have gained acceptance with no evidence of increased incidence of NEC. Early experience indicates such feedings may in fact be protective against NEC in nonasphyxiated preterm infants as well as exert other potential benefits.

Medical treatment of confirmed NEC consists of discontinuation of all oral feedings, institution of abdominal decompression via nasogastric suction, administration of IV antibiotics, and correction of extravascular volume depletion, electrolyte abnormalities, acid-base imbalances, and hypoxia. Replacing oral feedings with parenteral fluids decreases the need for oxygen and circulation to the bowel. Serial abdominal radiographic films (every 4 to 6 hours in the acute phase) are taken to monitor for possible progression of the disease to intestinal perforation.

Prognosis.   With early recognition and treatment, medical management is increasingly successful. If there is progressive deterioration under medical management or evidence of perforation, surgical resection and anastomosis are performed. Extensive involvement may necessitate surgical intervention and establishment of an ileostomy, jejunostomy, or colostomy. Sequelae in surviving infants include short-gut syndrome (see Chapter 24), colonic stricture with obstruction, fat malabsorption, and failure to thrive secondary to intestinal dysfunction. A variety of surgical interventions for NEC are available and depend on the extent of bowel necrosis, associated illness factors, and infant stability. Intestinal transplantation has been successful in some former preterm infants with NEC-associated short-gut syndrome who had already developed life-threatening total parenteral nutrition–related complications. Transplantation may be a life-saving option for infants who previously faced high morbidity and mortality (Vennarecci and others, 2000).

Nursing Considerations

Nursing responsibilities begin with early recognition. The nurse is a key factor in the prompt recognition of the early warning signs of NEC. Because the signs are similar to those observed in many other disorders of the newborn, nurses must constantly be aware of the possibility of this disease in infants who are at high risk for developing NEC (Box 9-12).

When the disease is suspected, the nurse assists with diagnostic procedures and implements the therapeutic regimen. Vital signs, including blood pressure, are monitored for changes that might indicate bowel perforation, septicemia, or cardiovascular shock, and measures are instituted to prevent possible transmission to other infants. It is especially important to avoid rectal temperatures because of the increased danger of perforation. To avoid pressure on the distended abdomen and to facilitate continuous observation, infants are often left undiapered and positioned supine or on the side.

> ### ⚠ NURSING ALERT
>
> Observe for indications of early development of NEC by checking the appearance of the abdomen for distention (measuring abdominal girth, measuring residual gastric contents before feedings, and listening for the presence of bowel sounds) and performing all routine assessments for high-risk neonates.

Conscientious attention to nutritional and hydration needs is essential, and antibiotics are administered as prescribed. The time at which oral feedings are reinstituted varies considerably but is usually at least 7 to 10 days after diagnosis and treatment. Feeding is usually re-established using human milk, if available. Some infants may benefit from the use of an elemental formula such as Pregestimil.

Because NEC is an infectious disease, one of the most important nursing functions is control of infection. Strict handwashing is the primary barrier to spread, and confirmed multiple cases are isolated. Persons with symptoms of a gastrointestinal disorder should not care for these or any other infants.

The infant who requires surgery requires the same careful attention and observation as any infant with abdominal surgery, including ostomy care (as applicable). This disorder is one of the most common reasons for performing ileostomies on newborns. Throughout the medical and surgical management of infants with NEC, the nurse is continually alert to signs of complications, such as septicemia, disseminated intravascular coagulation, hypoglycemia, and other metabolic derangements.

HIGH RISK RELATED TO MATERNAL CONDITIONS

The health of the fetus and newborn may be affected by a number of maternal conditions; essentially, any condition affecting the mother also has the potential for negatively impacting the health of the newborn. *Pregnancy-induced hypertension* or *HELLP (hemolysis, elevated liver enzymes, low platelets) syndrome* may cause premature delivery, intrauterine growth retardation, asphyxia, and death if not detected early and appropriate interventions implemented. It is not within the scope of this text to elaborate on the pathophysiology and treatment of these conditions; however, the reader is referred to any one of the excellent

---

BOX 9-12 ■ Clinical Manifestations of Necrotizing Enterocolitis

NONSPECIFIC CLINICAL SIGNS
Lethargy
Poor feeding
Hypotension
Vomiting
Apnea
Decreased urinary output
Unstable temperature
Jaundice

SPECIFIC SIGNS
Distended (often shiny) abdomen
Blood in the stools or gastric contents
Gastric retention
Localized abdominal wall erythema or induration
Bilious vomitus

maternity texts available for a detailed discussion of these conditions.

INFANTS OF DIABETIC MOTHERS

Before insulin therapy, few women with diabetes were able to conceive; for those who did, the mortality rate for both mother and infant was high. The morbidity and mortality of infants of diabetic mothers (IDMs) have been significantly reduced as a result of effective control of maternal diabetes and an increased understanding of fetal disorders. Because infants born to women with gestational diabetes mellitus are at risk for the same complications as IDMs, the following discussion of IDMs includes infants born to women with gestational diabetes mellitus.

The severity of the maternal diabetes affects infant survival. Severity of maternal diabetes is determined by the duration of the disease before pregnancy, age of onset, extent of vascular complications, and abnormalities of the current pregnancy, such as pyelonephritis, diabetic ketoacidosis, pregnancy-induced hypertension, and noncompliance. The single most important factor influencing fetal well-being is the euglycemic status of the mother. It has been found that reasonable metabolic control that begins before conception and continues during the first weeks of pregnancy can prevent malformation in an IDM. Elevated levels of hemoglobin A1c during the first trimester appear to be associated with a higher incidence of congenital malformations.

Hypoglycemia may appear a short time after birth and in IDMs is associated with increased insulin activity in the blood (see also p. 272). The serum glucose level that corresponds to clinical hypoglycemia have not been well defined. Because some infants experience metabolic complications at higher levels than previously thought, it is generally recommended that serum glucose levels be maintained above 47 mg/dL (2.6 mmol/L) to 50 mg/dL (2.8 mmol/L) in both term and preterm infants, regardless of the presence or absence of clinical symptoms (McGowan, Hagedorn, and Hay, 2002; Ogata, 1999).

Hypoglycemia in the IDM is related to hypertrophy and hyperplasia of the pancreatic islet cells, and thus is a transient state of hyperinsulinism.

High maternal blood glucose levels during fetal life provide a continual stimulus to the fetal islet cells for insulin production (glucose easily passes the placental barrier from maternal to fetal side; insulin, however, does not cross the placental barrier). This sustained state of hyperglycemia promotes fetal insulin secretion that ultimately leads to excessive growth and deposition of fat, which probably accounts for the infants who are large for gestational age, or macrosomic. When the neonate's glucose supply is removed abruptly at the time of birth, the continued production of insulin soon depletes the blood of circulating glucose, creating a state of hyperinsulinism and hypoglycemia within 0.5 to 4 hours, especially in infants of mothers with class C diabetes or beyond (class D through R). Precipitous drops in blood glucose levels can cause serious neurologic damage or death.

IDMs have a characteristic appearance (Box 9-13). Infants of mothers with advanced diabetes may be small for gestational age, may have intrauterine growth retardation (IUGR), or may be appropriate for gestational age because of the maternal vascular (placental) involvement. There is

BOX 9-13 ■ Clinical Manifestations of Infants of Diabetic Mothers

Large for gestational age
Very plump and full faced
Abundant vernix caseosa
Plethora
Listlessness and lethargy
Large placenta and umbilical cord (Wharton's jelly)
Possibly meconium-stained at birth

an increase in congenital anomalies in IDMs in addition to a high susceptibility to hypoglycemia, hypocalcemia, hypomagnesemia, polycythemia, hyperbilirubinemia, cardiomyopathy, hypomagnesemia, and RDS. Hyperinsulinemia and hyperglycemia in the diabetic mother may be a factor in reducing fetal surfactant synthesis, thus contributing to the development of RDS. Although large, these infants may be delivered before term as a result of maternal complications or increased fetal size.

Therapeutic Management

The most effective management of IDMs is careful monitoring of serum glucose levels and observation for accompanying complications such as RDS. The infants are examined for the presence of any anomalies or birth injuries, and blood studies for initial determinations of glucose, calcium, hematocrit, and bilirubin are obtained on a regular basis. Recent studies confirm the importance of maintaining serum glucose levels above 50 mg/dL (2.8 mmol/L) in hyperinsulinemic infants with hypoglycemia to prevent serious neurologic sequelae (Cowett and Loughead, 2002; Schwartz, 1997).

Because the hypertrophied pancreas is so sensitive to blood glucose concentrations, the administration of oral glucose may trigger a massive insulin release, resulting in rebound hypoglycemia. Therefore, feedings of breast milk or formula begin within the first hour after birth, provided that the infant's cardiorespiratory condition is stable (do not feed infant with RDS). Approximately half of these infants do very well and adjust without complications. Infants born to mothers with uncontrolled diabetes may require IV dextrose infusions. Oral and IV intake may be titrated to maintain adequate blood glucose levels. Frequent blood glucose determinations are needed for the first 2 to 4 days of life to assess the degree of hypoglycemia present at any given time. Testing blood taken from the heel with reagent strips and portable reflectance meters (e.g., Glucometer) is a simple and effective screening evaluation that can then be confirmed by laboratory examination.

Nursing Considerations

The nursing care of IDMs involves early examination for congenital anomalies, signs of possible respiratory or cardiac problems, maintenance of adequate thermoregulation, early introduction of carbohydrate feedings as appropriate, and monitoring of serum blood glucose levels. The latter is of particular importance because many hypoglycemic infants may remain asymptomatic. IV glucose infusion requires careful monitoring of the site and the neonate's reaction to therapy; high glucose concentrations (>12.5%)

should be infused via a central line instead of a peripheral site. Because macrosomic infants are at risk for problems associated with a difficult delivery, they are monitored for birth injuries such as brachial plexus injury and palsy, fractured clavicle, and phrenic nerve palsy. Additional monitoring of the infant for associated problems (polycythemia, hypocalcemia, poor feeding, and hyperbilirubinemia) with this condition is also a vital nursing function.

There is some preliminary evidence that IDMs have an increased risk of acquiring diabetes in childhood or early adulthood; therefore nursing care should also focus on healthy lifestyle and prevention later in life with IDMs.

DRUG-EXPOSED INFANTS*

Narcotics, which have a low molecular weight, readily cross the placental membrane and enter the fetal system. Illicit substances may also be transmitted to the newborn through breast milk. When the mother is a habitual user of opiates, especially heroin or methadone, the unborn child may also become chemically dependent or passively addicted to the drug, which places such infants at risk during the perinatal and early neonatal periods. *Neonatal abstinence syndrome (NAS)* is the term used to describe the set of behaviors exhibited by the infant exposed to chemical substances in utero.

Clinical Manifestations

Most infants who are exposed to drugs in utero may demonstrate no immediate untoward effects and appear normal at birth but may begin to exhibit signs of drug withdrawal within 12 to 24 hours if the mother has been taking heroin by itself. If mothers have been taking methadone, the signs appear somewhat later—anywhere from 1 or 2 days to 2 to 3 weeks or more after birth. The clinical manifestations may fall into any one or all of the following categories: CNS, gastrointestinal, respiratory, and autonomic nervous system signs (Kandall, 1999). The manifestations become most pronounced between 48 and 72 hours of age and may last from 6 days to 8 weeks, depending on the severity of the withdrawal (Box 9-14). Although these infants suck avidly on fists and display an exaggerated rooting reflex, they are poor feeders with uncoordinated and ineffectual sucking and swallowing reflexes.

Not all infants of heroin-addicted mothers will show signs of withdrawal. Because of irregular and varying degrees of drug use, quality of drug, and mixed drug usage by the mother, some infants display mild or variable manifestations. Most manifestations are the vague, nonspecific signs characteristic of all infants in general; therefore, it is important to differentiate between drug withdrawal and other disorders before specific therapy is instituted. Other conditions (e.g., hypocalcemia, hypoglycemia, sepsis) often coexist with the drug withdrawal.

---

*It is important to note that the term *addiction* is often associated with behaviors whereby the person seeks the drug(s) to experience a high, euphoria, escape from reality, or satisfy a personal need. Newborns who have been exposed to drugs in utero are not addicted in a behavioral sense, yet they may experience mild to strong physiologic signs as a result of the exposure. Therefore, to say that an infant born to a mother who uses substances is addicted is incorrect; *drug-exposed newborn* is a better term, which implies intrauterine drug exposure.

BOX 9-14 ■ Signs of Withdrawal in the Neonate

NEUROLOGIC
Irritability
Seizures
Hyperactivity
High-pitched cry
Tremors
Exaggerated Moro reflex
Hypertonicity of muscles

GASTROINTESTINAL
Poor feeding
Diarrhea
Dehydration
Vomiting
Frantic, uncoordinated sucking
Gastric residuals

AUTONOMIC
Diaphoresis
Fever
Mottled skin
Nasal stuffiness

MISCELLANEOUS
Disrupted sleep patterns
Diaphoresis
Tachypnea (>60 respirations/min)
Excoriations (knees, face)
Temperature instability

In one recent report, newborns born to substance-abusing (cocaine) mothers had significant growth deficits in birth weight, head circumference, and length in comparison to newborns of nonabusing mothers. In addition, infants born to mothers who smoked had growth failure in all three parameters as well and a dose-effect relationship was observed, whereas infants born to mothers with heavy alcohol intake had only decreased weight and length (Bada and others, 2002). Additional signs often seen in drug-exposed newborns include loose stools, tachycardia, fever, projectile vomiting, crying, nasal stuffiness, and generalized perspiration, which is unusual in newborns.

Infants who do not display the signs of fetal alcohol syndrome (FAS) but are born to mothers who are also heavy alcohol drinkers have significantly more tremors, hypertonia, restlessness, excessive mouthing movements, crying, and inconsolability than infants of substance-abusive mothers who do not consume alcohol during pregnancy. An added concern regarding substance abuse is that many of the mothers often use several drugs, such as tranquilizers, sedatives, amphetamines, phencyclidine, marijuana, and other psychotropic agents.

Diagnostic Evaluation

Newborn urine, hair, or meconium sampling may be required to identify drug exposure and implement appropriate early interventional therapies aimed at minimizing the consequences of intrauterine drug exposure. Meconium sampling for fetal drug exposure is reported to provide more screening accuracy than urine, since drug metabolites accumulate in meconium (Kandall, 1999). Urine toxicology screening has less accuracy since it reflects only recent substance intake by the mother (Huestis and Choo, 2002). Meconium and hair testing for drug metabolites have the advantages of being noninvasive, more accurate, and easy to collect.

Therapeutic Management

The treatment of the drug-exposed infant initially consists of early identification through maternal history, presenting symptoms of NAS, or toxicology screening when substance abuse is strongly suspected. Early identification and intervention are essential to prevent further adverse effects; early discharge from the birth institution should be postponed until further assessment of the maternal situation may occur and a treatment plan of care can be established for the mother and infant. Drug therapies to decrease withdrawal effects include parenteral or oral administration of phenobarbital, chlorpromazine, clonidine, diazepam, methadone, and morphine. A combination of these drugs may be necessary to treat infants exposed to multiple drugs in utero, and careful attention should be given to possible adverse effects of the treatment drugs (Johnson, Gerada, and Greenough, 2003).

Prognosis.   The prognosis for drug-exposed infants depends on the type and amount of drug(s) taken by the mother and the stage(s) of fetal development in which the drug was taken. The overall mortality of infants born to narcotic-addicted mothers is increased, but with early recognition, proper treatment, and long-term follow-up, the morbidity and mortality associated with drug exposure are decreased.

Often, drug-exposed infants will exhibit poor brain and body growth at birth; however, at times, infants will not exhibit any signs that indicate exposure to harmful agents and their condition may therefore be overlooked until symptoms appear later in life. Drug-exposed infants may have chronic feeding problems, irritability, abnormal neurologic responses, abnormal parent-infant interactions, developmental and cognitive delays, learning disabilities, and behavioral problems, including attention deficit hyperactivity disorder.

Nursing Considerations

One of the key factors in the treatment of drug-exposed neonates is early identification of substance abuse in the pregnant female so treatment can be initiated and side effects minimized. This is especially problematic from a social and legal standpoint because the pregnant female is often aware of the consequences of admitting to substance abuse and may therefore be less likely to readily admit to the problem for fear of social and legal repercussions. If the mother has had good prenatal care, the practitioner is aware of the problem, and therapy may have been instituted before delivery. However, a number of mothers deliver their infants without the benefit of adequate care, and the condition is unknown to health care personnel at the time of delivery. The degree of withdrawal is closely related to the amount of drug the mother has habitually taken, the length of time she has been taking the drug, and the drug level of the mother at the time of delivery. The most severe symptoms are observed in the infants of mothers who have taken large amounts of drugs over a long period. In addition, the nearer to the time of delivery that the mother takes the drug, the longer it takes the child to develop withdrawal, and the more severe the manifestations. The infant may not exhibit withdrawal symptoms until 7 to 10 days after delivery, by which time most newborns have been discharged from the birth center, and caregivers are less likely to recognize signs of irritability and poor feeding as withdrawal, thus predisposing the newborn to abuse or neglect. The infant may be at further risk for subsequent abuse or neglect because of home conditions that preclude adequate newborn care and follow-up.

After the presence of NAS is identified in an infant, nursing care is directed toward treatment of the presenting signs, decreasing stimuli that may precipitate hyperactivity and irritability (e.g., dimming the lights, decreasing noise levels), providing adequate nutrition and hydration, and promoting maternal-infant relationships. Appropriate individualized developmental care is implemented to facilitate self-consoling and self-regulating behaviors. Irritable and hyperactive infants have been found to respond to physical comforting, movement, and close contact. Wrapping infants snugly and rocking and holding them tightly limits their ability to self-stimulate. Arranging nursing activities to reduce the amount of disturbance helps to decrease exogenous stimulation.

Breast-feeding is encouraged in mothers who are not using illicit substances, are negative for HIV infection, and are compliant with a methadone program; breast-feeding promotes maternal-infant bonding, and small quantities of methadone passed through breast milk have not proved to be harmful.

The *Neonatal Abstinence Scoring System* has been developed to monitor infants in an objective manner and evaluate the infant's response to clinical and pharmacologic interventions (Kandall, 1999; Finnegan, 1985). This system is also designed to assist nurses and other health care workers in evaluating the severity of the infant's withdrawal symptoms. Another tool that may be used to evaluate withdrawal behavior and treatment in newborns is the **Neonatal Withdrawal Inventory** developed by Zahrodny and others (1998); it is important to note that neither of these tools is specific to preterm infants and may not be representative of withdrawal behaviors in such infants (Marcellus, 2002).

The **Neonatal Intensive Care Unit Network Neurobehavioral Scale (NNNS)** is a comprehensive neurologic and behavioral assessment tool that may be used to identify newborns at risk as a result of intrauterine drug exposure. The tool measures stress/abstinence, state, neurologic status, and muscle tone in the context of the newborn's medical condition at the time of examination. The NNNS may be used for medically stable newborns who are at least 30 weeks' gestation and up to 48 weeks' corrected or conceptional age (Lester, Tronick, and Brazelton, 2004).

Loose stools, poor intake, and regurgitation after feeding predispose these infants to malnutrition, dehydration, and electrolyte imbalance. Frequent weighing, careful monitoring of intake and output and electrolytes, and additional caloric supplementation may be necessary. In addition, these infants burn up energy with continual activity and increase oxygen consumption at the cellular level.

Hyperactive infants must be protected from skin abrasions on the knees, toes, and cheeks that are caused by rubbing on bed linens while in a prone position (awake). Monitoring and recording the activity level and its relationship to other activities, such as feeding and preventing complications, are important nursing functions.

A valuable aid to anticipating problems in the newborn is recognizing substance abuse in the mother. Unless the mother is enrolled in a methadone rehabilitation program, she seldom risks calling attention to her habit by seeking prenatal care. Consequently, infants and mothers are exposed to the additional hazards of obstetric and medical complications. Moreover, the nature of heroin addiction makes the user susceptible to disorders such as infection (hepatitis B, HIV), foreign body reaction, and the hazards of inadequate nutrition and preterm birth. Methadone treatment does not prevent withdrawal reaction in neonates, but the clinical course may be modified. Also, the intensive psychologic support of mothers is a factor in the treatment and reduction of perinatal mortality. Experience has indicated that mothers are usually anxious and depressed, lack confidence, have a poor self-image, and have difficulty with interpersonal relationships. They may have a psychologic need for the pregnancy and an infant.

Initial symptoms or the recurrence of withdrawal symptoms may develop after discharge from the hospital; therefore, it is important to establish rapport and maintain contact with the family so that they return for treatment if this occurs. The demands of the drug-exposed infant on the caregiver are enormous and nonrewarding in terms of positive feedback. The infants are difficult to comfort, and they cry for long periods, which can be especially trying for the caregiver after the infant's discharge from the hospital. Long-term follow-up to evaluate the status of the infant and family is very important. Sudden infant death syndrome and HIV infection are observed more commonly in infants born to users of methadone and heroin.

There are many problems in relation to the disposition of infants of drug-dependent mothers. Those who advocate separation of mothers and children argue that the mothers are not capable of assuming responsibility for their infant's care, that childcare is frustrating to them, and that their existence is too disorganized and chaotic. Others encourage the maternal-infant bond and recommend a protected environment such as a therapeutic community, a halfway house, or continuous ongoing, supportive services in the home after discharge. Careful evaluation and the cooperative efforts of a variety of health professionals are required whether the choice is foster home placement or supportive follow-up care of mothers who keep their infants.

Cocaine Exposure

Cocaine, the number one illicit drug used in the United States, has multiple modes of use. However, use of the relatively inexpensive and easily administered "crack" form is increasing alarmingly, especially among women of childbearing age (Eyler and Behnke, 1999). Because crack vaporizes at relatively low temperatures, it is smoked and absorbed in large quantities through pulmonary vasculature. The drug readily crosses the placenta, placing the fetus at risk (Malanga and Kosofsy, 1999).

Cocaine is a CNS stimulant and peripheral sympathomimetic. Legally it is classified as a narcotic, but it is not an opioid. The effects on the fetus are secondary to maternal effects—increased BP, decreased uterine blood flow, and increased vascular resistance. Consequently, the fetus suffers decreased blood flow and oxygenation because of placental and fetal vasoconstriction. The difficulties encountered by cocaine-exposed infants are compounded when the mother is taking the drug in conjunction with other illicit drugs (Askin and Diehl-Jones, 2001). Researchers have concluded that variables such as the mother's lack of prenatal care; poor nutrition; and use of tobacco and alcohol, as well as other drugs, during pregnancy compound the effects of cocaine exposure in the infant (Tronick and Beeghly, 1999).

Infants may appear normal, or they may show neurologic problems at birth that may continue during the neonatal period. Fortunately, these findings are transient, and there has been little evidence of permanent sequelae. Either of two types of behavior may emerge as a result of cocaine effects on fetal development: neurobehavioral depression or excitability. The behaviors of the depressed infant include lethargy, poor suck, hypotonia, weak cry, and difficulty in arousing. The behaviors of the excitable neonate may include a high-pitched cry, hypertonicity, rigidity, irritability, inability to be consoled, and intolerance to a change in routine (Chiriboga and others, 1999; Richardson, Hamel, and Goldschmidt, 1996). Other behaviors may include frequent startling, poor awake state, sleeping difficulties, and persistent primitive reflexes. Some infants develop late onset of symptoms (2 to 8 weeks). They may become irritable and hypertonic, experience sleep-awake disruptions, and demonstrate an inability to tolerate change; they may also be slightly febrile. However, these findings have been refuted in other studies (Eyler and Behnke, 1999; Tronick and Beeghly, 1999).

The adverse effects on the cocaine-exposed neonate are related to dose-response. The higher the dose, the more effects are noted, such as intrauterine growth retardation, hypertonia, and decreased fetal head growth (Chiriboga and others, 1999).

Sequelae of prenatal cocaine exposure include a smaller head circumference, decreased birth length, and decreased weight. Head growth may be one of the best predictors of long-term development (Bateman and Chiriboga, 2000). Other neonatal effects of cocaine exposure include increased incidence of gastroschisis, genitourinary anomalies, and periventricular and intraventricular hemorrhage. Long-term sequelae for newborns exposed to cocaine include lower language, motor, and cognitive scores in some studies (Singer and others, 2002; Koren and others, 1998); however, in one study there were no significant differences in the expressive, receptive, and total language scores (Hurt and others, 1997). Arendt and others (1999) noted that the fine and gross motor development indexes in 2-year-old children who were exposed to cocaine prenatally were lower than in the control group. Some researchers noted that the exposed children may be affected emotionally rather than intellectually. In a study of first-grade students, Delaney-Black and others (1998) concluded that the children who were exposed to cocaine prenatally were rated by their teachers as having more behavior problems than the control group.

Scores on the Brazelton Neonatal Assessment Scale have shown infants to be low in responding appropriately to arousal, auditory, and visual stimuli (Eyler, Behnke, and Conlon, 1998). However, other studies have not found significant differences (Frank and others, 1998; Richardson, Hamel, and Goldschmidt, 1996; Tronick and others, 1996).

Therapeutic Management. Treatment of these infants is similar to that for other drug-exposed infants—reduction of external stimuli, supportive treatment aimed at alleviating symptoms, and, at times, mild sedation.

Nursing Considerations. Nursing care of cocaine-exposed infants is the same as that for other drug-exposed infants. Because they have increased flexor tone, these infants respond to swaddling in a semiflexed position (Askin and Diehl-Jones, 2001). Positioning, infant massage, and limited tactile stimulation have been shown to be effective interventions. Effects of the drug from breast milk have been reported (Kandall, 1999); therefore, mothers should be cautioned regarding this hazard to their infants.

Referral to early intervention programs, including child health care, parental drug treatment, individualized developmental care, and parenting education, is essential in promoting the optimum outcome for these children. Many studies indicate that there is little or no significance between the cocaine-exposed and nonexposed groups; however, both groups score significantly lower than published norms. Because these children often live in an impoverished environment, both groups are at high risk for cognitive delays, lack of child health care, and inadequate nutrition and would benefit from an early intervention program (Tronick and Beeghly, 1999). A "one-stop shopping" model at one location affords comprehensive care for mothers and children, not just for drug treatment, but also for the social and medical problems that exist (Tanney and Lowenstein, 1997).

MATERNAL INFECTIONS

The range of pathologic conditions produced by infectious agents is large, and the difference between the maternal and fetal effects caused by any one agent is also great. Some maternal infections, especially during early gestation, can result in fetal loss or malformations because the ability of the fetus to handle infectious organisms is limited and the fetal immunologic system is unable to prevent the dissemination of infectious organisms to the various tissues.

Not all prenatal infections produce teratogenic effects. Furthermore, the clinical picture of disorders caused by transplacental transfer of infectious agents is not always well defined. Some microbial agents can cause remarkably similar manifestations, and it is not uncommon to test for all when a prenatal infection is suspected. This is the so-called TORCH complex, an acronym for:

T	*Toxoplasmosis*
O	*Other* (e.g., hepatitis B)
R	*Rubella*
C	*Cytomegalovirus infection*
H	*Herpes simplex*

To determine the causative agent in a symptomatic infant, tests are performed to rule out each of these infections. The *O* category may involve testing for several viral infections (e.g., hepatitis B, varicella zoster, measles, mumps, HIV, syphilis, human papillomavirus, and human parvovirus). Although this acronym has received substantial criticism because it does not cover the entire spectrum of congenital infections (Klein and Remington, 2001), it is still used in clinical settings. Bacterial infections are not included in the TORCH workup, because they are usually identified by clinical manifestations and readily available laboratory tests. Gonococcal conjunctivitis (ophthalmia neonatorum) and chlamydial conjunctivitis have been significantly reduced by prophylactic measures at birth (see Chapter 8). The major maternal infections, their possible effects, and specific nursing considerations are outlined in Table 9-13.

Nursing Considerations

One of the major goals in care of infants suspected of having an infectious disease is identification of the causative organism. Until the diagnosis is established, standard precautions are implemented according to institutional policy. In suspected cytomegalovirus and rubella infections, pregnant personnel are cautioned to avoid contact with the infant.

TABLE 9-13 ■ Infections Acquired From Mother Before, During, or After Birth

FETAL OR NEWBORN EFFECT	COMMENTS AND NURSING CONSIDERATIONS†
HUMAN IMMUNODEFICIENCY VIRUS (HIV)	
No significant difference between infected and uninfected infants at birth in some instances	Transmitted: transplacentally; during vaginal delivery; potentially in breast milk
Embryopathy reported by some observers:	Recommended treatment: administer zidovudine (ZDV) alone or zidovudine and lamivudine until delivery to HIV-positive mother; untreated mother may be treated at delivery with a two-dose regimen of nevirapine; administer nevirapine to newborn after delivery; in newborn whose mother is on ZDV, same may be given after birth
Depressed nasal bridge	
Mild upward or downward obliquity of eyes	
Long palpebral fissures with blue sclerae	Cesarean section in HIV-positive mother is recommended to reduce transmission
Patulous lips	Chemoprophylaxis against *Pneumocystis carinii* pneumonia (PCP) in HIV-exposed infants: drug of choice is trimethoprim sulfamethoxazole (Bactrim, Septra)
Ocular hypertelorism	
Prominent upper vermilion border	Documented routine HIV education and routine testing with consent for all pregnant women in the United States is recommended
CHICKENPOX (VARICELLA-ZOSTER VIRUS [VZV])	
Intrauterine exposure—congenital varicella syndrome: limb dysplasia, microcephaly, cortical atrophy, chorioretinitis, cataracts, cutaneous scars, other anomalies, auditory nerve palsy, mental retardation	Transmitted: first trimester (fetal varicella syndrome); perinatal period (infection)
	Treatment: exposed infants—varicella zoster immune globulin (VZIG) to infants born to mothers with onset of disease within 5 days before or 2 days after delivery (7 days before and 7 days after in United Kingdom)
Severe symptoms (rash, fever) and higher mortality in infant whose mother develops varicella 5 days before to 2 days after delivery	Isolation precautions 21 days after birth (if hospitalized)
	Prevention: universal immunization of all children with varicella (Var) vaccine

TABLE 9-13 ■ Infections Acquired From Mother Before, During, or After Birth*—cont'd

FETAL OR NEWBORN EFFECT	COMMENTS AND NURSING CONSIDERATIONS†
CHLAMYDIA INFECTION (CHLAMYDIA TRACHOMATIS)	
Conjunctivitis, pneumonia	Transmitted: last trimester or perinatal period Standard ophthalmic prophylaxis for gonococcal ophthalmia neonatorum (topical antibiotics, silver nitrate, or povidone-iodine) is not effective in treatment or prevention of chlamydia ophthalmia Treatment: oral erythromycin 14 days
COXSACKIEVIRUS (GROUP B ENTEROVIRUS–NONPOLIO)	
Poor feeding, vomiting, diarrhea, fever; cardiac enlargement, arrhythmias, congestive heart failure, lethargy, seizures, meningeal involvement Mimics bacterial sepsis	Transmitted: peripartum Treatment: supportive; IVIG in neonatal infections
CYTOMEGALOVIRUS (CMV)	
Variable manifestation from asymptomatic to severe Microcephaly, cerebral calcifications, chorioretinitis Jaundice, hepatosplenomegaly Petechial or purpuric rash Neurologic sequelae: seizure disorders, sensorimotor deafness, mental retardation	Infection acquired at birth, shortly thereafter, or via human milk is not associated with clinical illness Transmitted: throughout pregnancy Affected individuals excrete virus Virus detected in urine or tissue by electron microscopy Avoid kissing affected child Pregnant women should avoid close contact with known cases Treatment: IV antivirals such as ganciclovir given to newborn
ERYTHEMA INFECTIOSUM (PARVOVIRUS B19)	
Fetal hydrops and death from anemia and heart failure, early exposure Anemia from later exposure No teratogenic effects established Ordinarily, low risk of ill effect to fetus	Transmitted: transplacentally First trimester infection most serious effects Pregnant health care workers should not care for patients who might be highly contagious (e.g., child with sickle cell anemia, aplastic crisis) Routine exclusion of pregnant women from workplace where disease is occurring is not recommended
GONOCOCCAL DISEASE (NEISSERIA GONORRHOEAE)	
Ophthalmitis Neonatal gonococcal arthritis, septicemia, meningitis	Transmitted: last trimester or perinatal period Apply prophylactic medication to eyes at time of birth Obtain smears for culture Treatment: penicillin
HEPATITIS B VIRUS (HBV)	
May be asymptomatic at birth Acute hepatitis, changes in liver function	Transmitted: transplacentally; contaminated maternal fluids or secretions during delivery Treatment: hepatitis B immune globulin (HBIG) to all infants of HBsAG-positive mothers within 12 hours of birth; in addition, administer hepatitis B vaccine at separate site Prevention: universal immunization of all infants with Hep B vaccine (see Immunizations, Chapter 10)
HERPES, NEONATAL (HERPES SIMPLEX VIRUS)	
Cutaneous lesions: vesicles at 6 to 10 days of age; may be no lesions Disseminated disease resembles sepsis; encephalitis in 60%-70% Visceral involvement: granulomas Early nonspecific signs: fever, lethargy, poor feeding, irritability, vomiting May include hyperbilirubinemia, seizures, flaccid or spastic paralysis, apneic episodes, respiratory distress, lethargy, or coma	History of genital infection in mother or partner in 50% of cases Transmitted: intrapartum either ascending or direct contact, especially primary infection Cesarean sections sometimes a preventive measure for mothers with active lesions Vaginal delivery of infants of mothers with recurrent infection thought to be at lower risk Suggest infants room-in with mother in private room Treatment: acyclovir (intravenous) in newborn

*This table is not an exhaustive representation of all perinatally transmitted infections. For further information regarding specific diseases or treatment not listed here, the reader is referred to American Academy of Pediatrics, Committee on Infectious Diseases: *2003 Red Book report of the Committee on Infectious Diseases,* ed 26, Elk Grove Village, Il, The Academy.

†Isolation precautions depend on institutional policy (see Infection Control, Chapter 22).

Continued

TABLE 9-13 ■ **Infections Acquired From Mother Before, During, or After Birth*—_cont'd_**

FETAL OR NEWBORN EFFECT	COMMENTS AND NURSING CONSIDERATIONS†
LISTERIOSIS *(LISTERIA MONOCYTOGENES)*	
Maternal infection associated with abortion, preterm delivery, and fetal death Preterm birth, sepsis, and pneumonia are seen in early-onset disease; late-onset disease usually manifests as meningitis	Transmitted: transplacentally, by ascending infection or exposure at delivery
RUBELLA, CONGENITAL (RUBELLA VIRUS)	
Eye defects: cataracts (unilateral or bilateral), microphthalmia, retinitis, glaucoma CNS signs: microcephaly, seizures, severe mental retardation Congenital heart defects: patent ductus arteriosus Auditory: high incidence of delayed hearing loss Intrauterine growth retardation Hyperbilirubinemia, meningitis, thrombocytopenia, hepatomegaly	Transmitted: first trimester; early second trimester Pregnant women should avoid contact with all affected persons, including infants with rubella syndrome Emphasize vaccination of all unimmunized prepubertal children, susceptible adolescents, and women of childbearing age (nonpregnant) Caution women against pregnancy for at least 3 months after vaccination
SYPHYLIS, CONGENITAL *(TREPONEMA PALLIDUM)*	
Stillbirth, prematurity, hydrops fetalis May be asymptomatic at birth and in first few weeks of life or may have multisystem manifestations: hepatosplenomegaly, lymphadenopathy, hemolytic anemia, and thrombocytopenia Copper-colored maculopapular cutaneous lesions (usually after first few weeks of life), mucous membrane patches, hair loss, nail exfoliation, snuffles (syphilitic rhinitis), profound anemia, poor feeding, pseudoparalysis of one or more limbs, dysmorphic teeth (older child)	Transmitted: transplacentally; can be anytime during pregnancy or at birth Most severe form of syphilis Treatment: IV penicillin Diagnostic evaluation dependent on maternal serology testing and infant symptoms (see American Academy of Pediatrics, Committee on Infectious Diseases, 2003)
TOXOPLASMOSIS *(TOXOPLASMA GONDII)*	
May be asymptomatic at birth (70%-90% of cases) or maculopapular rash, lymphadenopathy, hepatosplenomegaly, jaundice, thrombocytopenia Hydrocephaly, cerebral calcifications, chorioretinitis (classic triad) Microcephaly, seizures, mental retardation, deafness Encephalitis, myocarditis, hepatosplenomegaly, anemia, jaundice, diarrhea, vomiting, purpura	Transmitted: throughout pregnancy Predominant host for organism is cats May be transmitted through cat feces, poorly cooked or raw infected meats Caution pregnant women to avoid contact with cat feces (e.g., emptying cat litter boxes) Treatment if not fetal infection: sulfonamides (Septra, Bactrim), pyrimethamine (Daraprim), folinic acid (leukovorin) Treatment if fetal infection: Spiramycin

*This table is not an exhaustive representation of all perinatally transmitted infections. For further information regarding specific diseases or treatment not listed here, the reader is referred to American Academy of Pediatrics, Committee on Infectious Diseases, Pickering L, editor: *2003 Red Book report of the Committee on Infectious Diseases,* ed 26, Elk Grove Village, Il, The Academy.
†Isolation precautions depend on institutional policy (see Infection Control, Chapter 22).

Herpes simplex is easily transmitted from one infant to another; therefore, risk of cross-contamination is reduced or eliminated by wearing gloves for patient contact. The American Academy of Pediatrics' *Red Book: Report of the Committee on Infectious Diseases* (2003) provides guidelines for the type and duration of precautions for most bacterial and viral exposures. Careful handwashing is the most important nursing intervention in reducing the spread of any infection.

Specimens need to be obtained for laboratory examinations, and the infant and parents need to be prepared for diagnostic procedures. When possible, long-term disabilities are prevented by early evaluation and implementation of therapy. The family is taught any special handling techniques needed for the care of their infant and signs of complications or possible sequelae. If sequelae are inevitable, the family will need assistance in determining how they can best cope with the problems, such as assistance with home care, referral to appropriate agencies, or placement in an institution for care. The major goal of nursing care is prevention of these disorders with provision of adequate prenatal care for the expectant mother and precautions regarding exposure to teratogenic infections.

CONGENITAL ANOMALIES*

Congenital anomalies, or *birth defects,* can be identified prenatally, at birth, or at any point after birth. About 2% to 3% of all births are associated with a major congenital anomaly. An even greater number of children will begin to exhibit manifestations of a genetic disorder at later stages of development (Box 9-15).

A few congenital defects are clearly caused by a genetic contribution such as a single-gene defect or a chromosome abnormality, others appear to be consistent with multifactorial inheritance, whereas other defects are produced by intrauterine environment factors, such as maternal diabetes; however, the exact cause is unknown for almost half of all congenital anomalies.

The types of malformations that can result from genetic or prenatal environmental causes can be *major structural abnormalities* with serious medical, surgical, or quality-of-life consequences, or they can be *minor anomalies* or *normal variants* with no serious consequences, such as a sacral dimple, an extra nipple, or a single simian crease of the hand. Malformations can occur in isolation, such as congenital heart defect, or multiple anomalies may be present. A recognized pattern of malformations resulting from a single specific cause is called a *syndrome* (e.g., Turner syndrome, FAS).

Genetic diseases can usually be classified into one of the following three broad categories according to the mechanisms that produce the observed effect. The categories of inheritance are *chromosomal,* *single-gene disorder,* and *multifactorial.* The normal number of chromosomes in the human is 46, with 23 received from the father and 23 from the mother. Any change in the normal number may result in a chromosome disorder. Single-gene or mendelian disorders are caused by an abnormality in a single-gene on a chromosome. Multifactorial inheritance is due to a combination of genetic and environmental factors specific to the pregnancy.

The classification of the genetic disorder has important implications for knowing:

- What is the disorder? Diagnosis
- What caused it? Etiology
- What does it mean? Prognosis
- What can be done? Therapy
- Will it happen again? Recurrence risk
- Is testing available for future pregnancies? Prenatal diagnosis

Establishing a diagnosis helps the family and health care team be aware of the findings that may be seen with the disorder and to initiate early intervention strategies. Accurate genetic counseling for the parents and family members can be provided after a diagnosis is established. For example, children with DiGeorge or 22q11 deletion syndrome may

---

*Susan Fernbach, BSN, RN, revised this section.

BOX 9-15 ■ Assessment Clues to Genetic Disorders*

Major or minor birth defects (anomalies) and dysmorphic features—Cardiac defect, ear or eye abnormalities, micrognathia, forehead prominence, low-set hairline on forehead or nape of neck, wide-set eyes, epicanthal folds, low-set ears

Growth abnormalities—Short stature, overgrowth, asymmetric growth, intrauterine growth retardation, postnatal growth delay

Skeletal abnormalities—Limb abnormalities, asymmetry, scoliosis, hyperextensible joints, hypotonic or hypertonic muscle tone, pectus excavatum, finger or joint abnormalities

Vision or hearing problems—Coloboma, cat's eye, hearing loss, vision loss

Metabolic disorders—Unusual odor of breath, urine, or stool; coarse facial features

Sexual development abnormalities—Ambiguous genitalia, small penis, delayed onset of puberty, primary amenorrhea, precocious sexual development, large testicles

Skin disorders—Unusual pigmentation, café-au-lait spots, dry and scaly skin, skin tumors, sparse hair, absent or unusual teeth

Recurrent infection or immune deficiency—Ear infections, pneumonia

Developmental and speech delays or loss of milestones:
Cognitive delays—Learning disabilities, mild to severe mental retardation
Behavioral disorders—Hyperactivity, attention deficit disorder, autistic-like behavior, aggressive behavior

*Suggests genetic etiology if two or more findings are present.

---

be identified and diagnosed because of the combination of velopharyngeal incompetence and cardiac defects. After the diagnosis of a chromosome microdeletion disorder is made, evaluation for immune function and renal abnormalities can be initiated. Cognitive, speech, and language delays are commonly seen in children with this disorder and enrollment in early childhood intervention programs should be arranged as soon after diagnosis as possible.

CHROMOSOMAL ABNORMALITIES

An *abnormality* is defined as a deviation from that which is normal or typical. *Chromosomal abnormalities* are deviations in either structure or number of chromosomes, and the consequences in either situation can usually be readily observed in the affected individual. A *structural abnormality* involves loss, addition, rearrangement, or exchange of some of the genes of a chromosome. Deviations in chromosomal number involve the gain or loss of a chromosome and are designated with the suffix *-somy.* A cell that contains one less than the normal number of chromosomes (46) is called a *monosomy* because of the loss of one member of a chromosome pair; a cell containing one more than the normal number of chromosomes that results from the addition of an extra member to a normal pair is called a *trisomy.* Most chromosomal abnormalities result from abnormal cell division during germ cell formation or early cell division in the zygote. Others are caused by a *translocation* in which a segment of one chromosome breaks off and attaches to another chromosome. An individual with a balanced translocation is usually normal in appearance and function because

TABLE 9-14 ■ Common Autosomal Abnormalities

CHROMOSOMAL ABNORMALITY AND NOMENCLATURE	AVERAGE INCIDENCE (LIVE BIRTH)*	MAJOR CLINICAL MANIFESTATIONS
CRI-DU-CHAT SYNDROME		
Deletion of short arm of No. 5 chromosome—46,XY or XX,5p–	1:50,000	Distinctive weak, high-pitched, mewlike cry resembling the cry of a cat; small head; hypertelorism; failure to thrive; severe mental retardation—profound with age
TRISOMY 13 (PATAU SYNDROME)		
Trisomy of No. 13 chromosome—47,XY or XX, +13	1:4000-15,000	Multiple anomalies, including cleft lip and palate (frequently bilateral); ear malformations; microphthalmia; polydactyly; eye defects; mental retardation; early death
TRISOMY 18 (EDWARDS SYNDROME)		
Trisomy of No. 18 chromosome—47,XY or XX, +18	1:3500-8000	Deformed and low-set ears; micrognathia; rocker-bottom feet; overlapping (index over third) fingers; prominent occiput; hypertelorism; failure to thrive and early death; mental retardation
TRISOMY 21 (DOWN SYNDROME)		
Trisomy of No. 21 chromosome—47,XY or XX, +21 (trisomy); 46,XY +14;21 (translocation); 46,XY/47,XY 21+ (mosaic)	1:700†	Brachycephaly with flat occiput; epicanthal folds; small ears, nose, and mouth with protruding tongue; muscular hypotonia; broad, short hands with stubby fingers and transverse palmar crease; broad, stubby feet with wide space between big and second toes; cardiac defects; mental retardation; variable life expectancy

*Data from Nora JJ, Fraser FC: *Medical genetics: principles and practice,* ed 3, Philadelphia, 1989, Lea & Febiger.
†Risk related to maternal age: age 30 years = 1:1500; age 35 years = 1:300; age 40 years = 1:100; age 45 years = 1:25.

no genetic material is gained or lost. However, the translocation can be passed to offspring in an unbalanced form, resulting in spontaneous abortion or a child with *congenital abnormalities.* Therefore referral for genetic counseling is recommended for individuals found to have a translocation.

Both numeric and structural abnormalities of autosomes (any chromosome that is not a sex chromosome) and sex chromosomes account for a variety of disorders of infancy and childhood. A few are associated with a group of characteristics that clearly indicate the precise chromosomal anomaly (Table 9-14). The most common is Down syndrome, which is usually caused by a trisomy of chromosome 21 (see Chapter 19 for a further discussion of Down syndrome). The other known viable autosomal trisomies involve chromosomes 18 and 13, and triploidy, which is a trisomy of every pair. Although the prognosis for survival after birth is poor, some children have lived for several years. Abnormalities of sex chromosomes are discussed in Chapter 17.

Single-Gene Defects. Single-gene disorders are caused by a mutation or change in a single gene on a chromosome or the matched gene pair on both chromosomes. For example, cystic fibrosis is caused when two matched pairs of genes on chromosomes 7 carry the cystic fibrosis gene mutation. However, Marfan syndrome occurs when a mutation in the fibrillin gene occurs on one chromosome 15. Single-gene disorders are individually rare, but collectively play a significant role in human disease. It is estimated that 6% to 8% of hospitalized children have a single-gene disorder.

Multifactorial Inheritance. Some congenital anomalies are caused by multifactorial inheritance. This means that several abnormal genes in combination with environmental factors contribute to the congenital anomaly. Cleft lip and palate, neural tube defects, and congenital heart defects are some examples of conditions caused by multifactorial inheritance

DEFECTS CAUSED BY CHEMICAL AGENTS

Prenatal environmental influences from chemicals such as alcohol, medications, or drugs; infectious disease; or radiation or other environmental influences may be regarded as nongenetic causes of congenital anomalies because these effects can produce congenital structural, functional, or growth defects. An agent that produces congenital malformations or increases their incidence is called a *teratogen.*

The relationship of the fetal and maternal circulations allows for the interchange of chemical substances across the placental membrane. Many drugs have been suspected of producing congenital malformations, and some have been definitely implicated. Some of the most recognized teratogenic drugs include alcohol, tobacco, antiepileptic medications, isotretinoin (Accutane), lithium, cocaine, and diethylstilbestrol (Table 9-15).

The extent to which chemical agents affect the unborn child depends on the interplay of several factors—the nature of the agent and its accessibility to the fetus, the gestational age at which exposure occurred, the level and duration of the dosage, and the genetic makeup of the fetus. For example, fetal exposure to valproic acid in the first 3 months of

TABLE 9-15 ■ Congenital Effects of Maternal Alcohol Ingestion and Tobacco Smoking

FETAL OR NEWBORN EFFECTS	COMMENTS AND NURSING CONSIDERATIONS
ALCOHOL (FETAL ALCOHOL SYNDROME [FAS] OR ALCOHOL-RELATED BIRTH DEFECTS [ARBD])	
Varies—infant may not display physical features; involves three main categories: (1) growth failure in utero, including microcephaly; (2) midfacial dysmorphic features; (3) central nervous system involvement including cognitive impairment, irritability, hyperactivity, hypertonia, and behavioral problems.	Quantity of alcohol consumed is not the determinant; rather, it is the amount consumed in excess of the liver's ability to detoxify alcohol. Free alcohol has an affinity for brain tissue, thus CNS symptoms. Ethanol by-products also contribute to toxicity as well as other substances consumed in addition to alcohol and poor maternal self-care. Effects of alcohol on CNS are not reversible. FAS (ARBD) is the leading cause of preventable mental retardation in the United States.
Facial features: hypoplastic maxilla, micrognathia, short palpebral fissures, thinned upper lip, hypoplastic philtrum, short, upturned nose. One or a combination of these features may present in infancy or later.	Early intervention with mother is aimed at minimizing fetal effects, education, and involvement in prevention and treatment counseling. Early intervention with newborn focuses on reducing the effects of alcohol exposure on growing child, especially in relation to cognitive deficits and learning disabilities.
Children or adults who demonstrate cognitive, behavioral, and psychosocial problems without physical features and growth delay are referred to as having FAE (fetal alcohol effects) or alcohol-related neurodevelopmental disorder (ARND).	Treatment in neonatal period is similar to that of drug-exposed infants and should involve extensive assessment and individualized developmental care.
Affected infants may display nonspecific signs such as irritability, lethargy, difficulty establishing respirations, seizures, tremors, poor suck reflex, abdominal distention. Birth defects may occur but are less common.	Provide resources to help decrease or eliminate alcohol intake: March of Dimes: *During your pregnancy: tips to giving up alcohol;* website: www.marchofdimes.com
Diagnosis is made more difficult by lack of a single biologic marker and may be made based on maternal history of alcohol ingestion.	Further information is available at NOFAS (National Organization on Fetal Alcohol Syndrome), 216 G Street, NE, Washington, DC 20002; (202) 785-4585; www.nofas.org; and Fetal Alcohol Syndrome Branch, Division of Birth Defects, Child Development and Disability and Health, Centers for Disease Control and Prevention, Atlanta, www.cdc.gov/ncbdd/fas.
MATERNAL TOBACCO SMOKING	
Associated with significant birth weight deficits; positive dose-response relationship related to size of fetus.	Counseling regarding fetal and postnatal effects should be made available to all pregnant women, and they are encouraged to stop smoking. Smoking cessation during pregnancy decreases chance of fetal complications. Encourage pregnant woman to enroll in a smoking cessation program.
Two active substances—nicotine and cotinine—are higher in newborns of mothers who smoke than in mothers who do not. Postnatal growth deficits occur as well as deficits in emotional and behavioral development in the growing child.	Evaluate polydrug use in conjunction with smoking. Women should be counseled regarding risks to fetus. Increased incidence of perinatal complications leading to preterm birth including abruption placentae, placenta previa, and premature rupture of membranes.
Maternal smoking is associated with an increased risk of Sudden Infant Death Syndrome, respiratory tract illnesses in childhood, and childhood learning deficits.	Provide resources to help eliminate smoking: *During your pregnancy: tips to quit* is available from the March of Dimes: www.marchofdimes.com

pregnancy may result in congenital anomalies such as neural tube defects, congenital heart defects, and distinctive facial features.

Nursing Considerations

Expectant mothers are cautioned against ingesting any medication without first consulting a practitioner. To help ensure that fewer women will inadvertently take some chemical that might be harmful to the fetus, labels on medications are now required to include information regarding the possible teratogenic effects of the drug. All women of childbearing age should be educated regarding the effects of chemicals, especially alcohol, on the unborn fetus. FAS is an irreversible condition but is completely preventable. The

March of Dimes* and **Centers for Disease Control and Prevention†** have information about prevention tips, and the **Genetic Alliance‡** has information about support groups for families of children with FAS. Genetic counseling is recommended for women who have a concern about a possible teratogen during pregnancy.

***March of Dimes,** 1275 Mamarek Avenue, White Plains, NY 10605; (888) MODIMES; website: www.marchofdimes.com.
†**Centers for Disease Control and Prevention;** website: www.cdc.gov.
‡**Genetic Alliance,** 4301 Connecticut Avenue NW, Suite 404, Washington, DC 20008; website: www.geneticalliance.org.

INBORN ERRORS OF METABOLISM

Inborn errors of metabolism (IEMs) constitute a large number of inherited diseases caused by the absence or deficiency of a substance essential to cellular metabolism, usually an enzyme. When the normal metabolic process is interrupted as a result of a missing enzyme, an accumulation of substances precedes the interruption, the end product of the process is absent, or the process takes an alternate metabolic pathway. The consequence is manifested as an illness. Most IEMs are characterized by abnormal protein, carbohydrate, or fat metabolism.

Newborn screening for IEMs varies from state to state, but all test for PKU and congenital hypothyroidism and the majority test for galactosemia.* The purpose of screening is to identify children who may have a condition that benefits from early identification and treatment to prevent mental retardation. The screening test is most reliable if the blood sample is taken after the infant has ingested a source of protein for 24 hours. Because of early discharge of newborns, recommendations for screening include (1) collecting the initial specimen as close as possible to discharge or no later than 7 days, (2) obtaining a subsequent sample by 2 weeks of age if the initial specimen is collected before the newborn is 24 hours old, and (3) designating a primary care provider to all newborns before discharge for adequate newborn screening follow-up (American Academy of Pediatrics, 1996a). A new screening test, tandem mass spectrometry, has the potential for identifying more than 20 inborn errors of metabolism, in addition to the standard IEMs. With tandem mass spectrometry earlier identification of IEMs may prevent further developmental delays and morbidities in affected children.

A major concern is that a significantly large number of infants are *not* rescreened for PKU after early discharge and are at risk for a missed or delayed diagnosis of PKU. Special consideration must be given to screening infants born at home who have no hospital contact. It is always necessary to confirm the screening results with diagnostic testing.

CONGENITAL HYPOTHYROIDISM

Congenital hypothyroidism (CH) may have a number of etiologies and can be either permanent or transient. However, no matter what the cause, the manifestations (Box 9-16) and management are similar. In some conditions the thyroid deficiency is severe and manifestations develop early; in others, the symptoms may be delayed for months or years.

Results of screening tests in the United States indicate that CH occurs in approximately 1 of every 3600 to 5000 newborns (American Academy of Pediatrics, 1996a). Infants with Down syndrome have a much higher rate of either permanent or transient forms of the disorder. Also, a higher incidence of other congenital abnormalities has been observed in infants with CH. Many preterm infants have hypothyroidism (hypothyroxinemia) at birth as a result of hypothalamic and pituitary immaturity. However, this type is transient and requires no treatment.

Diagnostic Evaluation

Diagnosis is aimed at early identification of the disorder to prevent the serious effects on mental development resulting from delayed treatment. Neonatal screening consists of an initial filter paper blood spot thyroxine (T_4) measurement followed by measurement of thyroid-stimulating hormone (TSH) in specimens with low T_4 values.

---

*Because newborn screening varies by state and policies change frequently, a good resource is the **National Newborn Screening & Genetics Resource Center** website: http://genes-r-us.uthscsa.edu.

BOX 9-16 ■ Clinical Manifestations of Congenital Hypothyroidism

BIRTH*	6-9 WEEKS†	OLDER CHILD
Poor feeding	Depressed nasal bridge	Short stature
Lethargy	Short forehead	Obesity
Prolonged jaundice (>2 weeks)	Puffy eyelids	Varying degrees of intellectual deficits
Respiratory difficulties	Large tongue	Abnormal tendon reflexes
Cyanosis	Thick, dry, mottled skin	Slow, awkward movements
Constipation	Coarse, dry, lusterless hair	
Bradycardia	Abdominal distention	
Hoarse cry	Umbilical hernia	
Large anterior/posterior fontanels	Hyporeflexia	
Postterm	Bradycardia	
Birth weight >4000 g	Hypothermia	
	Hypotension	
	Anemia	
	Widely patent cranial sutures	

*Clinical manifestations may not be obvious at birth, possibly because of maternal transfer of thyroid hormone to fetus. Manifestations may be delayed in infants with certain types of familial hypothyroidism and in breast-fed infants (may show once weaned).
†If untreated; classical features.

Tests are mandatory in all 51 US states and territories. Although a blood sample obtained by heel stick for the spot test is best obtained between 2 and 6 days of age, specimens are usually taken within the first 24 to 48 hours or before discharge as part of a concurrent screen for other metabolic defects. Early screening can result in overdiagnosis (false-positives) but is preferable to missing the diagnosis.

Screening results that show a low level of T_4 (<6 μg/dL) and a high level of TSH (>60 μU/mL) indicate CH and the need for further tests to determine the cause of the disease (see Appendix E for values). Additional tests include serum measurement of T_4, triiodothyronine (T_3), resin uptake, free T_4, and thyroid-bound globulin. Tests of thyroid gland function (thyroid scan and uptake) usually involve oral administration of a radioactive isotope of iodine (^{131}I) and measurement of iodine uptake by the thyroid, usually within 24 hours. In CH, protein-bound iodine, T_4, T_3, and free T_4 levels are low and thyroid uptake of ^{131}I is decreased. Skeletal radiography is used to assess age.

In the newborn, thyroid function studies are elevated in comparison with values in older children; therefore, it is important to document the timing of the tests. In preterm and sick full-term infants thyroid function tests are usually lower than in the healthy full-term infant; a repeat T_4 and TSH may be evaluated after 30 weeks (corrected age) in newborns born before that time and after resolution of the acute illness in the sick full-term infant.

Therapeutic Management

Treatment involves lifelong thyroid hormone replacement therapy as soon as possible after diagnosis to abolish all signs of hypothyroidism and reestablish normal physical and mental development. The drug of choice is synthetic levothyroxine sodium (Synthroid or Levothroid). Regular measurement of thyroxine levels is important in ensuring optimum treatment. Bone-age surveys are also performed to ensure optimum growth.

Prognosis. If treatment is started shortly after birth, normal physical growth and intelligence are possible. The most significant factor adversely affecting eventual intellectual development appears to be inadequate treatment, which may be related to noncompliance.

Nursing Considerations

The most important nursing objective is early identification of the disorder. Nurses caring for neonates must be certain that screening is performed, especially in infants who are preterm, discharged early, or born at home. Approximately 10% of cases are detected only by a second screening at 2 to 6 weeks of age. Nurses in community health need to be aware of the earliest signs of the disorder. Parental remarks about an unusually "quiet and good" baby as well as demonstrated symptoms such as prolonged jaundice, constipation, and umbilical hernia should lead to a suspicion of hypothyroidism, which requires a referral for specific tests.

After the diagnosis is confirmed, parents need an explanation of the disorder and the necessity of lifelong treatment. The child should be referred to a pediatric endocrinologist for care. The importance of compliance with the drug regimen for the child to achieve normal growth and

development must be stressed (Harrell and Murray, 1998). Because the drug is tasteless, it can be crushed and added to formula, water, or food. If a dose is missed, twice the dose should be given the next day. Unless there are maternal contraindicative factors, breast-feeding is acceptable in infants with hypothyroidism. Parents also need to be aware of signs indicating overdose, such as a rapid pulse, dyspnea, irritability, insomnia, fever, sweating, and weight loss. Ideally, they should know how to count the pulse and be instructed to withhold a dose and consult their practitioner if the pulse rate is above a certain value. Signs of inadequate treatment are fatigue, sleepiness, decreased appetite, and constipation.

If the diagnosis was delayed past early infancy, the chance of permanent mental retardation is great. Parents need the same guidance in caring for their child as do others who have an offspring with cognitive impairment (see Chapter 19). They need an opportunity to discuss their feelings regarding late recognition of the disorder. Although treatment will not reverse the intellectual deficit, it may prevent further damage. Genetic counseling is important for the rare families where the etiology of CH is thyroid dyshormonogenesis, which is inherited in an autosomal recessive manner (see Genetic Evaluation and Counseling, p. 301).

PHENYLKETONURIA

PKU, an inborn error of metabolism inherited as an autosomal-recessive trait, is caused by a deficiency or absence of the enzyme needed to metabolize the essential amino acid *phenylalanine.* The disorder is detected in 1 in 13,500 to 19,000 live births (Hellekson, 2001) and primarily affects Caucasian children, with the incidence highest in those living in the United States or Northern Europe. It is very rare in the African, Jewish, and Japanese populations.

Classic PKU is at one end of a spectrum of conditions known as *hyperphenylalaninemia.* Because rarer forms are a result of a deficiency in other enzymes and are diagnosed and treated differently, the following discussion of PKU is limited to the severe, classic form.

In PKU the hepatic enzyme *phenylalanine hydroxylase,* which normally controls the conversion of phenylalanine to tyrosine, is deficient. This results in the accumulation of phenylalanine in the bloodstream and urinary excretion of abnormal amounts of its metabolites, the phenyl acids (Fig. 9-17). One of these *phenylketones, phenylacetic acid,* gives urine the characteristic musty odor associated with the disease. Another is *phenylpyruvic acid*, which is responsible for the term *phenylketonuria.*

Tyrosine, the amino acid produced by the metabolism of phenylalanine, is absent in PKU. Tyrosine is needed to form the pigment melanin and the hormones epinephrine and thyroxine. Decreased melanin production results in similar phenotypes of most individuals with PKU—blond hair, blue eyes, and fair skin that is particularly susceptible to eczema and other dermatologic problems. Children with a genetically darker skin color may be red-haired or brunette.

Clinical manifestations in untreated PKU include failure to thrive, frequent vomiting, irritability, hyperactivity, and unpredictable, erratic behavior. Mental retardation is thought to be caused by the accumulation of phenylalanine and presumably by decreased levels of the neurotransmitters

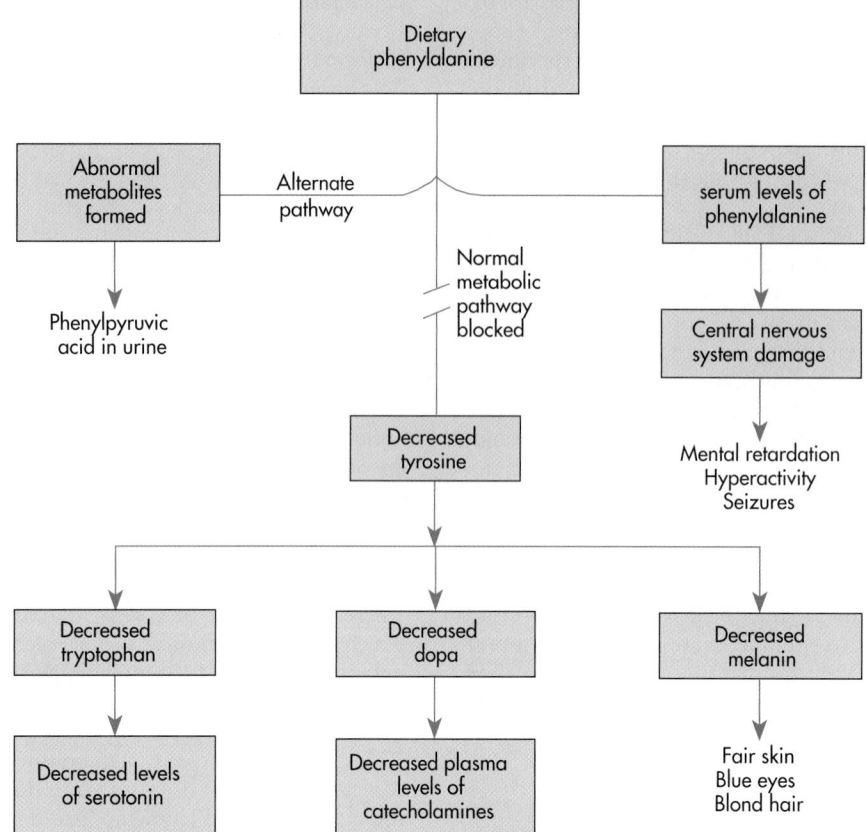

FIG. 9-17 ■ Metabolic error and consequences in phenylketonuria.

dopamine and tryptophan, which affect the normal development of the brain and CNS, resulting in defective myelinization, cystic degeneration of the gray and white matter, and disturbances in cortical lamination. Older children commonly display bizarre or schizoid behavior patterns such as fright reactions, screaming episodes, head banging, arm biting, disorientation, failure to respond to strong stimuli, and catatonia-like positions.

Diagnostic Evaluation*

The objective in diagnosing or treating the disorder is to prevent mental retardation. Every newborn in the United States should be screened for PKU. The most commonly used test for screening newborns is the *Guthrie blood test,* a bacterial inhibition assay for phenylalanine in the blood. *Bacillus subtilis,* present in the culture medium, grows if the blood contains an excessive amount of phenylalanine. If performed properly, this test detects serum phenylalanine levels greater than 4 mg/dL (normal value is 1.6 mg/dL), but it will not quantify the results. Other methods for testing include quantitative fluorometric assay and tandem mass spectrometry, which will give an absolute value. Only fresh heel blood, not cord blood, can be used for the test.

---

*Always refer patient to a genetic metabolic specialist. For a reference list visit the **American Society of Human Genetics** website: www.ashg.org.

> ⚠ **NURSING ALERT**
>
> Avoid "layering" the blood specimen on the special Guthrie paper. Layering is placing one drop of blood on top of the other or overlapping the specimen. This practice results in a falsely high reading or false positive, which will initiate the newborn screening department to call the family and physician to arrange for a diagnostic blood phenylalanine test to be ordered to determine if the newborn is truly affected with PKU. Best results are obtained by collecting the specimen with a pipette from the heel stick and spreading the blood uniformly over the blot paper.

Because of the possibility of variant forms of hyperphenylalaninemia, PKU cofactor variant screen should be performed an all children diagnosed with PKU.

Therapeutic Management*

Treatment of PKU is restricting phenylalanine in the diet. Because the genetic enzyme is intracellular, systemic administration of phenylalanine hydroxylase is of no value. Pheny-

---

*American Society of Human Genetics, 9650 Rockville Pike, Bethesda, MD 20814; (301) 634-7300, (866) HUM-GENE; www.ashg.org

An important resource for treatment guidelines for PKU is *NIH Consensus Development Panel on Phenylketonuria: screening and management,* October 2000. A resource for dietary management is Acosta PB and Yannicelli S: *The Ross Metabolic Formula System Nutrition Support Protocols,* ed 4, 2001, Ross (Abbott), Columbus, OH 43215-1744; (800) 986-8755; www.ross.com.

lalanine cannot be eliminated, because it is an essential amino acid in tissue growth. Therefore, dietary management must meet two criteria: (1) meet the child's nutritional need for optimum growth and (2) maintain phenylalanine levels within a safe range (2 to 6 mg/dL in neonates up to 12 years, 2 to 10 mg/dL through adolescence, and 2 to 15 mg/dL in adults) (NIH Consensus Development Panel on Phenylketonuria, 2000).

Professionals agree that infants with PKU who have blood phenylalanine levels higher than 10 mg/dL should be started on treatment to establish metabolic control as soon as possible, ideally by the time the neonate is 7 to 10 days of age (NIH Consensus Development Panel on Phenylketonuria, 2000). The daily amounts of phenylalanine are individualized for each child and require frequent changes on the basis of appetite, growth and development, and blood phenylalanine and tyrosine levels.

Because all natural food proteins contain phenylalanine and will be limited, the diet must be supplemented with a specially prepared PKU metabolic formula that does not contain any phenylalanine (e.g., Phenex-1 for infants or Phenex-2 for children and adults†). The PKU formula is essential in the low phenylalanine diet to provide the appropriate protein, vitamins, minerals, and calories for optimal growth and development. Because tyrosine becomes an essential amino acid, the PKU formula usually supplies an adequate amount, but in some cases additional supplementation may be needed. (Avoid using the PKU formula alone, because it is an incomplete nutritional source.) Although measuring phenylalanine in the diet will not be as accurate, partial breast-feeding may be possible with close monitoring of phenylalanine levels. Early breast-feeding in infants with PKU before diagnosis was shown to be a positive factor in the neurodevelopmental performance of the same children during the school-age years (Riva and others, 1996).

To achieve optimal metabolic control and outcome, a restricted-Phe diet, including medical foods and low-protein products, most likely will be medically required for virtually all individuals with classical PKU for their entire life (NIH Consensus Development Panel on Phenylketonuria, 2000). To evaluate the effectiveness of dietary treatment, frequent monitoring of blood phenylalanine and tyrosine levels is necessary.

Phenylalanine levels greater than 6 mg/dL in mothers with PKU affect the normal embryologic development of the fetus, including mental retardation, cardiac defects and LBW (NIH Consensus Development Panel on Phenylketonuria, 2000). It is recommended that phenylalanine levels below 6 mg/dL be achieved at least 3 months before conception in women with PKU (NIH Consensus Development Panel on Phenylketonuria, 2000).

Prognosis.   Although many individuals with treated PKU manifest no cognitive and behavioral deficits, many comparisons of individuals with PKU to controls show lower performance on IQ tests, with larger differences in other cognitive domains however their performance is still in the average range. Evidence for differences in behavioral ad-justment is inconsistent despite anecdotal reports suggesting greater risk for internalizing psychopathology and attention disorders (NIH Consensus Development Panel on Phenylketonuria, 2000). Total bone mineral density is considerably lower in children who are on a low-phenylalanine diet, even though calcium, phosphorous, and magnesium intakes are higher than normal.

Nursing Considerations

The principal nursing considerations involve teaching the family regarding the dietary restrictions. Although the treatment may sound simple, the task of maintaining such a strict dietary regimen is very demanding, especially for older children and adolescents. In addition, mothers of children with PKU may have to spend many hours preparing special foods such as low-phenylalanine snacks, and other foods. However, in a recent study mothers of children with PKU reported experiencing considerably less stress than those with mitochondrial disease (Read, 2003). Foods with low phenylalanine levels (e.g., vegetables; fruits; juices; some cereals, breads, and starches) must be measured to provide the prescribed amount of phenylalanine. High-protein foods, such as meat and dairy products, are eliminated from the diet. The sweetener aspartame (NutraSweet) should be avoided because it is composed of two amino acids: aspartic acid and phenylalanine and if used will decrease the amount of natural phenylalanine that is prescribed for the day. However, medications that use aspartame as the sweetener may be used in instances where no other nonaspartame medications are available, because the content of the artificial sweetener is minimal or can be counted in the total daily phenylalanine allowance.

Maintaining the diet during infancy presents few problems. Solid foods such as cereal, fruits, and vegetables are introduced as usual to the infant. Difficulties arise as the child gets older. A decreased appetite and refusal to eat may reduce intake of the calculated phenylalanine requirement. The child's increasing independence may inhibit absolute control of what he or she eats. Either factor can result in decreased or increased phenylalanine levels. During the school years, peer pressure becomes a major force in deterring the child from eating the prescribed foods or abstaining from high-protein foods such as milkshakes or ice cream. Limitations of this diet are best illustrated by an example: a quarter-pound hamburger may provide a 2-day phenylalanine allowance for a school-age child.

The assistance of a registered nutritionist is essential. Parents need a basic understanding of the disorder and practical suggestions regarding food selection and preparation.* Meal planning is based on weighing the food on a gram scale, or a less accurate method is the exchange list. As soon as children are old enough, usually by early preschool, they should be involved in the daily calculation, menu planning, and formula preparation. Using a computer, voice-activated calculator, cards, or colored beads can help children keep track of the daily allowance of phenylalanine foods. A system of goal setting, self-monitoring, contracts, and rewards can promote compliance in adolescents.

---

*A helpful resource is *Low Protein Cookery for Phenylketonuria*, ed 3, Schuett V, editor: 114 N. Murray Street, Madison, WI 53715, 1997, University of Wisconsin Press; (608) 262-8782; email: uwiscpress@uwpress.wisc.edu; www.wisc.edu/wisconsinpress/books/0407.htm.

---

†Ross Laboratories, Columbus, Oh.

Preparation of the PKU formula can present some challenges. The formula tends to be lumpy, so preparing the powder with a small amount of water to make a paste then adding the rest of the required liquid mixture helps alleviate this problem. A blender or mixer dissolves the powder more easily; a rechargeable hand mixer can be used when traveling. Although the taste is virtually impossible to camouflage, there are many new products on the market today. Some of the complete formulas are chocolate, vanilla, strawberry, and orange flavored. There are also incomplete formulas available that do not contain the vitamins and minerals that are plain tasting and can be added to cold foods instead of mixing as a formula. There are also formula bars, which are convenient for the active adolescent. One other product available is formula capsules, but if this product is used the patient will need to take at least 20 or more capsules per day.

*Family Support.** In addition to the problem related to a child with a chronic disorder (see Chapter 18), the parents have the burden of knowing that they are carriers of the defect. Genetic counseling is especially important to inform the parents that prenatal testing is now available to detect the presence of the defective gene in heterozygotes. Counseling is also important for adults with PKU to inform them that all of their offspring will be carriers for PKU (see Genetic Evaluation and Counseling, p. 301, and Family Focus box).

GALACTOSEMIA

Galactosemia is a rare autosomal-recessive disorder that affects approximately 1 of 50,000 births. It involves an inborn error of carbohydrate metabolism in which the hepatic enzyme *galactose 1-phosphate uridyltransferase (GALT)* is absent. This enzyme is one of three needed for the conversion of galactose to glucose. There is considerable genetic

---

*National support groups include the **National Coalition for PKU and Allied Disorders** www.pku-allieddisorders.org; and the Children's PKU Network at www.pkunetwork.org. The **Children's PKU Network** offers a variety of support services (3790 Via de la Valle, Suite 116E, Del Mar, CA 92014) (858)509-0767; email: PKUnetwork@aol.com; website: www.pkunetwork.org.

variability in enzyme deficiency, with some children having partial transferase activity.

As galactose accumulates in the blood, several organs are affected. Hepatic dysfunction leads to cirrhosis, resulting in jaundice in the infant by the second week of life. The spleen subsequently becomes enlarged as a result of portal hypertension. Cataracts are usually recognizable by 1 or 2 months of age; cerebral damage, manifested by the symptoms of lethargy and hypotonia, is evident soon afterward. Infants with galactosemia appear normal at birth, but within a few days of ingesting milk (which has a high lactose content), they begin to vomit and lose weight. *Escherichia coli* sepsis is also a common presenting clinical sign (American Academy of Pediatrics, 1996a). Death during the first month of life is not infrequent in untreated infants.

Diagnostic Evaluation

Diagnosis is made on the basis of the infant's history, physical examination, galactosuria, increased levels of galactose in the blood, and decreased levels of GALT activity in erythrocytes. The infant may display characteristics of malnutrition; signs of dehydration, decreased muscle mass, and body fat may be evident (Askin and Diehl-Jones, 2003). Newborn screening for this disease is required in most states. Heterozygotes can also be identified, because heterozygotic individuals have significantly lower levels of the essential enzyme.

Therapeutic Management

During infancy, treatment consists of eliminating all milk and lactose-containing formula, including breast milk. During infancy, lactose-free formulas are used, with soy-protein formula being the feeding of choice (American Academy of Pediatrics, 1998).

As the infant progresses to solids, only foods low in galactose should be consumed. Food lists should be given to the family to ensure appropriate foods are chosen.

If galactosemia is suspected, supportive treatment and care are implemented, including monitoring for hypoglycemia, liver failure, bleeding disorders, and *E. coli* sepsis.

Prognosis. Follow-up studies of children treated from birth or within the first 2 months of life after symptoms appear have found long-term complications, such as ovarian dysfunction, cataracts, abnormal speech, cognitive impairment, growth retardation, and motor delay (Lashley, 2002). These findings have revealed that eliminating sources of galactose does not significantly improve the outcome. New therapeutic strategies, such as enhancing residual transferase activity, replacing depleted metabolites, or using gene replacement therapy, are needed to improve the prognosis for these children.

Nursing Considerations*

Nursing interventions are similar to those for PKU, except that dietary restrictions are easier to maintain because many more foods are allowed. However, reading food labels very

---

*Information and support for parents can be found at the **American Liver Foundation** (www.liverfoundation.org) and **Parents of Galactosemic Children, Inc.,** 885 Del Sol Street, Sparks, NV 89436; (775) 626-5811; website: www.galactosemia.org.

carefully for the presence of any form of lactose, especially dairy products, is mandatory.

GENETIC EVALUATION AND COUNSELING

Genetic counseling is a communication process concerned with the human problems associated with the occurrence, or risk of occurrence, of a genetic disorder in a family. It involves relaying information about the diagnosis, treatment options, the recurrence risk, and the availability of prenatal diagnosis. With the completion of the Human Genome Project, the international project to determine the total genetic information in humans, a new era of human genetics is evident. It is hoped that there will be a better understanding of specifically how genetic variation contributes to health and disease. It is essential that nurses study the basic principles of heredity and understand how heredity contributes to the disorders as well as be aware of the types of genetic testing available (Table 9-16).

Nurses frequently encounter children with genetic diseases and families in which there is a risk that a disorder may be transmitted to or occur in an offspring. It is a responsibility of nurses to be alert to situations in which persons could benefit from a genetic evaluation and counseling (see Guidelines box), to be aware of the local genetic resources, to aid the family in finding services, and to offer support and care for children and families affected by genetic conditions. Local genetic clinics can be located through several sites; for example, the **Gene Clinics** (www.genetests.org), a publicly funded medical genetics information resource developed for physicians and other health care providers, is available at no cost to all interested persons. Another resource is the **National Society of Genetic Counselors** (www.nsgc.org), which lists genetic counselors by states in the United States.

Maintaining contact with the family or referring the family to an agency that can provide a sustained relationship, usually the public health agency in their locality, is one of the most important aspects in the care of the patient and family. In a disorder that requires conscientious diet management, such as PKU or galactosemia, it is important to make certain that the family understands and follows the advice. A vital role for nurses is to advocate for the child and family as they make their way through the various specialty clinics. This is especially important for families who are more vulnerable because of cognitive, hearing, language, or financial issues and those who otherwise may have difficulty accessing health services. Nurses can reinforce the genetic information or arrange for additional genetic counseling if a family has additional questions or misunderstandings.

One of the current ethical concerns is the testing of healthy children for carrier status of a genetic condition that either will not have adverse consequences until adulthood or only has reproductive implications. The American Academy of Pediatrics' (2001) policy statement does not support the broad use of carrier testing or screening in children or adolescents. When there is no clear medical benefit to testing in childhood, the child should be permitted the opportunity as an adult to choose whether or not to be tested. Genetic counseling is recommended to help the family weigh all of the issues.

TABLE 9-16 ■ Types of Genetic Testing

TEST/METHOD	SPECIMEN	INDICATION	COMMENTS
Chromosome analysis (karyotyping)	Blood, skin, amniocytes, bone marrow	Detection of chromosomal abnormality, sex determination, cancer classification	Almost 100% accuracy for whole or partial chromosome abnormality; will not detect microdeletions/duplication (submicroscopic chromosome segments), single-gene defects, or multifactorial disorders
Fluorescence in situ hybridization (FISH)	Blood, skin, amniocytes, bone marrow	Detection of microdeletion/duplications of chromosome segments (not visible by chromosome analysis)	A technique that is a cross between chromosome analysis and single-gene DNA tests
Direct DNA mutation detection (polymerase chain reaction, Southern blot, gene sequencing)	Blood, skin, amniocytes	Detection of gene mutation(s) in affected individual for diagnosis, in unaffected carrier, or for presymptomatic diagnosis	Gene location must be mapped, and disease-producing mutations must be characterized; can test single individual
Indirect DNA linkage studies (restriction length fragment polymorphisms, microsatellites, genetic markers)	Blood	Prediction of carrier, or presymptomatic status based on inheritance of same chromosome segment as in known affected individual	Must test several family members, including one or two confirmed affected individuals, for testing to be valid
Biochemical	Blood, skin, amniotic fluid, muscle biopsy, urine, stool, cerebrospinal fluid	Detection of metabolic pathway errors, enzyme defects, prenatal neural tube/ventral wall defect	Results may be difficult to interpret if partial pathway error or modified substrate is present
Maternal serum alpha-fetoprotein levels screen for neural tube/ventral wall defects

GUIDELINES

Common Indications for Referral

1. Previous child with multiple congenital anomalies, mental retardation, or an isolated birth defect, such as neural tube defect, cleft lip, and palate
2. Family history of a hereditary condition, such as cystic fibrosis, fragile X syndrome, or diabetes
3. Prenatal diagnosis for advanced maternal age or other indication
4. Consanguinity
5. Teratogen exposure, such as to occupational chemicals, medications, alcohol
6. Repeated pregnancy loss or infertility
7. Newly diagnosed abnormality or genetic condition
8. Before undertaking genetic testing and after receiving results, particularly when testing for susceptibility to late-onset disorders, such as cancer or neurological disease
9. As follow-up for a positive newborn test, as with PKU, or a heterozygote screening test, such as Tay-Sachs

From Nussbaum, R, McInnes, R. Willard, H: *Thompson & Thompson genetics in medicine,* ed 6, Philadelphia, 2001, WB Saunders.

PSYCHOLOGIC ASPECTS OF GENETIC DISEASE

The diagnosis of a genetic disorder in a child can be a life-altering experience for families. They may have to reassess their perception of "self" and the loss of the dream of the perfect baby. Parents may change educational, employment and reproductive plans after the diagnosis of a genetic disorder in their child.

Families may need to have the genetic information repeated several times. Families may also encounter ethical or moral dilemmas regarding genetic evaluation and testing options, as well as potential involvement of other family members. Nurses are pivotal caregivers in assessing the family's understanding of the genetic disorder, psychologic responses, and coping mechanisms. Nurses may help families by providing support and attempting to alleviate possible feelings of guilt, and by helping the family make the best possible adjustment to the disorder.

It is important to stress that there is nothing shameful about an inherited or congenital defect and to emphasize any appropriate remedy. The thought of a hereditary disorder often creates intrafamily strife, hostility, and marital disharmony, sometimes to the point of family disintegration. Relatives may change reproductive plans after the diagnosis of a genetic disorder in a member, or the decision to reproduce may be postponed indefinitely on the basis of a disorder in a relative, even a remote one. Although people may understand the information on an intellectual level, they may still harbor fears on an emotional level. Nurses can help the family to identify their personal strengths as well as offer them information about local and national support groups. (**The Genetic Alliance,** www.geneticalliance.org, is a nonprofit organization that has a database of support groups for genetic conditions.) Finally, it is important to keep in mind that the infant or child has the same basic needs after the diagnosis of a genetic disorder as he or she had before the diagnosis.

KEY POINTS

- Birth injuries are usually transient and may involve soft tissue, bone, or nervous tissue.
- High-risk neonates are those newborn infants, regardless of gestational age or birth weight, who have a greater than average chance of morbidity or mortality because of conditions or circumstances that are superimposed on the normal course of events associated with birth and adjustment to extrauterine life.
- Newborns of all gestational ages have the capacity to feel pain, and adequate pain control, especially during painful procedures or surgery, can reduce morbidity and mortality.
- Nurses must be proactive in the assessment and management of neonatal pain.
- Appropriate developmental care for preterm infants focuses on individualized neurobehavioral assessment, planning, diagnosis, intervention, and reevaluation to foster appropriate growth and maturation in a potentially harmful environment.
- Parents are encouraged to interact with their high-risk infant and gradually assume care of the infant as allowed by the infant's condition.
- Because of their immature physical status, preterm infants need special attention to promote respiratory efforts, maintain body temperature, maintain fluid and electrolyte balance, prevent infection, and provide adequate nutrition for growth.
- Hyperbilirubinemia is a common problem in the newborn that results from red blood cell breakdown that exceeds the ability of the immature liver to metabolize and excrete.
- Preterm infants are subject to a number of complications, including apnea, sepsis, respiratory distress syndrome, necrotizing enterocolitis, and intraventricular hemorrhage.
- Sepsis is a serious condition with generalized nonspecific manifestations that requires immediate intervention involving systemic antibiotics and observation for associated complications.
- Maternal conditions that may pose health risks in the neonatal period include maternal diabetes, infections, and substance abuse.
- Prenatal maternal testing for HIV is recommended so maternal pharmacologic treatment may be instituted to prevent transmission of the virus to the unborn infant; early identification and perinatal treatment significantly decreases the transmission to the newborn.
- Some of the most significant IEMs in the neonatal period include congenital hypothyroidism, phenylketonuria, and galactosemia. Specific population-based newborn screening for IEMs should take place in situations where the incidence of other IEMs is prevalent. Mental retardation can result if these conditions are undiagnosed and untreated.
- Chromosomal disorders are caused by abnormalities in either chromosome structure or number.
- Genetic counseling is directed toward providing individuals and families with information needed to make decisions about a course of action appropriate to them.
- Although no cure for genetic disease is presently available, various therapeutic measures are used to modify the basic defect.

References

Als H and others: Individualized developmental care for the very low birth weight preterm infant: medical and neurofunctional effects, *JAMA* 272(11):853-858, 1994.

Altimier L, Lutes L: Cobedding multiples, *Newborn Infant Nurs Rev* 1(4):205-206, 2001.

American Academy of Pediatrics, Committee on Fetus and Newborn, Committee on Drugs, Section on Anesthesiology, Section on Surgery, Canadian Pediatric Society, Fetus and Newborn Committee: Prevention and management of pain and stress in the neonate, *Pediatrics* 105(2):454-460, 2000.

American Academy of Pediatrics, Committee on Genetics: Newborn screening facts, *Pediatrics* 98(3):473-481, 1996a.

American Academy of Pediatrics, Committee on Bioethics: Ethical issues with genetic testing in pediatrics, *Pediatrics* 107(6):1451-1455, 2001.

American Academy of Pediatrics, Committee on Infectious Diseases, Pickering L, editor: *Red Book: Report of the Committee on Infectious Diseases,* ed 26, Elk Grove, Il, 2003, The Academy.

American Academy of Pediatrics, Committee on Injury and Poison Prevention and Committee on Fetus and Newborn: Safe transportation of premature and low birth weight infants, *Pediatrics* 97(5):758-760, 1996b.

American Academy of Pediatrics, Committee on Injury and Poison Prevention: Selecting and using the most appropriate car safety seats for growing children: guidelines for counseling parents, *Pediatrics* 109(3):550-553, 2002.

American Academy of Pediatrics, Committee on Nutrition: Soy protein-based formulas: recommendations for infant feedings, *Pediatrics* 101(1):148-153, 1998.

American Academy of Pediatrics, Provisional Committee for Quality Improvement and Subcommittee on Hyperbilirubinemia: Practice parameter: management of hyperbilirubinemia in the healthy term newborn, *Pediatrics* 94(4):558-562, 1994.

American Academy of Pediatrics: Safe transportation of newborns at hospital discharge, *Pediatrics* 104(4):986-987, 1999.

American Academy of Pediatrics, Subcommittee on Hyperbilirubinemia: Clinical Practice Guideline: Management of hyperbilirubinemia in the newborn infant 35 or more weeks of gestation, *Pediatrics* 114(1):297-316, 2004.

American Academy of Pediatrics, Task Force on Infant Positioning: Positioning and sudden infant death syndrome (SIDS): update, *Pediatrics* 98(6):1216-1218, 1996c.

American Academy of Pediatrics and American College of Obstetricians and Gynecologists: *Guidelines for perinatal care,* ed 5, Elk Grove Village, Il, 2002, The Academy and College.

Anand K, Hickey P: Pain and its effects in the human neonate and fetus, *N Engl J Med* 317(21):1321-1329, 1987.

Anand KJ, Grunau RE, Oberlander TF: Developmental character and long-term consequences of pain in infants and children, *Child Adolesc Psychiatr Clin North Am* 6(4):703-724, 1997.

Anand KJ: Clinical importance of pain and stress in preterm neonates, *Biol Neonate* 73(1):1-9, 1998.

Anand KJ and others: Analgesia and sedation in preterm infants who require ventilatory support: results from the NOPAIN trial: Neonatal Outcome and Prolonged Analgesia in Neonates, *Arch Pediatr Adolesc Med* 153(4):331-338, 1999.

Anand KJS and International Evidence-Based Group for Neonatal Pain: Consensus statement for the prevention and management of pain in the newborn, *Arch Pediatr Adolesc Med* 155(2):173-180, 2001.

Anderson GC: Kangaroo care of the premature infant. In Goldson E, editor: *Nurturing the premature infant: developmental interventions in the neonatal intensive care nursery,* New York, 1999, Oxford University Press.

Arendt R and others: Motor development of cocaine-exposed children at age two years, *Pediatrics* 103(1):86-92, 1999.

Askin DF, Diehl-Jones B: Cocaine: effects of in utero exposure on the fetus and newborn, *J Perinat Neonat Nurs* 14(4):83-102, 2001.

Askin DF, Diehl-Jones B: Liver. part III: pathophysiology of liver dysfunction, *Neonat Netw* 22(3):5-15, 2003.

Bada HS and others: Gestational cocaine exposure and intrauterine growth: maternal lifestyle study, *Obstet Gynecol* 100(5 part 1): 916-924, 2002.

Ballantyne M and others: Validation of the premature infant pain profile in the clinical setting, *Clin J Pain* 15(4):297-303, 1999.

Barba B and others: Pain memory in full-term newborn, *J Pain Symptom Manage* 6:206, 1991.

Bateman DA, Chiriboga CA: Dose-response effect of cocaine on newborn head circumference, *Pediatrics* 106(3):e33, 2000.

Behrman RE, Shiono PH: Neonatal risk factors. In Fanaroff AA, Martin RJ, editors: *Neonatal-perinatal medicine: diseases of the fetus and infant,* ed 7, St Louis, 2002, Mosby.

Bhutani VK, Johnson L, Sivieri EM: Predictive ability of a predischarge hour-specific serum bilirubin for subsequent significant hyperbilirubinemia in healthy term and near-term newborns, *Pediatrics* 103(1):6-14, 1999.

Bhuttani VK and others: Noninvasive measurement of total serum bilirubin in a multiracial newborn population to assess the risk of severe hyperbilirubinemia, *Pediatrics* 106(2):e16, 2000.

Bildner J, Krechel SW: Increasing staff nurse awareness of postoperative pain management in the NICU, *Neonat Netw* 15(1):11-16, 1996.

Blackburn S: Hyperbilirubinemia and neonatal jaundice, *Neonat Netw* 14(7):15-25, 1995.

Blackburn ST: *Maternal, fetal, and neonatal physiology: a clinical perspective,* ed 2, Philadelphia, 2003, WB Saunders.

Blake WW, Murray JA: Heat balance. In Merenstein GB, Gardner SL, editors: *Handbook of neonatal intensive care,* ed 5, St Louis, 2002, Mosby.

Blass EM, Watt LB: Sucking- and sucrose-induced analgesia in human newborns, *Pain* 83(3):611-623, 1999.

Briscoe L, Clark S, Yoxall CW: Can transcutaneous bilirubinometry reduce the need for blood tests in jaundiced full term babies? *Arch Dis Child Fetal Neonatal Ed* 86(3):F190-F192, 2002.

Buehler D and others: Effectiveness of individualized developmental care for low risk preterm infants: behavioral and electrophysiologic evidence, *Pediatrics* 96(5):923-932, 1995.

Burd RS, Tobias JD: Ketorolac for pain management after abdominal surgical procedures in infants, *South Med* 95(3):331-333, 2002.

Canadian Pediatric Society: Approach to the management of hyperbilirubinemia in term newborn infants, *J Paediatr Child Health* 4(2):161-164, 1999.

Centers for Disease Control and Prevention: Prevention of perinatal group B streptococcal disease: revised guidelines, *MMWR* 51(RR11):1-22, 2002.

Chiriboga CA and others: Drug-response effect on fetal cocaine exposure on newborn neurologic function, *Pediatrics* 103(1):79-85, 1999.

Cifuentes J, Segars AH, Carlo W: Respiratory system management and complications. In Kenner C, Lott J, editors: *Comprehensive neonatal nursing: a physiologic perspective,* ed 3, Philadelphia, 2003, WB Saunders.

Conde-Agudelo A, Diaz-Rossello JL, Belizan JM: Cochrane neonatal review: kangaroo mother care to reduce morbidity and mortality in low birthweight infants, 2000; available at http://www.nichd.nih.gov/ cochraneneonatal/Vickers/Vickers.htm.

Cowett RM, Loughead JL: Neonatal glucose metabolism: differential diagnoses, evaluation, and treatment of hypoglycemia, *Neonat Netw* 21(4):9-19, 2002.

Davis PG, Henderson-Smart DJ: Nasal continuous positive airways pressure immediately after extubation for preventing morbidity in preterm infants, *Cochrane Database Syst Rev* 2003(2):CD000143, 2003.

Delaney-Black V and others: Prenatal cocaine exposure and child behavior, *Pediatrics* 102(4):945-950, 1998.

DellaPorta K, Aforismo D, Butler-O'Hara M: Co-bedding of twins in the neonatal intensive care, *Pediatr Nurs* 24(6):529-531, 1998.

Dickenson AH, Rahman W: Mechanisms of chronic pain and the developing nervous system. In McGrath PJ, Finley GA, editors: *Chronic and recurrent pain in children and adolescents*, Seattle, 1999, IASP Press.

Dohil MA, Baugh WP, Eichenfield LF: Vascular and pigmented birthmarks, *Pediatr Clin North Am* 47(4):783-812, 2000.

Doyle JJ and others: Hematology. In Avery GB, Fletcher MA, MacDonald MG, editors: *Neonatology: pathophysiology and management of the newborn*, ed 5, Philadelphia, 1999, Lippincott Williams & Wilkins.

Engle WD and others: Assessment of a transcutaneous device in the evaluation of neonatal hyperbilirubinemia in a primarily Hispanic population, *Pediatrics* 110(1 Pt 1):61-67, 2002.

Evans JC: Physiology of acute pain in preterm infants, *Newborn Infant Nurs Rev* 1(2):75-84, 2001.

Evans RA, Thureen PJ: Early feeding strategies in preterm & critically ill neonates, *Neonat Netw* 20(7):7-18, 2001.

Eyler FD, Behnke M: Early development of infants exposed to drugs prenatally, *Clin Perinatol* 26(1):107-150, 1999.

Eyler FD, Behnke M, Conlon M: Birth outcome from a prospective, matched study of prenatal crack/cocaine use. II. Interactive and dose effects on neurobehavioral assessment, *Pediatrics* 101(2):237-241, 1998.

Finnegan LP: Neonatal abstinence. In Nelson N, editor: *Current therapy in neonatal perinatal medicine 1985-1986*, Toronto, 1985, BC Decker.

Fitzgerald M: Pain in infancy: some unanswered questions, *Pain Rev* 2(1):77-91, 1995.

Fitzgerald M, Millard C, McIntosh N: Cutaneous hypersensitivity following peripheral tissue damage in newborn infants and its reversal with topical anaesthesia, *Pain* 39(1):31-36, 1989.

Franck LS: A national survey of the assessment and treatment of pain and agitation in the neonatal intensive care unit, *J Obstet Gynecol Neonatal Nurs* 16(6):387-393, 1987.

Frank CG, Cooper SC, Merenstein G: Jaundice. In Merenstein GB, Gardner SL, editors: *Handbook of neonatal intensive care*, ed 5, St Louis, 2002, Mosby.

Frank DA, and others: Heavily cocaine exposed children show positive effects of early intervention on Bayley Scales of Infant Development (abstract), *Pediatr Res* 43:214A, 1998.

Furdon S and others: Outcome measures after standardized pain management strategies in postoperative patients in the NICU, *J Perinat Neonat Nurs* 12(1):58-69, 1998.

Garas T and others: Perinatal morbidity: a comparison of vacuum delivery and spontaneous delivery, *Obstet Gynecol* 97(4 suppl 1):S64, 2001.

Gardner SL, Hauser P, Merenstein GB: Grief and perinatal loss. In Merenstein GB, Gardner SL, editors: *Handbook of neonatal intensive care*, ed 5, St Louis, 2002, Mosby.

Gardner SL, Snell BJ, Lawrence RA: Breastfeeding the neonate with special needs. In Merenstein GB, Gardner SL, editors: *Handbook of neonatal intensive care*, ed 5, St Louis, 2002, Mosby.

Gartner LM: Neonatal jaundice, *Pediatr Rev* 15(11):422-432, 1994.

Gibbins S, Stevens B. State of the art: pain assessment and management in high-risk infants, *Newborn Infant Rev* 1(2):85-89, 2001.

Glass P: The vulnerable neonate and the neonatal intensive care environment. In Avery GB, Fletcher MA, MacDonald MG, editors: *Neonatology: pathophysiology and management of the newborn*, ed 4, Philadelphia, 1994, JB Lippincott.

Gradin M and others: Pain reduction at venipuncture in newborns: oral glucose compared with local anesthetic cream, *Pediatrics* 110(6):1053-1057, 2002.

Gray L, Philbin MK: Measuring sound in hospital nurseries, *J Perinatol* 20(8 pt 2):S100-S104, 2000.

Gray L, Watt L, Blass EM: Skin-to-skin contact is analgesic in healthy newborns, *Pediatrics* 105(1):110-111, 2000; available at www.pediatrics.org/cgi/content/full/105/1/e14.

Grunau RV and others: Early pain experience: child and family factors as precursors of somatization: a prospective study of extremely premature and full-term children, *Pain* 56(3):353-359, 1994.

Hadjistavropoulos HD and others: Judging pain in infants: behavioural, contextual, and developmental determinants, *Pain* 73(3):319-324, 1997.

Harrell G, Murray PD: Diagnosis and management of congenital hypothyroidism, *J Perinat Neonat Nurs* 11(4):75-83, 1998.

Hellekson KL: Practice guidelines: NIH consensus statement on phenylketonuria, *Am Fam Physician* 63(7):1430-1432, 2001.

Hengst JM: The role of C-reactive protein in the evaluation and management of infants with suspected sepsis, *Adv Neonat Care* 3(1):3-13, 2003.

Holditch-Davis D, Blackburn ST, VandenBerg K: Newborn and infant neurobehavioral development. In Kenner C, Lott J, editors: *Comprehensive neonatal nursing: a physiologic perspective*, Philadelphia, 2003, WB Saunders.

Horii KA, Lane AT: Evidence-based use of emollients in neonates, *Newborn Infant Nurs Rev* 1(1):21-24, 2001.

Huestis MA, Choo RE: Drug abuses's smallest victims: in utero drug exposure, *Forensic Sci Int* 128(1-2):20-30, 2002.

Hummel P, Puchalski M: Assessment and management of pain in infancy, *Newborn Infant Nurs Rev* 1(2):114-122, 2001.

Hunter J: The neonatal intensive care unit. In Case-Smith J, editor: *Occupational therapy for children*, ed 4, St Louis, 2001, Mosby.

Hurt H and others: A prospective education of early language development in children with in utero cocaine exposure and in control subjects, *J Pediatr* 130(2):310-312, 1997.

Hussain K, Sharief N: Dermal injury following the use of fiberoptic phototherapy in an extremely premature infant, *Clin Pediatr* 35(8):421-422, 1996.

Jansen JL: A bereavement model for the intensive care nursery, *Neonat Netw* 22(3):17-23, 2003.

Johnson CB: Head, eyes, ears, nose, mouth and neck assessment. In Tappero EP, Honeyfield ME, editors: *Physical assessment of the newborn: a comprehensive approach to the art of physical assessment*, ed 3, Petaluma, Calif, 2003, NICU Ink.

Johnson K, Gerada C, Greenough A: Treatment of neonatal abstinence syndrome, *Arch Dis Child Fetal Neonatal Ed* 88(1):F2-F5, 2003.

Johnston CC and others: A cross-sectional survey of pain and pharmacological analgesia in Canadian neonatal intensive care units, *Clin J Pain* 13(4):308-312, 1997.

Kandall SR: Treatment strategies for drug-exposed neonates, *Clin Perinatol* 26(1):231-243, 1999.

Kimberlin DW: Herpes simplex virus infections in the neonatal period, *Infect Med* 19(10):462-474, 2002.

Kinsella JP, Abman SH: Recent developments in inhaled nitric oxide therapy of the newborn, *Curr Opin Pediatr* 11(2):121-125, 1999.

Kinsella JP, Abman SH: Inhaled nitric oxide: current and future uses in neonates, *Semin Perinatol* 24(6):387-395, 2000.

Kinsella JP and others: Inhaled nitric oxide in premature infants with severe hypoxaemic respiratory failure: a randomised controlled trial, *Lancet* 354(9184):1047-1048, 1999.

Kirkpatrick JM, Alexander J, Cain RM: Recovering urine from diapers: are test results accurate? *MCN* 22(2):96-102, 1997.

Kliegman RM: Commentaries: experimental validation of neonatal feeding practices, *Pediatrics* 103(2):492-493, 1999.

Klein JO, Remington JS: Current concepts of infections of the fetus and newborn. In Remington JS, Klein JO, editors: *Infectious diseases of the fetus and newborn infant*, Philadelphia, 2001, WB Saunders.

Koren G, Nulman I, Rovet J, Greenbaum R, Loebstein M, Einarson T. and others: Long-term neurodevelopmental risks in children exposed in utero to cocaine: the Toronto adoption study, *Ann NY Acad Sci* 846:306-312, 1998.

Krechel SW, Bildner J: CRIES: a new neonatal postoperative pain measurement score: initial testing of validity and reliability, *Pediatr Anaesth* 5(1):53-61, 1995.

Langland J, Langland P: Pain in the neonate and fetus (letter), *N Engl J Med* 318:1398, 1988.

Lashley FR: Newborn screening: new opportunities and new challenges, *Newborn Infant Nurs Rev* 2(4):228-242, 2002.

Lawrence RA, Lawrence RM: *Breastfeeding: a guide for the medical profession*, ed 5, St Louis, 1999, Mosby.

Lester BM, Tronick EZ, Brazelton TB: The Neonatal Intensive Care Unit Network Neurobehavioral Scale procedures, *Pediatrics* 113 (3 suppl):641-667, 2004.

Luchtman-Jones L, Schwartz AL, Wilson DB: The blood and hematopoietic system. In Fanaroff AA, Martin RJ, editors: *Neonatal-perinatal medicine: diseases of the fetus and infant*, ed 6, St Louis, 1997, Mosby.

Ludington-Hoe SM, Swinth JY: Developmental aspects of kangaroo care, *J Obstet Gynecol Neonatal Nurs* 25(8):691-703, 1996.

Lund CH, Kuller JM: Assessment and management of the integumentary system. In Kenner C, Lott JW, editors: *Comprehensive neonatal nursing*, ed 3, Philadelphia, 2003, WB Saunders.

Lutes L: Personal communication, March 1998.

MMWR Weekly: Enterobacter sakazakii infections associated with the use of powdered infant formula–Tennessee, 2001, *MMWR* 51(14):98-300, 2002.

Malanga CJ, Kosofsy BE: Mechanism of action of drugs of abuse on the developing fetal brain, *Clin Perinatol* 26(1):17-37, 1999.

Maisels MJ: Jaundice. In Avery GB, Fletcher MA, MacDonald MG, editors: *Neonatology: pathophysiology and management of the newborn*, ed 5, Philadelphia, 1999, JB Lippincott.

Mangurten HH: Birth injuries. In Fanaroff AA, Martin RJ, editors: *Neonatal-perinatal medicine: diseases of the fetus and infant*, ed 7, St Louis, 2002, Mosby.

Marcellus L: Care of substance-exposed infants: the current state of practice in Canadian hospitals, *J Perinat Neonat Nurs* 16(3):51-68, 2002.

Margileth A: Dermatologic conditions. In Avery GB, Fletcher MA, MacDonald MG, editors: *Neonatology: pathophysiology and management of the newborn*, ed 5, Philadelphia, 1999, Lippincott Williams & Wilkins.

Martinez JC and others: Control of severe hyperbilirubinemia in full-term newborns with the inhibitor of bilirubin production Sn-mesoporphyrin, *Pediatrics* 103(1):1-5, 1999.

McCance K, Huether S: *Pathophysiology: the biological basis for disease in infants and children*, ed 3, St Louis, 1998, Mosby.

McGowan JE, Hagedorn MI, Hay WH: Glucose homeostasis. In Merenstein GB, Gardner SL, editors: *Handbook of neonatal intensive care*, ed 5, St Louis, 2002, Mosby.

McLaughlin CR and others: Neonatal pain: a comprehensive survey of attitudes and practices, *J Pain Symptom Manage* 8(1):7-16, 1993.

Merenstein GB, Gardner SL: *Handbook of neonatal intensive care*, ed 5, St Louis, 2002, Mosby.

Merrill J, Ballard R: Pulmonary surfactant for neonatal respiratory disorders, *Curr Opin Pediatr* 15(2):149-154, 2003.

Moise KJ: Management of rhesus alloimmunization in pregnancy, *Obstet Gynecol* 100(3):600-611, 2002.

Moolenaar RL and others: A prolonged outbreak of *Pseudomonas aeruginosa* in a neonatal intensive care unit: did staff fingernails play a role in disease transmission? *Infect Control Hosp Epidemiol* 21(2):80-85, 2000.

Moran M and others: Maternal kangaroo (skin-to-skin) care in the NICU beginning 4 hours postbirth, *Am J Matern Child Nurs* 24:74-79, 1999.

Morton JA: Strategies to support extended breastfeeding of the premature infant, *Adv Neonat Care* 2(5):267-282, 2002.

Neal JL: RhD isoimmunization and current management modalities, *J Obstet Gynecol Neonatal Nurs* 30(6):589-607, 2001.

NIH Consensus Development Panel on Phenylketonuria: *Phenylketonuria (PKU): screening and management*, Consensus Statements (NIH Development Program) 2000; available at http://consensus.nih.gov/cons/113/113_intro.htm.

Ogata ES: Carbohydrate homeostasis. In Avery GB, Fletcher MA, MacDonald MG, editors: *Neonatology: pathophysiology and management of the newborn*, ed 5, Philadelphia, 1999, JB Lippincott.

Paige PL, Carney PR: Neurologic disorders. In Merenstein GB, Gardner SL, editors: *Handbook of neonatal intensive care*, ed 5, St Louis, 2002, Mosby.

Penticuff J: Neonatal nursing ethics: toward a consensus, *Neonat Netw* 5:7-16, 1987.

Perry E and others: Blood pressure increases, birth weight-dependent stability boundary, and intraventricular hemorrhage, *Pediatrics* 85:727-732, 1990.

Pokela M: Pain relief can reduce hypoxemia in distressed neonates during routine treatment procedures, *Pediatrics* 93(3):379-383, 1994.

Polak JD, Ringler N, Daugherty B: Unit-based procedures: impact on the incidence of nosocomial infections in the newborn intensive care unit, *NINR* 4(1):38-45, 2004.

Porter ML, Dennis BL: Hyperbilirubinemia in the term newborn, *Am Fam Physician* 65(4):599-606, 613-614, 2002.

Porter FL, Grunau RE, Anand KJS: Long-term effects of pain in infants, *J Dev Behav Pediatr* 20(4):253-261, 1999.

Premji SS and others: Evidence-based feeding guideline for very low birthweight infants, *Adv Neonat Care* 2(1):5-18, 2002.

Putta LV, Spencer JP: Assisted vaginal delivery using the vacuum extractor, *Am Fam Physician* 62(6):1316-1320, 2000.

Ramenghi LA, Evans DJ, Levene MI: Sucrose analgesia: absorptive mechanism or taste perception? *Arch Dis Child Fetal Neonatal Ed* 80:F146-F147, 1999.

Read CY: The demands of biochemical genetic disorders: a survey of mothers of children with mitochondrial disease or phenylketonuria, *J Pediatr Nurs* 18(3):181-186, 2003.

Richardson GA, Hamel SC, Goldschmidt L: The effects of cocaine use on neonatal neurobehavioral status, *Neurotoxicol Teratol* 18(5):519-528, 1996.

Riva E and others: Early breastfeeding is linked to higher intelligence quotient scores in dietary treated phenylketonuric children, *Acta Paediatr* 85(1):56-58, 1996.

Rollnik JD and others: Botulinum toxin treatment of cocontractions after birth-related brachial plexus lesions, *Neurology* 55(1):112-114, 2000.

Ross MG, Fresquez M, El-Haddad MA: Impact of FDA advisory on reported vacuum-assisted delivery and morbidity, *J Fetal Matern Med* 9(6):321-326, 2001.

Ruchala PL, Seibold L, Stemsterfer K: Validating assessment of neonatal jaundice with transcutaneous bilirubin measurement, *Neonat Netw* 15(4):33-37, 1996.

Sadiq HF and others: Inhaled nitric oxide in the treatment of moderate persistent pulmonary hypertension of the newborn: a randomized controlled, multicenter trial, *J Perinatol* 23(2):98-103, 2003.

Sauer PJ, Dane HJ, Visser HK: New standards for neutral thermal environment of healthy very low birthweight infants in one week of life, *Arch Dis Child* 59(1):18-22, 1984.

Saugstad OD and others: Resuscitation of newborn infants with 21% or 100% oxygen: follow-up at 18 and 24 months, *Pediatrics* 112(2):296-300, 2003.

Schanler RJ and others: Feeding strategies for premature infants: randomized trial of gastrointestinal priming and tube-feeding method, *Pediatrics* 103(2):434-439, 1999.

Schwartz RP: Neonatal hypoglycemia: how low is too low? *J Pediatr* 131(2):171-173, 1997.

Sexson W and others: Auditory conditioning in the critically ill neonate to enhance interpersonal relationships, *J Perinatol* 6:20-23, 1986.

Shapiro CR: Pain in the neonate: assessment and intervention, *Neonat Netw* 8(1):7-21, 1989.

Shapiro CR: Nurses' judgments of pain in term and preterm newborns, *J Obstet Gynecol Neonatal Nurs* 22(1):41-47, 1993.

Shaw N: Assessment and management of the hematologic system. In Kenner C, Lott J, editors: *Comprehensive neonatal nursing: a physiologic perspective,* ed 3, Philadelphia, 2003, WB Saunders.

Singer LT and others: Cognitive and motor outcomes of cocaine-exposed infants, *JAMA* 287(15):1952-1960, 2002.

Stevens B and others: Premature Infant Pain Profile: development and initial validation, *Clin J Pain* 12(1):13-22, 1996.

Stevens B, Johnson C, Franck L: The efficacy of developmentally sensitive interventions and sucrose for relieving pain in very low birth weight infants, *Nurs Res* 48(1):35-43, 1999.

Stevens B, Yamada J, Ohlsson A: Sucrose for analgesia in newborn infants undergoing painful procedures, *Cochrane Database Syst Rev* 2001(4):CD001069, 2001.

Stevens DK and others: Prediction of hyperbilirubinemia in near-term and term infants, *J Perinatol* 21(suppl 1):S63-S72, 2001.

Symington A, Pinelli J: Developmental care for promoting development and preventing morbidity in preterm infants (Cochrane Review). In *The Cochrane Library,* Issue 1, 2003, Oxford, Update Software.

Szlachetka DM: Kasabach-Merritt syndrome: a case review, *Neonat Netw* 17(1):7-15, 1998.

Taddio A and others: Effect of neonatal circumcision on pain response during subsequent routine vaccination, *Lancet* 349(9052):599-603, 1997.

Taddio A and others: A systematic review of lidocaine-prilocaine cream (EMLA) in the treatment of acute pain in neonates, *Pediatrics* 101(2):E1, 1998.

Taddio A and others: Conditioning and hyperalgesia in newborns exposed to repeated heel lances, *JAMA* 288(7):857-861, 2002.

Tanney MR, Lowenstein V: One-stop shopping: description of a model program to provide primary care to substance-abusing women and their children, *J Pediatr Health Care* 11(1):20-25, 1997.

Tappero E: Musculoskeletal system assessment. In Tappero E, Honeyfield MA: *Physical assessment of the newborn,* ed 3, Santa Rosa, Calif, 2003, NICU Ink.

Tronick EZ, Beeghly M: Prenatal cocaine exposure, child development, and the compromising effects of cumulative risk, *Clin Perinatol* 26(1):151-171, 1999.

Tronick EZ and others: Late dose-response effects of prenatal cocaine exposure on neurobehavioral performance, *Pediatrics* 98(1):78-83, 1996.

Update: fatal air bag–related injuries to children—United States, 1993-1996, *MMWR* 45(49):1073-1076, 1997.

Van Acker J and others: Outbreak of necrotizing enterocolitis associated with *Enterobacter sakazakii* in powdered milk formula, *J Clin Microbiol* 39(1):293-297, 2001.

Vanderhoof SL, Doidge WW, Maughan T: Flashlamp-pumped pulsed dye laser treatment of vascular birthmarks, *AORN J* 67(6):1214-1223, 1998.

Vennarecci G and others: Intestinal transplantation for short gut syndrome attributable to necrotizing enterocolitis, *Pediatrics* 105(2):1-5, 2000.

Vento M and others: Oxidative stress in asphyxiated term infants resuscitated with 100% oxygen, *J Pediatr* 142(3):240-246, 2003.

Vogtman C, Mockel A, Tillig E: Warming therapy in a heated cot using a heated gel mattress, *Neonat Intensive Care* 9(4):15-19, 1996.

Vohra S and others: Effect of polyethylene occlusive skin wrapping on heat loss in very low birth weight infants at delivery: a randomized trial, *J Pediatr* 134(5):547-551, 1999.

Volpe JJ: *Neurology of the newborn,* ed 4, Philadelphia, 2001, WB Saunders.

Wilson D: Starting neonatal IVs: practical tips, *Mother Baby J* 5(1):11-19, 2000.

Witt C: Skin assessment. In Tappero EP, Honeyfield ME, editors: *Physical assessment of the newborn,* ed 3, Petaluma, Calif, 2003, NICU Ink.

Wong DL: *Physiological responses, facial expressions, and cry of infants during immunization in relation to their pain history,* Ann Arbor, Mich, 1992, University Microfilm (order no. 9321617).

Woo EK: Device errors: biliblanket phototherapy light, *Nursing* 28(8):79, 1998.

Yeo KL, Perlman M, Hao YMP: Outcomes of extremely premature infants related to their peak serum bilirubin concentrations and exposure to phototherapy, *Pediatrics* 102(6):1426-1431, 1998.

Zahorodny W and others: The neonatal withdrawal inventory: a simplified score of newborn withdrawal, *J Dev Behav Pediatr* 19(2):89-93, 1998.

Zenk KE: *Neonatal medications and nutrition,* Petaluma, Calif, 2000, NICU Ink.

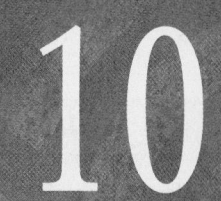

Health Promotion of the Infant and Family

DAVID WILSON

10

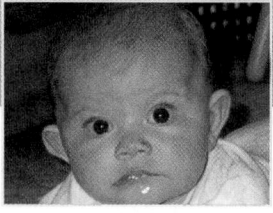

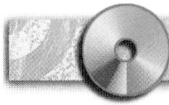 Remember to check out your companion CD-ROM

http://evolve.elsevier.com/Wong/essentials/

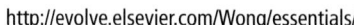

CHAPTER OUTLINE

RELATED TOPICS and ADDITIONAL RESOURCES

For additional information, please view "Growth and Development" in *Whaley and Wong's Pediatric Nursing Video Series,* St Louis, 1996, Mosby (800) 426-4545; website: www.elsevierhealth.com.
The Wong Update series on the Internet at www.elsevierhealth.com/WOW routinely includes information on changes in immunization information.

PROMOTING OPTIMAL GROWTH AND DEVELOPMENT

BIOLOGIC DEVELOPMENT

At no other time in life are physical changes and developmental achievements so dramatic as during infancy. All major body systems undergo progressive maturation, and there is concurrent development of skills that increasingly allows infants to respond to and cope with the environment. Acquisition of these fine and gross motor skills occurs in an orderly head-to-toe and center-to-periphery (cephalocaudal-proximodistal) sequence.

Proportional Changes

During the first year *growth* is very rapid, especially during the initial 6 months. Infants gain 150 to 210 g (5 to 7 ounces) weekly until approximately age 5 to 6 months, when the birth weight has at least doubled. An average weight for a 6-month-old child is 7.26 kg (16 pounds). Weight gain slows during the second 6 months. By 1 year of age the infant's birth weight has tripled, for an average weight of 9.75 kg (21.5 pounds). Infants who are breast-fed beyond 4 to 6 months of age typically gain less weight than those who are bottle-fed, yet head circumference is more than adequate. Dewey (2001) attributes the decreased weight gain seen in breast-fed infants to self-regulation of energy intake.

Height increases by 2.5 cm (1 inch) a month during the first 6 months and also slows during the second 6 months. Increases in length occur in sudden spurts, rather than in a slow, gradual pattern. Average height is 65 cm (25.5 inches) at 6 months and 74 cm (29 inches) at 12 months. By 1 year the birth length has increased by almost 50%. This increase occurs mainly in the trunk, rather than in the legs, and contributes to the characteristic physique of the infant (see Fig. 5-3).

Head growth is also rapid. During the first 6 months head circumference increases approximately 1.5 cm (0.6 inch) per month but decreases to only 0.5 cm (0.2 inch) monthly during the second 6 months. The average size is 43 cm (17 inches) at 6 months and 46 cm (18 inches) at 12 months. By 1 year, head size has increased by almost 33%. Closure of the cranial sutures occurs, with the posterior fontanel fusing by 6 to 8 weeks of age and the anterior fontanel closing by 12 to 18 months of age (the average age being 14 months).

Expanding head size reflects the growth and differentiation of the *nervous system.* By the end of the first year the brain has increased in weight about two and one half times. Maturation of the brain is exhibited in the dramatic developmental achievements of infancy (see Table 10-2). Primitive reflexes are replaced by voluntary, purposeful movement, and new reflexes that influence motor development appear.

The *chest* assumes a more adult contour, with the lateral diameter becoming larger than the anteroposterior diameter. The chest circumference approximately equals the head circumference by the end of the first year. The *heart* grows less rapidly than does the rest of the body. Its weight is usually doubled by 1 year of age in comparison with body weight, which triples during the same period. The size of the heart is still large in relation to the chest cavity; its width is approximately 55% of the chest width.

Maturation of Systems

Other organ systems also change and grow during infancy. The *respiratory rate* slows somewhat (see inside back cover) and is relatively stable. Respiratory movements continue to be abdominal. Several factors predispose the infant to more severe and acute respiratory problems. The close proximity of the trachea to the bronchi and its branching structures rapidly transmits an infectious agent from one anatomic location to another. The short, straight eustachian tube closely communicates with the ear, allowing infection to ascend from the pharynx to the middle ear. In addition, the inability of the immune system to produce *immunoglobulin A (IgA)* in the mucosal lining provides less protection against infection in infancy than during later childhood.

The *heart rate* slows (see inside back cover), and the rhythm is often *sinus arrhythmia* (rate increases with inspiration and decreases with expiration). Blood pressure also changes during infancy (see inside back cover). Systolic pressure rises during the first 2 months as a result of the increasing ability of the left ventricle to pump blood into the systemic circulation. Diastolic pressure decreases during the first 3 months, then gradually rises to values close to those at birth. Fluctuations in blood pressure occur during varying states of activity and emotion.

Significant *hematopoietic changes* occur during the first year (see Appendix E). Fetal hemoglobin (HgbF) is present for the first 5 months, with adult hemoglobin steadily increasing through the first half of infancy. Fetal hemoglobin results in a shortened survival of red blood cells and thus a decreased number of red blood cells. A common result at 2 to 3 months of age is *physiologic anemia.* High levels of fetal hemoglobin are thought to depress the production of erythropoietin, a hormone released by the kidney that stimulates red blood cell production.

Maternally derived iron stores are present for the first 5 to 6 months and gradually diminish, which also accounts for lowered hemoglobin levels toward the end of the first 6 months. The occurrence of physiologic anemia is not affected by an adequate supply of iron. However, when erythropoiesis is stimulated, iron supplies are necessary for the formation of hemoglobin.

The *digestive processes* are relatively immature at birth. Although term newborn infants have some limitations in digestive function, studies indicate that human milk has properties that partially compensate for decreased digestive enzymatic activity, thus enabling the breast-fed infant to receive optimal nutrition during the first several months of life. Saliva is secreted in small amounts, but the majority of the digestive processes do not begin functioning until age 3 months, when drooling is common because of the poorly coordinated swallowing reflex. The enzyme *ptyalin* (also called *amylase*) is present in small amounts but usually has little effect on the foodstuffs because of the small amount of time the food stays in the mouth. Gastric digestion in the stomach consists primarily of the action of hydrochloric acid and rennin, an enzyme that acts specifically on the casein in milk to cause the formation of curds—coagulated semisolid particles of milk. The curds cause the milk to be retained in the stomach long enough for digestion to occur.

Digestion also takes place in the duodenum, where pancreatic enzymes and bile begin to break down protein and fat. Secretion of the pancreatic enzyme *amylase,* which is needed for digestion of complex carbohydrates, is deficient until about the fourth to sixth month of life. *Lipase* is also limited, and infants do not achieve adult levels of fat absorption until 4 to 5 months of age. *Trypsin* is secreted in sufficient quantities to catabolize protein into polypeptides and some amino acids.

The immaturity of the digestive processes is evident in the appearance of stools. During infancy, solid foods (e.g., peas, carrots, corn, raisins) are passed incompletely broken down in the feces. An excess quantity of fiber easily disposes the child to loose, bulky stools.

During infancy the stomach enlarges to accommodate a greater volume of food. By the end of the first year the infant is able to tolerate three meals a day and an evening bottle and may have one or two bowel movements daily. However, with any type of gastric irritation the infant is vulnerable to diarrhea, vomiting, and dehydration (see Chapter 24).

The *liver* is the most immature of all the gastrointestinal organs throughout infancy. The ability to conjugate bilirubin and secrete bile is achieved after the first couple of weeks of life. However, the capacities for gluconeogenesis, formation of plasma protein and ketones, storage of vitamins, and deaminization of amino acids remain relatively immature for the first year of life.

Maturation of the suckling, sucking, and swallowing reflexes and the eruption of *teeth* (see Teething, p. 327) parallel the changes in the gastrointestinal tract and prepare the infant for the introduction of solid foods.

The *immunologic system* undergoes numerous changes during the first year. The full-term newborn receives significant amounts of maternal IgG, which, for approximately 3 months, confers immunity against antigens to which the mother was exposed. During this time the infant begins to synthesize IgG; approximately 40% of adult levels are reached by 1 year of age. Significant amounts of IgM are produced at birth, and adult levels are reached by 9 months of age. Secretory IgA is not present at birth but is found in saliva and tears by 2 to 5 weeks. IgA is present in large amounts in colostrum; this is believed to have a protective role in the gastrointestinal tract against many bacteria such as *Escherichia coli* and viruses such as poliovirus. The function and quantity of T-lymphocytes, lymphokines, and complement is reduced in early infancy, thus preventing optimal response to certain bacteria and viruses. The production of IgA, IgD, and IgE is much more gradual, and maximum levels are not attained until early childhood.

During infancy, *thermoregulation* becomes more efficient; the ability of the skin to contract and of muscles to shiver in response to cold increases. The peripheral capillaries respond to changes in ambient temperature to regulate heat loss. The capillaries constrict in response to cold, conserving core body temperature and decreasing potential evaporative heat loss from the skin surface. The capillaries dilate in response to heat, decreasing internal body temperature through evaporation, conduction, and convection. Shivering *(thermogenesis)* causes the muscles and muscle fibers to contract, generating metabolic heat, which is distributed throughout the body. Increased adipose tissue during the first 6 months insulates the body against heat loss.

A shift in the *total body fluid* occurs; at birth 75% of the infant's body weight is water, and there is an excess of extracellular fluid. As the percentage of body water decreases, so does the amount of extracellular fluid—from 40% at term to 20% in adulthood. The high proportion of extracellular fluid, which is composed of blood plasma, interstitial fluid, and lymph, predisposes the infant to a more rapid loss of total body fluid and, consequently, dehydration.

The immaturity of the *renal structures* also predisposes the infant to dehydration. Complete maturity of the kidney occurs during the latter half of the second year, when the cuboidal epithelium of the glomeruli becomes flattened. Before this time the filtration capacity of the glomeruli is reduced. Urine is voided frequently and has a low specific gravity (1.000 to 1.010).

Auditory acuity is at adult levels during infancy. Visual acuity begins to improve, and binocular fixation is established. *Binocularity,* or the fixation of two ocular images into one cerebral picture *(fusion),* begins to develop by 6 weeks of age and should be well established by age 4 months. *Depth perception (stereopsis)* begins to develop by age 7 to 9 months but may exist earlier as an innate safety mechanism against accidental falling.

Fine Motor Development

Fine motor behavior includes the use of the hands and fingers in the prehension (grasp) of an object. Grasping occurs during the first 2 to 3 months as a reflex and gradually becomes voluntary. At 1 month of age the hands are predominantly closed, and by 3 months they are mostly open. By this time infants

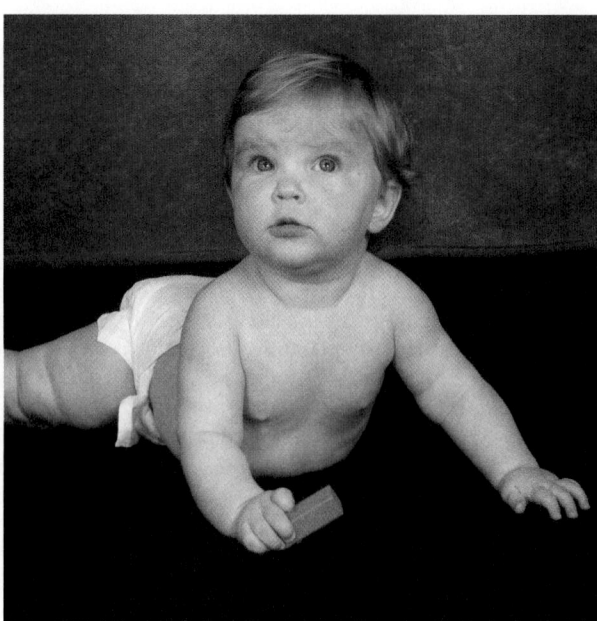

FIG. 10-1 ■ Crude pincer grasp at 8 to 10 months. (Photo by Paul Vincent Kuntz, Texas Children's Hospital.)

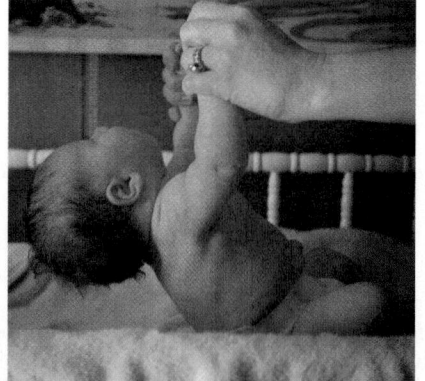

A

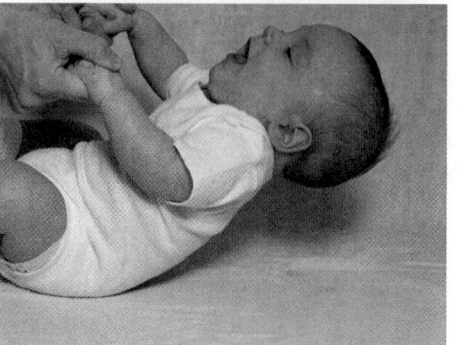

B

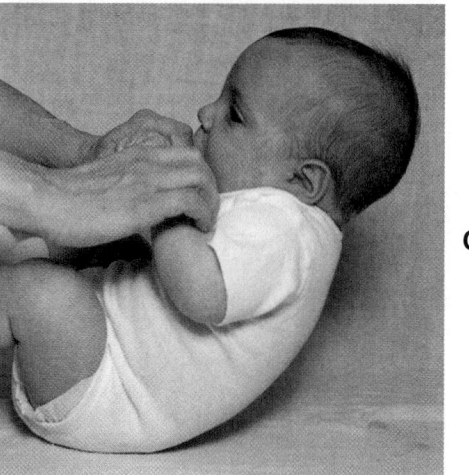

C

FIG. 10-2 ■ Head control while pulled to sitting position. **A,** Complete head lag at 1 month. **B,** Partial head lag at 2 months. **C,** Almost no head lag at 4 months.

demonstrate a desire to grasp an object, but they "grasp" it more with the eyes than with the hands. If a rattle is placed in the hand, the infant will actively hold onto it. By 4 months of age the infant regards both a small pellet and the hands and then looks from the object to the hands and back again. By 5 months the infant is able to voluntarily grasp an object.

Gradually the palmar grasp (using the whole hand) is replaced with a pincer grasp (using the thumb and index finger). By 8 to 9 months of age the infant uses a crude pincer grasp and by 11 months has progressed to a neat pincer grasp (Fig. 10-1).

By 6 months of age infants have increased manipulative skill. They hold their bottle, grasp their feet and pull them to their mouth, and feed themselves a cracker. By 7 months they transfer objects from one hand to the other, use one hand for grasping, and hold a cube in each hand simultaneously. They enjoy banging objects and will explore the movable parts of a toy.

By 10 months of age the pincer grasp is sufficiently established to enable infants to pick up a raisin and other finger foods. They can deliberately let go of an object and will offer it to someone. By 11 months they put objects into a container and like to remove them. By age 1 year, infants try to build a tower of two blocks but fail.

Gross Motor Development

Head Control.   The full-term newborn can momentarily hold the head in midline and parallel when the body is suspended ventrally and can lift and turn the head from side to side when prone (see Fig. 8-6). This is not the case when the infant is lying prone on a pillow or soft surface; infants do not have the head control to lift their head out of the depression of the object and therefore risk suffocation in the prone position early in infancy (see Sudden Infant Death Syndrome, Chapter 11). Marked head lag is evident when

the infant is pulled from a lying to a sitting position. By 3 months of age infants can hold their head well beyond the plane of the body. By 4 months of age infants can lift the head and front portion of the chest approximately 90 degrees above the table, bearing their weight on the forearms. Only slight head lag is evident when the infant is pulled from a lying to a sitting position, and by 4 to 6 months head control is well established (Figs. 10-2 and 10-3).

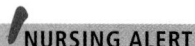

NURSING ALERT

Any child who displays head lag at 6 months of age **should have a developmental/neurologic evaluation.**

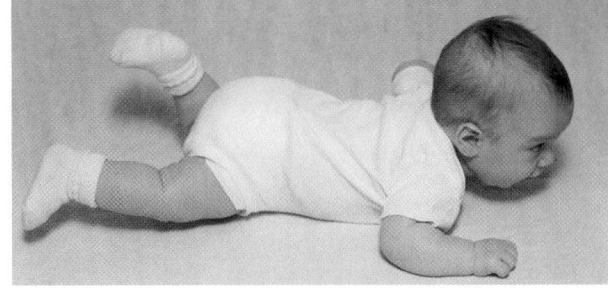

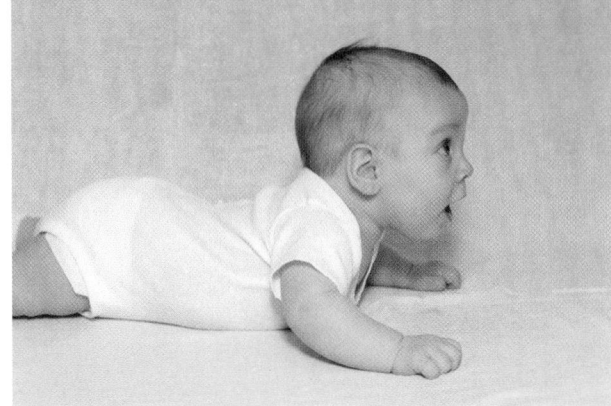

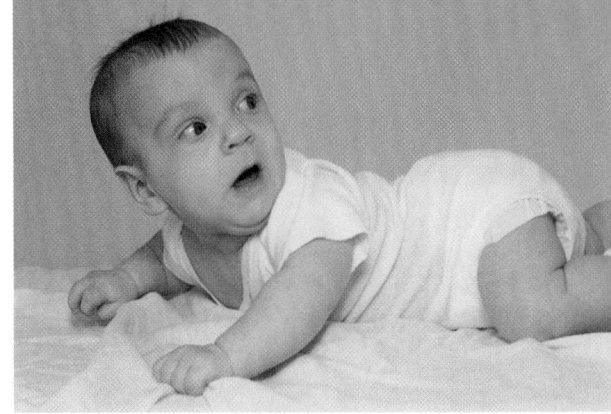

FIG. 10-3 ■ Head control while prone. **A,** Infant momentarily lifts head at 1 month. **B,** Infant lifts head and chest 90 degrees and bears weight on forearms at 4 months. **C,** Infant lifts head, chest, and upper abdomen and can bear weight on hands at 6 months. Note how this position facilitates turning from abdomen to back.

Rolling Over.   Newborns may roll over accidentally be-cause of their rounded back. The ability to willfully turn from the abdomen to the back occurs around 5 months, and the ability to turn from the back to the abdomen occurs at approximately 6 months. Infants put to sleep on their side may easily roll over to a prone (face-down) position, thus placing them at higher risk for sudden infant death syndrome (SIDS). It is therefore important to place infants in a supine position for sleep. While the infant is awake, a prone position is acceptable to enhance achievement of milestones such as head control, crawling, creeping, and turning over. It is noteworthy that the parachute reflex (Fig. 10-4), which elicits a protective response to falling, appears at approximately 7 months.

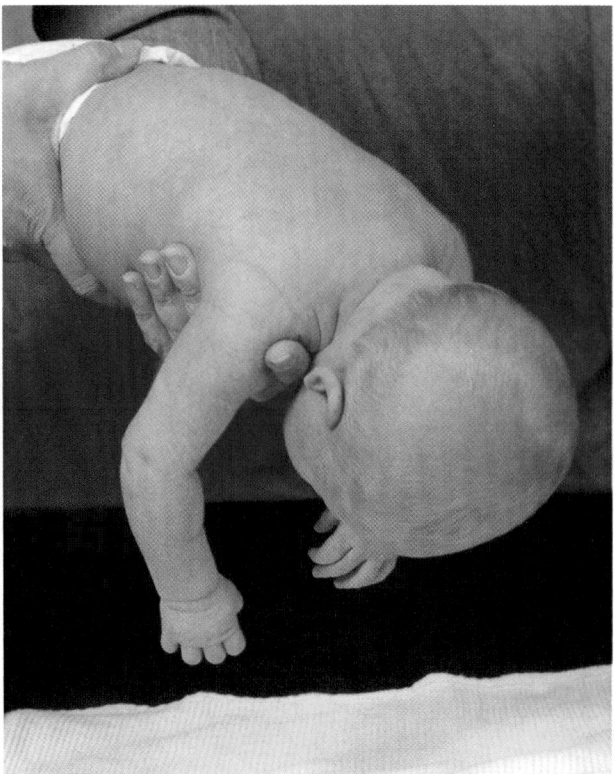

FIG. 10-4 ■ Parachute reflex. (Photo by Paul Vincent Kuntz, Texas Children's Hospital.)

! NURSING ALERT

In the first several months before the infant can roll over the head should be positioned on alternating sides to prevent positional plagiocephaly (when asleep in the supine position or awake and supine) (see Chapter 11).

Sitting.   The ability to sit follows progressive head con-trol and straightening of the back (Fig. 10-5). For the first 2 to 3 months the back is uniformly rounded. The convex cervical curve forms at approximately 3 to 4 months of age, when head control is established. The convex lumbar curve appears when the child begins to sit, at about age 4 months. As the spinal column straightens, the infant can be propped in a sitting position. By age 7 months infants can sit alone, leaning forward on their hands for support. By age 8 months they can sit well while unsupported and begin to explore their surroundings in this position rather than in a lying position. By 10 months they can maneuver from a prone to a sitting position.

Locomotion.   Locomotion involves acquiring the ability to bear weight, propel forward on all four extremities, stand upright with support and, finally, walk alone (Fig. 10-6). Following a cephalocaudal pattern, infants 4 to 6 months old have increasing coordination in their arms. Initial loco-motion results in infants propelling themselves backward by pushing with the arms. By 6 to 7 months of age they are able to bear all their weight on their legs with assistance. *Crawl-ing* (propelling forward with belly on floor) progresses to

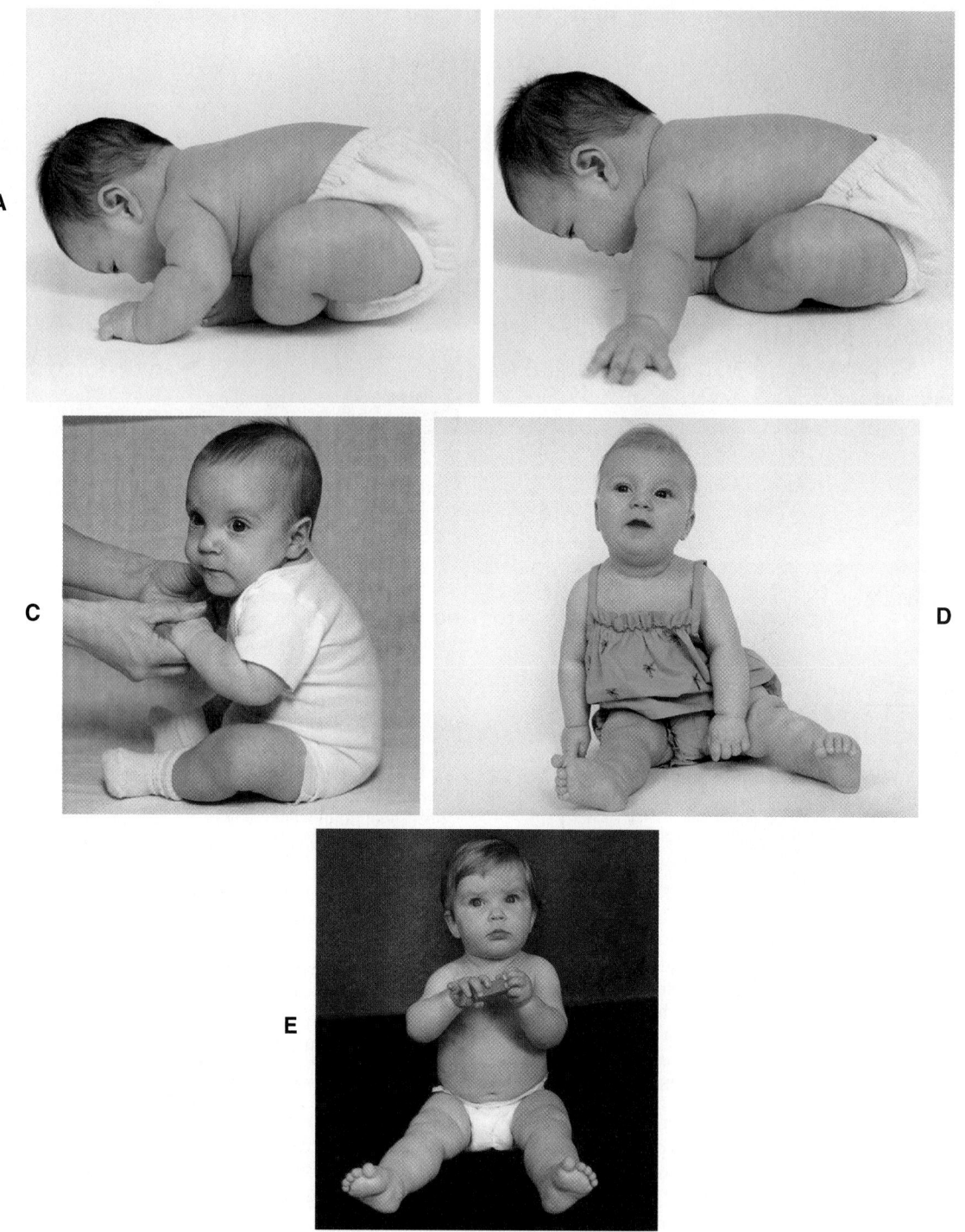

FIG. 10-5 ■ Development of sitting. **A,** Back is completely rounded, and infant has no ability to sit upright at 1 month. **B,** At 2 months, exhibits more control; back is still rounded, but infant can try to pull up with some head control. **C,** Back is rounded only in lumbar area, and infant is able to sit erect with good head control at 4 months. **D,** Infant can sit alone, leaning on hands for support, at 7 months. **E,** Infant sits without support at 8 months. Note the transferring of objects that occurs at 7 months. (**B, D,** and **E** photos by Paul Vincent Kuntz, Texas Children's Hospital.)

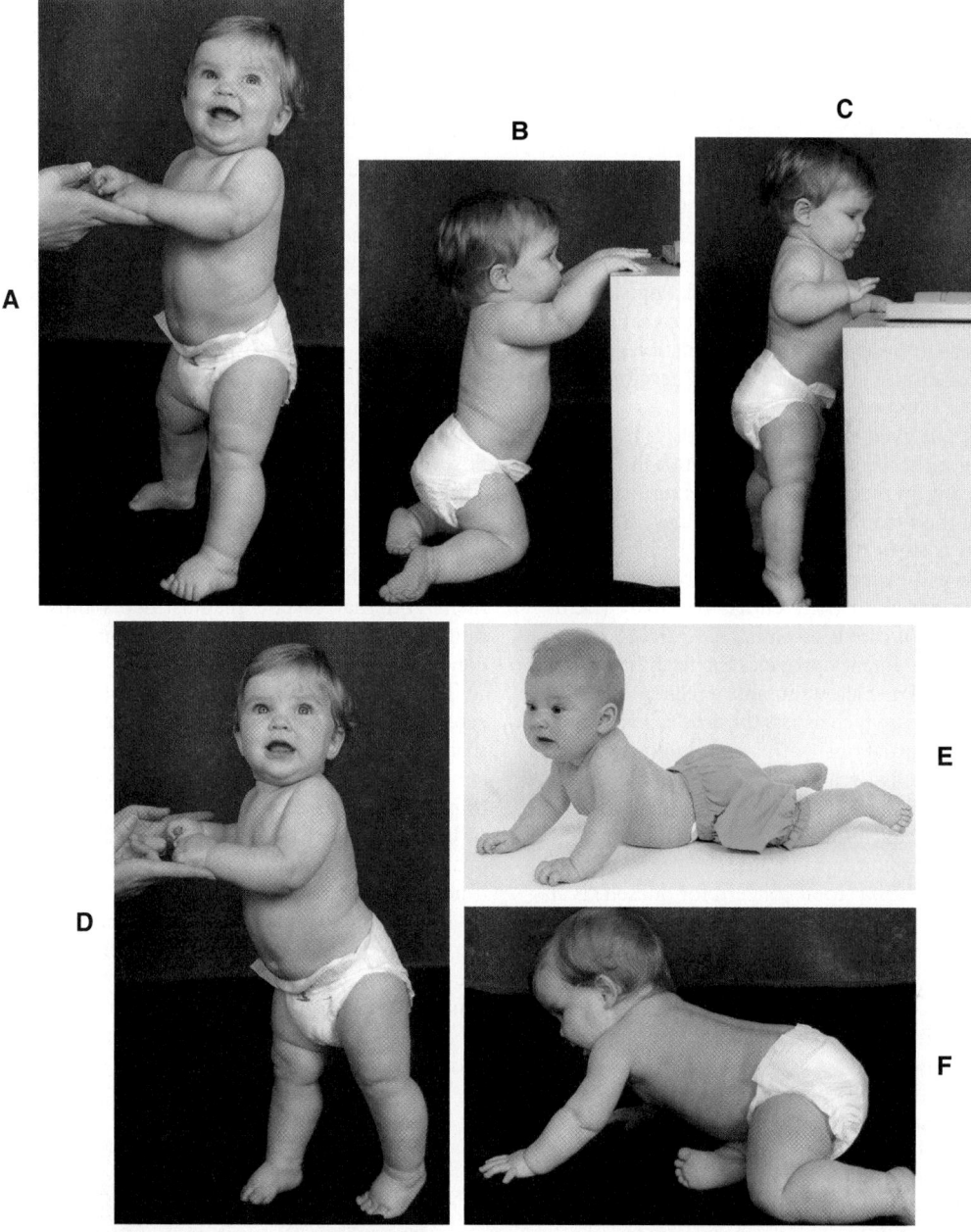

FIG. 10-6 ■ Development of locomotion. **A,** Infant bears full weight on feet by 7 months. **B,** Infant can maneuver from sitting to kneeling position. **C,** Infant can stand holding onto furniture at 9 months. **D,** While standing, infant takes deliberate step at 10 months. **E,** Infant crawls with abdomen on floor and pulls self forward, and then **F,** creeps on hands and knees at 9 months. (Photos by Paul Vincent Kuntz, Texas Children's Hospital.)

creeping on hands and knees (with belly off floor) by 9 months. At this time they stand while holding onto furniture and can pull themselves to the standing position, but they are unable to maneuver back down except by falling. By 11 months they walk while holding onto furniture or with both hands held, and by age 1 year they may be able to walk with one hand held. A number of infants attempt their first independent steps by their first birthday.

> **! NURSING ALERT**
>
> An infant who does not pull to a standing position by 11 to 12 months of age should be further evaluated for possible developmental dysplasia of the hip (see Chapter 31). Although there is considerable variation among infants for the achievement of these milestones, they provide guidelines for early intervention.

PSYCHOSOCIAL DEVELOPMENT
Developing a Sense of Trust (Erikson)

Erikson's phase I (birth to 1 year) is concerned with *acquiring a sense of trust* while *overcoming a sense of mistrust.* The trust that develops is a trust of self, of others, and of the world. Infants "trust" that their feeding, comfort, stimulation, and caring needs will be met. The crucial element for the achievement of this task is the quality of both the parent (caregiver)–child relationship and the care the infant receives. The provision of food, warmth, and shelter by itself is inadequate for the development of a strong sense of self. The infant and parent must jointly learn to satisfactorily meet their needs in order for mutual regulation of frustration to occur. When this synchrony fails to develop, mistrust is the eventual outcome.

Failure to learn "delayed gratification" leads to mistrust. Mistrust can result either from too much or too little frustration. If parents always meet their children's needs before the children signal their readiness, infants will never learn to test their ability to control the environment. If the delay is prolonged, infants will experience constant frustration and eventually mistrust others in their efforts to satisfy them. Therefore consistency of care is essential.

The trust acquired in infancy provides the foundation for all succeeding phases. Trust allows infants a feeling of physical comfort and security, which assists them in experiencing unfamiliar, unknown situations with a minimum of fear. Erikson has divided the first year of life into two oral/social stages. During the first 3 to 4 months, food intake is the most important social activity in which the infant engages. The newborn can tolerate little frustration or delay of gratification. Primary *narcissism* (total concern for oneself) is at its height.

However, as bodily processes such as vision, motor movements, and vocalization become better controlled, infants use more advanced behaviors to interact with others. For example, rather than cry, infants may put their arms up to signify a desire to be held.

The next social modality involves a mode of reaching out to others through *grasping.* Grasping is initially reflexive, but even as a reflex it has a powerful social meaning for the parents. The reciprocal response to the infant's grasping is the parents' holding on and touching. There is pleasurable tactile stimulation for both the child and the parents.

Tactile stimulation is extremely important in the total process of acquiring trust. The degree of mothering skill, the quantity of food, or the length of sucking does not determine the quality of the experience. Rather, it is the total nature of the quality of the interpersonal relationship that influences the infant's formulation of trust.

During the second stage the more active and aggressive modality of *biting* occurs. Infants learn that they can hold onto what is their own and can more fully control their environment. During this stage infants may be confronted with one of their first conflicts. If they are breast-feeding, they quickly learn that biting causes the mother to become upset and withdraw the breast. Yet biting also brings internal relief from teething discomfort and a sense of power or control.

This conflict may be solved in a variety of ways. The mother may wean the infant from the breast and begin bottle-feeding, or the infant may learn to bite substitute "nipples," such as a pacifier, and retain pleasurable breast-feeding. The successful resolution of this conflict strengthens the mother-child relationship because it occurs at a time when infants are recognizing the mother as the most significant person in their life.

COGNITIVE DEVELOPMENT
Sensorimotor Phase (Piaget)

The theory most commonly used to explain *cognition,* or the ability to know, is that of Piaget. The period from birth to 24 months is termed the *sensorimotor phase* and is composed of six stages; however, because this discussion is concerned with ages birth to 12 months, only the first four stages are discussed. The last two stages occur during the toddler period of 12 to 24 months and are discussed in Chapter 12.

During the sensorimotor phase infants progress from reflex behaviors to simple repetitive acts to imitative activity. Three crucial events take place during this phase. The first event involves *separation,* in which infants learn to separate themselves from other objects in the environment. They realize that others besides themselves control the environment and that certain readjustments must take place for mutual satisfaction to occur. This coincides with Erikson's concept of the formation of trust.

The second major accomplishment is achieving the concept of *object permanence,* or the realization that objects that leave the visual field still exist. A typical example of the development of object permanence is when infants are able to pursue objects they observe being hidden under a pillow or behind a chair (Fig. 10-7). This skill develops at approximately 9 to 10 months of age, which corresponds to the time of increased locomotion skills.

The last major intellectual achievement of this period is the ability to use *symbols,* or *mental representation.* The use of symbols allows the infant to think of an object or situation without actually experiencing it. The recognition of symbols is the beginning of the understanding of time and space.

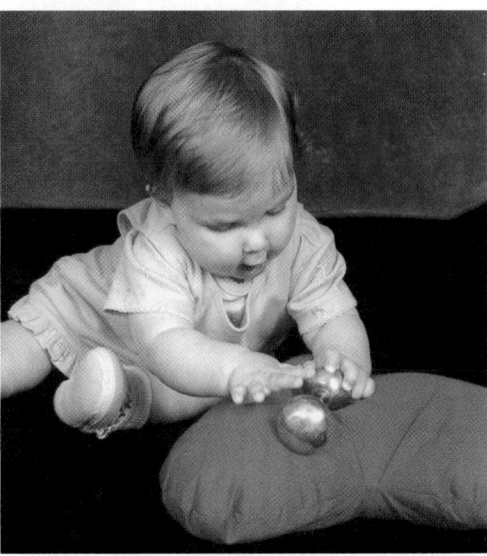

FIG. 10-7 ■ Nine-month-old is able to find hidden object under pillow. (Photo by Paul Vincent Kuntz, Texas Children's Hospital.)

The first stage, from birth to 1 month, is identified by the infant's *use of reflexes.* At birth the infant's individuality and temperament are expressed through the physiologic reflexes of sucking, rooting, grasping, and crying. The repetitious nature of the reflexes is the beginning of associations between an act and a sequential response. When infants cry because they are hungry, a nipple is put in the mouth, and they suck, feel satisfaction, and sleep. They are assimilating this experience while perceiving auditory, tactile, and visual cues. This experience of perceiving certain patterns, or "ordering," provides a foundation for the subsequent stages.

The second stage, *primary circular reactions,* marks the beginning of the replacement of reflexive behavior with voluntary acts. During the period from 1 to 4 months, activities such as sucking or grasping become deliberate acts that elicit certain responses. The beginning of accommodation is evident. Infants incorporate and adapt their reactions to the environment and recognize the stimulus that produced a response. Previously they would cry until the nipple was brought to the mouth. Now they associate the nipple with the sound of the parent's voice. They accommodate this new piece of information and adapt by ceasing to cry when they hear the voice—before receiving the nipple. What is taking place is a realization of causality and a recognition of an orderly sequence of events. The environment is taken in with all of the senses and with whatever motor ability is present.

The *secondary circular reactions* stage is a continuation of primary circular reactions and lasts until 8 months of age. In this stage the primary circular reactions are repeated and prolonged for the response that results. Grasping and holding now become shaking, banging, and pulling. Shaking is performed to hear a noise, not solely for the pleasure of shaking. The quality and quantity of an act become evident. "More" or "less" shaking produces different responses. Causality, time, deliberate intention, and separateness from the environment begin to develop.

Three new processes of human behavior occur. *Imitation* requires the differentiation of selected acts from several events. By the second half of the first year, infants can imitate sounds and simple gestures. *Play* becomes evident as they take pleasure in performing an act after they have mastered it. Much of infants' waking hours is absorbed in sensorimotor play. *Affect* (outward manifestation of emotion and feeling) is seen as infants begin to develop a sense of permanency. During the first 6 months infants believe that an object exists only for as long as they can visually perceive it. In other words: out of sight, out of mind. Affect to external objects is evident when the object continues to be present or remembered even though it is beyond the range of perception. Object permanence is a critical component of parent-child attachment and is seen in the development of stranger anxiety at 6 to 8 months of age (see p. 317).

During the fourth sensorimotor stage, *coordination of secondary schemas and their application to new situations,* infants use previous behavioral achievements primarily as the foundation for adding new intellectual skills to their expanding repertoire. This stage is largely transitional. Increasing motor skills allow for greater exploration of the environment. They begin to discover that hiding an object does not mean that it is gone but that removing an obstacle will reveal the object. This marks the beginning of intellectual reasoning. Furthermore, they can experience an event by observing it, and they begin to associate symbols with events (e.g., "bye-bye" with "Mommy/Daddy goes to work"), but the classification is purely their own. In this stage they learn from the object itself; this is in contrast to the second stage, in which infants learn from the type of interaction between objects or individuals. Intentionality is further developed in that infants now actively attempt to remove a barrier to the desired (or undesired) action (Fig. 10-7). If something is in their way, they attempt to climb over it or push it away. Previously an obstacle would cause them to give up any further attempt to achieve the desired goal.

DEVELOPMENT OF BODY IMAGE

The development of body image parallels sensorimotor development. Infants' kinesthetic and tactile experiences are the first perceptions of their body, and the mouth is the principal area of pleasurable sensations. Other parts of the body are primarily objects of pleasure—the hands and fingers to suck and the feet to play with. As physical needs are met, they feel comfort and satisfaction with their body. Messages conveyed by the caregivers reinforce these feelings. For example, when infants smile, they receive emotional satisfaction from others who smile back.

Achieving the concept of object permanence is basic to the development of self-image. By the end of the first year infants recognize that they are distinct from their parents. At the same time, there is increasing interest in their image, especially in the mirror (Fig. 10-8). As motor skills develop, they learn that parts of the body are useful; for example, the hands bring objects to the mouth, and the legs help them move to different locations. All of these achievements transmit messages to them about themselves. Therefore it is

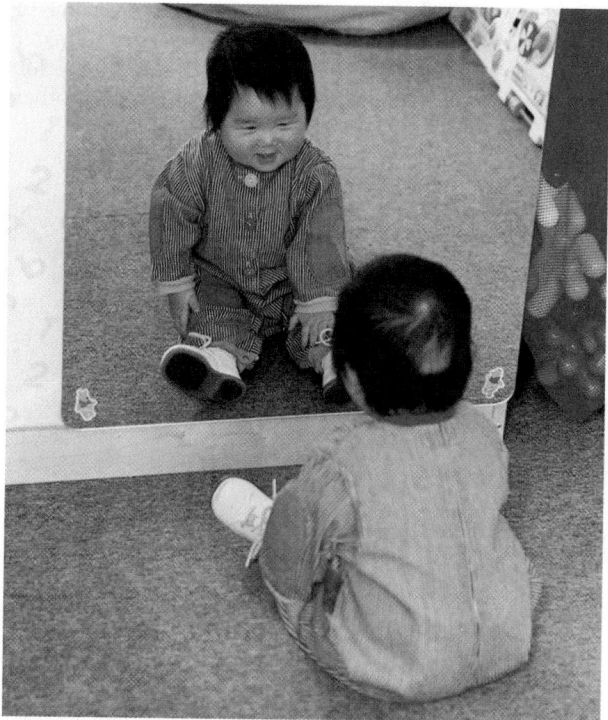

FIG. 10-8 ■ Nine-month-old infant enjoying own image in mirror.

important to transmit positive messages to infants about their bodies.

SOCIAL DEVELOPMENT

Infants' social development is initially influenced by their reflexive behavior, such as the grasp, and eventually depends primarily on the interaction between them and the principal caregivers. *Attachment* to the parent is increasingly evident during the second half of the first year. In addition, tremendous strides are made in communication and personal-social behavior. Whereas crying and reflexive behavior are methods to meet one's needs in the neonatal period, the social smile is an early step in social communication. This has a profound effect on family members and is a tremendous stimulus for evoking continued responses from others. By 4 months infants laugh aloud.

Play is a major socializing agent and provides stimulation needed to learn from and interact with the environment. By age 6 months infants are very personable. They play games such as peekaboo when their head is hidden in a towel, they signal their desire to be picked up by extending their arms, and they show displeasure when a toy is removed or their face is washed.

Attachment

The importance of human physical contact to infants cannot be overemphasized. Parenting is not an instinctual ability but a learned, acquired process. The attachment of parent and child, which often begins before birth and assumes even more importance at birth (see Chapter 8), continues during the first year (Fig. 10-9). In the following discussion of attachment, the term *mother* is used in the broad context of the consistent caregiver with whom the child relates more than anyone else. However, in society's changing social climate and sex-role stereotypes, this person may very well be the father or a grandparent. Studies on paternal-infant attachment demonstrate that stages similar to maternal attachment occur and that fathers are more involved in child care when mothers are employed (although mothers continue to do the majority of infant care). Additional research has shown that inexperienced, first-time fathers are as capable as experienced fathers of developing a close attachment with their infants.

Attachment progresses during infancy, with the child assuming an increasingly significant role. Two components of cognitive development are required for attachment: (1) the ability to discriminate the mother from other individuals, and (2) the achievement of object permanence. Both of these processes prepare the infant for an equally important aspect of attachment—separation from the parent. Separation-individuation should occur as a harmonious, parallel process with emotional attachment.

During the formation of attachment to the parent, the infant progresses through four distinct but overlapping stages. For the first few weeks infants respond indiscriminately to anyone. Beginning at approximately 8 to 12 weeks of age, they cry, smile, and vocalize more to the mother than to anyone else but continue to respond to others, whether familiar or not. At approximately 6 months of age, infants show a distinct preference for the mother. They follow her more, cry when she leaves, enjoy playing with her more, and feel most secure in her arms. About 1 month after showing attachment to the mother, many infants begin attaching to other members of the family, most often the father.

Infants acquire other developmental behaviors that influence the attachment process. These include (1) differential crying, smiling, and vocalization (more to the mother than to anyone else); (2) visual-motor orientation (looking more at the mother, even if she is not close); (3) crying when the mother leaves the room; (4) approaching through locomotion (crawling, creeping, or walking); (5) clinging (especially in the presence of a stranger); and (6) exploring away from the mother while using her as a secure base.

Reactive attachment disorder is a psychologic and developmental problem that stems from maladaptive or absent attachment between the infant and parent and may persist into childhood and even adulthood. Signs of reactive attachment disorder are usually seen before age 5 in infants who had insecure attachments to the mother or other primary caretaker. The child may manifest behaviors such as not being cuddly with parents, failing to make eye contact with significant others, having poor impulse control, and being destructive to self and others. Maltreated and orphaned children often are diagnosed with this complex disorder. Without early intervention, some of these children fail to develop a conscience and suffer from an antisocial personality disorder that may lead to criminal acts.

Separation Anxiety. Between ages 4 and 8 months the infant progresses through the first stage of separation-individuation and begins to have some awareness of self and mother as separate beings. At the same time, object permanence is developing, and the infant is aware that the parent can be absent. Therefore separation anxiety develops and is manifested through a predictable sequence of behaviors.

During the early second half of the first year, infants protest when placed in their crib, and a short time later they object when the mother leaves the room. Infants may not notice the mother's absence if they are absorbed in an activity. However, when they realize her absence, they protest. From this point on, they become very alert to her activities

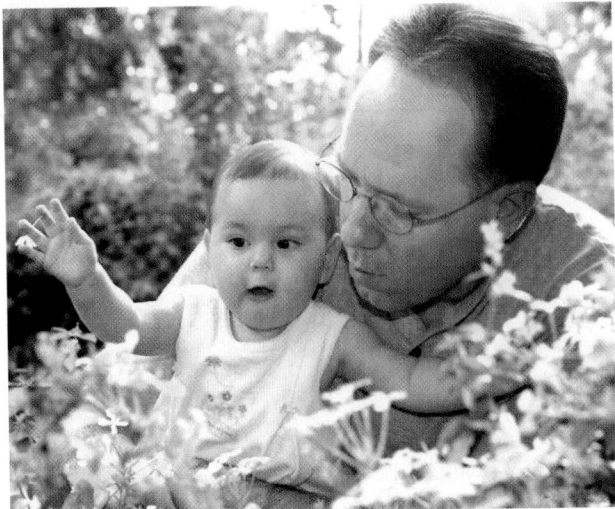

FIG. 10-9 ■ Infancy is an important time for attachment to significant others (Photo by Paul Vincent Kuntz, Texas Children's Hospital.)

and whereabouts. By 11 to 12 months they are able to anticipate her imminent departure by watching her behaviors, and they begin to protest *before* she leaves. At this point many parents learn to postpone alerting the child to their departure until just before leaving.

Stranger Fear.   As infants demonstrate attachment to one person, they correspondingly exhibit less friendliness to others. Between ages 6 and 8 months, fear of strangers and stranger anxiety become prominent and are related to infants' ability to discriminate between familiar and nonfamiliar people. Behaviors such as clinging to the parent, crying, and turning away from the stranger are common.

> **NURSING ALERT**
>
> Be alert to parents' reports about maternal postpartum depression and infant crying, because these concerns may indicate a stressed mother-infant relationship.

Language Development

The infant's first means of verbal communication is crying. Crying as a biologic sign conveys a message of urgency and signals displeasure, such as hunger. However, crying is also a social event that affects the development of the parent-infant relationship—either by its absence, which usually has a positive effect on parents, or its presence, which may evoke a negative response or persuade parents to minister to the child's physical or emotional needs.

In the first few weeks of life, crying has a reflexive quality and is mostly related to physiologic needs. Infants cry for 1 to 1.5 hours a day up to 3 weeks of age and then build up to 2, and even 4, hours by 6 weeks. Crying tends to decrease by 12 weeks. It is thought that the increase in crying for no apparent reason during the first few months may be related to the discharge of energy and the maturational changes in the central nervous system. During the end of the first year, infants cry for attention, from fear (especially stranger fear), and from frustration, usually in response to their developing but inadequate motor skills.

Vocalizations heard during crying eventually become syllables and words (e.g., the "mama" heard during vigorous crying). Infants vocalize as early as 5 to 6 weeks of age by making small throaty sounds. By 2 months they make single vowel sounds such as *ah, eh,* and *uh.* By 3 to 4 months the consonants *n, k, g, p,* and *b* are added, and the infants coo, gurgle, and laugh aloud. By 8 months they imitate sounds, add the consonants *t, d,* and *w,* and combine syllables (e.g., "dada"), but they do not ascribe meaning to the word until 10 to 11 months of age (see Family Focus box).

> **FAMILY FOCUS**
>
> ### Child's Developing Language Skills
>
> During the acquisition of new language skills the child temporarily may stop using other recently learned sounds or words. This is often distressing for parents, who have waited in anticipation for the words "dada" or "mama," because these sounds are commonly replaced by other vocalizations and may not be repeated for several weeks. Nurses can reassure parents that the child will again say these special words, and with increased meaning.

By 9 to 10 months they comprehend the meaning of the word "no" and obey simple commands. By age 1 year they can say three to five words with meaning.

Play

Play during infancy represents the various social modalities observed during cognitive development. The activity of infants is primarily narcissistic and revolves around their own body. As discussed under Development of Body Image (p. 315), body parts are primarily objects of play and pleasure.

During the first year, play becomes more sophisticated and interdependent. From birth to 3 months, infants' responses to the environment are global and largely undifferentiated. Play is dependent; pleasure is demonstrated by a quieting attitude (1 month), a smile (2 months), or a squeal (3 months). From 3 to 6 months, infants show more discriminate interest in stimuli and begin to play alone with a rattle or a soft stuffed toy or with someone else. There is much more interaction during play. By 4 months of age they laugh aloud, show preference for certain toys, and become excited when food or a favorite object is brought to them. They recognize an image in a mirror, smile at it, and vocalize to it.

By 6 months to 1 year, play involves sensorimotor skills. Actual games such as peekaboo and pat-a-cake are played. Verbal repetition and imitation of simple gestures occurs in response to demonstration. Play is much more selective, not only in terms of specific toys, but also in terms of "playmates." Although play is solitary or one-sided, infants choose with whom they will interact. At 6 to 8 months they usually refuse to play with strangers. Parents are definite favorites, and infants know how to attract their attention. At 6 months they extend the arms to be picked up, at 7 months cough to make their presence known, at 10 months pull the parent's clothing, and at 12 months call them by name. This represents a tremendous advance from the newborn who signaled biologic needs by crying to express displeasure.

Stimulation is as important for psychosocial growth as food is for physical growth. Knowledge of developmental milestones allows nurses to guide parents regarding proper play for infants. It is not sufficient to place a mobile over a crib and toys in a playpen for a child's optimum social, emotional, and intellectual development. Play must provide interpersonal contact and recreational and educational stimulation. Infants need to be *played with,* not merely *allowed to play.* Although the type of play infants engage in is called ***solitary,*** this is a figurative, not literal, term to denote one-sided play. The type of toys given to the child is much less important than the quality of personal interaction that occurs.

Table 10-1 lists play activities appropriate for the developmental level of the infant in view of motor, language, and personal-social achievements. Although the activities are grouped according to the major mode of stimulation provided, there is overlap in many instances. In addition, play activities suggested for one age-group may be appropriate for older infants but inappropriate for younger infants.

TEMPERAMENT

The infant's temperament or behavioral style influences the type of interaction that occurs between the child and parents, especially the mother, and other family members (see general discussion of temperament in Chapter 5). In assessing a child's temperament, it is the parents' perception of the

TABLE 10-1 ■ Play During Infancy

AGE (months)	VISUAL STIMULATION	AUDITORY STIMULATION	TACTILE STIMULATION	KINETIC STIMULATION
SUGGESTED ACTIVITIES				
Birth-1	Look at infant at close range Hang bright, shiny object within 20-25 cm (8-10 inches) of infant's face and in midline Hang mobiles with black-and-white designs	Talk to infant; sing in soft voice Play music box, tape, or compact disc Have ticking clock or metronome nearby	Hold, caress, cuddle Keep infant warm May like to be swaddled	Rock infant; place in cradle Use stroller for walks
2-3	Provide bright objects Make room bright with pictures or mirrors Take infant to various rooms while doing chores Place infant in infant seat for vertical view of environment (use a safe surface)	Talk to infant Include in family gatherings Expose to various environmental noises other than those of home Use rattles, wind chimes	Caress infant while bathing, at diaper change Comb hair with a soft brush Give massage	Use infant swing Take in car for rides Exercise body by moving extremities in swimming motion Use cradle gym
4-6	Place infant in front of unbreakable mirror Give brightly colored toys to hold (small enough to grasp)	Talk to infant; repeat sounds infant makes Laugh when infant laughs Call infant by name Place rattle or bell in hand	Give infant soft squeeze toys of various textures Allow to splash in bath Place nude on soft, furry rug and move extremities	Use swing or stroller Bounce infant in lap while holding in standing position Support infant in sitting position; let infant lean forward to balance self Place infant on floor to crawl, roll over, sit
6-9	Give infant large toys with bright colors, movable parts, and noisemakers Play peekaboo, especially hiding face in a towel Make funny faces to encourage imitation Give ball of yarn or string to pull apart	Call infant by name Repeat simple words such as "dada," "mama," "bye-bye" Speak clearly Name parts of body, people, and foods Tell infant what you are doing Use "no" only when necessary Give simple commands Show how to clap hands, bang a drum	Let infant play with fabrics of various textures Have bowl with foods of different sizes and textures to feel Let infant "catch" running water Encourage "swimming" in large bathtub or shallow pool Give wad of sticky tape to manipulate	Hold upright to bear weight and bounce Pick up, say "up" Put down, say "down" Place toys out of reach; encourage infant to get them Play pat-a-cake
9-12	Show infant large pictures in books Take infant to places where there are animals, many people, different objects (shopping center) Play ball by rolling it to child, demonstrate "throwing" it back Demonstrate building a two-block tower	Read infant simple nursery rhymes Point to body parts and name each one Imitate sounds of animals	Give infant finger foods of different textures Let infant mess and squash food Let infant feel cold (ice cube) or warm objects, say what temperature each is Let infant feel a breeze (fan blowing)	Give large push-pull toys Place furniture in a circle to encourage cruising Turn in different positions
SUGGESTED TOYS				
Birth-6	Nursery mobiles Unbreakable mirrors See-through crib bumpers Contrasting colored sheets	Music boxes Musical mobiles Crib dangle bells Small-handled clear rattle	Stuffed animals Soft clothes Soft or furry quilt Soft mobiles	Rocking crib/cradle Weighted or suction toy Infant swing
6-12	Various colored blocks Nested boxes or cups Books with rhymes and bright pictures Strings of big beads Simple take-apart toys Large ball Cup and spoon Large puzzles Jack-in-the box	Rattles of different sizes, shapes, tones, and bright colors Squeaky animals and dolls Records with light, rhythmic music	Soft, different-texture animals and dolls Sponge toys, floating toys Squeeze toys Teething toys Books with textures/objects, such as fur and zipper	Activity box for crib Push-pull toys Wind-up swing

child and the degree of fit between their expectations and the child's actual temperament that are important. The more dissonance or lack of harmony between the child's temperament and the parent's ability to accept and deal with the behavior, the more risk for subsequent parent-child conflicts.

Although most behavioral researchers agree there is a strong biologic component to temperament, researchers also suggest that temperament may be modified by the environment, particularly the family (Wilson and others, 2000). Family interaction with the infant is perceived as a circular process wherein each family member affects each other and the family as a unit. With these concepts in mind, the nurse has an important role in helping the family understand the infant's temperament as it relates to family dynamics and the eventual well-being of the child and family unit (Wilson and others, 2000).

The Revised Infant Temperament Questionnaire (RITQ) (Carey and McDevitt, 1978) can be used as a screening tool with parents. The questionnaire focuses on nine temperament variables, but the 95 questions relate specifically to activities such as sleep, feeding, play, diapering, and dressing. The scores from the RITQ help identify the child's temperamental style. Use of the RITQ is well accepted by parents and should be accompanied by an adequate explanation of the results. In discussing the results, it is best to avoid descriptors such as "difficult" by describing such infants in terms of characteristics such as "intense" or "less predictable." The Early Infancy Temperament Questionnaire is a 76-item parent questionnaire that was adapted from the RITQ to specifically evaluate temperament characteristics of infants 1 to 4 months old, whereas the RITQ is best suited for infants 4 months old and older (Medoff-Cooper, Carey, and McDevitt, 1993).

With knowledge of the infant's temperament, nurses are better able to (1) provide parents with background information that will help them see their child in a better perspective, (2) offer a more organized picture of their child's behavior and possibly reveal distortions in their perceptions of the behavior, and (3) guide parents regarding appropriate childrearing techniques.

Childrearing Practices Related to Temperament

Most parents realize that their infant is born with unique characteristics, and few parents of difficult infants need to be told of the challenge of caring for them. However, very few parents are aware of the significance of the temperamental characteristics and of constructive approaches to dealing with them. The following are examples of interventions that promote more positive parenting of infants with different temperament styles.*

"Difficult" children may respond better to scheduled feedings and structured caregiving routines than to demand feedings and frequent changes in daily routines. These children sleep less and may need more structured approaches to bedtime to prevent bedtime problems. "Highly distractible" children may require additional soothing measures such as

---

*Recommended resources for parents are *The Difficult Child* by S.K. Turecki and L. Tonner (2000, Bantam Books; www.randomhouse.com) and *Know Your Child: An Authoritative Guide for Today's Parents* by S. Chess and A. Thomas (1996, Jason Aronson, Inc.; www.aronson.com).

swinging, rocking, or being carried in a pack that the parent wears across the chest or back. Children with "high activity" levels require vigilant watching, and parents need to take extra precautions in safeguarding the home. These children benefit from increased opportunities for gross motor activity to constructively channel their energy.

The child who is "slow to warm up" may demonstrate more stranger fear than other children and may require gradual and frequent preparation for new situations, such as substitute child care. Even the "easy child" can present problems in that the parents may need reminders to feed the child who sleeps for prolonged intervals and rarely cries. They may need to "retrain" the child because of the ease of developing habits such as keeping the child up late or sleeping with the youngster, which may later become troublesome.

Appropriate counseling based on awareness of the child's temperament can greatly enhance the quality of interaction between parents and infant. Even just letting parents know that "difficult" traits are innate can relieve feelings of guilt and incompetence (see Family Focus box).

Because of the complexity of the developmental process during the first 12 months, Table 10-2 is presented to help organize and clarify the data already discussed. Although all milestones are important, some represent essential integrative aspects of development that lay the foundation for achievement of more advanced skills. These essential milestones are designated by a square (■) in the table. The table represents the average monthly age at which various skills are attained. It must be remembered that, although the sequence is the same, the rate will vary among children.

FAMILY FOCUS

Difficult Temperament and Preterm Infants

Parents typically rate preterm, low-birth-weight infants as being more difficult than full-term infants (Langkamp, Kim, and Pasco, 1998; Hughes and others, 2002). Parents are often concerned that the difficult temperament is permanent and results from the many negative and painful hospital experiences. The family can be reassured that although these infants may be difficult to parent for the first 6 months of corrected age (chronologic age minus amount of prematurity), over time the infants tend to become less difficult (Medoff-Cooper, 1995). Another study found that preterm infants were rated by their mothers at 4 and 9 months of age in relation to temperament. The preterm infants at 9 months were still significantly perceived as more difficult in comparison with full-term infants at the same ages (Langkamp and Pascoe, 2001). Further research is needed to clarify the relationship between preterm infant temperament, extent of illness at birth, and family and environmental influences. Many of the studies indicating that preterm infants are more difficult to console were performed before wide-scale implementation of individualized developmental care for such infants; kangaroo care and assisting the infant in self-regulation behaviors may in fact change current thought. One study found that healthy low-birth-weight infants who experienced kangaroo care (skin-to-skin contact) versus infants who received standard medical/nursing care, had higher scores for consolability and state orientation, and lower intensity ratings (Ohgi and others, 2002). By enabling the preterm infant to experience more positive caretaking and less stressful stimuli, such infants may be found in the future to be less temperamental.

TABLE 10-2 ■ **Growth and Development During Infancy**

AGE (months)	PHYSICAL	GROSS MOTOR	FINE MOTOR
1	Weight gain of 150-210 g (5-7 ounces) weekly for first 6 months Height gain of 2.5 cm (1 inch) monthly for first 6 months Head circumference increases by 1.5 cm (½ inch) monthly for first 6 months Primitive reflexes present and strong Doll's eye reflex and dance reflex fading Obligatory nose breathing (most infants)	■ Assumes flexed position with pelvis high but knees not under abdomen when prone (at birth, knees flexed under abdomen) ■ Can turn head from side to side when prone; lifts head momentarily from bed (see Fig. 10-3, *A*) Has marked head lag, especially when pulled from lying to sitting position (see Fig. 10-2, *A*) Holds head momentarily parallel and in midline when suspended in prone position Assumes asymmetric tonic neck flex position when supine When held in standing position, body is limp at knees and hips In sitting position, back is uniformly rounded, absence of head control	Hands predominantly closed Grasp reflex strong Hand clenches on contact with rattle
2	Posterior fontanel closed Crawling reflex disappears	■ Assumes less flexed position when prone-hips flat, legs extended, arms flexed, head to side Less head lag when pulled to sitting position (see Fig. 10-2, *B*) Can maintain head in same plane as rest of body when held in ventral suspension When prone, can lift head almost 45 degrees off table When moved to sitting position, head is held up but bends forward (see Fig. 10-5, *B*) Assumes symmetric tonic neck flex position intermittently	Hands often open Grasp reflex fading
3	Primitive reflexes fading	Able to hold head more erect when sitting, but still bobs forward Has only slight head lag when pulled to sitting position Assumes symmetric body positioning Able to raise head and shoulders from prone position to a 45-degree to 90-degree angle from table; bears weight on forearms When held in standing position, able to bear slight fraction of weight on legs Regards own hand	■ Actively holds rattle but will not reach for it Grasp reflex absent Hands kept loosely open Clutches own hand; pulls at blankets and clothes
4	Drooling begins Moro, tonic neck, and rooting reflexes have disappeared	■ Has almost no head lag when pulled to sitting position (see Fig. 10-5, *C*) ■ Balances head well in sitting position (see Fig. 10-5, *C*)	■ Inspects and plays with hands; pulls clothing or blanket over face in play Tries to reach objects with hand but overshoots Grasps object with both hands

■ Milestones that represent essential integrative aspects of development that lay the foundation for the achievement of more advanced skills.

SENSORY	VOCALIZATION	SOCIALIZATION/COGNITION
■ Able to fixate on moving object in range of 45 degrees when held at a distance of 20-25 cm (8-10 inches) Visual acuity approaches 20/100* Follows light to midline Quiets when hears a voice	Cries to express displeasure Makes small, throaty sounds Makes comfort sounds during feeding	Is in sensorimotor phase—stage I, use of reflexes (birth-1 month), and stage II, primary circular reactions (1-4 months) Watches parent's face intently as she or he talks to infant
Binocular fixation and convergence to near objects beginning When supine, follows dangling toy from side to point beyond midline Visually searches to locate sounds Turns head to side when sound is made at level of ear	■ Vocalizes, distinct from crying Crying becomes differentiated Coos Vocalizes to familiar voice	■ Demonstrates social smile in response to various stimuli
■ Follows objects to periphery (180 degrees) ■ Locates sound by turning head to side and looking in same direction Begins to have ability to coordinate stimuli from various sense organs	■ Squeals aloud to show pleasure Coos, babbles, chuckles Vocalizes when smiling "Talks" a great deal when spoken to Less crying during periods of wakefulness	Displays considerable interest in surroundings Ceases crying when parent enters room Can recognize familiar faces and objects, such as feeding bottle Shows awareness of strange situations
Able to accommodate to near objects Binocular vision fairly well established Can focus on a 1.25 cm (½ inch) block Beginning eye-hand coordination	Makes consonant sounds *n, k, g, p, b* ■ Laughs aloud Vocalization changes according to mood	Is in stage III, secondary circular reactions Demands attention by fussing; becomes bored if left alone Enjoys social interaction with people Anticipates feeding when sees bottle or mother if breast-feeding Shows excitement with whole body, squeals, breathes heavily

*Degree of visual acuity varies according to vision measurement procedure used.

Continued

TABLE 10-2 ■ Growth and Development During Infancy—*cont'd*

AGE (months)	PHYSICAL	GROSS MOTOR	FINE MOTOR
4—*cont'd*		Back less rounded, curved only in lumbar area Able to sit erect if propped up Able to raise head and chest off surface to angle of 90 degrees (see Fig. 10-3, *B*) Assumes predominant symmetric position ■ Rolls from back to side	Plays with rattle placed in hand, shakes it, but cannot pick it up if dropped Can carry objects to mouth
5	Beginning signs of tooth eruption Birth weight doubles	No head lag when pulled to sitting position When sitting, able to hold head erect and steady Able to sit for longer periods when back is well supported Back straight When prone, assumes symmetric positioning with arms extended ■ Can turn over from abdomen to back When supine, puts feet to mouth	■ Able to grasp objects voluntarily Uses palmar grasp, bidextrous approach Plays with toes Takes objects directly to mouth Holds one cube while regarding a second one
6	Growth rate may begin to decline Weight gain of 90-150 g (3-5 ounces) weekly for next 6 months Height gain of 1.25 cm (½ inch) monthly for next 6 months ■ Teething may begin with eruption of two lower central incisors ■ Chewing and biting occur	When prone, can lift chest and upper abdomen off surface, bearing weight on hands (see Fig. 10-3, *C*) When about to be pulled to a sitting position, lifts head Sits in high chair with back straight Rolls from back to abdomen When held in standing position, bears almost all of weight Hand regard absent	Resecures a dropped object Drops one cube when another is given Grasps and manipulates small objects Holds bottle Grasps feet and pulls to mouth
7	Eruption of upper central incisors	When supine, spontaneously lifts head off surface ■ Sits, leaning forward on both hands (see Fig. 10-5, *D*) When prone, bears weight on one hand Sits erect momentarily Bears full weight on feet (see Fig. 10-6, *A*) When held in standing position, bounces actively	■ Transfers objects from one hand to the other (see Fig. 10-5, *E*) Has unidextrous approach and grasp Holds two cubes more than momentarily Bangs cubes on table Rakes at a small object
8	Begins to show regular patterns in bladder and bowel elimination Parachute reflex appears (see Fig. 10-4)	■ Sits steadily unsupported (see Fig. 10-5, *E*) Readily bears weight on legs when supported; may stand holding onto furniture Adjusts posture to reach an object	Has beginning pincer grasp using index, fourth, and fifth fingers against lower part of thumb Releases objects at will Rings bell purposely Retains two cubes while regarding third cube Secures an object by pulling on a string Reaches persistently for toys out of reach

■ Milestones that represent essential integrative aspects of development that lay the foundation for the achievement of more advanced skills.

SENSORY	VOCALIZATION	SOCIALIZATION/COGNITION
		Shows interest in strange stimuli Begins to show memory
Visually pursues a dropped object Is able to sustain visual inspection of an object Can localize sounds made below ear	Squeals Makes cooing vowel sounds interspersed with consonant sounds (e.g., *ah-goo*)	Smiles at mirror image Pats bottle or breast with both hands More enthusiastically playful, but may have rapid mood swings Is able to discriminate strangers from family Vocalizes displeasure when object is taken away Discovers parts of body
Adjusts posture to see an object Prefers more complex visual stimuli Can localize sounds made above ear Will turn head to the side, then look up or down	▪ Begins to imitate sounds ▪ Babbling resembles one-syllable utterances—*ma, mu, da, di, hi* Vocalizes to toys, mirror image Takes pleasure in hearing own sounds (self-reinforcement)	Recognizes parents; begins to fear strangers Holds arms out to be picked up Has definite likes and dislikes Begins to imitate (cough, protrusion of tongue) Excites on hearing footsteps ▪ Briefly searches for a dropped object (object permanent beginning) Frequent mood swings—from crying to laughing with little or no provocation
▪ Can fixate on very small objects Responds to own name Localizes sound by turning head in a curving arch Beginning awareness of depth and space Has taste preferences	▪ Produces vowel sounds and chained syllables—*baba, dada, kaka* Vocalizes four distinct vowel sounds "Talks" when others are talking	▪ Increasing fear of strangers; shows signs of fretfulness when parent disappears Imitates simple acts and noises Tries to attract attention by coughing or snorting Plays peek-a-boo Demonstrates dislike of food by keeping lips closed Exhibits oral aggressiveness in biting and mouthing Demonstrates expectation in response to repetition of stimuli
	Makes consonant sounds *t, d,* and *w* Listens selectively to familiar words Utterances signal emphasis and emotion Combines syllables, such as *dada*, but does not ascribe meaning to them	Increasing anxiety over loss of parent, particularly mother, and fear of strangers Responds to word "no" Dislikes dressing, diaper change

Continued

TABLE 10-2 ■ Growth and Development During Infancy—*cont'd*

AGE (MONTHS)	PHYSICAL	GROSS MOTOR	FINE MOTOR
9	Eruption of upper lateral incisor may begin	Creeps on hands and knees Sits steadily on floor for prolonged time (10 minutes) Recovers balance when leans forward but cannot do so when leaning sideways ■ Pulls self to standing position and stands holding onto furniture (see Fig. 10-6, *B* to *C*)	■ Uses thumb and index finger in crude pincer grasp (see Fig. 10-1) Preference for use of dominant hand now evident Grasps third cube Compares two cubes by bringing them together
10	Labyrinth-righting reflex is strongest when infant is in prone or supine position, is able to raise head	Can change from prone to sitting position Stands while holding onto furniture, sits by falling down Recovers balance easily while sitting While standing, lifts one foot to take a step (see Fig. 10-6, *D*)	Crude release of an object beginning Grasps bell by handle
11	Eruption of lower lateral incisor may begin	When sitting, pivots to reach toward back to pick up an object ■ Cruises or walks holding onto furniture or with both hands held	Explores objects more thoroughly (e.g., clapper inside bell) Has neat pincer grasp Drops object deliberately for it to be picked up Puts one object after another into a container (sequential play) Able to manipulate an object to remove it from tight-fitting enclosure
12	■ Birth weight tripled ■ Birth length increased by 50% Head and chest circumference equal (head circumference 46 cm [18 inches]) Has total of six to eight deciduous teeth Anterior fontanel almost closed Landau reflex fading Babinski reflex disappears Lumbar curve develops; lordosis evident during walking	■ Walks with one hand held Cruises well ■ May attempt to stand alone momentarily; may attempt first step alone Can sit down from standing position without help	Releases cube in cup Attempts to build two-block tower but fails Tries to insert a pellet into a narrow-necked bottle but fails Can turn pages in a book, many at a time

■ Milestones that represent essential integrative aspects of development that lay the foundation for the achievement of more advanced skills.

COPING WITH CONCERNS RELATED TO NORMAL GROWTH AND DEVELOPMENT
Separation and Stranger Fear

A number of fears can appear during infancy. However, the fear that causes parents the most concern is fear related to strangers and separation. Although erroneously interpreted by some as a sign of undesirable, antisocial behavior, stranger fear and separation anxiety are important components of a strong, healthy parent-child attachment. Nevertheless, this period can present difficulties for the parent and child. Parents may be more confined to the home because baby-sitters are violently protested by the infant. To accustom the infant to new people, parents are encouraged to have close friends or relatives visit often. This provides for other persons with whom the child is comfortable and who can give parents time for themselves.

Infants also need opportunities to safely experience strangers. Usually toward the end of the first year, infants begin to venture away from the parent and demonstrate curiosity about strangers. If allowed to explore at their own rate, many infants eventually "warm up." If parents hold the

SENSORY	VOCALIZATION	SOCIALIZATION/COGNITION
Localizes sounds by turning head diagonally and directly toward sound Depth perception increasing	Responds to simple verbal commands Comprehends "no-no"	Parent (mother) is increasingly important for own sake Shows increasing interest in pleasing parent Begins to show fears of going to bed and being left alone Puts arms in front of face to avoid having it washed
	■ Says "dada," "mama" with meaning Comprehends "bye-bye" May say one word (e.g., "hi," "bye," "no")	Inhibits behavior to verbal command of "no-no" or own name Imitates facial expressions; waves bye-bye Extends toy to another person but will not release it ■ Develops object permanence Repeats actions that attract attention and cause laughter Pulls clothes of another to attract attention Plays interactive games such as pat-a-cake Reacts to adult anger; cries when scolded Demonstrates independence in dressing, feeding, locomotive skills, and testing of parents Looks at and follows picture in a book
	Imitates definite speech sounds	Experiences joy and satisfaction when a task is mastered Reacts to restrictions with frustration Rolls ball to another on request Anticipates body gestures when a familiar nursery rhyme or story is being told (e.g., holds toes and feet in response to "This little piggy went to market") Plays games up-down, "so big," or peek-a-boo Shakes head for "no"
Discriminates simple geometric forms (e.g., circle) Amblyopia may develop with lack of binocularity Can follow rapidly moving object Controls and adjusts response to sound; listens for sound to recur	■ Says three to five words besides "dada," "mama" Comprehends meaning of several words (comprehension always precedes verbalization) Recognizes objects by name Imitates animal sounds Understands simple verbal commands (e.g., "Give it to me," "Show me your eyes")	Shows emotions such as jealousy, affection (may give hug or kiss on request), anger, fear Enjoys familiar surroundings and explores away from parent Is fearful in strange situation; clings to parent May develop habit of "security blanket" or favorite toy Has increasing determination to practice locomotor skills ■ Searches for an object even if it has not been hidden, but searches only where object was last seen

child away from their face, the infant can observe while maintaining close physical contact.

The best approach for the stranger (who may be the nurse) is to talk softly, meet the child at eye level (to appear smaller), maintain a safe distance from the infant, and avoid sudden, intrusive gestures, such as holding the arms out and smiling broadly.

Parents also may wonder whether they should encourage the child's clinging, dependent behavior, especially if there is pressure from others who view this as "spoiling" (see following discussion). Parents need to be reassured that such behavior is healthy, desirable, and necessary for the child's optimal emotional development. If parents can reassure the infant of their presence, the infant will learn to realize that they are still there even if not physically present. Talking to infants when leaving the room, allowing them to hear one's voice on the telephone, and using transitional objects (e.g., a favorite blanket or toy) reassures them of the parent's continued presence.

Alternate Childcare Arrangements

For many parents, especially working mothers, the need for locating safe and competent childcare facilities for the infant is an increasingly difficult problem—one that is compounded by the number of mothers working outside the home. Over the past 30 years there has been a marked shift in childcare arrangements, with fewer children being cared for at home and more children being cared for in group centers or other settings.

The basic types of care are *in-home care,* either in the parents' or caregivers' home (family day care), and *center-based care,* usually in a day care center. *In-home care* may consist of a full-time baby-sitter who lives in the home, a full-time baby-sitter who comes to the home, cooperative arrangements such as exchange baby-sitting, or family day care. A licensed *family day care home* typically provides care and protection for up to five children for part of a 24-hour day and does not include informal arrangements such as exchange baby-sitting or caregivers in the child's own home. The five children include the family day care provider's own children younger than 5 years of age living in the home. Unfortunately, many family day care homes operate without a license and may care for large numbers of infants without adequate staff and facilities.

Center-based care usually refers to a licensed day care facility that provides care for six or more children, for 6 or more hours in a 24-hour day. *Work-based group care* is another option that is becoming increasingly popular as employers recognize the benefit of providing quality and convenient child care to their employees. *Sick-child care* may also be available for times when the youngster is ill. Such programs are often located in community hospitals or in work settings.

A major nursing responsibility is guiding parents in locating suitable facilities that have a well-qualified staff. State licensing agencies can help parents identify day care centers that accept children of specific age-groups and are convenient to home and work. Their records are available to the public and provide reports from the health, safety, and fire departments; periodic evaluations from the licensing agency; complaints filed against the center; and qualification of the center's employees. State-licensed programs are supposed to abide by established standards, which represent the minimum requirements and safeguards. However, enforcement of the standards is sometimes inadequate. Early childhood programs may also belong to a voluntary accreditation system, the National Academy of Early Childhood Programs, which serves as a model for optimum care.* References from other parents are also helpful, provided that

they have investigated the center carefully and have remained involved with the agency's activities.

Guidelines for selecting child care facilities are discussed in Chapter 13 under Preschool and Kindergarten Experience. The same conscientious attention should be applied to locating competent baby-sitters. References from other employers are essential, and there is no substitute for observing the interaction between the individual and the child. Although very young infants need little if any preparation for the introduction of a new caregiver, older infants may benefit from a gradual placement to reduce stranger anxiety. At all times the parent should have the right to visit the child, and regular conferences should be established to review the child's progress.

Limit Setting and Discipline

As infants' motor skills advance and mobility increases, parents are faced with the need to set safe limits to protect the child and establish a positive and supportive parent-child relationship (see Nurse's Role in Injury Prevention, p. 354). Although there are numerous disciplinary techniques, some are more appropriate for this age than others. An effective approach used in disciplining a child is the use of time-out. The basic principles are the same as those discussed in Chapter 3, except that the place for time-out needs to be commensurate with the child's abilities. For example, the playpen is better for most infants than a chair. Although parents may be concerned with instituting discipline during infancy, it is important to stress that the earlier effective disciplinary methods are employed, the easier it is to continue these approaches.

Parents must recognize the infant's cognitive and behavioral limitations; adequate protection from hazards must be implemented because infants and toddlers do not understand a cause-and-effect relationship between dangerous objects and physical harm. Additionally, parents may need reassurance that their infant's behavior is exploratory in nature, not oppositional (at this age) and primarily centered on the infant's basic needs of warmth, love, food, security, and comfort. Parents may verbalize that comforting the infant too much or meeting its needs will result in a spoiled child; there is no substantial evidence that meeting the infant's basic needs will result in such behaviors later in life. Children will innately test limits and explore during the exploratory phase of growth; instead of discouraging exploration, safe alternatives should be provided, dangerous household items should be put away, and children should be given consistent discipline and nurturing. Effective teaching for injury prevention optimally begins in infancy by helping parents understand the nature of their child's normal development. It must be reiterated continually that infants cry because a need is not being met, not to intentionally irritate an adult. The fussy or irritable infant is a potential victim of shaken baby syndrome (or other bodily harm), since adults and caretakers may not understand the nature of the infant's crying.

Thumb Sucking and Use of a Pacifier

Sucking is the infant's chief pleasure and may not be satisfied by breast- or bottle-feeding. It is such a strong need that infants who are deprived of sucking, such as those with a cleft lip repair, will suck on their tongue. Some newborns are born with sucking blisters on their hands from in utero

---

*Information about the accreditation criteria and procedures of the **National Academy of Early Childhood Programs** is available from the **National Association for the Education of Young Children,** 1509 16th Street NW, Washington, DC 20036; (800) 424-2460 or (202) 232-8777; fax: (202) 328-1846; website: www.naeyc.org. These criteria are excellent guidelines for evaluating childcare facilities. Other resources are *Child Care: Choosing the Best for Your Family,* available from the **American Academy of Pediatrics,** 141 Northwest Point Boulevard, Elk Grove Village, IL 60007; (888) 227-1770; fax: (847) 228-1281; website: www.medem.com, then enter Medical Library for pamphlet titles; and *Parent's Guide to Day Care,* available from the **National Association of Pediatric Nurse Associates and Practitioners (NAPNAP),** 1101 Kings Highway North, Suite 206, Cherry Hill, NJ 08034-1912; (877) 662-7627 or (856) 667-1773; fax: (856) 667-7187; website: www.napnap.org.

sucking activity. The benefits of nonnutritive sucking in preterm infants have been documented, such as increased weight gain, decreased length of stay, and improved pain management (Pickler and Frankel, 1995; Pinelli and Symington, 2000; Pinelli, Symington, and Ciliska, 2002).

Problems arise when parents are concerned about the sucking of the fingers, thumb, or pacifier and attempt to restrain this natural tendency. Before giving advice, nurses should investigate the parents' feelings and base guidance on this information.

During infancy and early childhood there is no need to restrain nonnutritive sucking of the fingers. Malocclusion may occur if thumb sucking persists past 4 years of age, or 6 years as indicated by some authorities (Johns, Miller, and Hochstetler, 1998; Van Norman, 2001), or when the permanent teeth erupt. Others have linked pacifier use in infancy and a higher incidence of malocclusion regardless of pacifier type (regular or orthodontic) (Nowak and Warren, 2000). Pacifiers may be relinquished earlier than thumbs because they are less readily available.

There are studies linking the early introduction of a pacifier with early termination of breast-feeding, decreased exclusive breast-feeding, and early weaning from the breast; other studies have shown a weak correlation between early weaning from breastfeeding and pacifier use. Biancuzzo (1999) suggests that health care workers maintain a commonsense approach to pacifier usage and breast-feeding. Parents should be informed of the relationship between pacifier use and early termination of breast-feeding so that an informed decision can be made. Furthermore, pacifier use should not replace actual feeding or suckling; prohibiting pacifier use will not ensure an increase in the length of breast-feeding, and there should be an emphasis on allowing the infant to control the pace, frequency, and termination of feeding rather than allowing the pacifier (or anything else) to become the focus of the interaction.

The use of a pacifier in infants has also been suggested as a causative factor in the increase in episodes of acute otitis media (Niemela, Uhari, and Mottonen, 1995); however, a later study showed a significant decrease in the incidence of acute otitis media when a pacifier was used only at bedtime (Niemela and others, 2000). The effect of continual pacifier use on early speech and language development is unknown, but the pacifier may decrease the child's desire to imitate

sounds and affect intelligibility. Parents need to be alerted that continual dependency on a pacifier may influence social and speech development.

If the child uses a pacifier, safety considerations in purchasing one must be stressed. Parents should be cautioned against altering a pacifier, thus making it more dangerous (see Aspiration of Foreign Objects, p. 349). To decrease dependence on nonnutritive sucking in young infants, sucking pleasure can be increased by prolonging feeding time. A small-holed, firm nipple causes stronger sucking and slower feeding. Also, the parent's excessive use of the pacifier to calm the child should be explored. It is not unusual for parents to place a pacifier in the infant's mouth as soon as crying begins, thus reinforcing a pattern of distress-relief.

At the time of this writing, there is no evidence that pacifier use and nonnutritive sucking in preterm infants has any effect on the initiation and length of breast-feeding. Nonnutritive sucking should not be withheld from preterm infants, especially when performed in conjunction with the use of concentrated sucrose for pain management.

Thumb sucking reaches its peak at age 18 to 20 months and is most prevalent when the child is hungry or tired. Persistent thumb sucking in a listless, apathetic child always warrants investigation. It may be a sign of an emotional problem between parent and child or of boredom, isolation, and lack of stimulation.

Teething

One of the more difficult periods in the infant's (and parents') life is the eruption of the deciduous (primary) teeth, often referred to as teething. The age of tooth eruption shows considerable variation among children, but the order of their appearance is fairly regular and predictable (Fig. 10-10). The first primary teeth to erupt are the lower central incisors, which appear at approximately 6 to 8 months of age. These are followed closely by the upper central incisors.

> **NURSING TIP**
>
> A quick guide to assessment of deciduous teeth during the first 2 years is: age of the child in months − 6 = number of teeth. For example: 8 months of age − 6 = 2 teeth at this time.

Teething is a physiologic process; some discomfort is common as the crown of the tooth breaks through the pe-

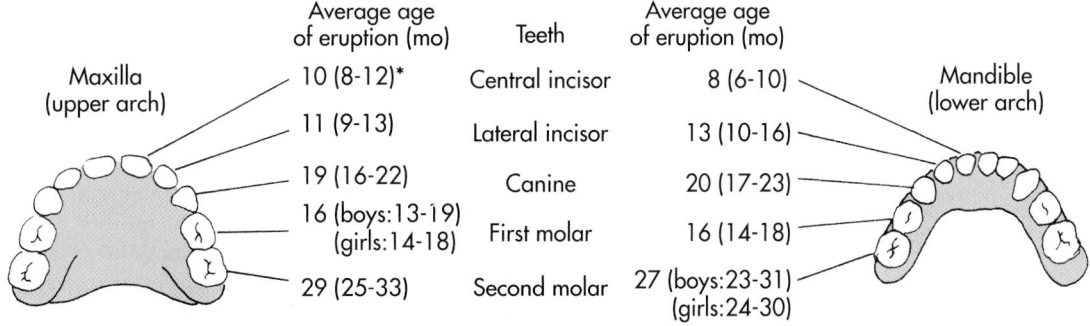

FIG. 10-10 ■ Sequence of eruption of primary teeth. *Range represents ±1 standard deviation, or 67% of subjects studied. (Data from McDonald RE, Avery DR: *Dentistry for the child and adolescent,* ed 6, St Louis, 1994, Mosby.)

riodontal membrane. Some children show minimum evidence of teething, such as drooling, swollen gums, increased finger sucking, or biting on hard objects. Others are very irritable, have difficulty sleeping, and refuse to eat. Generally, signs of illness such as fever (higher than 102° F), vomiting, or diarrhea are not symptoms of teething but of illness and may warrant further investigation. However, as many parents report, a low-grade temperature is common in the 4- to 19-day period before and on the day of tooth eruption.

Because teething pain is a result of inflammation, cold is soothing. Giving the child a frozen teething ring or an ice cube wrapped in a washcloth helps relieve the inflammation. Several nonprescription topical anesthetic ointments are available, such as Baby Ora-Jel. The active ingredient in most of them is benzocaine. If such products are used, parents are advised to apply them correctly. In the event of persistent irritability that affects sleeping and feeding, systemic analgesics such as acetaminophen or ibuprofen (age appropriate) can be given; however, parents should know that this is a temporary measure.

> **NURSING ALERT**
>
> The use of teething powders or procedures such as cutting or rubbing the gums with aspirin are discouraged, because ingestion of the powder, infection or irritation of the tissue, or aspiration of the aspirin can occur. Hard candy may cause accidental choking or aspiration and should be avoided at this age.

Infant Shoes

Many parents are unaware of the type of shoes that are appropriate for the older infant and buy expensive infant shoes because of misleading advertising claims. Inflexible shoes that have hard soles can be detrimental by delaying walking, aggravating intoeing or outtoeing, and impeding the development of supportive foot muscles. Therefore, counseling parents regarding footwear should begin when infants are 6 months old—well before they are walking.

It is helpful to begin by explaining to parents that changes in the feet occur during infancy and early childhood as locomotion and weight bearing progress. At birth the feet are flat because the arches are protected by fat pads on the soles of the feet. As the bones in the arches develop, the pads disappear and the feet begin to assume a mature shape. A normal arch is determined by proper alignment of all the bones and development of the surrounding musculature, not by the height of the arch.

When children begin walking, the main reason for shoes is *protection*. To provide protection, the shoe should retain its fit, be made of durable material with a smooth interior and few construction seams to irritate the skin, and be soft and flexible, especially in the toe area. A high-top shoe is not necessary for support but may be helpful in keeping the foot in the shoe.

A good shoe conforms to the anatomic shape of the foot, with a rounded toe and sufficient toe room. During weight bearing there should be at least the space of half the width of the thumbnail, or 1.25 cm (0.5 inch), between the end of the longest toe and the shoe. Roomy and square-toed socks allow for proper growth and alignment.

Inexpensive but well-constructed athletic shoes or soft-leather moccasin-type shoes are suggested as adequate footgear for walking infants.

Even if the shoes are fitted properly, frequent changes are needed to accommodate the infant's rapidly growing feet. Shoe size changes at approximately 3-month intervals between 12 to 36 months; during this time the child's foot should be measured every 3 months. Curled toes when shoes are removed and redness and irritation of the skin on the bottom of the toes indicate the need for a larger size.

PROMOTING OPTIMAL HEALTH DURING INFANCY

NUTRITION

Ideally, discussion of optimal nutrition should begin prenatally with the decision to breast- or bottle-feed the infant. The choice for either is highly individual and is discussed in Chapter 8. This section is primarily concerned with infant nutrition during the next 12 months, when growth needs and developmental milestones ready the child for the introduction of solid foods.

There is concern that, despite adequate availability of optimal nutrient sources, infants are not being fed appropriately. These practices may have far-reaching long-term health consequences for infants. It has been shown that infant health practices have an impact upon the child's life. Certain chronic health conditions have been linked to feeding practices in infancy (Calamaro, 2000; Hobbie, Baker, and Bayerl, 2000). Nurses must continue to be proactive in teaching parents about what constitutes appropriate infant nutrition and nutritional habits, which provide the opportunity to grow and develop into a healthy child and adult.

The use of complementary and alternative medicine has recently gained increased awareness by health professionals, particularly in relation to therapies used in children that may not be as beneficial as touted in various media sources. One concern is the intake of megavitamins and herbs by children; parents may assume that the word "natural" in reference to ingredients, means the product is safe, when this may not be the case. It is important for nurses to be aware of the effects, availability, and practice of complementary therapies and to be able to cogently discuss their use in children with the parents (Loman, 2003).

The First 6 Months

Human milk is the most desirable complete diet for the infant during the first 6 months. The normal infant receiving breast milk from a well-nourished mother usually requires no specific vitamin or mineral supplements, with the exception of iron by 4 to 6 months of age (when fetal iron stores are depleted). Daily supplements of vitamin D and vitamin B_{12} may be indicated if the mother's intake of these vitamins is inadequate (see Vitamin Disturbances, Chapter 11). The American Academy of Pediatrics (2003a) has recently issued a recommendation that all infants (including those exclusively breast-fed) receive a daily supplement of 200 IU of vitamin D beginning in the first 2 months of life to prevent rickets and vitamin D deficiency. If the infant is being exclusively breast-fed after 4 to 6 months, iron supplementation is recommended to offset the decrease in iron available in human milk at this time and to enhance erythropoiesis. Infants who are breast-fed or bottle-fed do not require additional fluids, especially water or juice, during the first 4 months of life. Excessive intake of water in infants may result in water intoxication, failure to thrive, and hyponatremia.

Employed mothers can continue breast-feeding with guidance and encouragement. Mothers are encouraged to set realistic goals for employment and breast-feeding, with accurate information regarding the costs, risks, and benefits of available feeding options. Many mothers may find that a program of breast pumping when away from home and bottle-feeding the infant the expressed milk with or without formula supplementation is successful. Expressed breast milk may be stored in the refrigerator (4° C [39° F]) without danger of bacterial contamination for up to 5 days (Lawrence and Lawrence, 1999). Although feeding the infant at home may occur on a demand basis, pumping milk away from home may be needed every 3 to 4 hours to maintain adequate supply. Breast milk may be expressed by hand or pump (manual or electric) and stored in an appropriate air-tight glass or plastic container. Expressed breast milk may be frozen (0° F [−18° C] or lower) for up to 12 months, but care should be taken to prevent the typical freezer burn. Health care workers and new mothers may find the booklet *Working and Breastfeeding—Can You Do It? Yes, You Can!* by Johnson & Johnson helpful.*

In addition to efficient breast pumping, mothers also need childcare by a trusted individual or agency and support and assistance from significant others. As with all breast-feeding mothers, these women must have proper nutrition and rest for adequate lactation. Maternal fatigue is considered the biggest threat to successful breast-feeding in employed mothers (Corbett-Dick and Bezek, 1997).

NURSING ALERT

To prevent oral burns from uneven warming of the milk, breast milk should never be thawed or rewarmed in a microwave oven. To thaw the frozen milk, either place the container under a lukewarm water bath (less than 40.5° C [105° F]) or place in the refrigerator overnight.

An acceptable alternative to breast-feeding is commercial iron-fortified formula. As with human milk, it supplies all of the nutrients needed by the infant for the first 6 months.

Unmodified whole cow's milk, low-fat cow's milk, skim milk, other animal milks, and imitation milks are not acceptable as a major source of nutrition for infants because of poor digestibility, an increased risk of contamination, and a lack of components needed for appropriate growth. Whole milk can cause iron deficiency anemia in infants, possibly as a result of occult gastrointestinal blood loss. Pasteurized whole cow's milk is deficient in iron, zinc, and vitamin C and has a high renal solute load, which makes it undesirable

for infants less than 12 months of age (American Academy of Pediatrics, 2004).

NURSING ALERT

Dietary fat should not be restricted. Substituting skim or low-fat milk is unacceptable, because the essential fatty acids are inadequate and the solute concentration of protein and electrolytes, such as sodium, is too high.

NURSING ALERT

Although microwaving of bottles and baby food is not recommended, it remains a common practice. Guidelines have been developed for microwave heating of refrigerated formula, and these should be given to the family (see Family Home Care box).

The amount of formula per feeding and the number of feedings per day vary among infants. Infants on demand feeding usually determine their own feeding schedule, but some infants may need a more planned schedule based on average feeding patterns to ensure sufficient nutrients. In general, the number of feedings decreases from six at 1 month of age to four to five at 6 months. Regardless of the number of feedings, the total amount of formula ingested will usually level off at about 32 ounces (960 mL) per day. Parents should be cautioned concerning the excessive use of juices and nonnutritive drinks such as fruit-flavored drinks or carbonated beverages (soda, or pop) during this period. Many juices and nonnutritive drinks, although readily available to consumers, do not provide sufficient caloric intake for infants less than 12 months of age; such drinks may replace the nutrients in milk (formula) and lead to growth or health problems. Also, water supplementation is not recommended for healthy infants, because it may lead to water intoxication (American Academy of Pediatrics, 2004).

FAMILY HOME CARE

Microwave Heating of Refrigerated Infant Formula

Before heating:
   Heat only 4 ounces or more.
   Heat only *refrigerated* formula.
   Always stand the bottle up.
   Always leave the bottle top uncovered to allow heat to escape.
Heating instructions (full power):
   Heat 4-ounce bottles for no more than 30 seconds.
   Heat 8-ounce bottles for no more than 45 seconds.
Serving instructions:
   Always replace nipple assembly; invert 10 times (vigorous shaking is unnecessary).
   Formula should be cool to the touch; formula warm to the touch may be too hot to serve.
   Always test formula; place several drops on your tongue or on the back of the hand (not the inside wrist)

Modified from Sigman-Grant M, Bush G, Anantheswaran R: Microwave heating of infant formula: a dilemma resolved, *Pediatrics* 90(3):414, 1992.

---

*Developed by **National Healthy Mothers, Healthy Babies Coalition,** 121 S. Washington Street, Suite 300, Alexandria, VA, 22314; (703) 836-6110; website: www.hmhb.org.

NURSING ALERT

If infants are being fed powdered or concentrated formula, they may receive a substantial amount of lead from tap water, placing them at risk for lead poisoning. Bottled water for mixing powdered or concentrated formula is a relatively safe alternative to tap water.

NURSING ALERT

Whole milk should not be introduced to infants until after 1 year of age (American Academy of Pediatrics, 2004).

The addition of solid foods before 4 to 6 months of age is not recommended. During the early months solid foods are not compatible with the ability of the gastrointestinal tract and nutritional needs of the infant. Feeding solids to young infants exposes them to food antigens that may produce food protein allergy. Developmentally, infants are not ready for solid food. The extrusion (protrusion) reflex is strong and causes food to be pushed out of the mouth. Despite these recommendations, and lacking evidence-based information to support such practices, many parents introduce solids as early as 2 weeks of age. In such cases, rice cereal is often added to the formula to help the infant sleep better at night or to enhance weight gain (Calamaro, 2000; Wilson and Bowman, 2000); however, this practice is not substantiated by any scientific evidence. Fruit juices are not required during the first 6 months; there are no studies demonstrating benefits of giving fruit juices, yet parents perceive this practice as beneficial.

The Second 6 Months

During the second half of the first year, human milk or formula continues to be the primary source of nutrition. Fluoride supplementation should begin, depending on the infant's intake of fluoride (in formula mixed with tap water) (see Dental Health, p. 334). If breast-feeding is discontinued, a commercial iron-fortified formula should be substituted. Follow-up or transition formulas specially marketed for older infants offer no special advantages over other infant formulas and provide excessive protein (American Academy of Pediatrics, 2004).

The major change in feeding habits is the addition of solid foods to the infant's diet. Physiologically and developmentally, the infant 4 to 6 months of age is in a transition period. By this time the gastrointestinal tract has matured sufficiently to handle more complex nutrients and is less sensitive to potentially allergenic foods. Tooth eruption is beginning and facilitates biting and chewing. The extrusion reflex has disappeared, and swallowing is more coordinated to allow the infant to accept solids easily. Head control is well developed, which permits infants to sit with support and purposely turn the head away to communicate disinterest in food. Voluntary grasping and improved eye-hand coordination gradually allow infants to pick up finger foods and feed themselves. Their increasing sense of independence is evident in their desire to hold the bottle and try to "help" during feeding.

Selection and Preparation of Solid Foods

The choice of solid foods to introduce first is variable but should meet the reasons for feeding solids, such as supplying nutrients not found in formula or breast milk. Iron-fortified infant cereal is generally introduced first because of its high iron content (7 mg/3 tablespoons of prepared dry cereal). Commercially prepared ready-to-serve dry cereals for infants include rice, barley, oatmeal, and high-protein cereals; rice is usually suggested as an initial food because of its easy digestibility and low allergenic potential. Cereals such as cream of farina are not used, because infant commercial cereals are a better source of iron. Some of the commercial baby cereals are combined with fruit. There is little nutritional benefit from these preparations, and they are more expensive. New foods should be added one at a time; therefore, parents should avoid cereal combinations when beginning a new grain.

Infant cereal (iron fortified) is mixed with formula until whole milk is given. If the infant is breast-fed, the cereal is mixed with expressed breast milk or water. After 6 months of age, fruit juices can be mixed with the dry cereal; the vitamin C content of the juice enhances the absorption of iron in the cereal. Because of their benefit as a source of iron, infant cereals should be continued until the child is 18 months of age.

The addition of solid foods to the exclusively breast-fed infant's diet does not significantly increase overall caloric intake or weight gain (Dewey, 2001).

Fruit juice can be offered from a cup for its rich source of vitamin C and as a substitute for milk for one feeding a day. Large quantities of certain juices (e.g., apple, pear, prune, sweet cherry, peach, grape) are avoided because they may cause abdominal pain, diarrhea, or bloating in some children. White grape juice is reported to be better absorbed and safe for infants this age (less than 6 oz per day) without causing gastrointestinal distress. Some studies have shown that excessive fruit juice consumption (12 or more oz per day) in young children increases the likelihood of short stature and childhood obesity (Dennison, Rockwell, and Baker, 1997) and nonorganic failure to thrive (Smith and Lifshitz, 1994); however, Skinner and others (1999) found no association between growth failure and the consumption of 12 ounces or more of 100% fruit juices in children 24 to 36 months of age. In addition, some researchers have found fruit juice, particularly apple juice, to exacerbate colic and diarrhea, possibly because of carbohydrate malabsorption (Duro and others, 2002; Moukarzel, Lesicka, and Ament, 2002). It is recommended that fruit juice intake not exceed 4 to 6 ounces per day and that juices not be given to infants less than 4 to 6 months old (American Academy of Pediatrics, 2001a). Because vitamin C is naturally destroyed by heat, juice is not warmed. Juice containers are always kept covered and refrigerated to prevent further vitamin loss.

NURSING ALERT

Offer fruit juice from a cup, rather than a bottle, to prevent the development of nursing caries (see Low-Cariogenic Diet, Chapter 12).

The addition of other foods is arbitrary. A common sequence is to introduce strained fruits followed by vegetables and, finally, meats; however, some clinicians prefer to add vegetables before fruit. If foods are introduced early, citrus fruits, meats, and eggs are delayed until after 6 months of age because of their potential to result in allergy.

At 6 months, foods such as a cracker or zwieback can be offered as a type of finger and teething food. By 8 to 9 months, junior foods and nutritious finger foods such as a firmly cooked vegetable, raw pieces of fruit (except grapes), or cheese can be given. By 1 year, well-cooked table foods are served.

Commercially prepared baby foods are the most commonly used types of food served to infants in the United States. They are convenient and contain no added salt or sugar, but can be relatively expensive. An alternative is to prepare baby foods at home, which is a simple and inexpensive process. Fruits and vegetables can be steamed in a small amount of water and pureed in a blender or food processor. Many of them, such as ripe banana, can be mashed fine with a fork. Fruits such as apples or pears require little or no water in the cooking process. Vegetables such as carrots, potatoes, or string beans require additional water in the cooking and blending process.

Preferably, home-prepared infant foods should be fresh or frozen, because canned foods, other than those prepared for infants, may contain excessive sodium or sugar. If sweetening is needed, refined sugar can be used, but honey is avoided because of the risk of infant botulism. There is no evidence that the addition of salt to foods such as vegetables increases the infant's acceptance of the new food.

Low-calorie foods should be avoided in infants and toddlers unless a strictly medically prescribed diet is required. The infant's growth during this phase is crucial to future development, and curtailing dietary fat should be done with great caution. Many parents may be concerned that their child is getting too much dietary fat; in such cases the primary practitioner should be consulted before dietary substitutions are made. On the other hand, making an infant or toddler finish a bottle or "clean up the plate" may lead to unhealthy eating habits (see Obesity, Chapter 17).

Introduction of Solid Foods

When the spoon is first introduced, infants often push it away and appear dissatisfied. Some patience and skill are required to overcome this initial response. A small-bowled, straight, long-handled spoon, similar to a demitasse spoon, allows a small portion of food to be placed toward the back of the tongue. Food that is placed on the front of the tongue and pushed out is simply scooped up and refed. As infants become accustomed to the spoon, they will more eagerly accept the food and eventually open the mouth in anticipation (or keep it closed in dislike). Because the first introduction of food is a new experience, spoon feeding should be attempted after ingestion of some breast milk or formula to associate this activity with a pleasurable and satisfying experience. Trying to introduce a food after the entire milk feeding is usually useless because the infant is satiated and has no inclination to try something new.

After several spoon feedings, food can be introduced at the beginning of a meal. It is best to introduce many foods during the first year, when the infant is more likely to eat them because of a hearty appetite resulting from a rapid growth rate. During the toddler years eating becomes less of an adventure, and strong food preferences become evident.

One food item is introduced at intervals of 4 to 7 days to allow for identification of food allergies. New foods are fed in small amounts, from 1 teaspoon to a few tablespoons. As the amount of solid food increases, the quantity of milk is decreased to less than 1 L daily to prevent overfeeding.

Because feeding is a learning process, as well as a means of nutrition, new foods are given alone to allow the child to learn new tastes and textures. Food should not be mixed in the bottle and fed through a nipple with a large hole. This deprives the child of the pleasure of learning new tastes and developing a discriminating palate. It can also cause problems with poor chewing of food later in life because of lack of experience. Guidelines for the introduction of new foods are given in the Family Home Care box.*

Introducing solid foods can be an exciting time for parent and child. Most infants are good eaters and enjoy eating from a spoon and later feeding themselves. However, the transition from "parent doing it" to "baby doing it" can be a trying experience, particularly for those who value a clean house or who view cleaning up the mess as a waste of time. The infant's first, second, and often twentieth try at self-feeding or cup feeding is a sloppy experience. Finger foods such as soft fruits or vegetables are just as good playthings as food; they can be squeezed, smeared, squashed, and thoroughly painted on oneself, others, and the surrounding environment. However, all of this is part of learning, and mastery follows many accidents.

If parents find this experience distressing, a few suggestions may prove helpful. The feeding area should have a floor that can be easily wiped and is relatively far from walls, upholstered furniture, or drapes. A handheld portable vacuum is helpful in cleaning up crumbs. Messes are confined to one area if the child is seated in a high chair rather than allowed to crawl or walk around while drinking or eating. Infants should be expected to get themselves covered with food; therefore, a large bib (plastic can be wiped easily but needs to be removed after feeding) should be used, as well as washable clothes that are easily removed. In a carpeted eating area a bedsheet or washable drop cloth can be spread under the high chair to save on cleanup time and avoid frustration; one can expect the infant to drop food at this stage. High chairs can be thoroughly cleaned in a shower. Outdoor dining provides an excellent opportunity for practicing with a cup, spoon, or fingers because accidents are simple to hose or sweep away. Children cannot be pressured into eating neatly or developing table manners before manipulative skill is acquired.

Weaning

Defined as the process of giving up one method of feeding for another, *weaning* usually refers to relinquishing the breast or bottle for a cup. In Western societies this is generally regarded as a major task for infants and is often seen as a potentially traumatic experience. It is psychologically significant because the infant is required to give up a major source of oral pleasure and gratification.

---

*A recommended resource is Starting Solids: a Guide for Parents and Child Care Providers, available from the **National Association of Pediatric Nurse Associates and Practitioners (NAPNAP),** 1101 Kings Highway North, Suite 206, Cherry Hill, NJ 08034-1912; (877) 662-7627 or (856) 667-1773; fax: (856) 667-7187; website: www.napnap.org.

There is no one time for weaning that is best for every child, but generally most infants show signs of readiness during the second half of the first year. They have learned that good things come from a spoon. Their increasing desire for freedom of movement may lessen their desire to be held close for feedings. They are acquiring more control over their actions and can easily manipulate a cup to their lips (even if it is held upside down!). Imitation becomes a powerful motivator by age 8 or 9 months, and they enjoy using a cup or glass like others do.

Weaning should be gradual by replacing one bottle- or breast-feeding at a time. The nighttime feeding is usually the last feeding to be discontinued. It is advisable never to begin allowing a child to take a bottle of milk to bed—this is a major cause of nursing caries in deciduous teeth. If breast-feeding is terminated before 5 or 6 months of age, weaning should be to a bottle to provide for the infant's continued sucking needs. If discontinued later, weaning can be directly to a cup, especially by age 12 to 14 months. Any sweet liquid, such as fruit juice, should be given in a cup.

SLEEP AND ACTIVITY

Sleep patterns vary among infants, with active infants typically sleeping less than placid children. Generally, by 3 to 4 months of age most infants have developed a nocturnal pattern of sleep that lasts 9 to 11 hours. The total daily sleep is approximately 15 hours. The number of naps per day varies, but infants may take one or two naps by the end of the first year. Breast-fed infants usually sleep for less prolonged periods, with more frequent waking, especially during the night, than do bottle-fed infants. Because of the trend toward breast-feeding, sleep norms such as those previously described, which were based primarily on bottle-fed infants, may not be relevant.

 FAMILY HOME CARE

Feeding During the First Year

BIRTH TO 6 MONTHS (BREAST- OR BOTTLE-FEEDING)
Breast-Feeding
Most desirable complete diet for first half of year.*
Requires supplements of vitamin D (400 units) if mother's diet is inadequate.

Formula
Iron-fortified commercial formula is a complete food for the first half of the year.*
Requires fluoride supplements (0.25 mg) when the concentration of fluoride in the drinking water is below 0.3 parts per million (ppm) after 6 months of age.
Evaporated milk formula requires supplements of vitamin C, iron, and fluoride (in accordance with the fluoride content of the local water supply after 6 months of age).

6 TO 12 MONTHS (SOLID FOODS)
May begin to add solids by 5 to 6 months of age.
First foods are strained, pureed, or finely mashed.
Finger foods such as teething crackers, raw fruit, or vegetables can be introduced by 6 to 7 months.
Chopped table food or commercially prepared junior foods can be started by 9 to 12 months.
With the exception of cereal, the order of introducing foods is variable; a recommended sequence is weekly introduction of other foods, beginning with fruit, then vegetables, and then meat.
As the quantity of solids increases, the amount of formula should be limited to approximately 960 mL (32 ounces) daily, and fruit juice to less than 180 mL (6 ounces) daily.

Method of Introduction
Introduce solids when infant is hungry.
Begin spoon feeding by pushing food to back of tongue because of infant's natural tendency to thrust tongue forward.
Use small spoon with straight handle; begin with 1 or 2 teaspoons of food; gradually increase to 2 to 3 tablespoons per feeding.

Introduce one food at a time, usually at intervals of 4 to 7 days, to identify food allergies.
As the amount of solid food increases, decrease the quantity of milk to prevent overfeeding.
Never introduce foods by mixing them with the formula in the bottle.

Cereal
Introduce commercially prepared iron-fortified infant cereals and administer daily until 18 months.
Rice cereal is usually introduced first because of its low allergenic potential.
Can discontinue supplemental iron once cereal is given.

Fruits and vegetables
Applesauce, bananas, and pears are usually well tolerated.
Avoid fruits and vegetables marketed in cans that are not specifically designed for infants because of variable and sometimes high lead content and addition of salt, sugar, or preservatives.
Offer fruit juice only from a cup, not a bottle, to reduce the development of "nursing caries."

Meat, fish, and poultry
Avoid fatty meats.
Prepare by baking, broiling, steaming, or poaching.
Include organ meats such as liver, which has a high iron, vitamin A, and vitamin B complex content.
If soup is given, be sure all ingredients are familiar to child's diet.
Avoid commercial meat/vegetable combinations because protein is low.

Eggs and cheese
Serve egg yolk hard boiled and mashed, soft cooked, or poached.
Introduce egg white in small quantities (1 teaspoon) toward end of first year to detect an allergy.
Use cheese as a substitute for meat and as finger food.

*Breast-feeding or commercial formula feeding for up to 12 months of age is recommended. After 1 year, whole cow's milk can be given.

Most infants are naturally active and need no encouragement to be mobile. However, problems can arise when devices such as playpens, strollers, commercial swings, and mobile walkers are used excessively. These items restrict movement and prevent infants from exploring and developing gross motor skills. Contrary to popular belief, mobile walkers do not enhance coordination and are dangerous if tipped over or placed near stairs. The American Academy of Pediatrics (2001b) recommended a ban on the sale of infant walkers because of the large number of injuries. Newer models of infant walkers have been designed to decrease infant injuries (see Falls, p. 351).

NURSING ALERT

Formal infant exercise programs do not provide any long-term benefit to normal infants, and the possibility for damage to the infant's skeletal system exists. For these reasons, such programs are not recommended (American Academy of Pediatrics, 1988).

Sleep Problems

Concerns regarding sleep are common during infancy. Sometimes these concerns are as basic as parents' questioning if the infant needs additional sleep. In this case it is best to investigate the reason for their concern, stressing the individual needs of each child. Infants who are active during wakeful periods and growing normally are sleeping a sufficient amount of time.

However, there are a number of more serious concerns that require intervention. Sleep disturbances of physiologic origin are rare with the exception of colic, which is discussed in Chapter 11 The more common sleep disturbances are a learned pattern or developmental characteristic of some infants (Table 10-3). Although many families may report sleep problems typical of these patterns, interventions are offered only when the pattern is disruptive to the family (see Cultural Awareness box).

Sleep problems in early infancy have also been positively correlated with higher maternal depression scores (Hiscock and Wake, 2001; Hawkins-Walsh, 2003); therefore, nurses must discuss infant sleep problems with the mother (and family) in addition to other developmental aspects of newborn care.

When a sleeping problem is presented, a careful assessment is essential. Charting sleep habits both before and after interventions is also an important strategy. Questions regarding the frequency and duration of waking, the usual bedtime routine, the number of nighttime feedings, the perceived problem (e.g., how much disruption the behavior generates), and the attempted interventions are important in planning effective approaches designed for the specific sleep problem. A common suggestion given for any type of

TABLE 10-3 ■ Selected Sleep Disturbances During Infancy and Early Childhood

DISORDER/DESCRIPTION	MANAGEMENT
NIGHTTIME FEEDING	
Child has a prolonged need for middle-of-night bottle- or breast-feeding	Increase daytime feeding intervals to 4 hours or more (may need to be done gradually)
Child goes to sleep at breast or with a bottle	Offer last feeding as late as possible at night; may need to gradually reduce amount of formula or length of breast-feeding
Awakenings are frequent (may be hourly)	Offer no bottles in bed
Child returns to sleep after feeding; other comfort measures (e.g., rocking or holding) are usually ineffective	Put to bed awake
	When child is crying, check at progressively longer intervals each night; reassure child but do not hold, rock, take to parent's bed, or give bottle or pacifier
DEVELOPMENTAL NIGHT CRYING	
Child age 6 to 12 months with undisturbed nighttime sleep now awakes abruptly; may be accompanied by nightmares	Reassure parents that this phase is temporary
	Enter room immediately to check on child but keep reassurances brief
	Avoid feeding, rocking, taking to parent's bed, or any other routine that may initiate trained night crying
REFUSAL TO GO TO SLEEP	
Child resists bedtime and comes out of room repeatedly	Evaluate if hour of sleep is too early (child may resist sleep if not tired)
Nighttime sleep may be continuous, but frequent awakenings and refusal to return to sleep may occur and become a problem if parent allows child to deviate from usual sleep pattern	Assist parents in establishing consistent before-bedtime routine and enforcing consistent limits regarding child's bedtime behavior
	If child persists in leaving bedroom, close door for progressively longer periods
	Use reward system with child to provide motivation
TRAINED NIGHT CRYING (INAPPROPRIATE SLEEP ASSOCIATIONS)	
Child typically falls asleep in place other than own bed (e.g., rocking chair or parent's bed) and is brought to own bed while asleep; on awakening, cries until usual routine is instituted (e.g., rocking)	Put child in own bed when awake
	If possible, arrange sleeping area separate from other family members
	When child is crying, check at progressively longer intervals each night; reassure child but do not resume usual routine

Modified from Ferber R: Behavioral "insomnia" in the child, *Psychiatr Clin North Am* 10(4):641-653, 1987.

Continued

TABLE 10-3 ■ Selected Sleep Disturbances During Infancy and Early Childhood—*cont'd*

DISORDER/DESCRIPTION	MANAGEMENT
NIGHTTIME FEARS	
Child resists going to bed or wakes during the night because of fears	Evaluate if hour of sleep is too early (child may fantasize when nothing to do but think in dark room)
Child seeks parent's physical presence and falls asleep easily with parent nearby, unless fear is overwhelming	Calmly reassure the frightened child; keeping a night-light on may be helpful
	Use reward system with child to provide motivation to deal with fears
	Avoid patterns that can lead to additional problems (e.g., sleeping with child or taking child to parent's room)
	If child's fear is overwhelming, consider desensitization (e.g., progressively spending longer periods of time alone; consult professional help for protracted fears)
	Distinguish between nightmares and sleep terrors (confused partial arousals).

Modified from Ferber R: Behavioral "insomnia" in the child, *Psychiatr Clin North Am* 10(4):641-653, 1987.

CULTURAL AWARENESS

The Family Bed

Co-sleeping, or sharing the "family bed," in which parents allow the children to sleep with them, is a relatively common and accepted practice, especially among African-American, Hispanic, and Asian families, such as the Japanese (Schachter and others, 1989). Other groups that are adopting co-sleeping include (1) single parents, whose need for company may encourage this practice; (2) working parents, who desire the closeness at night that was lost during the day; and (3) parents who have had an issue about sleep or separation in their own past (Brazelton, 1990). There is no scientific evidence to support infant co-sleeping with the mother as a preventive measure against the occurrence of SIDS (American Academy of Pediatrics, 2000). There is evidence of an increase in the number of infant deaths by suffocation associated with bed sharing and the use of adult beds, particularly in infants less than 3 months old (Drago and Dannenberg, 1999). Other studies have correlated higher incidences of SIDS and infant co-sleeping with maternal smoking, co-sleeping with multiple family members, soft bedding, and unintentional asphyxiation resulting from adult intoxication (Hauck and others, 2003; Person, Lavezzi, and Wolf, 2002; American Academy of Pediatrics, 2000). Population-based studies of infant co-sleeping and SIDS are currently in progress, and until there is evidence-based data to support or abandon the practice, parents should carefully evaluate the options available for sharing the family bed with infants, particularly under known high-risk conditions that place the infant at risk for asphyxia, albeit intentional or otherwise.

---

sleep problem—"let the child cry until he or she falls asleep"—is very difficult to implement and is inappropriate for certain conditions. After the parents relent and console the child, they have only reinforced the crying.

An equally effective and more atraumatic approach to night crying, known as *graduated extinction,* is to let the child cry for progressively longer times between brief parental interventions that consist only of reassurance—not rocking, holding, or using a bottle or pacifier. For example, the parents may check on the child every 5 minutes (of crying) during the first night and progressively extend this interval by 5 minutes on successive nights (Ferber and Kryger, 1995).

Families who cannot tolerate unexpected crying spells while everyone else is asleep can try the two-step approach. Graduated extinction is used during naps and at bedtime until the parents retire. If the child cries during the night, the parents use comforting measures. However, after the child is partially trained, step 2 is initiated—the use of graduated extinction at all times.

The best way to prevent sleep problems is to encourage parents to establish bedtime rituals that do not foster problematic patterns. One of the most constructive is placing infants awake in their own crib. When infants are accustomed to falling asleep somewhere else, such as in their parent's arms, and then being transferred to their crib, they awaken in unfamiliar surroundings and are unable to fall asleep until the routine is repeated. Also, the bed should be used for sleeping only—not as a playpen. It is advisable not to hang playthings over or on the bed; in this way the child associates the bed with sleep, not with activity. Although the interventions described previously and in Table 10-3 are usually successful, it is much easier to prevent the problem with appropriate counseling during the early months of the infant's life.*

DENTAL HEALTH

Good dental hygiene begins as soon as the primary teeth erupt. The teeth and gums are initially cleaned by wiping with a damp cloth; toothbrushing is too harsh for the tender gingiva. The caregiver can stabilize the infant by cradling the child with one arm and using the free hand to cleanse the teeth. Oral hygiene can be made pleasant by singing or talking to the infant. There are no clear guidelines regarding when toothbrushing should begin; however, it is recommended that the infant have an oral health examination by 6 months of age from a qualified pediatric health practitioner. Infants at high risk for dental caries should be seen by a dentist between 6 months and 1 year of age (American Academy of Pediatrics, 2003b). It is generally recommended that a small, soft-bristled toothbrush be used as more teeth erupt and the infant adjusts to the rou-

---

*An excellent resource for parents is *Solve Your Child's Sleep Problems* by Richard Ferber (1986, Simon & Schuster Trade; [800] 223-2336; website: www.simonsays.com). Also available in Spanish.

tine of cleaning. Water is preferred to toothpaste, which the infant will swallow (and if the toothpaste is fluoridated, the infant will ingest excessive amounts of fluoride).

Fluoride, an essential mineral for building caries-resistant teeth, is needed beginning at 6 months of age if the infant does not receive water with an adequate fluoride content. The American Academy of Pediatrics (1998) and the American Academy of Pediatric Dentists no longer recommend fluoride supplementation from birth to 6 months. The fluoride dosage has been decreased from earlier recommendations because of an increased occurrence of dental fluorosis from excessive fluoride ingestion. The latest recommendation is to give children 6 months to 3 years of age 0.25 mg fluoride daily if water fluoride content is less than 0.3 ppm (parts per million) (American Academy of Pediatrics, 2004).

Dietary considerations are also important because habits begun during infancy tend to continue into later years. Foods with concentrated sugar are used sparingly (if at all) in the infant's diet. The practice of coating pacifiers with honey or using commercially available hard-candy pacifiers is discouraged. Besides being cariogenic, honey also may cause infant botulism, and parts of the candy pacifier can be aspirated (see Aspiration of Foreign Objects, p. 349). Parents need to be counseled regarding the detrimental effects of frequent and prolonged bottle- or breast-feeding during sleep, when the sweet milk or other fluid, such as juice, bathes the teeth, producing nursing caries. In addition, carbonated beverages should be avoided in infancy. (See also Chapter 12 for a more extensive discussion of dental care, including nursing caries.)

IMMUNIZATIONS

One of the most dramatic advances in pediatrics has been the decline of infectious diseases during the twentieth century because of the widespread use of immunization for preventable diseases. Although many of the immunizations can be given to individuals of any age, the recommended primary schedule begins during infancy and, with the exception of boosters, is completed during early childhood. Therefore, the discussion of childhood immunizations for diphtheria, tetanus, pertussis (DTaP using acellular pertussis); polio; measles, mumps, rubella (MMR); *Haemophilus influenzae* type b (Hib); hepatitis B virus (HBV); pneumococcal conjugate vaccine (PCV); and chickenpox (Var) is included under health promotion during infancy. Selected vaccines generally reserved for children considered at high risk for the disease are discussed here and as appropriate throughout the text. (See also Communicable Diseases, Chapter 14, for a discussion of several of the diseases for which vaccines are available.)

Schedule for Immunizations

In the United States two organizations—the **Advisory Committee on Immunization Practices of the Centers for Disease Control and Prevention** and the **Committee on Infectious Diseases of the American Academy of Pediatrics**—govern the recommendations for immunization policies and procedures. In Canada, recommendations are from the **National Advisory Committee on Immunization** under the authority of the Minister of National Health and Welfare. The policies of each committee are *recommendations,* not rules, and they change as a result of advances in the field of immunology. Nurses need to keep informed of the latest advances and changes in policy (see Community Focus box).

In the United States the recommended age for beginning primary immunizations of infants is within 2 weeks of birth or, in special circumstances, at birth (Table 10-4). Children born prematurely should receive the full dose of each vaccine at the appropriate chronologic age. Recommended schedules for children not immunized during infancy are included in Table 10-5. Table 10-6 describes immunization schedules for Canadian children.

Children who began primary immunizations at the recommended age but fail to receive all of the doses do not need to begin the series again but instead receive only the missed doses. For situations in which there is doubt that the child will return for immunizations according to the optimum schedule, any of the recommended vaccines can be administered simultaneously. Parenteral vaccines are given in separate syringes in different injection sites (American Academy of Pediatrics, 2003c). The product brand names, routes of administration, and manufacturers for the principal childhood vaccinations are listed in Table 10-10.

Recommendations for Routine Immunizations

Hepatitis B virus.   Hepatitis B virus (HBV) is a significant pediatric disease because HBV infections that occur during childhood and adolescence can lead to fatal consequences from cirrhosis or liver cancer during adulthood. Up to 90% of infants infected perinatally and 25% to 50% of children infected before age 5 years become HBV carriers. In addition, the incidence of HBV infection increases rapidly during adolescence (American Academy of Pediatrics, 2003c). It is recommended that newborns receive the vaccine before hospital discharge if the mother is Hepatitis B surface antigen (HBsAg) negative. Monovalent Hep B should be given as the birth dose, whereas combination vaccine containing Hep B may be given for subsequent doses in the series. Both full-term and preterm infants born to mothers whose HBsAg status is positive or unknown should receive hepatitis B vaccine and hepatitis B immune globulin (HBIG) 0.5 mL within 12 hours of birth at two different injection sites. In the event that the preterm infant is given a dose at birth, the current recommendation is that the infant be given the full series (three additional doses) at 1, 2, and 6 months of age. The American Academy of Pediatrics (2003c) also encourages immunization of all children by age 11 years.

The vaccine is given intramuscularly in the vastus lateralis in newborns or in the deltoid for older infants and children. Regardless of age, the dorsogluteal site is avoided because it has been associated with low antibody seroconversion rates, indicating a reduced immune response (Zuckerman, Cockcroft, and Zuckerman, 1992). No data exist regarding the seroconversion when the ventrogluteal site is used. The vaccine can be safely administered simultaneously at a separate site with DTaP, MMR, and Hib vaccines.

Hepatitis A.   Hepatitis A virus (HAV) is now recognized as a significant child health problem, particularly in communities with unusually high infection rates. HAV is spread

COMMUNITY FOCUS

Keeping Current on Vaccine Recommendations

It is much easier to keep current if you know where to look for the official recommendations of the **American Academy of Pediatrics (AAP)** and the **Centers for Disease Control and Prevention's (CDC) Advisory Committee on Immunization Practices (ACIP)**. The primary sources are publications and the Internet. You can also contact each organization to request information:

American Academy of Pediatrics
141 Northwest Point Boulevard
PO Box 747
Elk Grove Village, IL 60009
(888) 227-1770
Fax: (847) 228-1281
Website: www.aap.org

Centers for Disease Control and Prevention
1600 Clifton Road NE
Atlanta, GA 30333
(404) 639-3311
Information Hotline: (800) 232-2522 or (800) 232-7468
International Travel Hotline: (877) 394-8747
Spanish Hotline: (800) 232-0233
Website: www.cdc.gov; National Immunization Program at CDC: www.cdc.gov/nip/

The American Academy of Pediatric's **Report of the Committee on Infectious Diseases**, known as the **Red Book**, is an authoritative source of information on vaccines and other important pediatric infectious diseases. However, it lacks an in-depth review and reference list of controversial issues. The recommendations in the *Red Book* first appear in the journal **Pediatrics** or the **AAP News**. Typically, the most recent immunization schedule appears in the January issue of the journal.

A publication of the CDC, **Morbidity and Mortality Weekly Report (MMWR),** contains comprehensive reviews of the literature, as well as important background data regarding vaccine efficacy and side effects. To receive an electronic copy, send an e-mail message to listserv@listserv.cdc.gov. The body content should read: SUBscribe mmwr-toc. Electronic copy also is available from the CDC's website at www.cdc.gov/ or from the CDC's file transfer protocol server at ftp.cdc.gov. To subscribe for a paper copy, contact:

Superintendent of Documents
U.S. Government Printing Office
Washington, DC 20402
(202) 512-1800.

Immunization Gateway: Your Vaccine Fact-Finder at www.immunofacts.com provides direct links to all of the best vaccine resources on the Internet.

Vaccine information statements (VISs) are available by calling your state or local health department. They can also be downloaded from the **Immunization Action Coalition's** website at www.immunize.org/vis/ or the CDC's website at www.cdc.gov/nip/publications/vis/. Several language translations are available. The Immunization Action Coalition has various publications for parents and older children (adolescents) on different immunizations and in several languages.

by the fecal-oral route, from person-to-person contact, and by ingestion of contaminated food or water, but rarely by blood transfusion. The illness has an abrupt onset with fever, malaise, anorexia, nausea, abdominal discomfort, dark urine, and jaundice being the most common clinical signs of infection. In children younger than 6 years of age, who represent approximately one third of all cases of HAV, the disease may be asymptomatic, and jaundice is rarely evident. Children living in communities with high infection rates should be immunized with either HAVRIX or VAQTA vaccine, given by the intramuscular route in the deltoid. These vaccines are recommended for children 2 years of age and older, in two doses administered at least 6 months apart. States in which hepatitis A is mandatory are Arizona, Oklahoma, Alaska, New Mexico, South Dakota, Idaho, Nevada, Oregon, Utah, California, and Washington (Prevention of Hepatitis A, 1999). For further information see footnote "8" in Table 10-4.

Diphtheria. Diphtheria vaccine is commonly administered (1) in combination with tetanus and pertussis vaccines (DTaP) or DTaP and Hib vaccines for children younger than 7 years of age; (2) in combination with a conjugate *H. influenzae* type B vaccine (see Table 10-4); (3) in a combined vaccine with tetanus (DT) for children younger than 7 years of age who have some contraindication to receiving pertussis vaccine; (4) in smaller doses (15% to 20% of that in DTaP or DT) with tetanus vaccine (Td) for use in children age 7 years and older; (5) in a combined vaccine with hepatitis B, tetanus, pertussis, and inactivated poliovirus vaccine for use during the primary series in infants; or (6) as a single antigen when combined antigen preparations are not indicated. Although the diphtheria vaccine does not produce absolute immunity, protective antitoxin persists for 10 years or more when given according to the recommended schedule, and boosters are given every 10 years for life.

Tetanus. Three forms of tetanus vaccine—tetanus toxoid, tetanus immune globulin (TIG) (human), and tetanus antitoxin (usually horse serum)—are available. Tetanus toxoid is used for routine primary immunization, usually in one of the combinations listed for diphtheria, and provides protective antitoxin levels for 10 years or more.

For wound management, passive immunity is available with TIG. In persons with a history of two previous doses of tetanus toxoid, a booster dose of the toxoid can be given. Separate syringes and different sites are used when tetanus toxoid and TIG are given concurrently. Table 10-7 presents a summary of the recommended procedure for tetanus prophylaxis in wound management.

Pertussis. Pertussis vaccine is recommended for all children 6 weeks through 6 years of age (up to the seventh birthday) who have no neurologic contraindications to its use. It is not given to children 7 years or older because the risk of receiving the vaccine increases as the incidence, severity, and fatality of the disease decrease.

Two forms of pertussis vaccine are available in the United States. The ***whole-cell pertussis vaccine*** is prepared from inactivated cells of *Bordetella pertussis* and contains multiple antigens. In contrast, the ***acellular pertussis*** vaccine con-

Text continued on p. 340.

TABLE 10-4 ■ Recommended Childhood and Adolescent Immunization Schedule: United States, 2004[1]

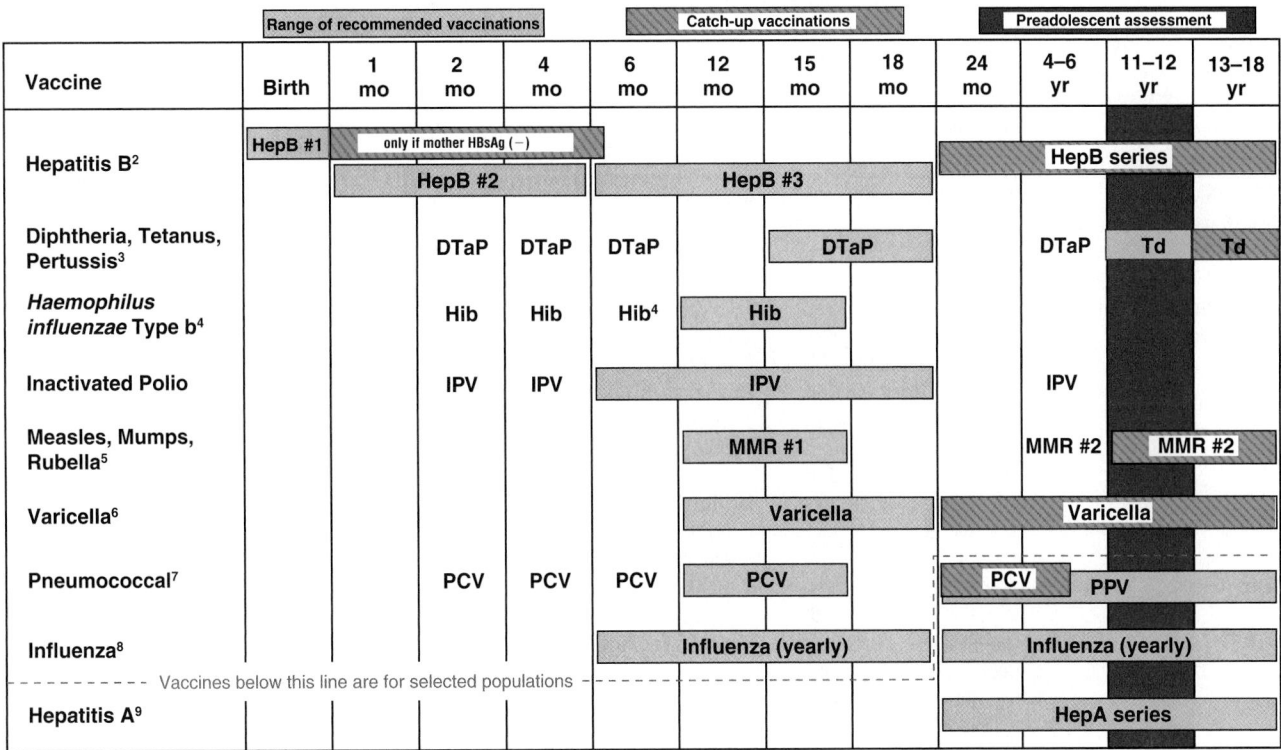

Vaccine	Birth	1 mo	2 mo	4 mo	6 mo	12 mo	15 mo	18 mo	24 mo	4–6 yr	11–12 yr	13–18 yr
Hepatitis B[2]	HepB #1	only if mother HBsAg (−)									HepB series	
		HepB #2				HepB #3						
Diphtheria, Tetanus, Pertussis[3]		DTaP	DTaP	DTaP		DTaP				DTaP	Td	Td
Haemophilus influenzae Type b[4]		Hib	Hib	Hib[4]		Hib						
Inactivated Polio		IPV	IPV		IPV					IPV		
Measles, Mumps, Rubella[5]						MMR #1				MMR #2	MMR #2	
Varicella[6]						Varicella					Varicella	
Pneumococcal[7]		PCV	PCV	PCV	PCV					PCV	PPV	
Influenza[8]					Influenza (yearly)					Influenza (yearly)		
— — — Vaccines below this line are for selected populations — — —												
Hepatitis A[9]										HepA series		

Legend: ▨ Range of recommended vaccinations ▨ Catch-up vaccinations ■ Preadolescent assessment

1. Indicates the recommended ages for routine administration of currently licensed childhood vaccines, as of December 1, 2003, for children through age 18 years. Any dose not given at the recommended age should be given at any subsequent visit when indicated and feasible. ▨ Indicates age-groups that warrant special effort to administer those vaccines not given previously. Additional vaccines may be licensed and recommended during the year. Licensed combination vaccines may be used whenever any components of the combination are indicated and the vaccine's other components are not contraindicated. Providers should consult the manufacturers' package inserts for detailed recommendations. Clinically significant adverse events that follow vaccination should be reported to the Vaccine Adverse Event Reporting System (VAERS). Guidance on how to obtain and complete a VAERS form is available at http://www.vaers.org or by telephone, 800-822-7967.

2. **Hepatitis B vaccine (HepB).** All infants should receive the first dose of HepB vaccine soon after birth and before hospital discharge; the first dose also may be given by age 2 months if the infant's mother is HBsAg-negative. Only monovalent HepB vaccine can be used for the birth dose. Monovalent or combination vaccine containing HepB may be used to complete the series; 4 doses of vaccine may be administered when a birth dose is given. The second dose should be given at least 4 weeks after the first dose except for combination vaccines, which cannot be administered before age 6 weeks. The third dose should be given at least 16 weeks after the first dose and at least 8 weeks after the second dose. The last dose in the vaccination series (third or fourth dose) should not be administered before age 24 weeks. Infants born to HBsAg-positive mothers should receive HepB vaccine and 0.5 mL hepatitis B immune globulin (HBIG) within 12 hours of birth at separate sites. The second dose is recommended at age 1-2 months. The last dose in the vaccination series should not be administered before age 24 weeks. These infants should be tested for HBsAg and anti-HBs at age 9-15 months. Infants born to mothers whose HBsAg status is unknown should receive the first dose of the HepB vaccine series within 12 hours of birth. Maternal blood should be drawn as soon as possible to determine the mother's HBsAg status; if the HBsAg test is positive, the infant should receive HBIG as soon as possible (no later than age 1 week). The second dose is recommended at age 1-2 months. The last dose in the vaccination series should not be administered before age 24 weeks.

3. **Diphtheria and tetanus toxoids and acellular pertussis vaccine (DTaP).** The fourth dose of DTaP may be administered at age 12 months provided that 6 months have elapsed since the third dose and the child is unlikely to return at age 15-18 months. The final dose in the series should be given at age ≥4 years. **Tetanus and diphtheria toxoids (Td)** is recommended at age 11-12 years if at least 5 years have elapsed since the last dose of tetanus and diphtheria toxoid-containing vaccine. Subsequent routine Td boosters are recommended every 10 years.

4. *Haemophilus influenzae* type b (Hib) conjugate vaccine. Three Hib conjugate vaccines are licensed for infant use. If PRP-OMP (PedvaxHIB(r) or ComVax(r) [Merck]) is administered at ages 2 and 4 months, a dose at age 6 months is not required. DTaP/Hib combination products should not be used for primary vaccination in infants at ages 2, 4, or 6 months but can be used as boosters after any Hib vaccine. The final dose in the series should be given at age ≥12 months.

5. **Measles, mumps, and rubella vaccine (MMR).** The second dose of MMR is recommended routinely at age 4-6 years but may be administered during any visit provided that at least 4 weeks have elapsed since the first dose and that both doses are administered beginning at or after age 12 months. Those who have not received the second dose previously should complete the schedule by the visit at age 11-12 years.

6. **Varicella vaccine (VAR).** Varicella vaccine is recommended at any visit at or after age 12 months for susceptible children (i.e., those who lack a reliable history of chickenpox). Susceptible persons aged ≥13 years should receive 2 doses given at least 4 weeks apart.

7. **Pneumococcal vaccine.** The heptavalent **pneumococcal conjugate vaccine (PCV)** is recommended for all children aged 2-23 months and for certain children aged 24-59 months. The final dose in the series should be given at age ≥12 months. **Pneumococcal polysaccharide vaccine (PPV)** is recommended in addition to PCV for certain high-risk groups. See *MMWR* 49(RR-9):1-35, 2000.

8. **Influenza vaccine.** Influenza vaccine is recommended annually for children aged ≥6 months with certain risk factors (including but not limited to asthma, cardiac disease, sickle cell disease, HIV, and diabetes), health care workers, and other persons (including household members) in close contact with persons in groups at high risk (see *MMWR* 52[RR-16], 2004), and can be administered to all others wishing to obtain immunity. In addition, healthy children aged 6-23 months and close contacts of healthy children aged 0-23 months are recommended to receive influenza vaccine because children in this age-group are at substantially increased risk for influenza-related hospitalizations. For healthy persons aged 5-49 years, the intranasally administered live-attenuated influenza vaccine (LAIV) is an acceptable alternative to the intramuscular trivalent inactivated influenza vaccine (TIV). See *MMWR* 52(RR-13):1-8, 2003. Children receiving TIV should be administered a dosage appropriate for their age (0.25 mL if 6-35 months or 0.5 mL if ≥3 years). Children aged ≤8 years who are receiving influenza vaccine for the first time should receive 2 doses (separated by at least 4 weeks for TIV and at least 6 weeks for LAIV). Additional information about vaccines, including precautions and contraindications for vaccination and vaccine shortages, is available at http://www.cdc.gov/nip or from the National Immunization Information Hotline, at 800-232-2522 (English) or 800-232-0233 (Spanish). Approved by the **Advisory Committee on Immunization Practices** (http://www.cdc.gov/nip/acip), the **American Academy of Pediatrics** (http://www.aap.org), and the **American Academy of Family Physicians** (http://www.aafp.org).

9. **Hepatitis A vaccine.** Hepatitis A vaccine is recommended for children and adolescents in selected states and regions, and for certain high-risk groups. Consult local public health authority and *MMWR* 48(RR-12):1-37, 1999. Children and adolescents in these states, regions, and high-risk groups who have not been vaccinated against hepatitis A can begin the hepatitis A vaccination series during any visit. The two doses in the series should be administered at least 6 months apart.

TABLE 10-5 ■ Catch-Up Immunization Schedule for Children and Adolescents Who Start Late or Who are >1 Month Behind

CATCH-UP SCHEDULE FOR CHILDREN AGES 4 MONTHS THROUGH 6 YEARS

DOSE ONE (minimum age)	MINIMUM INTERVAL BETWEEN DOSES			
	DOSE ONE TO DOSE TWO	DOSE TWO TO DOSE THREE	DOSE THREE TO DOSE FOUR	DOSE FOUR TO DOSE FIVE
DTaP (6 weeks)	4 weeks	4 weeks	6 months	6 months[1]
IPV (6 weeks)	4 weeks	4 weeks	4 weeks[2]	
HepB[3] (birth)	4 weeks	8 weeks (and 16 weeks after first dose)		
MMR (12 months)	4 weeks[4]			
Varicella (12 months)				
Hib[5] (6 weeks)	4 weeks: if first dose given at age <12 months / 8 weeks (as final dose): if first dose given at age 12 to 14 months / No further doses needed: if first dose given at age ≥15 months	4 weeks[6]: if current age <12 months / 8 weeks (as final dose)[6]: if current age ≥12 months and second dose given at age <15 months / No further doses needed: if previous dose given at age ≥15 months	8 weeks (as final dose): this dose only necessary for children ages 12 months to 5 years who received 3 doses before age 12 months	
PCV[7]: (6 weeks)	4 weeks: if first dose given at age <12 months and current age <24 months / 8 weeks (as final dose): if first dose given at age ≥12 months or current age 24 to 59 months / No further doses needed: for healthy children if first dose given at age ≥24 months	4 weeks: if current age <12 months / 8 weeks (as final dose): if current age ≥12 months / No further doses needed: for healthy children if previous dose given at age ≥24 months	8 weeks (as final dose): this dose only necessary for children ages 12 months to 5 years who received 3 doses before age 12 months	

CATCH-UP SCHEDULE FOR CHILDREN AGES 7 THROUGH 18 YEARS

MINIMUM INTERVAL BETWEEN DOSES		
DOSE ONE AND DOSE TWO	DOSE TWO TO DOSE THREE	DOSE THREE TO BOOSTER DOSE
Td: 4 weeks	Td: 6 months	Td[8]: 6 months: if first dose given at age <12 months and current age <11 years / 5 years: if first dose given at age ≥12 months and third dose given at age <7 years and current age ≥11 years / 10 years: if third dose given at age ≥7 years
IPV[9]: 4 weeks	IPV[9]: 4 weeks	IPV[2,9]
HepB: 4 weeks	HepB: 8 weeks (and 16 weeks after first dose)	
MMR: 4 weeks		
Varicella[10]: 4 weeks		

NOTE: A vaccine series does not require restarting, regardless of the time that has elapsed between doses.
1. **DTaP:** The fifth dose is not necessary if the fourth dose was given after the 4th birthday.
2. **IPV:** For children who received an all-IPV or all-OPV series, a fourth dose is not necessary if third dose was given at age ≥4 years. If both OPV and IPV were given as part of a series, a total of four doses should be given, regardless of the child's current age.
3. **HepB:** All children and adolescents who have not been immunized against hepatitis B should begin the hepatitis B vaccination series during any visit. Providers should make special efforts to immunize children who were born in, or whose parents were born in, areas of the world where hepatitis B virus infection is moderately or highly endemic.
4. **MMR:** The second dose of MMR is recommended routinely at age 4 to 6 years, but may be given earlier if desired.
5. **Hib:** Vaccine is not generally recommended for children age ≥ 5 years.
6. **Hib:** If current age <12 months and the first 2 doses were PRP-OMP (PedvaxHIB or ComVax), the third (and final) dose should be given at age 12 months and at least 8 weeks after the second dose.
7. **PCV:** Vaccine is not generally recommended for children age ≥5 years.
8. **Td:** For children age 7 to 10 years, the interval between the third and booster dose is determined by the age when the first dose was given. For adolescents aged 11-18 years, the interval is determined by the age when the third dose was given.
9. **IPV:** Vaccine is not generally recommended for persons age ≥18 years.
10. **Varicella:** Give two-dose series to all susceptible adolescents age ≥13 years.
Reporting Adverse Reactions
Report adverse reactions to vaccines through the federal Vaccine Adverse Event Reporting System. For information on reporting reactions following vaccines, please visit www.vaers.org or call the 24-hour national toll-free information line at 800-822-7967.
Disease Reporting
Report suspected cases of vaccine-preventable diseases to your state or local health department.

For additional information about vaccines, including precautions and contraindications for immunization and vaccine shortages, please visit the National Immunization Program website at www.cdc.gov/nip or call the National Immunization Information Hotline at 800-232-2522 (English) or 800-232-0233 (Spanish).
American Academy of Pediatrics, Committee on Infectious Diseases, Pickering L, editor: *2003 Red Book: report of the Committee on Infectious Diseases,* ed 26, Elk Grove Village, Il, 2003, The Academy; American Academy of Pediatrics, Committee on Infectious Diseases: Recommended childhood immunization schedule—United States—2004, *Pediatrics*

TABLE 10-6 ■ Routine Immunization Schedule for Infants and Children: Canada, 2002

AGE AT VACCINATION	DTaP[1]	IPV	Hib[2]	MMR	Td[3] OR dTap[10]	Hep B[4] (3 DOSES)	V	PC	MC
Birth									
2 months	X	X	X			Infancy or preadolescence (9-13 years)		X[8]	X[9]
4 months	X	X	X					X	X
6 months	X	(X)[5]	X					X	X
12 months				X			X[7]	X	
18 months	X	X	X	(X)[6] or					or
4-6 years				(X)[6]					
14-16 years					X[10]				X[9]

ROUTINE IMMUNIZATION SCHEDULE FOR CHILDREN <7 YEARS OF AGE NOT IMMUNIZED IN EARLY INFANCY

TIMING	DTaP[1]	IPV	Hib	MMR	Td[3] OR dTap[10]	Hep B[4] (3 DOSES)	V	P	M
First visit	X	X	X[11]	X[12]		X	X[7]	X[8]	X[9]
2 months later	X	X	X	(X)[6]		X		(X)	(X)
2 months later	X	(X)[5]						(X)	
6-12 months later	X	X	(X)[11]			X			
4-6 years of age[13]	X	X							
14-16 years of age					X				

ROUTINE IMMUNIZATION SCHEDULE FOR CHILDREN ≥7 YEARS OF AGE NOT IMMUNIZED IN EARLY INFANCY

TIMING	DTaP[10]	IPV	MMR	Hep B[4] (3 DOSES)	V	M
First visit	X	X	X	X	X	X[9]
2 months later	X	X	X[6]	X	(X)[7]	
6-12 months later	X	X		X		
10 years later	X					

From *Canadian immunization guide* ed 6, 2002, Health Canada. Reproduced with permission of the Minister of Public Works and Government Services, Canada, 2004.

NOTES:

1. DTaP (diphtheria, tetanus, acellular or component pertussis) vaccine is the preferred vaccine for all doses in the vaccination series, including completion of the series in children who have received ≥1 dose of DPT (whole-cell) vaccine.

2. Hib schedule shown is for PRP-T or HbOC vaccine. If PRP-OMP is used, give at 2, 4, and 12 months of age.

3. Td (tetanus and diphtheria toxoid), a combined adsorbed "adult type" preparation for use in people ≥7 years of age, contains less diphtheria toxoid than preparations given to younger children and is less likely to cause reactions in older people.

4. Hepatitis B vaccine can be routinely given to infants or preadolescents, depending on the provincial/territorial policy; three doses at 0, 1, and 6 month intervals are preferred. The second dose should be administered at least 1 month after the first dose, and the third at least 2 months after the second dose. A two-dose schedule for adolescents is also possible.

5. This dose is not needed routinely, but can be included for convenience.

6. A second dose of MMR is recommended, at least 1 month after the first dose for the purpose of better measles protection. For convenience, options include giving it with the next scheduled vaccination at 18 months of age or with school entry (4 to 6 years) vaccinations (depending on the provincial/territorial policy), or at any intervening age that is practicable. The need for a second dose of mumps and rubella vaccine is not established but may benefit (given for convenience as MMR). The second dose of MMR should be given at the same visit as DTaP IPV (±Hib) to ensure high uptake rates.

7. Children aged 12 months to 12 years should receive one dose of varicella vaccine. Individuals ≥13 years of age should receive two doses at least 28 days apart.

8. Recommended schedule, number of doses, and subsequent use of 23 valent polysaccharide pneumococcal vaccine depend on the age of the child when vaccination is begun.

9. Recommended schedule and number of doses of meningococcal vaccine depend on the age of the child.

10. dTap adult formulation with reduced diphtheria toxoid and pertussis component.

11. Recommended schedule and number of doses depend on the product used and age of the child when vaccination is begun. Not required past age 5.

12. Delay until subsequent visit if child is <12 months of age.

13. Omit these doses if the previous doses of DTaP and polio were given after the fourth birthday.

DTaP, Diphtheria, tetanus, pertussis (acellular) vaccine; *IPV*, inactivated poliovirus vaccine; *Hib*, *Haemophilus influenzae* type b conjugate vaccine; *MMR*, measles, mumps and rubella vaccine; *Td*, tetanus and diphtheria toxoid, adult type with reduced diphtheria toxoid; *dTap*, tetanus and diphtheria toxoid, acellular pertussis, adolescent/adult type with reduced diphtheria and pertussis components; *Hep B*, hepatitis B vaccine; *V*, varicella; *PC*, pneumococcal conjugate vaccine; *MC*, meningococcal C conjugate vaccine; *P*, pneumococcal vaccine; *M*, meningococcal vaccine.

TABLE 10-7 ■ **Guide to Tetanus Prophylaxis in Routine Wound Management**

HISTORY OF ABSORBED TETANUS TOXOID (DOSES)	CLEAN, MINOR WOUNDS		ALL OTHER WOUNDS*	
	Td†	TIG¶	Td†	TIG¶
Unknown or <3	Yes	No	Yes	Yes
≤3‡	No§	No	No‖	No

Data from American Academy of Pediatrics, Committee on Infectious Diseases, Pickering L, editor: *2003 Red Book: report of the Committee on Infectious Diseases,* ed 26, Elk Grove Village, Il, 2003, The Academy.

*Such as, but not limited to, wounds contaminated with dirt, feces, soil, and saliva; puncture wounds, avulsions, and wounds resulting from missiles, crushing, burns, and frostbite.

†For children <7 years old: DTaP (DT, if pertussis vaccine is contraindicated) is preferred to tetanus toxoid alone. For persons 7 years of age or older, Td is preferred to tetanus toxoid alone.

‡If only three doses of *fluid* toxoid have been received, then a fourth dose of toxoid, preferably an adsorbed toxoid, should be given.

§Yes, if 10 years since last dose.

‖Yes, if 5 years since last dose. (More frequent boosters are not needed and can accentuate side effects.)

¶Equine tetanus antitoxin should be used, if available, when TIG is not available.

tains one or more immunogens derived from the *B. pertussis* organism. The highly purified acellular vaccine is associated with fewer local and systemic reactions than those occurring with the whole-cell vaccine in children of similar age. The acellular pertussis vaccine is recommended by the American Academy of Pediatrics (2003c) for the first three immunizations and is usually given at 2, 4, and 6 months of age with DTaP. Five forms of acellular pertussis vaccine are currently licensed for use in infants: Daptacel, Acel-Imune, Tripedia, Certiva, Infanrix (diphtheria, tetanus toxoid, and acellular pertussis conjugate), and PEDIARIX (diphtheria, tetanus, hepatitis B, and inactivated poliovirus vaccine).

NURSING ALERT

For several decades pertussis vaccine was considered a rare cause of serious, permanent brain damage or death. After reviewing studies, experts have concluded that whole-cell pertussis vaccine has not been proved to cause neurologic damage. Previous contraindications to whole-cell pertussis vaccination are now considered precautions.

Polio. An all-inactivated poliovirus (IPV) schedule for routine childhood polio vaccination is now recommended; oral poliovirus (OPV) is no longer used in the United States. All children should receive four doses of IPV at 2 months, 4 months, 6 to 18 months, and 4 to 6 years of age (American Academy of Pediatrics, 2003c).

The change from the exclusive use of OPV to the exclusive use of IPV is related to the rare risk of *vaccine-associated polio paralysis* from OPV. The exclusive use of IPV eliminates the risk of this paralysis.

Measles. The measles (rubeola) vaccine is given at 12 to 15 months of age. During the course of measles outbreaks, the vaccine can be given any time after 6 months of age, followed by a second inoculation after age 12 months.

Because of continued outbreaks of measles among unvaccinated preschool-age children and among vaccinated school-age children and college students, a second measles immunization is recommended at 4 to 6 years of age (at school entry) but may be administered at any time as long as 4 weeks have passed since the first dose and provided that

both doses are administered at or after the age of 12 months. Otherwise the child may be revaccinated by 11 to 12 years of age.

Mumps. Mumps virus vaccine is recommended for children at 12 to 15 months of age and is typically given in combination with measles and rubella. It should not be administered to infants younger than 12 months because persisting maternal antibodies can interfere with the immune response.

Because of recent outbreaks of the disease, especially in children 10 to 19 years of age, mumps immunization is recommended for all individuals born after 1957 who may be susceptible to mumps (i.e., those who have no history of having had the disease or vaccine and when there is no laboratory evidence of immunity).

Rubella. Rubella is a relatively mild infection in children, but in a pregnant woman the actual infection presents serious risks to the developing fetus. Therefore, the aim of rubella immunization is actually protection of the unborn child rather than the recipient of the immunization.

Rubella immunization is recommended for all children at 12 to 15 months of age and is administered in a combined form with measles and mumps vaccine. Increased emphasis should also be placed on vaccinating all unimmunized prepubertal children and susceptible adolescents and adult women in the childbearing age-group.

Because the live attenuated virus may cross the placenta and theoretically present a risk to the developing fetus, rubella vaccine is not given to any pregnant woman. Although this is standard practice, current evidence from women who received the vaccine while pregnant and delivered unaffected offspring indicates that the risk to the fetus is negligible. In addition, there is no reported danger of administering rubella vaccine to a child if the mother is pregnant.

Hib. Hib conjugate vaccines provide protection against a number of serious infections caused by Hib, especially bacterial meningitis, epiglottitis, bacterial pneumonia, septic arthritis, and sepsis (Hib is not associated with the viruses that cause influenza, or "flu"). Several Hib vaccines are available, three of which may be given to infants (PRP-OMP [PedvaxHIB], Comvax, and ActHIB). Some Hib vaccines are combination vaccines, such as Comvax (Hib and HBV) (see Table 10-10). These conjugate vaccines connect Hib to a nontoxic form of another organism, such as meningococcal protein or diphtheria protein. There is no antibody response to these nontoxic proteins, but they significantly improve the antibody response to Hib, especially in infants. The use of combination vaccines provides equivalent immunogenicity and decreases the number of injections an infant receives; however, it is important that they be given to the appropriate-age child.

The DTaP/Hib combination vaccine (TriHIBit) should not be used for the first 3 doses at 2, 4, or 6 months but may be used as a booster thereafter.

When possible, the Hib conjugate vaccine used at the first vaccination should be used for all subsequent vaccinations in the primary series. All Hib vaccines are administered by intramuscular injection using a separate syringe and at a separate site from any concurrent vaccinations.

NURSING ALERT

The use of meningococcal and diphtheria proteins in combination vaccines does not mean the child has received adequate immunization for meningococcal or diphtheria illnesses; the child must be given the appropriate vaccine for that specific disease.

Varicella.   Administration of the cell-free live-attenuated varicella vaccine (Varivax) is recommended for healthy children 12 to 18 months of age. A single dose of 0.5 mL should be given by subcutaneous injection. From the age of 19 months to the thirteenth birthday, a single dose of varicella vaccine may be given at any time to children who may be susceptible, either by lack of proof of varicella vaccination, serologic testing, or a reliable history of varicella infection (American Academy of Pediatrics, 2003c). The vaccine should be kept frozen in the lyophilized form (stable particles that readily go into solution) and used within 30 minutes of being reconstituted to ensure viral potency (American Academy of Pediatrics, 2003c).

Varicella vaccine may be administered simultaneously with MMR. However, separate syringes and injection sites should be used. If they are not administered simultaneously, the interval between administration of varicella vaccine and MMR should be at least 1 month. Varicella vaccine may also be given simultaneously with DTaP, IPV, HBV, or Hib (American Academy of Pediatrics, 2003c).

Pneumococcal (Prevnar).   A seven-valent *Streptococcus pneumoniae* conjugate vaccine (PCV7 or PCV) has now been approved for use in all children 2 months to 23 months old. Streptococci pneumococci are responsible for a number of bacterial infections in children younger than age 2 years, which may cause serious morbidity and mortality. Among these are generalized infections such as septicemia and meningitis, and localized infections such as otitis media, sinusitis, and pneumonia. The vaccine is administered at 2, 4, and 6 months, with a fourth dose at 12 months of age. The vaccine is also recommended for children 24 to 59

months with conditions such as cardiac disease, pulmonary diseases (excluding asthma), immunodeficiency (human immunodeficiency virus, asplenia, sickle cell), diabetes mellitus, renal failure, leukemia, and malignancies (MMWR, 2000). PCV is also recommended for children 24 to 59 months old who attend group day care. The vaccine may be administered at the same time as other vaccines but in a separate syringe and at a separate site; it is given as an intramuscular injection (MMWR, 2000).

The pneumococcal polysaccharide vaccine (PPV) is also recommended after two doses of PCV (2 months apart and PPV given no sooner than 2 months after second dose of PCV) in children 24 to 59 months old with cardiac disease, pulmonary disease, immunodeficiencies, renal failure, sickle cell disease, nephrotic syndrome, asplenia, leukemia, and solid organ transplantation (MMWR, 2000).

Influenza.   The influenza vaccine is now recommended for children 6 months and older with risk factors including but not limited to the following: asthma, cardiac disease, human immunodeficiency virus, sickle cell disease, diabetes, and households with individuals at high risk. Influenza vaccine may be given to any healthy children 6 to 23 months old because this age-group is at particular risk. The vaccine is usually started in the fall before the flu season begins and is repeated yearly because different strains of influenza may be predominant each year. The intramuscular vaccine is administered as two separate doses 2 weeks apart in first-time recipients younger than 8 years old. The dose is 0.25 mL for children 6 to 35 months old and 0.5 mL for those over 3 years. The vaccine may be given at the same time as other immunizations but in a separate syringe and at a separate site (American Academy of Pediatrics, 2003c). A new preparation of the vaccine, FluMist, has been released by the Food and Drug Administration (Bechtel, 2003). The vaccine is given nasally as two doses 6 weeks apart. Although it is an alternative to the injection, there is a cost increase and insurance companies may not cover the cost of the nasal vaccine.

Recommendations for Selected Immunizations

Several additional vaccines are recommended for children at high risk for particular diseases. Most of these children have chronic disorders or impaired immune systems that make them more susceptible to certain infections than the general population. Selected immunizations are presented in Table 10-8. Others, such as the rabies vaccine, are discussed elsewhere in this text.

Reactions

Vaccines for routine immunizations are among the safest and most reliable drugs available. However, minor side effects do occur after many of the immunizations and, rarely, a serious reaction may result from the vaccine.

With inactivated antigens, such as DTaP, side effects are most likely to occur within a few hours or days of administration and are usually limited to local tenderness, erythema, and swelling at the injection site; low-grade fever; and behavioral changes (drowsiness, fretfulness, eating less, prolonged or unusual cry). Local reactions tend to be less

TABLE 10-8 ■ Recommendations for Selected Nonmandated Vaccines

DESCRIPTION	ADMINISTRATION/PRECAUTION
MENINGOCOCCAL POLYSACCHARIDE VACCINE (MENOMUNE)	
Affords protection against *Neisseria meningitidis:* serogroups A, C, Y, and W-135. Recommended for children 2 years of age and older with terminal complement deficiencies and anatomic or functional asplenia, incoming college students in dormitories, and military recruits.	Subcutaneous injection. Duration of protection unknown. Safety during pregnancy not established.
LYME DISEASE VACCINE	
Affords protection against infection with the spirochete *Borrelia burgdorferi,* which causes Lyme disease (LD) Recommended for individuals 15 to 70 years of age who are at high risk for LD from significant exposure to tick habitats in endemic areas (northeast and north-central United States) and for those who have been infected with LD; safety has been demonstrated in children 4 to 18 years of age, and thus may be used in children in Lyme epidemic areas.	Intramuscular injection in deltoid muscle. Administered on 0-, 1-, and 12-month schedule. Doses two and three should be given several weeks before *B. burgdorferi* season, which usually begins in April.

ATRAUMATIC CARE

Immunizations

To minimize local reactions from vaccines:

Select a needle of adequate length (1 inch [2.5 cm] in infants) to deposit the antigen deep in the muscle mass.

Inject into the vastus lateralis or ventrogluteal muscle; the deltoid may be used in children 18 months of age or older or in infants receiving HBV vaccine.

Use an air bubble to clear the needle after injecting the vaccine (theoretically beneficial but unproved).

To minimize pain:

Apply the topical anesthetic eutectic mixture of local anesthetic (EMLA) to the injection site and cover with an occlusive dressing for 2.5 hours (or apply an EMLA patch, which requires no occlusive dressing).

Apply a vapocoolant spray (i.e., ethyl chloride or Fluori-Methane) directly to the skin or to a cotton ball, which is placed on the skin for 15 seconds immediately before the injection.

In preschool children, use distraction, such as telling the child to "take a deep breath and blow and blow and blow until I tell you to stop."

NOTE: Changing the needle on the syringe after drawing up the vaccine and before injecting it has not been shown to decrease local reactions. In children 4 to 6 years of age, the administration of sequential injections or simultaneous injections of vaccines did not alter their perceptions of distress, but parents preferred the simultaneous method (Horn and McCarthy, 1999).

severe when the deltoid rather than the vastus lateralis site is used and when a needle of sufficient length to deposit the vaccine in the muscle is used (see Atraumatic Care box). Rarely, more severe reactions may occur, especially with pertussis (see Table 10-9). Reactions to DTaP tend to be more severe if they occurred with a previous immunization.

Hib vaccine is one of the safest vaccines available but may be associated with low-grade fever and mild local reactions at the site of injection, which resolve rapidly. Fever (temperature higher than 38.5° C [101.3° F]) may rarely occur.

Unlike the inactivated antigens, live attenuated virus vaccines such as MMR multiply for days or weeks, and unfavorable reactions and "vaccine-associated" disorders can occur for 30 to 60 days. These reactions are usually mild, although reactions to rubella tend to be more troublesome in older children and adults.

Studies in the United States and in various European countries (Denmark, Finland) have found no association between the MMR vaccine and the incidence of autism (Dales, Hammer, and Smith, 2001; Campion, 2002).

Contraindications/Precautions

Nurses need to be aware of the reasons for withholding immunizations—both for the child's safety in terms of avoiding reactions and for the child's maximum benefit from receiving the vaccine. Unfounded fears and lack of knowledge regarding contraindications can needlessly prevent a child from having protection from life-threatening diseases. Issues that have surfaced regarding vaccines include the misconception that administering combination vaccines may overload the child's immune system; the combined vaccines have undergone rigorous study in relation to side effects and immunogenicity rates following administration. Parents must be given appropriate information regarding vaccine safety, benefits, and risks so they can make informed decisions regarding vaccinations for their children (Koslap-Petraco and Parsons, 2003). The advantages of widespread media via television and the Internet are that information is readily available at any given moment; the disadvantage may rest in the fact that information—rather, misinformation—from sources is also readily available and may influence parents to make decisions that may have deleterious consequences on their children's health. The contraindications to the usual childhood vaccines are presented in Table 10-9.

TABLE 10-9 ■ **Contraindications and Precautions to Vaccinations**[a]

TRUE CONTRAINDICATIONS AND PRECAUTIONS	NOT CONTRAINDICATIONS (VACCINES MAY BE ADMINISTERED)
GENERAL FOR ALL VACCINES (DTaP, IPV, MMR, Hib, HEPATITIS B, Var, PCV, HEPATITIS A, INFLUENZA)	
Contraindications	
Anaphylactic reaction to a vaccine contraindicates further doses of that vaccine	Mild to moderate local reaction (soreness, redness, swelling) following a dose of an injectable antigen
Anaphylactic reaction to a vaccine constituent contraindicates the use of vaccines containing that substance	Mild acute illness with or without low-grade fever
Moderate or severe illnesses with or without a fever	Current antimicrobial therapy
	Convalescent phase of illnesses
	Prematurity (same dosage and indications as for normal, full-term infants)
	Recent exposure to an infectious disease
	History of penicillin or other nonspecific allergies or family history of such allergies
DIPHTHERIA, TETANUS, PERTUSSIS, OR ACELLULAR PERTUSSIS (DTAP)	
Contraindications	
Encephalopathy within 7 days of administration of previous dose of DTaP	Temperature of <40.5° C (105° F) after a previous dose of DTaP
	Family history of seizures[b]
	Family history of sudden infant death syndrome
	Family history of an adverse event after DTaP administration
Precautions[b]	
Fever of ≥40.5° C (105° F) within 48 hours after vaccination with a prior dose of DTaP	
Collapse or shocklike state (hypotonic-hyporesponsive episode) within 48 hours of receiving a prior dose of DTaP	
Seizures within 3 days of receiving a prior dose of DTaP[c]	
Persistent, inconsolable crying lasting 3 hours within 48 hours of receiving a prior dose of DTaP	
INACTIVATED POLIO VIRUS (IPV)	
Contraindication	
Anaphylactic reaction to neomycin or streptomycin	Breast-feeding
	Diarrhea
Precaution[b]	
Pregnancy	
MEASLES, MUMPS, RUBELLA (MMR)[d]	
Contraindications	
Pregnancy	Tuberculosis or positive PPD skin test
Known altered immunodeficiency (hematologic and solid tumors, congenital immunodeficiency, and long-term immunosuppressive therapy)	Simultaneous TB skin testing[e]
	Breast-feeding
	Pregnancy of mother of recipient
	Immunodeficient family member or household contact
	Infection with HIV
	Nonanaphylactic reactions to eggs or neomycin

Modified from American Academy of Pediatrics, Committee on Infectious Diseases, Pickering L, editor: *2003 Red Book: report of the Committee on Infectious Diseases*, ed 26, Elk Grove Village, Il, 2003, The Academy.

[a]This information is based on the recommendations of the Advisory Committee on Immunization Practices (ACIP) and those of the Committee on Infectious Diseases (*Red Book* Committee) of the American Academy of Pediatrics (AAP). Sometimes these recommendations vary from those contained in the manufacturer's package inserts. For more detailed information, providers should consult the published recommendations of the ACIP, AAP, and the manufacturer's package inserts.

[b]The events or conditions listed as precautions, although not contraindications, should be carefully reviewed. The benefits and risks of administering a specific vaccine to an individual under the circumstances should be considered. If the risks are believed to outweigh the benefits, the vaccination should be withheld; if the benefits are believed to outweigh the risks (e.g., during an outbreak or foreign travel), the vaccination should be administered. Whether and when to administer DTaP to children with proven or suspected underlying neurologic disorders should be decided on an individual basis. It is prudent on theoretic grounds to avoid vaccinating pregnant women.

[c]Acetaminophen given before administering DTaP and thereafter every 4 hours for 24 hours should be considered for children with a personal or family history of convulsions in siblings or parents.

[d]No data exist to substantiate the theoretic risk of a suboptimal immune response from the administration of OPV and MMR within 30 days of each other.

Continued

TABLE 10-9 ■ Contraindications and Precautions to Vaccinations—*cont'd*

TRUE CONTRAINDICATIONS AND PRECAUTIONS	NOT CONTRAINDICATIONS (VACCINES MAY BE ADMINISTERED)
MEASLES, MUMPS, RUBELLA (MMR)[d]—CONT'D	
Precautions[b]	
Recent immunoglobulin administration	
Immunoglobulin products and MMR should not be given simultaneously; if unavoidable, give at different sites and revaccinate or test for seroconversion in 3 months; if immunoglobulin is given first, MMR should not be given for at least 3 to 6 months, depending on the dose; if MMR is given first, immunoglobulin should not be given for 2 weeks	
Thrombocytopenia/thrombocytopenia purpura	
HAEMOPHILUS INFLUENZAE TYPE B (HIB)	
Contraindication	
Nonidentified	History of Hib disease
HEPATITIS B VIRUS (HBV)	
Contraindication	
Anaphylactic reaction to common baker's yeast	Pregnancy
VARICELLA (Var)	
Contraindications	
Immunocompromised individuals (e.g., human immunodeficiency virus, acute lymphocytic leukemia)	Breast-feeding
Pregnancy	
PNEUMOCOCCAL	
Allergy to vaccine components	
Acute, moderate, or severe illness with or without fever	Minor illnesses with or without fever
	Mild upper respiratory tract infection
	Allergic rhinitis
INFLUENZA*	
Acute febrile illness	
Egg hypersensitivity	

*See James JM and others: Safe administration of influenza vaccine to patients with egg allergies, *J Pediatr* 133:624-628, 1998.

Modified from American Academy of Pediatrics, Committee on Infectious Diseases, Pickering L, editor: *2003 Red Book: report of the Committee on Infectious Diseases*, ed 26, Elk Grove Village, Il, 2003, The Academy.

[a]This information is based on the recommendations of the Advisory Committee on Immunization Practices (ACIP) and those of the Committee on Infectious Diseases (*Red Book* Committee) of the American Academy of Pediatrics (AAP). Sometimes these recommendations vary from those contained in the manufacturer's package inserts. For more detailed information, providers should consult the published recommendations of the ACIP, AAP, and the manufacturer's package inserts.

[b]The events or conditions listed as precautions, although not contraindications, should be carefully reviewed. The benefits and risks of administering a specific vaccine to an individual under the circumstances should be considered. If the risks are believed to outweigh the benefits, the vaccination should be withheld; if the benefits are believed to outweigh the risks (e.g., during an outbreak or foreign travel), the vaccination should be administered. Whether and when to administer DTaP to children with proven or suspected underlying neurologic disorders should be decided on an individual basis. It is prudent on theoretic grounds to avoid vaccinating pregnant women.

[c]Acetaminophen given before administering DTaP and thereafter every 4 hours for 24 hours should be considered for children with a personal or family history of convulsions in siblings or parents.

[d]No data exist to substantiate the theoretic risk of a suboptimal immune response from the administration of OPV and MMR within 30 days of each other.

Administration

The principal precautions in administering immunizations include proper storage of the vaccine to protect its potency and institution of recommended procedures for injection. The nurse must be familiar with the manufacturer's directions for storage and reconstitution of the vaccine. For example, if the vaccine is to be refrigerated, it should be stored on a center shelf, not on the door, where frequent temperature increases from opening the refrigerator can alter the vaccine's potency. For protection against light, the vial can be wrapped in aluminum foil. Periodic checks are established to ensure that no vaccine is used after its expiration date.

The DTaP vaccines contain the adjuvant alum to retain the antigen at the injection site and prolong the stimulatory effect. Because subcutaneous or intracutaneous injection of the adjuvant can cause local irritation, inflammation, or abscess formation, attention to excellent intramuscular injection technique must be used (see Atraumatic Care box, p. 342, and Table 10-10).

One of the most important features of injecting vaccines is adequate penetration of the muscle for deposition of the

TABLE 10-10 ■ Product Brand Names, Manufacturers/Distributors, and Route of Administration for Principal Childhood Vaccine Types

PRODUCT	BRAND NAME/MANUFACTURER/DISTRIBUTOR	TYPE
DTaP Diphtheria and tetanus toxoids and acellular pertussis vaccine	Acel-Imune (WLV) Certiva (NAV, distributed by ALI) Infanrix (SBB, distributed by SB) Tripedia (CON, distributed by PMC) TriHIBit* (ActHIB Hib reconstituted with Tripedia DTaP; distributed by PMC)	IM
DTaP-Hib Diphtheria and tetanus toxoids and acellular pertussis and *Haemophilus influenzae* type b vaccine		IM
DTwP Diphtheria and tetanus toxoids and whole-cell pertussis vaccine	Tri-Immunol† (WLV)	IM
DTwP-Hib Diphtheria and tetanus toxoids and whole-cell pertussis and *Haemophilus influenzae* type B vaccine	ActHIB Hib reconstituted with DTwP (CON; distributed by PMC) Tetramune (WLV)	IM
HepA Hepatitis A vaccine	Havrix (SBB, distributed by SB) Vaqta (MRK)	IM
HepB Hepatitis B vaccine	Engerix-B (SBB, distributed by SB) Recombivax HB (MRK)	IM
Hib *Haemophilus influenzae* type b conjugate vaccine		IM
HbOC—Oligosaccharides conjugated to diphtheria CRM$_{197}$ toxin protein	HibTITER (WLV)	
PRP-OMP—Polyribosylribitol phosphate polysaccharide conjugated to a meningococcal outer membrane protein	PedvaxHIB (MRK)	
PRP-T—Polyribosylribitol phosphate polysaccharide conjugated to tetanus toxoid	ActHIB (PMSV, distributed by CON, PMC) OmniHIB (PMSV, distributed by SB)	
PRP-D—Polyribosylribitol phosphate polysaccharide conjugated to diphtheria toxoid	ProHIBiT (CON, distributed by PMC)	
Hib-HepB Haemophilus influenzae type b and hepatitis B vaccine	Comvax (Hib component = PRP-OMP) (MRK)	IM
IPV Trivalent inactivated polio vaccine (killed Salk type)	IPOL (PMSV, distributed by CON, PMC)	IM or SQ
MMR Measles, mumps, rubella vaccine	M-M-R II (MRK)	SQ
PCV Pneumococcal conjugate vaccine	Varivax (MRK)	Oral
PPV Pneumococcal polysaccharide vaccine	PEDIARIX (DTaP, Hep B, IPV) (SBB) Prevnar (Wyeth)	SQ
TIV (Influenza) Trivalent inactivated influenza vaccine—Aventis Pasteur	DAPTACEL (Aventis Pasteur)	IM

Modified from American Academy of Pediatrics: Combination vaccines for childhood immunization: recommendations of the Advisory Committee on Immunization Practices (ACIP), the American Academy of Pediatrics (AAP), and the American Academy of Family Physicians (AAFP), *Pediatrics* 103(5):1072, 1999.
ALI, Ross Products Division, Abbott Laboratories, Inc.; *CON,* Connaught Laboratories, Inc.; *MRK,* Merck & Co., Inc.; *NAV,* North American Vaccine, Inc.; *PMC,* Pasteur Mérieux Connaught; *PMSV,* Pasteur Mérieux Sérums & Vaccins, S.A.; *SBB,* SmithKline Beecham Biologicals; *SB,* SmithKline Beecham Pharmaceuticals; *WLV,* Wyeth-Lederle vaccines; *IM,* intramuscular injection; *SQ,* subcutaneous injection.
*TriHIBit is licensed only for the fourth dose, recommended at age 15 to 18 months, in the vaccination series.
†Manufacture discontinued.

drug intramuscularly and not subcutaneously. The use of appropriate needle length is an essential component of administering vaccines. In one study, the use of a longer needle (25 mm versus 16 mm; 23 gauge versus 25 gauge, respectively) significantly decreased the incidence of localized edema and tenderness when vaccines were administered to a group of infants (Diggle and Deeks, 2000) (see Chapter 22, Intramuscular Administration).

The total series requires several injections, and every attempt is made to rotate the sites and administer the injections as painlessly as possible (see discussion on intramuscular injections in Chapter 22). When two or more injections are given at separate sites, the order of injections is arbitrary. Some practitioners suggest injecting the less painful one first. Some believe this is DTaP, whereas others suggest the MMR or Hib vaccine. Still others advocate injecting at two sites simultaneously (requiring two operators). One study found that children between the ages of 4 and 6 years rated sequential injections for immunizations vs simultaneous injections as being equally stressful (Horn and McCarthy, 1999). Parents in the study preferred simultaneous immunization injections.

Because allergic reactions can occur after injection of vaccines, appropriate precautions are taken (see Anaphylaxis, Chapter 25).

Because nurses often administer vaccines, they may have the responsibility for adequately informing parents of the nature, prevalence, and risks of the disease; the type of immunization product to be used; the expected benefits and the risk of side effects of the vaccine; and the need for accurate immunization records. Referring to immunizations as "baby shots" and limiting the discussion to vague statements about the vaccines are unacceptable practices.

Another important nursing responsibility is accurate documentation. Each child should have an immunization record for parents to keep, especially for families who move frequently. A survey of the accuracy of parental recall of children's immunizations found that parents underestimated the number of polio, DTaP, and MMR vaccines. The accuracy rate was not related to ethnic background, education level, or insurance coverage. Although immunization rates have increased significantly, health professionals should use every opportunity to encourage complete immunization of all children (see Community Focus box). Blank immunization records may be downloaded from a number of websites including the Immunization Action Coalition (www.immunize.org), which has vaccine information and records in a number of languages.

The following information is documented on the medical record: day, month, and year of administration; manufacturer and lot number of vaccine; and the name, address, and title of the person administering the vaccine. Additional data to record are the site and route of administration and evidence that the parent or legal guardian gave informed consent before the immunization was administered. Any adverse reactions after the administration of any vaccine are reported to the **Vaccine Adverse Event Reporting System.** *

An additional source of vaccine information that must be given to parents (by law; National Childhood Vaccine Injury Act, 1986) before the administration of given vaccines is the *vaccine information statement (VIS)* for the particular vaccine being administered. Practitioners are required to fully inform families of the risks and benefits of the vaccines. VISs are designed to provide updated information to the adult vaccinee or parents/legal guardians of children being vaccinated regarding the risks and benefits of each vaccine. Questions regarding the information in the VISs should be answered by the practitioner. VISs are available for the following vaccines: *anthrax, DTaP, Td, MMR, IPV, varicella, Hib, influenza, meningococcal, pneumococcal (PCV and PPV),* and *hepatitis A and B.* An updated VIS should be provided, and documentation in the patient's chart should include that the VIS was given and the publication of the VIS. VISs are available from state or local health depart-

---

*For information call (800) 822-7967; website: www.fda.gov/cber/vaers/vaers.htm.

COMMUNITY FOCUS

Improving Immunization Among Children and Adolescents

Strategies that may increase compliance include giving parents vaccine information at the time of the newborn's discharge, mailing reminder cards, making immunization services readily available, removing barriers to vaccination (such as long waiting times and appointment-only systems), and taking every opportunity to immunize children when they enter a health care facility (such as emergency departments, clinics, private offices, and hospitals).

Despite improving vaccination rates among infants and young children, **adolescents** are often incompletely immunized. An immunization update is an important part of adolescent preventive care, especially at 11 to 12 years of age. With the exception of pregnant teenagers, all adolescents should receive a second dose of the **measles, mumps,** and **rubella (MMR) vaccine** unless they have documentation of two MMR vaccinations after the first 12 months of life. All adolescents who have not previously completed the three-dose series of the **hepatitis B (HBV) vaccine** should initiate or complete the series at age 11 to 12 years.

Adolescents ages 11 to 12 years should receive a booster dose of **diphtheria-tetanus (Td) vaccine** if they have received the primary series of vaccinations and if no dose has been received during the previous 5 years. Unvaccinated adolescents who lack a reliable history of chickenpox should receive the **varicella virus vaccine** at age 11 to 12 years.

Hepatitis A vaccine should be given to adolescents who are traveling or living in countries where the hepatitis A virus is endemic or in communities with high rates of hepatitis A, chronic liver disease, intravenous drug users, or males who have sex with other males. Adolescents who have chronic disorders or underlying medical conditions that place them at high risk for complications associated with the disease, such as influenza, should receive the appropriate vaccines (see p. 341).

---

ments or the following websites: Immunization Coalition—www.immunize.org/vis/ and Centers for Disease Control and Prevention—www.cdc.gov/nip/publications/vis/.

In response to the concerns of manufacturers, practitioners, and parents of children with serious vaccine-associated injuries, the **National Childhood Vaccine Injury Act** of 1986 and the **Vaccine Compensation Amendments** of 1987 were passed. Basically, these laws are designed to provide fair compensation for children who are inadvertently injured and provide greater protection from liability for vaccine manufacturers and providers.

INJURY PREVENTION

Injuries are a major cause of death during infancy, especially for children 6 to 12 months old. According to a recent Canadian survey (Pickett and others, 2003) the top leading causes of injury to infants were falls, ingestion injuries, and burns. Constant vigilance, awareness, and supervision are essential as the child gains increased locomotor and manipulative skills that are coupled with an insatiable curiosity about the environment. Table 10-11 lists the major developmental achievements of each period during infancy and the appropriate injury prevention plan.

TABLE 10-11 ■ Injury Prevention During Infancy

AGE: BIRTH-4 MONTHS

Major Developmental Accomplishments

Involuntary reflexes, such as the crawling reflex, may propel infant forward or backward, and the startle reflex may cause the body to jerk.

May roll over

Increasing eye-hand coordination and voluntary grasp reflex

Injury Prevention

Aspiration

Not as great a danger to this age-group, but should begin practicing safeguarding early (see under Age: 4-7 Months)

Never shake baby powder directly on infant; place powder in hand and then on infant's skin; store container closed and out of infant's reach

Hold infant for feeding; do not prop bottle

Know emergency procedures for choking

Use pacifier with one-piece construction and loop handle.

Suffocation/drowning

Keep all plastic bags stored out of infant's reach; discard large plastic garment bags after tying in a knot

Do not cover mattress with plastic

Use firm mattress and loose blankets; no pillows

Make sure crib design follows federal regulations and mattress fits snugly—crib slats 2.375 inches (6 cm) apart*

Position crib away from other furniture and away from radiators

Do not tie pacifier on a string around infant's neck

Remove bibs at bedtime

Never leave infant alone in bath

Do not leave infant under 12 months alone on adult or youth mattress or "beanbag" type pillows

Falls

Always raise crib rails

Never leave infant on a raised, unguarded surface

When in doubt as to where to place child, use floor

Restrain child in infant seat and never leave child unattended while the seat is resting on a raised surface

Avoid using a high chair until child can sit well with support

Poisoning

Not as great a danger to this age-group, but should begin practicing safeguards early (see under Age: 4-7 Months)

Poisoning

Not as great a danger to this age-group, but should begin practicing safeguards early (see under Age: 4-7 Months)

Burns

Install smoke detectors in home

Use caution when warming formula in microwave oven; always check temperature of liquid before feeding

Check bathwater

Do not pour hot liquids when infant is close by, such as sitting on lap

Beware of cigarette ashes that may fall on infant

Do not leave infant in sun for more than a few minutes; keep exposed areas covered

Wash flame-retardant clothes according to label directions

Use cool-mist vaporizers

Do not leave child in parked car

Check surface heat of car restraint before placing child in seat

Motor vehicles

Transport infant in federally approved, rear-facing car seat,† preferably in back seat

Do not place infant on seat (of car) or in lap

Do not place child in a carriage or stroller behind a parked car

Do not place infant or child in front passenger seat with an air bag

Bodily damage

Avoid sharp, jagged objects

Keep diaper pins closed and away from infant

AGE: 4-7 MONTHS

Major Developmental Accomplishments

Rolls over

Sits momentarily

Grasps and manipulates small objects

Resecures a dropped object

Has well-developed eye-hand coordination

Can focus on and locate very small objects

Mouthing is very prominent

Can push up on hands and knees

Crawls backward

Injury Prevention

Aspiration

Keep buttons, beads, syringe caps, and other small objects out of infant's reach

Keep floor free of any small objects

Do not feed infant hard candy, nuts, food with pits or seeds, or whole or circular pieces of hot dog

Exercise caution when giving teething biscuits, because large chunks may be broken off and aspirated

Do not feed infant while child is lying down

Inspect toys for removable parts

Keep baby powder, if used, out of reach

Avoid storing large quantities of cleaning fluid, paints, pesticides, and other toxic substances

Discard used containers of poisonous substances

Do not store toxic substances in food containers

Discard used button-size batteries; store new batteries in safe area

Know telephone number of local poison control center (usually listed in front of telephone directory)

---

*Information on many items such as cribs or walkers available from U.S. Consumer Product Safety Commission, (800) 638-CPSC; website: www.cpsc.gov/.

†See footnote on p. 351.

Continued

TABLE 10-11 ■ Injury Prevention During Infancy—*cont'd*

AGE: 4-7 MONTHS—CONT'D
Injury Prevention—*cont'd*
Suffocation
Keep all latex balloons out of reach
Remove all crib toys that are strung across crib or playpen when child begins to push up on hands or knees or is 5 months old.

Falls
Restrain in a high chair
Keep crib rails raised to full height

Poisoning
Make sure that paint for furniture or toys does not contain lead
Place toxic substances on a high shelf or in locked cabinet
Hang plants or place on high surface rather than on floor

Burns
Keep faucets out of reach
Place hot objects (cigarettes, candles, incense) on high surface
Limit exposure to sun; apply sunscreen

Motor vehicles
See under Age: Birth-4 Months

Bodily damage
Give toys that are smooth and rounded, preferably made of wood or plastic
Avoid long, pointed objects as toys
Avoid toys that are excessively loud
Keep sharp objects out of infant's reach

AGE 8-12 MONTHS
Major Developmental Accomplishments
Crawls/creeps
Stands, holding onto furniture
Stands alone
Cruises around furniture
Walks
Climbs
Pulls on objects

Throws objects
Is able to pick up small objects; has pincer grasp
Explores by putting objects in mouth
Dislikes being restrained
Explores away from parent
Increasing understanding of simple commands and phrases

Injury Prevention
Aspiration
Keep lint and small objects off floor, furniture, and out of reach of children
Take care in feeding solid table food to ensure that very small pieces are given
Do not use beanbag toys or allow child to play with dried beans
See also under Age: 4-7 Months

Suffocation/drowning
Keep doors of ovens, dishwashers, refrigerators, coolers, and front-loading clothes washers and dryers closed at all times
If storing an unused appliance, such as a refrigerator, remove the door
Supervise contact with inflated balloons; immediately discard popped balloons, and keep uninflated balloons out of reach
Fence swimming pools
Always supervise when near any source of water, such as cleaning buckets, drainage areas, toilets
Keep bathroom doors closed
Eliminate unnecessary pools of water
Keep one hand on child at all times when in tub

Falls
Avoid walkers, especially near stairs*
Ensure that furniture is sturdy enough for child to pull self to standing position and cruise
Fence stairways at top and bottom if child has access to either end*
Dress infant in safe shoes and clothing (soles that do not "catch" on floor, tied shoelaces, pant legs that do not touch floor)
Avoid walkers, especially near stairs
Ensure that furniture is sturdy enough for child to pull self to standing position and cruise

Poisoning
Administer medications as a drug, not as a candy
Do not administer medications unless so prescribed by a practitioner
Replace medications and poisons immediately after use; replace caps properly if a child-protector cap is used
Have syrup of ipecac in home; use only if advised

Burns
Place guards in front of or around any heating appliance, fireplace, or furnace
Keep electrical wires hidden or out of reach
Place plastic guards over electrical outlets; place furniture in front of outlets
Keep hanging tablecloths out of reach (child may pull down hot liquids or heavy or sharp objects)

*Information on many items such as cribs or walkers available from U.S. Consumer Product Safety Commission, (800) 638-CPSC; website: www.cpsc.gov/.

Aspiration of Foreign Objects

Asphyxiation by foreign material in the respiratory tract, combined with mechanical suffocation, is one of the leading causes of fatal injury in children younger than 1 year of age. In at least one study, choking was the fourth leading cause of death in infants (Brenner and others, 1999). The size, shape, and consistency of foods or objects are important determinants of fatal obstruction. For example, small spheric or cylindric and pliable objects (less than 3.2 cm, or 1.25 inches) are more likely to completely obstruct the airway. Unfortunately, common household items can be deadly to infants.

As soon as infants have the ability to find their mouth, they are vulnerable to aspiration of small objects, such as those left within reach or removable parts of objects that may on initial inspection appear safe. All toys must be carefully inspected for potential danger. Rattles, for example, have small beads in them to produce noise. A broken or cracked rattle can be dangerous because the beads can easily be aspirated while the infant has the toy in the mouth. Stuffed animals are another potentially dangerous toy if any of the parts, such as the eyes or nose, are removable buttons or plastic pieces. An active infant can grab a low-hanging mobile and quickly chew off a small piece. As soon as the infant crawls or plays on the floor, the floor must be kept free of any small articles that can be picked up and swallowed, such as coins.

When infant *clothes* are purchased, the type of closure is important. A front button can easily be pulled off and swallowed. Safety pins for diapers are kept closed and away from the dressing table. Even though a young infant may not search for them, practicing this good habit from the beginning prevents future injuries.

Food items are the second most common cause of aspiration, and the most common offenders are hot dogs, candy, nuts, and grapes. When new foods are given to the child, nuts, hard candies, marshmallows, large amounts of peanut butter, or fruits with pits or seeds are avoided. When traveling (especially in airplanes) or entertaining, snack foods such as peanuts and popcorn are kept away from young children. If given to young children, hot dogs must be cut into small, irregular pieces rather than served whole or sliced into sections, because their size (diameter), round shape, and consistency allow for complete occlusion of the airway. Perhaps the most dangerous foods are dried beans, which, if aspirated, enlarge when they come in contact with the wet mucosa and block the airway.

Pacifiers can also be dangerous because the entire object may be aspirated if it is small, or the nipple and shield may become detached from the handle and become lodged in the pharynx. Improvised pacifiers, such as those made in hospitals from a padded nipple, also present dangers. The nipple may separate from the plastic collar and be aspirated. In addition, parents may continue to offer this pacifier to the infant at home. To prevent the hazards of improvised pacifiers, hospitals should use only safe commercial types. Pacifiers should not be altered from their original shape to encourage or discourage usage. Candy pacifiers pose dangers because the candy portion can dislodge from the circular base and be aspirated. To be safe, pacifiers should have:

- Sturdy, one-piece construction with material that is nontoxic, flexible, and firm but not brittle
- An easily grasped handle
- A mouthguard that cannot be separated from the nipple, has two ventilating holes, and is too large to be aspirated
- No detachable ribbon or string
- A label warning against tying the pacifier around the infant's neck

Using a syringe to accurately measure and dispense oral liquid medications to young children has become common practice. However, the *syringe cap* is a potential aspiration hazard. As a precaution, keep parts of medication devices out of the reach of children and be certain the cap is removed before dispensing medication.

Even safety devices can be dangerous. To prevent tampering, items (such as baby food jars) may be covered with a plastic oversleeve. The *tear-down strip* can be aspirated and is very difficult to locate because it is clear.

Another hazardous substance if aspirated is *baby powder*, which is usually a mixture of talc (hydrous magnesium silicate) and other silicates. Although the use of talc has been discouraged, it is a common baby care product that can cause severe and often fatal aspiration pneumonia. One of the factors involved in talc aspiration is the similar appearance of baby powder containers and nursing bottles. Talc containers often become favorite playthings and are placed in the mouth. Improperly using powder by sprinkling it directly on the skin creates a cloud of talc dust that is easily inhaled. Parents are advised of the danger of baby powder and are discouraged from using it. If they prefer to use a powder, a cornstarch preparation can be substituted (see Diaper Dermatitis, Chapter 30). Whenever a powder is used, it is placed in the hand and then applied to the skin, never shaken directly from the container to the skin. The container is kept closed and immediately stored in a safe place, especially away from curious toddlers, who often imitate caregiving activities and may accidentally shake it on the infant.

Suffocation

Mechanical suffocation includes suffocation by covering of the airway (i.e., mouth and nose), by pressure on the throat and chest, and by exclusion of air, such as by refrigerator entrapment. Nonfood items cause the majority of deaths in young children. *Latex balloons*, whether partially inflated, uninflated, or popped, are the leading cause of pediatric choking deaths from children's products. They should be kept away from infants and young children. Even the practice of inflating latex gloves to amuse children in health care settings may pose a danger, especially if the child is latex sensitive. Future deaths may be avoided by changing balloon design and materials and substituting Mylar or paper balloons.

In addition, the accessibility of the plastic linings of diapers used on the infant or on dolls is especially dangerous to young children.

The *bed* or *crib* poses a number of hazards. An infant who is placed in a bed under tucked-in blankets and sheets can be caught under them and unable to wriggle free. Baby pillows filled with plastic foam beads that make them resemble small beanbags are dangerous; very young infants are suffocated when the pillow contours to the face and blocks the airway. There are potential dangers in adults sleeping with a small infant because of the possibility of the adult rolling over and smothering the child. The incidence of accidental infant suffocation by an adult when bed sharing increased during the period from 1980 to 1997 (Drago and Dannenberg, 1999). The most common causes of infant suffocation were wedging between a bed or mattress and a wall and oronasal obstruction by a plastic bag.

> **❗NURSING ALERT**
>
> Encourage adults to:
> - Blow up balloons for children
> - Supervise children's balloon play
> - Pick up and dispose of broken balloon pieces
> - Warn older children of dangers of chewing or sucking on balloons
> - Substitute Mylar or paper balloons for latex balloons

Infant strangulation may occur if the infant's head becomes caught between the crib slats and mattress or objects close to the crib. Suffocation deaths are not confined to cribs; ill-fitting mattresses in adult or youth beds, bunk beds, and waterbeds have also been reported. According to U.S. federal regulation, the distance between crib slats should not be more than 2.375 inches (approximately 6 cm), roughly the width of three adult fingers. Mattresses and bumper pads should fit snugly against the slats. A general rule is that the mattress is too small if two adult fingers can be placed between the mattress and crib or bed side. A temporary solution is to place large, rolled towels in the space to create a snug fit.

Corner post extensions on cribs are another source of strangulation. Children have died when their clothing caught on raised corner posts as they climbed out of the crib. Voluntary manufacturing standards state that corner post extensions not exceed 0.0625 inch. However, the safety of any extension is questionable. Decorative extensions need to be removed from cribs. Ideally, information regarding correct crib design should be given prenatally, before parents have purchased or borrowed a crib.*

Mesh-sided playpens and cribs can result in death if the sides are left in the lowered position. Infants have suffocated when they fell off the edge of the mattress and the head or chest was compressed between the floorboard and mesh side. Parents should be advised of this danger and encouraged to always keep the sides locked securely in the up position whenever the child is in the playpen or crib.

The crib should be positioned away from large furniture, because children who crawl out of the crib may become caught between the two objects. Cribs should also be located away from windows, where drape or blind cords can become wrapped around the infant's neck.

Another cause of suffocation is *plastic bags.* Large plastic bags used over garments are very lightweight and can easily and quickly be wrapped around the head of an active infant or pressed against the face. For this reason, pillows and mattresses should not be covered with plastic. Older infants may play with a plastic bag and accidentally pull it over their heads. Because plastic is nonporous, suffocation occurs in a matter of minutes.

Cords (drapery or window blinds) either located near the infant or tied around the infant's neck can potentially cause strangulation. Bibs are removed at bedtime, and objects such as pacifiers are never hung on a string around the infant's neck. This is a common practice in some cultures that can be remedied by tying a *short* string to a pacifier and pinning the string to the child's shirt.

Toys that have strings attached, such as a telephone, or toys that are tied to cribs or playpens can be hazards because the string can become wrapped around the child's neck or the child can become entrapped in the toy. As a precaution, all cords should be less than 30 cm (12 inches) long. Crib toys should be hung high enough that the infant cannot become entangled in them and should no longer be used after the child is able to reach them.

If applied too loosely or left unfastened, restraining straps can be a hazard. For example, a child may slide off a high chair beneath the tray and become strangled on the loose strap. All straps should be fastened securely.

Motor Vehicle Injuries

Automobile injuries are the leading cause of accidental death in children older than 1 year of age (Motor-vehicle occupant injury, 2001). However, a significant number of infants are injured or die from improper restraint within the vehicle, most often from riding on the lap of another occupant. Reports indicate that child restraint use decreases with increasing age of children and increasing number of occupants. Lack of proper child restraint continues to be a major factor in fatal accidents involving children. All infants must be secured in a U.S. federally approved restraint rather than held or placed on the seat of the car. There is no safe alternative.

Infant restraints are designed either as an infant-only model (Fig. 10-11) or as a convertible infant-toddler model. Either restraint is a semireclined seat that faces the *rear* of the car. A rear-facing car seat provides the best protection for the disproportionately heavy head and weak neck of a young child. This position minimizes the stress on the neck by spreading the forces of a frontal crash over the entire back, neck, and head; the spine is supported by the back of the car seat. If the seat were faced forward, the head would whip forward because of the force of the crash, creating enormous stress on the neck.

The restraint is anchored to the vehicle with the vehicle's seat belt, and the restraint has a harness system for securing the infant. Some harness systems require a clip to keep the shoulder straps correctly positioned. Newer vehicles (manufactured after 1999) have tether straps or anchors that attach to the top of a car seat to better anchor the seat and minimize forward movement in the event of an accident (see

---

*A number of parent education pamphlets—such as *Crib Safety Tips* and *Is Your Used Crib Safe?*—are available in English and Spanish from the **U.S. Consumer Product Safety Commission,** Publication Request, Washington, DC 20207 (800) 638-2772; website: www.cpsc.gov. Additional free information is available from the **Danny Foundation,** 3158 Danville Boulevard, PO Box 680, Alamo, CA 94507; (800) 83-DANNY; website: www.dannyfoundation.org.

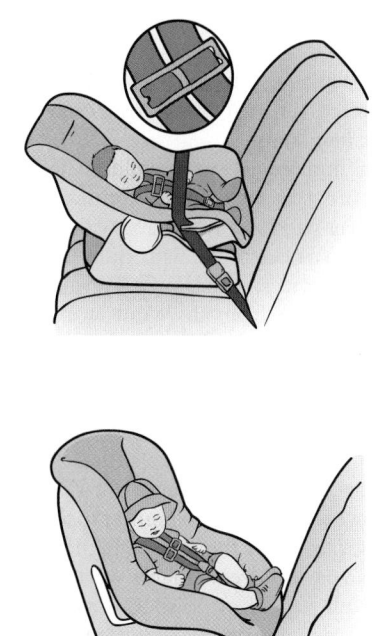

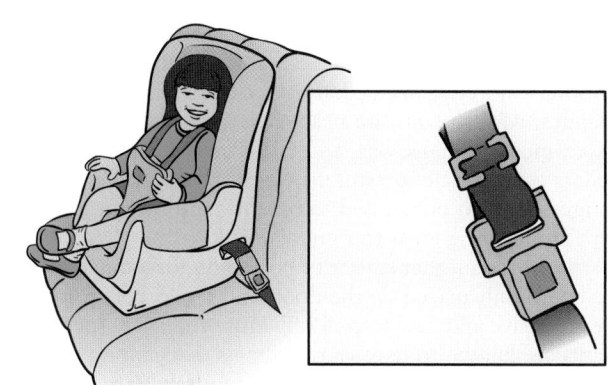

FIG. 10-11 ■ Federally approved infant car restraint. **A,** Rear-facing infant-only safety seat. **B,** Convertible seat in rear-facing position for use with infants. **C,** Convertible seat in forward-facing position for older infants and children. *Inset:* Use of locking clip.

Chapter 12, Fig. 12-11). The LATCH system provides car seat anchors between the front cushion and backrest so the seat belt does not have to be used. Some automobiles have tether anchors for rear-facing infant-only seats as well. Although many infant restraints can be recliners, they are used in the car only in the position specified by the manufacturer.

! NURSING ALERT

Infants should face the rear from birth to 20 pounds and as close to 1 year of age as possible. If the child weighs 20 pounds but is not 1 year old, the rear-facing position is still recommended.

Severe injuries and deaths in children have occurred from air bags deploying on impact in the front passenger seat. The back seat is the safest area of the car for children. If the back seat is not an option, an infant restraint may be positioned in the front seat provided that the seat belt can be locked into position and there is no passenger-side air bag. If there is a passenger-side air bag and the child has special health care needs or constant observation is recommended by the practitioner and no other adult is available to ride in the back seat with the child, an on/off switch may be installed to prevent the air bag from deploying and injuring the child riding in the front seat. Another condition that may arise is the use of vehicles without a back seat; in such cases it is best that the front passenger seat be placed as far back as possible and appropriate child safety restraint employed. With advanced technology new smart airbags will include features that make them a safer alternative for children (Kamerling, 2002).

For restraints to be effective, they must be used properly. Dressing the infant in an outfit with sleeves and legs allows the harness to hold the child securely in the seat. A small blanket or towel rolled tightly can be placed on either side of the head to minimize movement and keep the infant's hips against the back of the seat. Padding between the infant's legs and crotch is added to prevent slouching. Thick, soft padding is not placed under the infant or behind the back because during the impact the padding will compress, leaving the harness straps loose. Preterm infants being discharged home should be placed in an appropriate car seat restraint as it would be placed in the car and the infant's oxygen saturations monitored for a brief period to detect any potential problems with airway occlusion (for further discussion of car seat restraints, see Chapter 12).

! NURSING ALERT

Rear-facing infant safety seats must not be placed in the front seats of cars equipped with an air bag on the passenger side. If an infant safety seat is placed in the passenger seat with an air bag, the child could be seriously injured if the air bag is released, because rear-facing infant seats extend closer to the dashboard.*

Falls

Falls are most common after 4 months of age when the infant has learned to roll over, but they can occur at any age. The best advice is to never place a child of any age unattended on a raised surface that has no type of guardrails.

When in doubt, the safest place is the floor. Even though young infants cannot climb over a partially raised crib rail, it is best to form a habit of raising the rail all the way, because someday that infant will be able to climb out.

---

*An air bag safety fact sheet is available from the **American Academy of Pediatrics,** 141 Northwest Point Boulevard, Elk Grove Village, IL 60009; (888) 227-1770; fax: (847) 228-1281; websites: www.aap.org; for car seats, www.aap.org/family/famshop.htm; and the **Insurance Institute for Highway Safety,** 1005 N. Glebe Road, Suite 800, Arlington, VA 22201; (703) 247-1500; fax: (703) 247-1588; website: www.highwaysafety.org; the **National Highway Traffic Safety Administration,** website: www.nhtsa.org, also contains child passenger safety and air bag safety information for parents.

Crib sides should have a latching device that cannot be easily released.

Another danger area for falling is the *changing table,* which is usually high and narrow. Although these tables have a restraining belt, children are never left unattended, even when restrained. The best way to avoid needing to leave is to arrange the area with all necessary articles within easy reach so that the child is always in full sight of the caregiver. During the latter half of the first year, infants usually resist dressing and diapering and may be difficult to manage; therefore changing clothes may need to take place on a larger safe surface such as a clean floor.

Infant seats, high chairs, mobile walkers, and swings present additional opportunities for falls. If the *infant seat* is placed on a table, the child should never be left unrestrained or unattended. The same rule is essential for other baby equipment, particularly when the child has learned to crawl and to stand up. Small infants can slip through a high chair if a protective harness is not used. The danger of falls from being unrestrained also applies to shopping carts. *High chairs* are designed for older infants who can sit well and who are tall enough to have the tray at the level of their chest or abdomen. *Infant walkers* (mobile) are responsible for a number of different types of injuries that occur because the walker tipped over or fell down stairs. Parents need to be warned of these dangers and encouraged to keep a constant vigil on their child's activities; the use of older-model mobile walkers should be discouraged. The American Academy of Pediatrics (2001b) does not recommend the use of mobile infant walkers. In response to the large number of accidents and deaths associated with mobile infant walkers, several manufacturers made modifications on these products to prevent falls down stairs. The new models should have a label or sign indicating "meets new safety standard," must be wider than 36 inches, and must have a braking mechanism to stop the walker. Mobile infant walkers may still pose a risk for climbing up to reach dangerous objects and should be carefully supervised. One alternative is to use a stationary play station with a seat similar to a walker. There is no evidence that infant walkers help infants walk sooner when used.

After infants are mobile, they should not be allowed to crawl unsupervised on any raised surface, near stairs, or near any water reservoir. Gates should be used at the *bottom* and *top of stairs,* because both present dangers to the crawling and climbing infant. However, certain types of gates can present hazards. Freestanding enclosures constructed of crisscrossed wood slats that expand and contract can trap the head or neck when children attempt to climb over them. If these types of gates are used, they must be securely fastened to prevent mobility of the slats.

As children begin to pull themselves to a standing position, *heavy objects,* such as unsturdy furniture or any freestanding item (e.g., wrought iron fish tank stands, stereo equipment or television), can be extremely dangerous if pulled down on top of the child. To prevent injury from furniture tipping over, televisions should be placed on lower furniture and as far back as possible. Angle braces or anchors can secure furniture to walls.

Even when the environment is made safe, infants may sometimes literally trip over their own feet from *clothing.*

Slippery socks; hard, slick soles on shoes or rubber soles that can catch, especially on a carpet; and long pants or pajama bottoms can easily upset a child's balance. Such dangers need to be pointed out to parents, especially when infants are taking their first steps.

An alarming number of small children fall out of windows and are hurt; this is especially common with window ledges such as bay windows that have wide ledges for children to sit upon. Window screens should not be perceived as fall-prevention devices; rather, window guards should be installed to prevent falls from any window, regardless of the height. Furniture should be kept away from windows so children cannot climb onto the furniture and access the window (Feury, 2003).

Poisoning

Poisoning is one of the major causes of death in children younger than 5 years of age. The highest incidence occurs in the 2-year-old group, with the second highest incidence occurring in 1-year-old children. Infants who do not crawl are relatively free from danger of poisonous agents by virtue of immobility. However, after locomotion begins, danger from poisoning is present almost everywhere. There are more than 500 toxic substances in the average home, with approximately one third of all poisonings occurring in the kitchen.

The major reason for ingestion of poisons is *improper storage.* To protect the infant, toxic agents should not be placed on a low shelf, table, or floor. Drugs that are kept in a purse pose additional dangers; if the handbag is given to infants to play with, they may open it and ingest the drug. Another unrecognized hazard occurs during diaper changes, when infants are near many toxic substances such as ointments, creams, oils, and talc. Parents may even hand infants a potentially poisonous object to quiet them. Such dangers need to be stressed to parents, and toys need to be kept at diapering areas to minimize risks.

Plants are another source of poisoning for infants. Plants are commonly placed on the floor, and the leaves or flowers are attractive and easy to pull off. More than 700 species of plants are known to have caused illness or death.

Another danger is ingestion of the *button-sized batteries* used in devices such as hearing aids, calculators, watches, and cameras. Because they are bright and shiny, they are attractive to children. However, they can cause severe morbidity, even death, if lodged in the esophagus. The strong alkali in a battery can leak and cause a severe caustic burn. As a precaution, small batteries must be safely stored and discarded where young children cannot easily retrieve them.

Not all poisonings result from ingestion—*inhalation* is another possible route, such as inhaling chlorine vapors from household cleaning or pool supplies. Passive cocaine toxicity has occurred in young children exposed to freebase cocaine ("crack") smoking by adults.

The production of methamphetamines, a common central nervous system stimulant also known as ice, speed, or crystal, involves the use of a number of chemicals that may be toxic alone (contact or ingestion) or during the production (cooking) of the drug itself. Methamphetamine labs are common in household areas wherein children may be exposed to harmful inhalants. Mobile methamphetamine labs are also common, and children may be similarly exposed to dangerous chemicals. Methamphetamine use and exposure has been shown to cause developmental problems and short- and long-term permanent brain damage, particularly in children. Reports of the number of children exposed daily to methamphetamine labs in the United States and Canada are alarming; such children are also at high risk for abuse and neglect because their caretakers are preoccupied with production, sale, and use of the drug (Mecham and Melini, 2002). Children should be protected from environments in which inhaled toxins exist (for a discussion of passive or second-hand tobacco smoke, see Chapter 23).

The only sure way to prevent poisoning is to remove toxic agents, which means placing containers out of the infant's reach or contact. Because crawling infants soon become climbing toddlers, it is best to keep all toxic agents, especially drugs, in a locked cabinet. Special plastic hooks can be attached to the inside of cabinet doors to keep them securely closed. Firm thumb pressure is required to unlatch the hook, and small children are usually unable to manipulate them. Locks are best, but for frequently used cleaning agents, such as those often kept under a kitchen sink, hooks are a practical alternative.

With several hundred toxic substances in each house, locking up all potentially toxic substances can present a problem; however, careful planning can help. A large surplus of cleaning agents, furniture polishes, laundry additives, paints, insecticides, and solvents should be avoided. Used poison containers should be promptly discarded and not used to store another poison without adequately marking the package. Potentially hazardous substances should not be stored in any type of food container. A popular container used to store toxic liquids is a soda, or pop, bottle. A child who is unaware of the dangerous contents is a vulnerable victim for poisoning. Parents should know the location of local poison control centers and call them in the event of a suspected poisoning. Emergency measures for poisoning are discussed in Chapter 14.

Burns

Scalding from water that is too hot; excessive sunburn; and burns from house fires, electrical wires, sockets, and heating elements such as radiators, registers, and floor furnaces cause a significant number of deaths and many more injuries in infants. The infant's skin is particularly sensitive to irritation, and the mechanisms for temperature perception are not completely developed. As a general precaution, all homes should have smoke alarms installed near the bedroom areas and on each level of the building.

Scald burns from *hot tap water* can be prevented by lowering the water heater to a safe temperature of 49° C (120° F). In addition, the bathwater should be checked before the infant is immersed. Scalds can also occur from bathing infants in the kitchen sink when the garbage disposal, occluded with debris, causes the draining dishwasher effluent to back up into the sink. The temperature of the effluent from a dishwasher is typically that of the maximum water temperature of the household water heater, but many dishwashers are equipped with heating elements that heat water to a temperature that is even higher. As a precaution, instruct caregivers to avoid bathing small children in the kitchen sink while the dishwasher is running.

If formula or food is warmed in a *microwave oven,* it must be checked before feeding because the container may remain cool while the contents are hot. Another danger is explosion of the bottle from the buildup of steam. Because of these dangers, microwaving infant formula or food should be avoided or done using the guidelines in the Family Home Care box on p. 329. The handles of cooking utensils should be turned toward the back of the stove. When the infant is underfoot, pouring hot liquids and cooking with hot oil are avoided. Hanging tablecloths are also placed out of the infant's reach to prevent pulling hot items off the table.

Sunburn can be a source of a first- or second-degree burn. Exposure to direct sunlight should be avoided for the first 6 months. When infants are in the sun, the body, especially the face and head, should be covered. Sunscreen can be used on older infants but should be used on small areas of the body and sparingly in infants younger than 6 months (American Academy of Pediatrics, 1999) (see Sunburn, Chapter 30). Although dark-skinned infants burn less readily, their thin skin also can become sunburned and needs protection.

Electrical outlets should be covered with protective plastic caps that prevent the child from sucking on the outlet or putting objects such as hairpins into it. Live wires are placed out of reach so that curious infants cannot chew on them and break the rubber coating. Infants should not be allowed to play near television sets, stereo units, or other appliances, whether these units are turned on or off, because infants cannot determine when the appliance is safe.

Any *heat-producing element* should have a guard placed in front of it. Fireplaces should be well screened because they are very appealing and within easy access. Small, portable heaters should be placed on a high surface. Floor furnaces should have barrier gates to prevent children from crawling or walking over them. Burning cigarettes, candles, and incense should be kept out of reach, and infants should not be held by a smoking adult because falling ashes are a hazard, especially to the eyes. Heated-mist vaporizers are a source of burns and should not be used. If humidity is needed, only cool-mist vaporizers are safe.

By law, all infant sleepwear must be flame-retardant. Unfortunately, this does not apply to all *infant clothing.* Flame-retardant fabric must never be viewed as the ultimate protection against burns. Repeated washing reduces the flame-retardant properties, and the use of soap or bleach destroys the protection. If sleepwear is home sewn, parents are advised to look for specially treated, flame-retardant fabric.

Another type of thermal injury occurs when children are exposed to excessive heat during confinement in poorly ventilated *vehicles.* The practice of leaving the windows open a couple of inches is not protective. The nurse should caution parents never to leave children in parked cars, especially when the automobile is in direct sunlight.

Children can also be burned by overheated metal hardware and vinyl seats in cars parked in the sun. As a precaution, the surface heat of car restraints should be determined before placing children in them. Covering the restraints and hardware (such as metal latches on seat belts) may be necessary to prevent skin burns. An additional safeguard is buying a light-colored restraint, which absorbs less heat.

Drowning

Drowning in this age-group can occur in just an inch or two of water. Consequently, infants should *always* be supervised in a bathtub, hot tub, or near a source of water such as a swimming pool, lake, toilet, or bucket. In a survey of drownings most infants younger than age 1 year drowned in a toilet, bathtub, or bucket (Lassman, 2002); 5-gallon buckets are particularly dangerous because the child may inadvertently fall in head first and, because of the weight of the upper body at this age, cannot withdraw from the bucket. Organized swimming instruction is not recommended for children younger than 4 years of age, because it may lead to a false sense of security. No infant can be expected to learn the elements of water safety or to react appropriately in an emergency. Therefore, all young children need to be considered at risk when near water. Infants and toddlers are also at increased risk of infection and seizures from swallowing large amounts of water.

Bodily Damage

Injuries can occur in numerous ways. Sharp, jagged-edged objects can cause wounds in the skin. Long-pointed articles, such as the common toothpick or fork, can be poked into the eye or ear, causing serious damage. Such articles should be safely stored away from the infant's reach; forks are best avoided for self-feeding until the child has mastered the spoon, usually by age 18 months.

In addition to hazards such as aspiration, small articles can be placed in the ear or nose, and excessive noise from toys can result in sensorineural hearing loss. Although toys with the highest noise levels are model airplanes, air guns, and toy cap guns, even common squeaking toys used by young children may be harmful if placed close to the ear.

Even clothes and hair can present dangers to infants who cannot call attention to the problem. For example, constriction injuries can occur from excessively tight bands on socks, as well as fibers of hair or thread wrapped tightly around appendages, usually toes or fingers.

A disturbing trend is the increasing amount of infant deaths attributed to homicide. In one study 6.4% of 10,370 infant injury deaths occurred as a result of homicide (Brenner and others, 1999). Specific interventions must be set in place to protect infants from harm, especially in preventable situations.

Another commonly unrecognized danger to infants is animal attacks. As newcomers to the home, infants can provoke jealousy in animals such as dogs or cats or play with pets unaware of the danger. Parents must be constantly vigilant to protect the child from household pets and farm animals (see Animal Bites, Chapter 30).

Nurse's Role in Injury Prevention

The task of injury prevention begins to be appreciated only when the potential environmental dangers to which infants are vulnerable are considered. Nurses must be aware of the possible causes of injury in each age-group for *anticipatory* preventive teaching to occur. For example, the guidelines for injury prevention during infancy presented in Table 10-11 should be discussed *before* the child reaches the susceptible age-group. Preventive teaching ideally occurs during pregnancy. Two thirds of all injuries to children occur in the home, and therefore the importance of safety cannot be overemphasized. The Family Home Care box on p. 355 summarizes a home safety checklist that can be presented to parents to increase their awareness of danger areas in the home and assist them in implementing safety devices and practices *before* their absence can inflict injury on infants. In addition, displays such as a safety demonstration board can be helpful in familiarizing parents with inexpensive commercial devices that can be used in the home to prevent injuries.

Injury prevention requires protection of the child and education of the caregiver. Nurses in ambulatory care settings, health maintenance centers, or visiting nurse agencies are in a most favorable position for injury education. This does not exclude nurses in inpatient facilities, who could use visiting times as an excellent opportunity for discussing this topic. Although early postpartum discharge may be restrictive for parent teaching, this is an excellent opportunity to introduce the family to infant safety and safety for other children as well. Parents should be encouraged to take an infant cardiopulmonary resuscitation class to deal effectively with potential problems. This tool further empowers the parents to raise their new infant in the best environment possible.

One approach to teaching injury prevention is to relate why children in various age-groups are prone to specific types of injuries. Stressing prevention is just as important as emphasizing the *why* of the injury. However, injury prevention must also be practical. Asking parents for their ideas leads to realistic suggestions that can be followed. For instance, bathroom cleaning agents, cosmetics, and personal care items can be placed on a top shelf in the linen closet, and towels or sheets can be stored on the lower shelves and floor.

If an injury has occurred, the nurse should not be too quick to admonish the parent. Injuries do not always indicate neglect. It is a difficult task to watch children carefully without overprotecting or unnecessarily confining them. Small falls help children learn the dangers of heights. Touching a hot object once can emphasize to the child the pain of a burn. Allowing children to explore while maintaining consistent, age-appropriate limits is sound advice.

Parents need to remember that infants and young children cannot anticipate danger or understand when it is or is not present. A dead electrical wire may present no actual harm, but if the child is allowed to play with it, a poor behavior is enforced and will be practiced when the child encounters a live wire. Although it is always wise to explain why something is dangerous, it must be remembered that small children need to be physically removed from the situation.

It is not easy to teach safety, supervise closely, and refrain from saying "no" a hundred times a day. Parents become acutely aware of this dilemma as soon as the infant learns to crawl. Preventing injuries to children is usually the first reason for limit setting and discipline, but limits are also set to prevent damage to valuable household objects. When small children are in the home, dangerous objects must be removed or guarded and valuable articles placed out of reach.

When children are taught the meaning of "no," they should also be taught what "yes" means. Children should be praised for playing with suitable toys, their efforts at behaving or listening should be reinforced, and innovative and

FAMILY HOME CARE

Child Safety Home Checklist

SAFETY: FIRE, ELECTRICAL, BURNS

❑ Guards in front of or around any heating appliance, fireplace, or furnace (including floor furnace)*

❑ Electrical wires hidden or out of reach*

❑ No frayed or broken wires; no overloaded sockets

❑ Plastic guards or caps over electrical outlets, furniture in front of outlets*

❑ Hanging tablecloths out of reach, away from open fires*

❑ Smoke detectors tested and operating properly

❑ Kitchen matches stored out of child's reach*

❑ Large, deep ashtrays throughout house (if used)

❑ Small stoves, heaters, and other hot objects (cigarettes, candles, coffee pots, slow cookers) placed where they cannot be tipped over or reached by children

❑ Hot water heater set at 49° C (120° F) or lower

❑ Pot handles turned toward back of stove, center of table

❑ No loose clothing worn near stove

❑ No cooking or eating hot foods or liquids with child standing nearby or sitting in lap

❑ All small appliances, such as iron, turned off, disconnected, and placed out of reach when not in use

❑ Cool, not hot, mist vaporizer used

❑ Fire extinguisher available on each floor and checked periodically

❑ Electrical fuse box and gas shutoff accessible

❑ Family escape plan in case of a fire practiced periodically; fire escape ladder available on upper-level floors

❑ Telephone number of fire or rescue squad and address of home with nearest cross street posted near phone

SAFETY: SUFFOCATION AND ASPIRATION

❑ Small objects stored out of reach*

❑ Toys inspected for small removable parts or long strings*

❑ Hanging crib toys and mobiles placed out of reach

❑ Plastic bags stored away from young child's reach, large plastic garment bags discarded after tying in knots*

❑ Mattress or pillow not covered with plastic or in manner accessible to child*

❑ Crib design according to federal regulations (crib slats less than 2.375 inches [6 cm] apart) with snug-fitting mattress*†

❑ Crib positioned away from other furniture or windows*

❑ Portable playpen gates up at all times while in use*

❑ Accordion-style gates not used*

❑ Bathroom doors kept closed and toilet seats down*

❑ Faucets turned off firmly*

❑ Pool fenced with locked gate

❑ Proper safety equipment at poolside

❑ Electric garage door openers stored safely and garage door adjusted to rise when door strikes object

❑ Doors of ovens, trunks, dishwashers, refrigerators, and front-loading clothes washers and dryers kept closed*

❑ Unused appliance, such as a refrigerator, securely closed with lock or doors removed*

❑ Food served in small, noncylindric pieces*

❑ Toy chests without lids or with lids that securely lock in open position*

❑ Buckets and wading pools kept empty when not in use*

❑ Clothesline above head level

❑ At least one member of household trained in basic life support (cardiopulmonary resuscitation) including first aid for choking

SAFETY: POISONING

❑ Toxic substances, including batteries, placed on a high shelf, preferably in locked cabinet

❑ Toxic plants hung or placed out of reach*

❑ Excess quantities of cleaning fluid, paints, pesticides, drugs, and other toxic substances not stored in home

❑ Used containers of poisonous substances discarded where child cannot obtain access

❑ Telephone number of local poison control center and address of home with nearest cross street posted near phone

❑ Medicines clearly labeled in childproof containers and stored out of reach

❑ Household cleaners, disinfectants, and insecticides kept in their original containers, separate from food and out of reach

❑ Smoking in areas away from children

SAFETY: FALLS

❑ Nonskid mats, strips, or surfaces in tubs and showers

❑ Exits, halls, and passageways in rooms kept clear of toys, furniture, boxes, or other items that could be obstructive

❑ Stairs and halls well lighted, with switches at both top and bottom

❑ Sturdy handrails for all steps and stairways

❑ Nothing stored on stairways

❑ Treads, risers, and carpeting in good repair

❑ Glass doors and walls marked with decals

❑ Safety glass used in doors, windows, and walls

❑ Gates on top and bottom of staircases and elevated areas, such as porch, fire escape*

❑ Guardrails on upstairs windows with locks that limit height of window opening and access to areas such as fire escape*

❑ Crib side rails raised to full height; mattress lowered as child grows*

❑ Restraints used in high chairs, walkers, or other baby furniture; preferably walkers not used*

❑ Scatter rugs secured in place or used with nonskid backing

❑ Walks, patios, and driveways in good repair

SAFETY: BODILY INJURY

❑ Knives, power tools, and unloaded firearms stored safely or placed in locked cabinet

❑ Garden tools returned to storage racks after use

❑ Pets properly restrained and immunized for rabies

❑ Swings, slides, and other outdoor play equipment kept in safe condition

❑ Yard free of broken glass, nail-studded boards, other litter

❑ Cement birdbaths placed where young child cannot tip them over*

*Safety measures are specific for homes with young children. All safety measures should be implemented in homes where children reside and visit frequently, such as those of grandparents or baby-sitters.

†Federal regulations are available from U.S. Consumer Product Safety Commission, (800) 638-CPSC; website: www.cpsc.gov.

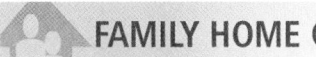

FAMILY HOME CARE

Guidance During Infant's First Year

FIRST 6 MONTHS

Teach car safety with use of federally approved restraint, facing rearward, in the middle of the back seat—not in a seat with an air bag.

Understand each parent's adjustment to newborn, especially mother's postpartal emotional needs.

Teach care of infant and help parents to understand his or her individual needs and temperament and that the infant expresses wants through crying.

Reassure parents that infant cannot be spoiled by too much attention during the first 4 to 6 months.

Encourage parents to establish a schedule that meets needs of child and themselves.

Help parents understand infant's need for stimulation in environment.

Support parents' pleasure in seeing child's growing friendliness and social response, especially smiling.

Plan anticipatory guidance for safety.

Stress need for immunization.

Prepare for introduction of solid foods.

SECOND 6 MONTHS

Prepare parents for child's "stranger anxiety."

Encourage parents to allow child to cling to them and avoid long separation from either.

Guide parents concerning discipline because of infant's increasing mobility.

Encourage use of negative voice and eye contact rather than physical punishment as a means of discipline.

Encourage showing most attention when infant is behaving well, rather than when infant is crying.

Teach injury prevention because of child's advancing motor skills and curiosity.

Encourage parents to leave child with suitable caregiver to allow some free time.

Discuss readiness for weaning.

Explore parents' feelings regarding infant's sleep patterns.

---

creative recreational toys should be provided for them. Infants love to tear paper and avidly pursue books, magazines, or newspapers left on the floor. Instead of always scolding them for destroying a valued book, child-safe books (such as those constructed of fabric) can be kept available for them to play with. If they enjoy pots and pans, a cabinet can be arranged with safe utensils for them to explore.

One additional factor must be stressed concerning injury prevention and education. Children are imitators; they copy what they see and hear. *Practicing safety teaches safety,* which applies to parents and their children and to nurses and their clients. Saying one thing but doing another confuses children and can lead to difficulties as the child grows older.

ANTICIPATORY GUIDANCE—CARE OF FAMILIES

Childrearing is no easy task; it presents challenges to both new parents and "seasoned" parents. With society's changing roles and mores, combined with a highly mobile popu-

lation, there is little stability for traditional role models and time-honored methods of raising children. As a result, parents look to professionals for guidance. Nurses are in an advantageous position to render assistance and suggestions. Every phase of a child's life has its particular traumas-toilet training for toddlers, unexplained fears for preschoolers, and identity crises for adolescents. For parents of an infant some challenges center around dependency, discipline, increased mobility, and safety. Major areas for parental guidance during the first year are listed in the Family Home Care box at left.

KEY POINTS

- Biologic development of the child encompasses proportional changes; sensory changes, including binocularity, depth perception, and visual preference; maturation of biologic systems; fine motor development; and gross motor development.

- Erikson's theory of psychosocial development (birth to 1 year) is concerned with acquiring a sense of trust while overcoming a sense of mistrust.

- Piaget's theory of cognitive development, as it applies to the infant, focuses on the sensorimotor phase, which includes the use of reflexes, primary circular reactions, secondary circular reactions, and coordination or secondary schemata and their application to new situations.

- Development of body image begins in infancy; by 1 year of age infants recognize that they are distinct from their parents.

- Social development of the infant is guided by attachment, language development, personal-social behavior, and participation in play.

- Temperament influences the type of interaction that occurs between the child and parents and siblings.

- Parents are faced with many concerns, including infant fears, day care, limit setting and discipline, thumb sucking and pacifier use, teething, and choice of infant shoes.

- Breast milk or formula is the most desirable food for the infant during the first 6 months, followed by gradual introduction of solid food during the second 6 months. Whole milk is not recommended until after 12 months.

- Common sleep problems that develop during infancy—and that are easily prevented—are associated with night crying and feeding. Nurses should instruct the parents, after careful assessment, in strategies to deal with the specific problem.

- Cleaning the teeth regularly and appropriate dietary intake promote good dental health.

- Recommended routine immunizations include those for hepatitis B virus, hepatitis A (in some states), diphtheria, tetanus, pertussis, polio, measles, mumps, rubella, chickenpox, pneumococcal conjugate vaccine, and *Haemophilus influenzae* type b.

- Recommended immunizations for selected groups of children are influenza virus, Lyme, hepatitis A, and meningococcal vaccines.

- Because injuries are a major cause of death during infancy, parents should be alerted to aspiration of foreign objects, suffocation, falls, poisoning, burns, motor vehicle injuries, and bodily damage, as well as preventive actions needed to make the environment safe for infants.

References

American Academy of Pediatrics: Prevention of rickets and vitamin D deficiency: new guidelines for vitamin D intake, *Pediatrics* 111(4): 908-910, 2003a.

American Academy of Pediatrics, Committee on Environmental Health: Ultraviolet light: a hazard to children, *Pediatrics* 104(2): 328-333, 1999.

American Academy of Pediatrics, Committee on Infectious Diseases, Pickering L, editor: *2003 Red Book: report of the Committee on Infectious Diseases,* ed 26, Elk Grove Village, Il, 2003c, The Academy.

American Academy of Pediatrics, Committee on Infectious Diseases: Recommended childhood and adolescent immunization schedule—United States, January-June, 2004, *Pediatrics* 113(1):142-143, 2004.

American Academy of Pediatrics, Committee on Injury and Poison Prevention: Injuries associated with infant walkers, *Pediatrics* 108(3):790-792, 2001b.

American Academy of Pediatrics, Committee on Nutrition: *Pediatric nutrition handbook,* ed 5, Elk Grove Village, Il, 2004, The Academy.

American Academy of Pediatrics, Committee on Nutrition: The use and misuse of fruit juice in pediatrics, *Pediatrics* 107(5):1210-1213, 2001a.

American Academy of Pediatrics, Committee on Sports Medicine: Infant exercise programs, *Pediatrics* 82(5):800, 1988.

American Academy of Pediatrics, Section on Pediatric Dentistry: Oral health risk assessment timing and establishment of the dental home, *Pediatrics* 111(5):1113-1116, 2003b.

American Academy of Pediatrics, Task Force on Infant Sleep Position and Sudden Infant Death Syndrome: Changing concepts of sudden infant death syndrome: implications for infant sleeping environment and sleep position, *Pediatrics* 105(3):650-656, 2000.

Bechtel B: Intranasal influenza vaccine granted approval by FDA, *Infect Dis Child* 16(7):3, 9, 2003.

Biancuzzo M: *Breastfeeding the newborn: clinical strategies for nurses,* St Louis, 1999, Mosby.

Brazelton T: Parent-infant cosleeping revisited, *Brazelton Center Newslett* vol 2, Boston, 1990.

Brenner RA and others: Deaths attributable to injuries in infants, United States, 1983-1991, *Pediatrics* 103(5):968-974, 1999.

Calamaro CJ: Infant nutrition in the first year of life: tradition or science? *Pediatr Nurs* 26(2):211-215, 2000.

Campion EW: Suspicions about the safety of vaccines, *N Engl J Med* 347(19):1474-1475, 2002.

Carey WB, McDevitt SC: Revision of the infant temperament questionnaire, *Pediatrics* 61(5):735-739, 1978.

Corbett-Dick P, Bezek SK: Breastfeeding promotion for the employed mother, *J Pediatr Health Care* 11(1):12-19, 1997.

Dales L, Hammer SJ, Smith NJ: Time trends in autism and in MMR immunization coverage in California, *JAMA* 285(9):1183-1185, 2001.

Dennison BA, Rockwell HL, Baker SL: Excess fruit juice consumption by preschool-aged children is associated with short stature and obesity, *Pediatrics* 99(1):15-22, 1997.

Dewey KG: Nutrition, growth, and complementary feeding of the breastfed infant, *Pediatr Clin North Am* 48(1):87-104, 2001.

Diggle L, Deeks J: Effect of needle length on incidence of local reactions to routine immunizations in infants aged 4 months: randomized controlled trial, *BMJ* 321(7266):931-993, 2000.

Drago DA, Dannenberg AL: Infant mechanical suffocating deaths in the United States, 1980-1997, *Pediatrics* 103(5):e59, 1999.

Duro D and others: Association between infantile colic and carbohydrate malabsorption from fruit juices in infancy, *Pediatrics* 109(5): 797-805, 2002.

Ferber R, Kryger M: *Principles and practice of sleep medicine in the child,* Philadelphia, 1995, WB Saunders.

Feury KJ: Injury prevention: where are the resources? *Orthop Nurs* 22(2):124-130, 2003.

Hauck FR and others: Sleep environment and the risk of sudden infant death syndrome in an urban population: the Chicago Infant Mortality Study, *Pediatrics* 111(5 part 2):1207-1214, 2003.

Hawkins-Walsh E: A behavioural infant sleep intervention resolved sleep problems, *Evidence-Based Nurs* 6(1):10-12, 2003.

Hiscock H, Wake M: Infant sleep problems and postnatal depression: a community-based study, *Pediatrics* 107(6):1317-1322, 2001.

Hobbie C, Baker S, Bayerl C: Parental misunderstanding of basic infant nutrition: misinformed feeding choices, *J Pediatr Health Care* 14(1):26-31, 2000.

Horn MI, McCarthy AM: Children's responses to sequential versus simultaneous immunization injections, *J Pediatr Health Care* 13(1): 18-23, 1999.

Hughes MB and others: Temperament characteristics of premature infants in the first year of life, *J Dev Behav Pediatr* 23(6):430-435, 2002.

Johns RM, Miller L, Hochstetler J: Mother and baby dental care, *Mother Baby J* 3(3):15-22, 1998.

Kamerling SN: Airbags & children: making correct choices in child passenger restraints, *MCN* 27(5):264-273, 2002.

Koslap-Petraco MB, Parsons T: Communicating the benefits of combination vaccines to parents and health care providers, *J Pediatr Health Care* 17(2):53-57, 2003.

Langkamp DL, Kim Y, Pascoe JM: Temperament of preterm infants at 4 months of age: maternal ratings and perceptions, *J Dev Behav Pediatr* 19(6):391-396, 1998.

Langkamp DL, Pascoe JM: Temperament of pre-term infants at 9 months of age, *Amb Child Health* 7(3/4):203-212, 2001.

Lassman J: Water safety, *J Emerg Nurs* 28(3):241-243, 2002.

Lawrence RA, Lawrence RM: *Breastfeeding: a guide for the medical profession,* ed 5, St Louis, 1999, Mosby.

Loman DG: The use of complementary and alternative health care practices among children, *J Pediatr Health Care* 17(2):58-63, 2003.

Mecham N, Melini J: Unintentional victims: development of a protocol for the care of children exposed to chemicals at methamphetamine laboratories, *Pediatr Emerg Care* 18(4):327-332, 2002.

Medoff-Cooper B: Infant temperament: implications for parenting from birth through 1 year, *J Pediatr Nurs* 10(3):141-145, 1995.

Medoff-Cooper B, Carey WB, McDevitt SC: The early infancy temperament questionnaire, *J Dev Behav Pediatr* 14(4):230-235, 1993.

MMWR: Preventing pneumococcal disease among infants: recommendations of the Advisory Committee on Immunization Practices, *MMWR* 49(RR09):1-38, 2000.

Motor-vehicle occupant injury: strategies for increasing use of child safety seats, increasing use of safety belts, and reducing alcohol-impaired driving, *MMWR* 50 (RR7):1-13, 2001.

Moukarzel AA, Lesicka H, Ament ME: Irritable bowel syndrome and nonspecific diarrhea in infancy and childhood—relationship with juice carbohydrate malabsorption, *Clin Pediatr* 41(3):145-150, 2002.

Niemela M, Uhari M, Mottonen M: A pacifier increases the risk of recurrent acute otitis media in children in day care centers, *Pediatrics* 96(5 pt 1):884-888, 1995.

Niemela M and others: Pacifier as a risk factor for acute otitis media: a randomized, controlled trial of parental counseling, *Pediatrics* 106(3):483-488, 2000.

Nowak AJ, Warren JJ: Infant oral health and oral habits, *Pediatr Clin North Am* 47(5):1043-1066, 2000.

Oghi S and others: Comparison of kangaroo care and standard care: behavioral organization, development, and temperament in healthy, low-birth-weight infants through 1 year, *J Perinatol* 22(5):374-379, 2002.

Person TL, Lavezzi WA, Wolf BC: Cosleeping and sudden unexpected death in infancy, *Arch Pathol Lab Med* 126(3):343-345, 2002.

Pickett W and others: Injuries experienced by infant children: a population-based epidemiological analysis, *Pediatrics* 111(4 pt 1): e365-370, 2003.

Pickler R, Frankel H: The effect of non-nutritive sucking on preterm infants' behavioral organization and feeding performance, *Neonat Netw* 14(2):83, 1995.

Pinelli J, Symington A: Non-nutritive sucking for promoting physiologic stability and nutrition in preterm infants, *Cochrane Database Syst Rev* 2000(2):CD 001071, 2000.

Pinelli J, Symington A, Ciliska D: Nonnutritive sucking in high-risk infants: benign intervention or legitimate therapy? *JOGNN* 31(5): 582-591, 2002.

Prevention of hepatitis A through active or passive immunization: recommendations of the Advisory Committee on Immunization Practices (ACIP), *MMWR* 48(RR12):1-37, 1999.

Schachter F and others: Cosleeping and sleep problems in Hispanic-American urban young children, *Pediatrics* 84(3):522-530, 1989.

Skinner JD and others: Fruit juice is not related to children's growth, *Pediatrics* 103(1):58-64, 1999.

Smith MM, Lifshitz F: Excess fruit juice consumption as a contributing factor in nonorganic failure to thrive, *Pediatrics* 93(3):438-443, 1994.

Van Norman RA: Why we can't afford to ignore prolonged digit-sucking, *Contemp Pediatr* 18(6):61-81, 2001.

Wilson D, Bowman C: Infant nutrition: building blocks for the future, Mother Baby J 5(4):17-21, 2000.

Wilson ME and others: Family dynamics, parental-fetal attachment and infant temperament, *J Adv Nurs* 31(1):204-210, 2000.

Zuckerman JN, Cockcroft A, Zuckerman AJ: Site of injection for vaccination, *BMJ* 305(6862):1158, 1992.

Health Problems of Infants

DAVID WILSON

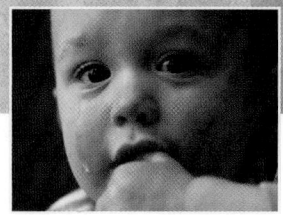
http://evolve.elsevier.com/Wong/essentials/

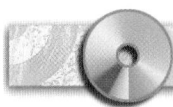
Remember to check out your companion CD-ROM

CHAPTER OUTLINE

RELATED TOPICS and ADDITIONAL RESOURCES

 IN TEXT

 CD COMPANION

Case Study—Health Problems of Infants
Guidelines—Feeding Children With
   Nonorganic Failure to Thrive
Clinical Manifestations of Cow's-Milk
   Sensitivity
Nursing Care Plan
NCLEX-Style Review Questions

 WEBSITE

WebLinks
NCLEX-Style Review Questions

 WONG'S CLINICAL MANUAL
OF PEDIATRIC NURSING, 6/E

Community and Home Care
   Instructions—Apnea Monitoring, CPR
Nursing Care Plan

- Identify children at increased risk of developing nutritional disturbances.
- Outline a nutritional counseling plan for vitamin or mineral deficiency or excess.
- Outline a dietary plan for parents when the infant is sensitive to milk.
- List measures that can be used to alleviate colic.
- Plan nursing care that meets the physical and emotional needs of the nonorganic failure-to-thrive child and parent.
- Provide nursing care that meets the immediate and long-term needs of the family who has lost a child from sudden infant death syndrome.
- Identify the stresses and needs of the family whose child is home monitored for apnea.

NUTRITIONAL DISTURBANCES

VITAMIN DISTURBANCES

Although true vitamin deficiencies are rare in the United States, subclinical deficiencies are commonly seen in population subgroups in which either maternal or child dietary intake of foods containing adequate amounts of vitamins is imbalanced. Vitamin D–deficiency rickets, once rarely seen because of vitamin D–fortified milk, has increased. Populations at risk include (1) children breast-fed by mothers with an inadequate intake of vitamin D or who are breast-fed longer than 6 months without adequate maternal vitamin D intake or supplementation; (2) children who are exposed to minimal sunlight because of their particular clothing, religious, or cultural beliefs, housing in areas of high pollution, or dark skin pigmentation; (3) those with diets that are low in sources of vitamin D and calcium; and (4) individuals who use milk products not supplemented with vitamin D (e.g., yogurt, raw cow's milk) as the primary source of milk. Thus the American Academy of Pediatrics (2003a) now recommends that infants who are exclusively breast-fed begin to receive 200 IU of vitamin D by age 2 months. Furthermore, children who have minimal sun exposure, do not consume at least 500 mL of vitamin D–fortified milk, or are not taking a vitamin supplement with vitamin D, should take vitamin D supplements daily to prevent rickets and vitamin D deficiency. The 200 IU of vitamin D may be obtained by taking a multivitamin supplement containing 400 IU vitamin D per mL or per tablet (American Academy of Pediatrics, 2003a). Inadequate maternal ingestion of cobalamin (vitamin B_{12}) may contribute to infant neurologic impairment when exclusive breast-feeding (past 6 months) is the only source of the infant's nutrition (MMWR, 2003).

Children may also be at risk secondary to disorders or their treatment. For example, vitamin deficiencies of the fat-soluble vitamins A and D may occur in malabsorptive disorders. Preterm infants may develop rickets in the second month of life as a result of inadequate intake of vitamin D, calcium, and phosphorous. Children receiving high doses of salicylates, such as for rheumatoid arthritis, may have impaired vitamin C storage. Environmental tobacco smoke exposure has been implicated with decreased concentrations of ascorbate in children; therefore increased intake of sources of vitamin C should be encouraged even in children minimally exposed to environmental tobacco smoke (Preston and others, 2003). Children with chronic illnesses resulting in anorexia, decreased food intake, or possible nutrient malabsorption as a result of multiple medications should be carefully evaluated for adequate vitamin and mineral intake in some form (parenteral or enteral).

Vitamin A deficiency correlates with increased morbidity and mortality in children with measles. Complications from diarrhea and infections are often increased in infants and children with vitamin A deficiency. The American Academy of Pediatrics (2003b) recommends that vitamin A supplementation be considered in children hospitalized with measles and associated complications (diarrhea, croup, pneumonia), especially children between the ages of 6 months and 2 years.

Of particular concern is the overuse of vitamins as a part of *complementary and alternative medicine.* One recent survey found that a relatively small group of parents routinely gave their children megavitamin therapy; however, the researcher recommends further research to ascertain a more realistic number of children using multivitamin preparations (Loman, 2003). There is concern among health care workers that terms often used to market supplements such as megavitamins may mislead parents regarding the actual benefits (or harm) of such therapies. The intention herein is not to discredit the use of complementary and alternative medicine such as vitamin supplements; rather, it is to ensure safety and efficacy in children who may experience inadvertent harm. The use of various herbal therapies, or intake of herbs, is also becoming more popular; many of these have been a part of medicine since early days and are beneficial in some cases. Herbs known to have adverse effects in children include ephedra, comfrey, and pennyroyal; some herbs may not be harmful taken alone but may counteract or potentiate prescription medications when taken together (Loman, 2003). Parents should be fully cognizant of the use of herbs to ensure that there is more benefit than potential harm in the ingredient being used. Health care workers also need to be knowledgeable of the benefits or potential harm in herbs to appropriately counsel parents and address their concerns. Little research has been performed in children on many over-the-counter herbal medicines (Westerdahl, 1999), yet some herbs are known to cause harm in children (Kemper and Gardiner, 2004; Lanski and others, 2003 Loman, 2003). Parents should be cautioned not to exceed the upper limits of vitamin intake according to the new Dietary Reference Intakes (See DRIs, p. 371, and RDAs in Appendix F).*

---

*Helpful websites for health care and consumer information concerning herbs are: **National Center for Complementary and Alternative Medicine:** www.nccam.nih.gov; **American Botanical Council:** www.herbalgram.org; and **Herb Research Foundation:** www.herbs.org.

An excessive dose of a vitamin is generally defined as 10 or more times the recommended dietary allowance, although the fat-soluble vitamins, especially A and D, tend to cause toxic reactions at lower doses. With the addition of vitamins to commercially prepared foods, the potential for hypervitaminosis has increased, especially when combined with the excessive use of vitamin supplements. Hypervitaminosis of A and D presents the greatest problems, because these fat-soluble vitamins are stored in the body. Vitamin D is the most likely of all vitamins to cause toxic reactions in relatively small overdoses. The water-soluble vitamins, primarily niacin, B_6, and C, can also cause toxicity. Poor outcomes in infants have been associated with megavitamin therapy, namely a fatal hypermagnesemia, as a result of high doses of magnesium oxide (McGuire, Kulkarni, and Baden, 2000), and severe anemia and thrombocytopenia resulting from megadoses of vitamin A (Perrotta and others, 2002).

One vitamin supplement that is recommended for all women of childbearing age is a daily dose of 0.4 mg of folic acid, the usual recommended dietary allowance (RDA). Folic acid taken before conception and during early pregnancy can reduce the risk of neural tube defects such as spina bifida by as much as 70%. Drugs such as oral contraceptives and antidepressants may decrease folic acid absorption; thus adolescent females taking such medications should consider supplementation.

Deficiencies and excesses of vitamins A, B complex, C, D, E, and K are summarized in Table 11-1, and the RDAs are listed in Appendix F. General nursing considerations are discussed below, and specific interventions are presented in Table 11-1.

MINERAL DISTURBANCES

A number of minerals are essential nutrients. The *macrominerals* refer to those with daily requirements greater than 100 mg and include calcium, phosphorus, magnesium, sodium, potassium, chloride, and sulfur. *Microminerals*, or *trace elements*, have daily requirements of less than 100 mg and include several essential minerals and those whose exact role in nutrition is still unclear. The greatest concern with minerals is deficiency, especially iron, calcium, phosphorus, magnesium, and zinc. Low levels of zinc can cause nutritional failure to thrive. *Text continues on p. 366*

TABLE 11-1 ■ Vitamins and Their Nutritional Significance

PHYSIOLOGIC FUNCTIONS/SOURCES	RESULTS OF DEFICIENCY OR EXCESS	NURSING CONSIDERATIONS
VITAMIN A (RETINOL)* **Functions** Necessary component in formation of pigment rhodopsin (visual purple) Formation and maintenance of epithelial tissue Normal bone growth and tooth development Needed for growth and spermatogenesis Involved in thyroxine formation Antioxidant	**Deficiency** Night blindness Keratinization (hardening and scaling) of epithelium Xerophthalmia (hardening and scaling of cornea and conjunctiva) Phrynoderma (toad skin) Drying of respiratory, gastrointestinal, and genitourinary tracts Defective tooth enamel Retarded growth Impaired bone formation Decreased thyroxine formation Decreased resistance to infections	Encourage foods rich in vitamin A, such as whole cow's milk. As milk consumption decreases, encourage foods rich in vitamin A. Ensure adequate intake in preterm infants. Advise parents of safe use of supplements in child with measles.
Sources *Natural form*—Liver, kidney, fish oils, milk and nonskim milk products, egg yolk *Provitamin A (carotene)*—Carrots, sweet potatoes, squash, apricots, spinach, collards, broccoli, cabbage, artichokes	**Excess** *Early signs*—Irritability, anorexia, pruritus, fissures at corners of nose and lips *Later signs*—Hepatomegaly, jaundice, retarded growth, poor weight gain, thickening of the cortex of long bones with pain and fragility, hard tender lumps in extremities and occiput of the skull Can cause birth defects if excessive maternal intake NOTE: Overdose results from ingestion of large quantities of the vitamin only, not the provitamin; large amounts of carotene (carotenemia) cause yellow or orange discoloration of the skin (not the sclera, urine, or feces as in jaundice) but none of the above symptoms.	Emphasize correct use of vitamin supplements and potential hazards of excess. Investigate child's dietary habits to calculate approximate intake; if excessive, remove supplemental source (e.g., daily feeding of liver). Advise parents of the benign nature of carotenemia; treatment is avoidance of excess pigmented fruits or vegetables, especially carrots; skin color returns to normal in 2 to 6 weeks.

*Fat soluble.

Continued

TABLE 11-1 ■ Vitamins and Their Nutritional Significance—*cont'd*

PHYSIOLOGIC FUNCTIONS/SOURCES	RESULTS OF DEFICIENCY OR EXCESS	NURSING CONSIDERATIONS
VITAMIN B₁ (THIAMIN)‡		
Functions	**Deficiency**	
Coenzyme (with phosphorus) in carbohydrate metabolism	*Gastrointestinal*—Anorexia, constipation, indigestion	
Needed for healthy nervous system	*Neurologic*—Apathy, fatigue, emotional instability, polyneuritis, tenderness of calf muscles, partial anesthesia, muscle weakness, paresthesia, hyperesthesia, decreased or absent tendon reflexes, convulsions, coma (in infants)	
Digestion and normal appetite	*Cardiovascular*—Palpitations, cardiac failure, peripheral vasodilation, edema	
Sources	**Excess**	**Vitamin B complex**
Pork, beef, liver, legumes, nuts, whole or enriched grains and cereals, green vegetables,† fruits, milk, brown rice	Headache	Encourage foods rich in B vitamins.
	Irritability	Stress proper cooking and storage techniques to preserve potency, such as minimum cooking of vegetables in small amount of liquid, storage of milk in opaque container.
	Insomnia	
	Rapid pulse	
	Weakness	Advise against fad diets that severely restrict groups of food, such as vegetarianism (vegans or macrobiotics).
		Explore need for vitamin supplements when dieting, when using goat milk exclusively for infant feeding (deficient in folic acid), or when the breast-feeding mother is a strict vegetarian (vitamin B₁₂).
		Emphasize correct use of vitamin supplements and potential hazards of excess.
VITAMIN B₂ (RIBOFLAVIN)‡		
Functions	**Deficiency**	Same as vitamin B complex
Coenzyme (with phosphorus) in carbohydrate, protein, and fat metabolism	Ariboflavinosis	
	Lips—Cheilosis (fissures at corners of lips), perlèche (inflammation at corners of lips)	
Maintains healthy skin, especially around mouth, nose, and eyes	*Tongue*—Glossitis	
	Nose—Irritation and cracks at nasal angle	
	Eyes—Burning, itching, tearing, photophobia, corneal vascularization, cataracts	
	Skin—Seborrheic dermatitis, delayed wound healing and tissue repair	
Sources	**Excess**	
Milk and its products, eggs, organs (liver, kidney, heart), enriched cereals, some green leafy vegetables,† legumes	Paresthesia, pruritus	
NIACIN (NICOTINIC ACID, NICOTINAMIDE)‡		
Functions	**Deficiency**	Same as vitamin B complex
Coenzyme (with riboflavin) in protein and fat metabolism	Pellagra	If used as hypolipidemic agent, stress safe dosage to prevent child's accidental ingestion.
	Oral—Stomatitis, glossitis	
Needed for healthy nervous system and skin and for normal digestion	*Cutaneous*—Scaly dermatitis on exposed areas	
	Gastrointestinal—Anorexia, weight loss, diarrhea, fatigue	
May lower cholesterol	*Neurologic*—Apathy, anxiety, confusion, depression, dementia	
	Death	

*Fat soluble.
†Green leafy vegetables include spinach, broccoli, kale, turnip greens, mustard greens, collards, dandelion greens, and beet greens.
‡Water soluble.

TABLE 11-1 ■ Vitamins and Their Nutritional Significance—*cont'd*

PHYSIOLOGIC FUNCTIONS/SOURCES	RESULTS OF DEFICIENCY OR EXCESS	NURSING CONSIDERATIONS
Sources Meat, poultry, fish, peanuts, beans, peas, whole or enriched grains (except corn and rice) Milk and its products are sources of tryptophan (60 mg tryptophan = 1 mg niacin).	**Excess** Release of histamine, a vasodilator (flushing, decreased blood pressure, increased cerebral blood flow; aggravates asthma) Dermatologic problems (pruritus, rash, hyperkeratosis, acanthosis nigricans) Increased gastric acidity (aggravates peptic ulcer disease) Hepatotoxicity Increased serum uric acid levels Elevated plasma glucose levels Certain cardiac arrhythmias	
VITAMIN B$_6$ (PYRIDOXINE)‡ **Functions** Coenzyme in protein and fat metabolism Needed for formation of antibodies and hemoglobin Needed for utilization of copper and iron Aids in conversion of tryptophan to niacin	**Deficiency** Scaly dermatitis, weight loss, anemia, retarded growth, irritability, convulsions, peripheral neuritis	Same as vitamin B complex Stress proper cooking and storing techniques to preserve potency. Cook food covered in small amount of water. Do not soak food in water. Store in light-resistant container.
Sources Meats, especially liver and kidney, cereal grains (wheat, corn), yeast, soybeans, peanuts, tuna, chicken, salmon	**Excess** Peripheral nervous system toxicity (unsteady gait, numb feet and hands, clumsiness of hands, sometimes perioral numbness) May cause peptic ulcer disease or seizures	
FOLIC ACID (FOLACIN; REDUCED FORM CALLED FOLINIC ACID OR CITROVORUM FACTOR)‡ **Functions** Coenzyme for single-carbon transfer (purines, thymine, hemoglobin) Necessary for formation of red blood cells May prevent neural tube defects (i.e., myelomeningocele)	**Deficiency** Macrocytic anemia, bone marrow depression, glossitis, intestinal malabsorption	Same as vitamin B complex Stress proper cooking and storing techniques to preserve potency: Cook food covered in small amount of water. Do not soak food in water. Store in light-resistant container. Women of childbearing age should supplement to prevent neural tube defects.
Sources Green leafy vegetables,† cabbage, asparagus, liver, kidneys, nuts, eggs, whole grain cereals, legumes, bananas	**Excess** Rare because megadoses not available over the counter May cause insomnia and irritability	
VITAMIN B$_{12}$ (COBALAMIN)‡ **Functions** Coenzyme in protein synthesis; indirect effect on formation of red blood cells (particularly on formation of nucleic acids and folic acid metabolism) Needed for normal functioning of nervous tissue	**Deficiency** Pernicious anemia (one form of deficiency from absence of intrinsic factor in gastric secretions) General signs of severe anemia Lemon-yellow tinge to skin Spinal cord degeneration Delayed brain growth	Same as vitamin B complex
Sources Meat, liver, kidney, fish, shellfish, poultry, milk, eggs, cheese, nutritional yeast, sea vegetables	**Excess** Rare	

*Fat soluble.

†Green leafy vegetables include spinach, broccoli, kale, turnip greens, mustard greens, collards, dandelion greens, and beet greens.

‡Water soluble.

Continued

TABLE 11-1 ■ Vitamins and Their Nutritional Significance—*cont'd*

PHYSIOLOGIC FUNCTIONS/SOURCES	RESULTS OF DEFICIENCY OR EXCESS	NURSING CONSIDERATIONS
BIOTIN‡ **Functions** Coenzyme in carbohydrate, protein, and fat metabolism Interrelated with functions of other B vitamins	**Deficiency** Deficiency is uncommon because synthesized by bacterial flora.	Same as vitamin B complex
Sources Liver, kidney, egg yolk, tomatoes, legumes, nuts	**Excess** Unknown	
PANTOTHENIC ACID‡ **Functions** Coenzyme in carbohydrate, protein, and fat metabolism Synthesis of amino acids, fatty acids, and steroids	**Deficiency** Deficiency is uncommon because of its multiple food sources and synthesis by bacterial flora	Same as vitamin B complex
Sources Liver, kidney, heart, salmon, eggs, vegetables, legumes, whole grains	**Excess** Minimum toxicity (occasional diarrhea and water retention)	
VITAMIN C (ASCORBIC ACID)‡ **Functions** Essential for collagen formation Increases absorption of iron for hemoglobin formation Enhances conversion of folic acid to folinic acid Affects cholesterol synthesis and conversion of proline to hydroxyproline Probably a coenzyme in metabolism of tyrosine and phenylalanine May play role in hydroxylation of adrenal steroids May have stimulating effect on phagocytic activity of leukocytes and formation of antibodies Antioxidant agent (spares other vitamins from oxidation)	**Deficiency** Scurvy *Skin*—Dry, rough, petechiae, perifollicular hyperkeratotic papules (raised areas around hair follicles) *Musculoskeletal*—Bleeding muscles and joints, pseudoparalysis from pain, swelling of joints, costochondral beading (scorbutic rosary) *Gums*—Spongy, friable, swollen, bleed easily, bluish red or black, teeth loosen and fall out *General disposition*—Irritable, anorexic, apprehensive, in pain, refuses to move, assumes semi-froglike position when supine (scorbutic pose) Signs of anemia Decreased wound healing Increased susceptibility to infection	Encourage foods rich in vitamin C. Investigate infant's diet for sources of vitamin, especially when cow's milk is principal source of nutrition. Stress proper cooking and storing techniques to preserve potency: Wash vegetables quickly; do not soak in water. Cook vegetables in covered pot with minimum water and for short time; avoid copper or cast iron cookware. Do not add baking soda to cooking water. Use fresh fruits and vegetables as soon as possible; store in refrigerator. Store juice in airtight, opaque container. Wrap cut fruit or eat soon after exposing to air. In caring for child with scurvy: Position for comfort and rest. Handle very gently and minimally. Administer analgesics as needed. Prevent infection. Provide good oral care. Provide soft, bland diet. Emphasize rapid recovery when vitamin is replaced. Emphasize correct use of vitamin supplement and potential hazards of excess. Identify groups at risk for vitamin C supplements (e.g., those with thalassemia or those receiving anticoagulant or aminoglycoside antibiotic therapy).

‡Water soluble.

TABLE 11-1 ■ Vitamins and Their Nutritional Significance—*cont'd*

PHYSIOLOGIC FUNCTIONS/SOURCES	RESULTS OF DEFICIENCY OR EXCESS	NURSING CONSIDERATIONS
Sources Citrus fruits, strawberries, tomatoes, potatoes, cabbage, broccoli, cauliflower, spinach, papaya, mango, cantaloupe, watermelon, enriched fruit juice	**Excess** Diarrhea Increased excretion of uric acid and acidification of urine (may cause urate precipitation and formation of oxalate stones) Hemolysis Impaired leukocytosis activity Damage to beta cells of pancreas and decreased insulin production Reproductive failure "Rebound scurvy" from withdrawal of large amounts	

VITAMIN D₂ (ERGOCALCIFEROL) AND D₃ (CHOLECALCIFEROL)*

Functions Absorption of calcium and phosphorus and decreased renal excretion of phosphorus	**Deficiency** Rickets *Head*—Craniotabes (softening of cranial bones, prominence of frontal bones), deformed shape (skull flat and depressed toward middle), delayed closure of fontanels *Chest*—Rachitic rosary (enlargement of costochondral junction of ribs), Harrison groove (horizontal depression in lower portion of rib cage), pigeon chest (sharp protrusion of sternum) *Spine*—Kyphosis, scoliosis, lordosis Abdomen—Pot belly, constipation *Extremities*—Bowing of arms and legs, knock knee, saber shins, instability of hip joints, pelvic deformity, enlargement of epiphyses at ends of long bones *Teeth*—Delayed calcification, especially of permanent teeth *Rachitic tetany*—Seizures	Encourage foods rich in vitamin D, especially fortified cow's milk. In breast-fed infants, encourage use of vitamin D supplements if maternal diet inadequate or if infant exposed to minimal sunlight. In caring for child with rickets: Maintain good body alignment. Reposition frequently to prevent decubiti and respiratory infection. Handle very gently and minimally. Prevent infection. Institute seizure precautions. Have 10% calcium gluconate available in case of tetany. Observe for possibility of overdose from supplements. If prescribed, supervise proper use of orthopedic splints and braces. Same as vitamin A; may include low-calcium diet during initial therapy
Sources Direct sunlight Cod liver oil, herring, mackerel, salmon, tuna, sardines Enriched food sources—Milk, milk products, enriched cereals, margarine, breads, many breakfast drinks	**Excess** *Acute*—Vomiting, dehydration, fever, abdominal cramps, bone pain, convulsions, coma *Chronic*—Lassitude, mental slowness, anorexia, failure to thrive, thirst, urinary urgency, polyuria, vomiting, diarrhea, abdominal cramps, bone pain, pathologic fractures *Calcification of soft tissue*—Kidneys, lungs, adrenal glands, vessels (hypertension), heart, gastric lining, tympanic membrane (deafness) Osteoporosis of long bones Elevated serum levels of calcium and phosphorus	

*Fat soluble.

Continued

TABLE 11-1 ■ Vitamins and Their Nutritional Significance—*cont'd*

PHYSIOLOGIC FUNCTIONS/SOURCES	RESULTS OF DEFICIENCY OR EXCESS	NURSING CONSIDERATIONS
VITAMIN E (TOCOPHEROL)*		
Functions	**Deficiency**	Initiate early feeding in premature infants; may need supplementation.
Production of red blood cells and protection from hemolysis	Hemolytic anemia from hemolysis caused by shortened life of red blood cells, especially in premature infants; focal necrosis of tissues	
Muscle and liver integrity	Causes infertility in rats but not in humans (does not increase human male virility or potency)	
Coenzyme factor in tissue respiration		
Minimizes oxidation of polyunsaturated fatty acids and vitamins A and C in intestinal tract and tissues		
Sources	**Excess**	
Vegetable oils, wheat germ oil, milk, egg yolk, fish, whole grains, nuts, legumes, spinach, broccoli	Little is known; less toxic than other fat-soluble vitamins	
VITAMIN K*		
Functions	**Deficiency**	Administer prophylactically to all newborns. Other indications include intestinal disease, lack of bile, prolonged antibiotic therapy; may be used in management of blood-clotting time when anticoagulants such as warfarin (Coumadin) and dicumarol (bishydroxycoumarin), which are vitamin K antagonists, are used.
Catalyst for production of prothrombin and blood-clotting factors II, VII, IX, and X by the liver	Hemorrhage	
Sources	**Excess**	
Pork, liver, green leafy vegetables,† cabbage, tomatoes, egg yolk, cheese	Hemolytic anemia in individuals who are deficient in glucose-6-phosphate dehydrogenase	

*Fat soluble.
†Green leafy vegetables include spinach, broccoli, kale, turnip greens, mustard greens, collards, dandelion greens, and beet greens.

The regulation of mineral balance in the body is a complex process. Dietary extremes of mineral intake can cause a number of mineral-mineral interactions that could result in unexpected deficiencies or excesses. For example, excessive amounts of one mineral, such as zinc, can result in a deficiency of another mineral, such as copper, even if sufficient amounts of copper are ingested. Thus megadose intake of one mineral may cause an inadvertent deficiency of another essential mineral by blocking its absorption in the blood or intestinal wall, or by competing with binding sites on protein carriers needed for metabolism.

Deficiencies can also occur when various substances in the diet interact with minerals. For example, iron, zinc, and calcium can form insoluble complexes with **phytates** or **oxalates** (substances found in plant proteins), which impair the bioavailability of the mineral. This type of interaction is important in vegetarian diets because plant foods such as soy are high in phytates. Contrary to popular opinion, spinach is not an ideal source of iron or calcium because of its high oxalate content.

Deficiencies and excesses of the essential macrominerals and microminerals are summarized in Table 11-2. General nursing considerations are discussed on p. 371, and specific interventions are discussed in the table.

Text continues on p. 371

BOX 11-1 ■ Factors That Affect Iron Absorption

IINCREASE

Acidity (low pH)—Administer iron between meals (gastric hydrochloric acid)

Ascorbic acid (vitamin C)—Administer iron with juice, fruit, or multivitamin preparation

Vitamin A

Calcium

Tissue need

Meat, fish, poultry

Cooking in cast iron pots

DECREASE

Alkalinity (high pH)—Avoid any antacid preparation

Phosphates—Milk is unfavorable vehicle for iron administration

Phytates—Found in cereals

Oxalates—Found in many fruits and vegetables (plums, currants, green beans, spinach, sweet potatoes, tomatoes)

Tannins—Found in tea, coffee

Tissue saturation

Malabsorptive disorders

Disturbances that cause diarrhea or steatorrhea

Infection

TABLE 11-2 ■ Minerals and Their Nutritional Significance

PHYSIOLOGIC FUNCTIONS/SOURCES	RESULTS OF DEFICIENCY OR EXCESS	NURSING CONSIDERATIONS
CALCIUM* **Functions** Bone and tooth development and maintenance (in combination with phosphorus) Muscle contractions, especially the heart Blood clotting Absorption of vitamin B$_{12}$ Enzyme activation Nerve conduction Integrity of intracellular cement substances and various membranes	**Deficiency** Rickets Tetany Impaired growth, especially of bones and teeth Osteoporosis	Encourage foods rich in calcium, especially dairy products. Caution that oxalates in leafy vegetables (spinach), oxalates in chocolates, and a high phosphorus intake (especially from carbonated beverages) can decrease calcium absorption. Discourage use of whole cow's milk in newborns because the phosphorus/calcium ratio favors excretion of calcium. Advise against fad diets, especially those that restrict dairy products. Emphasize correct use of calcium supplements, especially the possible interaction between megadoses of calcium and resulting deficiency states of other minerals.
Sources Dairy products, egg yolk, sardines, canned salmon with bones, green leafy vegetables† (except spinach), soybeans, dried beans, peas	**Excess** Drowsiness, extreme lethargy Impaired absorption of other minerals (iron, zinc, manganese) Calcium deposits in tissues (renal failure)	
CHLORIDE* **Functions** Acid-base and fluid balance Enzyme activation in saliva Component of hydrochloric acid in stomach	**Deficiency** Acid-base disturbances (hypochloremic alkalosis, dehydration); occurs mostly in combination with sodium loss	Deficiency and excess are unusual; most diets supply adequate chloride (usually in combination with sodium). Disease states such as excessive vomiting can necessitate chloride replacement.
Sources Salt, meat, eggs, dairy products, many prepared and preserved foods	**Excess** Acid-base disturbance	
CHROMIUM† **Functions** Involved in glucose metabolism and energy production	**Deficiency** Possible abnormal glucose metabolism	No specific recommendations are needed.
Sources Meat (liver, dark meat of chicken), cheese, whole-grain breads and cereals, legumes, peanuts, brewer's yeast, vegetable oils	**Excess** Unknown	
COPPER† **Functions** Production of hemoglobin Essential component of several enzyme systems	**Deficiency** Anemia, leukopenia, neutropenia	Deficiency from inadequate food sources is less likely than from excess intake of other minerals, especially zinc and possibly iron; therefore emphasize the correct use of any vitamin supplement. Caution against cooking acid foods in unlined copper pots, which can lead to chronic and toxic accumulation of copper
Sources Organ meats, oysters, nuts, seeds, legumes, corn oil margarine	**Excess** Severe vomiting and diarrhea Hemolytic anemia	

*Macrominerals—required intake >100 mg/day.
†Microminerals or trace elements—required intake <100 mg/day.

TABLE 11-2 ■ Minerals and Their Nutritional Significance—*cont'd*

PHYSIOLOGIC FUNCTIONS/SOURCES	RESULTS OF DEFICIENCY OR EXCESS	NURSING CONSIDERATIONS
FLUORIDE† **Functions** Formation of caries-resistant teeth Strong bone development	**Deficiency** Increased susceptibility to tooth decay	In areas with optimally fluoridated water, encourage sufficient intake to supply recommended amount of fluoride. In areas of unfluoridated water or when ready-to-use formula, bottled water, or breast milk is used, stress the importance of fluoride supplements. In areas with excess fluoride in the water, consider the use of bottled water in drinking and cooking to reduce the fluoride intake to safe levels. Fluoride has the narrowest range of safe and adequate intake; therefore stress the importance of storing supplements in a safe area.
Sources Fluoridated water and foods or beverages prepared with fluoridated water, fish, tea, commercially prepared chicken for infants	**Excess** Fluorosis (mottling or pitting of enamel) Severe bone deformities	
IODINE† **Functions** Production of thyroid hormone Normal reproduction	**Deficiency** Goiter (enlarged thyroid from decreased thyroxine formation)	Encourage use of iodized salt for individuals living far from the sea. If iodine preparations are in the home, stress the importance of safe storage.
Sources Seafood, kelp, iodized salt, sea salt, enriched bread, milk (from dairy processing)	**Excess** Unknown from food sources; may occur from ingestion of iodine preparations, such as saturated solutions of potassium iodide	
IRON† **Functions** Formation of hemoglobin and myoglobin Essential part of several enzymes and proteins	**Deficiency** Anemia (See Chapter 26.)	Discourage excessive milk consumption, especially more than 1 liter per day (milk is a very poor source of iron). If iron supplements are prescribed, teach parents factors that affect absorption (Box 11-1). Stress the importance of storing iron supplements in a safe area.
Sources Liver, especially pork, followed by calf, beef, and chicken; kidney, red meat, poultry, shellfish, whole grains, iron-enriched infant formula and cereal, enriched cereals and bread, legumes, nuts, seeds, green leafy vegetables (except spinach), dried fruits, potatoes, molasses, tofu, prune juice	**Excess** Hemosiderosis (excess iron storage in various tissues of the body, especially the spleen, liver, lymph glands, heart, and pancreas) Hemochromatosis (excess iron storage with cellular damage)	

*Macrominerals—required intake >100 mg/day.
†Microminerals or trace elements—required intake <100 mg/day.

TABLE 11-2 ■ Minerals and Their Nutritional Significance—*cont'd*

PHYSIOLOGIC FUNCTIONS/SOURCES	RESULTS OF DEFICIENCY OR EXCESS	NURSING CONSIDERATIONS
MAGNESIUM* **Functions** Bone and tooth formation Production of proteins Nerve conduction to muscles Activation of enzymes needed for carbohydrate and protein metabolism	**Deficiency** Tremors, spasm Irregular heartbeat Muscular weakness Lower extremity cramps Convulsions, delirium	
Sources Whole grains, nuts, soybeans, meat, green leafy vegetables* (uncooked), tea, cocoa, raisins	**Excess** Nervous system disturbances caused by imbalance in calcium/magnesium ratio	Deficiency and excess are unusual, except in disease states such as prolonged vomiting or diarrhea or kidney dysfunction, where replacement may be needed.
MANGANESE† **Functions** Activation of enzymes involved in reproduction, growth, and fat metabolism Normal bone structure Nervous system functioning	**Deficiency** Unknown	No specific recommendations are needed.
Sources Nuts, whole grains, legumes, green vegetables, fruit	**Excess** Unknown	
MOLYBDENUM† **Functions** Essential component of several oxidative enzymes	**Deficiency** Very rare; diagnosed in patients on complete total parenteral alimentation	No specific recommendations are needed.
Sources Legumes, whole grains, organs, some dark green vegetables	**Excess** Produces secondary copper deficiency (growth failure, anemia, disturbed bone development)	
PHOSPHORUS* **Functions** Bone and tooth development (in combination with calcium) Involved in numerous chemical reactions, including protein, carbohydrate, and fat metabolism Acid-base balance	**Deficiency** Weakness, anorexia, malaise, bone pain	Dietary deficiency is uncommon, although prolonged use of antacids can produce deficiency, in which case supplementation is recommended. To preserve calcium/phosphorus ratio in newborns, discourage use of whole cow's milk.
Sources Dairy products, eggs, meat, poultry, legumes, carbonated beverages	**Excess** Produces secondary calcium deficiency from disturbed calcium/phosphorus ratio	
POTASSIUM* **Functions** Acid-base and fluid balance (major extracellular fluid areas) Nerve conduction Muscular contraction, especially the heart Release of energy	**Deficiency** Cardiac arrhythmias Muscular weakness Lethargy Kidney and respiratory failure Heart failure	Dietary deficiency and excess are unlikely, although disease states such as prolonged nausea and vomiting or the use of diuretics can result in hypokalemia; in such instances, encourage replacement with supplements of rich food sources, such as bananas.
Sources Bananas, citrus fruit, dried fruits, meat, fish, bran, legumes, peanut butter, potatoes, coffee, tea, cocoa	**Excess** Cardiac arrhythmias Respiratory failure Mental confusion Numbness of extremities	

*Macrominerals—required intake >100 mg/day.
†Microminerals or trace elements—required intake <100 mg/day.

Continued

TABLE 11-2 ■ Minerals and Their Nutritional Significance—*cont'd*

PHYSIOLOGIC FUNCTIONS/SOURCES	RESULTS OF DEFICIENCY OR EXCESS	NURSING CONSIDERATIONS
SELENIUM†		
Functions	**Deficiency**	
Antioxidant, especially protective of vitamin E	Keshan disease (cardiomyopathy in children; found in China)	Deficiency and excess are uncommon in North America, although selenium deficiency can occur in patients receiving prolonged total parenteral alimentation; in these instances, supplementation is required.
Protects against toxicity of heavy metals		
Associated with fat metabolism		
Sources	**Excess**	
Seafood, organs, egg yolk, whole grains, chicken, meat, tomatoes, cabbage, garlic, mushrooms, milk	Eye, nose, and throat irritation	
	Increased dental caries	
	Liver and kidney degeneration	
SODIUM*		
Functions	**Deficiency**	
Acid-base and fluid balance (major extracellular fluid cation)	Dehydration	Deficient intake is very rare, although losses secondary to nausea, vomiting, excessive sweating, and use of diuretics can occur and require replacement.
	Hypotension	
Cell permeability; absorption of glucose	Convulsions	Encourage parents to limit excessive use of salt in preparing foods and to limit commercial foods with high sodium content, such as smoked meats.
Muscle contraction	Muscle cramps	
Sources	**Excess**	
Table salt, seafood, meat, poultry, numerous prepared foods	Edema	
	Hypertension	
	Intracranial hemorrhage	
SULFUR*		
Functions	**Deficiency**	
Essential component of cell protein, especially of hair and skin	Unknown	No specific recommendations are needed.
Enzyme activation		
Associated with energy metabolism		
Detoxification of certain chemical reactions		
Sources	**Excess**	
Dairy products, eggs, meat, fish, nuts, legumes	Unknown	
ZINC†		
Functions	**Deficiency**	
Component of about 100 enzymes	Loss of appetite	Encourage food sources rich in zinc, especially protein.
Synthesis of nucleic acids and protein in immune system and coagulation	Diminished taste sensation	Caution that fiber, phytates, oxalates, tannins (in tea or coffee), iron, and calcium adversely affect zinc absorption.
	Delayed healing	
Release of vitamin A from liver	*Skin lesions*—Erythematous, crusted lesions around body orifices	Recognize groups at risk for zinc deficiency, such as vegetarians and Hispanics, whose diets may have restricted or low meat content and high fiber and phytate content, and patients with malabsorption syndromes.
Improved wound healing with vitamin C	Alopecia	
Normal taste sensitivity	Diarrhea	
	Growth failure	
	Retarded sexual maturity	Emphasize correct use of zinc supplements and the possible interaction with other minerals.
Sources	**Excess**	
Seafood (especially oysters), meat, poultry, eggs, wheat, legumes	Vomiting and diarrhea	
	Malaise, dizziness	
	Anemia, gastric bleeding	
	Impaired absorption of calcium and copper	

*Macrominerals—required intake >100 mg/day.
†Microminerals or trace elements—required intake <100 mg/day.

VEGETARIAN DIETS

Vegetarian diets are becoming more popular in the United States because people are concerned about hypertension, obesity, cardiovascular disease, and cancer of the stomach, intestine, and colon. A survey of adolescent vegetarians indicated that this group was more likely than nonvegetarians to meet the Healthy People 2010 objectives for overall nutrient consumption (Perry and others, 2002). Although there are many health benefits to vegetarian diets in adults, the importance of such diets and their relationship to potential nutritional deficiencies in children cannot be overemphasized. The stricter the vegetarian diet, the more difficult it becomes to ensure adequate nutrition for infants and children. The major types of vegetarianism are:

- **Lacto-ovo vegetarians,** who exclude meat from their diet but consume dairy products and rarely fish
- **Lactovegetarians,** who exclude meat and eggs but drink milk
- **Pure vegetarians (vegans),** who eliminate any food of animal origin, including milk and eggs
- **Zen macrobiotics,** who are even more restrictive than pure vegetarians; small amounts of fruits, vegetables, and legumes are allowed
- **Semi-vegetarians,** who consume a lacto-ovo vegetarian diet with some fish and poultry; this is an increasingly popular form of vegetarianism and poses little or no nutritional risk to infants unless dietary fat and cholesterol intake is severely restricted. Many individuals who are concerned about healthy diets subscribe to vegetarian diets that may not be typified by the above categories. Therefore, during nutritional assessment it is necessary to clearly list exactly what the diet includes and excludes.*

The major deficiencies in the stricter vegetarian diets are inadequate protein for growth; inadequate calories for energy and growth; poor digestibility of many of the bulky natural, unprocessed foods, especially for infants; and deficiencies of vitamin B_6, niacin, riboflavin, vitamin D, iron, calcium, and zinc. Strict vegetarian diets also require supplements of vitamin B_{12} and vitamin D. Vitamin D is essential if exposure to sunlight is inadequate (<5 to 15 minutes per day on the hands, arms, and face) or in persons who are dark-skinned or who live in northern latitudes or cloudy or smoky areas.

Iron deficiency anemia and rickets may also be seen in children on strict vegetarian and macrobiotic diets as a result of consuming plant foods such as unrefined cereals, which impair the absorption of iron, calcium, and zinc.

Nursing Considerations

Identification of nutrient imbalance is the initial nursing goal and requires assessment based on a dietary history and physical examination for signs of deficiency or excess (see Nutritional Assessment, Chapter 6). After assessment data are collected, this information is evaluated against standard intakes to identify areas of concern. The most widely used standard is the *RDAs,* developed by the **National Academy**

of Sciences, Food and Nutrition Board. The RDAs are not average requirements but recommendations intended to meet the physiologic needs of almost every healthy person. To meet the needs of those with the highest requirements, the RDAs will exceed most people's requirements. Therefore children consuming less than the RDAs are not necessarily consuming an inadequate diet, but they are more likely at risk for deficiency than those who are consuming nutrients in amounts equal to the RDAs.

In the past 20 years, scientific knowledge regarding the role of nutrients in health promotion and disease prevention has advanced dramatically. As a result, the Institute of Medicine has developed new guidelines for nutritional intake referred to as the *Dietary Reference Intakes (DRIs).* This is a generic term that encompasses not only the RDAs but also three additional reference values: Estimated Average Requirement, Adequate Intakes, and the Tolerable Upper Intake Level. These contemporary values allow the practitioner the expanded capability of evaluating nutrient intakes based not solely upon the traditional RDAs. The Estimated Average Requirement is the intake value that is estimated to meet the requirement defined by a specified indicator of adequacy in 50% of an age- and gender-specific group. At this level of intake, the remaining 50% of the specified group would not have met its required nutrient needs. The Adequate Intake is established only when there is no RDA available and is based on observed intakes of the nutrient by a group of healthy persons. The *Tolerable Upper Intake Level* is the maximum level of a nutrient that is unlikely to pose risks for adverse health effects to almost all the individuals in the group for whom it is designed; it is not meant to be a recommended level of intake. The new guidelines also present information about lifestyle factors that may affect nutrient function such as caffeine intake and exercise, and how the nutrient may be related to chronic disease; the goal is to prevent chronic diseases related to nutritional intake. An important factor in the development of the DRIs that impacts children, particularly infants 0 to 6 months, is that the Adequate Intakes are based on the nutrient intake of term healthy breast-fed infants (by well-nourished mothers) which now represents the gold standard for infant nutrition in this age-group. This represents a major change in infant nutrition recommendations; specific needs to meet the nutrient requirements for formula-fed infants were not included in DRI reports (Devaney and Barr, 2002; Institute of Medicine, 2000).*

Several organizations have published dietary advice for the public. The *Dietary Guidelines for Americans* encourage eating a variety of foods, maintaining ideal body weight, consuming adequate starch and fiber, and limiting intake of fat, cholesterol, sugar, salt, and alcohol. The *Food Guide Pyramid For Young Children* (Fig. 11-1), which replaces the basic four food groups, is used to convey nutrition information to the public and applies to children as young as 2 years of age.

The new Food Guide Pyramid includes pictures aimed at younger children. The different food groups and servings

---

*Further information regarding vegetarian diets may be found at the **Vegetarian Resource Group (VRG),** PO Box 1463, Baltimore, MD 21203; (410) 366-VEGE; website: www.vrg.org

*Further information may be found regarding the newer nutrient DRI groups at website: www4.nas.edu.

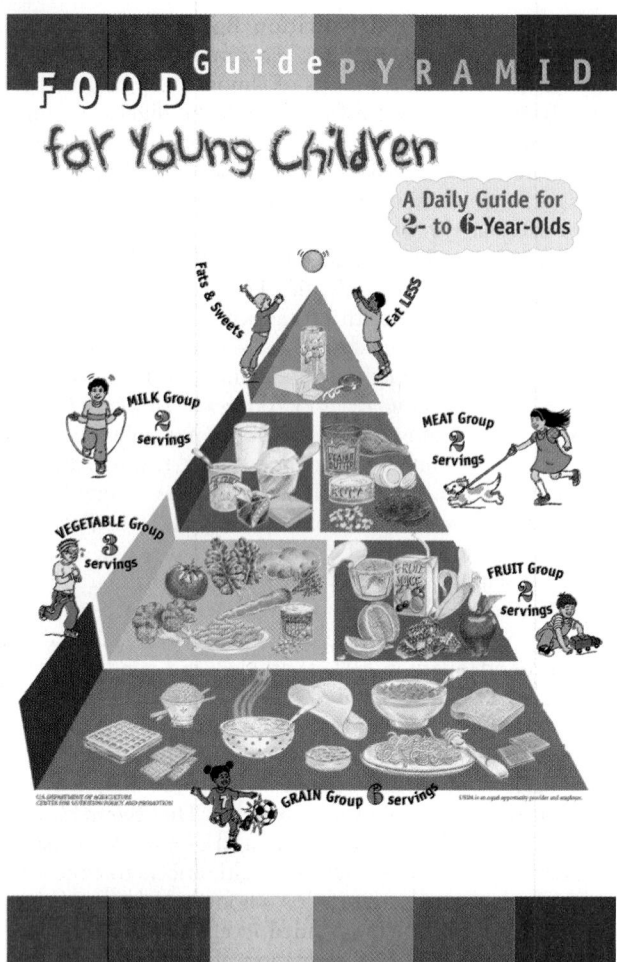

FOOD Guide PYRAMID
for Young Children

A Daily Guide for
2- to 6-Year-Olds

Eat LESS

Fats & Sweets

MILK Group
2 servings

MEAT Group
2 servings

VEGETABLE Group
3 servings

FRUIT Group
2 servings

GRAIN Group 6 servings

U.S. DEPARTMENT OF AGRICULTURE
CENTER FOR NUTRITION POLICY AND PROMOTION

USDA is an equal opportunity provider and employer.

FIG. 11-1 ■ Food Guide Pyramid for Young Children. (Courtesy U.S. Department of Agriculture Center for Nutrition Policy and Promotion, 1999.)

are the same, yet the foods are made to appear more realistic than the previous Food Guide Pyramid. The names of the groups have also been reduced for children to better understand. The tip of the pyramid emphasizes a decrease in the consumption of fats and sweets.

!**NURSING ALERT**

When solid foods are introduced, the safety and digestibility of the selections must be considered. Raw fruits with seeds, vegetables, and nuts are hazardous for infants and young children because of the danger of aspiration. Beans, grain cereals, and vegetables should be served well-cooked and mashed during infancy.

The number of servings and serving sizes are important components of the Food Guide Pyramid. Suggested serving sizes for the five food groups are listed in Box 11-2. Young children need the same variety of foods as older children but may need less than the 1600 calories provided by the suggested minimum number of servings in each food group. To meet their caloric needs, adjustments are made by using the minimum number of servings and smaller serving sizes. However, it is important that children have the equivalent of at least 2 cups of milk per day. Adolescents, who require increased calories for growth, should have at least 3 cups of

BOX 11-2 ■ Food Guide Pyramid: Sample Serving Sizes

Grain group—1 slice of bread; 1 ounce of ready-to-eat cereal; $\frac{1}{2}$ cup of cooked cereal, rice, or pasta
Vegetable group—1 cup of raw leafy vegetable; $\frac{1}{2}$ cup of other vegetable, cooked or chopped raw; $\frac{3}{4}$ cup of vegetable juice
Fruit group—1 medium apple, banana, or orange; $\frac{1}{2}$ cup of chopped, cooked, or canned fruit; $\frac{3}{4}$ cup of fruit juice
Milk group—2 cups of milk or yogurt, $1\frac{1}{2}$ ounces of natural cheese, 1 ounce of processed cheese
Meat group—2-3 ounces of cooked lean meat, poultry, or fish; $\frac{1}{2}$ cup of cooked dry beans, 1 egg, or 2 tablespoons of peanut butter count as 1 ounce of lean meat

milk per day and more fruits, and may require the maximum number of suggested servings. Current recommendations for fat intake for children older than 2 years of age are that no more than 30% of calories should come from fat and the remainder of calories should come from carbohydrates and protein (see also Hyperlipidemia [Hypercholesterolemia], Chapter 25).

Because one of the best assurances of nutritional adequacy is eating a variety of foods, families need guidelines for selecting foods that provide essential nutrients without exceeding energy requirements. With a varied diet most children do not need vitamin or mineral supplements. Unfortunately, there are no restrictions on the availability of toxic doses of vitamins or minerals. Nurses need to inquire about alternative therapies that include vitamin or mineral supplements and inform families of the potential dangers from excess vitamins or minerals. The idea that "more is better" is probably best dispelled by a simple explanation of the body's inability to use more than the needed requirement.

!**NURSING ALERT**

Educate childbearing adolescent females about the need for folic acid to prevent neural tube birth defects. It is easily obtained from a well balanced diet or a daily multivitamin supplement (Table 11-1).

Achieving a nutritionally adequate vegetarian diet requires careful planning and knowledge of nutrient sources. For children the lacto-ovo vegetarian diet is nutritionally adequate; however, the vegan diet requires supplementation with vitamins D and B_{12} for children ages 2 to 12 years. Infants should be breast-fed for the first 6 months and preferably for 1 year, be fed solid foods after about 4 months, and receive iron-fortified cereal for at least 18 months. The **American Dietetic Association** (1997) recommends iron supplementation in infants exclusively breast-fed after 4 to 6 months by vegetarian mothers and no dietary fat restrictions in vegetarian children younger than 2 years. The use of vitamin C juices with foods high in iron will further improve iron absorption.

However, breast milk from vegetarian mothers can be deficient in vitamin B_{12}; supplementation of both mother and child is advisable. If whole fortified cow's or human milk or commercial infant formula is not given, fortified soy milk is recommended. A variety of foods should be introduced during the early years to ensure a more well-balanced intake.

Mothers who continue exclusive or partial breast-feeding past 6 months should have a careful evaluation of their particular vegetarian diet to ensure adequate intake of nutrients

To ensure sufficient protein in the diet, foods with incomplete proteins (those that do not have all of the essential amino acids) should be eaten with other foods that supply the missing amino acids. The three basic combinations of foods consumed by vegetarians that generally provide the appropriate amounts of essential amino acids are:

1 Grains (cereal, rice, pasta) and legumes (beans, peas, lentils, peanuts)
2 Grains and milk products (milk, cheese, yogurt)
3 Seeds (sesame, sunflower) and legumes

PROTEIN AND ENERGY MALNUTRITION

Malnutrition continues to be a major health problem in the world today, particularly in children younger than 5 years of age. Lack of food, however, is not always the primary cause for malnutrition. In many developing and underdeveloped nations, diarrhea is a major factor. Additional factors are bottle-feeding (in poor sanitary conditions), inadequate knowledge of proper child care practices, parental illiteracy, economic and political factors, and simply the lack of adequate food for children.. The most extreme forms of malnutrition, or protein and energy malnutrition (PEM), are kwashiorkor and marasmus.

In the United States milder forms of PEM are seen, although the classic cases of marasmus and kwashiorkor may also occur. Unlike developing countries, where the main reason for PEM is inadequate food, in the United States PEM occurs primarily in children with chronic illnesses or inadvertent malnourishment as a consequence of caretaker knowledge inadequacy (see Failure to Thrive, pp. 378-381).

Kwashiorkor

Kwashiorkor has been defined in the past as primarily a deficiency of protein with an adequate supply of calories. A diet consisting mainly of starch grains or tubers provides adequate calories in the form of carbohydrates but an inadequate amount of high-quality proteins. There is evidence supporting a multifactorial etiology, including cultural, psychologic, and infective factors that may jointly or singly interact to place the child at risk for kwashiorkor. Taken from the Ga language (Ghana), the word *kwashiorkor* means "the sickness the older child gets when the next baby is born" and aptly describes the syndrome that develops in the first child, usually between 1 and 4 years of age, when weaned from the breast after the second child is born.

The child with kwashiorkor has thin, wasted extremities and a prominent abdomen from edema (ascites). The edema often masks the severe muscular atrophy, making the child appear less debilitated than he or she actually is. The skin is scaly and dry and has areas of depigmentation. Several dermatoses may be evident, partly resulting from the vitamin deficiencies. Permanent blindness often results from the severe lack of vitamin A. Mineral deficiencies are common, especially iron, calcium, and zinc. The hair is thin, dry, coarse, and dull. Depigmentation is common, and patchy alopecia may occur.

Diarrhea commonly occurs from a lowered resistance to infection and produces electrolyte imbalance. A large number of fatalities in children with kwashiorkor has occurred in those who developed human immunodeficiency virus (HIV) infection, many of whom were breast-fed. Protein deficiency increases the child's susceptibility to infection, which eventually results in death. Behavioral changes are evident as the child grows progressively more irritable, lethargic, withdrawn, and apathetic. Fatal deterioration may be caused by diarrhea and infection or as the result of circulatory failure.

Marasmus

Marasmus results from general malnutrition of both calories and protein. It is a common occurrence in underdeveloped countries during times of drought, especially in cultures where adults eat first; the remaining food is often insufficient in quality and quantity for the children.

Marasmus is usually a syndrome of physical and emotional deprivation and is not confined to geographic areas where food supplies are inadequate. It may be seen in children with failure to thrive in whom the cause is not solely nutritional but primarily emotional. Marasmus may be seen in infants as young as 3 months of age if breast-feeding is not successful and there are no suitable alternatives. *Marasmic-kwashiorkor* is a form of PEM in which clinical findings of both kwashiorkor and marasmus are evident; the child has edema, severe wasting, and stunted growth.

Marasmus is characterized by gradual wasting and atrophy of body tissues, especially of subcutaneous fat. The child appears to be very old, with flabby and wrinkled skin, unlike the child with kwashiorkor, who appears more rounded from the edema. Fat metabolism is less impaired than in kwashiorkor, so that deficiency of fat-soluble vitamins is usually minimal or absent.

The child is fretful, apathetic, withdrawn, and so lethargic that prostration frequently occurs. Intercurrent infection with debilitating diseases such as tuberculosis, parasitosis, HIV, and dysentery is common.

Therapeutic Management

The treatment of PEM includes providing a diet with high-quality proteins, carbohydrates, vitamins, and minerals. When PEM occurs as a result of diarrhea (see also Diarrhea, Chapter 24), three management goals are identified: (1) rehydration with an oral rehydration solution that also replaces electrolytes, (2) medications such as antibiotics and antidiarrheals, and (3) provision of adequate nutrition either by breast-feeding or a proper weaning diet. When the child is too ill to tolerate oral fluids, intravenous administration of fluids, electrolytes, minerals, and vitamins will be required to prevent death. Additional management of PEM is aimed at restoring or replacing essential vitamins and minerals, namely vitamin E, vitamin A, selenium, and zinc, which have been shown to have significant roles in infection and congestive heart failure related to PEM.

Nursing Considerations

Provision of essential physiologic needs, such as protection from infection, adequate hydration, skin care, and restoration of physiologic integrity, is paramount. Because children are usually weak and withdrawn, they depend on others for feeding. Poor skin integrity increases the chance of infections and further skin breakdown. Tube feedings may be required in infants too weak to breast- or bottle-feed. Oral rehydration with an approved oral rehydration solution is commonly used in cases of PEM where diarrhea and infection are not immediately life-threatening.

A larger problem is the prevention of these conditions through education concerning the importance of proper nutrition, whether breast-feeding or bottle-feeding, when being weaned to semisolid foods. There are reported cases of kwashiorkor in children in the United States as a result of ingestion of improper types of nutrients; in both cases, toddlers were being fed a health food milk alternative and very few solids (Carvalho and others, 2001). It is imperative that nurses be at the forefront in educating and reinforcing healthy nutrition habits in parents of small children to prevent malnutrition. Because children with marasmus may suffer from emotional starvation as well, care should be consistent with care of the child with failure to thrive (pp. 380-381).

FOOD SENSITIVITY

Food sensitivity is a general term that includes any type of adverse reaction to food or food additives. Food sensitivities can be divided into two broad categories:

1 **Food allergy or hypersensitivity,** which refers to reactions involving immunologic mechanisms, usually immunoglobulin E (IgE); the reactions may be immediate or delayed and mild or severe, such as an anaphylactic reaction.
2 **Food intolerance,** which refers to reactions involving known or unknown nonimmunologic mechanisms; lactose intolerance is an example of a reaction that looks like allergy but is due to deficiency of the enzyme lactase.

However, this classification is not universally accepted; therefore, the terms *food sensitivity, hypersensitivity, allergy,* and *intolerance* are often used interchangeably.

Food allergy is caused by exposure to **allergens,** usually proteins (but not the smaller amino acids) that are capable of inducing IgE antibody formation ("sensitization") when ingested. *Sensitization* refers to the initial exposure of an individual to an allergen, resulting in an immune response; subsequent exposure induces a much stronger response that is clinically apparent. Consequently, food hypersensitivity typically occurs after the food has been ingested one or more times. The most common food allergens are listed in Box 11-3.

Allergies in general demonstrate a genetic component: children who have one parent with allergy have a 50% or greater risk of developing allergy; children who have both parents with allergy have up to a 100% risk of developing allergy. Allergy with a hereditary tendency is referred to as *atopy.* Some infants with atopy can be identified at birth from elevated levels of IgE in cord blood.

Deaths have been reported in children who suffered an anaphylactic reaction to food. Onset of the reactions occurred shortly after ingestion, usually within seconds or minutes. In most of the children the reactions did not begin with skin signs such as hives, red rash, or flushing, but rather as an acute asthma attack. Additional clinical features that individuals with acute anaphylactic food reactions have include (1) asthma, (2) accidental ingestion of the food allergen, (3) immediate symptoms, and (4) a prior allergic reaction to the food (Burks, 2000). Other symptoms of anaphylaxis to food allergens include wheezing, cough, dyspnea, urticaria, abdominal cramps,

BOX 11-3 ■ Hyperallergenic Foods/Sources

Milk*—Ice cream, butter, margarine (if it contains dairy products), yogurt, cheese, pudding, baked goods, wieners, bologna, canned creamed soups, instant breakfast drinks, powdered milk drinks, milk chocolate

Eggs*—Mayonnaise, creamy salad dressing, baked goods, egg noodles, some cake icing, meringue, custard, pancakes, French toast, root beer

Wheat*—Almost all baked goods, wieners, bologna, pressed or chopped cold cuts, gravy, pasta, some canned soups

Legumes—Peanuts,* peanut butter or oil, beans, peas, lentils

Nuts*—Some chocolates, candy, baked goods, cherry soda (may be flavored with a nut extract), walnut oil

Fish or shellfish*—Cod liver oil, pizza with anchovies, Caesar salad dressing, any food fried in same oil as fish

Soy*—Soy sauce, teriyaki or Worcestershire sauce, tofu, baked goods using soy flour or oil, soy nuts, soy infant formulas or milk, soybean paste, tuna packed in vegetable oil, many margarines

Chocolate—Cola beverages, cocoa, chocolate-flavored drinks

Buckwheat—Some cereals, pancakes

Pork, chicken—Bacon, wieners, sausage, pork fat, chicken broth

Strawberries, melon, pineapple—Gelatin, syrups

Corn—Popcorn, cereal, muffins, cornstarch, corn meal, corn bread, corn tortilla

Citrus fruits—Orange, lemon, lime, grapefruit; any of these in drinks, gelatin, juice, or medicines

Tomatoes—Juice, some vegetable soups, spaghetti, pizza sauce, catsup

Spices—Chili, pepper, vinegar, cinnamon

*Most common allergens.

vomiting, diarrhea, a drop in systemic blood pressure or shock, and, in small preverbal children, restlessness, urticaria, irritability, listlessness, and unresponsiveness. A grading system of clinical signs and symptoms associated with food anaphylaxis has been proposed to measure the severity of the reaction (Sampson, 2003). Children with suspected food anaphylaxis should be watched closely because a biphasic response has been recorded in a number of cases in which there is an immediate response, apparent recovery, then acute recurrence of symptoms. The most common foods causing anaphylaxis are peanut, tree nut, fish, and shellfish (Pongracic, 2000).

The spectrum of food allergy symptoms may include clinical manifestations that involve the skin (urticaria), gastrointestinal tract, and respiratory tract. Oral allergy syndrome occurs when a food allergen is ingested (commonly fruits and vegetables) and there is subsequent edema and pruritus involving the lips, tongue, palate, and throat; recovery from symptoms is usually rapid. Immediate gastrointestinal hypersensitivity is an IgE-mediated reaction to a food allergen, and reactions include nausea, abdominal pain, cramping, diarrhea, vomiting, anaphylaxis, or all of these (Burks, 2000). Additional food hypersensitivities seen in young children include allergic eosinophilic gastritis, allergic eosinophilic gastroenterocolitis, dietary protein enterocolitis (or milk protein intolerance), and dietary protein proctitis (Burks, 2000).

Parents, teachers, and day care workers should be educated regarding signs and symptoms of food allergies.

Those with food sensitivity should avoid unfamiliar foods, as well as restaurants and fast-food establishments that do not disclose food ingredients. Peanut allergy warnings are now standard on products that contain peanut fragments from the manufacturing process but hidden ingredients remain an issue for children with food hypersensitivity.

Although the reason is unknown, many children "outgrow" their food allergies; children may outgrow milk and egg allergies, but peanut allergies may persist. Children who are allergic to more than one food may develop tolerance to each food at different times. Because of the tendency to lose the hypersensitivity, allergic foods should be reintroduced into the diet after a period of abstinence (usually a year or more) to evaluate if the food can be safely added to the diet. However, foods that are associated with severe anaphylactic reactions, will continue to present a lifelong risk and must be avoided. Because children with food allergies (usually two or more) are at risk for inadequate nutrient intake and growth failure, it is recommended that they have an annual nutritional assessment to prevent such problems (Christie and others, 2002).

Breast-feeding is now considered to be a primary consideration for avoiding atopy in families with known food sensitivities; however, there is some evidence that cow's milk protein is transferred via breast milk. The breast-feeding mother is encouraged to avoid foods such as peanuts, tree nuts, fish, and shellfish during the first 6 months of breast-feeding. In addition, supplementation, if required, is best with hydrolysated or amino acid formulas, *not soy* formulas. The strategies listed in the Guidelines box are those recommended by most authorities for infants with a family history of atopy.*

! NURSING ALERT

Children with extremely sensitive food allergies should wear medical identification such as a bracelet and have an injectable epinephrine cartridge readily available and know how to use it. It is also helpful for the child to have a copy of the individualized written treatment plan on hand for prompt diagnosis and treatment (such plans can be downloaded from www.foodallergy.org and completed by the practitioner).

Cow's-Milk Allergy

Cow's-milk allergy (also referred to as cow's-milk protein allergy [CMPA]) is a multifaceted disorder representing adverse systemic and local gastrointestinal reactions to cow's-milk protein. (This discussion is centered on cow's-milk protein found in commercial infant formulas; whole milk is not recommended for infants younger than the age of 12 months.) The hypersensitivity may be manifested within the first 4 months of life through a variety of signs and symp-

---

*Further information for parents of infants with food allergies is available from the **American Academy of Allergy, Asthma, and Immunology,** 611 East Wells Street, Milwaukee, WI 52202; (800) 822-2762, website: www.aaaai.org. Additional helpful websites for information on food allergy include Medline Plus Health Information (sponsored by NIH): http://medlineplus.gov/; **The Food Allergy & Anaphylaxis Network:** www.foodallergy.org ; and the **National Institute of Allergy and Infectious Diseases:** www.niaid.nih.org

---

⸂ GUIDELINES

Preventing Atopy in Children
IDENTIFY CHILDREN AT RISK
Family history of allergy
Increased IgE in cord blood and postnatal serum
Dry, flaky skin

PRENATAL PRECAUTIONS (LAST TRIMESTER)
Avoid any known food allergens
Avoid milk and other dairy products, peanuts, and eggs
Minimize ingestion of other hyperallergenic foods (see Box 11-3)

POSTNATAL PRECAUTIONS
Breast milk (preferred) or casein/whey hydrolysate formula (e.g., Nutramigen, Pregstimil, Alimentum) or amino acid formula such as Neocate exclusively for at least 6 months
No solid food for first 6 months
No cow's milk or soy formula for 12 months
No egg, fish, corn, citrus, peanuts, nuts, or chocolate for 12 months
One new food added at 5-day intervals to identify possible reaction

ENVIRONMENTAL CONTROL
Limited exposure to dust mites, molds, furry animals, latex products, and cigarette smoke

Data from Johnstone D: Strategy for intervention of food allergy in infants, *Int Pediatr* 4(4):319-325, 1989; Zeiger R and others: Effectiveness of dietary manipulation in the prevention of food allergy in infants, part 2, *J Allergy Clin Immunol* 78(1 pt 2):224-238, 1986; Wood RA: Prospects for the prevention of allergy in children, *Curr Opin Pediatr* 8(6):601-605, 1995.

BOX 11-4 ■ Common Clinical Manifestations of Cow's-Milk Sensitivity

GASTROINTESTINAL	RESPIRATORY	OTHER SIGNS AND SYMPTOMS
Diarrhea	Rhinitis	Eczema
Vomiting	Bronchitis	Excessive crying
Colic	Asthma	Pallor (from anemia
Abdominal pain	Wheezing	secondary to
	Sneezing	chronic blood
	Coughing	loss in gastrointestinal tract)
	Chronic nasal discharge	

---

toms (Box 11-4) that may appear within several minutes of milk ingestion or after a period of several days. The diagnosis may initially be made from the history, although the history alone is not diagnostic; the timing and diversity of clinical manifestations vary greatly. For example, cow's-milk allergy may be manifested as colic (see discussion on p. 377), chronic constipation, gastroesophageal reflux, or sleeplessness in an otherwise healthy infant. The incidence of CMPA is reported to range from 2% to 7.5% in developed countries, although the percentage may appear to be higher because of parental report of symptoms rather than actual confirmation of CMPA (Host, 2002; Salvatore and Vandenplas, 2002).

Diagnostic Evaluation.

A number of diagnostic tests may be performed, including stool analysis for blood (both frank and occult bleeding can occur from the colitis), serum IgE levels, skin-prick or scratch testing, and radioallergosorbent test (measures IgE antibodies to specific allergens in serum by radioimmunoassay). Both skin and radioallergosorbent testing help identify the offending food, but the results are not always conclusive. The CAP System FEIA test is reported to have a 95% or greater predictive value in identifying children with allergies to egg, milk, peanut, and fish; use of this test would negate the need for the double-blind placebo-controlled food challenge in many children (Sampson, 2001).

The most definitive diagnostic strategy is elimination of milk, followed by challenge testing after improvement of symptoms. Challenge testing involves reintroducing small quantities of milk in the diet to detect resurgence of symptoms; at times challenge testing involves the use of a placebo so that the parent is unaware of or "blind" to the timing of allergen ingestion. A double-blind placebo-controlled food challenge is the gold standard for diagnosing food allergies such as CMPA, yet is not used very often for diagnosing cow's milk protein allergy (Baron, 2000).

Therapeutic Management.

Treatment of cow's-milk allergy is elimination of all dairy products. For infants fed cow's-milk formula, this primarily involves changing the formula to a casein hydrolysate milk formula (Pregestimil, Nutramigen, or Alimentum), in which the protein has been broken down (or "predigested") into its amino acids through enzymatic hydrolysis. Another choice is the amino acid–based formula, NEOCATE. Soy-based formula is **not** recommended because of cross-reactivity to soy (American Academy of Pediatrics, 1998). Goat's milk is not an acceptable substitute because it cross-reacts with cow's-milk protein, is deficient in folic acid, and is unsuitable as the only source of calories. Infants who are breast-fed but have symptoms of cow's-milk hypersensitivity are treated by eliminating all dairy products from the lactating mother's diet, although there is some evidence that restricting maternal dairy intake is not necessary. If maternal dairy intake is restricted, these women need vitamin D and calcium supplementation to prevent deficiency. Infants are maintained on the dairy-free diet for a year or more, depending on the type of reaction and severity, at which time very small quantities of milk are reintroduced.

Nursing Considerations.

The principal nursing objectives are identification of potential milk allergy and appropriate counseling of parents regarding substitute formulas. The protein hydrolysate formulas tend to be less palatable than milk-based formulas. Consequently, reluctance to accept the new formula may be a problem. This can be overcome by introducing the formula gradually over a few days using 1 ounce of new formula to 7 ounces of old formula, then 2 to 6 ounces, 3 to 4, and as needed, or by adding nonnutritive flavor packets available in a number of different flavors (Ross Laboratories). Parents also need to be reassured that the infant will receive complete nutrition from the new formula and will suffer no ill effects from the absence of cow's milk. Carnation Good Start, a whey protein hydrolysate, is not appropriate for CMPA because some children may react to it (Anderson, 1997).

After solid foods are started, parents need guidance in avoiding all associated milk products, although many children reportedly outgrow cow's-milk protein sensitivity by 3 to 4 years of age (Sicherer, 2001) (see Box 11-3). Carefully reading all food labels helps avoid ingesting prepared foods containing milk products.

Lactose Intolerance

Lactose intolerance refers to at least three different entities that involve a deficiency of the enzyme *lactase,* which is needed for the hydrolysis or digestion of lactose in the small intestine; lactose is hydrolyzed into glucose and galactose. *Congenital lactase deficiency* occurs soon after birth after the newborn has consumed lactose-containing milk (human milk or commercial formula). This inborn error of metabolism involves the complete absence or severely reduced presence of lactase, is rare, and requires lifelong lactose-free or extremely reduced lactose diet.

Late-onset lactase deficiency, sometimes referred to as *primary lactase deficiency,* is the most common type of lactose intolerance and is manifested usually around 3 to 7 years of age, although the time of onset is variable. Ethnic groups with a high incidence of lactase deficiency include Asians, southern Europeans, Arabs, Israelis, and African Americans.

Lactose intolerance *(secondary lactase deficiency)* may occur secondary to damage of the intestinal lumen, which decreases or destroys the enzyme lactase. Cystic fibrosis, sprue, kwashiorkor, or infections such as giardiasis, HIV, or rotavirus may cause a temporary or permanent lactose intolerance.

The primary symptoms of lactose intolerance include abdominal pain, bloating, flatulence, and diarrhea, and severity may range from mild to severe. The onset of symptoms occurs within 30 minutes to several hours of lactose consumption. Lactose intolerance is often perceived as an allergy, and, in several studies, reports of acute gastrointestinal symptoms ascribed to lactose intolerance, measurement of lactase activity is normal (Goldberg, Folta, and Must, 2002).

Lactose intolerance may be diagnosed on the basis of the history and improvement with a lactose-reduced diet. The breath hydrogen test is used to positively diagnose the condition. Breath samples in lactose-deficient individuals will yield a higher percentage of hydrogen (20 parts per million or more above baseline).

Treatment of lactose intolerance is elimination of offending dairy products; however, some advocate decreasing amounts of dairy products rather than total elimination, especially in small children (Goldberg, Folta, and Must, 2002). In infants, soy-based formula can be substituted for cow's-milk formula or human milk (American Academy of Pediatrics, 1998). Most people are able to tolerate small amounts of lactose even in the presence of deficient lactase activity (Goldberg, Folta, and Must, 2002) and should be encouraged to continue their intake of dairy products in small amounts to obtain much-needed nutrients. Milk taken

FAMILY HOME CARE

Controlling Symptoms of Lactose Intolerance

In infants substitute soy-based formula for cow's-milk formula or human milk.

Limit milk consumption to one glass at a time.

Drink milk with other foods rather than alone.

Eat hard cheese, cottage cheese, or yogurt instead of drinking milk.

Use enzyme tablets (Lactaid, Lactrase, Dairy Ease) to metabolize the lactose in milk or supplement the body's own lactase (add tablets to milk or sprinkle on dairy products such as ice cream).

Eat small amounts of dairy foods daily to help colonic bacteria adapt to ingested lactose.

at meals may be better tolerated than when taken alone (see Family Home Care box.) Pretreated milk (with microbial-derived lactase) is reported to be effective in improving lactose absorption. Because dairy products are a major source of calcium and vitamin D, supplementation of these nutrients is needed to prevent deficiency. Yogurt contains inactive lactase enzyme, which is activated by the temperature and pH of the duodenum; this lactase activity substitutes for the lack of endogenous lactase. Fresh yogurt may be tolerated better than frozen yogurt; hard cheeses, lactase-treated dairy products, and lactase tablets taken with dairy products are also viable options. An important distinction between lactose intolerance and food hypersensitivity is that lactose intolerance will not manifest as an anaphylactic-type reaction.

Nursing Considerations.   Nursing care is similar to the interventions discussed for cow's milk allergy: explaining the dietary restrictions to the family; identifying alternate sources of calcium such as yogurt; explaining the importance of supplementation; and discussing sources of lactose, especially hidden sources such as its use as a bulk agent in certain medications, and ways of controlling the symptoms (see Family Home Care box). Parents are advised to check with the pharmacist regarding this possibility when obtaining medication.

FEEDING DIFFICULTIES

REGURGITATION AND "SPITTING UP"

The return of small amounts of food after a feeding is a common occurrence during infancy. It should not be confused with actual vomiting, which can be associated with a number of disturbances that may be insignificant or serious. It is usually benign, although persistent regurgitation necessitates medical evaluation to rule out gastroesophageal reflux (see Chapter 24). For clarification the following terms are defined:

- **Regurgitation**—Return of undigested food from the stomach, usually accompanied by burping
- **Spitting up**—Dribbling of unswallowed formula from the infant's mouth immediately after a feeding

The normal occurrence of regurgitation or spitting up should be explained to parents, especially to those who are unduly concerned about it. Regurgitation can be reduced by some simple measures, such as frequent burping during and after feeding, minimum handling during and after feeding, and positioning the child on the right side with the head slightly elevated after feeding. The inconvenience of spitting up can be managed with the use of absorbent bibs on the infant and protective cloths on the parent.

Sometimes frequent dribbling of formula causes excoriation of the corners of the mouth, chin, and neck. Keeping the area dry promotes healing but can be difficult to maintain. Helpful suggestions include applying a thin film of petrolatum or A and D Ointment to the affected areas after cleansing and using absorbent nonplastic-lined terry-cloth bibs, which are changed frequently.

PAROXYSMAL ABDOMINAL PAIN (COLIC)

Colic is reported to occur in 5% to 30% of all infants (Neu and Robinson, 2003), yet has no particular affinity in regard to the gender, race, or socioeconomic status of the infant and family (Ellett, 2003). The condition is generally described as paroxysmal abdominal pain or cramping that is manifested by loud crying and drawing the legs up to the abdomen. Other definitions include variables such as duration of cry greater than 3 hours a day, occurring more than 3 days per week, and parental dissatisfaction with the child's behavior. Some studies report an increase in symptoms (fussiness and crying) in the late afternoon or evening; however, in some infants the onset of symptoms occurs at another time. Colic is more common in young infants under the age of 3 months than in older infants, and infants with "difficult" temperaments are more likely to be colicky. Despite the obvious behavioral indications of pain, the child tolerates breast milk or some type of infant formula well, gains weight, and usually thrives. There is no evidence of a residual effect of colic on older children, except perhaps a strained parent-child relationship in some cases; in other words, infants who are colicky grow up to be normal children and adults.

Among the theories that have been investigated as potential causes are too rapid feeding, overeating, swallowing excessive air, improper feeding technique (especially in positioning and burping), and emotional stress or tension between parent and child. Although all of these may occur, there is no evidence that one factor is consistently present. In some infants colic may be a sign of cow's-milk protein allergy or cow's-milk intolerance, and eliminating cow's milk products from the infant's diet and the diet of lactating mothers can reduce the symptoms; in some infants soy milk may cause the same discomfort as cow's milk. Parental smoking, strained parent-infant interaction, lactase deficiency, difficult infant temperament, difficulty regulating emotions, central nervous system immaturity, and neurochemical dysregulation in the brain have also been proposed as potential causes of colic (Ellett, 2003; Neu and Robinson, 2003; Friedman, 1996). A positive association between consumption of fruit juices (carbohydrate malabsorption) and colic has been demonstrated in some cases (Duro and others, 2002). The final consensus of most experts who study colic is that it is multifactorial in nature and that no single treatment for every colicky infant will be effective in alleviating the symptoms.

Therapeutic Management

Management of colic should begin with an investigation of possible organic causes, such as CMPA. If a sensitivity to cow's milk is strongly suspected, a trial substitution of another formula such as a casein hydrolysate (Nutramigen, Alimentum, Pregestimil), whey hydrolysate, or amino acid (Neocate) is warranted. Soy formulas are avoided because of the possibility of sensitivity to soy protein as well.

The use of drugs, including sedatives, antispasmodics, antihistamines, and antiflatulents, is sometimes recommended. The most commonly used sedatives are phenobarbital, hydroxyzine hydrochloride (Atarax), and chloral hydrate. Simethicone (Mylicon) may also help allay the symptoms of colic. However, in most controlled studies none of these drugs completely reduce the symptoms of colic. Herbal (chamomile) tea offered at the onset of crying and up to three times daily has been proved to be effective in relieving the symptoms of colic (Weizman and others, 1993). The addition of lactase to infant formula has produced mixed results as far as abatement of overall symptoms.

Nursing Considerations

The initial step in managing colic is to take a thorough, detailed history of the usual daily events. Areas that should be stressed include (1) the infant's diet; (2) the diet of the breast-feeding mother; (3) the time of day when crying occurs; (4) the relationship of the crying to feeding time; (5) the presence of specific family members during the crying and habits of family members, such as smoking; (6) activity of the mother or usual caregiver before, during, and after the crying; (7) characteristics of the cry (duration, intensity); (8) measures used to relieve the crying and their effectiveness; and (9) the infant's stooling, voiding, and sleeping patterns. Of special emphasis is a careful assessment of the feeding process via demonstration by the parent.

If milk sensitivity is suspected, bottle-feeding and breast-feeding mothers should follow a milk-free diet for a minimum of 3 to 5 days in an attempt to reduce symptoms in the infant. Mothers need to be cautioned that some nondairy creamers may contain calcium caseinate, a cow's milk protein. If a milk-free diet is helpful, lactating mothers may need calcium supplements to meet the body's requirement. Bottle-fed infants may improve with the same dietary modifications as for the child with cow's-milk protein allergy (see p. 375).

One nursing intervention that is important and appropriate (before and after organic cause has been eliminated) is reassurance of both parents that they are not doing anything wrong and that the infant is not experiencing any physical or emotional harm. Parents, especially mothers, become easily frustrated with the infant's crying and perceive this as a sign that there is something horribly wrong. An empathetic, gentle, and reassuring attitude, in addition to suggestions about remedies for treatment, will help allay parents' anxieties, which are usually exacerbated by loss of sleep and preoccupation over the infant's welfare. Other support persons and extended family members may be enlisted to help support the parents during this time of difficulty.

When no cause can be identified, helping parents understand the infant's crying behavior and modifying parent interventions to promptly attend to the infant's needs can de-

FAMILY HOME CARE

Managing the Colicky Infant

Place infant prone over a covered hot-water bottle, heated towel, or covered heating pad.

Massage infant's abdomen.

Respond immediately to the crying.

Change infant's position frequently; walk with child's face down and with body across parent's arm, with parent's hand under infant's abdomen, applying gentle pressure (Fig. 11-2).

Use a front carrier for transporting infant.

Swaddle infant tightly with a soft, stretchy blanket.

Place infant in an electric (or wind-up) infant swing.

Take infant for car rides or outside for a change in environment.

Use bottles that minimize air swallowing (curved bottle or inner collapsible bag).

Use a commercial device* in the crib that stimulates the vibration and sound of a car ride or plays soothing "noise," in utero sounds, or music.†

Provide smaller, frequent feedings; burp infant during and after feedings using the shoulder position or sitting upright, and place infant in an upright seat after feedings.

Introduce a pacifier for added sucking.

In breast-fed infants, mother should avoid all milk products for a trial period.

If household members smoke, avoid smoking near infant; preferably confine smoking activity to outside of home.

Give appropriate dose of acetaminophen elixir or suppository if suggested by health professional; not recommended for daily use.

If nothing reduces the crying, place infant in crib and allow to cry; periodically hold and comfort child and put down again.

Maintain a brief diary of the time of day the crying starts; events going on in household; time, amount and type of last feeding; length of crying; and characteristics of cry—although this will not stop the crying, it may help the practitioner identify a possible cause

*Sweet Dreems, Inc., Sleep Tight Order Department, 4710 East Walnut Street, Westerville, OH 43081; (800) NO COLIC, (800) 662-6542.

†Suggested infant relaxation music: "Heartbeat Lullabies" by Terry Woodford. Available from Baby-Go-To-Sleep Center, Audio Therapy Innovations, Inc., PO Box 550, Colorado Springs, CO 80901; (800) 537-7748; website: www.babygotosleep.com.

crease the length of fussiness and crying (Dihigo, 1998). Other approaches for managing colic are listed in the Family Home Care box. Parents are encouraged to try as many of these approaches as possible, because not all are effective for every infant. Research is in progress on an Infant Colic Scale, which will assist in narrowing the cause of infant colic (Ellett, 2003). Meanwhile, the researcher suggests that a problem-solving discussion with the parents, in addition to acknowledgment that the infant has colic, is an optimal strategy for helping parents manage the infant with colic until a cure is found (Ellett, 2003).

FAILURE TO THRIVE

Failure to thrive (FTT) is a sign of inadequate growth resulting from inability to obtain or use calories required for growth. FTT has no universal definition, although one of the more common parameters is a weight (and sometimes height) that falls below the 5th percentile for the child's age. Growth

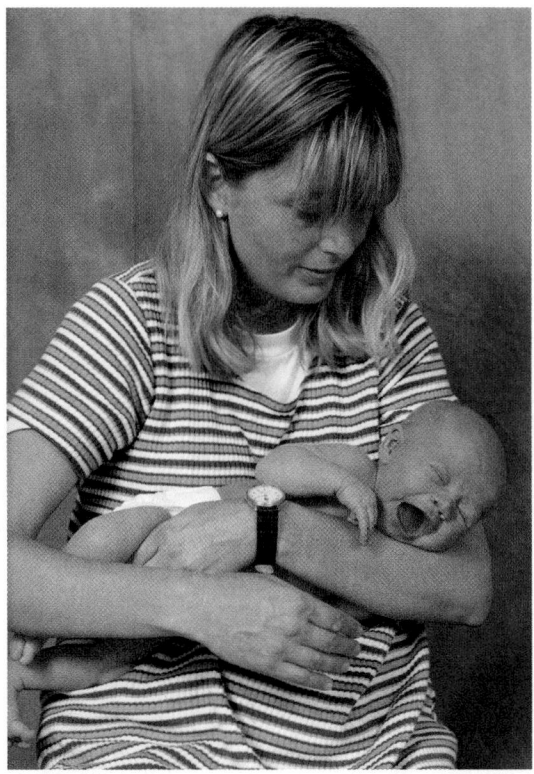

FIG. 11-2 ■ The "colic carry" may be comforting to an infant with colic. (Photo by Paul Vincent Kuntz, Texas Children's Hospital.)

measurements alone are not used to diagnose children with FTT. Rather, the finding of a pattern of persistent deviation from established growth parameters is cause for concern.

Three general categories of failure to thrive are the following:

1 **Organic failure to thrive**—Result of a physical cause, such as congenital heart defects, neurologic lesions, microcephaly, chronic renal failure, gastroesophageal reflux, malabsorption syndrome, endocrine dysfunction, cystic fibrosis, or acquired immunodeficiency syndrome.

2 **Nonorganic failure to thrive (NFTT)**—A definable cause that is unrelated to disease. NFTT is most often the result of psychosocial factors, such as inadequate nutritional information by the parent; deficiency in maternal care or a disturbance in maternal-child attachment; or a disturbance in the child's ability to separate from the parent, leading to food refusal to maintain attention.

3 **Idiopathic failure to thrive**—Unexplained by the usual organic and environmental etiologies but may also be classified as NFTT. Both categories of NFTT account for the majority of cases of FTT.

Traditionally the category of NFTT has implied a disturbance in the parent-child interaction. However, this is not always the case. Many other factors can lead to inadequate infant caloric intake, such as the following:

■ **Poverty**—Lack of funds to buy sufficient food; may dilute formula to extend available supply

■ **Health or childrearing beliefs**—Use of fad diets; excessive concern with preventing conditions such as obesity, hypercholesterolemia, or nursing caries; strict use of scheduled feedings

■ **Inadequate nutritional knowledge**—Cultural confusion of newly arrived immigrants who are unaware of appropriate food selections in American markets; parents with cognitive impairment

■ **Family stress**—Overwhelming involvement with another chronically ill child; any number of other stresses (financial, marital, excessive parenting and employment responsibilities, depression, chemical abuse, acute grief)

■ **Feeding resistance**—Result of nonoral nutritional therapy early in life

■ **Insufficient breast milk**—Result of a number of different causes (fatigue, illness, poor release of milk, insufficient glandular tissue, lack of maternal confidence)

In these instances parent education and provision of necessary supports (financial or psychosocial) are successful in correcting the reason for the malnutrition. Dealing with families in which a child has NFTT because of a parent-child disturbance is much more difficult and is the focus of the nursing care discussion. It has also been pointed out that growth failure in childhood may be a combination of both NFTT (possibly disturbed parent-infant interaction or nonnurturing environment) and organic failure to thrive (child's difficult disposition) and that malnutrition itself often makes the child's behavior less interactive, thus further contributing to the ongoing paradigm of growth failure (Careaga and Kerner, 2000).

Diagnostic Evaluation

Diagnosis is initially made from evidence of growth retardation and caloric deprivation. If the onset of FTT is fairly recent (versus chronic), the weight, but not the height, is below accepted standards (usually the 5th percentile); if FTT is long-standing, both weight and height are depressed, indicating chronic malnutrition. Additional diagnostic procedures include a complete health and dietary history, physical examination for evidence of organic causes, developmental assessment, and a family assessment. Other tests are selected *only* as indicated to rule out organic problems. To prevent the overuse of diagnostic procedures, NFTT should be considered *early* in the differential diagnosis. To avoid the social stigma of NFTT during the early investigative phase, many health care workers use the term ***growth delay*** (or ***failure***) until the actual cause is established.

Therapeutic Management

Regardless of the cause of FTT, the treatment is directed at reversing the malnutrition and the underlying cause. The goal is to provide sufficient calories to support "catch-up" growth—a rate of growth greater than the expected rate for age. Any coexisting medical problems are treated.

In most cases of NFTT a multidisciplinary team of physician, nurse, dietitian, gastroenterologist, child-life specialist, and social worker or mental health professional is needed to deal with the multiple psychologic problems. Efforts are made to relieve any additional stresses on the family, such as referrals to welfare agencies or supplemental food programs.

Prognosis

The prognosis for NFTT is related to the cause. If the parents have simply been ignorant of the infant's needs, teaching may remedy the child's limited caloric intake and permanently

BOX 11-5 ■ Clinical Manifestations of Failure to Thrive

Growth failure—below 5th percentile in weight only or weight and height
Developmental delays—social, motor, adaptive, language
Apathy
Poor hygiene
Withdrawn behavior
Feeding or eating disorders, such as vomiting, anorexia, pica, rumination
No fear of strangers (at age when stranger anxiety is normal)
Avoidance of eye contact
Wide-eyed gaze and continual scan of the environment ("radar gaze")
Stiff and unyielding or flaccid and unresponsive
Minimal smiling

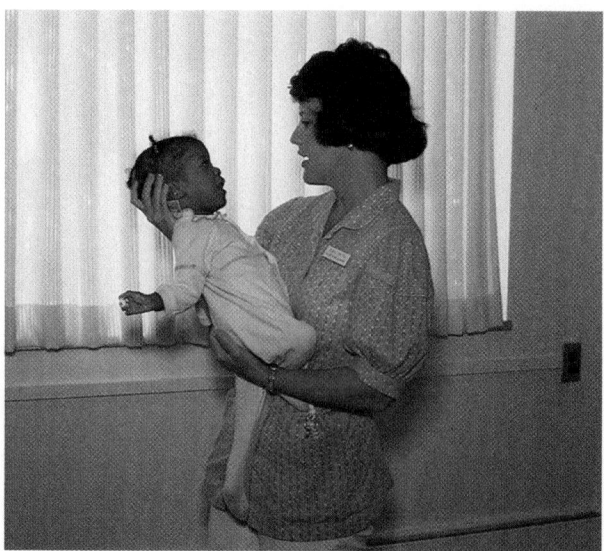

FIG. 11-3 ■ A consistent nurse is important in developing trust in infants with failure to thrive.

reverse the growth failure. Inadequate or decreased feeding periods by the infant's primary caretaker are often observed to be the cause of NFTT in conjunction with family disorganization. When family dysfunction is extensive, the prognosis is uncertain. Factors related to poor prognosis are severe feeding resistance, lack of awareness in and cooperation from the parent(s), low family income, low maternal educational level, adolescent parent, and early age of onset of NFTT.

Nursing Considerations

Nurses play a critical role in the diagnosis of NFTT through their assessment of the child, parents, and family interaction. Knowledge of the characteristics of children with NFTT and their families is essential in helping identify these children and hastening the confirmation of a correct diagnosis (Box 11-5). Accurate assessment of initial weight and height and daily weight, as well as recording of all food intake, is mandatory. The feeding behavior of the child is documented, as is parent-child interaction during feeding, other caregiving activities, and play. An excellent feeding observation instrument is the *Nursing Child Assessment Satellite Training Feeding Scale,* which is designed to assess the feeding interaction of infants up to 12 months of age (Barnard and others, 1993).*

Another tool that may be used is the 25-item observational scale, the *Feeding Checklist,* which was developed specifically for the purpose of observing mother-infant dyads with NFTT. The checklist has helped nurses and other health care professionals in the objective assessment of key aspects of infant and toddler feeding situations related to NFTT (MacPhee and Schneider, 1996).

A feature of many children with NFTT is their irregularity (low rhythmicity) in activities of daily living. Some of these children typify the "difficult" temperament pattern. However, another type is the passive, sleepy, lethargic infant who does not wake up for feedings. Parents who have been

---

*Training is required to use the Feeding Scale, and information on the training program is available from Jean F. Kelly, PhD, Director, **Nursing Child Assessment Satellite Training,** WJ-10, University of Washington, Seattle, WA 98195; (206) 543-8528; e-mail: ncast@u.washington.edu.

advised of "demand feeding schedules" may be unsure of whether to wake the child or let the child sleep. Because of their inexperience and lack of guidance, parents may develop a pattern of infrequent feeding that is inadequate to meet the infant's nutritional needs. Such a pattern is particularly detrimental with the breast-feeding infant, in whom frequent nursing is essential to an adequate milk supply.

Some parents are at increased risk for attachment problems because of (1) isolation and social crisis; (2) inadequate support systems, such as teenage and single mothers; and (3) poor parenting role models as a child. Other factors that should be considered are lack of education; physical and mental health problems such as physical and sexual abuse, depression, or drug dependence; immaturity, especially in adolescent parents; and lack of commitment to parenting, such as giving priority to other ventures such as entertainment or employment. Often these parents and their families are under stress and in multiple chronic emotional, social, and financial crises.

Because part of the difficulty between parent and child is dissatisfaction and frustration, the child should have a primary core of nurses (Fig. 11-3). The nurses caring for the child can learn to perceive the child's cues and reverse the cycle of dissatisfaction, especially in the area of feeding. Because these children are not ill with any physical disorder but are debilitated from general malnutrition, they should be placed in a room with noninfectious children of a similar age. Depending on the cause of NFTT, children may be treated on an outpatient basis.

Because many of these children are responding to stimuli that have led to the negative feeding patterns, the first goal is to structure the feeding environment to encourage eating. General guidelines for the feeding process are outlined in the Guidelines box.

Four primary goals in the nutritional management of FTT are to (1) correct nutritional deficiencies and achieve ideal weight for height, (2) allow for catch-up growth, (3) restore optimum body composition, and (4) educate the

GUIDELINES

Feeding Children With Failure to Thrive

Provide a primary core of staff to feed the child. The same nurses are able to learn the child's cues and respond consistently.

Provide a quiet, unstimulating atmosphere. A number of these children are very distractible, and their attention is diverted with minimal stimuli. Older children do well at a feeding table; younger children should always be held.

Maintain a calm, even temperament throughout the meal. Negative outbursts may be commonplace in this child's habit formation. Limits on eating behavior definitely need to be provided, but they should be stated in a firm, calm tone. If the nurse is hurried or anxious, the feeding process will not be optimized.

Talk to the child by giving directions about eating. "Take a bite, Lisa" is appropriate and directive. The more distractible the child, the more directive the nurse should be to refocus attention on feeding. Positive comments about feeding are actively given.

Be persistent. This is perhaps one of the most important guidelines. Parents often give up when the child begins negative feeding behavior. Calm perseverance through 10 to 15 minutes of food refusal will eventually diminish negative behavior. Although forced feeding is avoided, "strictly encouraged" feeding is essential.

Maintain a face-to-face posture with the child when possible. Encourage eye contact and remain with the child throughout the meal.

Introduce new foods slowly. Often these children have been exclusively bottle-fed. If acceptance of solids is a problem, begin with pureed food and, once accepted, advance to junior and regular solid foods.

Follow the child's rhythm of feeding. The child will set a rhythm when the previous conditions are met.

Develop a structured routine. Disruption in their other activities of daily living has great impact on feeding responses, so bathing, sleeping, dressing, and playing, as well as feeding, are structured. The nurse should feed the child in the same way and place as often as possible. The length of the feeding should also be established (usually 30 minutes).

parents or primary caregivers regarding the child's nutritional requirements and appropriate feeding methods (Corrales and Utter, 1999; Maggioni and Lifshitz, 1995). To increase caloric intake in formula-fed infants, supplements such as Polycose or medium-chain triglycerides may be added slowly. Other carbohydrate additives include rice cereal and vegetable oil. Because vitamin and mineral deficiencies may occur, multivitamin supplementation, including zinc and iron, is recommended. Breast-fed infants with NFTT may require caloric supplementation which may be accomplished by adding 1 teaspoon of 24 kcal/ounce formula to 3 ounces of breast milk. The consumption of fruit juices should be minimized in infants under 6 months. Usually only in extreme cases of malnourishment are tube feedings or intravenous therapy required.

Besides attending to the physical needs of the child, the interdisciplinary team must plan care for appropriate developmental stimulation. After an approximate developmental age is established, a planned program of play is begun. Ideally a child-life specialist is involved to implement and su-

pervise the stimulation program. Every effort is made to teach the parent how to play and interact with the child.

Nursing care of these children involves a "family systems" approach. In other words, for the entire family to become healthy, each member must be helped to change. Care of the parents is aimed at helping them increase their feelings of self-esteem through positive, successful parenting skills. Initially this necessitates providing an environment in which they feel welcomed and accepted. Because these parents are often distrustful of authority figures, it may take some time before they develop any trust toward the nurse. One approach is to empathize with the parent about the difficulties of childrearing. For example, the nurse may state that many parents find adjusting to parenthood a trying time or that the demands of caring for an infant can become overwhelming.

Teaching infant care techniques to the parents is begun through example and demonstration, not by lecturing. As the nurse perceives the infant's cues, these are emphasized to the parents. For example, during a feeding the nurse might comment that the infant is still hungry because the child sucks vigorously and looks at the nurse. When the infant is satisfied, the nurse points out that the infant is signaling this by releasing the strong suck, closing the eyes, and breathing deeply and more slowly. By example, the child is gently placed in the crib for a nap.

Plans are made to implement these interventions at home. A home health referral is made, and if a foster grandparent was included, this person should also visit the family. Social agencies that can provide financial or housing assistance to lessen the stress of everyday life are also contacted.

DISORDERS OF UNKNOWN ETIOLOGY

SUDDEN INFANT DEATH SYNDROME

Sudden infant death syndrome (SIDS) is defined as the sudden death of an infant younger than 1 year of age that remains unexplained after a complete postmortem examination, including an investigation of the death scene and a review of the case history. In the United States mortality from SIDS has declined more than 40% since 1992: 1.3 deaths per 1000 live births in 1991 versus 0.65 deaths per 1000 live births in 1999 (American Academy of Pediatrics, 2000; CDC, 2001). The dramatic decrease is attributed to the "Back to Sleep" campaign* (see following section). SIDS is the third leading cause of death in children between the ages of 1 month and 1 year and claimed the lives of almost 2500 infants in 1998 (Guyer and others, 1999). Table 11-3 summarizes the major epidemiologic characteristics of SIDS.

Etiology

Numerous theories have been proposed regarding the etiology of SIDS; however, the cause remains unknown. The most compelling hypothesis is that SIDS is related to a

---

*"Back to Sleep" materials may be ordered by calling (800) 505-CRIB, faxing requests to (301) 496-7101, or writing to NICHD/Back to Sleep, 31 Center Drive, Room 2A32, Bethesda, MD 20892-2425; website: www.nichd.nih.gov/publications/pubskey.cfm?from=sids.

TABLE 11-3 ■ Epidemiology of SIDS

FACTORS	OCCURRENCE
Incidence	0.65:1000 live births (1999)
Peak age	2 to 4 months; 95% occur by 6 months
Sex	Higher percentage of males affected
Time of death	During sleep
Time of year	Increased incidence in winter
Racial	Greater incidence in Native Americans, African Americans, and Hispanics
Socioeconomic	Increased occurrence in lower socioeconomic class
Birth	Higher incidence in: Preterm infants, especially infants of low birth weight; Multiple births*; Neonates with low Apgar scores; Infants with central nervous system disturbances and respiratory disorders such as bronchopulmonary dysplasia (chronic lung disease); Increasing birth order (subsequent siblings as opposed to firstborn child); Infants with a recent history of illness
Sleep habits	Prone position; use of soft bedding; overheating (thermal stress); co-sleeping with adult, especially on sofa
Feeding habits	Lower incidence in breast-fed infants
Siblings	May have greater incidence
Maternal	Young age; cigarette smoking, especially during pregnancy; poor prenatal care; substance abuse (heroin, methadone, cocaine)

*Although a rare event, simultaneous death of twins from sudden infant death syndrome can occur.

brainstem abnormality in the neurologic regulation of cardiorespiratory control. Abnormalities include prolonged sleep apnea, increased frequency of brief inspiratory pauses, excessive periodic breathing, and impaired arousal responsiveness to increased carbon dioxide or decreased oxygen. However, sleep apnea is not the cause of SIDS. The vast majority of infants with apnea do not die, and only a minority of SIDS victims have documented *apparent life-threatening events (ALTEs)* (see Apnea of Infancy, p. 385). Numerous studies indicate that there is no association between SIDS and diphtheria, tetanus, and pertussis vaccines.

Maternal smoking, both prenatally and postnatally, has been proposed as a possible cause of SIDS, as has poor prenatal care and low maternal age (Leach and others, 1999). Increased nicotine concentrations were found in infants who died of SIDS compared with a group of controls, regardless of whether smoking was reported (McMartin and others, 2002). Co-sleeping, or bed sharing, has been reported to have a possible association with SIDS, especially in cases of maternal smoking. The American Academy of Pediatrics (2000) recommends that adults follow the same safeguards in the bed as in the crib. In addition, the bed sharer (who should only be parents) should not smoke or use substances such as alcohol or drugs that may impair arousal. Unlike cribs, which are designed to meet safety standards for infants, adult beds or sofas are not so designed and may carry a risk of accidental entrapment and suffocation. One survey found a high association between infant deaths, nonstandard beds, and bed sharing; a large percentage of infants were found dead on their backs when bed-sharing was in effect, suggesting suffocation (Unger and others, 2003).

Suffocation hazards included wedging between a mattress or bed and wall and oronasal obstruction by a plastic bag (Drago and Dannenberg, 1999). The prone sleeping position was found to be higher among African-American infants dying of SIDS in Chicago than among Caucasians (Hauck and others, 2002). Another survey revealed that non–college educated, lower income families, and Hispanics were less likely to place the infant to sleep on the back at age 3 months (Corwin and others, 2003). Another postulated cause of SIDS is prolonged Q-T interval; however, at this time there is no strong evidence to support this as a cause. Overheating has been proposed as a potential cause of SIDS; therefore, infants should be dressed in light clothing and the room temperature kept at a comfortable range for a lightly dressed adult; overbundling the infant should be avoided.

The most compelling data come from studies that link sleep habits with an increased risk of SIDS. Sleeping in the prone position may cause oropharyngeal obstruction or affect the thermal balance or arousal state. Rebreathing of carbon dioxide by the prone infant and impaired arousal from active and quiet sleep when sleeping prone have both been suggested as a potential mechanism for the cause of death.

The American Academy of Pediatrics (2000) recommends that healthy infants be placed to sleep in the supine (on the back) position. There is an increased risk of SIDS in infants placed in the side-lying position, primarily because of their ability to turn to a prone position; therefore, the side-lying sleep position is no longer recommended. In the event that the side sleeping position is used, the infant's dependent arm should be placed forward to prevent rolling over onto the prone position. Soft bedding such as pillows or quilts should not be used under the infant for bedding. Bedding items such as stuffed animals or towels should be removed from the crib while the infant is asleep to prevent possible asphyxia.

Most preterm infants being discharged from the hospital should be placed in the supine sleep position unless there are factors that predispose to airway obstruction.

Although the etiology is unknown, autopsies reveal consistent pathologic findings such as pulmonary edema and intrathoracic hemorrhages that confirm the diagnosis of SIDS. Consequently, autopsies should be performed on all infants suspected of dying of SIDS, and the findings should be shared with the parents as soon as possible after the death.

Whether subsequent siblings of one SIDS infant are at increased risk for SIDS is unclear. Even if the increased risk is correct, families have a 99% chance that their subsequent child will *not* die of SIDS. Home monitoring is not recommended for this group of children, but it is often used by practitioners and may even be requested by parents. Monitoring is best initiated on an individual basis.

FAMILY HOME CARE

Infant Sleep Position and SIDS

For decades nurses have been taught to place newborns and infants on their tummies or sides to sleep in order to prevent aspiration and subsequent asphyxia. Nurses instructed parents to do the same. In the early 1990s, however, research data from New Zealand suggested that infants placed prone to sleep were more likely to die of SIDS than those who were placed in a nonprone (supine) position. "Nonsense, that cannot be!" those of us who worked with newborns and infants said. In 1992 the Back to Sleep campaign was initiated to encourage physicians, nurses, and other health professionals to inform parents about placing newborns and infants in a side-lying or nonprone position to sleep to decrease the risk of SIDS. This recommendation was later amended to propose that infants be placed only in a supine sleep position because infants placed in the side-lying position might roll over to a prone position and be at greater risk for SIDS. Since 1992, the incidence of SIDS in the United States has decreased by more than 40% to an all-time low of 0.7 per 1000 live births (American Academy of Pediatrics, 2003c). In 1992 SIDS was the leading cause of death in infants less than 1 year old; SIDS is now the third leading cause of death, preceded by congenital anomalies and prematurity (Moon, 2001). Yet research indicates that approximately 20% of all infants younger than age 6 months are still being placed in a side-lying or prone position to sleep despite findings in New Zealand, Great Britain, Australia, and the United States that the supine sleeping position has not been associated with an increase in the number of asphyxiation events or deaths in this age-group (American Academy of Pediatrics, 2003c). Additional research from Australia supports the theory that supine sleeping does not increase the incidence of mortality as a result of gastric contents being aspirated into the trachea (Byard and Beal, 2000).

Recent research from 94 Iowa hospitals indicates that a large number of newborns are still being placed in side-lying sleep positions; 51.4% of those surveyed indicated that the rationale for placing the newborn on the side was out of fear of asphyxiation (Hein and Pettit, 2001). Parents who hear physicians and nurses encourage them to place the infant supine at home may be confused by witnessing hospital workers placing infants prone or in side-lying positions in the nursery or mother-infant care unit. It is imperative that research be evaluated carefully, and while it is true that old habits die hard, it is time for nurses to be the front-line proponents for saving the lives of thousands of infants yearly by helping parents and caregivers understand the importance of preventing SIDS by putting infants to sleep on their back—at home, in the hospital nurseries, and in day care facilities.

Nursing Considerations

Nurses have a vital role in the prevention of SIDS by educating families about the risk of prone sleeping position in infants from birth to 6 months of age, using appropriate bedding surfaces, parental smoking around the infant, and the dangers of sharing an adult bed with the infant. It has been reported that as many as 20% of all infants this age are still placed to sleep in the prone position (Willinger and others, 2000). Nurses must be proactive in further decreasing the incidence of prone sleeping and other potential threats to healthy infants; postpartum discharge planning, newborn discharge teaching and newborn-care classes, fol-

low-up home visits, well-baby clinic visits, and immunization visits provide an excellent opportunity to educate parents and caregivers in these matters. (See Family Home Care box.)

One concern of many health care workers has been that infants placed on the back to sleep will aspirate emesis or mucus; one survey found no increase in infant deaths, aspiration, asphyxia, or respiratory failure as a result of supine sleep positioning over a 3-year period (Malloy, 2002). A recent study indicated that 20% of SIDS cases occurred in day care settings out of the home; therefore, it is important that infant sleep position be discussed with day care workers as well (Moon, Patel, and Shaefer, 2000).

Loss of a child from SIDS presents several crises with which the parents must cope. In addition to grief and mourning the death of their child, the parents must face a tragedy that was sudden, unexpected, and unexplained. The psychologic intervention for the family must deal with these additional variables. This discussion focuses primarily on the objectives of care for families experiencing SIDS, rather than on the process of grief and mourning, which is explored in Chapter 18.

> ### ! NURSING ALERT
>
> Research findings have important implications for practices that may reduce the risk of SIDS, such as avoiding smoking during pregnancy and near the infant; encouraging the supine sleeping position; avoiding soft, moldable mattresses, blankets, and pillows; discouraging bed sharing; encouraging breast-feeding; and avoiding overheating during sleep. The infant's head position should be varied to prevent flattening of the skull (*positional plagiocephaly*) (see Family Focus box and Figure 11-4).

Finding the Infant.   Usually it is the mother who finds the child dead in the crib. Typically the child is in a disheveled bed, with blankets over the head, and huddled in a corner. Frothy, blood-tinged fluid fills the mouth and nostrils, and the infant may be lying face down in the secretions, suggesting that he or she bled to death. The diaper is wet and full of stool, which is consistent with a cataclysmic type of death. The hands may be clutching the sheets, as if the child were in distress before death. The initial appearance of the child combined with the shock of such an unexpected event adds to the horror that the parents must face.

The parent who finds the infant initially must deal with her or his initial shock, panic, grief, questions of the other siblings, and the decision of where to find help. The first persons to arrive may be the police and ambulance attendants. Hopefully, they will handle the situation by asking few questions; giving no indication of wrongdoing, abuse, or neglect; making sensitive judgments concerning any resuscitation efforts for the child; and comforting the members of the family as much as possible. These individuals should be properly informed about SIDS to recognize its characteristic signs and tell parents that their child probably died of a condition called sudden infant death syndrome, which cannot be predicted or prevented. A compassionate, sensitive approach to the family during the very first few

FAMILY FOCUS

The Misshapen Head

Since the Back to Sleep campaign in 1992 advocating nonprone sleeping for infants, an increase in the incidence of positional *plagiocephaly* has been observed. Because the infant's sutures are not closed, the skull is very pliable and when the infant is placed on the back to sleep, the posterior occiput flattens over time; a typical bald spot will develop, which is usually transient. As a result of prolonged pressure on one side of the skull, that side becomes misshapen; facial asymmetry may develop. The sternocleidomastoid muscle may tighten on the preferential side and torticollis may also develop. Treatment of torticollis and plagiocephaly initially involve exercises to loosen the tight muscle and switching head position sides during feeding, carrying and sleep. If the plagiocephaly is not resolved within 4 to 8 weeks of physical therapy, a customized helmet may be worn to decrease the pressure on the affected side of the skull (Biggs, 2003). If there is a lack of improvement with physical therapy or a molded helmet over a given period, the infant may be referred to a pediatric neurosurgeon or craniofacial surgeon (American Academy of Pediatrics, 2003d). Minor skull flattening is not considered significant, but efforts should be taken to educate parents regarding changing head positions during sleep. To prevent plagiocephaly it is recommended that the infant's head position be altered during sleep time. Infants should be placed prone on a firm surface during awake time, which is encouraged to prevent plagiocephaly and to encourage development of upper shoulder girdle strength; the latter helps in the progressive development of movements such as rolling over and starting to rise up on all fours, which are precursors to crawling and eventually walking. Because the supine sleeping position has resulted in a significant decrease in loss of infant lives from SIDS, no changes in this stance appear to be on the horizon. The increased incidence of misshapen heads in infants as a result of supine sleeping can easily be prevented by changing certain infant care habits so the infant's skull shape remains intact and subsequent development progresses. Parents should not become alarmed at the development of plagiocephaly to the extent that they abandon supine sleeping position for the infant but should consult with the practitioner for further advice.

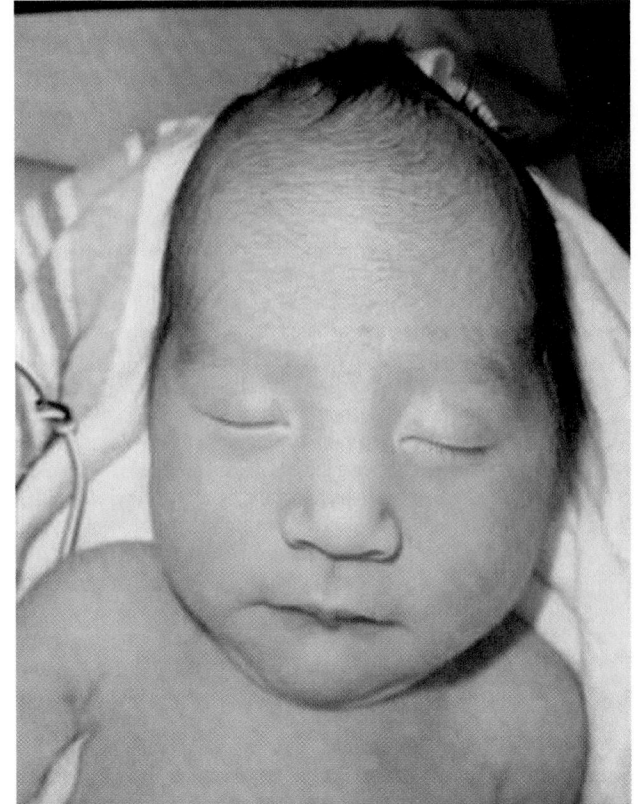

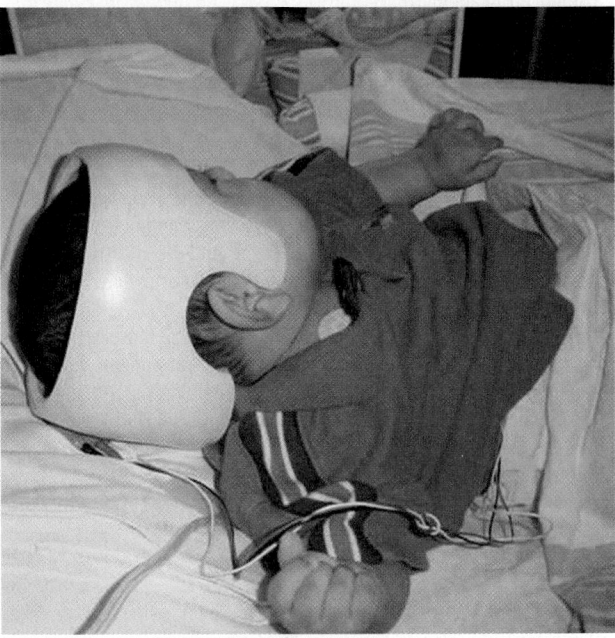

FIG. 11-4 ■ **A,** Plagiocephaly. **B,** Helmet used to correct plagiocephaly. (Courtesy Dr. Gerardo Cabrera-Meza, Deptartment of Neonatology, Baylor College of Medicine, Houston, Tex.)

minutes can help spare them some of the overwhelming guilt and anguish that commonly follow this type of death.

Arriving at the Emergency Department. The first contact that nurses typically have with these families is in the emergency department, when the infant is seen by a physician to be pronounced dead. Usually there is no attempt at resuscitation. During the time in the emergency department several aspects warrant special consideration. Parents are asked only factual questions, such as when they found the infant, how he or she looked, and whom they called for help. Any remarks that may suggest responsibility, such as why did they not go in earlier, did they not hear the infant cry out, was the head buried in a blanket, or were the other siblings jealous of this child, are avoided.

If statements were made that were misguided, such as "This looks like suffocation," they can be corrected before parents harbor them in their minds as indications of their guilt. The discussion of an autopsy should be presented at this time, emphasizing that a diagnosis cannot be confirmed until the postmortem examination is completed. If the

mother was breast-feeding, she needs information about abrupt discontinuation of lactation.

Another important aspect of compassionate care for these parents is allowing them to say good-bye to their child. Because the parents leave the hospital without their infant, it is helpful to accompany them to the car or arrange for someone else to take them home. A debriefing session may help health care workers who dealt with the family and deceased infant to deal with feelings that are often engendered when a SIDS victim is brought into the acute care facility.

Returning Home. When the parents return home, they should be visited by a competent, qualified professional as soon after the death as possible. Printed material that contains excellent information about SIDS (available from several qualified organizations*) should be provided.

Ideally the number of visits and plans for subsequent intervention need to be flexible. For example, the siblings may initially appear accepting of the explanation and well-adjusted but may later refuse to go to sleep or ask questions about graves or funerals, indicating their need for further help in dealing with the death. Parents facing the question of a subsequent child will need support. Both the birth of a subsequent child and the survival of that child, especially past the age of death of the previous child, are important transitional stages for parents.

Because the mourning process continues for at least a year or more, referrals to other parents who have lost a child to SIDS should be considered. The practitioner should be available to answer parents' questions regarding the infant's death, which may persist for months to years later until there is some resolution of the loss of the child.

APNEA OF INFANCY

Apnea of infancy (AOI) generally refers to pathologic apnea in infants of more than 37 weeks' gestation. The clinical presentation of AOI is an *ALTE* (previously referred to by the inaccurate and misleading expression "near-miss SIDS") that is described as:

- Frightening to the observer, who fears the child died or would have died without vigorous intervention
- Some combination of:
  - Apnea—Cessation of breathing for 20 seconds or more
  - Color change—Cyanosis or pallor, but sometimes plethora
  - Marked change in muscle tone—Usually marked hypotonia
  - Choking or gagging

AOI can be a symptom of many disorders, including sepsis, seizures, upper airway abnormalities, gastroesophageal reflux, hypoglycemia or other metabolic problems, impaired regulation of breathing during sleep or feeding, or a result of intentional poisoning by a caregiver. Abnormal physical properties of pulmonary surfactant have been identified in some children with recurrent ALTE. However, in about half the cases no cause is identified. Infants with a history of ALTEs are at increased risk for SIDS, but these children

constitute less than 7% of all SIDS victims. A diagnosis of AOI is made when no identifiable cause for the ALTE is found. Results from the Collaborative Home Infant Monitoring Evaluation study found that apnea and bradycardia occurred at conventional and extreme alarm thresholds in all groups of infants studied: siblings of SIDS infants, infants with ALTEs, symptomatic (of apnea and bradycardia) and asymptomatic preterm infants weighing less than 1750 g at birth, and healthy term infants. The researchers concluded that many infants experience apnea and bradycardia in each of these groups yet do not die. Furthermore, it was reported that apnea does not appear to be an immediate precursor to SIDS and that cardiorespiratory monitoring is not an effective tool for identifying infants at greater risk for SIDS (American Academy of Pediatrics, 2003c).

Diagnostic Evaluation

It is recommended that any infant experiencing an ALTE be admitted to an appropriate acute care center for evaluation of the event, which involves a detailed history and physical examination. The most widely used test for evaluating apneic events is continuous recording of cardiorespiratory patterns (cardiopneumogram or pneumocardiogram). Four-channel (or multichannel pneumogram) pneumocardiograms monitor heart rate, respirations (chest impedance), nasal airflow, and oxygen saturation. A more sophisticated test, polysomnography ("sleep study"), also records brain waves, eye and body movements, esophageal manometry, and end-tidal carbon dioxide measurements. However, none of these tests can predict risk. Some children with normal results may still have subsequent apneic episodes.

Therapeutic Management

Treatment usually involves continuous home monitoring of cardiorespiratory rhythms. The criteria for discontinuing the monitoring is based on the infant's clinical condition. A general guideline for discontinuation is when infants with ALTEs have gone 1 or 2 months without a significant number of episodes requiring intervention. Newer home apnea monitors allow download of information that assists the practitioner in the decision about when home monitoring may be discontinued. It is imperative to keep in mind however that the home apnea monitor will not predict or prevent SIDS deaths. (See Family Home Care Box.)

Nursing Considerations

The diagnosis of AOI engenders great anxiety and concern in parents, and the institution of home monitoring presents additional physical and emotional burdens. Parents of infants on home apnea monitors report experiencing emotional distress, especially depression and hostility, during the first few weeks after hospital discharge (Abendroth and others, 1999). If monitoring is required, the nurse can be a major source of support to the family in terms of education about the equipment, observation of the infant's status, and immediate intervention during apneic episodes, including *cardiopulmonary resuscitation (CPR)*. To help the family cope with the numerous procedures it must learn, adequate preparation before discharge and written instructions are essential. In the first few weeks after discharge, parents may benefit by having a practitioner readily available to answer

---

*American Sudden Infant Death Syndrome (SIDS) Institute, 6065 Roswell Road, Suite 876, Atlanta, GA 30328; (800) 232-SIDS (in Georgia, [800] 847-SIDS); website: www.sids.org; **The Sudden Infant Death Syndrome Alliance,** 1314 Bedford Avenue, Suite 210, Baltimore, MD 21208; (800) 221-SIDS; website: www.sidsalliance.org; **National SIDS Resource Center,** 2070 Chain Bridge Road, Suite 450, Vienna, VA 22182; (866) 866-7437 (free) or (703) 821-8955; website: www.sidscenter.org.

FAMILY HOME CARE

Using Apnea Monitors

Use the monitor as instructed by the practitioner or home monitor equipment company.

Do not adjust the monitor to eliminate false alarms. Adjustments could compromise the monitor's effectiveness.

Place the monitor on a firm surface away from the crib and drapes; plug power cord directly into a wall socket with a three-pronged outlet.

Do not sleep in the same bed as the monitored infant.

Keep pets and children away from the monitor and infant.

Keep the monitor away from possible electrical interferences such as appliances (e.g., electric blankets, televisions, air conditioners, remote telephones).

Check the monitor several times a day to be sure the alarm is working and that it can be heard from room to room. Be sure the caregiver can reach the monitor quickly (in less than 30 seconds).

Periodically check the monitor's breath detection indicator and battery or charger connections.

Be aware that strong signals from nearby radio and television stations, airports, ham radios, cellular phones, or police stations could interfere with the monitor. Check for interference if the monitor is to be operated in these areas.

Read the monitor's user manual carefully; report problems promptly.

Inform community utility and rescue squads of home monitoring as appropriate.

Keep emergency numbers near phones in the home.

Practice safety precautions:

Remove leads when infant is not attached to the monitor.

Unplug the power cord from the electrical outlet when the cord is not plugged into the monitor.

Use safety covers on electrical outlets to prevent children from inserting objects into a socket.

Data primarily from FDA: *Safety Alert: Important Tips for Apnea Monitor Users,* Rockville, Md, 1990, Department of Health and Human Services.

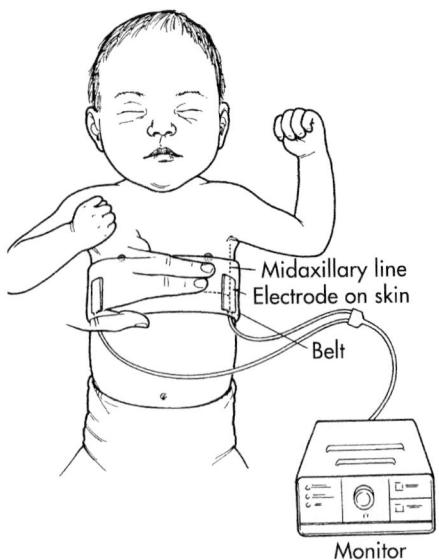

FIG. 11-5 ■ Placement of electrodes or belt for apnea monitoring.

NURSING ALERT

If the infant is apneic, gently stimulate the trunk by patting or rubbing it. If the infant is prone, turn to the back and flick the feet. If there is still no response, begin CPR. Never vigorously shake the child. No more than 15 to 20 seconds are spent on stimulation before implementing CPR.

questions regarding false alarms and for other technical assistance.

Several types of home monitors are available, and are set up by either a home monitor equipment company or nursing staff. Nurses, especially those involved in the care at home, must become familiar with the equipment, including its advantages and disadvantages. Safety is a major concern because monitors can cause electrical burns and electrocution. The following precautions are recommended:

- Remove leads from infant when not attached to monitor.
- Unplug power cord from electrical outlet when cord is not plugged into monitor.
- Use safety covers on electrical outlets to discourage children from inserting objects into a socket.

Siblings should also be supervised when near the infant and taught that the monitor is not a toy. Other safety practices include informing local utility and rescue squads of the home monitoring in case of an emergency. Telephone numbers for these services should be posted near all telephones in the home.

Caregivers need detailed information regarding proper attachment of the electrodes to the infant's chest with impedance monitors that detect chest movement. The electrodes are placed in the midaxillary line, at a space one or two fingerbreadths below the nipple. For home use, electrodes attached to a belt that is placed around the child's trunk are preferred (Fig. 11-5). The belt is positioned so that the electrodes contact the skin in the same area. Monitors may have memory chips that allow for event recording, which can be an effective tool in evaluating the use of the monitor, events immediately before and after the event, and reported frequency of alarms.

Monitors are effective only if they are used. They do not prevent death but alert the caregiver to the ALTE in time to intervene. The need to use the monitor and to respond appropriately to alarms must be stressed. Noncompliance can result in the infant's death.

Family Support. Although AOI is not a chronic illness, many of the stresses observed during the monitoring period are characteristic of those of families with chronically ill children. Parents report increased stress, including concern for the child's survival, fear of incompetency in assuming home responsibility, inadequate respite care, social isolation, constant work, and fatigue. Siblings are affected, as is the affected child, who may be characterized as "spoiled" and having developmental delays. To deal with these potential effects, nurses need to use the same interventions as those discussed for children with chronic illness (see Chapter 18 and be aware of the need for referral when difficulties are suspected).

To lessen the continuous responsibility of monitoring, other family members such as grandparents should be taught how to manipulate the equipment, read and interpret the signals, and administer CPR. They are encouraged to stay with the infant for regular periods to allow parents a respite. Support groups of other families who have successfully completed monitoring can also be of benefit.

KEY POINTS

- Common nutritional disturbances of infancy may result from vitamin and mineral deficiency or excess, some types of vegetarian diets, protein and calorie malnutrition, and food intolerance.

- Food consumption varies among vegetarians; therefore, a detailed dietary intake is essential for planning adequate intakes, particularly in children and pregnant and lactating women.

- Protein-energy malnutrition may occur as a complication of underlying disease, lack of parental education about infant nutrition, inappropriate management of food allergy, or incorrect preparation of formula.

- Food intolerance encompasses food allergies and food sensitivities, the most serious of which are cow's milk allergy and lactose intolerance.

- Treatment of colic may involve change in feeding practices, correction of a stressful environment, behavior modification, and support of the parent.

- Failure to thrive may be classified as organic, resulting from some physical cause, or nonorganic, resulting from psychosocial factors involving the child and caregiver (e.g., maternal deprivation), environmental causes (e.g., inadequate parental knowledge of child feeding), or unexplained causes.

- SIDS is the third leading cause of death in children between the ages of 1 month and 1 year.

- Evidence linking SIDS to the prone sleeping position has led to the recommendation that healthy infants sleep supine.

- The primary nursing responsibility in care associated with sudden infant death and other conditions of unknown etiology is emotional support of the family.

- Children with apnea of infancy receive home monitoring to alert the family to an apparent life-threatening event.

- Home monitors do not prevent SIDS.

References

Abendroth D and others: Do apnea monitors decrease emotional distress in parents of infants at high risk for cardiopulmonary arrest? *J Pediatr Health Care* 13(2):50-57, 1999.

American Academy of Pediatrics, Clinical Report: Prevention and management of positional skull deformities in infants, *Pediatrics* 112(1):199-202, 2003d.

American Academy of Pediatrics, Committee on Fetus and Newborn: Apnea, sudden infant death syndrome, and home monitoring, *Pediatrics* 111(4):914-917, 2003c.

American Academy of Pediatrics, Committee on Infectious Diseases, Pickering L, editor: *2003 Red book: report of the Committee on Infectious Diseases,* ed 26, Elk Grove Village, Il, 2003b, The Academy.

American Academy of Pediatrics: Prevention of rickets and vitamin D deficiency: new guidelines for vitamin D intake, *Pediatrics* 111(4):908-910, 2003a.

American Academy of Pediatrics, Committee on Nutrition: Soy protein–based formulas: recommendations for its use in infant feeding, *Pediatrics* 101(1):148-153, 1998.

American Academy of Pediatrics, Task Force on Infant Sleep Position and Sudden Infant Death Syndrome: Changing concepts of sudden infant death syndrome: implications for infant sleeping environment and sleep position, *Pediatrics* 105(3):650-656, 2000.

American Dietetic Association: ADA reports: position of the American Dietetic Association: vegetarian diets, *J Am Diet Assoc* 97(11):1317-1321, 1997.

Anderson JA: Milk, eggs, and peanuts: food allergies in children, *Am Fam Physician* 56(5):1365-1373, 1997.

Barnard K and others: Measurement and meaning of parent-child interaction. In Morrison F, Lord C, Keating D, editors: *Applied developmental psychology,* vol 3, New York, 1993, Academic Press.

Baron ML: Assisting families in making appropriate feeding choices: cow's milk protein allergy versus lactose intolerance, *Pediatr Nurs* 26(5):516-520, 2000.

Biggs WS: Diagnosis and management of positional head deformity, *Am Fam Physician* 67(9):1953-1956, 2003.

Burks W: Diagnosis of allergic reactions to food, *Pediatr Ann* 29(12):744-752, 2000.

Byard RW, Beal SM: Gastric aspiration and sleeping position in infancy and early childhood, *J Paediatr Child Health* 36(4):403-405, 2000.

Careaga MG, Kerner JA: A gastroenterologist's approach to failure to thrive, *Pediatr Ann* 29(9):558-567, 2000.

Carvalho NF and others: Severe nutritional deficiencies in toddlers resulting from health food milk alternatives, *Pediatrics* 107(4):e46, 2001.

Centers for Disease Control and Prevention, National Vital Statistics Reports: Deaths: final data for 1999, Centers for Disease Control and Prevention, National Center for Health Statistics *Natl Vital Stat Rep* 49(8):1-114, 2001.

Christie L and others: Food allergies in children affect nutrient intake and growth, *J Am Diet Assoc* 102(11):1648-1651, 2002.

Corrales KM, Utter SL: Failure to thrive. In Samour PQ, Helm KK, Lang CE, editors: *Handbook of pediatric nutrition,* ed 2, Gaithersburg, Md, 1999, Aspen Publications.

Corwin MJ and others: Secular changes in sleep position during infancy: 1995-1998, *Pediatrics* 111(1):52-60, 2003.

Devaney BL, Barr SI: DRI, EAR, RDA, AI, UL: making sense of this alphabet soup, *Pediatr Basics* 97(winter):2-9, 2002.

Dihigo SK: New strategies for the treatment of colic: modifying the parent/infant interaction, *J Pediatr Health Care* 12(5):256-262, 1998.

Drago DA, Dannenberg AL: Infant mechanical suffocation deaths in the United States, 1980-1997, *Pediatrics* 103(5):e59, 1999.

Duro D and others: Association between infantile colic and carbohydrate malabsorption from fruit juices in infancy, *Pediatrics* 109(5):797-805, 2002.

Ellett MLC: What is known about colic? *Gastroenterol Nurs* 26(2):60-65, 2003.

Friedman EH: Infantile colic, *Arch Pediatr Adolesc Med* 150(6):770-771, 1996.

Goldberg JP, Folta SC, Must A: Milk: can a "good" food be so bad? *Pediatrics* 110(4):826-831, 2002.

Guyer B and others: Annual summary of vital statistics—1998, *Pediatrics* 104(6):1229-1246, 1999.

Hauck FR and others: The contribution of prone sleeping position to the racial disparity in sudden infant death syndrome: the Chicago infant mortality study, *Pediatrics* 110(4):772-780, 2002.

Hein HA, Petit SF: Back to sleep: good advice for parents but not for hospitals? *Pediatrics* 107(3):537-539, 2001.

Host A: Frequency of cow's milk allergy in childhood, *Ann Allergy Asthma Immunol* 89(6 suppl 1):33-37, 2002.

Institute of Medicine, Food and Nutrition Board: *Dietary Reference Intakes: applications in dietary assessment,* National Academy Press, Washington, DC, 2000.

Kemper KJ, Gardiner P: Herbal medicines. In Behrman RE, Kliegman RM, Jenson HB, editors: *Nelson textbook of pediatrics,* ed 17, Philadelphia, 2004, WB Saunders.

Lanski SL and others: Herbal therapy in a pediatric emergency department population: expect the unexpected, *Pediatrics* 111(5 pt 1):981-985, 2003.

Leach CEA and others: Epidemiology of SIDS and explained sudden infant deaths, *Pediatrics* 104(4):e43, 1999.

Loman DG: The use of complementary and alternative health care practices among children, *J Pediatr Health Care* 17(2):58-63, 2003.

MacPhee M, Schneider J: A clinical tool for nonorganic failure-to-thrive feeding interactions, *J Pediatr Nurs* 11(1):29-39, 1996.

Maggioni A, Lifshitz F: Nutritional management of failure to thrive, *Pediatr Clin North Am* 42(4):791-809, 1995.

Malloy MH: Trends in postneonatal aspiration deaths and reclassification of sudden infant death syndrome: impact of the "Back to Sleep" program, *Pediatrics* 109(4):661-665, 2002.

McGuire JK, Kulkarni MS, Baden HP: Fatal hypermagnesemia in a child treated with megavitamin/megamineral therapy, *Pediatrics* 105(2):414, 2000.

McMartin KI and others: Lung tissue concentrations of nicotine in sudden infant death syndrome, *J Pediatr* 140(2):205-209, 2002.

MMWR: Neurologic impairment in children associated with maternal dietary deficiency of cobalamin—Georgia, 2001, *MMWR* 52(4):61-64, 2003.

Moon RY: Are you talking to parents about SIDS? *Contemp Pediatr* 18(3):122-129, 2001.

Moon RY, Patel KM, Shaefer SJM: Sudden infant death syndrome in child care settings, *Pediatrics* 106(2):295-300, 2000.

Neu M, Robinson JA: Infants with colic: their childhood characteristics, *J Pediatr Nurs* 18(1):12-20, 2003.

Perrotta S and others: Infant hypervitaminosis A causes severe anemia and thrombocytopenia: evidence of a retinol-dependent bone marrow cell growth inhibition, *Blood* 99(6):2017-2022, 2002.

Perry CL and others: Adolescent vegetarians: how well do their dietary patterns meet the Healthy People 2010 objectives? *Arch Pediatr Adolesc Med* 156(5):426-427, 2002.

Pongracic JA: Is it food allergy? *Contemp Pediatr* 17(12):101-122, 2000.

Preston AM and others: Influence of environmental tobacco smoke on vitamin C status in children, *Am J Clin Nutr* 77(1):167-172, 2003.

Salvatore S, Vandenplas Y: Gastroesophageal reflux and cow milk allergy: is there a link? *Pediatrics* 110(5):972-984, 2002.

Sampson HA: Utility of food-specific IgE concentrations in predicting symptomatic food allergy, *J Allergy Clin Immunol* 107(5):891-896, 2001.

Sampson HA: Anaphylaxis and emergency treatment, *Pediatrics* 111(6):1601-1608, 2003.

Sicherer SH: Diagnosis and management of childhood food allergy, *Curr Prob Pediatr* 21(2):39-57, 2001.

Unger B and others: Racial disparity and modifiable risk factors among infants dying suddenly and unexpectedly, *Pediatrics* 111(2):E127-E131, 2003.

Weizman Z and others: Efficacy of herbal tea preparation in infantile colic, *J Pediatr* 122(4):650-652, 1993.

Westerdahl J: Botanicals in pediatrics. In Samour PQ, Helm KK, Lang CE, editors, *Handbook of pediatrics,* ed 2, Gaithersburg, Md, 1999, Aspen.

Willinger M and others: Factors associated with caregiver's choice of infant sleep position, 1994-1998: the National Infant Sleep Position study, *JAMA* 283(16):2135-2142, 2000.

Health Promotion of the Toddler and Family

CHRISTINE CHORDAS

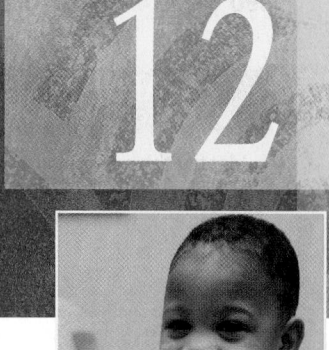

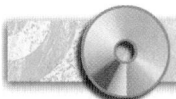 Remember to check out your companion CD-ROM

http://evolve.elsevier.com/Wong/essentials/

RELATED TOPICS and ADDITIONAL RESOURCES

For additional information, please view "Growth and Development" in *Whaley and Wong's Pediatric Nursing Video Series,* St Louis, 1996, Mosby; (800) 426-4545; website: www.elsevierhealth.com.

PROMOTING OPTIMAL GROWTH AND DEVELOPMENT

The term *terrible twos* has often been used to describe the toddler years, the period from 12 to 36 months of age. It is a time of intense exploration of the environment as children attempt to find out how things work and how to control others through temper tantrums, negativism, and obstinacy. Although this can be a challenging time for parents and child as each learns to know the other better, it is an extremely important period for developmental achievement and intellectual growth.

BIOLOGIC DEVELOPMENT
Proportional Changes

Growth slows considerably during toddlerhood. The average *weight* gain is 1.8 to 2.7 kg (4 to 6 pounds) per year. The average weight at 2 years is 12 kg (27 pounds). The birth weight is quadrupled by 2.5 years of age. The rate of increase in height also slows. The usual increment is an addition of 7.5 cm (3 inches) per year and occurs mainly in elongation of the legs rather than the trunk. The average *height* of a 2-year-old is 86.6 cm (34 inches). In general, adult height is about twice the 2-year-old child's height. Accurate measurement of height and weight during the toddler years should reveal a steady growth curve that is *steplike* in nature rather than linear (straight), which is characteristic of the growth spurts during the early childhood years.

The rate of increase in *head circumference* slows somewhat by the end of infancy, and head circumference is usually equal to chest circumference by 1 to 2 years of age. The usual total increase in head circumference during the second year is 2.5 cm (1 inch). Then the rate of increase slows until at age 5 years the increase is less than 1.25 cm (0.5 inch) per year. The anterior fontanel closes between 12 and 18 months of age.

Chest circumference continues to increase in size and exceeds head circumference during the toddler years. Its shape also changes as the transverse, or lateral, diameter exceeds the anteroposterior diameter. After the second year the chest circumference exceeds the abdominal measurement, which, in addition to the growth of the lower extremities, gives the child a taller, leaner appearance. However, the toddler retains a squat, "pot-bellied" appearance because of the less well developed abdominal musculature and short legs. The legs retain a slightly bowed or curved appearance during the second year from the weight of the relatively large trunk.

Sensory Changes

Visual acuity of 20/40 is considered acceptable during the toddler years. Full binocular vision is well developed, and any evidence of persistent strabismus requires professional attention as early as possible to prevent amblyopia. Depth perception continues to develop but, because of the child's lack of motor coordination, falls from heights continue to be a persistent danger.

The senses of *hearing, smell, taste,* and *touch* become increasingly well developed, coordinated with each other, and associated with other experiences. All of the senses are used to explore the environment. Toddlers will visually inspect an object by turning it over; they may taste it, smell it, and touch it several times before they are satisfied with their investigation. They will shake it to see if it makes noise and vigorously test its durability.

Another example of the integrated function of the senses is the toddler's development of specific *taste preferences.* The child is much less likely than infants to try a new food because of its appearance or smell, not just its taste.

Maturation of Systems

Most of the physiologic systems are relatively mature by the end of toddlerhood. Volume of the *respiratory tract* and growth of associated structures continue to increase during early childhood, lessening some of the factors that predisposed the child to frequent and serious infections during infancy. The internal structures of the ear and throat continue to be short and straight, and the lymphoid tissue of the tonsils and adenoids continues to be large. As a result, otitis media, tonsillitis, and upper respiratory tract infections are common. The respiratory and heart rates slow, and the blood pressure increases (see inside back cover). Respirations continue to be abdominal.

Under conditions of moderate variation in temperature, the toddler rarely has the difficulties of the young infant in maintaining *body temperature.* The mature functioning of the renal system serves to conserve fluid under times of stress, decreasing the risk of dehydration.

The *digestive processes* are fairly complete by the beginning of toddlerhood. The acidity of the gastric contents continues to increase and has a protective function, since it is capable of destroying many types of bacteria. Stomach capacity increases to allow for the usual schedule of three meals a day.

One of the more prominent changes of the gastrointestinal system is the voluntary control of elimination. With complete myelination of the spinal cord, control of the anal and urethral sphincters is gradually achieved. The physiologic ability to control the sphincters probably occurs somewhere between ages 18 and 24 months. Bladder capacity also increases considerably. By 14 to 18 months of age the child is able to retain urine for up to 2 hours or longer.

The *defense mechanisms* of the skin and blood, particularly phagocytosis, are much more efficient in toddlers than in infants. The production of antibodies is well established. However, many young children demonstrate a sudden increase in colds and minor infections when they enter preschool or other group situations, such as day care, because of their exposure to pathogens.

Rapid growth in *neurobehavioral organization* contributes to greater regularity of sleep-wake cycles, the diminishing of crying and unexplained fussiness, and the enhanced predictability in mood. Valuable stimulants of early brain development include the various interactions (talking, singing, and playing) between the toddler and caregivers. Adequate nutrition, protection from environmental toxins (lead), various drugs, and stress and promoting good health care all contribute to healthy brain growth.

Gross and Fine Motor Development

The major *gross motor skill* during the toddler years is the development of locomotion. By 12 to 13 months of age toddlers walk alone using a wide stance for extra balance, and by 18 months they try to run but fall easily. Between 2 and 3 years of age, refinement of the upright, biped position is evident in improved coordination and equilibrium. At age 2 years, toddlers can walk up and down stairs, and by age 2.5 years they can jump, using both feet, stand on one foot for a second or two, and manage a few steps on tiptoe. By the end of the second year they can stand on one foot, walk on tiptoe, and climb stairs with alternate footing.

Fine motor development is demonstrated in increasingly skillful manual dexterity. For example, by age 12 months toddlers are able to grasp a very small object but are unable to release it at will. At 15 months they can drop a pellet into a narrow-necked bottle. Casting or throwing objects and retrieving them become almost obsessive activities at about 15 months. By 18 months of age toddlers can throw a ball overhand without losing their balance. By 2 years of age toddlers use their hands to build towers and by 3 years of age draw circles on paper.

Mastery of gross and fine motor skills is evident in all phases of the child's activity, such as play, dressing, language comprehension, response to discipline, social interaction, and propensity for injuries. Activities occur less in isolation and more in conjunction with other physical and mental abilities to produce a purposeful result. For example, the toddler walks to reach a new location, releases a toy to pick it up or to choose a new one, and scribbles to look at the image produced. The possibilities of the exploration, investigation, and manipulation of the environment—and its hazards—are endless.

PSYCHOSOCIAL DEVELOPMENT

Toddlers are faced with the mastery of several important tasks. If the need for basic trust has been satisfied, they are ready to give up dependence for control, independence, and autonomy. Some of the specific tasks to be dealt with include:

- Differentiation of self from others, particularly the mother
- Toleration of separation from parent
- Ability to withstand delayed gratification
- Control over bodily functions
- Acquisition of socially acceptable behavior
- Verbal means of communication
- Ability to interact with others in a less egocentric manner

Mastery of these goals is only begun during late infancy and the toddler years, and such tasks as developing interpersonal relationships with others may not be completed until adolescence. However, crucial foundations for successful completion of such developmental tasks are laid during these early formative years.

Developing a Sense of Autonomy (Erikson)

According to Erikson, the developmental task of toddlerhood is acquiring a sense of *autonomy* while overcoming a sense of *doubt* and *shame.* As infants gain trust in the predictability and reliability of their parents, environment, and interaction with others, they begin to discover that their behavior is their own and that it has a predictable, reliable effect on others. However, although they realize their will and control over others, they are confronted with the conflict of exerting autonomy and relinquishing the much-enjoyed dependence on others. Exerting their will has definite negative consequences, whereas retaining dependent, submissive behavior is generally rewarded with affection and approval. However, continued dependency creates a sense of doubt regarding their potential capacity to control their actions. This doubt is compounded by a sense of shame for feeling this urge to revolt against others' will and a fear that they will exceed their own capacity for manipulating the environment. Skillful monitoring and balance of controls by parents allows a growing rate of realistic successes and the emergence of autonomy.

Just as the infant has the social modalities of grasping and biting, the toddler has the newly gained modality of holding on and letting go. To hold on and let go is evident with the use of the hands, mouth, eyes, and, eventually, the sphincters, when toilet training is begun. These social modalities are expressed constantly in the child's play activities, such as casting or throwing objects; taking objects out of boxes, drawers, or cabinets; holding on tighter when someone says, "No, don't touch"; and spitting out food as taste preferences become very strong.

Several characteristics, especially negativism and ritualism, are typical of toddlers in their quest for autonomy. As toddlers attempt to express their will, they often act with *negativism,* the persistent negative response to requests. The words "no" or "me do" can be the sole vocabulary. Emotions become very strongly expressed, usually in rapid mood swings. One minute, toddlers can be engrossed in an activity, and the next minute they might be violently angry because they are unable to manipulate a toy or open a door. If scolded for doing something wrong, they can have a temper tantrum and almost instantaneously pull at the parent's legs to be picked up and comforted. Understanding and coping with these swift changes is often difficult for parents.

Many parents find the negativism exasperating and, instead of dealing constructively with it, give in to it, which further threatens children in their search for learning acceptable methods of interacting with others (see Temper Tantrums and Negativism, pp. 399-401).

In contrast to negativism, which frequently disrupts the environment, *ritualism,* the need to maintain sameness and reliability, provides a sense of comfort. Toddlers can venture out with security when they know that familiar people, places, and routines still exist. One can easily understand why change, such as hospitalization, represents such a threat to these children. Without the comfortable rituals, there is little opportunity to exert autonomy. Consequently, dependency and regression occur (see Regression, p. 401).

Erikson focuses on the development of the *ego,* which may be thought of as reason or common sense, during this phase of psychosocial development. There is a struggle as the child deals with the impulses of the *id* and attempts to tolerate frustration and learn socially acceptable ways of interacting with the environment. The *ego* is evident as the child is able to tolerate delayed gratification.

There is also a rudimentary beginning of the *superego,* or conscience, which is the incorporation of the morals of society and the process of acculturation. With the development of the ego, children further differentiate themselves from others and expand their sense of trust within themselves. But as they begin to develop awareness of their own will and capacity to achieve, they also become aware of their ability to fail. This ever-present awareness of potential failure creates doubt and shame. Successful mastery of the task of autonomy necessitates opportunities for self-mastery while withstanding the frustration of necessary limit setting and delayed gratification. Opportunities for self-mastery are present in appropriate play activities, toilet training, the crisis of sibling rivalry, and successful interactions with significant others (Fig. 12-1).

COGNITIVE DEVELOPMENT
Sensorimotor and Preconceptual Phase (Piaget)

The period from 12 to 24 months of age is a continuation of the final two stages of the sensorimotor phase. During this time the cognitive processes develop rapidly and at times seem similar to those of mature thinking. However, reasoning skills are still quite primitive and need to be understood to effectively deal with the typical behaviors of a child of this age.

Tertiary Circular Reactions. In the fifth stage of the sensorimotor phase (13 to 18 months of age), the child uses active experimentation to achieve previously unattainable goals. Newly acquired physical skills are increasingly important for the function they serve rather than for the acts themselves. The child incorporates the old learning of secondary circular reactions with new skills and applies the combined knowledge to new situations, with emphasis on the results of the experimentation. In this way there is the beginning of rational judgment and intellectual reasoning. During this stage there is further differentiation of oneself from objects. This is evident in the child's increasing ability to venture away from the parent and to tolerate longer periods of separation.

Awareness of a causal relationship between two events is apparent. After flipping a light switch, toddlers are aware that a reciprocal response occurs. However, they are not able to transfer that knowledge to new situations. Therefore, every time they see what appears to be a light switch, they must reinvestigate its function. Such behavior demonstrates the beginning of categorizing data into distinct classes and subclasses. There are innumerable examples of this type of behavior as toddlers continuously explore the same object each time it appears in a new place.

Because classification of objects is still rudimentary, the appearance of an object denotes its function. For example, if the child's toys are stored in a paper bag or large container, that toy receptacle is no different from the garbage pail or laundry basket. If allowed to turn over the toy receptacle, the child will just as quickly do the same to other similar containers because, in the child's mind, there is no difference. Expecting the child to judge which receptacles are permissible to explore and which are not is inappropriate for this age-group. Instead, the forbidden object, such as the garbage pail, should be placed out of reach.

The discovery of objects as objects leads to the awareness of their spatial relationships. Children are able to recognize different shapes and their relationship to each other. For example, they can fit slightly smaller boxes into each other (nesting) and can place a round object into a hole, even if the board is turned around, upside down, or reversed. Children are also aware of space and the relationship of their body to dimensions such as height. They will stretch, stand on a low stair or stool, and pull a string to reach an object.

Object permanence has also advanced. Although they still cannot find an object that has been invisibly displaced or moved from under one pillow to another without their seeing the change, toddlers are increasingly aware of the existence of objects behind closed doors, in drawers, and under tables. Parents are usually acutely aware of this developmental achievement and find high places and locked cabinets the only places inaccessible to toddlers.

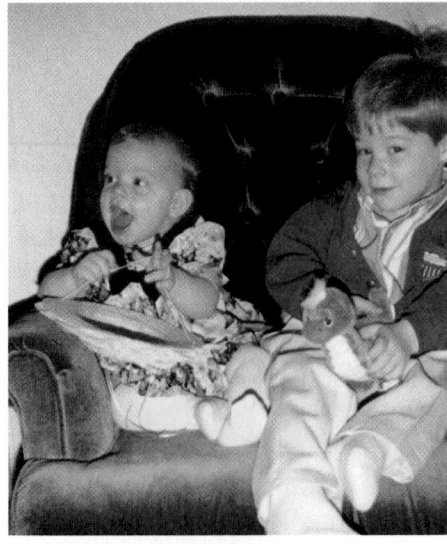

FIG. 12-1 ■ Toddlers begin socializing with significant others such as siblings as a part of development.

Invention of New Means Through Mental Combinations.   From ages 19 to 24 months the child is in the final sensorimotor stage. During this stage the child completes the more primitive, autistic thought processes of infancy and is prepared for the more complex mental operations that occur during the phase of preoperational thought. One of the most dramatic achievements of this stage is in the area of object permanence. Children will now actively search for an object in several potential hiding places. In addition, they can infer a cause when only experiencing the effect. They can infer that an object was hidden in any number of places even if they only saw the original hiding place.

Imitation displays deeper meaning and understanding. There is greater symbolization to imitation. The child is acutely aware of others' actions and attempts to copy them in gestures and in words. *Domestic mimicry* (imitating household activities) and sex-role behavior become increasingly common during this period and during the second year. Identification with the parent of the same sex becomes apparent by the second year and represents the child's intellectual ability to differentiate different models of behavior and to imitate them appropriately (Fig. 12-2).

The conception of time is still embryonic, but children have some sense of timing in terms of anticipation, memory, and the limited ability to wait. They may listen to the command, "Just a minute," and behave appropriately. However, their sense of timing is exaggerated—1 minute can seem like an hour. Toddlers' limited attention spans also indicate their sense of immediacy and concern for the present.

Preconceptual Phase.   At approximately 2 years of age the child enters the preconceptual phase of cognitive development, which lasts until about age 4 years. The preconceptual phase is a subdivision of the preoperational phase, which spans ages 2 to 7 years. The preconceptual phase is primarily one of transition that bridges the purely self-satisfying behavior of infancy and the rudimentary socialized behavior of latency. *Preoperational thought* implies that children cannot think in terms of *operations*—the ability to manipulate objects in relation to each other in a logical fashion. Rather, toddlers think primarily on the basis of their perception of an event. Problem solving is based on what they see or hear directly rather than on what they recall about objects and events. Several characteristics are unique to preoperational thought (Box 12-1).

Within the second year the child increasingly uses language symbolically and is concerned with the "why" and "how" of things. For example, a pencil is "something to write with," and food is "something to eat." However, such mental symbolization is closely associated with prelogical reasoning. For instance, a needle is "something that hurts." Such painful experiences take on new significance because memory is associated with the specific event, and fears are likely to develop, such as resistance to people who wear white uniforms or rooms that look like the practitioner's office. Because of the vulnerability of these early years, it is essential to prepare children for any new experience, whether it is a new baby-sitter or a visit to the dentist.

SPIRITUAL DEVELOPMENT

Toddlers learn about God through the words and the actions of those closest to them. They have only a vague idea of God and religious teachings because of their immature cognitive processes; however, if God is spoken about with reverence, young children associate God with something special. They begin to assimilate behaviors associated with the divine (folding hands in prayer). Routines such as saying prayers before meals or at bedtime can be very important and comforting. Near the end of toddlerhood, when children use preoperational thought, there is some advancement of their understanding of God. Religious teachings, such as reward or fear of punishment (heaven or hell) and moral development (see Chapter 5), may influence their behavior (Fosarelli, 2003).

DEVELOPMENT OF BODY IMAGE

As in infancy, the development of body image closely parallels cognitive development. Developing psychologic understanding provides greater self-awareness, and young children learn to answer the question "Who am I." During the second year, children recognize themselves in a mirror and make verbal references about themselves ("Me big"). With increasing motor ability, toddlers recognize the usefulness of body parts and gradually learn their respective names. They also learn that certain parts of the body have various meanings; for example, during toilet training the genitals become significant and cleanliness is emphasized. By 2 years of age there is recognition of gender differences and reference to self by name and then by pronoun. Gender identity is developed by age 3 years. Also by this time the child begins to remember events with reference to their personal significance, forming an autobiographic memory that helps to establish a continuous identity throughout life's events (Thompson, 2001).

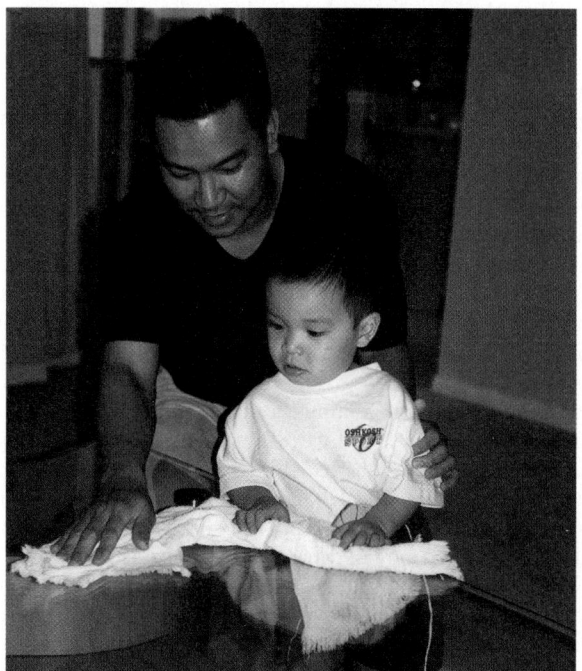

FIG. 12-2 ■ Domestic mimicry is common during toddlerhood.

BOX 12-1 ■ Characteristics of Preoperational Thought

Egocentrism—Inability to envision situations from perspectives other than one's own
Example: If a person is positioned between the toddler and another child, the toddler, who is facing the person, will explain that both children can see the middle person's face. The young child is unable to realize that the other person views the middle person from a different perspective, the back.
Implication: Avoid moralizing about "why" something is wrong if it requires an understanding of someone else's feelings or opinion. Telling a child to stop hitting because hitting hurts the other person is often ineffective because, to the aggressor, it feels good to hit someone else. Instead, emphasize that hitting is not allowed.

Transductive—Reasoning from the particular to the particular
Example: Child refuses to eat a food because something previously eaten did not taste good.
Implication: Accept child's reasoning; offer refused food at different time.

Global organization—Reasoning that changing any one part of the whole changes the entire whole
Example: Child refuses to sleep in room because location of bed is changed.
Implication: Accept child's reasoning; use same bed position or introduce change slowly.

Centration—Focusing on one aspect rather than considering all possible alternatives
Example: Child refuses to eat a food because of its color, even though its taste and smell are acceptable.
Implication: Accept child's reasoning.

Animism—Attributing lifelike qualities to inanimate objects
Example: Child scolds stairs for making child fall down.
Implication: Join child in the "scolding." Keep frightening objects out of view.

Irreversibility—Inability to undo or reverse the actions initiated physically
Example: When told to stop doing something, such as talking, child is unable to think of positive activity.
Implication: State requests or instructions positively (e.g., "Be quiet.").

Magical—Believing that thoughts are all-powerful and can cause events
Example: Child wishes someone died; then if the person dies, child feels at fault because of the "bad" thought that made the death happen.
Calling children "bad" because they did something wrong makes children feel as if they are bad.
Implication: Clarify that thoughts do not make things happen and that child is not responsible.
Use "I" messages rather than "you" messages to communicate thoughts, feelings, expectations, or beliefs without imposing blame or criticism. Emphasize that the act is bad, not the child.

Inability to conserve—Inability to understand the idea that a mass can be changed in size, shape, volume, or length without losing or adding to the original mass (instead, children judge what they see by the immediate perceptual clues given to them)
Example: If two lines of equal length are presented in such a way that one appears longer than the other, child will state that one line is longer even if child measures both lines with a ruler or yardstick and finds that each has the same length.
Implication: Change the most obvious perceptual clue to reorient child's view of what is seen. For example, give medicine in a small medicine cup, rather than a large cup, because the child will imagine that the large vessel contains more liquid. If child refuses the medicine in the small cup, pour it into a large cup, because the liquid will appear to be less in a tall, wide container.
Give a large, flat cookie rather than a thick, small one, or do the reverse with meat or cheese; child will usually eat larger size of favorite food and smaller size of less favorite food.

After they begin preoperational thought, toddlers can use symbols to represent objects, but their thinking may lead to inaccuracies. For example, if someone who is pregnant is called "fat," they will describe all "fat" women as having babies. There is a beginning recognition of words used to describe physical appearance, such as "pretty," "handsome," or "big boy." Such expressions eventually influence how children view their own bodies.

Although there has been little research done on body-image development in young children, it is evident that body integrity is poorly understood and that intrusive experiences are threatening (Dahlquist and others, 2002). For example, toddlers forcefully resist procedures such as examining the ear or mouth and taking a rectal temperature. Toddlers also have unclear body boundaries and may associate nonviable parts, such as feces, with essential body parts. This can be seen in a toddler who is upset by flushing the toilet and watching the stool disappear.

Nurses can assist parents in fostering a positive body image in their child by encouraging them to avoid negative labels, such as "skinny arms" or "chubby legs"—self-perceptions that can last a lifetime. Body parts, especially those related to elimination and reproduction, should be called by their correct names. Respect for the body should be practiced.

DEVELOPMENT OF GENDER IDENTITY

Just as toddlers explore their environment, they also explore their bodies and find that touching certain body parts is pleasurable. Genital fondling (masturbation) can occur and involves manual stimulation, as well as posturing movements against objects, and sucking on fingers and toes. Other demonstrations of sensual activities include rocking, swinging, and hugging people and toys. During the activity the child may perspire, and the activity may be difficult to interrupt. If performed in public, the behavior should be ignored. The child should be taught that it is more acceptable to perform the behavior in private (Meyer, 2002).

Children in this age-group are learning vocabulary associated with anatomy, elimination, and reproduction. Certain associations between words and functions become significant and can influence future sexual attitudes. For example, if parents refer to the genitals as dirty, especially in the context of elimination, this association between "genitals" and "dirty" may be transferred to sexual functions.

Sex-role differences become obvious to children and are evident in much of their imitative play. A sense of maleness or femaleness, *gender identity,* is formed by age 3 years. Early attitudes are formed about affectionate behaviors between adults from observing parental and other adult sexual/sensual activities. (See also Sex Education, Chapter 13.) The quality of relationships with parents is important to the child's capacity for sexual and emotional relationships later in life (DeLamater and Friedrich, 2002).

SOCIAL DEVELOPMENT

A major task of the toddler period is differentiation of self from significant others, usually the mother. The differentiation process consists of two phases: *separation,* the children's emergence from a symbiotic fusion with the mother, and *individuation,* those achievements that mark children's assumption of their individual characteristics in the environment. Although the process begins during the latter half of infancy, the major achievements occur during the toddler years.

Toddlers have an increased understanding and awareness of object permanence and some ability to withstand delayed gratification and tolerate moderate frustration. As a result, toddlers react differently to strangers than do infants. The appearance of unfamiliar persons does not represent such a significant threat to their attachment to mother. They have learned from experience that parents exist when physically absent. Repetition of events such as going to bed without the parents but waking to find them there again reinforces the reliability of such brief separations. Consequently, toddlers are able to venture away from their parents for brief periods of time because of the security of knowing that the parents will be there when they return.

Transitional objects, such as a favorite blanket or toy, provide security for children, especially when they are separated from parents, dealing with a new stress, or just fatigued (Fig. 12-3). Security objects often become so important to toddlers that they refuse to have them taken away. Such behavior is normal; there is no need to discourage this tendency. During separations, such as day care, hospitalization, or even staying overnight with a relative, transitional objects should be provided to minimize any feelings of fear or loneliness.

Learning to tolerate and master brief periods of separation is an important developmental task of children in this age-group. In addition, it is a necessary component of parenting, since brief periods of separation allow parents to recuperate their energy and patience and to minimize directing their irritations and frustrations at the children.

Language

The most striking characteristic of language development during early childhood is the increasing level of comprehension. Although the number of words acquired—from about 4 at 1 year of age to approximately 300 at age 2 years—is notable, *the ability to comprehend and understand speech is much greater than the number of words the child can say.* Bilingual children can also achieve their early linguistic milestones in each of the languages at the same time and produce a substantial number of semantically corresponding words in each of their two languages from the very first words or signs (Petitto and others, 2001).

At age 1 year the child uses one-word sentences or holophrases. The word "up" can mean "pick me up" or "look up there." For the child the one word conveys the meaning of a sentence, but to others it may mean many

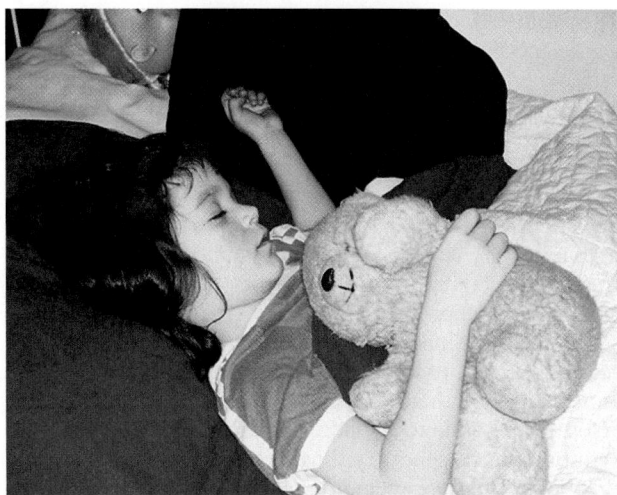

FIG. 12-3 ■ Transitional objects, such as a warm and fuzzy stuffed animal, are sources of security to a toddler.

things or nothing. At this age about 25% of the vocalizations are intelligible. By the age of 2 years the child uses multiword sentences by stringing together two or three words, such as the phrases, "mama go bye-bye" or "all gone," and approximately 65% of the speech is understandable. By 3 years the child puts words together into simple sentences, begins to master grammatical rules, and acquires five to six new words daily.

Gestures precede or accompany each of the language milestones up to 30 months of age (putting phone to ear, pointing). After language develops enough, gestures phase out and the pace of word learning increases (Bates and Dick, 2002).

Personal-Social Behavior

One of the most dramatic aspects of development in the toddler is personal-social interaction. Personal-social behaviors are evident in such areas as dressing, feeding, playing, and establishing self-control. Parents frequently wonder why their manageable, docile, lovable infant has turned into a determined, strong-willed, volatile-tempered little tyrant. In addition, the tyrant of the terrible twos can swiftly and unpredictably revert back to the adorable infant. All of this is part of "growing up" as toddlers acquire a more sophisticated awareness that others' feelings and desires can be different from their own. Through interactions with caregivers, the child is able to explore these differences and their consequences.

Toddlers are developing skills of independence, which are evident in all areas of behavior. By 15 months children feed themselves, drink well from a covered cup, and manage a spoon with considerable spilling. By 24 months they use a spoon well and by 36 months may be using a fork. Between ages 2 and 3 years they eat with the family and like to help with chores such as setting the table or removing dishes from the dishwasher, but they lack table manners and may find it difficult to sit through the family's entire meal.

In dressing, toddlers also demonstrate strides in independence. The 15-month-old child helps by putting the arm or foot out for dressing and pulls shoes and socks off. The

18-month-old child removes gloves, helps with pullover shirts, and may be able to unzip. By age 2 years the toddler removes most articles of clothing and puts on socks, shoes, and pants without regard for right or left and back or front. Help is still needed to fasten clothes.

Toddlers also begin to develop concern for the feelings of others and develop an understanding of how adult expectations for behavior apply to specific situations (causing a sibling to cry while playing rough) (Thompson, 2001). As their understanding is fostered, they are able to develop control. Age-appropriate discipline contributes to healthy social and emotional development. Positive reinforcement, redirecting, and time-out are appropriate for most toddlers. It is recognized that social and emotional problems can develop in the youngest children. Early screening and intervention promotes more positive developmental outcomes as the young child grows and develops.

Play

Play magnifies the toddler's physical and psychosocial development. Interaction with people becomes increasingly important. The solitary play of infancy progresses to *parallel play*—the toddler plays alongside, not with, other children. Although sensorimotor play is still prominent, there is much less emphasis on the exclusive use of one sensory modality. The toddler inspects the toy, talks to the toy, tests its strength and durability, and invents several uses for it. Imitation is one of the most distinguishing characteristics of play and enriches children's opportunity to engage in fantasy. With less emphasis on gender-stereotyped toys, play objects such as dolls, carriages, dollhouses, dishes, cooking utensils, child-size furniture, trucks, and dress-up clothes (Fig. 12-4) are suitable for both genders; however, boys may be more interested than girls in activities related to trucks, trailers, men, and logs, whereas girls may prefer doll-related activities (Lyytinen and others, 1999).

Increased locomotive skills make push-pull toys, straddle trucks or cycles, a small gym and slide, balls of various sizes, and rocking horses appropriate for the energetic toddler. Finger paints, thick crayons, chalk, blackboard, paper, and puzzles with large, simple pieces use the child's developing fine motor skills. Interlocking blocks in various sizes and shapes provide hours of fun and, during later years, are useful objects for creative and imaginative play. The most educational toy is the one that fosters the interaction of an adult with a child in supportive, unconditional play. Toys are never substitutes for the attention of devoted caregivers, but toys can enhance these interactions (Glassy and Romano, 2003).

Certain aspects of play are related to emerging linguistic abilities. Talking is a form of play for toddlers, who enjoy musical toys such as age-appropriate cassette tape players, "talking" dolls and animals, and toy telephones. Appropriate children's television programs are excellent for children in this age-group, who learn to associate words with visual images. However, total media time should be limited to 1 to 2 hours of quality programming per day (American Academy of Pediatrics, 2001a). Toddlers also enjoy "reading" stories from a picture book and imitating the sounds of animals.

Tactile play is also important for the exploring toddler. Water toys, a sandbox with pail and shovel, finger paints,

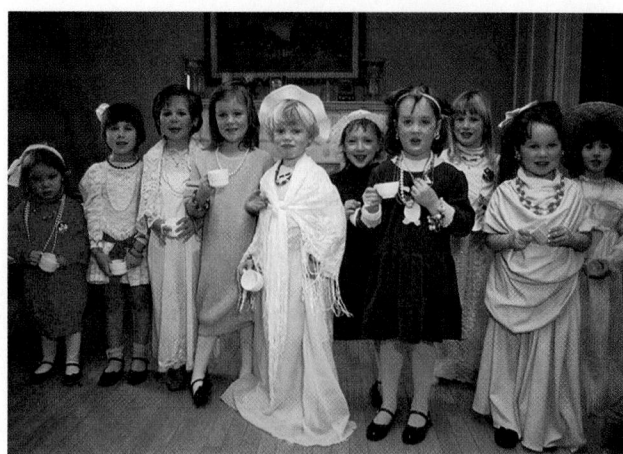

FIG. 12-4 ■ Young children enjoy dressing up.

soap bubbles, and clay provide excellent opportunities for creative and manipulative recreation. Adults sometimes forget the fascination of feeling slippery cream, such as whipped cream or pudding, catching air bubbles, squeezing and reshaping clay, or smearing paints. These types of unstructured activities are as important as educational play to allow children freedom of expression.

Selection of appropriate toys must involve safety factors, especially in relation to size and sturdiness. The oral activity of toddlers makes them at risk for aspirating small objects or ingesting toxic substances. Parents need to be especially vigilant of toys played with in other children's homes or those of older siblings. Toys are a potential source of serious bodily damage to toddlers, who may have the physical strength to manipulate them but not the knowledge to appreciate their danger (see Family Home Care box: Toy Safety, Chapter 5).

Table 12-1 summarizes the major features of growth and development for the age-groups of 15, 18, 24, and 30 months.

COPING WITH CONCERNS RELATED TO NORMAL GROWTH AND DEVELOPMENT
Toilet Training

One of the major tasks of toddlerhood is toilet training. Anticipatory guidance and clinical intervention for families surrounding toilet training should begin to be discussed during routine well-child visits prior to the child's developmental readiness to toilet train. Preparation and education reveals and allays misconceptions, leads to the development of appropriate expectations, and provides information, guidance, and support to parents for managing this potentially frustrating process.

Voluntary control of the anal and urethral sphincters is achieved sometime after the child is walking, probably between ages 18 and 24 months. However, complex psychophysiologic factors are required for readiness. The child must be able to recognize the urge to let go and hold on and be able to communicate this sensation to the parent. In addition, there is probably some necessary motivation in the desire to please the parent by holding on, rather than pleasing oneself by letting go.

Usually, physiologic and psychologic readiness is not complete until 18 to 24 months of age. By this time, the child has mastered the majority of essential gross motor skills, can communicate intelligibly, is less in conflict with self-assertion and negativism, and is aware of the ability to control the body and please the parent. Helping parents identify the right time to initiate training can alleviate stress and anxiety for the child that could prolong the toilet training process. There is not a universal right age to begin toilet training or an absolute deadline to complete training. One of the most important responsibilities of nurses is to help parents identify the readiness signs in their child (see Guidelines box).*

Nighttime bladder control normally takes several months to years after daytime training begins. This is because the sleep cycle needs to mature so the child can awake in time to urinate. Few children will have night wetting episodes after daytime dryness is totally achieved; however, those children who do not have nighttime dryness by the age of 6 years are likely to require intervention (Mercer, 2003).

Bowel training is usually accomplished before bladder training because of its greater regularity and predictability. There is a stronger sensation for defecation than for urination, and the sensation of defecation can be brought to the child's attention. A well-balanced diet that includes dietary fiber helps keep stool soft and supports the development and maintenance of regular bowel movements.

A number of techniques can be helpful when initiating training. One is the selection of a potty chair or use of the toilet. A freestanding potty chair allows children a feeling of security. Another option is a portable seat attached to the regular toilet, which may ease the transition from potty chair to regular toilet. Placing a small bench under the feet helps to stabilize the child's position. It is probably best to keep the potty chair in the bathroom and to let the child observe the excreta being flushed down the toilet to associate these activities with usual practices. If a potty chair seat is not available, having the child sit *facing* the toilet tank provides added support. Boys may begin toilet training in the stand-up position or by sitting on a potty chair or toilet (Fig. 12-5). Imitating one's father during the preschool years is a powerful motivating force.

Practice sessions should be limited to 5 or 10 minutes, a parent should stay with the child, and sanitary habits should be employed after every session. Allow the child time to become familiar with the potty chair. Let the child sit on it first fully clothed before removing the clothing. Dressing children in easily removed clothing; using training pants, "pull-on" diapers, or panties; and encouraging imitation by watching others are other helpful suggestions.

When the child begins to show regular daytime dryness, parents may experiment with underwear during the day. Daytime accidents are common, particularly during periods of intense activity. Young children become so engrossed in play activity that if they are not reminded, they will wait until it is too late to reach the bathroom. Therefore, frequent reminders and trips to the toilet are necessary.

As the child masters each step of toileting (discussion, undressing, going, wiping, dressing, flushing, and hand-washing), he or she gains a sense of accomplishment that should be reinforced by parents. If the parent-child relationship becomes strained, both may need a break to focus on enjoyable activities together. Regression may coincide with a stressful family situation or if the child is being pushed too hard and too fast. Regression is a normal part of toilet training and does not mean failure but should be viewed as a temporary setback to a more comfortable place for the child.

Day care providers also play a role in the support and education of parents regarding toilet training practices. It is important for parents to inform all caregivers of their individual family values and the child's specific needs when planning for training away from home. Ensuring consistency in care of the toddler, as well as ensuring healthy practices in a sanitary environment, allows for safe and effective toilet practices in all settings.

Sibling Rivalry

The natural jealousy and resentment of children toward a new child in the family or toward other children in the family when a parent turns his or her attention from them and interacts with their brother or sister is referred to as *sibling rivalry.*

The arrival of a new infant represents a crisis for even the best-prepared toddlers. It is not the infant that toddlers hate or resent but the changes that this additional sibling produces, especially the separation from mother during the birth. The parents now share their love and attention with someone else, the usual routine is disrupted, and toddlers may lose their crib or room—all at a time when they thought they were in control of their world. Sibling rivalry tends to be most pronounced in the firstborn, who experiences *dethronement* (loss of sole parental attention). It also seems to be most difficult for young children, particularly in terms of mother-child interaction.

Preparation of children for the birth of a sibling is quite individual, but age dictates some important considerations. Time for toddlers is a vague concept. Tomorrow could be yesterday or next week, and a month from now could be never. Preparing children too soon for the birth may lessen their interest by the time the event occurs. A good time to start talking about the baby is when toddlers become aware of the pregnancy and the changes taking place in the home in anticipation of the new member.

Toddlers need to have a realistic idea of what the newborn will be like. Telling them that a new playmate will come home soon sets up unrealistic expectations. Rather, parents should stress the activities that will take place when the baby arrives home, such as diapering, bottle- or breast-feeding, bathing, and dressing. At the same time, parents should emphasize which routines will stay the same, such as reading stories or going to the park. If toddlers have had no contact with an infant, it is a good idea to introduce them to one, if feasible. Providing a doll on which toddlers can imitate parental behaviors is another excellent strategy. They can tend to the doll's needs (diapering, feeding) at the same time the parent is performing similar activities for the infant. A new sibling in the home is stressful, so any additional stresses for the toddler should be avoided or minimized.

---

*A helpful book is *Guide to Toilet Training,* available from American Academy of Pediatrics (888) 227-1770; website: aap.org/bookstore.

TABLE 12-1 ■ Growth and Development During the Toddler Years

AGE (MONTHS)	PHYSICAL	GROSS MOTOR	FINE MOTOR
15	Steady growth in height and weight Head circumference 48 cm (19 inches) Weight 11 kg (24 pounds) Height 78.7 cm (31 inches)	Walks without help (usually since age 13 months) Creeps up stairs Kneels without support Cannot walk around corners or stop suddenly without losing balance Assumes standing position without support Cannot throw ball without falling	Constantly casting objects to floor Builds tower of two cubes Holds two cubes in one hand Releases a pellet into a narrow-necked bottle Scribbles spontaneously Uses cup well but often rotates spoon
18	Physiologic anorexia from decreased growth needs Anterior fontanel closed Physiologically able to control sphincters	Runs clumsily; falls often Walks up stairs with one hand held Pulls and pushes toys Jumps in place with both feet Seats self on chair Throws ball overhand without falling	Builds tower of three or four cubes Release, prehension, and reach well developed Turns pages in a book two or three at a time In a drawing, makes stroke imitatively Manages spoon without rotation
24	Head circumference 49-50 cm (19.5-20 inches) Chest circumference exceeds head circumference Lateral diameter of chest exceeds anteroposterior diameter Usual weight gain of 1.8-2.7 kg (4-6 pounds) Usual gain in height of 10-12.5 cm (4-5 inches) Adult height approximately double height at 2 years of age May have achieved readiness for beginning daytime control of bowel and bladder Primary dentition of 16 teeth	Goes up and down stairs alone with two feet on each step Runs fairly well, with wide stance Picks up object without falling Kicks ball forward without overbalancing	Builds tower of six or seven cubes Aligns two or more cubes like a train Turns pages of book one at a time In drawing, imitates vertical and circular strokes Turns doorknob, unscrews lid
30	Birth weight quadrupled Primary dentition (20 teeth) completed May have daytime bowel and bladder control	Jumps with both feet Jumps from chair or step Stands on one foot momentarily Takes a few steps on tiptoe	Builds tower of eight cubes Adds chimney to train of cubes Good hand-finger coordination; holds crayon with fingers rather than fist In drawing, imitates vertical and horizontal strokes; makes two or more strokes for cross; draws circles

For example, moving the toddler to a regular bed or to a different room should be done well in advance of the infant's arrival.

Pregnancy is an abstraction for toddlers. They need concrete illustrations of how the baby is growing inside the mother. It is an excellent opportunity for introducing aspects of reproduction and sexuality. Seeing simple pictures of the uterus and fetus and feeling the fetus move help the child feel involved in the experience. Children also benefit from classes for siblings that may be part of prenatal sessions (Storr and Robinson, 1998).

When the new baby arrives, toddlers keenly feel the changed focus of attention. Visitors may initiate problems when they inadvertently shower the infant with attention and presents while neglecting the older child. Parents can minimize this by alerting visitors to the toddler's needs, having small presents on hand for the toddler, and including the child in the visit as much as possible. The toddler

SENSORY	LANGUAGE	SOCIALIZATION
Able to identify geometric forms; places round object into appropriate hole Binocular vision well developed Displays an intense and prolonged interest in pictures	Uses expressive jargon Says four to six words, including names "Asks" for objects by pointing Understands simple commands May use head-shaking gesture to denote "no" Uses "no" even while agreeing to the request Uses common gestures such as putting cup to mouth when empty	Tolerates some separation from parent Less likely to fear strangers Beginning to imitate parents, such as cleaning house (sweeping, dusting), folding clothes May discard bottle Manages spoon but rotates it near mouth Kisses and hugs parents; may kiss pictures in a book
	Says 10 or more words Points to a common object, such as a shoe or ball, and to two or three body parts Forms word combinations Forms gesture-word combinations (points while naming) Forms gesture-gesture combinations	Expresses emotions; has temper tantrums Great imitator (domestic mimicry) Takes off gloves, socks, and shoes, and unzips zippers Temper tantrums may be more evident Beginning awareness of ownership ("my toy") May develop dependency on transitional objects, such as "security blanket"
Accommodation well developed in geometric discrimination; able to insert square block into oblong space	Has a vocabulary of approximately 300 words Uses two-or three-word phrases Uses pronouns "I," "me," "you" Understands directional commands Gives first name; refers to self by name Verbalizes need for toileting, food, or drink Talks incessantly Able to remember and imitate arbitrary sequences of manual actions/gestures	Stage of parallel play Has sustained attention span Temper tantrums decreasing Pulls people to show them something Increased independence from parent Dresses self in simple clothing Develops visual recognition and verbal self-reference ("Me big.") Develops awareness that feelings and desires of others may be different and begins to explore implications and consequences
	Gives first and last name Refers to self by appropriate pronoun Uses plurals Names one color	Separates more easily from parent In play, helps put things away; can carry breakable objects; pushes with good steering Begins to notice sex differences; knows own sex May attend to toilet needs without help except for wiping Emotions expand to include pride, shame, guilt, embarrassment

can also help with the care of the newborn by getting diapers and doing other small tasks (Fig. 12-6).

How children exhibit jealousy is complex. Some will overtly hit the infant, push the child off the mother's lap, or pull the bottle or breast from the infant's mouth. More often the expressions of hostility and resentment are more subtle and covert. Toddlers may verbally express a wish that the infant "go back inside mommy," or they will revert to more infantile forms of behavior, such as demanding a bottle, soiling their underpants, clinging for attention, using baby talk, or aggressively acting out toward others. For this reason, infants must be protected by parental supervision of the interaction between the siblings.

Temper Tantrums

Temper tantrums are nearly universal during toddlerhood as independence is established and more complex tasks are attempted that may overwhelm the child emotionally. Tod-

GUIDELINES

Assessing Toilet Training Readiness

PHYSICAL READINESS

Voluntary control of anal and urethral sphincters, usually by 18 to 24 months of age

Ability to stay dry for 2 hours; decreased number of wet diapers; waking dry from nap

Regular bowel movements

Gross motor skills of sitting, walking, and squatting

Fine motor skills to remove clothing

MENTAL READINESS

Recognizes urge to defecate or urinate

Verbal or nonverbal communicative skills to indicate when wet or has urge to defecate or urinate

Cognitive skills to imitate appropriate behavior and follow directions

PSYCHOLOGIC READINESS

Expresses willingness to please parent

Able to sit on toilet for 5 to 10 minutes without fussing or getting off

Curiosity about adults' or older sibling's toilet habits

Impatience with soiled or wet diapers; desire to be changed immediately

PARENTAL READINESS

Recognizes child's level of readiness

Willing to invest the time required for toilet training

Absence of family stress or change, such as a divorce, moving, new sibling, or imminent vacation

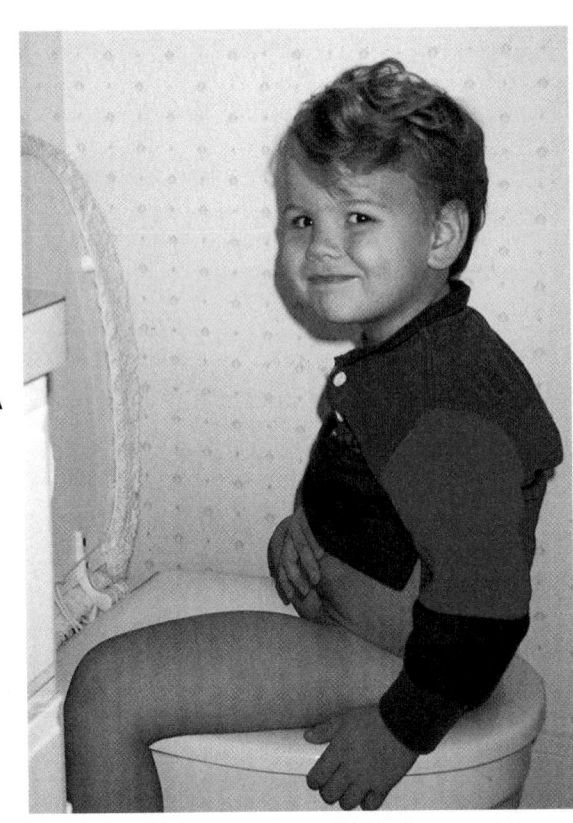
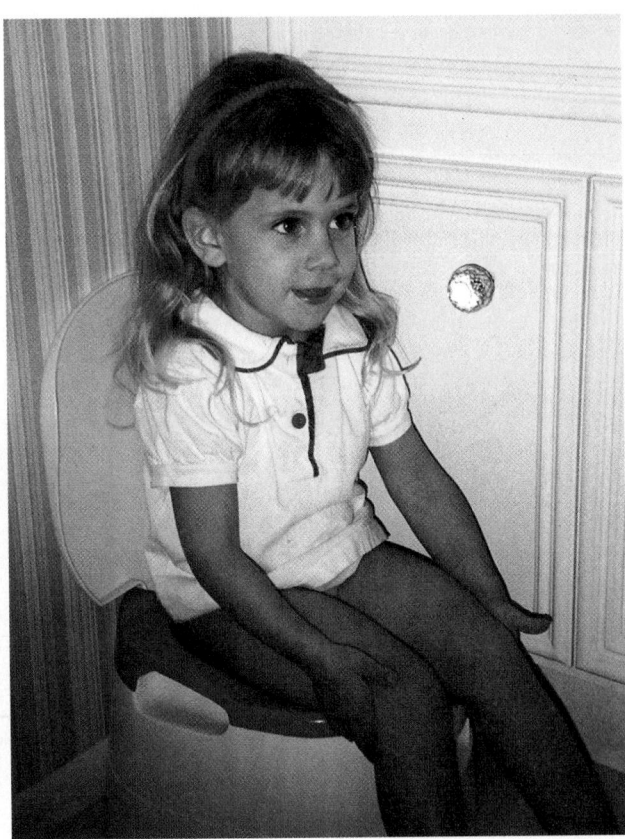

FIG. 12-5 ■ **A,** Sitting in reverse fashion on a regular toilet provides additional security to a young child. **B,** Children may begin toilet training sitting on a small toilet.

dlers may assert their independence by violently objecting to discipline. They may lie down on the floor, kick their feet, and scream at the top of their lungs. Some have learned the effectiveness of holding their breath until the parent relents. Although holding one's breath may cause fainting from the lack of oxygen, the accumulation of carbon dioxide will stimulate the respiratory control center, resulting in no physical harm.

The best approach toward tapering temper tantrums requires consistency and developmentally appropriate expectations and rewards. Ensuring consistency among all caregivers in expectations, prioritizing what rules are important,

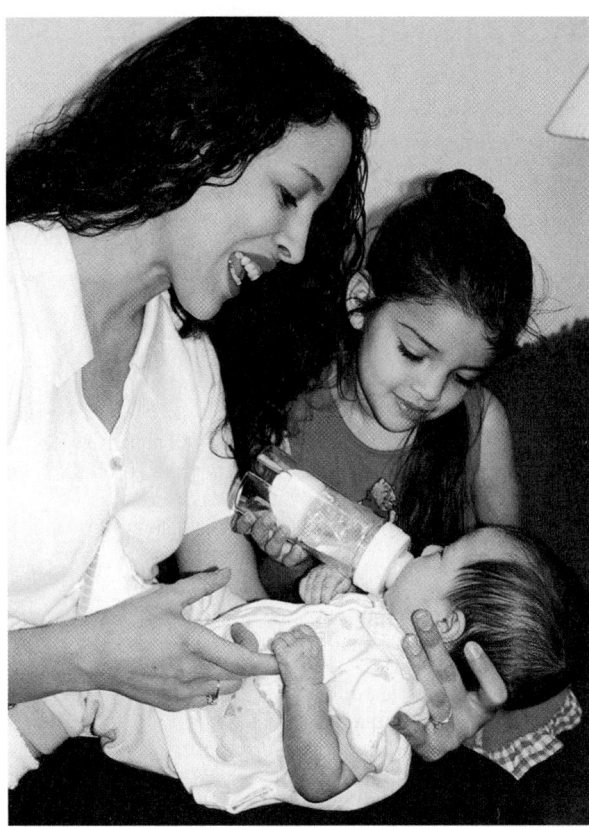

FIG. 12-6 ■ To minimize sibling rivalry, parents should include the toddler during caregiving activities.

and developing consequences that are reasonable for the child's level of development help manage the behavior. For example, a popular time for a tantrum is before bed. Active toddlers often have trouble slowing down and, when placed in bed, resist staying there. Parents can reinforce consistency and expectations by stating, "After this story it is bedtime." Starting at 18 months, time-outs work well for managing temper tantrums.

During tantrums ignore the behavior, provided the behavior is not injurious to the child, such as violently banging the head on the floor. Continue to be present to provide a feeling of control and security to the child once the tantrum has subsided. At this time a toy or a favorite activity can be substituted for the request. (See also Limit Setting and Discipline, Chapter 3.) During periods of no tantrums practice developmentally appropriate positive reinforcement.

Negativism

One of the more difficult aspects of rearing children in this age-group is their persistent "no" response to every request. The negativism is not an expression of being stubborn or insolent, but a necessary assertion of self-control. Children test limits to gain understanding of the world and to learn to modify their behavior to fit the expectations of society. Negativism begins to subside as most children prepare to enter kindergarten.

One method of dealing with the negativism is to reduce the opportunities for a "no" answer. Asking the child, "Do you want to go to sleep now?" is an almost certain example of a question that will be answered with an emphatic "no." Instead, tell the child that it is time to go to sleep and proceed accordingly. In their attempt to exert control, children like to make choices. When confronted with appropriate choices, such as "You may have a peanut butter and jelly sandwich or chicken noodle soup for lunch," they are more likely to choose one rather than automatically say no. However, if their response is negative, parents should make the choice for the child.

Regression

The retreat from one's present pattern of functioning to past levels of behavior is referred to as *regression.* It usually occurs in instances of discomfort or stress when one attempts to conserve psychic energy by reverting to patterns of behavior that were successful in earlier stages of development. Regression is common in toddlers, because almost any additional stress hinders their ability to master present developmental tasks. Any threat to their autonomy, such as illness, hospitalization, separation, or adjustment to a sibling, represents a need to revert to earlier forms of behavior, such as increased dependency; refusal to use the potty chair; temper tantrums; demand for the bottle, stroller, or crib; and loss of newly learned motor, language, social, and cognitive skills.

At first, such regression appears acceptable and comfortable for children. The loss of newly acquired achievements is frightening and threatening, because children are aware of their helplessness. Parents become concerned about regressive behavior and frequently, in their efforts to deal with it, force the child to cope with an additional source of stress—the pressure to live up to expected standards. Brazelton (1999) suggests that these predictable times of regression, or *touchpoints,* are an opportunity to prepare parents for the next step in their child's development.

When regression does occur, the best approach is to ignore it while praising existing patterns of appropriate behavior. Regression is a child's way of saying, "I can't cope with this present stress and perfect this skill as well, but I will if given patience and understanding." For this reason, it is advisable not to attempt new areas of learning when an additional crisis is present or expected, such as beginning toilet training shortly before a sibling is born or attempting new areas of learning during a brief period of hospitalization.

PROMOTING OPTIMAL HEALTH DURING TODDLERHOOD

NUTRITION

During the period from 12 to 18 months of age, the growth rate slows, decreasing the child's need for calories, protein, and fluid. However, the protein (1.2 g/kg) and caloric (102 kcal/kg) requirements are still relatively high to meet the demands for muscle tissue growth and high activity level (Picciano and others, 2000). The need for minerals such as iron, calcium, and phosphorus is still high, particularly when one considers the poor food habits of children in this age-group and the increased mineralization within bones.

At approximately 18 months of age, most toddlers manifest this decreased nutritional need with a decreased appetite, a phenomenon known as *physiologic anorexia*. They become picky, fussy eaters with strong taste preferences. They may eat large amounts one day and almost nothing the next. Toddlers are increasingly aware of the nonnutritive function of food: the pleasure of eating, the social aspect of mealtime, and the control of refusing food. They are influenced by factors other than taste when choosing food. If a family member refuses to eat something, toddlers are likely to imitate that response. If the plate is overfilled, they are likely to push it away, overwhelmed by its size. If food does not appear or smell appetizing, they will probably not agree to try it. In essence, mealtime is more closely associated with psychologic components than with nutritional ones.

Developmentally, by 12 months of age most children are eating the same food prepared for the rest of the family. Some may have mastered using a cup with occasional spilling, although most cannot adeptly use a spoon until 18 months of age or later and generally prefer using their fingers.

Nutritional Counseling

Eating habits established in the first 2 or 3 years of life tend to have lasting effects on subsequent years. If food is used as a reward or sign of approval, a child may overeat for nonnutritive reasons. If food is forced and mealtime is consistently unpleasant, the usual pleasure associated with eating may not develop. Mealtimes should be enjoyable rather than times for discipline or family arguments. The social aspect of mealtime may be distracting for young children; therefore an earlier feeding hour may be appropriate. Young children are unable to sit through a long meal and become restless and disruptive. This is particularly common when children are brought to the table just after active play. Calling them in from play 15 minutes before mealtime allows them ample opportunity to get ready for eating while settling down their active minds and bodies.

The method of serving food also takes on more importance during this period. Toddlers need to have a sense of control and achievement in their abilities. Giving them large, adult-size portions can overwhelm them. In general, what is eaten is much more significant than how much is consumed. Small amounts of meat and vegetables supply greater food value than a large consumption of bread or potato. Serving sizes need to be appropriate for age (Box 12-2). Young children tend to like less spicy, bland food, although this is a culturally determined preference. Substitutions can be provided for foods that they do not enjoy, although this practice should not cater to all of their desires. Frequent nutritious snacks can replace a meal. "Grazing"—nibbling and snacking—is a good way to ensure proper nutrition, provided that appropriate foods are offered.

NURSING TIP Serving Size for Young Children

- A general guide to the serving size of food is 1 tablespoon of solid food per year of age or one fourth to one third of the adult portion size.
- Use the tablespoon guide for easily measured foods such as vegetables or rice.
- Use the fraction guide for bread or milk.

BOX 12-2 ■ Sample Menu for Toddlers Based on Food Guide Pyramid*

Breakfast	½ cup dry, unsweetened cereal
	½ cup orange juice
	4 oz low-fat milk†
Snack	½ -1 whole banana
Lunch	1 tbsp peanut butter
	2 tsp all-fruit preserves
	1 slice whole-wheat bread
	2 tbsp peas
	4 oz low-fat milk†
Snack	2 graham crackers
	4 oz low-fat milk†
Dinner	1 chicken leg, roasted without skin
	¼-½ cup macaroni and cheese
	2 tbsp green beans, cooked
	2 tbsp carrots, cooked
	4-6 oz low-fat milk†
Snack	½ cup frozen yogurt

TOTAL SERVINGS	
Bread, cereal, rice, pasta	6-7
Vegetable	3
Fruit (vitamin A and C sources)	3-4
Milk, yogurt, cheese, pudding	2-3
Meat, poultry, fish, dried beans, eggs, nuts	2

*Use fats, oils, and sweets sparingly. Increase fluids with servings of water. Serving sizes are minimums for nutritional adequacy. Many children eat more.
†Substitute whole milk if child is younger than 24 months.

The ritualism of this age also dictates certain principles in feeding practices. Toddlers like the same dish, cup, or spoon every time they eat. They may reject a favorite food simply because it is served in a different utensil. If one food touches another, they often refuse to eat it. Mixed foods, such as stews or casseroles, are rarely favorites. Because toddlers are unpredictable in their table manners, it is best to use plastic dishes and cups, for both economy and safety. For some children a regular mealtime schedule also helps satisfy their desire and need for predictability and ritualism.

Most children by 12 months of age are eating the same food prepared for the rest of the family. However, mastication skills continue to mature, putting children at risk for choking. Large round foods should be avoided (hot dogs, grapes, peas, carrots, popcorn, fruit gel snacks). Active play while eating should be discouraged to prevent choking. Appetite and food preferences are sporadic. Often the interest in food parallels a growth spurt, so that periods of good eating are interspersed with phases of poor eating. If exposed to the same food every day, a young toddler does not get the exposure to learn how to manage the complex sensory information needed to eat new, more difficult foods (vegetables with a different texture versus pureed, slippery fruits). To help prevent "food jags" it is recommended to present food in various physical forms. The child may need to progress to eating new foods in a step-like fashion: visually tolerating the food, interacting with the food, smelling the food, touching the food, tasting and then eating the food.

Dietary Guidelines

Dietary guidelines are necessary to promote adequate energy and nutrient intake to support physical, emotional, psychologic, and cognitive development.

Nutrition during toddlerhood is a transition as a young toddler is weaned off milk/formula–based diets. Milk consumption decreases to 16 to 24 ounces/day. Larger volumes can contribute to iron deficiency anemia. Iron deficiency anemia is a significant health concern during the second year of life because whole cow's milk is low in iron and interferes with iron absorption. Iron deficiency anemia has been associated with impaired mental status and psychomotor development during the first 2 years of life. Iron-fortified cereals and iron-rich foods are recommended for all children beyond 6 months of age. Provide an iron-rich diet that includes heme and non-heme–iron sources (red meats, poultry, fish, green leafy vegetables, dried fruit, beans) and limit whole-milk consumption. Iron supplementation may be necessary in some cases.

Calcium and vitamin D are essential for healthy bone development. Adequate intake of calcium for the child 1 to 3 years of age is 500 mg. Whole milk, cheese, yogurt, legumes (beans), and vegetables (broccoli, collard greens, kale) are good sources for calcium. Popular calcium-fortified foods include waffles, cereals and cereal bars, orange juice, and some white breads. Adequate vitamin D intake is essential to prevent rickets; it is now recommended that children and adolescents have an intake of at least 200 IU of vitamin D daily. Mutivitamin preparations containing 400 IU of vitamin D (per tablet or milliliter) are adequate if food intake is poor; single vitamin D vitamin tablets contain too much vitamin D for children at this time (American Academy of Pediatrics, 2003a). Sources of vitamin D include fish, fish oils, and egg yolks. Fortified cereals, dairy products, and meat are also good sources of zinc and vitamin E.

It is recommended that toddlers have two fruit servings each day. Vitamin C enhances iron absorption. Toddlers should consume approximately 5 to 6 oz of juice per day. It tastes good to toddlers and is readily available. A 6-oz glass of fruit juice equals one fruit serving; however, juices lack the fiber of whole fruit and should not be a substitution for whole fruit. High intake of juice can contribute to diarrhea, overnutrition or undernutrition, and the development of caries (American Academy of Pediatrics, 2001b).

Fat restriction is not appropriate for toddlers. Thirty percent of calories should come from fat. The use of whole milk is recommended.

SLEEP AND ACTIVITY

Total sleep decreases only slightly during the second year and averages about 12 hours a day. Most children take one nap a day, and by the end of the second or third year many relinquish this habit. Children reach an adult pattern of sleep by 3 years of age (Howard and Wong, 2001).

Sleep problems are common, especially going to bed and falling asleep, and are a response to fears and awareness of separation. Fears can be provoked by a child's daily stressors such as pressure to toilet train, moves, sibling birth, experiencing a loss, or separation from parents.

Establishing a regular bedtime and routine is helpful, and providing transitional objects, such as a favorite stuffed animal or blanket, can help ease the child's insecurity at bedtime (see Fig. 12-3). Toddlers no longer sleeping in a crib may come out of their rooms after being put to bed. Limit prolonged bedtime rituals by defining a length of time and set of activities (one more story, one more drink). Toddlers who are too immature to respond to the measures identified may need their doorway gated.

A toddler's activity level is high, and there is rarely a problem with too little physical exercise, provided inappropriate restrictions are not instituted. With increasing numbers of young children being cared for outside the home, attention to the kinds of activity provided is important. For example, children with high activity levels may benefit from an environment in which outdoor play is encouraged. Neurodevelopment is necessary for the developing child to participate in activities. For example, the American Academy of Pediatrics (2000) recommends that children are not developmentally ready for swimming lessons until after 4 years of age.

DENTAL HEALTH
Regular Dental Examinations

The American Academy of Pediatrics (2003b), now recommends that every child have an oral health examination by a practitioner by 6 months of age; if the child is in a high-risk category for caries, it is recommended that an initial visit to a dentist or pedodontist (pediatric dentist) occur by age 6 months or within 6 months of the eruption of the first tooth. Initial visits to the dentist should be nontraumatizing. Because toddlers react negatively to new and potentially frightening experiences, the initial visit can center around meeting the dentist, seeing the equipment, and sitting in the chair. If the child is cooperative, the dentist may just look at the teeth but reserve a more thorough examination for another visit. Modeling, in which the child observes procedures performed on the parent or a cooperative sibling, can also be effective.

Removal of Plaque

Oral hygiene measures should be implemented as noted above to remove *plaque,* soft bacterial deposits that adhere to the teeth and cause *dental caries* (decay or cavities) and *periodontal* (gum) *disease.* Poor oral hygiene and poor dietary habits are associated with the development of caries in children.

The most effective methods for plaque removal are brushing and flossing. Several brushing techniques exist, although there is no universal agreement regarding the best method. One that is suitable for cleaning the primary teeth is the scrub method. The tips of the bristles are placed firmly at a 45-degree angle against the teeth and gums and moved back and forth in a vibratory motion. The ends of the bristles should be wiggling but not moving forcefully back and forth, which can damage the gums and enamel. All the surfaces of the teeth are cleaned in this manner except the lingual (inner) surfaces of the anterior teeth. To clean these surfaces, the toothbrush is placed vertical to the teeth and moved up and down. Only a few teeth are brushed at one time, using six to eight strokes for each section. A systematic approach is used so that all surfaces are thoroughly cleaned (Fig. 12-7).

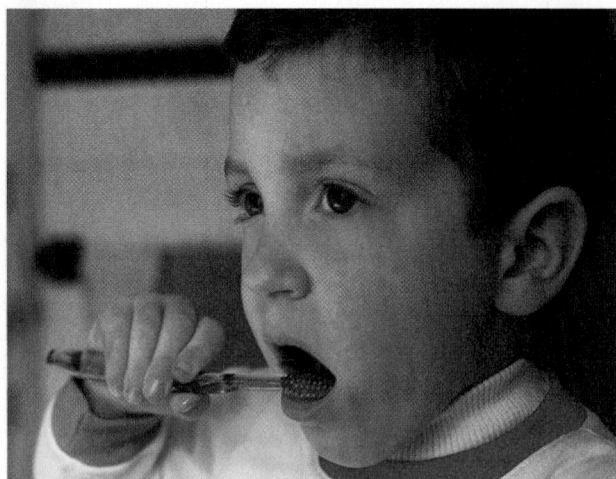

FIG. 12-7 ■ Young children can participate in toothbrushing, but parents need to brush all of the child's teeth thoroughly.

For young children the most effective cleaning is done by parents (Fig. 12-8). Several positions can be used that facilitate access to the mouth and help stabilize the head for comfort:

- Stand with child's back toward adult. (When done in front of a bathroom mirror, both child and adult can see what is being done in the mirror.)
- Sit on a couch or bed with child's head resting in adult's lap.
- Sit on the floor or a stool with child's head resting between adult's thighs.

With all positions, use one hand to cup the chin and one to brush the teeth. For easier access to back teeth, hold the mouth partially open.

NURSING TIP

- To encourage children to open their mouth, ask them to "tweet like a bird" to brush the front teeth and to "roar like a lion" to brush the back teeth.
- Sing, tell stories, or talk to children during teeth cleaning to prevent boredom.

For effective cleaning, a small toothbrush with soft, rounded, multitufted nylon bristles that are short and uniform in length is recommended. Nylon bristles dry more rapidly after use and retain their shape better than natural bristles. Toothbrushes are replaced as soon as the bristles are frayed or bent. With young children, brushing may be more easily accomplished using only water, because many children dislike the foam from toothpaste and the foam interferes with visibility. There is also the danger of swallowing fluoridated toothpaste (see following discussion under Fluoride). Introduce toothpaste around 2 years of age. When using toothpaste, children should select the flavor they like to encourage the brushing habit. Use a pea-sized amount of toothpaste (apply across the narrow width of the toothbrush, rather than along its length, to decrease the chance of applying an excessive amount).

After the teeth have been cleaned, flossing with dental floss is done to remove plaque and debris from between the teeth and below the gum margin, where brushing is ineffective. Because young children do not have the dexterity to manipulate the floss, parents are taught the procedure.

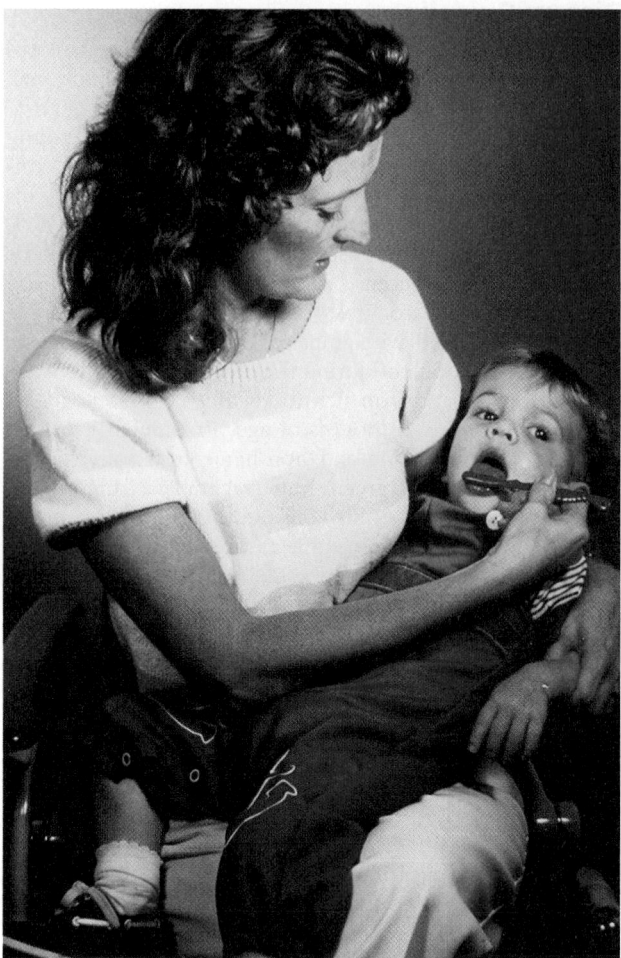

FIG. 12-8 ■ The most effective cleaning of teeth is done by parents.

A disclosing agent is helpful in identifying those areas of the teeth where plaque accumulates. It also helps motivate children to clean their teeth because plaque is difficult to see. After cleaning, the mouth is inspected to ensure that all traces of plaque have been removed. Where plaque remains, the teeth are rebrushed.

Ideally, the teeth should be cleaned after each meal and especially before bedtime, and the child should be given nothing to eat or drink after the night brushing except water. At those times when brushing is impractical, the "swish-and-swallow" method of cleaning the mouth is taught: with a mouthful of water the child rinses the mouth and swallows, repeating the procedure three or four times.*

Fluoride

Fluoride supplementation should be considered for any child over the age of 6 months whose drinking water is deficient in fluoride. Supplementation based on fluoride concentration of water supply <0.3 parts per million is 0.25 mg for a child 6 months to 3 years of age (American Academy of Pediatric Dentistry, 1999).

*More detailed information can be obtained by contacting the **American Academy of Pediatric Dentistry** website: www.aapd.org

TABLE 12-2 ■ Fluoride Supplementation*

	WATER FLUORIDE CONTENT (ppm)†		
AGE	0.3	0.3-0.6	>0.6
Birth-6 months	0	0	0
6 months-3 years	0.25	0	0
3-6 years	0.50	0.25	0
6-16 years	1.00	0.50	0

From Dental Care, *Pediatr Rev* 22(1):13-15, 2001.
*Fluoride daily doses are given in milligrams.
†Parts per million (ppm).

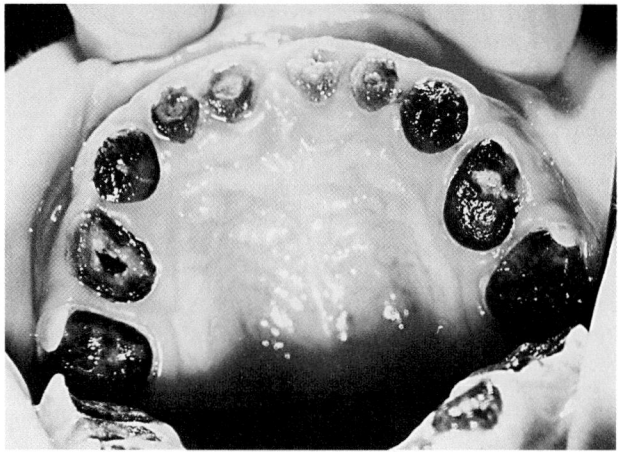

FIG. 12-9 ■ Nursing caries. (Courtesy Bruce Carter, DDS, Texas Children's Hospital, Houston, TX.)

Fluoride, a mineral, is found in water, foods, or drinks in which fluoridated water was used as part of the processing system. Because the water fluoridation process and manufacturing of fluoride toothpaste are almost impossible to standardize in the United States, the dosage of fluoride supplements has been lowered to reduce the incidence of fluorosis (Table 12-2). Increased fluoride ingestion leads to enamel protein retention, hypomineralization of the enamel and dentin, and disturbance of crystal formation. The effects caused by this change range from barely discernible white fiberlike lines or spots to gray-brown stains or pitted areas.

Low-Cariogenic Diet

Diet is critical to developing good teeth because the carious process depends primarily on fermentable sugars, especially sucrose. Refined table sugar, honey, molasses, corn syrup, and dried fruits such as raisins are highly cariogenic.

Ideally, such foods should be eliminated. However, because this is impractical, some suggestions can be helpful. First, *the frequency with which sugar is consumed is more important than the total amount eaten.* Therefore, when sweets are eaten, they are less damaging if consumed immediately after a meal rather than as a snack between meals. When sweets are served as the dessert, the teeth can be cleaned afterward, decreasing the amount of time the sugar is in the mouth.

Second, the form of sugar is important. The more cariogenic foods are those that are sticky or hard, because they remain in the mouth longer. Consequently, sucking on lollipops is more cariogenic than eating a chocolate bar. Sometimes the source of the sugar is "hidden," such as in numerous prescription and nonprescription drugs and in many popular cereals, including the "all-natural" variety. Reading food labels is essential in eliminating sources of sucrose.

FYI

Some snacks do not contribute to tooth decay. Aged cheeses, such as cheddar, may alter the pH and retard bacterial growth. Sugarless gum chewed after eating may actually protect against cavities by stimulating saliva that neutralizes acid. The artificial sweeteners saccharin, aspartame, and Splenda are noncariogenic; sorbitol has low cariogenic potential.

A special form of tooth decay in children between 18 months and 3 years of age is *nursing caries* (also called *nursing bottle caries* or *bottle-mouth caries*), which occurs when the child is routinely given a bottle of milk or juice at nap or bedtime or uses the bottle as a pacifier while awake. Frequent nocturnal breast-feeding for prolonged periods also leads to extensive destruction of the teeth. The practice of coating pacifiers in honey can also contribute to caries and may be a potential source of botulism poisoning. As the sweet liquid pools in the mouth, the teeth are bathed for several hours in this cariogenic environment. The maxillary (upper) incisors and molars are affected most, because the mandibular (lower) incisors are protected by the lower lip, tongue, and saliva (Fig. 12-9). Severely decayed teeth may require the application of stainless steel bands to preserve the spacing until the permanent teeth erupt.

Prevention involves eliminating the bedtime bottle completely, feeding the last bottle before bedtime, substituting a bottle of water for milk or juice, not using the bottle as a pacifier, and never coating pacifiers in sweet substances. Juice in bottles, especially commercially available ready-to-use bottles, is discouraged; beverages are especially damaging because the sugar is more readily converted to acid. Juice should always be offered in a cup to avoid prolonging the bottle-feeding habit. Toddlers should be encouraged to drink from a cup at the first birthday and weaned from a bottle by 14 months of age. Nurses are in an excellent position to counsel parents regarding the dangers of this habit and other aspects of dental care.*

INJURY PREVENTION

Injuries cause more deaths in children between the ages of 1 and 4 years than in any other childhood age-group except adolescence. The injury death rate has remained relatively

---

*Sources of information about nursing caries and other aspects of child dental health include the **National Institute of Dental and Craniofacial Research,** Building 31, 31 Center Drive, MFC-2290, Bethesda, MD 20892-2290; (301) 496-4261; website: www.nidr.nih.gov; **Academy of Pediatric Dentistry,** 211 E. Chicago Avenue, Suite 700, Chicago, IL 60611; (312) 337-2169 or (800) 544-2174 (outside Illinois); website: www.aapd.org; **American Dental Association,** 211 E. Chicago Avenue, Chicago, IL 60611; (312) 440-2500 or (800) 621-8099 (outside Illinois); website: www.ada.org; and **Canadian Dental Association,** 1815 Alta Vista Drive, Ottawa, Ontario K1G 3Y6; (613) 523-1770 or (800) 267-6354; website: www.cda-adc.ca/.

unchanged during the past decade; however, the corresponding rates from all other causes of death combined have declined significantly. Traumatic injury is the leading cause of childhood hospitalization, and infants and younger children are at higher risk because of small size and inability to protect themselves (Dowd, Keenan, and Bratton 2002). Child protection (adapting environment, society regulations and laws) and parent and child education are key determinants in injury prevention.

A major factor in the critical increase of injuries during early childhood is the unrestricted freedom achieved through locomotion combined with an unawareness of danger within the environment. Specific categories of injuries and appropriate prevention are best understood by associating them with the major developmental achievements of young children

(Table 12-3). The discussions of injuries in Chapters 1 and 10 are also relevant to safety concerns at this age.

Motor Vehicle Injuries

Motor vehicle injuries cause more accidental deaths in all pediatric age-groups after age 1 year than any other type of injury or disease and are responsible for almost one half of all accidental deaths among children ages 1 to 4 years. Many of the deaths are caused by injuries within the car when restraints have not been used or have been used improperly. Approved restraints properly installed and applied can reduce the majority of fatalities and injuries (American Academy of Pediatrics, 2003c).

Nurses have a responsibility for educating parents regarding the importance of car restraints and their proper use.

TABLE 12-3 ■ Injury Prevention During Early Childhood

DEVELOPMENTAL ABILITIES RELATED TO RISK OF INJURY	INJURY PREVENTION

Walks, runs, and climbs
Able to open doors and gates
Can ride tricycle
Can throw ball and other objects
	Motor vehicles
	Use federally approved car restraint; if restraint is not available, use lap belt
	Supervise child while playing outside
	Do not allow child to play on curb or behind a parked car
	Do not permit child to play in pile of leaves, snow, or large cardboard container in trafficked area
	Supervise tricycle riding; wear helmet
	Limit playing in driveways with parked cars or provide physical barriers limiting access.
	Lock fences and doors if not directly supervising children
	Teach child to obey pedestrian safety rules:
	    Obey traffic regulations; cross only at crosswalks and only when traffic signal indicates it is safe
	    Stand back a step from the curb until it's time to cross
	    Look left, right, and left again and check for turning cars before crossing street
	    Use sidewalks; when there is no sidewalk, walk on the left, facing traffic
	    Wear light colors at night and attach fluorescent material to clothing

Able to explore if left unsupervised Has great curiosity Helpless in water; unaware of its danger; depth of water has no significance	**Drowning** Supervise closely when near any source of water, including buckets Never, under any circumstance leave unsupervised in bathtub Keep bathroom doors closed and lid down on toilet Have fence around swimming pool and lock gate* Teach swimming and water safety (age appropriate)
Able to reach heights by climbing, stretching, and standing on toes Pulls objects Explores any holes or opening Can open drawers and closets Unaware of potential sources of heat or fire Plays with mechanical objects	**Burns** Turn pot handles toward back of stove Place electric appliances, such as coffee maker and popcorn machine, toward back of counter Place guardrails in front of radiators, fireplaces, or other heating elements Store matches and cigarette lighters in locked or inaccessible area; discard carefully Place burning candles, incense, hot foods, and cigarettes out of reach Do not let tablecloth hang within child's reach Do not let electric cord from iron or other appliance hang within child's reach Cover electrical outlets with protective plastic caps Keep electrical wires hidden or out of reach Install smoke and carbon monoxide alarms; change batteries every 6 months Develop a fire escape plan for the entire family and have drills Do not allow child to play with electrical appliance, wires, or lighters Stress danger of open flames; teach what "hot" means Always check bathwater temperature; adjust water heater temperature to 120° F (48.9° C) or lower; do not allow children to play with faucets Apply a sunscreen when child is exposed to sunlight (all year round)

*Detailed guidelines for safety barriers for pools may be found at http://www.cpsc.gov/CPSCPUB/PUBS/Pool.pdf; accessed January 13, 2004.

TABLE 12-3 ■ Injury Prevention During Early Childhood—*cont'd*

DEVELOPMENTAL ABILITIES RELATED TO RISK OF INJURY	INJURY PREVENTION
Explores by putting objects in mouth Can open drawers, closets, and most containers Climbs Cannot read labels Does not know safe dose or amount	**Poisoning** Place all potentially toxic agents out of reach or in a locked cabinet, including cosmetics, personal care items, cleaning products, pesticides, medications Caution against eating nonedible items, such as plants Replace medications or poisons immediately; replace child-guard caps properly Administer medications as a drug, not as a candy Do not store large surplus of toxic agents Promptly discard empty poison containers; never reuse to store a food item or other poison Teach child not to play in trash containers Never remove labels from containers of toxic substances Have syrup of ipecac in home; use only if advised Know number and location of nearest poison control center (usually listed in front of telephone directory)
Able to open doors and some windows Goes up and down stairs Depth perception unrefined	**Falls** Use window guards—do not rely on screens to stop falls Place gates at top and bottom of stairs Keep doors locked or use child-proof doorknob covers at entry to stairs, high porch, or other elevated area, including laundry chute Ensure safe and effective barriers on porches, balconies, bleachers, decks Remove unsecured or scatter rugs Apply nonskid decals in bathtub or shower Keep crib rails fully raised and mattress at lowest level Place carpeting under crib and in bathroom Keep large toys and bumper pads out of crib or playpen (child can use these as "stairs" to climb out), then move to youth bed when child is able to climb out of crib Avoid using mobile walker, especially near stairs Dress in safe clothing (soles that do not "catch" on floor, tied shoelaces, pant legs that do not touch floor) Keep child restrained in vehicle; never leave unattended in vehicle or shopping cart Never leave child unattended in high chair Supervise at playgrounds; select play areas with soft ground cover and safe equipment
Puts things in mouth May swallow hard or inedible pieces of food	**Choking and suffocation** Avoid large, round chunks of meat, such as whole hot dogs (slice lengthwise into short pieces) Avoid fruit with pits, fish with bones, dried beans, hard candy, chewing gum, nuts, popcorn, grapes, marshmallows Choose large, sturdy toys without sharp edges or small removable parts Discard old refrigerators, ovens, and so on; if storing an old appliance, remove the door Keep automatic garage door transmitter in inaccessible place Select safe toy boxes or chests without heavy, hinged lids Keep Venetian blind cords out of child's reach Remove drawstrings from clothing Avoid contact with round hollow, semirigid plastic items such as half a plastic ball
Still clumsy in many skills Easily distracted from tasks Unaware of potential danger from strangers or other people	**Bodily damage** Avoid giving sharp or pointed objects—such as knives, scissors, or toothpicks—especially when walking or running Do not allow lollipops or similar objects in mouth when walking or running Teach safety precautions (e.g., to carry knife or scissors with pointed end away from face) Store all dangerous tools, garden equipment, and firearms in locked cabinet Be alert to danger of supervised animals and household pets Use safety glass on large glassed areas, such as sliding glass doors Teach child name, address, and phone number and to ask for help from appropriate people (cashier, security guard, policeman) if lost; have identification on child (shown in clothes, inside shoe) Teach stranger safety: 　Avoid personalized clothing in public places 　Never go with a stranger 　Tell parents if anyone makes child feel uncomfortable in any way 　Always listen to child's concerns regarding others' behavior 　Teach child to say "no" when confronted with uncomfortable situations

Car Restraints. Five types of restraints are available: (1) infant-only devices, (2) convertible models for both infants and toddlers, (3) boosters, (4) safety belts, and (5) devices for children with special needs (see Chapter 18). The infant-type restraints are discussed in Chapter 10; the convertible restraints and boosters are included here. The *convertible restraint* is suitable for infants in the rearward-facing position and for toddlers in the forward-facing position (Fig. 12-10). The transition point for switching to the forward-facing position is defined by the manufacturer but is generally at a body weight of at least 9 kg (20 pounds) and 1 year of age. Infants who weigh 20 pounds before 1 year of age should continue to ride rear-facing (American Academy of Pediatrics, 2003c). A convertible safety seat is positioned semireclined and facing the rear of the car for a child younger than 1 year weighing less than 20 pounds. The seat is positioned upright and facing forward for an older and heavier child (up to 40 pounds). Convertible safety seats should be used until the child weighs at least 40 pounds. Convertible restraints use different types of harness systems: a five-point harness that consists of a strap over each shoulder, one on each side of the pelvis, and one between the legs (all five come together at a common buckle); a padded shield that uses shoulder straps attached to a shield that is held in place by a crotch strap; or a T-shield that has retracting shoulder straps attached to a flat chest shield with a rigid stalk that attaches to a restraint between the legs.

> ⚠ **NURSING ALERT**
>
> Safety belts should be worn low on the hips, snug, and not on the abdominal area. Children should be taught to sit up straight to allow for proper fit. The shoulder belt is used *only* if it does not cross the child's neck or face.

Booster seats, also known as belt-positioning devices, allow proper use of the shoulder harness and provide an artificial pelvis to serve as the anchor points for the lap belt. Booster seats are used for children who are less than 4 feet, 9 inches tall and weigh more than 40 pounds, typically between 4 and 8 years old. A booster seat should be used until the child is able to sit against the back of the seat with

feet hanging down and legs bent at the knees. The belt-positioning booster model raises a child higher in the seat, moving the shoulder part of the belt off the neck and the lap portion of the belt off the abdomen onto the pelvis. Booster seats must be used with the lap and shoulder belts and should never be used in a position with an active front air bag; a rear seat use is recommended (Ebel and Grossman, 2003). A shield booster model uses a large plastic shield slipped into place in front of the child. The shields have been found to be unsafe for children weighing more than 40 pounds and must be removed when the child reaches this weight. Both the National Highway Traffic Safety Administration and the American Academy of Pediatrics (2003c) recommend that children use a harness-type seat instead of a shield booster when possible; however, if used, the plastic shield must be removed.

Some older model restraints require the use of a top anchor (tether) strap to prevent the child from pitching forward in a crash. If the tether strap is not used, up to 90% of the restraint's protection is lost. Instructions for proper installation of the tether strap and permanent bracket are included with the car restraint. Cars with free-sliding latch-plates on the lap/shoulder belt require the use of a metal locking clip to keep the belt in a tight-holding position. The locking clip is threaded onto the belt above the latchplate (see inset, Fig. 12-10). If parents have newer cars with automatic lap/shoulder belts, they need to have additional lap belts installed to properly secure the restraint.

Children should use specially designed car restraints until they weigh at least 60 pounds or are 8 years old (American Academy of Pediatrics, 2003c). Children who outgrow the convertible restraint may still be able to ride safely in a booster seat until the midpoint of the head is higher than the vehicle seat back. If a car safety seat is not available, the lap belt provides more protection than no restraint (except for infants, where there is no safe alternative to approved restraint devices). Shoulder-only automatic belts are designed to protect adults. Children should use the manual shoulder belts in the rear seat. Air bags do not take the place of child safety seats or seat belts and can be lethal to young children. The safest area of the car for children is the back seat. Children who must ride in the passenger side of the front seat with an air bag should be positioned as far back as possible.

Built-in seats are available in some cars and vans. They may be used for children who are at least 1 year of age and weigh at least 20 pounds. Built-in seats eliminate installation problems. However, weight and height limits vary. Reinforce that owners verify with vehicle manufacturers details about built-in seats.

For any restraint to be effective, it must be used consistently and properly. Examples of misuse include misrouting the vehicle seat belt through the restraint, failing to use the vehicle seat belt to secure the restraint, failing to use a tether strap, failing to use the restraint's harness system, and incorrectly positioning the child, especially facing infants forward instead of rearward. To address these issues, nurses must stress correct use of car restraints and rules that ensure compliance (see Family Home Care box). Children riding in car safety seats are generally much better behaved than children left unrestrained, which can be a major benefit to

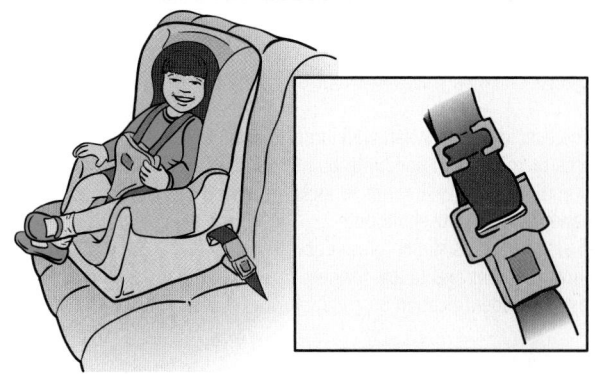

FIG. 12-10 ■ Convertible seat in forward-facing position for toddlers and children. *Inset,* Use of locking clip.

FAMILY HOME CARE

Using Car Safety Seats

Read manufacturer's directions and follow them exactly.

Anchor safety seat securely to car's seat and apply harness snugly to child.

Do not start the car until everyone is properly restrained.

Always use the restraint, even for short trips.

If child begins to climb out or undo the harness, firmly say, "No." It may be necessary to stop the car to reinforce the expected behavior. Use rewards, such as stars or stickers, to encourage cooperative behavior.

Encourage child to help attach buckles, straps, and shields, but always double-check fastenings.

Decrease boredom on long trips. Keep soft toys in the car for quiet play; talk to child; point out objects and teach child about them. Stop periodically. If child wishes to sleep, make sure child stays in the restraint.

Insist that others who transport children also follow these safety rules.

FYI

The LATCH (Lower Anchors and Tethers for CHildren) universal child safety seat system was implemented as a requirement starting in the fall of 2002 for all new automobiles and child safety seats. This system provides a uniform anchorage consisting of two lower anchorages and one upper anchorage in the rear seat of the vehicle. New child safety seats will have a hook, buckle, strap, or other tether that attaches to the anchorage (Fig. 12-11). Seat belts will no longer be used to anchor child safety seats in newer vehicles. The first phase requires all new cars to have an upper anchorage. By fall of 2002, all new cars must have had the entire LATCH system installed.

parents and should be emphasized as an additional advantage of restraints.*

Other Car-Related Injuries.   Injuries may also occur during sudden stops when objects are left unrestrained. On sudden impact, a loose ball becomes a projectile missile. Therefore, all items should be secured or stored in the trunk or behind a barrier such as netting in vans and wagons.

Children older than 3 years of age are often involved in pedestrian traffic injuries. Because of their gross motor skills of walking, running, and climbing and their fine motor skills of opening doors and fence gates, they are likely to be in hazardous areas when unsupervised. Unaware of danger

*American Academy of Pediatrics, 141 Northwest Point Boulevard, PO Box 927, Elk Grove Village, IL 60007; (888) 227-1770; website: www.aap.org; and local division of traffic safety or US Department of Transportation, National Highway Traffic Safety Administration, 400 Seventh Street SW, Washington, DC 20590; (800) 424-9393; website: www.nhtsa.dot.gov.

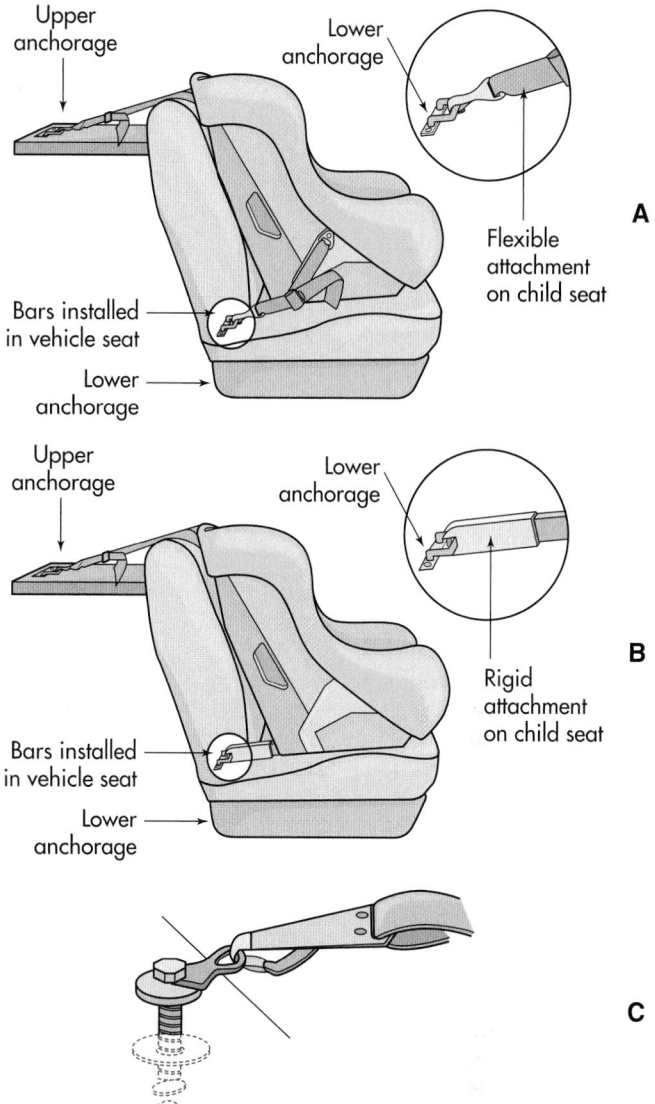

FIG. 12-11 ■ LATCH (Lower Anchors and Tethers for CHildren) universal child safety seat system. **A,** Flexible two-point attachment with top tether. **B,** Rigid two-point attachment with top tether. **C,** Top tether. (Courtesy US Department of Transportation, National Highway Traffic Safety Administration.)

and unable to approximate the speed of a car, they are hit by moving vehicles. Running after a ball, riding a tricycle, and playing behind a parked car are common activities that may result in a vehicular tragedy. Toddlers playing in driveways or farmyards are at risk of a run-over injury caused by vehicles in reverse gear (backing up). A precaution when children are playing in driveways is attaching to the tricycle a pole with a bright flag that is high enough to be visible through an automobile's back window. Another safeguard is the use of a device that beeps when the vehicle is driven in reverse to alert children to the oncoming car, van, tractor, or truck. Preventing vehicular injuries involves protecting and educating children and adults about the danger of moved or parked vehicles.

One type of injury that has become more commonplace occurs when children crawl into an open trunk and pull it closed; asphyxia may occur in such cases; therefore, car trunks should not be left open when children are not being supervised. Some cars are equipped with a safety switch that can be activated from inside the trunk to open a closed trunk door.

Preventing vehicular injuries involves protecting and educating children about the danger of moving or parked vehicles. Although preschool children are too young to be trusted to always obey, the parent should emphasize looking for moving vehicles before crossing the street, recognizing the stop and go colors of traffic lights, and following traffic officers' signals. Physical barriers limiting children from playing near vehicles help prevent these injuries (Mayr and others, 2001). Most important, what is preached must be practiced. Children learn through imitation, and consistency reinforces learning.

Drowning

Drowning, not including drowning from water transportation, ranks second among boys and third among girls ages 1 to 4 years as a cause of accidental death. With well-developed skills of locomotion, toddlers are able to reach potentially dangerous areas, such as bathtubs, toilets, buckets, swimming pools, hot tubs, and lakes. The toddler's intense drive for exploration and investigation, combined with an unawareness of the danger of water and her or his helplessness in water, makes drowning always a viable threat. It is also one category of injuries that results in death within minutes, diminishing the chance for rescue and survival. Adult supervision of children when near any source of water is essential; teaching swimming and water safety can be helpful but cannot be regarded as sufficient protection. Pool fencing, although critical, does not always deter the fast-moving child (see Table 12-3).

Burns

Burns rank second among girls and third among boys in this age-group as a cause of accidental death. Toddlers' ability to climb, stretch, and reach objects above their head makes any hot surface a potential source of danger. Scalds from children pulling pots on top of themselves are a major source of burns. As a precaution, pot handles should be turned toward the back of the stove. Ideally, the knobs for controlling the range burners should be out of reach, not on the front panel where nimble fingers can turn them on and accidentally touch the hot burner. Oven doors should be closed whenever the oven is turned on or when it is cooling. The outside of doors of automatic self-cleaning ovens may become hot and, if touched, could cause a burn. Microwave ovens present much less of a burn hazard to toddlers because the outside remains cool, and they are often inaccessible, although foods heated in microwaves can scald children (Wolf, Adler, and Hauben, 2001).

Other sources of heat, such as radiators, fireplaces, accessible furnaces, kerosene heaters, or wood-burning stoves, should have guards placed in front of them. The tops of some of these heaters are designed to become hot enough to boil water to provide humidity. They are hazardous if touched or if the pan of water is spilled. Portable electric heaters must be placed in a high area, well out of reach of climbing young children. Hair curling irons may also be easily reached and can burn hands of curious toddlers.

Hot objects such as candles, incense, cigarettes, pots of tea or coffee, or irons must be placed away from children. The flame of a candle and the smoke of a cigarette invite investigation. Ashtrays with a center well are preferred to prevent the cigarette from falling off the rim, and adults should try not to smoke, cook, or drink hot liquids when children are physically close. If tablecloths are used, the edges should be placed out of reach to prevent injuries from both burns and falling objects.

Flame burns represent one of the most fatal types of burns and commonly occur when children play with matches and accidentally set themselves (and the home) on fire. To prevent flame burns, matches and lighters must be stored safely away from children, and parents need to teach children the dangers of playing with such objects. In addition, all homes should have smoke detectors installed to alert the occupants of a fire. A safety plan for immediate escape is also essential.

Electrical burns also represent an immediate danger to children. With preschoolers' ability to manipulate small, thin objects, they are able to insert hairpins or other conductive articles into electrical sockets. Young toddlers may explore outlets and wires by mouthing them. Since water is an excellent conductor, the chance for a severe circumoral electrical burn is great. Electrical outlets should have protective guards plugged into them when not in use (Fig. 12-12) or

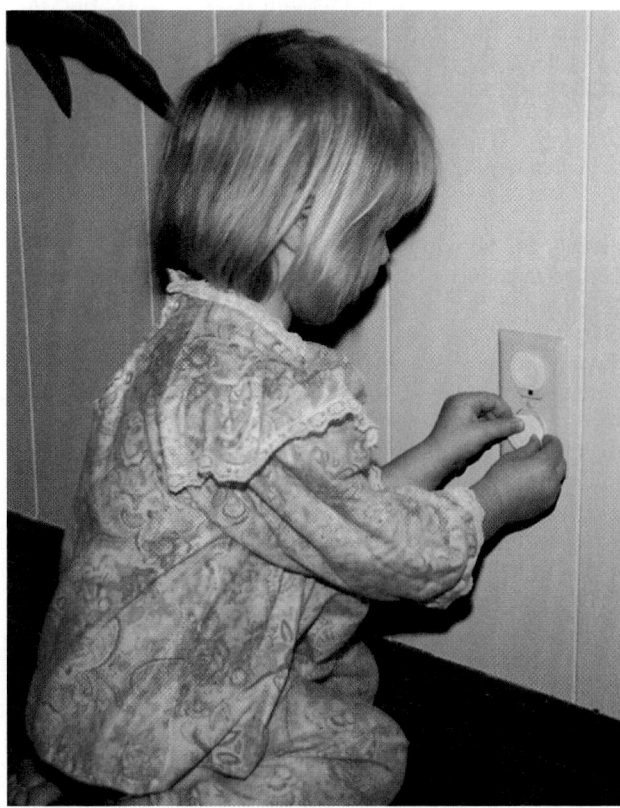

FIG. 12-12 ■ Special plastic caps in electrical sockets prevent young fingers from exploring dangerous areas.

be made inaccessible by having furniture placed in front of them when feasible. Children should not be allowed to play with electrical cords or appliances, which should be kept out of reach as much as possible.

Scald burns are the most common type of thermal injury in children. A scalding burn is often caused by high-temperature tap water, which children come in contact with as a result of turning on the hot-water faucet, falling into a bathtub of hot water, pulling hot pots onto themselves, or deliberate abuse. Always supervising youngsters when they are near tap water and checking bathwater temperatures are methods of prevention. Limiting household water temperatures to less than 49° C (120° F) is also recommended. At this temperature it takes 10 minutes of exposure to the water to cause a full-thickness burn. Conversely, water temperatures of 54° C (130° F), the usual setting of most water heaters, expose household members to the risk of full-thickness burns within 30 seconds. Nurses can help prevent such burns by advising parents of this common household danger and recommending that they readjust the water heater to a safe temperature. A meat or candy thermometer is a convenient way to measure water temperature. An easy-to-read hot-water gauge that changes color to show water temperatures between 120° and 150° is also available; it shows a "hot," "cool," or "OK" water temperature. A special device can also be added to the faucet that reduces the water flow once the set temperature is reached.

Sunburns are a year-round concern. Children spend a large amount of time outdoors year round. Their increased mobility makes it difficult to prevent sun exposure. Sunburn can be prevented by applying a sunscreen with a sun protection factor (SPF) of 15 or greater, dressing in protective clothing (wide-brimmed hat, protective cotton clothing with a tight weave), and avoiding sun exposure between 10 AM and 2 PM.

Poisoning

Toddlers are at the highest risk for poisoning. Mouthing activity continues to be prevalent after 1 year of age, and exploring objects by tasting them is part of children's curious investigation. Many household products, medications, and plants can be poisonous if swallowed, if in contact with the skin or eyes, or if inhaled (Shannon, 2003). Although in many instances poisoning does not result in mortality, it may cause significant morbidity, such as esophageal stricture from lye ingestion. Toddlers are able to climb most heights, open most drawers or closets, and unscrew most lids. By trial and error, younger children also manage to undo tops of bottles, plastic containers, aerosol cans, and jars, including those with child-resistant lids. In addition, pharmacists often transfer drugs to regular containers for the elderly, who may have difficulty with child-resistant lids. Newer forms of drugs, such as transdermal patches and cough-suppressant lozenges, have created additional dangers, since they are not packaged with safety caps and the lozenges look like candy.

The major reason for poisoning is improper storage (Fig. 12-13). The guidelines suggested in Chapter 10 apply to children in this age-group as well. However, unlike the infant, who was confined to certain heights and unable to un-

latch inventive locks, young children manage to find access to many high-level, tight-security places. For this age-group only a locked cabinet is safe.

Emergency and preventive measures for accidental poisoning are discussed in Chapter 14. Parents should have ready access to the telephone number for the poison control center and be prepared to act on the advice of the center.*

Falls

Falls are still a hazard to children in this age-group, although by the later part of early childhood, gross and fine motor skills are well developed, decreasing the incidence of falls down stairs or from chairs. However, playground injuries are common. Children need to be taught safety at

---

*The national toll-free telephone number for poison control centers is **(800) 222-1222.** This number provides everyone in the US with free access—24 hours a day, 7 days a week—to their regional poison center. For some tips on preventing poisoning in your home, see the TIPP slip, "Protect your Child . . . Prevent Poisoning," available online: http://www.aap.org/family/poistipp.htm.

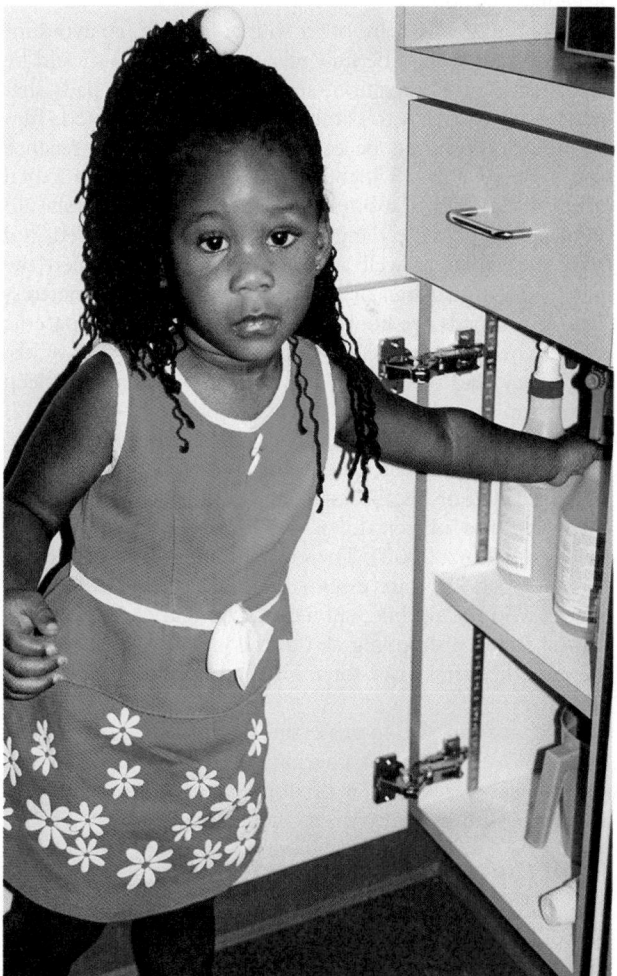

FIG. 12-13 ■ Children are most likely to ingest substances that are on their level, such as cleaning agents stored under sinks, rat poison, plants, or diaper pail deodorants.

play areas, such as no horseplay on high slides or jungle gyms, *sitting* on swings, and staying away from moving swings (Purvis and Hirsch, 2003). Passive prevention includes placement of grass, sand, or wood chips under play equipment. Swing seats should be made of plastic, canvas, or rubber and have smooth or rounded edges. Slides should not exceed an incline of 30 degrees, have evenly spaced rungs for climbing, and have protective "tunnels."

The climbing and running of the typical toddler are complicated by the child's total neglect for and lack of appreciation of danger. Gates must be placed at both ends of stairs. Accessible windows that are left open must have window guards, not screens, to prevent falls to the ground below. Falling from open windows is a major cause of accidental death in urban, lower socioeconomic groups. Doors leading to stairwells or porches must be locked, since preschoolers can easily open them. A convenient type of lock is a sliding bar or hook that can be attached to the door and frame at a level higher than the child can reach. Falling from balconies, porches, decks, and bleachers are all possible for the active toddler. Rails need to be sized appropriately because most children younger than 6 years can slip through a 6-inch opening and none older than 1 year can usually pass through a 4-inch opening (American Academy of Pediatrics, 2001c).

Cribs and vehicles are other sources of falls. To avoid injury, crib rails should be fully raised, the mattress should be kept at the lowest position, and toys or bumper pads that may be used as steps to climb out should be removed. Ideally, the floor should be carpeted. Once children reach a height of 89 cm (35 inches), they should sleep in a bed rather than a crib. If a bunk bed is selected, parents should be aware of possible dangers: falls from the top bed and from the ladder as well as head entrapment between the mattress and guardrail or between the supporting mattress slats. If the beds are constructed of tubular metal, parents should check for breaks or cracks in the metal and welds, which may lead to collapse and injury. Children who sleep on the top bunk should be 6 years or older.

Children who are unrestrained can fall from high chairs, shopping carts, carriages, car seats, and strollers if not properly restrained or because of a change in balance created by weighting the object down with heavy objects (Powell, Jovtis, and Tanz, 2002). Therefore, proper restraint and adequate supervision are essential. Children, especially older infants who are mobile, should not be placed in an infant seat on top of a shopping cart as the infant seat may fall off the cart; the safest place for an infant seat is inside the cart's bed.

Clothing can also increase the chance of falling. Simple safety measures, such as checking clothing and shoes and keeping shoelaces tied with double knots or using self-adhering closures, can prevent accidents.

Aspiration and Suffocation

Foreign body aspiration is most common during the second year of life. Usually by 1 year of age children chew well, but they may have difficulty with large pieces of food, such as meat and whole hot dogs, and with hard foods, such as nuts or dried beans. Young children cannot discard pits from fruit or bones from fish. It takes practice to learn how to chew gum without swallowing it. Gel snacks (also known as Gel-ly drops or fruit poppers) can also be difficult to manage and can be aspirated. Therefore the same precautions as discussed for infants regarding food selection must be implemented (see Chapter 10).

Play objects for toddlers must still be chosen with an awareness of danger from small parts. Large, sturdy toys without sharp edges or removable parts are safest. Small plastic toys such as Legos can cause choking or can be aspirated; such plastic items often do not appear on radiographic films. Balloons, coins, paper clips, pins, bells, button batteries, pull-tabs on cans, thumbtacks, nails, screws, jewelry (especially pierced earrings), and all types of pins are common household objects that can cause significant harm if swallowed or aspirated. Because of the danger of aspiration, parents should be taught emergency procedures for choking (see Airway Obstruction, Chapter 23).

Another cause of death by traumatic injury is from electrically operated garage doors. Young children playing in the garage may become trapped under the door. Although the automatic doors (only available in models built since 1993) should reverse when striking an object, they may not do so when hitting a flexible object or one that is very close to the ground. Precautions include placing controls where they are inaccessible to children, such as high on a wall and in a locked car, and instructing children not to run under a closing garage door. Periodically the door should be checked to determine if it returns after striking an object and if the limit settings meet manufacturer recommendations. Additional safety precautions include having an automatic eye near ground level of the door frame, which prevents the door from closing when an object is detected at the door opening. Suffocation from causes seen during infancy is less frequent, but old refrigerators, ovens, and other large appliances are an ever-present threat. Toddlers can climb inside these appliances and, if they close the door behind them, can be trapped inside. Discarding old appliances or removing all doors during storage prevents such tragic deaths. Toddlers may also suffocate when unsafe toy box lids accidentally close on their head or neck. Parents should be advised of this danger and encouraged to buy storage chests with lightweight, removable covers.

Hollow, semirigid hemispherical or ellipsoidal objects (toys, compartments of toys, containers) can form suction and cupping around a small child's face, causing complete airway obstruction. Several different types of objects have been involved with incidents, including toys, components of toys, and containers (Nakamura Pollack-Nelson, and Chidekel, 2003) (Fig. 12-14).

Children can become entangled on a cornerpost extension near or at the corner of a crib. Catch points in the corners of cribs have been eliminated; however, knobs and vertical protrusions not in cribs may also be hazardous. Strangulation can result from entanglement from these protrusions (Ridenour, 2002).

Because some of the older heating systems and hot water heaters may emit carbon monoxide, which is undetectable by human smell, houses should have a carbon monoxide detector in addition to a smoke detector.

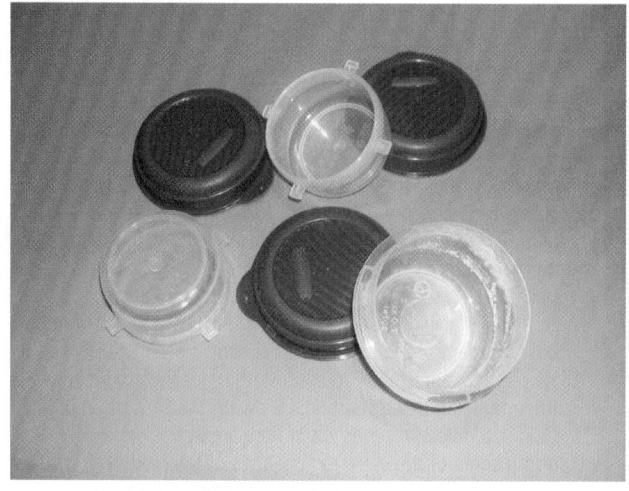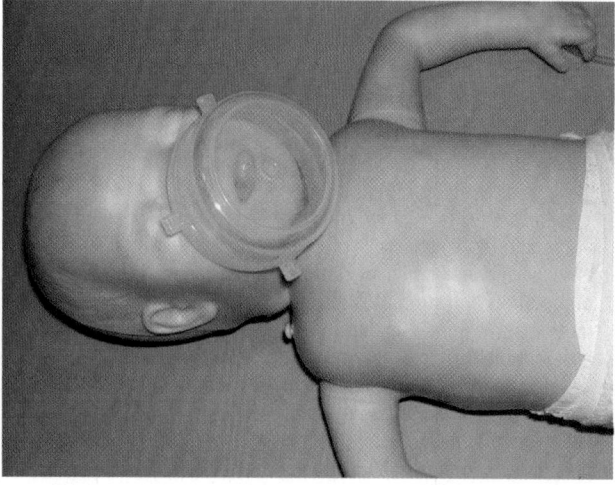

FIG. 12-14 ■ **A,** Round cup-shaped objects that may cause suction asphyxia in toddlers. **B,** Simulation of a hollow cup covering child's face (doll used).

Bodily Damage

Toddlers are still clumsy in many of their skills and can seriously harm themselves when walking while holding a sharp or pointed object or having food or objects such as spoons in their mouths. Preventing such occurrences is the best approach with toddlers. With preschoolers, teaching safety is most important. The child should be taught that when walking with a pointed object such as a knife or scissors, the pointed end is held away from the face. Dangerous garden or workshop equipment and all firearms should be stored in a locked cabinet (Crawley-Coha, 2002). Power lawn mowers and weed eaters are especially dangerous because they can throw rocks and other solid items (projectiles), and young children should not be allowed in an area where such tools are in use; nor should they be taken for a ride on a mower or allowed to operate the device (Robertson, 2003). Safety education should include respect for firearms and their proper and appropriate use, including nonpowder guns, such as air guns and rifles, which cause serious penetrating injuries (Darras, 2002). In addition, the child should be warned of and protected against potential danger from animal bites, which are quite common in toddlers, who do not understand the potential harm inherent in some animals (see Bodily Damage, Chapter 10, and Animal Bites, Chapter 30).

Toys can be a source of danger, and safety must be a prime consideration when selecting toys (see Family Home Care box: Toy Safety, Chapter 5). Most toys have age ranges written on them to designate their safety, but this information must be used with knowledge of the specific child's readiness.

Household safety should be practiced and includes the usual precautions recommended for any age-group (see Family Home Care box: Child Safety Home Checklist, Chapter 10). An additional safeguard for young children is the use of safety glass in doors, windows, and tabletops and the application of decals on glassed areas to lessen the likelihood of running through glass. Also, children should not be allowed to run, jump, wrestle, or play ball near glass structures.

Terrorism/Violence

During a time of national conflict and struggle, terrorism, violence, and fear inflict young minds. Emergency preparedness and anticipatory guidance are the responsibility of all health care professionals. The immature emotional and physical developmental stage of toddlers makes them unable to distinguish reality from fantasy. Fears and anxiety can be exhibited in separation anxiety and sleep problems. Children who recently mastered toileting may develop secondary enuresis. Providing easy, clear answers to questions at an age-appropriate level and allaying children's fears fosters security and comfort. Supporting a sense of control and developmentally appropriate activities, limiting television viewing, and ensuring a feeling of safety in home and community can assist children with coping with such crises. The websites for the American Academy of Pediatrics, the US Department for Homeland Security, and the American Red Cross offer a wealth of information for clinicians, families and children.

ANTICIPATORY GUIDANCE—CARE OF FAMILIES

Understanding toddlers is fundamental to successful childrearing. Nurses, particularly those in ambulatory or child health centers, are in a favorable position to assist parents in meeting the tasks and needs of children in this age-group. Prevention yields better results than treatment. Anticipatory guidance is paramount if one wishes to prevent future problems (see Family Home Care box). Advice is sometimes not the sole answer. Actual assistance, such as being available for home visiting or telephone consulting, should be part of the nurse's flexible repertoire of interventions. Whether parents are experiencing the rearing dilemmas of a first or a subsequent child, they benefit from sharing their feelings, frustrations, and satisfactions. They need adult companionship, freedom from childrearing responsibilities, and periodic separations from their children. Part of a nurse's responsibility is to provide opportunities for parents to express their feelings and to meet their physical, mental, and spiritual needs.

👪 FAMILY HOME CARE

Guidance During Toddler Years

AGES 12 TO 18 MONTHS

Prepare parents for expected behavioral changes of toddler, especially negativism and ritualism.

Assess present feeding habits and encourage gradual weaning from bottle and increased intake of solid foods.

Stress expected feeding changes of physiologic anorexia, presence of food fads and strong taste preferences, need for scheduled routine at mealtimes, inability to sit through an entire meal, and lack of table manners.

Assess sleep patterns at night, particularly habit of a bedtime bottle, which is a major cause of dental caries, and procrastination behaviors that delay hour of sleep.

Prepare parents for potential dangers of the home, particularly motor vehicle injuries, poisoning, and falling injuries; give appropriate suggestions for safeproofing the home. Discuss need for firm but gentle discipline and ways in which to deal with negativism and temper tantrums; stress positive benefits of appropriate discipline.

Emphasize importance for both child and parents of brief, periodic separations.

Discuss new toys that use developing gross and fine motor, language, cognitive, and social skills.

Emphasize need for dental supervision, types of basic dental hygiene at home, and food habits that predispose to caries; stress importance of supplemental fluoride.

AGES 18 TO 24 MONTHS

Stress importance of peer companionship in play.

Explore need for preparation for additional sibling; stress importance of preparing child for new experiences.

Discuss present discipline methods, their effectiveness, and parents' feelings about child's negativism; stress that negativism is important aspect of developing self-assertion and independence and is not a sign of spoiling.

Discuss signs of readiness for toilet training; emphasize importance of waiting for physical and psychologic readiness.

Discuss development of fears, such as darkness or loud noises, and of habits, such as security blanket or thumb sucking; stress normalcy of these transient behaviors.

Prepare parents for signs of regression in time of stress.

Assess child's ability to separate easily from parents for brief periods of separation under familiar circumstances.

Allow parents opportunity to express their feelings of weariness, frustration, and exasperation; be aware that it is often difficult to love toddlers at times when they are not asleep!

Point out some of the expected changes of the next year, such as longer attention span, somewhat less negativism, and increased concern for pleasing others.

AGES 24 TO 36 MONTHS

Discuss importance of imitation and domestic mimicry and need to include child in activities.

Discuss approaches toward toilet training, particularly realistic expectations and attitude toward accidents.

Stress uniqueness of toddlers' thought processes, especially through their use of language, poor understanding of time, causal relationships in terms of proximity of events, and inability to see events from another's perspective.

Stress that discipline still must be quite structured and concrete and that relying solely on verbal reasoning and explanation leads to injuries, confusion, and misunderstanding.

Discuss investigation of preschool or day care center toward completion of second year.

KEY POINTS

- The toddler stage, extending from 12 to 36 months, is a period of intense exploration of the environment.

- Biologic development during the toddler years is characterized by the acquisition of fine and gross motor skills that allow children to master a wide variety of activities.

- Although most of the physiologic systems are mature by the end of toddlerhood, development of certain areas of the brain is still occurring, allowing for greater intellectual capacity.

- Locomotion is the major gross motor skill acquired during toddlerhood, followed by increased eye-hand coordination.

- Specific tasks in the psychosocial development of a toddler include differentiating self from others, tolerating separation from parent, coping with delayed gratification, controlling bodily functions, acquiring socially acceptable behavior, communicating verbally, and interacting with others in a less egocentric manner.

- According to Erikson the major developmental task of toddlerhood is acquiring a sense of autonomy while overcoming a sense of doubt and shame.

- In Piaget's sensorimotor and preconceptual phases of development, the toddler experiments by incorporating the old learning of secondary circular reactions with new skills and applies this knowledge to new situations. There is the beginning of rational judgment, an understanding of causal relationships, and discovery of objects as objects. Preconceptual thought is characterized by egocentricism, centration, global organization of thought processes, animism, and irreversibility.

- Language is the major cognitive achievement in toddlerhood.

- The most striking characteristic of language development during early childhood is the increasing level of comprehension.

- Development of body image occurs with increasing motor ability, at which point toddlers recognize the importance and capacity of body parts.

- The two phases of differentiation of self from significant others are separation and individuation.

- Parental concerns during the toddler years include toilet training, coping with sibling rivalry, limit setting and discipline, dealing with temper tantrums, negativism, and regression.

- Effective discipline techniques for toddlers include reward, ignoring or extinction, and time-out.

- Nutrition is important at this stage because eating habits established in toddlerhood tend to have lasting effects in subsequent years.

- Regular dental examinations, fluoride supplementation, removal of plaque, and provision of a low-cariogenic diet promote optimum dental health.

- Because of increased locomotion, toddlers are at high risk for sustaining injuries. Fatal injuries are primarily a result of motor vehicle accidents, drownings, and burns.

References

American Academy of Pediatrics: Car safety seats: A guide for families 2003, www.aap.org/family/carseatguide.htm, 2003c.

American Academy of Pediatrics, Committee on Injury and Poison Intervention: Falls from heights: windows, roofs, and balconies, *Pediatrics* 107(5):1188-1191, 2001c.

American Academy of Pediatrics, Committee on Nutrition: The use and misuse of fruit juice in pediatrics, *Pediatrics* 107(5):1210-1213, 2001b.

American Academy of Pediatrics, Committee on Public Health: Children, adolescents, and television, *Pediatrics* 107(2):423-426, 2001a.

American Academy of Pediatrics, Committee on Sports Medicine and Fitness and Committee on Injury and Poison Prevention: Swimming programs for infants and toddlers, *Pediatrics* 105(4):868-870, 2000.

American Academy of Pediatrics, Section on Pediatric Dentistry: Oral health risk assessment timing and establishment of the dental home, *Pediatrics* 111(5):1113-1116, 2003b.

American Academy of Pediatrics: Prevention of rickets and vitamin D deficiency: new guidelines for vitamin D intake, *Pediatrics* 111(4):908-910, 2003a.

American Academy of Pediatric Dentistry: Oral health policies, *Pediatr Dent* 21:18-37, 1999.

Bates E, Dick F: Language, gesture, and the developing brain, *Dev Psychobiol* 40:293-310, 2002.

Brazelton TB, How to help parents of young children: the touchpoints model, *J Perinatol* 19(6 pt 2):S6-7, 1999.

Crawley-Coha T: Childhood injury: a status report, part 2, *J Pediatr Nurs* 17(2):133-138, 2002.

Dahlquist LM and others: Distraction for children of different ages who undergo repeated needle sticks, *J Pediatr Oncol Nurs* 19(1): 22-34, 2002.

Darras KM: Firearm safety: an essential primary care issue, *Adv Nurs Pract* 10(2):51-54, 2002.

DeLamater J, Friedrich WN: Human sexual development, *J Sex Res* 39(1): 10-14, 2002.

Dowd DM, Keenan HT, Bratton SL: Epidemiology and prevention of childhood injuries, *Crit Care Med* 30(11):S385-392, 2002.

Ebel BE, Grossman DC: Crash proof kids? An overview of current motor vehicle child occupant safety strategies, *Curr Prob Pediatr Adolesc Health Care* 33: 38-55, 2003.

Fosarelli P: Children and the development of faith: implications for pediatric practice, *Contemporary Pediatr* 20(1):85-98, 2003.

Glassy D, Romano J, and the Committee on Early Childhood, Adoption, and Dependent Care: Selecting appropriate toys for young children: the pediatrician's role, *Pediatrics* 111(4):911-913, 2003.

Howard BJ, Wong J: Sleep disorders, *Pediatr Rev* 22(10):327-342, 2001.

Lyytinen P and others: The development and predictive relations of play and language across the second year, *Scand J Psychol* 40:177-186, 1999.

Mayr JM and others: Vehicles reversing or rolling backwards: an underestimated hazard, *Inj Prev* 7:327-328, 2001.

Mercer R: Treating nocturnal enuresis, *Adv Nurs Pract* 11(2):26-31, 2003.

Meyer TL: Unveiling the secrecy behind masturbation, *Pediatr Rev* 23(4):148-149, 2002.

Nakamura SW, Pollack-Nelson C, Chidekel AS: Suction-type suffocation incidents in infants and toddlers, *Pediatrics* 111(1):e12-e16, 2003.

Petitto LA and others: Bilingual signed and spoken language acquisition from birth: implications for the mechanisms underlying early bilingual language acquisition, *J Child Lang* 28(2):453-496, 2001.

Picciano MF and others: Nutritional guidance is needed during dietary transition in early childhood, *Pediatrics* 106(1):109-114, 2000.

Powell EC, Jovtis E, Tanz RR: Incidence and description of stroller related injuries to children, *Pediatrics* 110(5):e62, 2002.

Purvis JM, Hirsch SA: Playground injury prevention, *Clin Orthop* 409:11-19, 2003.

Ridenour MV: How do children climb out of cribs, *Percept Mot Skills* 95:363-366, 2002.

Robertson WW: Power lawnmower injuries, *Clinic Orthop* 409:37-42, 2003.

Shannon M: Primary care: Ingestion of toxic substances by children, *N Engl J Med* 342(3):186-191, 2003.

Storr GB, Robinson P: Preparing kids for the new baby, *Can Nurs* 94(3):33-34, 1998.

Thompson RA: Caring for infants and toddlers, *Future Child* 11(1):21-33, 2001.

Wolf Y, Adler N, Hauben DJ: Exploding microwaved eggs—revisited, *Burns* 27:853-855, 2001.

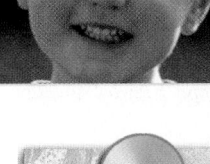

13

Health Promotion of the Preschooler and Family

DAVID WILSON

Remember to check out your companion CD-ROM

http://evolve.elsevier.com/Wong/essentials/

CHAPTER OUTLINE

RELATED TOPICS and ADDITIONAL RESOURCES

IN TEXT

 CD COMPANION

Critical Thinking Exercise—Imitative Play
Case Study—Sleep Problems
NCLEX-Style Review Questions

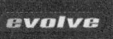 WEBSITE

WebLinks
NCLEX-Style Review Questions

WONG'S CLINICAL MANUAL OF PEDIATRIC NURSING, 6/E

Guidelines for helping parents deal with sleep problems

For additional information, please view "Growth and Development" in *Whaley and Wong's Pediatric Nursing Video Series,* St Louis, 1996, Mosby; (800) 426-4545; website: www.elsevierhealth.com.

PROMOTING OPTIMAL GROWTH AND DEVELOPMENT

The combined biologic, psychosocial, cognitive, spiritual, and social achievements during the *preschool period* (3 to 5 years of age) prepare preschoolers for their most significant change in lifestyle—entrance into school. Their control of bodily functions, experience of brief and prolonged periods of separation, ability to interact cooperatively with other children and adults, use of language for mental symbolization, and increased attention span and memory ready them for the next major period—the school years. Successful achievement of previous levels of growth and development is essential for preschoolers to refine many of the tasks that were mastered during the toddler years.

BIOLOGIC DEVELOPMENT

The rate of physical growth slows and stabilizes during the preschool years. The average *weight* is 14.6 kg (32 pounds) at 3 years, 16.7 kg (36.75 pounds) at 4 years, and 18.7 kg (41.25 pounds) at 5 years. The average weight gain per year remains approximately 2.3 kg (5 pounds).

Growth in *height* also remains steady at a yearly increase of 6.75 to 7.5 cm (2.5 to 3 inches) and generally occurs in elongation of the legs rather than of the trunk. The average height is 95 cm (37.25 inches) at 3 years, 103 cm (40.5 inches) at 4 years, and 110 cm (43.25 inches) at 5 years.

Physical proportions no longer resemble those of the squat, potbellied toddler. The preschooler is slender but sturdy, graceful, agile, and posturally erect. There is little difference in physical characteristics according to gender, except as dictated by such factors as dress and hairstyle.

Most organ systems can adjust to moderate stress and change. During this period most children are toilet trained. For the most part, motor development consists of increases in strength and refinement of previously learned skills, such as walking, running, and jumping. However, muscle development and bone growth are still far from mature. Excessive activity and overexertion can injure delicate tissues. Good posture, appropriate exercise, and adequate nutrition and rest are essential for optimal development of the musculoskeletal system.

Gross and Fine Motor Behavior

Walking, running, climbing, and jumping are well established by age 36 months. Refinement in eye-hand and muscle coordination is evident in several areas. At age 3 the preschooler rides a tricycle, walks on tiptoe, balances on one foot for a few seconds, and broad jumps. By age 4 the child skips and hops proficiently on one foot (Fig. 13-1) and catches a ball reliably. By age 5 the child skips on alternate feet, jumps rope, and begins to skate and swim.

Fine motor development is evident in the child's increasingly skillful manipulation, such as in drawing and dressing. These skills provide readiness for learning and independence for entry into school.

PSYCHOSOCIAL DEVELOPMENT
Developing a Sense of Initiative (Erikson)

After preschoolers have mastered the tasks of the toddler period, they are ready to face the developmental endeavors of the preschool period. Erikson asserts that the chief psy-

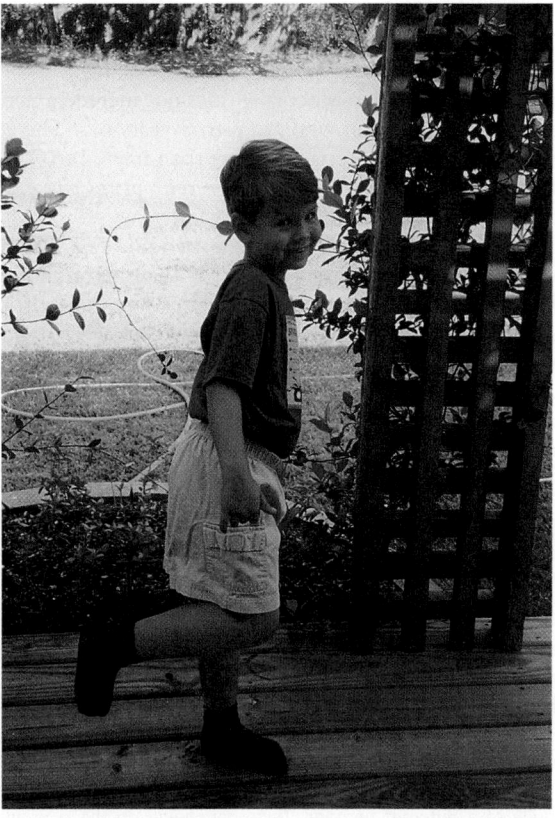

FIG. 13-1 ■ A 4-year-old child has sufficient balance to walk or hop on one foot.

chosocial task of this period is acquiring a sense of *initiative.* Children are in a stage of energetic learning. They play, work, and live to the fullest and feel a real sense of accomplishment and satisfaction in their activities. Conflict arises when children overstep the limits of their ability and inquiry and experience a sense of *guilt* for not having behaved appropriately. Feelings of guilt, anxiety, and fear may also result from thoughts that differ from expected behavior.

A particularly stressful thought is wishing one's parent dead. As a sense of rivalry or competition develops between the child and same-sex parent, the child may think of ways to get rid of the interfering parent. In most situations this rivalry is resolved by strongly identifying with the same-sex parent and peers during the school years. However, if that parent dies before the identification process is completed, the preschooler can be overwhelmed with feelings of guilt for having wished and therefore "caused" the death. Clarifying for children that wishes cannot and do not make events occur is essential in helping them overcome their guilt and anxiety.

Development of the *superego,* or *conscience,* has its beginnings toward the end of the toddler years and is a major task for preschoolers (see Cultural Awareness box). Learning right from wrong and good from bad is the beginning of morality (see Moral Development).

COGNITIVE DEVELOPMENT

One of the tasks related to the preschool period is readiness for school and scholastic learning. Many of the thought processes of this period are crucial for achieving such readiness, and it is intentional that the child begins school between ages 5 and 6 rather than at an earlier age.

Preoperational Phase (Piaget)

Piaget's cognitive theory actually does not include a period specifically for children who are 3 to 5 years old. The *preoperational phase* comprises the age span from 2 to 7 years and is divided into two stages: the *preconceptual phase,* ages 2 to 4, and the phase of *intuitive thought,* ages 4 to 7. One of the main transitions during these two phases is the shift from totally egocentric thought to social awareness and the ability to consider other viewpoints. However, egocentricity is still evident. (For a review of the characteristics of preoperational thought, see Chapter 12.)

Language continues to develop during the preschool period. Speech remains primarily a vehicle of egocentric communication. Preschoolers assume that everyone thinks

as they do and that a brief explanation of their thinking makes the entire thought understood by others. Because of this self-referenced, egocentric verbal communication, it is frequently necessary to explore and understand the young child's thinking through other nonverbal approaches. For children in this age-group, the most enlightening and effective method is *play,* which becomes the child's way of understanding, adjusting to, and working out life's experiences.

Preschoolers increasingly use language without comprehending the meaning of words, particularly concepts of right and left, causality, and time. Children may use the concepts correctly but only in the circumstances in which they have learned them. For example, they may know how to put on shoes by remembering that the buckle is always on the outside of the foot. However, if different shoes have no buckles, they cannot reason which shoe fits which foot. In other words, they do not understand the concept of *right and left.*

Superficially, *causality* resembles logical thought. Preschoolers explain a concept as they heard it described by others, but their understanding is limited. An example is the concept of time. Because *time* is still incompletely understood, the child interprets it according to his or her own frame of reference, such as "A long time means until Christmas." Consequently, time is best explained in relationship to an event, such as "Your mother will visit you after you finish your lunch." Avoiding words such as "yesterday," "tomorrow," "next week," or "Tuesday" to express when an event is expected to occur and associating time with usual expected daily occurrences help children learn about temporal relationships while increasing their trust in others' predictions.

Preschoolers' thinking is often described as *magical thinking.* Because of their egocentrism and transductive reasoning, they believe that thoughts are all-powerful. Such thinking places them in the vulnerable position of feeling guilty and responsible for bad thoughts, which may coincide with the occurrence of a wished event. Their inability to logically reason the cause and effect of illness or an injury makes it especially difficult for them to understand such events.

> **! NURSING ALERT**
>
> Counseling children whose parents are going through a divorce or separation should involve a discussion with the child about her or his role—because of magical thinking, the child may believe he or she wished the other parent away. The child should be reassured that this is not the case.

Preschoolers believe in the power of words and accept their meaning literally. An example of this type of thinking is calling children "bad" because they did something wrong. In the preschooler's mind calling them bad means they are a bad person; thus it is better to say that their actions were bad rather than call them bad so this does not become ingrained into their sense of self-worth.

MORAL DEVELOPMENT
Preconventional or Premoral Level (Kohlberg)

Young children's development of moral judgment is at the most basic level. There is little, if any, concern for why something is wrong. They behave because of the freedom

---

CULTURAL AWARENESS

Learning Sociocultural Mores

Developing a conscience implies learning the sociocultural mores of the family's heritage. Depending on the type of attitudes conveyed, children will learn not only appropriate behaviors, but also tolerant, biased, or prejudicial values concerning their ethnic, religious, and social background and those of other groups. Much of this influence may remain dormant until they associate with children or adults of a different heritage. Then, depending on the particular group, they may be accepted or ostracized for their attitudes.

or restriction that is placed on actions. In the *punishment and obedience orientation,* children (ages about 2 to 4 years) judge whether an action is good or bad depending on whether it results in reward or punishment. If children are punished for it, the action is bad. If they are not punished, the action is good, regardless of the meaning of the act. For example, if parents allow hitting, the child will perceive that hitting is good because it is not associated with punishment.

From approximately 4 to 7 years of age children are in the stage of *naive instrumental orientation,* in which actions are directed toward satisfying their needs and less frequently the needs of others. They have a very concrete sense of justice. Reciprocity or fairness involves the philosophy of "You scratch my back, and I'll scratch yours," with no thought of loyalty or gratitude (Thomas, 1996).

SPIRITUAL DEVELOPMENT

Children's knowledge of faith and religion is learned from significant others in their environment, usually from the parents' religious practices (Kenny, 1999). However, young children's understanding of spirituality is influenced by their cognitive level. Preschoolers have a concrete concept of a God with physical characteristics, who is often like an imaginary friend. They understand simple Bible stories and memorize short prayers, but their understanding of the meaning of these rituals is limited. Preschoolers benefit from concrete representations of religious practices, such as picture Bible books, and small statues, such as those of the Nativity scene. They will imitate the religious practices of their parents without fully understanding the significance of these acts.

Development of the conscience is strongly linked to spiritual development. At this age children are learning right from wrong and behaving correctly to avoid punishment. Wrongdoing provokes feelings of guilt, and preschoolers often misinterpret illness as a punishment for real or imagined transgressions. When children feel an overwhelming sense of guilt about their wrongdoings it affects their concept of who they are in relation to God; if they perceive themselves as being unloved and unaccepted by parents or their environment, they in turn will not be able to perceive God as a loving God (Steen and Anderson, 1995), but rather as a strict disciplinarian. Thus it is important that parents discipline the child consistently yet demonstrate unconditional love to help the preschooler lay a healthy foundation for faith and spirituality. It is important that children view God as one who bestows unconditional love, rather than as a judge of good or bad behavior. Praying to God and observing religious traditions (e.g., prayers before meals or bedtime) can help children through stressful periods, such as hospitalization. In many religious faiths, cultural practices and religion are closely intertwined (McEvoy, 2003) and are an important part of the child and family's life. (See Community Focus box.)

DEVELOPMENT OF BODY IMAGE

The preschool years play a significant role in the development of body image. With increasing comprehension of language, preschoolers recognize that individuals have undesirable and desirable appearances. They recognize differences in skin color and racial identity and are vulnerable to learning prejudices and biases. They are aware of the meaning of words such as "pretty" or "ugly," and they reflect the opinions of others regarding their own appearance. By 5 years of age children compare their size with their peers' and can become conscious of being large or short, especially if others refer to them as "so big" or "so little" for their age. In one study, negative associations between weight status and self-concept were identified in girls as young as 5 years (Davison and Birch, 2001).

Despite the advances in body-image development, preschoolers have poorly defined body boundaries and little knowledge of their internal anatomy. Intrusive experiences are frightening, especially those that disrupt the integrity of the skin, such as injections and surgery. There is a fear that if the skin is "broken," all of their blood and "insides" can leak out. Therefore bandages are critical to "keeping everything from coming out."

DEVELOPMENT OF SEXUALITY

Sexual development during these years is a very important phase to a person's overall sexual identity and beliefs. Preschoolers are forming strong attachments to the opposite-sex parent while identifying with the same-sex parent. Sex-typing, or the process by which an individual develops the behavior, personality, attitudes, and beliefs appropriate for his or her culture and sex, occurs through several mechanisms during this period. Probably the most powerful mechanisms are childrearing practices and imitations. Studies increasingly demonstrate that gender identification is a result of complex prenatal and postnatal psychologic factors, as well as biologic or genetic factors, and that most children are aware of their gender and the expected sets of related behaviors by 1.5 to 2.5 years of age.

As sexual identity is developing beyond gender recognition, modesty may become a concern, as well as fears of mutilation. There is sex-role imitation, and "dressing up like Mommy (or Daddy)" is an important activity. Attitudes and responses of others to role-playing can condition the child to views of self or others. For example, comments such as "Boys shouldn't play with dolls" can influence a boy's self-concept of masculinity (Finan, 1997).

Sexual exploration may be more pronounced now than ever before, particularly in terms of exploring and manipu-

COMMUNITY FOCUS

Spiritual Assessment

The mnemonic B-E-L-I-E-F was developed by McEvoy (2000) for pediatric nurses to initiate discussions with parents and children about their faith or religious values and beliefs. The components of the assessment tool are:

Belief system
Ethics or values
Lifestyle
Involvement in a spiritual community (church, synagogue, mosque)
Education
Future events

The tool may be used to develop a culturally sensitive dialog regarding spiritual matters and practices that affect the child and family.

lating the genitals. Questions about sexual reproduction may come to the forefront in the preschooler's search for understanding (see Sex Education, p. 423 and in Chapters 15 and 16).

SOCIAL DEVELOPMENT

During the preschool period the *individuation-separation process* is completed. Preschoolers have overcome much of the anxiety associated with strangers and the fear of separation of earlier years. They relate to unfamiliar people easily and tolerate brief separations from parents with little or no protest. However, they still need parental security, reassurance, guidance, and approval, especially when entering preschool or elementary school. Prolonged separation, such as that imposed by illness and hospitalization, is difficult, but preschoolers respond very well to anticipatory preparation and concrete explanation. They can cope with changes in daily routine much better than can toddlers; however, they may develop more imaginary fears. Preschoolers gain security and comfort from familiar objects, such as toys, dolls, or photographs of family members. They are able to work through many of their unresolved fears, fantasies, and anxieties through play, especially if guided with appropriate play objects (e.g., dolls, puppets) that represent family members, medical and nursing staff, and other children.

Language

During the preschool years language becomes more sophisticated and complex. Both cognitive ability and environment—particularly, consistent role models—influence vocabulary, speech, and comprehension (Huttenlocher, 1998). Language becomes a major mode of communication and social interaction, and its development during the preschool period sets the stage for later success in school (Needlman, 2004) (see Fig. 13-2). Vocabulary increases dramatically, from 300 words at age 2 to more than 2100 words at the end of 5 years. Sentence structure, grammatical usage, and intelligibility also advance to a more adult level. Through language preschool children learn to express feelings of frustration or anger without acting them out.

Children between the ages of 3 and 4 form sentences of about three to four words and include only the most essential words to convey a meaning. Such speech is often termed *telegraphic* for its brevity in length. Three-year-old children ask many questions and use plurals, correct pronouns, and the past tense of verbs. They name familiar objects, such as animals, parts of the body, relatives, and friends. They can give and follow simple commands. They talk incessantly, regardless of whether anyone is listening or answering them. They enjoy musical or talking toys or dolls and imitate new words proficiently.

From ages 4 to 5 years preschoolers use longer sentences of four to five words and use more words to convey a message, such as prepositions, adjectives, and a variety of verbs. They follow simple directional commands, such as "Put the ball on the chair," but can carry out only one request at a time. They answer questions such as "What do you do when you are hungry?" by describing the appropriate action. The pattern of asking questions is at its peak, and children usually repeat the question until they receive an answer.

By the end of age 5 years children can use all parts of speech correctly, except for deviations from the rule. They can define simple things by describing their use, shape, or general category of classification, rather than simply describing their outward appearance. For example, they define a ball as "round," "something you bounce," or "a toy," rather than by its color. They can give some opposites, such as "If Mommy is a woman, Daddy is a man." By the time they are 6 years old, they can describe an object according to its composition, such as "A spoon is made of metal."

Personal-Social Behavior

The pervasive ritualism and negativism of toddlerhood gradually diminish during the preschool years. Although self-assertion is still a major theme, preschoolers demonstrate their sense of autonomy differently. They are able to verbalize their request for independence and perform independently because of their much-refined physical and cognitive development. By 4 or 5 years of age they need little if any assistance with dressing, eating, or toileting (Fig. 13-3). They can also be trusted to obey warnings of danger, although 3- or 4-year-old children may exceed their boundaries at times.

They are also much more sociable and willing to please. They have internalized many of the standards and values of the family and culture. However, by the end of early childhood they begin to question parental values and compare them with those of their peer group and other authority figures; as a result, they may be less willing to abide by the family's code of conduct. Preschoolers become increasingly aware of their position and role within the family. Although this is a more secure age for experiencing the addition of another sibling, relinquishing the position of first or youngest is still difficult and requires appropriate preparation (see Sibling Rivalry, Chapter 12).

Play

Various types of play are typical of this period, but preschoolers especially enjoy *associative play*—group play in similar or identical activities but without rigid organization or rules. Play should provide for physical, social, and mental development.

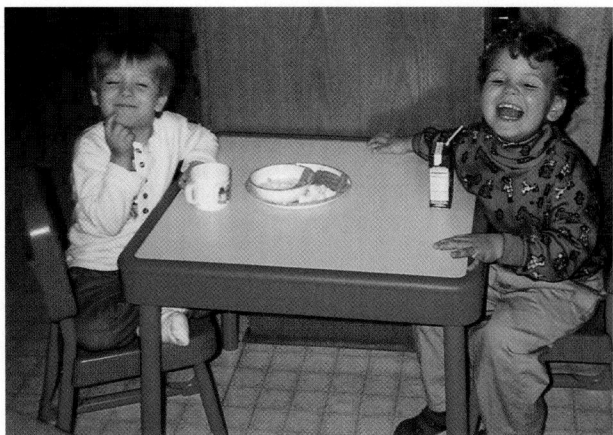

FIG. 13-2 ■ Preschool children enjoy friends and often use nonverbal messages to communicate.

Play activities for physical growth and refinement of motor skills include jumping, running, and climbing. Tricycles, scooter trucks, wagons, gym and sports equipment, sandboxes, wading pools, and winter sleds can help develop muscles and coordination. Activities such as swimming and skating teach safety as well as muscle development and coordination. Children involved in the work of play do not require expensive toys and gadgets to keep them entertained but often find common household items such as a broom handle or even items adults consider junk (sticks, rocks, dirt, and sand) to play with. The imaginative mind of the preschooler enjoys playing for play's sake.

Manipulative, constructive, creative, and educational toys provide for quiet activities, fine motor development, and self-expression. Easy construction sets, large blocks of various sizes and shapes, a counting frame, alphabet or number flash cards, paints, crayons, simple carpentry tools, musical toys, illustrated books, simple sewing or handicraft sets, large puzzles, and clay are suitable toys (see Fig. 13-4). Electronic games and computer programs are especially valuable in helping children learn basic skills, such as letters and simple words.

Probably the most characteristic and pervasive preschool activity is *imitative, imaginative,* and *dramatic play.* Dress-up clothes, dolls, housekeeping toys, dollhouses, play-store toys, telephones, farm animals and equipment, village sets, trains, trucks, cars, planes, hand puppets, and doctor and nurse kits provide hours of self-expression (Fig. 13-5). Probably at no other time is the reproduction of adult behavior so faithful and absorbing as in 4- and 5-year-old children. During this time gender stereotyping is also part of the child's development; the notion that men can become nurses, women can become doctors, and so on, becomes ingrained in the child's set of life expectations, especially if they are reinforced by the parents or significant-other adults. Toward the end of the preschool period, children are less satisfied with make-believe or pretend objects and enjoy actually doing the activity, such as cooking and carpentry.

Television and videotapes also have their places in children's play, although each should be only one part of children's total repertoire of social and recreational activities. Parents and other caregivers should supervise selection of programs, preview programs for appropriateness, and sched-

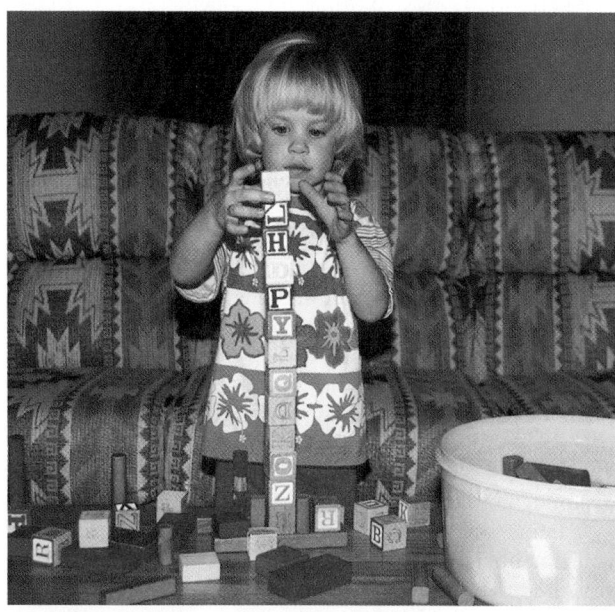

FIG. 13-4 ■ Preschoolers enjoy a sense of accomplishment from activities such as building blocks.

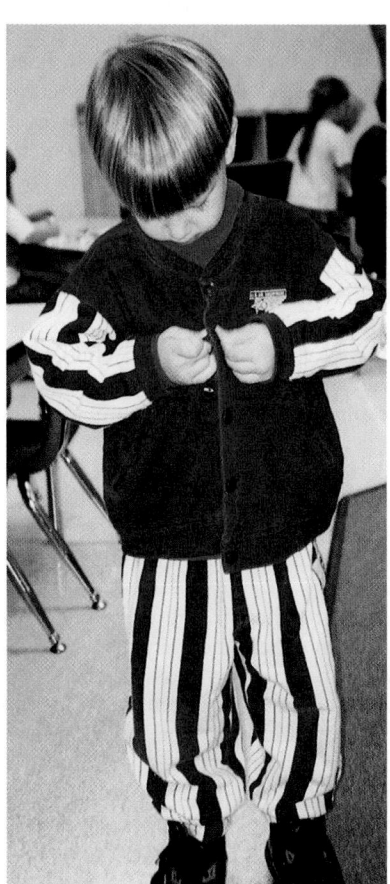

FIG. 13-3 ■ Most preschoolers are able to dress themselves but need help with more difficult items of clothing.

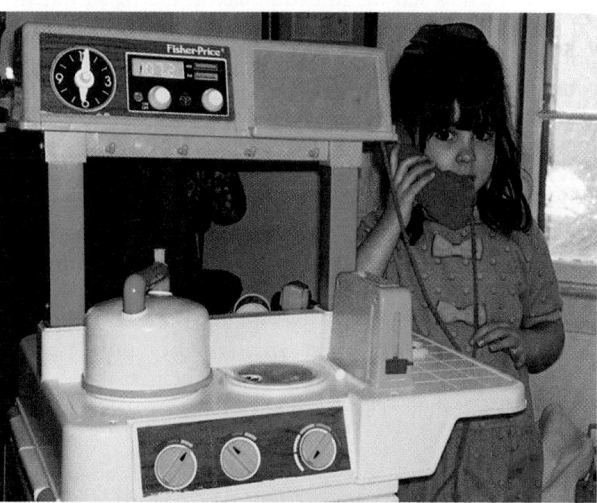

FIG. 13-5 ■ Imaginative and dramatic play is typical of preschoolers, who enjoy fantasy.

ule hours for television viewing (Vessey, Yim-Chiplis, and MacKenzie, 1998). Children also enjoy and learn from educational programs; television can become an interactive activity when adults view programs with children and discuss program content. (See discussion on television, including Parent Guidelines, in Chapter 5.) In one study, viewing educational programs as preschoolers was associated with higher grades, reading more books, greater emphasis on achievement, increased creativity, and less aggression in adolescent years (Anderson and others, 2001). The researchers emphasize that the quality of television viewing appeared more important than the amount viewed.

Play is so much a part of the young child's life that reality and fantasy become blurred. The make-believe is reality during play and only becomes fantasy when the toys are put away or the dress-up clothes are removed. It is no wonder that *imaginary playmates* are so much a part of this age period.

The appearance of imaginary companions usually occurs between the ages of 2.5 and 3 years, and for the most part such playmates are relinquished when the child enters school. There seems to be a relationship between the level of intelligence and the presence of the imaginary companion. More intelligent children tend to have more vivid and complex pretend playmates.

Imaginary companions serve many purposes: they become friends in times of loneliness, they accomplish what the child is still attempting, and they experience what the child wants to forget or remember. It is not unusual for the "friend" to have a myriad of vices and to be blamed for wrongdoing. Sometimes the child hopes to escape punishment by saying, "My friend George broke the glass." At other times the child may fantasize that the companion misbehaved and play the role of parent. This becomes a way of assuming control and authority in a safe situation.

Parents often worry about the imaginary playmates, not realizing how normal and useful they are. Parents need to be reassured that children's fantasy is a sign of health that helps them differentiate between make-believe and reality. Parents can acknowledge the presence of the imaginary companion by calling him or her by name and even agreeing to simple requests such as setting an extra place at the table, but they should not allow the child to use the playmate to avoid punishment or responsibility. For example, if the child blames the companion for messing up a room, parents need to state clearly that the child is the only one they see and therefore the child is responsible for cleaning up.

Children also benefit from play that occurs between them and a parent. *Mutual play* fosters development from birth through the school years and provides enriched opportunities for learning. Through mutual play parents can provide tactile and kinesthetic experiences, can maximize verbal and language abilities, and can offer praise and encouragement for exploration of the world. In addition, mutual play encourages positive interactions between the parent and child, strengthening their relationship (Gottesman, 1999).*

---

*Recommended books for suggestions on mutual play include *Quick and Fun Learning Activities* books, by Teacher Created Material, Inc., 6421 Industry Way, Westminster, CA 92683; (714) 891-7895 or (800) 858-7339; website: www.teachercreated.com.

Table 13-1 summarizes the major developmental achievements for children 3, 4, and 5 years old.

COPING WITH CONCERNS RELATED TO NORMAL GROWTH AND DEVELOPMENT
Preschool and Kindergarten Experience

Some children are home-schooled, but many children attend some type of early childhood program, usually preschool or a day care center. Group care has become commonplace with the large number of mothers presently employed outside the home (see Alternate Childcare Arrangements, Chapter 10). The effects of early education and stimulation on children have increasingly gained recognition and importance. (For a discussion of the effects of day care on young children, see Working Mothers, Chapter 3.) Because social development widens to include age-mates and other significant adults, preschool provides an excellent vehicle for expanding children's experiences with others. It also is an excellent preparation for entrance into elementary school.

In preschool or day care centers children are exposed to opportunities for learning group cooperation, adjusting to various sociocultural differences, and coping with frustration, dissatisfaction, and anger. If activities are tailored to provide mastery and achievement, children increasingly have feelings of success, self-confidence, and personal competence. Whether or not structured learning is imposed is less important than the social climate, type of guidance, and attitude toward the children that is fostered by the teacher or leader. With a teacher who is aware of preschoolers' developmental abilities and needs, children will learn from the activity that is provided. Most programs incorporate a daily schedule of quiet play, active outdoor activity, group activities such as games and projects, creative or free play, and snack and rest periods. Preschool is particularly beneficial for children who lack a peer-group experience, such as an only child, and for children from impoverished homes. It also is an excellent preparation for kindergarten.

One of the issues that parents face is the child's readiness for preschool or kindergarten. There are no absolute indicators for school readiness, but the child's social maturation, especially attention span, is as important as his or her academic readiness. Using a developmental screening tool that addresses cognitive (especially language), social, and physical milestones can identify children who may benefit from diagnostic testing. Developmental screening focuses on the potential to learn and differs from readiness testing, which stresses the specific skills the child has acquired (Glascoe, 2001).

Nurses and other health care workers can be helpful in guiding parents in selecting enriched social and educational early intervention programs and schools. Careful selection of early childhood education is intrinsic to future learning and development. Licensed and regulated programs are mandated to abide by established standards, which represent minimum requirements and safeguards. The importance of regulation is to protect children from harm and to promote the conditions essential for a child's healthy development and learning, and to provide a variety of firsthand experiences and learning activities either directly to children or through parent participation (National Association for the Education of Young Children, 1995). The National Association for the Education of Young Children serves as the model for optimal care of small children.*

Areas for parents to evaluate include the facility's daily program, teacher qualifications, staff-to-student ratio, discipline policy, environmental safety precautions, provision of meals, sanitary conditions, adequate indoor/outdoor space per child, and fee schedule. References from other parents help evaluate a facility, but personal observation of the facility is recommended. Encourage parents to meet the director and some of the employees at a few facilities to make an informed choice.

Important in selecting childcare centers is an evaluation of the facility's health practices. Substantial evidence shows that children in day care centers, especially those younger than 3 years of age, have more illnesses, especially diarrhea, hepatitis A, meningitis, otitis media, respiratory tract infections, and cytomegalovirus than children not in day care centers (Rovers and others, 1999).

Nurses play an important role in infection control. Not only can they advise parents regarding the evaluation of a facility's sanitary practices, but they can also take an active part in educating staff in measures to minimize transmission of infection (Lafontaine and Bedard, 1997). For example, in centers caring for children who are not toilet trained, reducing environmental contamination with urine and feces is an important infection control issue (Fig. 13-6).

Children need preparation for the preschool or kindergarten experience.† For young children it represents a change from their usual home environment and prolonged separation from parents.

Before the child begins the school experience, the parents should present the idea as exciting and pleasurable. Talking to the child about activities such as painting, building with blocks, or enjoying swings and other outdoor equipment allows the child to fantasize about the forthcoming event in a positive manner. When the first day of school arrives, the parents should behave confidently. Such behavior requires parents to have resolved their own feelings regarding the experience.

Parents should introduce their child to the teacher and the facility. In some instances it is helpful to remain for at least some part of the first day until the child is comfortable and at ease. Other specific actions that can help lessen separation anxiety include providing the school with detailed information about the child's home environment, such as familiar routines, favorite activities, food preferences, names of siblings or pets, and personal habits. Such information helps the child feel familiar in the strange surroundings. When schools automatically request this information, the parent has a valuable clue to evaluating the quality of the

program, because the request represents the staff's awareness of each child's needs. Transitional objects, such as a favorite toy, may also help the child bridge the gap from home to school.

Sex Education

Preschoolers have experienced a tremendous amount of information during their short lifetimes. Although their thinking may not be mature, they search constantly for explanations and reasons that are logical and reasonable to them. The word "why" seems to supplant the word "no," which was common in toddlerhood. It is only natural that as they learn about "me," they will also want to know "why me" and "how me." Questions such as "Where do babies come from?" are as casual as "What makes it rain?" or "Who is that?" It is the *way* in which questions about procreation are answered that conditions children, even the youngest, to separate these questions from others about their world.

Two rules govern answering sensitive questions about topics such as sex. The first is to *find out what children know and think.* By investigating the theories children have produced as a reasonable explanation, parents can not only give correct information, but also help children understand why their explanation is inaccurate. Another reason for ascertaining what the child thinks before offering any information is that the "unasked for" answer may be given. For example, 4-year-old Sally asked her father, "Where did I come from?" Both parents quickly took this inquiry as a clue for offering sex education. After the explanation, Sally exclaimed, "I don't know about all that! All I know is Mary came from New York and I want to know where I was born."

The second rule for giving information is to *be honest.* It is true that much of the correct information will be forgotten or misunderstood by the preschooler, but what is more important is that the correct information can be restated until the child absorbs and comprehends the facts. Even though the correct anatomic words may be hard to pronounce or even more difficult to remember, they become foundational content for explaining other concepts later on.

Honesty does not imply imparting to children every fact of life or allowing excessive permissiveness in sexual curiosity. When children ask one question, they are looking for one

---

*Information about the accreditation criteria and procedures of the National Academy of Early Childhood Programs is available from the **National Association for the Education of Young Children,** 1509 16th Street NW, Washington, DC 20036; (202) 232-8777 or (800) 424-2460; www.naeyc.org. These criteria are excellent guidelines for evaluating preschools or day care centers.

†Recommended books for preparing young children for day care or school include *Going to Day Care* (1985) and *When Your Child Goes to School* by Fred Rogers (out of print) (GP Putnam's Sons).

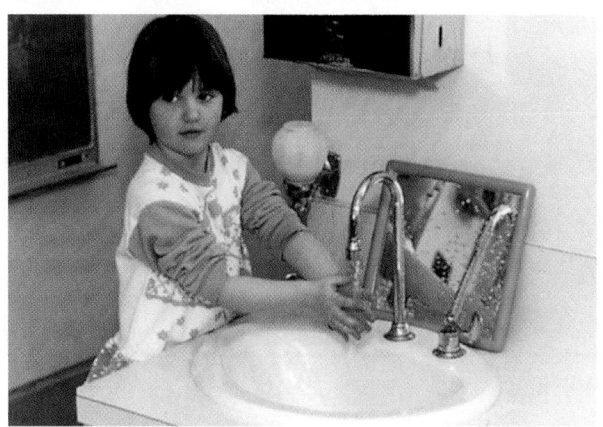

FIG. 13-6 ■ Thorough handwashing is the single most effective method of preventing infection.

TABLE 13-1 ■ **Growth and Development During Preschool Years**

AGE (YEARS)	PHYSICAL	GROSS MOTOR	FINE MOTOR	LANGUAGE
3	Usual weight gain of 1.8-2.7 kg (4-6 pounds) Average weight of 14.6 kg (32 pounds) Usual gain in height of 7.5 cm (3 inches) per year Average height of 95 cm (37.5 inches) May have achieved night-time control of bowel and bladder	Rides tricycle Jumps off bottom step Stands on one foot for a few seconds Goes up stairs using alternate feet; may still come down using both feet on step Broad jumps May try to dance, but balance may not be adequate	Builds tower of 9 or 10 cubes Builds bridge with three cubes Adeptly places small pellets in narrow-necked bottle In drawing, copies a circle, imitates a cross, names what has been drawn, cannot draw stick figure but may make circle with facial features	Has vocabulary of about 900 words Uses primarily "telegraphic" speech Uses complete sentences of three or four words Talks incessantly regardless of whether anyone is paying attention Repeats sentence of six syllables Asks many questions
4	Pulse and respiration rates decrease slightly Growth rate is similar to that of previous year Average weight of 16.7 kg (36.75 pounds) Average height of 103 cm (40.5 inches) Length at birth is doubled Maximum potential for development of amblyopia	Skips and hops on one foot Catches ball reliably Throws ball overhead Walks down stairs using alternate footing	Uses scissors successfully to cut out picture following outline Can lace shoes but may not be able to tie bow In drawing, copies a square, traces a cross and diamond, adds three parts to stick figure	Has vocabulary of 1500 words or more Uses sentences of four or five words Questioning is at peak Tells exaggerated stories Knows simple songs May be mildly profane if associates with older children Obeys four prepositional phrases, such as "under," "on top of," "beside," "in back of," or "in front of" Names one or more colors Comprehends analogies, such as, "If ice is cold, fire is ____"
5	Pulse and respiration rates decrease slightly Average weight of 18.7 kg (41.5 pounds) Average height of 110 cm (43.25 inches) Eruption of permanent dentition may begin Handedness is established (about 90% are right-handed)	Skips and hops on alternate feet Throws and catches ball well Jumps rope Skates with good balance Walks backward with heel to toe Jumps from height of 12 inches and lands on toes Balances on alternate feet with eyes closed	Ties shoelaces Uses scissors, simple tools, or pencil very well In drawing, copies a diamond and triangle; adds seven to nine parts to stick figure; prints a few letters, numbers, or words, such as first name	Has vocabulary of about 2100 words Uses sentences of six to eight words, with all parts of speech Names coins (e.g., nickel, dime) Names four or more colors Describes drawing or pictures with much comment and enumeration Knows names of days of week, months, and other time-associated words Knows composition of articles, such as "A shoe is made of ____" Can follow three commands in succession

SOCIALIZATION	COGNITION	FAMILY RELATIONSHIPS
Dresses self almost completely if helped with back buttons and told which shoe is right or left Pulls on shoes Has increased attention span Feeds self completely Can prepare simple meals, such as cold cereal and milk Can help to set table; can dry dishes without breaking any May have fears, especially of dark and going to bed Knows own gender and gender of others Play is parallel and associative; begins to learn simple games, but often follows own rules; begins to share	Is in preconceptual phase Is egocentric in thought and behavior Has beginning understanding of time; uses many time-oriented expressions, talks about past and future as much as about present, pretends to tell time Has improved concept of space, as demonstrated by understanding of prepositions and ability to follow directional command Has beginning ability to view concepts from another perspective	Attempts to please parents and conform to their expectations Is less jealous of younger sibling; may be opportune time for birth of additional sibling Is aware of family relationships and sex-role functions Boys tend to identify more with father or other male figure Has increased ability to separate easily and comfortably from parents for short periods
Very independent Tends to be selfish and impatient Aggressive physically as well as verbally Takes pride in accomplishments Has mood swings Shows off dramatically, enjoys entertaining others Tells family tales to others with no restraint Still has many fears Play is associative Imaginary playmates are common Uses dramatic, imaginative, and imitative devices Sexual exploration and curiosity demonstrated through play, such as being "doctor" or "nurse"	Is in phase of intuitive thought Causality is still related to proximity of events Understands time better, especially in terms of sequence of daily events Unable to conserve matter Judges everything according to one dimension, such as height, width, or order Immediate perceptual clues dominate judgment Is beginning to develop less egocentrism and more social awareness May count correctly but has poor mathematic concept of numbers Obeys because parents have set limits, not because of understanding of right or wrong	Rebels if parents expect too much, such as impeccable table manners Takes aggression and frustration out on parents or siblings Do's and don'ts become important May have rivalry with older or younger siblings; may resent older sibling's privileges and younger sibling's invasion of privacy and possessions May "run away" from home Identifies strongly with parent of opposite sex Is able to run simple errands outside the home
Less rebellious and quarrelsome than at age 4 years More settled and eager to get down to business Not as open and accessible in thoughts and behavior as in earlier years Independent but trustworthy, not foolhardy; more responsible Has fewer fears; relies on outer authority to control world Eager to do things right and to please; tries to "live by the rules" Has better manners Cares for self totally, occasionally needing supervision in dress or hygiene Not ready for concentrated close work or small print because of slight farsightedness and still unrefined eye-hand coordination Play is associative; tries to follow rules but may cheat to avoid losing	Begins to question what parents think by comparing them with age-mates and other adults May notice prejudice and bias in outside world Is more able to view other's perspective, but tolerates differences rather than understanding them May begin to show understanding of conservation of numbers through counting objects regardless of arrangement Use time-oriented words with increased understanding Very cautious about factual information regarding world	Gets along well with parents May seek out parent more often than at age 4 years for reassurance and security, especially when entering school Begins to question parents' thinking and principles Strongly identifies with parent of same sex, especially boys with their fathers Enjoys activities such as sports, cooking, and shopping with parent of same sex

answer. When they are ready, they will ask about the other "unfinished" parts of the story. Sooner or later they will wonder how the "sperm meets the egg" and "how the baby gets out," but (during this period) it is best to wait until they ask.

Regardless of whether children are given sex education, they will engage in games of sexual curiosity and exploration. At about 3 years of age children are aware of the anatomic differences between the sexes and are very concerned with how the other "works." This is not really "sexual" curiosity, because many children are still unaware of the reproductive function of the genitals. Their curiosity is for the eliminative function of the anatomy. Little boys wonder how girls can urinate without a penis, so they watch girls go to the bathroom. Because they cannot see anything but the stream of water coming out, they want to observe further for what makes it come out. "Doctor play" is often a game invented for just such investigation. Little girls are no less curious about boys' anatomy. It is very intriguing to have a closer inspection of this "thing" that girls do not have.

One question that parents often have is how to handle such sexual curiosity. A positive approach is to neither condone nor condemn the sexual curiosity but to express that if children have questions, they should ask the parents; then the parents should encourage them to engage in some other activity. In this way children can be helped to understand that there are ways that their sexual curiosity can be satisfied other than through playing investigative games. This in no way condemns the act but stresses alternate methods to seek solutions and answers. Allowing children unrestricted permissiveness only intensifies their anxiety and concern, because exploring and searching usually yield little evidence to satisfy their curiosity.

Many excellent books on sex education are available for preschool children at public libraries, and the **Sexuality Information and Education Council of the United States (SIECUS),*** local chapters of the **Planned Parenthood Federation of America,†** and the **American Academy of Pediatrics‡** have bibliographies of suggested reading material. Parents should read the book themselves *before* giving or reading it to a child.

Another concern for some parents is *masturbation,* or self-stimulation of the genitals. This occurs at any age for a variety of reasons and, if not excessive, is normal and healthy. It is most common at 4 years of age and during adolescence. For preschoolers it is a part of sexual curiosity and exploration. If parents are concerned about masturbation in their children, it is essential for nurses to investigate the circumstances associated with the activity, because it may be an expression of anxiety, boredom, or unresolved conflicts. For example, a boy who repeatedly touches his penis is not masturbating for pleasure but may be reassuring himself that it is intact. Also, children who openly and publicly masturbate are inviting a reaction, such as discipline, punishment, or criticism. They may be overwhelmed by

their sexual feelings and will ask others to help them channel them into more constructive outlets. Because masturbation, as with other forms of sex play, is a private act, parents should emphasize this to children as part of teaching them socially acceptable behavior.

Fears

The greatest number and variety of real and imagined fears are present during the preschool years and include fear of the dark, being left alone (especially at bedtime), animals (particularly large dogs and snakes), ghosts, sexual matters (castration), and objects or persons associated with pain (Muris, Merckelbach, and Prins, 2000). The exact cause of children's fears is unknown. Parents often become perplexed about handling the fears because no amount of logical persuasion, coercion, or ridicule will send away the ghosts, boogeymen, monsters, and devils. Prolonged or inappropriate television viewing by preschoolers may increase fears and anxieties because of the inability to separate reality-based experiences from fantasy, which is often portrayed in television and video game media. Preschool boys are known to imitate and act out violent behavior viewed on television (Villani, 2001; Krug and Mikus, 1999). The preschooler who fears sitting on the toilet seat may relate to a television program wherein a toilet became a monster and swallowed a child. This, of course, is fantasy or *animism,* yet preschoolers may not be able to separate fantasy from reality or to adequately verbalize their fears. Fear of annihilation is very common in preschoolers. Their fear of losing body parts with certain medical procedures such as an intravenous insertion or cast application on a limb is a very real threat to their existence.

The best way to help children overcome their fears is by actively involving them in finding practical methods to deal with the frightening experience. This may be as simple as keeping a night-light on in the child's bedroom for assurance that no monsters lurk in the dark. Exposing children to the feared object in a safe situation also provides a type of conditioning, or *desensitization.* For instance, children who are afraid of dogs should never be forced to approach or touch one, but they may be gradually introduced to the experience by watching other children play with the animal. This type of modeling, demonstrating fearlessness in others, can be very effective if the child is allowed to progress at his or her own rate.

Usually by 5 or 6 years of age children relinquish these old fears. Explaining the developmental sequence of fears and their gradual disappearance may help parents feel more secure in handling preschoolers' fears. Sometimes fears do not subside with simple measures or developmental maturation. When children experience severe fears that disrupt family life, professional help is required.

Stress

Although for parents the preschool years generally are less troublesome than toddlerhood, this period of life presents children with many unique stresses. Some, such as fears, are innate and stem from preschoolers' unique understanding of the world. Others are imposed, such as beginning school. Although minimal amounts of stress are beneficial during the early years to help children develop effective coping

---

*130 West 42nd Street, Suite 350, New York, NY 10036; (212) 819-9770; website: www.siecus.org.

†National office: 434 West 33rd Street, New York, NY 10001; (212) 541-7800 or (800) 829-7732; website: www.plannedparenthood.org.

‡141 Northwest Point Boulevard., Elk Grove Village, IL 60007; (888) 227-1770; fax: (847) 228-1281; website: www.aap.org.

skills, excessive stress is harmful. Young children are especially vulnerable because of their limited capacity to cope. Expression of frustration, fear, or anxiety is further exacerbated by inadequate expressive language.

To help parents deal with stress in their child's life, they must be aware of signs of stress (see Stress in Childhood, Chapter 5) and be helped to identify the source. In addition, any number of other stresses may be present, such as the birth of a sibling, marital discord, divorce and separation, relocation, or illness.

The best approach to dealing with stress is prevention—monitoring the amount of stress in children's lives so that levels exceeding their coping ability do not occur. In many instances structuring children's schedules to allow rest and preparing them for change, such as entering school, are sufficient measures.

Aggression

The term *aggression* refers to behavior that attempts to hurt a person or destroy property. Aggression differs from anger, which is a temporary emotional state, but anger may be expressed through aggression. Aggression is influenced by a complex set of biologic, sociocultural, and familial variables. Factors that tend to increase aggressive behavior are gender, frustration, modeling, and reinforcement. Hyperaggressive behavior in preschoolers is characterized by unprovoked physical attacks on other children and adults, destruction of others' property, frequent intense temper tantrums, extreme impulsivity, disrespect, and noncompliance.

There is evidence that males are more overtly aggressive than females (Stormshak and others, 2000). *Frustration,* or the continual thwarting of self-satisfaction by disapproval, humiliation, punishment, or insults, can lead children to act out against others as a means of release. Especially if they fear parents, these children will displace their anger on others, particularly peers and other authority figures. This type of aggression often applies to the child who is well behaved at home but a discipline problem at school or a bully among playmates.

Modeling, or imitating the behavior of significant others, is a powerful influencing force in preschoolers. Children who see their parents as verbally or physically abusive are observing behavior that they come to know as acceptable (Hart and others, 1998). Another aspect of modeling is the "double standard" for acceptable conduct. For example, in some families, aggression is synonymous with masculinity, and boys are encouraged to defend themselves. Television is also a significant source for modeling at this age. Therefore, parents need encouragement to supervise television programs viewed by their preschool children. The American Academy of Pediatrics (2001a) offers a list of recommendations for healthy television viewing.

Reinforcement can also shape aggressive behavior. Sometimes the reward for aggression is negative (e.g., punishment), yet reinforcing because it brings attention. For example, children who are ignored by a parent until they hit a sibling or the parent learn that this act garners attention.

When extreme behaviors such as aggression are present in children, parents are concerned about the need for professional help. Generally the difference between "normal" and "problematic" behavior is not the behavior itself but its *quantity* (number of occurrences), *severity* (interference with social or cognitive functioning), *distribution* (different manifestations), *onset* (when behavior started), and *duration* (at least 4 weeks).*

Speech Problems

The most critical period for speech development occurs between 2 and 4 years of age. During this period children are using their rapidly growing vocabulary faster than they can produce the words. This failure to master sensorimotor integrations results in *stuttering* or *stammering* as children try to say the word they are already thinking about. This dysfluency in speech pattern is a *normal* characteristic of language development (Ambrose and Yairi, 1999) and usually resolves provided that caregivers speak clearly and do not complete the child's sentences and overcorrect mistakes. When parents or other significant persons place undue emphasis or stress on this pattern of dysfluency, an abnormal speech pattern may develop. The best therapy for speech problems is prevention and early detection. Common causes of speech problems are hearing loss, developmental delay, and a lack of verbal stimulation (American Academy of Pediatrics, 2003). Referral for further evaluation and treatment may be necessary to prevent a problem from interfering with learning. Anticipatory preparation of parents for expected developmental norms may allay caregiver concerns.

Children pressured into producing sounds ahead of their developmental level may develop *dyslalia* (articulation problems) or revert to using infantile speech. Prevention involves discussing with parents the usual achievement of speech production during childhood. The *Denver Articulation Screening Examination* is an excellent tool for assessing articulation skills in the child and for explaining to parents the expected progression of sounds (see Appendix C).

PROMOTING OPTIMAL HEALTH DURING THE PRESCHOOL YEARS†

NUTRITION

Nutritional requirements for preschoolers are fairly similar to those for toddlers. The requirement for calories per unit of body weight continues to decrease slightly to 90 kcal/kg, for an average daily intake of 1800 calories. Fluid requirements may also decrease slightly to about 100 mL/kg daily but depend on the activity level, climatic conditions, and state of health. The protein requirements are 1.2 g/kg, for an average daily consumption of 24 g. A diet that is moderately reduced in fat may be recommended for healthy preschool children. The American Academy of Pediatrics, Committee on Nutrition (1998) recommends that by 5 years of age saturated fatty acid consumption should be less than 10% of total caloric intake. There is increasing evidence that the incidence of coronary heart disease, obesity, and

---

*A helpful site for resources dealing with child behavior is Developmental-Behavioral Pediatrics Online Community website: www.dbpeds.org.

†For a more comprehensive understanding, the reader is urged to review the material presented in Chapter 12 under Promoting Optimal Health During Toddlerhood.

chronic health problems such as diabetes mellitus can be influenced by early eating patterns. Preschoolers may have a decreased fat intake with substitutes such as soy-enriched foods without affecting overall growth (Endres and others, 2003; Johnson, 2000). In a Healthy Start intervention study a group of preschool children consumed meals with 10% less saturated fat and maintained adequate total energy intake; interventions were aimed at counseling cooks in the Head Start Centers to prepare foods with less saturated fats (Williams and others, 2002). Parents and others who provide soy substitutes should ensure that the products are vitamin enriched and low in fat content because all soy products may not have a lower fat content and may be deficient in some nutrients (Endres and others, 2003). It is important that the diet contain adequate nutrients such as calcium. Milk and dairy products are excellent sources of calcium and vitamin D (fortified). Low-fat milk may be substituted so the quantity of milk may remain the same but fat intake limited overall.

In children older than 2 years of age, intake of fiber, fruits, and vegetables should equal the child's age plus 5 in grams/day. This translates into five servings of fruits and vegetables each day (Johnson, 2000). The amount of fruit juice intake should not exceed 6 ounces per day (approximately one serving) for children ages 1 to 6 (American Academy of Pediatrics, 2001b). Intake of carbonated beverages in young children is known to contribute large amounts of nonnutritive calories that may displace or preclude intake of nutrients necessary for growth. A high intake of soda at 5 years was associated with a significantly increased risk of dental caries in comparison with children with low or no soda intake (Marshall and others, 2003). In one study children at 5 years of age consumed more carbonated beverages and fruit drinks (non–100% fruit juice) than the recommended 4 to 6 oz/day of 100% fruit juice (Rampersaud, Bailey, and Kauwell, 2003). Parents should be educated regarding nonnutritious fruit drinks that usually contain less than 10% fruit juice yet are often advertised as healthy and nutritious; sugar content is increased dramatically and often precludes an adequate intake of milk by the child. Nutritious mid-morning and mid-afternoon snacks may be given to preschoolers without affecting their overall daily intake of protein and energy or mealtime intake (Wilson, 1999). The USDA (1999) Food Guide Pyramid for Young Children (see Fig. 11-1) is appropriate for preschoolers. The foods depicted are those commonly eaten by children in this age-group, and the illustrations emphasize the importance of physical activity. Parents and caregivers can provide opportunities for children to learn to like a variety of nutritious foods by exposing them to these foods. The importance of role modeling by parents cannot be overemphasized in regard to food intake and dietary habits; if the parent will not eat a particular food or if dietary habits are poor in the adults, children are likely to develop the same habits.

NURSING ALERT

Obesity has increased over the last two decades in young children. Efforts to provide a healthy diet and to encourage physical activity should begin early to help children achieve optimal health.

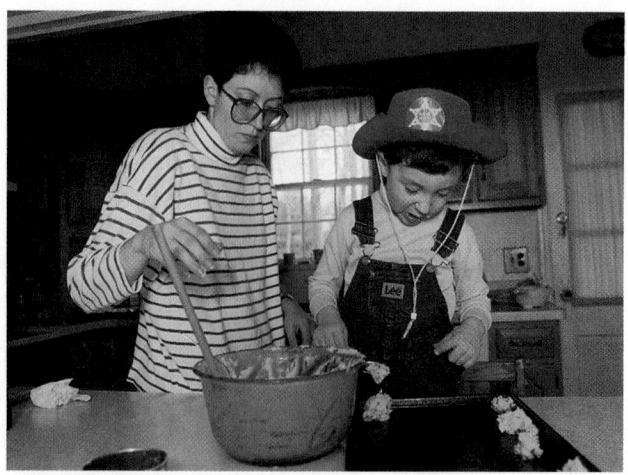

FIG. 13-7 ■ Preschool-age children enjoy helping adults and are more likely to try new foods if they can assist in the preparation.

Some preschoolers still have food habits that are typical of toddlers, such as food fads and strong taste preferences. When children reach 4 years of age, they seem to enter another period of finicky eating, which is generally characteristic of the more rebellious and rowdy behavior of children in this age-group. Just as with the toddler, small portions should be offered of each item being served. Large portions tend to overwhelm the child and lead to less intake. The practice of having the child remain at the table until the "plate is clean" should be avoided because this may contribute to overeating and the development of poor eating habits that may contribute to poor health later in life. By age 5 years children are more agreeable to trying new foods, especially if they are encouraged by an adult who allows them to help with food preparation or experiment with a new taste or different dish (Fig. 13-7). Mealtimes can become battlegrounds if parents expect perfect table manners.* Usually the 5-year-old child is ready for the "social" side of eating, but the 3- or 4-year-old child still has difficulty sitting quietly through a long family meal.

The amount and variety of foods consumed by young children vary greatly from day to day. Consequently, parents sometimes worry about the quantity of food preschoolers consume. In general, the quality is much more important than the quantity, a fact that should be stressed during nutritional counseling. Some evidence suggests that children self-regulate their caloric intake. If they eat less at one meal, they will compensate at another meal or will snack.

One approach toward lessening this parental concern is advising parents to keep a weekly record of everything the child eats. In particular, the need for measuring the amount of food, such as setting aside a half-cup of vegetables, and serving the child from this premeasured amount is stressed to provide a more accurate estimate of food intake at each meal. When parents look at the food chart at the end of the week, they are usually amazed at how much the child has consumed. In general, preschoolers consume only slightly more than toddlers, or about half an adult's portion.

---

*An excellent resource for parents related to meal times with toddlers and preschoolers is Satter E: *How to Get Your Child to Eat but Not Too Much,* Palo Alto, Calif, (1987, Bull Publishing); available at www.amazon.com.

SLEEP AND ACTIVITY

Sleep patterns vary widely, but the average preschooler sleeps about 12 hours a night and infrequently takes daytime naps. Waking during the night is common throughout early childhood and may be related to social rather than developmental factors (Thiedke, 2001). Motor activity levels continue to be high and allow preschoolers to explore their environment, begin learning physical games and sports, and interact with others. Sedentary activities, such as television, are increasingly appealing and can become an unhealthy substitute for active play.

Preschoolers' increased gross motor abilities and coordination provide them with the opportunity to engage in many physical activities, if only at a novice level. Whether young children should begin formalized training in an activity at this early age is controversial. Training programs must consider the child's physical and psychologic immaturity. Readiness to participate in organized sports should be determined individually. The decision should be based on the child's (not the parent's) motivation and enjoyment. The American Academy of Pediatrics (2000) encourages free play, a variety of physical activities, a noncompetitive atmosphere, and emphasis on fun and safety.

Sleep Problems

The preschool years are a prime time for sleep disturbances. As toddlers and preschoolers cope with autonomy, separation, and object permanence, they begin to have more sleep problems (Thiedke, 2001). Some have trouble going to sleep, especially after so much activity and stimulation during the day. Others may develop bedtime fears, wake during the night, or have nightmares or sleep terrors. Still others may prolong the inevitable through elaborate rituals.

Recommendations for handling a sleep disturbance are offered only *after* a thorough assessment of the problem has been completed. Cultural traditions may dictate sleep practices that are contrary to certain well-accepted professional recommendations; therefore, parents may not perceive a particular sleep practice as a problem (see Cultural Awareness box).

Interventions differ greatly; for example, **nightmares** (frightening dreams that are followed by full waking) and **sleep terrors** (partial arousal from deep, nondreaming sleep) require very different approaches (see Table 13-2).

For children who delay going to bed, a recommended approach involves counseling parents about the importance of a consistent bedtime ritual. Attention-seeking behavior is ignored, and the child is not taken into the parents' bed or allowed to stay up past a reasonable hour. Other measures that may be helpful include keeping a light on in the room, providing transitional objects such as a favorite toy, or leaving a drink of water by the bed.

Helping children slow down *before* bedtime also contributes to less resistance to going to bed. One approach is to establish limited rituals that signal readiness for bed, such as a bath or story. Parents can reinforce the pattern by stating, "After this story it is bedtime," and consistently carrying out the routine. If extra stimulation, such as having visitors arrive at bedtime, is disruptive to children's routine, it is advisable to settle children in bed beforehand. Television viewing before bedtime may cause bedtime resistance and delay sleep onset.

CULTURAL AWARENESS

Co-Sleeping

Although many experts recommend that infants and children be trained to always sleep in their own crib or bed, co-sleeping, or the "family bed" (in which parents allow the children to sleep with them or the siblings to sleep together in one bed), is a relatively common and accepted cultural practice, especially among African-American, Hispanic, and Asian families, such as the Japanese (Latz, Wolf, and Lozoff, 1999). Other groups that are adopting co-sleeping include (1) single parents, whose need for company may encourage this practice; (2) working parents, who desire the closeness at night that was lost during the day; and (3) parents who have had an issue about sleep or separation in their own past (Anderson, 2000). There is some concern among health care professionals that the incidence of sudden infant death syndrome (SIDS) may be increased with bed-sharing, especially when parental smoking, maternal obesity, and use of an atypical adult bed are involved (see Chapter 11). Co-sleeping may be a practical solution to limited numbers of bedrooms or beds in lower socioeconomic families. In a longitudinal study measuring the effects of co-sleeping at 6 and 18 years, bedsharing in early childhood was found to correlate positively with increased cognitive competence in 6 year olds. Co-sleeping was not associated with sleep problems, sexual pathology, or any other problematic consequences at 6 and 18 years, respectively. At 18 years children who had practiced bedsharing experienced no particular measurable positive effects of the experience. The researchers caution health care workers about warning parents to avoid bedsharing to prevent SIDS and further question the safety of solitary sleep (Okami, Weisner, and Olmstead, 2002). Parents who are considering adopting the practice of bedsharing should be made aware that this is a difficult habit for the child to break in the future. There appear to be no advantages to bedsharing in relation to decreasing SIDS deaths (some believed that bedsharing might prevent SIDS), and there may be disadvantages if co-sleepers are not cautious.

DENTAL HEALTH

By the beginning of the preschool period the eruption of the deciduous teeth is complete. Dental care is essential to preserve these temporary teeth and to teach good dental habits (see Chapter 12). Although preschoolers' fine motor control is improved, they still require assistance and supervision with brushing twice daily, and flossing should be performed by parents. Professional care and prophylaxis, especially fluoride supplements, should be continued. Routine dental care should be well established during preschool years and is recommended at 6- to 12-month intervals depending on the family history, the child's dental development, and the presence or absence of dental caries (Martof, 2001). For children cared for away from home, parents are encouraged to monitor the dental care provided by others, including keeping cariogenic foods to a minimum in the diet. Trauma to teeth during this period is not uncommon, and prompt evaluation by a dentist is warranted if oral trauma occurs. Preservation of the space previously occupied by an avulsed tooth is necessary for proper eruption of the secondary tooth.

INJURY PREVENTION

Because of improved gross and fine motor skills, coordination, and balance, preschoolers are less prone to falls than are toddlers. They tend to be less reckless, listen more to

TABLE 13-2 ■ Comparison of Nightmares to Sleep Terrors

NIGHTMARES	SLEEP TERRORS
Description	
A scary dream; takes place during rapid eye movement (REM) sleep and is followed by full waking	A partial arousal from very deep (state IV, non-REM) sleep
Time of Distress	
After the dream is over, child wakes and cries or calls, not during the nightmare itself	During the terror itself, child screams and thrashes; afterward is calm
Time of Occurrence	
In the second half of the night, when dreams are most intense	Usually 1 to 4 hours after falling asleep, when non-REM sleep is deepest
Child's Behavior	
Crying in younger children, fright in all; these behaviors persist even though the child is awake	Initially child may sit up, thrash, or run in a bizarre manner, with eyes bulging, heart racing, and profuse perspiring; may cry, scream, talk, or moan; there is apparent fright, anger, or obvious confusion, which disappears when child is fully awake
Responsiveness to Others	
Child is aware of and reassured by another's presence	Child is not very aware of another's presence, is not comforted, and may push person away and scream and thrash more if held or restrained
Return to Sleep	
May be considerably delayed because of persistent fear	Usually rapid; often difficult to keep child awake
Description of Dream	
Yes (if old enough)	No memory of a dream or of yelling or thrashing
Interventions	
Accept dream as real fear	Observe child for a few minutes, *without interfering,* until child becomes calm or wakes fully
Sit with child; offer comfort, assurance, and sense of protection	
Avoid taking child to own bed	Intervene only if necessary to protect child from injury
Consider professional counseling for recurrent nightmares unresponsive to above approaches	Guide child back to bed if needed
	Stress to parents that sleep terrors are a normal, common phenomenon in preschoolers that requires relatively little intervention.

Modified from Ferber R: *Solve your child's sleep problems,* New York, 1985, Simon & Schuster.

 FAMILY HOME CARE

Guidance During Preschool Years

AGE 3 YEARS

Prepare parents for child's increasing interest in widening relationships.

Encourage enrollment in preschool.

Emphasize importance of setting limits.

Prepare parents to expect exaggerated tension reduction behaviors, such as need for "security blanket."

Encourage parents to offer child choices when child vacillates.

Prepare parents to expect marked changes at 3.5 years, when child becomes less coordinated (motor and emotional), becomes insecure, and exhibits emotional extremes.

Prepare parents for normal dysfluency in speech and advise them to avoid focusing on the pattern.

Prepare parents to expect extra demands on their attention as a reflection of child's emotional insecurity and fear of loss of love.

Warn parents that equilibrium of 3-year-old will change to aggressive, out-of-bounds behavior of 4-year-old.

Inform parents to anticipate more stable appetite with more food selections.

Stress need for protection and education of child to prevent injury (see Injury Prevention, Chapter 12).

AGE 4 YEARS

Prepare parents for more aggressive behavior, including motor activity and offensive language.

Prepare parents to expect resistance to parental authority.

Explore parental feelings regarding child's behavior.

Suggest some kind of respite for primary caregivers, such as placing child in preschool for part of the day.

Prepare parents for child's increasing sexual curiosity.

Emphasize importance of realistic limit setting on behavior and appropriate discipline techniques.

Prepare parents for highly imaginative 4-year-old who indulges in "tall tales" (to be differentiated from lies) and for child's imaginary playmates.

Prepare parents to expect nightmares or an increase in them and suggest that parents make sure child is fully awakened from a frightening dream.

Provide reassurance that a period of calm begins at 5 years of age.

AGE 5 YEARS

Inform parents to expect tranquil period at 5 years.

Help parents to prepare child for entrance into school environment.

Make sure immunizations are up to date before entering school.

Suggest that nonemployed mothers (or fathers if appropriate) consider own activities when child begins school.

Suggest swimming lessons for child.

parental rules, and are aware of potential dangers, such as hot objects, sharp instruments, and dangerous heights. Putting objects in the mouth as part of exploration has all but ceased, although accidental poisoning is still a danger and playground injuries increase. Pedestrian motor vehicle injuries increase because of activities such as playing in the parking lot, driveway, or street; riding tricycles, bicycles, and other play vehicles and running after balls; or forgetting safety regulations when crossing streets.

In general the guidelines suggested for injury prevention in Table 12-3 apply to children in this age-group as well. However, emphasis is now on *education* concerning safety and potential hazards, in addition to appropriate protection. This period is an excellent time to start enforcing the use of safety items such as bicycle helmets to prevent head trauma; children are less likely to warm to the idea later in life because of peer pressure. Because preschoolers are great imitators, it is especially essential that parents set a good example by "practicing what they preach." Children quickly observe discrepancies in what they are told to do and what they see others do. Establishing habits at this time, such as wearing bicycle helmets, can create long-term safety behaviors.

ANTICIPATORY GUIDANCE—CARE OF FAMILIES

The preschool years present fewer childrearing difficulties than do earlier years, and this stage of development is facilitated by appropriate anticipatory guidance in the areas already discussed (see Family Home Care box). There is a shift in childrearing practices from protection to education. Whereas injury prevention previously focused on safeguarding the immediate environment, with less emphasis on reasoning, now the protective guardrails or electrical outlet caps may be substituted with verbal explanations of why danger exists and how to avoid it with appropriate judgment and understanding.

During this period an emotional transition between parent and child is also occurring. Although children are still attached to their parents and accepting of all parental values and beliefs, they are nearing the period of life when they will question previous teachings and prefer the companionship of peers. Entry into school marks a separation from home for parents, as well as for children. Parents need help in adjusting to this change, particularly if the mother (or other primary caregiver) has focused daily activity primarily on home responsibilities. All family members must adjust to changes, which is part of the process of growth and development.

KEY POINTS

- The preschool years comprise the period from 3 to 5 years of age, a time that is considered critical for emotional and psychologic development.

- Biologic development in the preschool period is characterized by mature body systems and refinement in gross and fine motor behavior, as evidenced by participation in activities such as running, riding a tricycle, and drawing.

- According to Erikson, acquiring a sense of initiative is the chief psychosocial task of the preschooler. Development of the superego occurs during this period, and conscience begins to emerge.

- According to Piaget, the preschool age is characterized by intuitive or prelogical thinking and a move toward logical thought processes through advanced, complex learning, language, and understanding of causality.

- The seeds of moral development are planted during the preschool period. According to Kohlberg, children are in the stage of naive instrumental orientation, in which they are concerned with satisfying their own needs and less frequently the needs of others.

- Social development includes further individuation-separation, more sophisticated language, greater independence, and more complex, imaginative forms of play.

- Areas of special concern to parents during the preschool period are preschool and kindergarten experience, sex education, fears, stress, and speech problems.

- In selecting an early learning program, parents should inquire about daily programs, teacher qualifications, accreditation, student-staff ratio, safety, meals, fees, and health practices.

- Two rules that govern answering questions about sex and other sensitive issues are to find out what the child knows and to be honest.

- Fears constitute a great part of the preschool period; objects, potential annihilation, and parent-induced fears are common sources.

- Preschool aggression may result from frustration, modeling behavior, and reinforcement.

- Hesitancy or dysfluency in speech patterns is a normal characteristic of language development. Speech problems can occur when parents express excessive concern over this pattern.

- Health promotion continues to be directed toward proper nutrition, adequate sleep, proper dental care, and injury prevention.

References

Ambrose NG, Yairi E: Normative disfluency data for early childhood stuttering, *J Speech Lang Hear Res* 42(4):895-909, 1999.

American Academy of Pediatrics, Committee on Nutrition: The use and misuse of fruit juices in pediatrics, *Pediatrics* 107(5):1210-1213, 2001b.

American Academy of Nutrition, Committee on Nutrition: *Pediatric nutrition handbook*, ed 4, Elk Grove Village, Il, 1998, The Academy.

American Academy of Pediatrics: Hearing assessment in infants and children: recommendations beyond neonatal screening, *Pediatrics* 111(2):436-440, 2003.

American Academy of Pediatrics, Committee on Public Education: Children, adolescents, and television, *Pediatrics* 107(2):423-426, 2001a.

American Academy of Pediatrics, Committee on Sports Medicine and Fitness and Committee on School Health: Physical fitness and activity in schools, *Pediatrics* 105(5):1156-1157, 2000.

Anderson DR and others: Early childhood television viewing and adolescent behavior: the recontact study, *Monogr Soc Res Child Dev* 66(1):I-VIII, 1-147, 2001.

Anderson JE: Co-sleeping: can we ever put the issue to rest? *Contemp Pediatr* 107(6):98-120, 2000.

Davison KK, Birch LL: Weight status and self-concept in young girls, *Pediatrics* 107(1):46-53, 2001.

Endres J and others: Soy-enhanced lunch acceptance by preschoolers, *J Am Diet Assoc* 103(3):346-351, 2003.

Finan SL: Promoting healthy sexuality: guidelines for infancy through preschool, *Nurse Pract* 22(10):79-80, 83-86, 88, 1997.

Glascoe FP: Are referrals on developmental screening tests really a problem? *Arch Pediatr Adolesc Med* 155(1):54-59, 2001.

Gottesman MM: Playing to learn: the work of children and their parents, *J Pediatr Health Care* 13(5):259-262, 1999.

Hart CH and others: Overt and relational aggression in Russian nursery-school-aged children: parenting style and marital linkages, *Dev Psychol* 34(4):687-697, 1998.

Huttenlocher J: Language input and language growth, *Prev Med* 27(2):195-199, 1998.

Johnson RK: Changing eating and physical activity patterns of U.S. children, *Proc Nutr Soc* 59(2):295-301, 2000.

Kenny G: Assessing children's spirituality: what is the way forward? *Br J Nurs* 8(1):28, 30-32, 1999.

Krug EF, Mikus KC: The preschool years. In Levine MD, Carey WB, Crocker AC, editors, *Developmental-behavioral pediatrics*, ed 3, Philadelphia, 1999, WB Saunders.

Lafontaine G, Bedard L: The prevention of infections in child daycare centers: potential influential factors, *Can J Public Health* 88(4):250-254, 1997.

Latz S, Wolf AW, Lozoff B: Cosleeping in context: sleep practices and problems in young children in Japan and the United States, *Arch Pediatr Adolesc Med* 153(4):339-346, 1999.

Marshall TA and others: Dental caries and beverage consumption in young children, *Pediatrics* 112(3):e177-e183, 2003.

Martof A: Consultation with the specialist: dental care, *Pediatr Rev* 22(1):13-15, 2001.

McEvoy M: An added dimension to the pediatric health maintenance visit: the spiritual history, *J Pediatr Health Care* 14(5):216-220, 2000.

McEvoy M: Culture and spirituality as an integrated concept in pediatric care, *MCN* 28(1):39-43, 2003.

Muris P, Merckelbach H, Prins E: How serious are common childhood fears? II. The parents' point of view, *Behav Res Ther* 38(3):813-818, 2000.

National Association for the Education of Young Children: Position statement on school readiness, 1995; available at www.naeyc.org.

Needlman R: Growth and development: Preschool years. In Behrman RE, Kliegman RM, Jenson HB, editors. *Nelson textbook of pediatrics*, ed 17, Philadelphia, 2004, WB Saunders.

Okami P, Weisner T, Olmstead R: Outcome correlates of parent-child bedsharing: an eighteen-year longitudinal study, *J Dev Behav Pediatr* 23(4):244-253, 2002.

Rampersaud GC, Bailey LB, Kauwell GPA: National survey beverage consumption data for children and adolescents indicate the need to encourage a shift toward more nutritive beverages, *J Am Diet Assoc* 103(1):97-100, 2003.

Rovers MM and others: Day-care and otitis media in young children: a critical review, *Eur J Pediatr* 158(1):1-6, 1999.

Steen S, Anderson B: Ages & stages of spiritual development, *J Christian Nurs* 12(2):6-11, 1995.

Stormshak EA and others: Parenting practices and child disruptive behavior problems in early elementary school, *J Clin Child Psychol* 29(1):17-29, 2000.

Thiedke CC: Sleep disorders and sleep problems in childhood, *Am Fam Physician* 63(2):277-284, 2001.

Thomas RM: *Comparing theories of child development*, ed 4, Pacific Grove, Calif, 1996, Brooks-Cole.

US Department of Agriculture, Center for Nutrition Policy and Promotion: Tips for using the Food Guide Pyramid for young children 2 to 6 years old, *Program Aid 1647*, 1999; available atwww.usda.gov/cnpp.

Vessey JA, Yim-Chiplis PK, MacKenzie NR: Effects of television viewing on children's development, *Pediatr Nurs* 23(5):483-485, 1998.

Villani S: Impact of media on children and adolescents: a 10-year review research, *J Am Acad Child Adolesc Psychiatry* 40(4):392-401, 2001.

Williams CL and others: Healthy start: outcome of an intervention to promote a heart healthy diet in preschool children, *J Am Coll Nutr* 21(1):62-71, 2002.

Wilson JF: Preschoolers' mid-afternoon snack intake is not affected by lunchtime food consumption, *Appetite* 33(3):319-327, 1999.

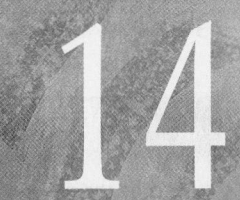

14

Health Problems of Toddlers and Preschoolers

KIMBERLY CHILDERS

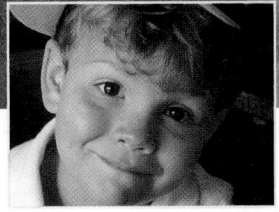

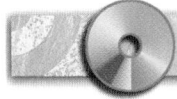
Remember to check out your companion CD-ROM

http://evolve.elsevier.com/Wong/essentials/

CHAPTER OUTLINE

RELATED TOPICS and ADDITIONAL RESOURCES

INFECTIOUS DISORDERS

COMMUNICABLE DISEASES

The incidence of childhood communicable diseases has declined greatly since the advent of immunizations. Serious complications resulting from such infections have been further reduced with the use of antibiotics and antitoxins. However, infectious diseases do occur, and nurses must be familiar with the infectious agent to recognize the disease and to institute appropriate preventive and supportive interventions (Table 14-1). (See also Chapter 30 for a discussion of nursing care for dermatologic conditions.)

Nursing Considerations

● Assessment

Identification of the infectious agent is of primary importance to prevent exposure to susceptible individuals. Nurses in ambulatory care settings, childcare centers, and schools are often the first persons to see signs of a communicable disease, such as a rash or sore throat. The nurse must operate under a high index of suspicion for common childhood diseases to identify potentially infectious cases and to recognize diseases that require medical intervention. An example is the common complaint of sore throat. Although most often a symptom of a minor viral infection, it can signal diphtheria or a streptococcal infection, such as scarlet fever. Each of these bacterial conditions requires appropriate medical treatment to prevent serious sequelae.

When a communicable disease is suspected, it is important to assess: (1) recent exposure to a known case; (2) *prodromal symptoms* (symptoms that occur between early manifestations of the disease and its overt clinical syndrome) or evidence of constitutional symptoms, such as a fever or rash (see Table 14-1); (3) immunization history; and (4) history of having the disease. Immunizations are available for many diseases, and infection usually confers lifelong immunity; therefore, the possibility of many infectious agents can be eliminated based on these two criteria.

● Nursing Diagnoses

Several nursing diagnoses are prominent in the nursing care of the child with a communicable disease. Others specific to individual cases may also be evident. The most common nursing diagnoses are presented in the Nursing Care Plan on pp. 446-447.

● Planning

The principal nursing goals, in addition to identification of the communicable disease (see Assessment) are:

1 Child will not spread the infection to others.
2 Child will not experience complications.
3 Child will have minimal discomfort.
4 Child and family will receive adequate emotional support.

● Implementation

Prevent Spread. Prevention consists of two components: prevention of the disease and control of its spread to others. Primary prevention rests almost exclusively on immunization. (The nurse's role in immunization of children is discussed in Chapter 10.)

Control measures to prevent spread of disease should include techniques to reduce risk of cross-transmission of infectious organisms between patients and to protect health care workers from organisms harbored by patients. If the child is hospitalized, the facility's policies for infection control are followed (see Chapter 22). The most important procedure is handwashing. Persons directly caring for the child or handling contaminated articles must wash their hands before care of another patient. The child is instructed to practice good handwashing technique after toileting and before eating. For those diseases spread by droplets, the nurse instructs parents in measures to reduce airborne transmission. The child who is old enough should use a tissue to cover the face during coughing or sneezing; otherwise, the parent should cover the child's mouth with a tissue and then discard it. The usual hygiene measures of not sharing eating and drinking utensils are stressed to the family.

> **! NURSING ALERT**
>
> If a child is admitted to the hospital with an undiagnosed exanthema, strict isolation is instituted until a diagnosis is confirmed. Childhood communicable diseases requiring isolation are diphtheria, chickenpox, measles, tuberculosis, adenovirus, *Haemophilus influenzae* type b, influenza, mumps, *Mycoplasma pneumoniae*, pertussis, plague, streptococcal pharyngitis, pneumonia, or scarlet fever (American Academy of Pediatrics, 2003a).

Prevent Complications. Although most children recover without difficulty, certain groups are at risk for serious, even fatal, complications from communicable diseases, especially the viral diseases of chickenpox and erythema infectiosum (EI). Children with immunodeficiency—those receiving steroid or other immunosuppressive therapy, those with a generalized malignancy such as leukemia or lymphoma, or those with an immunologic disorder—are at risk for viremia from replication of the *varicella-zoster virus (VZV)** in the blood. VZV is so named because it causes two distinct diseases: *varicella (chickenpox)* and *zoster (herpes zoster or shingles)*. Varicella occurs primarily in children younger than 15 years of age. However, it leaves the threat of herpes zoster, an intensely painful varicella that is localized to a single dermatome (body area innervated by a particular segment of the spinal cord). Immunocompromised patients and healthy infants younger than 1 year of age (who also have reduced immunity) are at a higher risk for reactivation of VZV causing herpes zoster, probably as a result of a deficiency in cellular immunity (Chen and others, 2002).

Children with hemolytic disease, such as sickle cell disease, are at risk for aplastic anemia from EI. The *human parvovirus (HPV)* infects and lyses red blood cell precursors, thus interrupting the production of red blood cells. Therefore, the virus may precipitate a severe aplastic crisis in patients who need increased red blood cell production to maintain normal red blood cell volumes. Because the fetus depends on a high rate of red blood cell production and has an immature immune system, it may develop severe anemia as a result of HPV infection in the mother.

NURSING ALERT

High-risk children who have signs of these communicable diseases are referred to the practitioner immediately. School nurses are responsible for warning parents about recent outbreaks of these communicable diseases to prevent susceptible children's exposure to known cases.

Prevention of complications from diseases such as diphtheria and scarlet fever necessitates compliance with antibiotic therapy. With oral preparations the need to complete the entire course of therapy is stressed (see Compliance, Chapter 22). The use of varicella-zoster immune globulin (VZIG) should be strongly considered in high-risk children after exposure to chickenpox to prevent the development of varicella. The antiviral agent acyclovir (Zovirax) may be used to treat varicella infections; it is effective in decreasing the number of lesions, shortening the duration of fever, and decreasing itching, lethargy, and anorexia. Acyclovir should be considered for otherwise healthy, nonpregnant individuals older than 12 years of age; children with chronic cutaneous or pulmonary conditions; those receiving chronic salicylate therapy; and those receiving short, intermittent, or aerosolized courses of corticosteroids (American Academy of Pediatrics, 2003a). Immunocompromised children should receive acyclovir by intravenous infusion (American Academy of Pediatrics, 2003a).

Recent evidence suggests that vitamin A supplementation reduces both morbidity and mortality in measles and that all children with severe measles should be given vitamin A sup-

*Educational materials may be obtained from the **Varicella Zoster Virus Research Foundation,** 40 East 72nd Street, New York, NY 10021; or GlaxoSmithKline, 3030 Cornwallis Road, Research Triangle Park, NC 27709; (919) 248-3000 or (888) 825-5249; website: www.gsk.com.

plements (Stalkup, 2002). A single oral dose of 200,000 IU for children at least 1 year old (use half that dose for children 6 to 12 months of age) is recommended. The higher dose may be associated with vomiting and headache for a few hours. The dose should be repeated the next day and at 4 weeks for children with ophthalmologic evidence of vitamin A deficiency (American Academy of Pediatrics, 2003a).

NURSING ALERT

Although the risk of vitamin A toxicity from these doses (they are 100 to 200 times the recommended dietary allowance) is very low, nurses should instruct parents on safe storage of the drug. Ideally, vitamin A should be dispensed in the age-appropriate unit dose to prevent excessive administration and possible toxicity.

Provide Comfort.   Many communicable diseases cause skin manifestations that are bothersome to the child. The chief discomfort from most rashes is itching, and measures such as cool baths (usually without soap) and lotions (e.g., calamine) are helpful.

NURSING ALERT

When lotions with active ingredients such as diphenhydramine in Caladryl are used, they are applied sparingly, especially over open lesions, where excessive absorption can lead to drug toxicity. These lotions should be avoided in children who are simultaneously receiving oral diphenhydramine.

To avoid overheating, which increases itching, children should wear lightweight, loose, nonirritating clothing and keep out of the sun. If the child persists in scratching, the nails are kept short and smooth; mittens and clothes with long sleeves or legs may be needed. For severe itching, antipruritic medication, such as diphenhydramine (Benadryl) or hydroxyzine (Atarax), may be required, especially when the child has trouble sleeping because of itching.

An elevated temperature is common, and both antipyretic medicine (acetaminophen or ibuprofen) and environmental manipulation are implemented (see Controlling Elevated Temperature, Chapter 22). The acetaminophen is effective in lowering the fever but does not significantly reduce the symptoms of itching, anorexia, abdominal pain, fussiness, or vomiting.

A sore throat, another frequent symptom, is managed with lozenges, saline rinses (if the child is old enough to cooperate), and analgesics. Because most children are anorectic during an illness, bland foods and increased liquids are usually preferred. During the early stages of the disease, children voluntarily curtail their activity, and although bed rest is beneficial, it should not be imposed unless specifically indicated (e.g., with pertussis). During periods of irritability, quiet activity (e.g., reading, music, television, videos, puzzles, coloring) helps distract children from the discomfort.

Support Child and Family.   Most communicable diseases are benign, but may produce considerable concern and anxiety for parents. Often the occurrence of a disease such as chickenpox is the first time the child is acutely uncomfortable. Parents need assistance to cope with manifestations of the

Text continued on p. 444

TABLE 14-1 ■ Communicable Diseases of Childhood

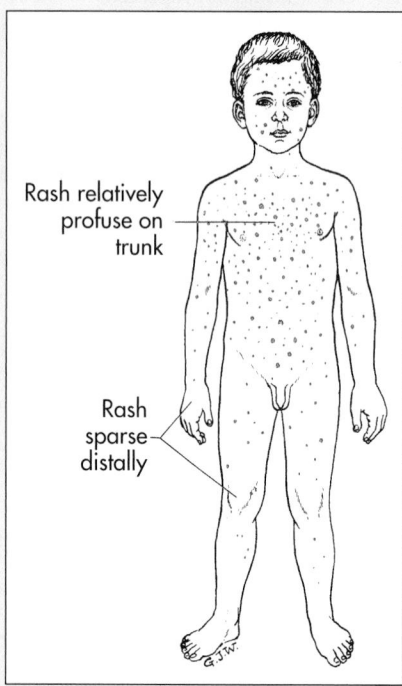

Rash relatively profuse on trunk

Rash sparse distally

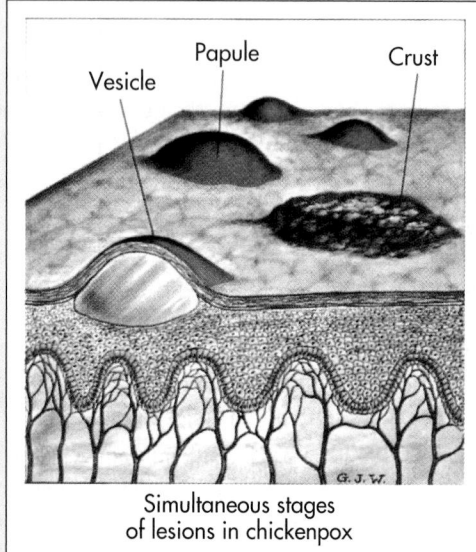

Vesicle Papule Crust

Simultaneous stages of lesions in chickenpox

DISEASE

CHICKENPOX (VARICELLA) (Fig.14-1)
Agents: Varicella-zoster virus (VZV)
Source: Primary secretions of respiratory tract of infected persons; to a lesser degree, skin lesions (scabs not infectious)
Transmissions: Direct contact, droplet (airborne) spread, and contaminated objects
Incubation period: 2-3 weeks, usually 14-16 days
Period of communicability: Probably 1 day before eruption of lesions (prodromal period) to 6 days after first crop of vesicles when crusts have formed

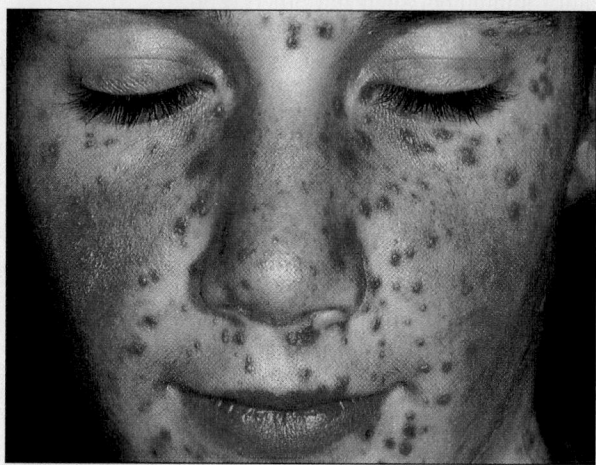

FIG. 14-1 ■ Chickenpox (varicella). (Clinical view from Habif TP: *Clinical dermatology: a color guide to diagnosis and therapy,* ed 4, St Louis, 2004, Mosby.)

DIPHTHERIA
Agent: *Corynebacterium diphtheriae*
Source: Discharges from mucous membranes of nose and nasopharynx, skin, and other lesions of infected person
Transmission: Direct contact with infected person, a carrier, or contaminated articles
Incubation period: Usually 2-5 days, possibly longer
Period of communicability: Variable; until virulent bacilli are no longer present (identified by three negative cultures); usually 2 weeks but as long as 4 weeks

CLINICAL MANIFESTATIONS	THERAPEUTIC MANAGEMENT/ COMPLICATIONS	NURSING CONSIDERATIONS
Prodromal stage: Slight fever, malaise, and anorexia for first 24 hours; rash highly pruritic; begins as macule, rapidly progresses to papule and then vesicle (surrounded by erythematous base, becomes umbilicated and cloudy, breaks easily and forms crusts); all three stages (papule, vesicle, crust) present in varying degrees at one time **Distribution:** Centripetal, spreading to face and proximal extremities but sparse on distal limbs and less on areas not exposed to heat (i.e., from clothing or sun) **Constitutional signs and symptoms:** Elevated temperature from lymphadenopathy, irritability from pruritus	**Specific:** Antiviral agent acyclovir (Zovirax); varicella-zoster immune globulin (VZIG) after exposure in high-risk children **Supportive:** Diphenhydramine hydrochloride or antihistamines to relieve itching; skin care to prevent secondary bacterial infection **Complications:** Secondary bacterial infections (abscesses, cellulitis, necrotizing fasciitis, pneumonia, sepsis) Encephalitis Varicella pneumonia (rare in normal children) Hemorrhagic varicella (tiny hemorrhages in vesicles and numerous petechiae in skin) Chronic or transient thrombocytopenia	Maintain strict isolation in hospital Isolate child in home until vesicles have dried (usually 1 week after onset of disease), and isolate high-risk children from infected children Administer skin care: give bath and change clothes and linens daily; administer topical calamine lotion; keep child's fingernails short and clean; apply mittens if child scratches Keep child cool (may decrease number of lesions) Lessen pruritus; keep child occupied Remove loose crusts that rub and irritate skin Teach child to apply pressure to pruritic area rather than scratching it If older child, reason with child regarding danger of scar formation from scratching Avoid use of aspirin
Vary according to anatomic location of pseudomembrane **Nasal:** Resembles common cold, serosanguineous mucopurulent nasal discharge without constitutional symptoms; may be frank epistaxis **Tonsillar/pharyngeal:** Malaise; anorexia; sore throat; low-grade fever; pulse increased above expected for temperature within 24 hours; smooth, adherent, white or gray membrane; lymphadenitis possibly pronounced ("bull's neck"); in severe cases, toxemia, septic shock, and death within 6-10 days **Laryngeal:** Fever, hoarseness, cough, with or without previous signs listed; potential airway obstruction, apprehensive, dyspneic retractions, cyanosis	Antitoxin (usually intravenously); preceded by skin or conjunctival test to rule out sensitivity to horse serum Antibiotics (penicillin or erythromycin) Complete bed rest (prevention of myocarditis) Tracheostomy for airway obstruction Treatment of infected contacts and carriers **Complications:** Myocarditis (second week) Neuritis	Maintain strict isolation in hospital Participate in sensitivity testing; have epinephrine available Administer complete care to maintain bed rest Use suctioning as needed Observe respiration for signs of obstruction Administer humidified oxygen if prescribed

Continued

TABLE 14-1 ■ Communicable Diseases of Childhood—*cont'd*

DISEASE

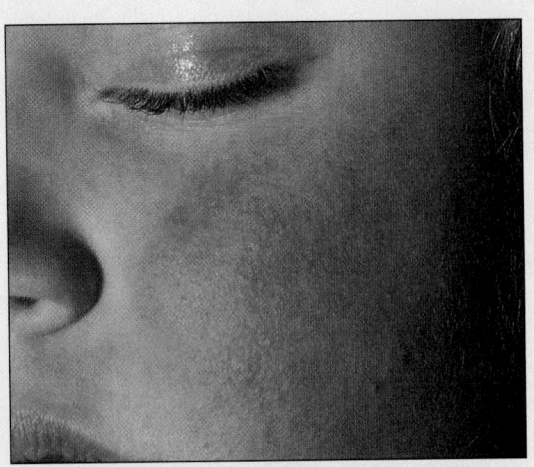

FIG. 14-2 ■ Erythema infectiosum. (From Habif TP: *Clinical dermatology: a color guide to diagnosis and therapy,* ed 4, St Louis, 2004, Mosby.)

ERYTHEMA INFECTIOSUM (FIFTH DISEASE) (Fig. 14-2)
Agent: Human parvovirus B19 (HPV)
Source: Infected persons
Transmission: Unknown; possibly respiratory secretions and blood
Incubation period: 4-14 days, may be as long as 21 days
Period of communicability: Uncertain but before onset of symptoms in children with aplastic crisis

EXANTHEM SUBITUM (ROSEOLA) (Fig. 14-3)
Agent: Human herpesvirus type 6 (HHV-6)
Source: Unknown
Transmission: Unknown (virtually limited to children between 6 months and 3 years of age)
Incubation period: Usually 5-15 days
Period of communicability: Unknown

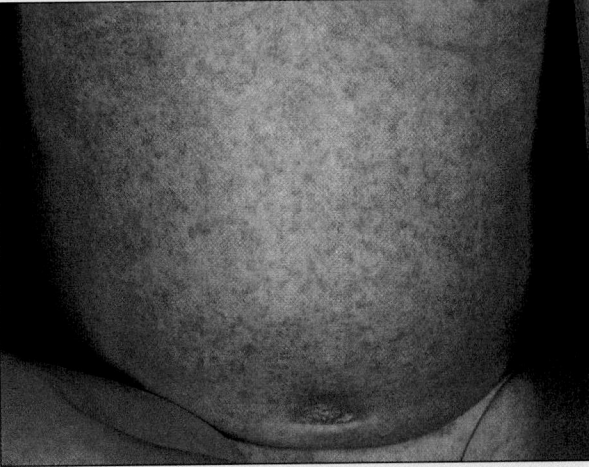

FIG. 14-3 ■ Roseola infantum. (From Habif TP: *Clinical dermatology: a color guide to diagnosis and therapy,* ed 4, St Louis, 2004, Mosby.)

CLINICAL MANIFESTATIONS	THERAPEUTIC MANAGEMENT/ COMPLICATIONS	NURSING CONSIDERATIONS

Rash appears in three stages:
  I—Erythema on face, chiefly on cheeks, "slapped face" appearance; disappears by 1-4 days
  II—About 1 day after rash appears on face, maculopapular red spots appear, symmetrically distributed on upper and lower extremities; rash progresses from proximal to distal surfaces and may last a week or more
  III—Rash subsides but reappears if skin is irritated or traumatized (sun, heat, cold, friction)
In children with aplastic crisis, rash is usually absent and prodromal illness includes fever, myalgia, lethargy, nausea, vomiting, and abdominal pain
	Symptomatic and supportive: Antipyretics, analgesics, anti-inflammatory drugs
	Possible blood transfusion for transient aplastic anemia
	Complications: Self-limited arthritis and arthralgia (arthritis may become chronic) (Moore, 2000)
	May result in fetal death if mother infected during pregnancy
	Aplastic crisis in children with hemolytic disease or immunodeficiency
	Myocarditis (rare)
		Isolation of child not necessary, except hospitalized child (immunosuppressed or with aplastic crises) suspected of HPV infection is placed on respiratory isolation and standard precautions
		Pregnant women: need not be excluded from workplace where HPV infection is present; should not care for patients with aplastic crises; explain low risk of fetal death to those in contact with affected children

Persistent high fever for 3-4 days in child who appears well Precipitous drop in fever to normal with appearance of rash **Rash:** Discrete rose-pink macules or maculopapules appearing first on trunk, then spreading to neck, face, and extremities; nonpruritic, fades on pressure, lasts 1-2 days **Associated signs and symptoms:** Cervical/postauricular lymphadenopathy, inflamed pharynx, cough, coryza	Nonspecific Antipyretics to control fever **Complications:** Recurrent febrile seizures (possibly from latent infection of central nervous system that is reactivated by fever) Encephalitis (rare)	Teach parents measures for lowering temperature (antipyretic drugs) If child is prone to seizures, discuss appropriate precautions, possibility of recurrent febrile seizures (Stoeckle, 2000)

Continued

TABLE 14-1 ■ **Communicable Diseases of Childhood—*cont'd***

DISEASE

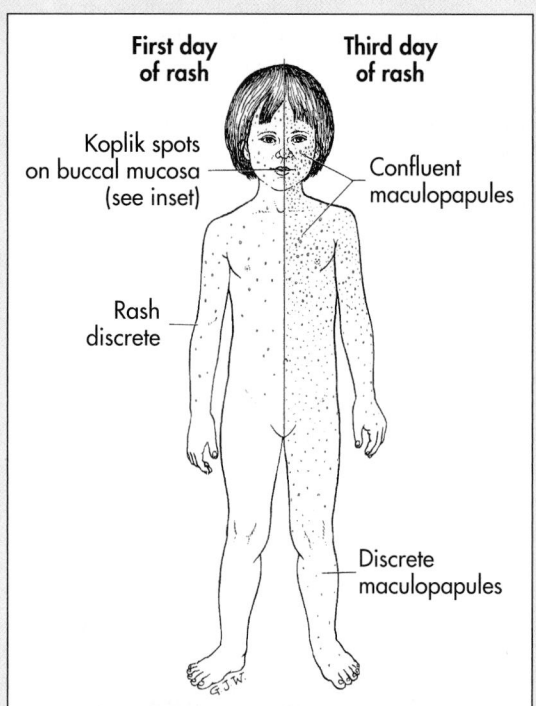

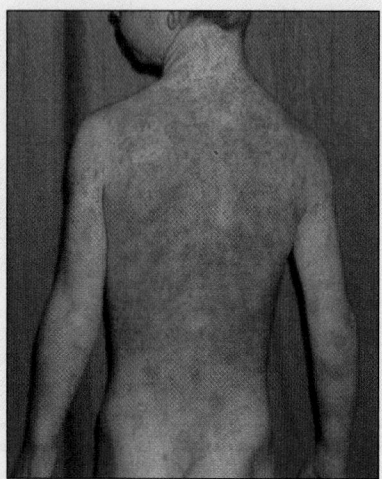

FIG. **14-4** ■ Measles (rubeola). (Clinical view from Seidel HM and others: *Mosby's guide to physical examination,* ed 4, St Louis, 1999, Mosby; Koplik spots from Zitelli BJ, Davis HW: *Atlas of pediatric physical diagnosis,* ed 3, St Louis, 1997, Mosby.)

MEASLES (RUBEOLA) (Fig. 14-4)
Agent: Virus
Source: Respiratory tract secretions, blood, and urine of infected person
Transmission: Usually by direct contact with droplets of infected person
Incubation period: 10-20 days
Period of communicability: From 4 days before to 5 days after rash appears but mainly during prodromal (catarrhal) stage

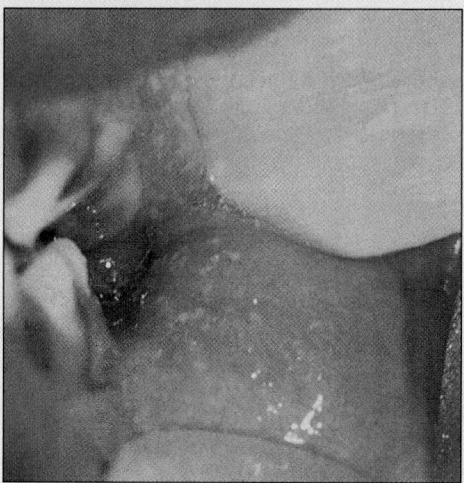

Koplik spots

MUMPS
Agent: Paramyxovirus
Source: Saliva of infected persons
Transmission: Direct contact with or droplet spread from an infected person
Incubation period: 14-21 days
Period of communicability: Most communicable immediately before and after swelling begins

PERTUSSIS (WHOOPING COUGH)
Agent: *Bordetella pertussis*
Source: Discharge from respiratory tract of infected persons

CLINICAL MANIFESTATIONS	THERAPEUTIC MANAGEMENT/ COMPLICATIONS	NURSING CONSIDERATIONS
Prodromal (catarrhal) stage: Fever and malaise, followed in 24 hours by coryza, cough, conjunctivitis, Koplik spots (small, irregular red spots with a minute, bluish white center first seen on buccal mucosa opposite molars 2 days before rash); symptoms gradually increase in severity until second day after rash appears, when they begin to subside **Rash:** Appears 3-4 days after onset of prodromal stage; begins as erythematous maculopapular eruption on face and gradually spreads downward; more severe in earlier sites (appears confluent) and less intense in later sites (appears discrete); after 3-4 days assumes brownish appearance, and fine desquamation occurs over area of extensive involvement **Constitutional signs and symptoms:** Anorexia, malaise, generalized lymphadenopathy	Vitamin A supplementation (see p. 435) **Supportive:** Bed rest during febrile period; antipyretics Antibiotics to prevent secondary bacterial infection in high-risk children **Complications:** Otitis media Pneumonia Bronchiolitis Obstructive laryngitis and laryngotracheitis Encephalitis	Isolation until fifth day of rash; if hospitalized, institute respiratory precautions Maintain bed rest during prodromal stage; provide quiet activity **Fever:** Instruct parents to administer antipyretics; avoid chilling; if child is prone to seizures, institute appropriate precautions **Eye care:** Dim lights if photophobia present; clean eyelids with warm saline solution to remove secretions or crusts; keep child from rubbing eyes; examine cornea for signs of ulceration **Coryza/cough:** Use cool-mist vaporizer; protect skin around nares with layer of petrolatum; encourage fluids and soft, bland foods **Skin care:** Keep skin clean; use tepid baths as necessary
Prodromal stage: Fever, headache, malaise, and anorexia for 24 hours, followed by "earache" that is aggravated by chewing **Parotitis:** By third day, parotid gland(s) (either unilateral or bilateral) enlarges and reaches maximum size in 1-3 days; accompanied by pain and tenderness	**Symptomatic and supportive:** Analgesics for pain and antipyretics for fever Intravenous fluid may be necessary for child who refuses to drink or vomits because of meningoencephalitis **Complications:** Sensorineural deafness Postinfectious encephalitis Myocarditis Arthritis Hepatitis Epididymo-orchitis Sterility (extremely rare in adult males) Meningitis	Isolation during period of communicability; institute respiratory precautions during hospitalization Maintain bed rest during prodromal phase until swelling subsides Give analgesics for pain; if child is unwilling to chew medication, use elixir form Encourage fluids and soft, bland foods; avoid foods requiring chewing Apply hot or cold compresses to neck, whichever is more comforting To relieve orchitis, provide warmth and local support with tight-fitting underpants (stretch bathing suit works very well)
Catarrhal stage: Begins with symptoms of upper respiratory tract infection, such as coryza, sneezing, lacrimation, cough, and low-grade fever; symptoms continue for 1-2 weeks, when dry, hacking cough becomes more severe	Antimicrobial therapy (e.g., erythromycin) Administration of pertussis immune globulin	Isolation during catarrhal stage; if hospitalized, institute respiratory precautions Maintain bed rest as long as fever present

Continued

TABLE 14-1 ■ **Communicable Diseases of Childhood**—*cont'd*

DISEASE

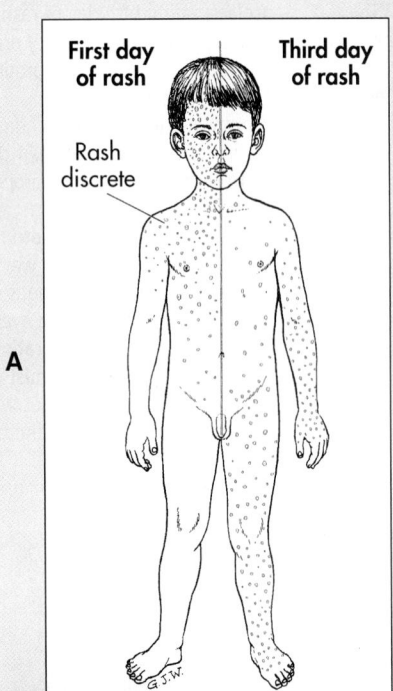

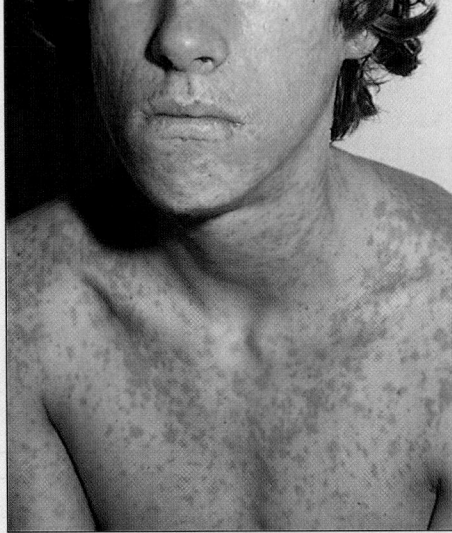

FIG. 14-5 ■ Rubella (German measles), **A,** Progression of rash, **B,** Clinical view. (From Zitelli BJ, Davis HW: *Atlas of pediatric physical diagnosis,* ed 4, St Louis, 2002, Mosby; courtesy Dr. Michael Sherlock.)

PERTUSSIS (WHOOPING COUGH)—*cont'd*

Transmission: Direct contact or droplet spread from infected person; indirect contact with freshly contaminated articles

Incubation period: 6-20 days, usually 7-10 days

Period of communicability: Greatest during catarrhal stage before onset of paroxysms

POLIOMYELITIS

Agent: Enteroviruses, three types: type 1—most frequent cause of paralysis, both epidemic and endemic; type 2—least frequently associated with paralysis; type 3—second most frequently associated with paralysis

Source: Feces and oropharyngeal secretions of infected persons, especially young children

Transmission: Direct contact with persons with apparent or inapparent active infection; spread is via fecal-oral and pharyngeal-oropharyngeal routes

Incubation period: Usually 7-14 days, with range of 5-35 days

Period of communicability: Not exactly known; virus is present in throat and feces shortly after infection and persists for about 1 week in throat and 4-6 weeks in feces

RUBELLA (GERMAN MEASLES) (Fig. 14-5)

Agent: Rubella virus

Source: Primarily nasopharyngeal secretions of person with apparent or inapparent infection; virus also present in blood, stool, and urine

Incubation period: 14-21 days

Period of communicability: 7 days before to about 5 days after appearance of rash

Constitutional signs and symptoms: Occasionally low-grade fever, headache, malaise, and lymphadenopathy

CLINICAL MANIFESTATIONS	THERAPEUTIC MANAGEMENT/ COMPLICATIONS	NURSING CONSIDERATIONS
Paroxysmal stage: Cough most often occurs at night and consists of short, rapid coughs followed by sudden inspiration associated with a high-pitched crowing sound or "whoop"; during paroxysms, cheeks become flushed or cyanotic, eyes bulge, and tongue protrudes; paroxysm may continue until thick mucous plug is dislodged; vomiting frequently follows attack; stage generally lasts 4-6 weeks, followed by convalescent stage	**Supportive treatment:** Hospitalization required for infants, children who are dehydrated, or those who have complications Bed rest Increased oxygen intake and humidity Adequate fluids Intubation possibly necessary **Complications:** Pneumonia (usual cause of death) Atelectasis Otitis media Seizures Hemorrhage (subarachnoid, subconjunctival, epistaxis) Weight loss and dehydration Hernia Prolapsed rectum	Provide restful environment and reduce factors that promote paroxysms (dust, smoke, sudden change in temperature, chilling, activity, excitement); keep room well ventilated Encourage fluids; offer small amount of fluids frequently; refeed child after vomiting Provide high humidity (humidifier or tent); suction gently but often to prevent choking on secretions Observe for signs of airway obstruction (increased restlessness, apprehension, retractions, cyanosis) Involve public health nurse if child cared for at home
May be manifested in three different forms: **Abortive or inapparent**—Fever, uneasiness, sore throat, headache, anorexia, vomiting, abdominal pain; lasts a few hours to a few days **Nonparalytic**—Same manifestations as abortive but more severe, with pain and stiffness in neck, back, and legs **Paralytic**—Initial course similar to nonparalytic type, followed by recovery and then signs of central nervous system paralysis	Treatment is supportive Complete bed rest during acute phase Assisted respiratory ventilation in case of respiratory paralysis Physical therapy for muscles following acute stage **Complications:** Permanent paralysis Respiratory arrest Hypertension Kidney stones from demineralization of bone during prolonged immobility	Maintain complete bed rest Administer mild sedatives as necessary to relieve anxiety and promote bed rest Participate in physiotherapy procedures (use of moist hot packs and range-of-motion exercises) Position child to maintain body alignment and prevent contractures or decubiti; use footboard Encourage child to move; administer analgesics for maximum comfort during physical activity Observe for respiratory paralysis (difficulty in talking, ineffective cough, inability to hold breath, shallow and rapid respirations); report such signs and symptoms to practitioner; have tracheostomy tray at bedside
Prodromal stage: Absent in children, present in adults and adolescents; consists of low-grade fever, headache, malaise, anorexia, mild conjunctivitis, coryza, sore throat, cough, and lymphadenopathy; lasts 1-5 days, subsides 1 day after appearance of rash **Rash:** First appears on face and rapidly spreads downward to neck, arms, trunk, and legs; by end of first day, body is covered with discrete, pinkish red maculopapular exanthema; disappears in same order as it began and is usually gone by third day	No treatment necessary other than antipyretics for low-grade fever and analgesics for discomfort **Complications:** Rare (arthritis, encephalitis, or purpura); most benign of all childhood communicable diseases; greatest danger is teratogenic effect on fetus	Reassure parents of benign nature of illness in affected child Use comfort measures as necessary Isolate child from pregnant women

Continued

TABLE 14-1 ■ Communicable Diseases of Childhood—*cont'd*

DISEASE

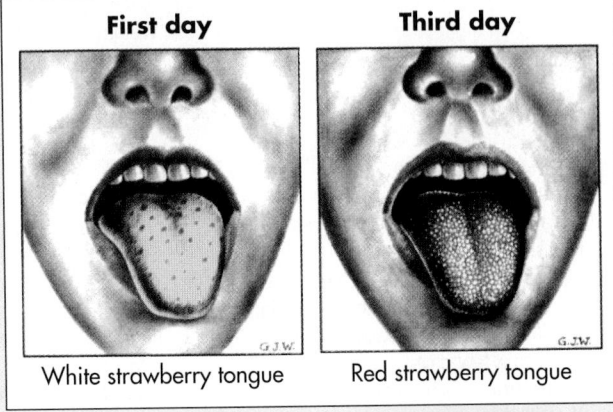

First day of rash

Flushed cheeks
White strawberry tongue (see inset)
Increased density on neck
Transverse lines (Pastia sign)
Increased density in groin

Third day of rash

Circumoral pallor
Red strawberry tongue (see inset)
Increased density in axilla
Positive blanching test (Schultz-Charlton)

First day — White strawberry tongue
Third day — Red strawberry tongue

FIG. 14-6 ■ Scarlet fever.

SCARLET FEVER (Fig. 14-6)
Agent: Group A β-hemolytic streptococci
Source: Usually from nasopharyngeal secretions of infected persons and carriers
Transmission: Direct contact with infected person or droplet spread; indirectly by contact with contaminated articles or ingestion of contaminated milk or other food
Incubation period: 2-5 days, with range of 1-7 days
Period of communicability: During incubation period and clinical illness, approximately 10 days; during first 2 weeks of carrier phase, although may persist for months

---

illness, such as intense itching. Sometimes a visiting nurse may be beneficial to help the family develop a plan of care and encourage compliance with treatments.

The family and child need reassurance that recovery is generally rapid. However, visible signs of the dermatosis may be present for some time after the child is well enough to resume usual activities. When the disease involves noticeable signs, such as the crusts of chickenpox, the child may benefit from preparation before returning to school. For example, the parent can discuss the child's physical appearance with the teacher or school nurse and request that they explain the child's condition to classmates.

> **NURSING ALERT**
>
> The occurrence of a communicable disease provides the opportunity to ask parents about the child's immunization status and reinforce the benefits of vaccines for children.

● *Evaluation*

The effectiveness of nursing interventions is determined by continual reassessment and evaluation of care based on the following observational guidelines and expected outcomes:

1 Observe or inquire about family members' use of control measures; observe for signs of disease in household contacts.

2 Monitor vital signs, especially temperature; inquire about the identification of high-risk contacts and appropriate isolation of the contact; observe or inquire about compliance with antibiotic or antiviral therapy.
3 Inquire about effectiveness of comfort measures.
4 Interview family and child regarding their feelings and concerns, especially when child returns to school.

The *expected outcomes* are described in the Nursing Care Plan on pp. 446-447.

CONJUNCTIVITIS

Acute conjunctivitis (inflammation of the conjunctiva) occurs from a variety of causes that are typically age-related. In newborns conjunctivitis can occur from infection during birth, most often from *Chlamydia trachomatis* (inclusion conjunctivitis) or *Neisseria gonorrhoeae*. These organisms, as well as herpes simplex virus (HSV), cause serious ocular damage. In infants recurrent conjunctivitis may be a sign of nasolacrimal (tear) duct obstruction. In children the usual causes are viral, bacterial, allergic, or related to a foreign body. Bacterial infection accounts for most instances of acute conjunctivitis in children. Diagnosis is made primarily from the clinical manifestations (Box 14-1), although cultures of purulent drainage may be needed to identify the specific cause.

CLINICAL MANIFESTATIONS	THERAPEUTIC MANAGEMENT/ COMPLICATIONS	NURSING CONSIDERATIONS
Prodromal stage: Abrupt high fever, pulse increased out of proportion to fever, vomiting, headache, chills, malaise, abdominal pain **Enanthema:** Tonsils enlarged, edematous, reddened, and covered with patches of exudates; in severe cases appearance resembles membrane seen in diphtheria; pharynx is edematous and beefy red; during first 1-2 days tongue is coated and papillae become red and swollen (white strawberry tongue); by fourth or fifth day white coat sloughs off, leaving prominent papillae (red strawberry tongue); palate is covered with erythematous punctate lesions **Exanthema:** Rash appears within 12 hours after prodromal signs; red pinhead-sized punctate lesions rapidly become generalized but are absent on face, which becomes flushed with striking circumoral pallor; rash is more intense in folds of joints; by end of first week desquamation begins (fine, sandpaper-like on torso; sheetlike sloughing on palms and soles), which may be complete by 3 weeks or longer	Treatment of choice is full course of penicillin (or erythromycin in penicillin-sensitive children) Antibiotic therapy for newly diagnosed carriers (nose or throat cultures positive for streptococci) **Supportive measures:** Bed rest during febrile phase, analgesics for sore throat **Complications:** Otitis media Peritonsillar and retropharyngeal abscess Sinusitis Glomerulonephritis Carditis, polyarthritis (uncommon)	Institute respiratory precautions until 24 hours after initiation of treatment Ensure compliance with oral antibiotic therapy (intramuscular benzathine penicillin G [Bicillin] may be given if parents' reliability in giving oral drugs is questionable) Maintain bed rest during febrile phase; provide quiet activity during convalescent period Relieve discomfort of sore throat with analgesics, gargles, lozenges, antiseptic throat sprays, and inhalation of cool mist Encourage fluids during febrile phase; avoid irritating liquids (citrus juices) or rough foods; when child is able to eat, begin with soft diet Advise parents to consult practitioner if fever persists after beginning therapy Discuss procedures for preventing spread of infection

Therapeutic Management

Treatment of conjunctivitis depends on the cause. Viral conjunctivitis is self-limiting, and treatment is limited to removal of the accumulated secretions. Bacterial conjunctivitis is usually treated with topical antibacterial agents. Drops may be used during the day and an ointment at bedtime because the ointment preparation remains in the eye longer. Ointments are usually not used in the daytime because they blur vision.

Nursing Considerations

Nursing goals include keeping the eye clean and properly administering ophthalmic medication. Accumulated secretions are always removed by wiping from the inner canthus downward and outward, away from the opposite eye. Warm, moist compresses, such as a clean washcloth wrung out with hot tap water, are helpful in removing the crusts. Compresses are *not* kept on the eye, because an occlusive covering promotes bacterial growth. Medication is instilled immediately after the eyes have been cleaned and according to correct procedure (see Chapter 22).

Prevention of infection in other family members is an important consideration with bacterial conjunctivitis. The child's washcloth and towel are kept separate from those used by others. Tissues used to clean the eye are discarded. The child should refrain from rubbing the eye and is instructed in good handwashing technique.

NURSING ALERT

Signs of serious conjunctivitis include reduction or loss of vision, ocular pain, photophobia, exophthalmos (bulging eyeball), decreased ocular mobility, corneal ulceration, and unusual patterns of inflammation (e.g., the perilimbal flush associated with iritis or localized inflammation associated with scleritis). If a patient has any of these signs, refer him or her immediately for further evaluation (Lederman and Lederman, 2003).

STOMATITIS

Stomatitis is inflammation of the oral mucosa, which may include the buccal (cheek) and labial (lip) mucosa, tongue, gingiva, palate, and floor of the mouth. It may be infectious or noninfectious and may be caused by local or systemic factors. In children aphthous stomatitis and herpetic stomatitis are typically seen.

Aphthous stomatitis (aphthous ulcer, canker sore) is a benign but painful condition whose cause is unknown. Its onset is usually associated with mild traumatic injury (biting the cheek, hitting the mucosa with a toothbrush, or a mouth appliance rubbing on the mucosa), allergy, or emotional stress. The lesions are painful, small, whitish ulcerations surrounded by a red border. They are distinguished from other types of stomatitis by healthy adjacent tissues,

NURSING CARE PLAN The Child With a Communicable Disease

NURSING DIAGNOSIS ■ **Risk for infection related to susceptible host and infectious agents**

PATIENT GOAL 1: Will not become infected

NURSING INTERVENTIONS/*RATIONALES*

Be highly suspicious of infectious diseases, especially in susceptible children

Identify high-risk children (e.g., those with an immunodeficiency or hemolytic disease) to whom communicable disease may be fatal; in case of an outbreak, advise parents to confine child to the home *to avoid exposure*

Participate in public education and service programs regarding prophylactic immunizations, method of spread of communicable diseases, proper preparation and handling of food and water supplies, control of animal vectors in regard to reservoirs of disease (not a factor in childhood communicable disease but in other infectious illness such as malaria), or screening programs to identify streptococcal infections

EXPECTED OUTCOME

Susceptible children do not contract the disease

PATIENT GOAL 2: Will not spread disease

NURSING INTERVENTIONS/*RATIONALES*

Institute appropriate infection control practices (see Chapter 22)

Make referral to public health nurse when necessary *to ensure appropriate procedures in the home*

Work with families *to ensure compliance with therapeutic regimens*

Identify close contacts who may require prophylactic treatment (e.g., specific immune globulin or antibiotics)

Report disease to local health department if appropriate

EXPECTED OUTCOME

Infection remains confined to original source

PATIENT GOAL 3: Will exhibit no evidence of complications

NURSING INTERVENTIONS/*RATIONALES*

Ensure compliance with therapeutic regimen (e.g., bed rest, antiviral therapy, antibiotics, adequate hydration)

Avoid giving aspirin to children with viral illness *because of the possible risk of Reye syndrome*

Institute seizure precautions if febrile convulsions are a possibility

Monitor temperature; *unexpected elevations may signal an infection*

Maintain good body hygiene *to reduce risk of secondary infection of lesions*

Offer small, frequent sips of water or favorite drinks *to ensure adequate hydration* and soft, bland foods (gelatin, pudding, ice cream, soups), *because many children are anorectic during an illness;* feed again after vomiting; observe for signs of dehydration

EXPECTED OUTCOME

Child exhibits no evidence of complications such as infection or dehydration

*Dependent nursing action

NURSING DIAGNOSIS ■ **Pain related to skin lesions, malaise**

PATIENT GOAL 1: Will experience minimal discomfort

NURSING INTERVENTIONS/*RATIONALES*

Use cool-mist vaporizer, gargles, and lozenges *to keep mucous membranes moist*

Apply petrolatum to chapped lips or nares

Cleanse eyes with physiologic saline solution *to remove secretions or crusts*

Keep skin clean; change bedclothes and linens at least daily

Administer oral hygiene

Keep child cool *because overheating increases itching*

Give cool baths and apply lotion such as calamine *to decrease itching*

Assess need for pain medication (see Chapter 21)

Employ nonpharmacologic pain reduction techniques (see Chapter 21)

*Administer analgesics, antipyretics, and antipruritics as needed

EXPECTED OUTCOMES

Skin and mucous membranes are clean and free of irritants

Child exhibits minimal evidence of discomfort (specify)

NURSING DIAGNOSIS ■ **Impaired social interaction related to isolation from peers**

PATIENT GOAL 1: Will have some understanding of reason for isolation

NURSING INTERVENTIONS/*RATIONALES*

Explain reason for confinement and use of any special precautions *to increase child's understanding of restrictions*

Allow child to play with mask and gown (if used) *to facilitate positive coping*

EXPECTED OUTCOME

Child demonstrates understanding of restrictions

PATIENT GOAL 2: Will have opportunity to participate in suitable activities

NURSING INTERVENTIONS/*RATIONALES*

Always introduce self to child; allow to see face before donning protective clothing, if required

Provide diversionary activity

Encourage parents to remain with child during hospitalization *to decrease separation and provide companionship*

Encourage contact with friends via telephone

Prepare child's peers for altered physical appearance, such as with chickenpox, *to encourage peer acceptance*

EXPECTED OUTCOMES

Child engages in suitable activities and interactions

Peers accept child

NURSING CARE PLAN The Child With a Communicable Disease—*cont'd*

NURSING DIAGNOSIS ■ **Risk for impaired skin integrity related to scratching from pruritus**

PATIENT GOAL 1: Will maintain skin integrity

NURSING INTERVENTIONS/*RATIONALES*

Keep nails short and clean *to minimize trauma and secondary infection*

Apply mittens or elbow restraints *to prevent scratching*

Dress in lightweight, loose, and nonirritating clothing *because overheating increases itching*

Cover affected areas (long sleeves, pants, one-piece outfit) *to prevent scratching*

Bathe in cool water with no soap or apply cool compresses

Apply soothing lotions (sparingly on open lesions *because absorption of drug is increased) to decrease pruritus*

Avoid exposure to heat or sun, *which can aggravate rash* (e.g., chickenpox)

EXPECTED OUTCOME
Skin remains intact

NURSING DIAGNOSIS ■ **Altered family processes related to child with an acute illness**

PATIENT (FAMILY) GOAL 1: Will receive adequate emotional support

NURSING INTERVENTIONS/*RATIONALES*

Inform parents of treatment options, especially acyclovir for varicella

Reinforce family's effort to carry out plan of care

Provide assistance when necessary, such as visiting nurse *to help with home care*

Keep family aware of child's progress *to encourage optimistic attitude*

Stress rapidity of recovery in most cases *to decrease anxiety*

EXPECTED OUTCOMES
Family continues to comply with expectations
Family seeks needed support

BOX 14-1 ■ Clinical Manifestations of Conjunctivitis

BACTERIAL CONJUNCTIVITIS ("PINK EYE")
Purulent drainage
Crusting of eyelids, especially on awakening
Inflamed conjunctiva
Swollen lids

VIRAL CONJUNCTIVITIS
Usually occurs with upper respiratory tract infection
Serous (watery) drainage
Inflamed conjunctiva
Swollen lids

ALLERGIC CONJUNCTIVITIS
Itching
Watery to thick, stringy discharge
Inflamed conjunctiva
Swollen lids

CONJUNCTIVITIS CAUSED BY FOREIGN BODY
Tearing
Pain
Inflamed conjunctiva
Usually only one eye affected

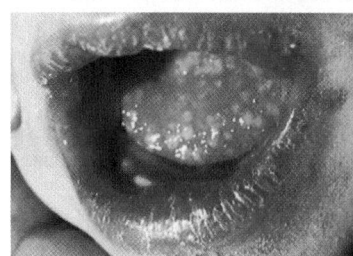

FIG. 14-7 ■ Primary gingivostomatitis. (From Thompson JM and others: *Clinical nursing*, St Louis, 1986, Mosby.)

on the mucosa, causing severe pain (Fig. 14-7). Cervical lymphadenitis often occurs, and the breath has a distinctly foul odor. The disease can last 5 to 14 days with varying degrees of severity.

Therapeutic Management

Treatment for both types of stomatitis is aimed at relief of symptoms, primarily pain. Acetaminophen is usually sufficient for mild cases, but with more severe HGS, stronger analgesics such as codeine may be needed. A mixture of equal parts of diphenhydramine (Benadryl) elixir and Maalox, applied topically, provides mild analgesia, antiinflammatory action, and a protective coating for the lesions. Sucralfate can also be used as a coating agent for oral mucus membranes (Zempsky and Schechter, 2000). Specific treatment for children with severe cases of HGS is the use of acyclovir (Zovirax) (Patel and Sciubba, 2003).

Nursing Considerations

The chief nursing goals for children with stomatitis are relief of pain and prevention of spread of the herpes virus. Analgesics and topical anesthetics are used as needed to provide relief, especially before meals to encourage food and fluid

absence of vesicles, and no systemic illness. The ulcers persist for 4 to 12 days and heal uneventfully.

Herpetic gingivostomatitis (HGS) is caused by HSV, most often type 1, and may occur as a primary infection or recur in a less severe form known as recurrent herpes labialis (commonly called "cold sores" or "fever blisters"). The primary infection usually begins with a fever; the pharynx becomes edematous and erythematous; and vesicles erupt

intake. Drinking bland fluids through a straw is helpful in avoiding the painful lesions. Mouth care is encouraged; the use of a very soft bristle toothbrush or disposable foam-tipped toothbrush provides gentle cleaning near ulcerated areas.

Careful handwashing is essential when caring for children with HGS. Because the infection is autoinoculable, children should keep their fingers out of the mouth; contaminated hands can infect other body parts. Very young children may require elbow restraints to ensure compliance. Articles placed in the mouth are cleaned thoroughly. Newborns and individuals with immunosuppression should not be exposed to infected children.

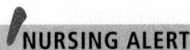
NURSING ALERT

When examining herpetic lesions, wear gloves. The virus easily enters breaks in the skin and can cause herpetic whitlow of the fingers.

Because herpes infection is often associated with sexual transmission, the nurse should explain to parents and older children that HGS is usually caused by type 1 HSV, the type not associated with sexual activity.

INTESTINAL PARASITIC DISEASES

Intestinal parasitic diseases, including helminths (worms) and protozoa, constitute the most frequent infections in the world. In the United States the incidence of intestinal parasitic disease, especially giardiasis, has increased among young children who attend day care centers. Young children are especially at risk because of typical hand-mouth activity and uncontrolled fecal activity.

Intestinal parasitic diseases in humans are caused by various infecting organisms. This discussion is limited to the two most common parasitic infections among children in the United States: giardiasis and pinworms. Table 14-2 de-

TABLE 14-2 ■ Selected Intestinal Parasites

CLINICAL MANIFESTATIONS	COMMENTS
ASCARIASIS—*ASCARIS LUMBRICOIDES* (COMMON ROUNDWORM)	
Light infections: asymptomatic	Transferred to mouth by way of contaminated food, fingers, or toys
Heavy infections: anorexia, irritability, nervousness, enlarged abdomen, weight loss, fever, intestinal colic	Largest of the intestinal helminths
Severe infections: intestinal obstruction, appendicitis, perforation of intestine with peritonitis, obstructive jaundice, lung involvement—pneumonitis	Affects principally young children 1-4 years of age
	Prevalent in warm climates
HOOKWORM DISEASE—*NECATOR AMERICANUS*	
Light infections in well-nourished individuals: no problems	Transmitted by discharging eggs on the soil, which are picked up, causing infection from direct skin contact with contaminated soil
Heavier infections: mild to severe anemia, malnutrition	Wearing shoes is recommended, although children playing in contaminated soil expose many skin surfaces
May be itching and burning followed by erythema and a papular eruption in areas to which the organism migrates	
STRONGYLOIDIASIS—*STRONGYLOIDES STERCORALIS* (THREADWORM)	
Light infection: asymptomatic	Transmission is same as for hookworm except autoinfection common
Heavy infection: respiratory signs and symptoms; abdominal pain, distention; nausea and vomiting; diarrhea—large, pale stools, often with mucus	Older children and adults affected more often than young children
Threat to life in children with weakened immunologic defenses	Severe infections may lead to severe nutritional deficiency
VISCERAL LARVA MIGRANS—*TOXOCARA CANIS* (DOGS); INTESTINAL TOXOCARIASIS—*TOXOCARA CATI* (CATS)	
Depends on reactivity of infected individual	Transmitted by direct contamination of hands from contact with dog, cat, or objects or by ingestion of soil
May be asymptomatic except for eosinophilia	Dogs and cats should be kept away from areas where children play; sandboxes are especially important transmission areas
Specific diagnosis difficult	Periodic deworming of diagnosed dogs and cats
	Control of dog and cat population
TRICHURIASIS—*TRICHURIS TRICHIURA* (WHIPWORM)	
Light infections: asymptomatic	Transmitted from contaminated soil, vegetables, toys, and other objects
Heavy infections: abdominal pain and distention, diarrhea	Most frequent in warm, moist climates
	Occurs most often in undernourished children living in unsanitary conditions

scribes the outstanding features of selected helminths that belong to the family of nematodes.

GENERAL NURSING CONSIDERATIONS

Nursing responsibilities related to intestinal parasitic infections involve assistance with identification of the parasite, treatment of the infection, and prevention of initial infection or reinfection. Identification of the organism is accomplished by laboratory examination of substances containing the worm, its larvae, or ova. Most are identified by examining fecal smears from the stools of persons suspected of harboring the parasite. Fresh specimens are best for revealing parasites or larvae; therefore, collected specimens should be taken directly to the laboratory for examination. If this is not feasible, the specimen is placed in a container with a preservative. Parents need clear instructions on obtaining an adequate sample and the number of samples required. (See Stool Specimens, Chapter 22.) In most parasitic infections, examination of other family members, especially children, may be carried out to identify those who are similarly affected.

After the diagnosis is confirmed and appropriate treatment is planned, parents need further explanation and reinforcement. Compliance in terms of drug therapy and other measures, such as thorough handwashing, are essential for eradication of the parasite. The family needs to understand the nature of transmission and that in some cases the medication must be repeated in 2 weeks to 1 month to kill organisms hatched since initial treatment.

The nurse's most important function is preventive education of children and families regarding hygiene and health habits. Thorough handwashing before eating or handling food and after using the toilet is the most important precautionary method. Other preventive practices are listed in the Family Home Care box.

FAMILY HOME CARE

Preventing Intestinal Parasitic Disease

Always wash hands and fingernails with soap and water before eating and handling food and after toileting.

Avoid placing fingers in mouth and biting nails.

Discourage children from scratching bare anal area.

Use superabsorbent disposable diapers to prevent leakage.

Change diapers as soon as soiled and dispose of diapers in closed receptacle out of children's reach.

Do not rinse diapers in toilet.

Disinfect toilet seats and diaper-changing areas; use dilute household bleach (10% solution) or Lysol and wipe clean with paper towels.

Drink water that is specially treated, especially if camping.

Wash all raw fruits and vegetables and food that has fallen on the floor.

Avoid growing foods in soil fertilized with human excreta.

Teach children to defecate only in a toilet, not on the ground.

Keep dogs and cats away from playgrounds or sandboxes.

Avoid swimming in pools frequented by diapered children.

Wear shoes outside.

GIARDIASIS

Giardiasis is caused by the protozoan *Giardia lamblia* (also called *Giardia intestinalis*, *Giardia duodenalis*, and *Lamblia intestinalis*). It is the most common intestinal parasitic pathogen in the United States. Childcare centers are common sties for urban giardiasis, and the children may pass cysts for months. Giardia should also be considered in those with a history of recent travel to an endemic area (Pickering, 2004).

The potential for transmission is great, because the cysts—the nonmotile stage of the protozoa—can survive in the environment for months. Chief modes of transmission are person to person; water, especially mountain lakes, streams, and pools frequented by diapered infants; food; and animals, especially puppies. In children, person-to-person transmission is the most likely cause. Although individuals infected with giardiasis may be asymptomatic, common symptoms include abdominal cramps and diarrhea (Box 14-2).

Diagnosis of giardiasis may be made by microscopic examination of stool specimens or duodenal fluid, or by identification of *G. lamblia* antigens in these specimens by techniques such as enzyme immunoassay (EIA). Because the *Giardia* organisms live in the upper intestine and are excreted in a highly variable pattern, repeated microscopic examination of stool specimens may be required to identify trophozoites (active parasites) or cysts. Duodenal specimens are obtained by direct aspiration, biopsy, or the *string* test. In the string test, the child swallows a gelatin capsule with a nylon string attached. Several hours later, the string is withdrawn and the contents are sent for laboratory analysis. With the availability of EIA techniques to identify *Giardia* antigens in stool specimens, other tests are being used less often.

Therapeutic Management

The drugs available for treatment of giardiasis are quinacrine (Atabrine), furazolidone (Furoxone), and metronidazole (Flagyl). The drug of choice is furazolidone, unless cost is a factor, in which case quinacrine is substituted. Quinacrine is less than one-tenth the cost of furazolidone, and its long-term

BOX 14-2 ■ Clinical Manifestations of Giardiasis

Infants and young children:
  Diarrhea
  Vomiting
  Anorexia
  Failure to thrive
Children older than 5 years of age:
  Abdominal cramps
  Intermittent loose stools
  Constipation
  Stools may be malodorous, watery, pale, and greasy
Most infections resolve spontaneously in 4 to 6 weeks
Rarely, chronic form occurs:
  Intermittent loose, foul-smelling stools
  Possibility of abdominal bloating, flatulence, sulfur-tasting belches, epigastric pain, vomiting, headache, and weight loss

safety is established over the use of metronidazole. For pregnant women who need treatment, paromomycin may be used first, followed by metronidazole if the initial treatment is unsuccessful (Mileno, 2003). Unfortunately, quinacrine has the highest frequency of side effects, especially nausea and vomiting; temporary yellow staining of the skin, sclera, and urine; and a very bitter taste.

Nursing Considerations

The most important nursing consideration is prevention of giardiasis, especially among children and staff of day care centers. Attention to meticulous sanitary practices, especially during diaper changes, is essential (see Family Home Care box and Fig. 14-8). Nurses can play an important role in educating day care staff regarding appropriate sanitation practices (see Preschool and Kindergarten Experience, Chapter 13).

After children are infected, family education regarding drug administration is essential. Parents often need suggestions for encouraging the child to take quinacrine. If other household members are infected, the nurse should inquire about their understanding and management of the disease.

To decrease the side effects of quinacrine and increase its palatability, crush tablets and mix them with a strong flavoring such as jam or syrup and administer the drug with or after meals

ENTEROBIASIS (PINWORMS)

Enterobiasis, or pinworms, caused by the nematode *Enterobius vermicularis,* is the most common helminthic infection in the United States. It is universally present in temperate climatic zones and may infect more than 30% of all children at any one time. Crowded conditions, such as in classrooms and day care centers, favor transmission.

Infection begins when the eggs are ingested or inhaled (the eggs float in the air). The eggs hatch in the upper intestine, then mature and migrate through the intestine. After mating, adult females migrate out the anus and lay eggs (American Academy of Pediatrics, 2003). The movement of the worms on skin and mucous membrane surfaces causes intense itching. As the child scratches, eggs are deposited on the hands and underneath the fingernails. The typical hand-to-mouth activity of youngsters makes them especially prone to reinfection. Pinworm eggs persist in the indoor environment for 2 to 3 weeks, contaminating anything they contact, such as toilet seats, doorknobs, bed linen, underwear, and food. Except for the intense rectal itching associated with pinworms, the clinical manifestations (Box 14-3) are nonspecific.

Diagnostic Evaluation

Diagnosis is most commonly made from the tape test (see Nursing Considerations). Repeated tests to collect eggs may be necessary, and if there is a possibility that other family members may be infected, a tape test should be performed on them.

Therapeutic Management

The drugs available for treatment of pinworms include mebendazole (Vermox), pyrantel pamoate (Antiminth), piperazine phosphate, and pyrvinium pamoate (Povan). The drug of choice is mebendazole, which is safe, effective, and convenient, with few side effects. However, it is not recommended for children younger than 2 years of age. If pyrvinium pamoate is prescribed, parents are advised that the drug stains stool and vomitus bright red, as well as clothing or skin that comes in contact with the drug. Because pinworms are easily transmitted, all household members are treated. The drugs should be repeated in 2 weeks to prevent reinfection.

Nursing Considerations

Nursing care is directed at identifying the parasite, eradicating the organism, and preventing reinfection. Parents need clear, detailed instructions for the *tape test.* A loop of transparent (not "frosted" or "magic") tape, sticky side out, is placed around the end of a tongue depressor, which is then firmly pressed against the child's perianal area. A

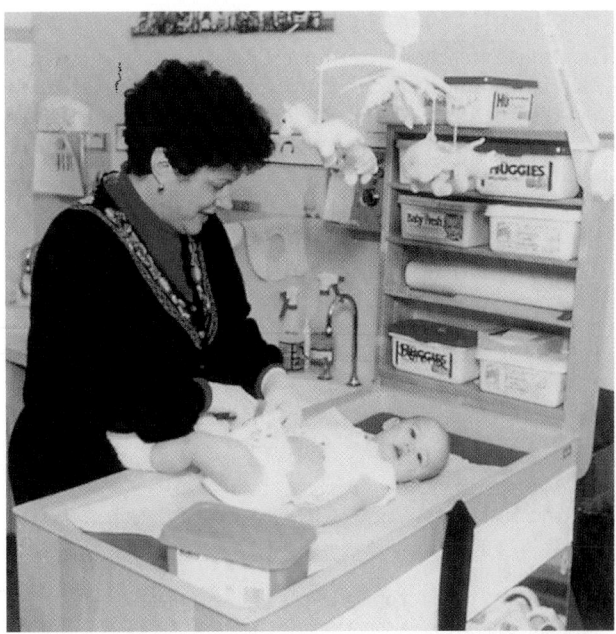

FIG. 14-8 ■ Prevention of giardiasis, especially in day care centers, requires sanitary practices during diaper changes, such as discarding paper diapers in a covered receptacle, changing paper covers on the diaper-changing surface, and having facilities for handwashing nearby. NOTE: Soiled cloth diapers and clothing should be stored in a plastic bag for transport home.

BOX 14-3 ■ Clinical Manifestations of Pinworms

Intense perianal itching (principal symptom); evidence of itching in young children includes the following:
  General irritability
  Restlessness
  Poor sleep
  Bed-wetting
  Distractibility
  Short attention span
Perianal dermatitis and excoriation secondary to itching
If worms migrate, possible vaginal and urethral infection

convenient, commercially prepared tape is also available for this purpose. Pinworm specimens are collected in the morning as soon as the child awakens and *before* the child has a bowel movement or bathes. The procedure may need to be performed more than once before eggs are collected. Parents are instructed to place the tongue blade in a glass jar or loosely in a plastic bag so that it can be brought in for microscopic examination. For specimens collected in the hospital, practitioner's office, or clinic, the tape is placed smoothly on a glass slide, sticky side down, for examination.

Adherence to the drug regimen is usually excellent, because the duration of treatment is typically only one dose. However, the family is reminded of the need to take a second dose in 2 weeks. Posting a reminder on the refrigerator door or bathroom mirror is helpful.

To prevent reinfection, washing all clothes and bed linens in hot water and vacuuming the house may be recommended. However, there is little documentation on the effectiveness of these measures, because pinworms survive on many surfaces. Helpful suggestions include handwashing after toileting and before eating, keeping the child's fingernails short to minimize the chance of ova collecting under the nails, dressing children in one-piece sleeping outfits, and daily showering rather than tub bathing. Families should be informed that recurrence is common. Repeated infections should be treated in the same manner as the first one.

INGESTION OF INJURIOUS AGENTS

Since the passage of the Poison Prevention Packaging Act of 1970, which requires that certain potentially hazardous drugs and household products be sold in child-resistant containers, the incidence of poisonings in children has decreased dramatically. However, despite these advances, poisoning remains a significant health concern, with most cases occurring in children younger than 6 years of age. Although pharmaceuticals such as analgesics, cough and cold preparations, topical preparations, antibiotics, vitamins, gastrointestinal preparations, hormones, and antihistamines are frequently the agents of poisonings, children may be poisoned by a variety of substances. The most frequently ingested poisons include (Litovitz and others, 2000; Powers, 2000):

- Cosmetics and personal care products (perfume, cologne, aftershave)*
- Cleaning products (hypochlorite ["household"] bleach, pine oil disinfectants)
- Plants (nontoxic gastrointestinal irritants, oxalates; Box 14-4: Poisonous and Nonpoisonous Plants)
- Foreign bodies, toys, and miscellaneous substances (desiccants, thermometers, bubble-blowing solutions)

More than 90% of poisonings occur in the home, although a significant number take place elsewhere, such as in a grandparent's or friend's home, in a school, or in a health care facility.

---

*The most common substances in each category are in parentheses. Substances ingested are not necessarily most toxic but often represent ready availability.

The following five commonly used and easily available drugs (first four are over-the-counter products) can cause serious or fatal consequences if as little as ¼ teaspoon or ½ tablet is ingested: methyl salicylate, camphor, topical imidazolines (sympathomimetics such as those contained in Visine, Afrin, Otrivin, and Clear Eyes), benzocaine, and diphenoxylate-atropine (Lomotil and others). Stress to parents the importance of keeping such drugs away from children. If these agents are ingested, advise parents to seek medical treatment immediately. Emesis should not be induced at home.

The developmental characteristics of young children predispose them to poisoning by ingestion. Infants and toddlers explore their environment through oral experimentation. Because the sense of taste is not discriminating at this age, many unpalatable substances are ingested. In addition, toddlers and preschoolers are developing autonomy and initiative, which increase their curiosity and noncompliant behavior. Imitation is also a powerful motivator, especially when combined with lack of awareness of danger.

This section is primarily concerned with the immediate emergency treatment of ingestion of injurious agents. Specific

BOX 14-4 ■ Poisonous and Nonpoisonous Plants

POISONOUS PLANTS	TOXIC PARTS	NONPOISONOUS PLANTS
Apple	Leaves, seeds	African violet
Apricot	Leaves, stem, seed pits	Aluminum plant
Azalea	All parts	Asparagus fern
Buttercup	All parts	Begonia
Cherry (wild or cultivated)	Twigs, seeds, foliage	Boston fern
Daffodil	Bulbs	Christmas cactus
Dumb cane, Dieffenbachia	All parts	Coleus
Elephant ear	All parts	Gardenia
English ivy	All parts	Grape ivy
Foxglove	Leaves, seeds, flowers	Jade plant
Holly	Berries and leaves	Piggyback begonia
Hyacinth	Bulbs	Piggyback plant
Ivy	Leaves	Prayer plant
Mistletoe*	Berries, leaves	Rubber tree
Oak tree	Acorn, foliage	Snake plant
Philodendron	All parts	Spider plant
Plum	Pit	Swedish ivy
Poinsettia†		Wax plant
Poison ivy, poison oak	Leaves, stems, sap, fruit, stems, smoke from burning plants	Weeping fig
		Zebra plant
Pothos	All parts	
Rhubarb	Leaves	
Tulip	Bulbs	
Water hemlock	All parts	
Wisteria	Seeds, pods	
Yew	All parts	

*Eating one or two berries or leaves is probably nontoxic.
†Mildly toxic if ingested in massive quantities.

BOX 14-5 ■ Selected Poisonings in Children

CORROSIVES (STRONG ACIDS OR ALKALIS)
Drain, toilet, or oven cleaners
Electric dishwasher detergent (liquid, because of higher pH, is more hazardous than granular)
Mildew remover
Batteries
Clinitest tablets
Denture cleaners
Bleach

Clinical Manifestations
Severe burning pain in mouth, throat, and stomach
White, swollen mucous membranes; edema of lips, tongue, and pharynx (respiratory obstruction)
Violent vomiting (hemoptysis)
Drooling and inability to clear secretions
Signs of shock
Anxiety and agitation

Comments
Household bleach is a frequently ingested corrosive but rarely causes serious damage
Liquid corrosives cause more damage than granular preparations

Treatment
Inducing emesis is contraindicated (vomiting redamages the mucosa)
Dilute corrosive with water or milk (usually no more than 120 mL [4 ounces])
Do not neutralize. Neutralization can cause an exothermic reaction (which produces heat and causes increased symptoms or produces a thermal burn in addition to a chemical burn)
Maintain patent airway if needed
Administer analgesics
Do not allow oral intake
Esophageal stricture may require repeated dilations or surgery

HYDROCARBONS
Gasoline
Kerosene
Lamp oil
Mineral seal oil (found in furniture polish)
Lighter fluid
Turpentine
Paint thinner and remover (some types)

Clinical Manifestations
Gagging, choking, and coughing
Nausea
Vomiting
Alterations in sensorium, such as lethargy
Weakness
Respiratory symptoms of pulmonary involvement
    Tachypnea
    Cyanosis
    Retractions
    Grunting

Comments
Immediate danger is aspiration (even small amounts can cause bronchitis and chemical pneumonia)
Gasoline, kerosene, lighter fluid, mineral seal oil, and turpentine cause severe pneumonia

Treatment
Inducing emesis is generally contraindicated
Gastric decontamination and emptying are questionable, even when the hydrocarbon contains a heavy metal or pesticide; if gastric lavage must be performed, a cuffed endotracheal tube should be in place before lavage because of a high risk of aspiration
Symptomatic treatment of chemical pneumonia includes high humidity, oxygen, hydration, and antibiotics for secondary infection

ACETAMINOPHEN
Clinical Manifestations
Occurs in four stages:
1. Initial period (2 to 4 hours after ingestion)
    Nausea
    Vomiting
    Sweating
    Pallor
2. Latent period (24 to 36 hours)
    Patient improves
3. Hepatic involvement (may last up to 7 days and be permanent)
    Pain in right upper quadrant
    Jaundice
    Confusion
    Stupor
    Coagulation abnormalities
4. Patients who do not die in hepatic stage gradually recover

Comments
Most common drug poisoning in children
Occurs from acute ingestion
Toxic dose is 150 mg/kg or greater in children
Because of multiple formulations and concentrations, chronic acetaminophen toxicity is a significant problem
Parents should be counseled to read product packaging carefully and to consult a health care professional to avoid inappropriate dosing (Abruzzi and Stork, 2002)

Treatment
Antidote *N*-acetylcysteine (NAC) (Mucomyst) can usually be given orally but is first diluted in fruit juice or soda because of the antidote's offensive odor
Given as 1 loading dose and usually 17 maintenance doses in different dosages
May be given intravenously, but use is investigational

ASPIRIN (ACTEYLSALICYLIC ACID [ASA])
Clinical Manifestations
Acute poisoning
    Nausea
    Disorientation
    Vomiting
    Dehydration
    Diaphoresis
    Hyperpnea
    Hyperpyrexia
    Oliguria
    Tinnitus
    Coma
    Convulsions
Chronic poisoning
    Same as above but subtle onset (often mistaken for viral illness)
    Dehydration, coma, and seizures may be more severe
    Bleeding tendencies

BOX 14-5 ■ Selected Poisonings in Children—*cont'd*

Comments
May be caused by acute ingestion (severe toxicity occurs with 300 to 500 mg/kg)

May be caused by chronic ingestion (i.e., more than 100 mg/kg/day for 2 or more days); can be more serious than acute ingestion

Time to peak serum salicylate level can vary with enteric aspirin or the presence of concretions (bezoars)

Treatment
Hospitalization for severe toxicity

Emesis, lavage, activated charcoal, or cathartic

Lavage will not remove concretions of ASA

Activated charcoal is important early in ASA toxicity

Sodium bicarbonate transfusions to correct metabolic acidosis, and urinary alkalinization may be effective in enhancing elimination, urinary alkalinization is very difficult to achieve.

Be aware of the risk for fluid overload and pulmonary edema

External cooling for hyperpyrexia

Anticonvulsants

Oxygen and ventilation for respiratory depression

Vitamin K for bleeding

In severe cases, hemodialysis (not peritoneal dialysis) may be used

IRON
Mineral supplement or vitamin containing iron

Clinical Manifestations
Occurs in five stages:

1. Initial period (0.5 to 6 hours after ingestion; if child does not develop gastrointestinal symptoms in 6 hours, toxicity is unlikely)
   Vomiting
   Hematemesis
   Diarrhea
   Hematochezia (bloody stools)
   Gastric pain
2. Latency (2 to 12 hours)
   Patient improves
3. Systemic toxicity (4 to 24 hours after ingestion)
   Metabolic acidosis
   Fever
   Hyperglycemia
   Bleeding
   Shock
   Death (may occur)
4. Hepatic injury (48 to 96 hours)
   Seizures
   Coma
5. Rarely, pyloric stenosis develops at 2 to 5 weeks

Comments
Factors related to frequency of iron poisoning include:

Widespread availability

Packaging of large quantities in individual containers

Lack of parental awareness of iron toxicity

Resemblance of iron tablets to candy (e.g., M&Ms)

Toxic dose is based on the amount of elemental iron in various salts (sulfate, gluconate, fumarate), which ranges from 20% to 33%; ingestions of 60 mg/kg are considered dangerous

Treatment
Emesis or lavage

For toxic doses lavage may be necessary for all chewable tablets or liquids if spontaneous vomiting has not occurred

Chelation therapy with deferoxamine in severe intoxication (may turn urine a red to orange color)

If intravenous deferoxamine is given too rapidly, hypotension, facial flushing, rash, urticaria, tachycardia, and shock may occur; stop the infusion, maintain the intravenous line with normal saline, and notify the practitioner immediately

PLANTS
Plants listed in Box 14-4

Clinical Manifestations
Depends on type of plant ingested

May cause local irritation of oropharynx and entire gastrointestinal tract

May cause respiratory, renal, and central nervous system symptoms

Topical contact with plants can cause dermatitis

Comments
Some of most frequently ingested substances

Rarely cause serious problems, although some plant ingestions can be fatal

Can also cause choking and allergic reactions

Treatment
Induce emesis

Wash from skin or eyes

Supportive care as needed

---

management of corrosive, hydrocarbon, acetaminophen, salicylate, plant, and iron poisoning is summarized in Box 14-5. Because of the importance of lead poisoning among young children, ingestion of lead is discussed separately. Appropriate suggestions for poison prevention are discussed on p. 455 and in Chapter 12.

PRINCIPLES OF EMERGENCY TREATMENT

A poisoning may or may not require emergency intervention, but in every instance medical evaluation is necessary to initiate appropriate action. Parents are advised to call the **Poison Control Center (PCC)** *before* initiating any intervention. The local PCC telephone number (usually listed in the front of the telephone directory) should be posted near each phone in the house.* (See Critical Thinking Exercise and Emergency Treatment box.)

Based on the initial telephone assessment, the PCC counsels the parents to begin treatment at home or to take the child to an emergency facility. When a call is taken, the name and telephone number of the caller is recorded to reestablish contact if the connection is interrupted. Because

---

*Also available by calling (800) 222-1222 or online at **American Association of Poison Control Centers:** www.aapcc.org.

CRITICAL THINKING EXERCISE

Poisoning

Mrs. Berry, a neighbor, calls you. She is very upset because her 2-year-old son has eaten several chewable multivitamins with iron. She asks you if she should give her son syrup of ipecac. What should you advise her to do?

QUESTIONS

1. Evidence—Is there sufficient evidence to formulate an answer for Mrs. Berry?
2. Assumptions—Describe some underlying assumptions about the following:
   a. What is the best initial response when a child ingests a potentially poisonous substance?
   b. What is syrup of ipecac?
   c. What are the dangers involved in the use of syrup of ipecac?
3. What is the priority for nursing care at this time?
4. Does the evidence support your conclusion?
5. What alternative perspectives might you have?

ANSWERS

1. Yes, there is sufficient evidence to formulate an answer for Mrs. Berry.
2. a. When a child ingests a poisonous substance, the initial goal is to remove the poison. Specific actions that are taken to remove poisons include inducing vomiting, administering activated charcoal to adsorb the toxin, and performing gastric lavage.
   b. Syrup of ipecac is an emetic that induces vomiting by producing an irritant effect on the gastric mucosa. In the past, syrup of ipecac was recommended for home treatment of some cases of ingestion. However, ipecac is no longer recommended for routine home treatment of poisoning.
   c. Syrup of ipecac is contraindicated when a corrosive substance or a hydrocarbon has been ingested or in cases when a child is comatose or having seizures.
3. The first priority for nursing care is to advise Mrs. Berry to call the Poison Control Center immediately to obtain guidance. Each ingestion is treated individually, and information from the Poison Control Center is essential to determine the most appropriate action. The most toxic ingredient in a chewable multivitamin is iron, which produces symptoms after several hours. Therefore, treatment, if needed, should begin long before symptoms appear.
4. Yes, there is sufficient information to formulate an answer for Mrs. Berry.
5. This situation is very straightforward, and the response is easily derived from the information. No other alternative perspectives are apparent at this time.

---

most poisonings are managed in the home, expert advice is essential in minimizing adverse effects. When the exact quantity or type of ingested toxin is not known, admission to a hospital for laboratory evaluation and surveillance is critical during the time after ingestion.

Assessment

The first and most important principle in dealing with a poisoning is to treat the child first, not the poison. This necessitates an immediate concern for life support. Vital signs are taken and respiratory or circulatory support is instituted as needed. The victim's condition is routinely reevaluated. Be-

EMERGENCY TREATMENT
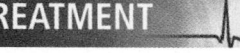

Poisoning

1. Assess the victim:
   Take vital signs; reevaluate routinely.
   Initiate cardiorespiratory support if needed.
   Treat other symptoms, such as seizures.
2. Terminate exposure:
   Empty mouth of pills, plant parts, or other material.
   Flush eyes continuously with normal saline (room-temperature tap water at home) for 15 to 20 minutes.
   Flush skin and wash with soap and a soft cloth; remove contaminated clothes, especially if a pesticide, acid, alkali, or hydrocarbon is involved.
   Bring victim of an inhalation poisoning into fresh air.
   Give one sip of water to dilute ingested poison.
3. Identify the poison:
   Question the victim and witnesses.
   Look for environmental cues (empty container, nearby spill, odor on breath) and save all evidence of poison (container, vomitus, urine).
   Be alert to signs and symptoms of potential poisoning in absence of other evidence, including symptoms of ocular or dermal exposure.
   Call Poison Control Center or other competent emergency facility for immediate advice regarding treatment.
4. Remove poison and prevent absorption:
   Place child in side-lying, sitting, or kneeling position with head below chest to prevent aspiration.
   Administer activated charcoal if ordered (unless used repeatedly, usual dose is 1 g/kg unless amount of toxin is known).

---

cause shock is a complication of several types of household poisons, particularly corrosives, measures to reduce the effects of shock, such as elevation of the legs and head to the level of the heart to promote venous drainage and provision of warmth and rest, are important. Maintenance of respiratory function may require insertion of an airway or mechanical ventilation.

The emergency department nurse's responsibility is to be prepared for immediate intervention with all of the necessary equipment. Because time and speed are critical factors in recovery from serious poisonings, anticipation of potential problems and complications means the difference between life and death.

Gastric Decontamination

In general, the immediate treatment is to remove the ingested poison by adsorbing the toxin with activated charcoal, performing gastric lavage, or increasing bowel motility (catharsis). Because of continuing controversy regarding the use of these methods, each toxic ingestion should be treated individually (Abruzzi and Stork, 2002). Specific antidotes may be administered for certain poisonings. *Syrup of ipecac,* an emetic that exerts its action through irritation of the gastric mucosa and by stimulation of the vomiting center, is no longer recommended for immediate treatment at home. The American Academy of Pediatrics (AAP), 2003b) recommends that existing ipecac in the home should be disposed of safely and that the first action for a caregiver of a child who may have ingested a toxic substance is to consult the local PCC. If the Poison Control Center cannot be reached, the child should be taken to the nearest emergency department.

! NURSING ALERT

Syrup of ipecac is contraindicated in cases of ingestion of corrosive substances and in the child who is comatose or having seizures. In children who have ingested hydrocarbons, ipecac is contraindicated if the risk of aspiration outweighs the benefit of gastric evacuation. Ipecac may cause prolonged vomiting (enduring as long as 12 hours), which makes it relatively contraindicated in ingestions that may cause sedation, coma, or seizures (Powers, 2000).

No emetic or other substance should be given at home without consultation with a PCC or physician.

If the child is admitted to an emergency facility, *gastric lavage* may be performed to empty the stomach of the toxic agent. Lavage is indicated for young infants in whom ipecac is contraindicated; if the patient is comatose or convulsing or requires a protected airway; or if the ingested poison is rapidly absorbed (strychnine or cyanide). The use of lavage in petroleum distillate poisoning remains controversial because of the danger of aspiration. When lavage is performed, the largest-diameter tube that can be inserted is used to facilitate passage of gastric contents.

Another method of decontaminating the stomach is the use of *activated charcoal,* an odorless, tasteless, fine black powder that adsorbs many compounds, creating a stable complex. In the future, activated charcoal may replace syrup of ipecac as the home remedy of choice (Ford, 2001), but the AAP (2003b) believes it is premature to recommend the administration of activated charcoal in the home. Activated charcoal is mixed with water or a saline cathartic to form a slurry. Slurries are neither gritty nor distasteful but resemble black mud. To increase the child's acceptance of activated charcoal, the nurse should mix it with diet soda and serve it through a straw in an opaque container with a cover (such as a disposable coffee cup and lid) or an ordinary cup covered with aluminum foil or placed inside a small paper bag. Potential complications from the use of activated charcoal include aspiration (usually in patients with impaired gag reflexes), constipation, and intestinal obstruction (in multiple doses). Cathartics, such as sorbitol, sodium, or magnesium, may be administered to stimulate evacuation of the bowel, thus decreasing systemic absorption of the poison and aiding in the removal of the charcoal. Many commercial preparations of activated charcoal contain cathartics. However, the use of cathartics is controversial.

In a minority of poisonings, specific *antidotes* are available to counteract the poison. They are highly effective and should be available in all emergency facilities. The supply of antidotes should be checked routinely and replaced as used or according to expiration dates. Among the more frequently employed antidotes are *N*-acetylcysteine for acetaminophen poisoning, oxygen for carbon monoxide inhalation, naloxone for opioid overdose, flumazenil (Romazicon) for benzodiazepine (Valium, Versed) overdose, Digibind for digoxin toxicity, and antivenin for certain poisonous bites.

FAMILY FOCUS

Poisoning

A poisoning is more than a physical emergency for the child—it usually represents an emotional crisis for the parents, particularly in terms of guilt, self-reproach, and insecurity in the parenting role. The emergency department is no place to admonish the family for negligence, lack of appropriate supervision, or failure to injury-proof the home. Rather, it is a time to calm and support the child and parents, while unaccusingly exploring the circumstances of the injury. If the nurse prematurely attempts to discuss ways of preventing such an incident from recurring, the parents' anxiety will block out any suggestions or offered guidance. Therefore, it is preferable for the nurse to delay the discussion until the child's condition is stabilized or, if the child is discharged immediately after emergency treatment, to make a public health referral or send a packet of information.

Prevention of Recurrence

The ultimate objective is to prevent poisonings from occurring or recurring. One effective counseling method is first to discuss the difficulties of constantly watching and safeguarding young children (see Family Focus box). In this way the challenging task of raising children can lead to a discussion of injury prevention as part of the parental role. This approach also incorporates contributory causes for the incident, such as inadequate support systems, marital discord, discipline techniques (especially use of physical punishment), and maternal distress. A visit to the home, especially after a repeat poisoning situation, is recommended as part of the follow-up care to assess hazards, including family factors, and to evaluate appropriate injury-proofing measures. One method of identifying risk areas is to ask specific questions or to have the parent complete a questionnaire designed to isolate factors that predispose children to poisoning.

Another approach is to encourage parents to bend down to the child's eye level and survey the home environment for potential hazards. Have the parents try to open cabinets and reach shelves to access poisons.

Passive measures (those that do not require active participation) have been the most successful in preventing poisoning and include child-resistant closures and limiting the number of tablets in one container. However, these measures alone are not sufficient to prevent poisoning, because most toxic agents in the home do not have safety closures. Therefore, *active measures* (those that require participation) are essential. Guidelines for preventing the occurrence or recurrence of a poisoning are listed in the Guidelines box.

HEAVY METAL POISONING

Heavy metal poisoning can occur from the ingestion of a variety of substances, the most common being lead. Other sources that are important in terms of children are iron and mercury. *Mercury toxicity,* a rare form of heavy metal poisoning, has occurred in children from a variety of sources, such as broken thermometers or thermostats, broken fluorescent lights, and interior latex house paint (Etzel, 2000). Elemental mercury (also called metallic mercury or quicksilver) is nontoxic if ingested and if the gastrointestinal tract

GUIDELINES

Poison Prevention

Assess possible contributing factors in occurrence of injury, such as discipline, parent-child relationship, developmental ability, environmental factors, and behavior problems.

Institute anticipatory guidance for possible future injuries based on child's age and maturational level.

Refer to visiting nurse agency to evaluate home environment and need for injury-proofing measures.

Provide assistance with environmental manipulation when necessary, such as lead removal.

Educate parents regarding safe storage of toxic substances.

Advise parents to take drugs out of sight of children.

Teach children the hazards of ingesting nonfood items.

Advise parents against using plants for teas or medicine.

Discuss problems of discipline and children's noncompliance and offer strategies for effective discipline.

Instruct parents regarding correct administration of drugs for therapeutic purposes and to discontinue drug if there is evidence of mild toxicity.

Advise parents to contact the Poison Control Center or practitioner immediately when a poisoning occurs.

Post number of regional Poison Control Center with emergency phone list by telephone.

Include by the telephone the home address with nearest cross street in case an ambulance is needed. (In an emergency, family members may not remember the house address, and baby-sitters may not be aware of the information.)

BOX 14-6 ■ Sources of Lead*

Lead-based paint in deteriorating condition
Lead solder
Lead crystal
Battery casings
Lead fishing sinkers
Lead curtain weights
Lead bullets
Some of these may contain lead:
  Ceramic ware
  Water
  Pottery
  Pewter
  Dyes
  Industrial factories
  Vinyl mini-blinds
  Playground equipment
  Collectible toys
  Artists' paints
  Pool cue chalk
Occupations and hobbies involving lead:
  Battery and aircraft manufacturing
  Lead smelting
  Brass foundry work
  Radiator repair
  Construction work
  Bridge repair work
  Painting contracting
  Mining
  Ceramics work
  Stained-glass making
  Jewelry making

*The U.S. Consumers Product Safety Commission issues alerts and recalls for products that contain lead and that may unexpectedly pose a hazard to young children.

is healthy (e.g., has no fistulas). However, mercury is volatile at room temperature and enters the bloodstream after it is inhaled, causing toxicity (tremors, memory loss, insomnia, gingivitis, diarrhea, anorexia, weight loss). The classic form of mercury poisoning is called *acrodynia* (or "painful extremities").

! NURSING ALERT

Mercury thermometers are no longer recommended for use because, if broken, the inhaled vapors can cause toxicity. To prevent inhalation, spilled mercury must be cleaned up quickly, using disposable towels and rubber gloves and washing the hands well after removing the spill.

Heavy metals have an affinity for certain essential tissue chemicals, which must remain free for adequate cell functioning. When metals are bound to these substances, cellular enzyme systems are inactivated. Treatment involves *chelation,* use of a chemical compound that combines with the metal for rapid and safe excretion.

LEAD POISONING

Poisoning from lead has been a problem throughout history and throughout the world. In the United States the problem began in the early 1900s when white lead was added to paints and when tetraethyl lead was added to gasoline as an antiknock compound. Lead content in paint was decreased in 1950, and in 1978 the use of lead in household paint was banned. The greatest problems remaining for young children are the presence of deteriorating lead-based paint in many older homes and the soil in yards that has a high lead

content. Chipping, flaking, and chalking lead-based paint contributes to the environmental dust found in households. Normal hand-to-mouth behavior, coupled with the presence of lead dust in the environment, is the most common method of poisoning (Jacob and others, 2000).

Independent risk factors for having an elevated blood lead level include poverty, age less than 6 years, African-American ethnicity, and dwelling in the city (Markowitz, 2000). Any child, however, is at risk for becoming lead poisoned if hazardous conditions for lead are present in their environment.

Causes of Lead Poisoning

Although there are numerous sources of lead (Box 14-6), in most instances of acute childhood lead poisoning, the source is nonintact lead-based paint in an older home or lead-contaminated bare soil in the yard. Microparticles of lead gain entrance into a child's body through ingestion or inhalation and, in the case of an exposed pregnant woman, by placental transfer. Inhalation exposure usually occurs during renovation and remodeling activities in the home, while ingestion happens during normal day-to-day play and mouthing activities. Sometimes a child will actually swallow loose chips of lead-based paint because it has a sweet taste. Water and food may also be contaminated with lead.

Nurses must be aware of their patients' cultural and ethnic practices and product use. Substances used as natural

CULTURAL AWARENESS

Sources of Lead

In some cultures the use of traditional ethnic remedies that contain lead may increase children's risk of lead poisoning. These remedies include:

Azarcon (Mexico)—For digestive problems; a bright orange powder; usual dose is 0.25 to 1 teaspoon, often mixed with oil, milk, or sugar or sometimes given as a tea; sometimes a pinch is added to a baby bottle or tortilla dough for preventive purposes

Greta (Mexico)—A yellow-orange powder, used in the same way as azarcon

Paylooah (Southeast Asia)—Used for rash or fever; an orange-red powder given as 0.5 teaspoon straight or in a tea

Surma (India)—Black powder applied to the inner lower eyelid that is used as a cosmetic to improve eyesight

Unknown ayurvedic (Tibet)—Small, gray-brown balls used to improve slow development; two balls are given orally three times a day.

Tamarindo jellied, fruit candy (Mexico)—Fruit candy packaged in ceramic jars (which are lead-contaminated).

Lozeena (Iraq)—A bright orange powder used by Iraqis to color meat and rice.

Modified from Lead poisoning associated with use of traditional ethnic remedies—California, 1991-1992, *MMWR* 42(27):521-524, 1993; Lead poisoning associated with imported candy and powdered food coloring—California and Michigan, *MMWR* 47(48):1041-1043, 1998.

therapies have been found to contain lead (see Cultural Awareness box).

Pathophysiology and Clinical Manifestations

Lead can affect any part of the body, including the renal, hematologic, and neurologic systems (Fig. 14-9). Of most concern for young children is the developing brain and nervous system, which is more vulnerable than that of an older child or adult. Lead in the body moves via an equilibration process between the blood, the soft tissues and organs, and the bones and teeth. At the cellular level it competes with molecules of calcium, interfering with the regulating action of calcium. The inorganic lead found in lead-based paint is not fat-soluble and consequently should not cross the blood-brain barrier. However, it does so by impairing the endothelial cells there. Lead interferes with several neurotransmitter mechanisms in the brain. Massive body burdens of lead can lead to cerebral edema and encephalopathy.

Lead can also interfere with the binding of iron onto the heme molecule. This sometimes creates a picture of anemia, even though the child is not iron deficient. Lead toxicity to the erythrocytes leads to the release of the enzyme erythrocyte protoporphyrin (EP). Because EP is not sensitive to blood lead levels of less than about 16 to 25 μg/dL, it is no longer used as a screening test. However, elevation of the EP level (above 35 μg/dL of whole blood) is a good indicator of toxicity from lead and reflects the length of exposure and body burden of lead in the individual child.

Diagnostic Evaluation

Children with lead poisoning rarely have symptoms, even at levels requiring chelation therapy. A diagnosis of lead poisoning is based only on the lead testing of a venous blood specimen from a venipuncture. The level of concern for an elevated blood lead level has dropped from 80 μg/dL in 1950 to 10 μg/dL today.

Anticipatory Guidance

Anticipatory guidance lends support to primary prevention efforts. The Centers for Disease Control and Prevention (CDC) (1997a) recommends that the following information be made available to families beginning during prenatal care, at 3 to 6 months, and at 1 year of age:

- Hazards of lead-based paint in older housing
- Ways to control lead hazards safely
- Hazards accompanying repainting and renovation of homes built before 1978
- Other exposure sources, such as traditional remedies, that might be relevant for a family

Screening for Lead Poisoning

When primary prevention fails, the secondary prevention effort of screening for elevated blood lead levels can identify children much earlier than in the past. The most recent CDC guidelines (1997a, 1997b) recommend either universal screening or targeted screening, depending on the risk factors and blood lead level surveillance information available for the area.

Universal screening should be done at ages 1 and 2 years. Any child between the ages of 3 and 6 years who has not been previously screened should also be tested. Any child with risk factors should be screened more often.

Targeted screening is acceptable when an area has been determined by existing data to have less risk. Children should be screened when they live in a high-risk geographic area or are members of a group determined to be at risk (e.g., Medicaid recipients), or if their family cannot answer "no" to the following personal risk questions:

- Does your child live in or regularly visit a house that was built before 1950?
- Does your child live in or regularly visit a house built before 1978 with recent or ongoing renovations or remodeling within the past 6 months?
- Does your child have a sibling or playmate who has or did have lead poisoning?

Therapeutic Management

The degree of concern, urgency, and need for medical intervention changes as the lead level increases. Education is one of the most important elements of the treatment process. The CDC (1997a) has identified several areas that should be discussed with the family of every child who has an elevated blood lead level (10 μg/dL and above):

- The child's blood lead level and what it means
- Potential adverse health effects of an elevated blood lead level
- Sources of lead exposure and suggestions on how to reduce exposure
- The importance of wet cleaning to remove lead dust on floors, window sills, and other surfaces
- The importance of good nutrition, particularly adequate amounts of calcium and iron
- The need for follow-up testing to monitor the child's blood lead level
- Results of an environmental investigation when applicable
- The hazards of improper removal of lead paint (dry sanding, scraping, or open-flame burning)

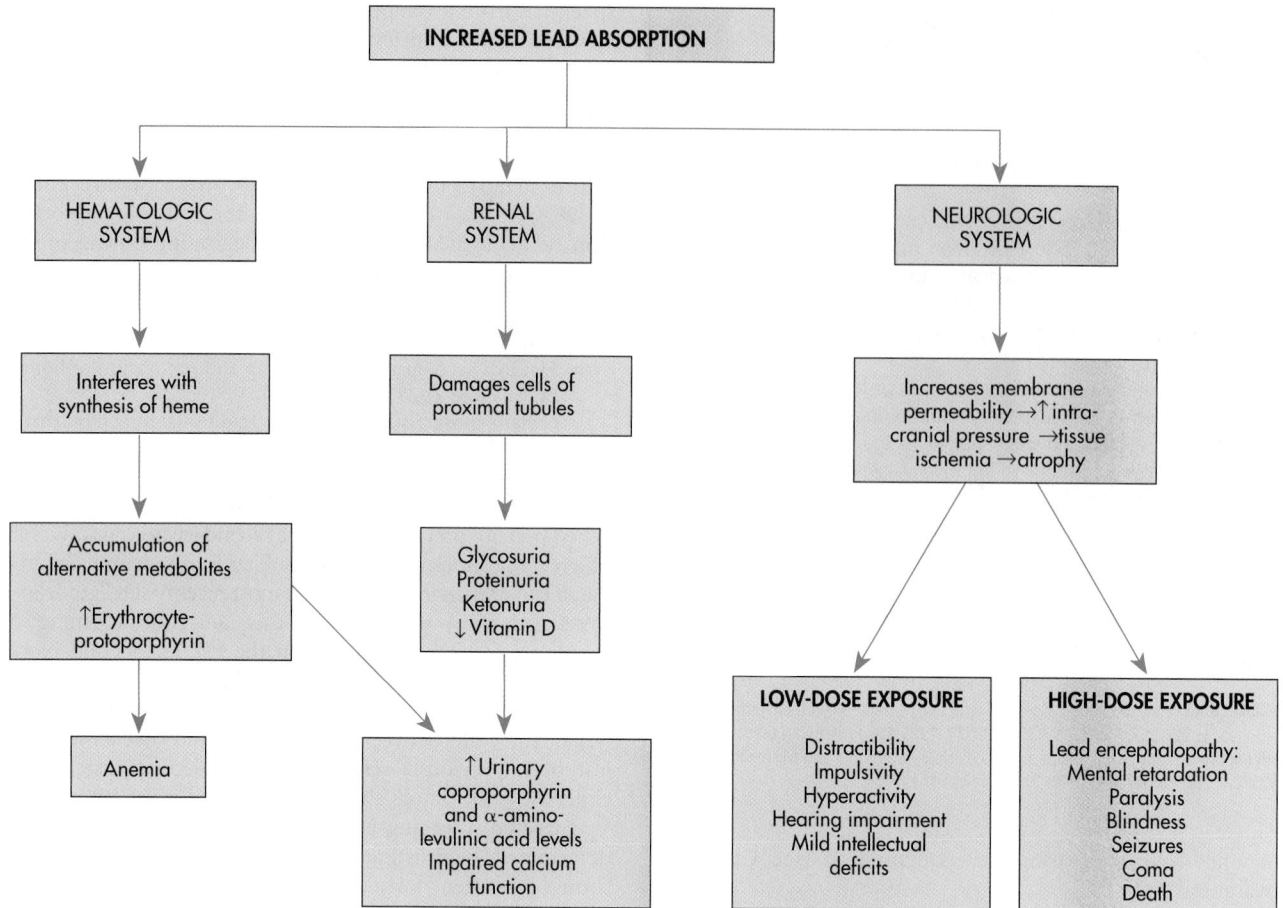

FIG. 14-9 ■ Main effects of lead on body systems.

Treatment actions vary depending on the child's blood lead level. Based on a diagnosis from a venous blood lead level test, the CDC (1997a) recommends the following actions:

BLOOD LEAD LEVEL (μg/dL)	ACTION
<10	Reassess or rescreen in 1 year. If exposure status changes, do this sooner.
10-14	Provide family with lead poisoning education, follow-up testing, and social service referral if necessary.
15-19	Provide family with lead poisoning education, follow-up testing, and social service referral as needed; if blood lead level persists, initiate actions for blood lead level of 20 to 44 μg/dL.
20-44	Provide coordination of care, clinical management, environmental investigation, and lead hazard control.
45-69	Within 48 hours, provide coordination of care and clinical management, including *chelation therapy* (medication that removes lead from the blood and, to some extent, in other places in the body), environmental investigation, and lead hazard control. The child must not remain in a lead hazardous environment if resolution is to occur.
≥70	*Immediately* provide medical treatment and chelation therapy, and begin coordination of care, clinical management, environmental investigation, and lead hazard control.

Chelation Therapy. Medical treatment and chelation therapy for the child with lead poisoning varies from practice to practice. However, when a child has a venous blood lead level of 45 μg/dL and above, two chelating agents are used consistently: calcium disodium edetate (CaNa$_2$EDTA or EDTA) and succimer (Chemet, meso-2,3 dimercaptosuccinic acid [DMSA]). With a blood lead level of 70 μg/dL or greater, British antilewisite (BAL, dimercaprol, dimercaptopropanol) is used in conjunction with EDTA. All of the agents have potential toxic side effects and contraindications. Renal, hepatic, and hematologic parameters must be monitored.

Because of the equilibration process between blood, soft tissues, and other sites in the body, there is often a rebound of the blood lead level after chelation. After the body burden of lead is reduced enough to stabilize the blood lead level, rebound will cease. Multiple chelations may be necessary. Adequate hydration is essential during therapy because the chelates are excreted via the kidneys.

BAL must not be used in the presence of a glucose-6-phosphate dehydrogenase deficiency (G6PD) or peanut allergy, nor should it be given in conjunction with iron. It is never used as a single-agent therapy, only in conjunction with EDTA. It must be given only at a deep intramuscular site. EDTA should be given intravenously over several hours and, when necessary to restrict fluids, may be given intramuscularly.

COMMUNITY FOCUS

Reducing Blood Lead Levels

Make sure child does not have access to peeling paint or chewable surfaces painted with lead-based paint, especially window sills and wells.

If a house was built before 1960 (possibly before 1980) and has hard-surface floors, wet mop them at least once per week. Wipe other hard surfaces (e.g., window sills, baseboards). If there are loose paint chips in an area, such as a window well, use a wet disposable cloth to pick up and discard them. Do not vacuum hard-surfaced floors or window sills or wells, because this spreads dust. Use vacuum cleaners with agitators to remove dust from rugs rather than vacuum cleaners with suction only. If a rug is known to contain lead dust and cannot be washed, it should be discarded.

Wash and dry child's hands and face frequently, especially before eating.

Wash toys and pacifiers frequently.

If soil around home is or is likely to be contaminated with lead (e.g., if home was built before 1960 or is near a major highway), plant grass or other ground cover; plant bushes around outside of house so that child cannot play there.

During remodeling of older homes, be sure to follow correct procedures. Be certain children and pregnant women are not in the home, day or night, until process is completed. After deleading, thoroughly clean house using cleaning solution to damp mop and dust before inhabitants return.

In areas where lead content of water exceeds the drinking water standard and a particular faucet has not been used for 6 hours or more, "flush" the cold-water pipes by running the water until it becomes as cold as it will get (30 seconds to greater than 2 minutes). The more time water has been sitting in pipes, the more lead it may contain.

Use only cold water for consumption (drinking, cooking, and especially for making infant formula). Hot water dissolves lead more quickly than cold water and thus contains higher levels of lead. May use first-flush water for nonconsumption uses.

Have water tested by a competent laboratory. This action is especially important for apartment dwellers; flushing may not be effective in high-rise buildings or in other buildings with lead-soldered central piping.*

Do not store food in open cans, particularly if cans are imported.

Do not use pottery or ceramic ware that was inadequately fired or is meant for decorative use for food storage or service. Do not store drinks or food in lead crystal.

Avoid folk remedies or cosmetics that contain lead.

Make sure that home exposure is not occurring from parental occupations or hobbies. Household members employed in occupations such as lead smelting should shower and change into clean clothing before leaving work. Construction and lead abatement workers may also bring home lead contaminants.

Make sure child eats regular meals, because more lead is absorbed on an empty stomach.

Make sure child's diet contains sufficient iron and calcium and not excessive fat.

Modified from Centers for Disease Control and Prevention: *Preventing lead poisoning in young children,* Atlanta, 1991, CDC.

*For more information, contact the county or state department of health or environment for information on local water quality. For general information on lead, call the **National Lead Information Center** (National Safety Council), 1019 19th Street NW, Suite 401, Washington, DC 20036-5105; (800) 424-LEAD; website: www.nsc.org/ehc/lead.htm or **Alliance to End Childhood Lead Poisoning;** (202)-543-1147; website: www.qec/p.org.

Succimer is given orally over a 19-day course of treatment. The capsule is opened and sprinkled on a small amount of food or may be swallowed whole. Adverse effects include nausea, vomiting, diarrhea, loss of appetite, rash, elevated liver function tests, and neutropenia. Because the chelates are excreted via the kidneys, adequate hydration is essential.

Prognosis. The central nervous system is the focus of the most dramatic effects of lead exposure. Massive amounts of lead cause lead encephalopathy. Seizures, coma, and even death were known to occur in the days before children's exposure to lead was identified early.

Children with smaller amounts of lead poisoning who do not develop encephalopathy are still at risk for neurologic impairment (Markowitz, 2000). They are more likely to have a decrease in intellectual functions, to develop learning problems, and to manifest behavior problems than children who have not had lead poisoning (Finkelstein, Markowitz, and Rosen, 1998).

Nursing Considerations

The primary nursing goal in lead poisoning is to prevent the child's initial or further exposure to lead. For children with low-level exposure, this requires identifying the sources of lead in the environment. Careful history taking is the most useful and most valuable tool and should concentrate on the personal risk questions (see p. 457). Suggestions for reducing lead in the child's environment are listed in the Community Focus box.

Children who must undergo chelation therapy are prepared for the injections and allowed to express their pain and anger. Playing with syringes and aggressive play (e.g., pounding clay, throwing beanbags) provides an excellent outlet for children and their frustrations. Children also deserve an explanation of the need for the treatment, particularly that it is not a punishment for eating lead or paint. During home or chelation therapy, parents need to understand the importance of giving the drug as prescribed.

Chelating agents are administered deeply into a large muscle mass (see Atraumatic Care box). To lessen the pain from CaNa$_2$EDTA, the local anesthetic procaine is injected with the drug. Rotation of sites is essential to prevent the formation of painful areas of fibrotic tissue. Because CaNa$_2$EDTA and lead are toxic to the kidneys, records are kept of intake and output, and the results of urinalysis are assessed to monitor renal functioning. Because of the risk of seizures, appropriate precautions are instituted at the bedside of children with high blood lead levels (BLLs).

ATRAUMATIC CARE

Lead Chelation Therapy

To lessen the pain from intramuscular injection of $CaNa_2EDTA$, the local anesthetic procaine is injected with the drug. Apply eutectic mixture of local anesthetic (i.e., EMLA) cream over the puncture site 2.5 hours before the injection of EDTA and BAL. Administer intravenous EDTA whenever possible.

! NURSING ALERT

$CaNa_2EDTA$ is never given in the absence of an adequate urinary output. Children receiving the drug intramuscularly must be able to maintain adequate oral intake of fluids.

Discharge planning for children with lead poisoning must include thorough education of families regarding safety from lead hazards, clear instructions regarding medication administration and follow-up, and confirmation that the child will be discharged to a home without lead hazards. Although caution must be used to avoid alarming parents unnecessarily, it is important that they know the risk implications for their child's behavior and cognitive functions. Nurses should observe the development and behavior of children who are hospitalized. Any concerns that are identified should be thoroughly evaluated. Referral to a child development or speech and language specialist may be indicated.

As in any situational crisis, parents need support and understanding if their child is treated for lead poisoning. Many families at the highest risk for lead poisoning have the fewest resources to comply with measures such as relocation or deleading the home. Appropriate referrals are essential.

CHILD MALTREATMENT

The broad term *child maltreatment* includes intentional physical abuse or neglect, emotional abuse or neglect, and sexual abuse of children, usually by adults. It is one of the most significant social problems affecting children. In 2002, Child Protective Service (CPS) agencies in the United States confirmed that just under one million children were victims of child maltreatment. Of the confirmed cases, 20% suffered physical abuse, 10% sexual abuse, 60% neglect, 7% emotional abuse, and 20% other forms of maltreatment.† In 2002, estimates indicated that 1400 children died as a result of child abuse and neglect (National Clearinghouse on Child Abuse and Neglect Information, 2004). Reported statistics only partially represent the actual incidence of child maltreatment, because many cases are believed to go unreported.*

CHILD NEGLECT

Child neglect is the most common form of maltreatment. About half of all reported cases are associated with depriva-

---

*Additional information is available from the Clearinghouse on Child Abuse and Neglect Information, 330 C Street SW, Washington, DC, 20477; (703) 835-7565 or 1-800-FYI-3366; www.calib.com/nc-canch.

†These numbers add up to more than 100% because some children are victims of more than one type of maltreatment.

tion of necessities, and more than one third of deaths from maltreatment are in this group. Neglect is generally defined as the failure of a parent or other person legally responsible for the child's welfare to provide for the child's basic needs and an adequate level of care.

Little is known about the etiology of neglect, although it appears that many of the risk factors identified in physical abuse apply to neglect as well (see following discussion). Ignorance of the child's needs and a lack of resources are important contributing factors. For example, neglectful parents often demonstrate poor parenting skills. They may be unaware that an infant needs to be fed every 3 to 4 hours, may not know what to feed the child, and may have insufficient funds to buy food. The most serious lack of knowledge is failure to recognize emotional nurturing as an essential need of children. (See also Failure to Thrive, Chapter 11.)

Types of Neglect

Neglect takes many forms and can be classified broadly as physical or emotional maltreatment. *Physical neglect* involves the deprivation of necessities, such as food, clothing, shelter, supervision, medical care, and education. *Emotional neglect* generally refers to failure to meet the child's needs for affection, attention, and emotional nurturance.

It may also include lack of intervention for or fostering of maladaptive behavior, such as delinquency or substance abuse. *Emotional abuse,* an even more difficult aspect of maltreatment to define, refers to the deliberate attempt to destroy or significantly impair a child's self-esteem or competence. Emotional abuse may take the following forms: rejecting, isolating, terrorizing, ignoring, corrupting, verbally assaulting, or overpressuring the child (Nelms, 2001).

PHYSICAL ABUSE

The deliberate infliction of physical injury on a child, usually by the child's care giver, is termed *physical abuse.* Minor physical injury is responsible for more reported cases of maltreatment than major physical injury, but major physical abuse causes more deaths. Despite the importance of the problem, a universally accepted definition of what constitutes minor and major physical abuse does not exist. Rather, each state in the United States defines abuse according to its individual reporting laws.

Munchausen Syndrome by Proxy

One of the more unusual and perplexing types of abuse, usually physical, is Munchausen syndrome by proxy (MSP), which refers to illness that one person fabricates or induces in another person (Paulk, 2001; Hall and others, 2000). In children it is usually the mother who fabricates signs and symptoms of illness in her child, the proxy, to gain attention from the medical staff. MSP can take many forms, such as adding maternal blood to the child's urine to simulate hematuria, presenting a fictitious medical history, chronic poisoning of the child, or suffocating the child to cause apnea and seizures. Alleging that the child has been sexually abused by someone else to gain recognition as the child's protector is another form of MSP.

Such cases are often very difficult to confirm and require a high index of suspicion to protect the children. Warning signs of MSP include:

- Unexplained, prolonged, recurrent, or extremely rare illness
- Discrepancies between clinical findings and history
- Illness unresponsive to treatment
- Signs and symptoms occurring only in parent's presence
- Parent knowledgeable about illness, procedures, and treatments
- Parent very interested in interacting with health team members
- Parent very attentive toward child (refuses to leave hospital)
- Family members with similar symptoms

Consequences for children with MSP can be serious. They often undergo needless and painful medical procedures and treatments. The parent's actions may induce a serious illness in children—one that is fatal in almost 10% of the cases (Hall and others, 2000; Souid, Keith, and Cunningham, 1998). Children may develop chronic invalidism, accepting the illness story and believing themselves to be ill. Finally, they may develop MSP as an adult. Even when some of these children are removed from the home, they continue to suffer severe psychologic trauma. Other siblings remaining in the home may become substitute victims.

Factors Predisposing to Physical Abuse

The exact cause of child abuse is not known, although three factors—parental characteristics, characteristics of the child, and environmental characteristics—influence the potential for abuse. However, no single factor or group of factors is predictive of abuse. Rather, the interaction of these factors is thought to increase the risk of abuse occurring in a particular family.

Parental Characteristics. Extensive research has focused on parental characteristics that distinguish abusive parents from nonabusive parents. Although some studies provide conflicting evidence, it is not generally recognized that parental history of abuse or neglect during childhood is a significant risk factor for child abuse (Johnson, 2004; Murray, Baker and Lewin, 2000). Although physical punishment tends to occur in abusive parents' childhood, most of the parents were not physically abused as children. However, abusive parents who report that they were severely punished as children are much more likely to injure their own children. If the abuse was not overt physical violence, abusive parents typically recall their punishment as unfair and severe, and they characterize their relationship with their parents as negative. Abusive parents tend to have difficulty coping with stress and in controlling anger expression (Rodriguez and Green, 1997).

Another finding is that abusive families are often more socially isolated and have fewer supportive relationships than nonabusive parents. Children of teenage mothers are more at risk of abuse than those of older mothers (Murray, Baker and Lewin, 2000; McCullough and Scherman, 1998). With little or no available support system and the presence of concurrent stresses imposed by the child or environment, these parents are extremely vulnerable to additional crises of any nature and literally strike out at the child as a method of releasing their increasing frustration and anxiety.

Other factors identified in abusive parents include low self-esteem and less adequate maternal functioning. Although inadequate knowledge of childrearing is often cited

as a characteristic of abusive parents, research findings do not consistently support this belief. However, this does not mean that these parents cannot benefit from learning more constructive ways of rearing their children, especially nonviolent discipline methods.

Characteristics of the Child. The child also unintentionally contributes to the abusive situation. In families of two or more children, usually only one child is the victim of abuse. This child's temperament, position in the family, additional physical needs if ill or disabled, activity level, and degree of sensitivity to parental needs all contribute to the potential for physical abuse. For example, one child may not be abused if he or she fits into the "easy-child pattern," whereas another sibling with a difficult temperament may add to the parent's stress sufficiently to precipitate an abusive act. However, temperament alone is not the critical factor; rather, it is the "fit" or compatibility between the child's temperament and the parent's ability to deal with that behavioral style.

Occasionally the abused child is illegitimate, unwanted, brain damaged (especially in situations where the parents cannot accept the retardation), hyperactive, or physically disabled. Sometimes children are abused because they remind the parent of someone the parent dislikes, such as a younger brother or sister who received all of the attention from their own parents. Premature infants may be at risk for maltreatment because of the failure of parent-child bonding during early infancy. Often a difficult pregnancy, labor, or delivery is a predisposing factor in abuse, especially when the infant is born prematurely or with congenital anomalies.

Although one child is usually the victim in an abusive family, removing that child from the home often places the other siblings at risk for abuse. Child maltreatment usually is not confined to one child because of a disturbed parent-child relationship but is a result of a family in distress. Therefore, no child is safe if left in the abusive environment unless the parents can be helped to learn new parenting skills and to meet their needs and release their frustration through alternatives other than attacking their children.

Environmental Characteristics. The environment is a significant part of the potential abusive situation. Typically the environment is one of chronic stress, including problems of divorce, poverty, unemployment, poor housing, frequent relocation, alcoholism, and drug addiction. Increased exposure between children and parents, such as that which occurs in crowded living conditions, also increases the likelihood of abuse.

Although most reporting of abuse has been from lower socioeconomic populations, child abuse is not a problem of any one societal group. It spans all educational, social, and economic levels. Stresses imposed by poverty predispose lower socioeconomic families to abusive situations, and abuse in these groups is more apt to be reported. However, concealed crises may also be present in upper-class families. For example, a wealthy family experiencing major life changes, such as rehousing, the birth of an additional child, or marital discord, may have sufficient environmental stressors imposed on them to produce a potentially abusive situation. Wealthy families may be so overinvolved with commitments outside the home that abuse may be inflicted by substitute caregivers. Nurses need to be aware of all these factors to identify the less obvious examples of child abuse and neglect.

SEXUAL ABUSE

Sexual abuse is one of the most devastating types of child maltreatment, and estimates indicate that it has increased significantly during the past decade. Child sexual abuse constitutes approximately 10% of officially substantiated child maltreatment cases. Some of the apparent increase can be attributed to increased awareness (Putnam, 2003).

As with all forms of child maltreatment, no universal definition for sexual abuse exists. The Child Abuse and Prevention Act (Public Law 100-235) defines *sexual abuse* as "the use, persuasion, or coercion of any child to engage in sexually explicit conduct (or any simulation of such conduct) for producing any visual depiction of such conduct, or rape, molestation, prostitution, or incest with children."

Sexual abuse includes the following types of sexual maltreatment (see also Sexual Assault, Chapter 17):

Incest—Any physical sexual activity between family members; blood relationship is not required (abusers can include stepparents, nonrelated siblings, grandparents, uncles, and aunts); does not include sexual relations between legally sanctional partners, such as spouses

Molestation—A vague term that includes "indecent liberties," such as touching, fondling, kissing, single or mutual masturbation, or oral-genital contact

Exhibitionism—Indecent exposure, usually exposure of the genitals by an adult male to children or female adults

Child pornography—Arranging and photographing, in any media, sexual acts involving children, alone or with adults or animals, regardless of consent by the child's legal guardian; also may denote distribution of such material in any form with or without profit

Child prostitution—Involving children in sex acts for profit and usually with changing partners

Pedophilia—Literally means "love of child" and does not denote a type of sexual activity but the preference of an adult for prepubertal children as the means of achieving sexual excitement

Characteristics of Abusers and Victims

Anyone, including siblings and mothers, can be sexual abusers, but a typical abuser is a male whom the victim knows. Offenders come from all levels of society. Some are prominent persons in the community, and some, especially in the case of pedophiles (also called "child molesters"), are in positions where they work closely with children, such as teaching or coaching.

Pornography and prostitution may involve strangers, as well as the children's own parents. There are no typical characteristics of these offenders, although the abused children tend to be runaways—young adolescents who engage in these activities to obtain money for food, shelter, drugs, and alcohol. Incestuous relationships between father or stepfather and daughter are generally prolonged, and the victims are usually reluctant to report the situation because of fear of retaliation and fear that they will not be believed. Typically,

incestuous relationships begin later than other forms of child abuse. The eldest daughter is usually abused, but in her absence another sister is substituted. Sibling incest may also occur (Adler and Schutz, 1995). Sexual abuse by relatives with a strong emotional bond with the victim is the most devastating to the child (Fischer and McDonald, 1998).

Boys are also victims of both intrafamilial and extrafamilial abuse. Male victims are much less likely to report abuse, and they may suffer much greater emotional harm from incestuous relationships, especially between mother and son, than female victims (Moody, 1999). Boys are likely to be subjected to anal penetration and oral-genital contact, to have subtle physical findings, and to be abused by a father, stepfather, or mother's boyfriend.

Initiation and Perpetuation of Sexual Abuse

The cycle of sexual abuse often starts innocently unless it involves an isolated attack, such as rape. Often offenders spend time with the victims to gain their trust before initiating any sexual contact. Most victims are then pressured into being an accessory to the sexual activity through various means (Box 14-7) and may be unaware that sexual activity is part of the offer. Children may not reveal the truth for fear that their parents would not believe them if they told, especially if the offender is a trusted member of the family. Some fear that they will be blamed for the situation, and many young children with limited vocabulary have difficulty describing the activity when they do have the courage or opportunity to reveal the abuse.

Seductiveness by the child does not initiate incest. Most young girls experiment in seduction, especially during the preschool years, but the father's response normally differentiates this playfulness from overt sexual invitation. Although the reasons for incest are complicated and can occur in various family types, it does not occur in healthy families. Most incestuous relationships are directly tied to sexual maladjustment and estrangement between husband and wife. Most begin following the cessation of sexual relationships with the usual partner. Most fathers experience little guilt, and many wives at some level are aware of the incestuous affair. The wife may react by tolerating the situation or may resort to use of denial; some remain unaware of the activity. Consequently, the home offers little protection to young victims because abusers have easy access to their vic-

BOX 14-7 ■ Methods Used to Pressure Children Into Sexual Activity

The child is offered gifts or privileges.

The adult misrepresents moral standards by telling the child that it is "okay to do."

Isolated and emotionally and socially impoverished children are enticed by adults who meet their needs for warmth and human contact.

The successful sex offender pressures the victim into secrecy regarding the activity by describing it as a "secret between us" that other people may take away if they find out.

The offender plays on the child's fears, including fear of punishment by the offender, fear of repercussions if the child tells, and fear of abandonment or rejection by the family.

tims and the children feel they cannot reveal their secret to other family members. However, not all incestuous relationships follow this pattern of silence. Reports of father-daughter incest during child custody conflicts have become more common and have raised serious concerns regarding the possibility of false accusation. Rather than tolerating or denying the child's sexual abuse, the other parent (usually the mother) is typically the chief accuser.

NURSING CARE OF THE MALTREATED CHILD

● Assessment

A critical responsibility of health professionals is identifying abusive situations as early as possible. The characteristics that may predispose members of some families to commit abuse can serve as a framework for assessing vulnerability but are never predictive of actual abuse. A thorough physical examination and a careful, detailed history are the diagnostic tools needed to identify abuse. Nurses have a special role because they may be the first person to see the child and parent and are the consistent caregivers if the child is hospitalized (see Guidelines box).

> **NURSING ALERT**
>
> Nurses must be aware of their biases regarding child abuse. Studies show that nurses are less likely to report abuse when the child is female and from a middle-income, as opposed to lower-income, family (Pillitteri and others, 1992); are significantly less comfortable dealing with sexual abuse, abuse of infants, and fathers as the abusers (Seidl and others, 1993); and experience greater discomfort when dealing with abusers of children with disabilities than with abusers of children without disabilities (Stanton and others, 1994).

Evidence of Maltreatment.   Recognition of abuse or neglect necessitates a familiarity with both physical and behavioral signs that suggest maltreatment (Box 14-8). No one indicator can be used to diagnose maltreatment. It is a pattern or combination of indicators that should arouse suspicion and further investigation. In addition, signs of possible abuse must be coupled with an understanding of diseases, such as bleeding disorders, osteogenesis imperfecta, or sudden infant death syndrome (SIDS), and cultural practices, such as cupping or coin rubbing (see Health Practices,

Chapter 4), that may mimic physical abuse. Unintentional injuries may also be wrongly diagnosed as abuse, such as burns from metal buckles on car seats, lacerations from seat belts, or retinal hemorrhage after cardiopulmonary resuscitation. Normal variants, such as mongolian spots and congenital anomalies of genitalia, can be mistaken for abuse.

Not all forms of physical abuse have obvious signs. Violent shaking of children *(shaken baby syndrome [SBS])* can cause fatal intracranial trauma without signs of external head injury (Castiglia, 2001). Nurses should suspect SBS in infants younger than 1 year of age who present with subdural or retinal hemorrhages in the absence of external signs of trauma (Castiglia, 2001).

> **NURSING ALERT**
>
> Stress to parents the dangers of shaking infants (shaking can cause SBS). Advise against shaking as a method of burping or waking infant, tossing infant in air, or shaking infant when feeling angry or tense.

If abuse is suspected, nurses play an important role in monitoring the parent's activities to identify instances of causing the children's symptoms. Using a hidden video camera to document the parent's behavior is becoming a more common diagnostic procedure, but the parent's right of privacy must be considered (Hall and others, 2000).

Neglect and Emotional Abuse.   Neglect from deprivation of necessities is easier to identify than emotional neglect or abuse because physical signs are usually evident. Emotional maltreatment may be readily suspected, but it is very difficult to substantiate. Physical signs are often nonspecific, and nurses must rely on behavioral indicators, which range from depression to acting-out behavior, to help identify a possibly abusive situation. Any persistent and unexplained change in the child's behavior is an important clue to possible emotional abuse.

BOX 14-8 ■ Warning Signs of Abuse

Physical evidence of abuse or neglect, including previous injuries

Conflicting stories about the "accident" or injury from the parents or others

Cause of injury blamed on sibling or other party

An injury inconsistent with the history, such as a concussion and broken arm from falling off a bed

History inconsistent with child's developmental level, such as a 6-month-old turning on the hot water

A complaint other than the one associated with signs of abuse (e.g., a chief complaint of a cold when there is evidence of first- and second-degree burns)

Inappropriate response of caregiver, such as an exaggerated or absent emotional response; refusal to sign for additional tests or agree to necessary treatment; excessive delay in seeking treatment; absence of the parents for questioning

Inappropriate response of child, such as little or no response to pain; fear of being touched; excessive or lack of separation anxiety; indiscriminate friendliness to strangers

Child's report of physical or sexual abuse

Previous reports of abuse in the family

Repeated visits to emergency facilities with injuries

⚖ GUIDELINES

Talking With Children Who Reveal Abuse

Provide a private time and place to talk.

Do not promise not to tell; tell them that you are required by law to report the abuse.

Do not express shock or criticize their family.

Use their vocabulary to discuss body parts.

Avoid using any leading statements that can distort their report.

Reassure them that they have done the right thing by telling.

Tell them that the abuse is not their fault, that they are not bad or to blame.

Determine their immediate need for safety.

Let the child know what will happen when you report.

Sexual Abuse. Identifying instances of sexual abuse is particularly difficult because, often, few if any obvious physical indications of the activity exist. Also, many individuals are hesitant to believe children and are unwilling to report incidents. Even health professionals are sometimes at fault when they perform cursory physical examinations of the genitalia and ignore behavior or verbal comments that suggest abuse. When sexual abuse is suspected, other children in the family should be evaluated, because multiple victims are not uncommon.

Unfortunately, there is no typical profile of the victim, and there must be a high index of suspicion to identify these children. Physical signs vary and may include any of those listed for sexual abuse. The victim may exhibit various behavioral manifestations. Unfortunately, none of these behaviors is diagnostic. When abused children exhibit these behaviors, the signs may be incorrectly attributed to the normal stresses of childhood, especially in older school-age children or adolescents. Even signs considered most predictive of sexual abuse, such as certain genital findings, sexually inappropriate behavior for age, enactment of adult sexual activity, and intense focus on sexual activity (e.g., masturbation), do not always indicate that sexual abuse has occurred. Conversely, abused children may not demonstrate more knowledge of sexual activity than nonabused children. However, one difference in the abused children's explanation of sexual activity may be unusual affective responses. For example, abused children may have an increased incidence of sleep disorders, temper tantrums, and depression (Calam and others, 1998).

Many genital findings that have been reported as conclusive or highly suspect for sexual abuse, such as vaginal opening greater than 4 mm, hymenal tears and synechiae (tissue bands) inside the vagina, reflex anal dilation, and condylomata acuminata (anogenital or venereal warts), may be found in unabused prepubertal children (Brodeur and Monteleone, 1994). Results of a physical examination will be normal in 80% of child victims of sexual abuse (Lahoti, 2001).

History Pertaining to the Incident.

In addition to observable evidence of abuse, the type of history revealed by the parents or other caregiver, such as the baby-sitter or mother's boyfriend, is a significant factor. Areas of the history that should arouse suspicion of abuse are summarized in Box 14-9.

> **NURSING ALERT**
>
> Incompatibility between the history and the injury is probably the most important criterion on which to base the decision to report suspected abuse.

An important point to remember when taking a history is that maltreated children rarely betray their parents by admitting to the abuse they received. If questioned, they will repeat the same story as the parents and try to defend their parents' actions. If the interviewer directly accuses the parents of abuse, the child may accept responsibility for the act in an attempt to vindicate the parents. Whether children respond in this way out of fear is uncertain. However, children do fear losing whatever security and love they have.

Between abusive acts, children may receive some measure of attention and love from the parents. If they betray the parents, they may lose this and be uncertain or fearful of the consequences, such as foster care. Preserving the present situation may be less frightening than the unknown future.

The *disclosure of sexual abuse* occurs in several ways: it is observed by others, resulting in a direct confrontation; the child tells someone; visible clues are observed (such as an accumulation of coins, gifts, or candy); or the child appears disheveled, demonstrates physical or behavioral signs and symptoms, or becomes pregnant. Children usually describe the experience in terms of whether it was unpleasant or hurt or was pleasurable (usually a response to hand-genital contact); some indicate no reaction. Young children often feel no guilt or shame because the act is pleasurable and they are unaware of its inappropriateness.

> **NURSING ALERT**
>
> When children report potentially sexually abusive experiences, their reports need to be taken seriously, but also cautiously to avoid alarming the child or falsely accusing someone.

Children's reports of sexual abuse may vary from contradictory stories to unwavering versions of the experience. Stories that sound contradictory may reflect the child's experiences in several instances of abuse. Also, children who repeatedly tell identical facts may have been prompted to do so. Increasing evidence suggests that the types of interrogation children are exposed to after reports of sexual abuse shape their thinking. To avoid biasing the interaction, nurses must be very skillful interviewers when questioning children who may be victims of abuse. Medical records should include verbatim statements made by the child and interviewer that reflect appropriate non-leading questions and statements (Horner, 2001; McClain and others, 2000).

Parental Behaviors.

Certain behavioral responses of the parents to their child and to the interviewer should alert the nurse to the possibility of maltreatment. Although no one pattern of behavior is characteristic of these parents, some responses include the following. Abusive parents have difficulty showing concern toward their child. They are unable to comfort the child and give no indication of realizing how the child may feel, physically or emotionally. Instead, they are critical of and angry with the child for being injured. They maintain that the child is responsible for the injury, and if asked any question regarding their responsibility of protecting or supervising the child, they become hostile and aggressive. They act as if the child's injury is an assault on them. Their entire perception of the incident is in terms of how it affects them, not the child, which is an indication of their preoccupation with their own needs and of their inability to give any support to others.

During the child's hospitalization they may not become involved in the child's care and may show little concern for his or her progress, eventual discharge, or need for follow-up care. However, if they are pressured during interrogation, they immediately demand to take the child home, regardless of the child's readiness for discharge.

Families respond to sexual abuse with a wide variety of emotional reactions, which range from not believing the

BOX 14-9 ■ Clinical Manifestations of Potential Child Maltreatment

PHYSICAL NEGLECT
Suggestive Physical Findings
Failure to thrive
Signs of malnutrition, such as thin extremities, abdominal disten-
tion, lack of subcutaneous fat
Poor personal hygiene
Unclean or inappropriate dress
Evidence of poor health care, such as delayed immunization, un-
treated infections, frequent colds
Frequent injuries from lack of supervision

Suggestive Behaviors
Dull and inactive; excessively passive or sleepy
Self-stimulatory behaviors, such as finger sucking or rocking
Begging or stealing food
Absenteeism from school
Drug or alcohol addiction
Vandalism or shoplifting

EMOTIONAL ABUSE AND NEGLECT
Suggestive Physical Findings
Failure to thrive
Feeding disorders
Enuresis
Sleep disorders

Suggestive Behaviors
Self-stimulatory behaviors, such as biting, rocking, sucking
During infancy, lack of social smile and stranger anxiety
Withdrawal
Unusual fearfulness
Antisocial behavior, such as destructiveness, stealing, cruelty
Extremes of behavior, such as overcompliant and passive, or ag-
gressive and demanding
Lags in emotional and intellectual development, especially lan-
guage
Suicide attempts

PHYSICAL ABUSE
Suggestive Physical Findings
Bruises and welts (may be in various stages of healing)
On face, lips, mouth, back, buttocks, thighs, or areas of torso
Regular patterns descriptive of object used, such as belt buckle,
hand, wire hanger, chain, wooden spoon, squeeze or pinch
marks
May be present in various stages of healing
Burns
On soles of feet, palms of hands, back, or buttocks
Patterns descriptive of object used, such as round cigar or ciga-
rette burns; sharply demarcated areas from immersion in
scalding water; rope burns on wrists or ankles from being
bound; burns in the shape of an iron, radiator, or electric
stove burner
Absence of "splash" marks and presence of symmetric burns
Stun gun injury: lesions circular, fairly uniform (up to 0.5 cm),
and paired about 5 cm apart (Frechette and Rimsza, 1992)
Fractures and dislocations
Skull, nose, or facial structures
Injury may denote type of abuse, such as spiral fracture or dislocation from twisting of an extremity or whiplash from
shaking the child

Multiple new or old fractures in various stages of healing
Lacerations and abrasions
On backs of arms, legs, torso, face, or external genitalia
Unusual symptoms, such as abdominal swelling, pain, and vom-
iting from punching
Descriptive marks such as from human bites or pulling out of
hair
Chemical
Unexplained repeated poisoning, especially drug overdose
Unexplained sudden illness, such as hypoglycemia from insulin
administration

Suggestive Behaviors
Wary of physical contact with adults
Apparent fear of parents or going home
Lying very still while surveying environment
Inappropriate reaction to injury, such as failure to cry from pain
Lack of reaction to frightening events
Apprehensive when hearing other children cry
Indiscriminate friendliness and displays of affection
Superficial relationships
Acting-out behavior, such as aggression, to seek attention
Withdrawal behavior

SEXUAL ABUSE
Suggestive Physical Findings
Bruises, bleeding, lacerations, or irritation of external genitalia,
anus, mouth, or throat
Torn, stained, or bloody underclothing
Pain on urination or pain, swelling, and itching of genital area
Penile discharge
Sexually transmitted disease, nonspecific vaginitis, or venereal warts
Difficulty in walking or sitting
Unusual odor in the genital area
Recurrent urinary tract infections
Presence of sperm
Pregnancy in young adolescent

Suggestive Behaviors
Sudden emergence of sexually related problems, including exces-
sive or public masturbation, age-inappropriate sexual play,
promiscuity, or overtly seductive behavior
Withdrawn behavior, excessive daydreaming
Preoccupied with fantasies, especially in play
Poor relationships with peers
Sudden changes, such as anxiety, loss or gain of weight, clinging
behavior
In incestuous relationships, excessive anger at mother for not pro-
tecting daughter
Regressive behavior, such as bed-wetting or thumb sucking
Sudden onset of phobias or fears, particularly fears of the dark,
men, strangers, or particular settings or situations (e.g., undue
fear of leaving the house or staying at the day care center or
the baby-sitter's house)
Running away from home
Substance abuse, particularly of alcohol or mood-elevating drugs
Profound and rapid personality changes, especially extreme de-
pression, hostility, and aggression (often accompanied by social
withdrawal)
Rapidly declining school performance
Suicidal attempts or ideation

Nurse Credentialling
HEALTH AND COMMUNITY STUDIES DIVISION

child to being very supportive. Parents and other family members may display the same type of emotional responses as the victim, such as inability to eat or sleep, and somatic complaints, such as headache. In the acute emotional phase, parents have a need to blame someone. The three common targets are the offender, the child, and the parents themselves. The parents frequently express anger at the child for "stupid" behavior and may even restrict the child's privileges as punishment. When the victim is a girl, the parents may question her sexual provocation of the event. Self-blaming parents assume full responsibility, believing that they have been inadequate parents or should not have allowed the child to go out. When a baby-sitter or trusted relative is involved in the assault and the child's complaint has not been believed until gross evidence is presented, the parents are often devastated by guilt.

Child Behaviors.   Abused children's responses to their parents or the injury may also support the suspicion of abuse. Although no one pattern is typical, extremes of behavior may be observed. Children may be very unresponsive to the parent or excessively clinging and intolerant of separation. They may be overattached to the abusive parent, possibly in the hope of preventing any upset that may precipitate anger and another attack. During care of the injury, children may be passive and accepting of the discomfort or uncooperative and fearful of any physical contact. Some children maintain a wary watchfulness of all strangers; some shy away from strangers as if frightened; others are unusually affectionate and outgoing.

● *Nursing Diagnoses*

A number of nursing diagnoses are prominent in the nursing care of the maltreated child and family, and others specific to individual cases become evident. The most common nursing diagnoses are outlined in the Nursing Care Plan on p. 469.

● *Planning*

The main nursing goals related to child maltreatment are as follows:

1 Child will be protected from further abuse.
2 Child and family will receive adequate support.
3 Hospitalized child and family, including foster parents if appropriate, will be prepared for discharge.
4 Child will not experience any maltreatment.

● *Implementation*

Protect Child From Further Abuse.   Initially, identification of instances of suspected abuse or neglect is essential. The nurse may come in contact with abused children in an emergency department, practitioner's office, home, day care center, or school.

NURSING ALERT

The priority is to remove the child from the abusive situation to prevent further injury.

All states and provinces in North America have laws for mandatory reporting of child maltreatment. Suspected child abuse is reported to the local authorities.* Referrals

GUIDELINES

Recording Assessment Data in Suspected Abuse

HISTORY OF INJURY

1. Date, time, and place of occurrence
2. Sequence of events with recorded times
3. Presence of witnesses, especially person caring for child at time of incident
4. Time lapse between occurrence of injury and initiation of treatment
5. Interview with child when appropriate, including verbal quotations and information from drawing or other play activities
6. Interview with parent, witnesses, or other significant persons, including verbal quotations
7. Description of parent-child interactions (verbal interactions, eye contact, touching, parental concern)
8. Name, age, and condition of other children in home (if possible)

PHYSICAL EXAMINATION

1. Location, size, shape, and color of bruises; approximate location, size, and shape on drawing of body outline
2. Distinguishing characteristics, such as a bruise in the shape of a hand; round burn (possibly caused by cigarette)
3. Symmetry or asymmetry of injury; presence of other injuries
4. Degree of pain; any bone tenderness
5. Evidence of past injuries; general state of health and hygiene
6. Developmental level of child; perform screening test (see Developmental Assessment, Chapter 7)

usually come to the state child welfare department and are assigned to a caseworker in an agency such as **CPS**. After a referral has been made, a caseworker is assigned to investigate the report. Based on the findings, the child is left in the home or temporarily removed.

A court proceeding may be necessary before the child can be placed outside the home or when parental rights are to be terminated. When the courts are involved, they usually require firsthand testimony by the referring parties. Nurses may be subpoenaed to appear in court, or their notes may be introduced as evidence in court hearings. Accurate and factual documentation is essential. Behaviors are described, not interpreted, and are recorded daily to establish a progress record (see Guidelines box). Conversations among the nurse, child, and parent are recorded verbatim as much as possible.

Support Child.   Frequently, children suspected of abuse are hospitalized for medical management of their injuries. The type of care needed by the sexually abused child depends on the circumstances of the abuse. It varies from reassurance and support when the abuse involves exhibitionism to long-term counseling in incestuous situations. In interviewing these children, the nurse must be very careful to avoid biasing the child's retelling of the events. Some experts suggest that health professionals limit the interview to

---

*Telephone numbers are usually listed under "Child Abuse" in the business white pages of the local directory, or call the emergency child abuse hotline: (800) 422-4453 ([800] 4-A-CHILD).

the child's physical and mental health concerns and leave topics of the family's social, legal, or other problems to the police or CPS personnel (McClain and others, 2000). When the sexually abused child has been physically harmed, the care is consistent with that provided to a rape victim (see Chapter 17). Regardless of the type of abuse, the child's needs are the same as those of any hospitalized child. The child should be treated as a child with the usual physical needs, developmental tasks, and play interests, not as a dramatic victim of abuse. The nurse is the child's advocate in this goal. The nurse also encourages the child's relationship with the parents.

Do Not Become a Substitute Parent.

The nurse does not become a substitute parent to the exclusion of the child's natural parents. Such behavior only intensifies the parents' feelings of inadequacy, worthlessness, and isolation. It does not help them understand their child or promote their trust in health professionals. The goal of the *consistent* nurse-child relationship is to provide a role model for the parents in helping them to relate positively and constructively to their child and to foster a therapeutic environment for the child in his or her reprieve from the abusing situation.

Support Family.

One of the most difficult, yet essential, components of success with abusive parents is the quality of the *therapeutic relationship.* It must be one of genuine concern and treatment, not one of accusation and punishment. Nurses must examine their personal feelings toward these parents, particularly when sexual abuse is present. A therapeutic approach is to view the parent as the patient and the child as the victim of abuse. Unless the nurse's attitude is positive, abusive parents will not be motivated to change, because they will not be working with a trusting person who demonstrates the kind of behavior that is being asked of them.

When parental ignorance of childrearing practices has played a part in the abuse, the nurse can educate the parent regarding children's physical and emotional needs. Because of the parents' own childrearing, they may not be aware of nonviolent methods of discipline, such as time-out. They may also need help in dealing with their frustration so that they do not vent anger on the child. Because these parents may be sensitive to criticism or domination and already possess a very low self-esteem, teaching is implemented through demonstration and example rather than through lecturing. Any competent parenting abilities they demonstrate are praised to promote their sense of parental adequacy.

Care of the family also depends on the circumstances of the *sexual abuse.* With a nonparent offender the family may be more able to support the child than if incest were involved. Family members are encouraged to express their feelings of anger, guilt, shame, or embarrassment but are also cautioned to avoid displacing such feelings on the child. For example, it is easy for parents to admonish the child with a statement such as "We told you never to go with strangers," which makes the child feel responsible.

Family members are advised to encourage the child to resume normal activities and observe the child for signs of distress (see Posttraumatic Stress Disorder, Chapter 17).

Children express their feelings primarily through behavior. Parents should be alert for changes in behavior that indicate distress resulting from the incident, such as remaining in the house, refusing to go to school, changes in sleeping patterns, and frequency of dreams and nightmares. Children are encouraged to talk about these feelings and nightmares, because the more they talk about the experience, the more they are able to gain control over it.

Referral to appropriate agencies is also essential. Most abusive parents tend to live in poverty, and the daily stresses imposed by their lifestyle are overwhelming. Resources for financial aid, improved housing, and childcare should be sought. Self-help groups also provide important services. Groups such as **Parents Anonymous*** (a group for parents who have abused or fear that they may abuse their child, but only in terms of physical abuse, not sexual abuse) and **Parents United International, Inc.†** (a group devoted to helping sexually abused families) are very accepting and nonjudgmental.

There is no way to predict which families will be successfully rehabilitated. With father-daughter incest, however, the best results occur when the father accepts full responsibility for the act, the mother acknowledges her role in failing to protect the child, and the child is able to understand and forgive the parents and develop a positive self-image despite the traumatic experience.

Plan for Discharge.

Discharge planning should begin as soon as the legal disposition for placement has been decided, which may be temporary foster home placement, return to the parents, or permanent termination of parental rights. The latter is the most drastic solution, but it is necessary in situations of repeated, life-threatening abuse. Whenever children are sent to a foster home or juvenile institution, they must be allowed an opportunity to express their feelings. No matter how severe the abuse, they usually mourn the loss of their parents. They need help to understand why they must not return home and that this new home is in no way a punishment. Whenever possible, foster parents are encouraged to visit in the hospital, and the nurse should take an active role in helping these new parents understand the child. It is unfortunate that some abused children live in torment as they are sent from one foster home to another, sometimes enduring worse circumstances than those that existed in their original home. Only through constant evaluation of the placement residence and the child's adjustment to a new environment can the vicious circle of abuse, abandonment, and neglect be stopped.

Prevent Abuse.

Prevention of child maltreatment has been an extremely difficult goal. Programs aimed at identifying potential abusers and instituting supportive intervention before the occurrence of an abusive act have met with variable success (Flournoy, 1996). However, nurses have played an important role in such programs. For example, home visiting by nurses to primiparas who were either

---

*675 West Foothill Boulevard, Suite 220, Claremont, CA 91711; (909) 621-6181; website: www.parentsanonymous/natl.org.
†PO Box 952, San Jose, CA 95108; (408) 453-7616.

FAMILY HOME CARE

Preventing or Dealing With Sexual Abuse of Children

Sexual assault of children is much more common than most people realize. It may be preventable if children have good preparation. *To provide protection and preparation:*

Pay careful attention to who is around children. (Unwanted touch may come from someone liked and trusted.)

Back up a child's right to say "no."

Encourage communication by taking seriously what children *say.*

Take a second look at signals of potential danger.

Refuse to leave children in the company of those not trusted.

Include information about sexual assault when teaching about safety.

Provide specific definitions and examples of sexual assault.

Remind children that even "nice" people sometimes do mean things.

Urge children to tell about *anybody* who causes them to be uncomfortable.

Prepare children to deal with bribes and threats, as well as possible physical force.

Virtually eliminate secrets between children and parents.

Teach children how to say "no," ask for help, and control who touches them and how.

Model self-protective and limit-setting behavior for children.

Should it ever become necessary to *help a child recover from a sexual assault:*

Listen carefully to understand children.

Support the child for telling through praise, belief, sympathy, and lack of blame.

Know local resources and choose help carefully.

Provide opportunities to talk about the assault.

Provide opportunities for the entire family to go through a recovery process.

Sexual assault affects everyone. *To help deal with this social problem:*

Provide care and support to those who have been victimized.

Recognize that offenders do not change without intervention.

Organize neighborhood programs to support each other's efforts to protect children.

Encourage schools to provide information about sexual assault as a problem of health and safety.

Organize community groups to support educational treatment and law enforcement programs.

Modified from Adams C, Fay J: *No more secrets: protecting your child from sexual assault,* San Luis Obispo, Calif, 1981, Impact.

---

teenagers, unmarried, or of low socioeconomic status was noted to be an effective preventive measure (Eckenrode and others, 2000; McMillian, 2000). The nurses provided information on normal child growth and development and routine health care needs, served as informal support persons, and referred families to appropriate services when a need for assistance was identified.

Such programs provide models that can be used to reduce factors that increase the risk of abuse. Nurses in a variety of settings can implement similar activities. For example, nurses in prenatal clinics can prepare expectant families for adjustment to parenthood. Nursery and postpartum nurses can foster the attachment process by encouraging parents to hold and look at their infant. Nurses in neonatal intensive care units can minimize the effects of separation by encouraging parents to visit and can help parents to become comfortable caring for their child. Nurses in ambulatory settings can teach parents appropriate methods of bathing, feeding, toileting, disciplining, and preventing injuries, while stressing the normal needs and developmental characteristics of children. Nurses must be sensitive to parental needs for attention, reassurance, and reinforcement, and refer parents to community services and self-help groups.

Unlike preventive efforts for neglect and physical abuse, which have been aimed at the potential offender, *prevention of child sexual abuse* has centered on education of children to protect themselves. Much controversy surrounds the effectiveness of these programs. The main issue is whether young children should be expected to participate in their own protection. Clearly, sexual abuse prevention is more than teaching children to say "no" or to recognize their right not to be touched in "private places." It is equally important to teach children safety in terms of potential risk situations. Several suggestions for parents regarding protecting and educating children against possible molestation are presented in the Community Focus box.

The nurse is frequently in a position to discuss the topic of abuse with parents and to provide guidelines.

Books are available for parents that describe sexual abuse and its prevention.* Supporting parental qualities of respect, affection, empathy, and ability to set boundaries, and providing quality childcare and education comprise the true preventive approach to sexual abuse (Flournoy, 1996). Helpful games such as "What if the baby-sitter wants to wrestle and hug but tells you to keep it a secret?" can be used to explore dangerous situations in advance and help children learn the importance of saying "no." They need reassurance that no matter what the other person says or does, the parents want to know about it and will not punish them. Even if children participate in the activity before telling the parents, they must be reassured that it was not their fault.

In addition, parents need to be made aware that "nice" people, including friends and relatives, can be offenders; parents should carefully observe how others act toward the child. A sudden change in the child's behavior and a response such as "I don't like Uncle anymore" are clues to investigate the relationship. In the event of any doubt, further solitary encounters with this person and the child should be prevented. It is sometimes to the child's great misfortune that parents do not take certain comments seriously, such as "He hugs me too tight" or "I don't want to go with him." Casual parental

---

*Sources of information are **Prevent Child Abuse America,** Publishing Department, 200 South Michigan Avenue, Suite 1700, Chicago, IL 60604-4357; (312) 663-3520 or (800) Children; website: www.childabuse.org; **Kempe Children's Center,** 1825 Marion Street, Denver, CO 80218; (303) 864-5250, website: www.kempecenter.org; **American Association for Protecting Children, American Humane Association,** 63 Inverness Drive East, Englewood, CO 80112; (800) 227-4645 (outside Colorado) or (303) 792-9900; and **National Clearing House on Child Abuse and Neglect Information,** 330 C Street SW, Washington, DC 20447; (800) 394-3366; website: www.calib.com/nccanch.

NURSING DIAGNOSIS ■ **Risk for trauma related to characteristics of child, care giver(s), environment**

PATIENT GOAL 1: Will experience no further abuse or neglect

NURSING INTERVENTIONS/*RATIONALES*

Implement measures to prevent abuse:
 Report suspicions to appropriate authorities
 Assist in removing child from unsafe environment and establishing a safe environment
 Establish protective measures for the hospitalized child as indicated *to prevent continued abuse in* hospital
Refer family to social agencies for assistance with finances, food, clothing, housing, and health care *to help prevent neglect*
Keep factual, objective records *for documentation,* including:
 Child's physical condition
 Child's behavioral response to parents, others, and environment
 Interviews with family members
Collaborate efforts of multidisciplinary team *to continually evaluate progress of child in foster home or in return to own family*
Be alert for signs of continued abuse or neglect
Help parents identify those circumstances that precipitate an abusive act and alternative ways to deal with the release of anger other than attacking child
Refer for alternative placement when indicated *to prevent further injury or neglect*

EXPECTED OUTCOME

Child experiences no further injury or neglect

NURSING DIAGNOSIS ■ **Fear/anxiety related to negative interpersonal interaction, repeated maltreatment, powerlessness, potential loss of parents**

PATIENT GOAL 1: Will experience reduction or relief of anxiety and stress

NURSING INTERVENTIONS/*RATIONALES*

Provide consistent caregiver and therapeutic environment during hospitalization *to relieve child's stress and to be a role model for family*
Demonstrate acceptance of child while not expecting same in return
Show attention while not reinforcing inappropriate behavior, *because all children have this need*
Plan appropriate activities for attention with nurse, other adults, and other children; use play *to work through relationships*
Praise child's abilities, *which promotes self-esteem*
Treat child as one who has a specific physical problem for hospitalization, not as "abused" victim
Avoid asking too many questions, *because this can upset child and interfere with other professionals' interrogations*
Use play, especially family or dollhouse activity, *to investigate type of relationships perceived by child*
Provide one consistent person to whom child relates regarding events of abuse *so that child is not overwhelmed*
Help child grieve for loss of parents if their rights are terminated *because child may be very attached to parents despite abuse*
Encourage child to talk about feelings toward parents and future placement *to facilitate coping*
Encourage introduction to foster parents before placement if possible *to give child time to adjust*

EXPECTED OUTCOMES

Child exhibits minimal or no evidence of distress
Child engages in positive relationships with caregivers
Child grieves for loss of parent

NURSING DIAGNOSIS ■ **Altered parenting related to child, caregiver, or situational characteristics that precipitate abusive behavior**

PATIENT (FAMILY) GOAL 1: Will exhibit evidence of positive interaction with children

NURSING INTERVENTIONS/*RATIONALES*

Identify families at risk for potential abuse *so that appropriate intervention is instituted*
Promote parental attachment to child, *because all children have this need*
Emphasize childrearing practices, especially effective methods of discipline, *because parents may lack knowledge about nonviolent discipline methods*
Increase parents' feeling of adequacy and self-esteem
Encourage support systems *that lessen stress and total responsibility of childcare on one or both parents*
Teach children to recognize situations that place them at risk for sexual abuse and teach assertive responses *to discourage abuse*

EXPECTED OUTCOME

Families exhibit evidence of positive interaction with children

PATIENT (FAMILY) GOAL 2: Will receive adequate support

NURSING INTERVENTIONS/*RATIONALES*

Provide "mothering" by directing attention to parent, taking over childcare responsibilities until parent feels ready to participate, and focusing on parent's needs *so that parents can eventually meet child's needs*
Convey an attitude of genuine concern, not one of accusation and punishment, *because this only serves to further alienate family*
Refer parents to special support groups or counseling *for long-term support*
Help identify a support group for parents, such as extended family or nearby neighbors; help these significant others understand their important role in also preventing further abuse
Refer to social agencies that can provide assistance in areas such as financial support, adequate housing, and employment

EXPECTED OUTCOMES

Parents demonstrate appropriate parenting activities
Parents seek group and individual support
Parents receive assistance with problems

PATIENT (FAMILY) GOAL 3: Will exhibit knowledge of normal growth and development

NURSING INTERVENTIONS/*RATIONALES*

Teach realistic expectations of child's behavior and capabilities
Emphasize alternate methods of discipline, such as reward, time-out, consequences, and verbal disapproval, *so that parents learn nonviolent discipline methods*
Suggest methods of handling developmental problems or goals, such as toddler negativism, toilet training, and independence, *because these situations may precipitate abuse*
Teach through demonstration and role modeling, rather than lecture; avoid authoritarian approach, *because family may be sensitive to criticism or domination and lack self-esteem*

EXPECTED OUTCOME

Parents demonstrate an understanding of normal expectations for their child

statements such as "He just loves you" or "You do whatever adults tell you to do" can place children in jeopardy. Health professionals must alert parents to such dangers and guide them toward an appreciation of the problem, providing concrete guidelines toward child education and protection.

● Evaluation

Continual reassessment and evaluation of care based on the following observational guidelines determine the effectiveness of nursing interventions:

1 Observe child for additional physical and behavioral evidence of abuse; observe child's reactions to health professionals; if child is hospitalized, check staffing patterns for schedule of consistent group of nurses caring for child.
2 Interview parents regarding their knowledge of children's physical and development needs.
3 Interview child regarding feelings about returning home or placement outside the home.
4 Investigate community programs aimed at preventing child maltreatment.

The **expected outcomes** are described in the Nursing Care Plan on p. 469.

KEY POINTS

- Common infectious disorders during early childhood include communicable diseases, intestinal parasitic infections, conjunctivitis, and stomatitis.

- Nursing goals in the treatment of a communicable disease are identification, prevention of transmission, provision of comfort, and prevention of complications.

- Intestinal parasitic diseases constitute the most common infections in the world; giardiasis and enterobiasis are the most widespread parasitic infections among children in the United States.

- Although the incidence of poisoning has decreased in the last 30 years as a result of more stringent packaging regulations, childhood poisoning remains a serious health concern.

- The major principles of emergency treatment for poisoning are assessment, supportive measures, gastric decontamination, family support, and prevention of recurrence.

- Communication with the area Poison Control Center is essential in the treatment of any poisoning.

- Acetaminophen poisoning is the most common drug poisoning among children and occurs primarily from acute overdose.

- The most important factor contributing to lead poisoning is its availability in the child's environment. Lead-based paint is the most toxic source of lead.

- Because of increasing awareness of the detrimental effects of low levels of lead on the developing nervous system, acceptable blood lead levels have been decreasing and now are at less than 10 μg/dL.

- Child maltreatment may take the form of physical abuse or neglect, emotional abuse or neglect, or sexual abuse.

- Parental, child, and environmental characteristics are criteria that may predispose children to maltreatment.

- Identification of abuse entails securing evidence of maltreatment, taking a history pertaining to the incident, and assessing parental and child behaviors.

- The reported incidence of sexual abuse has increased in the last decade; common forms are incest, molestation, rape, exhibitionism, child pornography, child prostitution, and pedophilia.

References

Abruzzi G, Stork CM: Pediatric toxicological concerns, *Emerg Med Clin North Am* 20(1):223-247, 2002.

Adler NA, Schutz J: Sibling incest offenders, *Child Abuse Negl* 19(7):811-819, 1995.

American Academy of Pediatrics, Committee on Infectious Diseases, Pickering L, editor: *2003 Red Book: report of the Committee on Infectious Diseases*, ed 26, Elk Grove Village, Il, 2003a, The Academy.

American Academy of Pediatrics, Committee on Injury, Violence, and Poison Prevention: Poison treatment in the home, *Pediatrics* 112(5):1182-1185, 2003b.

Brodeur AE, Monteleone JA: *Child maltreatment, a clinical guide and reference*, St Louis, 1994, Mosby.

Calam R and others: Psychological disturbances and child sexual abuse: a follow-up study, *Child Abuse Negl* 22(9):901-913, 1998.

Castiglia R: Shaken baby syndrome, *J Pediatr Health Care* 15(2):78-80, 2001.

Centers for Disease Control and Prevention: *Preventing lead poisoning in young children*, Atlanta, 1997a, CDC.

Centers for Disease Control and Prevention: *Screening young children for lead poisoning: guidance for state and local public health officials*, Atlanta, 1997b, CDC.

Chen TM and others: Clinical manifestations of varicella-zoster virus infection, *Dermatologic Clin* 20(2):267-282, 2002.

Eckenrode J and others: Preventing child abuse and neglect with a program of nurse home visitation: the limiting effects of domestic violence, *JAMA* 284(11):1385-1391, 2000.

Etzel R: The "fatal four' indoor air pollutants, *Pediatr Ann* 29(6):344-350, 2000.

Frechette A, Rimsza ME: Stungun injury: a new presentation of the battered child syndrome, *Pediatrics* 89(5):898-901, 1992.

Finkelstein Y, Markowitz ME, Rosen JF: Low-level lead induced neurotoxicity in children: an update on central nervous system effects, *Brain Res Brain Res Rev* 27:168-176, 1998.

Fischer DG, McDonald WL: Characteristics of intrafamilial and extrafamilial child sexual abuse, *Child Abuse Negl* 22(9):915-929, 1998.

Flournoy J: Incest prevention: the role of the pediatric nurse practitioner, *J Pediatr Health Care* 10(6):246-254, 1996.

Ford M, Delaney KA: Activated charcoal alone. In Ford MD: *Clinical toxicology*, St Louis, 2001, WB Saunders.

Hall D and others: Evaluation of covert video surveillance in the diagnosis of Munchausen by proxy: lessons from 41 cases, *Pediatrics* 105(6):1305-1312, 2000.

Hornor G: Repeated sexual abuse allegations: a problem for primary care providers, *J Pediatr Health Care,* 15(2):71-76, 2001.

Jacob B and others: The effect of low level blood on hematological parameters in children, *Environ Res* 82(2):150-159, 2000.

Johnson, CF: Abuse and neglect of children. In Behrman RE, Kliegman RM, Jenson HB: *Nelson textbook of pediatrics*, ed 17, Philadelphia, 2004, WB Saunders.

Lahoti SL and others: Evaluating the child for sexual abuse, *Am Fam Physician* 63(5):883-892, 2001.

Lederman C, Lederman M: Ophthalmologic emergencies. In Crain EF, Gershel JC: *Clinical manual of emergency pediatrics*, ed 4, New York, 2003, McGraw-Hill.

Litovitz T and others: 1999 Annual report of the American Association of Poison Control Centers toxic exposure surveillance system, *Am J Emerg Med* 18(5):517-574, 2000.

Markowitz M: Lead poisoning, *Pediatr Rev* 21(10):327-335, 2000.

McClain N and others: Evaluation of sexual abuse in the pediatric patient, *J Pediatr Health Care* 14(3):93-102, 2000

McCullough M, Scherman A: Family of origin interaction and adolescent mothers' potential for child abuse, *Adolescence* 33(130):375-384, 1998.

McMillian H: Child maltreatment: what we know in the year 2000, *Can J Psychiatry* 45(8):702-709, 2000.

Mileno MD: Intestinal parasites. In Rakel RE, Bope ET: *Conn's current therapy,* ed 55, St Louis, 2003, WB Saunders.

Moody CW: Male child sexual abuse, *J Pediatr Health Care* 13(3): 112-119, 1999.

Murry S, Baker A, Lewin L: Screening families with young children for child maltreatment potential, *Pediatr Nurs* 26(1):47-65, 2000.

National Clearinghouse on Child Abuse and Neglect Information: Child maltreatment 2002: Summary of key findings, 2004, The Clearinghouse. Retrieved May 6, 2004 from http://nccanch.acf. hhs.gov/general/stats/index.cfm.

Nelms BC: Emotional abuse: helping prevent the problem, *J Pediatr Health Care* 15(3):103-104, 2001.

Patel NJ, Sciubba J: Oral lesions in young children, *Pediatr Clin North Am* 50(2):469-481, 2003.

Paulk D: Munchausen syndrome by proxy, *Clin Rev* 11(8):51-56, 2001.

Pickering LK: Giardiasis and balantidiasis. In Behrman RE, Kliegman R, Jenson HB: *Nelson textbook of pediatrics,* ed 17, Philadelphia, 2004, WB Saunders.

Pillitteri A and others: Parent gender, victim gender, and family socioeconomic level influences on the potential reporting by nurses of physical child abuse, *Issues Compr Pediatr Nurs* 15:239-247, 1992.

Powers K: Diagnosis and management of common toxic ingestions and inhalations, *Pediatr Ann* 29(6):330-342, 2000.

Putnam FW: Ten year update review: child sexual abuse, *J Am Acad Child Adolesc Psychiatry* 42(3):269-278, 2003.

Rodriquez CM, Green AJ: Parenting stress and anger expression as predictors of child abuse potential, *Child Abuse Negl* 21(4):367-377, 1997.

Seidl AH and others: Nurses' attitudes toward the child victims and the perpetrators of emotional, physical, and sexual abuse, *Issues Child Abuse Accus* 5(1):28-38, 1993.

Souid AD, Keith DV, Cunningham AS: Munchausen syndrome by proxy, *Clin Pediatr* 37(8):497-503, 1998.

Stalkup JR: A review of measles virus, *Dermatol Clin* 20(2):209-215, 2002.

Stanton M and others: Nurses' attitudes toward emotional, sexual, and physical abusers of children with disabilities, *Rehabil Nurs* 19(4):214-218, 1994.

Stoeckle M: The spectrum of human herpes virus 6 infection: from roseola infantum to adult disease, *Ann Rev Med* 51:423-430, 2000.

Wang CT, Daro D: *Current trends in child abuse reporting and fatalities: the results of the 1997 annual fifty state survey,* Chicago, 1998, Prevent Child Abuse America.

Zempsky WT, Schechter NL: Acute pain in children, *Pediatr Clin North Am* 47(3):601-615, 2000.

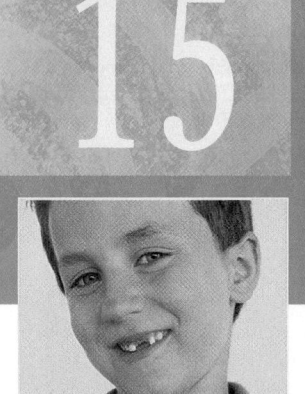

15

Health Promotion of the School-Age Child and Family

MARILYN L. WINKELSTEIN

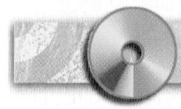 Remember to check out your companion CD-ROM

http://evolve.elsevier.com/Wong/essentials/

CHAPTER OUTLINE

RELATED TOPICS and ADDITIONAL RESOURCES

 IN TEXT

 CD COMPANION

Case Study—Injury Prevention
NCLEX-Style Review Questions

 WEBSITE

WebLinks
NCLEX-Style Review Questions

**WONG'S CLINICAL MANUAL
OF PEDIATRIC NURSING, 6/E**

Guidelines for Car Seat Safety

PROMOTING OPTIMAL GROWTH AND DEVELOPMENT

The segment of the life span that extends from age 6 to approximately age 12 has a variety of labels, each of which describes an important characteristic of the period. These middle years are most often referred to as *school-age* or the *school years.* This period begins with entrance into the school environment, which has a significant impact on development and relationships.

Physiologically the middle years begin with the shedding of the first deciduous tooth and end at puberty with the acquisition of the final permanent teeth (with the exception of the wisdom teeth). Before 5 or 6 years of age, children have progressed from helpless infants to sturdy, complicated individuals with an ability to communicate, conceptualize in a limited way, and become involved in complex social and motor behaviors. Physical growth is also rapid during the preschool-age years. In contrast, the period of middle childhood, between the rapid growth of early childhood and the prepubescent growth spurt, is a time of gradual growth and development with more even progress in both physical and emotional aspects.

BIOLOGIC DEVELOPMENT

During middle childhood, growth in height and weight assumes a slower but steady pace as compared with the earlier years. Between ages 6 and 12, children will grow an average of 5 cm (2 inches) per year to gain 30 to 60 cm (1 to 2 feet) in height and will almost double their weight, increasing 2 to 3 kg (4.5 to 6.5 pounds) per year. The average 6-year-old child is about 116 cm (45 inches) tall and weighs about 21 kg (46 pounds); the average 12-year-old child is about 150 cm (59 inches) tall and weighs approximately 40 kg (88 pounds). During this period, girls and boys differ very little in size, although boys tend to be slightly taller and somewhat heavier than girls. Toward the end of the school-age years, both boys and girls begin to increase in size, although most girls begin to surpass boys in both height and weight, to the acute discomfort of both girls and boys.

Proportional Changes

School-age children are more graceful than they were as preschoolers, and they are steadier on their feet. Their body proportions take on a slimmer look, with longer legs, varying body proportion, and a lower center of gravity. Posture improves over that of the preschool period to facilitate locomotion and efficiency in using the arms and trunk. These proportions make climbing, bicycle riding, and other activities easier. Fat gradually diminishes, and its distribution patterns change, contributing to the thinner appearance of the child during the middle years.

Accompanying the skeletal lengthening and fat diminution is an increase in the percentage of body weight represented by muscle tissue. By the end of this age period, both boys and girls double their strength and physical capabilities and their steady and relatively consistent development of coordination increases their poise and skill. However, this increased strength can be misleading. Although strength increases, muscles are still functionally immature when compared with those of the adolescent, and they are more readily damaged by muscular injury caused by overuse.

The most pronounced changes that indicate increasing maturity in children are a decrease in head circumference in relation to standing height, a decrease in waist circumference in relation to height, and an increase in leg length related to height. These observations often provide a clue to a child's degree of physical maturity and have proved useful in predicting readiness for meeting the demands of school. There appears to be a correlation between physical indications of maturity and success in school.

Facial Changes. Specific physiologic and anatomic characteristics are typical of children in middle childhood. Facial proportions change as the face grows faster in relation to the remainder of the cranium. The skull and brain grow very slowly during this period and increase little in size. Because all of the primary (deciduous) teeth are lost during this age span, middle childhood is sometimes known as the *age of the loose tooth* (Fig. 15-1). The early years of middle childhood, when the new secondary (permanent) teeth appear too large for the face, are known as the *ugly duckling stage.*

Maturation of Systems

Maturity of the gastrointestinal system is reflected in fewer stomach upsets, better maintenance of blood glucose levels, and an increased stomach capacity, which permits retention of food for longer periods. The school-age child does not need to be fed as carefully, as promptly, or as frequently as the preschool-age child. Caloric needs are less than they were in the preschool years.

Physical maturation is evident in other body tissues and organs. *Bladder capacity,* although differing widely among individual children, is generally greater in girls than in boys.

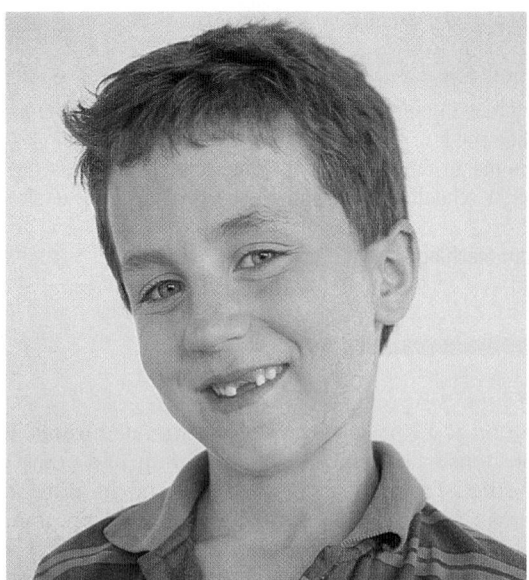

FIG. 15-1 ■ Middle childhood is the stage of development when deciduous teeth are shed.

The *heart* grows more slowly during the middle years and is smaller in relation to the rest of the body than at any other period of life. Heart and respiratory rates steadily decrease and blood pressure increases during ages 6 to 12 (see inside back cover).

The *immune system* becomes more competent in its ability to localize infections and to produce an antibody-antigen response. However, children have several infections in the first 1 to 2 years of school because of increased exposure to other children.

Bones continue to ossify throughout childhood but yield to pressure and muscle pulls more readily than mature bones. Children need ample opportunity to move around, but they should observe caution in carrying heavy loads. For example, they should shift books or tote bags from one arm to the other. Backpacks distribute weight more evenly than tote bags.

Wider differences between children are observed at the end of middle childhood than at the beginning. These differences become increasingly apparent and, if they are extreme or unique, may create emotional problems. The associated characteristics of height and weight relationships, rapid or slow growth, and other important features of development should be explained to children and their families. Physical maturity is not necessarily correlated with emotional and social maturity. Seven-year-old children who look like 10-year-old children will, in fact, think and act like 7-year-old children. To expect behaviors appropriate for the older age is unrealistic and can be detrimental to their development of competence and self-esteem. Conversely, to treat 10-year-old children who look young physically as though they were younger is an equal disservice to them.

Prepubescence

Preadolescence is the period of approximately 2 years that begins at the end of middle childhood and ends with the thirteenth birthday. Because puberty signals the beginning of the development of secondary sex characteristics, *prepubescence* typically occurs during preadolescence.

Toward the end of middle childhood the discrepancies in growth and maturation between boys and girls become apparent. On the average, there is a difference of approximately 2 years between girls and boys in the age of onset of pubescence. This is a period of rapid growth in height and weight, especially for girls.

There is no universal age at which children assume the characteristics of prepubescence. The first physiologic signs appear at about 9 years of age (particularly in girls) and are usually clearly evident in 11- to 12-year-old children. Although preadolescent children do not want to be different, variability in physical growth and physiologic changes between children of the same sex and between the two sexes is often striking at this time. This variability, especially in relation to the onset of secondary sexual characteristics, is of great concern to the preadolescent. Either early or late appearance of these characteristics is a source of embarrassment and uneasiness to both sexes.

Preadolescence is a period of time when considerable overlapping of developmental characteristics of both middle childhood and early adolescence occurs. However, there are several unique characteristics that set this period apart from others. Generally, the earliest age at which puberty begins is 10 years in girls and 12 years in boys, although there has been an increase in the number of girls reaching puberty at age 9. The average age of puberty is 12 years in girls and 14 years in boys. Boys experience little visible sexual maturation during preadolescence.

PSYCHOSOCIAL DEVELOPMENT

Freud described middle childhood as the *latency period,* a time of tranquility between the Oedipal phase of early childhood and the eroticism of adolescence. During this time children experience relationships with same-sex peers following the indifference of earlier years and preceding the heterosexual fascination that occurs for most boys and girls in puberty.

Developing a Sense of Industry (Erikson)

Successful mastery of Erikson's first three stages of psychosocial development are important in terms of development of a healthy personality (Erikson, 1963). Successful completion of these stages requires a loving environment within a stable family unit. These experiences prepare the child to engage in experiences and relationships beyond the intimate family group.

A *sense of industry,* or a *stage of accomplishment,* is achieved somewhere between age 6 and adolescence. School-age children are eager to develop skills and participate in meaningful and socially useful work. They acquire a sense of personal and interpersonal competence, receive the systematic instruction prescribed by their individual cultures, and develop the skills needed to become useful, contributing members of their social communities.

Interests expand in the middle years, and with a growing sense of independence, children want to engage in tasks that can be carried through to completion (Fig. 15-2). They gain satisfaction from independent behavior in exploring and manipulating their environment and from interaction with peers. Often the acquisition of skills provides a way to achieve success in social activities. Reinforcement in the form of grades, material rewards, additional privileges, and recognition provides encouragement and stimulation.

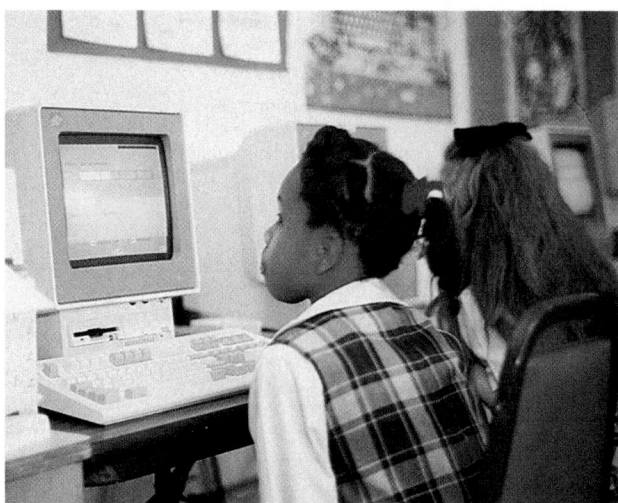

FIG. 15-2 ■ School-age children are motivated to complete tasks working alone.

A sense of accomplishment also involves the ability to cooperate, to compete with others, and to cope effectively with people. Middle childhood is the time when children learn the value of doing things with others and the benefits derived from division of labor in the accomplishment of goals. Peer approval is a strong motivating power.

The danger inherent in this period of development is the occurrence of situations that might result in a sense of *inferiority.* Children with physical and mental limitations may be at a disadvantage for acquisition of certain skills. When the reward structure is based on evidence of mastery, children who are incapable of developing these skills are at risk for feeling inadequate and inferior. However, even children without chronic disabilities may experience feelings of inadequacy in some areas. No child is able to do everything well, and children must learn that they will not be able to master every skill they attempt. All children, even children who usually have positive attitudes toward work and their own abilities, will feel some degree of inferiority when they encounter specific skills that they cannot master.

Children need and want real achievement. When they have access to tasks that need to be done, that they are able to do well despite individual differences in their innate capacities and emotional development, and for which they are suitably rewarded, children achieve a sense of industry.

COGNITIVE DEVELOPMENT (PIAGET)

When children enter the school years, they begin to acquire the ability to relate a series of events to mental representations that can be expressed both verbally and symbolically. This is the stage Piaget describes as *concrete operations,* when children are able to use thought processes to experience events and actions. The rigid, egocentric view of the preschool years is replaced by mental processes that allow children to see things from another's point of view.

During this stage, children develop an understanding of relationships between things and ideas. They progress from making judgments based on what they see *(perceptual thinking)* to making judgments based on what they reason *(conceptual thinking).* They are able to master symbols and

to use their memories of past experiences to evaluate and interpret the present.

One cognitive task of school-age children is mastering the concept of *conservation* (Fig. 15-3). At an early age (about 5 to 7 years), children grasp the concept of reversibility of numbers as a basis for simple mathematics problems (e.g., $2 + 4 = 6$ and $6 - 4 = 2$). They learn that simply altering their arrangement in space does not change certain properties of the environment, and they are able to resist perceptual cues that suggest alterations in the physical state of an object. For example, they recognize that changing the shape of a substance such as a lump of clay does not alter its total mass. They no longer perceive a tall, thin glass of water as containing a greater volume than a short, wide glass; they can distinguish between the weight of items regardless of their size. They recognize that size is not necessarily related to weight or volume. There is a developmental sequence in children's capacity to conserve matter. Conservation of mass usually is accomplished first, weight some time later, and volume last.

School-age children also develop *classification* skills. They can group and sort objects according to the attributes they share, place things in a sensible and logical order, and hold a concept in mind while making decisions based on that concept. Another characteristic of middle childhood that children derive enjoyment from is classifying and ordering their environment. They become occupied with collections of objects, such as stickers, stamps, shells, dolls, cars, and stones. They may even begin to order friends and relationships (e.g., first best friend, second best friend).

They develop the ability to understand relational terms and concepts, such as bigger and smaller; darker and paler; heavier and lighter; to the right of and to the left of; first, last, and intermediate relationships; and more than and less than. They view family relationships in terms of reciprocal roles (e.g., to be a brother, one must have a sibling).

School-age children learn the alphabet and the world of symbols called words that can be arranged in terms of structure and their relationship to the alphabet. They learn to tell time, to see the relationship of events in time (history) and places in space (geography), and to combine time and space relationships (geology and astronomy).

The *ability to read* is acquired during the school years and becomes the most significant and valuable tool for independent inquiry. Children's capacity to explore, imagine, and expand their knowledge is enhanced by reading.

MORAL DEVELOPMENT (KOHLBERG)

As children move from egocentrism to more logical patterns of thought, they also move through stages in the development of conscience and moral standards. Young children do not believe that standards of behavior come from within themselves but that rules are established and set down by others. During the preschool years children adopt and internalize the moral values of their parents. They learn standards for acceptable behavior, act according to these standards, and feel guilty when they violate them. Although children of 6 or 7 years of age know the rules and behaviors expected of them, they do not understand the reasons behind them. Rewards and punishments guide their judgment; a "bad act" is one that breaks a rule or does harm. Young children believe that what other people tell them to do is right and that what they themselves think is wrong.

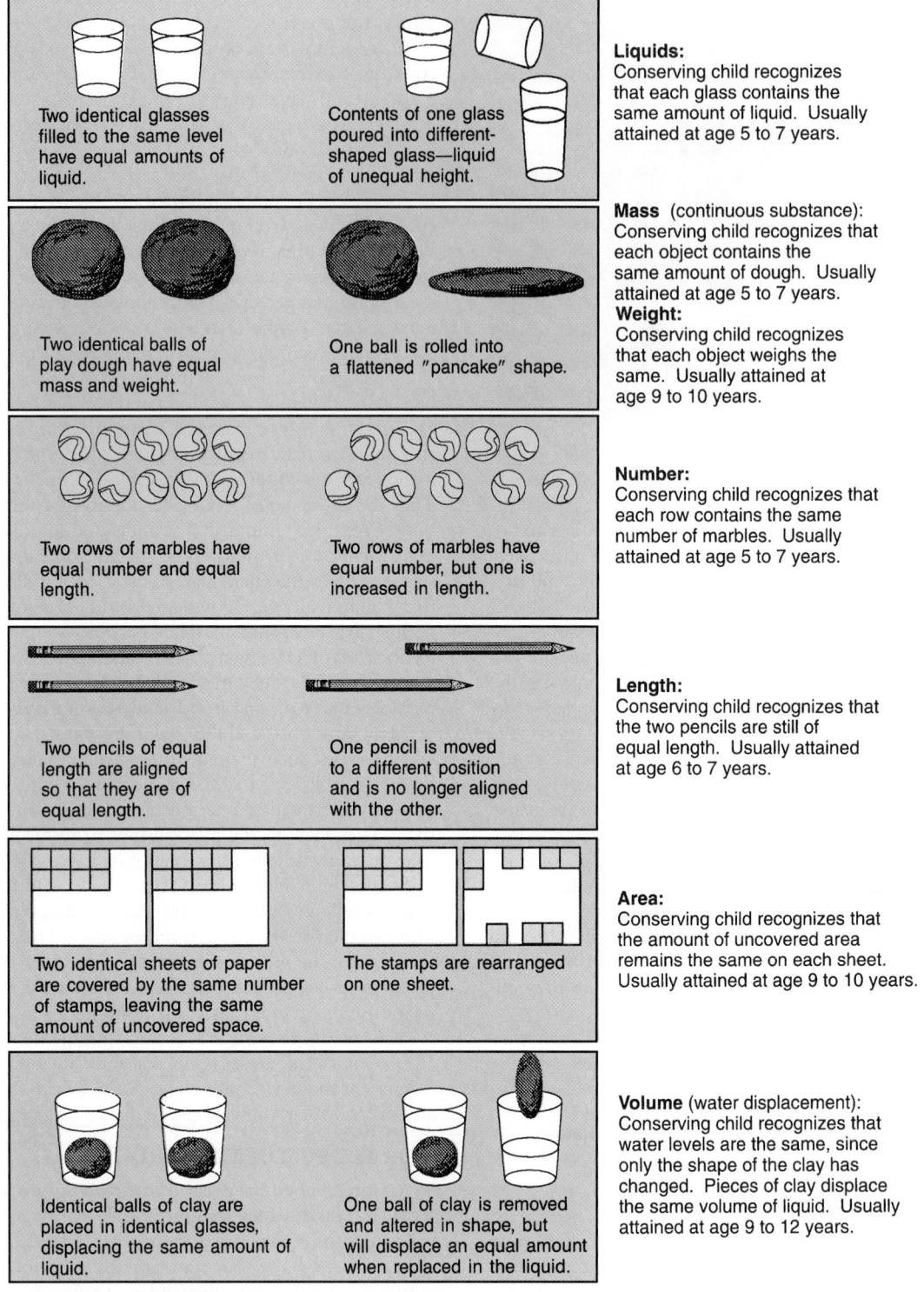

Liquids:
Conserving child recognizes that each glass contains the same amount of liquid. Usually attained at age 5 to 7 years.

Two identical glasses filled to the same level have equal amounts of liquid.

Contents of one glass poured into different-shaped glass—liquid of unequal height.

Mass (continuous substance):
Conserving child recognizes that each object contains the same amount of dough. Usually attained at age 5 to 7 years.
Weight:
Conserving child recognizes that each object weighs the same. Usually attained at age 9 to 10 years.

Two identical balls of play dough have equal mass and weight.

One ball is rolled into a flattened "pancake" shape.

Number:
Conserving child recognizes that each row contains the same number of marbles. Usually attained at age 5 to 7 years.

Two rows of marbles have equal number and equal length.

Two rows of marbles have equal number, but one is increased in length.

Length:
Conserving child recognizes that the two pencils are still of equal length. Usually attained at age 6 to 7 years.

Two pencils of equal length are aligned so that they are of equal length.

One pencil is moved to a different position and is no longer aligned with the other.

Area:
Conserving child recognizes that the amount of uncovered area remains the same on each sheet. Usually attained at age 9 to 10 years.

Two identical sheets of paper are covered by the same number of stamps, leaving the same amount of uncovered space.

The stamps are rearranged on one sheet.

Volume (water displacement):
Conserving child recognizes that water levels are the same, since only the shape of the clay has changed. Pieces of clay displace the same volume of liquid. Usually attained at age 9 to 12 years.

Identical balls of clay are placed in identical glasses, displacing the same amount of liquid.

One ball of clay is removed and altered in shape, but will displace an equal amount when replaced in the liquid.

FIG. 15-3 ■ Common examples that demonstrate the child's ability to conserve (ages are only approximate).

Consequently, children 6 or 7 years old may interpret accidents or misfortunes as punishment for "bad" acts.

Older school-age children are able to judge an act by the intentions that prompted it rather than just its consequences. Rules and judgments become less absolute and authoritarian, and begin to be founded on the needs and desires of others. For older children, a rule violation is likely to be viewed in relation to the total context in which it appears. The situation, as well as the morality of the rule itself, influences reactions. Although younger children judge an act only according to whether it is right or wrong, older children take into account a different point of view. They are able to understand and accept the concept of treating others as they would like to be treated.

SPIRITUAL DEVELOPMENT

Children at this age think in concrete terms, but are avid learners and have a great desire to learn about their God. They picture God as human and use adjectives such as "loving" and "helping" to describe their deity. They are fascinated by the concepts of hell and heaven, with a developing conscience and concern about rules. They may fear going to hell for misbehavior. School-age children want and expect to be punished for misbehavior and, when given the option, tend to choose a punishment that "fits the crime." However, they may view illness or injury as a punishment for a real or imagined misdeed. The beliefs and ideals of family and religious persons are more influential than those of their peers in matters of faith.

School-age children begin to learn the difference between the natural and the supernatural but have difficulty understanding symbols. Consequently, religious concepts must be presented to them in concrete terms. Prayer or other religious rituals comfort them, and if these activities are a part of their daily lives, they can help them cope with threatening situations. Their petitions to their God in prayers tend to be for tangible rewards. Although younger children expect their prayers to be answered, as they get older, they begin to recognize that this does not always occur and become less concerned when prayers are not answered. They are able to discuss their feelings about their faith and how it relates to their lives (see Cultural Awareness box).

SOCIAL DEVELOPMENT

One of the most important socializing agents in the school-age years is the peer group. In addition to parents and the schools, the peer group conveys a substantial amount of material to its members. Peer groups have a culture of their own, with secrets, mores, and codes of ethics that promote feelings of solidarity and detachment from adults. Through peer relationships children learn ways to deal with dominance and hostility, how to relate to persons in positions of leadership and authority, and how to explore ideas and the physical environment.

Peer group identification is an important factor in gaining independence from parents. The aid and support of the group provides the child with enough security to risk the moderate parental rejection brought about by small victories in the development of independence.

A child's concept of the appropriate sex role is influenced by relationships with peers. During the early school years there are few gender differences in the play experiences of children. Both girls and boys share games and other activities. However, in the later school years the differences in the play of boys and girls becomes more marked.

Social Relationships and Cooperation

Daily relationships with peers provide important social interactions for school-age children. For the first time, children join group activities with unrestrained enthusiasm and steady participation. Previous interactions were limited to short periods under considerable adult supervision. With increased skills and wider opportunities, children become

CULTURAL AWARENESS

Religious Orientation

Many schools and communities have a Judeo-Christian orientation toward prayer, holidays, and values. This may result in conflict and discomfort for children of other religious or ethnic groups. Sensitivity must be exercised so as not to offend and confuse children from other religious backgrounds, such as the Buddhist, Hindu, and Muslim faiths.

involved with one or more peer groups in which they can gain status as respected members.

Valuable lessons are learned from daily interaction with age-mates. First, children learn to appreciate the numerous and varied points of view that are represented in the peer group. As children interact with peers who see the world in ways that are somewhat different from their own, they become aware of the limits of their own point of view. Because age-mates are peers and are not forced to accept each other's ideas as they are expected to accept those of adults, other children have a significant influence on decreasing the egocentric outlook of the child. Consequently, children learn to argue, persuade, bargain, cooperate, and compromise to maintain friendships.

Second, children become increasingly sensitive to the social norms and pressures of the peer group. The peer group establishes standards for acceptance and rejection, and children are often willing to modify their behavior to be accepted by the group. The need for peer approval becomes a powerful influence toward conformity. Children learn to dress, talk, and behave in a manner acceptable to the group. A variety of roles, such as class joker or class hero, may be assumed by individual children to gain approval from the group.

Third, the interaction among peers leads to the formation of intimate friendships between same-sex peers. The school-age period is the time when children have "best friends" with whom they share secrets, private jokes, and adventures; they come to one another's aid in times of trouble. In the course of these friendships children also fight, threaten each other, break up, and reunite. These relationships, in which the child experiences love and closeness for a peer, may be important as a foundation for relationships in adulthood (Fig. 15-4).

Clubs and Peer Groups.   One of the outstanding characteristics of middle childhood is the formation of formalized groups, or clubs. A prominent feature of these groups is the rigid rules imposed on the members. There is exclusiveness in the selection of persons who have the privilege of joining. Acceptance in the group is often determined on a pass-fail basis according to social or behavioral criteria. Conformity is the core of the group structure. There are often secret codes, shared interests, and special modes of dress, and each child must abide by a standard of behavior established by the members. Conforming to the rules provides children with feelings of security and relieves them of the responsibility of making decisions. By merging their identities with those of their peers, children are able to move from the family group to an outside group as a step toward seeking further independence. Peer groups and

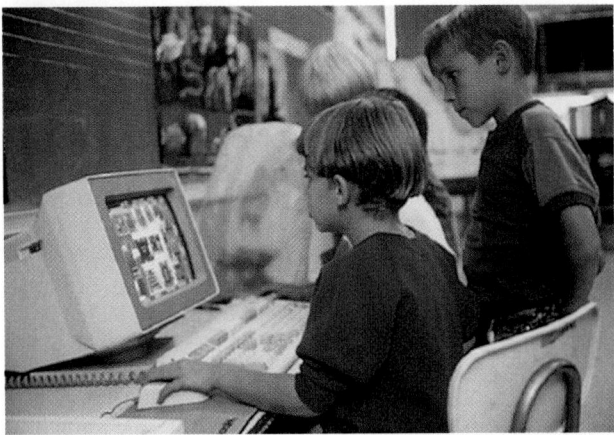

FIG. 15-4 ■ School-age children enjoy engaging in activities with a "best friend."

clubs allow children to substitute conformity to a peer group for conformity to a family at a time when children are still too insecure to function independently.

During the early school years, groups are usually small and loosely organized, with changing membership and no formal structure. The prolonged cohesiveness characteristic of groups or cliques in later school years is not obvious. In general, girls' groups are less formalized than boys' are, and although there may be a mixture of both sexes in the early school years, the groups of later school years are composed predominantly of children of the same sex. Common interests are the basis around which the group is structured.

Peer-group identification and association are essential to a child's socialization. Poor relationships with peers and a lack of group identification can contribute to bullying. *Bullying* is the repetitive, persistent use of verbal or nonverbal behaviors by one or more peers to inflict physical, or psychologic abuse (Olweus, 1997). Bullying occurs most frequently at school during unstructured times such as recess or lunch. Bullies may be from any ethnic, racial, or socioeconomic group. They are generally defiant toward adults, antisocial, and likely to break school rules. They have little anxiety, strong self-esteem, and may come from homes in which physical punishment is used and parental involvement and warmth are lacking. Boys who bully tend to use physical force, whereas girls who bully employ psychologic methods such as ostracism or rumors. Bullying by boys is more common than by girls. Children who are targeted for bullying often have characteristics different from the group norm (i.e., children who are short, obese, have facial deformities, attention deficit hyperactivity disorder, mental retardation or other developmental disabilities) (Vessey, Carlson, and David, 2003). The long-term consequences of bullying are significant. Chronic bullies seem to continue their behaviors into adulthood, negatively influencing their ability to develop and maintain relationships. Victims of bullying often fear school and can develop school phobia or long-term problems of depression and low self-esteem (Muscari, 2002). School personnel play an important role in developing proactive strategies to deal with bullies and by promoting a safe environment where bullying is not tolerated (Cavendish and Salomone, 2001).

There are also dangers in peer-group attachments that are too strong. Peer pressures force some children to take risks or engage in behaviors that are against their better judgment. Peer-group activities that result in unlawful or criminal *gang violence* are increasing in the United States, and gang violence is an important factor contributing to the problem of school violence (Kettl, 2001).

Relationships With Families

Although the peer group is influential and necessary to normal child development, parents are the primary influence in shaping the child's personality, setting standards for behavior, and establishing value systems. Family values usually take precedence over peer value systems. Although children may reject parental values while testing the new values of the peer group, ultimately they retain and incorporate into their own value systems the parental values they have found to be of worth.

In the middle school years, children want to spend more time in the company of peers and they often prefer peer-group activities to family activities. This can be very disturbing to parents. Children become intolerant and critical of parents and their ways when they deviate from those of the group. They discover that parents can be wrong, and they begin to question their knowledge and authority. Parents are no longer considered to be all-knowing or all-powerful.

Although increased independence is the goal of middle childhood, children are not ready to abandon parental control. They need and want restrictions placed on their behavior, and they are not prepared to cope with all the problems of their expanding environment. They feel more secure knowing that there is an authority figure to implement controls and restrictions. Children may complain loudly about restrictions and try to break down parental barriers, but they are uneasy if they succeed in doing so. They respect adults who prevent them from acting on every urge. Children view this behavior as an expression of love and concern for their welfare.

Children also need their parents as adults, not as pals. Sometimes parents, hurt at their children's rejection, attempt to maintain their love and gratitude by assuming the role of "pals." Children need the stable, secure strength provided by mature adults to whom they can turn during troubled relationships with peers or stressful changes in their world. With a secure base in a loving family, children are able to develop the self-confidence and maturity needed to break loose from the group and stand independently.

Play

Play takes on new dimensions that reflect a new stage of development in the school years. Play involves increased physical skill, intellectual ability, and fantasy, and children form groups and cliques and develop a sense of belonging to a team or club.

Rules and Rituals. The need for conformity in middle childhood is strongly manifested in the activities and games of school-age children. In the preschool years, children's games were either invented for them or played in the company of a friend or an adult. Now children begin to see the need for rules, and their games have fixed and unvarying rules that may be bizarre and extraordinarily rigid (especially those made up by the group). Conformity and ritual permeate their play and are also evident in their behavior and language. Childhood is full of chants and taunts, such as "Eeeny, meeny, miney, mo," "Last one is a rotten egg," and "Step on a crack, break your mother's back." Children derive a sense of pleasure and power from such sayings, which have been handed down with few changes through generations.

Team Play. A more complex form of play that evolves from the need for peer interaction is the team game and sports. The rules of team games may require the presence of a referee, umpire, or person of authority so that the rules can be followed more accurately. Team play teaches children to modify or exchange personal goals for goals of the group; it also teaches them that division of labor is an effective strategy for attaining a goal. Children learn about competition and the importance of winning—an attribute highly valued in the United States.

Team play can also contribute to children's social, intellectual, and skill growth. Children will work hard to develop the skills needed to become team members, to improve their contribution to the group, and to anticipate the consequences of their behavior for the group. Team play helps to stimulate cognitive growth because children are called on to learn many complex rules, make judgments about those rules, plan strategies, and assess the strengths and weaknesses of members of their own team and members of the opposing team.

Quiet Games and Activities. Although play at this age is highly active, school-age children also enjoy quiet and solitary activities. The middle years are the time for collections, which constitute another ritual. Young school-age children's collections are an odd assortment of unrelated objects in messy, disorganized piles. Collections of later school years are more orderly, selective, and organized in scrapbooks, on shelves, or in boxes.

School-age children become fascinated with complex board, card, or computer games that they can play alone, with a best friend, or a group. As in all games, adherence to the rules is fanatic. There is usually much discussion and argument, but any disagreements are easily resolved through reading the rules of the game.

The newly acquired skill of reading becomes increasingly satisfying as school-age children expand their knowledge of the world through books (Fig. 15-5). School-age children never tire of stories, and as with preschool children, they love to have stories read aloud. Sewing, cooking, carpentry, gardening, and creative activities such as painting are other activities enjoyed. Many creative skills such as music and art, as well as athletic skills such as swimming, horseback riding, dancing, and skating, are learned during these years and continue to be enjoyed into adolescence and adulthood (Fig. 15-6).

Ego Mastery. Play affords children the means to acquire mastery over themselves, their environment, and others. Through play, children can feel as big, as powerful, and as skillful as their imaginations will allow. They can also feel in control and attain vicarious mastery and power over whomever and whatever they choose. Schoolchildren still need the opportunity to use large muscles in exuberant outdoor play and the freedom to exert their newfound autonomy and initiative. They need space in which to exercise large muscles and to deal with tensions, frustrations, and hostility. Physical skills practiced and mastered in play help them to develop a feeling of personal competence, which contributes to a sense of accomplishment and provides status in their peer group.

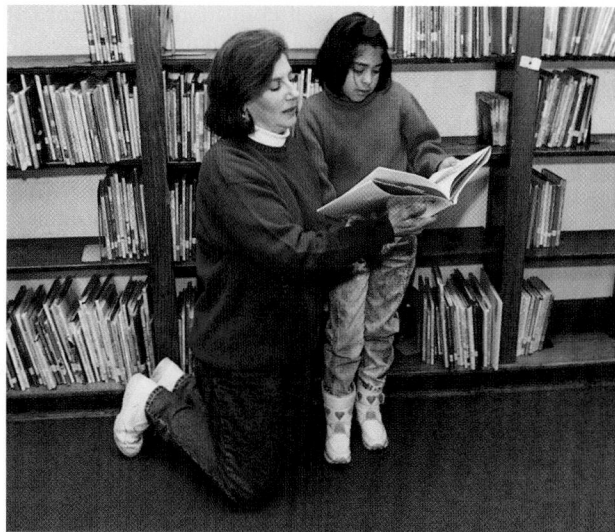

FIG. 15-5 ■ Selecting a book with the assistance of an adult.

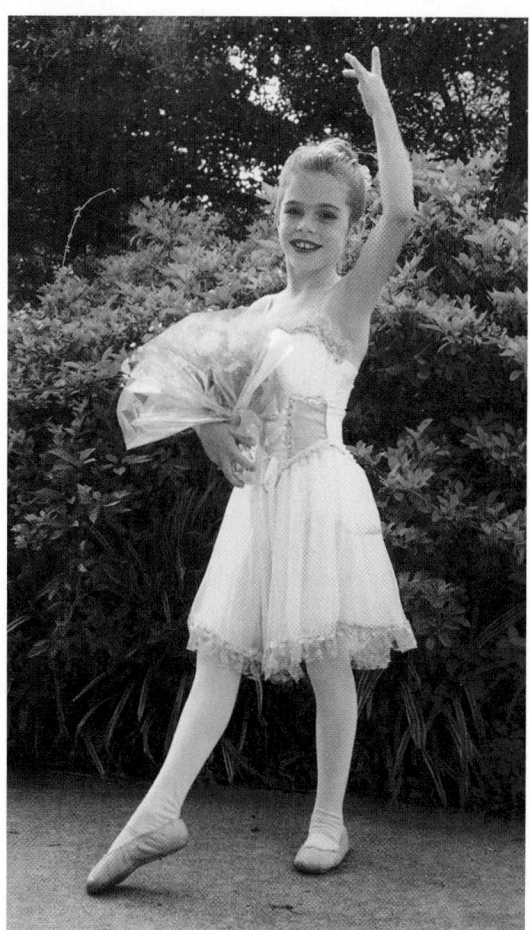

FIG. 15-6 ■ School-age children take pride in learning new skills.

DEVELOPING A SELF-CONCEPT

The term *self-concept* refers to a conscious awareness of self-perceptions, such as one's physical characteristics, abilities, values, self-ideals and expectancy, and an idea of self in relation to others. It also includes one's body image, sexuality, and self-esteem. Although primary caregivers continue to exert influence on children's self-evaluation, the opinions of peers and teachers provide valuable input during middle childhood. With the emphasis on skill building and broadened social relationships, children are continually engaged in the process of self-evaluation.

Significant adults can often manage to unobtrusively manipulate the environment so that children experience success. Each small success increases a child's self-image. The more positive children feel about themselves, the more confident they will be in trying for success in the fu-

ture. All children profit from feeling that they are in some way special to a significant adult. A positive self-concept makes children feel likable, worthwhile, and capable of significant contributions. These feelings lead to self-respect, self-confidence, and happiness. Negative feelings lead to self-doubt.

Developing a Body Image

School-age children have a relatively accurate and positive perception of their physical selves, but in general they like

TABLE 15-1 ■ Growth and Development During School-Age Years

AGE (YEARS)	PHYSICAL AND MOTOR	MENTAL
6	Height and weight gain continues slowly Weight: 16-23.6 kg (35.5-58 pounds); height: 106.6-123.5 cm (42-48 inches) Central mandibular incisors erupt Loses first tooth Gradual increase in dexterity Active age; constant activity Often returns to finger feeding More aware of hand as a tool Likes to draw, print, color Vision reaches maturity	Develops concept of numbers Can count 13 pennies Knows whether it is morning or afternoon Defines common objects such as fork and chair in terms of their use Obeys triple commands in succession Knows right and left hands Says which is pretty and which is ugly of a series of drawings of faces Describes the objects in a picture rather than simply enumerating them Attends first grade
7	Begins to grow at least 5 cm (2 inches) in height per year Weight: 17.7-30 kg (39-66.5 pounds); height: 111.8-129.7 cm (44-51 inches) Maxillary central incisors and lateral mandibular incisors erupt More cautious in approaches to new performances Repeats performances to master them Jaw begins to expand to accommodate permanent teeth	Notices that certain items are missing from pictures Can copy a diamond Repeats three numbers backward Develops concept of time; reads ordinary clock or watch correctly to nearest quarter hour; uses clock for practical purposes Attends second grade More mechanical in reading; often does not stop at the end of a sentence, skips words such as "it," "the," and "he"
8-9	Continues to gain 5 cm (2 inches) in height per year Weight: 19.6-39.6 kg (43-87 pounds); height: 117-141.8 cm (46-56 inches) Lateral incisors (maxillary) and mandibular cuspids erupt Movement fluid; often graceful and poised Always on the go; jumps, chases, skips Increased smoothness and speed in fine motor control; uses cursive writing Dresses self completely Likely to overdo; hard to quiet down after recess More limber; bones grow faster than ligaments	Gives similarities and differences between two things from memory Counts backward from 20 to 1; understands concept of reversibility Repeats days of the week and months in order; knows the date Describes common objects in detail, not merely their use Makes change out of a quarter Attends third and fourth grades Reads more; may plan to wake up early just to read Reads classic books, but also enjoys comics More aware of time; can be relied on to get to school on time Can grasp concepts of parts and whole (fractions) Understands concepts of space, cause and effect, nesting (puzzles), conservation (permanence of mass and volume) Classifies objects by more than one quality; has collections Produces simple paintings or drawings
10-12	*Boys:* Slow growth in height and rapid weight gain; may become obese in this period Weight: 24.3-58 kg (54-128 pounds); height: 127.5-162.3 cm (50-64 inches) Posture is more similar to an adult's; will overcome lordosis *Girls:* Pubescent changes may begin to appear; body lines soften and round out Remainder of teeth will erupt and tend toward full development (except wisdom teeth)	Writes brief stories Attends fifth to seventh grades Writes occasional short letters to friends or relatives on own initiative Uses telephone for practical purposes Responds to magazine, radio, or other advertising Reads for practical information or own enjoyment—stories or library books of adventure or romance, animal stories

their physical selves less as they grow older. The head appears to be the most important part of the school-age child's perceived image of self, with hair and eye color the characteristics used most frequently to describe the physical self.

Body image is influenced, but not solely determined, by significant others. The number of significant others influencing one's perception of the physical self increases with age. Children are acutely aware of their own body, the bodies of their peers, and those of adults. They are also aware of deviations from the norm. It is important that children learn about bodily functions and that adults provide correct information.

Physical impairments, such as hearing or visual defects, ears that "stick out," or birthmarks, assume great importance. Increasing awareness of these differences, especially when accompanied by unkind comments and taunts from others, may cause a child to feel inferior and less desirable. This is especially true if the defect interferes with the child's ability to participate in games and activities. Table 15-1 summarizes the major developmental achievements of the school-age years.

ADAPTIVE	PERSONAL-SOCIAL
At table, uses knife to spread butter or jam on bread At play, cuts, folds, pastes paper toys; sews crudely if needle is threaded Takes bath without supervision; performs bedtime activities alone Reads from memory; enjoys oral spelling game Likes table games, checkers, simple card games Giggles a lot Sometimes steals money or attractive items Has difficulty owning up to misdeeds Tries out own abilities	Can share and cooperate better Has great need for children of own age Will cheat to win Often engages in rough play Often jealous of younger brother or sister Does what adults are seen doing May have occasional temper tantrums Is a boaster Is more independent, probably influence of school Has own way of doing things Increases socialization
Uses table knife for cutting meat; may need help with tough or difficult pieces Brushes and combs hair acceptably without help May steal Likes to help and have a choice Is less resistant and stubborn	Is becoming a real member of the family group Takes part in group play Boys prefer playing with boys; girls prefer playing with girls Spends a lot of time alone; does not require a lot of companionship
Makes use of common tools such as hammer, saw, screwdriver Uses household and sewing utensils Helps with routine household tasks such as dusting, sweeping Assumes responsibility for share of household chores Looks after all of own needs at table Buys useful articles; exercises some choice in making purchases Runs useful errands Likes pictorial magazines Likes school; wants to answer all the questions Is afraid of failing a grade; is ashamed of bad grades Is more critical of self Takes music and sport lessons	Is easy to get along with at home Likes the reward system Dramatizes Is more sociable Is better behaved Is interested in boy-girl relationships but will not admit it Goes about home and community freely, alone or with friends Likes to compete and play games Shows preference in friends and groups Plays mostly with groups of own sex but is beginning to mix Develops modesty Compares self with others Enjoys organizations, clubs, and group sports
Makes useful articles or does easy repair work Cooks or sews in small way Raises pets Washes and dries own hair Is responsible for a thorough job of cleaning hair, but may need reminding to do so Is sometimes left alone at home for an hour or so Is successful in looking after own needs or those of other children left in his or her care	Loves friends; talks about them constantly Chooses friends more selectively; may have a "best friend" Enjoys conversation Develops beginning interest in opposite sex Is more diplomatic Likes family; family really has meaning Likes mother and wants to please her in many ways Demonstrates affection Likes father, who is admired and may be idolized Respects parents

COPING WITH CONCERNS RELATED TO NORMAL GROWTH AND DEVELOPMENT
School Experience

The school serves as the agent for transmitting the values of the society to each succeeding generation of children. School is also the setting for relationships with peers. After the family, schools are the second most important socializing agent in the lives of children.

Entrance into school causes a sharp break in the structure of the child's world. For many children it is their first experience in conforming to a group pattern imposed by an adult who is not a parent and who has responsibility for too many children to be constantly aware of each child as an individual. Children want to go to school and usually adapt to the new conditions with little difficulty. Successful adjustment is related to the physical and emotional maturity of the child and to the parent's readiness to accept the separation associated with school entrance. Unfortunately, some parents express their unconscious attempts to delay the child's maturity by clinging behavior, particularly with their youngest child.

By the time they enter school, most children have a fairly realistic concept of what school involves. They receive information regarding the role of a student from parents, siblings, playmates, and the media. In addition, most children have had some experience with day care, preschool, or kindergarten. Middle-class children have fewer adjustments to make and less to learn about expected behavior, because schools tend to reflect dominant middle-class customs and values. If the child has attended a preschool program, the focus of the preschool program also affects the child's adjustment. Some preschool programs provide custodial care only, whereas others emphasize emotional, social, and intellectual development.

Classmates have a significant impact on the socialization of children. School is the first time that most children become members of a large group of individuals their own age. Peer relationships become increasingly important and influential as children proceed through school. The specific influence exerted by the peer group depends on the background, interests, and abilities of the individual child.

Teachers.   Children respond best to teachers who possess the characteristics of a warm, loving parent. Teachers in the early grades perform many of the activities formerly assumed by the parent, such as recognizing the child's personal needs (e.g., the need to go to the bathroom, need for help with clothing) and helping to develop their social behavior (e.g., manners).

Teachers, like parents, are concerned about the psychologic and emotional welfare of the child. Although the functions of teachers and parents differ, both place constraints on behavior and both are in a position to enforce standards of conduct. However, the teacher's primary responsibility involves stimulating and guiding children's intellectual development, as opposed to providing for their physical welfare beyond the school setting.

Teachers serve as models that children try to emulate. Children seek their teachers' approval and avoid their disapproval. The teacher is a very significant person in the life of the early schoolchild, and hero worship of a teacher may extend into late childhood and preadolescence. Teachers who make supportive statements that reassure or commend children, use accepting and clarifying statements that help children refine ideas and feelings, and provide assistance that aids children with their own problem solving contribute to the development of a positive self-concept in the school-age child.

Parents.   Parents share responsibility for helping children achieve their maximum potential. There are numerous ways that parents can supplement the school program (see Family Home Care box). Cultivating responsibility is the goal of parental assistance. Being responsible for schoolwork helps children learn to keep promises, meet deadlines, and succeed at their jobs as adults. Responsible children may occasionally ask for help (e.g., with a spelling list), but usually they prefer to think through their work by themselves. Excessive pressure or lack of encouragement from parents may inhibit the development of these desirable traits.

Latchkey Children

The term *latchkey children* is used to describe children in elementary school who are left to care for themselves before or after school without the supervision of an adult. The increasing numbers of single-parent families and working mothers, together with the lack of available childcare, have created a stress-provoking situation for many school-age children. Some of these children may have a chronic illness as well.

Inadequate adult supervision after school leaves children at greater risk for injury and delinquent behavior. In some instances outside activities are curtailed and relationships with peers may be significantly diminished. Latchkey children may feel more lonely, isolated, and fearful than children who have someone to care for them. To cope with their fears and anxieties while alone, these children may devise strategies such as hiding, playing the television at loud volume, or using pets as a comfort.

Many communities and persons concerned about the welfare of latchkey children are trying to help these children and their parents to deal with this potentially serious problem. Some communities and employers have implemented after-school programs or telephone "hotlines" that provide check-in and reassurance for children. Nurses should be aware of these community services and encourage parents to teach self-help skills to these children.

Limit Setting and Discipline

Many factors influence the amount and manner of discipline and limit setting imposed on school-age children. Some of these factors are: the psychosocial maturity of the parents, the childhood and childrearing experiences of the parents, the temperament of the children, the context of the children's misconduct, and the response of the children to rewards and punishments. When children develop an ability to see a situation from the point of view of another, they are also able to understand the effects of their reactions on others and themselves.

Disciplinary techniques should help children control their own behavior. Reasoning is an effective technique for middle school–age children. With advancing cognitive skills

FAMILY HOME CARE

Helping Children in School

GENERAL GUIDELINES

Be supportive—through companionship, share ideas and thoughts.

Be positive—every child should experience some success each day.

Share an interest in reading—use the library; discuss books they are reading.

Support and encourage activity rather than passivity.

Encourage originality—help children make their own projects from discarded articles or other available materials.

Foster the development of hobbies and collections.

Encourage children to wonder and reflect during free time.

Encourage family experiences and trips to places of interest.

Encourage questions—help children discover sources for information or places to explore and investigate.

Stimulate creative thinking and problem solving—help children try out new solutions to problems without fear of making mistakes.

Use rewards rather than punishment.

SPECIFIC GUIDELINES

Meet the teacher at the beginning of school and plan to visit the school to see what is taught and expected.

Send the child to school every day—teachers are concerned when parents make other plans for their children; it conveys the impression that school is unimportant.

Demonstrate an interest in what the child is learning.

Demonstrate an interest in content and growth more than in grades.

Make it clear to the child that schoolwork is between the child and the teacher; teacher and child should set goals for better school performance to allow the child to feel responsible for school successes and failures.

Take advantage of situations that support and reinforce school learning.

Share information with teachers that will help them understand the child better.

Communicate with the teacher if there appears to be a problem—avoid waiting for a scheduled conference.

Provide a quiet, well-lighted area for study that is safe from interruption; do not allow television or radio.

Avoid dictating a study time, but do enforce rules, such as no television until homework is done; accept the child's word that work is complete.

Help with homework should focus on explaining the question, not giving the answer.

Teach the child to break large tasks (e.g., a report) into smaller, manageable tasks spread over the allotted time rather than attempt the entire project the night before it is to be completed.

Limit home tutoring to special circumstances, such as when the teacher requests parental assistance after a child's prolonged absence.

Request special help for children with learning problems.

Support the school staff by showing respect for both the school system and the teacher, at least in the child's presence.

---

they are able to benefit from more complex disciplinary strategies. For example, withholding privileges, requiring compensation, imposing penalties, and contracting can be used with great success. Problem solving is the best approach to limit setting, and children themselves can be included in the process of determining appropriate disciplinary measures.

Dishonest Behavior

During middle childhood, children may engage in what is considered to be antisocial behavior. Lying, stealing, and cheating may become manifest in previously well-behaved children. Such behaviors are disturbing and challenging to parents.

Lying can occur for a number of reasons. By the time children enter school, they still "tell stories," and often they exaggerate a story or situation as a means of impressing their family or friends. However, during middle childhood, children become able to distinguish between fact and fantasy. If children do not develop this characteristic, parents need to teach them what is real and what is make-believe.

Young children may lie to escape punishment or to get out of some difficulty even when their misbehavior is very evident. Older children may lie to meet expectations set by others to which they have been unable to measure up. However, most children know that lying and cheating are wrong, and they are very concerned when it is observed in their friends. They are quick to tell on others when they detect cheating.

Parents need to be reassured that all children lie sometimes and that sometimes children may have difficulty separating fantasy from reality. Parents should be helped to understand the importance of being truthful in their relationships with children.

Cheating is most common in young children 5 to 6 years of age. They find it difficult to lose at a game or contest, so they may cheat to win. They have not yet acquired the realization that this behavior is wrong, and they do it almost automatically. This behavior usually disappears as they mature. However, because children model observed behaviors, parents need to be aware of their own behavior. When parents set examples of honesty, children are more likely to conform to these standards.

As with other ethically related behavior, *stealing* is not an unexpected event in the younger child. Between 5 and 8 years of age, children's sense of property rights is limited, and they tend to take something simply because they are attracted to it or to take money for what it will buy. They are equally likely to give away something valuable that belongs to them. When young children are caught and punished, they are penitent—they "didn't mean to" and "promise never to do it again"—but it is quite likely that they will repeat the performance the following day. Often they not only steal but also lie about their behavior or attempt to justify it with excuses. It is seldom helpful to trap children into admission by asking directly if they committed the offense. Children do not take responsibility for these behaviors until the end of middle childhood.

Children steal for several reasons. Young children may lack a sense of property rights or attempt to acquire a specific object to bribe favors from other children. A strong desire to own a coveted item, and a desire for revenge to "get back at someone" (usually a parent for unfair treatment) are additional reasons for stealing. Older children may steal to supplement an inadequate allowance. However, stealing can be an indication that something is seriously wrong or lacking in the child's life. For example, children may steal to make up for love or another satisfaction that they feel is lacking. In most situations it is wise not to attempt to attach a hidden or deep meaning to the stealing. An admonition, together with an appropriate and reasonable punishment, such as having the older child pay back the money or return the stolen items, usually takes care of most cases. Most children can be taught to respect the property rights of others with little difficulty despite numerous temptations and opportunities. If children's personal rights are respected, they are likely to respect the rights of others. Some children simply need more time to learn the rules regarding private property.

Stress and Fear

Children today experience significant amounts of stress, and for some children, this stress can cause long-term adjustment and health problems. Stress in childhood comes from a variety of sources such as conflict within the family, interpersonal relationships, poverty, and chronic illness. The school environment itself may be a source of stress. Competing with classmates for grades and teacher recognition, and test or performance anxiety are common sources of school-related stress (Lau, 2002). When parents and teachers stress achievement and performance extensively, children experience emotional distress, and some children may actually develop school phobia (an exaggerated fear associated with attending school).

The increasing violence in society has also spilled over into the school setting. In the present information age, in which tragedy is broadcast daily in the media, children come to school knowing more about the latest world events than any previous generation of children. In addition, today's children are often personally aware of violence in their families or communities. Many children know other children who have been killed or children who have brought weapons to school. School-age children are also the victims of teasing, bullying, and physical abuse in the school environment (Nansel and others, 2003)

To help children cope with stress, parents, teachers, and health care providers must recognize signs that indicate a child is undergoing stress, identify the source of the stress promptly, and refer those children who need specialized treatment.

> ### NURSING ALERT
>
> The nurse who observes the following signs of stress in a child should explore the situation further:
> Stomach pains or headache
> Sleep problems
> Bed-wetting
> Changes in eating habits
> Aggressive or stubborn behavior
> Reluctance to participate
> Regression to earlier behaviors (e.g., thumb sucking)

Children 7 to 12 years of age are capable of identifying their own physiologic responses to stress with terms that have meaning to them. Some words or phrases used by children to describe their body's reaction to stress include "tight muscles," "hot or red in the face," "tingling," "chills or goose bumps," "shakiness," "heart beating fast," "headache," and "stomachache" (Sharrer and Ryan-Wenger, 2002). Children should be taught to recognize these signs as indicators of stress and to use techniques to manage their stress. Parents can help children to problem solve and to develop a plan to cope with stress. When an effective strategy has been developed for one situation, parents can show the child how to transfer the coping strategy or technique to other situations. Age-appropriate chores are an excellent way to teach children to face problems and learn to solve them (Lau, 2002). As children accept responsibility for chores and accomplish specific tasks, they develop strength of character, a sense of personal competence, and a willingness to accept new challenges.

In addition to stress, school-age children experience a wide variety of fears, including fear of the dark, excessive worry about past behavior, self-consciousness, social withdrawal, and an excessive need for reassurance. These fears are considered normal for children this age. During the middle-school years, children become less fearful of body safety than they were as preschoolers, but they still fear being hurt, kidnapped, or having to undergo surgery. They also fear death and are fascinated by all the aspects of death and dying. The fears of noises, darkness, storms, and dogs lessen, but new fears related predominantly to school and family bother children during this time.

PROMOTING OPTIMAL HEALTH DURING THE SCHOOL YEARS

NUTRITION

Although caloric needs are diminished in relation to body size during middle childhood, resources are being laid down at this time for the increased growth needs of adolescence. Parents as well as children need to be aware of the value of a balanced diet to promote growth because children usually eat what their family members eat. The quality of the child's diet depends on the family's pattern of eating.

Likes and dislikes established at an early age continue in middle childhood, although preferences for single foods subside, and children develop a taste for a variety of foods. However, the easy availability of fast-food restaurants, the influence of the mass media, and the temptation of "junk food" make it easy for children to fill up on empty calories. Foods that do not promote growth, such as sugars, starches, and excess fats, are common in the school-age child's diet. The easy availability of high-calorie foods, combined with the tendency toward more sedentary activities, has also contributed to an epidemic of childhood obesity. This problem is discussed further in Chapter 17.

Parents are unable to monitor what their children eat when they are away from home. A parent may pack a lunch for school but be unaware of how much is eaten, traded, sold, or thrown away. Nutrition education can and should be integrated in the curriculum throughout the school years. The Food and Drug Administration's Food Guide Pyramid, elements of a wholesome diet, and how food products are grown, processed, and prepared are important aspects of nutrition education. However, the school cafeteria may not always provide healthy, nutritious meals. The school nurse can take an active role in nutrition education by working with teachers to plan and implement units on nutrition instruction and by working with parents and children to give nutritional guidance.

SLEEP AND REST

The amount of sleep and rest required during middle childhood is highly individualized. The amount of sleep depends on the child's age, activity level, and state of health. The growth rate slows in the school-age years, and less energy is expended in growth than during preceding years.

School-age children usually do not require a nap, and they sleep approximately 9.5 hours at night. Although fewer bedtime problems occur during these years, occasional difficulties are still associated with the bedtime ritual. Usually children 6 or 7 years old exhibit few problems, and encouraging quiet activity before bedtime, such as coloring or reading, facilitates the task of going to bed. However, most children in middle childhood must be reminded frequently to go to bed; 8- to 9-year-old children and 11-year-old children are particularly resistant. Often these children are unaware that they are tired. However, if they are allowed to remain up later than usual, they are fatigued the following day. Sometimes, bedtime resistance can be resolved by allowing a later bedtime as the child gets older. Twelve-year-old children usually offer no resistance at bedtime; some even retire early to read a book or listen to music.

EXERCISE AND ACTIVITY

The improved capabilities and adaptability of the school-age child permit greater speed and effort in motor activities. Larger, stronger muscles permit longer and increasingly strenuous play without exhaustion. School-age children acquire the coordination, timing, and concentration that are required to participate in adult-type activities, but they may lack the strength, stamina, and control of the adolescent and adult. They can engage in a greater amount of physical activity during the school years. However, parents, teachers and coaches must remember that, although children this age are large and appear to be strong, they may not be ready for strenuous competitive athletics.

All growing children need regular exercise and opportunities for satisfying experiences that meet individual likes and dislikes. Appropriate activities during the school-age years include running, jumping rope, swimming, roller skating, in-line skating, ice skating, dancing, and bicycle riding. Positive reinforcement achieved by experiencing increasingly smooth, rhythmic, and efficient use of the body conditions the child toward regular physical activity. Exercise is essential for muscle development and tone, refinement of balance and coordination, increased strength and endurance, and stimulation of body functions and metabolic processes. Children need ample space to run, jump, skip, and climb, in addition to safe indoor and outdoor facilities and equipment. Most children have abundant energy and need little encouragement to engage in physical activity. Children with disabling conditions or those who hesitate to become involved in active play (such as obese children) require special assessment and help so that activities that appeal to them, and that are compatible with their limitations while also meeting their developmental needs, can be determined.

Sports

Considerable controversy surrounds the trend toward early participation in competitive athletics and the amount and type of competitive sports that are appropriate for children in the elementary grades. The current view is that virtually every child is suited for some sport, and authorities do not discourage participation if children are matched to the type of sport appropriate to their abilities and to their physical and emotional constitution. School-age children enjoy competition. However, teachers and coaches must understand the physical limitations of children this age and teach them the proper techniques and safety measures needed to avoid injuries. Hopefully, even the most unskilled and noncompetitive child can participate in safe, appropriate activities (Fig. 15-7). Common activities for school-age children include baseball, soccer, gymnastics, and swimming. Equipment must be maintained in safe condition, and protective apparatus should be worn to prevent serious injury (see Traumatic Injury, Chapter 31).

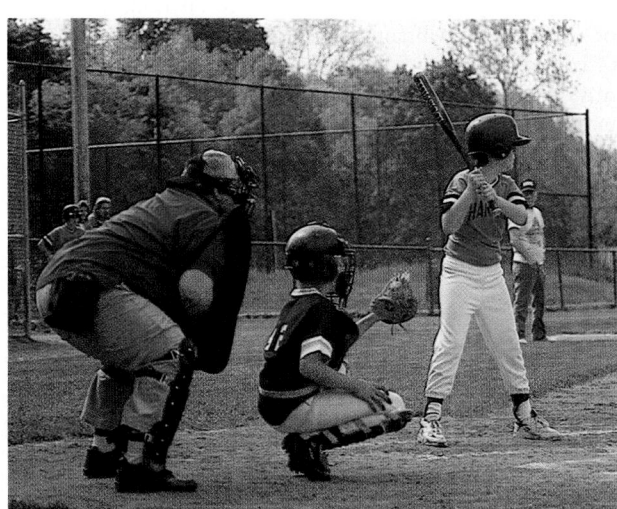
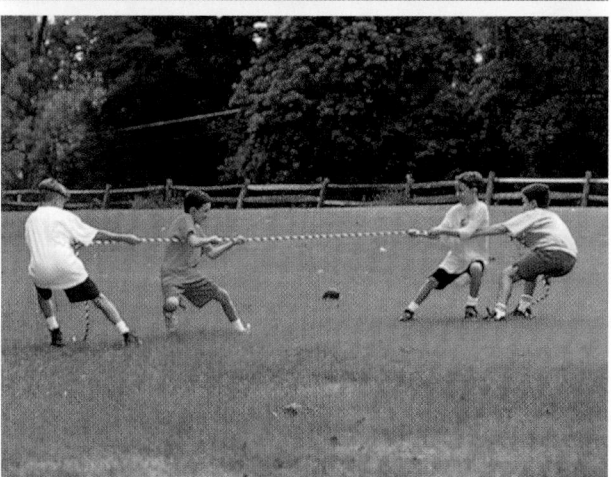

FIG. 15-7 ■ The activities engaged in by school-age children vary according to interest and opportunity. **A,** Little League competitors. **B,** Playing tug-of-war.

During the school-age years girls have the same basic body structure as boys and have a similar response to systematic exercise training. However, at puberty, boys become larger and have more muscle mass, and at this stage, it is usually recommended that girls compete only against other girls. Before puberty there is no essential difference in strength and size between girls and boys, making these precautions unnecessary.

Preadolescence is a time to teach fundamental motor skills; develop fitness in a practical, safe, and gradual manner; and promote healthy attitudes and values. Activities should include both practice sessions and unstructured play; the actual game or event should be managed in a manner that stresses mastery of the sport and enhancement of self-image rather than winning or pleasing others. All children should have an opportunity to participate, and special ceremonies should recognize all participants, not just individuals who excel in sports or athletics.

Acquisition of Skills

School-age children demonstrate increasing fine motor abilities and complex artistic skills. Handedness is well established by the beginning of the school years, and children make great strides in writing and drawing during this period. It is a time of energetic and vibrant creative productivity. With the tools of language and reading, children create poems, stories, and plays. With more advanced fine motor skills, they are able to master an unlimited variety of handicrafts, such as ceramics, needlework, wood carving, and beadwork. They avidly pursue these skills in solitude, with a friend, or in programs offered through organized groups such as boys' or girls' clubs or special interest groups that use crafts or other activities as a means to occupy, entertain, and educate children.

School-age children are capable of assuming responsibility for their own needs, although their distaste for soap and water and "dress" clothes is legendary. School-age children can and want to assume their share of household tasks, which usually are related to the male and female roles that have been defined by their culture. Many children also assume responsibility for tasks outside the home, such as baby-sitting, mowing lawns, or paper routes.

DENTAL HEALTH

The first permanent (secondary) teeth erupt at about 6 years of age, beginning with the 6-year molar, which erupts posterior to the deciduous molars. Other permanent teeth appear in approximately the same order as eruption of the primary teeth (see Teething, Chapter 10) and follow shedding of the deciduous teeth (Fig. 15-8). With the appearance of the second permanent (12-year) molar, most permanent teeth are present. Permanent dentition is more advanced in girls than in boys.

Because the permanent teeth erupt during the school-age years, dental hygiene and regular attention to dental caries are important parts of health supervision during this period (see Dental Health, Chapter 12). Correct brushing techniques should be taught or reinforced, and the role that fermentable carbohydrates play in production of dental caries should be emphasized. It is important to be alert to possible malocclusion problems that may result from irregular eruption of permanent teeth and that may impair function. Regular dental

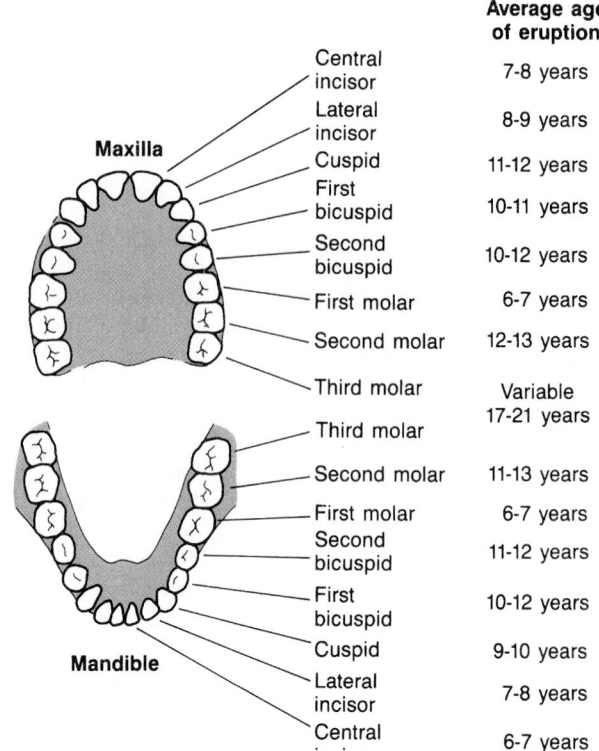

	Average age of eruption
Central incisor	7-8 years
Lateral incisor	8-9 years
Cuspid	11-12 years
First bicuspid	10-11 years
Second bicuspid	10-12 years
First molar	6-7 years
Second molar	12-13 years
Third molar	Variable 17-21 years
Third molar	
Second molar	11-13 years
First molar	6-7 years
Second bicuspid	11-12 years
First bicuspid	10-12 years
Cuspid	9-10 years
Lateral incisor	7-8 years
Central incisor	6-7 years

FIG. 15-8 ■ Sequence of eruption of secondary teeth. (Data from McDonald RE, Avery DR: *Dentistry for the child and adolescent,* ed 6, St Louis, 1994, Mosby.)

supervision and continued fluoride supplementation are essential integral parts of the health maintenance program.

The most effective means of preventing dental caries is proper oral hygiene. Children should be taught to perform their own dental care with the supervision and guidance of the parents. Parents should learn the correct brushing technique with their children, and they should monitor their child's efforts until the child can assume full responsibility.

Teeth should be brushed after meals, after snacks, and at bedtime. Children who brush their teeth frequently and become accustomed to the feel of a clean mouth at an early age usually maintain the habit throughout life. For the school-age child with mixed and permanent dentition, the best toothbrush is one with soft nylon bristles and an overall length of about 21 cm (6 inches). Several methods of brushing have been described and recommended for children, but there is no conclusive evidence that one method is superior to another. Thorough cleaning is more important than the specific technique used. The dentist should assess factors, such as the manipulative skills and special needs of the child, and suggest the most appropriate brushing technique and regimen. Flossing follows brushing. Parents should perform the flossing until children acquire the manual dexterity required for flossing (usually at about 8 or 9 years of age).

Dental Problems

Limited or inadequate dental care results in the most common dental problems (dental caries, malocclusion, and periodontal disease). Trauma, especially tooth evulsion, is another important dental problem. All of these conditions benefit from early intervention to prevent tooth loss.

Dental caries (cavities) is the principal oral problem in children and adolescents. Reducing the incidence and consequences of dental caries is extremely important in childhood. If untreated, dental caries can result in total destruction of the involved teeth. The ages of greatest vulnerability are 4 to 8 years for the primary dentition and 12 to 18 years for secondary or permanent dentition.

Dental caries is a multifactorial disease involving susceptible teeth, cariogenic microflora, and an appropriate oral environment. The incidence of lesions and the likelihood of progressive invasion vary considerably and depend on a number of factors being present in the right combination. Oral inspection is an integral part of the nursing assessment of the child. If there is any evidence of dental caries or other unhealthy dental state, the child should be referred for dental services. An alarming number of children do not receive regular dental supervision, and a significant number reach adulthood without dental examinations or treatment by a dentist.

Periodontal disease, an inflammatory and degenerative condition involving the gums and tissues supporting the teeth, often begins in childhood and accounts for a significant amount of tooth loss in adulthood. The more common periodontal problems are *gingivitis* (simple inflammation of the gums) and *periodontitis* (inflammation of the gums and loss of connective tissue and bone in the supporting structures of the teeth).

Gingivitis, the most prevalent periodontal disease, is a reversible inflammatory disease that begins in early childhood and is most often associated with the buildup of plaque on the teeth. Changes take place in the plaque bacteria, in both the type and number of organisms, causing them to release destructive exotoxins, enzymes, and other noxious agents. These substances produce an inflammatory reaction in the gingival tissues, causing the gums to become red, edematous, tender, and subject to bleeding at the slightest irritation. Management is directed toward prevention by conscientious brushing and flossing, including the use of fluoride. The child should see the dentist at any signs of inflammation or irritation.

Malocclusion occurs when teeth of the upper and lower dental arches do not approximate in the proper relationships. As a result, the physiologic function of chewing is less effective and the cosmetic effect is displeasing. Teeth that are uneven, crowded, or overlapping are unable to meet their counterparts in the opposite jaw in the appropriate relationships and may be predisposed to disease in later years.

Orthodontic treatment is most successful when it is started in the late school-age or early teenage years, after the last primary teeth have been shed and before growth ceases. However, referral should be made as soon as malocclusion is evident, because some deformities can be corrected at an earlier age.

Dental injury may occur in childhood and includes fractures of varying degrees of severity, chipping, dislocation, or evulsion. All tooth injuries require prompt treatment by a competent dentist to prevent permanent displacement or loss. Delayed examination and diagnosis of tooth damage can result in infection or pulp involvement. Because it can

EMERGENCY TREATMENT

Evulsed Tooth

Recover tooth.

Hold tooth by crown; avoid touching root area.

If tooth is dirty, rinse it gently under running water or saline; be sure to insert stopper in sink or basin (to avoid tooth loss).

Insert tooth into socket.

Have child maintain tooth in place.

Transport child to dentist immediately.

Avoid sudden stops or sharp turns to prevent dislodging tooth.

If Reluctant to Reimplant Tooth:

Place evulsed tooth in suitable medium for transport:

  a. Cold milk

  b. Saliva—under child's or parent's tongue

If child is holding tooth in the mouth, avoid sudden stops to prevent swallowing tooth.

DON'T FORGET TO TAKE TOOTH.

affect the remaining teeth, replacement of the lost tooth is needed to maintain normal alignment and position of the other teeth.

A tooth that is *evulsed* (exarticulated, or "knocked out") should be replanted by the child, parent, or nurse and stabilized as soon as possible so that the blood supply to the tooth can be reestablished and the tooth kept alive (see Emergency Treatment box). If the tooth is replaced within 30 minutes, there is a 70% chance that it will become reattached and the roots will not resorb or the crown will not exfoliate. Evulsed primary teeth are usually not reimplanted.

As with all injuries to the mouth, an evulsed tooth causes a large amount of bleeding, which is frightening to children and their families; therefore, the nurse or anyone faced with dental trauma should be prepared to cope with the emotionality that accompanies tooth evulsion. A calm approach and gentle reassurance to the child are successful strategies to reduce anxiety.

SEX EDUCATION

Many children experience some form of sex play during or before preadolescence as a response to normal curiosity, not as a result of love or sexual urges. Children are experimentalists by nature, and sex play is incidental and transitory. Any adverse emotional consequences or guilt feelings depend on how the behavior is managed by the parents, if it is discovered, or whether children view their actions as wrong in the eyes of significant persons, particularly the parents.

The child's attitude toward sex is acquired indirectly at a very early age. Initial curiosity about differences in body structure between boys and girls and between children and adults arises in the preschool years. Middle childhood is an ideal time for formal sex education, and many authorities believe that the topic is best presented from a lifespan approach. Information about sexual maturation and the process of reproduction helps to minimize the child's uncertainty, embarrassment, and feelings of isolation that often accompany puberty.

An important component of ongoing sex education is effective communication with parents. If parents either repress the child's sexual curiosity or avoid dealing with it, the sexual information that the child receives may be acquired almost entirely from peers. When peers are the primary source of sexual information, it is transmitted and exchanged in secret conversation and contains a large amount of misinformation.

Nurse's Role in Sex Education

No matter where nurses practice, they can provide information on human sexuality to both parents and children. To discuss the topic adequately, nurses must have an understanding of the physiologic aspects of sexuality, knowledge of the cultural and societal values, and an awareness of their own attitudes, feelings, and biases about sexuality.

When sexual information is presented to school-age children, sex should be treated as a normal part of growth and development. Questions should be answered honestly, matter-of-factly, and to the same extent as questions about other topics. Answers should be at the child's level of understanding. There may be times when boys and girls should be taught content separately.

Children need help to differentiate sex and sexuality. Exercises on clarifying values, identifying role models, engaging in problem-solving skills, and practicing responsibility are important to prepare children for early adolescence and puberty. In addition, children need explanations of sexual information that is provided via the media or jokes. Information concerning human immunodeficiency virus (HIV) infection should be presented in simple, accurate terms and should focus on how HIV is transmitted.

Preadolescents need precise and concrete information that will allow them to answer questions such as "What if I start my period in the middle of class?" or "How can I keep people from telling I have an erection?" It is important to tell children what they want to know and what they can expect to happen as they become mature sexually.

During encounters with parents, nurses can be open and available for questions and discussion. They can set an example by the language they use in discussing body parts and their function and by the way in which they deal with problems that have emotional overtones, such as exploratory sex play and masturbation. Parents need help to understand normal behaviors and to view sexual curiosity in their children as a part of the developmental process. Assessing the parents' level of knowledge and understanding of sexuality provides cues to their need for supplemental information that will prepare them for the increasingly complex explanations they will need to provide as their children grow older.

SCHOOL HEALTH

Child health maintenance is ultimately the responsibility of the parents; however, the public schools and health departments in the United States have contributed to the improvement of child health by providing a healthful school environment, health services, and health education that emphasizes sound health practices. Most of these functions constitute major components of community health services and involve large amounts of public funds and large numbers of health professionals, including nurses.

A school health program is involved in ongoing health maintenance through assessment, screening, and referral activities. Routine health services provided by most schools include health appraisal, emergency care, safety education, communicable disease control, counseling, and follow-up care. Health education of schoolchildren is directed toward providing knowledge of health and influencing habits, attitudes, and conduct in relation to health and injury prevention.

Traditionally, school nurses were viewed as the individuals who detected diseases in the school, and the people who applied bandages and cared for students who were ill or injured. Although these functions remain important parts of the school nurse's job, the role of the school nurse has expanded considerably in recent years. Today, school nurses manage and coordinate all the care required by regular students and students with special health care needs. In many settings, school health services have enlarged into family health centers that meet the needs of not only school-age children, but also their families and the community. In these settings, school nurse practitioners provide health care that includes assessment of physical, psychomedical, psychoeducational, behavioral, and learning problems as well as comprehensive well-child care (American Academy of Pediatrics, 2001b).

The passage of Public Laws 94-142 and 99-457 mandated the integration of children with chronic illness or disability into regular classrooms. School nurses are responsible for the medical and nursing needs of these children while the children are in the school setting. School nurses develop, implement, and evaluate individualized health care plans for these children. Unfortunately, not all schools have a school nurse, and the use of unlicensed assistive personnel (UAP) is increasing. In many schools, nurses are faced with the task of delegating to and supervising UAP (Rhodes, 1997; Delegation of School Health Services to Unlicensed Assistive Personnel, 1995). Delegation and supervision of UAP requires skillful nursing assessment and professional judgment.

INJURY PREVENTION

Because school-age children have developed more refined muscular coordination and control and can apply their cognitive capacities to their behavior, the number of injuries in middle childhood are diminished compared with the number in early childhood. The most common cause of severe injury and death in school-age children is motor vehicle accidents—either as a pedestrian or passenger. It is important that nurses continue to emphasize three automobile safety measures that have been found to reduce the severity of injuries: effective car restraint systems, door-lock mechanisms, and appropriate passenger-seating locations in the motor vehicle. The American Academy of Pediatrics (2002) advises health professionals and parents that the rear vehicle seat is the safest place for children of any age to ride in an automobile.

The school-age child's desire for riding bicycles increases the risk of injury on streets. Other serious injuries include accidents on skateboards, roller skates, in-line skates, skis, and other sports equipment. All-terrain vehicles (ATVs), popular with children younger than 16 years of age, are unstable, difficult to handle, and responsible for an increasing number of childhood injuries. The American Academy of Pediatrics (2000) views ATVs as a major health hazard for children and opposes their use by children younger than 16 years of age.

Most injuries occur in or near the home or school. The most effective means of prevention is education of the child and family regarding the hazards of risk taking and the improper use of equipment. Safety helmets, protective eye and mouth shields, and protective padding are strongly recommended for children engaging in active sports, even though they may not be required equipment. Falls from bicycles, ATVs, and skating devices are the cause of a significant number of head injuries in school-age children. Because head injury is the major cause of bicycle-related fatalities, the most important aspect of bicycle safety is to encourage the rider to wear a protective helmet (Fig. 15-9) (American Academy of Pediatrics, 2001a).

Physically active school-age children are also highly susceptible to cuts and abrasions, and the incidence of childhood fractures, strains, and sprains is high. Trampoline injuries are highest in children 5 through 14 years and account for numerous fractures, sprains, and head injuries. The American Academy of Pediatrics (1999) recommends against the use of trampolines in the home environment, routine physical education classes, or outdoor playgrounds. Injuries of a serious nature are discussed elsewhere in the book: burns (Chapter 30), eye trauma (Chapter 19), near-drowning (Chapter 28), and head injuries (Chapter 28). The prevalence of injuries depends on the dangers present in the environment, the protection offered by adults, and the behavior patterns of the chil-

dren. Table 15-2 lists characteristics of the school-age child that make them prone to injury and suggestions for injury prevention. Family Home Care boxes provide guidelines for bicycle, skateboard, and in-line skate safety and guidance during the school years.

FAMILY HOME CARE

Bicycle Safety

Always wear a properly fitted bicycle helmet that is approved by the **U.S. Consumer Product Safety Commission (SPSC);** encourage parents to look for the CPSC approval sticker on the inside liner of the helmet.

Replace a helmet every 5 years or sooner if manufacturer recommends it. **Never use a damaged or outgrown helmet.**

Ride bicycles with traffic and away from parked cars.

Ride single file.

Walk bicycles through busy intersections only at crosswalks.

Give hand signals well in advance of turning or stopping.

Keep as close to the curb as practical.

Watch for drain grates, potholes, soft shoulders, loose dirt, or gravel.

Keep both hands on handlebars, except with signaling.

Never ride double on a bicycle.

Do not carry packages that interfere with vision or control; do not drag objects behind bike.

Watch for and yield to pedestrians.

Watch for cars backing up or pulling out of driveways; be especially careful at intersections.

Look left, right, then left before turning into traffic or roadway.

Never hitch a ride on a truck or other vehicle.

Learn rules of the road and respect for traffic officers.

Obey all local ordinances.

Wear shoes that fit securely while riding.

Wear light colors at night and attach fluorescent material to clothing and bicycle.

Be certain the bicycle is the correct size for rider.

Equip bicycle with proper lights and reflectors.

Have bicycle inspected to ensure good mechanical condition.

Children riding as passengers must wear appropriate-size helmets in specially designed protective seats.

Modified from American Academy of Pediatrics, Committee on Injury and Poison Prevention: Bicycle helmets, *Pediatrics* 108(4):1030-1032, 2001.

FAMILY HOME CARE

Skateboard and In-Line Skate Safety

Children younger than 5 years of age should not use skateboards or in-line skates. They are not developmentally prepared to protect themselves from injury.

Children who ride skateboards or in-line skates should wear helmets and other protective equipment, especially on knees, wrists, and elbows, to prevent injury.

Skateboards and in-line skates should never be used near traffic. Their use should be prohibited on streets and highways. Activities that bring skateboards together (e.g., "catching a ride") are especially dangerous.

Some types of use, such as riding homemade ramps on hard surfaces, may be particularly hazardous.

Modified from American Academy of Pediatrics, Committee on Injury and Poison Prevention: Skateboard injuries, *Pediatrics* 95(4):611-612, 1995.

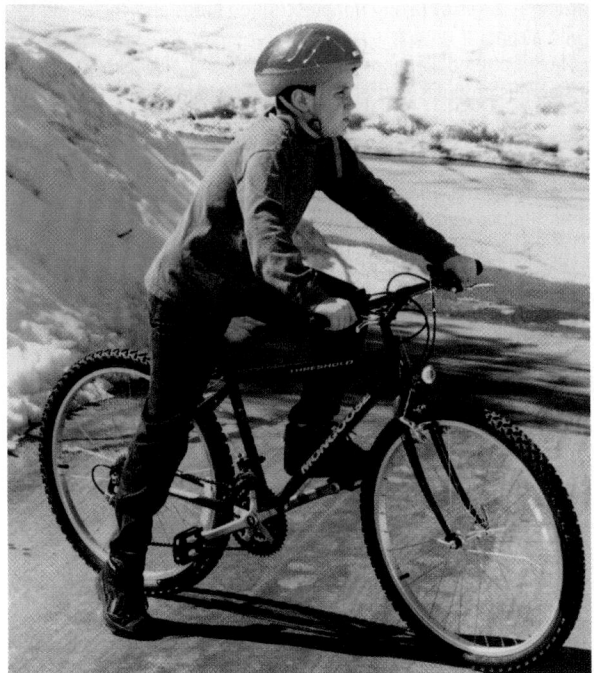

FIG. 15-9 ■ The right size bike is important; the child should be able to sit on the bike and place the balls of both feet on the ground. The foot should comfortably reach and manipulate the pedal in the down position. Wearing a protective helmet is mandatory. The helmet should be positioned on the head so it sits low on the forehead and parallel to the ground when the head is held upright. It should not rock back and forth or shift from side to side. The strap should be fastened securely under the chin.

TABLE 15-2 ■ Injury Prevention During School-Age Years

DEVELOPMENTAL ABILITIES RELATED TO RISK OF INJURY	INJURY PREVENTION
Is increasingly involved in activities away from home Is excited by speed and motion Is easily distracted by environment Can be reasoned with	**Motor vehicle accidents** Educate child regarding proper use of seat belts while a passenger in a vehicle Maintain discipline while a passenger in a vehicle (e.g., keep arms inside, do not lean against doors, do not interfere with driver) Remind parents and children that no one should ride in the bed of a pickup truck Emphasize safe pedestrian behavior Insist on wearing safety apparel (e.g., helmet) when applicable, such as riding bicycle, motorcycle, moped, or all-terrain vehicle (see Family Home Care box, p. 489)
Is apt to overdo May work hard to perfect a skill Has cautious, but not fearful, gross motor actions Likes swimming	**Drowning** Teach child to swim Teach basic rules of water safety Select safe and supervised places to swim Check sufficient water depth for diving Swim with a companion Use an approved flotation device in water or boat Advocate for legislation requiring fencing around pools Learn cardiopulmonary resuscitation (CPR)
Has increasing independence Is adventuresome Enjoys trying new things	**Burns** Make sure smoke detectors are in homes Set water heaters to 48.9° C (120° F) to avoid scald burns Instruct child in behavior in areas involving contact with potential burn hazards (e.g., gasoline, matches, bonfires or barbecues, lighter fluid, firecrackers, cigarette lighters, cooking utensils, chemistry sets); avoid climbing or flying kite around high-tension wires Instruct child in proper behavior in the event of fire (e.g., fire drills at home and school) Teach child safe cooking (use low heat; avoid any frying; be careful of steam burns, scalds, or exploding foods, especially from microwaving)
Adheres to group rules May be easily influenced by peers Has strong allegiance to friends	**Poisoning** Educate child regarding hazards of taking nonprescription drugs and chemicals, including aspirin and alcohol Teach child to say "no" if offered illegal or dangerous drugs or alcohol Keep potentially dangerous products in properly labeled receptacles, preferably out of reach

Has increased physical skills
Needs strenuous physical activity
Is interested in acquiring new skills and perfecting attained skills
Is daring and adventurous, especially with peers
Frequently plays in hazardous places
Confidence often exceeds physical capacity
Desires group loyalty and has strong need for friends' approval
Attempts hazardous feats
Accompanies friends to potentially hazardous facilities
Delights in physical activity
Is likely to overdo
Growth in height exceeds muscular growth and coordination
	Bodily damage
	Help provide facilities for supervised activities
	Encourage playing in safe places
	Keep firearms safely locked up except during adult supervision
	Teach proper care of, use of, and respect for devices with potential danger (e.g., power tools, firecrackers)
	Teach children not to tease or surprise dogs, invade their territory, take dogs' toys, or interfere with dogs' feeding
	Stress eye, ear, or mouth protection when using potentially hazardous objects or devices or when engaging in potentially hazardous sports
	Do not permit use of trampolines except as part of supervised training
	Teach safety regarding use of corrective devices (glasses); if child wears contact lenses, monitor duration of wear to prevent corneal damage
	Stress careful selection, use, and maintenance of sports and recreation equipment, such as skateboards and in-line skates (see Family Home Care box, p. 489)
	Emphasize proper conditioning, safe practices, and use of safety equipment for sports or recreational activities
	Caution against engaging in hazardous sports, such as those involving trampolines
	Use safety glass and decals on large glassed areas, such as sliding glass doors
	Use window guards to prevent falls
	Teach name, address, and phone number and emphasize that child should ask for help from appropriate people (e.g., cashier, security guard, police) if lost; have identification on child (e.g., sewn in clothes, inside shoe)
	Teach stranger safety:
	    Avoid personalized clothing in public places
	    Caution child to never go with a stranger
	Have child tell parents if anyone makes child feel uncomfortable in any way
	Always listen to child's concerns regarding others' behavior
	Teach child to say "no" when confronted with uncomfortable situations.

FAMILY HOME CARE

Guidance During School Years

AGE 6 YEARS

Prepare parents to expect strong food preferences and frequent refusal of specific food items.

Prepare parents to expect increasingly ravenous appetite.

Prepare parents for emotionality as child experiences erratic mood changes.

Help parents anticipate continued susceptibility to illness.

Teach injury prevention and safety, especially bicycle safety.

Encourage parents to respect child's need for privacy and to provide a separate bedroom for child, if possible.

Prepare parents for child's increasing interests outside the home.

Help parents understand the need to encourage child's interactions with peers

AGES 7 TO 10 YEARS

Prepare parents to expect improvement in health with fewer illnesses, but warn them that allergies may increase or become apparent.

Prepare parents to expect an increase in minor injuries.

Emphasize caution in selecting and maintaining sports equipment and reemphasize safety.

Prepare parents to expect increased involvement with peers and interest in activities outside the home.

Emphasize the need to encourage independence while maintaining limit setting and discipline.

Prepare mothers to expect more demands at 8 years.

Prepare fathers to expect increasing admiration at 10 years; encourage father-child activities.

Prepare parents for prepubescent changes in girls.

AGES 11 TO 12 YEARS

Help parents prepare child for body changes of pubescence.

Prepare parents to expect a growth spurt in girls.

Make certain child's sex education is adequate with accurate information.

Prepare parents to expect energetic but stormy behavior at 11 years, becoming more even-tempered at 12 years.

Encourage parents to support child's desire to "grow up" but to allow regressive behavior when needed.

Prepare parents to expect an increase in child's masturbation.

Instruct parents that the amount of rest the child needs may increase.

Help parents educate child regarding experimentation with potentially harmful activities.

HEALTH GUIDANCE

Help parents understand the importance of regular health and dental care for the child.

Encourage parents to teach and model sound health practices, including diet, rest, activity, and exercise.

Stress the need to encourage children to engage in appropriate physical activities.

Emphasize providing a safe physical and emotional environment.

Encourage parents to teach and model safety practices.

ANTICIPATORY GUIDANCE—CARE OF FAMILIES

Parents of the school-age child must share their child's time with the increasingly important peer group. Experiences with the peer group prepare school-age children for the broader world of relationships and increased independence from their parents. Parents must learn to provide support as unobtrusively as possible without feeling rejected, hurt, or angry. The nurse can help parents of the school-age child by providing anticipatory guidance and reassurance throughout this period (see Family Home Care box).

KEY POINTS

- Middle childhood, also known as the school years, is the period of life that extends from 6 to 12 years of age.
- Although growth is slower than in previous years, there is a steady gain in height and weight, with maturation of body systems; primary teeth are lost and replaced by permanent teeth.
- A major task during the middle school years is developing a sense of industry or accomplishment (Erikson).
- Piaget's period of concrete operations refers to the school-age period, when children are able to use their thought processes to experience events and actions, and make judgments based on what they reason.
- The child develops a conscience and is able to understand and adhere to rules and standards set by others.
- Entertaining different points of view, becoming sensitive to social norms, and forming peer friendships are important features of social development during the school years.
- Cooperative play, team activities, and the acquisition of skills are prime elements of play during the school years; rules and rituals assume greater importance.
- Parental concerns during middle childhood are beginning separation from the family unit, dishonest behavior, and school achievement.
- The availability of junk foods, irregular family meals, and schedules of working parents often hamper optimal nutrition.
- Dental care is important during this time; dental problems include caries, periodontal disease, malocclusion, and dental injury.
- Increased socialization and media exposure make the school years an ideal time for sex education.
- School health ideally offers programs that include health appraisal, emergency care, safety education, communicable disease control, counseling, guidance, and health education with adjustment to individual student needs.
- Injury prevention is directed toward safety education, provision of safe play areas and equipment, and well-supervised sports activities.

References

American Academy of Pediatrics, Committee on Injury and Poison Prevention: All terrain vehicle injury prevention: two-, three- and four-wheeled unlicensed motor vehicles, *Pediatrics* 105(6):1352-1354, 2000

American Academy of Pediatrics, Committee on Injury and Poison Prevention: Bicycle helmets, *Pediatrics* 108(4):1030-1032, 2001a.

American Academy of Pediatrics, Committee on Injury and Poison Prevention: Selecting and using the most appropriate car safety seats for growing children: guidelines for counseling parents, *Pediatrics* 109(3):550-553, 2002.

American Academy of Pediatrics, Committee on Injury and Poison Prevention and Committee on Sports Medicine and Fitness: Trampolines at home, school, and recreational centers, *Pediatrics* 103(5 pt 1):1053-1056, 1999.

American Academy of Pediatrics, Committee on School Health: School health centers and other integrated school health services, *Pediatrics* 107(1):198-201, 2001b.

Cavendish R, Salomone C: Bullying and sexual harassment in the school setting, *J Sch Nurs* 17(1):25-31, 2001.

Delegation of School Health Services to Unlicensed Assistive Personnel: A position paper of the National Association of State School Nurse Consultants, *J Sch Nurs* 11(4):13-16, 1995.

Erikson EH: *Childhood and society,* ed 2, New York, 1963, WW Norton.

Kettl P: Biological and social causes of school violence. In Shafii M, Shafii S, editors: *School violence assessment, management prevention,* Washington, DC, 2001, American Psychiatric Publishing.

Lau BWK: Stress in children: can nurses help? *Pediatr Nurs* 28(1):13-19, 2002.

Muscari ME: Sticks and stones: the NP's role with bullies and victims, *J Pediatr Health Care* 16(1):22-28, 2002.

Nansel TR and others: Relationships between bullying and violence among US youth, *Arch Pediatr Adolesc Med* 157(4):348-353, 2003

Olweus D: Bully/victim problems in school: facts and intervention, *Eur J Psych Educ* 12:495-510, 1997.

Rhodes AM: Liability for unlicensed assistive personnel, part I, *MCN* 22:269, 1997.

Sharrer VW, Ryan-Wenger NA: School-age children's self-reported stress symptoms, *Pediatr Nurs* 28(1):21-27, 2002.

Vessey JA, Carlson K, David J: Helping children who are being teased and bullied, *Nurs Spectrum* 13:16-18, 2003.

16

Health Promotion of the Adolescent and Family

LINDA M. KOLLAR

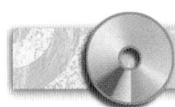 Remember to check out your companion CD-ROM

http://evolve.elsevier.com/Wong/essentials/

CHAPTER OUTLINE

RELATED TOPICS and ADDITIONAL RESOURCES

 IN TEXT

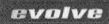

PROMOTING OPTIMAL GROWTH AND DEVELOPMENT

Adolescence is a period of transition between childhood and adulthood—a time of rapid physical, cognitive, social, and emotional maturing as the boy prepares for manhood and the girl prepares for womanhood (see Cultural Awareness box). The precise boundaries of adolescence are difficult to define, but this period is customarily viewed as beginning with the gradual appearance of secondary sex characteristics at about 11 or 12 years of age and ending with cessation of body growth at 18 to 20 years.

Several terms are used to refer to this stage of growth and development. *Puberty* refers to the maturational, hormonal, and growth process that occurs when the reproductive organs begin to function and the secondary sex characteristics develop. This process is sometimes divided into three stages: *prepubescence,* the period of about 2 years immediately before puberty when the child is developing preliminary physical changes that herald sexual maturity; *puberty,* the point at which sexual maturity is achieved, marked by the first menstrual flow in girls but by less obvious indications in boys; and *postpubescence,* a 1- to 2-year period following puberty during which skeletal growth is completed and reproductive functions become fairly well established. *Adolescence,* which literally means, "to grow into maturity," is generally regarded as the psychologic, social, and maturational process initiated by the pubertal changes. It involves three distinct subphases: *early adolescence* (ages 11 to 14), *middle adolescence* (ages 15 to 17), and *late adolescence* (ages 18 to 20). The term *teenage years* is used synonymously with *adolescence* to describe ages 13 through 19.

BIOLOGIC DEVELOPMENT

The physical changes of puberty are primarily the result of hormonal activity under the influence of the central nervous system, although all aspects of physiologic functioning are mutually interacting. The obvious physical changes are noted in increased physical growth and in the appearance and development of secondary sex characteristics; less obvious are physiologic alterations and neurogonadal maturity, accompanied by the ability to procreate. Physical distinction between the sexes is made on the basis of distinguishing characteristics. *Primary sex characteristics* are the external and internal organs that carry out the reproductive functions (e.g., ovaries, uterus, breasts, penis). *Secondary sex characteristics* are the changes that occur throughout the body as a result of hormonal changes (e.g., voice alterations, development of facial and pubertal hair, fat deposits), but that play no direct part in reproduction.

Hormonal Changes of Puberty

The events of puberty are caused by hormonal influences and controlled by the anterior pituitary (adenohypophysis) in response to a stimulus from the hypothalamus. Stimulation of the gonads has a dual function: (1) production and release of gametes—production of sperm in the male and maturation and release of ova in the female—and (2) secretion of sex-appropriate hormones—estrogen and progesterone from the ovaries (female) and testosterone from the testes (male).

Sex Hormones. The ovaries, testes, and adrenals secrete sex hormones. These hormones are produced in varying amounts by both sexes throughout the lifespan. The adrenal cortex is responsible for the small amounts secreted before the pubescent years, but the sex hormone production that accompanies maturation of the gonads is responsible for the biologic changes observed during puberty.

Estrogen, the feminizing hormone, is found in low quantities during childhood. This hormone is secreted in slowly increasing amounts until about age 11 years. In males this gradual increase continues through maturation. In females the onset of estrogen production in the ovary causes a pronounced increase that continues until about 3 years after the onset of menstruation, at which time it reaches a maximum level that continues throughout the reproductive life of the female.

Androgens, the masculinizing hormones, are also secreted in small and gradually increasing amounts up to about 7 or 9 years of age, at which time there is a more rapid increase in both sexes, especially boys, until about age 15 years. These hormones appear to be responsible for most of the rapid growth changes of early adolescence. With the onset of testicular function, the level of androgens (principally *testosterone*) in males increases over that in females and continues to increase until a maximum is attained at maturity.

Sexual Maturation

The visible evidence of sexual maturation is achieved in an orderly sequence, and the state of maturity can be estimated on the basis of the appearance of these external manifestations. The age at which these changes are observed and the time required to progress from one stage to another may vary among children. The time from the appearance of breast buds to full maturity may be 1.5 to 6 years for adolescent girls. It may take 2 to 5 years for male genitalia to reach adult size. The stages of development of secondary sex characteristics and genital development have been defined as a guide for estimating sexual maturity and are referred to as the *Tanner stages.* The usual sequence of appearance of maturational changes is presented in Box 16-1.

Sexual Maturation in Girls.   In most girls the initial indication of puberty is the appearance of breast buds, an event known as *thelarche,* which occurs between 9 and 13.5 years of age (Fig. 16-1). This is followed in approximately 2 to 6 months by growth of pubic hair on the mons pubis, known as *adrenarche* (Fig. 16-2). In a minority of normally developing girls, however, pubic hair may precede breast development.

The initial appearance of menstruation, or *menarche,* occurs about 2 years after the appearance of the first pubescent changes, approximately 9 months after attainment of peak height velocity and 3 months after attainment of peak

weight velocity. Menarche has been related to a critical gain in body fat content (more fat content, earlier menarche), although this is controversial. The normal age range of menarche is usually 10.5 to 15 years, with the average age being 12 years 9.5 months for North American girls. Ovulation and regular menstrual periods usually occur 6 to 14 months after menarche. Girls may be considered to have *pubertal delay* if breast development has not occurred by age 13 or if menarche has not occurred within 4 years of the onset of breast development.

Sexual Maturation in Boys.   The first pubescent changes in boys are testicular enlargement accompanied by thinning, reddening, and increased looseness of the scrotum (Fig. 16-3). These events usually occur between 9.5 and 14 years of age. Early puberty is also characterized by the initial appearance of pubic hair. Penile enlargement begins, and testicular enlargement and pubic hair growth continue throughout midpuberty. During this period there is also increasing muscularity, early voice changes, and development of early facial hair. Temporary breast enlargement and tenderness, *gynecomastia,* are common during midpuberty, occurring in up to one third of boys. The spurts in height and weight occur concurrently toward the end of midpuberty. For most boys, breast enlargement disappears within 2 years. By late puberty there is a definite increase in the length and width of the penis, testicular enlargement continues, and first ejaculation occurs. Axillary hair develops, and facial hair extends to cover the anterior neck. Final voice changes occur secondary to the growth of the larynx. Concerns about *pubertal delay* should be considered for boys who exhibit no enlargement of the testes or scrotal changes by 13.5 to 14 years of age, or if genital growth is not complete 4 years after the testicles begin to enlarge.

Physical Growth

A constant phenomenon associated with sexual maturation is a dramatic increase in growth. The final 20% to 25% of height is achieved during puberty, and most of this growth occurs during a 24- to 36-month period—the adolescent *growth spurt.* This accelerated growth occurs in all children but, as in other areas of development, is highly variable in age of onset, duration, and extent. The growth spurt begins earlier in girls, usually between ages 9.5 and 14.5 years; on the average it begins between ages 10.5 and 16 years in boys. During this period, the average boy gains 10 to 30 cm (4 to 12 inches) in height and 7 to 30 kg (15 to 65 pounds) in weight. The average girl, in whom the growth spurt is slower and less extensive, gains 5 to 20 cm (2 to 8 inches) in height and 7 to 25 kg (15 to 55 pounds) in weight. Growth in height typically ceases 2 to 2.5 years after menarche in girls and at age 18 to 20 years in boys.

This increase in size is acquired in a characteristic sequence. Growth in length of the extremities and neck precedes growth in other areas, and because these parts are the first to reach adult length, the hands and feet appear larger than normal during adolescence. Increases in hip and chest breadth take place in a few months, followed several months later by an increase in shoulder width. These changes are followed by increases in length of the trunk and depth of the chest. This sequence of changes is responsible for the

BOX 16-1 ■ Usual Sequence of Maturational Changes

GIRLS	BOYS
Breast changes	Enlargement of testicles
Rapid increase in height and weight	Growth of pubic hair, axillary hair, hair on upper lip, hair on face and elsewhere on body (facial hair usually appears about 2 years after appearance of pubic hair)
Growth of pubic hair	
Appearance of axillary hair	
Menstruation (usually begins 2 years after first signs)	
Abrupt deceleration of linear growth	Rapid increase in height
	Changes in the larynx and consequently the voice (usually take place along with growth of penis)
	Nocturnal emissions
	Abrupt deceleration of linear growth

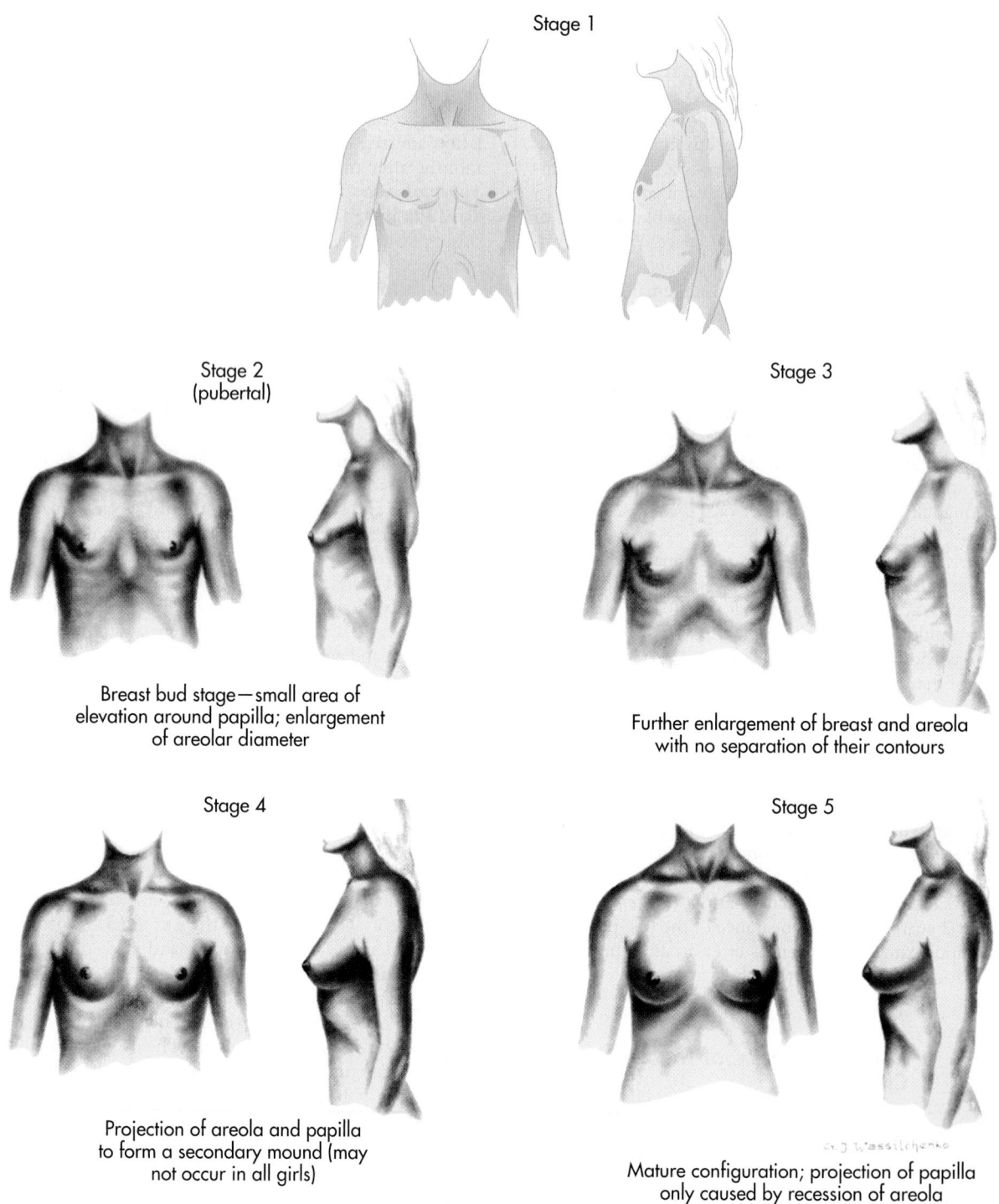

FIG. 16-1 ■ Development of the breast in girls—average age span: 11 to 13 years. (Modified from Marshall WA, Tanner JM: *Arch Dis Child* 44:291, 1969; Daniel WA, Paulshock BZ: A physician's guide to sexual maturity, *Patient Care* May 13, 122-124, 1979.)

characteristic long-legged, gawky appearance of the early adolescent child.

Sex Differences in General Growth Patterns. Sex differences in general growth and distribution patterns are apparent in skeletal growth, muscle mass, adipose tissue, and skin. Skeletal growth differences between boys and girls are apparently a function of hormonal effects at puberty and are evident primarily in limb length. The earlier cessation of growth in girls is caused by epiphyseal unity under the potent effect of estrogen secretion, and the hormonal effect on female bone growth is much stronger than the similar ef-

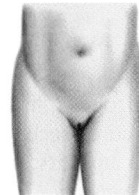

Stage 1 (prepubertal)

No pubic hair; essentially the same as during childhood; no distinction between hair on pubis and over the abdomen

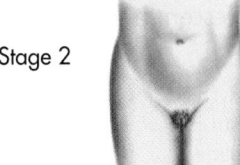

Stage 2

Sparse growth of long, straight, downy, and slightly pigmented hair extending along labia; between stages 2 and 3 begins to appear on pubis

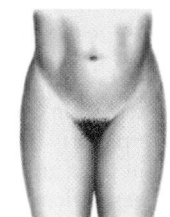

Stage 3

Hair darker, coarser, and curly and spread sparsely over entire pubis in the typical female triangle

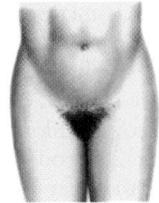

Stage 4

Pubic hair denser, curled, and adult in distribution but less abundant and restricted to the pubic area

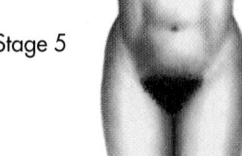

Stage 5

Hair adult in quantity, type, and pattern with spread to inner aspect of thighs

FIG. 16-2 ■ Growth in pubic hair in girls—average age span for stages 2 through 5: 11 to 14 years. (Modified from Marshall WA, Tanner JM: *Arch Dis Child* 44:291, 1969; and Daniel WA, Paulshock BZ: A physician's guide to sexual maturity, *Patient Care* May 13, 122-124, 1979.)

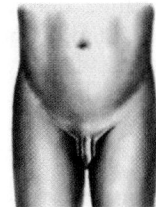

Stage 1 (prepubertal)

No pubic hair; essentially the same as during childhood; no distinction between hair on pubis and over the abdomen

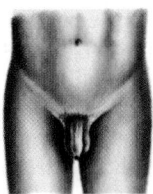

Stage 2 (pubertal)

Initial enlargement of scrotum and testes; reddening and textural changes of scrotal skin; sparse growth of long, straight, downy, and slightly pigmented hair at base of penis

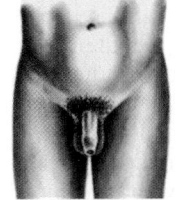

Stage 3

Initial enlargement of penis, mainly in length; testes and scrotum further enlarged; hair darker, coarser, and curly and spread sparsely over entire pubis

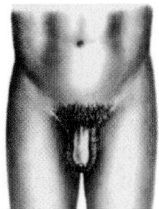

Stage 4

Increased size of penis with growth in diameter and development of glans; glans larger and broader; scrotum darker; pubic hair more abundant with curling but restricted to pubic area

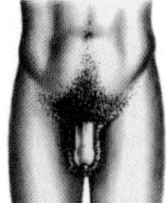

Stage 5

Testes, scrotum, and penis adult in size and shape; hair adult in quantity and type with spread to inner surface of thighs

FIG. 16-3 ■ Developmental stages of secondary sex characteristics and genital development in boys—average age span, 12 to 16 years. (Modified from Marshall WA, Tanner JM: *Arch Dis Child* 44:291, 1969; Daniel WA, Paulshock BZ: A physician's guide to sexual maturity, *Patient Care* May 13, 122-124, 1979.)

fect of testosterone in boys. In boys the prolonged growth period before puberty and the less rapid epiphyseal closure are reflected in their greater overall height and longer arms and legs. Other skeletal differences are increased shoulder width in boys and broader hip development in girls.

Hypertrophy of the laryngeal mucosa and enlargement of the larynx and vocal cords occur in both boys and girls to produce voice changes. Girls' voices become slightly deeper and considerably fuller, but the effect in boys is striking. The change in the voice of adolescent boys occurs between Tanner stages 3 and 4, with the voice often shifting uncontrollably from deep to high tones in the middle of a sentence. The change is associated with not only a lengthening of the vocal cords, but also an increase in the structure and mass of the vocal folds (Harries and others, 1998).

Growth of lean body mass, principally muscle, which tends to occur after the bone growth spurt, takes place steadily during adolescence. Lean body mass is both quantitatively and qualitatively greater in boys than in girls at comparable stages of pubertal development. Muscle development, under the influence of androgenic hormones, increases steadily. Muscles become remarkably well developed in boys, whereas in girls, muscle mass increase is proportionate to general tissue growth.

Nonlean body mass, primarily fat, is also increased but follows a less orderly pattern. There may be a transient increase in subcutaneous fat just before the skeletal growth spurt, especially in boys. This is followed 1 to 2 years later by a modest to marked decrease, which is again more marked in boys. Later, variable amounts of fat are deposited to fill out and contour the mature physique in patterns characteristic of the adolescent's sex, particularly in the regions over the thighs, hips, and buttocks and around the breast tissue. It should be noted, however, that pediatric obesity is steadily on the increase in the United States, and obesity can change the timing of puberty. Early maturers (beginning puberty 1.5 to 3.3 years earlier) are shorter and have a greater body mass index than mid-onset or late maturers (Biro and others, 2001).

Hormonal influences during puberty cause acceleration in growth and maturation of the skin and its structural appendages. Sebaceous glands become extremely active at this time, especially those on the genitals and in the "flush areas" of the body (i.e., face, neck, shoulders, upper back, and chest). This increased activity and the structural nature of the glands are extremely important in the pathogenesis of a common problem of puberty: acne (see Chapter 30). The eccrine sweat glands, present almost everywhere on the human skin, become fully functional and respond to emotional as well as thermal stimulation. Heavy sweating appears to be more pronounced in boys than in girls. The apocrine sweat glands, nonfunctional in childhood, reach secretory capacity during puberty. Unlike the eccrine sweat glands, the apocrine glands are limited in distribution and grow in conjunction with hair follicles in the axillae, around the areola of the breast, around the umbilicus, on the external auditory canal, and in the genital and anal regions. Apocrine glands secrete a thick substance as a result of emotional stimulation that, when acted on by surface bacteria, becomes highly odoriferous.

Body hair assumes very characteristic distribution patterns and changes texture during puberty. Under the influence of gonadal and adrenal androgens, hair coarsens, darkens, and lengthens at sites related to secondary sex characteristics. Pubic and axillary hair appears in both sexes, although pubic hair is more extensive in males than in females. Beard, mustache, and body hair on the chest, upward along the linea alba, and sometimes on other areas (e.g., back and shoulders) appears in males and is androgen-dependent. Extremity hair appears in varying amounts in both males and females but is also more prolific in the male.

Physiologic Changes

A number of physiologic functions are altered in response to some of the pubertal changes. The size and strength of the heart, blood volume, and systolic blood pressure increase, whereas the pulse rate and basal heat production decrease (see inside back cover). Blood volume, which has increased steadily during childhood, reaches a higher value in boys than in girls, a fact that may be related to the increased muscle mass in pubertal boys. Adult values are reached for all formed elements of the blood. Respiratory rate and basal metabolic rate, decreasing steadily throughout childhood, reach the adult rate in adolescence. Respiratory volume and vital capacity are increased, and to a far greater extent in males than in females. During this period, physiologic responses to exercise change drastically: performance improves, especially in boys, and the body is able to make the physiologic adjustments needed for normal functioning after exercise is completed. These capabilities are a result of the increased size and strength of muscles and the increased level of cardiac, respiratory, and metabolic functioning.

PSYCHOSOCIAL DEVELOPMENT
Developing a Sense of Identity (Erikson)

Traditional psychosocial theory holds that the developmental crisis of adolescence leads to the formation of a sense of identity (Erikson, 1963). Throughout childhood, individuals have been going through the process of identification as they concentrate on various parts of the body at specific times. During infancy children identify themselves as being separate from the mother; during early childhood they establish a gender-role identification with the appropriate-sex parent; and in later childhood they establish who they are in relation to others. In adolescence they come to see themselves as distinct individuals, somehow unique and separate from every other individual.

The early period of adolescence begins with the onset of puberty and extends to relative physical and emotional stability at or near graduation from high school. During this time the adolescent is faced with the crisis of *group identity vs. alienation.* In the period that follows, the individual strives to attain autonomy from the family and develop a sense of *personal identity* as opposed to *role diffusion.* A sense of group identity appears to be essential to the development of a sense of personal identity. Young adolescents must resolve questions concerning relationships with a peer group before they are able to resolve questions about who they are in relation to family and society.

Group Identity.   During the early stage of adolescence pressure to belong to a group is intensified. Teenagers find it essential to have a group to which they feel they can belong and that provides them with status. Belonging to a crowd helps adolescents to establish the differences between themselves and their parents. They dress as the group dresses and wear makeup and hairstyles according to group criteria, all of which are different from those of the parental generation. Language, music, and dancing reflect a culture that is exclusive to the adolescent. When adults begin to emulate these fashions and interests, the style changes immediately. The evidence of adolescent conformity to the peer group and nonconformity to the adult group provides teenagers with a frame of reference in which they can display their own self-assertion while they reject the identity of their parents' generation. To be different is to be unaccepted and alienated from the group.

Individual Identity. The quest for personal identity is part of the ongoing identification process. As youngsters establish identity within a group, they also attempt to incorporate multiple body changes into a concept of the self. Body awareness is part of self-awareness. In their search for identity, adolescents consider the relationships that have developed between themselves and others in the past, as well as the directions they hope to take in the future.

Significant others hold expectations for the behavior of the adolescent. Often these expectations or demands are persistent enough to result in certain decisions that might be made differently or not at all if the individual could be solely responsible for identity formation. It is all too easy to slip into the roles that are expected by these external influences without incorporating personal goals or questioning these decisions. Thus individuals may become what parents or others wish them to be based on these premature decisions. Young persons might form a negative identity when society or their culture provides them with a self-image that is contrary to the values of the community. Labels such as "juvenile delinquent," "hoodlum," or "failure" are applied to certain adolescents, who then accept and live up to these labels with behaviors that validate and strengthen them.

The process of evolving a personal identity is time-consuming and fraught with periods of confusion, depression, and discouragement. Determining an identity and a place in the world is a critical and perilous feature of adolescence (see Critical Thinking Exercise). However, as the pieces are gradually shifted and settled into place, a positive identity eventually emerges. Role diffusion results when the individual is unable to formulate a satisfactory identity from the multiplicity of aspirations, roles, and identifications.

Sex-Role Identity. Adolescence is the time for consolidation of a sex-role identity. During early adolescence the peer group begins to communicate expectations regarding heterosexual relationships, and as development progresses, adolescents encounter expectations for mature sex-role behavior from both peers and adults. Expectations vary from culture to culture, among geographic areas, and among socioeconomic groups.

Emotionality. Adolescents vacillate in their emotional states between considerable maturity and childlike behavior. One minute they are exuberant and enthusiastic; the next minute they are depressed and withdrawn. Unpredictable, but essentially normal, mood swings are common during this time. As the tension is relieved, emotion is brought un-

?? CRITICAL THINKING EXERCISE ??

Discussing the Future

Jeremy, age 17, will be graduating from high school in the spring. His mother, a single parent, tells you that she is concerned because graduation is quickly approaching and Jeremy has made no plans for what he will do with his life after graduation. Whenever Jeremy mentions the topic, his mother tells him, "This is what you must do," and begins to outline the steps he must take. Jeremy just walks away. She asks, "What should I do?" What advice should you give Jeremy's mother?

QUESTIONS

1. Evidence—Is there sufficient evidence to draw any conclusions about what advice the nurse should give Jeremy's mother?
2. Assumptions—Describe an underlying assumption about each of the following issues:
   a. Adolescents and the search for personal identity
   b. The influence of others on the adolescent's search for personal identity
   c. Ways to communicate with adolescents
3. What implications and priorities for nursing care can be drawn at this time?
4. Does the evidence objectively support your argument (conclusion)?
5. Are there alternative perspectives to your arguments? What are they?

ANSWERS

1. Yes, there is sufficient information to arrive at a conclusion about what advice to give Jeremy's mother.
2. a. During adolescence, teens consider all their past relationships as they attempt to form their own personal identity. They attempt to formulate a satisfactory identity from a multiplicity of roles, aspirations and identifications. The process of developing this identity is time-consuming and can be associated with confusion and discouragement.
   b. If significant others are too persistent and demand that adolescents make specific decisions or behave in definite ways, adolescents often make premature decisions and accept roles that do not incorporate their own personal goals or aspirations.
   c. Parents who communicate well with their teens have an open, nonjudgmental, nondictatorial manner. They demonstrate that they are available and willing to listen to their teenagers. However, they also wait until the teenager opens the discussion, and then they listen attentively and allow the teen to explore their issues.
3. The nursing priority in this situation is to have the mother become more aware that Jeremy is not likely to discuss his concerns on a timetable, and that it is important for her to respect his point of view. Although Jeremy wants his mother's guidance and support, he does not want to be told what to do, and he needs an opportunity to express his own feelings and views. An example of appropriate advice to give Jeremy's mother might be: "Be open and available to Jeremy. Tell him what you think, but *not what to do.*"
4. Yes, the information about how teens formulate a personal identity and the principles of effective parent communication allow the nurse to formulate this response.
5. If Jeremy's mother changes her behavior and Jeremy still does not want to communicate and continues to withdraw from conversation, after a significant period of time, the nurse might explore the possibility of counseling for Jeremy and his mother. Jeremy could be suffering from depression or some other condition that causes him to withdraw from conversation and interaction with his mother.

der control and individuals retreat to review what has happened, to attempt to master their anger, and to grow in their ability to control their emotions and gain from the new experience. Because of these mood swings, adolescents are frequently labeled as unstable, inconsistent, and unpredictable. Little things can cause an emotional upheaval and, depending on the teenager's interpretation, can mean a great deal.

Teenagers are better able to control their emotions in later adolescence. They can approach problems more calmly and rationally, and although they are still subject to periods of sadness, their feelings are less vulnerable and they begin to demonstrate the more mature emotions of later adolescence. Whereas early adolescents react immediately and emotionally, older adolescents can control their emotions until socially acceptable times and places for expression present themselves. They are still subject to heightened emotion, and when it is expressed, their behavior reflects feelings of insecurity, tension, and indecision.

COGNITIVE DEVELOPMENT (PIAGET)

Cognitive thinking culminates with the capacity for *abstract thinking*. This stage, the period of *formal operations*, is Piaget's fourth and last stage. Adolescents are no longer restricted to the real and actual, which was typical of the period of concrete thought; now they are also concerned with the possible. They think beyond the present. Without having to center attention on the immediate situation, they can imagine a sequence of events that might occur, such as college and occupational possibilities; how things might change in the future, such as relationships with parents; and the consequences of their actions, such as dropping out of school. At this time their thoughts can be influenced by logical principles rather than just their own perceptions and experiences. They become increasingly capable of scientific reasoning and formal logic.

Adolescents are capable of mentally manipulating more than two categories of variables at the same time. For example, they can consider the relationship between speed, distance, and time in planning a trip. They can detect logical consistency or inconsistency in a set of statements and evaluate a system or set of values in a more analytic manner. For instance, they question the parent who insists on honesty in the youngster but at the same time cheats on an income tax report or expense account.

In adolescence, young people begin to think about both their own thinking and the thinking of others. They wonder what opinion others have of them, and they are able to imagine the thoughts of others. With this capacity comes the ability to differentiate between others' thoughts and their own and to interpret the thoughts of others more accurately. They are able to understand that few concepts are absolute or independent of other influencing factors. As they become aware that other cultures and communities have different norms and standards from their own, it becomes easier for them to accept members of these other cultures, and the decision to behave in their own culture in an accepted manner becomes a more conscious commitment.

MORAL DEVELOPMENT (KOHLBERG)

Although younger children merely accept the decisions or point of view of adults, adolescents, to gain autonomy from adults, must substitute their own set of morals and values.

When old principles are challenged but new independent values have not yet emerged to take their place, young people search for a moral code that preserves their personal integrity and guides their behavior, especially in the face of strong pressure to violate the old beliefs. Their decisions involving moral dilemmas must be based on an *internalized set of moral principles* that provides them with the resources to evaluate the demands of the situation and to plan actions that are consistent with their ideals.

Late adolescence is characterized by serious questioning of existing moral values and their relevance to society and the individual. Adolescents can easily take the role of another. They understand duty and obligation based on reciprocal rights of others, as well as the concept of justice that is founded on making amends for misdeeds and repairing or replacing what has been spoiled by wrongdoing. However, they seriously question established moral codes, often as a result of observing that adults verbally ascribe to a code but do not adhere to it.

SPIRITUAL DEVELOPMENT

As youngsters move toward independence from parents and other authorities, some begin to question the values and ideals of their families. Others cling to these values as a stable element in their lives as they struggle with the conflicts of this turbulent period. Adolescents need to work out these conflicts for themselves, but they also need support from authority figures or peers for their resolution.

Adolescents are capable of understanding abstract concepts and of interpreting analogies and symbols. They are able to empathize, philosophize, and think logically. Most teens search for ideals and speculate about illogical statements and conflicting ideologies. Their tendency toward introspection and emotional intensity often makes it difficult for others to know what they are thinking. They tend to keep their thoughts private, fearing that no one will understand these feelings that they perceive to be unique and special. However, they may reveal deep spiritual concerns. They need support and encouragement in their struggle for understanding and the freedom to question without censure.

Greater levels of religiosity and spirituality are associated with fewer high-risk behaviors and more health-promoting behaviors (Brown, 2001). Nurses play an important role for teens by providing an opportunity to discuss issues regarding spirituality.

SOCIAL DEVELOPMENT

To achieve full maturity, adolescents must free themselves from family domination and define an identity independent of parental authority. However, this process is fraught with ambivalence on the part of both teenagers and their parents. Adolescents want to grow up and to be free of parental restraints, but they are fearful as they try to comprehend the responsibilities that are linked with independence. Feelings of immortality and exemption from the consequences of risk-taking behavior, although viewed as negative, can serve an important developmental function at this time. These feelings give adolescents the courage to separate from their parents and become independent. Part of this emancipation involves developing social relationships outside the family that help teenagers to identify their role in society. Adolescence is a time of intense sociability and often a time of equally intense loneliness. Acceptance by peers, a few close friends, and the secure love of a supportive family are requisites for interpersonal maturation.

Relationships With Parents

During adolescence the parent-child relationship changes from one of protection-dependency to one of *mutual affection and equality.* The process of achieving independence often involves turmoil and ambiguity as both parent and adolescent learn to play new roles and work toward this end while, at the same time, resolving the often painful series of rifts essential to establishing the ultimate relationship.

Most behavior observed in the adolescent is related to the struggle for independence and the external restrictions and checks that are placed on this spontaneous maturation process. On the one hand, adolescents are accepted as maturing preadults. They are allowed privileges heretofore denied, and they are provided with increasing responsibilities. On the other hand, because of their unpredictability and insecurity in evaluating situations and making sound judgments, they must conform to regulations and restrictions set by adults. This state of affairs is particularly exemplified by the struggle between parents and adolescents concerning the nightly curfew.

As teenagers assert their rights for grown-up privileges, they frequently create tensions within the home. They resist parental control, and conflicts can arise from almost any situation or any subject. Favorite topics of dispute include use of the telephone, manners, dress, chores and duties, homework, disrespectful behavior, friendships, dating, money, automobiles, drinking or drugs, and time schedules. Present in these areas of conflict are the overriding arguments that "Everyone else has one" or is allowed the desired item or privilege and the ever-present assertions that "You don't understand me or trust me" and "You always treat me like a baby." Spoken or unspoken, parents' reactions consist of "Is this all the thanks I get for what I have done for you?"

Teenagers' earliest attempts to achieve emancipation from parental controls are manifested in a period of rejection of the parents. They absent themselves from home and family activities and spend an increasing amount of time with the peer group. They confide less in their parents, but parents continue to play an important role in the personal and health-related decision making of adolescents.

With advancing adolescence, teenagers become more competent, and with this competence comes a need for more autonomy. Although they may be psychologically prepared for independence, they are often thwarted in their efforts by lack of money or other parental barriers. Conflict arises in relation to the teenager's outside activities and the elements of privacy and trust. Parental supervision remains important throughout adolescence and may have a direct influence on adolescent sexual and substance use behavior. Parents should be guided toward an authoritative style of parenting in which authority is used to guide the adolescent while allowing developmentally appropriate levels of freedom and providing clear, consistent messages regarding expectations (Baker and others, 1999). However, to gain the trust of adolescents, parents must respect their youngster's privacy, as well as show an honest and sincere interest in what the adolescent believes and feels (see Family Focus box).

 FAMILY FOCUS

Communication With Teens: The Art of Listening

Conflicts between parents and their adolescents are often a result of a very natural characteristic of parenthood: the desire to protect one's offspring—from harm or from simply doing something "stupid" or embarrassing or something they may later regret. Teenagers sometimes "bounce" their thoughts and ideas off adults. At times they really want some feedback; at other times they simply want to elicit a reaction.

I found it easy to listen openly, thoughtfully, and without interrupting when my teenagers' friends discussed troublesome topics. However, one day, when one of my own teenagers had a similar conversation with me, the parent part kicked in. I felt responsible and spoke my piece on the spot.

This brought communication to a halt and resulted in defensiveness. It was a long time before my child tried to talk to me about anything controversial again.

The next time one of my teenagers started a similar conversation, I decided to try to trick myself.

Throughout the entire conversation, I told myself over and over again to act as if this were not my teenager, but rather someone else's child. I found this actually worked quite well, and I was able to listen without interrupting. I continue to use the system, sometimes with more success than at other times.

Mother of four

Relationships With Peers

Although parents remain the primary influence in their lives, for the majority of teenagers, peers assume a more significant role in adolescence than they did during childhood. The peer group serves as a strong support to teenagers, individually and collectively, providing them with a sense of belonging and a feeling of strength and power. The peer group forms the transitional world between dependence and autonomy.

Peer Group. Adolescents are usually social, gregarious, and group-minded. Thus the peer group has an intense influence on adolescents' self-evaluation and behavior. To gain acceptance by a group, younger teenagers tend to conform completely in such things as mode of dress, hairstyle, taste in music, and vocabulary. Teenagers use the peer group as a yardstick of what is normal.

The school is psychologically important to adolescents as a focus of social life. Teenagers usually distribute themselves into a relatively predictable social hierarchy. They know to which groups they and others belong. A sense of school connectedness has been found to predict decreased risk-taking behaviors in adolescents (Resnick and others, 1997). School connectedness is correlated with caring teachers and the absence of prejudice or discrimination from peers. A sense of school connectedness is less dependent on class size, attendance, academic preparation, and parental involvement (Maes and Lievens, 2003).

Within the larger groups are smaller, distinct, and rather exclusive crowds or cliques of selected close friends who are emotionally attached to each other. The selection is based on common tastes, interests, and background. Although cliques may become formalized, most remain informal and small. However, each has an identifying feature that proclaims its difference from others and its solidarity within itself, in much the same manner as the adolescent generation as a whole sets itself apart from the adult generation. Cliques are usually made up of one sex, and girls tend to be more cliquish than boys and to have a greater need for close friendships (Fig. 16-4). Within the intimacy of the group, adolescents gain support in learning about themselves, consideration for the feelings of others, and increased ego development and self-reliance.

To belong is of utmost importance; thus, adolescents behave in a way that will ensure their establishment in a group. Adolescents are highly susceptible to social approval, acceptance, and demands. To be ignored or criticized by peers creates feelings of inferiority, inadequacy, and incompetence.

Best Friends. Personal friendships of the one-on-one variety usually develop between same-sex adolescents. This relationship is closer and more stable than it is in middle childhood, and it is important in the quest for identity. A best friend is the best audience on whom to try out possible roles and identities that an adolescent wants to test. Best friends may try a role together, each providing support for the other. Each cares about what the other thinks and feels. Because a sense of intimacy grows within a permanent relationship, the stability of this same-sex friendship is an important link in the progress toward an intimate relationship in young adulthood.

Heterosexual Relationships

During adolescence, relationships with members of the opposite sex take on new importance (Fig. 16-5). Although there seems to be a trend toward earlier dating, on the *average,* dating activities begin in the seventh and eighth grades and are usually "crowd" dates at organized school functions. For example, a group of girls just happen to be around a certain group of boys at most activities. During high school, crowd dates are still popular, but there is more pairing off of couples. Double-dating and then single-pair dating follow group dating. Most adolescents are dating to some degree by the time they leave high school.

The type and degree of seriousness of heterosexual relationships vary. The initial stage is usually noncommittal, extremely mobile, and seldom characterized by any deep romantic attachments. Crushes, those strong feelings of attachment to an important or well-liked adult who embodies the qualities considered most valuable by the adolescent, are common in early adolescence and constitute one of the earliest "love" attachments. The behavioral sequencing in sexual development is from less to more intimate forms of behavior with another person.

Middle adolescence is the time when teenagers begin to develop romantic relationships and when most teenagers begin sexual experimentation. Early and middle adolescents choose their partners based on physical and personality characteristics that are acceptable to their peer group. Through these relationships and experimentation, early and middle adolescents begin to explore and understand romantic feelings and experiences. As teenagers move into late adolescence, the partner choice is more likely to be based on individual characteristics and interests.

Sexual Activity. Sexuality and sexual activity is an area that should be addressed with each adolescent in a confidential manner. Messages to postpone sexual involvement must begin by the middle school period. Although sexual activity rates have decreased for older teens, the percentage of teens younger than 15 years of age who are engaging in sexual activity has increased. Among teenagers who have initiated sexual intercourse at an age younger than 14 years,

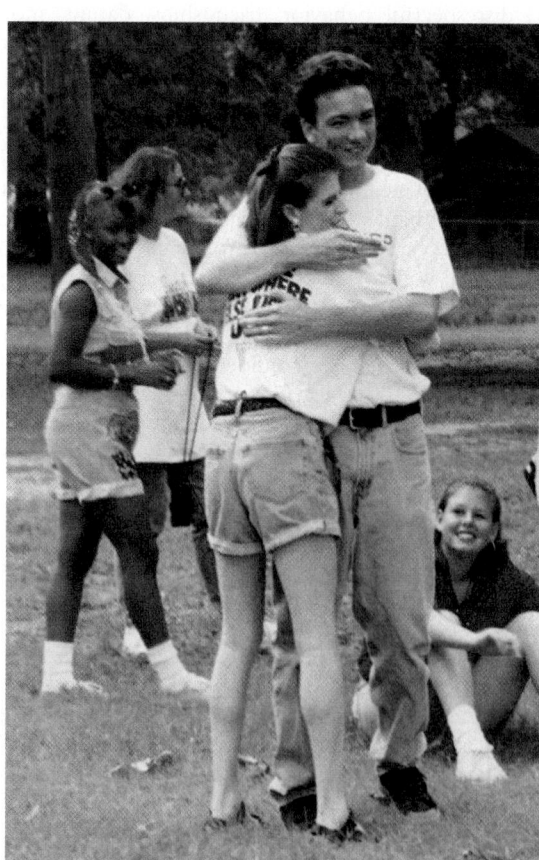

FIG. 16-5 ■ Heterosexual relationships are an important part of adolescence.

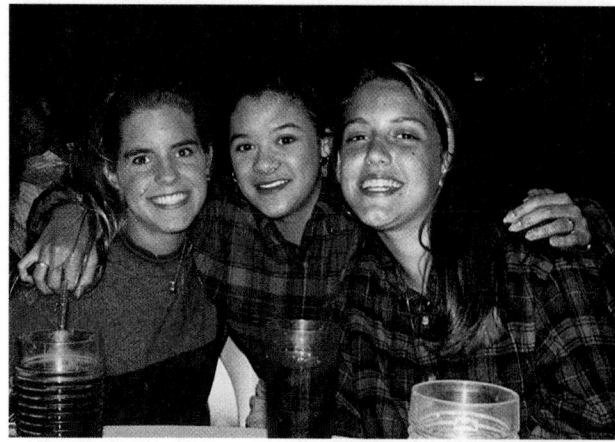

FIG. 16-4 ■ Teenagers like to gather in small groups.

the incidence of sexual abuse is very high. However, by 17 years of age, more than 50% of teenagers have had volitional sexual intercourse (Alan Guttmacher Institute, 1998).

Adolescents report the pressure to have sex is only exceeded by the pressure to drink. This pressure to engage in sexual activity is strongest for those who have already been sexually active and for males. Teens engage in a wide range of sexual activity including kissing and petting, oral sex, and vaginal and rectal sex. Teens remain uninformed about sexually transmitted disease transmission, contraception, and access to confidential care (Hoff, Greene, and Davis, 2003). Many adolescents feel uncomfortable bringing up sexual health issues with their health care provider. They prefer to have the provider approach the subject in a clear and direct manner. Discomfort on the part of the provider about sexuality issues will present a barrier for teens in need of accurate health information.

Adolescents become involved in sexual relationships for a wide variety of reasons: to obtain pleasurable sensations, to satisfy sexual drives, to satisfy curiosity, as a conquest, as an expression of affection, or because they are not able to withstand pressures to conform. Often the urge to belong to and gain reassurance from a group and the wish to really belong to someone provoke a series of increasingly intimate physical contacts with a favored boyfriend or girlfriend.

Homosexuality in Adolescents

During adolescence, youths develop a sexual identity. This process becomes incredibly complicated when the sexual identity is not heterosexual. Retrospective studies of gay men and lesbians indicate that adolescence is when individuals become aware of same-sex attraction. Gay men become aware of same-sex attraction at a younger mean age than women. Homosexual and bisexual youths face tremendous challenges to growing up and becoming mentally and physically healthy when confronted with antihomosexual attitudes and values. These adolescents are at increased risk for health-damaging behaviors, not because of the sexual behavior itself, but because of society's reaction to the behavior (Saewyc and others, 1998). Behaviors that place homosexual and bisexual youths at risk for poor health outcomes include early initiation of sexual activity (usually heterosexual), substance abuse, suicide and suicidal ideation, running away from home, and engaging in behaviors that result in sexually transmitted diseases. Nurses should view gay and lesbian youth within the broader context of general adolescent development. The goal is not to identify all gay and lesbian youth but to provide a safe environment for appropriate health care (Garofalo and Katz, 2001) (see Critical Thinking Exercise).

Interests and Activities

Adolescents spend a large amount of time engaging in leisure-time activities. As teenagers progress through the developmental stages of adolescence, these leisure-time activities move from being family centered to being peer centered. In addition to providing teenagers with fun and enjoyment, leisure-time activities assist in the development of social, physical, and cognitive skills. Leisure-time activities also allow teenagers the opportunity to learn to set priorities and structure their time (Fig. 16-6).

Today, many adolescents must learn to juggle their time between school, leisure-time activities, and the responsibilities of a job. Adolescent work experiences provide many benefits, including time management, teamwork skills, and increased income. However, many jobs available to teenagers

??? CRITICAL THINKING EXERCISE ???

Discussing Sexual Orientation With Adolescents

John, a 17-year-old adolescent, comes into the school-based clinic and tells the nurse practitioner that he thinks he is homosexual. What is the most appropriate response for the nurse practitioner?

QUESTIONS

1. Evidence—Is there sufficient evidence to draw any conclusions about John's sexual orientation at this time?
2. Assumptions—Describe an underlying assumption about each of the following issues:
   a. Sexual orientation in adolescents
   b. Society's reaction to homosexuality
   c. Health care professionals and sexuality
3. What implications and priorities for nursing care can be drawn at this time?
4. Does the evidence support your argument (conclusion)?
5. Are there alternative perspectives to your arguments? What are they?

ANSWERS

1. Yes, there are sufficient data to arrive at a conclusion about how to respond to John.
2. a. Studies of gay men and lesbians indicate that adolescence is the time when individuals become aware of same-sex attraction. Homosexual and bisexual youths are at risk for health-damaging behaviors such as early initiation of sexual behavior, substance abuse, suicide, and running away from home.
   b. Homosexual and bisexual youths are often confronted with the antihomosexual attitudes and values of society. It is this reaction of society that makes it difficult for homosexual and bisexual youths to grow up and become healthy physically and mentally.
   c. Health professionals who work with adolescents should consider the adolescent's increasing independence and responsibility while ensuring confidentiality.
3. The nurse's first priority in this situation is to give John permission to discuss his feelings about this topic. He has come to the nurse practitioner to discuss this matter, and he probably feels comfortable sharing this information with her. The nurse practitioner needs to be open and nonjudgmental in her interactions with John. He needs to know that the nurse practitioner will maintain confidentiality, appreciate his feelings, and remain sensitive to his need to talk about this topic. An example of an appropriate response for the nurse practitioner might be: "John, tell me more about how you came to this conclusion."
4. Yes, the information about sexual orientation in adolescence and the role of the health care professional support this conclusion.
5. It might be appropriate for the nurse to gather information about John's support system and to determine the attitudes and values of John's family and peer group toward homosexuality.
   In addition to establishing a trusting relationship and effective communications with John, the nurse practitioner should make sure that John has a safe environment.

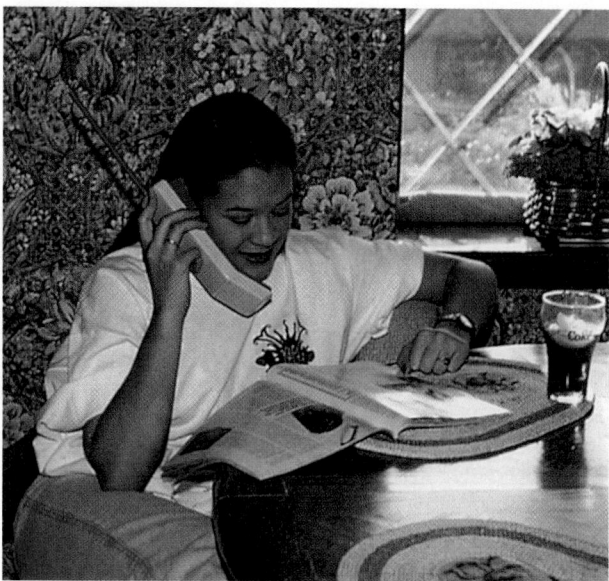

FIG. 16-6 ■ The telephone, especially the portable phone, provides teenagers with hours of conversation with same-sex and opposite-sex friends.

do not provide opportunities to apply the skills they learn in school, and jobs often have high demands for quick work with low rewards. Very few apprentice opportunities are available for teenagers. It is generally recommended that adolescents limit their work to no more than 20 hours per week during the school year.

DEVELOPMENT OF SELF-CONCEPT AND BODY IMAGE

The sudden growth that takes place in early adolescence creates feelings of confusion for adolescents. They have lost the security of a familiar body and feel uncomfortable with their altered body. Consequently, they may try to either hide their body or advertise it, or they may alternate between the two extremes. Teenagers are acutely aware of their appearance as they begin to acquire images of themselves as adults, but they see discrepancies between their ideal and actual skills and abilities.

Adolescents are continually comparing themselves with their peers and making judgments about their own normality based on these observations. Pubertal children feel most comfortable when they are just like their friends and agemates. Perceived defects or deviations from the group average are threatening to their idealized image. Any blemish is likely to be magnified out of proportion, and any delay of the visible evidence of maturity is cause for worry. Unfortunately, this is also the time when the hormonal effect of the sebaceous glands produces acne, which creates problems for many youngsters. To the adolescent, even the most insignificant pimple may be viewed as a gross disfigurement. The advent of chronic disease or a permanent physical disability has very special significance during adolescence and creates additional stresses for both youngsters with the condition and health care providers.

It has been determined that the body image established during adolescence is the one that individuals retain throughout life. Much of adolescents' search for identity takes place before a mirror as they try to read from the reflected features just who they are and what they look like to other people. Adolescents practice facial expressions and postures, try out hair arrangements, worry about a pimple, and in other ways attempt to assess the best means to achieve a maximum effect—to reveal the "true self."

The self-concept becomes more differentiated as adolescents acquire a more complex picture of themselves, one that takes situational factors into account. The self-concept gradually becomes more individualized and more distinct from the concepts of others. Although younger teenagers describe themselves in terms of similarities with peers, as adolescence advances, young people describe themselves in terms of their special characteristics.

Responses to Puberty

The response to the physical changes of pubertal growth and development is manifested differently depending on the stage of development. During early adolescence, young adolescents become preoccupied with the rapid changes in their body and are very interested in the anatomy, physiology, and function of their sexual organs. Boys must also confront the sexual feelings and tensions that accompany puberty, and the appearance of nocturnal emissions may be puzzling, troublesome, or embarrassing events. Unless the boy has been prepared in advance, he may find it difficult to discuss his feelings with his parents and may turn to his friends for information and guidance. Many girls also find the rapid changes in their body to be sources of concern. Some girls perceive the increase in weight and associated fat deposition as evidence of obesity and may indulge in fad diets. Although many girls look forward to menstruation and take this event in stride, others may find the first menstrual period a distressing and frightening event. All teenagers, regardless of gender, are very concerned with the question "Am I normal?" To answer this question, they compare their body with the bodies of their peers and with images in the media. This leads to a great deal of uncertainty about their appearance and attractiveness.

If an adolescent does not enter puberty at the same time as his or her peers, considerable inner conflict may occur. Early-maturing girls and boys, as well as late-maturing boys, have higher rates of risk-taking behaviors than their on-time peers (Graber and others, 1997; Hayward and others, 1997). Nurses who work with adolescents must provide teaching and health care interventions that are appropriate for the chronologic and cognitive development of the adolescent rather than the physical maturation.

As growth and development proceed through middle adolescence, the rapid body changes diminish, and the adolescent has time to try to make the body more attractive. Adolescents strive to achieve the perfect body within their own cultural norms. The "right" clothes and hairstyle become very important. By late adolescence the heightened concern with body image has ended and is replaced with a general comfort with the body.

■ ■ ■

The changes that occur during the early, middle, and late phases of adolescence are summarized in Table 16-1.

TABLE 16-1 ■ Growth and Development During Adolescence

EARLY ADOLESCENCE (11-14 years)	MIDDLE ADOLESCENCE (15-17 years)	LATE ADOLESCENCE (18-20 years)
GROWTH		
Rapidly accelerating growth Reaches peak velocity Secondary sex characteristics appear	Growth decelerating in girls Stature reaches 95% of adult height Secondary sex characteristics well advanced	Physically mature Structure and reproductive growth almost complete
COGNITION		
Explores newfound ability for limited abstract thought Clumsy groping for new values and energies Comparison of "normality" with peers of same sex	Developing capacity for abstract thinking Enjoys intellectual powers, often in idealistic terms Concern with philosophic, political, and social problems	Established abstract thought Can perceive and act on long-range options Able to view problems comprehensively Intellectual and functional identity established
IDENTITY		
Preoccupied with rapid body changes Trying out of various roles Measurement of attractiveness by acceptance or rejection of peers Conformity to group norms	Modifies body image Very self-centered; increased narcissism Tendency toward inner experience and self-discovery Has a rich fantasy life Idealistic Able to perceive future implications of current behavior and decisions; variable application	Body image and gender-role definition nearly secured Mature sexual identity Phase of consolidation of identity Stability of self-esteem Comfortable with physical growth Social roles defined and articulated
RELATIONSHIPS WITH PARENTS		
Defining independence-dependence boundaries Strong desire to remain dependent on parents while trying to detach No major conflicts over parental control	Major conflicts over independence and control Low point in parent-child relationship Greatest push for emancipation; disengagement Final and irreversible emotional detachment from parents; mourning	Emotional and physical separation from parents completed Independence from family with less conflict Emancipation nearly secured
RELATIONSHIPS WITH PEERS		
Seeks peer affiliations to counter instability generated by rapid change Upsurge of close, idealized friendships with members of the same sex Struggle for mastery takes place within peer group	Strong need for identity to affirm self-image Behavioral standards set by peer group Acceptance by peers extremely important—fear of rejection Exploration of ability to attract opposite sex	Peer group recedes in importance in favor of individual friendship Testing of romantic relationships against possibility of permanent alliance Relationships characterized by giving and sharing
SEXUALITY		
Self-exploration and evaluation Limited dating, usually group Limited intimacy	Multiple plural relationships Internal identification of heterosexual, homosexual, or bisexual attractions Exploration of "self appeal" Feeling of "being in love" Tentative establishment of relationships	Forms stable relationships and attachment to another Growing capacity for mutuality and reciprocity Dating as a romantic pair May publicly identify as gay, lesbian, or bisexual Intimacy involves commitment rather than exploration and romanticism
PSYCHOLOGIC HEALTH		
Wide mood swings Intense daydreaming Anger outwardly expressed with moodiness, temper outbursts, and verbal insults and name-calling	Tendency toward inner experiences; more introspective Tendency to withdraw when upset or feelings are hurt Vacillation of emotions in time and range Feelings of inadequacy common; difficulty in asking for help	More constancy of emotion Anger more apt to be concealed

PROMOTING OPTIMAL HEALTH DURING ADOLESCENCE

The major causes of morbidity and mortality in adolescence are not diseases, but health-damaging behaviors. New sources of morbidity in adolescence include injury, depression, violence, sexually transmitted infections, and pregnancy. Health promotion for this age-group consists mainly of teaching and guidance to avoid risk-taking activities and health-damaging behaviors. Adolescence provides an opportunity for teenagers to incorporate healthy lifestyle behaviors that will benefit them not only during the teenage years, but also throughout the lifespan.

Effective health education for adolescents should incorporate a developmentally appropriate, multifaceted approach, but education alone is not enough to change behavior. Effective programs must include opportunities for skill building and must be comprehensive rather than problem focused and include a community-wide approach (Hamburg, 1997).

As teenagers progress through adolescence, they are able to assume additional responsibility for their own health, including maintaining health practices, taking prescribed medications, keeping appointments, and performing procedures when necessary. Health professionals who work with adolescents should consider the adolescent's increasing independence and responsibility while maintaining privacy and ensuring confidentiality (see Guidelines box and the Critical Thinking Exercise). Parents should also respect their teenager's independence and move toward the role of consultant about health issues while also maintaining some level of parental involvement throughout adolescence.

In response to changes in adolescent morbidity and mortality, the American Medical Association developed the *Guidelines for Adolescent Preventive Services (GAPS)*, which provide a framework for health care providers to use in their clinical practice. The following discussion provides information on specific GAPS topics and recommendations related to screening, guidance, and immunizations.

IMMUNIZATIONS

An immunization update is an important part of adolescent preventive care. Obtaining a record of the teenager's prior immunizations is important. Adolescents should receive a tetanus-diphtheria (Td) vaccine at the age of 11 to 12 years if a period of at least 5 years has elapsed since the last dose of diphtheria-tetanus-pertussis or acellular pertussis, or diphtheria-tetanus (DTP, DTaP, or DT) vaccine. Subsequent routine Td boosters are recommended every 10 years. With the exception of pregnant teenagers, all adolescents should receive a second measles-mumps-rubella (MMR) vaccine unless they have documentation of two MMR vaccinations during childhood but not before 12 months of age. All adolescents who have not previously received three doses of hepatitis B vaccine should be vaccinated against hepatitis B virus. All adolescents should also be assessed for previous history of varicella infection or vaccination. Vaccination with the varicella vaccine is recommended for those with no previous history. For adolescents older than age 13 years, the varicella vaccine is given in two doses 4 or more weeks apart. Hepatitis A vaccine should be

Interviewing Adolescents

Ensure confidentiality and privacy; interview adolescent without parents.

Show concern for adolescent's perspective: "First, I'd like to talk about your main concerns" and "I'd like to know what you think is happening."

Offer a nonthreatening explanation for the questions you ask: "I'm going to ask a number of questions to help me better understand your health."

Maintain objectivity; avoid assumptions, judgments, and lectures.

Ask open-ended questions when possible; move to more directive questions if necessary.

Begin with less sensitive issues and proceed to more sensitive ones.

Use language that both the adolescent and you understand. Clarify terms, such as "having sex."

Restate: reflect back to adolescents what they have said, along with feelings that may be associated with their descriptions.

given to adolescents living in communities with high rates of hepatitis A or those with risk factors for hepatitis A such as injectable drug use or high-risk sexual activity (American Academy of Pediatrics, 2000). College freshmen living in dormitories are at increased risk for meningococcal disease. Discussions for incoming college students and their parents should include encouragement to obtain the meningococcal immunization (Rosenstein, Fischer and Tappero, 2001). (See also Immunizations, Chapter 10.)

NUTRITION

The rapid and extensive increase in height, weight, muscle mass, and sexual maturity of adolescence is accompanied by increased nutritional requirements. Because nutritional needs are closely related to the increase in body mass, the peak requirements occur in the years of maximum growth, during which the body mass almost doubles. The caloric and protein requirements during this time are higher than at almost any other time of life. As a result of this increased anabolic need, the adolescent is highly sensitive to caloric restrictions.

The nutritional needs of adolescents are difficult to determine because of meager nutritional information on members of this age-group. This difficulty is further complicated by the influence of emotional and other stress factors affecting nutrient utilization and the psychologic factors that influence eating habits. In addition, the wide variations in growth rates during adolescence and the equally wide variations in ages at which these changes take place complicate attempts to set minimum dietary standards.

Adolescents usually have sufficient intake of protein to meet their needs, except those who limit their food intake because of economic problems or in an attempt to lose weight. There is a substantial increase in the need for the minerals calcium, iron, and zinc during periods of rapid growth: calcium for skeletal growth, iron for expansion of muscle mass and blood volume, and zinc for the generation of both skeletal and bone tissue. Girls with very heavy or frequent menses may be especially susceptible to iron defi-

?!? CRITICAL THINKING EXERCISE   ?!?

Respecting Privacy

Jamie, a 17-year-old girl, arrives at the adolescent clinic with her mother, Mrs. S., for a routine history and physical examination with the nurse practitioner. As the nurse practitioner walks with Jamie to an examination room, Mrs. S. whispers to the nurse practitioner, "I need to speak with you in private." How should the nurse practitioner respond to Mrs. S.'s request?

QUESTIONS

1. Evidence—Is there sufficient evidence to formulate a response to Jamie's mother?
2. Assumptions—Describe an underlying assumption about each of the following topics:
    a. The role of the adolescent in health care
    b. The role of the parents in the health of their adolescent
    c. Adolescents and confidentiality
3. What implications for nursing care should be established at this time?
4. Does the evidence support your conclusion?
5. Are there alternative perspectives that you should consider?

ANSWERS

1. Yes, there is sufficient evidence for the nurse to formulate a response to Jamie's mother.
2. a. As teenagers progress through adolescence, they are able to assume more responsibility for their own health. They can take prescribed medications, keep health care appointments, and discuss their care with health care professionals.
    b. Parents of adolescents should respect their teenager's independence while maintaining some level of parental involvement with their child. However, in matters of health care, they should gradually assume the role of a consultant and allow their child to take an increasingly more active role in relating to health professionals.
    c. Health professionals who work with adolescents must consider the adolescent's increasing independence and responsibility while also maintaining privacy and ensuring confidentiality. In most adolescent clinics, health care professionals meet with the adolescent and the parent together, followed by individual time with both the adolescent and the parent.
3. The first priority for nursing care at this point is to reassure both Jamie and her mother that they each will have an opportunity to express their concerns to the nurse practitioner. Because Jamie is the nurse practitioner's patient and the setting is an adolescent clinic, the nurse practitioner should speak with Jamie first after she has met briefly with Jamie and her mother together. An appropriate response by the nurse practitioner might be: "I would like to begin by speaking with both of you together, then spend some time with just you, Jamie, then with just you, Mrs. S." Knowing that her mother will also have an opportunity to express concerns, Jamie will likely be more open and may even say, "I know what my mother will tell you," and address the issue herself. This response will also demonstrate to Jamie that the nurse practitioner respects her privacy and will maintain confidentiality. If the nurse speaks with Jamie first, Jamie might feel that her privacy is being violated and become distrustful of both the nurse practitioner and her mother. In addition, if the nurse practitioner speaks with Mrs. S. first, Jamie is likely to become defensive and spend her time trying to draw from the nurse practitioner what her mother said.
4. Yes, the information about adolescent growth and development and the roles of adolescents, their parents, and the health care professional support this conclusion.
5. The nurse practitioner should remember the circumstances under which she or he would not be able to maintain confidentiality. For example, if either Jamie or her mother share information that indicates that Jamie is at risk for either a self-destructive behavior (e.g., a suicide attempt) or maltreatment by others (child abuse), the nurse practitioner would not be able to maintain confidentiality. However, this does not seem to be the case based on the evidence presented at this point.

---

ciency resulting from blood loss. Calcium intake from food sources is essential during adolescence to assist in the prevention of osteoporosis. Eventual bone mass is a balance between the amount of bone laid down during adolescence and the amount later lost with aging. Overall, osteoporosis is a result of genetic and environmental factors such as nutrition and exercise (Ralston, 1997). Dietary intervention should promote the regular consumption of breakfast and a balanced intake of a variety of foods.

Eating Habits and Behavior

Eating and attitudes toward food are primarily family-centered during early and middle childhood, and food habits are largely related to cultural and individual family preferences and patterns. With adolescence and the move toward independence, family influences on the child change. Children's interests, attitudes, and routines are altered as an in-

creasing number of meals are eaten away from home. These changes are largely a result of the high value that teenagers place on peer acceptability and sociability. Their peers easily influence their eating habits.

Pressure for time and commitments to activities adversely affect the teenager's eating habits. Omitting breakfast or eating a breakfast that is nutritionally poor in quality is frequently a problem. Snacks, usually selected on the basis of accessibility rather than nutritional merit, become more and more a part of the habitual eating pattern during adolescence (Fig. 16-7). Adolescents often eat an insufficient amount of fresh fruits and vegetables, especially those that are rich in ascorbic acid. Milk is usually passed over in favor of soft drinks.

Overeating or undereating during adolescence presents special problems. When they experience the normal increase in weight and fat deposition of the growth spurt, teenage

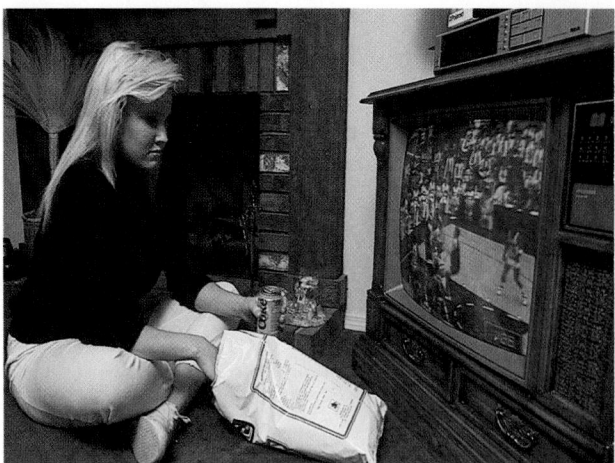

FIG. 16-7 ■ Snacking on empty calories is common among adolescents, especially during inactivity.

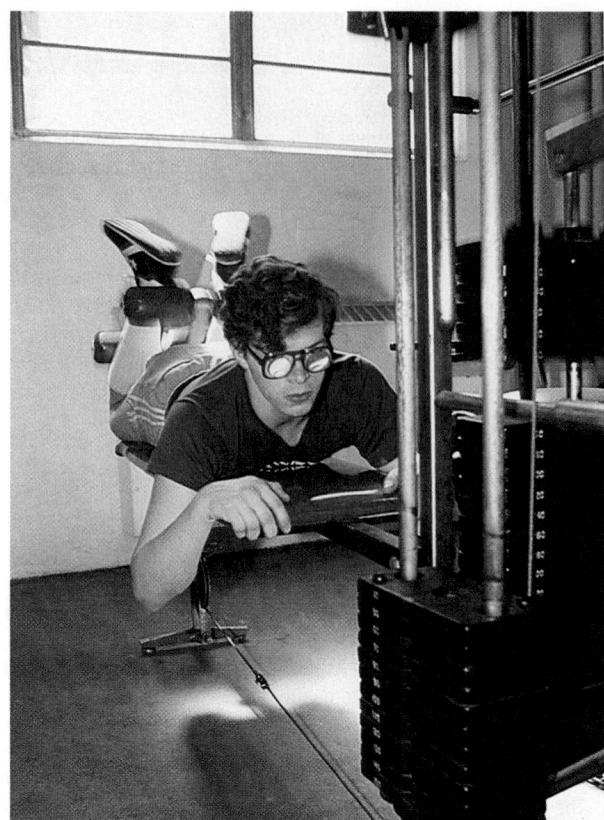

FIG. 16-8 ■ Adolescents should be encouraged to participate in activities that contribute to lifelong physical fitness.

girls often resort to dieting. The desire for a slim figure and a fear of becoming "fat" prompt teenage girls to embark on nutritionally inadequate reducing regimens that drain their energy and deprive their growing bodies of essential nutrients. They resort to diets on their own or with peers in an effort to conform. Many adopt current fad diets and are victims of food misinformation. Boys are less inclined to undereat. They are more concerned about gaining size and strength. However, they tend to eat foods high in calories but low in other essential nutrients.

Obesity is increasing among both children and adolescents in the United States. The obesity currently seen is not a result of metabolic disturbances, but of poor dietary habits and increasingly sedentary lifestyles. Childhood obesity often results in obesity in adulthood. The last two decades have revealed an increase in the overall portion size of foods. The largest portions for most foods are found at fast-food restaurants. However, portion sizes for desserts and hamburgers are the largest at home (Nielsen and Popkin, 2003). Lifestyle changes necessary for adolescents to lose weight require the involvement of family members who provide support and encourage active participation.

Nursing Considerations

Healthy dietary habits should be discussed with all adolescents. Adolescents need to learn about the Food Guide Pyramid (see Chapter 11); the relationships among dietary fat, weight status, and health; and food sources of fat, salt, and fiber (Seidell, 1999). Their food habits must be considered when planning nutritional education and guidance because they reflect many influences and conditions. Nurses in the school setting can assist in advocating for comprehensive nutritional services for preschool through grade 12 students. Comprehensive nutrition education with access to nutritious meals and snacks and physical activity at school will begin to reverse the trend of childhood obesity (Briggs, Safaii, and Beall, 2003).

To help teenagers select a nutritious diet, it is best to begin with their present diet and actively involve them in the process. Teenagers do not respond well to judgmental attitudes and dislike lectures, but they do respond when their

independence is respected and they are given the opportunity to make their own decisions regarding food choices.

In general, adolescents are body conscious and concerned about their appearance. Concrete messages about the relationship between an attractive appearance and the benefits of a healthy lifestyle are most effective. However, helping young persons arrive at a decision for change is more difficult than providing information. They respond best when the counselor provides straightforward information, uses instructional methods that actively involve them, talks *with* them and not *at* them, and listens to what they have to say.

SLEEP AND REST

Teenagers vary in their need for sleep and rest. Rapid physical growth, the tendency toward overexertion, and the overall increased activity of this age contribute to fatigue in adolescents. During growth spurts the need for sleep is increased. Their propensity for staying up late makes it very difficult to arise in the morning, and they may sleep late at every opportunity. Adequate sleep and rest at this time are important to a total health regimen.

EXERCISE AND ACTIVITY

Although today's youth are less fit than children 20 years ago, adolescents probably spend more time and energy practicing and participating in sports activities than members of any other age-group. Many adolescents participate in sports within school settings (Fig. 16-8). School-based, health-oriented physical education may provide both immediate effects of the activity and sustained effects through encouragement of lifelong activity patterns. Although daily physical education classes have decreased in schools in the last 10 years, the physical education classes that are held include more time spent in actual physical activity (Centers for Disease Control and Prevention, 2000).

The practice of sports, games, and even dancing contributes significantly to growth and development, the education process, and better health. These activities provide exercise for growing muscles, interactions with peers, and a socially acceptable means of enjoying stimulation and conflict. In addition, competitive activities help the teenager in the process of self-appraisal and the development of self-respect and concern for others. Because physical fitness appears to be a major influence on one's lifelong health status, children should be encouraged to participate in activities that contribute to lifelong physical fitness. Nurses can encourage participation as a way to promote health and build self-esteem. However, youngsters should not be encouraged to engage in physical activities that are beyond their physical or emotional capacity (see Health Problems Related to Sports Participation, Chapter 17).

DENTAL HEALTH

Dental health should not be neglected during adolescence, although the rate of caries formation is not as great as in childhood. Dental care is an aspect of preventive care that substantial proportions of children in the United States do not receive. Pit and fissure sealants are an underused safe and effective technique for dental caries prevention (Simonsen, 2002). Early adolescence is usually when corrective orthodontic appliances are worn, and these are frequently a source of embarrassment and concern to the youngster. Reassurance regarding the temporary nature of the annoyance and anticipation of an improved appearance help to make the inconvenience tolerable. It is also important to reinforce the orthodontist's directions regarding use and care of the appliances and to emphasize careful attention to toothbrushing during this time (see also Chapters 12 and 15).

PERSONAL CARE

The body-conscious teenager is highly amenable to discussion and counseling about personal care and hygiene. Body changes associated with puberty bring special needs for cleanliness. The hyperactive sebaceous glands and newly functioning apocrine glands make frequent bathing or showering a necessity, and underarm deodorants assume an important place in personal care. The adolescent discovers that hair requires more frequent shampooing, and girls often have questions about hair removal, use of cosmetics, and menstrual hygiene. Peer group discussions center around the advantages of particular products or methods. Adolescents are continually bombarded with messages from the media regarding the best way to enhance their popularity and attractiveness. Nurses are in a position to help them evaluate the relative merits of commercial products.

Vision

Regular vision testing is an important part of health care and supervision during adolescence. During adolescence, visual refractive difficulties reach a peak that is not exceeded until the fifth decade of life. The increased demands of schoolwork make adequate vision essential for academic success. Consequently, teenagers are more likely to be referred for visual evaluation. The need for corrective lenses can create psychologic problems for teenagers if they believe that glasses spoil their appearance or do not fit their body image. For those who can afford them, contact lenses may be a preferred solution. For some, the impact of a visual defect, no matter how slight, may be stressful.

Hearing

Considerable concern has focused on current teenage practices that cause hearing damage. Cochlear damage from relatively continuous exposure to the loud sound levels of rock music has been documented. The popularity of portable radios, stereo cassettes, and compact disc (CD) players with lightweight earphones are of particular concern to health care professionals. When these units are used for extended periods, permanent hearing loss can occur. Although appeals for more judicious use are not always successful, teenagers should be informed of the risk. Efforts directed toward legislating legal limits to the noise exposure that can be achieved through the sets may be another possible solution. (See Chapter 19 for a discussion of noise-related hearing loss.)

Posture

Many adolescents demonstrate altered posture. Rapid skeletal growth is often associated with slower muscular growth, and as a result, some teenagers may appear awkward or slump and fail to stand or sit upright. However, some postural defects of adolescence require early medical intervention. Scoliosis is a defect of the spine that occurs frequently in adolescence and is more common in girls than in boys (see Scoliosis, Chapter 31). The majority of the cases are idiopathic, and the defect presents as a painless curvature of the spine. Fortunately, most of these spinal curvatures will not require treatment. However, because there is no way to predict which curvatures will progress, all curvatures of the spine should be referred for further evaluation.

Body Art

Body art (piercing and tattooing) is used to assist with adolescent identity formation. The skin has become the latest source of parent/adolescent conflict. The adolescent often seeks body art as an expression of his or her personal identity and style. Tattoos are often obtained to mark significant life events such as new relationships, births, and deaths. Piercing the ear, nose, nipple, navel, penis, or tongue may sometimes create a health problem in the uninformed teenager. It is a nursing responsibility to caution girls and boys against the practice of having piercing performed by friends, parents, or themselves. Although in most cases there are few if any serious side effects, there is always a danger of complications such as infection, cyst or keloid formation, bleeding, dermatitis, or metal allergy. Using the same unsterilized needle to pierce body parts of multiple teenagers presents the same risk of human immunodeficiency virus (HIV) and hepatitis B virus transmission as occurs with other needle-sharing activities.

A qualified operator using proper sterile technique should perform the procedure. This is especially important if a youngster has a history of diabetes, allergies, or skin disorders. Adolescents should be informed about the approximate time for healing after body piercing and the care of the pierced area during and after healing. Some body sites need extra precautions. For example, cartilage (ear, nose) has a poor blood supply and heals slowly and scars easily; nipple piercing puts the adolescent at risk for breast abscess. Finally, migration of the piercing is common with naval and other flat skin surface piercing. Piercing guns should not be used for piercing anything other than the earlobe because guns place the piercing too deeply.

Nearly 15% of adolescents have at least one tattoo (Carroll and others, 2002). Professionals as well as amateur artists administer tattoos. The risk to the adolescent receiving a tattoo is low. The greatest risk is for the tattoo artist who comes in contact with the client's blood. Adolescents who are amateur tattoo artists benefit from discussions about universal precautions and the hepatitis B vaccination. Many states either have no regulations or do not enforce existing regulations of piercing and tattooing facilities. The state health department is a source of information about local regulatory requirements.

Suntanning

The quest for an attractive appearance leads many teenagers to excessive sunbathing and artificial means for suntanning. However, this practice has serious long-term risks, and the adolescent should be educated regarding the detrimental effects of sunlight on the skin (see Sunburn, Chapter 30). Long-term effects include premature aging of the skin, increased risk of skin cancer, and, in susceptible individuals, phototoxic reactions.

The increasing popularity of artificial suntanning has prompted concern from health professionals regarding the use of sunlamps and suntanning machines. The long-term effects of tanning machines are similar to those of the sun; dermatologists do not recommend suntanning by this means. Those who insist on using suntanning equipment should be warned that goggles must be worn in tanning booths to prevent serious corneal burning. Education on the use of sunscreens, including hypoallergenic products, with a sun protective factor (SPF) of at least 15 and a nonalcohol base without lanolin, parabens, or fragrance is important (Starr, 1999). Self-tanning creams safely stimulate the appearance of a tan; however, teens using these products should be cautioned that sun protection is still required. Targeting health education messages to adolescents and incorporating educational components relating to sun protection behaviors in school health curricula are essential (Hoffman, Rodrique, and Johnson, 1999). A large cross-sectional study of 12- to 18-year olds in the United States found that teens are not following these recommendations; 34% used sunscreen routinely in the past summer, and 14% used a tanning bed at least once (Geller and others, 2002).

STRESS REDUCTION

The multiple changes occurring in adolescence can result in great stress (Fig. 16-9 and Box 16-2). Adolescents are faced with pressures from peers that often involve flaunting adult authority and taking serious health risks. Health risks in-

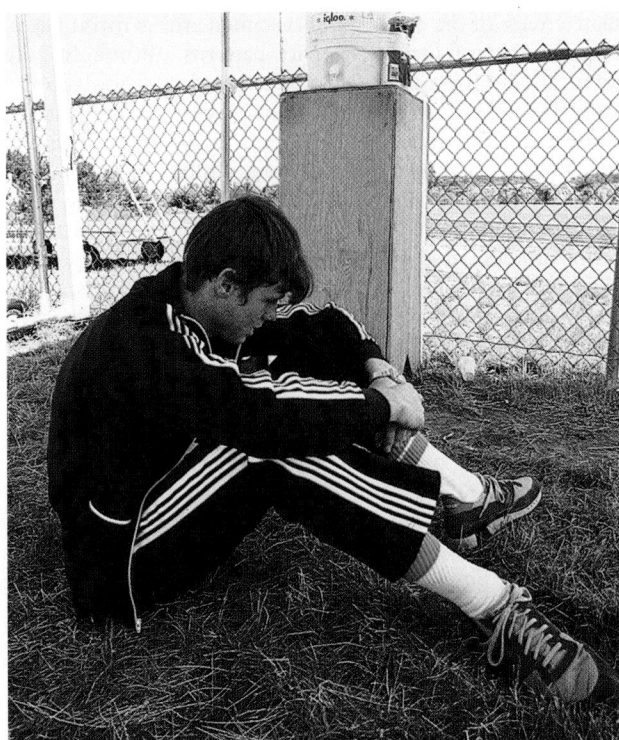

FIG. 16-9 ■ Adolescents use being alone as a method of coping with stress.

clude pressures for sexual experimentation and use of drugs, alcohol, and cigarettes, as well as potentially dangerous physical activities.

Early-maturing girls and late-maturing children are especially sensitive to the stresses of being different from their peers. Many feel intense anxiety over their identity. Both early- and late-maturing children feel out of place among their classmates, but slow-maturing children appear to suffer the most pronounced inner turmoil and may be hesitant to voice their concerns. Slow-maturing youngsters need support and reassurance that they are not abnormal and need only be patient until the time comes when they, too, will develop the characteristics for which they yearn.

SEXUALITY EDUCATION AND GUIDANCE

Contemporary adolescents are constantly exposed to sexual symbolism and erotic stimulation from the mass media. At the same time, the development of primary and secondary sex characteristics and the increased sensitivity of the genitals produce thoughts and fantasies about sexual relationships. Sexual aspects of interpersonal relationships become particularly important. Societal expectations push adolescents toward dating, and their own inner sex drive urges them toward exploration.

Our society continues to do a poor job of educating adolescents about pubertal growth and development. Omar, McElderry, and Zakharia (2003) found that 36% of males and 2% of females never were spoken to about pubertal development or sexuality issues. Girls received education at a mean age of 13 years and boys at an average age of 15 years. A large portion of their knowledge relating to sex is acquired from their peers, television, movies, and magazines.

BOX 16-2 ■ Areas of Stress in Adolescence

Body image
Sexuality conflicts
Scholastic pressures
Competitive pressures
Relationships with parents
Relationships with siblings
Relationships with peers
Finances
Decisions about present and future roles
Career planning
Ideologic conflicts

In addition, some information obtained from their parents may be inaccurate. As a result, the information they accumulate may be incomplete, inaccurate, riddled with cultural and moral judgments, and not very helpful.

The responsibility for providing sexuality education has been assumed by parents, schools, churches, community agencies such as **Planned Parenthood Federation of America, Inc.,*** and health professionals, especially nurses. Many adolescents perceive nurses, especially school nurses, as individuals who possess important information and who are willing to discuss sex with them. To be able to discuss the topic adequately, nurses must have not only an understanding of the physiologic aspects of sexuality and a knowledge of cultural and societal values, but also an awareness of their own attitudes, feelings, and biases about sexuality.

Comprehensive information about sexuality education is offered by the **Sexuality Information and Education Council of the United States (SIECUS)†** and the **Sex Information and Education Council of Canada (SIEC-CAN).‡** SIECUS maintains that every sexuality education program should present the topic from six aspects: biologic, social, health, personal adjustments and attitudes, interpersonal associations, and the establishment of values.

Whether nurses counsel young people on an individual basis, in mixed groups, or in groups segregated by gender makes little difference. Ideally, boys and girls should be able to discuss sexuality objectively with one another and in groups, but this is not always possible. The differences in the rate of maturation between boys and girls and between different members of the same sex often make it desirable to discuss certain aspects of sexuality in segregated groups. As a general rule, the need for separate discussion groups diminishes as young people progress toward maturity.

Sexuality education should consist of instruction concerning normal body functions and should be presented in a straightforward manner using correct terminology. When discussing sex and sexual activities, nurses should use simple but correct language, not street language, highly scientific terminology, or evasive jargon. Once the meanings of biologic

---

*810 Seventh Avenue, New York, NY 10019; (800) 230-PLAN; website: www.plannedparenthood.org.

†130 West 42nd Street, Suite 350, New York, NY 10036; (212) 819-9770; website: www.siecus.org.

‡850 Coxwell Avenue, East York, Ontario M4C 5R1, Canada; (416) 466-5304.

terms such as *uterus, testicles,* and *vagina* are understood, most teenagers prefer to use them in their discussions.

Many girls arrive at menarche with ambivalent attitudes, myths, and illogical beliefs. Even girls adequately prepared for menstruation do not always understand its relationship to the total process of reproduction. Many are under the incorrect impression that the "safe" time for sexual intercourse is midway between menstrual periods.

Teenagers' curiosity and desire for information extend beyond the need for anatomic and physiologic knowledge. They need to know more than the mechanics of conception, pregnancy, and birth. Adolescents, girls in particular, want answers to questions such as "What is it like?" "Does it hurt?" "What happens when . . . ?" and "Is it all right if you . . . ?" Boys are often concerned about the fallacy that a relationship exists between penis size and sexual function. They need reassurance that masturbation is a normal and common practice, that some degree of homosexuality is not unusual in early adolescence, and that oral-genital relations can be normal substitutes for intercourse.

Teenagers need to discuss intercourse, alternative methods of sexual satisfaction, and how to resist peer pressure. With the increased incidence of sexually transmitted diseases, especially HIV infection, the topic of "safe sex," especially abstinence or the use of condoms and abstinence, is essential. Role-playing can help teenagers learn effective approaches to dealing with difficult situations. Sex and sexuality cannot be taught without discussions of mature decision making, sexual responsibility, and values clarification.

Adolescents need role models and life experiences with delayed gratification. Most important, they need problem-solving experience and decision-making skills so that they can anticipate the positive and negative outcomes of a decision. With these types of assistance, teenagers can become sexually responsible young adults.

INJURY PREVENTION

Physical injuries are the greatest single cause of death in the adolescent age-group and claim more lives than all other causes combined. The most vulnerable ages are the years 15 to 24, when accidental injuries account for about 60% of deaths in boys and 40% of deaths in girls. These figures remain fairly constant from year to year and are significant because almost all fatal injuries are preventable.

During adolescence, peak physical, sensory, and psychomotor function gives teenagers a feeling of strength and confidence that they have never experienced before, and the physiologic changes of puberty give impetus to many basic instinctual forces. One manifestation of this is an increase in energy that simply must be discharged through action, often at the expense of logical thinking and other control mechanisms. Their propensity for risk-taking behavior plus feelings of indestructibility makes adolescents especially prone to injuries. Some of the developmental characteristics of teenagers and the common injuries associated with this age-group are outlined in Table 16-2.

Vehicle-Related Injuries

The adolescent's newly acquired ability to drive and the normal developmental need for independence and freedom make the automobile an attractive part of an adolescent's

TABLE 16-2 ■ Injury Prevention During Adolescence

DEVELOPMENTAL ABILITIES RELATED TO RISK OF INJURY	INJURY PREVENTION
Need for independence and freedom Testing independence Age permitted to drive a motor vehicle (varies) Inclination for risk taking Feeling of indestructibility Need for discharging energy, often at expense of logical thinking and other control mechanisms Strong need for peer approval May attempt hazardous feats Peak incidence for practice and participation in sports Access to more complex tools, objects, and locations Can assume responsibility for own actions	**Motor/nonmotor vehicles** *Pedestrian*—Emphasize and encourage safe pedestrian behavior At night, walk with a friend If someone is following you, go to nearest place with people Do not walk in secluded areas; take well-traveled walkways *Passenger*—Promote appropriate behavior while riding in a motor vehicle *Driver*—Provide competent driver education; encourage judicious use of vehicle; discourage drag racing, "playing chicken"; maintain vehicle in proper condition (brakes, tires, etc.) Teach and promote safety and maintenance of two-wheeled vehicles Promote and encourage wearing of safety apparel such as helmet, long trousers Reinforce the dangers of drugs, including alcohol, when operating a motor vehicle **Drowning** Teach nonswimmer to swim Teach basic rules of water safety Judicious selection of place to swim Sufficient water depth for diving Swimming with companion **Burns** Reinforce proper behavior in areas involving contact with burn hazards (gasoline, electric wires, fires) Advise regarding excessive exposure to natural or artificial sunlight (ultraviolet burn) Discourage smoking Encourage use of sunscreen **Poisoning** Educate in hazards of drug use, including alcohol **Falls** Teach and encourage general safety measures in all activities **Bodily damage** Promote acquisition of proper instruction in sports and use of sports equipment Instruct in safe use of and respect for firearms and other devices with potential danger (e.g., power tools, firecrackers) Provide and encourage use of protective equipment when using potentially hazardous devices Promote access to or provision of safe sports and recreational facilities Be alert for signs of depression (potential suicide) Discourage use of or availability of hazardous sports equipment (e.g., trampoline, surfboards) Instruct regarding proper use of corrective devices (e.g., glasses, contact lenses, hearing aids) Encourage and foster judicious application of safety principles and prevention

life. Forty percent of all teen deaths in the United States are the result of motor vehicle crashes (Centers for Disease Control and Prevention, 2003). Many factors contribute to the higher rate of crashes among teen drivers, including lack of driving experience and maturity, following too closely, driving too fast, having other teen passengers in the car, and using alcohol (Williams and Ferguson, 2002). Because there is a significant increase in the number of accidents when adolescents drive at night, many states have effectively enacted

driving curfews to curtail this risk. Nurses should educate teenagers and their parents about the risk of driving while drinking alcohol or when intoxicated, or of riding in an automobile with a drunk driver. Many families have developed a plan to arrange a no-questions-asked ride home to prevent an adolescent from riding with a drunk driver. Families should also require adolescents to log several hours of supervised practice driving before taking the car out alone. The major risk for death in a motor vehicle accident is failure to use a safety restraint. Teenage seatbelt use, especially among males, is lower than adult seatbelt use. Belt use as a passenger is low for teens even when the driver is an adult. Continued efforts to ensure teenage seatbelt use should be focused at the individual educational level as well as through tough enforcement laws (Williams, McCartt, and Geary, 2003).

Nonautomotive Vehicle Injuries.   The increasing use of motorized bicycles, all-terrain vehicles (ATVs), jet skis, and snowmobiles has caused an increase in injuries among young people who are below the legal age for driving automobiles. Many adolescents ride bicycles without helmets and without lights at night, and the overwhelming majority of deaths from bicycle injuries (primarily head injuries) involve teenagers.

Firearms

Firearms are the major cause of intentional fatal injuries in the United States. Adolescence is the peak age for being either a victim or an offender in an injury involving a firearm. Gun carrying among adolescents is on the rise and is not limited to the stereotypic inner-city youth. Family members and acquaintances are a common source of guns for young people. Gun availability in the general population is linked to increased gun death among children (Miller, Azrael, and Hemenway, 2002). Having a gun in the home increases the risk of adolescent suicide and homicide. All families should be assessed for the presence of a gun in the home and informed of the increased risk for suicide and homicide. When guns are present in the home, families must take preventive action to be sure that the guns are never loaded, that they are locked up in a safe place, and that ammunition is stored and locked up separately in a location where only appropriate adults have access to it.

Nonpowder Firearms.   Guns that do not use powder (e.g., air rifles, BB guns), although viewed as toys by many, account for almost as many injuries as powder guns. The regulations regarding nonpowder guns are relaxed; they can be purchased legally by youngsters and are labeled as suitable for children as young as 8 years of age. Few states regulate their use. Nurses should act as child advocates and urge passage of laws to regulate the sale of these potentially dangerous "toys."

Sports Injuries

Because the degree of physical maturation, size, coordination, and endurance varies greatly among adolescents of the same age, sports competition between young people who differ greatly in strength and agility is unfair and hazardous. Matching candidates for sports should be done relative to physical maturity, height, weight, and physical fitness and skills, particularly in a sport involving rigorous body contact. Age is a less important consideration.

Every sport has some potential for injury, whether one participates in serious competition or is actively engaged in the activity for pure enjoyment. Overuse injuries are common in adolescents and result in more time missed from the activity than fractures. A large number of severe or fatal injuries occur to youths who are not physically prepared for the

FAMILY HOME CARE

Guidance During Adolescence

ENCOURAGE PARENTS TO:
Accept adolescent as a unique individual.
Respect adolescent's ideas, likes and dislikes, and wishes.
Be involved with school functions and attend adolescent's performances, whether it be a sporting event or a school play.
Listen and try to be open to teenager's views, even when they disagree with parental views.
Avoid criticism about no-win topics.
Provide opportunity for choosing options and accept natural consequences of these choices.
Allow young persons to learn by doing, even when choices and methods differ from those of adults.
Provide adolescent with clear, reasonable limits.
Clarify house rules and consequences for breaking them.
Let society's rules and consequences teach responsibility outside the home.
Allow increasing independence within limitations of safety and well-being.
Be available but avoid pressing teenager too far.
Respect adolescent's privacy.
Try to share adolescent's feelings of joy or sorrow.
Respond to feelings, as well as words.
Be available to answer questions, give information, and provide companionship.
Try to make communication clear.
Avoid comparisons with siblings.
Assist adolescent in selecting appropriate career goals and preparing for adult role.
Welcome adolescent's friends into the home and treat them with respect.
Provide unconditional love.
Be willing to apologize when mistaken.

BE AWARE THAT ADOLESCENTS:
Are subject to turbulent, unpredictable behavior.
Are struggling for independence.
Are extremely sensitive to feelings and behavior that affect them.
May receive a different message than what was sent.
Consider friends extremely important.
Have a strong need "to belong."

activity. The increase in strength and vigor in adolescence may tempt youngsters to overextend themselves, especially boys who are urged on by teammates or are stimulated by the admiration of female observers. The range of injuries sustained in sports or recreational activities can involve any part of the body and extend from relatively minor cuts, bruises, and abrasions to totally incapacitating central nervous system injuries or death. The leading cause of serious sports injuries among boys is participation in football, whereas most girls are injured while participating in gymnastics.

Nursing Considerations

Injury prevention is an ongoing part of nursing responsibility throughout the childhood years. Anticipatory guidance to parents and children regarding the expected problems and hazards related to growth and development does not

FAMILY FOCUS

Family Rules for Adolescents

U.S. society does little to help adolescents mature and separate. Americans have remarkably few rites of passage that mark the stages of life. Few ceremonies and tests are practiced to determine eligibility for specific adult privileges. Obtaining a driver's license, graduating from high school, and reaching legal age for drinking are among the few that exist. U.S. society also does not have many generally agreed-on social dictums. When is the right age to begin dating? What is a reasonable curfew? Should an 18-year-old be allowed to stay out all night? There are few areas of general agreement. Every family makes up its own rules, influenced, but uninstructed, by the society at large. Many families have great difficulty with this process.

Modified from Prothrow-Stith D: *Deadly consequences: how violence is destroying our teenage population and a plan to begin solving the problem*, New York, 1993, HarperCollins.

end as children approach maturity. They need education in basic safety precautions, as well as instruction in skills required in the performance of activities such as sports, instruction in handling motor vehicles, using proper protective equipment, and properly maintaining equipment. During adolescence, however, health and safety education and guidance are more effective when the young people are involved directly. Parents and health professionals can emphasize the importance of safety during performance of activities and the proper conditioning and preparation for sports.

Prevention can occur on a variety of levels. Safety advocacy, changing public policy, and legislation can curtail injuries. Examples of such approaches are laws that mandate wearing seatbelts, mandatory helmet use while driving moving vehicles other than automobiles, keeping the legal drinking age at 21 years, and instituting curfews for teen drivers. In addition to improving the environment, health education for teenagers and significant adults is essential. Helping adolescents understand their need for engaging in risky behavior, exploring possible negative outcomes, and weighing possible alternatives are critical components of injury prevention.

ANTICIPATORY GUIDANCE—CARE OF FAMILIES

Both adolescents and their parents are often confused and perplexed about the changes and behavior of this stage of development. Parents need support and guidance to help them through this trying time. They need to understand the changes taking place and to accept the expected behaviors that accompany the process of detachment. Parents may need help to "let go," and to promote the changed relationship from one of dependence to one of mutuality (see Family Home Care and Family Focus boxes).

KEY POINTS

- The pubescent growth spurt that begins around age 10 in girls and age 12 in boys signals the beginning of adolescence.

- Biologic development during puberty is characterized by increased activity of the pituitary gland, which results in sexual maturity and the appearance of secondary sex characteristics.

- According to Erikson, the major developmental crisis of adolescence is establishing a sense of identity.

- Cognitive development in adolescence includes abstract thought, thinking beyond the present, logical reasoning, and a sense of idealism.

- Development of body image is closely tied to body changes and social interactions.

- According to Kohlberg's theory of moral development, adolescents begin to question existing moral values and learn to make choices.

- Spiritual development is characterized by the questioning of family values and ideals, a move to more philosophic thinking, and emphasis on personal religion.

- Adolescent relationships with parents may be strained, whereas the influence of the peer group increases and intimate relationships assume importance.

- Teenagers demonstrate a wide variety of interests, and their increased physical and cognitive skills allow them to engage in increasingly difficult and complex activities.

- Adolescents' emotions fluctuate.

- Nutritional needs, especially for calcium, zinc, and iron, may not be met by teenagers' eating habits, such as snacking and irregular mealtimes.

- Motor vehicle injuries are the primary cause of death from injury in the adolescent years.

References

Alan Guttmacher Institute: *Facts in brief: teen sex and pregnancy*, New York, 1998, The Institute.

American Academy of Pediatrics, Committee on Infectious Diseases: Recommended childhood immunization schedule—United States, January-December 2000, *Pediatrics* 105(1):148, 2000.

Baker JG and others: Relationship between perceived parental monitoring and young adolescent girls' sexual and substance use behaviors, *J Pediatr Adolesc Gynecol* 12:17-22, 1999.

Biro FM and others: Impact of timing of pubertal maturation on growth in black and white female adolescents: the National Heart, Lung, and Blood Institute Growth and Health Study, *J Pediatr* 138(5):636-643, 2001.

Briggs M, Safaii S, Beall DL: Nutrition services: an essential component of comprehensive school health programs, *J Am Diet Assoc* 103(4):505-514, 2003.

Brown J: Body and spirit: religion, spirituality and health among adolescents, *Adolesc Med* 12(3):509-523, 2001.

Carroll ST and others: Tattoos and body piercings as indicators of adolescent risk-taking behaviors, *Pediatrics* 109(6):1021-10217, 2002.

Centers for Disease Control and Prevention: Youth Risk Behavior Surveillance—United States, 1999, *MMWR* 49(SS-5):1-94, 2000.

Centers for Disease Control and Prevention: *Teen drivers, 2003;* available at: www.cdc.gov/ncipc/factsheets/teenmvh.htm.

Erikson EH: *Childhood and society*, ed 2, New York, 1963, WW Norton.

Garofalo R, Katz E: Healthcare issues of gay and lesbian youth, *Curr Opin Pediatr* 13:298-302, 2001.

Geller AC and others: Use of sunscreen, sunburning rates and tanning bed use among more than 10,000 U.S. children and adolescents, *Pediatrics* 109(6):1009-1014, 2002.

Graber JA and others: Is psychopathology associated with the timing of pubertal development? *J Am Acad Child Adolesc Psychiatry* 36:1768-1775, 1997.

Hamburg DA: Toward a strategy for healthy adolescent development, *Am J Psychiatry* 154(6):7-12, 1997.

Harries M and others: Changes in the male voice at puberty: vocal fold length and its relationship to the fundamental frequency of the voice, *J Laryngol Otol* 112(5):451-454, 1998.

Hayward C and others: Psychiatric risk associated with early puberty in adolescent girls, *J Am Acad Child Psychiatry* 36:255-262, 1997.

Hoff T, Greene L, Davis J: *National survey of adolescent and young adult sexual health knowledge, attitudes and experiences,* Menlo Park, Calif, 2003, Henry J Kaiser Family Foundation.

Hoffman RG, Rodrique JR, Johnson JH: Effectiveness of a school-based program to enhance knowledge of sun exposure: attitudes toward sun exposure and sunscreen use among children, *Child Health Care,* 28(1):69-86, 1999.

Maes L, Lievens J: Can the school make a difference? a multilevel analysis of adolescent risk and health behaviour, *Soc Sci Med* 56(3):517-529, 2003.

Miller M, Azrael D, Hemenway D: Firearm availability and unintentional firearm deaths, suicide and homicide among 5-14 year olds, *J Trauma* 52:267-275, 2002.

Nielsen SJ, Popkin BM: Patterns and trends in food portion sizes, 1977-1998, *JAMA* 289(4):450-453, 2003.

Omar H, McElderry D, Zakharia R: Educating adolescents about puberty: what are we missing? *Int J Adolesc Med Health* 15(1):79-83, 2003.

Ralston SH: What determines peak bone mass and bone loss, *Baillieres Clin Rheumatol* 11(3):479-494, 1997.

Resnick MD and others: Protecting adolescents from harm: findings from the National Longitudinal Study on Adolescent Health, *JAMA* 278:823-832, 1997.

Rosenstein NE, Fischer M, Tappero JW: Vaccine recommendations: challenges and controversies, *Infect Dis Clin North Am* 15(1): 155-169, 2001.

Saewyc EM and others: Gender differences in health and risk behaviors among bisexual and homosexual adolescents, *J Adolesc Health Care* 23:181-188, 1998.

Seidell JC: Obesity: a growing problem, *Acta Paediatr* 88(428 suppl):46-50, 1999.

Simonsen RJ: Pit and fissure sealant: review of the literature, *Pediatr Dent* 24(5):393-414, 2002.

Starr NB: Sun smarts: the essentials of sun protection, *J Pediatr Health Care* 13:136-138, 1999.

Williams AF, Ferguson SA: Rationale for graduated licensing and the risks it should address, *Inj Prevent* 6:9-16, 2002

Williams AF, McCartt AF, Geary L: Seatbelt use by high school students, *Inj Prevent* 9:25-28, 2003.

17

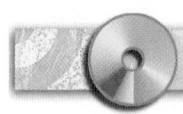

Health Problems of School-Age Children and Adolescents

MARILYN L. WINKELSTEIN

Remember to check out your companion CD-ROM

http://evolve.elsevier.com/Wong/essentials/

CHAPTER OUTLINE

RELATED TOPICS and ADDITIONAL RESOURCES

 IN TEXT

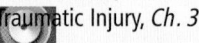

CD COMPANION

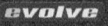 WEBSITE

 WONG'S CLINICAL MANUAL
 OF PEDIATRIC NURSING, 6/E

COMMON HEALTH PROBLEMS

INFECTIOUS MONONUCLEOSIS

Infectious mononucleosis is an acute, self-limiting infectious disease that is common among people younger than 25 years of age. The disease is characterized by an increase in the mononuclear elements of the blood and by general symptoms of an infectious process. The course is usually mild but occasionally can be severe or, rarely, accompanied by serious complications.

Etiology/Pathophysiology

The herpes-like Epstein-Barr virus is the principal cause of infectious mononucleosis. It appears in both sporadic and epidemic forms, but the sporadic cases are more common. The mechanism of spread has not been proved, but it is believed to be transmitted by direct intimate contact with oral secretions. It is mildly contagious, but the period of communicability is unknown. The incubation period following exposure is 4 to 6 weeks.

Diagnostic Tests

The onset of symptoms may be acute or insidious. The presenting symptoms vary greatly in type, severity, and duration (Box 17-1). The leukocyte count may be normal or low. Usually lymphocytic leukocytosis develops, and there is an increase in atypical leukocytes in the peripheral blood smear. The heterophil antibody test determines the extent to which the patient's serum will agglutinate sheep red blood cells. In infectious mononucleosis, a titer of 1:160 is considered diagnostic, although a rising titer during the early stages is the best indicator.

The *"spot test" (Monospot)* is a slide test of blood obtained by finger puncture that has high specificity. It is rapid, sensitive, inexpensive, and easy to perform, and has the advantage that it can detect significant agglutinins at lower levels, thus allowing earlier diagnosis.

Therapeutic Management

No specific treatment exists for infectious mononucleosis. Simple remedies ordinarily relieve the symptoms. A mild analgesic is often sufficient to relieve the headache, fever, and malaise. Bed rest is encouraged for fatigue but is not imposed for any specific period. Affected youngsters are instructed to regulate activities according to their own tolerance unless complicating factors are present. If the spleen is enlarged, activities in which children might receive a blow to the abdomen or chest are avoided.

A short course of oral penicillin is sometimes prescribed for sore throat, especially if β-hemolytic streptococci are present. However, administration of ampicillin frequently precipitates a maculopapular rash, and its use is contraindicated. If sore throat is severe, gargles, hot drinks, anesthetic troches, or analgesics, including opioids, are effective therapies. Although corticosteroids have been used to treat respiratory distress from tonsillar hypertrophy, hemolytic anemia, thrombocytopenia, and neurologic complications, routine use of steroids is not recommended (Barone and Krilov, 2001).

Prognosis. The course of this disease is usually self-limiting and uncomplicated. Acute symptoms often disappear within 7 to 10 days, and persistent fatigue subsides within 2 to 4 weeks. Some children need to restrict activities for 2 to 3 months, but the disease rarely extends for longer periods. Complications are uncommon, but can be serious and require appropriate management.

Nursing Considerations

Nursing responsibilities are directed toward providing comfort measures to relieve symptoms and toward helping affected youngsters and their families to determine appropriate

BOX 17-1 ■ Clinical Manifestations of Infectious Mononucleosis

EARLY SIGNS
Headache
Malaise
Fatigue
Chills
Low-grade fever
Loss of appetite
Puffy eyes

FULL-BLOWN DISEASE
Cardinal Features
Fever
Sore throat
Cervical adenopathy

Common Features
Splenomegaly (may persist for several months)
Palatine petechiae
Macular eruption (especially on trunk)
Exudative pharyngitis/tonsillitis
Hepatic involvement to some degree, often associated with jaundice

activities for the stage of the disease. Families often need diet counseling to select foods that contain sufficient calories to meet growth and energy needs but are easy to swallow. Every effort should be made to prevent a secondary infection. The child is advised to limit exposure to persons outside the family, especially during the acute phase of illness.

> **⚠ NURSING ALERT**
>
> Advise the family to seek medical evaluation of the youngster if:
> Breathing becomes difficult.
> Abdominal pain develops.
> Sore throat pain is so severe that the child is unable to eat or drink.

The illness and its associated weakness and fatigue can cause depression and resentment in vigorous, active teenagers. It is important to listen to concerns and to allow children to express their feelings and to vent their anger. Adolescents, in particular, need reassurance that the limitations are temporary and that social activity can be resumed after the acute phase. They also need to know that they will have sufficient autonomy to determine the extent of their capabilities and the rate of resumption of activities.

SMOKING

From 1997 until 2001, the percentage of young people who reported current cigarette use and frequent cigarette use decreased significantly (Grunbaum and others, 2002). Despite this decrease, however, a significant number of children and teenagers initiate or continue to smoke. The 2001 Youth Risk Behavior Survey indicated that 28.5% of senior high school students in the United States currently smoked cigarettes. Nationwide, 22% of young people initiate smoking by 13 years of age.

The hazards of smoking at any age are well known, and prevention of smoking is essential in childhood and adolescence. The age at which most children initiate or experiment with smoking is approximately 11 years, and most adults who are currently addicted to tobacco developed the habit in adolescence (Moolchan, Ernst, and Henningfield, 2000). In children and adolescents, smoking produces almost immediate effects of reduced lung function, "smoker's" cough, and respiratory difficulties. In addition, 24% to 50% of teens who start to smoke become nicotine dependent (Rojas and others, 1998). Research also indicates an association between current use of tobacco and the development of depression (Goodman and Capitman, 2000) and sleep problems (Patten and others, 2000) in adolescence. Cigarettes are considered to be a gateway drug, and teenagers who smoke are 11.4 times more likely to use illicit drugs (Gordon, 2000).

Etiology

Teenagers begin smoking for a variety of reasons (e.g., imitation of adult behavior, peer pressure, a desire to imitate behaviors portrayed in the movies and advertisements, a desire to control weight especially among females) (Strauss, 2000). Teenagers who do not smoke usually have family members and friends who do not smoke or who oppose smoking. Most teens who refrain from smoking have a de-

sire to succeed in academics or athletics (particularly high-performance sports, such as basketball, swimming, and track), and plans to go to college (see Community Focus box). Although smoking among college students has increased in recent years (Rigotti, Lee, and Wechsler, 2000), rates of smoking are highest among adolescents who do not complete high school.

Smokeless Tobacco

The term *smokeless tobacco* refers to tobacco products that are placed in the mouth but not ignited (e.g., snuff, chewing tobacco). This popular substitute for cigarettes poses a serious hazard to children and adolescents. These products have been proven to be carcinogenic, and regular use causes foul-smelling breath and dental problems such as periodontal degeneration and oral soft-tissue lesions. Use of smokeless tobacco can also lead to cigarette smoking.

Nursing Considerations

Prevention of regular smoking in teenagers is the most effective way to reduce the overall incidence of smoking. A variety of strategies have been used to prevent smoking. Because smoking is a social symbol, antismoking campaigns that address the norms of potential smokers without ridiculing or

---

 COMMUNITY FOCUS

Early Sexual Maturation, Alcohol, and Cigarettes

Cigarette smoking and the drinking of alcohol among adolescents are complex behaviors that are not explained by any one cause or factor. Some theorists and investigators believe there is a relationship between biologic maturation and these risk-taking behaviors. For example, young girls who are sexually mature at an earlier age than their peers are often attracted to older girls and boys who may engage in risk-taking behaviors. If older teens smoke, drink, and drive while under the influence of alcohol with no adverse consequences (e.g., no motor vehicle accidents), young girls may believe that they, too, will be safe while smoking, drinking, or riding in an automobile with friends who are drinking.

Although parents and nurses cannot influence the time of biologic maturation, they can identify young girls who are at risk for the initiation of risk-taking behaviors because of early puberty. Parents need to understand that an early-maturing daughter might be uncomfortable with her body, and they should take advantage of opportunities to build her self-esteem. Parental sensitivity to the importance of peer-group acceptance and parental support of a teenage daughter who feels left out or different are crucial. School nurses can provide anticipatory guidance to these girls and help them to role-play coping strategies for situations that involve offers to smoke and drink. In addition, school nurses can provide information about physical development during puberty and emphasize the fact that not all teenagers mature at the same time or rate.

Teachers, coaches, and church leaders can provide opportunities for these girls to "fit in" with their same-age peers through activities that stress mutual goals. For example, an early-maturing girl is typically taller than her age-mates and can be an asset in sports such as basketball and track-and-field events.

threatening their social group norms are more successful than programs that focus on the negative long-term effects of smoking. Youth-to-youth programs that emphasize the immediate personal and social consequences of smoking (e.g., unattractive stains on teeth and hands, unpleasant breath, and clothing or hair that smell of smoke) are effective in changing teenagers' attitudes toward smoking. When a significant number of influential peers "sell" their classmates on the idea that smoking is not popular, teens imitate their behavior. Teaching resistance to peer pressure to smoke is another effective strategy to prevent initiation of smoking in early adolescence. En-

forcing smoking bans in schools discourages smoking and promotes a smoke-free environment as the norm. Expanding these programs to include parents, mass media, youth groups, and community organizations strengthens the impact of school-based programs (see Community Focus box).

HEALTH PROBLEMS RELATED TO SPORTS PARTICIPATION

Every sport has the potential for injury to the participant—whether the youngster engages in serious competition or participates for enjoyment. Serious injury occurs most often during rough contact sports or to persons who are not physically prepared for the activity. Injuries also occur when the child or adolescent's body is not suited to the sport, when their muscles and body systems (respiratory and cardiovascular) are not conditioned to endure physical stress, or when they lack the insight and judgment to recognize that an activity exceeds their physical abilities. More injuries occur during recreational sports participation than during organized athletic competition.

The environment and the sports or recreational equipment can also present risks (Fig. 17-1). Children who participate in physical activity or sports do so in many different environments: indoors and outdoors, on floors, on the ground and snow, on or beneath water surfaces, and sometimes in free air space. Most of these activities also involve equipment.

Acute overload injuries are those that occur suddenly during an activity and produce immediate symptoms. A blow or overstretching, twisting, or sudden stress to tissues can cause these injuries. For descriptions and management of traumatic injuries see Chapter 31.

OVERUSE SYNDROMES

To excel in sports, the young athlete is forced to train longer, harder, and earlier in life than previously. The rewards are an increased level of fitness, better performances, faster times, and the satisfaction of attaining a personal goal. However, the risk of overuse injury is always present and is related to several factors: training errors, muscle-tendon imbalance, anatomic malalignment, incor-

---

COMMUNITY FOCUS

Nonsmoking Strategies

Nurses who work in schools, hospitals, and community agencies can take advantage of all opportunities to provide education about the dangers of smoking, to discourage smoking initiation by children and adolescents, to encourage smoking cessation, and to promote smoke-free environments. In particular, school nurses must be alert to the vulnerability of young preteens when they enter junior high school. These nurses are in an ideal position to assess stress, personal conflict, weight concerns, peer pressures, and other factors that place preteens at risk for smoking initiation. Nurses should serve as counselors to student, teacher, and parent groups and as advocates for antismoking legislative efforts. Several additional strategies are recommended.*

- Provide only brief information about long-term health consequences (e.g., cardiovascular, cancer risks).
- Discuss immediate physiologic consequences (e.g., changes in heart rate, blood pressure, respiratory symptoms, blood carbon monoxide concentrations).
- Mention alternatives to smoking that also establish a self-image that appears independent, mature, or sophisticated (e.g., establishing a weight-lifting regimen; jogging; dancing; joining a Boys or Girls Club; engaging in volunteer work for a hospital, political, religious, or community group).
- Mention the negative effects in detail (e.g., earlier wrinkling of skin; yellow stains on teeth and fingers; tobacco odor on breath, hair, and clothing).
- Mention the increasing ostracism of smokers by nonsmokers, both legal and informal, in the workplace and in public places.
- Mention the increasing evidence that secondhand smoke is injurious to the health of nonsmokers who are regularly exposed, especially small children.
- Acknowledge that many adults who were enticed to start smoking as teenagers because of its social benefits now wish they could stop smoking.
- Give cooperative adolescents effective arguments to deal with peer pressure (e.g., by not smoking, a teenager demonstrates independence and nonconformity, traits normally prized by youth).
- Request posters or pamphlets from local agencies (e.g., American Cancer Society, American Heart Association, American Lung Association) to display in prominent places at school.

*For information on smoking cessation, nurses can contact the **Nursing Center for Tobacco Intervention**, 1585 Neil Avenue, Columbus, OH 43210-1216; (614) 292-0653; fax: (614) 292-7976; website: www.con.ohio-state.edu/tobacco/. Information can also be obtained from **Stop Teenage Addiction to Tobacco (STAT)**, a national organization devoted to educating the public and professionals, at Northeastern University, 360 Huntington Avenue, 241 Cushing Hall, Boston, MA 02115; (617) 373-7828; e-mail: info@stat.org.

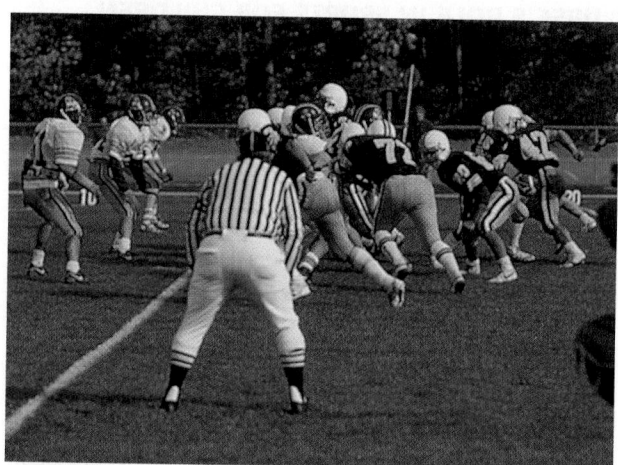

FIG. 17-1 ■ Football is an example of a strenuous collision sport.

rect footwear or playing surface, an associated disease state, and growth.

A common feature in overuse injuries is the *repetitive microtrauma* that occurs to a particular anatomic structure when the same movements are performed over a long period. The result is inflammation of the involved structure with complaints of chronic pain, tenderness, swelling, and disability. Examples of overuse syndromes include "Little League elbow" (tendinitis and osteochondritis from repetitive throwing), "tennis elbow" (lateral epicondylitis from repetitive elbow strain), and Osgood-Schlatter disease (traction apophysitis of the tibial tubercle).

Stress Fractures

Stress fractures occur as a result of repeated muscle contraction and are seen most often in repetitive weight-bearing sports such as running, gymnastics, and basketball. They occur less often in swimmers. The most common symptoms are a sharp, persistent, progressive pain or a deep, persistent, dull ache located over the bone. Sometimes there is pain on impact (heel strike), but the most important clinical sign is pain over the involved bony surface. Diagnosis is established on the basis of clinical observation, but occasionally a bone scan is performed.

Therapeutic Management

Inflammation is common in all overuse syndromes, and management is directed toward rest or alteration of activities, physical therapy, and medication. Rest is the primary therapy and is usually interpreted as reduced activity and the use of alternative exercise—*not* bed rest or immobilization with casting. The primary purpose is to alleviate the repetitive stress that initiated the symptoms. It is important to keep the youngster mobile, and training can be continued. Alternative exercise that maintains conditioning without aggravating the injury is selected. For example, pool running (treading water in the deep end of a pool) is an excellent alternative to running. Pool running uses the same movements as running without weight bearing. Other therapies include cryotherapy, cold whirlpools, and sometimes taping, bracing, splinting, or orthotics. Treatment is specific to the injury. Nonsteroidal antiinflammatory medications are prescribed to reduce pain and inflammation. Topical medications are of questionable value.

NURSE'S ROLE IN SPORTS FOR CHILDREN AND ADOLESCENTS

Nurses are often involved in sports activities in the areas of preparation and evaluation for activities, prevention of injury, treatment of injuries, and rehabilitation after injury. Selecting an appropriate sport for both recreation and competition is a joint effort of the youngster, parents, and health professionals. The best approach to counseling children and parents regarding sports participation is to encourage activities that are most likely to provide pleasure and physical benefits throughout childhood and into adulthood. Exposure to a variety of activities is better for young children than limiting them to one sport. Parents should be cautioned against overcommitting children to sports activities so they have time for other activities.

When children sustain athletic injuries, nurses are often responsible for instructions regarding care. Instructions (e.g., schedule for appointments, application of ice, any re-strictions in activity) should be clear and accompanied by written directions. The importance of taking medications as prescribed is emphasized, especially if medications are needed for an extended period and if adherence is an issue. Medications given an hour before practice or competition may be advantageous to children continuing their activities.

Prevention of sports injuries is the most important aspect of athletic programs. Children should be suited to the activity; the environment and the equipment must be safe. Children should be prepared for the sport, especially if it requires strenuous or continuous physical exertion. Nurses, coaches, and athletic trainers must collaborate to ensure that safety measures are implemented. Stretching exercises, warm-up and cool-down activities, and appropriate training are requirements for safe participation. Protective measures such as pads, taping, and wrapping are also important to prevent injury. Finally, nurses must be aware of environmental safety risks.

ALTERED GROWTH AND MATURATION

The absence of physical or sexual maturation at a time when other children are experiencing positive evidence of sexual development and its associated spurt in growth and physical strength is an important concern to both the parents and their affected child. Fortunately, in most instances the delay in development is a simple physiologic or *constitutional delay* that represents one end of the normal genetically influenced variation of pubertal growth. These children will go through a delayed but normal puberty and finally catch up, in their late teens, with their more rapidly developing agemates. Less benign causes of delayed development may be the result of endocrine disorders or chromosomal abnormalities. Delayed development can also be a result of chronic diseases (such as malabsorption or chronic asthma) that are serious enough to retard development or environmental factors (such as stress or poor nutrition).

The rate of maturation is important during the school years, but at puberty it assumes gigantic proportions to both teens and their parents. Girls or boys who lag behind their peers in physical maturation are painfully aware of their difference in growth. Adolescent girls with delayed maturation feel out of place among companions whose hips and breasts are developing, feel cheated if they have not yet menstruated, and feel left out when their friends giggle and talk about boys. Adolescent boys with delayed maturation feel weak and small compared with their more muscular companions with whom they can no longer compete. Slow-maturing youngsters need support and reassurance that they are not abnormal and that they will develop the physical characteristics they desire.

Serial measurements of growth are plotted periodically on standard growth charts to determine the pattern of growth and to compare the individual child with the norms for his or her age-group. When children are in the extremes of height ranges, it is important to compare their height with that of their parents and siblings.

TALL OR SHORT STATURE
Tall Stature

Despite the fact that the average height of both boys and girls is steadily increasing, there is a small group of children who, because of some organic disorder or a familial tendency, are excessively tall when compared with their peers. To boys, this may be a source of pride; to girls, it may cause intense anxiety and be a severe social handicap.

When the rate of height change before puberty suggests the probability of excessive adult height, treatment with hormones may be considered, although there is considerable controversy regarding the use of hormones for this purpose. The use of estrogens is effective in controlling height when therapy is initiated before menarche and before the end of the adolescent growth spurt that normally precedes menarche. The selection of children for hormonal therapy is made on the basis of a careful evaluation of physical, psychologic, and social factors.

Short Stature

Short stature is a nonspecific finding that may be the first manifestation of a serious disorder, or it may be of no consequence medically. On a worldwide scale, the most common cause of short stature or delayed development is inadequate nutrition. The major physical disorders that produce delayed development are chronic diseases, endocrine dysfunction, and syndromes of primary gonadal failure.

Chronic diseases can interfere with growth, but unless the illness is unduly prolonged, catch-up growth occurs. Diseases and disorders that cause some degree of growth delay include asthma, cystic fibrosis, gastrointestinal diseases (such as parasitic infections), malabsorption syndromes, cardiac anomalies, and chronic renal disturbances. The duration of the illness is more significant than the intensity in terms of the effect on growth, although the precise length of time necessary to affect growth permanently has not been determined.

Skeletal disorders that affect growth in stature are those described as dwarfism. Most disorders are caused by congenital defects and disorders, such as achondroplasia, and by inborn errors of metabolism, such as Hurler or Hunter syndrome.

Psychosocial, or *deprivation, dwarfism* is a stress-induced growth failure. It is defined as growth retardation in children older than 2 years of age that is caused by environmental (emotional) stress and is associated with a marked delay in physical growth, delayed developmental skills, and immature behavior. When these children are removed from the deprived environment, their growth proceeds at a normal or increased rate. (See also Failure to Thrive, Chapter 11, and Child Maltreatment, Chapter 14.)

Management involves continued medical observation, attention to general health and nutrition, and psychologic support. When growth delay is accompanied by poor self-esteem, many authorities recommend hormonal therapy. Testosterone in carefully regulated doses is effective in some cases. Growth hormone is capable of increasing height and is used to treat growth hormone deficiency (see Hypopituitarism, Chapter 29). Its use with children who have constitutional delay is highly controversial.

Nursing Considerations

Deviation from the normal course of puberty is a significant concern for affected adolescents. For some teens, this concern assumes monumental proportions. Most cases of delayed development are caused by simple constitutional delay of puberty, and the child can be assured that normal development will eventually take place.

One difficulty related to a size that is incongruent with chronologic and mental age is the manner in which others relate to the child. People often respond to children with short stature as though they are younger than their age. Consequently, these children may react with babyish or juvenile behavior, thus establishing a circular pattern of behavior and response. Conversely, children who are tall or physically advanced for their age are frequently treated as though they are more advanced than their years. They are often considered to be retarded or immature when they perform according to the normal behavioral expectations for their age.

Listening to distressed adolescents and conveying interest and concern are important interventions for these children and adolescents. Counseling and therapy are individualized for each youth. Encouraging these children to focus on the positive aspects of their bodies and personalities and to adopt sound health practices and practice good grooming fosters a more positive self-image.

SEX CHROMOSOME ABNORMALITIES

Most sex chromosome abnormalities are caused by an alteration in sex chromosome number (see Table 17-1). The majority of these conditions are due to nondisjunction. An alteration in the number of sex chromosomes usually does not produce the profound defects that are associated with the autosomal trisomies. Intelligence may be normal or low normal, or the child may have some learning disabilities. Moderate or severe mental retardation is less common.

Turner Syndrome

Turner syndrome is caused by absence of one of the X chromosomes. Most girls who have this disorder have one X chromosome missing from all cells (45,X). This disorder is often recognized at birth if the newborn has a webbed neck, low posterior hairline, widely spaced nipples, and edema of the hands and feet. It can also be diagnosed at puberty because of three features: short stature, sexual infantilism, and amenorrhea. Girls with Turner syndrome are generally infertile. They may also have difficulty with peer relationships and understanding social cues. They frequently exhibit behavioral problems, especially in relation to their immature, socially isolated behavior. Diagnosis is confirmed on the basis of a negative sex chromatin test.

Therapy is individualized for these girls and consists primarily of hormone treatment and psychologic counseling for both the child and the parents. Linear growth can be increased by the administration of growth hormone if therapy is begun early. Estrogen therapy is initiated during the usual time for puberty to promote the development of secondary sex characteristics. Responses to estrogen therapy vary from girl to girl, but gradual feminization is accomplished to some degree in most individuals.

Klinefelter Syndrome

Klinefelter syndrome, the most common of all sex chromosome abnormalities, is caused by the presence of one or more additional X chromosomes. Most males with this syndrome have a chromosome complement of 47,XXY. The disorder is seldom seen before puberty, at which time varying degrees of failure of adolescent virilization occur. Some males are not diagnosed until they appear for evaluation for

TABLE 17-1 ■ Common Sex Chromosome Abnormalities*

SYNDROME	CHROMOSOMAL NOMENCLATURE	PHENOTYPE	INCIDENCE (LIVE BIRTHS)	CLINICAL MANIFESTATIONS
Turner	45,X or 45X0	Female	1:2500 female births	Short stature; webbed neck; low posterior hairline; shield-shaped chest with widely spaced nipples; sterile; no development of secondary sex characteristics
Triple X, or superfemale	47,XXX (can also be 48,XXXX or 49,XXXXX)	Female	1:850-1250 female births	Normal female characteristics; usually tall; variable mental capacity and behavior; at risk for impaired language, learning difficulties; fertile
XYY male	47,XYY (can also be 48,XYYY or mosaic)	Male	1:900 male births	Usually normal sexual development; tendency to be tall with long head; poor coordination; may demonstrate aberrant behavior
Klinefelter	47,XXY (48,XXYY, 48,XXXY, 49,XXXXY, and so on, mosaics)	Male	1:850 male births	Tall with long legs; hypogenitalism; sterile; male secondary sex characteristics may be deficient; may demonstrate aberrant behavior; learning disabled; possible gynecomastia

*Data from Nora JJ, Fraser FC: *Medical genetics: principles and practice,* ed 3, Philadelphia, 1989, Lea & Febiger.

infertility. All have absence of sperm in the semen (azoospermia), small testes, and defective development of secondary sex characteristics. In 80% of these boys there is a chromatin-positive buccal smear, and the extra chromosome is apparent on chromosome analysis.

Cognitive impairment is a frequent clinical finding and appears to be related to the number of X chromosomes. Boys may also have gross motor skill difficulties, a developmental language delay, poor verbal skills, reduced auditory memory, shyness, passivity, behavioral problems, and school difficulties. Therapy is directed toward enhancing the masculine characteristics through administration of testosterone.

Nursing Considerations

The nursing care of children with Turner or Klinefelter syndrome is primarily supportive. Nurses assist in diagnosis, explain tests and therapies, and provide support and encouragement to the child and the family. Because both disorders render the individual unable to reproduce, psychologic counseling is an important aspect of care. Marriage and sexual relationships are possible, but alternative reproductive options, such as artificial insemination and adoption, should be discussed.

DISORDERS RELATED TO THE REPRODUCTIVE SYSTEM*

AMENORRHEA

Menarche, or the first menstrual period, occurs relatively late in female pubertal development. Although there is variation among girls in the onset and rate of progression of pubertal development, the sequence and tempo should be the same. When an adolescent presents with a complaint of ab-

sence of menses, a careful history of the timing of her pubertal development will help to determine if there is a need for further evaluation or if reassurance is all that is necessary.

Primary amenorrhea is an absence of secondary sex characteristics and no uterine bleeding by 14 to 15 years of age, or absence of uterine bleeding with secondary sex characteristics by 16 to 16.5 years of age. No uterine bleeding after attaining sexual maturity rating 5 (SMR 5) for 1 year, or after breast development for 4 years, is also considered primary amenorrhea (Neinstein, 2002). The etiology of primary amenorrhea may be anatomic, hormonal, genetic, or idiopathic. A thorough history and physical examination will provide clues to the etiology.

Secondary amenorrhea is defined as the absence of menses for 6 months or at least three cycles after menstruation was previously established. Irregular menstrual cycles are common within the first year or two after menarche. These early cycles may be anovulatory resulting in regular, irregular, or absent bleeding; however, cycle lengths greater than 90 days are rare and should be investigated (Timmreck and Reindollar, 2003). Girls with a later onset of menarche will take longer to establish regular ovulatory cycles. Pregnancy is the most common cause of secondary amenorrhea and should be ruled out in both types of amenorrhea, even if the adolescent denies sexual activity. When pregnancy has been ruled out, the history should be evaluated for evidence of stress, weight changes, and changes in the environment. Other common causes of amenorrhea in adolescents include hyperandrogenism, eating disorders, and exercise-induced amenorrhea (Hillard and Nelson, 2003).

DYSMENORRHEA

A certain amount of discomfort during the first day or two of the menstrual flow is extremely common. Most girls experience cramping, abdominal pain, backache, and leg ache, but in a few the pain is intolerable and incapacitating. *Primary dysmenorrhea* is painful menses not related to any pelvic dis-

---

*Linda M. Kollar, MSN, RN, revised this section.

ease. When the discomfort is related to endometriosis, infection, adhesions from peritonitis, or other pelvic disease, the complaint is termed *secondary dysmenorrhea.*

Primary dysmenorrhea usually begins at the time of menarche or within 6 to 12 months. The pain begins with menstrual flow or hours before the onset of bleeding each month, usually continuing for 48 to 72 hours. The exact etiology is widely debated. The pain is clearly related to ovulatory cycles. The overproduction of uterine prostaglandins has been implicated, and women with dysmenorrhea have higher levels of prostaglandins. Overproduction of vasopressin (a hormone that stimulates the contraction of muscular tissue) may also contribute to dysmenorrhea.

A careful history should include the onset of symptoms; the duration, type of pain, and relationship to menstrual flow; age at menarche; family history of dysmenorrhea; and sexual history. The nurse should also ask about previous treatment that has been tried, including dosages of medications. Associated symptoms such as nausea, vomiting, diarrhea, and leg and back pain are helpful for diagnosis and treatment. Depending on the results of the history, the physical examination may include a gynecologic examination.

Therapeutic Management

First-line treatment for adolescents with dysmenorrhea is the administration of nonsteroidal antiinflammatory drugs that block the formation of prostaglandins for 2 to 3 days of the menstrual cycle. The girl should be instructed to begin the medication at the first sign of cramping or bleeding. Girls with vomiting at the time of menstruation benefit from beginning the medication 1 to 2 days before the onset of their menses. The medications should be taken with food.

Cyclic estrogen therapy and oral contraceptives are also effective. Simple exercises such as pelvic rocking, assuming the knee-chest position, and breathing exercises may be beneficial. Encouraging adequate personal hygiene, participation in regular activities, and methods to decrease stress should be discussed with the adolescent.

A balanced diet and specific dietary changes that may be helpful include the elimination of caffeine from the diet and the addition of herbal teas. Many dietary and herbal treatments have been tried, including vitamins B_1, B_6, and E; omega-3 fatty acids; and magnesium. Vitamin B_1, 100 mg daily, is the only dietary treatment with a large clinical trial to demonstrate its effectiveness. Use of magnesium has shown promise in smaller studies (Wilson and Murphy, 2001).

Nursing Considerations

All adolescent girls need reassurance that menstruation is a normal function. When nurses are asked for advice regarding menstrual problems, they have a valuable opportunity to engage in health teaching concerning menstrual physiology and hygiene, as well as the importance of a well-balanced diet, exercise, and general health maintenance. Health teaching can dispel myths about menstruation and femininity. When assessment indicates a potential problem and the need for evaluation, referral to an appropriate practitioner, health service, or clinic may be necessary.

One of the most difficult experiences facing the adolescent girl is the gynecologic examination. Whether it is her first experience or not, she is often filled with apprehension.

Almost all adolescents are extremely self-conscious about their bodies and the changes taking place. They need continuing support in the form of anticipatory guidance regarding what to expect and suggestions of what to do to relax during the procedure. Usually the stressful experience of being placed in stirrups for the pelvic examination can be avoided. The adolescent girl who is relaxed may be examined in the supine position with hips and knees flexed and legs abducted. If a female nurse is not the examiner, it is essential for her to remain with the patient during the examination to offer support and guidance.

VAGINITIS

Vaginitis can be caused by physical, chemical, or infectious agents. Physical causes may include a forgotten tampon; chemical irritants include bubble bath, douching, deodorant pads, and tampons. Removal of the offending material or discontinuing use of the irritating substance is usually all that is necessary to treat physical or chemical vaginitis. Infectious vaginitis can be caused by *Candida* fungi (yeast), *Trichomonas* protozoa parasites, or bacteria. Diagnosis is confirmed with microscopic evaluation of vaginal secretions. Treatment varies depending on the infectious agent.

Health teaching is important in the prevention and management of vaginitis. Adolescent girls need reassurance that increased vaginal mucus can occur at the time of ovulation, before menstruation, or with sexual excitement. Many teenage girls mistake these variations as signs of infection. Girls should be taught to wipe from front to back after toileting and to realize that vaginitis can result from irritation, foreign objects, and sexual activity. Nurses should stress the importance of an evaluation to determine the exact cause.

DISORDERS OF THE MALE REPRODUCTIVE SYSTEM

Most obvious anomalies, such as hypospadias, hydrocele, phimosis, and cryptorchidism, have been identified, and corrective measures have been instituted during early childhood. The most frequent problems related to the reproductive organs in later childhood are (1) infections, such as urethritis (see Urinary Tract Infection, Chapter 27); (2) hematuria; (3) penile problems, such as nonretractable foreskin in uncircumcised males, carcinoma, and trauma; (4) scrotal conditions, such as varicocele (elongation, dilation, and tortuosity of the veins superior to the testicle); and (5) testicular torsion (a condition in which the testicle hangs free from its vascular structures, which can result in partial or complete venous occlusion with rotation). Tumors of the testes are not common, but when manifested in adolescence, they are generally malignant and demand immediate evaluation.

The usual presenting symptom for testicular cancer is a heavy, hard painless mass (either smooth or nodular) that is palpated on the testis. Treatment involves surgical removal of the affected testicle (orchiectomy) and possibly chemotherapy and radiation if metastasis has occurred.

Nursing Considerations

The adolescent boy is extremely self-conscious about his changing body and needs preparation for a genital examination. The most successful approach is to assume a matter-of-fact attitude toward the examination, explain precisely what will take place, and maintain a continuous commentary

⁇ CRITICAL THINKING EXERCISE ⁇

Testicular Self-Examination

At a recent faculty meeting, Paul, the pediatric nurse practitioner who runs the school-based health clinic, presented his plan for a class on testicular self-examination (TSE) to be delivered to the sophomore boys. Several teachers questioned the value of providing such a class when there is limited time to deliver content relating to "routine academic subjects." What important issues regarding testicular cancer and TSE should Paul use to justify providing this class to the sophomore boys?

QUESTIONS

1. Evidence—Is there sufficient evidence to justify teaching sophomore boys about TSE?
2. Assumptions—Describe the underlying assumption about each of the following:
   a. Detection of testicular cancers in adolescence
   b. Usual presenting symptom of testicular cancer
   c. Knowledge of genital anatomy among adolescent boys
   d. Ways to teach adolescent boys about their anatomy
3. What priorities for nursing care can be drawn at this time?
4. Does the evidence support your nursing intervention?
5. What alternative perspectives might you have?

ANSWERS

1. Yes. Although testicular cancer is not common in adolescence, when it does occur, it is generally malignant. Testicular cancer is very curable if detected early.
2. a. The best way to detect testicular tumors is by performing TSE every month.
   b. The usual presenting symptom for testicular cancer is a heavy, hard painless mass (either smooth or nodular) that is palpated on the testis.
   c. Adolescent boys are very self-conscious about their genital anatomy. However, as a pediatric nurse practitioner at the school-based clinic, Paul is in an excellent position to teach young men how to perform this exam. It is highly probable that he has already won their trust and confidence through his routine daily nursing activities, such as providing sports physicals and treating their episodic illnesses. Paul will be able to present the class in a manner that is respectful of the young boys, while also allaying their anxieties and providing them with an important health skill.
   d. The class should be presented in a matter-of-fact way, with an explanation of both the characteristics of the normal testicle as well as a description of abnormal findings.
3. The first priority is to make sure that all adolescent boys with health problems feel comfortable visiting the health suite and sharing their concerns with the nurse practitioner. The ultimate goal is to be sure that no adolescent boy with a potential testicular tumor fails to get an immediate assessment and referral for treatment.
4. Yes, the information about testicular cancer and the importance of detecting it early provide a definite rationale for the class.
5. If it is difficult to find the time for the class in the regular school health curriculum, Paul should suggest other options. Perhaps Paul could provide the information on TSE as part of an extra class that students volunteer to attend, or he could develop a self-learning packet that male students could complete when they visit the health suite.

about what is being done and the findings at each phase of the examination.

The routine health assessment of every adolescent boy should include teaching about testicular cancer and how to perform a testicular self-examination every month. This rare malignancy is curable if detected early. Nurses are in an ideal position to teach testicular self-examination, in a manner that is respectful of the adolescent boy's anxieties, and that promotes early treatment (see Critical Thinking Exercise).

The normal testicle is a firm organ with a smooth, egg-shaped contour; the epididymis is palpated as a raised swelling on the superior aspect of the testicle and should not be confused as an abnormality.

GYNECOMASTIA

The male breast, although not strictly part of the male reproductive system, responds to hormonal changes. Some degree of bilateral or unilateral breast enlargement occurs frequently in boys during puberty. It is estimated that approximately half of adolescent boys have transient gynecomastia, usually lasting less than 1 year, that subsides spontaneously with achievement of male development. A careful assessment of the pubertal stage at the onset of gynecomastia, medication history including anabolic steroids, and the exclusion of renal, liver, thyroid, and endocrine disorders or dysfunction allow the examiner to reassure the adolescent that the changes are pubertal gynecomastia and that no further assessment is indicated.

If the condition persists or is extensive enough to cause embarrassment or to produce doubts about gender identity in the young boy, plastic surgery may be indicated for cosmetic and psychologic considerations. Administration of testosterone has no effect on breast development or regression and may aggravate the condition.

Nursing Considerations

Treatment usually consists of assurance to the adolescent and his parents that this is a benign and temporary situation. Adolescents who are distressed about physical integrity and masculinity may benefit from the knowledge that this condition occurs in more than 50% of all adolescent boys.

HEALTH PROBLEMS RELATED TO SEXUALITY*

By the time adolescents finish high school, more than half of them have had sexual intercourse. There are many serious health consequences associated with adolescent sexual activity including unplanned pregnancy and sexually transmitted infections, increased number of partners over time, and incomplete education. Health professionals must understand the issues related to adolescent sexual activity and the psychosocial dynamics that influence them.

ADOLESCENT PREGNANCY

Although adolescent pregnancy remains a problem in the United States, pregnancy rates for 15- to 19-year-old adolescents decreased through the 1990s. This decrease is a result of increased abstinence among teenagers and, to a

---

*Linda M. Kollar, MSN, RN, revised this section.

larger extent, the result of changes in behavior of sexually experienced teenagers (Darroch and Singh, 1999). At the same time that this decrease has occurred for teens who are 15 to 19 years of age, the proportion of unmarried teens who have had sexual intercourse at age 14 and younger has increased appreciably. Nearly one in five adolescents has had sex before his or her fifteenth birthday. The younger a girl is at the time of her first intercourse, the more likely that intercourse will have been unwanted (Albert, Brown, and Flanigan, 2003).

The reduction in teen pregnancy is an important national goal because of the risk for negative outcomes for both the mother and the child. A wide range of factors put an adolescent at risk for pregnancy, including having sex with an older partner, the type of contraception used, living in poverty, having a mother who was a teen parent, school failure, and living in a poor community.

With better facilities available for care, the mortality for teenage pregnancies is decreasing, but morbidity remains high. Teenage girls and their unborn infants are at greater risk for complications of both pregnancy and delivery. The most frequent complications are premature labor and infants of low birth weight, high neonatal mortality, pregnancy-induced hypertension (PIH), iron deficiency anemia, fetopelvic disproportion, and prolonged labor. These obstetric difficulties seem to be related to the smaller maternal size rather than the younger age or developmental immaturity.

Although teenagers have special needs, the obstetric risk should be no greater than for any pregnant patient. When quality prenatal care is available early in the pregnancy, the progress and outcome of teenage pregnancies compare favorably with those of older women.

Nursing Considerations

A pregnant teenager needs careful assessment by the nurse to determine the level of social support available to her and possibly her partner. The adolescent needs to make many important decisions and may not have the life experience to know how to cope with this stress. Whenever possible, guidance from the adults in her life will be invaluable. Information about options to continue the pregnancy and parent the child, continue the pregnancy with adoption, or terminate the pregnancy with abortion should be given in a nonjudgmental manner. If the adolescent chooses to continue the pregnancy, prenatal care should be initiated as soon as possible. No matter what the teenager decides, nutrition information will be necessary.

CONTRACEPTION

Family planning services have developed and expanded during recent years, but the need for contraceptive services as part of the health care of adolescents remains great. By the time most adolescents approach the health care provider for a contraceptive method, they have been sexually active for 6 months to 1 year. Unfortunately, it is often a pregnancy scare that brings the adolescent to the health care provider to discuss contraception. Counseling about contraceptive options should be conducted in a manner that is consistent with the cognitive level of the adolescent. The adolescent should be given accurate information about the risks and benefits of each method before making a choice.

The choice of a safe and effective contraceptive method must be suited to the individual (Table 17-2). The choice is based on preference after the adolescent is informed of the benefits and disadvantages. Motivation is necessary for most methods. For example, the pill is very effective if used correctly, but the adolescent must remember to take the pill every day. For many young women, Depo-Provera is an ideal choice because it is extremely effective and is administered every 12 weeks. However, sexually active adolescents need to remember that contraceptive devices other than condoms do not prevent sexually transmitted diseases. Condom use is still important and must be discussed with all adolescents who seek contraceptive advice.

Nursing Considerations

Nurses are often involved in providing education about contraception. Such education is ideally combined with ongoing sex education. Although sexual abstinence is a highly desirable form of contraception for teenagers, it may be difficult for many adolescents to "just say no." Postponing sexual involvement requires effective communication and decision-making skills. Adolescents benefit from role-playing refusal skills and practice making decisions in a safe environment. Information about safe sex must be provided, and role-playing how to discuss condom use with a partner is very helpful to teenagers. Education concerning contraception should be provided in both oral and written form. All available methods, including their benefits, disadvantages, and side effects, should be discussed. Concrete, concise language must be used, demonstrations of how to use the contraceptive should be provided, and adolescents should repeat all instructions in their own words. If teenagers are using oral contraceptive pills (OCPs), they should be encouraged to use a daily activity as a reminder or cue to take the pill. A knowledgeable phone triage person should be available for questions and concerns. Parents or other important adults may be included in all discussions with the adolescent's permission.

SEXUALLY TRANSMITTED DISEASES

Sexually active adolescents are at increased risk for the acquisition of STDs. Physiologically, the adolescent girl's cervix has a large ectropion, which is composed of columnar epithelial cells that are much more susceptible to STDs, especially human papillomavirus (HPV) and chlamydia. The adolescent's immune system also contributes to the increased risk because the adolescent has not had an opportunity to develop resistance to these organisms (Neinstein, 2002). Behavioral factors contributing to increased risk include initiating sexual intercourse at an early age, high disease prevalence among sexual partners, and inconsistent use of barrier or other types of contraceptives. A listing of common sexually transmitted diseases is included in Table 17-3.

Human immunodeficiency virus (HIV) infections continue to rise among adolescents and women. Most HIV infections diagnosed among people in their twenties were acquired during adolescence (Centers for Disease Control and Prevention [CDC], 1996). Decreasing adolescent risk behavior for the acquisition of other STDs will help decrease the number of HIV infections among adolescents.

TABLE 17-2 ■ Advantages and Disadvantages of Contraceptive Methods in the Adolescent

METHOD	ADVANTAGES	DISADVANTAGES
Abstinence	100% effective in preventing sexually transmitted diseases (STDs) and pregnancy	Peer pressure to conform Relatively high failure rate from noncompliance
Withdrawal/coitus interruptus Withdrawal of penis before ejaculation	No medical visit necessary	High failure rate Some seminal fluid often released before ejaculation Ejaculate at vaginal orifice may enter vagina No STD protection
Calendar method Refrain from intercourse during fertile period (time of ovulation)	Teaches adolescent girls about their menstrual cycle Encourages couple participation	High failure rate Requires a regular, predictable menstrual cycle (irregular menses are common for first 2 years after menarche) No STD protection
Barrier methods Condom *Male:* Penile covering to trap sperm; spermicidal condoms increase effectiveness for pregnancy and STD prevention	Minimal side effects Easy to use Available without prescription Portability Provides protection against STDs	Requires consistent use Requires premeditated intent for sexual union May decrease sensation Misuse results in failure Small percentage of people have latex sensitivity/allergies Decreased spontaneity
Female: Inserted into vagina with base covering part of perineum; may be inserted 8 hours before intercourse	Female participation Made of polyurethane; no latex sensitivities	May be difficult to insert Coital dependent Noisy
Diaphragm Cervical covering to prevent sperm from reaching egg Must be used in conjunction with spermicidal jelly May be inserted 4-6 hours before intercourse If inserted early, should be checked for placement before coitus	Virgins can be fitted Low failure rate when used correctly Few contraindications May be reused	High failure rate in adolescents because of inconvenience of use Requires consistent use Requires fitting and instruction by medical personnel Requires premeditated intent for sexual union Requires body awareness and comfort with touching oneself for insertion Little STD protection May increase incidence of urinary tract infection
Lea's Shield Reusable vaginal contraceptive made of silicone; elliptical bowl placed in vagina up to 48 hours before sexual intercourse; removed 8 hours after intercourse	No latex allergies Reusable Very effective in nulliparous women Simple fitting	Less effective in women who have delivered a baby Requires prescription
Chemicals Spermicidal foam, jelly, cream, and suppositories Substance inserted into vagina to kill sperm	Available without prescription Inexpensive Easy to use No major health concerns	High failure rate unless combined with condom Possible for sperm to be ejaculated directly into uterine os, bypassing spermicide in vagina Must be used shortly before coitus; therefore requires interruption of sexual experience Repeated sexual union requires repeated application Requires premeditated intent for sexual union Messy Nonoxynol-9 associated with increased transmission of HIV to females
Oral contraceptives Estrogen and progesterone-like compounds Inhibit ovulation by blocking release of gonadotropins from anterior pituitary gland	99% effective if used correctly Exceedingly safe for adolescents Method of choice for most youngsters Administered by mouth Becomes a ritual not associated with sexual activity Regulates menses, decreases dysmenorrhea and acne, decreases menstrual flow Prevents ovarian and endometrial cancers Prevents functional ovarian cysts	Higher failure rate in adolescents than in older women Need to follow precise instructions; requires continued motivation, consistent use Requires prescription Price substantial for teenager No STD protection Possible side effects include headaches, missed or scanty periods, breakthrough bleeding Increased rates of chlamydia

TABLE 17-2 ■ Advantages and Disadvantages of Contraceptive Methods in the Adolescent—*cont'd*

METHOD	ADVANTAGES	DISADVANTAGES
Depo Provera Progestin that suppresses hormonal cycle and prevents ovulation Injection given every 3 months	No interruption of sex Invisible method	No STD protection Possible side effects include significant weight gain, decreased bone density, decreased high-density lipoproteins (HDLs), irregular menses or amenorrhea, decreased libido, depression Fertility may be delayed Must return to care provider every 3 months for injection
Lunelle **Medroxyprogesterone acetate plus estradiol cypionate** Monthly injectable; inhibits ovulation	99.9% effective if given on time each month Not associated with sexual activity Regular menstrual cycles Positive effects on lipids	Must come to health care provider monthly for injections Possible side effects include some weight gain, increase in acne, and mood changes
Ortho Evra Transdermal System 4.5-cm square patch with norelgestromin and ethinyl estradiol Hormonal patch applied to skin weekly for 3 weeks/month Suppresses ovulation, thickens cervical mucus and thins endometrium	88.2% effective in perfect users Simple to use Regular menstrual cycles Not associated with sexual activity Avoids first-pass metabolism, resulting in more constant levels	Not recommended for women >198 pounds Possible side effects include skin reaction at site, nausea, headache, dysmenorrhea, and breast tenderness Patch may be visible
Nuva Vaginal Ring **Etonogestrel plus ethinyl estradiol** Soft flexible transparent ring placed in vagina for 3 weeks Suppresses ovulation	99.3% effective Immediate return to ovulation at discontinuation May leave in place during sexual intercourse Avoids first-pass metabolism, resulting in more constant levels No spermicide needed No vaginal erosion No weight gain	Device may be felt by female or partner during sexual intercourse Device may fall out Possible side effects include headache, vaginitis, leukorrhea, nausea, and breakthrough bleeding May have late withdrawal bleeding requiring placement of ring during menses
Levonorgestrel Intrauterine System (Mirena) T-shape intrauterine device that releases 20 μg/d of levonorgestrel Inserted within 7 days of menses and remains in place for 5 years Thickens cervical mucus, inhibits sperm mobility and function	0.71 pregnancies/100 women years Effectively prevents fertilization, resulting in low rates of ectopic pregnancy Reduced length and quantity of menstrual bleeding Reduced dysmenorrhea No weight gain	Risk of perforation at time of insertion 2%-12% expulsion rate Not recommended in nulliparous women or women not in monogamous relationships Possible side effects include abdominal pain, headache, vaginal discharge, and breast pain
Emergency/postcoital contraception Progestin-only pill given within 72 hours *or* Combined estrogen-progestin pill containing ethinyl estradiol; given within 72 hours of unprotected sex and repeated 12 hours later Emergency contraception works in one of three ways: by suppressing or delaying ovulation, by preventing the meeting of sperm and egg, or by preventing implantation *or* Insertion of a copper-releasing intrauterine device (IUD) up to 7 days after unprotected intercourse	Useful in unplanned sexual intercourse or contraceptive failure May be given in advance for emergency use	No STD protection May cause nausea if combination method used Timing of next menstrual cycle may be changed

TABLE 17-3 ■ Selected Sexually Transmitted Diseases

MANIFESTATIONS	THERAPY	NURSING CONSIDERATIONS
GONORRHEA *(Neisseria gonorrhoeae)* **Male:** Urethritis—dysuria with profuse yellow discharge, frequency, urgency, nocturia—or pharyngitis **Female:** Cervicitis (postpubertal)—may be associated with discharge, dysuria, dyspareunia, vulvovaginitis (prepubertal), or pharyngitis	Single oral dose of ciprofloxacin followed by doxycycline for 7 days *or* Single-dose azithromycin if chlamydial infection is not ruled out *or* Single intramuscular dose of ceftriaxone	Instruct patient to abstain from sexual intercourse for 7 days after single-dose treatment Find and treat sexual contacts Educate young people regarding facts of the disease and its spread Encourage use of condoms in sexually active young people
CHLAMYDIA *(CHLAMYDIA TRACHOMATIS)* **Male:** Meatal erythema, tenderness, itching, dysuria, urethral discharge; or no symptoms **Female:** Mucopurulent cervical exudate with erythema, edema, congestion; or no symptoms	Azithromycin or doxycycline If pregnant: azithromycin	Same as above Rescreen women 3-4 months after treatment; repeat infection elevates risk for pelvic inflammatory disease (PID)
SYPHILIS *(Treponema pallidum)* Primary stage: Chancre—a hard, painless, red, sharply defined lesion with indurated base, raised border, eroded surface, and scanty yellow discharge; usually located on penis, vulva, or cervix Secondary stage: Systemic influenza-like symptoms and lymphadenopathy, rash; usually appears 1-3 weeks after healing of chancre	Penicillin	Viability of organism outside body is short Rapidly killed by oxygen, soap, common bacterial agents, and drying About 95% transmitted sexually; affected person most infectious during first year of disease May be transmitted to fetus Increased risk for HIV when open lesions are present
HERPES PROGENITALIS (Genital herpes simplex infection [HSV]) Small (usually painful) vesicles on genital area, buttocks, and thighs; itching usually initial symptom; when vesicles break, shallow, circular, extremely painful lesions remain	No known cure Acyclovir, famciclovir, or valacyclovir May need suppressive therapy for recurrences	Use of condoms to avoid spread or infection with other organisms Infection can be transmitted to infant during birth
TRICHOMONIASIS *(Trichomonas vaginalis)* Pruritus and edema of external genitalia; foul-smelling, greenish vaginal discharge; sometimes postcoital bleeding May be asymptomatic, especially in males	Oral metronidazole May be given in single dose	Patient should not consume alcohol while taking medication and for at least 48 hours following last dose Sexual partners should be treated
HUMAN PAPILLOMAVIRUS (HPV) Warts may be found on any part of male or female genitalia	Patient applied: Podofilox solution or imiquimod cream Provider applied: Podophyllin resin Freezing with liquid nitrogen Trichloroacetic acid Laser therapy or Intralesional interferon	An acceptable alternative is to forego treatment and await spontaneous resolution Treatments are usually painful; analgesics may be needed, and steroid cream may provide relief Male partners should inform female partner of need for Papanicolaou (Pap) testing
ACQUIRED IMMUNODEFICIENCY SYNDROME (HUMAN IMMUNODEFICIENCY VIRUS [HIV]) See Chapter 26	Numerous medications to delay progression of disease	See Chapter 26

Therapeutic Management

Effective treatment of both males and females with an STD involves administration of the appropriate therapeutic agent. Treatment of sexual partners is also an essential part of therapy. Adolescents need help to develop strategies to inform their partner and to abstain from sex until both have completed treatment.

A totally effective prophylaxis against infection is not yet available; therefore, preventive efforts must be directed toward finding and treating affected persons, locating and examining contacts of affected persons, educating young people regarding the facts of the disease and its spread, and encouraging the use of condoms in sexually active young people.

Nursing Considerations

Nursing responsibilities encompass all aspects of sexually transmissible disease education, confidentiality, prevention, and treatment. Part of the sex education of young people should include providing information about these diseases, including their symptoms and treatment, and dispelling the myths associated with their mode of transmission. Many vulnerable adolescents are uninformed or misinformed about STDs.

Primary prevention efforts, aimed at preventing STDs, include encouraging abstinence and postponing sexual involvement, encouraging condom use, and hepatitis B vaccination. Nurses play a role in secondary prevention by helping to identify early cases and referring adolescents for treatment. Nurses can also be involved in tertiary prevention by decreasing the medical and psychologic effects of STDs; conducting support groups for adolescents with HIV, herpes simplex virus (HSV), and HPV infections; and assisting pregnant adolescents in obtaining adequate prenatal screening and treatment of STDs.

PELVIC INFLAMMATORY DISEASE

Pelvic inflammatory disease (PID) is an infection of the upper female genital tract (endometrium and fallopian tubes), most commonly caused by STDs. Teenagers account for 16% to 20% of all cases of PID, which often result from untreated gonorrheal or chlamydial infections.

Presenting symptoms in the adolescent may be generalized, with fever, abdominal pain, urinary tract symptoms, and vague influenza-like manifestations, such as malaise, nausea, diarrhea, or constipation. A pelvic examination is indicated for every sexually active female who complains of lower abdominal pain to evaluate the possibility of PID.

PID is of major concern to nurses because of its devastating effects on the reproductive tract. Approximately 25% of females experiencing PID may have short-term complications, such as acute abscess formation in the fallopian tubes (tubo-ovarian abscess), or long-term complications, such as chronic pelvic pain, dyspareunia (painful coitus), or adhesion formation. Most significant, however, is the increased risk for ectopic pregnancy or infertility, which results from tubal scarring.

Prevention is the primary concern of health care professionals. Barrier contraceptive methods, such as condoms, seem to offer the best protection for preventing STDs and PID. Sexually active teenagers should be screened every 6 months to detect asymptomatic STDs, and treatment should be initiated to prevent PID and all associated complications. Reinfec-

BOX 17-2 ■ Definitions for Sexual Assaults

Sexual Assault: comprehensive term that includes various types of forced or inappropriate sexual activity. Sexual assault includes both physical and psychologic coercion as well as touch, penetration, and other sexual contact.

Rape: forced sexual intercourse that occurs by physical force or psychologic coercion. Rape includes vaginal, anal, or oral penetration by body parts or inanimate objects.

Acquaintance Rape (Date Rape): applied in those situations in which the assailant and victim know each other.

Statutory Rape: consensual sexual contact by a person 18 years of age or older with a person under the age of consent or unable to consent because of developmental disability. Age of consent varies by state.

tion with *Chlamydia* is associated with a higher incidence of PID. Females who have had a *Chlamydia* infection should be rescreened for *Chlamydia* 3 months after treatment.

SEXUAL ASSAULT

The adolescent age-group consistently has the highest rate of rape and other sexual assault when compared with any other age group. Female victims exceed males by a margin of 13.5 to 1. The majority of adolescent rapes and sexual assaults are perpetrated by either an acquaintance (older adolescents) or a relative (younger adolescents) (American Academy of Pediatrics, 2001). An understanding of the legal definitions of sexual assault, rape, acquaintance rape, and statutory rape is essential for the nurse to identify, treat, and manage adolescent victims (see Box 17-2).

Statutory rape laws have recently been revised in many states across the country. The motivation for tougher laws and greater enforcement is to decrease teen pregnancy, increase male responsibility, and decrease welfare dependency. Traditionally, statutory rape laws have been concerned with the protection of females. In the last 20 years, many laws have been rewritten to be gender neutral. However, prosecution of statutory rape remains more common when the victim is female. Statutory rape laws require reporting to child protective services or local law enforcement. One risk of strict statutory rape enforcement is that females may not seek health care for reproductive care, prenatal care, or domestic violence. Young people may not only fear for themselves, but also for their partner. There is also the threat and fear of repercussion from the older partner if the statutory rape is reported (Teare and English, 2002).

Nurses can obtain information about their state statutory rape reporting responsibilities from state or local child protective service agencies, legal counsel, rape crisis organizations, state or local law enforcement agencies, or the state nurses' association. The limits of confidentiality should be clearly reviewed with each adolescent patient before beginning the interview about sexual activity.

Diagnostic Evaluation

The rape victim may exhibit a variety of reactions (Box 17-3), and the circumstances of the initial medical evaluation may be frightening and stressful. The initial contact with the rape victim must be supportive because the interrogation and associated activities have the potential to add

BOX 17-3 ■ Clinical Manifestations of Rape Victims

MAY DISPLAY A VARIETY OF BEHAVIORS:
Hysterical crying
Giggling
Agitation
Feelings of degradation
Anger and rage
Helplessness
Nervousness
Rapid mood swings
Appear calm and controlled (masking inner turmoil)
Confused
Self-blame
Fear—of the rape and of injury

EVIDENCE OF PHYSICAL FORCE FROM:
Roughness
Nonbrutal beating (slapping)
Brutal beating (slugging, kicking, beating repeatedly with fists)
Choking or gagging

MEDICAL EXAMINATION PROVIDES EVIDENCE OF:
Penetration
Ejaculation
Use of force

to the trauma of the sexual assault. First of all, the victim needs to know that she (or he) is (1) all right and (2) not being blamed for the situation.

It is important to obtain a clear account of the circumstances of an alleged rape without forcing the victim to relive a very painful experience. Information includes date, time, location, and an accurate description of any type of sexual contact. The physical examination is carried out as soon as possible, because physical evidence deteriorates rapidly. The victim should not bathe or shower before the examination.

！NURSING ALERT

It is not uncommon for rape victims to delay seeking help, especially in cases of acquaintance or date rape. Nurses can be most supportive by acknowledging the painful and sometimes confusing feelings that surround such experiences and by focusing on the fact that the victim is seeking assistance now.

The young person is always told in advance in understandable terms exactly what to expect in the way of tests and procedures, and the explanation is accompanied by strong emotional support. The victim is examined thoroughly, including nongenital areas, for evidence of injury that might substantiate the use of force.

The forensic examination of a sexual assault victim must follow strict legal requirements. The medical record may provide key evidence for the legal case. Evaluation for sexually transmitted diseases is an important part of the evaluation. All potential infection sites are tested to detect gonorrhea, chlamydia and trichomoniasis. Blood samples for syphilis, hepatitis B virus (HBV), and human immunodeficiency virus (HIV) are obtained as a baseline. Syphilis and HBV tests are repeated in 6 weeks, and the HIV test is repeated in 3 to 6 months.

Prophylactic treatment for *Chlamydia* and gonorrhea is recommended. Female victims should be provided with emergency contraception. The recommendation for HIV prophylaxis varies depending on the geographic area, the circumstances of the assault, and the known HIV status of the perpetrator. The CDC (2002b) maintains updates and recommendations for treatment.

Therapeutic Management

Adolescents who have been raped arrive at the emergency department or practitioner's office under a variety of circumstances. They are usually brought by parents, friends, or police officers, but some may seek medical help on their own. It is advisable to obtain parental consent for examination, but the examination may be performed without parental consent if the adolescent is mature and the parents are unavailable. A female observer should be present during the history and examination of female victims who are examined by a male practitioner. Whether a parent should be present during the examination is determined on an individual basis. The parent's presence is usually encouraged if the parent is supportive and the young person agrees.

Rape Trauma Syndrome

The term *rape trauma syndrome* refers to the victim's reaction to a sexual assault. The syndrome involves two phases: (1) the acute phase of disorganization of lifestyle and (2) a long-term process of reorganization. These phases encompass behavioral, somatic, and psychologic reactions to the stressful event. Counseling should begin immediately upon the adolescent's entrance into the emergency room with follow-up within the first 24 hours. Early intervention has been shown to be effective in decreasing the extent of rape trauma syndrome (Patel and Minshall, 2001).

Nursing Considerations

Many of the approaches that have been described for the sexually abused child (see Chapter 14) apply to the adolescent. Sexual assault is a devastating experience with long-lasting effects. The primary goal of nursing care is to avoid inflicting further stress on the youngster, who is often angry, confused, frightened, embarrassed, and filled with self-blame. The nurse must do everything possible to reduce the stress of the interrogation and examination. Although most health professionals and law enforcement officers are sensitive to the needs of the youngster and attempt to make the process as nonstressful as possible, the nurse should be alert to cues that indicate the victim is being overstressed.

Follow-up care of the rape victim is essential and extends over a long period. Aside from the universal need for emotional support, the needs of rape victims vary widely and depend on the nature of the incident, when it took place, the physical and emotional injuries sustained by the victim, the legal actions being considered as a result, the resources available for informal support, and the anticipated reactions of persons in the informal support network (see Family Focus box).*

---

*For information about local organizations contact the **National Organization for Victim Assistance,** 1730 Park Road, NW, Washington, DC 20010; (800) TRY-NOVA or (202) 232-6682; website: www.try-nova.org.

FAMILY FOCUS

Supporting the Rape Victim's Parents

In addition to the needs of the adolescent rape victim, the nurse is also sensitive to the needs and reactions of the youngster's parents. Some will be angry and blame the adolescent; others will feel guilty and embarrassed. Many reactions can be expected at the time of the incident, ranging from despair to extreme agitation. Frequently the parents require as much support and reassurance as the victim. Agitated, angry, or incapacitated parents are unable to provide support for their youngster.

Meeting their needs can facilitate their ability to support the teenager during the crisis.

EATING DISORDERS

OBESITY

Few problems in childhood and adolescence are so obvious to others, so difficult to treat, and have such long-term effects on health as obesity. Several different definitions exist for obesity and overweight. *Obesity* is currently defined as an excessively high amount of body fat or adipose tissue in relation to lean body mass (CDC, 2002a). *Overweight* refers to the state of increased body weight in relation to height. Authorities recommend that the body mass index (BMI) measurement be used to screen for childhood obesity. The BMI measurement is strongly associated with subcutaneous and total body fat and also with skinfold thickness measurements. The CDC has standards available for tracking children's body mass index from 2 to 20 years of age (Lindeke, Rogers, and Finley, 2002).* Children with a BMI between the 85th and 95th percentiles are considered overweight, and obesity is defined by a BMI greater than the 95th percentile (Moran, 2003) .

Regardless of the definition used, the number of overweight children in the United States is increasing and may be approaching epidemic status (Shulman, 2004). In the 1999-2000 National Health and Nutrition Examination Survey, data indicated that 15% of children and teens between 6 and 19 years were overweight (Binns and Ariza, 2004; Ogden and others, 2002). The prevalence of childhood obesity in the United States is estimated to be 25% to 30% (Moran, 1999). Although obesity occurs across gender, racial, ethnic, and socioeconomic lines, obesity rates are higher among low-income youths and among African American, Hispanic, and Native American population groups. Increases in the number of overweight children and adolescents pose serious problems for society. Obesity is associated with numerous physical complications including type 2 diabetes mellitus, coronary artery disease, pulmonary dysfunction, arthritis, ischemic stroke, and some forms of cancer (Binns and Ariza, 2004; National Task Force on Prevention and Treatment of Obesity, 2000). Obesity is also a serious handicap to the social well-being of children and adolescents. Common emotional consequences of obesity include poor body image, low self-esteem, social isolation, and feelings of depression and rejection.

*Centers for Disease Control and Prevention growth charts, as well as instruction for nurses on accurate measurement and interpretation of children's growth, can be found at www.cdc.gov/growthcharts.

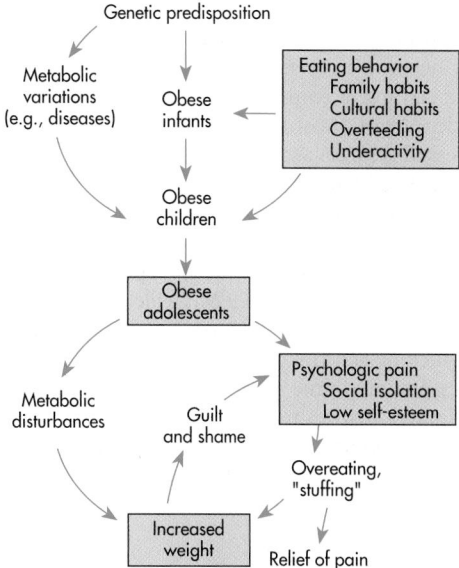

FIG. 17-2 ■ Complex relationships in obesity.

Etiology/Pathophysiology

Obesity in childhood and adolescence occurs as the result of several interrelated influences such as hypothalamic, hereditary, metabolic, social, cultural, and psychologic factors (Fig. 17-2). The complex interrelationships between hunger, satiety, the central nervous system, and metabolism continue to be investigated. Underlying diseases such as hypothyroidism, adrenal hypercorticoidism, hyperinsulinism, or dysfunction of the central nervous system are responsible for only a small number of cases of childhood obesity. Heredity is an important factor in the development of obesity. Identical twins reared apart tend to resemble their natural parents to a greater extent than they do their adoptive parents. However, it is impossible to distinguish between hereditary and environmental factors, because both may be operating in any situation when other family members are obese.

Investigators have proposed the following theories to explain the development of obesity:

Adipose cell theory. Obese children have larger adipose tissue cells that stay the same size once they reach a maximum, and their fat cells appear to increase in number during childhood.

Set point theory. Individuals have a programmed level or set point for body weight that remains relatively stable during adulthood. With increased caloric intake the metabolic rate increases to burn the excess; when intake is reduced, metabolism decreases to conserve energy.

Sociocultural factors also play a role in weight gain. Patterns of eating are learned in the culture, and the food preferences of the culture may contribute to the development of obesity. Many mothers consider plumpness a sign of health, view obesity as evidence of well-being, and foster weight gain as a desirable feature (Baughcum and others, 2000).

Psychologic factors may influence weight. In infancy, children experience relief from discomfort through feeding, and learn to associate eating with feelings of security and the comforting presence of the nurturing person. Eating is often associated with the feeling of being loved. Many parents use food as a positive reinforcer for desired behavior. This practice may become a habit, and the child may continue to use food as a reward, a comfort, and a means to deal with feelings of depression, hostility, boredom, or loneliness.

Decreased physical activity is clearly related to body fatness and an increased risk of obesity. Our society has changed to include more sedentary lifestyles. Children between 6 and 11 years of age spend an average of 26 hours per week watching television. This is as much time as they spend attending school (Dennison and Boyer, 2004; McArdle, Katch, and Katch, 2000). Other factors that lead to a sedentary lifestyle among children include apartment living, unsafe neighborhood environments, a limited time spent with parents in recreational activities, limited finances to participate in recreational activities, and limited opportunities to participate in extracurricular events that involve physical activity (McWhorter, Wallmann, and Alpert, 2003).

Diagnostic Evaluation

Many methods to determine weight status, such as magnetic resonance imaging, bioelectrical impedance, and underwater weighing, are very accurate, but expensive and invasive. Currently, clinicians rely on skinfold thickness (SFT), body fat distribution, and weight-height indices, especially the BMI, to assess weight. The BMI measurement expresses the relationship between height and weight (e.g., kilograms divided by meters squared [kg/m²]). BMI is easily calculated using growth charts available from the CDC. These charts are considered more accurate than the older weight-for-stature charts. Appropriate diagnostic tests should also be performed to rule out metabolic or endocrine disorders that can cause obesity.

Nursing Considerations

Assessment

Obtaining an accurate measurement of the child or adolescent's height and weight is an essential part of assessment. These measurements are necessary to calculate the BMI measurement. Children with a BMI greater than or equal to the 95th percentile for age and sex should receive an in-depth medical assessment. Children with a BMI in the 85th to 95th percentile range should be evaluated for secondary complications such as hypertension and hyperlipidemia. Evaluation should also include the height and weight history of the parents and siblings, as well as an assessment of eating habits, appetite and hunger patterns, and physical activities of the child. A psychosocial history is also important to determine the impact that the child's weight has on his or her quality of life.

Nursing Diagnoses

After a thorough assessment of the child or adolescent, several nursing diagnoses become apparent. The prominent diagnoses are outlined in Box 17-4.

Planning

The goals of a weight loss program include:

1 Child will follow a diet that provides loss of body weight without interfering with growth, normal activity, or psychologic well-being.
2 Child will engage in a regular exercise program.

BOX 17-4 ■ Nursing Diagnoses: The Child Who Is Obese

Activity intolerance
Activity intolerance, Risk for
Coping, Ineffective
Family processes, Interrupted
Nutrition: more than body requirements, Imbalanced
Nutrition: more than body requirements, Risk for imbalanced
Self-esteem, Chronic low
Self-esteem, Situational low
Self-esteem, Risk for situational low

---

3 Child will modify eating behavior.
4 Child and family will receive psychologic support.

Implementation

Motivation to lose weight is the key to success. Success is rarely achieved unless youngsters are motivated to lose weight and take some personal responsibility for their dietary habits and exercise program. Children who are forced by parents to seek help are seldom motivated and often become rebellious and unwilling to control dietary intake. An approach that focuses on healthy eating habits and enjoyable exercise for all members of the family is more likely to be successful.

Diet. The ideal diet for children and adolescents should meet the criteria outlined in Box 17-5. Because obesity is often a lifelong problem, it is important to provide children, adolescents, and their families with a diet that fosters healthier eating habits. Increasing dietary fiber and complex carbohydrates, modifying fat intake, and encouraging eating only in response to physical hunger cues are essential components of any diet. Recently, low-carbohydrate diets such as the "Atkins Diet" have been promoted for weight loss in adults and adolescents (Sondike and others, 2003). However, low-carbohydrate diets can result in ketosis, insulin resistance, and glucose intolerance. More research is needed to evaluate the long-term safety and efficacy of these diets for children and adolescents (Ariza, Greenberg, and Unger, 2004; Daniels, 2003). A healthy diet should include high-nutrient foods such as fruits, vegetables, whole grains, and low-fat dairy and protein products. Calories and fats should be kept to a healthy level, and extremes should be avoided. Children and adolescents should not become so food conscious that they believe fats and calories are bad and that they must avoid both high-calorie and high-fat foods. Diets that contain ordinary foods in controlled portions (not adult-sized portions) rather than those that avoid specific foods are most successful. Children and adolescents need advice on how to include their favorite foods in small amounts and how to select satisfying substitutes for favorite foods. Knowing the caloric values for a wide variety of foods and snacks and how to read food labels is helpful to children, adolescents, and family members. Snacking is an important part of the daily routine for children and adolescents. Vending machines at schools are often stocked with high-calorie, low-nutrient snacks that are easily accessible to children who have pocket money. Parents, nutritionists, and

BOX 17-5 ■ Essentials of an Ideal Weight-Management Program

Weight maintenance or steady, slow weight loss
Nutrient, energy, and growth needs met
Feelings of hunger avoided
Preservation of lean body mass
Increased physical activity
Absence of metabolic complications
Absence of psychiatric reactions

school nurses need to lobby for "treats" such as fruits, juices, and raw vegetables in school cafeterias and vending machines. Fast-food establishments, which are often located near schools, continue to present problems for children and adolescents who are attempting to lose weight.*

Children and adolescents should not initiate a reduction diet without health assessment and counseling (Schwimmer, 2004). Significant caloric restriction for children and adolescents who are still growing is usually not recommended. Restriction diets can cause delayed or stunted growth and are often ineffective for long periods of time. The potential dangers of exotic fad diets and crash dietary programs for growing children and adolescents should be emphasized. Successful dietary programs are those that are nutritionally sound, have sufficient satiety value, produce the desired weight loss, and involve nutrition education and social support.

Exercise.   Physical activity is necessary to bring about weight loss, to maintain weight loss, and to redistribute body fat into muscle. Regular physical activity or exercise progressively increased over the child or adolescent's usual activity is an integral part of a weight-reduction program. Initial goals for activity should be small and reasonable so the child does not fell overwhelmed. Physical activities should be those that stress self-improvement rather than competition. All children and teens need continued psychologic support and encouragement to participate in physical activities and exercise.

Behavioral Therapy.   The most successful method for treating obesity is diet and exercise combined with behavior modification, which emphasizes identification and elimination of inappropriate eating habits and problem-solving strategies to use in situations that encourage overeating. Self-monitoring is used to increase awareness of eating behavior, and attention is focused on the social and behavioral aspects surrounding food consumption. Children are encouraged to maintain an activity log, and parents are encouraged to prohibit eating in front of the television, to limit trips to fast-food restaurants, and to omit using food for comfort or as rewards.

Group Involvement.   Commercial groups or diet workshops composed primarily of adults may be helpful to some teenagers; however, a group composed of individuals their

own age is more effective for children and adolescents. Groups for youngsters who are obese include summer camps designed and conducted by health professionals, school groups organized and led by the school nurse, and groups associated with special clinics. These groups should focus on weight loss as well as the development of positive self-image. Nutrition education, diet planning, and discussions centered around improvement of social skills are essential components of these groups.

Medical Therapies.   There are currently no weight-loss medications approved by the Food and Drug Administration for use in the pediatric population (Moran, 2003). Appetite-suppressant drugs are no more effective than diet and exercise in maintaining weight loss, and the use of these drugs may become habit-forming. Surgical techniques that bypass a substantial portion of the intestine or occlude a large segment of the stomach to produce diet restriction and weight loss are not well studied and should be considered only in extreme circumstances when medical complications have developed.

Prevention.   Weight loss programs do not enjoy the success of therapeutic interventions for other disorders. Prevention of obesity should begin in early childhood with the development of healthy eating habits, regular exercise patterns, and a positive relationship between parents and children. Health care professionals should encourage frequent health visits for children who are overweight or obese and incorporate a dietary history and counseling into each health encounter.

● Evaluation

The effectiveness of nursing interventions is determined by continual reassessment based on the following observational guidelines and expected outcomes:

1 Assess weight at regular intervals (usually weekly); discuss the child or adolescent's feelings, reactions, and concerns; analyze daily logs of activities (eating, behavior, exercise).
2 Review exercise program with child or teenager.
3 Interview child or adolescent about the plan of care and progress toward short-term and long-term goals.

● Expected Outcomes

1 Eating patterns lead to weight loss; child or adolescent expresses feelings and concerns regarding problems.
2 Child or adolescent engages in preferred exercise and activities regularly.
3 Child or adolescent demonstrates an understanding of eating patterns.
4 Child or adolescent demonstrates steady weight loss (or weight maintenance in a growing child).

ANOREXIA NERVOSA

Anorexia nervosa (AN) is an eating disorder characterized by a refusal to maintain a minimally normal body weight and by severe weight loss in the absence of obvious physical causes. Approximately 5% of adolescent females in the United States have AN, and 5% to 10% of all cases occur in males (American Academy of Pediatrics, 2003). The average age of onset is 13 years, but the disorder can occur as early as 10 years of

---

*Information on the nutrient value of name-brand foods, including menu items from fast-food restaurants, is available from the **Nutrition Coordinating Center**, 1300 South Second Street, Suite 300, Minneapolis, MN 55414; (612) 626-9450; e-mail: nccservicecenter@epi.umn.ed; website: www.ncc.umn.edu.

age and as late as 25 years of age. Individuals with AN are described as perfectionists, academically high achievers, conforming, and conscientious. Typically, they have high energy levels, even with marked emaciation.

Etiology/Pathophysiology

The etiology of the disorder remains unclear. There is a distinct psychologic component, and the diagnosis is based primarily on psychologic and behavioral criteria. The dominant aspects of anorexia nervosa are a relentless pursuit of thinness and a fear of fatness, usually preceded by a period of mood disturbances and behavior changes. Weight loss may be triggered by a typical adolescent crisis such as the onset of menstruation or a traumatic interpersonal incident that precipitates serious, out-of-control dieting. Situations of severe family stress (such as parental separation or divorce) or circumstances in which the youngster perceives a lack of personal control (such as teasing at school, changing schools, or going to college) may precipitate a desire for control and the decision not to eat. Frequently, there is an exaggerated misinterpretation of the normal fat deposition characteristic of early adolescence, or anxiety because of comments that the adolescent is putting on weight. Society's emphasis and the media's focus on tall, thin individuals may also play a role. Another factor in some cases is childhood sexual abuse.

Diagnostic Evaluation

Diagnosis is made on the basis of clinical manifestations (Box 17-6) and conformity to the criteria established by the American Psychiatric Association (2000) (Box 17-7).

Therapeutic Management

Treatment involves three major thrusts: (1) reinstitution of normal nutrition or reversal of malnutrition, (2) resolution of disturbed patterns of family interaction, and (3) individual psychotherapy to correct deficits and distortions in psychologic functioning. Most adolescents are treated on an outpatient basis, but those with severe malnutrition or electrolyte, or psychiatric disturbances (severe depression or suicidal ideation) require hospitalization. An interdisciplinary team of dietitians, physicians, nurses, and counselors deliver the interventions.

Nutrition. The most important goal is to treat any life-threatening malnutrition and to restore dietary stability and weight gain. This may require the administration of tube feed-ings or intravenous fluids if the malnutrition is severe. In most cases, it is best to reintroduce food and snacks slowly in a stepwise manner. A reasonable goal is to reach an eventual intake of 2000 to 3000 kcal per day and a weight gain of 0.5 to 2 pounds per week (American Academy of Pediatrics, 2003). When restoring nutrition, health professionals must avoid the refeeding syndrome, which consists of cardiovascular, neurologic, and hematologic complications that occur when nutritional replacement is given too rapidly. This syndrome can be avoided with slow refeeding and the addition of phosphorus when total body phosphorus is depleted. Treatment goal weights are individualized and based on age, height, stage of puberty, premorbid weight, and previous growth charts. In girls who have reached menarche, resumption of menses is an objective measure of return to biologic health.

Dietary interventions are combined with psychotherapy to improve the underlying psychologic misconceptions about weight loss. Another aspect of treatment is to relieve the anxiety related to eating and the depression that accompanies the disorder. The administration of antianxiety or antidepressant medications is beneficial. However, when these drugs are used, patients should be carefully monitored for cardiovascular side effects.

Psychotherapy. Behavioral interventions are often necessary to encourage patients to accomplish the desired caloric intake and weight gain. Mental health interventions are essential. The ultimate goal is to have children and adolescents become more realistic in their self-appraisal and capable of living as competent individuals without manipulating their body and its functions. Individual psychotherapy is aimed at helping the young person resolve the adolescent

---

BOX 17-6 ■ Clinical Manifestations of Anorexia Nervosa

Severe and profound weight loss
Signs of altered metabolic activity:
Secondary amenorrhea (if menarche attained)
Primary amenorrhea (if menarche not attained)
Bradycardia
Lowered body temperature
Decreased blood pressure
Cold intolerance
Dry skin and brittle nails
Appearance of lanugo hair

BOX 17-7 ■ Diagnostic Criteria for Anorexia Nervosa

1. Refusal to maintain body weight over a minimal normal weight for age and height (e.g., weight loss leading to maintenance of body weight less than 85% of that expected; or failure to make expected weight gain during period of growth, leading to body weight less than 85% of that expected)
2. Intense fear of gaining weight or becoming fat, even though underweight
3. Disturbance of body image, undue influence of shape or weight on evaluation, or denial of the seriousness of the current low body weight
4. In postmenarchal females, amenorrhea (i.e., the absence of at least three consecutive menstrual cycles); a woman is considered to have amenorrhea if her periods occur only after hormone (e.g., estrogen) administration

Specify type:
Restricting type—no regular bingeing or purging behavior (i.e., self-induced vomiting or the misuse of laxatives, diuretics, or enemas).
Binge eating/purging type—during the current episode of anorexia nervosa, the person has regularly engaged in binge eating or purging behavior (i.e., self-induced vomiting or the misuse of laxatives, diuretics, or enemas).

From American Psychiatric Association: *Diagnostic and statistical manual of mental disorders,* ed 4 *(DSM-IV TR),* Washington, DC, 2000, The Association.

identity crisis, particularly as it relates to a distorted body image. If the disorder is related to a dysfunctional family situation, therapy is most successful when it is started soon after the onset of illness and directed toward disengagement and redirection of malfunctioning processes in the family.

Nursing Considerations

The psychogenic nature of AN makes treatment difficult and lengthy. Only about 25% of affected individuals attain full recovery; 50% improve, but may relapse during times of stress, and 25% do poorly despite adequate treatment (Schneider and Fisher, 2001).

Nurses who care for children or teens with AN should maintain a kind, supportive, yet firm manner. The child or adolescent requires sustained support and reassurance to cope with ambivalent feelings related to the body concept. Assistance is also needed to help teens view themselves as cooperative and reliable individuals worthy of receiving kindness. Encouraging education and activities that foster self-esteem facilitates the resocialization process and promotes social acceptance among peers.

It is important for nurses to be aware of the physical side effects of AN. Patients frequently limit their fluid intake. Urinary tract problems are common, and ketones and protein may be detected in the urine as a result of breakdown of fat and protein. Vital sign instability can be severe and can include orthostatic hypotension; the pulse becomes irregular, and the rate decreases markedly. Bradycardia and hypothermia can result in cardiac arrest (see Critical Thinking Exercise).

Health professionals, patients, and families can find assistance and information from several organizations. The **National Eating Disorders Organization*** provides information and support services for patients and families. The **National Association of Anorexia Nervosa and Associated Disorders, Inc. (ANAD)†** and the **American Anorexia/ Bulimia Association, Inc. (AABA),‡** provide counseling, referrals, and self-help programs.

BULIMIA

Bulimia is an eating disorder characterized by repeated episodes of binge eating. The binge behavior consists of secretive, frenzied consumption of large amounts of high-calorie (or "forbidden") foods during a brief period (usually less than 2 hours). The binge is counteracted by a variety of weight control methods (purging), including self-induced vomiting, diuretic and laxative abuse, and rigorous exercise. The frequency of bingeing can be anywhere from once per week to seven or eight times a day. Self-deprecating thoughts, a depressed mood, and awareness that the eating pattern is abnormal follow these binge/purge cycles.

The disorder is observed more frequently in older adolescent girls and young women. Affected individuals have been unsuccessful dieters, have low impulse control, and may have been self-conscious about being overweight in childhood.

---

*603 Stewart Street, Suite 803, Seattle, WA 98101; website: www. nationaleatingdisorders.org.
†PO Box 7, Highland Park, IL 60035; (847) 831-3438; e-mail: anad20.aol.com; website: www.anad.org.
‡410 East 76th Street, New York, NY 10021; (212) 734-1114; website: www.aabainc.org.

??? CRITICAL THINKING EXERCISE ???

Anorexia Nervosa

Jane is a 13-year-old whose grades have been excellent and whom the teachers describe as a "model student." Recently, Jane's teacher told the nurse practitioner that Jane's parents were in the middle of a "messy divorce." In addition, several of Jane's friends told the nurse practitioner that they are concerned about Jane because she "jogs" every day at lunchtime and seldom eats lunch with them. Jane told her friends that she gained weight over the winter months and that she is "jogging" because she wants to qualify for the track team this spring. At the time of her routine health interview and sports physical, the nurse practitioner notes that Jane's oral temperature is 96.8° F and that she weighs 34 kg. Jane has lost 9 kg since her last sports physical. When discussing her menstrual periods with the nurse practitioner, Jane states that she has not had her period for 3 months.

QUESTIONS

1. Evidence—Is there sufficient evidence to draw any conclusions about Jane's behavior?
2. Assumptions—Describe some underlying assumptions about the following:
   a. Personality characteristics of individuals with anorexia nervosa
   b. Factors influencing the development of anorexia nervosa
   c. Clinical manifestations of anorexia nervosa
   d. Treatment of anorexia nervosa
3. What implications for nursing care should be established for Jane at this time?
4. Does the evidence support your conclusion?
5. Are there alternative perspectives that you should consider?

ANSWERS

1. Using the clinical manifestations of anorexia nervosa (see Box 17-6) and the diagnostic criteria for anorexia nervosa (see Box 17-7), there is sufficient evidence to support the conclusion that Jane has anorexia nervosa.
2. a. Young adolescent females with anorexia nervosa are often high achievers or excellent students. They have an abundance of energy, a distorted body image, and a fear of gaining weight.
   b. A family crisis can influence anorexia nervosa. Jane's parents are currently in the middle of a divorce, and, in this type of situation, some teens feel they have no control over events in their life. Consequently, some adolescents take control by refusing to eat and developing anorexia nervosa.
   c. Jane is engaging in increased physical activity and is skipping lunch several days each week. On physical examination, she has a decreased body temperature (96.8° F), and she has lost 9 kg (or 18 pounds) in the past year (she is at less than 85% of her expected weight). She also told the nurse practitioner that she has not had her menstrual period for 3 months. These manifestations are all congruent with anorexia nervosa.
   d. Anorexia nervosa is treated by a team of health professionals who address the abnormal eating patterns as well as the altered body image of the individual with anorexia nervosa and the dysfunctional family dynamics that accompany this disorder.
3. Jane should be referred to a specialist who deals with adolescents with anorexia nervosa
4. Yes, the evidence supports the conclusion.
5. Because Jane has not had her menstrual period for 3 months, there is a possibility that Jane is pregnant. The nurse practitioner should obtain a pregnancy test to rule out the possibility of pregnancy.

They fall into two categories: (1) those who purge and (2) those who do not purge. Some women are of normal weight or (more often) slightly above normal weight. Other individuals with bulimia restrict their intake and become severely underweight. This type of bulimia is called *bulimorexia*.

Diagnostic Evaluation

The diagnosis may be first suspected from the presence of complications, including fluid and electrolyte disturbances from gastrointestinal losses, abdominal complaints from laxative abuse, erosion of tooth enamel and increased dental caries from vomited gastric acid, and throat complaints. The diagnosis is established on the basis of criteria established by the American Psychiatric Association (2000) (Box 17-8).

Therapeutic Management

Therapy is similar to management of AN. Hospitalization may be required for complications such as potassium depletion and esophageal damage. Intravenous fluids, potassium replacement, and cardiac monitoring are essential elements of care. Nutritional consultation and follow-up are essential. Behavior therapy may also be used.

Nursing Considerations

Nursing care is similar to the care of the patient with AN; acute care involves careful monitoring of fluid and electrolyte alterations and observation for signs of cardiac complications. The nurse may need to help the adolescent and family to structure the environment to reduce the bingeing

---

BOX 17-8 ■ Diagnostic Criteria for Bulimia

1. Recurrent episodes of binge eating. An episode of binge eating is characterized by both of the following:
   Eating, in a discrete period (e.g., within any 2-hour period), an amount of food that is definitely larger than most people would eat during a similar period and under similar circumstances
   A sense of lack of control over eating during the episode (e.g., a feeling that one cannot stop eating or control what or how much one is eating)
2. Recurrent inappropriate compensatory behavior to prevent weight gain, such as self-induced vomiting; misuse of laxatives, diuretics, enemas, or other medications; fasting; or excessive exercise
3. The binge eating and inappropriate compensatory behaviors both occur, on average, at least twice a week for 3 months
4. Self-evaluation is unduly influenced by body shape and weight
5. The disturbance does not occur exclusively during episodes of anorexia nervosa

Specify type:
Purging type: During the current episode of bulimia nervosa, the person has regularly engaged in self-induced vomiting or the misuse of laxatives, diuretics, or enemas.
Nonpurging type: During the current episode of bulimia nervosa, the person has used other inappropriate compensatory behaviors, such as fasting or excessive exercise, but has not regularly engaged in self-induced vomiting or the misuse of laxatives, diuretics, or enemas.

From American Psychiatric Association: *Diagnostic and statistical manual of mental disorders*, ed 4 *(DSM-IV TR)*, Washington, DC, 2000, The Association.

---

behavior. Relaxation techniques and telephone support networks are also helpful interventions for bingeing behavior.

DISORDERS WITH BEHAVIORAL COMPONENTS

ATTENTION DEFICIT HYPERACTIVITY DISORDER AND LEARNING DISABILITY

Attention deficit hyperactivity disorder (ADHD) refers to developmentally inappropriate degrees of inattention, impulsiveness, and hyperactivity. To be diagnosed as ADHD, the symptoms must have been present before age 7 years and must be present in at least two settings. In addition, the persistence of developmentally inappropriate and marked inattention must not be a symptom of another disorder (American Psychiatric Association, 2000). A *learning disability (LD)* refers to a heterogeneous group of disorders manifested by significant difficulties in the acquisition and use of listening, speaking, reading, writing, reasoning, or mathematical skills.

ADHD and LDs affect every aspect of the child's life but are most obvious in the classroom. Early identification of affected children is important because the characteristics of these disorders significantly interfere with the normal course of emotional and psychologic development. Many children develop maladaptive behavior patterns that impede psychosocial adjustment while they try to cope with cognitive dysfunction. Their behavior evokes negative responses from others, and repeated exposure to negative feedback adversely affects their self-concept. The characteristics of ADHD impact the child's written and adaptive skills, social status, and self-esteem (Myers, Eisenhauer, and Ryan, 2003).

Diagnostic Evaluation

The behaviors exhibited by the child with ADHD are not unusual aspects of behavior. The difference lies in the quality of motor activity and developmentally inappropriate inattention, impulsivity, and hyperactivity that the child displays. The manifestations may be numerous or few, mild or severe, and will vary with the developmental level of the child. Any given child will not have every symptom of the condition. The basic characteristics of ADHD are outlined in Box 17-9.

A comprehensive battery of tests is needed to confirm a learning disability. These include intelligence tests (many children have normal or above-average IQs), hand-eye coordination tests, and measurements of auditory and visual perception, comprehension, and memory. Often there is a wide gap between verbal and performance scores on IQ tests.

Therapeutic Management

Management of the child with ADHD usually involves multiple approaches that include family education and counseling, medication, proper classroom placement, environmental manipulation, and sometimes behavioral or psychotherapy for the child. Interventions for children with LD are primarily educational.

Medication. Stimulant medications or behavioral therapy are appropriate for the school-age child with ADHD (Clinical Practice Guideline, 2001). The most frequently prescribed medications are the psychostimulants, methylphenidate hydrochloride (Ritalin), and dextroamphetamine sulfate (Dexedrine). These medications increase dopamine and norepinephrine levels that lead to simulation of the inhibitory system of the central nervous system. Tricyclic antidepressants, bupropion, and alpha-2 agonists (clonidine and guanfacine) are second-line medications.

Recently, atomoxetine, a presynaptic norepinephrine transport inhibitor, became available for use in children (Aschenbrenner, 2003; Michelson and others, 2001). Regularly scheduled evaluations of the child are essential with all of these medications. Children taking stimulant medication may have side effects that include nervousness, insomnia, increased blood pressure, and decreased appetite with subsequent weight loss (see Critical Thinking Exercise). Long-term use of dextroamphetamine may result in suppression of growth

Environmental Manipulation.   In ADHD the child's environment is simplified by decreasing external stimuli and distractions, reducing alternatives, increasing consistency in routines, and encouraging desired patterns of behavior. Parents need help to develop firm but reasonable limits and to provide a stable and predictable environment with regular routines of sleeping, eating, working, and playing.

Classroom Education.   Special activities are designed to address learning deficits that involve visual perception, auditory perception, and other areas involving integration and coordination. The purpose of programs for children with learning disabilities is to assist them to move toward more successful achievement and personal adjustment in the regular classroom. According to Public Law 94-142, the Education for All Handicapped Children's Act, children with ADHD or LDs must receive free public education in the least restrictive environment (see Chapters 1 and 18).

Prognosis.   ADHD is relatively stable through early adolescence for most children. Some children experience decreased symptoms during late adolescence and adulthood, but a significant number of these children carry their symptoms into adulthood. The goal for children with LDs is to help them identify their areas of weakness and learn to compensate for them.

Nursing Considerations

Nurses are active participants in all aspects of management of the child with ADHD or LD. Nurses in the community work with families and school personnel on a long-term basis to help plan and implement therapeutic regimens and to evaluate the effectiveness of therapy. They should teach parents and children to take stimulant medication in the morning to maximize its effectiveness in the classroom and to decrease its insomnia-producing potential. If decreased appetite is a concern, giving the psychostimulant with or after meals rather

---

BOX 17-9 ■ Diagnostic Criteria for Attention Deficit Hyperactivity Disorder

A. Either (1) or (2):
  (1) Six (or more) of the following symptoms of ***inattention*** have persisted for at least 6 months to a degree that is maladaptive and inconsistent with developmental level:
  Inattention
  (a) Often fails to give close attention to details or makes mistakes in schoolwork, work, or other activities
  (b) Often has difficulty sustaining attention in tasks or play activities
  (c) Often does not seem to listen when spoken to directly
  (d) Often does not follow through on instructions and fails to finish schoolwork, chores, or duties in the workplace (not because of oppositional behavior or failure to understand instructions)
  (e) Often has difficulty organizing tasks and activities
  (f) Often avoids, dislikes, or is reluctant to engage in tasks that require sustained mental effort (such as schoolwork or homework)
  (g) Often loses things necessary for tasks or activities (e.g., toys, school assignments, pencils, books, tools)
  (h) Is often easily distracted by extraneous stimuli
  (i) Is often forgetful in daily activities
  (2) Six (or more) of the following symptoms of ***hyperactivity-impulsivity*** have persisted for at least 6 months to a degree that is maladaptive and inconsistent with developmental level:
  Hyperactivity
  (a) Often fidgets with hands or feet or squirms in seat
  (b) Often leaves seat in classroom or in other situations in which remaining seated is expected
  (c) Often runs about or climbs excessively in situations in which it is inappropriate (in adolescents or adults, may be limited to subjective feelings of restlessness)
  (d) Often has difficulty playing or engaging in leisure activities quietly
  (e) Is often "on the go" or often acts as if "driven by a motor"
  (f) Often talks excessively
  Impulsivity
  (g) Often blurts out answers before questions have been completed
  (h) Often has difficulty awaiting turn
  (i) Often interrupts or intrudes on others (e.g., butts into conversations or games)
B. Some hyperactive-impulsive or inattentive symptoms that caused impairment were present before age 7 years.
C. Some impairment from the symptoms is present in two or more settings (e.g., at school, work, at home).
D. There must be clear evidence of clinically significant impairment in social, academic, or occupational functioning.
E. The symptoms do not occur exclusively during the course of or are not accounted for by another mental disorder.

From American Psychiatric Association: *Diagnostic and statistical manual of mental disorders,* ed 4 *(DSM-IV),* Washington, DC, 1994, The Association.

??? CRITICAL THINKING EXERCISE ???

Attention Deficit Hyperactivity Disorder

Johnnie, age 8 years, is a third-grader who was recently diagnosed with attention deficit hyperactivity disorder (ADHD). He has been taking the drug methylphenidate (Ritalin) for about a month. In the short time that Johnnie has been on this medication, his math teacher has noticed an improvement in his performance in math class. He is receiving a grade of B instead of his previous grades of D on most math quizzes. The math teacher has also noted that Johnnie is socializing more with his class-mates and that he now has a "best friend" in math class. Johnnie usu-ally receives his Ritalin from the school nurse before lunch. Yesterday Johnnie's mother told the school nurse that he has not eaten his lunch for the past week and that he is not hungry.

What important issues regarding Johnnie's medication should the nurse consider in her discussions with Johnnie's mother?

QUESTIONS

1. Evidence—Is there sufficient evidence to draw conclusions about Johnnie's medication from his behavior?
2. Assumptions—Describe some underlying assumptions about the following:
   a. Pharmacologic action of methylphenidate in ADHD
   b. Side effects of methylphenidate
   c. Management of side effects
3. What implications for nursing care can be drawn at this time?
4. Does the evidence objectively support your conclusion?
5. Are there alternative perspectives to your arguments?

ANSWERS

1. Yes, there are sufficient data to arrive at a possible conclusion.
2. a. Methylphenidate is a stimulant that increases dopamine and norepinephrine levels that lead to stimulation of the inhibitory system of the central nervous system.
   b. Common side effects of methylphenidate include nausea, anorexia, decreased appetite, and insomnia.
   c. Although the absorption rate of methylphenidate is increased when the drug is taken with meals, side effects such as de-creased appetite may become more pronounced with this schedule of administration. Side effects can be alleviated by changing the times that the drug is administered or by switch-ing to a sustained time-release form of the drug that is taken once per day in the morning.
3. Although Johnnie seems to have responded favorably to his medica-tion and has demonstrated several positive effects of methylphenidate (improvement in math class and increasing self-confidence in social skills), the nurse should be concerned about the fact that Johnnie has not eaten his lunch for the past week and that he is not hungry. De-creased appetite is a negative side effect of methylphenidate.
4. Yes, the data indicate that Johnnie is currently experiencing a de-crease in his appetite. Because decreased appetite is a common side effect of methylphenidate, there is a high probability that this symp-tom is related to Johnnie's medication. However, adjusting or chang-ing the times the medication is administered can often alleviate this side effect. Another option is to ask Johnnie's doctor to switch his medication to a sustained time-release form of methylphenidate that can be given once per day in the morning.
5. It is possible that Johnnie's decreased appetite is due to some other factor and is not related to his medication. Therefore, the nurse should encourage the mother to communicate information about this side effect to Johnnie's primary care physician so that a more complete evaluation can be made.

FAMILY FOCUS

A Child's Perception of Taking Ritalin at School

I feel embarrassed by having to leave class early to go take my medication. The other kids always ask where I'm going and why. It would be better if we could leave class at the same time as every-one else, go take the medication, and then just be a little late to the next class. Students don't ask why people are late for class, only why they leave early. It also bothers me when kids tell other kids, "Go take a pill," and other mean things just because someone is acting up. What could nurses and teachers do to help? Most kids do not understand why other kids have to take medication. I think it would help if a nurse or teacher talked with the other kids and ex-plained why some children take the medication and how ADHD af-fects people. That way there would be more understanding among all the kids.

Marissa White, age 16

than before is helpful. Parents also benefit from practical, specific strategies that help children with ADHD, such as the need for structure and consistency in dressing, meals, sleep, and discipline (see Family Focus box).

Nurses must understand which type of LD a child has to provide direction for the child, parents, and teachers. Chil-dren with an auditory perceptual deficit are often unable to follow directions or to comprehend large amounts of verbal teaching. These children need diagrams, pictures, demonstra-tion, and written lists. Children with visual perceptual deficits may have difficulty reading, lining up numbers for mathe-matic operations, or judging distance. These children may have dyslexia (letter reversals) and do better with demonstra-tion and a verbal approach. Children with an integrative deficit may have difficulty sequencing data or storing and re-trieving sensory data. Multisensory techniques should be used, and comprehension should be checked frequently throughout instruction. Children with dysgraphia (difficulty with writing) often benefit from computers in the classroom, because their handwriting will *not* improve. They need to find alternatives to physical competition that requires coordination of movement (Selekman and Snyder, 2000).

ENURESIS

Enuresis (bed-wetting) is a common and troublesome dis-order that is defined as intentional or involuntary passage of urine into bed (usually at night) or into clothes during the day in children who are beyond the age when voluntary bladder control should normally have been acquired. The inappropriate voiding of urine must occur at least twice a week for at least 3 months, and the chronologic or devel-opmental age of the child must be at least 5 years (see Cul-tural Awareness box). The predominant symptom is ur-gency that is immediate and accompanied by acute discomfort, restlessness, and urinary frequency. Enuresis is more common in boys; nocturnal bed-wetting usually ceases between 6 and 8 years of age.

Organic causes that may be related to enuresis should be ruled out before psychogenic factors are considered. These in-clude structural disorders of the urinary tract; urinary tract in-

CULTURAL AWARENESS

Enuresis

The age at which children attain urinary continence varies widely. For example, white children in the United States tend to achieve continence earlier than African-American children. In addition, children in Great Britain and Sweden appear to attain continence slightly earlier than children in the United States, and in the extreme, the East African Digos often achieve bladder control by the age of 12 months. Therefore practitioners must be sensitive to the differences among groups before labeling a child enuretic (Rappaport, 1992).

FAMILY FOCUS

Helping Families Understand Encopresis

The prevailing attitude of nurses toward the family of a child with encopresis should be one of no-fault, thus relieving the guilt of both parents and child. Because parents and children are often reluctant to volunteer information, direct questioning about the soiling is more successful. Parents are usually relieved to know that other parents share this problem and are surprised to know that functional changes that take place as the condition develops make control of seepage impossible. Many parents complain that their children soil because they do not take time from play for a bowel movement. Actually, the children may be unaware of a prior sensation and unable to control the urge once it begins. They may be so accustomed to bowel accidents that they are unable to smell or feel it and even deny soiling when it occurs.

fection; neurologic deficits; disorders that increase the normal output of urine, such as diabetes; and disorders that impair the concentrating ability of the kidneys, such as chronic renal failure or sickle cell disease. A bladder volume of 300 to 350 mL is sufficient to hold a night's urine. (To determine a child's bladder capacity, have the child void in a measuring cup after holding urine for as long as possible. Normal bladder capacity [in ounces] is the child's age plus 2 [e.g., a 6-year-old's normal capacity is 8 ounces].) In other cases the enuresis is influenced by emotional factors, although it is doubtful that they are causative factors. Parents report that these children sleep more soundly than other children; however, the depth of sleep has not been identified as the cause of nocturnal enuresis. Enuresis has a strong familial tendency.

Therapeutic techniques used to manage enuresis include medications, bladder training, restriction or elimination of fluids after the evening meal, interruption of sleep to void, and various devices designed to establish a conditioned reflex response to waken the child at the initiation of voiding.

Three types of drugs are used to treat enuresis: tricyclic antidepressants, antidiuretics, and antispasmodics. The drug used most frequently to inhibit urination is the tricyclic antidepressant, imipramine (Tofranil). Another anticholinergic drug, oxybutynin, reduces uninhibited bladder contractions and may be helpful for children with daytime urinary frequency. Desmopressin (DDAVP) nasal spray, an analog of vasopressin, reduces nighttime urine output to a volume less than functional bladder capacity.

Nursing Considerations

No matter what techniques are used, the nurse can help both children and parents to understand the problem of enuresis, the treatment plan, and the difficulties they may encounter in the process. The nurse can also provide consistent support and encouragement to help sustain both the child and the parents through the inconsistent and unpredictable treatment process. Parents need to understand that punishment is contraindicated because of its negative emotional impact and limited success in reducing the behavior. Children need to believe that they are helping themselves, and they need to sustain feelings of confidence and hope.

ENCOPRESIS

Encopresis is the repeated voluntary or involuntary passage of feces of normal or near-normal consistency into places not appropriate for that purpose according to the individual's own sociocultural setting. The event must occur at

least once per month for at least 3 months, and the chronologic or developmental age of the child must be at least 4 years. The fecal incontinence must not be caused by any physiologic effect, such as a laxative, or a general medical condition.

Primary encopresis is identified by age 4 when the child has not achieved fecal continence. *Secondary encopresis* is fecal incontinence occurring in a child older than 4 years of age after a period of established fecal continence. The disorder is more common in boys than in girls.

One of the most common causes of encopresis is constipation, which may be precipitated by environmental change. Chronic, severe constipation has a tendency to impair the usual movement and contractions of the colon, which can lead to fecal obstruction. Abnormalities in the digestive tract can also lead to encopresis.

Children with encopresis often feel ashamed and may wish to avoid situations that might lead to embarrassment. School performance and attendance are affected as the child's offensive odor becomes a target for scorn and ridicule from classmates. Therapeutic management consists of determining the cause of the soiling and using appropriate interventions to correct the problem. Interventions may involve dietary changes, relief of a fecal impaction, or behavioral therapy. Frequently psychotherapeutic intervention with the child and the family may be necessary.

Nursing Considerations

The nursing care of the child with encopresis involves education and support of the family, as well as treatment of existing constipation. Education regarding the physiology of normal defecation, toilet training as a developmental process, and the treatment outlined for the particular family is essential to a successful outcome. Family counseling is directed toward reassurance that most problems resolve successfully, although relapses during periods of stress are possible (see Family Focus box).

POSTTRAUMATIC STRESS DISORDER

Posttraumatic stress disorder (PTSD) refers to the development of characteristic symptoms after exposure to an extremely traumatic experience or catastrophic event. The traumatic experience is typically life-threatening to self or a significant other and may involve grotesque mutilation or death, serious injury, or physical coercion (e.g., an assault, a natural disaster, sexual abuse, witnessing violence). It is important to note that PSTD is not limited to children who have lived in "war-torn" countries. Events such as automobile, school, or recreational accidents, and bullying have been identified as causes of PTSD (Sundelin-Wahlsten, Ahmad, and von Knorring, 2001). The characteristic symptoms are persistent reexperiencing of the traumatic event, avoidance of stimuli associated with the event or trauma, numbing of general responsiveness, and increased arousal.

The response to the event takes place in three stages. The *initial response* involves intense arousal, which usually lasts for a few minutes to 1 or 2 hours. The stress hormones are at the maximum as the individual prepares for "fight or flight." A prolonged arousal phase may indicate psychosis.

The *second phase,* which lasts approximately 2 weeks, is one in which defense mechanisms are mobilized. It is a period of quiescence in which the event appears to have produced no impression. The child feels numb, and stress hormone secretion is absent.. Defense mechanisms are less adaptive to specific situations and may not be what the situation demands. Denial that anything is wrong is a frequently observed defense mechanism.

The *third phase* is one of coping and consciously directed inquiry, which normally extends over 2 to 3 months. The victims want to know what happened and appear to be getting worse, when actually they are getting better. Numerous psychologic symptoms, such as depression, phobia, anxiety, and conversion reactions may be present. Children frequently display repetitive actions. They play out the situation over and over again in an attempt to come to terms with their fear. Flashbacks are common. This phase can be self-perpetuating, and a prolonged reaction can develop into an obsession with the traumatic event. Some traumatic effects remain indefinitely.

Nursing Considerations

Children need to deal with any traumatic event. Their reactions depend heavily on their social environment and the way in which their caretaking adults react to the event. In the second phase of the PTSD, the appropriateness of the defense mechanism must be assessed, and children must be assisted in application of their defense. If children do not engage in some catharsis, or if their defense phase is prolonged, they need referral for special psychologic help.

Coping is a learned response, and children in the third phase can be helped to deal with their fear. Children usually are willing to accept reasoning. Those who are assisted in their catharsis and allowed expression will survive without serious lasting effects. They should be encouraged to play out the stress and to discuss their feelings about the event. If they are unable to do this, they may become obsessed with the traumatic event and require professional help. Conversion reactions are common obsessive behaviors in children suffering from PTSD.

Children need professional help if any of the phases of PTSD are prolonged. Boys tend to have a prolonged defense phase more often than girls. Occasionally the event will be unrecognized, and the affected child will engage in

what is considered to be unusual behavior. Children exhibiting any sudden change in behavior need to be assessed for a traumatic event. When the change in behavior is traced to a traumatic event, treatment can be implemented.

SCHOOL PHOBIA

Children, other than beginning students, who resist going to school or who demonstrate extreme reluctance to attend school for a sustained period as a result of severe anxiety or fear of school-related experiences are said to have school phobia. The terms *school refusal* and *school avoidance* are also used to describe this behavior. School avoidance behaviors occur in both boys and girls and in children from all socioeconomic levels.

Physical symptoms are prominent and may affect any part of the body (e.g., anorexia, nausea, vomiting, diarrhea, dizziness, headache, leg pains, abdominal pains, even a low-grade fever). A striking feature of school phobia is the prompt subsiding of symptoms when it is evident that the child can remain at home. Another significant observation is absence of symptoms on weekends and holidays unless they are related to other places such as Sunday school or parties. Occasional mild reluctance is not uncommon among schoolchildren, but if the fear continues for longer than a few days it must be considered a serious problem.

Nursing Considerations

Treatment for school phobia depends on the cause. The primary goal is *to return the child to school.* The longer a child is permitted to stay out of school, the more difficult it is for the child to reenter. Parents must be convinced gently but firmly that *immediate* return is essential and that it is their responsibility to insist on school attendance.

A school reentry protocol may be necessary for the child with severe symptoms. In reentry programs, the child role-plays routines involved in getting ready for school and that occur at school. Relaxation techniques are also used. The child usually goes to school initially for a half-day and then progresses to a full day. Often the school nurse is asked to provide support to the parents and the teacher during the reentry process. If the problem persists, professional help is recommended.

RECURRENT ABDOMINAL PAIN

Recurrent abdominal pain (RAP) is a complaint that is often attributed to a psychogenic etiology, although it can be a symptom of either psychosomatic or organic disease. RAP is defined as three or more separate episodes of abdominal pain during a 3-month period similar to the "spastic" or "irritable" colon syndrome of adulthood. Children with RAP have real pain that is usually located in the periumbilical or epigastric area. On palpation the pain is likely to be experienced in the epigastric area or in the lower right or left quadrant and is accompanied by vague tenderness without muscle guarding. The pain is irregular in time, duration, and intensity and associated with either loose or pellet-formed stools. Other symptoms that may accompany the pain are headache, pallor, dizziness, dysuria, flushing, vomiting, diarrhea, and fatigue.

Children at risk for RAP tend to be high achievers who have extensive personal goals or whose parents have unusually high expectations. They are described as sensitive and overly concerned about what others think of them. They are uncomfortable with expressions of anger or argument, especially in those persons who are significant in their life. School attendance is adversely affected, and these children may exhibit poor learning performance. It is not uncommon for symptoms to be aggravated during school days.

Treatment involves providing reassurance and reducing or eliminating the symptoms. Hospitalization may be necessary, and the child frequently shows improvement in the hospital. Initial efforts are directed toward ruling out organic causes of the pain, relieving discomfort, and attempting to determine the situations that precipitate attacks. A high-fiber diet, psyllium bulk agents, lubricants such as mineral oil, and bowel training are emphasized. Other therapies include cognitive-behavioral therapy, biofeedback, and medications such as famotidine and propantheline bromide (an antispasmodic).

Nursing Considerations

After the diagnosis has been established, the parents and the child need an explanation of the pain, which can be compared to a skeletal muscle cramp or "charley horse." Reassurance that the symptoms are not unique to their child and that the pain can be expected to subside is helpful in relieving parental fears and anxieties.

The simple measure of having the child rest in a peaceful, quiet environment and providing comfort will often relieve the symptoms in a short time. A heating pad may also help ease the discomfort (see Nonpharmacologic Pain Management, Chapter 21). When pain is not relieved by these simple measures, the parents are taught how to administer antispasmodics, if prescribed. For example, if pain is precipitated by meals, having the child take the medication 20 to 30 minutes before mealtime may prevent an episode.

The most valuable assistance that the nurse can provide is support and reassurance to the family. When open communication is established and families appreciate the relationship between stress-provoking situations and the child's symptoms, the chance for remedial action is enhanced. Follow-up care and continued support are essential, because the symptoms tend to remit and exacerbate. The availability of a supportive health professional is a source of comfort to the child and family.

CONVERSION REACTION

Conversion reaction, also known as *hysteria, hysterical conversion reaction,* and *childhood hysteria,* is a psychophysiologic disorder with a sudden onset that can usually be traced to a precipitating environmental event. In childhood the disorder is observed with equal frequency in both sexes, but girls outnumber boys during adolescence.

The manifestations involve primarily the voluntary musculature and special senses. Symptoms include abdominal pain, fainting, pseudoseizures, paralysis, headaches, and visual field restriction. The most common symptom is seizure activity, which can be differentiated from symptoms of neurogenic origin by formal tests. A normal electroencephalogram indicates that the origin is not neurogenic. Many children with a conversion reaction have experienced a major family crisis (such as the loss of a parent or other significant person through death, divorce, or moving) before the onset of symptoms.

Nursing Considerations

Nursing care is similar to that for the child with recurrent abdominal pain. If significant personality problems are evident, psychiatric consultation is indicated.

CHILDHOOD DEPRESSION

Depression in childhood is often difficult to detect because children may be unable to express their feelings and tend to act out their problems and concerns. Some states of depression are of a temporary nature (e.g., acute depression precipitated by a traumatic event). This might include a period of hospitalization, loss of a parent through death or separation, or loss of a significant relationship with something (a pet), someone (a friend or family member), or a place (move from a familiar home, neighborhood, or city). Children with depression may demonstrate a variety of behaviors (see Box 17-10). Most responses in children are not sustained and can be modified with social and family support.

More serious and less common are the depressive responses to chronic stress and loss; these are frequently observed in children with chronic illness or disability when other family members have denial depression. There is no apparent precipitating event, but there is often a history of frequent disruptions in important relationships. Often, there is also a history of depressive illness in one or both parents. Manifestations in the child are similar to those observed in acute depression, but they occur more frequently and extend over a longer period.

Nursing Considerations

Depressed children are managed by a health team especially prepared in the care of children with mental disorders. Treatment is highly individualized and undertaken in the least restrictive environment. Suicidal children are admitted to the hospital for protection if the family is unable to provide constant monitoring. Pharmacotherapy may involve

---

BOX 17-10
Characteristics of Children With Depression

BEHAVIOR
Predominantly sad facial expression with absence or diminished range of affective response
Solitary play or work; tendency to be alone; disinterest in play
Withdrawal from previously enjoyed activities and relationships
Lowered grades in school; lack of interest in doing homework or achieving in school
Diminished motor activity; tiredness
Tearfulness or crying
Dependent and clinging or aggressive and disruptive

INTERNAL STATES
Utterance of statements reflecting lowered self-esteem, sense of hopelessness, or guilt
Suicidal ideations

PHYSIOLOGY
Constipation
Nonspecific complaints of not feeling well
Change in appetite resulting in weight loss or gain
Alterations in sleeping pattern, sleeplessness, or hypersomnia

tricyclic antidepressants or serotonin reuptake inhibitors (SRIs) such as fluoxetine (Prozac), trazodone (Desyrel), sertraline (Zoloft), paroxetine (Paxil), bupropion (Wellbutrin), and venlafaxine (Effexor). Nurses should be aware that depression is a problem that can easily be overlooked in the child and one that can interrupt normal growth and development. Recognizing depression and suicidal tendencies in depressed adolescents and making appropriate referrals is an important nursing function. Identification of the depressed child requires a careful history (health, growth and development, social, and family health), interviews with the child, and observations by the nurse, parents, and teachers. (See also Suicide, p. 544.)

CHILDHOOD SCHIZOPHRENIA

Childhood schizophrenia is a term that refers to severe deviations in ego functioning and is generally reserved for psychotic disorders that appear in children younger than 15 years of age. Childhood schizophrenia is a very rare illness among children in the general population, and among children with mental illness, only about 2 in every 1000 have childhood schizophrenia.

Childhood schizophrenia is characterized by symptoms that last for at least 6 months and that seriously interfere with the child's functioning in school, at home, or in other social situations. The basic disturbance is a lack of contact with reality and the subsequent development of a world of the child's own. Other areas of development that may be impaired include cognition, perception, emotion, language, and physical motor control. The most common manifestations involve language disturbances, impaired interpersonal relationships, and inappropriate affect (outward expression of emotion). Treatment involves management of the symptoms, prevention of relapse, and social and occupational rehabilitation of the young person. Antipsychotic drugs that are used to treat schizophrenia include haloperidol, chlorpromazine, and risperidone.

Nursing Considerations

Nursing of psychotic children is a highly specialized area. However, nurses should be alert to the possibility that schizophrenia can occur in children and refer children who consistently demonstrate abnormal behavior to a psychiatrist for evaluation. In addition, nurses will need to teach family members of children taking antipsychotic drugs to observe for possible side effects.

SERIOUS HEALTH PROBLEMS OF LATER CHILDHOOD AND ADOLESCENCE

SUBSTANCE ABUSE

Although experimentation with drugs during childhood and adolescence is widespread, most children and teens do not become high-risk users. Experimentation is limited to 1 adolescent in 5 for stimulants and inhalants, and less than 1 in 10 for hallucinogens, sedatives, and "crack" cocaine. Adolescents are the group at greatest risk for regular use of drugs; approximately 1% to 2% of teens use hard drugs regularly (US Department of Health and Human Services, 1999).

Drug abuse, misuse, and *addiction* are culturally defined and are voluntary behaviors. *Drug tolerance* and *physical dependence* are involuntary physiologic responses to the pharmacologic characteristics of the drugs, such as opioids and alcohol. Consequently, an individual can be addicted to a narcotic with or without being physically dependent. A person can also be physically dependent on a narcotic without being addicted (e.g., patients who use opioids to control pain).

Motivation

Most drug use begins with experimentation. The drug may be used only once, may be used occasionally, or may become part of a drug-centered lifestyle. Children and adolescents initiate drug use out of curiosity. For many youths, drugs produce a dreamy state of altered consciousness or a feeling of power, excitement, heightened acuity, or confidence. Others seek the visual hallucinatory experiences and sexual sensation that result from drug use. Many youngsters use drugs because their peers use them, or because they want to belong to a group. Some youths also turn to drugs because they are looking for a way to cope with stress, the social and technologic changes of the world, and their feelings of powerlessness.

Types of Drugs Abused

Any drug can be abused, and most are potentially harmful to youngsters still going through formative life experiences. Although rarely considered drugs by society, the chemically active substances most frequently abused are the xanthines and theobromines contained in chocolate, tea, coffee, and colas. Ethyl alcohol and nicotine are other drugs that are legal and socially sanctioned. Any of these substances can produce mild to moderate euphoric or stimulant effects and can lead to physical and psychologic dependence.

Drugs with mind-altering abilities that are available on the "street" and are of medical and legal concern are the hallucinogenic, narcotic, hypnotic, and stimulant drugs. In addition, health professionals are concerned about the use of alcohol and volatile substances that are inhaled to achieve altered sensation (such as gasoline, antifreeze, plastic model airplane cement, typewriter correction fluid, and organic solvents). Recently, abuse of prescription and synthetic drugs has become a concern for professionals who work with children and adolescents. Internet websites have also promoted the "safe use" of some psychoactive drugs and have supplied information on new "designer" drugs that are not detectable on a standard urine drug screening test (Wax, 2002).

Alcohol.   Acute or chronic abuse of alcohol (ethanol) is responsible for many acts of violence, suicide, accidental injury, and death. Alcohol drinking is likely to begin in the middle school years and increases with age. By 18 years of age, 80% to 90% of adolescents have tried alcohol. Ethanol is a depressant that reduces inhibitions against aggressive and sexual acting out. Severe physical and psychologic symptoms accompany abrupt withdrawal, and long-term use leads to slow tissue destruction, especially of the brain and liver cells. The most noticeable effects of alcohol occur within the central nervous system and include changes in cognitive and autonomic functions such as judgment, memory, learning ability, and other intellectual capacities. Young alcoholics often drink alone and cannot control their use of alcohol. They often rely on the substance as a defense against depression, anxiety, fear, or anger. Not all of these characteristics are observed in the youngster who is abusing alcohol, but if several signs are evident, the child or adolescent should be considered at risk. Referral to a health care professional and detoxification therapy may be necessary. Information about alcohol and answers to questions are available through the **Alcohol Hotline.*** Other groups that provide support and counseling for families are **Al-Anon, Ala-Teen, Ala-Tot,** and **Alcoholics Anonymous** (an organization that has listings in all local telephone directories.

Cocaine. Although cocaine is not pharmacologically considered a narcotic, it is legally categorized as such. Cocaine is available in two forms: water-soluble cocaine hydrochloride, which is administered by "snorting" or intravenous injection, and nonsoluble alkaloid (freebase) cocaine, which is used primarily for smoking. Crack, or "rock," is a purer, more menacing form of the drug. It can be produced cheaply and smoked in either water pipes or mentholated cigarettes. The use of cocaine has increased in recent years because of its availability and affordability; its association with persons in glamorous occupations; peer pressure; and its reputation as a sexually enhancing drug.

Cocaine creates a sense of euphoria, or an indefinable high. Withdrawal does not produce the dramatic symptoms observed in withdrawal from other substances. The effects are those commonly seen in depression, including lack of energy and motivation, irritability, appetite changes, psychomotor retardation, and irregular sleep patterns. More serious symptoms include cardiovascular manifestations and seizures. Physical withdrawal should not be confused with the so-called crash after a cocaine high, which consists of a long period of sleep. Answers to questions about the risks of using cocaine are available at the **National Cocaine Hotline,†** which also provides referrals to support groups and treatment centers.

Narcotics. Narcotic drugs include opiates such as heroin and morphine, and opioids (opiate-like drugs), such as hydromorphone (Dilaudid), fentanyl, meperidine (Demerol), and codeine. These drugs produce a state of euphoria by removing painful feelings and creating a pleasurable experience and a sense of success accompanied by clouding of the consciousness and a dreamlike state. Physical signs of narcotic abuse include constricted pupils, respiratory depression, and, often, cyanosis. Needle marks may be visible on the arms or legs in chronic users. Physical withdrawal from opiates is extremely unpleasant unless controlled with supervised tapering doses of the opioid or substitution of methadone.

Equally as important as the physical effects are the indirect consequences related to the illegal status of narcotic use and the problems associated with securing the drug (e.g., the time-consuming searches to obtain the drug and the often illegal methods used to meet the high cost of purchasing it). Health problems also result from self-neglect of physical needs (nutrition, cleanliness, dental care), overdose, contamination, and infection, including HIV infection and hepatitis B.

Central nervous system depressants include a variety of hypnotic drugs that produce physical dependence and withdrawal symptoms on abrupt discontinuation. They create a feeling of relaxation and sleepiness but impair general functioning. Drugs in this category include barbiturates, nonbarbiturates (such as methaqualone [Quaalude]), and alcohol. Barbiturates combined with alcohol produce a profound depressant effect.

Central Nervous System Stimulants.   Amphetamines and cocaine do not produce strong physical dependence and can be withdrawn without much danger. However, psychologic dependence is strong, and acute intoxication can lead to violent aggressive behavior or psychotic episodes characterized by paranoia, uncontrollable agitation, and restlessness. When combined with barbiturates, the euphoric effects are particularly addictive.

Methamphetamine can be snorted, injected, swallowed, or smoked and produces a burst of energy in its users, along with intense, alternating attacks of boldness and paranoia. It provokes excitement far more intense than that caused by crack and cocaine. The drug, with the street names "crank," "meth," and "crystal," is inexpensive and has a longer period of action than cocaine. Instead of a short (few minutes) high, as achieved with crack, a user can remain "up" for hours on a similar dose of crank.

Inhalants include glue "sniffing" and the inhalation of plastic cement, spray paint, and other volatile substances (e.g., gasoline, nitrous oxide, air dusters used to remove dust from computers and camera lenses). Youngsters breathe or place these substances into paper or plastic bags or soda cans from which they rebreathe the fumes to produce a feeling of euphoria and altered consciousness. These substances contain chemical solvents and are extremely hazardous. Dusters contain freon, a substance that can cause fatal cardiac arrhythmias. The use of inhalants is increasing, and inhalants are becoming a gateway drug for young children and preteens who often progress to other harder drugs such as marijuana, heroin, and cocaine. Many young children are unaware of the dangers of "sniffing" or "huffing." In addition to rapid loss of consciousness and respiratory arrest, these substances may cause visual scanning problems, language deficiencies, motor instability, memory deficits, and attention and concentration problems.

Mind-Altering Drugs.   Hallucinogens (psychedelic, psychotomimetic, psychotropic, or illusionogenic) are drugs that produce vivid hallucinations and euphoria. These drugs do not produce physical dependence, and they can be abruptly withdrawn without ill effect. However, the acute and long-term effects are variable, and in some individuals the dissociative behavior may be prolonged. Cannabis (marijuana, hashish) and lysergic acid diethylamide (LSD) are also included in this category of drugs.

Nursing Considerations Related to Therapeutic Management

Nurses who have contact with children and adolescents are in an excellent position to provide information about substance abuse and to serve as a patient advocate. The nurse most often encounters young drug abusers when they are

---

*800-ALCOHOL.
†800-COCAINE.

(1) experiencing overdose or withdrawal symptoms, (2) manifesting bizarre behavior or confusion secondary to drug ingestion, (3) worried that they are becoming or will become addicted, or (4) worried about a friend or family member who is addicted.

In particular, nurses who care for hospitalized adolescents need to know if these youths use drugs compulsively. Drug withdrawal can seriously complicate other illnesses. Nurses should be alert for any physical or behavioral clues that indicate the onset of withdrawal or the effects of drugs. Obstetric and nursery nurses may encounter drug dependence and withdrawal in newborn infants or compulsive drug-using mothers. School nurses and nurses who work in the community also play an essential role in identifying children, adolescents, and families with substance abuse problems. Early identification of children, adolescents, and families at risk for substance abuse problems is an essential aspect of prevention. Pediatric health care professionals also prevent substance abuse by creating trusting relationships so that children and adolescents feel comfortable asking questions about drugs and that health professionals can alert preadolescents and adolescents to websites and other aspects of society that encourage experimentation with drugs.

Acute Care.
Adolescents experiencing toxic drug effects or withdrawal symptoms are usually seen initially in the emergency department. Experienced emergency department personnel are familiar with the management of acute drug toxicity, and the signs, symptoms, and behavioral characteristics of a variety of substances. When the drug is questionable or unknown, knowledge of these factors facilitates management and treatment. Often, observation or description of the child or adolescent's behavior is more valuable than reports by patients or their friends

The treatment for drug toxicity or withdrawal varies according to the drug and the method used. Every effort is made to determine the type, the time of ingestion, the amount of drug taken, the mode of administration, and the factors related to the onset of presenting symptoms. It is helpful to know the individual's pattern of use. For example, if two types of drugs are involved, they may require different treatments. Gastric lavage may be employed when the drug has been ingested recently and the cough reflex is intact, but it is of little value when the drug has been administered by the intravenous ("mainlined") or intranasal ("sniffed") route. Because the actual content of most street drugs is highly questionable, other pharmaceutical agents are administered with caution, except perhaps the narcotic antagonists in cases of suspected opiate overdoses. It is also necessary to assess for possible trauma sustained while the patient was under the influence of the drug.

Long-Term Management.
A major factor in the treatment and rehabilitation of young drug users is careful assessment in the nonacute stage to determine the function that the drug plays in the youngster's life. The motivation phase is directed toward exploring the factors that influence drug use. It also involves establishing a feeling of self-worth and a commitment to self-help in the teen.

Rehabilitation begins when youngsters decide that they can and are willing to change. Rehabilitation involves fostering healthy interdependent relationships with caring and supportive adults and exploring alternate mechanisms for problem solving while simultaneously reducing or eliminating drug use. Persons working with troubled youth must be prepared for recidivism, or the tendency to relapse, and maintain a plan for reentry into the treatment process.

Family Support.
Most treatment programs for substance abusers are based on adult 12-step models such as Alcoholics Anonymous. Research is needed to determine whether these adult models are effective for adolescents. **Tough Love*** is one such program that is based on the conviction that parents have the right and responsibility to be the policymakers in the family, to set limits on the behavior of their children, and to take control of the household from out-of-control youngsters. The premise is that allowing teenagers to experience the negative consequences of their behavior will bring them closer to accepting help or changing their behavior. Another group that provides support and counseling for families experiencing substance abuse and seeking strategies to cope with their children is **Parents Anonymous.†**

Prevention.
Nurses play an important role in education efforts, as well as in individual observation, assessment, and therapy related to substance abuse. In recent years, a variety of educational programs have been applied with promising results. The most effective prevention strategies are those that are part of a broader, more general effort to promote overall health and success. Health-compromising behaviors are often interconnected and have common antecedents. Prevention efforts that focus on changing only one behavior (e.g., alcohol, other drug use) are less likely to be successful. Successful programs are those that have promoted parenting skills, social skills among distractible children, academic achievement, and skills to resist peer pressure.

Peer pressure is a powerful tool and can be used effectively in substance abuse prevention. A group that has had some success in reducing injury from drunk driving is **Students Against Driving Drunk (SADD).‡** Techniques used by this group include peer counseling, parental guidelines for teenage parties, and community awareness. Nurses should encourage the formation of SADD chapters in the high schools in their communities.

SUICIDE

Suicide is defined as the deliberate act of self-injury with the intent that the injury results in death. Most experts distinguish between suicidal ideation, suicide attempt (or parasuicide), and suicide.

Suicidal ideation involves a preoccupation with thoughts about committing suicide and may be a precursor to suicide.

---

*PO Box 1069, Doylestown, PA 18901; (215) 348-7090; website: www.toughlove.org

†675 West Foothill Boulevard, Suite 220, Claremont, CA 91711; (909) 621-6184. Another source of information: **National Clearinghouse for Alcohol and Drug Information,** PO Box 2345, Rockville, MD 20852; (800) 729-6686; email: info@health.org; website: www.health.org

‡PO Box 800, Marlboro, MA 01752; (508) 481-3568 or (800) 886-2972; website: www.saddonline.com.

Although it is not uncommon for adolescents to experience occasional suicidal thoughts, expressions of preoccupation with suicide should be taken seriously, and an assessment should be conducted for appropriate referral. A *suicide attempt* is intended to cause injury or death. The term *parasuicide* is used to refer to behaviors ranging from gestures to serious attempts to kill oneself. Parasuicide is a preferred term because it make no reference to intent and because a person's motive may be too difficult or complex to determine. However, all parasuicidal activity should be taken seriously.

NURSING ALERT

A history of a previous suicide attempt is a serious indicator for possible suicide completion in the future. Studies of adolescent suicides have found that as many as half of the adolescents had made previous attempts.

Recent results from the Youth Risk Behavior Survey, 2001, indicated that 8.8% of students nationwide had attempted suicide at least once during the 12 months preceding the survey (Grunbaum and others, 2002). This number represented a significant increase from 7.8% who reported attempts in 1999 (Division of Adolescent and School Health, 2000). Approximately 15% of the students in this survey reported that they had made a specific plan to attempt suicide in the 12 months preceding the survey. In the United States, the suicide rate for adolescents has increased dramatically in the last few decades. Suicide is currently the third leading cause of death during the teenage years, surpassed only by death from injury and homicide (see Chapter 1).

Etiology

Individual, family, and social/environmental factors have all been implicated in suicide. The single most important individual factor is the presence of an active psychiatric disorder (depression, bipolar disorder, psychosis, substance abuse, or conduct disorder). Comorbidity of an affective disorder and substance abuse also increases the risk for suicide. Alcohol use has been associated with more than 50% of suicides (American Academy of Pediatrics, 2000). Gay and lesbian adolescents are at particularly high risk for suicide completion, especially if raised in an environment in which they are denied support systems (see Community Focus box). Family factors influencing suicide include parental loss; family disruption; a family history of suicide, depression, substance abuse, or emotional disturbance; child abuse or neglect; unavailable parents; poor communication and isolation within the family; family conflict; and unrealistically high parental expectations or parental indifference with low expectations. Social/environmental factors include incarceration, isolation, acute loss of a boyfriend or girlfriend, lack of future options, and availability of firearms in the home.

Methods

Firearms are by far the most commonly used instruments in completed suicides among males and females (American Academy of Pediatrics, 2000). For adolescent males, the second and third most common means of suicide are hanging and overdose, respectively; for females the second and third most common means are overdose and strangulation, respectively.

COMMUNITY FOCUS

Suicide, Sexual Identity, and Sexual Orientation

A significant number of teenage suicides occur among homosexual youths. Gay or lesbian adolescents who live in families or communities that do not accept homosexuality are likely to suffer low self-esteem, self-loathing, depression, and hopelessness as a result of lack of acceptance from their family or community. Such internalization, without treatment and support, can lead to substance abuse and, eventually, suicide. Youths most at risk are those who struggle with gender identity issues such as gay identity formation at a young age, intrapersonal conflict regarding sexuality, and nondisclosure of orientation to others.

Supportive parents, friends, or relationships serve as protective factors against suicide. However, many gay, lesbian, and bisexual adolescents do not feel supported, understood, or accepted by their friends, parents, and families. Nurses who interact with adolescents must be aware of the association between suicide and adolescent homosexuality and gender nonconformity. School nurses may be the first individuals to discuss issues of sexual identity and orientation with adolescents or their families. In their professional capacity, nurses can also serve as support persons for these adolescents. Nurses can also provide guidance and resources to families so that they know and understand how best to nurture and support their child.

Nurses must also capitalize on opportunities or experiences that promote the healthy development of self-esteem in youths who choose nontraditional sexual orientation. Educational programs to raise the level of consciousness about the risk factors for and warning signs of suicide are one example. Another possibility could be programs conducted in or outside of school that are designed to foster peer relationships and competency in social skills among high-risk adolescents and young adults, such as support groups and social organizations for these young people.

The most common method of suicide attempt is overdose or ingestion of a potentially toxic substance, such as drugs. The second most common method of suicide attempt is self-inflicted laceration.

NURSING ALERT

Given what is known about youth suicide, nurses should ask parents, especially those with at-risk teenagers, if firearms are available in the house and, if so, recommend their removal. Parents must ensure that their children—especially those, who are depressed, have poor problem-solving skills, or use drugs or alcohol—do not have access to firearms. Parents must also be educated on the warning signs of suicide (Box 17-11).

Motivation

Suicidal ideation is not uncommon in adolescents. It represents numerous fantasies, such as relief from suffering, a means of gaining comfort and sympathy, or a means of revenge against those who have hurt them. Adolescents have the erroneous perception that the act of suicide will evoke remorse and pity and that they will be able to return and witness the grief. Angry children who are unable to punish directly those who have injured or insulted them may take revenge on those who love them through self-destruction

BOX 17-11 ■ Warning Signs of Suicide

Preoccupation with themes of death—focuses on morbid thoughts
Wants to give away cherished possessions
Talks of own death, desire to die
Loss of energy—loss of interest, listlessness
Exhaustion without obvious cause
Changes in sleep patterns—too much or too little
Increased irritability, argumentativeness, or stubbornness
Physical complaints—recurrent stomachaches, headaches
Repeated visits to physician, nurse practitioner, or emergency department for treatment of injuries
Reckless behavior
Antisocial behavior—engages in drinking, uses drugs, fights, commits acts of vandalism, runs away from home, becomes sexually promiscuous
Sudden change in school performance—lowered grades, cutting classes, dropping out of activities
Resists or refuses to go to school
Remains distant, sad, remote—flat affect, frozen facial expression
Describes self as worthless
Sudden cheerfulness following deep depression
Social withdrawal from friends, activities, interests that were previously enjoyed
Impaired concentration
Dramatic change in appetite

("They'll be sorry when they find me dead"; "They'll be sorry they were mean to me").

For adolescents who are severely depressed, suicide seems to be the only release from their despair. These youngsters rarely provide evidence of their intent, and frequently conceal their suicidal thoughts. Many adolescents, however, tell their peers of their suicidal thoughts or plans but avoid telling adults. Social isolation is a significant factor in distinguishing adolescents who will kill themselves from those who will not. It is also more characteristic of those who complete suicide than of those who make attempts or threats.

The frequency of *contagion,* or *copycat suicides* (i.e., an increase in youth suicide that occurs after the suicide of one teenager is publicized) is disturbing and may indicate that teenagers perceive suicide as "glamorous." In addition, young people may not realize the finality of suicide, because they have become desensitized from constantly viewing violence and death on television.

Diagnostic Evaluation

Depression is common among adolescents who attempt suicide. Depression is characterized by both subjective symptoms and objective signs that reflect the adolescent's sadness and despair. Adolescents describe feelings of sadness, despair, helplessness, hopelessness, boredom, loss of interest, and isolation. They may also feel self-reproach, self-deprecation, and guilt. Subjective symptoms of depression or specific changes in behavior place an adolescent at risk for suicide.

Therapeutic Management

Threats of suicide should always be taken seriously. There has been a tendency to dismiss a suicide attempt as an impulsive act resulting from a temporary crisis or depression. If a sui-

cide attempt fails to draw attention to their problems or makes them worse, the child or adolescent may conclude that suicide is the only answer. Children need to know that someone cares and must be provided with swift and efficient crisis intervention. Although ordinary practitioners can manage an acute depressive reaction without difficulty, the youngster who has made a serious attempt or has a specific plan for suicide should receive immediate attention and competent psychiatric care.

NURSING ALERT

Adolescents who express suicidal feelings and have a specific plan should be monitored at all times. They should not have access to firearms, prescription or over-the-counter drugs, belts, scarves, shoestrings, sharp objects, matches, or lighters. If they are intoxicated, they must be restrained or placed in a protective environment until a psychiatrist or psychologist can assess them.

Nursing Considerations

Care of the suicidal youngster includes early recognition, management, and prevention. The most important aspect of management is the recognition of warning signs that indicate a youngster is troubled and might attempt suicide. Health professionals must be alert to the signs of depression, and anyone who exhibits such behavior should be referred for thorough psychologic assessment. Depression is manifested differently in children and adolescents than in adults. In teens it may be masked by impulsive aggressive behaviors. Defiance, disobedience, behavior problems, and psychosomatic disturbances can indicate underlying depression, suicidal ideation, and impending suicide attempts.

NURSING ALERT

No threat of suicide should be ignored or challenged. Threats are a symptom that must be taken seriously. Too often, suicidal threats or minor attempts are confused with bids for attention. It is also a mistake to be lulled into a false sense of security when the adolescent's depression is apparently relieved. The improvement in attitude may mean that the youngster has made the decision and found the means to carry out the threat.

Peers or other confidants are valuable observers and excellent sources of information about potential suicide attempts. They may not be able to diagnose depression, but they are able to sense when a friend has undergone a marked personality change. It is important to emphasize that the peer who detects any changes in a friend is a potential rescuer and should not remain silent about the observations. Friendship does not imply collusion. A peer who believes that a friend may be suicidal should alert someone who can help (e.g., a parent, teacher, guidance counselor, school nurse).

Routine health assessments of adolescents should include questions that assess the presence of suicidal ideation or intent. The following questions can be asked (Greydanus and Pratt, 1995):

■ Do you consider yourself more a happy person, an unhappy person, or somewhere in the middle?
■ Have you ever been so unhappy or upset that you felt like being dead?

- Have you ever thought about hurting yourself?
- Have you ever developed a plan to hurt yourself or kill yourself?
- Have you ever attempted to kill yourself?

If children or adolescents express suicidal intent, nurses make a contract, asking them to sign an agreement that they will not attempt suicide during an agreed-on period and that they will call the 24-hour crisis line immediately if they feel that they cannot keep to their contract. The amount of time a youngster feels comfortable contracting is usually an indication of his or her risk and stability.

Because a suicide attempt is frequently an outgrowth of family distress, it is essential to intervene with the family. It is important to assess family interactions and to recognize disturbed relationships. The most effective approach is recognition of susceptible youngsters during the early stages of family distress so that family counseling can be started. Prevention must be directed toward improving childrearing practices through support and education of parents and changing societal conditions that generate defeat, despair, and maladaptive behavior.

Although confidentiality is an essential part of adolescent counseling, in the case of self-destructive behaviors confidentiality cannot be honored. Suicidal behavior is reported to the family and other professionals, and youngsters are informed that this will be done. Such action conveys an important message to the youth—that the professionals understand and care.

Many schools have instituted suicide prevention programs. These programs include services such as drop-in counseling and a peer-counseling telephone line. Information can also be obtained from the **American Association of Suicidology.***

KEY POINTS

- Smoking is a significant problem among teenagers; reasons for smoking include social pressures, mass media influence, and a need to develop a self-concept.

- Participation in sports predisposes children and adolescents to both acute injuries and overuse syndromes.

- Alterations in growth and maturation may be manifested as short or tall stature, precocious puberty, or delayed sexual development.

- Tools for assessment of growth include a family history, previous growth patterns, physical examination, bone age determination, and endocrine studies.

- The most frequent health problems related to the female reproductive system involve menstrual dysfunction.

- Health problems related to sexuality include pregnancy, sexual assault, and sexually transmitted diseases; prevention includes sex education and contraceptive counseling.

- Eating disorders observed in middle and late childhood include obesity, anorexia nervosa, and bulimia.

- Behavior problems in middle childhood can result from attention deficit hyperactivity disorder, enuresis, encopresis, school

phobia, recurrent abdominal pain, childhood depression, conversion reaction, and childhood schizophrenia.

- The substances abused by children and adolescents include alcohol, marijuana, narcotics, central nervous system depressants, central nervous system stimulants, inhalants, and mind-altering drugs.

- Signs of depression in children and adolescents are often subtle and require astute observation by parents and health professionals.

- Suicide, the deliberate act of self-injury with the intent to kill, is often associated with depression, substance abuse, difficulties in coping with stress, an affective disorder, or a disturbed family environment.

References

Albert B, Brown S, Flanigan C, editors: *14 and younger: the sexual behavior of young adolescents,* Washington, DC, 2003, National Campaign to Prevent Teen Pregnancy.

American Academy of Pediatrics, Committee on Adolescence: Suicide and suicide attempts in adolescents, *Pediatrics* 105(4):871-874, 2000.

American Academy of Pediatrics, Committee on Adolescence: Identifying and treating eating disorders, *Pediatrics* 111(1):204-211, 2003.

American Academy of Pediatrics, Committee on Adolescence: Care of the adolescent sexual assault victim, *Pediatrics* 107(6):1476-1479, 2001.

American Psychiatric Association: *Diagnostic and statistical manual of mental disorders,* ed 4 (DSM-IV TR), Washington, DC, 2000, The Association.

Ariza AJ, Greenberg RS, Unger R: Childhood overweight: management approaches in young children, *Pediatr Annu* 33(1):33-44, 2004.

Aschenbrenner DS: New drug for ADHD, *Am J Nurs* 103(4):63, 2003.

Barone SR, Krilov LR: Infectious mononucleosis and other Epstein-Barr virus infections. In Hoekelman RA and others, editors: *Primary pediatric care,* ed 4, St Louis, 2001, Mosby.

Baughcum AE and others: Maternal perceptions of overweight preschool children, *Pediatrics* 106(6):1380-1386, 2000.

Binns JH, Ariza AJ: Guidelines help clinicians identify risk factors for overweight in children, *Pediatr Annu* 33(1):19-22, 2004.

Centers for Disease Control and Prevention: *Defining overweight and obesity,* Atlanta, 2002a, National Center for Chronic Disease Prevention and Health Promotion.

Centers for Disease Control and Prevention: *Sexually transmitted diseases treatment guidelines,* 51(no RR-6):1-76, 2002b.

Centers for Disease Control and Prevention: *HIV/AIDS surveillance report,* Atlanta, 1996, The Centers.

Clinical Practice Guideline: Treatment of the school-aged child with attention-deficit/hyperactivity disorder, *Pediatrics* 108(4):1033-1044, 2001.

Daniels SR: Abnormal weight gain and weight management: are carbohydrates the enemy? *J Pediatr* 142(3):225-227, 2003.

Darroch JE, Sings S: *Why is teenage pregnancy declining? The roles of abstinence, sexual activity and contraceptive use,* New York, 1999, Alan Guttmacher Institute.

Dennison BA, Boyer PS: Risk evaluation in pediatric practice: aids in prevention of childhood overweight, *Pediatr Annu* 33(1):25-30, 2004.

Division of Adolescent and School Health, National Center for Chronic Disease Prevention and Health Promotion: Youth risk behavior surveillance—United States, 1999, *MMWR* 49(SS05):1-96, 2000.

Goodman E, Capitman J: Depressive symptoms and cigarette smoking among teens, *Pediatrics* 106(4):748-755, 2000.

Gordon SM: *Adolescent drug use: trends in abuse, treatment and prevention,* Wernersville, Pa, 2000, Caron Foundation.

Greydanus DE, Pratt HD: Emotional and behavioral disorders of adolescence, part 2, *Adolesc Health Update* 8(1):1-8, 1995.

*Suite 408, 4201 Connecticut Avenue NW, Suite 408, Washington, DC 20008; (202) 237-2280; website: www.suicidology.org.

Grunbaum JA and others: Youth risk behavior surveillance—United States, 2001, *MMWR* 51(SS04):1-64, 2002.

Hillard PA, Nelson LM: Adolescent girls, the menstrual cycle and bone health, *J Pediatr Endocrinol Metab* 16(suppl 3):673-681, 2003.

Lindeke LL, Rogers S, Finley L: An update on growth charts, old and new, *Pediatr Nurs* 28(2):138-141, 2002.

McArdle WD, Katch FI, Katch VL: *Essentials of exercise physiology,* ed 2, Philadelphia, 2000, Lippincott Williams & Wilkins.

McWhorter JW, Wallmann HW, Alpert PT: The obese child: motivation as a tool for exercise, *J Pediatr Health Care* 17(1):11-17, 2003.

Michelson D and others: Atomoxetine in the treatment of children and adolescents with attention-deficit/hyperactivity disorder: a randomized, placebo-controlled, dose-response study, *Pediatrics* 108:E83, 2001.

Moolchan ET, Ernst M, Henningfield JE: A review of tobacco smoking in adolescents: treatment implications, *J Am Acad Child Adolesc Psychiatry* 39(6):682-693, 2000.

Moran R: Evaluation and treatment of childhood obesity, *Am Fam Physician* 59(4):861-868, 1999.

Moran R: Breaking the cycle of childhood obesity, *Clin Advisor* 6(2):62-67, 2003.

Myers SM, Eisenhauer NJ, Ryan ME: ADHD: It is real, and it can be treated, *Clin Advisor* 6(3):15-25, 2003.

National Task Force on the Prevention and Treatment of Obesity: Overweight, obesity and health risk, *Arch Intern Med* 160:898, 2000.

Neinstein LS: *Adolescent health care: a practical guide,* ed 4, Philadelphia, 2002, Lippincott Williams & Wilkins.

Ogden CL and others: Prevalence and trends in overweight among US children and adolescents, 1999-2000, *JAMA* 288:1728-1732, 2002.

Patel M, Minshal L: Management of sexual assault, *Emerg Clin North Am* 19(3):817-831, 2001.

Patten CA and others: Depressive symptoms and cigarette smoking predict development and persistence of sleep problems in US adolescents, *Pediatrics* 106(2):E23, 2000.

Rappaport LA: Enuresis. In Levine M and others: *Developmental-behavioral pediatrics,* ed 2, Philadelphia, 1992, WB Saunders.

Rigotti NA, Lee JE, Wechsler H: US college student's use of tobacco products: results of a national survey, *JAMA* 284(6):699-705, 2000.

Rojas NL, Killen JD, Haydel KF, Robinson TN: Nicotine dependence among adolescent smokers, *Arch Pediatr Adolesc Med* 152(2):151-156, 1998.

Schneider MB, Fisher MM: Anorexia and bulimia nervosa. In Hoeckelman RA, editor: *Primary pediatric care,* ed 4, St Louis, 2001, Mosby.

Schwimmer JB: Managing overweight in older children and adolescents, *Pediatr Annu* 33(1):39-44, 2004.

Selekman J, Snyder M: Learning disabilities and/or attention deficit disorder. In Jackson P, Vessey JA, editors: *Primary care of children with chronic conditions,* ed 3, St Louis, 2000, Mosby.

Shulman ST: The overweight epidemic, *Pediatr Annu* 33(1):6, 2004.

Sondike S and others: Effects of a low-carbohydrate diet on weight loss and cardiovascular risk factors in overweight adolescents, *J Pediatr* 142(3):253-258, 2003.

Strauss RS: Childhood obesity and self-esteem, *Pediatrics* 105(1):E15. 2000.

Sundelin-Wahlsten V, Ahmad A, von Knorring A-L: Traumatic experiences and post-traumatic stress reactions in children from Kurdistan and Sweden, *Acta Paediatr* 90:563-568, 2001.

Teare C, English A: Nursing practice and statutory rape: effects of reporting and enforcement on access to care for adolescents, *Nurs Clin North Am* 37:393-404, 2002.

Timmreck LS, Reindollar RH: Contemporary issues in primary amenorrhea, *Obstet Gynecol Clin* 30:2, 2003.

US Department of Health and Human Services: *National household survey on drug abuse, 1999,* Washington, DC, 1999, Substance Abuse and Mental Health Services Administration.

Wax, PM: Just a click away: recreational drug web sties on the internet, *Pediatrics* 109(6):E96, 2002.

Wilson ML, Murphy PA: Herbal and dietary therapies for primary and secondary dysmenorrhea, *Cochrane Database Syst Rev* 3:CD002124, 2001.

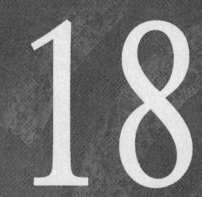

Chronic Illness, Disability, or End-of-Life Care for the Child and Family

MELODY BROWN-HELLSTEN

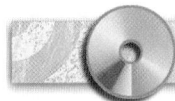

Remember to check out your companion CD-ROM

http://evolve.elsevier.com/Wong/essentials/

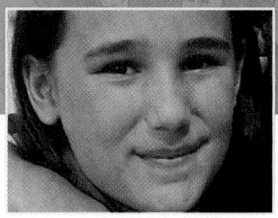

CHAPTER OUTLINE

RELATED TOPICS and ADDITIONAL RESOURCES

IN TEXT

Childhood Morbidity, *Ch. 1*
Communicating With Families, *Ch. 6*
Compliance, *Ch. 22*
Cultural/Religious Influences on Health Care, *Ch. 4*
Developmental Assessment, *Ch. 7*
Discharge Planning and Home Care: High-Risk Newborn, *Ch. 9*
General, *Ch. 21*
Family Assessment, *Ch. 6*
Family-Centered Care, *Ch. 1*
Family-Centered Care of the Child During Illness and Hospitalization, *Ch. 21*

Family-Centered Home Care, *Ch. 20*
Health Promotion: Infant, *Ch. 10;* Toddler, *Ch. 12;* Preschooler, *Ch. 13;* School-Age Child, *Ch. 15;* Adolescent, *Ch. 16*
Mortality, *Ch. 1*
Nursing Care of the High-Risk Newborn and Family, *Ch. 9*
Pain Management, *Ch. 21*
School Phobia, *Ch. 17*

CD COMPANION

Critical Thinking Exercise—Neonatal Loss
Case Study—The Dying Child

Guidelines—Promoting Normalization; Informing the Family of a Serious Condition; Assessing Coping Behaviors; Encouraging Expression of Emotion; Supporting Grieving Families
Nursing Care Plans
NCLEX-Style Review Questions

evolve WEBSITE

WebLinks
NCLEX-Style Review Questions

LEARNING OBJECTIVES
On completion of this chapter the reader will be able to:

- Identify the scope of and changing trends in care of children with special needs.
- Identify the major reactions of and effects on the family with a child with a special need.
- Define the stages of adjustment to the diagnosis of a chronic condition.

- Recognize the impact of the illness or disability on the developmental stages of childhood.
- Outline nursing interventions that promote the family's optimal adjustment to the child's chronic disorder.

- Outline nursing interventions that support the family at the time of death.
- Define the usual symptoms of normal grief.

PERSPECTIVES ON THE CARE OF CHILDREN WITH SPECIAL NEEDS

SCOPE OF THE PROBLEM

A number of terms and defining characteristics have been used to describe chronic illness and disability in children (Box 18-1). In recent years there have been continuing efforts to develop a definition that better identifies the numbers of children living with chronic conditions, as well as the impact on health and social services (Jackson, 2000). Currently children with special health care needs are defined as (Msall and others, 2003; Newacheck and others, 1998):

Children who have or are at increased risk for a chronic physical, developmental, behavioral, or emotional condition and who also require health and related services of a type or amount beyond that generally required by children.

Ongoing progress in medical and technologic disease management has contributed to the growing number of children with special health care needs. The number of US children with AIDS diagnosed each year had declined by 75% from 1992 to 2000 (Yogev and Chadwick, 2004). Technologic advances have substantially increased the survival of extremely- and very-low-birth-weight infants (Jackson, 2000). Children with disabilities are more likely to be in poor health than children without disabilities (Newacheck and Halfon, 1998). The result of such progress is an estimated 15% to 18% of the children in the United States living with a chronic

BOX 18-1 ■ Common Terms Regarding Children With Special Needs

Chronic illness—A condition that interferes with daily functioning for more than 3 months in a year, causes hospitalization of more than 1 month in a year, or (at time of diagnosis) is likely to do either of these
Congenital disability—A disability that has existed since birth but is not necessarily hereditary
Developmental delay—A maturational lag; an abnormal, slower rate of development in which a child demonstrates a functioning level below that observed in normal children of the same age
Developmental disability—Any mental and/or physical disability that is manifested before age 22 years and is likely to continue indefinitely
Disability—A functional limitation that interferes with a person's ability, for example, to walk, lift, hear, or learn
Handicap—A condition or barrier imposed by society, the environment, or one's own self; not a synonym for disability
Impairment—A loss or abnormality of structure or function
Technology-dependent child—A child between the ages of birth and 21 years with a chronic disability that requires the routine use of a medical device to compensate for the loss of a life-sustaining body function; daily ongoing care and/or monitoring is required by trained personnel

Adapted from Westbrook LE, Silver EJ, Stein RE: Implications for estimates of disability in children: a comparison of definitional components, *Pediatrics* 101(6):1025-1030, 1998; Newacheck PW, Halfon N: Prevalence and impact of disabling chronic conditions in childhood, *Am J Public Health* 88(4):610-617, 1998.

illness or disability and requiring specialized health care of a type or amount beyond that generally required by children (Perrin, 2004).

The most commonly occurring conditions causing disability are diseases of the respiratory tract and impairments of speech, special senses, and intelligence. Mental and nervous system disorders account for about one sixth of all childhood disability (Newacheck and Halfon, 1998).

The impact of chronic illness and disability in children is wide ranging. Chronic conditions in children present most families with additional tasks, responsibilities, and concerns (Ray, 2002). A child's activity level and developmental opportunities can be affected. Days can be lost from school. Children with chronic illness or disability may be at increased risk for behavior or emotional problems. Parents may lose days from work, experience financial strain, and be challenged both emotionally and physically as they cope with care of the child.

Siblings are also affected by having a "different" brother or sister and may simultaneously feel guilt and anger/jealousy toward their ill sibling. Additionally, secondary losses such as the ability to participate in extracurricular activities or social events occur because of routines imposed by the affected child's chronic condition.

TRENDS IN CARE
Developmental Focus

Focusing on the child's *developmental level* rather than chronologic age or diagnosis emphasizes the child's abilities and strengths rather than disabilities. Attention focuses on normalizing experiences, adapting the environment, and promoting coping skills. Nurses often are in vital positions to redirect attention from the pathologic model with its focus on weaknesses and problems to the developmental model to meet the unique needs of the child and family.

A developmental focus also considers family development. The life cycle of the family unit reflects changing ages and needs of family members, as well as changing external demands. A family member's serious illness or disability can cause significant stress or crisis at any stage of the family life cycle. Just as with individual development, family development may be interrupted or even regress to an earlier level of functioning. Nurses can use the concept of family development to plan meaningful interventions and evaluate care (see Developmental Theory, Chapter 3).

Family-Centered Care

Children's physical and emotional health, as well as cognitive and social functioning, are strongly influenced by how well their families function (Schor, 2003). The importance of family-centered care—a philosophy that considers the family as the constant in the child's life—is especially evident in the care of children with special needs (see also Family-Centered Care, Chapter 1). As parents learn about the youngster's health care needs, they often become experts in delivering care. Health care providers, including nurses, are adjuncts to the child's care and need to form partnerships with parents. Collaboration is essential to forming trusting and effective partnerships and has the goal of finding the best ways to meet the needs of the child and family. Collaborative relationships are characterized by communication, dialogue, active listening, awareness, and acceptance of differences (Schor, 2003).

Family–Health Care Provider Communication

The disclosure of a serious acute or chronic illness of a child is one of the most stressful aspects of communication between families and health care professionals. Often, parents have suspected for some time that there is something wrong with their child and feel that their concerns were minimized or ignored by health care professionals (Whitehead and Gosling, 2003; Thomlinson, 2002; Cohen, 1995). After a diagnosis is made, numerous studies have shown that parents are not always satisfied with the way in which information is given. Factors that influence parent dissatisfaction with communication include unsympathetic and brief diagnostic interviews, lack of privacy during diagnostic discussions, and not being provided the opportunity to ask questions. Conversely, parents report satisfaction when they perceive the health care providers providing information in an open and honest manner with respect for the parents' need for privacy and time to express emotions and ask questions (Davies, Davis, and Seibert, 2003). Similar factors are important in communication of changes in the child's condition throughout the course of the illness.

Providing information to families with a chronically ill child should be a process of repeated discussions to allow the family to process the information and their reactions to that information, and allow them to ask for clarification and further information. Nurses play an important role in ensuring that families' needs are met during discussions related to the child's diagnosis, condition, and treatment. This requires assessment regarding how much information the family is comfortable with, what they understand of the information already given to them, and how they are coping with the information both cognitively and emotionally. Nurses should ensure that the appropriate health care professionals address any concerns or further questions that families may have.

Establishing Therapeutic Relationships

Another important aspect of family-centered care of chronically ill children is establishing a therapeutic relationship with the child and family. Families, most often the mother, take on enormous responsibility in providing technical care and symptom management of their child's condition outside the health care institution (O'Brien and Wegner, 2002; Swallow and Jacoby, 2001). To build successful therapeutic relationships with families, it is necessary for nurses to recognize parents' expertise with regard to their child's condition and needs. Care conferences, especially multidisciplinary meetings that include the family and key health professionals, provide an opportunity for joint sharing of ideas and expression of feelings or concerns.

Individual discussions, especially with the case manager, primary nurse, clinical nurse specialist, or nurse practitioner, help establish a consistent and flexible plan of care that can prevent conflicts or deal with these conflicts before they disrupt care. In family-centered care, the goal is to maintain the integrity of the leadership role and support the family during times of crisis or stress.

The Role of Culture in Family-Centered Care

Issues of culture, ethnicity, and race affect access to services, utilization, and follow-through with referrals and recommendations (Zuvekas and Taliaferro, 2003; Wise and others, 2002; Wood and others, 2002). For some ethnic and minority populations, cultural understandings of illness and disability, the structure of family life, social roles for individuals who are disabled, and other factors related to the perception of children may differ from those of "mainstream" American culture. These factors may affect family needs and family choices regarding the care of their child with special needs.

Although culture cannot completely explain how an individual will think and act, understanding cultural perspectives can help the nurse anticipate and understand why families may make certain decisions. Cultural attributes such as values and beliefs regarding illness or disability and its causation, social roles for the ill or disabled, family structure, the role of children, childrearing practices, self versus group orientation, spirituality, and time orientation also affect a family's response to illness or disability in a child (Sterling and Peterson, 2003; Carter, 2002; Marshall and others, 2003; Rehm, 1999).

When parents are informed of their child's chronic illness, interpreters familiar with both culture and language should be used. Children, family members, and friends of the family should not be used as translators because their presence may prevent parents from an open discussion of the issues. When working with people of other cultural backgrounds, nurses must listen carefully with an initial goal of understanding and articulating the family's perspective. The ability to interpret the mainstream medical culture to the family is also important. Furthermore, every effort is made to incorporate traditional cultural beliefs of a family into treatment plans. Developing a plan of care in conjunction with the family, considering their preferences and priorities, is an important first step in formulating a plan of care that best meets the family's needs, no matter what their cultural background (Ahmann, 1994).

Shared Decision Making

Shared decision making among the child, family, and health care team is the desired result of open, honest, culturally sensitive communication and the establishment of a therapeutic relationship between the family and health care providers. In a shared decision-making model the health care professionals provide honest, clear information regarding diagnosis, prognosis, treatment options, and risk/benefit assessment. The patient and/or family then share information with the health care team regarding important family values, acceptable levels of discomfort or inconvenience, and the ability to comply with treatments being recommended (Charles, Gafni, and Whelan, 1997). This process allows for all options to be discussed with regard to their consequence risks and benefits to the child and family, the prognosis or expected course of the illness, and the impact on the family's resources (Box 18-2).

Normalization

Normalization refers to behaviors and intentions of the disabled to integrate into society by living life as persons without a disability would (Morse, Wilson, and Penrod, 2000). For the chronically ill or disabled child, such behaviors could include attending school, pursuing hobbies and recreational interests, and achieving employment and a level of independence in their life. For their families, it may en-

BOX 18-2 ■ Facilitating Shared Decision Making

Continually assess the impact of the child's illness and treatment on the family.
Provide honest, accurate information regarding the trajectory of the disease, anticipated complications, and prognostic information.
Discuss what the family desires for the child's quality of life.
Avoid personal opinion or judgment of the family's questions and decisions.

tail adapting the ill or disabled child's health and physical needs into the family routine (McDougal, 2002).

Children with chronic illness and disability and their families face numerous challenges in achieving "normalization." Families move between the "normal" of living with the experience of chronic childhood illness and the "normal" or the healthy outside world, and often redefine "normal" based on their particular experiences, needs, and circumstances (Nelson, 2002; Deatrick, Knafl, and Murphy-Moore, 1999).

Nurses can assist families with normalizing their lives by assessing social support systems, coping strategies, family cohesiveness, and family/community resources. Interventions should focus on encouraging families to reduce stress through delegation of care and family tasks, identifying ways to incorporate care into current routines, structuring the home environment to encourage the child's engagement in age-appropriate activities, and ensuring families have access to appropriate community support services. Being supportive of the child's illness and treatment and actively including the family in all aspects of care will improve their self-esteem and promote further development (Shepard and Mahon, 2000).

Home care represents the return to a system and set of priorities in which family values are as important in the care of a child with a chronic health problem as they are in the care of other children. Home care seeks to achieve goals that are consistent with the developmental model (Stein, 1985):

- Normalize the life of a child with special needs, including those with technologically complex care, in a family and community context and setting.
- Minimize the disruptive impact of the child's condition on the family.
- Foster the child's maximum growth and development.

With appropriate training and support, families provide complex procedures and treatments in the home. Parents are challenged to retain a homelike setting among monitors, ventilators, and other sophisticated equipment. Throughout the text, home care is discussed as appropriate for specific conditions. The process of transition from hospital to home is elaborated in Chapters 20 and 21.

Paralleling normalization and home care is the process of *mainstreaming,* or integrating children with special needs into regular classrooms. Just as the home is the natural environment for children, so school must also be included as an essential component of the children's overall physical, intellectual, and social development. Children who attend school have the advantages of learning and socializing with a wide group of peers. There is an increased focus on individualization as the academic needs of these children are planned along with those of the rest of the students.

A variety of supplemental programs have been designed in the school system to accommodate special needs, both at school age and younger, through early intervention, which consists of any sustained and systematic effort to assist children from birth to age 3 years who are young, disabled, and developmentally vulnerable. This change and increasing opportunities for normalization for children with special needs in large part have resulted from the passage of Public Law 94-142 (the Education of All Handicapped Children Act of 1975) and its 1990 amendments (Public Law 101-47b), which changed the name of the act to the Individuals with Disabilities Education Act (IDEA); Public Law 99-457 (the Education of the Handicapped Act Amendments of 1986, which directs states to develop and implement statewide comprehensive, coordinated, multidisciplinary interagency programs of early intervention services for infants and toddlers with disabilities, as well as support services for their families); and the Americans With Disabilities Act (ADA) of 1990 (see also Chapter 1). Nurses can provide parents with information about these laws and in some cases may participate in the development of individualized educational programs (IEPs) or individualized family service plans (IFSPs) for children with special needs.

Managed Care

Managed care programs have become the major form of health care provision in the United States (Jackson, 2000). The transition to this model of care both offers opportunities and presents challenges with respect to the care of children with special health care needs. Managed care may promote continuity and coordination of care. At the same time, some research has shown decreased access to pediatric specialists and health-related services in managed care environments.

Managing care for chronically ill children differs greatly from managing care for chronically ill adults in three major ways. First, the large number of rare disorders and low prevalence of children with such disorders makes it difficult to monitor the overall quality of care for the total population of chronically ill children. Second, the influence of the child's growth and development on aspects of onset, impact, treatment, and outcomes of chronic conditions varies with the different developmental stages. Third, children rely on adults for access to health care and follow-up with treatment regimens, making it necessary to manage the child's care in the context of the family (American Academy of Pediatrics, 1998; Kuhlthau and others, 1998).

THE FAMILY OF THE CHILD WITH SPECIAL NEEDS

A major goal in working with the family of a child with special needs is to support the family's coping and promote their optimal functioning throughout the child's life. Long-term, comprehensive, family-centered approaches extend beyond supporting the child and family during the critical periods of diagnosis and hospitalization. Rather, comprehensive care involves forming parent-professional partnerships that can support a family's adaptation to the many changes that may be necessary in day-to-day life, determine expectations of and for the child, and provide a long-term perspective (Box 18-3).

BOX 18-3 ■ Adaptive Tasks of Parents Having Children With Chronic Conditions

1. Accept the child's condition.
2. Manage the child's condition on a day-to-day basis.
3. Meet the child's normal developmental needs.
4. Meet the developmental needs of other family members.
5. Cope with ongoing stress and periodic crises.
6. Assist family members to manage their feelings.
7. Educate others about the child's condition.
8. Establish a support system.

From Canam C: Common adaptive tasks facing parents of children with chronic conditions, *J Adv Nurs* 18:46-53, 1993.

The impact of a child's medical or developmental condition is often experienced as a crisis at the time of diagnosis, which may be at the time of birth, following a long period of physical or psychologic testing, or immediately after a tragic injury. It may also begin before the diagnosis is made, when parents are aware that something is wrong with their child but before medical confirmation (Whitehead and Gosling, 2003; Thomlinson, 2002; Cohen, 1995).

The time of diagnosis is a critical time for parents. Several factors can make it particularly difficult, including a long duration of uncertainty in the diagnostic process and negative perceptions of chronic illness or disability (Cohen, 1995; Garwick and others, 1995). Planning the setting for informing parents, assessing the family's background knowledge and experience, choosing strategies that fit the family's situation, and evaluating the family's understanding of the information will encourage optimal support at the time of diagnosis.

IMPACT OF THE CHILD'S CHRONIC ILLNESS OR DISABILITY

Each family who has a child with special needs is affected by the experience. The effects on the parents and their responses are so critical that they directly influence the other members' reactions and the child's own coping.

Parents

Besides grieving for the loss of a perfect child, parents may or may not receive positive feedback from transactions with their child. Many parents feel satisfaction and fulfillment from the parenting role. For others, parenting may be a series of unrewarding experiences that contribute to parental feelings of inadequacy and failure (Box 18-4). These responses may be most evident in parents who are responsible for the child's care. For example, parents may become preoccupied with their ability to carry out certain procedures, overlooking the child's personal comfort and satisfaction or failing to offer praise for anything less than perfect cooperation or performance. They may pursue a frustrating activity until they achieve "success"—long after the child has become irritable and uncooperative. As a result, parents can become caught in a pattern of interaction that is mutually unrewarding and minimally productive. For these parents, several strategies may be helpful: education regarding what can reasonably be expected of their child, assistance in identifying the child's strengths, praise for a parental job well done, and finding respite care so that parents can renew their energies.

Parental Roles. Parenting a child with a chronic illness or disability is above and beyond that of raising a typical child. In addition to attending to the routine aspects of parenting, parents of chronically ill children take on the added responsibility of complex technical care and symptom management, advocacy, and seeking and coordinating health and social services for their ill/disabled child. These added responsibilities must then be balanced with the needs of other family members, extended family and friends, and personal health and obligations to minimize consequences to the overall functioning of the family (Ray, 2002).

Enormous demands may be placed on parental time, energy, and financial resources. Depending on the roles assumed by each partner, these responsibilities may be shared or shifted more heavily to one member. In a shared approach, parents often divide tasks in a very specific way, according to their skills or level of comfort. For example, the parent with patience for waiting may be the logical person to take the child for tests, examinations, and procedures. The parent who deals best with the sickness and side effects of treatment can ready the environment for the child's return home. It is important for nurses to realize that the absence of one parent from the hospital or clinic does not necessarily indicate that the shared parent pattern is not in effect. On the other hand, making efforts to involve both parents in decision making and in learning how to care for the child's special needs can reduce some of the burden of care often placed on mothers.

In other families, changing sex roles mean added responsibilities for one parent. For example, the working mother may feel the need to continue employment to help defray the expenses, but she also incurs the added burden of additional child/home responsibilities. Eventually marital conflicts arise as one partner views his or her responsibilities as unequal.

In addition, the partner who is not included in the caregiving activities may feel neglected because all of the atten-

tion is directed toward the child and resentful that he or she is not sufficiently informed to be competent in the care. Without active participation in the child's care, the parent has little appreciation of the time and energy involved in performing those activities. When this partner does attempt to participate, the other parent frequently criticizes the less skillful efforts. As a result, communication and support for each other may be adversely affected.

Although marital stress often increases, divorce rates in these families are not substantially higher than those for the general population. Research suggests that families of children with chronic conditions who adjust poorly are those who had problems before the illness. A couple's marital functioning before the birth or diagnosis of a child with special needs may well be the best predictor of long-term marital adjustment. Factors contributing to marital stress include decreased time spent in recreational activities, increased caregiving responsibilities, and fewer exchanges of affection (Quittner and others, 1998).

The nurse can assist parents in avoiding role conflicts by providing anticipatory guidance early on. Teaching should address stressors often identified as having an impact on the marriage: (1) the burden of care at home assumed by primarily one parent, (2) the financial burden, (3) the fear of the child dying, (4) pressure from relatives, (5) the hereditary nature of the disease (if applicable), and (6) fear of pregnancy. Other causes of tension may center on the inconveniences associated with care, such as long waits for an appointment, lack of parking near care facilities, or lack of overnight accommodations. Certainly, these last stressors are within health professionals' domain to minimize, if not eliminate.

Mother/Father Differences. Mothers and fathers in the same family often adjust and cope differently as parents of a child with special needs. Some mothers experience a peaks-and-valleys periodic crisis pattern, whereas most fathers tend to experience a steady, gradual recovery. Some research suggests that mothers of children with certain conditions may be more susceptible to psychologic distress and feeling worn out than fathers (Tong and others, 2002). Mothers are more likely to have to deal with forfeiting or delaying personal goals. Mothers often have greater needs for social support and positive reappraisal of the situation, whereas fathers are more likely to use self-controlling behaviors to cope (Goldbeck, 2001; Mastroyannopoulou and others, 1997).

The father of a child with special needs struggles with issues that may be quite distinct from those of the mother. He may feel that his role of protector is challenged because he does not know how to help and cannot protect the family from the seemingly overwhelming recurring problems. Dreams of lineage, ego fulfillment, and athletic and vocational achievement are threatened and in turn may threaten the father's self-esteem. Because the traditional paternal role, particularly with sons, emphasizes joint recreation over caregiving, fathers seem to have more difficulty adjusting to a son with special needs than to a daughter with special needs. With today's increased emphasis on fathers' involvement in the lives of their children, this loss is felt more profoundly than in the past. The extensive stresses in the family can leave the father feeling depressed, weak, guilty,

BOX 18-4 ■ Anticipated Parental Stress Points

Diagnosis of the condition—Requires considerable learning, as well as dealing with emotional response

Developmental milestones—Times that children normally achieve walking, talking, and self-care are delayed or impossible for the child

Start of schooling—Particularly stressful are situations in which appropriate schooling will not be in a regular class placement

Reaching the ultimate attainment—Situations, such as realizing that ambulation will be impossible or that the child will not learn to read, must be handled

Adolescence—Issues such as sexuality and independence become prominent

Future placement—Decisions about placement must be made when the child becomes an adult or when the parents can no longer care for the child

Death of the child

powerless, isolated, embarrassed, and very angry. Fearful that he will lose control or be viewed as weak or ineffectual, however, the father will often hide his feelings and display an outward confidence that may lead others to believe that everything is fine. Feelings are further exacerbated by a health care system that frequently excludes and disregards men. Too often the father feels like an afterthought in the care of his child (May, 1996).

Fathers worry about what the future holds for their children, as well as about their ability to manage the increasing financial burden. Some fathers escape in their work as a means for dulling the pain. Common coping strategies are problem oriented and include praying, getting information, looking at options, and weighing choices, in addition to withdrawal and being practical (Mastroyannopoulou and others, 1997).

Single-Parent Families.

Single-parent families are of special concern. The absence of a parent may result from divorce or death, or the parents may never have married. As the only parent of a child who may require extensive, sophisticated, and lifelong care, the single parent may feel an enormous burden. Available financial and emotional resources may already be stretched to the limit. A special effort should be made to assist the single parent in finding financial and support services that can ease the burden of care. Nurses can also assist the single parent in identifying helping roles that may be acceptable to relatives and friends.

Siblings

Results of studies on how siblings are affected by having a brother or sister with special needs are inconsistent. Generally, there is evidence that there is a negative effect on siblings of children with a chronic illness when compared with siblings of healthy children. This effect appears, however, to be decreasing in significance in recent years—most likely because of changes in public attitudes toward the ill and disabled (Sharpe and Rossiter, 2002). However, most investigators do agree that brothers and sisters of children with special needs are no more at risk for *severe* psychiatric problems than are siblings of children without chronic or disabling conditions.

There are a number of factors that increase the risk of negative effects for siblings of ill children. Responsibility for caregiving, differential treatment by parents, and limitations in family resources and recreational time are often the experience of siblings of ill/disabled children (Lobato and Kao, 2002). Some difficulties for siblings arise from the demands of the child's condition. For example, at diagnosis the child with special needs by necessity becomes the focus of parental attention and concern. Frequent hospitalizations or trips to the physician or clinic disrupt the family routine. Siblings are pushed to the background, often staying at the homes of family and friends. The child's condition may interfere with holiday celebrations, vacations, and other special events. Siblings may resent these intrusions, which frequently demand self-sacrifice. Their parents may be unable to attend their school functions, ball games, or other activities and at times may be physically and emotionally unavailable for them. The family's financial and emotional resources may be directed toward the child with special needs. When this occurs, there is often not only a decrease in normal family activities, but a decrease in personal items for the other children as well. Not

surprisingly, children with siblings who have chronic illnesses that affect day-to-day functioning appear to be more negatively affected than children of siblings with less intense daily assistance needs (Sharpe and Rossiter, 2002).

Many of the difficulties that siblings encounter are a result of the nature of the sibling relationship itself (see Chapter 3). It is within the sibling relationship that children learn to share, compete, and compromise with others close to them in status. The equality of this relationship is often lost when a brother or sister has special needs. The child with special needs is suddenly "out of tune," unable to contribute to the family or the sibling relationship in his or her usual way. Because identification is another characteristic of sibling relationships, some siblings believe that they, too, will "catch" the condition, a reasonable assumption in light of experiences with contagious diseases, such as chickenpox. Identification, combined with a young child's egocentric thinking, may lead a sibling to feel responsible for a brother or sister's condition. For example, siblings may believe that playing rough with their brother or sister or even thinking bad thoughts about the sibling caused the condition.

Most brothers and sisters experience mixed and sometimes contradictory feelings. They may feel left out of new family developments and changing roles, guilty that they escaped getting the condition, or sad when their brother or sister is unable to participate in a particular activity or event. Some siblings feel embarrassed and ashamed; having a child in the family who is ill, disfigured, or disabled marks the family as "different" (see Family Focus box). Some siblings worry about the health of the affected child (Faulkner, 1996). However, sibling relationships can show a rather usual pattern, consisting of both conflict and companionship. This suggests that although having an ill sibling can present challenges, the relationship may be important and possibly even enhanced between the ill child and his or her sibling (Sharpe and Rossiter, 2002) (Box 18-5).

An important factor in sibling adjustment and coping is information and knowledge regarding their brother or sister's illness/disability. What siblings piece together or overhear is often much worse than the truth. Oftentimes they imagine gruesome things regarding the experiences related to the illness, treatment, and hospitalization (Shepard and Mahon, 2000). Parents are usually in the best position to impart information, although they are often overwhelmed with the medical crisis at hand (Fleitas, 2000). Nurses can encourage parents to talk with the siblings about how they perceive their sick brother or sister and to be accepting of the siblings' feelings. Nurses can be ideal educators and

FAMILY FOCUS

Reflection of an Older Brother

My youngest sister, Kerry, was on an apnea monitor 3 years ago, when I was 15. I was never embarrassed about Kerry being on the monitor, except for the time it went off in church and everyone turned around to look at us.

Joey Bellino
Oldest sibling of an infant on an apnea monitor
Washington, DC

BOX 18-5 ■ Supporting Siblings of Children With Special Needs

PROMOTE HEALTHY SIBLING RELATIONSHIPS

Value each child individually and avoid comparisons. Remind each child of his or her positive qualities and contribution to other family members.

Help siblings see the differences and similarities between themselves and a child with special needs. Create a climate in which children can achieve successes without feeling guilty.

Teach siblings ways to interact with the child.

Seek to be fair in terms of discipline, attention, and resources; require the affected child to do as much for himself or herself as possible.

Let siblings settle their own differences; intervene only to prevent siblings from hurting one another.

Legitimize reasonable anger. Even children with special needs behave badly sometimes.

Respect a sibling's reluctance to be with or to include the child with special needs in activities.

HELP SIBLINGS COPE

Listen to siblings to let them know that their thoughts and suggestions are valued.

Praise siblings when they have been patient, have sacrificed, or have been particularly helpful. Do not expect siblings to always act in this manner.

Acknowledge the personal strengths siblings have and their ability to cope with stress successfully.

Provide age-appropriate information about the child's condition, and update when appropriate.

Let teachers know what is happening so they can be understanding and helpful.

Recognize special stress times for siblings and plan to minimize negative effects.

Schedule special time with siblings; have a friend or family member substitute when parent is unavailable.

Encourage siblings to join or help establish a sibling support group.

Use the services of professionals when needed. If parent feels that such a service is necessary, it should be provided in as vigorous a manner as a service for the child with special needs.

INVOLVE SIBLINGS

Seek out ways to realistically include siblings in the care and treatment of the child with special needs.

Limit caregiving responsibilities and give recognition when siblings perform them.

Develop a library of children's books on special needs.

Invite siblings to attend meetings to develop plans for the child with special needs (e.g., individualized educational program, individualized family service plan).

Discuss future plans with them.

Solicit their ideas on treatment and service needs.

Have them visit professionals who work with the child.

Help them develop competencies to teach the child new skills.

Provide opportunities for siblings to advocate for the child.

Allow siblings to set their own pace for learning and involvement.

Modified from Powell T, Ogle P: Brothers and sisters—a special part of exceptional families, Baltimore, 1985, Paul H Brooks; Spokane Washington Deaconess Medical Center, Pediatric Oncology Unit: Tips for dealing with siblings, Candlelighters Childhood Cancer Found Q Newslett 11(3,4):7, 1987; and Carlson J, Leviton A, Mueller M: Services to siblings: an important component of family-centered practice, ACCH Advocate 1(1):53-56, 1993.

counselors of siblings during the course of their brother's or sister's illness (Shepard and Mahon, 2000).

Extended Family Members and Society

In addition to parents and siblings, significant nonnuclear family members or friends may experience the effects of a child's chronic illness or disability. Although extended family relationships are often helpful to parents in rearing a child with special needs, they may also be sources of stress. For example, grandparents or other well-meaning relatives may attempt to reassure the parents that the child "will grow out of" his or her slowness at a time when parents are struggling to accept reality.

Most grandparents experience some ambivalence: they love their grandchild and yet feel personal disappointment. They often experience a double grief, both for their grandchild and for their child, the parent. The future is now unpredictable not only for the grandchild, but for the child's parents as well. Grandparents do not often acknowledge these emotions and are left to adapt on their own. Support groups for grandparents, although uncommon, can be beneficial.

Considerable stress can also arise from nonfamilial sources, such as friends, neighbors, or strangers. Inability to cope with comments about the disorder or curious stares by others may foster the tendency to isolate and protect the child within the home. The family needs guidance in preparing for these inevitable experiences. Encouraging parents to dress the child as much as possible like other children is one approach. Good grooming is very important in minimizing differences in appearance. Through role-playing, parents can practice responses to comments such as "Is your child retarded?" or "Has he always been crippled?" Through parent groups, family members can share experiences and learn from each other about dealing with probing questions or unkind remarks. Such interventions should include the siblings and the affected child, who also must face and deal with these events.

Parents have to decide how much and what to tell relatives, friends, baby-sitters, and teachers. Concerns about discrimination are very real for parents and must be balanced with the need to share information so that the child receives appropriate care. The nurse can raise the issue by asking parents if they have concerns about how to inform others of the child's condition. Nurses may be able to offer advice regarding essential safety teaching for others who will care for the child.

COPING WITH ONGOING STRESS AND PERIODIC CRISES

Professionals can help families cope with stress by providing anticipatory guidance, providing emotional support, assisting the family in assessing and identifying specific stressors, aiding the family in developing coping mechanisms and problem-solving strategies, and working collaboratively with parents so that they become empowered in the process.

Concurrent Stresses Within the Family

The ability to deal with the overwhelming stresses of a lifelong disability or illness is challenged further when additional stresses are present. Stressors may be situational or developmental. They may be related to marital difficulties, sibling needs, homelessness, or social isolation. Some families may simultaneously be struggling with a family member's alcohol or other drug problem. Even the more minor stresses, such as arranging care for siblings, managing the home, and traveling to distant treatment centers, can challenge a family's ability to cope successfully.

For most families, regardless of their income or insurance coverage, financial concerns exist. The costs of caring for a child with special needs can be overwhelming. Nurses and social workers can help a family review various options for financial assistance, including insurance, managed care, or health maintenance organization (HMO) policies; Medicaid; Supplemental Security Income (SSI); Women, Infants, and Children program (WIC); the state Program for Children with Special Health Needs; disease-related associations; and local philanthropic organizations.

Coping Mechanisms

Coping mechanisms are behaviors aimed at reducing the tension caused by a crisis. *Approach behaviors* are coping mechanisms that result in movement toward adjustment and resolution of the crisis. *Avoidance behaviors* result in movement away from adjustment or maladaptation to the crisis. Several approach and avoidance behaviors used in coping with a chronic illness or disability are listed in the Guidelines box at right. None of the indices can be used singly to assess the possible success or failure in resolving the crisis. Each behavior must be viewed in the context of all of the variables affecting the family. For example, the observation of several avoidance behaviors in an emotionally healthy family may denote significantly less risk to the successful resolution of the crisis than an equal number of avoidance behaviors in an individual who has few available supports.

Parental Empowerment

Empowerment can be seen as a process of recognizing, promoting, and enhancing competence. For parents of children with chronic conditions, empowerment may occur gradually as strength and capabilities are drawn on to master the child's care, manage family life, and plan for the future. Advocating for the child and developing parent-professional partnerships are part of taking charge (Ray, 2002).

ASSISTING FAMILY MEMBERS IN MANAGING THEIR FEELINGS

Although some previous research has postulated stages of adaptation to a chronic illness or disability, there is a great deal of individual variation in responses to the diagnosis, adjustments made, and time frames for coming to terms with a diagnosis. It is important that professionals recognize and respect a wide range of reactions and coping mechanisms. In fact, members of the family of a child with a chronic illness or disability may experience a number of difficult emotions, including fear, guilt, anger, resentment, and anxiety. Learning to manage these emotions promotes adaptive coping (see Guidelines box at right). Support from professionals, other family members, and friends can assist family members in managing their feelings. The following discussion examines some common phases of adjustment and emotional reactions.

Shock and Denial

The initial diagnosis of a chronic illness or disability is often met with intense emotion and is characterized by shock, disbelief, and sometimes denial, especially if the disorder is not obvious, such as in chronic illness. Denial as a defense mech-

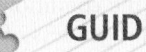

GUIDELINES

Assessing Coping Behaviors

APPROACH BEHAVIORS

Asks for information regarding diagnosis and child's present condition

Seeks help and support from others

Anticipates future problems; actively seeks guidance and answers

Endows the illness or disability with meaning

Shares burden of disorder with others

Plans realistically for the future

Acknowledges and accepts child's awareness of diagnosis and prognosis

Expresses feelings such as sorrow, depression, and anger and realizes reason for the emotional reaction

Realistically perceives child's condition; adjusts to changes

Recognizes own growth through passage of time, such as earlier denial and nonacceptance of diagnosis

Verbalizes possible loss of child

AVOIDANCE BEHAVIORS

Fails to recognize seriousness of child's condition despite physical evidence

Refuses to agree to treatment

Intellectualizes about the illness, but in areas unrelated to child's condition

Is angry and hostile to members of the staff, regardless of their attitude or behavior

Avoids staff, family members, or child

Entertains unrealistic future plans for child, with little emphasis on the present

Is unable to adjust to or accept a change in progression of disease

Continually looks for new cures with no perspective toward possible benefit

Refuses to acknowledge child's understanding of disease and prognosis

Uses magical thinking and fantasy, may seek "occult" help

Places complete faith in religion to point of relinquishing own responsibility

Withdraws from outside world; refuses help

Punishes self because of guilt and blame

Makes no change in lifestyle to meet needs of other family members

Resorts to excessive use of alcohol or drugs to avoid problems

Verbalizes suicidal intents

Is unable to discuss possible loss of child or previous experiences with death

anism is a necessary cushion to prevent disintegration and is a normal response to grieving for any type of loss. Probably all family members experience various degrees of adaptive denial as they learn of the impact that the diagnosis has on their lives.

Shock and denial can last from days to months, sometimes even longer. Examples of denial that may be exhibited at the time of diagnosis include the following:

1 Physician shopping
2 Attributing the symptoms of the actual illness to a minor condition
3 Refusing to believe the diagnostic tests
4 Delaying consent for treatment
5 Acting very happy and optimistic despite the revealed diagnosis

6 Refusing to tell or talk to anyone about the condition
7 Insisting that no one is telling the truth, regardless of others' attempts to do so
8 Denying the reason for admission
9 Asking no questions about the diagnosis, treatment, or prognosis

Generally, these mechanisms should be respected as short-term responses that allow individuals to distance themselves from the onslaught of a tremendous emotional impact and to collect and mobilize their energies toward goal-directed, problem-solving behaviors.

In some instances, various indicators of denial can actually be adaptive behaviors. Searching for another professional opinion may mean that parents cannot obtain answers to their questions or that they are looking for a different approach to treatment that better meets the needs of their child and family. Sometimes a delay in making decisions or a failure to ask questions simply reflects a lack of information.

In children, the importance of denial has repeatedly been demonstrated as a factor in their positive coping with the diagnosis. Denial allows the child to maintain hope in the face of overwhelming odds and to function adaptively and productively. Like hope, denial may be an adaptive mechanism for dealing with loss that persists until a family or patient is ready or needs other responses.

Denial is probably the least understood and most poorly dealt-with reaction. Health professionals typically label denial as "maladaptive" and act inappropriately by attempting to strip it away by repeated and sometimes blunt explanations of the prognosis. However, denial becomes maladaptive only when it prevents recognition of treatment or rehabilitative goals necessary for the child's optimal survival or development.

Adjustment

For most families, adjustment gradually follows shock and is usually characterized by an open admission that the condition exists. This stage may be accompanied by several responses, which are quite normal parts of the adaptation process. Probably the most universal of these feelings are *guilt* and *self-accusation.* Guilt is often greatest when the cause of the disorder is directly traceable to the parent, such as in genetic diseases or from accidental injury. However, it can occur even without any scientific or realistic basis for parental responsibility. Frequently the guilt stems from a false assumption that the disability is a result of personal failing or wrongdoing, such as not doing something correctly during pregnancy or the birth. Guilt may also be associated with cultural or religious beliefs. Some parents are convinced that they are being punished for some previous misdeed. Others may see the disorder as a sacrifice sent by God to test their religious strength and faith. With correct information, support, and time, most parents master guilt and self-accusation. The ability to master resentful and self-accusatory feelings of having "caused" the child's disorder is a crucial factor in determining the parents' acceptance of their child.

Children, too, may interpret their serious illness as retribution for past misbehavior. The nurse should be particularly sensitive to the child who passively accepts all painful procedures. This child may believe that such acts are inflicted as deserved punishment. It is vital that parents and health care professionals reassure children that their illness is not their fault.

Other common and normal reactions to a diagnosis are *bitterness* and *anger.* Anger directed inward may be evident as self-reproaching or punitive behavior, such as neglecting one's health and verbally degrading oneself. Anger directed outward may be manifested in either open arguments or withdrawal from communication and may be evident in the person's relationship with any number of individuals, such as the spouse, the child, and siblings. Passive anger toward the ill child may be evident in decreased visiting, refusal to believe how sick the child is, or inability to provide comfort. Among the most common targets for parental anger are members of the staff. Parents may complain about the nursing care, the insufficient time physicians spend with them, or the lack of skill of those who draw blood or start intravenous infusions.

Children are apt to respond with anger as well, and this includes the affected child, as well as the well siblings. Children are aware of the loss engendered by their illness or disability and may react angrily to the restrictions imposed or the feelings of being different. Siblings may also feel anger and resentment toward the ill child and parents for the loss of routine and parental attention. It is difficult for older children and almost impossible for younger children to comprehend the plight of the affected child. Their perception is of a brother or sister who has the undivided attention of their parents, is showered with cards and gifts, and is the focus of everyone's concern.

During the period of adjustment, four types of parental reactions to the child influence the child's eventual response to the disorder: *overprotection,* in which the parents fear letting the child achieve any new skill, avoid all discipline, and cater to every desire to prevent frustration (Box 18-6); *rejection,* in which the parents detach themselves emotionally from the child but usually provide adequate physical care or constantly nag and scold the child; *denial,* in which parents act is if the disorder does not exist or attempt to have the child overcompensate for it; and *gradual acceptance,* in which parents place necessary and realistic restrictions on the child, encourage self-care activities, and promote reasonable physical and social abilities.

Reintegration and Acknowledgment

For many families the adjustment process culminates in the development of realistic expectations for the child and reintegration of family life with the illness or disability in a manageable perspective. Because a large portion of this phase is one of grief for a loss, total resolution is not possible until the child dies or leaves home as an independent adult. Therefore one can regard adjustment as "increased comfort" with everyday living rather than a complete resolution.

This adjustment phase also involves social reintegration in which the family broadens its activities to include relationships outside of the home, with the child as an acceptable and participating member of the group. This last criterion often differentiates the reaction of gradual acceptance during the adjustment period from total acceptance, or perhaps is more descriptive of the acknowledgment process.

Many parents of children with chronic illnesses experience *chronic sorrow,* feelings of sorrow and loss that recur

BOX 18-6 ■ Characteristics of Parental Overprotection

Sacrifices self and rest of family for the child

Continually helps the child, even when the child is capable

Is inconsistent with regard to discipline or employs no discipline; frequently, different rules apply to the siblings

Is dictatorial and arbitrary, making decisions without considering the child's wishes, such as keeping the child from attending school

Hovers and offers suggestions; calls attention to every activity, overdoing praise

Protects the child from every possible discomfort

Restricts play, often because of fear that the child will be injured

Denies the child opportunities for growing up and assuming responsibility, such as learning to give own medications or perform treatments

Does not understand the child's capabilities and sets goals too high or too low

Monopolizes the child's time, such as sleeping with the child, permitting few friends, or refusing participation in social or educational activities

BOX 18-7 ■ Concept of Functional Burden

IMPACT OF THE CHILD WITH SPECIAL NEEDS

The child's need for medical and nursing care

The child's fixed deficits

The child's age-appropriate dependency in activities of daily living

The disruptions in the family routine caused by the care

The psychologic burden of the prognosis on the family

FAMILY RESOURCES AND ABILITY TO COPE

The family's physical resources

The family's emotional resources

The family's educational resources

The family's social supports and available help

The competing demands for family members' time and energy

Data from Stein REK: Home care: a challenging opportunity, *Child Health Care* 14(2):90-95, 1985.

in waves over time. As the child's condition progresses, parents experience repeated losses that present further decline and new caregiving demands. Consequently, families must be assessed on an ongoing basis and offered appropriate support and resources as the needs of the family change over time (Gravelle, 1997).

ESTABLISHING A SUPPORT SYSTEM

The diagnosis of a child with a serious health problem or disability is a major situational crisis that affects the entire family system. However, families can experience positive outcomes as they successfully deal with the many challenges that accompany a child with chronic illness or disability.

One nursing goal is to assess which families are at greater or lesser risk for succumbing to the effects of the crisis. Several variables—available support system, perception of the event, coping mechanisms, reactions to the child, available resources, and concurrent stresses within the family—influence the resolution of a crisis. Although most families cope well, the needs of families at risk are great. If they receive emotional support and guidance early, there is an increased likelihood that they will also cope successfully.

Although it is easy to assume that families of children with the most severe illnesses or disabilities would have the poorest adjustment, the severity of the condition reflects only one part of the overall picture. The level of adjustment is significantly influenced by the *functional burden* on the individual family (Stein, 1985). This concept considers the issues related to caring for and living with the child in relation to the family's resources and ability to cope (Box 18-7). The family of a child with multiple disabilities demanding complex care—yet having many resources and coping skills—may adjust more successfully to the child's situation than the family of a child with a less serious condition and few resources to counter the balance.

Intrafamilial resources, social support from friends and relatives, parent-to-parent support, parent-professional partnerships, and community resources interweave to provide a flexible web of support for the family of a child with a chronic condition.

THE CHILD WITH SPECIAL NEEDS

IMPACT OF CHRONIC ILLNESS OR DISABILITY ON THE CHILD

The child's reaction to chronic illness or disability depends to a great extent on his or her developmental level, temperament, and available coping mechanisms; on the reactions of family members or significant others; and to a lesser extent, on the condition itself. A child's conceptual understanding of his or her own illness is based not only on age and developmental level, but also on the duration and type of experience accumulated with the disease. Knowledge of these variables is essential in providing the kind of information and support needed by these children to cope with a sometimes overwhelming situation.

Developmental Aspects

The impact of a chronic illness or disability is influenced by the age at onset. Chronic illness affects children of all ages, but the developmental aspects of each age-group dictate particular stresses and risks for the child. The nurse must also recognize that children need to redefine their condition and its implications as they develop and grow. Children's developmental concepts of illness are discussed in Chapter 21. An understanding of these developmental factors facilitates planning care to support the child and minimize the risks.

Infant.   During infancy the child is engaged in the task of developing trust through an intimate, satisfying, consistent relationship with his or her parents. When illness or disability occurs, this relationship is potentially affected. For example, a visible defect can delay parent bonding as the parent mourns the loss of the perfect child. In addition, prolonged illness may impose separations that prevent the child and parent from normal attachment and deprive the infant of the nurturing relationship.

The illness itself affects the infant, especially because sensorimotor experiences are critical at this age. Illness and/or disability often impairs the child's motor abilities by confining the child to a crib and lessening contact with the environment. The messages transmitted to infants about their bodies are influenced by the amount of pain and discomfort they experience. Associating touch with pain can compromise the infant's ability to give and receive affection. Lack of pleasurable sensations can lead to an irritable and unhappy child. Consequently, parents may interpret the behaviors as evidence that they are not adequately meeting the child's physical and emotional needs, which further affects the parent-child relationship and the acquisition of trust. Nursing intervention can be important in helping parents work with the irritable child in a way that encourages understanding and caring.

Nurses should advocate for policies and practices that will best meet the needs of the infant and family. Twenty-four hour visitation in the neonatal intensive care unit and other infant units is of primary importance. Showing parents how to touch and hold the infant will promote their confidence and competence. "Kangaroo care" has been shown to be both safe and beneficial to the infant. Mothers who choose to breast-feed can be encouraged, with a private space provided for them to nurse or pump and storage facilities made available for breast milk. Sibling visitation can be facilitated.

Toddler. The toddler is in the stage of autonomy; the need for mastery of locomotor and language skills is paramount. The child learning to walk and talk progresses toward becoming a separate person, both physically and psychologically. However, illness or disability can hinder mobility and deprive the child of mastery. In addition, overprotective parents can magnify the problem by setting limits on the child's exploration and experimentation for fear of injury or exertion. Even the most basic self-help skills, such as feeding and dressing, may be done for the child. Age-appropriate tasks such as toilet training may be delayed. Within the constraints of illness or disability, maximum opportunities should be provided for independence in these and other areas.

Illness can impose separations that are detrimental to the toddler. As with the infant, separation is the most anxiety-producing event. A chronic illness or disability can necessitate repeated hospitalizations and painful procedures. If the need to preserve the parent-child relationship is not appreciated, the child may become depressed and eventually detach from the parent. Children seem to have a tremendous capacity to withstand stress, provided that their attachment to the parent is maintained. Parents of toddlers may begin to look for respite care or day care, which is often difficult to find for the child with special needs.* The *Americans With Disabilities Act (ADA)* requires day care providers to make "reasonable modifications" for equal access to program participation (Siegel, 1995). Special medical day care centers are being developed in certain areas (Ahmann and Scher, 1996; Monical, 1995).

*****Access to Respite Care and Help (ARCH)** is a national information center on respite programs: ARCH, c/o Chapel Hill Training Outreach Project, 800 Eastowne Drive, Chapel Hill, NC 27514; (919) 490-5577 or (800) 473-1727 ext. 243; fax: (919) 490-4905; website: www.chtop.com (look for ARCH icon).

Preschooler. The preschooler is in the stage of initiative; numerous tasks are achieved during this age that can be hampered by chronic illness and disability. Impairment can limit the preschooler's learning about the environment, especially in terms of social development. The chronically ill preschooler confined to the home may be slow to develop social skills useful in group or school settings.

One of the major tasks of this period is establishing sexual identity, and one of the principal methods is through imitation of gender-related activities. However, the child with special needs may have fewer opportunities to engage in such activity and may view the parent predominantly in the caregiving role, because this may be the focus of their relationship. Some families expect the mother to assume the care of the child while the father provides the financial base by working outside the home. This can limit the child's identification with the male role.

In addition to sexual identity, the child's body image is forming. Children's knowledge of their bodies is limited to what they see, feel, and use. If the child is chronically ill, body awareness is focused on the personal pain and anxiety it causes. The young child may lose control over newly acquired bowel and bladder function and feel embarrassed and inferior. The child with a disability may have difficulty forming a mental image of impaired body parts, such as paralyzed extremities. This poorly developed sense of body integrity makes children especially fearful of intrusive or mutilating experiences, which can be frequent during prolonged illness.

One of the more critical influences of chronic illness or disability on preschoolers is the feeling of guilt that they "caused" the condition by a real or imagined misdeed. This is probably less a factor if the child is born with the disorder than if it occurs during the preschool years. Such guilt can greatly affect the child's developing but fragile self-esteem. Unlike the child with a temporary physical impairment who has additional opportunities for achieving mastery and thus overcoming feelings of guilt and inferiority, the child with a chronic illness or disability experiences continual insults. Unless situations are structured for success, life can become a series of failures—of never being strong enough or good enough to compete with peers.

School-Age Child. The child of school age is striving to achieve a sense of accomplishment while overcoming a sense of inferiority. Successful mastery of this task depends on the child's ability to cooperate and compete with others. Consequently, physical impairments can greatly affect the ability to achieve and compete. For example, physical disability may hinder participation in sports, and repeated absences from school caused by illness can place the child at an academic disadvantage. To repeat a grade can saddle the child with feelings of shame, inadequacy, and inferiority. However, the decision to remain in the same grade can also enhance feelings of success because the work requirements may be easier and new classmates provide a second chance for forming friendships.

During this age there is a transition from relationships with family members to strong identification with peers. Peers increasingly influence school-age children's views of themselves and their self-esteem. Anything that labels children as "different" can affect their sense of belonging to the group (Vessey and Mebane, 2000). Nurses can help families to promote social competence in their children. For example, if children are helped to deal with their feelings of not being "normal and perfect" and to recognize their unique abilities, these children can cope very well. It is to be expected that not all children are able to master every task and that they will feel some degree of disappointment. If this is stressed to children with physical impairment, the burden to achieve is lessened.

Peer interaction is especially important in relation to cognitive development, social development, and maturation. Cognitive development is facilitated by interaction—by exploration of personal, social, and ethical values with peers, parents, and teachers. As school-age children identify more with the peer group and authority figures outside the home, there is a concurrent striving for independence from the family. However, the ill child may be forced into an extended period of dependency either from the disorder or from parental overprotectiveness. Attempts to demonstrate independence may be manifested as resentment toward the parents, refusal to comply with treatment, or risk-taking behavior such as cheating on the special diet. If parents can understand that these behaviors represent a normal phase of development, they may be more tolerant and able to find appropriate outlets for independence (e.g., increasing the child's responsibility for home care or increasing the child's control in non–disease-related activities).

Adolescent.   The impact of illness or disability can be most difficult during adolescence. The major task of the adolescent is to establish a personal identity. Pubertal changes must be integrated into the self-image while the teenager is gaining control and mastery over increased physical capabilities and sexuality. During early adolescence this takes place primarily within the peer group. Illness or injury at this time interferes with teenagers' sense of mastery and control over a changing body. They are different at a stage of development when being different is unacceptable to the peer group, which may view a disability in one member as a threat to the established uniformity by which all are measured. At no other time of life is an individual so vulnerable to the emotional stress of biologic impairment. In fact, adolescents with physical differences tend to blame most of their problems on the fact that they have something wrong with them. Appearance, skills, and abilities are highly valued by peers (Fig. 18-1); a teenager who is limited in any of these qualities is subject to rejection. This is especially marked when a physical disability interferes with sexual attractiveness.

The subject of sexuality related to the effects of the disorder is a prominent concern of adolescents, but they rarely initiate a discussion of this sensitive topic. Any probable interference in sexual function because of the disability should be discussed openly and candidly with the teenager (Lock, 1998).

Teenagers with special needs are faced with the task of incorporating their disabilities into the changing self-concept. The youngster who develops the illness or acquires the disability during the crucial adolescent years has more difficulty accomplishing this task than has the teenager who has been affected since childhood. It appears that the earlier the onset

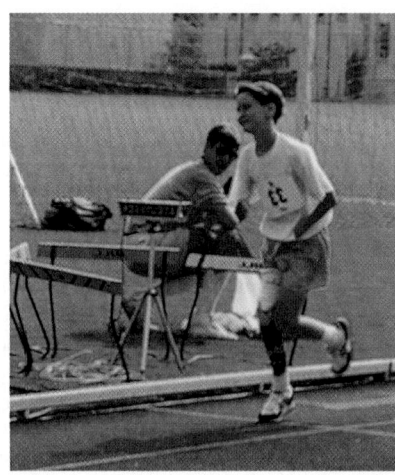

FIG. 18-1 ■ Children with any type of impairment should have the opportunity to develop their skills. (Courtesy Poyo/Hinton Photography.)

of a limiting condition, the better the individual is able to adapt to it. The youngster with a newly acquired disorder will have the additional task of grieving for a lost "perfection" while adjusting to the changes taking place as a natural course of events. He or she often feels rejected because of personal appearance or an inability to engage in activities expected of a healthy adolescent. The threat is greatest during middle adolescence, when the teenager has less available energy to cope with illness because emotional resources are being used to meet the normal demands of this developmental phase.

Adolescence is a time for achieving independence from the family and planning for future goals and responsibilities. Adolescents with long-term chronic illness may be less future directed and less independent than well peers (Perrin, 2004). Enforced dependency caused by physical impairment can exacerbate the parent-child conflicts surrounding independence. Lack of understanding from both parties can result in bitter feelings and intrafamilial turmoil. The tendency toward rebellion may be directed at the disorder and reflected in decreased compliance with treatment; denial of the disorder to preserve a sense of normalcy with peers; and risk-taking behavior that can place the teenager in jeopardy, such as driving a car despite a disorder that increases the chance of an injury. Such behaviors can further strain an already tense parent-child relationship. On the other hand, parents can promote independence by giving the adolescent a greater role in his or her own treatment regimen, encouraging the adolescent to develop a relationship with the health care team that is not mediated by parents, and promoting normalization principles.

Coping Mechanisms

Children's innate and learned coping mechanisms are very important in terms of their ability to deal with their disorder. Individual characteristics and the social support afforded the child are critically important influences on the child's ability to cope with stress. The better the family copes, the better the child is able to deal with the stressors imposed by the illness or disability. Individual characteristics associated with positive coping are female sex, early infancy or age older than 4 years, active or easy temperament, high self-esteem, above-average intelligence, and strong social skills.

Children with chronic conditions tend to use five distinct patterns of coping (Box 18-8). Children with more positive and accepting attitudes about their chronic illness use a more adaptive coping style characterized by optimism, competence, and compliance. They show fewer behavior problems at home and at school. The two maladaptive coping patterns—"Feels different and withdraws" and "Is irritable, moody, and acts out"—are associated with poorer adaptation; children using these strategies have poorer self-concepts, more negative attitudes about their conditions, and more behavior problems at home and at school.

Well-adapted children gradually learn to accept their physical limitations but find achievement in a variety of compensatory motor and intellectual pursuits. They function well at home, at school, and with peers. They have an understanding of their disorder that allows them to accept their limitations, assume responsibility for care, and assist in treatment and rehabilitation regimens. They express appropriate emotions, such as sadness, anxiety, and anger, at times of exacerbations but confidence and guarded optimism during periods of clinical stability (Fig. 18-2). They are able to identify with other similarly affected individuals, promoting positive self-images and displaying pride and self-confidence in their ability to master a productive, successful life despite the disability.

Hopefulness.   Children, particularly adolescents, are sensitive to the presence or absence of hope. Hopefulness is an internal quality that mobilizes humans into goal-directed action that may be satisfying and life sustaining. A sense of hopefulness can produce increased participation in health-seeking behaviors and an improved sense of well-being (Ritchie, 2001).

Health Education and Self-Care.   Health education is an intervention that promotes coping. Children need information about their condition, the therapeutic plan, and how the disease or the therapy might affect their particular situation. Children nearing puberty also need to understand the maturation process and how their disability may alter this event. For example, the youngster with Crohn disease should understand that this disorder is associated with growth failure and delayed puberty; the child with diabetes needs to know that hormonal changes and increased growth needs will alter food and insulin requirements at this time; and the sexually active girl with sickle cell anemia or systemic lupus erythematosus needs to be aware of the risks of pregnancy. The information should not be given all at once but should be timed appropriately to meet the changing needs of the youngsters, and it should be described and repeated as often as the situation demands it.

Developing the skills and judgment needed for participation in self-care of a chronic illness or disability is a process that occurs over time. Self-care requires negotiation between parent and child. Nurses can assist families by offering information on methods for instructing children of various ages in self-care (Faulkner, 1996). Answering each child's questions as they arise in an honest and age-appropriate manner and having family discussions about the illness or disability can foster a positive family environment for health education of the child.

Responses to Parental Behavior

The parents' behavior toward the child, especially in terms of childrearing, is one of the most important influencing factors in the child's adjustment. For example, children whose parents are overprotective tend to have marked dependency (especially on the mother), fearfulness, inactivity,

BOX 18-8 ■ Coping Patterns Used by Children With Special Needs

Develops competence and optimism. Accentuates the positive aspects of the situation and concentrates more on what he or she has or can do than on what is missing or on what he or she cannot do; is as independent as possible.

Feels different and withdraws. Sees self as being different from other children because of the chronic health condition; views being different as negative; sees self as less worthy than others; focuses on things he or she cannot do and sometimes overrestricts activities needlessly.

Is irritable, moody, and acts out. Uses proactive and self-initiated coping behaviors, although usually counterproductive in that the behaviors are not ego enhancing or socially responsible and do not result in desired outcomes; acts out irritability, which may or may not be associated with condition's symptoms.

Complies with treatment. Takes necessary medications, treatments; adheres to activity restrictions; also uses behaviors that indicate developing independence (e.g., assumes responsibility for taking medication).

Seeks support. Talks with adults, children, physicians, and nurses; develops plans to handle problems as they occur; uses downward comparison (i.e., realizes that others have it worse).

Modified from Austin J, Patterson J, Huberty T: Development of the Coping Health Inventory for children, *J Pediatr Nurs* 6(3):166-174, 1991.

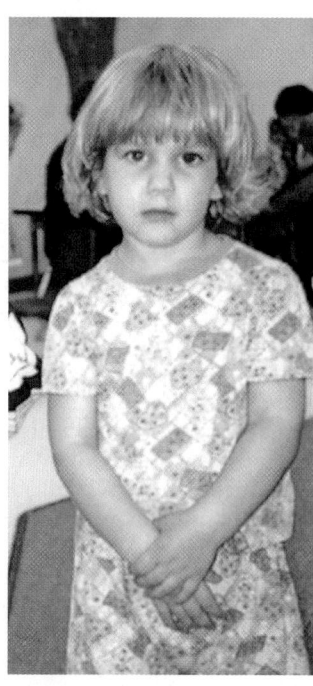

FIG. 18-2 ■ Periods of sadness and anger are appropriate in the child's adjustment to a chronic illness or disability, especially during exacerbations of the disorder.

and lack of outside interests. Children who are raised by overly solicitous and guilt-ridden parents are often overly independent, defiant, and risk takers. Children who are reared by parents who emphasize their deficits and tend to "hide" or isolate them appear as shy and lonely individuals who harbor resentful and hostile attitudes toward unaffected persons. In contrast, children who are reared by parents who establish reasonable limits tend to develop age-appropriate independence and achievement commensurate with their limitations. In addition, family organization and illness-related support and involvement of parents influence children's adjustment to chronic illness (Schor, 2003). They often display pride and confidence in their ability to cope successfully with the challenges imposed by their disorder. Anticipatory guidance by the nurse and encouragement of normalizing practices may assist parents in facilitating positive adjustment in their children.

Type of Illness or Disability

The type of illness or disability also influences the child's emotional response. Interestingly, children with *more* severe disorders often cope better than those with milder conditions. However, the presence of multiple conditions may place a child at risk for more behavioral problems (Newacheck and Halfon, 1998). Considering children's cognitive ability and their delay in achieving abstract thinking until adolescence, it is likely that an obvious condition is easier to accept because its limitations are concrete. For example, children who are blind or physically disabled are constantly reminded of their inability to run. However, children with cardiac defects not only live by rules they do not understand, but also only vaguely and occasionally sense their illness, such as when they try to run and experience dyspnea and fatigue. Therefore, some chronic illnesses pose special threats to children.

The onset of a disabling condition may generate a state of confusion for children, who may have trouble differentiating between actual bodily functions and their image of their bodies. They may also experience problems in identifying themselves and those extensions of self (e.g., wheelchairs, braces, crutches, other mechanical or prosthetic devices) and may have difficulty in accepting functional aids.

NURSING CARE OF THE FAMILY AND CHILD WITH SPECIAL NEEDS

Assessment

Because the nurse may meet a family during any phase of the adjustment process, several assessment areas are important. Knowledge of the family's available support system is essential and may include the marital relationship, nonmarital partners, extended family, colleagues and co-workers, friends, and professionals. The family's perception of the illness or disability is also an area that influences family adjustment. Assessment questions should focus on members' general knowledge of the condition even before the child's diagnosis was made, the influence of culture and religion on their thinking, imagined causes of the condition, and the effects of the child's disorder on the family.

Because the family's ability to cope with previous stresses influences the current situation, answers to questions about their usual coping skills are enlightening. Knowledge of

concurrent stresses, such as financial, marital or nonmarital, career, or unemployment, helps identify families who may have fewer resources to cope with the child's needs.

Finally, awareness of the family members' reactions to the child and the illness or disability is important. Sample questions that the nurse and family can use to evaluate the support system, perception of the illness, coping mechanisms, resources, and concurrent stresses are listed in Table 18-1. Because factors affecting the family's response may change at any point during the illness, assessment must be a continuous process.

Special challenges exist in assessing the child's feelings about having a disability. Chapter 6 presents several approaches to encourage a child to discuss feelings about the condition. The nurse should use a variety of communication techniques, such as drawing and play, as assessment tools rather than relying solely on parental reports. Often, children are neglected partners in their care, and their unique needs are not identified (Young and others, 2003; Dixon-Woods, Young, and Henry, 1999).

The needs of working parents and siblings also should be assessed, a goal that requires flexibility in scheduling appointments to include these important family members. When working parents know that their input is valuable, they will often change their work schedule to meet with a health professional. Because siblings can be of any age, the use of appropriate communication strategies for assessment must be considered. Nonverbal techniques such as those discussed in Chapter 6 should be considered for these children. Several instruments can be used to assist the family in assessing their overall functioning and support system (see Chapter 6).

Nursing Diagnoses

A number of nursing diagnoses are prominent in the nursing care of the family and child with special needs. Others specific to individual cases become evident, especially when the child's actual disorder is considered.

Planning

The nursing plan depends to a large extent on the child's actual illness or disability. However, the following are basic goals for all families and children with special needs:

1 Child and family will receive support at the time of diagnosis.
2 Family's emotional reactions will be accepted.
3 Child and family will cope with stresses of the situation.
4 Child and family will receive appropriate information about the condition.
5 Family will establish an environment of normalization for the child.
6 Family will establish realistic future goals.

Implementation

The main objective in working with the family is to help them to cope effectively with those stresses imposed by the child's special needs. To achieve this goal, the entire family should be considered in every aspect of the implementation process (see Family Focus box).

Provide Support at the Time of Diagnosis

This is a critical time for parents and can influence how they perceive their health care providers throughout care. Although they may not hear or remember all that is said to

TABLE 18-1 ■ Assessment of Factors Affecting Family Adjustment

FACTORS AFFECTING ADJUSTMENT	ASSESSMENT QUESTIONS
Available support system Status of marital relationship Alternate support systems Ability to communicate	Whom do you talk to when you have something on your mind? (If answer is not the spouse, ask for the reason.) When something is worrying you, what do you do? What helps you most when you are upset? Does talking seem to help when you feel upset?
Perception of the illness/disability Previous knowledge of disorder Influence of religion Imagined cause of disorder Effects of illness or disability on family	Have you ever heard the word (name of diagnosis) before? Tell me about it (if answer is yes). Has your religion or faith been of help to you? Tell me how (if answer is yes). What are your thoughts about the causes of the disorder? How has your child's illness or disability affected you and your family? How has your lifestyle changed?

Coping mechanisms
Reactions to previous crises
Reactions to the child
   Childrearing practices
   Attitudes
	Tell me one time you've had another crisis (problem, bad time) in your family. How did you solve that problem?
	Do you find yourself being a little more cautious with this child than with your other children?
	Do you feel as comfortable disciplining this child compared with your other children?
	How is this child different from the siblings or other children of similar age?
	Describe your child's personality. Is it easy, difficult, or in between?
	When you think of your child's future, what thoughts come to mind?

Available resources	What parts of your child's care are causing the most difficulty for you and/or your family? What services are available to help? What services do you need that presently are not available?
Concurrent stresses	What other problems are you facing now? (Be specific; ask about financial, marital, sibling, and extended family/friends concerns.)

FAMILY FOCUS

Identifying Family Needs

To ensure an effective plan of care, attention to family-identified needs and priorities is essential. For example, a family may have difficulty focusing on treatment issues if their current priority is obtaining enough food to feed their children.

them, they frequently sense a certain attitude of acceptance, rejection, hope, or despair that may influence their ability to absorb the shock and begin adapting to the family's altered future.

Parents should be encouraged to be together when they are informed of their child's condition, thus avoiding the problem of one parent having to interpret complex findings and deal with the initial emotional reaction of the other. The informing session should take place in a private, comfortable setting free of distractions and interruptions, in an atmosphere in which the parents feel free to express their emotions (Fig. 18-3). If their feelings can be expressed and acknowledged, the parents can be helped to deal openly with them. Their emotional needs are acknowledged by showing acceptance of such expressions as crying, sadness, anger, and disappointment. Emotional support is offered by having tissues available if a family member cries and demonstrating through facial and body language that indeed this is a difficult and painful period. Although touching is a powerful expression of empathy, it must be used wisely. For

example, it can prematurely terminate free expression of feelings, especially when combined with statements such as "Everything will be all right." Nurses should also be aware of cultural issues regarding touching (see Chapter 4).

Parents should receive the kind of information they desire. This can be assessed by asking the parent questions such as, "Do you prefer to hear detailed information?" Parents or other family members may have different preferences regarding the amount of information they wish to hear. Most parents want a clear, simple explanation of the diagnosis, a prediction of possible futures for the child, advice on what to do next, an opportunity to ask questions, a warm and sympathetic listener, and most important, time. Clarification of explanations is elicited with such questions as "Do you see what I mean?" or "Is this clear to you?" Technical terms are used with simple definitions. If the parents are unaware of the term, they are given written literature or at least a written summary of the diagnosis.

NURSING TIP

Develop a glossary of commonly used terms, acronyms, and "initials" to distribute to parents. The list can stand alone or become a part of patient or parent handbooks.

Finally, the informing conference should not end with the presentation of devastating news. Instead, the child's strengths, appealing behaviors, and potential for development are stressed, as are available rehabilitation efforts or treatment. Parents can be encouraged to view their experiences as a series of challenges that they are capable of handling, particularly with available professional feedback. The

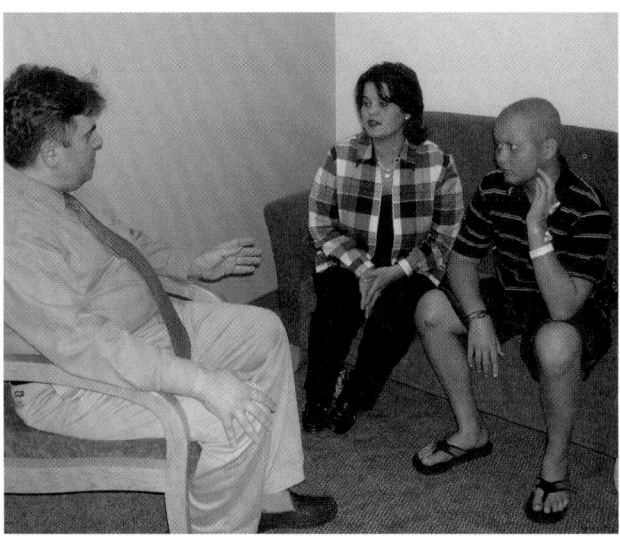

FIG. 18-3 ■ Informing session should take place in a private, comfortable setting free of distractions and interruptions.

parents are assured that the nurse will be available to answer questions and to provide further assistance as needed.

The preceding discussion relates primarily to the initial informing interview. However, because of the need for long-term follow-up, it is only one in a series of continuing discussions. In all interactions the family's input is solicited and incorporated into the plan of care. Some situations require consideration of special problems (see Guidelines box).

Accept Family's Emotional Reactions

One of the most supportive interventions is to accept the family's emotional reactions to the child's condition in as nonjudgmental a manner as possible. Although all families respond differently and in varying degrees of intensity, three responses are so common and often so poorly handled that they deserve special consideration.

Denial.   The nurse's response to denial is a critical component of the individual's continuing need for this defense mechanism. The most effective method of support is active listening. Silence neither reinforces nor rejects denial (or any other emotional reaction) but implies a willingness and acceptance of the person's need for this behavior. However, silence alone can be misinterpreted. For example, if the person demonstrates denial, such as by saying, "I am sure the doctors made a mistake," and the nurse responds silently and leaves, the person may infer disapproval, agreement, avoidance, or rejection from this behavior.

To be effective, silence and listening must be accompanied by physical and mental concentration and use of body language to communicate interest and concern. Direct eye contact, touch, physical closeness, and body posture, such as sitting and leaning slightly forward, demonstrate silent but effective communication. (See also Communication Techniques, Chapter 6.)

Guilt.   Because guilt is such a common response and can cause family members tremendous anxiety, they should be told directly that there is no known cause of the disorder (when appropriate) and that they are not to be blamed. Us-

ing the third-person technique is valuable in eliciting thoughts of guilt. For example, with children, an appropriate statement may be, "When people get sick, they often wonder if they did anything to make themselves sick." This allows children an opportunity to explore any feelings of responsibility they harbor.

If family members are expressing feelings of guilt, it is important to allow them to talk about their feelings rather than quickly trying to dispel them with long "scientific" explanations. Statements such as "If you believe you are responsible for Johnny's condition, then no wonder you feel so bad" acknowledge the family member's feelings. This step is frequently appreciated and necessary before the facts can be presented and absorbed. An effective method in lessening guilt is to *encourage the irrationality of thought.* For example, one mother stated that her son probably developed cancer by sitting too close to the television, which she could have prevented by being more strict. By following her reasoning and talking about how *many* children sit close to the television and how *few* of them ever have cancer, the nurse was able to help the mother realize that this activity was not a cause.

Anger.   Anger is one of the more difficult reactions to accept and deal with therapeutically. The responses to anger may be reciprocal anger, fear, acceptance, or encouragement. The first two reactions impede communication and express disapproval and rejection of the person. They most frequently occur when the listener views the anger as a personal assault. The last two responses allow the individual to express his or her feelings in an atmosphere of nonjudgmental acceptance. Two basic rules for dealing with the angry person are to avoid losing one's temper and to encourage the person to talk (see Guidelines box). One essential element in the successful implementation of this process is to wait for the person to respond to a statement before proceeding to the next step. Because the objective of each statement is for the person to speak freely, the responses should avoid "yes" or "no" types of answers.

Support Family's Coping Methods

For the family to meet the stresses of optimally adjusting to the child's condition, each member must be individually supported so that the family system is strong. Although the family can indefinitely support a member who is in need of assistance, its greatest strength lies in every member supporting each other. The nurse should bear in mind that the family member in greatest need is not necessarily the affected child but may be a parent or sibling who is dealing with stresses that require intervention.

Parents.   The nurse can provide support by being attentive to families' responses to their children. Mothers and fathers need to experience success, joy, and pride in their children to give the support they need. Children, too, require support for their interactions, adjustments, and efforts. They must be reinforced for attempts to get to know their care providers and to communicate their needs to them.

Nurses must examine their attitudes to determine their ability to engage in parent-professional partnerships. An essential characteristic is the belief that parents are equal to professionals and that parents are experts regarding their child (see Guidelines box).

GUIDELINES

Situations Requiring Special Consideration

Congenital anomaly. Tension in the delivery room conveys the sense that something is seriously wrong. Communication is often delayed while the physician is involved with the mother's care. The manner in which the infant is presented may well set the tone for the early parent-child relationship.

Clarify role with physician in regard to revealing information, to enable immediate parental support.

Explain to parents briefly in simple language what the defect is and something concerning the immediate prognosis before showing them the infant, when they are more apt to "hear" what is said.

Be aware of nonverbal communication. Parents watch facial expressions of others for signs of revulsion or rejection.

Present infant as something precious.

Emphasize well-formed aspects of infant's body.

Allow time and opportunity for parents to express their initial response.

Encourage parents to ask questions, and provide honest, straightforward answers without undue optimism or pessimism.

Cognitive impairment. Unless cognitive impairment (mental retardation) is associated with other physical problems, it is often easy for parents to miss clues to its presence or to make defensive excuses regarding the diagnosis.

Plan situations that help parents become aware of the problem.

Encourage parents to discuss their observations of child, but withhold diagnostic opinions.

Focus on what child can do and appropriate interventions to promote progress (e.g., infant stimulation programs) to involve parents in their child's care while helping them gain an awareness of child's disability.

Physical disability. If loss of motor or sensory ability occurs during childhood, the diagnosis is readily apparent. The challenge lies in helping the child and parents over the period of shock and grief and toward the phase of acceptance and reintegration.

Institute early rehabilitation (e.g., using a prosthetic limb, learning to read braille, learning to read lips).

Be aware that physical rehabilitation usually precedes psychologic adjustment.

When the cause of the disability is accidental, avoid implying that parents or child was responsible for the injury, yet allow them the opportunity to discuss feelings of blame.

Encourage expression of feelings (see Communication Techniques, Chapter 6).

Chronic illness. Realization of the true impact may take months or years. Conflict over parent's versus child's concerns may result

in serious problems. When condition is inherited, parents may blame themselves or child may blame parents.

Help each family member gain an appreciation of the other's concerns.

Discuss hereditary aspect of condition with parents at time of diagnosis to lessen guilt and accusatory feelings.

Encourage child to express feelings by using third-person technique (e.g., "Sometimes when a person has an illness that was passed on by the parents, that person feels angry or bitter toward them").

Multiple disabilities. The child or parent may require additional time for the shock phase and may be able to attend to only one diagnosis before hearing significant information regarding other disorders.

Acknowledge parents' understanding and acceptance of all diagnoses, especially when an obvious and more hidden disability coexists.

Appreciate the devastating consequences of more than one disability for a child, especially if they interfere with expressive-receptive abilities.

Terminal illness. Parents require much support to deal with their own feelings and guidance in how to tell the child the diagnosis. They may want to conceal the diagnosis from the child. They may believe that the child is too young to know, will not be able to cope with the information, or will lose hope and the will to live.

Approach the subject of disclosure in a positive way by asking, "How will you tell your child about the diagnosis?"

Help parents understand the disadvantages of not telling children (e.g., deprives them of the opportunity to discuss their feelings openly and ask questions, incurs the risk of them learning the truth from outside and sometimes less tactful sources, may lessen children's trust and confidence in their parents after they learn the truth).

Guide parents to see the potential problems involved in fostering a conspiracy.

Offer parents guidelines for how and what to tell children about their disease or the possibility of death. Explanations should be tailored to child's cognitive ability, be based on knowledge child already has, and be honest. Honesty must be tempered with concern for child's feelings.

Assure parents that telling a child the name of the illness and the reason for treatment instills hope, provides support from others, and serves as a foundation for explaining and understanding subsequent events.

Acknowledge that being honest is not always easy because the truth may prompt children to ask other distressing questions, such as "Am I going to die?" However, even this difficult question must be answered.

GUIDELINES

Encouraging Expression of Emotion

Describe the behavior: "You seem angry at everyone."

Give evidence of understanding: "Being angry is only natural."

Give evidence of caring: "It must be difficult to endure so many painful procedures."

Help focus on feelings: "Maybe you wonder why this happened to your child."

Because most mothers and fathers of children with special needs have little or no experience with children who have chronic or disabling conditions, the nurse can serve as a role model for appropriate interactions with the child. Above all, the nurse should ensure that the parents and siblings learn to perceive the child as a child first, with unique and individual needs. The nurse needs to convey a humanistic, accepting approach to the child to enable the parents to observe this acceptance. This attitude of liking, concern for, and acceptance of the child should begin in early infancy and continue throughout the child's life.

Communication among all family members is encouraged. Parent group sessions can help parents to verbalize thoughts and feelings to each other but often do not take into account siblings' or the child's viewpoint. Therefore, the nurse may need to set up a family session, such as during a home or clinic visit. Although the ideal situation is to have all of the members present at one time, this is often not possible. However, inviting members to participate at various visits is an appropriate alternative.

Parents can be encouraged to discuss their feelings toward the child, the impact of this event on their marriage, and associated stresses such as financial burdens. For most families, regardless of their income or insurance coverage, financial concerns exist. The costs of caring for a child with special needs can be overwhelming. In addition, the family wage earner may have to sacrifice job opportunities to remain close to a medical facility or to avoid losing insurance benefits.*

The nurse should regard fathers as able, effective parents, competent and capable of coping with the challenges they face. Every effort is made to include the father in visits, such as to the nursery, clinic, special school, and stimulation programs. The father should be included in the assessment process, with specific emphasis on having him describe the child's strengths and difficulties. It is not unusual to find two parents who have differing views of the child's abilities, especially in the area of developmental disabilities.

Numerous volunteer and community resources are available that provide assistance, rehabilitation, equipment, and funding for a variety of health problems.† National and local disease-oriented organizations may provide needed assistance and support to families that qualify. Many of these are discussed elsewhere in the text under the specific diagnosis. State and federal departments of health, mental health, social service, and labor may be able to help locate appropriate regional resources. For example, state **Programs for Children With Special Health Needs** (formerly Crippled Children's Services) provide financial assistance for children with many disabling conditions. Local and national sources of respite care and medical day care may be useful to families. Nurses should become acquainted with those in their communities and with vocational programs for special groups.

Although community resources may exist, it is often very difficult for parents to locate suitable services, and coordina-

GUIDELINES

Developing Successful Parent-Professional Partnerships

Promote primary nursing; in nonhospital settings designate a case manager.

Acknowledge parents' overall competence and their unique expertise with their child.

Respect parents' time as having value equal to that of other members of child's health care team.

Explain or define any medical, technical, or disciplinary-specific terms.

Tell families, "I am not sure" or "I don't know," when appropriate.

Facilitate family's effectiveness in team meetings (e.g., provide parents with same information as other participants).

tion among several agencies may be lacking. Fragmented care is one of the chief complaints from families. Consequently, community networking for improved services is essential. Although this topic is beyond the scope of the present discussion, nurses can become key figures in coordinating services.

Parent-to-Parent Support.   The support a parent receives from another parent is unique and unobtainable from any other source. A growing number of hospitals and clinics now have a parent on staff. The services these parents provide are particularly valuable for parents of children with special needs who are likely to experience frequent and lengthy hospitalizations, as well as numerous routine clinic visits.

Just being with another parent who has shared similar experiences is helpful. A parent of a child with the same diagnosis is not always necessary, because parents in the process of adjusting to a child with special needs—or finding respite services, educational or rehabilitative services, special equipment vendors, and financial counseling—tread a common path. If the agency does not have a parent staff position, the nurse can contact parent groups that will often send a representative. Another strategy is ask another parent to talk to the parents. The nurse should seek out a parent who is a good listener, has a nonjudgmental approach to differences in families, and possesses good advocacy and problem-solving skills.

The parent self-help group is another way to promote parent-to-parent support.* Group members feel less alone and have the opportunity to observe both coping and mastery role modeling from other members. Parents' groups are rich resources for information. Even if parents are unable to attend meetings, they can still benefit from group newsletters and other literature that often accompany membership. The nurse can foster parent participation in self-help groups by serving as a referral agent, a group advisory board member, a resource person, a group member, or an assistant in founding a group. Sometimes all that is required in starting a group is identifying one or two parents as leaders; sharing

---

*Information regarding financial issues is available from the **Federation for Children With Special Needs,** 95 Berkeley Street, Suite 104, Boston, MA 02116; (617) 482-2915.

†General sources of information are the **Clearinghouse for Disability Information,** Room 3132, Switzer Building, C Street SW, Washington, DC 20202-2524; **National Information Center for Children and Youth with Disabilities,** PO Box 1492, Washington, DC 20013; (202) 884-8200 or (800) 695-0285; website: www.nichcy.org; and **National Center for Children with Chronic Illness and Disability,** Box 721-UMHC, Harvard Street at E. River Road, Minneapolis, MN 55455; (612) 626-2820. A comprehensive list of books and pamphlets for parents and teachers is available from the **Easter Seals National Headquarters,** 230 W. Monroe Street, Suite 1800, Chicago, IL 60606; (312) 726-6200; website: www.easter-seals.org. In Canada: **Council of Canadians with Disabilities,** Suite 926, 294 Portage Avenue, Winnipeg, Manitoba R3C 0B9; (204) 947-0303; website: www.pcs.mb.ca/~ccd.

---

*Information about self-help groups and books and pamphlets are available from the **National Self-Help Clearinghouse,** 365 5th Avenue, Suite 3300, New York, NY 10016; website: www.selfhelpweb.org.

with them the names, telephone numbers, and addresses of other families who have expressed both an interest and a willingness to release their phone number and address; and guiding them in how to initiate a first meeting.*

Advocate for Empowerment. Nurses can advocate for methods that foster opportunities for parent empowerment. For example, nurses can suggest reimbursement for travel and child care, plus stipends to enable parents' voices to be heard at meetings and conferences. They can encourage parent membership on staff, committees, and boards. They can keep parents informed of pending legislation on child health issues or take action when parents inform them.

The Child. Through ongoing contacts with the child, the nurse (1) observes the child's responses to the disorder, ability to function, and adaptive behaviors within the environment and with significant others; (2) explores the child's own understanding of the nature of his or her illness or condition; and (3) provides support while the child learns to cope with his or her feelings. Children are encouraged to express their concerns rather than allowing others to express them for them, because open discussions may reduce anxiety.

Parents sometimes convey concern because children cannot express their anxieties. If children cannot or will not talk, they may have to play out their feelings. They can be provided with toys to express threatening or stressful emotions. The nurse may find that children respond best to drawing pictures or telling stories (see Chapter 6). Puppets can also be used. By demonstrating to parents how useful these techniques are, the nurse also helps them learn new ways of communicating with their child. For youngsters with extremely serious handicaps or persistent maladjustment, psychiatric evaluation and management may be needed.

One of the most important interventions is alleviating the child's feeling of being different and normalizing his or her life as much as possible (see Guidelines box). Whenever possible, the nurse should assist the family in assessing the child's daily routine for indications of normalizing practices. For example, the child who remains in a bedroom all day is in need of a restructured daily routine to provide activities in different parts of the house, such as eating in the kitchen or dining room with the family. Such children may also be deprived of social, recreational, and academic activities that can be recognized by applying normalization practices. For example, home and out-of-home health-related treatments should be planned at times that least interfere with normal daily activities.

Children who are concerned that their condition detracts from their physical attractiveness need attention focused on the normal aspects of appearance and capabilities. Health professionals must help strengthen and consolidate the self-image by emphasizing the normal, while at the same time allowing children to express anger, isolation, fear of rejection, feelings of sadness, and loneliness. They need positive reinforcement for compliance and any evidence of improvement. Anything that might improve attractiveness and contribute

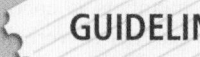

GUIDELINES

Promoting Normalization

Preparation. Prepare child in advance for changes that may occur from the illness or disability; for example, the child is told in advance of the possible side effects of drug therapy.

Participation. Include child in as many decisions as possible, especially those relating to his or her care regimen; for example, the child is responsible for taking medications or scheduling home treatments.

Sharing. Allow both family members and child's peers to be a part of the care regimen whenever possible; for example, the child is given his or her medication when the other siblings receive their vitamins; the parent cooks the same menu for the whole family; and if the child is invited to another's home, the parent advises the family of the child's dietary restrictions.

Control. Identify areas where child can be in control so that feelings of uncertainty, passivity, and helplessness are decreased; for example, the child identifies activities that are appropriate to his or her energy level and chooses to rest when fatigued.

Expectation. Apply the same family rules to the child with a chronic illness or disability as to the well siblings or peers; for example, the child is disciplined, expected to fulfill household responsibilities, and attends school in accordance with abilities.

to a positive self-image is employed, such as makeup for a teenager with a scar, clothing that disguises a prosthesis, or a hairstyle or wig to cover a deformity or lost hair.

Siblings. The presence of a child with special needs in a family may result in parents paying less attention to the other children. Siblings may respond by developing negative attitudes toward the child or by expressing anger in different forms. The nurse can help by using "anticipatory guidance," questioning the parents about what they believe is the best way to have siblings respond to the child and guiding them through ways to meet their other children's needs for attention. This questioning should take place before serious negative effects occur.

Siblings may also experience embarrassment associated with having a brother or sister with an illness or disability. Parents are then faced with the difficulty of responding to this embarrassment in an understanding and appropriate manner without punishing the siblings for how they feel. Parents should talk with the siblings about how they view their affected sibling. For example, siblings of a child who is retarded may express fears about their ability to bear normal children. Adolescents in particular may not be able to discuss these vital issues with their parents and may prefer to consult with the nurse. Many siblings benefit from sharing their concerns with other young people who are experiencing a similar situation.* Support groups for siblings can help decrease isolation, promote expression of feelings, and provide examples of effective coping skills.

Many parents express concern about when and how to inform the other children in the family about a sibling's dis-

---

*New Jersey Self-Help Clearinghouse,** (973) 6326-6789; website: www.groups.org.

*For information on the **Sibling Information Network,** contact the Information Network, CUAP, 991 Main Street, Suite 3A, East Hartford, CT 06108.

ability. The answer depends on each child's level of sophistication and understanding. However, it is usually best to inform the siblings before a neighbor or other nonfamily member does so. Uninformed siblings may fantasize or develop apprehensions that are out of proportion to the child's actual condition. Furthermore, if parents choose to be silent or deceptive about the issue, they are setting a negative precedent for the siblings to follow, rather than encouraging the siblings to cope with the experience in a healthy and nurturing way.

The nurse must be sensitive to the reactions of siblings and whenever possible intervene to promote more positive adjustment. For example, siblings often mention that they are expected to take on additional responsibilities to help the parents care for the child. It is not unusual for them to express a positive reaction to assuming the extra duties but a negative response to feeling unappreciated for doing so. Such feelings can often be minimized by encouraging siblings to discuss this with the parents and by suggesting to parents ways of showing gratitude, such as an increase in allowance, special privileges, and, most significantly, verbal praise (see Family Focus box).

Extended Family Members and Community.   The nurse must also be sensitive to the family's cues regarding sources of stress from extended members, such as grandparents. For example, the nurse may encourage the parents to invite the grandparents to be present during one of the child's visits to a clinic, during the diagnostic workup, or during a parent conference or to provide appropriate literature. Including grandparents in a discussion in which they can share their concerns may help them deal with their feelings, thus reducing stress on the entire family. Grandparents' feelings of blame and anger, as well as any "cure fantasies" they harbor, can be brought out in the open and discussed if necessary. Grandparents can be helped to understand the effects of their behavior on the family with an appropriate statement such as "Your daughter is currently experiencing a great deal of pain and anguish. We realize that this is difficult for you, as well as your daughter; however, you can be of tremendous help by being supportive toward her."

Considerable stress can also arise from nonfamilial sources, such as friends, neighbors, or strangers. Inability to cope with comments about the disorder or curious stares by others may foster the tendency to isolate and protect the child within the home. The family needs guidance in preparing for these inevitable experiences. Encouraging parents to dress the child as much as possible like other children is one approach. Good grooming is very important in minimizing differences in appearance. Through role-playing, parents can practice responses to comments such as "Is your child retarded?" or "Has he always been crippled?" Through parent groups, family members can share experiences and learn from each other how they successfully deal with probing questions or unkind remarks. Interventions should include the siblings and the affected child, who also must face and deal with these events. Nurses can teach young children about disabilities to familiarize them with the special needs and abilities of these individuals. For example, school nurses can simulate experiences such as having only one leg through role-playing, can use books or films, or can invite community guests with physical limitations to visit the class.

Educate About the Disorder and General Health Care

Educating the family about the disorder is actually an extension of revealing the diagnosis. Education involves not only supplying technical information, but also discussing how the condition will affect the child. Parents may be able to digest only so much information at a time. It may be helpful to provide essential information and then follow by asking, "What else would you like to know about your child's condition?" Responding to parents' questions and concerns ensures that their information needs are met.

Activities of Daily Living.   Parents also need guidance in how the condition may interfere with or alter activities of daily living, such as eating, dressing, sleeping, and toileting. One area frequently affected is nutrition. Common problems are undernutrition resulting from food being inappropriately restricted; loss of appetite, vomiting, or motor deficits that interfere with feeding; and overnutrition, usually caused by a caloric intake in excess of energy expenditure or boredom and lack of stimulation in other areas. Although the child requires the same basic nutrients as other children, the daily requirements may differ. Special nutritional considerations are discussed as appropriate throughout the text.

Safe Transportation.   Modifications may also be needed regarding car safety. Children with conditions such as low birth weight (see Discharge Planning and Home Care, Chapter 9) or orthopedic, neuromuscular, or respiratory problems often cannot safely use conventional car restraints. For example, children with hip spica casts cannot sit properly in child safety seats (see Congenital Hip Dysplasia, Chapter 31). Modifications can be made to some commercial models, and for older children a special vest is available that secures the child to the back seat in a lying-down position.*

If a child requires a wheelchair, the family should consult the wheelchair manufacturer for specific instructions regarding safe car transportation. Considerations for wheelchairs used with vehicle transportation must address securing both the wheelchair and the occupant in the wheelchair. Wheelchairs should be secured facing forward with tie downs at four points. The tie-down system should be dynamically crash tested, as should the occupant securement system that secures the child in the wheelchair. For example, use of trays would not be recommended for transportation. With children who must travel with additional medical equipment, this equipment (i.e., oxygen, monitors, or ventilators) should be anchored to the floor or underneath the vehicle seat or wheelchair. Soft padding should be added around the equipment to reduce movement. A second adult should be present to monitor the condition of a medically fragile child while traveling.

---

*Information on car safety restraints for children with special needs is available from the **Automotive Safety for Children Program**, Riley Hospital for Children, 575 West Drive, Room 004, Indianapolis, IN 46202; (800) 543-6227 or (317) 278-0399; website: www.preventinjury.org.

Primary Health Care. Children with special needs require all the usual health care recommended for any child. Attention to injury prevention, immunizations, dental health, and regular physical examinations is essential. Nurses can play an important role in reminding parents of these aspects of care that are so often neglected when the concern is focused on the child's specific illness or disability. Specific discussions of nutrition, sleep and activity, dental health, and injury prevention are presented in the chapters on health promotion for specific age-groups. Immunizations are discussed in Chapter 10.

Parents also need to be aware of the importance of communicating the child's condition in the event of a medical emergency. Young children are unable to give information about their disorder, and although older children may be reliable sources, after an accident they may be physically unable to speak. Therefore, all children with any type of chronic condition that may affect medical care should wear some type of identification, such as Medic-Alert bracelet,* or carry a card in their wallet that lists the medical condition and a phone number for emergency medical records and other personal information.

Children need information about their condition, the therapeutic plan, and how the disease or the therapy might affect their particular situation. Children nearing puberty also need to understand the maturation process and how their disability may alter this event. Information should not be given all at once but be timed appropriately to meet the changing needs of the youngsters, and it should be described and repeated as often as the situation demands. The subject of sexuality related to the effects of the disorder is a prominent concern of adolescents, but they rarely initiate a discussion of this sensitive topic. Any probable interference in sexual function because of the disability should be discussed openly and candidly with the teenager.

Promote Normal Development

Aside from knowledge of the condition and its effect on the child's abilities, the family must be guided toward fostering appropriate development in their child. Although each stage may take longer to achieve, parents are guided toward helping the child to fully realize his or her potential in preparation for the next developmental stage. Table 18-2 outlines developmental aspects of chronic illness or disability and supportive interventions. With appropriate planning and knowledge of strategies to improve the child's functional abilities, most children can live fulfilling and productive lives.

One important aspect of promoting normal development is to encourage the child's self-care abilities in both activities of daily living and the medical regimen. An assessment of the child's age and physical, emotional, and mental capacities, as well as the support and structure provided by the family, should be considered in determining the appropriate level of self-care in the medical regimen. Even toddlers can be involved in their own care by holding supplies for the parent during a procedure. Over time, children should be encouraged toward greater autonomy in the self-care arena.

*PO Box 1009, Turlock, CA 95381-1009; (800) ID-ALERT, website: www.medicalert.org.

Early Childhood. During infancy the child is achieving basic *trust* through a satisfying, intimate, consistent relationship with his or her parents. However, the affected child's early existence may be stressful, chaotic, and unsatisfying. Consequently, he or she may need more parental support and expressions of affection to achieve trust. Likewise, the parents require assistance in finding ways to meet the infant's needs, such as how to hold a rigid or flaccid infant, how to feed a child with tongue thrust or episodes of dyspnea, and how to stimulate a child who seems incapable of achieving any skills. If hospitalizations are frequent or prolonged, every effort is made to preserve the parent-child relationship (see also Chapter 21). Hospital policies should promote visitation by and involvement of families.

During early childhood the goal is to achieve separation from parents, autonomy, and initiative. However, the natural parental response to having a sick child is overprotection. Parents need help in realizing the importance of brief separations of the child from them and from others involved in the child's care and of providing social experiences outside the home whenever possible. Respite care, which provides temporary relief for family members, can be essential in allowing caregivers time away from the daily burdens.

Young children also need the opportunity to develop independence. Frequently the child is able to learn self-help skills, such as holding the bottle, finger feeding, and removing simple articles of clothing, but the parent continues to perform the act. The nurse can guide parents to the usual milestones expected from the child.

When the young child has a disability that interferes with motor development, intervention must be based on providing activities that allow maximum motor development. Also, the activity must take into account the child's need for social interaction, sense of control over the body, feeling of competence and achievement, and an outlet for aggression.

When a child is unable to perform a skill independently, functional aids should be used. With innovation, many adaptations can be implemented in children's environments to increase their mobility and independence and allow them to play like other children their age. For example, with slight modifications, a child with physical limitations may be able to ride a tricycle (Fig. 18-4).

Another critical component for normal child development is discipline. Discipline and guidance serve several purposes, such as providing children with boundaries on which to test out their behavior and teaching them socially acceptable behavior. Resentment and hostility can arise among siblings if different standards are applied to each child. The nurse's responsibility is to help parents learn successful methods of managing a child's behaviors before they become problems (see Chapter 3).

School Age. For school-age children the major tasks are entry into school and achieving a sense of *industry.* Although the importance of school in the life of all children is well known, school absences are significantly higher among children with chronic illness than among their healthy peers. The more school absences the child experiences, the more difficult it is to resume attendance, and "school pho-

TABLE 18-2 ■ Developmental Aspects of Chronic Illness or Disability on Children

DEVELOPMENTAL TASKS	POTENTIAL EFFECTS OF CHRONIC ILLNESS OR DISABILITY	SUPPORTIVE INTERVENTIONS
INFANCY		
Develop a sense of trust	Multiple caregivers and frequent separations, especially if hospitalized	Encourage consistent caregivers in hospital or other care settings
	Deprived of consistent nurturing	Encourage parental presence, "rooming in" during hospitalization, and participation in care
Bond/attach to parent	Delayed because of separation, parental grief for loss of "dream" child, parental inability to accept the condition, especially a visible defect	Emphasize healthy, perfect qualities of infant Help parents learn special care needs of infant for them to feel competent
Learn through sensorimotor experiences	Increased exposure to painful experiences over pleasurable ones	Expose infant to pleasurable experiences through all senses (touch, hearing, sight, taste, movement)
	Limited contact with environment from restricted movement or confinement	Encourage age-appropriate developmental skills (e.g., holding bottle, finger feeding, crawling)
Begin to develop a sense of separateness from parent	Increased dependency on parent for care Overinvolvement of parent in care	Encourage all family members to participate in care to prevent overinvolvement of one member Encourage periodic respite from demands of care responsibilities
TODDLERHOOD		
Develop autonomy	Increased dependency on parent	Encourage independence in as many areas as possible (e.g., toileting, dressing, feeding)
Master locomotor and language skills	Limited opportunity to test own abilities and limits	Provide gross motor skill activity and modification of toys or equipment, such as modified swing or rocking horse
Learn through sensorimotor experience; beginning preoperational thought	Increased exposure to painful experiences	Give choices to allow simple feeling of control (e.g., choice of what book to look at, what kind of sandwich to eat)
		Institute age-appropriate discipline and limit setting Recognize that negative and ritualistic behaviors are normal
		Provide sensory experiences (e.g., water play, sandbox play, finger painting)
PRESCHOOL		
Develop initiative and purpose	Limited opportunities for success in accomplishing simple tasks or mastering self-care skills	Encourage mastery of self-help skills Provide devices that make task easier (e.g., self-dressing)
Master self-care skills	Limited opportunities for socialization with peers; may appear "like a baby" to age-mates	Encourage socialization (e.g., inviting friends to play, day care experience, trips to park)
Begin to develop peer relationships	Protection within tolerant and secure family may cause child to fear criticism and withdraw	Provide age-appropriate play, especially associative play opportunities Emphasize child's abilities; dress appropriately to enhance desirable appearance
Develop sense of body image and sexual identification	Awareness of body may center on pain, anxiety, and failure	Encourage relationships with same-sex and opposite-sex peers and adults
	Sex-role identification focused primarily on mothering skills	Help child deal with criticisms; realize that too much protection prevents child from realities of world
Learn through preoperational thought (magical thinking)	Guilt (thinking he or she caused the illness/disability or is being punished for wrongdoing)	Clarify that cause of child's illness or disability is not his or her fault or a punishment
SCHOOL AGE		
Develop a sense of accomplishment	Limited opportunities to achieve and compete (e.g., many school absences, inability to join regular athletic activities)	Encourage school attendance; schedule medical visits at times other than school; encourage child to make up missed work
Form peer relationships	Limited opportunities for socialization	Educate teachers and classmates about child's condition, abilities, and special needs
Learn through concrete operations	Incomplete comprehension of the imposed physical limitations or treatment of the disorder	Encourage sports activities (e.g., Special Olympics) Encourage socialization (e.g., Girl Scouts, Campfire, Boy Scouts, 4-H Club; having a best friend or club membership)
		Provide child with knowledge about his or her condition
		Encourage creative activities (e.g., Very Special Arts)

Continued

TABLE 18-2 ■ Developmental Aspects of Chronic Illness or Disability on Children—cont'd

DEVELOPMENTAL TASKS	POTENTIAL EFFECTS OF CHRONIC ILLNESS OR DISABILITY	SUPPORTIVE INTERVENTIONS
ADOLESCENCE		
Develop personal and sexual identity	Increased sense of feeling different from peers and less able to compete with peers in appearance, abilities, special skills	Realize that many of the difficulties the teenager is experiencing are part of normal adolescence (rebelliousness, risk taking, lack of cooperation, hostility toward authority)
Achieve independence from family	Increased dependency on family; limited job/career opportunities	Provide instruction on interpersonal and coping skills
Form heterosexual relationships	Limited opportunities for heterosexual friendships; less opportunity to discuss sexual concerns with peers	Encourage socialization with peers, including peers with special needs and those without special needs
Learn through abstract thinking	Increased concern with issues such as why did he or she get the disorder, can he or she marry and have a family	Provide instruction on decision making, assertiveness, and other skills necessary to manage personal plans
	Decreased opportunity for earlier stages of cognition may impede achieving level of abstract thinking	Encourage increased responsibility for care and management of the disease or condition (e.g., assuming responsibility for making and keeping appointment [ideally alone], sharing assessment and planning stages of health care delivery, contacting resources)
		Encourage activities appropriate for age (e.g., attending mixed-sex parties, sports activities, driving a car)
		Be alert to cues that signal readiness for information regarding implications of condition on sexuality and reproduction
		Emphasize good appearance and wearing stylish clothes, use of makeup
		Understand that adolescent has same sexual needs and concerns as any other teenager
		Discuss planning for future and how condition can affect choices

bia" may result. The child should return to school as soon as possible after diagnosis or treatments.

Preparation for entry into or resumption of school is best accomplished through a team approach with the parents, child, schoolteacher, school nurse, and primary nurse in the hospital. Ideally, this planning should begin before hospital discharge, provided that the child is well enough to resume usual activities. A structured plan should be developed, with attention to those aspects of care that must be continued during school hours, such as administration of medication or other treatments.

Children also need preparation before entering or resuming school. Having a tutor in the hospital or home as soon as children are physically able helps them realize that school will continue and gives them time to consider this prospect (Fig. 18-5). They need to investigate possible answers to the many questions others will ask. One method of anticipatory preparation is to role-play, with the child as the "returned pupil" and the nurse or parent as "other schoolmates." If the child returns to school with some obvious physical change, such as hair loss, amputation, or visible scar, the nurse might also ask questions about these alterations to prompt preparatory responses from the child.

Classroom peers also need preparation, and a joint plan of the schoolteacher, nurse, and child is best. At a minimum, the classmates should be given a description of the child's condition, prepared for any visible changes in the child, and allowed an opportunity to ask questions. The child should have the option of attending this session. As the child's condition changes, particularly if the illness is potentially fatal, school personnel, including the students, need periodic appraisal of the child's status and preparation for what to expect.

Children with special needs are encouraged to maintain or reestablish relationships with peers and to participate according to their capabilities in any age-appropriate activities. Alternative activities may be substituted for those that are impossible or that place a strain on the child's condition. Programs such as the **Special Olympics*** offer children an opportunity to compete with their peers and to achieve athletic skill. Summer camps† allow children to associate with peers and develop a wide variety of skills. Children with spe-

---

*1350 New York Avenue, NW, Suite 500, Washington, DC 20005-1581; (202) 628-3630. Several pamphlets on sports and recreation for children with disabilities are available from the **Easter Seals National Headquarters,** 230 W. Monroe Street, Suite 1800, Chicago, IL 60606; (312) 726-6200; website: www.easter-seals.org; and the **American Alliance for Health, Physical Education, Recreation and Dance (AAHPERD),** 1900 Association Drive, Reston, VA 22091; (703) 476-3400; website: www.aahperd.org.
†A directory of camps for children with a variety of chronic illnesses or general physical disabilities is available for a fee from the **American Camping Association,** Publications Service, 5000 State Road, 67 N., Martinsville, IN 46151; (800) 428-CAMP.

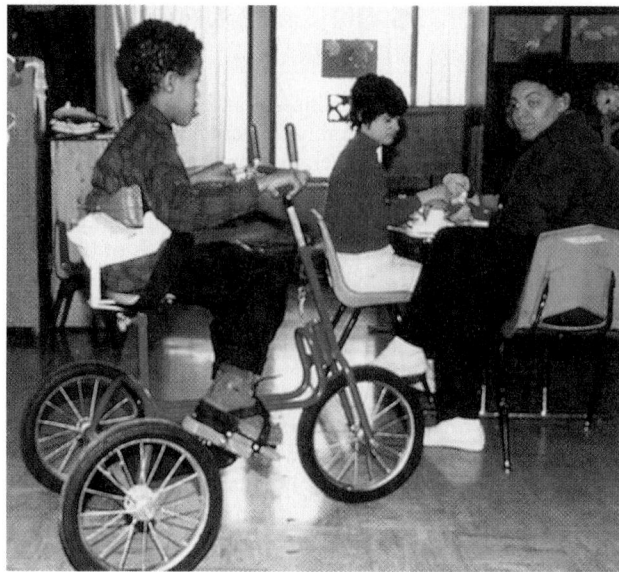

FIG. 18-4 ■ A modified tricycle with block pedals, self-adhesive straps for support, and modified seat and handle bars can help a child with disabilities gain mobility.

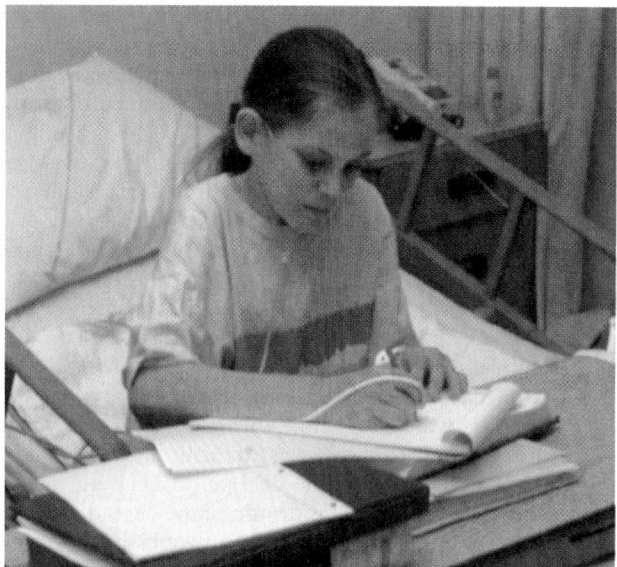

FIG. 18-5 ■ Children with special needs should continue their schooling as soon as their condition permits.

cial needs can derive enormous benefits from expressive activities, such as art, music, poetry, dance, and drama. With adaptive equipment and imagination, children can participate in a variety of activities. Organizations such as **VSA Arts** (Very Special Arts) offer children an opportunity to celebrate and share their accomplishments.* Children need the opportunity to interact with healthy peers, as well as to engage in activities with groups or clubs composed of similarly affected age-mates. Such organizations as ostomy clubs, diabetes clubs, and cerebral palsy groups share information and provide support related to the special problems the members face.

Adolescence.   Adolescence can be a particularly difficult period for the teenager and family. All of the needs discussed previously apply to this age-group as well. Developing *independence* or *autonomy,* however, is a major task for the adolescent as planning for the future becomes a prominent concern. Although the emphasis in the past has been on achieving independence from physical assistance, recent developments in the fields of special education, adolescent development, and family systems suggest redefining autonomy in terms of individuals' capacities to take responsibility for their own behavior, to make decisions regarding their own lives, and to maintain supportive social relationships. Given this understanding, even individuals with severe impairment can be viewed as autonomous if they perceive their own needs and take responsibility for meeting them, either directly or by engaging the assistance of others. As adolescents become more autonomous, the nurse can help

them articulate needs, participate in developing their own plan of care, and discover and express how others can be of greatest assistance.

Physical symptoms are high on the teenager's list of health-related concerns. Because adolescence is a time of enormous physical and emotional changes, it is important for the nurse to make a distinction between body changes that are related to disability and those that are a result of normal body development. It can be a great comfort for teenagers with disabling conditions to know that many of the changes they experience are normal developmental outcomes.

A sense of feeling different from peers can lead to loneliness, isolation, and depression. Participation in groups of teenagers with chronic conditions or disabilities can alleviate feelings of isolation and smooth the transition to a meaningful relationship with one person in adulthood.

Establish Realistic Future Goals

One of the most difficult adjustments is setting realistic future goals for the child and for those involved in his or her continued care. Sometimes the impact of this decision does not surface until the child finishes school or the parents approach retirement, when a crisis can arise because all of the family roles and relationships that maintained stability are now disrupted.

Planning for the future should be a gradual process. All along, the parents should cultivate realistic vocations for the child. For example, if children have physical disabilities, they are directed to intellectual, artistic, or musical pursuits. Children with developmental disabilities are taught manual skills. In this way, the child's development proceeds in the direction of self-support through gainful employment.

With prolonged survival, young people with chronic illnesses must deal with new decisions and problems, such as marriage, employment, and insurance coverage. With appropriate guidance, gainful employment, marriage, and a family are attainable goals. For those whose conditions are

---

*VSA Arts has affiliate chapters in all 50 states and in selected sites internationally; yearly festivals are held throughout the world. Information is available from **VSA Arts,** 1300 Connecticut Avenue NW, Suite 700, Washington, DC 20036; (202) 737-0645; website: www.vsarts.org.

genetic, counseling is needed regarding future offspring. Prospective spouses often benefit from an opportunity to discuss their feelings regarding marriage to an individual with continued health needs and possibly a limited lifespan. Health insurance coverage is a critical issue because some private carriers may no longer insure a young person who leaves home or may be unwilling to reinsure the person who is independent. Life insurance is another dilemma, especially when children have serious defects, such as congenital heart anomalies.

Unfortunately, vocational pursuits and completely independent living are not realistic goals for all persons. Persons with multiple or severe disabilities may require lifelong care and assistance. In these situations parents must look to the time when they will no longer be able to care for their child. Residential placement may be very difficult unless the family mutually participates in the decision-making and planning process. Placement outside the home should not be viewed as abandonment. Not infrequently it is the only way to preserve the family unit. The nurse should help the family investigate suitable placements, discuss their feelings regarding this decision, and help the family explore measures to maintain meaningful communication between family members.

● *Evaluation*

The effectiveness of nursing interventions is determined by continual reassessment and evaluation of care based on the following observational guidelines:

1 Observe family members' responses to the diagnosis and the types of questions or concerns they have.
2 Interview family regarding their knowledge and understanding of the child's condition; observe if they have instituted suggestions, such as use of identification devices for children with certain conditions.
3 Observe responses of professionals to reactions such as denial, guilt, and anger and whether supportive interventions are used with the family.
4 Observe family's communication patterns with each other and their ability to discuss feelings about issues such as the impact of the child's condition on the marriage or additional care responsibilities; investigate family's use of services, such as self-help groups or other community resources.
5 Perform a developmental screening test on young children and compare results with expected milestones for the child's abilities; investigate use of functional aids to assist children in developing to their potential; question family about the child's attendance at school and interaction with peers.
6 Interview family to determine whether their self-identified needs and concerns have been adequately addressed.

● *Expected Outcomes*

1 Parents verbalize feelings and concerns regarding the disease or disability.
2 Parents demonstrate an attitude of acceptance and adjustment.
3 Family demonstrates an understanding of the disease and treatment options.
4 Family members set realistic goals for themselves and the child.
5 Family demonstrates positive, growth-promoting behaviors for the child and other family members.

PERSPECTIVES ON CARE OF CHILDREN AT THE END OF LIFE

Although most childhood illnesses and many injuries and other trauma respond favorably to treatment, some do not. When a child and family face a prolonged and possibly terminal illness, health professionals are faced with the challenge of providing the best possible care to meet the physical, psychologic, spiritual, and emotional needs of the child and family during the uncertain course of the illness and at the time of death. When death is sudden and unexpected, nurses are challenged to respond to grief and shock in families and provide comfort and support in the absence of a prior relationship.

Many factors affect the causes of death that nurses are likely to encounter in children: developmental factors, medical advances and technology, and changing social patterns. In infants the leading causes of death are congenital anomalies, respiratory distress syndrome, disorders related to short gestation and low birth weight, and sudden infant death syndrome (Arias and others, 2003) (see Chapter 1). The leading causes of death in children 5 to 9 years of age include injuries (accidents), malignant neoplasms, congenital anomalies, homicide (and legal intervention), and heart disease. In children 10 to 14 years of age, suicide is the third leading cause of death after injuries (accidents) and malignant neoplasms. In youths 15 to 19 years of age, homicide (and legal intervention), suicide, malignant neoplasms, and heart disease follow accidents as the most prevalent causes of death (Minino and Smith, 2001).

A child who is diagnosed with a life-threatening illness or who is suffering serious, life-threatening trauma needs medical diagnosis and intervention, as well as nursing assessment and care—sometimes for a short time and sometimes over a lengthy period. When cure is no longer possible and life-prolonging measures are resulting in pain and distress to the child, parents need information about care options that are available to assist them in deciding how they want the remaining time with their child to be managed by the health care team. It is important that families be reassured that although their child cannot be cured, active care will continue to be provided to maintain the child's comfort. Support must be provided to assist the child and family during the dying process. As a result, nurses may care for children and families who are making the difficult transition from curative or restorative treatments to palliative care.

PRINCIPLES OF PALLIATIVE CARE

Palliative care involves a multidisciplinary approach to the management of a terminal illness or the dying process that focuses on symptom control and support rather than on cure or life prolongation in the absence of the possibility of a cure (Billings, 1998). The World Health Organization (1996) defines *palliative care* as the "active total care of patients whose disease is not responsive to curative treatment. Control of pain, of other symptoms, and of psychologic, social and spiritual problems is paramount. The goal of palliative care is the achievement of the best possible quality of life for patients and their families." Palliative care interventions do not serve to hasten death; rather, they provide pain and symptom management, attention to issues faced by the child and family with regard to death and dying, and promotion of optimal functioning and quality of life during the time the child has remaining. There are several principles that are hallmarks of palliative care.

The child and family are considered the unit of care. The death of a child is an extremely stressful event for a family because it is out of the natural order of things. Children represent health and hope, and their death calls into question the understanding of life. A multidisciplinary team of health care professionals consisting of social workers, chaplains, nurses, personal care aides, and physicians skilled in caring for dying patients assist the family by focusing care on the complex interactions between physical, emotional, social, and spiritual issues.

Palliative care seeks to create a therapeutic environment, as homelike as possible, if not in the child's own home. Through education and support of family members, an atmosphere of open communication is provided regarding the child's dying process and its impact on all members of the family.

DECISION MAKING AT THE END OF LIFE

Discussions concerning the possibility that a child's illness or condition is not curable and that death is an inevitable outcome causes everyone involved a great deal of stress. Physicians, other members of the health care team, and families must consider all information regarding the child's situation and make decisions that all parties agree to and that will have a profound impact on the child and family.

Ethical Considerations in End-of-Life Decision Making

A number of ethical concerns arise when parents and health care professionals are deciding on the best course of care for the dying child. Many parents and health care providers are concerned that not offering treatment that would cause potential pain and suffering, but might extend life, would be considered euthanasia or assisted suicide. To eliminate such concerns, it is necessary to understand the various terms. *Euthanasia* involves an action carried out by a person other than the patient to end the life of the patient suffering from a terminal condition. The intent of this action is based on the belief that the act is "putting the person out of his or her misery," and this action has also been called *mercy killing. Assisted suicide* occurs when someone provides the patient with the means to end his or her life and the patient uses that means to do so. The important distinction between these two actions involves who is actually acting to end the person's life.

The American Nurses Association (ANA) Code for Nurses (2001) does not support the active intent on the part of a nurse to end a person's life. However, it does permit the nurse to provide interventions to relieve symptoms in the dying client even when the interventions involve substantial risks of hastening death. When the prognosis for a patient is poor and death is the expected outcome, it is ethically acceptable to withhold or withdraw treatments that may cause pain and suffering and provide interventions that promote comfort and quality of life. Therefore, providing palliative care for patients is the ethically correct choice in such a circumstance.

Physician/Health Care Team Decision Making

Decisions by physicians regarding care are often made on the basis of the progression of the disease or amount of trauma, the availability of treatment options that would provide cure from disease or restoration of health, the impact of such treatments on the child, and the child's overall prognosis (Davis and Eng, 1998). When the physician discusses this information openly with families, a shared decision-making process can occur and decisions can be made regarding *"do not resuscitate" (DNR) orders* and care that is focused on the comfort of the child and family during the dying process. Unfortunately, many families are not given the option of terminating treatment and pursuing care that is focused on comfort and quality of life when cure is unlikely, and staff may be reluctant to raise the question of DNR orders. This occurs for a number of reasons, including the belief that not being able to "save" a child is a "failure." Also, the physician and other members of the health care team may lack knowledge of and experience with the principles of palliative care (Field and Behrman, 2003; Sumner, 2003; Sahler and others, 2000).

Parental Decision Making

Rarely are families prepared to cope with the numerous decisions that must be made when a child is dying. When the death is unexpected, as in the case of an accident or trauma, the confusion of emergency services and possibly an intensive care setting presents challenges to parents as they are asked to make very difficult choices. If the child has experienced either a life-threatening illness such as cancer or lived with a chronic illness that has now reached its terminal phase, parents are often unprepared for the reality of their child's impending death (see Family Focus box). Numerous studies have found that families facing the impending death of a child depend on information provided to them by the health care team, particularly an honest appraisal of the child's prognosis, to make difficult decisions regarding care options for their child (Wolfe, Friebert, and Hilden, 2002; Hinds and others, 2001; James and Johnson, 1997).

As the group of health professionals who are most involved with families, nurses are in an excellent position to ensure that families are presented with the options available to them. The nurse's first responsibility is to explore the family's wishes. This is best done in concert with the physician, but at times may need to be initiated by the nurse. Statements such as "Tell me about your thoughts for the type of care you want your child to receive when he is dying" or "Have you considered the types of interventions you would like us to use when your child is near death?" can begin discussion of this sensitive but critical aspect of terminal care.

The Dying Child

Children need honest and accurate information about their illness, treatments, and prognosis; this information needs to be given in clear, simple language. In most situations this best occurs as a gradual process over time, characterized by increasingly open dialogue between parents, professionals, and the child (Young and others, 2003). Providing an atmosphere of open communication early in the course of an illness facilitates answering difficult questions as the child's condition worsens. Providing appropriate literature about the disease, as well as the experience of illness and possible death, is also helpful. Exactly how and when to involve children in decisions regarding care during their dying process and death is a very individual matter. The age or developmental level of the child is an important consideration in the process (Table 18-3). In general, parents should be asked how they would like their child to be told of their prognosis, and should be included in their care. Some parents may request that their child not be told that he or she is dying, even if the child asks. This often places health care providers in a difficult situation. Children, even at a young age, are very perceptive. Despite not being "told" outright that they are dying, they realize that there is something seriously wrong and that it involves them. Often, helping parents understand that honesty and shared decision making between them and their child at this time is very important to the child's emotional health, as well as the emotional health of the family, will encourage parents to allow discussion of dying with their child. Parents may require professional support and guidance in this process from a nurse, social worker, or child life specialist who has a good relationship with the child and family.

If given the opportunity, children will tell others how much they want to know. Asking questions such as "If the disease came back, would you want to know?" "Do you want others to tell you everything, even if the news isn't good?" or "If someone were not getting better (or more directly, "were dying"), do you think they would want to know?" helps children set the limits of how much truth they can accept and cope with. Children need time to process many feelings and much information so that they can assimilate and hopefully accept the inevitable fact of mortality.

Care of the dying adolescent requires the nurse to become knowledgeable about any possible delays or alterations in the normal growth and development. Legal and ethical issues also come to the forefront with respect to the age at which an adolescent should have autonomy in decision making with regard to care and treatment. Effective communication between the patient, family, and health care team is an important part of optimal care for the dying adolescent (Freyer 2004).

Treatment Options for Terminally Ill Children

Based on the outcome of the decision by the child and family regarding their wishes for care, there are several options for care that the family may choose.

Hospital.   Families may choose to remain in the hospital to receive care if the child's illness or condition is unstable and home care is not an option or the family is uncomfortable with providing care at home. If a family chooses to remain at the hospital for terminal care, the setting should be made as homelike as possible. Families should be encouraged to bring familiar items from the child's room at home. In addition, there should be a consistent and coordinated plan of care for the child and family's comfort.

Home Care.   Some families may prefer to take their child home and receive services from a home care agency. Generally, these services entail periodic nursing visits to administer a treatment or provide medications, equipment, or supplies. The child's care continues to be directed by the primary physician. Home care is often the option chosen by physicians and families because of the traditional view that a child must be considered to have a life expectancy of less than 6 months to be referred to hospice care. Fortunately, a number of hospice organizations are expanding their services to children based on the presence of a life-limiting disease process for which cure is not possible, rather than on the sole criteria of a limited 6-month prognosis.

Hospice Care.   Parents should be offered the option of caring for their child at home during the final phases of an illness with the assistance of a hospice organization. ***Hospice*** is a community health care organization that specializes in the care of dying patients by combining the hospice philosophy with the principles of palliative care. Hospice philosophy regards dying as a natural process and care of dying patients as including management of the physical, psychologic, social, and spiritual needs of the patient and family. Care is provided by a multidisciplinary group of professionals in the patient's home or an inpatient facility that employs the hospice philosophy. Hospice care for children was introduced in the 1970s, and a number of community hospice organizations now accept children into their care (Davies, Davis, and Sibert, 2003; Forrester, 2003; Winkler and Mardegian, 2001; Faulkner and Armstrong-Daily, 1997). Collaboration

FAMILY FOCUS

Family of the Dying Child

No matter whether you have a PhD or many children, when your child dies, it is a new experience and nothing can prepare you for it. Like so many things in life, experience is the best teacher.

Three of our children have died, and by the time the third was dying, we handled many things differently. We learned a lot about dignity and the rights of the child and family. For example, at first, we didn't know that we had a right to have our child die at home. We also didn't understand pain medications and that if children are taking these medicines and are still in agony, they have not overdosed on the medication.

We learned a lot about case management. With our first two children, lots of different people were making decisions and disagreeing about what was best and what should be done. No one had primary authority. With our third child, one doctor took a primary role. Any questions and problems were handled by one person. I could call him 24 hours a day. It made a lot of difference, and I felt our concerns and needs were better heard and respected.

The nurses caring for our third child at home enabled me to step back and just be his mommy. When I could do this, I realized that we were fighting so hard for his life that we weren't really letting him die. His nurses had worked with him for a long time and really loved him. It was hard for them when we decided to let him die. In his last several days we wanted a lot of family time with our son, and I think the nurses felt left out. Something about their reaction to our increased time with him in the last few days made us feel guilty. If we had all been able to communicate a little more openly, I would have understood that they needed more time with him at the end, too. Everyone's needs could have been met.

Jeni Stepanek
Mother
Upper Marlboro, Md

between the child's primary treatment team and the hospice care team is essential to the success of hospice care. Families may continue to see their primary care physicians as they choose.*

Hospice care is based on a number of important concepts that significantly set it apart from hospital care. First, family members are the principal caregivers and are supported by a team of professional and volunteer staff. Second, the priority of care is comfort. The child's physical, psychologic, social, and spiritual needs are considered. Pain and symptom control are primary concerns, and no extraordinary efforts are used to attempt a cure or prolong life. Third, the needs of the family are considered to be as important as those of the patient. Fourth, hospice is concerned with the family's postdeath adjustment, and care may continue for a year or more.

The goal of hospice care is for children to live life to the fullest without pain, with choices and dignity, in the fa-

*National Hospice and Palliative Care Organization, 1700 Diagonal Road, Suite 625, Alexandria, VA 22314; (703) 837-1500; fax: (703) 837-1233; website: www.nho.org; and Children's Hospice International, 901 North Pitt Street, Suite 230, Alexandria, VA 22314; (703) 684-0330 or (800) 24-CHILD; website: www.chionline.org.

TABLE 18-3 ■ Children's Understanding of and Reactions to Death

CONCEPTS OF DEATH	REACTIONS TO DEATH	INTERVENTIONS
INFANTS AND TODDLERS		
Death has least significance to children younger than 6 months of age	With the death of someone else, they may continue to act as though the person is alive	Help parents deal with their feelings, allowing them more emotional reserve to meet the needs of their children
After parent-child attachment and the development of trust is established, the loss, even if temporary, of the significant person is profound	As children grow older, they will be increasingly able and willing to let go of the dead person	Encourage parents to remain as near to child as possible, yet be sensitive to parents' needs
Prolonged separation during the first several years is thought to be more significant in terms of future physical, social, and emotional growth than at any subsequent age	Ritualism is important; a change in lifestyle could be anxiety producing	Maintain as normal an environment as possible to retain ritualism
Toddlers are egocentric and can only think about events in terms of their own frame of reference—living	This age-group reacts more to the pain and discomfort of a serious illness than to the probable fatal prognosis	If a parent has died, encourage having consistent caregiver for child
Their egocentricity and vague separation of fact and fantasy make it impossible for them to comprehend absence of life	This age-group also reacts to parental anxiety and sadness	Promote primary nursing
Instead of understanding death, this age-group is affected more by any change in lifestyle		
PRESCHOOL CHILDREN		
Believe their thoughts are sufficient to cause death; the consequence is the burden of guilt, shame, and punishment	If they become seriously ill, they conceive of the illness as a punishment for their thoughts or actions	Help parents deal with their feelings, allowing them more emotional reserve to meet the needs of their children
Their egocentricity implies a tremendous sense of self-power and omnipotence	May feel guilty and responsible for the death of a sibling	Help parents to understand behavioral reactions of their children
Usually have some connotation of its meaning	Greatest fear concerning death is separation from parents	Encourage parents to remain near the child as much as possible, to minimize the child's great fear of separation from parents
Death is seen as a departure, a kind of sleep	May engage in activities that seem strange or abnormal to adults	If a parent has died, encourage having a consistent caregiver for child
May recognize the fact of physical death but do not separate it from living abilities	Because of their fewer defense mechanisms to deal with loss, young children may react to a less significant loss with more outward grief than to the loss of a very significant person	Promote primary nursing
Death is seen as temporary and gradual; life and death can change places with one another	The loss is so deep, painful, and threatening that the child must deny it for the time being to survive its overwhelming impact	
No understanding of the universality and inevitability of death	Behavior reactions such as giggling, joking, attracting attention, or regressing to earlier developmental skills indicate children's need to distance themselves from tremendous loss	

Continued

TABLE 18-3 ■ **Children's Understanding of and Reactions to Death—***cont'd*

CONCEPTS OF DEATH	REACTIONS TO DEATH	INTERVENTIONS
SCHOOL-AGE CHILDREN		
Still associate misdeeds or bad thoughts with causing death and feel intense guilt and responsibility for the event Because of their higher cognitive abilities, they respond well to logical explanations and comprehend the figurative meaning of words Have a deeper understanding of death in a concrete sense Particularly fear the mutilation and punishment they associate with death Personify death as the devil, a monster, or the bogeyman May have naturalistic/physiologic explanations of death By age 9 or 10, children have an adult concept of death, realizing that it is inevitable, universal, and irreversible	Because of their increased ability to comprehend, they may have more fears, for example: 　The reason for the illness 　Communicability of the disease to themselves or others 　Consequences of the disease 　The process of dying and death itself Their fear of the unknown is greater than their fear of the known The realization of impending death is a tremendous threat to their sense of security and ego strength Likely to exhibit fear through verbal uncooperativeness rather than actual physical aggression Very interested in postdeath services May be inquisitive about what happens to the body	Help parents deal with their feelings, allowing them more emotional reserve to meet the needs of their children Encourage parents to remain near child as much as possible, yet be sensitive to parents' needs Because of children's fear of the unknown, anticipatory preparation is very important Because the developmental task of this age is industry, interventions of helping children maintain control over their bodies and increasing their understanding allow them to achieve independence, self-worth, and self-esteem and avoid a sense of inferiority Encourage children to talk about their feelings and provide aggressive outlets Encourage parents to honestly answer questions about dying rather than avoiding or fabricating euphemisms Encourage parents to share their moments of sorrow with their children Provide preparation for postdeath services
ADOLESCENTS		
Have a mature understanding of death Still very much influenced by "remnants" of magical thinking and are subject to guilt and shame Likely to see deviations from accepted behavior as reasons for their illness	Straddle transition from childhood to adulthood Have the most difficulty in coping with death Least likely to accept cessation of life, particularly if it is their own Concern is for the present much more than for the past or the future May consider themselves alienated from their peers and unable to communicate with their parents for emotional support, feeling alone in their struggle Adolescents' orientation to the present compels them to worry about physical changes even more than the prognosis Because of their idealistic view of the world, they may criticize funeral rites as barbaric, money making, and unnecessary	Help parents deal with their feelings, allowing them more emotional reserve to meet the needs of their children Avoid alliances with either parent or child Structure hospital admission to allow for maximum self-control and independence Answer adolescents' questions honestly, treating them as mature individuals and respecting their needs for privacy, solitude, and personal expressions of emotions Help parents understand their child's reactions to death/dying, especially that concern for present crises, such as loss of hair, may be much greater than for future ones, including possible death

miliar environment of their home, and with the support of their family. Hospice care is covered under state Medicaid programs, as well as by most insurance plans. The service provides home nursing visits, as well as visits from social workers, chaplains, and, in some cases, physicians. Medications, medical equipment, and any necessary medical supplies are all provided by the hospice organization providing care.

With children, the home has been the more common environment for implementing the hospice concept; it benefits the family in a variety of ways. Children who are dying are allowed the opportunity to remain with those they love and with whom they feel secure. Many children who were

thought to be in imminent danger of death have gone home and lived longer than expected. Siblings can feel more involved in the care and often have more positive perceptions of the death. Parental adaptation is often more favorable, as is shown by their perceptions of how the experience at home affected their marriage, social reorientation, religious beliefs, and views on the meaning of life and death.

If the home is chosen for hospice care, the child may or may not die in the home. Reasons for final admission to a hospital vary but may be related to the parents' or siblings' wish to have the child die outside the home; exhaustion on the part of the caregivers; and physical problems such as sudden, acute pain or respiratory distress.

NURSING CARE OF THE CHILD AND FAMILY AT THE END OF LIFE

Regardless of where the child is cared for during the terminal stage of illness, both the child and the family usually experience the following fears: (1) fear of pain and suffering, (2) fear of dying alone (child) or of not being present when the child dies (parent), and (3) fear of actual death. Nurses can assist families by lessening their fears through attention to the care needs of the child and family (see Nursing Care Plan, below).

FEAR OF PAIN AND SUFFERING

The presence of unrelieved pain in a terminally ill child can have very detrimental effects on the quality of life experienced by the child and family. Parents have reported that having their child in pain was unendurable and resulted in feelings of helplessness and a sense that they must be present and vigilant to get the necessary pain medications. Persistent pain also has an impact on the family as a whole. Nurses can alleviate the fear of pain and suffering by providing interventions aimed at treating the pain and symptoms associated with the terminal process in children.

NURSING CARE PLAN   The Child Who Is Terminally Ill or Dying

NURSING DIAGNOSIS ■ **Altered growth and development related to terminal illness or impending death**

PATIENT GOAL 1: Will receive adequate support during terminal phase

NURSING INTERVENTIONS/*RATIONALES*

Encourage family to remain near child as much as possible *to provide support through their presence*

Encourage child to talk about feelings; help family as they encourage child to express feelings

Provide safe, acceptable outlets for aggression

Answer questions as honestly as possible while maintaining a positive, hopeful approach

Explain all procedures and therapies, especially physical effects child will experience

Help child distinguish between consequences of therapies and manifestations of disease process

Structure hospital environment to allow for maximum self-control and independence within the limitations imposed by child's developmental level and physical condition

Respect child's need for privacy without neglecting child

Provide for presence of customary support systems

EXPECTED OUTCOMES

Child expresses feelings freely

Child demonstrates an understanding of symptoms

PATIENT GOAL 2: Will exhibit minimal or no evidence of physical discomfort

NURSING INTERVENTIONS/*RATIONALES*

Appreciate that pain control is essential component of physical and emotional care during terminal stage

Provide pain relief around the clock *to prevent the recurrence of pain*

Encourage family to provide comfort measures child prefers (e.g., rocking, stroking)

Avoid excessive noise or light *that may irritate child*

Place all commodities within easy reach *to increase child's control and lessen need for excessive movement*

Use gentle, minimal physical manipulation

Avoid pressure (bedclothes, sheets) on painful areas

Experiment with using heat or cold on painful areas *(use cautiously because of easy skin breakdown)*

Whenever possible, make use of procedures (e.g., noninvasive temperature monitoring) *to minimize discomfort*

Change position frequently; if difficult for child, coordinate with pain relief from analgesics *to make moving easier and less distressing*

Avoid pressure on bony prominences or painful sites (water bed, flotation mattress); ensure good body alignment *to prevent skin breakdown*

Keep fresh air circulating in room (open window, use small fan)

Use pillows or other supports to prop child in comfortable position

Carry child (if possible) to other areas for diversion if desired

Place absorbent pads under hips *because child may be* incontinent

Help child to toilet if desired

Limit care to essentials

    May need to forego usual hygienic measures such as bath or clothing change but provide comfort measures (e.g., mouth care, wiping forehead, gentle back rub)

*Administer anticholinergic drugs (atropine or scopolamine) *to reduce secretions (lessens "death rattle," which can be distressing to family)*

EXPECTED OUTCOME

Child exhibits minimal or no evidence of physical discomfort

PATIENT GOAL 3: Will receive adequate emotional support at time of dying

NURSING INTERVENTIONS/*RATIONALES*

Preserve child's physical closeness with family members (e.g., parent may want to rock child in chair, lie next to child in bed)

Teach family about supportive interventions

Talk to child even though child may not appear to be awake

Position self and others where child can easily see face (e.g., sit at head of bed)

Speak to child in clear, distinct voice; avoid whispering

Avoid conversation about child in child's presence *to reduce anxiety/fear*

Offer calm reassurance and orient child to surroundings when awake

Phrase questions for "yes" or "no" answers *to conserve energy*

Avoid repeated measurements of vital signs, *which only disturb child*

Play favorite music *(may soothe child)*

EXPECTED OUTCOME

Child appears calm and relaxed

---

*Dependent nursing action.

Continued

NURSING CARE PLAN The Child Who Is Terminally Ill or Dying—*cont'd*

NURSING DIAGNOSIS ▪ Altered nutrition: less than body requirements related to loss of appetite, disinterest in food

PATIENT GOAL 1: Will receive optimal nutrition

NURSING INTERVENTIONS/*RATIONALES*
Offer any food and fluids child requests
Provide small meals and snacks several times a day
Avoid excessive encouragement to eat or drink
Avoid foods with strong odors *because they may cause nausea*
Provide pleasant environment for eating
Serve foods that require the least energy to eat (soups, shakes)
Feed slowly *to conserve energy*
*Administer antiemetic as prescribed if nausea/vomiting is a problem
Provide mouth care before and after eating; lubricate lips with petrolatum *to prevent cracking and promote comfort*

EXPECTED OUTCOME
Child consumes some nutrients

NURSING DIAGNOSIS ▪ Fear/anxiety related to diagnosis, tests, therapies, and prognosis

PATIENT GOAL 1: Will experience reduction of anxiety

NURSING INTERVENTIONS/*RATIONALES*
Limit interventions to palliation only; discuss need for nonpalliative treatment with family and physician
Explain all procedures and other aspects of care to child *to reduce anxiety/fear*
Remain with child or provide for constant attendance
Determine what child has been told about prognosis *so this information can be reinforced*
Determine what family wants child to know about prognosis
Emphasize importance of honesty
Answer child's questions as openly and honestly as possible
Involve parents in child's care
Remain nonjudgmental regarding child's behavior

EXPECTED OUTCOME
Child discusses fears without evidence of stress

NURSING DIAGNOSIS ▪ Anticipatory grieving related to potential loss of a child

PATIENT (FAMILY) GOAL 1: Will receive adequate support

NURSING INTERVENTIONS/*RATIONALES*
Discuss the grieving process with family *so that family better understands normalcy of feelings*
Provide opportunities for family to express emotions
Help parents deal with their feelings, *allowing them more emotional reserve to meet the needs of their children*
Encourage parents to remain as near to child as possible, yet be sensitive to parents' needs

*Dependent nursing action.

Provide information regarding child's status and anticipated reactions *to decrease anxiety/fear*
Help parents to understand behavioral reactions of their children, especially that concern for present crisis, such as loss of hair, may be much greater than for future ones, including possible death
Facilitate family's assistance with child's care
Provide comfort measures for child and family
Encourage family to maintain own health care needs
Provide as much privacy as possible
Assist family in assessing their need for referral services (e.g., hospice services, specific organizations for grieving families)
Encourage parents to answer questions about dying honestly rather than avoiding questions or using euphemisms
Encourage parents to share their moments of sorrow with their children
Discuss with parents appropriate involvement of siblings
Identify religious and cultural beliefs related to death (e.g., prayer, rites, rituals)
Provide preparation for postdeath services
Discuss with family their preferences for care if death is imminent
Arrange for appropriate spiritual care in accordance with family's beliefs or affiliations
Maintain contact with family
Provide support for families who choose home care for their child
See Guidelines box, p. 585.

EXPECTED OUTCOMES
Family expresses fear, concerns, and any special desires for terminal child
Family demonstrates an understanding of child and his or her needs (specify)
Family members avail themselves of services as desired
See also:
   Nursing Care Plan: The Child in the Hospital, Chapter 21
   Nursing Care Plan: The Family of the Ill or Hospitalized Child, Chapter 21

PATIENT (FAMILY) GOAL 2: Will exhibit no evidence of loneliness

NURSING INTERVENTIONS/*RATIONALES*
Offer calm reassurance to child
Reassure child of the love of others
Continue to set some limits for child *to provide a sense of security*
Spend time with child when not directly involved in care
Reinforce to child that what is happening is not child's fault *to decrease feelings of guilt*
Involve child in routine activities as tolerated
Maintain a "normal" atmosphere
Play favorite music and read stories to child
Orient child to surroundings when child is awake
Phrase questions for "yes" or "no" answers when possible *to conserve child's energy*

EXPECTED OUTCOME
Child exhibits no evidence of loneliness

NURSING CARE PLAN   The Child Who Is Terminally Ill or Dying—*cont'd*

NURSING DIAGNOSIS ■ **Anticipatory grieving related to imminent death of a child**

PATIENT (FAMILY) GOAL 1: Will receive adequate support

NURSING INTERVENTIONS/*RATIONALES*

Be available to family
Inform family of what to expect at time of death
Convey an attitude of caring for both child and family
Encourage at least one family member to stay with child
Help family to provide care of child as they desire without forcing involvement
*Administer medications or other agents as prescribed *to reduce unpleasant manifestations*
    Oxygen *for respiratory distress*
    Antiepileptics *for seizures*
    Anticholinergic drugs *to reduce secretions ("death rattle")*
    Analgesics *for pain*
    Stool softeners/laxatives *for constipation*
    Antiemetics *for nausea/vomiting*
Help and encourage family to express feelings appropriately
Encourage family to meet their own physical needs
Provide privacy
Provide for physical comfort of family
Provide emotional support and comfort to family
Encourage family to talk to child

*Dependent nursing action.

Involve family and other children in decision making whenever possible, especially regarding alternatives for terminal care (hospital, home, hospice)
Support and assist family in giving explanations to other family members regarding child's status
Maintain nonjudgmental attitude toward behavior of family members

EXPECTED OUTCOMES

Family members discuss their feelings
Family members are actively involved in child's care

PATIENT (FAMILY) GOAL 2: Will receive adequate support for home care

NURSING INTERVENTIONS/*RATIONALES*

Teach family physical care of child
Provide family with means for contacting health professionals at any time (e.g., phone numbers)
Maintain daily contact with family (e.g., telephone call, home visit)
Refer to community agencies as appropriate *for ongoing support*
Reassure family that they can readmit child to the hospital at any time
Help plan with family what to do when child dies and what to expect

EXPECTED OUTCOMES

Family demonstrates ability to provide care for child
Family is in contact with appropriate support groups

Pain/Symptom Management

Pain control for children in the terminal stages of illness or injury must be given the highest priority. Despite ongoing efforts to educate physicians and nurses on pain management strategies in children, studies have reported that children continue to be undermedicated for their pain (Wolfe and others, 2000). Nearly all children experience some amount of pain in the terminal phase of their illness. The current standard for treating children's pain is according to the World Health Organization's analgesic stepladder (1996). This approach promotes tailoring the pain interventions to the child's level of reported pain. Children's pain should be assessed frequently, and medications adjusted as necessary. Pain medications should be given on a regular schedule, and extra doses for "breakthrough pain" should be available to maintain comfort. Opioid drugs such as morphine should be given for severe pain, and the dose should be increased as necessary to maintain optimal pain relief. Techniques such as distraction, relaxation techniques, and guided imagery (Lambert, 1999) should be combined with drug therapy to provide the child and family with strategies to control pain (see Chapter 21 for further discussion of pain management strategies).

In addition to pain, children experience a variety of additional symptoms during their terminal course as a result of their disease process or as a side effect of medicines used to manage pain or other symptoms. These symptoms include fatigue, nausea and vomiting, constipation, anorexia, dyspnea, congestion, seizures, anxiety, depression, restlessness,

agitation, and confusion (Wolfe, Fiebert, and Hilden, 2002; Hellsten and others, 2000). Each of these symptoms should be aggressively managed with appropriate medications or treatments, as well as interventions such as repositioning, relaxation, massage, and other measures to maintain the child's comfort and quality of life.

Occasionally, children require very high doses of opioids to control pain. There are several reasons why this occurs. The child on long-term opioid pain management can become *tolerant* of the drug, meaning that it is necessary to give more drug to maintain the same level of pain relief. This should not be confused with *addiction*, which is a psychologic dependence on the side effects of opioids. Addiction is not a factor in managing terminal pain in children. Other obvious reasons for requiring increased doses of opioids include progression of disease and other physiologic experiences of pain. It is important to understand that there is no maximum dose that can be given to control pain. However, nurses often express concern that administering doses of opioids that exceed what they are familiar with will hasten the child's death. The principle of double effect (Box 18-9) addresses such concerns. It provides an ethical standard that supports the use of interventions that have the intention of relieving pain and suffering even though there is a foreseeable possibility that death may be hastened (Rousseau, 2001). However, in cases in which the child is terminally ill and in severe pain, using large doses of opioids and sedatives to manage pain is justified when there are no other treatment options available that would relieve the pain but make the risk of death less likely (Hawryluck and Harvey, 2000). See Chapter 21 for an extensive discussion of pain assessment and management.

Parents' and Siblings' Need for Education and Support

Parents are the primary caregivers when the child is at home, and nurses providing care to the child and family need to teach the family about the medications being given to the child, as well as how to administer medications and use nonpharmacologic techniques. Parents should also be kept informed of all medications and treatments given to a child in the hospital, and they should be allowed to participate in the child's care to the extent that they desire. This empowers parents and provides a sense of control over the child's comfort and well-being, reducing their fear that their child will be in pain or suffering as the child is dying.

Siblings may feel isolated and displaced during the time that their brother or sister is dying. Parents devote the majority of their time to the care and comfort of the dying child, causing siblings to feel left out of the parent–sick child relationship. Siblings may become resentful of their sick sibling and begin to feel guilty or shameful about such feelings. Nurses can assist the family by helping the parents identify ways to involve siblings in the caring process, perhaps by bringing some supply or favorite toy, game, or food item. Parents should also be encouraged to schedule some time to spend with the other children where their focus is on them. Helping parents identify a trusted friend or family member that can sit with the ill child for a short period will allow them to attend to their own needs or those of their other children.

FEAR OF DYING ALONE OR OF NOT BEING PRESENT WHEN THE CHILD DIES

When a child is being cared for at home, the burden of care experienced by parents and family members can be great. Often, as the child's condition declines, family members begin the "death vigil." Rarely is a child left alone for any length of time. This can be exhausting for family members, and nurses can assist the family by helping them arrange "shifts" so that friends or family members can be present with the child and allow others to rest. If the family has limited resources, community organizations such as hospice or churches often have volunteers who are willing to visit and sit with children. It is important that whoever is sitting with the child be aware of when the parent(s) would like to be notified to return to the child's bedside (Fig. 18-6).

When a child is dying in the hospital, parents should be given full access to the child at all times. If parents need to leave for a period, they should be provided with a pager or other means of immediate communication and alerted if staff members note any change in the child that may indicate imminent death. Nurses should advocate for parents' presence in intensive care and emergency departments and attend to the parents' needs for food, drinks, comfortable chairs, blankets, and pillows.

FEAR OF ACTUAL DEATH
Home Deaths

The majority of children receiving hospice care die at home, often in their own room with family, pets, and other loved possessions around them. The physical process of dying can be very distressing to parents, because often the child has slowly become less alert in the days before the actual death. The nurse can assist the family by providing them with information about what changes will occur as the child progresses through the dying process (Box 18-10). During this time, nursing visits often become more frequent and longer in duration to provide the family with additional support as the death nears. The most distressing change for parents to observe is the change in the respiratory pattern. In the final hours of life, the dying patient's respiration may become labored, with deep breaths and long periods of apnea, referred to as Cheyne-Stokes respirations. Families should be reassured that this is not distressing to the child and that it is a normal part of the dying process. However, the use of opioids can slow the respirations to make the child breathe more easily, and scopolamine, usually applied as a topical patch, can help reduce noisy respirations known as the

BOX 18-9 ■ Ethical Principle of Double Effect

An action that has one good (intended) and one bad (unintended but foreseeable) effect is permissible if the following conditions are met:
  The action itself must be good or indifferent. Only the good consequences of the action must be sincerely intended.
  The good effect must not be produced by the bad effect.
  There must be a compelling or proportionate reason for permitting the foreseeable bad effect to occur.

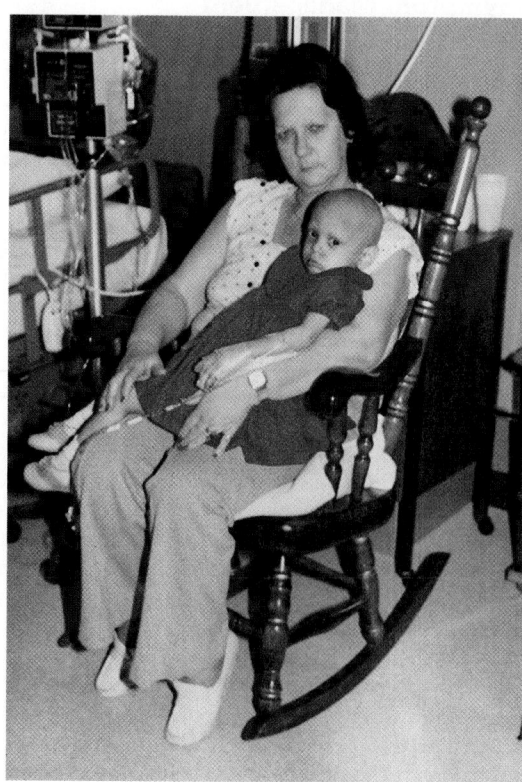

FIG. 18-6 ■ For the dying child there is no greater comfort than the security and closeness of a parent.

"death rattle." Noisy respirations are more likely to occur if the child is overhydrated.

All families have the option of admitting their child to the hospital if they feel unable to deal with the death. The child who dies at home must be pronounced dead; hospice programs typically have provisions so that this may proceed smoothly. In some circumstances the police may be notified, with an explanation of the circumstances to prevent unnecessary concern regarding abuse. Providing the police with the number of the responsible practitioner is usually all that is necessary to confirm the cause of death.

Hospital Deaths

Children dying in the hospital of terminal illnesses who are receiving supportive care interventions will experience a similar process. Again, increased nursing presence and attendance to the child and family's needs provide comfort and support for many families.

Death resulting from accident or trauma or acute illness in settings such as the emergency department or intensive care unit often requires the active withdrawal of some form of life-supporting intervention, such as a ventilator or bypass machine. These situations often raise difficult ethical issues (Sine and others, 2001), and parents are often less prepared for the actual moment of death. Nurses can assist these parents by providing detailed information about what will happen as supportive equipment is withdrawn, ensuring that appropriate pain medications are administered to prevent pain during the dying process, and allowing the parents time before the start of the withdrawal to be with and speak to their child. It is important that the nurse attempt to control the environment around the family at this time by providing privacy, asking if they would like to play music, softening lights and monitor noises, and arranging for any religious or cultural rituals that the family may want performed.

After the child's death, the family should be allowed to remain with the body and hold or rock the child if they desire. After the nurse has removed all tubes and equipment

from the body, parents should be given the option of assisting with the preparation of the body, such as bathing and dressing. It is important for the nurse to determine if the family has any specific needs because many cultures have adapted specific methods for coping and mourning death and impeding these practices may interfere with the grieving process (Clements and others, 2003).

At some point the nurse should discuss if the family has made preparations for the burial service and if the staff can help in any way. Parents often have concerns about the funeral, such as siblings' involvement in the death rituals. Although no absolute answers exist regarding the question of siblings attending the funeral or burial services, the general consensus is that the surviving children benefit from being involved in these events. However, children need preparation for postdeath services. They should be told what to expect, particularly how the deceased person will look if the coffin is open; allowed their private time to say good-bye; and permitted to stay as long as they wish. Ideally, the parents should prepare the siblings. If the parents' grief prevents this communication, a significant family member or friend should substitute (see Family Focus box).

ORGAN OR TISSUE DONATION/AUTOPSY

Many states have legislated a mandatory request for organ/tissue donation when a child dies. For some families this may be a meaningful act—one that benefits another human being despite the loss of their child. Unfortunately, initiating a discussion about tissue donation is often very stressful for staff, and there may be confusion regarding whose responsibility this is. In centers in which transplants are performed, a full-time transplant coordinator is usually available to inform the family about organ donation and to take care of details. If such services are not available, the staff needs to

---

BOX 18-10 ■ Physical Signs of Approaching Death

Loss of sensation and movement in the lower extremities, progressing toward the upper body
Sensation of heat, although body feels cool
Loss of senses:
    Tactile sensation decreases
    Sensitive to light
    Hearing is last sense to fail
Confusion, loss of consciousness, slurred speech
Muscle weakness
Loss of bowel and bladder control
Decreased appetite/thirst
Difficulty swallowing
Change in respiratory pattern:
    Cheyne-Stokes respirations (waxing and waning of depth of breathing with regular periods of apnea)
    "Death rattle" (noisy chest sounds from accumulation of pulmonary and pharyngeal secretions)
Weak, slow pulse; decreased blood pressure

FAMILY FOCUS

Children Need to Say Good-Bye

As a nurse/grief counselor, I conduct grief workshops with children who have experienced the death of someone special. Children often communicate their feelings of being excluded through drawings. They may draw a picture of the dying person in a hospital bed that is raised too high for them to see the person's face clearly. Sometimes children reveal that they did not get to say good-bye because a family member told them, for example, "You don't want to see your grandma this way. She is too sick for you to visit." If the special person died at home, the children had to stay in their room when the funeral home staff took away the body.

I have learned never to underestimate the importance of allowing children to be involved with the dying person and the significance of a child's loss. Once, when I asked a 6-year-old girl to draw a picture with the theme. "This is what I was doing when my _____ died," she drew a picture and completed the sentence with "when my home died." Her grandmother had been like her mother; to the child, her home was gone. We need to give children the choice of being included in the family's activities of saying good-bye.

Barbara Bilderback, MS, MA, RN
Bereavement Supervisor, Saint Francis Hospice
Tulsa, Okla

determine which members should discuss this topic with the family. Ideally, the person who knows the family best, knows when the death is expected, or has the opportunity to spend time with the family when the death is unexpected takes the role. Often nurses are in an optimal position to suggest tissue donation after consultation with the attending physician. When possible, the topic should be raised before death occurs. The request should be made in a private and quiet area of the hospital and should be simple and direct, with questions such as "Are you a donor family?" or "Have you ever considered organ donation?"

Most states have "required request" laws that mandate that the hospital make a request for tissue donation from the family of the deceased, especially if the patient is brain dead. A written consent from the family is required before donation can proceed. When requests for organ donation are made, health care practitioners must address common misunderstandings families have about brain death and organ donation (Franz and others, 1997). Training health care professionals on sensitive approaches to requests for organ donation has been shown to increase families' willingness to consent to organ donation (Hardy and others 2002; Evanisko and others, 1998). The option to donate organs should always be separate from the communication of impending or actual death.

Nurses need to be aware of common questions about organ donation to help families make an informed decision. Healthy children who die unexpectedly are excellent candidates for organ donation. Children with cancer, chronic disease, or infection or who have suffered prolonged cardiac arrest may not be suitable candidates, although this is individually determined. The nurse should inquire if organ donation was discussed with the child or if the child ever expressed such a wish. Any number of body tissues or organs can be donated (skin, corneas, bone, kidney, heart, liver, pancreas), and their removal does not mutilate or desecrate the body or cause any suffering. The family may have an open casket, and there is no delay in the funeral. There is no cost to the donor family, but organ donation does not eliminate funeral or cremation responsibilities. Most religions permit organ donation as long as the recipient benefits from the transplant, although Orthodox Judaism forbids it.

In cases of unexplained death, violent death, or suspected suicide, autopsy is required by law. In other instances it may be optional, and parents should be informed of this choice. The procedure, as well as forms that require signing, should be explained. The family should know that the child can be in an open casket following an autopsy.

GRIEF AND MOURNING

The crisis of loss does not end with the child's death. In many ways it only begins. Unfortunately, the child's death often marks the close of the family's contacts with health professionals involved in the care. Consequently, many of these families never receive the support and guidance that could assist them in resolving the loss. Fortunately, hospice programs recognize this need and provide regular follow-up after the death.

When death is the expected or possible outcome of a disorder, the child and family members experience the behavioral reactions of anticipatory grief. Anticipatory grief may be manifested in varying behaviors and intensities and may

include denial, anger, depression, and other psychologic and somatic symptoms.

When death occurs—whether expected or unexpected—acute grief develops within hours to days. Acute grief is a definite syndrome with psychologic and somatic symptoms that cause intense distress (Box 18-11). Anticipatory guidance may assist grieving family members. Health professionals should emphasize that grief reactions such as hearing the dead person's voice, feeling distant from others, or seeking reassurance that they did everything possible for the lost person are normal, necessary, and expected. They in no way signify poor coping, insanity, or an approaching mental breakdown. On the contrary, such behaviors signify that the survivor is working through the acute grief. They are a necessary part of satisfactory resolution of the loss. These reactions are part of the process of resuming or restructuring a meaningful role in the social environment.

After the death, the lengthy process of grief work or mourning begins and extends into a period of adjustment to the loss, with eventual attachment to new people and the development of new interests. Contrary to the common belief that mourning is completed in a year, research indicates that resolution of grief may take years and that there may be an *intensification* of grief during the early years. The time since a child's death is not necessarily a factor in reducing the intensity of grief for families (Murphy and others, 2003; Davis and Eng, 1998). Anticipatory guidance regarding the

BOX 18-11 ■ Symptomatology of Normal Grief

SENSATIONS OF SOMATIC DISTRESS
Feeling of tightness in the throat
Choking, with shortness of breath
Marked tendency toward sighing
Empty feeling in the abdomen
Lack of muscular power
Intense subjective distress described as tension or mental pain

PREOCCUPATION WITH IMAGE OF THE DECEASED
Hears, sees, or imagines that the dead person is present
Slight sense of unreality
Feeling of emotional distance from others
May believe that he or she is approaching insanity

FEELINGS OF GUILT
Searches for evidence of failure in preventing the death
Accuses self of negligence or exaggerates minor omissions

FEELINGS OF HOSTILITY
Loss of warmth toward others
Tendency toward irritability and anger
Wishes to not be bothered by friends or relatives

LOSS OF USUAL PATTERNS OF CONDUCT
Restlessness, inability to sit still, aimless moving about
Continual searching for something to do or what he or she thinks should be done
Lack of capacity to initiate and maintain organized patterns of activity

Modified from Lindermann E: Symptomatology and management of acute grief, *Am J Psychiatry* 101:141-143, 1944.

mourning process may be helpful to families so that they can recognize the normalcy of their experiences.

It is important to recognize that some family members may experience "complicated" grief. Complicated grief reactions (more than a year after the loss) include such symptoms as intense intrusive thoughts, pangs of severe emotion, distressing yearnings, feeling excessively alone and empty, unusual sleep disturbance, and maladaptive levels of loss of interest in personal activities. Bereaved persons experiencing such prolonged and complicated grief should be referred to an expert in grief and bereavement counseling.

A child's death can also challenge the marital relationship in several ways. Maternal and paternal reactions often differ (Birenbaum and others, 1996; Moriarty and others, 1996; Vance and others, 1995). Different grieving styles between the couple may hinder communication and support for each other. Differing needs and expectations can place a strain on the marriage.

At times family members may need assistance in their grieving (see Guidelines box). Mothers, in particular, often feel a great sense of loneliness and emptiness, and part of their resolving the grief is finding a substitute role that is fulfilling and rewarding. Nurses can be instrumental in this process by (1) preparing the mother for anticipating the *normal* feelings of emptiness, loneliness, and sometimes even failure; (2) helping her reevaluate her role as parent and spouse, stressing that giving up the lost child must occur before she can reestablish emotional relationships; (3) encouraging her to explore fulfilling activities that use her special interests, talents, and qualifications; and (4) supporting her as her role changes, particularly assisting with communication between affected family members.

Nurses should also be aware of behaviors that indicate siblings' difficulty with resolving their grief, such as persistent blame and guilt, patterns of overactivity with aggressive and destructive outbursts, compulsive caregiving, persistent anxieties (e.g., fear of another family death or of their own), excessive clinging to the parent, difficulty with forming new relationships, problems at school, or delinquency (e.g., stealing). Providing anticipatory guidance to parents regarding behaviors to watch for may be helpful. Even siblings as young as 2 years of age can experience survivor guilt. In these situations professional assistance may be required, and the nurse can provide appropriate referral.

Communication with the bereaved family is essential, but often there is a feeling of not knowing what to say and of helplessness in offering words of comfort. The most supportive approach is to avoid judging the family's reactions or offering advice or rationalizations and to focus on feelings. Perhaps the most valuable supportive measure the nurse can perform for families is to listen. Families understand that no words will relieve their pain; all they want is acceptance, understanding, and respect for their grief. A plan for regular follow-up with bereaved families can be beneficial.

It is important for families to understand that mourning takes a long time. Whereas acute grief may last only weeks or months, resolving the loss is measured in years. Holidays and anniversaries can be particularly difficult, and people who previously had been supportive may now expect the family to have "adjusted." Consequently, prolonged mourning is often silent and lonely.

GUIDELINES

Supporting Grieving Families*

GENERAL

Stay with the family; sit quietly if they prefer not to talk; cry with them if desired.

Accept the family's grief reactions; avoid judgmental statements (e.g., "You should be feeling better by now").

Avoid offering rationalizations for the child's death (e.g., "You should be glad your child isn't suffering anymore").

Avoid artificial consolation (e.g., "I know how you feel," or "You are still young enough to have another baby").

Deal openly with feelings such as guilt, anger, and loss of self-esteem.

Focus on feelings by using a feeling word in the statement (e.g., "You're still feeling all the pain of losing a child").

Refer the family to an appropriate self-help group or for professional help if needed.

AT THE TIME OF DEATH

Reassure the family that everything possible is being done for the child, if they want lifesaving interventions.

Do everything possible to ensure the child's comfort, especially relieving pain.

Provide the child and family with the opportunity to review special experiences or memories in their lives.

Express personal feelings of loss or frustrations (e.g., "We will miss him so much," "We tried everything; we feel so sorry that we couldn't save her").

Provide information that the family requests and be honest.

Respect the emotional needs of family members, such as siblings, who may need brief respites from the dying child.

Make every effort to arrange for family members, especially parents, to be with the child at the moment of death, if they want to be present.

Allow the family to stay with the dead child for as long as they wish and to rock, hold, or bathe the child.

Provide practical help when possible, such as collecting the child's belongings.

Arrange for spiritual support, based on the family's religious beliefs; pray with the family if no one else can stay with them.

POSTDEATH

Attend the funeral or visitation if there was a special closeness with the family.

Initiate and maintain contact (e.g., sending cards, telephoning, inviting them back to the unit, making a home visit).

Refer to the dead child by name; discuss shared memories with the family.

Discourage the use of drugs or alcohol as a method of escaping grief.

Encourage all family members to communicate their feelings rather than remaining silent to avoid upsetting another member.

Emphasize that grieving is a painful process that often takes years to resolve.

*"Family" refers to all significant persons involved in the child's life, such as the parents, siblings, grandparents, or other close relatives or friends.

Many families never receive the support and guidance that could help them resolve the loss. At a minimum, one follow-up phone call or meeting with the family should be arranged. Families can also be referred to self-help groups. When such groups are not available, nurses can be instrumental in networking families or facilitating parent and sibling groups. Formal bereavement programs or bereavement counseling can be helpful as well.

For more information on end of life care, visit these websites:

Americans for Better Care of the Dying
www.abcd-caring.com
City of Hope Pain/Palliative Care Resources Center
mayday.coh.org
End-of-Life Physician Education Resource Center
www.eperc.mcw.edm
Growth House
www.growthhouse.org
Last Acts
www.lastacts.org

NURSES' REACTIONS TO CARING FOR DYING CHILDREN

The death of a patient is one of the most stressful aspects of critical care or oncology nursing (see Family Focus box).* Nurses experience reactions to a fatal illness that are very similar to the responses of family members, including denial, anger, depression, guilt, and ambivalent feelings.

Strategies that can assist the nurse in maintaining the ability to work effectively in these settings include maintaining good general health, developing well-rounded interests, using distancing techniques such as taking time off when needed, developing and using professional and personal support systems, cultivating the capacity for empathy, focusing on the positive aspects of the caregiver role, and basing nursing interventions on sound theory and empiric

---

*Other sources of publications on life-threatening illness and death are **The Compassionate Friends,** PO Box 3696, Oak Brook, IL 60522-3696; (630) 990-0010; e-mail: nationaloffice@compassionatefriends.org; **Centering Corporation,** 1531 N. Saddle Creek Road, Omaha, NE 68104; (402) 553-1200; website: www.centering.org; **Children's Hospice International,** 2202 Mt. Vernon Avenue, Suite 3-C, Alexandria, VA 22314; (800) 24-CHILD; e-mail: chiorg@aol.com; website: www.chionline.org; and **National Cancer Institute, Cancer Information Service,** Building 21, Room 10A29, Bethesda, MD 20892-2580; (800) 422-6237.

FAMILY FOCUS

A Dying Child: A Nurse's Perspective

Claire was unresponsive with slow, gasping breathing. Her mother asked me what I thought was happening. I replied honestly, "Your baby is dying because of her brain tumor." The mother put her arms around me and cried. We arranged for Claire to be baptized.
Honesty. As painful as the loss of a child is, my job is to assist the family through this experience. Although I usually wait until a private moment, such as driving home, I found tears streaming down my face as family and friends gathered for Claire's baptism. I went into the kitchen to compose myself, only to find several of my colleagues crying as well. Saying good-bye to a dying child will always be a difficult but shared experience.

Jeanne O'Connor Egan, RN, MSN
Pediatric Clinical Specialist, Children's Hospital
Washington, DC

---

observations. Attending shared-remembrance rituals assists some nurses in resolving grief (Davies and Eng, 1998). Similarly, attending the funeral services can be a supportive act for both the family and the nurse and in no way detracts from the professionalism of care.

KEY POINTS

- Trends in the treatment of children with chronic illness or disability have focused on developmental age, the child's strengths and uniqueness, family-centered care, establishment of normalization, early discharge, home care, mainstreaming, and early intervention.

- In response to the child with chronic illness or disability, parents may be affected by feelings of inadequacy and failure; excessive demands on time, energy, and financial resources; and strain on the marital relationship.

- Families' reactions to disability or chronic illness are manifested in the following stages: shock and denial, adjustment, reintegration, and acknowledgment.

- The child's reaction to illness or disability depends on the child's developmental level, coping mechanisms, others' reactions, and the illness itself.

- Assessment of the family's adjustment to a child's chronic illness, disability, or death includes the availability of a support system, their perception of the event, their coping mechanisms, concurrent stressors, and their response to the child.

- To help parents cope with their child's chronic illness or disability, nurses must offer attentiveness, humanistic support, solicitation of suggestions for care, facilitation of communication, verbalization of feelings, and referral to volunteer and community agencies.

- Supporting the child involves encouraging self-expression, alleviating feelings of being different, and strengthening the child's self-image.

- Children's concept of death is determined by their cognitive ability and their experience with life-threatening illness.

- Young children see death as temporary and reversible and mainly fear separation.

- School-age children view death as irreversible but not necessarily inevitable and may fear mutilation.

- Children beyond 9 to 10 years of age realize that death is irreversible, universal, and inevitable but may resist the thought of their own death.

- Siblings have special needs, including the need for information, reassurance about their own health status, assurance that they are not responsible for the illness or death, and support for their own grieving process.

- Special needs of the family facing the unexpected death of a child include support while awaiting news of the child's status; a sensitive pronouncement of death; acknowledgment of feelings of denial, guilt, and anger; an opportunity to view the body; closure; and referrals for support.

- Special decisions at the time of dying and death may involve hospital or hospice care, the child's right to die, visualization of the body, tissue donation and autopsy, and siblings' attendance at the funeral.

- Acute grief is a syndrome with intense and distressing psychologic and somatic symptoms that appear at the time of death.

- Mourning is a prolonged, painful process that consists of four phases: shock and disbelief, expression of grief, disorganization and despair, and reorganization.

- In dealing with stress related to the dying patient, the nurse can cope successfully through self-awareness, consciousness raising, knowledge and practice, an available support system, and maintenance of general good health, and by focusing on the positive rewards of involvement with dying children and their families.

References

Ahmann E: "Chunky stew": appreciating cultural diversity while providing health care for children, *Pediatr Nurs* 20(3):320-324, 1994.

Ahmann E, Scher A: Alternatives to home care for medically fragile children. In Ahmann E, editor: *Home care for the high risk infant: a family centered approach,* Gaithersburg, Md, 1996, Aspen.

American Academy of Pediatrics, Committee on Children with Disabilities: Managed care and children with special health care needs: a subject review, *Pediatrics* 102(3):657-660, 1998.

American Nurses Association: *Code of ethics for nurses with interpretive statements,* Washington, DC, 2001, ANA Publishing.

Arias E, MacDorman MF, Strobino DM, Guyer B: Annual summary of vital statistics—2002, *Pediatrics* 112(6):1215-1230, 2003.

Billings JA: What is palliative care? *J Palliat Med* 1(1):73-81, 1998.

Birenbaum LK and others: Health status of bereaved parents, *Nurs Res* 45(2):105-109, 1996.

Carter B: Chronic pain in childhood and the medical encounter: professional ventriloquism and hidden voices, *Qual Health Res* 12:28-41, 2002.

Charles C, Gafni A, Whelan T: Shared decision making in the medical encounter: what does it mean? *Soc Sci Med* 44:681-692, 1997.

Clements PT and others: Cultural perspectives of death, grief, and bereavement, *J Psychosoc Nurs Ment Health Serv* 41(7):18-26, 2003.

Cohen MH: The stages of the prediagnostic period in chronic life-threatening childhood illness: a process analysis, *Res Nurs Health* 18(1):39-48, 1995.

Davies R, Davis B, Sibert J: Parents' stories of sensitive and insensitive care by paediatricians in the time leading up to and including diagnostic disclosure of a life-limiting condition in their child, *Child Care Health Dev* 29(1):77-82, 2003.

Davis B, Eng B: Special issues in bereavement and staff support. In Doyle D, Hanks GWC, MacDonald N, editors: *Oxford textbook of palliative medicine,* ed 2, Oxford, 1998, Oxford.

Deatrick JA, Knafl KA, Murphy-Moore C: Clarifying the concept of normalization, *Image J Nurs Sch* 31:209-214, 1999.

Dixon-Woods M, Young B, Henry D: Partnerships with children, *Br J Med* 319:778-780, 1999.

Evanisko MJ and others: Readiness of critical care physicians and nurses to handle requests for organ donation, *Am J Crit Care* 7(1):4-12, 1998.

Faulkner KW, Armstrong-Dailey A: Care of the dying child. In Pizzo PA, Poplack DG, editors: *Principles and practice of pediatric oncology,* Philadelphia, 1997, Lippincott-Raven.

Faulkner MS: Family responses to children with diabetes and their influence on self-care, *J Pediatr Nurs* 11(2):82-93, 1996.

Field MJ, Behrman RE: Educating health care professionals. In Field MJ, Behrman RE, editors: *When children die: improving palliative and end-of-life care for children and their families,* Washington, DC, 2003, National Academies Press.

Fleitas J: When Jack fell down . . . Jill came tumbling after: siblings in the web of illness and disability, *MCN* 25:267-273, 2000.

Forrester L: One to one care in children's hospice, *Nurs Times* 99(16):44-45, 2003.

Franz HG and others: Explaining brain death: a critical feature of the donation process, *J Transplant Coord* 7(1):14-21, 1997.

Freyer DR: Care of the dying adolescent: special considerations, *Pediatrics* 113(2):381-388, 2004.

Garwick AW and others: Breaking the news: how families first learn about their child's chronic condition, *Arch Pediatr Adolesc Med* 149(9):991-997, 1995.

Goldbeck L: Parental coping with the diagnosis of childhood cancer: gender effects, dissimilarity within couples, and quality of life, *Psychooncology* 10:325-335, 2001.

Gravelle AM: Caring for a child with a progressive illness during the complex chronic phase: parents' experience of facing adversity, *J Adv Nurs* 25:738-745, 1997.

Hardy DR and others: Pediatric organ donation and transplantation, *Pediatrics* 109(5):982-984, 2002.

Hawryluck LA, Harvey WR: Analgesia, virtue, and the principle of double effect, *J Palliative Care* 16(suppl):S24-S30, S24-S30, 2000.

Hellsten MB, Hockenberry M, Lamb D and others: *End-of-life care for children,* Austin, Tex, 2000, Texas Cancer Council.

Hinds PS and others: End-of-life decision making by adolescents, parents, and healthcare providers in pediatric oncology: research to evidence-based practice guidelines, *Cancer Nurs* 24:122-134, 2001.

Jackson PL: The primary care provider and children with chronic conditions. In Jackson PL, Vessey PA: *Primary care of the child with a chronic condition,* ed 3, St Louis, 2000, Mosby.

James L, Johnson B: The needs of parents of pediatric oncology patients during the palliative care phase, *J Pediatr Oncol Nurs* 14(2):83-95, 1997.

Kuhlthau K and others: Assessing managed care for children with chronic conditions, *Health Aff* 17(4):42-52, 1998.

Lambert S: Distraction, imagery, and hypnosis techniques for management of children's pain, *J Child Fam Nurs* 2(1):5-15, 1999.

Lobato DJ, Kao BT: Integrated sibling-parent group intervention to improve sibling knowledge and adjustment to chronic illness and disability, *J Pediatr Psychol* 27:711-716, 2002.

Lock J: Psychosexual development in adolescents with chronic medical illness, *Psychosomatics* 39:340-349, 1998.

Marshall ES and others: "This is a spiritual experience": perspectives of Latter-Day Saint families living with a child with disabilities, *Qual Health Res* 13:57-76, 2003.

Mastroyannopoulou K and others: The impact of childhood non-malignant life threatening illness on parents: gender differences and predictors of parental adjustment, *J Child Psychol Psychiatry* 38(7):823-829, 1997.

May J: Fathers: the forgotten parent, *Pediatr Nurs* 22(3):243-246, 271, 1996.

McDougal, J: Promoting normalization in families with preschool children with type 1 diabetes, *J Specialty Pediatr Nurs* 7(3):113-120, 2002.

Minino AM, Smith BL: Deaths: preliminary data for 2000, *Natl Vital Stat Rep* 49:1-40, 2001.

Monical W: Daycare for children who are medically fragile, *Except Parent* 25(2):27-31, 1995.

Moriarty H and others: Differences in bereavement reactions within couples following the death of a child, *Res Nurs Health* 19:461-469, 1996.

Morse JM, Wilson S, Penrod J: Mothers and their disabled children: refining the concept of normalization, *Health Care Woman Int* 21(8):659-676, 2000.

Msall ME and others: Functional disability and school activity limitations in 41,300 school-age children: relationship to medical impairments, *Pediatrics* 111:548-553, 2003.

Murphy SA and others: Bereaved parents outcomes 4 to 60 months after their child's death by accident, suicide, or homicide: a comparative study demonstrating differences, *Death Studies* 27(1):39-61, 2003.

Nelson AM: A metasynthesis: mothering other-than-normal children, *Qual Health Res* 12:515-530, 2002.

Newacheck PW, Halfon N: Prevalence and impact of disabling chronic conditions in childhood, *Am J Public Health* 88(4):610-617, 1998.

Newacheck PW and others: An epidemiologic profile of children with special health care needs, *Pediatrics* 102(1):117-123, 1998.

O'Brien ME, Wegner CB: Rearing the child who is technology dependent: perceptions of parents and home care nurses, *J Spec Pediatr Nurs* 7:7-15, 2002.

Perrin JM: Chronic illness in childhood. In Behrman RE, Kleigman RM, Jensen HB, editors: *Nelson textbook of pediatrics,* ed 17, Philadelphia, 2004, WB Saunders.

Quittner AL and others: Role strain in couples with and without a child with a chronic illness: associations with marital satisfaction, intimacy, and daily mood, *Health Psychol* 17(2):112-124, 1998.

Ray LD: Parenting and childhood chronicity: making visible the invisible work, *J Pediatr Nurs* 17(6):424-38, 2002.

Rehm RS: Religious faith in Mexican-American families dealing with chronic childhood illness, *Image J Nurs Sch* 31:33-38, 1999.

Ritchie MA: Self-esteem and hopefulness in adolescents with cancer, *J Pediatr Nurs* 16:35-42, 2001.

Rousseau P: Ethical and legal issues in palliative care, *Prim Care* 28:391-400, 2001.

Sahler O and others: Medical education about end-of-life care in the pediatric setting: principles, challenges, and opportunities, *Pediatrics* 105:575-584, 2000.

Schor EL: Family pediatrics: report of the Task Force on the Family, *Pediatrics* 111:1541-1571, 2003.

Sharpe D, Rossiter L: Siblings of children with a chronic illness: a meta-analysis, *J Pediatr Psychol* 27:699-710, 2002.

Shepard MP, Mahon MM: Chronic conditions and the family. In Jackson PL, Vessey JA: *Primary care of the child with a chronic condition,* ed 3, St Louis, 2000, Mosby.

Siegel RD: Child care and the ADA, *Except Parent* 25(2):34, 1995.

Sine D and others: Pediatric extubation: "pulling the tube," *J Palliative Med* 4:519-524, 2001.

Stein REK: Home care: a challenging opportunity, *Child Health Care* 14(2):90-95, 1985.

Sterling YM, Peterson JW: Characteristics of African American women caregivers of children with asthma, *MCN* 28:32-38, 2003.

Sumner LH: Lighting the way: improving the way children die in America, *Caring* 22:14-18, 2003.

Swallow VM, Jacoby A: Mothers' evolving relationships with doctors and nurses during the chronic childhood illness trajectory, *J Adv Nurs* 36:755-764, 2001.

Thomlinson EH: The lived experience of families of children who are failing to thrive, *J Adv Nurs* 39:537-545, 2002.

Tong H and others: Physical functioning in female caregivers of children with physical disabilities compared with female caregivers of children with a chronic medical condition, *Arch Pediatr Adolesc Med* 156:1138-1142, 2002.

Vance JC and others: Psychological changes in parents eight months after the loss of an infant from stillbirth, neonatal death, or sudden infant death syndrome—a longitudinal study, *Pediatrics* 96(5):933-938, 1995.

Vessey, JA, Mebane, DJ: Chronic conditions and child development. In Jackson PL, Vessey JA, *Primary care of the child with a chronic condition,* ed 3, St Louis, 2000, Mosby.

Whitehead LC, Gosling V: Parent's perceptions of interactions with health professionals in the pathway to gaining a diagnosis of tuberous sclerosis (TS) and beyond, *Res Dev Disabil* 24:109-119, 2003.

Winkler WD, Mardegian CA: Completing the continuum of care: the growth of a pediatric hospice program, *Caring* 20:22-25, 2001.

Wise PH and others: Chronic illness among poor children enrolled in the temporary assistance for needy families program, *Am J Public Health* 92:1458-1461, 2002.

Wolfe J and others: Symptoms and suffering at the end of life in children with cancer, *N Engl J Med* 342(5):326-333, 2000.

Wolfe J, Friebert S, Hilden J: Caring for children with advanced cancer: integrating palliative care, *Pediatr Clin North Am* 49:5, 2002.

Wood PR and others: Relationships between welfare status, health insurance status, and health and medical care among children with asthma, *Am J Public Health* 92:1446-1452, 2002.

World Health Organization: Cancer pain relief and palliative care, Geneva, Switzerland, 1996, The Organization.

Yogev R, Chadwick EG: Acquired immunodeficiency syndrome. In Behrman RE, Kleigman RM, Jensen HB, editors: *Nelson textbook of pediatrics,* ed 17, Philadelphia, 2004, WB Saunders.

Young B and others: Managing communication with young people who have a potentially life threatening chronic illness: qualitative study of patients and parents, *BJM* 326:1-5, 2003.

Zuvekas SH, Taliaferro GS: Pathways to access: health, insurance, the health care delivery system and racial/ethnic disparities, 1996-1999, *Health Aff* 22(2):139-53, 2003.

Impact of Cognitive or Sensory Impairment on the Child and Family

ROSALIND BRYANT

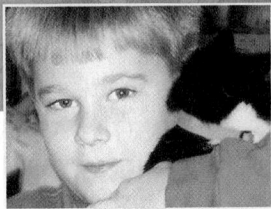

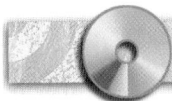 Remember to check out your companion CD-ROM

http://evolve.elsevier.com/Wong/essentials/

RELATED TOPICS and ADDITIONAL RESOURCES

COGNITIVE IMPAIRMENT

GENERAL CONCEPTS

Cognitive impairment is a general term that encompasses any type of mental difficulty or deficiency. In this chapter the term is used synonymously with *mental retardation (MR)*. Although the needs and concerns of the family are a primary focus throughout the chapter, the reader is encouraged to review Chapter 18, which details the family's adjustment to disabilities in general.

The definition of MR in children comprises three components that include intellectual functioning, functional strengths and weaknesses, and age younger than 18 years at time of diagnosis. Intellectual functioning is measured by the intelligence quotient (IQ) of 70 to 75 or below. In addition, the child must demonstrate functional impairment in at least 2 of 10 different adaptive skill areas: communication, self-care, home living, social skills, leisure, health and safety, self-direction, functional academics, community use, and work (Daily, 2000; Fredericks and Williams, 1998). The development of an MR classification system by the **American Association of Mental Retardation (AAMR)** allows for identification of the individual's specific needs in four established dimensions of care. These dimensions are found in Box 19-1. Careful evaluation to identify the needs of individuals with MR is focused on promoting habilitation for each person. It is anticipated that the functional capabilities of children with MR will improve over time when support is provided.

Diagnosis and Classification

The diagnosis of MR is usually made after a period of suspicion, by professionals or the family, that the child's developmental progress is delayed. In some cases it is confirmed at birth because of recognition of distinct syndromes, such as Down syndrome. At the other extreme, the diagnosis is made when problems such as speech delays arouse concern. In all cases a high index of suspicion for developmental delay and behavioral signs (Box 19-2) is necessary for early diagnosis; routine developmental screening (see Chapter 7) can assist in early identification. Delays are typically seen in gross and fine motor and speech development, although the latter is most predictive.

Results of standardized tests are used in making the diagnosis of MR. Tests for assessing adaptive behaviors include the Vineland Social Maturity Scale and the AAMR Adaptive Behavior Scale. Informal appraisal of adaptive behavior may be made by those fully acquainted with the child (e.g., teachers, parents, other care providers). Frequently these observations lead parents to seek evaluation of the child's development.

A more useful approach for clinical application is classification based on educational potential or symptom severity. For educational purposes the term *educable mentally retarded (EMR)* corresponds to the mildly retarded group, which constitutes about 85% of all people with MR. *Trainable mentally retarded (TMR)* generally applies to children with moderate levels of cognitive impairment and accounts for about 10% of the MR population (First, McQueen, and Pincus, 1996) (Table 19-1). Although nurses may be familiar with the approximate range of IQ for classifying severity, they should refrain from using numbers as the criterion for assessing or evaluating the child's abilities, because numbers are of little value in counseling parents or training these children.

Etiology

The causes of severe MR are primarily genetic, biochemical, and infectious. Although the etiology is unknown in the majority of cases, familial, social, environmental and organic causes may predominate. General categories of events that

---

BOX 19-1 ■ Dimensions of Care for Mental Retardation

Dimension I: Intellectual functioning and adaptive skills
Dimension II: Psychologic/emotional considerations
Dimension III: Physical/health/etiology considerations
Dimension IV: Environmental considerations

BOX 19-2 ■ Early Behavioral Signs Suggestive of Cognitive Impairment

Nonresponsiveness to contact
Poor eye contact during feeding
Diminished spontaneous activity
Decreased alertness to voice or movement
Irritability
Slow feeding

From Crocker A, Nelson R: Mental retardation. In Levine M, Carey WB, Crocker AC, editors: *Developmental-behavioral pediatrics*, ed 3, Philadelphia, 1999, WB Saunders.

may lead to retardation include (Kabra and Gulati, 2003; Gurrieri and others, 1999):

- Infection and intoxication, such as congenital rubella, syphilis, maternal drug consumption (e.g., excessive alcohol), chronic lead ingestion, or kernicterus
- Trauma or physical agent (i.e., injury to the brain suffered during the prenatal, perinatal, or postnatal period)
- Inadequate nutrition and metabolic disorders, such as phenylketonuria
- Gross postnatal brain disease, such as neurofibromatosis and tuberous sclerosis
- Unknown prenatal influence, including cerebral and cranial malformations, such as microcephaly and hydrocephalus
- Chromosomal abnormalities resulting from radiation, viruses, chemicals, parental age, and genetic mutations
- Gestational disorders, including prematurity, low birth weight, and postmaturity
- Psychiatric disorders that have their onset during the child's developmental period up to age 18 years, such as autism
- Environmental influences, including evidence of a deprived environment associated with a history of MR among parents and siblings
- Chromosomal abnormalities, such as Down syndrome and fragile X syndrome

NURSING CARE OF CHILDREN WITH COGNITIVE IMPAIRMENT

Assessment

Nurses play a major role in identifying children with cognitive impairment. In the newborn and early infancy periods, few signs are present, with the exception of Down syndrome (p. 596). After this age, however, delayed developmental milestones are the major clues to MR. In addition, nurses must have a high index of suspicion for early behavior patterns that may suggest cognitive impairment (see Box 19-2) and be aware of stereotypes that may delay diagnosis, such as "retarded children have to look dumb." Parental concerns, such as delayed development compared with siblings, need to be taken seriously. All children should receive regular developmental assessment, and the nurse is often the person responsible for performing such assessments (see Chapter 7). When delays are found, the nurse must use sensitivity and discretion in revealing this finding to parents.

Nursing Diagnoses

A number of nursing diagnoses are prominent in the nursing care of the child with cognitive impairment and the child's family; other diagnoses specific to individual cases become evident. The most common nursing diagnoses are outlined in the Nursing Care Plan on p. 597.

TABLE 19-1 ■ Classification of Mental Retardation

LEVEL (IQ)*	PRESCHOOL (BIRTH-5 YEARS)—MATURATION AND DEVELOPMENT	SCHOOL AGE (6-21 YEARS)—TRAINING AND EDUCATION	ADULT (21 YEARS AND OLDER)—SOCIAL AND VOCATIONAL ADEQUACY
Mild: 50-55 to approximately 70-75	Often not noticed as retarded by casual observer but is slower to walk, feed self, and talk than most children; follows same sequence in development as normal children	Can acquire practical skills and useful reading and arithmetic to a third- to sixth-grade level with special education; can be guided toward social conformity; achieves mental age of 8-12 years	Can usually achieve social and vocational skills adequate to self-maintenance; may need occasional guidance and support when under unusual social or economic stress; can adjust to marriage but not childrearing
Moderate: 35-40 to 50-55	Noticeable delays in motor development, especially in speech; responds to training in various self-help activities	Can learn simple communication, elementary health and safety habits, and simple manual skills; does not progress in functional reading or arithmetic; achieves mental age of 3-7 years	Can perform simple tasks under sheltered conditions; participates in simple recreation; travels alone in familiar places; usually incapable of self-maintenance
Severe: 20-25 to 35-40	Marked delay in motor development; little or no communication skills; may respond to training in elementary self-care (e.g., self-feeding)	Usually walks, barring specific disability; has some understanding of speech and some response; can profit from systematic habit training; achieves mental age of toddler	Can conform to daily routines and repetitive activities; needs continuing direction and supervision in protective environment
Profound: below 20-25	Gross retardation; minimum capacity for functioning in sensorimotor areas; needs total care	Obvious delays in all areas of development; shows basic emotional responses; may respond to skillful training in use of legs, hands, and jaws; needs close supervision; achieves mental age of young infant	May walk; needs complete custodial care; has primitive speech; usually benefits from regular physical activity

*Data from American Psychiatric Association: *Diagnostic and statistical manual of mental disorders*, ed 4 *(DSM-IV TR)*, Washington, DC, 2000, The Association.

● *Planning*

The goals of nursing care for the child with MR and family are as follows:

1 Child will be educated using effective teaching strategies.
2 Child's optimal development will be promoted.
3 Child will learn self-care skills.
4 Family will plan for future care.
5 Child will be cared for appropriately during hospitalization.

● *Implementation*

Educate Child and Family. To teach children with cognitive impairment, it is necessary to investigate their learning abilities and deficits. This is important for the nurse who may be involved in a home care type of program or who may be caring for the child in a health care setting. The nurse who understands how these children learn can effectively teach them basic skills or prepare them for various health-related procedures.

Children with cognitive impairment have a marked deficit in their ability to discriminate between two or more stimuli because of difficulty in recognizing the relevance of specific cues. However, these children can learn to discriminate if the cues are presented in an exaggerated, concrete form and if all extraneous stimuli are eliminated. For example, the use of colors to emphasize visual cues or the use of singing or rhymes to stress auditory cues can help them learn. Their deficit in discrimination also implies that concrete ideas are learned much more effectively than abstract ideas. Therefore demonstration is preferable to verbal explanation, and learning should be directed toward mastering a skill rather than understanding the scientific principles underlying a procedure.

Another cognitive deficit is in short-term memory. Whereas children of average intelligence can remember several words, numbers, or directions at one time, children with MR are less able to do so. Therefore they need simple, one-step directions. Learning through a step-by-step process requires a ***task analysis,*** in which each task is separated into its necessary components and each step is taught completely before proceeding to the next activity.

One critical area of learning that has had a tremendous impact on education for cognitively impaired individuals is ***motivation.*** Programs based on the motivational principles of behavior modification, employing positive reinforcement for specific tasks or behaviors, have demonstrated marked improvement in children's ability to learn. Advances in technology have greatly aided in providing reinforcement, especially in children who are severely retarded and who may have physical disabilities that limit their range of capabilities. For example, with the use of specially designed switches, children are given control of some event in the environment, such as turning on the television (Fig. 19-1). The television picture becomes reinforcement for activating the switch. Repetitive use of these switches provides an early, simplistic association with a technical device that may progress to increasingly more complex aids.

Early intervention programs have been widely promoted for children with developmental disabilities, and there is considerable evidence that these programs are valuable for cog-

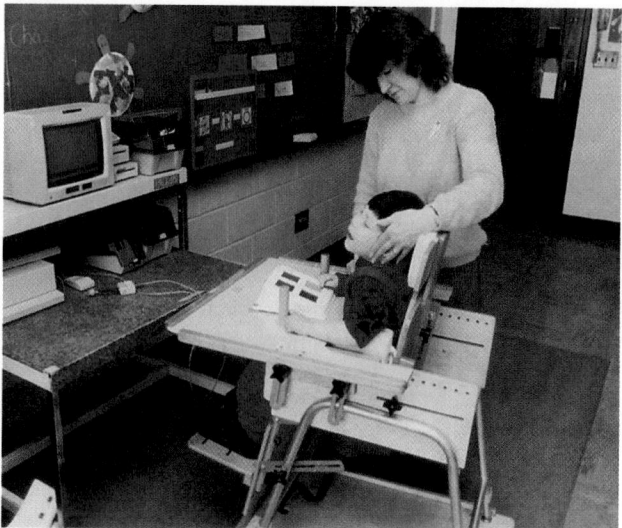

FIG. 19-1 ■ A push panel allows a child with cognitive impairment to turn a computer on and off.

nitively impaired children. Nurses working with these families need to be aware of the types of programs in their community. Under Public Law 101-476, the Individuals With Disabilities Education Act of 1990, states are encouraged to provide full early intervention services and are required to provide educational opportunities for all children with disabilities from birth to 21 years of age. Services may be provided under state **Programs for Children with Special Health Needs** (formerly **Crippled Children's Program**) or **Head Start,** or by private organizations such as **National Down Syndrome Society,*** **National Easter Seals,†** or the **Association of Retarded Citizens of the United States.‡** Parents should inquire about these programs by contacting the appropriate agencies. The child's education should begin as soon as possible, not at 5 or 6 years of age. As children grow older, their education should be directed toward vocational training that prepares them for as independent a lifestyle as possible within their scope of abilities.

Teach Child Self-Care Skills. When a child with cognitive impairment is born, parents need assistance in promoting normal developmental skills that are almost automatically learned by other children. These include self-care skills such as feeding, toileting, dressing, and grooming. Teaching these skills requires a basic knowledge of the developmental sequence in learning the skills demonstrated by children of average intelligence. For example, children with subaverage intelligence would not be expected to dress themselves as early as unaffected youngsters.

---

*Information on early intervention programs in each state is available from the **National Down Syndrome Society,** 666 Broadway, 8th floor, New York, NY 10012-2317; (800) 221-4602; fax: (212) 979-2873; website: www.ndss.org.
†230 West Monroe, Suite 1800, Chicago, IL 60606-4802; (800) 221-6827; TTY: (312) 726-4258; fax: (312) 726-1494; website: www.easter-seals.com.
‡1010 Wayne Avenue, Suite 650, Silver Spring, MD 20910; (301) 565-3842; fax: (301) 565-5342; website: www.thearc.org.

Teaching self-care skills also necessitates a working knowledge of the individual steps needed to master a skill. For example, before beginning a self-feeding program, a task analysis is performed. After a task analysis, the child is observed in a particular situation, such as eating, to determine what skills are possessed and the child's developmental readiness to learn the task. Family members are included in this process because their "readiness" is as important as the child's. Numerous self-help aids are available to facilitate independence and can be most helpful in eliminating some of the difficulties of learning, such as using a plate with suction cups to prevent accidental spills.*

Promote Child's Optimal Development. Optimal development involves more than achieving independence. It requires appropriate guidance for establishing acceptable social behavior and personal feelings of self-esteem, worth, and security. These attributes are not simply learned through a stimulation program. Rather, they must arise from the genuine love and caring that exist among family members. However, families need guidance in providing an environment that fosters optimal development. Often it is the nurse who can provide assistance in these areas of child-rearing.

Another important area for promoting optimal development and self-esteem is ensuring the child's physical well-being. Any congenital defects should be repaired, such as cardiac, gastrointestinal, or orthopedic anomalies. Plastic surgery may be considered when the child's appearance may be substantially improved. Dental health is very significant, and orthodontic and restorative procedures can improve facial appearance immensely.

Play/Exercise. Children who are cognitively impaired have the same needs for recreation and exercise as other children. However, because of the child's slower development, parents may be less aware of the need to provide such activities. Therefore the nurse guides parents toward selection of suitable play and exercise activities. Because play has been discussed for children in each age-group in earlier chapters, only the exceptions are presented here (Fig. 19-2).

The type of play is based on the child's developmental age, although the need for sensorimotor play may be prolonged for several years. Parents should use every opportunity to expose the child to as many different sounds, sights, and sensations as possible. Appropriate play includes musical mobiles, stuffed toys, water play, floating toys, a rocking chair or horse, a swing, bells, and rattles. The child should be taken on outings, such as trips to the grocery store or shopping center; other people should be encouraged to visit in the home; and the child should be related to directly, such as by cuddling, holding, rocking, talking to the child in the *en face* (face-to-face) position, and giving "rides" on the parents' shoulders.

Toys are selected for their recreational and educational value. For example, a large inflatable beach ball is a good

*A resource for a variety of self-help equipment is **Sammons/Preston/Rolyan,** An AbilityOne Corporation, 4 Sammons Court, Bolingbrook, IL 60440; (800) 323-5547. In Canada: (800) 665-9200, fax: 800-547-4333; website: www.sammonspreston.com.

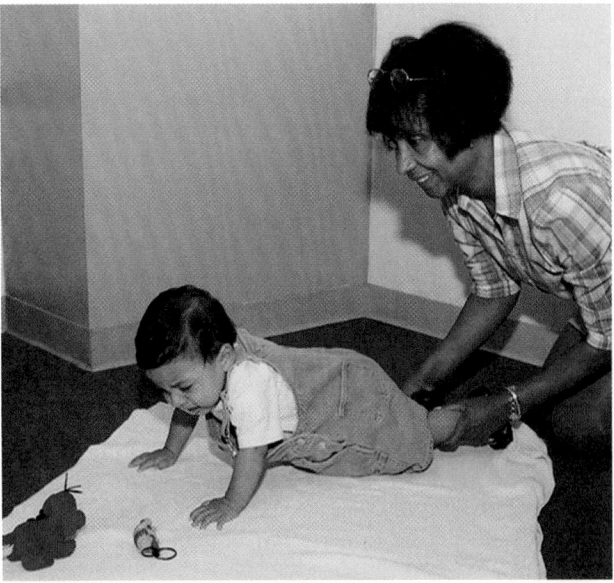

FIG. 19-2 ■ Placing an attractive object outside of the child's reach encourages crawling movements. (Courtesy James DeLeon, Texas Children's Hospital.)

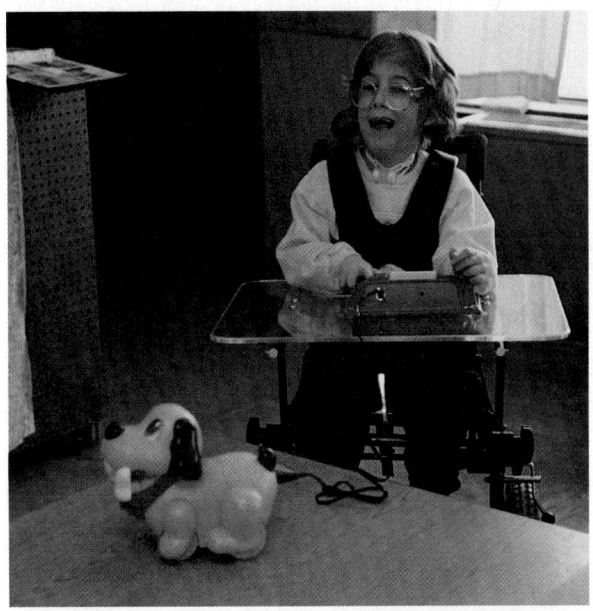

FIG. 19-3 ■ A manual switch allows a child with cognitive impairment to play with a battery-operated toy.

water toy; it encourages interactive play and can be used to learn motor skills, such as balance, rocking, kicking, and throwing. A doll with removable clothes and different types of closures can help the child learn dressing skills. Musical toys that mimic animal sounds or respond with social phrases are excellent ways of encouraging speech. Toys should be simple in design so that the child can learn to manipulate them without help. For children with severe cognitive and physical impairment, electronic switches can be used to allow them to operate toys (Fig. 19-3).

Suitable activities for physical activity are based on the child's size, coordination, physical fitness and maturity, motivation, and health (Fig. 19-4). Some children may have physical problems that prevent participation in certain sports, such as atlantoaxial instability in children with Down syndrome (p. 596). These children often have greater success in individual and dual sports than in team sports and enjoy themselves most with children of the same developmental level. The **Special Olympics, Inc.,*** provides these children with a unique competitive opportunity.

Safety is a major consideration in selecting recreational and exercise activities. For example, toys that may be appropriate developmentally may present dangers to a child who is strong enough to break them or use them incorrectly.

Communication. Verbal skills are typically delayed more than other physical skills. Speech requires hearing and interpretation *(receptive skills)* and facial muscle coordination *(expressive skills).* Because both types of skills may be impaired, these children need frequent audiometric testing and should be fitted with hearing aids if this is indicated. In addition, they may need help in learning to control their facial muscles. For example, some children may need tongue exercises to correct the tongue thrust or gentle reminders to keep the lips closed.

Nonverbal communication may be appropriate for some of these children, and various devices are available. For the child without associated physical disabilities, a talking picture board is helpful. For children with physical limitations, several adaptations or types of communication devices are

---

*1325 G Street NW, Suite 500, Washington, DC 20005; (800) 700-8585 or (202) 628-3630; fax: (202) 824-0200; website: www.specialolympics.org. (Website includes listing of state offices.) In Canada: **Canadian Special Olympics,** 60 St. Clair Avenue E., Suite 700, Toronto, Ontario M4T 2N5; (416) 927-9050; fax: (416) 927-8475; website: www.cso.on.ca.

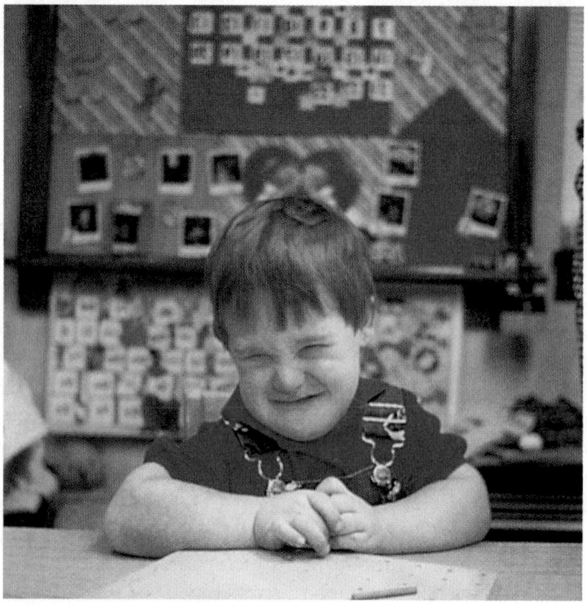

available to facilitate selection of the appropriate picture or word (Fig. 19-5). Some children may be taught sign language or *Blissymbols*—a highly stylized system of graphic symbols that represent words, ideas, and concepts. Although the symbols require education to learn their meaning, no reading skill is needed. The symbols are usually arranged on a board, and the person points or uses some type of selector to convey a message.

Discipline. Discipline must begin early. Limit-setting measures need to be simple, consistently applied, and appropriate for the child's mental age. Control measures are based primarily on teaching a specific behavior rather than on understanding the reasons behind it. Stressing moral lessons is of little value to a child who lacks the cognitive skills to learn from self-criticism or from a lesson based on previous wrong-doing. Behavior modification, especially reinforcement of desired actions, and time-out are appropriate forms of behavior control.

Socialization. Acquiring social skills is a complex task, as is learning self-care procedures. Active rehearsal with role-playing and practice sessions and positive reinforcement for desired behavior have been the most successful approaches. Parents should be encouraged early to teach their child socially acceptable behavior: waving goodbye, saying "hello" and "thank you," responding to his or her name, greeting visitors but not being overly affectionate, and sitting modestly. The teaching of socially acceptable sexual behavior is especially important to minimize sexual exploitation. Parents also need to expose the child to strangers so that he or she can practice manners, because there is no automatic transfer of learning from one situation to another.

Dressing and grooming are also important aspects of socialization. A child who is dressed in age-appropriate clothing and is well groomed is much more likely to be accepted

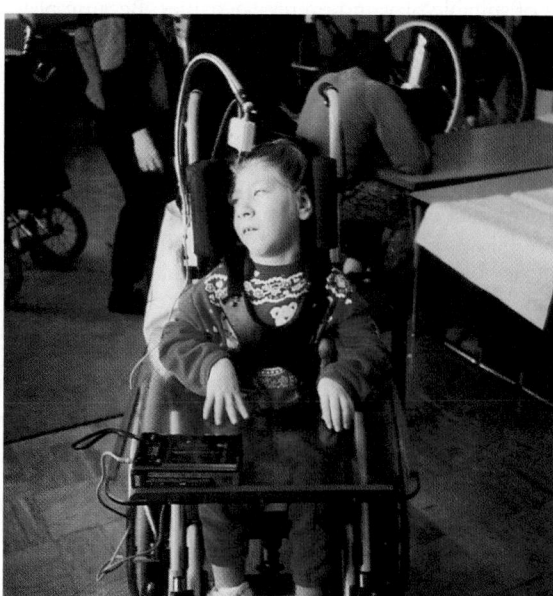

FIG. 19-4 ■ Play activities for children with cognitive impairments need to be appropriate for their abilities.

FIG. 19-5 ■ A child with cognitive and physical impairments can play a tape recorder by moving a device near her head.

and to develop good self-esteem. Clothes should be clean, up-to-date, and well fitted. Many attractive outfits can be adapted with self-adhering fasteners and elastic openings to facilitate self-dressing.

Children of all ages need peer relationships, and these children are no exception. As soon as possible, parents should enroll the child in appropriate preschool programs. Not only do these programs provide education and training, but they also offer an opportunity for social experiences among the children. As children grow older, they should have peer experiences similar to those of other children, including group outings, sports, and organized activities, such as Boy Scouts, Girl Scouts, or Special Olympics. They are encouraged to form a close relationship with a best friend of the same developmental age (American Academy of Pediatrics, 2000).

Sexuality.   Adolescence may be a particularly difficult time for the family, especially in terms of the child's sexual behavior, possibility of pregnancy, future plans to marry, and ability to be independent. Frequently, little anticipatory guidance has been offered parents to prepare the child for physical and sexual maturation. The nurse can help in this area by providing parents with information about sexuality education that is geared to the child's developmental level. For example, the adolescent female needs a *simple* explanation of menstruation and instructions on personal hygiene during the menstrual cycle.

These adolescents also need practical sexual information regarding anatomy, physical development, and conception.* Because of their easy persuasion and lack of judgment, they need a well-defined, concrete code of conduct. The subtleties of social sexual behavior are less beneficial than specific instructions for handling certain situations. For example, a girl should be firmly told never to go alone anywhere with any person she does not know well. A boy should be warned about intimate advances from other males. To protect him or her from abusive sexual activities, parents must closely observe their teenager's activities and associates.

The question of contraceptive protection for these adolescents is often a parental concern. Permanent contraception through sterilization is a special dilemma because of moral and ethical questions, as well as psychologic effects on the adolescent. State laws vary; some allow no sterilization, and others permit review of sterilization requests.

Parents of these adolescents are often very concerned about the advisability of marriage between two individuals with significant cognitive impairment. There is no conclusive answer; each situation must be judged individually. In some instances marriage is possible, but parenthood is usually not desirable because of the complexity of childrearing and the potential problem of perpetuating mental deficiency. The nurse should discuss this topic with parents and

---

*Sources of information on sexuality and conception are the **Association for Retarded Citizens of the United States** (see footnote, p. 592) and the **Planned Parenthood Federation of America,** 434 West 33rd Street, New York, NY 10001; (212) 541-7800 or (800) 829-7732; fax: (212) 245-1845; website: www.plannedparenthood.org.

with the prospective couple, stressing suitable living accommodations and contraceptive methods to prevent pregnancy. If children are conceived, these parents require specialized assistance in learning to meet the needs of their offspring (Greene, in press).

Help Family Adjust to Future Care.   Not all families are able to cope with home care of their affected child, especially one who is severely or profoundly retarded and/or multidisabled. Older parents may not be able to assume care responsibilities after they reach retirement or older age. For these parents, the decision regarding residential placement is a difficult one, and the availability of such facilities varies widely. The nurse working with a family should help them investigate and evaluate various programs, in addition to assisting them in their adjustment to the decision for placement.

Care for Child During Hospitalization.   Caring for the child during hospitalization can be a special challenge. Frequently, nurses are unfamiliar with children who are cognitively impaired, and they may cope with their feelings of insecurity and fear by ignoring or isolating the child. Not only is this approach nonsupportive, but it may also be destructive for the child's sense of self-esteem and optimal development, and it may hamper the parents' ability to cope with the stress of the experience. One method that successfully avoids this nontherapeutic approach is the use of the mutual participation model in planning the child's care. Parents are encouraged to stay with their child but should not be made to feel as if the responsibility is totally theirs.

When the child is admitted, a detailed history is taken (see Chapter 21), especially in terms of all self-care activity. During the interview the child's developmental age is assessed. It is best to avoid directly asking about IQ levels, because this may make the parents uncomfortable and often tells little about the child's actual abilities. Questions are approached positively. For example, rather than asking, "Is your child toilet trained yet?" the nurse may state, "Tell me about your child's toileting habits." The assessment should also focus on any special devices the child uses, effective measures of limit setting, unusual or favorite routines, and any behaviors that may require intervention. For example, if the parent states that the child engages in self-stimulatory or self-injurious activities, the nurse inquires about events that precipitate them and techniques that the parents use to manage them (Bosch and Ringdahl, 2001).

The child's functional level of eating and playing, ability to express needs verbally, progress in toilet training, and relationship with objects, toys, and other children are also assessed. The child is encouraged to be as independent as possible in the hospital.

Realizing that the child may be lonely in the hospital, the nurse makes certain that toys and other activities are provided. The child is placed in a room with other children of approximate developmental age, preferably a room with two beds, to avoid overstimulation. The nurse discusses with the other parents the child's abilities and introduces the parents and children to each other. By the nurse's example of treating the child with dignity and respect, others who may be fearful of what they do not understand are encouraged to accept the child.

Procedures are explained to the child through methods of communication that are at the appropriate cognitive level. Generally, explanations should be simple, short, and concrete, emphasizing what the child will experience *physically*. Demonstration either through actual practice or with visual aids is always preferable to verbal explanation. The nurse repeats instructions often and evaluates the child's understanding by asking questions such as "What will it feel like?" "What will the doctor look like?" "Show me how you must lie," or "Where will the dressing be?" Parents are included in preprocedural teaching for their own learning and to help the nurse learn effective methods of communicating with the child.

During hospitalization the nurse should also focus on growth-promoting experiences for the child. For example, hospitalization may be an excellent opportunity to emphasize to parents abilities that the child does have but has not had the opportunity to practice, such as self-dressing.

It may also be an opportunity for social experiences with peers, group play, or new educational and recreational activities. For example, one child who had the habit of screaming and kicking demonstrated a definite decrease in those behaviors after he learned to pound pegs and use a punching bag. Through social services the parents may become aware of specialized programs for the child. Hospitalization may also offer parents a respite from everyday care responsibilities and an opportunity to discuss their feelings with a concerned professional.

Assist in Measures to Prevent Retardation. Besides having a responsibility to families with a child with MR, nurses also need to be involved in programs aimed at preventing MR. Many of the familial, social, and environmental factors known to cause mild retardation are preventable. Counseling and education can reduce or eliminate such factors (e.g., poor nutrition, cigarette smoking, chemical abuse, which increase the risk of prematurity and intrauterine growth retardation). Consequently, the major interventions are directed at improving maternal health and educating women regarding the dangers of chemicals, including alcohol, during pregnancy and lead during childhood. Other preventive strategies that play an important role include adequate prenatal care; optimal medical care of high-risk newborns; rubella immunization; genetic counseling and prenatal screening, especially in terms of Down or fragile X syndrome; use of folic acid supplements during the childbearing years and during pregnancy to prevent neural tube defects; newborn screening for treatable inborn errors of metabolism, such as congenital hypothyroidism, phenylketonuria, and galactosemia; and early appropriate therapies and rehabilitation services for children with developmental disabilities.

● Evaluation

The effectiveness of nursing interventions is determined by continual reassessment and evaluation of care based on the following observational guidelines:

1 Observe techniques used to teach child and child's success in ability to learn; inquire if child is enrolled in early stimulation program.
2 Interview family regarding provision of appropriate socialization, discipline, and play for child; observe

child's ability to communicate with others; if possible, interview child regarding feelings of self-worth.
3 Observe those activities of daily living that child can completely or partially perform.
4 Interview family regarding any plans for future care and their awareness of community services.
5 Check patient record for evidence of nursing admission history, especially for self-help activities; observe parent's involvement in child's care; observe social interaction of child and family with other patients.
6 Investigate community programs aimed at preventing retardation and inquire as to nursing involvement in these efforts.

The *expected outcomes* are described in the Nursing Care Plan on p. 597.

DOWN SYNDROME

Down syndrome is the most common chromosomal abnormality of a generalized syndrome, occurring in 1 in every 800 to 1000 live births (National Down Syndrome Society, 2003c; Grech, 2001). It occurs slightly more often in whites than in blacks, although the incidence is unchanged in various socioeconomic classes.

Etiology

The cause of Down syndrome is not known, but evidence from cytogenetic and epidemiologic studies supports the concept of multiple causality. Approximately 95% of all cases of Down syndrome are attributable to an extra chromosome 21 (group G), thus the name *nonfamilial trisomy 21* (National Down Syndrome Society, 2003d; Grech, 2001). Although children with trisomy 21 are born to parents of all ages, there is a statistically greater risk in older women, particularly those older than 35 years of age. For example, in women 35 years of age the chance of conceiving a child with Down syndrome is about 1 in 400 live births, but in women age 40 it is about 1 in 110. However, the majority (about 80%) of infants with Down syndrome are born to women younger than age 35. In less than 5% of cases, paternal age is a factor, especially in men 55 years of age or older (National Down Syndrome Society, 2003c; Hixon and others, 1998).

About 3% to 4% of the cases may be caused by *translocation* of chromosomes 15 and 21 or 22. This type of genetic aberration is usually hereditary and is not associated with advanced parental age. From 1% to 2% of affected persons demonstrate *mosaicism,* which refers to cells with both normal and abnormal chromosomes. The degree of physical and cognitive impairment is related to the percentage of cells with the abnormal chromosome makeup.

Diagnostic Evaluation

Down syndrome can usually be diagnosed by the clinical manifestations alone (Box 19-3 and Fig. 19-6), but a chromosome analysis should be done to confirm the genetic abnormality.

Several physical problems are associated with Down syndrome. Many of these children have congenital heart malformations, the most common being septal defects. Respiratory tract infections are very prevalent and, when combined with cardiac anomalies, are the chief cause of death, particularly during the first year of life. Hypotonicity of chest and ab-

NURSING CARE PLAN   The Child With Mental Retardation

NURSING DIAGNOSIS ■ **Altered growth and development related to impaired cognitive functioning**

PATIENT GOAL 1: Will achieve optimal growth and development potential

NURSING INTERVENTIONS/*RATIONALES*

Involve child and family in an early infant stimulation program *to help maximize child's development*

Assess child's developmental progress at regular intervals; keep detailed records to distinguish subtle changes in functioning *so that plan of care can be revised as needed*

Help family determine child's readiness to learn specific tasks, *because readiness may not be easily recognized*

Help family set realistic goals for child *to encourage successful attainment of goals and self-esteem*

Employ positive reinforcement for specific tasks or behaviors *because this improves motivation and learning*

Encourage learning of self-care skills as soon as child is ready

Reinforce self-care activities *to facilitate optimal development*

Encourage family to investigate special day care programs and educational classes as soon as possible

Emphasize that child has same needs as other children (e.g., play, discipline, social interaction)

Before adolescence, counsel child and parents regarding physical maturation, sexual behavior, marriage, and childrearing

Encourage optimal vocational training

EXPECTED OUTCOMES

Child and family are actively involved in infant stimulation program

Family applies developmental concepts and continues activities in home care of child

Child performs activities of daily living at optimal capacity

Family investigates integrated educational programs

Appropriate limit-setting, recreation, and social opportunities are provided

Adolescent issues are explored as appropriate

PATIENT GOAL 2: Will achieve optimal socialization

NURSING INTERVENTIONS/*RATIONALES*

Emphasize that child has same need for socialization as other children

Encourage family to teach child socially acceptable behavior (e.g., saying "hello" and "thank you," manners, appropriate touch)

Encourage grooming and age-appropriate dress *to encourage acceptance by others and self-esteem*

Recommend programs that provide peer relationships and experiences (e.g., mainstreaming, Boy Scouts, Girl Scouts, Special Olympics) *to promote optimum socialization*

Provide adolescent with practical sexual information and a well-defined, concrete code of conduct *because child's easy persuasion and lack of judgment may place child* at risk

EXPECTED OUTCOMES

Child behaves in socially acceptable manner

Child has peer relationships and experiences

Child does not experience social isolation

NURSING DIAGNOSIS ■ **Altered family processes related to having a child with MR**

PATIENT (FAMILY) GOAL 1: Will receive adequate support

NURSING INTERVENTIONS/*RATIONALES*

Inform family as soon as possible at or after birth, *because family may suspect a problem and need immediate* support

Have both parents present at informing conference *to avoid problem of one parent having to relay complex information to the other parent and deal with the initial emotional reaction of the other*

Give family written information about the condition, when possible (e.g., a specific syndrome or disease), *for family to refer to later*

Discuss with family members benefits of family-centered home care; allow them opportunities to investigate all residential alternatives before making a decision

Encourage family to meet other families with a similarly affected child *so that they can receive additional support*

Refrain from giving definitive answers about the degree of retardation; stress the potential learning abilities of these children, especially with early intervention, *to encourage hope*

Demonstrate acceptance of child through own behavior *because parents are sensitive to the affective attitude of the professional*

Emphasize normal characteristics of child *to help family see child as an individual with strengths, as well as weaknesses*

Encourage family members to express their feelings and concerns *because this is part of the adaptation process*

EXPECTED OUTCOMES

Family expresses feelings and concerns regarding the birth of a child with MR and its implications

Family members make realistic decisions based on their needs and capabilities

Family members demonstrate acceptance of child

PATIENT (FAMILY) GOAL 2: Will be prepared for long-term care of child

NURSING INTERVENTIONS/*RATIONALES*

As child grows older, discuss with parents alternatives to home care, especially as parents near retirement or old age, *so that appropriate long-term care can be provided*

Encourage family to consider respite care as needed *to facilitate family's ability to cope with child's long-term care*

Help family investigate residential settings (e.g., small group homes or supervised apartments), *because this may be needed for child's optimal care*

Encourage family to include affected member in planning and to continue meaningful relationships and ongoing support after placement

Encourage the young adult to enter workforce or volunteer workshop settings or participate in community-supported employment

Refer to agencies that provide support and assistance

EXPECTED OUTCOMES

Family identifies realistic goals for future care of child

Family avails themselves and child of supportive services

BOX 19-3 ■ Clinical Manifestations of Down Syndrome

HEAD
*Separated sagittal suture
Brachycephaly
Skull rounded and small
Flat occiput
Enlarged anterior fontanel
Sparse hair (variable)

FACE
Flat profile

EYES
*Oblique palpebral fissures (upward, outward slant)
Inner epicanthal folds
Speckling of iris (Brushfield spots)
Short, sparse eyelashes
Blepharitis

NOSE
*Small
*Depressed nasal bridge (saddle nose)

EARS
Small
Short pinna (vertical ear length)
Overlapping upper helices
Narrow canals

MOUTH
*High, arched, narrow palate
Small osseous orbit

Protruding tongue; may be fissured at lip and furrowed on surface
Hypoplastic mandible
Downward curve (especially noted when crying)
Mouth kept open

TEETH
Delayed eruption
Alignment abnormalities common
Microdontia
Periodontal disease

CHEST
Shortened rib cage
Twelfth rib anomalies
Pectus excavatum/carinatum

NECK
*Skin excess and lax
Short and broad

ABDOMEN
Protruding
Muscles lax and flabby
    Diastasis recti
    Umbilical hernia

GENITALIA
Small penis
Cryptorchidism
Bulbous vulva

HANDS
Broad, short
Stubby fingers
Incurved little finger (clinodactyly)
Transverse palmar crease
Characteristic dermal ridge patterns
Distally located axial triradius
Increased ulnar loops on fingers

FEET
*Wide space between big and second toes
*Plantar crease between big and second toes
Broad, stubby, short

MUSCULOSKELETON
Short stature
*Hyperflexibility
*Muscle weakness
Hypotonia
Atlantoaxial instability

SKIN
Dry, cracked, and frequent fissuring
Cutis marmorata (mottling)

OTHER
Reduced birth weight

*Most common findings in modified chart (Pueschel, 1999).

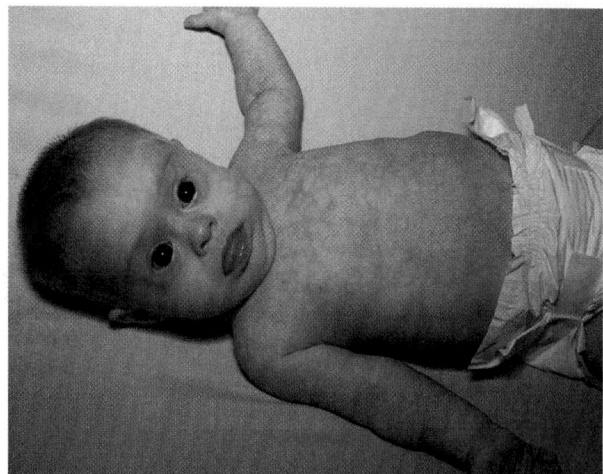

FIG. 19-6 ■ Down syndrome in infant. Note small, square head with upward slant to the eyes, flat nasal bridge, protruding tongue, mottled skin, and hypotonia.

dominal muscles and dysfunction of the immune system probably predispose to the development of respiratory tract infection. Other physical problems include thyroid dysfunction, especially congenital hypothyroidism, and an increased incidence of leukemia.

Therapeutic Management

Although no cure exists for Down syndrome, a number of therapies are advocated, such as surgery to correct serious congenital anomalies and possibly the physical stigmata, although the latter is controversial. These children also benefit from regular medical care. Evaluation of sight and hearing is essential, and treatment of otitis media is required to prevent auditory loss, which can influence cognitive function. Periodic testing of thyroid function is recommended, especially if growth is severely delayed. Children participating in sports that may involve stress on the head and neck, such as gymnastics, diving, butterfly stroke in swimming, high jump, and soccer, should be evaluated radiologically for *atlantoaxial instability.* Symptoms of the disorder include neck pain, weakness, and torticollis. Affected children are at risk for spinal cord compression.

> **NURSING ALERT**
>
> Report immediately any child with the following signs of spinal cord compression:
> Persistent neck pain
> Loss of established motor skills and bladder or bowel control
> Changes in sensation

Prognosis.   Life expectancy for those with Down syndrome has improved in recent years but remains lower than for the general population. More than 80% survive to age

ETHICAL CASE STUDY

Ethical Decision Making Model*	Elena is a 3-month-old girl with Down syndrome who has an atrioventricular septal defect (AVSD). Elena and her family recently came to the United States from Romania. The cardiologist following Elena in Romania had not recommended surgery to repair the AVSD. Since arriving in the United States, Elena has been experiencing increased symptoms of heart failure. The new pediatrician that the parents were referred to discussed surgical repair of the AVSD. Elena's parents expressed surprise that reparative surgery was an option, indicating that the cardiologist in Romania felt surgery would be of no benefit to a child with Down syndrome. In addition, they were told that Elena would not live past 1 year of age and thus had not anticipated raising a child with Down syndrome. The father expressed concern about being able to pay for such an expensive operation, stating that, in Romania, surgery would not be considered in a child with Down syndrome. During the discussion with the pediatrician, the mother sat quietly crying while holding the infant.
Evaluate the issue	In recent years, there has been increased discussion in the literature of refusals to perform interventions on individuals with learning disabilities (Coats, 2001; Keenan and others, 1999). This has prompted concern that individuals with disabilities may not receive equal access to health care. Although the life expectancy of children with Down syndrome remains between 5 and 10 years less than the overall population with disabilities, there is still a reasonable life expectancy for these individuals (Glasson and others, 2002; Keenan and others, 1999). There is continued discussion in the literature regarding the restrictions of socialized medicine in industrialized countries as well as the inadequacies of medical care in less-developed countries. These difficult choices, because of resource-limited medical care, are often not made in the best interest of the child and family.

A second major concern often raised is whether there are increased risks associated with surgery for infants with Down syndrome. Recent studies show no differences in survival after major surgery in children with Down syndrome compared with children with a normal genotype (Al-Hay and others, 2002). |
Treat all involved with respect	Of major importance in this case is listening to the concerns raised by the family. It is important to understand that the parents realize for the first time since the birth of their child that surgery could be of benefit. Nonjudgmental support is essential. The parents need time to evaluate the situation. It is important to consider the mother's feelings as well as those of the father, although culture may determine that the father is the primary decision maker in relation to such matters. Cultural values related to quality of life for a child with Down syndrome must be explored with both parents and extended family.
Hear all sides	Differences in health care practices in other countries may contribute to the dilemma in ethical cases such as Elena. For example, publicity regarding a heart transplant refusal in England a few years ago brought new attention to the concern as to how to maximize access to care for the largest number of individuals when resources are limited (Palmer, 1999). This case brought renewed concern that a decreased state of health could be accepted for children with Down syndrome and other disabilities. Nurses must critically evaluate their beliefs regarding what is considered quality of life to be of support to all families who seek care and advice regarding the future of a child with a disability such as Down syndrome.
Initiate action	The first step in this case is to educate the family on the risks and benefits of surgery for an AVSD repair in a child with Down syndrome. Discussions with the family should be coordinated by the health care team. Consideration of the family's support network in the United States is important. Assessment of the family's resources and ability to provide financial support for the surgery must be considered in light of restrictions placed on many hospitals. The implications for the child's life without surgical intervention must be discussed with the family. The family should be given time to ask questions and to consult with other family members and friends. The family needs support for the realization that Elena has a good chance of surviving to an adult age.
Consider the outcome	The family has been told since Elena's birth that she will not survive past the first year of life. The recent news that Elena has a chance of surviving if she receives surgical intervention is a shock to the family. Although having no previous experience with Western medicine, the family needs time to realize that their child has a greater chance of surviving. Surgery to repair the AVSD can change the outcome for this child. The family's awareness that children with Down syndrome have access to modern surgical interventions in the United States is an important ethical issue that the health care team must discuss.

55 years and beyond. As the prognosis continues to improve for these individuals, it will be important to provide for their long-term health care, social, and leisure needs (National Down Syndrome Society, 2003b; Van Riper, 2003). (See Ethical Case Study.)

Nursing Considerations

Support Family at Time of Diagnosis. Because of the unique physical characteristics, the infant with Down syndrome is usually diagnosed at birth, and parents should be informed of the diagnosis at this time. Parents usually prefer that both of them be present during the informing interview so that they can support one another emotionally.

They appreciate receiving reading material about the syndrome* and being referred to others for help or advice, such as parent groups or professional counseling.

---

*Sources of information include the **Association for Retarded Citizens of the United States** (see footnote, p. 592); the **American Association on Mental Retardation,** 444 North Capitol Street Northwest, Suite 846, Washington, DC 20001-1512; (800) 424-3688 or (202) 387-1968; fax: (202) 387-2193; website: www.aamr.org; the **National Down Syndrome Society,** 666 Broadway, 8th floor, New York, NY 10012-2317; (800) 221-4602; fax: (212) 979-2873; website: www.ndss.org; and the **National Down Syndrome Congress,** 1370 Center Drive, Suite 102, Atlanta, GA 30338; (800) 232-6372 or (770) 604-9500; website: www.ndsccenter.org.

After parents are aware of the diagnosis, they are confronted with the crisis of losing their perfect or dream child and grieving for and accepting their reality child. Consequently, the parents' responses to the child may greatly influence decisions regarding future care. Whereas some families willingly want to take the child home, others consider immediate residential placement. The nurse must carefully answer questions regarding developmental potential. Institutionalization is no longer an option. For families unable or unready to choose taking the newborn home, specialized foster care or adoption are other options (see Critical Thinking Exercise).

Assist Family in Preventing Physical Problems. Many of the physical characteristics of Down syndrome present nursing problems. The hypotonicity of muscles and hyperextensibility of joints complicate positioning. The limp, flaccid extremities resemble the posture of a rag doll; as a result, holding the infant is difficult and cumbersome. Sometimes parents perceive this lack of molding to their bodies as evidence of inadequate parenting. The extended body position promotes heat loss because more surface area is exposed to the environment. Parents are encouraged to swaddle or wrap the infant tightly in a blanket before picking up the child to provide security and warmth. The nurse also discusses with parents their feelings concerning attachment to the child, emphasizing that the child's lack of clinging or molding is a physical characteristic, not a sign of detachment or rejection.

Decreased muscle tone compromises respiratory expansion. In addition, the underdeveloped nasal bone causes a chronic problem of inadequate drainage of mucus. The constant stuffy nose forces the child to breathe by mouth, which dries the oropharyngeal membranes, increasing the susceptibility to upper respiratory tract infections. Measures to lessen these problems include clearing the nose with a bulb-type syringe, rinsing the mouth with water after feedings, increasing fluid intake, and using a cool-mist vaporizer to keep the mucous membranes moist and the secretions liquefied. Other helpful measures include changing the child's position frequently; performing postural drainage with percussion if necessary, practicing good handwashing, and properly disposing of soiled articles such as tissues. If antibiotics are ordered, the importance of completing the full course of therapy for successful eradication of the infection and prevention of growth of resistant organisms is stressed.

Inadequate drainage resulting in pooling of mucus in the nose also interferes with feeding. Because the child breathes by mouth, sucking for any length of time is difficult. When eating solids, the child may gag on the food because of mucus in the oropharynx. Parents are advised to clear the nose before each feeding, give small, frequent feedings, and allow opportunities for rest during mealtime.

The protruding tongue also interferes with feeding, especially of solid foods. Parents need to know that the tongue thrust is not an indication of refusal to feed, but a physiologic response. Parents are advised to use a small but long, straight-handled spoon to push the food toward the back and side of the mouth. If food is thrust out, it is refed.

Dietary intake needs supervision. Decreased muscle tone affects gastric motility, predisposing the child to constipa-

CRITICAL THINKING EXERCISE

Diagnosis of Down Syndrome

The parents of Melissa, a newborn diagnosed as having Down syndrome, ask the nurse, "What are we supposed to do with her?" They further state that they already have three other children at home.

QUESTIONS

1. Evidence: Is there sufficient evidence to draw conclusions about the parents' concerns regarding their newborn daughter?
2. Assumptions: Describe an underlying assumption about each of the following:
   a. Newborn diagnosed with Down syndrome
   b. Parental care of a newborn with Down syndrome
   c. Newborn with Down syndrome and older siblings
3. What priorities for the nursing response should be established?
4. Does the evidence support your nursing intervention?
5. What alternative perspectives might you have?

ANSWERS

1. Yes. Shocked parents with three children are notified their newborn has Down syndrome.
2. a. Melissa is a developmentally delayed newborn who requires time-consuming care.
   b. Melissa will develop a variety of medical problems causing a huge financial expense.
   c. Melissa will always require parent/sibling supervision and care.
3. The first priority is to allow the parents to express their feelings of grief, anger, sadness, and guilt regarding the birth of a mentally retarded child.
   The nurse should not take anything for granted or give definite suggestions regarding retarded children.
   The nurse should demonstrate acceptance of the child because parents are sensitive to the professional's attitude.
4. Yes. The parents' response suggest unexpressed feelings of anger, loss, sadness, and confusion.
5. The nurse should guide the parents toward appropriate resources when asked, such as written information and organizations.
   The nurse may ask the pediatrician and the social worker to talk with the parents.
   Emphasize normal characteristics of the child to help the parents see the child as an individual.
   Encourage parents to meet other families with a similarly affected child for additional support.

tion. Dietary measures such as increased fiber and fluid promote evacuation. The child's eating habits may need careful scrutiny to prevent obesity. Height and weight measurements should be obtained on a serial basis, especially during infancy. Because these children's growth is slower than that of the general pediatric population's trends, special growth charts developed for these children should be used (American Academy of Pediatrics, 2001; Cohen, 1999).

During infancy the child's skin is pliable and soft. However, it gradually becomes rough and dry and is prone to cracking and infection. Skin care involves the use of minimum soap and application of lubricants. Lip balm is applied to the lips, especially when the child is outdoors, to prevent excessive chapping.

Assist in Prenatal Diagnosis and Genetic Counseling.
Prenatal diagnosis of Down syndrome is possible through chorionic villus sampling and amniocentesis because chromosome analysis of fetal cells can detect the presence of trisomy or translocation. However, analysis will not identify sporadic cases in young women when there is no indication for prenatal testing. Testing for low maternal serum alphafetoprotein, high chorionic gonadotropin, low unconjugated estriol levels, and maternal serum fetal cell markers may identify an affected fetus in women who can then undergo amniocentesis (National Down Syndrome Society, 2003; Yang and others, 2003).

Prenatal testing and genetic counseling should be offered to women of advanced maternal age or who have a family history of the disorder. If prenatal testing indicates the fetus is affected, the nurse must allow the parents to express their feelings concerning elective abortion and support their decision to terminate or proceed with the pregnancy.

FRAGILE X SYNDROME

Fragile X syndrome is the most common inherited cause of MR and the second most common genetic cause of MR after Down syndrome. It has been described in all ethnic groups and races; the incidence of affected males is 1 in 3600; the incidence of affected females is 1 in 4000 to 1 in 6000; and the incidence of carrier females is 1 in 246 to 1 in 468 (National Fragile X Foundation, 2002; Crawford, 2001).

The syndrome is caused by an abnormal gene on the lower end of the long arm of the X chromosome. Chromosome analysis may demonstrate a *fragile site* (a region that fails to condense during mitosis and is characterized by a nonstaining gap or narrowing) in the cells of affected males and females and in carrier females. This fragile site has been determined to be caused by a gene mutation that results in excessive repeats of nucleotide in a specific deoxyribonucleic acid (DNA) segment of the X chromosome. The number of repeats in a normal individual is between 6 and 50. An individual with 50 to 200 base-pair repeats is said to have a *permutation* and is therefore a carrier. When passed from a parent to a child, these base-pair repeats can expand from 200 or more, which is termed a *full mutation.* This expansion occurs only when a carrier mother passes the mutation to her offspring; it does not occur when a carrier father passes the mutation to his daughters.

The inheritance pattern has been termed *X-linked dominant with reduced penetrance.* It is in distinct contrast to the classic X-linked recessive pattern in which all carrier females are normal, all affected males have symptoms of the disorder, and no males are carriers. Consequently, genetic counseling of affected families is more complex than that for families with a classic X-linked disorder, such as hemophilia. Prenatal diagnosis of the fragile X gene mutation is now possible with direct DNA testing in a family with an established history, using amniocentesis or chorionic villus sampling (CDC, 2002; Welch and Williams, 1999). Both affected sexes are fertile and therefore capable of transmitting the fragile X disorder.

Clinical Manifestations

The classic trend of physical findings in adult men with fragile X syndrome consists of a long face with a prominent jaw (prognathism); large, protruding ears; and large testes

---

BOX 19-4 ■ Clinical Manifestations of Fragile X Syndrome

PHYSICAL FEATURES

Long, wide, and/or protruding ears
Long, narrow face with prominent jaw
In postpubertal males, enlarged testicles
Long palpebral fissures
High, arched palate
Strabismus
Increased head circumference
Mitral valve prolapse/aortic root dilation
Hypotonia
Hyperextensible finger joints
Transpalmar crease
Pes planus (flat feet)

BEHAVIORAL FEATURES

Mild to severe cognitive impairment (occasionally, normal intelligence with learning disabilities)
Speech delay; speech may be rapid, with stuttering and repetition of words
Short attention span, hyperactivity
Mouthing beyond expected age for behavior
Hypersensitivity to taste, sounds, touch
Intolerance to change in routine
Autistic-like behaviors
May exhibit aggressive behavior

(macro-orchidism). In prepubertal children, however, these features may be less obvious, and behavioral manifestations may initially suggest the diagnosis (Box 19-4). In carrier females the clinical manifestations are extremely varied.

Therapeutic Management

No cure exists for fragile X syndrome. Medical treatment may include the use of serotonin agents such as carbamazepine (Tegretol) or fluoxetine (Prozac) to control violent temper outbursts and the use of central nervous system (CNS) stimulants or clonidine (Catapres) to improve attention span and decrease hyperactivity. The use of folic acid, which affects the metabolism of CNS transmitters, is controversial.

All affected children require early speech and language therapy, occupational therapy, and special education assistance. Without appropriate intervention, a progressive decline in IQ can occur.

Prognosis. Individuals with fragile X syndromes are expected to live a normal lifespan. Their cognitive impairment may be improved by behavioral and educational interventions.

Nursing Considerations

Because cognitive impairment is a fairly consistent finding in individuals with fragile X syndrome, the care given to these families is the same as for any child with MR. Because the disorder is hereditary, genetic counseling is necessary to inform parents and siblings of the risks of transmission. In addition, any male or female with unexplained or nonspecific mental impairment should be referred for genetic testing and, if needed, counseling. Families with a member affected by the disorder should be referred to the **National Fragile X Foundation.***

SENSORY IMPAIRMENT

HEARING IMPAIRMENT

Hearing impairment is one of the most common disabilities in the United States. An estimated 2 in 1000 infants are born with permanent hearing loss (Applebaum, 1999). For infants admitted to the neonatal intensive care unit, the incidence rises sharply to approximately 2 to 4 per 100 neonates (Cunningham and Cox, 2003; American Academy of Pediatrics, 1999). There are about 1 million children with hearing impairment ranging in age from birth to 21 years in the United States, and almost a third of these children have other disabilities, such as visual or cognitive deficits.

Definition and Classification

Hearing impairment is a general term indicating disability that may range in severity from mild to profound and includes the subsets of deaf and hard-of-hearing. *Deaf* refers to a person whose hearing disability precludes successful processing of linguistic information through audition, with or without a hearing aid. *Hard-of-hearing* refers to a person who, generally with the use of a hearing aid, has residual hearing sufficient to enable successful processing of linguistic information through audition. Other terms, such as *deaf and dumb, mute,* or *deaf-mute,* are unacceptable. Hearing-impaired persons are not dumb and, if mute, have no physical speech defect other than that caused by the inability to hear.

Hearing defects may be classified according to etiology, pathology, or symptom severity. Each is important in terms of treatment, possible prevention, and rehabilitation.

Etiology. Hearing loss may be caused by a number of prenatal and postnatal conditions. These include a family history of childhood hearing impairment, anatomic malformations of the head or neck, low birth weight, severe perinatal asphyxia, perinatal infection (cytomegalovirus, rubella, herpes, syphilis, toxoplasmosis, bacterial meningitis), chronic ear infection, cerebral palsy, Down syndrome, or administration of ototoxic drugs (Holte, 2003; Berrettini and others, 1999).

In addition, high-risk neonates who are surviving formerly fatal prenatal or perinatal conditions may be susceptible to hearing loss from the disorder or its treatment.

For example, sensorineural hearing loss may be a result of continuous humming noises or high noise levels associated with incubators, oxygen hoods, or intensive care units, especially when combined with the use of potentially ototoxic antibiotics.

Environmental noise is a special concern. Sounds loud enough to damage sensitive hair cells of the inner ear can produce irreversible hearing loss. Very loud, brief noise, such as gunfire, can cause immediate, severe, and permanent loss of hearing. Longer exposure to less intense but still hazardous sounds, such as music, can also produce hearing loss (Segal and others, 2003; Roizen, 1999). The exact sound level that produces hearing loss is unknown.

Pathology. Disorders of hearing are divided according to the location of the defect. *Conductive* or *middle-ear hearing loss* results from interference of transmission of sound to the middle ear. It is the most common of all types of hearing loss and most frequently is a result of recurrent serous otitis media. Conductive hearing impairment involves mainly interference with loudness of sound.

Sensorineural hearing loss, also called *perceptive* or *nerve deafness,* involves damage to the inner ear structures or the auditory nerve. The most common causes are congenital defects of inner ear structures or consequences of acquired conditions, such as kernicterus, infection, administration of ototoxic drugs, or exposure to excessive noise. Sensorineural hearing loss results in distortion of sound and problems in discrimination. Although the child hears some of everything going on around him or her, the sounds are distorted, severely affecting discrimination and comprehension.

Mixed conductive-sensorineural hearing loss results from interference with transmission of sound in the middle ear and along neural pathways. It frequently results from recurrent otitis media and its complications.

Central auditory imperception includes all hearing losses that do not demonstrate defects in the conductive or sensorineural structures. They are usually divided into organic or functional losses. In the *organic type* of central auditory imperception, the defect involves the reception of auditory stimuli along the central pathways and the expression of the message into meaningful communication. Examples are *aphasia,* the inability to express ideas in any form, either written or verbally; *agnosia,* the inability to interpret sound correctly; and *dysacusis,* difficulty in processing details or discrimination among sounds.

In the *functional type* of hearing loss, no organic lesion exists to explain a central auditory loss. Examples of functional hearing loss are conversion hysteria (an unconscious withdrawal from hearing to block remembrance of a traumatic event), infantile autism, and childhood schizophrenia.

TABLE 19-2 ■ Intensity of Sounds Expressed in Decibels

DECIBELS	REPRESENTATIVE SOUND
0	Softest sound normal ear can hear
10	Heartbeat, rustling of leaves
20	Whisper at 1.8 meter (5 feet)
30-45	Normal conversation
60	Noise in average restaurant
70-80	Street noises
80	Loud radio in home
90-100	Train
120	Thunder, rock music
140	Thunder, rock music
>140	Pain threshold

*PO Box 190488-0488, San Francisco, CA 94119; (800) 688-8765 or (925) 938-9300; fax: (925) 938-9315; website: www.fragilex.org.

Symptom Severity.   Hearing impairment is expressed in terms of a *decibel (dB),* a unit of loudness (Table 19-2); hearing is measured at various frequencies, such as 500, 1000, and 2000 cycles/second, the critical listening speech range. Hearing impairment can be classified according to *hearing threshold level* (the measurement of an individual's hearing threshold by means of an audiometer) and the degree of symptom severity as it affects speech (Table 19-3). These classifications offer only general guidelines regarding the effect of the impairment on any individual child, because children differ greatly in their ability to use residual hearing.

Therapeutic Management

Conductive Hearing Loss.   Treatment of hearing loss depends on the cause and type of hearing impairment. Many conductive hearing defects respond to medical or surgical treatment, such as antibiotic therapy for acute otitis media or insertion of tympanostomy tubes for chronic otitis media. When the conductive loss is permanent, hearing can be improved with the use of a hearing aid to amplify sound.

The nurse should be familiar with the types, basic care, and handling of hearing aids, especially when the child is hospitalized.* Types of aids include those worn in or behind the ear, models incorporated into an eyeglass frame, or types worn on the body with a wire connection to the ear (Fig. 19-7). One of the most common problems with a hearing aid is *acoustic feedback,* an annoying whistling sound usually caused by improper fit of the ear mold. Sometimes the whistling may be at a frequency that the child cannot hear but that is annoying to others. In this case, if children are old enough, they are told of the noise and asked to readjust the aid.

> **NURSING TIP**
>
> To reduce or eliminate whistling from a hearing aid, try reinserting the aid, making certain that no hair is caught between the ear mold and the canal, cleaning the ear mold or ear, or lowering the volume of the aid.

As children grow older, they may be self-conscious about the device. Every effort is made to make the aid inconspicuous, such as an appropriate hairstyle to cover behind-the-ear or in-the-ear models, attractive frames for glasses, and placement of the on-the-body type where it is not seen, such as under a blouse or sweater. Children are given responsibility for the care of the device as soon as they are able, because fostering independence is a primary goal of rehabilitation.

> **⏷ NURSING ALERT**
>
> When parents express concern about their child's hearing and speech development, refer the child for a hearing evaluation. Absence of well-formed syllables ("da," "na," "yaya") by 11 months of age should result in immediate referral.

Sensorineural Hearing Loss.   Treatment for sensorineural hearing loss is much less satisfactory. Because the defect is not one of intensity of sound, hearing aids are of less value

TABLE 19-3 ■ Classification of Hearing Loss Based on Symptom Severity

HEARING LEVEL (DB)	EFFECT
Slight: 16-25	Has difficulty hearing faint or distant speech
	Usually is unaware of hearing difficulty
	Likely to achieve in school but may have problems
	No speech defects
Mild to moderate: 26-55	May have speech difficulties
	Understands face-to-face conversational speech at 3-5 feet
Moderately severe: 56-70 (hard of hearing)	Unable to understand conversational speech unless loud
	Considerable difficulty with group or classroom discussion
	Requires special speech training
Severe: 71-90 (deaf)	May hear a loud voice if nearby
	May be able to identify loud environmental noises
	Can distinguish vowels but not most consonants
	Requires speech training
Profound: 91 (deaf)	May hear only loud sounds
	Requires extensive speech training

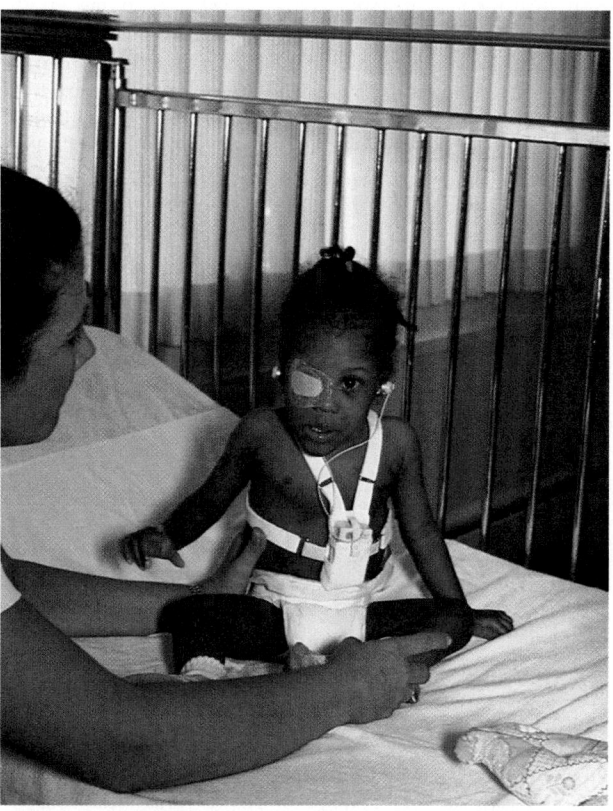

FIG. 19-7 ■ On-the-body hearing aids are convenient for young children, such as this child with severe bilateral hearing loss. Note eye patching for strabismus.

in this type of defect. The use of *cochlear implants** (a surgically implanted prosthetic device) provides a sensation of hearing for individuals who have severe or profound hearing loss (Waltzman, Roland Jr., and Cohen, 2002; Slattery and Fayad, 1999). Children with sensorineural hearing loss have lost or damaged some or all of their hair cells or auditory nerve fibers. Often these children cannot benefit from conventional hearing aids because they only amplify sound that cannot be processed by a damaged inner ear. A cochlear implant bypasses the hair cells to directly stimulate surviving auditory nerve fibers so that they can send signals to the brain. These signals can be interpreted by the brain to produce sound and sensations (Allegretti, 2002).

Multichanneled implants are now available. This more sophisticated device stimulates the auditory nerve at a number of locations with differently processed signals. This type of stimulation gives a person the opportunity to use the pitch information present in speech signals, allowing the person to better understand speech.

The trend is toward early use of cochlear implants, usually by 18 months of age, to give the child maximum opportunity to develop listening, language, and speaking skills.

Nursing Considerations

● *Assessment*

Assessment of children for hearing impairment is a critical nursing responsibility. Early detection of hearing loss, preferably within the first 3 to 6 months of life, is essential to improve the language and educational outcomes of those with hearing impairments (Holte, 2003; Yoshinaga-Itano and others, 1998). To accomplish this goal, the current recommendation is universal newborn hearing screening before discharge from the newborn nursery (Cunningham and Cox, 2003; American Academy of Pediatrics, 1999). This discussion focuses on developmental and behavioral indexes associated with hearing impairment. Auditory testing is presented in Chapter 7.

Infancy. At birth the nurse can observe the neonate's response to auditory stimuli, as evidenced by the startle reflex, head turning, eye blinking, and cessation of body movement. The infant may vary in the intensity of the response, depending on the state of alertness. However, a consistent absence of a reaction should lead to suspicion of hearing loss. Box 19-5 summarizes other clinical manifestations of hearing impairment in the infant.

Childhood. The child who is profoundly deaf is much more likely to be diagnosed during infancy than the less severely affected one. If the defect is not detected during early childhood, it likely will become evident during entry into

---

Cochlear Implant Association, Inc., 5335 Wisconsin Avenue NW, Suite 440, Washington, DC 20015; (202) 895-2781; fax: (202) 895-2782; website: www.cici.org; **Hearing Enrichment Language Program of the Hough Ear Institute,** 3434 NW 56th Street, Oklahoma City, OK 73112; (405) 945-7186; fax: (405) 945-7188; website: www.oraldeafed.org; **Auditory-Verbal International, Inc. (AVI),** 2121 Eisenhower Avenue, Suite 402, Alexandria, VA 22314; voice: (703) 739-1049; TDD: (703) 739-0874; fax: (703) 739-0395.

BOX 19-5 ■ Clinical Manifestations of Hearing Impairment

INFANTS
Lack of startle or blink reflex to a loud sound
Failure to be awakened by loud environmental noises
Failure to localize a source of sound by 6 months of age
Absence of babble or inflections in voice by age 7 months
General indifference to sound
Lack of response to the spoken word; failure to follow verbal directions
Response to loud noises as opposed to the voice

CHILDREN
Use of gestures rather than verbalization to express desires, especially after age 15 months
Failure to develop intelligible speech by age 24 months
Monotone quality, unintelligible speech, lessened laughter
Vocal play, head banging, or foot stamping for vibratory sensation
Yelling or screeching to express pleasure, annoyance (tantrums), or need
Asking to have statements repeated or answering them incorrectly
Responding more to facial expression and gestures than to verbal explanation
Avoidance of social interaction; often puzzled and unhappy in such situations; prefer to play alone
Inquiring, sometimes confused facial expression
Suspicious alertness, sometimes interpreted as paranoia, alternating with cooperation
Frequently stubborn because of lack of comprehension
Irritable at not making themselves understood
Shy, timid, and withdrawn
Often appear "dreamy," "in a world of their own," or exhibit inattentiveness

---

school, when the child has difficulty in learning. Unfortunately, some of these children are mistakenly placed in special classes for students with learning disabilities or MR. Therefore it is essential that the nurse suspect a hearing impairment in any child who demonstrates the behaviors listed in Box 19-5.

Of primary importance is the effect of hearing impairment on speech development. A child with a mild conductive hearing loss may speak fairly clearly but in a loud, monotone voice. A child with a sensorineural defect usually has difficulty in articulation. For example, inability to hear higher frequencies may result in the word *spoon* being pronounced "poon." Children with articulation problems need to have their hearing tested.

!NURSING ALERT

Stress to parents the importance of storing batteries for hearing aids in a safe location and teaching children or supervising young children not to remove the battery from the hearing aid. Ingestion of batteries is most often of those from hearing aids, including the child's own aid.

● *Nursing Diagnoses*

A number of nursing diagnoses are prominent in the nursing care of the child with hearing impairment and the child's family; other diagnoses specific to individual cases become evident. The most common nursing diagnoses are outlined in the Nursing Care Plan on pp. 608-609.

● Planning

The goals of nursing care for the child with hearing impairment and family are as follows:

1 Child will achieve optimal development through enhancement of the communication process and socialization.
2 Child and family will receive support.
3 Child will receive appropriate care during hospitalization.

● Implementation

Promote the communication process. The nurse's initial role in rehabilitation is to encourage the family to participate in an auditory training program.* Rehabilitation training consists of learning appropriate methods to improve communication, such as lipreading, sign language, speech language, and therapy.

Lipreading.

Even though the child may become an expert at lipreading, only about 40% of the spoken word is understood, and less if the speaker has an accent, mustache, or beard. Exaggerating pronunciation or speaking in an altered rhythm further lessens comprehension. Parents can help the child understand the spoken word by using the suggestions in the Guidelines box. The child learns to supplement the spoken word with sensitivity to visual cues, primarily body language and facial expression (e.g., tightening the lips, muscle tension, eye contact).

Cued Speech.

This method of communication is an adjunct to straight lipreading. It uses hand signals to help the child with a hearing impairment distinguish between words that look alike when formed by the lips (e.g., "mat," "bat"). It is most often used by children with hearing impairments who are using speech rather than those who are nonverbal.

Sign Language.

Sign language, such as *American Sign Language (ASL)* or *British Sign Language (BSL),* is a visual gestural language that uses hand signals that roughly correspond to specific words and concepts in the English language. Family members are encouraged to learn signing because using or watching hands requires much less concentration than lipreading or talking. Also, a symbol method enables some children to learn more and to learn faster.

*Home training correspondence programs are sponsored by the **John T. Tracy Clinic,** 806 West Adams Boulevard, Los Angeles, CA 90007; (800) 522-4582; TTY: (213) 747-2924; fax: (213) 749-1651; website: www.johntracyclinic.org. Other sources of information on several aspects of hearing loss and on the International Parents' Organization are the **Alexander Graham Bell Association for the Deaf,** 3417 Volta Place NW, Washington, DC 20007; voice: (202) 337-5220 TTY: (202) 337-5221; fax: (202) 337-8314; website: www.agbell.org; and **Canadian Hearing Society,** 271 Spadina Road, Toronto, Ontario M5R 2V3; voice: (416) 964-9595; TTY: (416) 964-9595; fax: (416) 928-2525; website: www.chs.ca.

Speech Language Therapy.

The most formidable task in the education of a child who is profoundly hearing impaired is learning to speak. Speech is learned through a multisensory approach, using visual, tactile, kinesthetic, and auditory stimulation. Parents are encouraged to participate fully in the learning process.

Additional Aids.

Everyday activities present problems for older children with hearing impairment. For example, they may not be able to hear the telephone, doorbell, or alarm clock. Several commercial devices are available to help them adjust to these dilemmas. Flashing lights can be attached to a telephone or doorbell to signal its ringing. Trained hearing ear dogs can provide great assistance because they alert the person to sounds, such as someone approaching, a moving car, a signal to wake up, or a child's cry. Special *teletypewriters* or *telecommunications devices for the deaf (TDD or TTY)* help people with impaired hearing communicate with each other over the telephone; the typed message is conveyed via the telephone lines and displayed on a small screen.*

Any audiovisual medium presents dilemmas for these children, who can see the picture but cannot hear the message. However, with *closed captioning* a special decoding device is attached to the television, and the audio portion of a program is translated into subtitles that appear on the screen.†

As children learn to compensate for their lack of hearing, they become extremely perceptive to visual and vibratory changes. Children often know when another person wants to talk to them because the person will walk close by but not pass. They learn to be alert to other people approaching them by seeing their shadows or feeling the vibrations of their footsteps. They are acutely aware of facial expressions and may comprehend the unspoken word more quickly than the spoken word.

Socialization.

Because socialization is extremely important to the child's development, the nurse discusses with the family methods of fostering social contact. If children attend a special school for the deaf, they are able to socialize with peers in that setting. Classmates become a potential source of close friendships because they communicate more easily among themselves. Parents are encouraged to promote these relationships whenever possible.

Children with a hearing impairment may need special help with school or social activities. For those children wearing hearing aids, background noise should be kept to a minimum. Because many of these children are able to attend regular classes, the teacher may need assistance in adapting methods of teaching for the child's benefit. The school nurse is often in an optimal position to emphasize methods of facilitated communication, such as lipreading

*Directory listings stating "TDD or TTY only" before a phone number indicate that regular telephone use is not possible; "TDD or TTY and voice" indicates that both TDD/TYY users and speaking/hearing people can use the telephone number.

†Additional information is available from the **National Captioning Institute, Inc.,** 1900 Gallows Road, Suite 3000, Vienna, VA 22182; (703) 917-7600; fax: (703) 917-9878; website: www.ncicap.org.

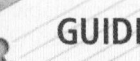

GUIDELINES

Facilitating Lipreading

Attract child's attention before speaking; use light touch to signal speaker's presence.

Stand close to child.

Face child directly or move to a 45-degree angle.

Stand still; do not walk back and forth or turn away to point or look elsewhere.

Establish eye contact and show interest.

Speak at eye level and with good lighting on speaker's face.

Be certain nothing interferes with speech patterns, such as chewing food or gum.

Speak clearly and at a slow and even rate.

Use facial expression to assist in conveying messages.

Keep sentences short.

Rephrase message if child does not understand the words.

(see Guidelines box). Because group projects and audiovisual teaching aids may hinder the child's learning, these educational methods should be carefully evaluated.

In a group setting it is helpful for the other members to sit in a semicircle in front of the child. Because one of the difficulties in following a group discussion is that the child is unaware of who will speak next, someone should point out each speaker. Speakers can also be given numbers, or their names can be written down as each person talks. If one person writes down the main topic of the discussion, the child is able to follow lipreading more closely. Such suggestions can increase the child's ability to participate in sports, organizations such as Boy Scouts or Girl Scouts, and group projects.

Support Child and Family. After the diagnosis of hearing impairment is made, parents need extensive support to adjust to the shock of learning about their child's disability and an opportunity to realize the extent of the hearing loss. If the hearing loss occurs during childhood, the child also requires sensitive, supportive care during the long and often difficult adjustment to this sensory loss. Early rehabilitation is one of the best strategies for fostering adjustment. However, progress in learning communication may not always coincide with emotional adjustment. Depression or anger is common, and such feelings are a normal part of the grieving process. (See also Chapter 18 for an extensive discussion of the emotional support of the child and family.)

Care for Child During Hospitalization. The needs of the hospitalized child with impaired hearing are the same as those of any other child, but the disability presents special challenges to the nurse (see Critical Thinking Exercise). For example, verbal explanations must be supplemented with tactile and visual aids, such as books or actual demonstration and practice. Children's understanding of the explanation needs to be constantly reassessed. If their verbal skills are poorly developed, they can answer questions through drawing, writing, or gesturing. For example, if the nurse is attempting to clarify where a spinal tap is done, the child is asked to point to where the procedure will be done on the body. Because these children often need more time to grasp the full meaning of an explanation, the nurse needs to be patient, allowing ample time for understanding.

When communicating with the child, the nurse should use the same principles as those outlined for facilitating lipreading. Ideally, nurses without foreign accents should be assigned to the child. The child's hearing aid is checked to ensure that it is working properly. If it is necessary to awaken the child at night, the nurse gently shakes the child or turns on the hearing aid before arousing the child. The nurse always makes sure that the child can see him or her before any procedures, even routine ones such as changing a diaper or regulating an infusion, are performed. It is important to remember that the child may not be aware of one's presence until alerted through visual or tactile cues.

Ideally, parents are encouraged to room with the child. However, it must be conveyed to them that this is not to serve as a convenience to the nurse but as a benefit to the child. Although the parents' aid can be enlisted in familiarizing the child with the hospital and explaining procedures, the nurse also talks directly to the youngster, encouraging expression of feelings about the experience. If there is difficulty in understanding the child's speech, an effort is made to become familiar with his or her pronunciation of words. Parents often can be helpful by explaining the child's usual speech habits. Nonverbal communication devices that employ pictures or words that the child can point to are also available (see p. 605). Such boards can also be made by drawing pictures or writing the words of common needs on cardboard, such as *parent, food, water,* or *toilet.*

The nurse has a special role as child advocate with the child and is in a strategic position to alert other health team members and other patients to the child's special needs regarding communication. For example, the nurse should accompany other practitioners on visits to the child's room to ensure that they speak to the child and that the child understands what is said. Caregivers sometimes forget that the child has the abilities to perceive and learn despite a hearing loss, and consequently they communicate only with the parents. As a result, the child's needs and feelings remain unrecognized and unmet.

Because children with impaired hearing may have difficulty in forming social relationships with other children, the child is introduced to roommates and encouraged to engage in play activities. The hospital setting can provide growth-promoting opportunities for social relationships. With the assistance of a child-life specialist, the child can learn new recreational activities, experiment with group games, and engage in therapeutic play. The use of puppets, dollhouses, role-playing with dress-up clothes, building with a hammer and nails, finger painting, playing with syringes, and water play can help the child express feelings that previously were suppressed.

Assist in Measures to Prevent Hearing Impairment. A primary nursing role is prevention of hearing loss. Because the most common cause of impaired hearing is chronic otitis media, it is essential that appropriate measures be instituted to treat existing infections and prevent recurrences (see Chapter 23). Children with histories of ear or respiratory infections or any other condition known to in-

??? CRITICAL THINKING EXERCISE   ???

Hearing Impairment

Four-year-old Jason has a severe congenital hearing impairment. Jason has been admitted to the outpatient surgery postanesthesia care unit (PACU) after a herniorrhaphy and regional block. As he emerges from anesthesia, he becomes more and more agitated.

QUESTIONS

1. Evidence—Is there sufficient evidence to draw conclusions about Jason's postsurgical increasing agitation?
2. Assumptions—Describe an underlying assumption about each of the following:
   a. Severe congenital hearing impairment in a preschool child
   b. Preschooler with severe congenital hearing impairment and awakening in the PACU after surgery
   c. Preschooler with severe congenital hearing impairment and awakening from herniorrhaphy and postregional block
3. What priorities for nursing care should be established for Jason?
4. Does the evidence support your nursing intervention?
5. What alternative perspectives might you have?

ANSWERS

1. Yes. Jason is severely hearing impaired and awakening in an unfamiliar environment after a surgical procedure. Jason awakens in an unfamiliar environment with monitors, intravenous line, and other equipment that may create fear, anxiety, and agitation.
2. a. Jason's inability to hear and communicate promotes frustration and fear.
   b. Jason's increasing agitation may be due to not having his hearing aid.
   c. Jason, who is status postregional block for herniorrhaphy, is unable to clearly verbalize or use sign language to express needs.
3. The first priority is to establish communication with Jason by directly facing him to facilitate lip reading, touching him to get his attention, and correctly placing his hearing aids if available.
   Determine his usual means of communicating and encourage expression of feelings/questions regarding environment, equipment, and procedures.
   Explain procedures before performing using gestures, objects, or pictures and speak slowly and clearly.
   Allow ample time for child to show understanding of explanations.
   Decrease environmental noise.
   Listen closely as the child speaks and focus on his pronunciation of words.
4. Yes. Jason's behavior does not suggest the transitory confusion associated with the initial emergence from anesthesia. Rather, it suggests that he became increasingly frustrated as he became aware of his environment with the inability to communicate his desires and feelings. Although pain is a possibility and needs to be evaluated, regional blocks are typically given during surgery to keep children comfortable until after they are discharged.
5. It would be appropriate to make a referral to the child-life therapist (CLT) during the hospitalization. The CLT would encourage Jason to express his feelings, fears, and anxieties regarding surgery, the hospital environment, equipment, and procedures through therapeutic play.

---

crease the risk of hearing impairment should receive periodic auditory testing.

To prevent the causes of hearing loss that begin prenatally and perinatally, pregnant women need counseling regarding the necessity of early prenatal care, including genetic counseling for known familial disorders; avoidance of all ototoxic drugs, especially during the first trimester; tests to rule out syphilis, rubella, or blood incompatibility; medical management of maternal diabetes; strict control of alcohol intake; and adequate dietary intake. The necessity of routine immunization during childhood to eliminate the possibility of acquired sensorineural loss from rubella, mumps, or measles (encephalitis) is stressed.

Exposure to excessive noise pollution is a well-established cause of sensorineural hearing loss. The nurse should routinely assess the possibility of environmental noise pollution and advise children and parents of the potential danger. When individuals engage in activities associated with high-intensity noise, such as flying model airplanes, target shooting, or snowmobiling, they should wear ear protection such as earmuffs or earplugs (not ordinary dry cotton). However, any protection is better than none. Even common household equipment, such as lawn mowers, power vacuum cleaners, and cordless telephones, can be hazardous.

⚑ NURSING ALERT

Suspect hazardous noise if the listener experiences (1) difficulty in communication while hearing the sound, (2) ringing in the ears (tinnitus) after exposure to the sound, or (3) muffled hearing after leaving the sound.

● Evaluation

The effectiveness of nursing interventions is determined by continual reassessment and evaluation of care based on the following observational guidelines:

1 Observe techniques used to communicate with child; inquire if child is enrolled in an auditory training program; inquire about socialization opportunities for child (i.e., who are child's friends, what are his or her extracurricular activities).
2 Interview family regarding their adjustment to the sensory impairment; observe family members' relationship with child; interview child regarding feelings about the sensory impairment and its effect on activities of daily living (especially important if impairment is recent).
3 Observe types of preparation and communication used to prepare child for hospitalization or procedures; ob-

serve parents' involvement in child's care; observe interaction of child and family with other patients.

4 Investigate community programs aimed at preventing or detecting hearing loss and inquire as to nursing involvement in these efforts.

The *expected outcomes* are described in the Nursing Care Plan below.

VISUAL IMPAIRMENT

Visual impairment is a common problem during childhood. In the United States the prevalence of blindness and serious visual impairment in the pediatric population is estimated at 30 to 64 children per 100,000 population. Another 100 children per 100,000 have less serious impairment (Davidson, 1999). The nurse's role is clearly one of assessment, prevention, referral, and, in some instances, rehabilitation.

Definition and Classification

Visual impairment is a general term that refers to visual loss that cannot be corrected with regular prescription lenses. However, more useful definitions for classifying visual impairments include the following. *School vision* (also known as *partially sighted*) refers to visual acuity between 20/70 and 20/200. The child should be able to obtain an education in the usual public school system with the use of normal-sized print. Near vision is almost always better than distance vision.

NURSING CARE PLAN The Child With Hearing Impairment

NURSING DIAGNOSIS ■ **Sensory/perceptual alterations (auditory) related to hearing impairment**

PATIENT GOAL 1: Will experience maximum hearing potential

NURSING INTERVENTIONS/RATIONALES

Help family investigate audiologists *to locate a specialist in pediatrics*

Discuss types of hearing aids and their proper care *to ensure maximum benefit*

Stress to family importance of storing hearing aid batteries safely and of teaching children (or supervising young children) not to remove the battery *to prevent ingestion or aspiration of batteries*

Help child focus on all sounds in the environment and talk about them *to maximize listening skills*

For older child, discuss methods of camouflaging the aid *to make it less conspicuous*

For child with sensorineural loss, emphasize benefit of early use of cochlear implant

EXPECTED OUTCOMES

Child acquires and uses hearing aid properly

Child does not ingest or aspirate hearing aid battery

Family is aware of benefit of cochlear implant

NURSING DIAGNOSIS ■ **Impaired verbal communication related to inability to hear auditory cues**

PATIENT GOAL 1: Will engage in communication process within limits of impairment

NURSING INTERVENTIONS/RATIONALES

Encourage family to attend the rehabilitation program *to continue learning in the home*

Teach language that serves a useful purpose *for communication*

Encourage use of language and books in the home *to stimulate verbal communication and promote normal development*

Encourage spontaneous language and correct speech *to promote speech development*

EXPECTED OUTCOMES

Family continues communication practices in home environment

Family provides stimulation to child

PATIENT GOAL 2: Will demonstrate ability to lipread

NURSING INTERVENTIONS/RATIONALES

Test child for visual problems *that may interfere with learning to lipread or use sign language*

Teach family and others involved with child (e.g., teacher) behaviors that facilitate lipreading (see Guidelines box on p. 606) *to promote communication process*

EXPECTED OUTCOMES

Child communicates with others in manner taught (specify)

Persons communicating with child use good communication techniques

---

NURSING DIAGNOSIS ■ **Altered growth and development related to impaired communication**

PATIENT GOAL 1: Will achieve optimal independence level for age

NURSING INTERVENTIONS/RATIONALES

Help family apply normal childrearing practices to this child *to promote optimal development*

Emphasize importance of attaining independence in self-care

Provide child with devices that foster independence (e.g., hearing ear dog, special signaling aids for telephone or doorbell)

Discuss with family importance of discipline and limit setting, *because all children have these needs*

EXPECTED OUTCOMES

Child performs activities of daily living appropriate to level of development

Appropriate discipline and limit setting are provided

PATIENT GOAL 2: Will have opportunity to participate in activities for play and socialization

NURSING INTERVENTIONS/RATIONALES

Guide family in selection of toys *to maximize auditory, visual, and tactile senses*

Encourage child to participate in group activities (e.g., Scouting, sports) *to promote socialization*

Help child follow group discussion by pointing out the speaker and arranging the group in a semicircle *to facilitate hearing and/or lipreading*

NURSING CARE PLAN   The Child With Hearing Impairment—*cont'd*

Help child develop friendships among hearing and deaf peers *to promote socialization*

Recommend closed-captioned television *for child's enjoyment*

EXPECTED OUTCOMES

Child engages in activities appropriate to developmental level

Child has peer relationships and experiences

PATIENT GOAL 3: Will be provided educational opportunities within a regular classroom

NURSING INTERVENTIONS/*RATIONALES*

Discuss with teacher and children ways of communicating effectively with child (e.g., through facilitating lipreading) *to facilitate child's education*

Promote socialization with classmates *to encourage enjoyment of education*

EXPECTED OUTCOMES

Child attends school regularly

Child communicates with others in the classroom

NURSING DIAGNOSIS ■ **Altered family processes related to diagnosis of deafness of a child**

PATIENT (FAMILY) GOAL 1: Will adjust to child's hearing loss

NURSING INTERVENTIONS/*RATIONALES*

Anticipate grief reaction as part of adjustment to loss

Provide opportunities for family to express feelings and concerns *to promote adjustment*

Help family deal with feelings regarding previous responses to child when true nature of the problem was unknown *to minimize feelings of guilt*

Help family realize extent of child's disability and its tremendous influence on speech and language development

Discuss advantages and limitations of amplification devices with different types of hearing loss *so that family can make informed decisions*

Encourage formal rehabilitation as soon as possible *to foster normal growth and development of child*

EXPECTED OUTCOMES

Family expresses feelings and concerns regarding child's loss of hearing

Family demonstrates an understanding of the implications of hearing loss

Family becomes involved in appropriate programs

PATIENT (FAMILY) GOAL 2: Will receive emotional support

NURSING INTERVENTIONS/*RATIONALES*

Be available to family *for assistance and support*

Encourage family members to discuss their feelings regarding the disability *to enhance coping*

Stress child's abilities rather than disability *to promote child's optimal development*

Become familiar with techniques used for communication if following the family on a long-term basis

Refer family to appropriate community agencies for medical, psychiatric, educational, vocational, or financial assistance *to ensure that their overall needs are met*

Involve parents in local parent groups for deaf children *for continuing support*

EXPECTED OUTCOMES

Family expresses feelings and concerns about the disability and its ramifications

Family members avail themselves of available resources

PATIENT (FAMILY) GOAL 3: Will demonstrate attachment to child

NURSING INTERVENTIONS/*RATIONALES*

Help family identify clues other than verbal ones that signify infant's communication with them *because communication is an important part of attachment process*

Encourage family to stimulate child with visual and tactile cues *because auditory cues are absent or diminished*

Stress importance of continuing to talk to child even though child may not hear their voices *to promote normalization*

EXPECTED OUTCOME

Parents and child demonstrate a positive relationship

NURSING DIAGNOSIS ■ **Risk for injury related to environmental hazards, infection**

PATIENT (OTHERS) GOAL 1: Will not acquire or have greater hearing loss

NURSING INTERVENTIONS/*RATIONALES*

Infancy

Encourage immunization at appropriate age *to prevent acquired sensorineural hearing loss from childhood diseases*

Minimize noise levels in intensive care unit *because this is associated with hearing loss*

Prevent ear infection; detect early *because this is the most common cause of impaired hearing*

Ensure newborn hearing screen completed and referral made as needed to prevent speech/communication deficits

Childhood

Assess hearing ability of infants and children receiving ototoxic antibiotics *for early detection*

Promote compliance with treatment regimens for otitis media *because this is a common cause of impaired hearing*

Discuss with parents measures to prevent otitis media (see Chapter 23)

Evaluate auditory ability of children prone to chronic ear or respiratory problems *for early detection of impaired hearing*

Assess sources of excessive noise in child's environment; institute appropriate measures to decrease sound levels (e.g., turn music lower, use ear protection) *because exposure to excessive noise is a cause of sensorineural hearing loss*

Participate in immunization programs for children *to prevent childhood diseases that may result in hearing loss*

EXPECTED OUTCOMES

Infant or child does not develop hearing loss

Child is not exposed to excessive noise levels

Child is properly immunized

BOX 19-6 ■ Types of Visual Impairment

REFRACTIVE ERRORS

Myopia

Nearsightedness—Ability to see objects clearly at close range but not at a distance

Pathophysiology

Results from eyeball that is too long, causing image to fall in front of retina

Clinical Manifestations

Rubs eyes excessively

Tilts head or thrusts head forward

Has difficulty in reading or doing other close work

Holds books close to eyes

Writes or colors with head close to table

Clumsy; walks into objects

Blinks more than usual or is irritable when doing close work

Is unable to see objects clearly

Does poorly in school, especially in subjects that require demonstration, such as arithmetic

Dizziness

Headache

Nausea after close work

Treatment

Corrected with biconcave lenses that focus rays on retina

May be corrected with laser surgery

Hyperopia

Farsightedness—Ability to see objects at a distance

Pathophysiology

Results from eyeball that is too short, causing image to focus beyond retina

Clinical Manifestations

Because of accommodative ability, child can usually see objects at all ranges

Most children normally hyperopic until about 7 years of age

Treatment

If correction is required, use convex lenses to focus rays on retina

May be corrected with laser surgery

Astigmatism

Unequal curvatures in refractive apparatus

Pathophysiology

Results from unequal curvatures in cornea or lens that cause light rays to bend in different directions

Clinical Manifestations

Depends on severity of refractive error in each eye

May have clinical manifestations of myopia

Treatment

Corrected with special lenses that compensate for refractive errors

May be corrected with laser surgery

Anisometropia

Different refractive strength in each eye

Pathophysiology

May develop amblyopia as weaker eye is used less

Clinical Manifestations

Depends on severity of refractive error in each eye

May have clinical manifestations of myopia

Treatment

Treated with corrective lenses, preferably contact lenses, to improve vision in each eye so they work as a unit

May be corrected with laser surgery

AMBLYOPIA

Lazy eye—Reduced visual acuity in one eye

Pathophysiology

Results when one eye does not receive sufficient stimulation

Each retina receives different images, resulting in diplopia (double vision)

Brain accommodates by suppressing less intense image

Visual cortex eventually does not respond to visual stimulation, with resultant loss of vision in that eye

Clinical Manifestations

Poor vision in affected eye

Legal blindness, visual acuity of 20/200 or less and/or a visual field of 20 degrees or less in the better eye, is useful only as a legal definition, not as a medical diagnosis. It allows special considerations with regard to taxes, entrance into special schools, eligibility for aid, and other benefits.

Etiology

Visual impairment can be caused by a number of genetic and prenatal or postnatal conditions. These include perinatal infections (herpes, chlamydia, gonococci, rubella, syphilis, toxoplasmosis), retinopathy of prematurity, trauma, postnatal infections (meningitis), and disorders such as sickle cell disease, juvenile rheumatoid arthritis, Tay-Sachs disease, albinism, and retinoblastoma. In many instances, such as with refractive errors, the cause of the defect is unknown.

Refractive errors are the most common types of visual disorders in children. The term *refraction* means bending and refers to the bending of light rays as they pass through the lens of the eye. Normally, light rays enter the lens and fall directly on the retina. However, in refractive disorders the light rays either fall in front of the retina *(myopia)* or

beyond it *(hyperopia).* Other eye problems, such as strabismus, may or may not include refractive errors, but they are very important because, if untreated, they result in blindness from amblyopia. These, along with other less frequent visual disorders, are summarized in Box 19-6. In addition to these disorders, other visual problems can be a result of infection or trauma.

Trauma. Trauma is a common cause of blindness in children. Injuries to the eyeball and adnexa (supporting or accessory structures, such as eyelids, conjunctiva, or lacrimal glands) can be classified as penetrating or nonpenetrating. *Penetrating wounds* are most often a result of sharp instruments, such as sticks, knives, or scissors; propulsive objects, such as firecrackers, guns, bows and arrows, or slingshots; or a powerful contusion by a blunt object, which may occur during a fight or from a serious car accident. *Nonpenetrating injuries* may be a result of foreign objects in the eyes, lacerations, a blow from a blunt object such as a ball (baseball, softball, basketball, racquet sports) or fist, or thermal or chemical burns.

BOX 19-6 ■ Types of visual impairment—*cont'd*

Treatment
Preventable if treatment of primary visual defect, such as anisometropia or strabismus, begins before 6 years of age

STRABISMUS
"Squint" or cross-eye—Malalignment of eyes
Estropia—Inward deviation of eye
Exotropia—Outward deviation of eye
Pathophysiology
May result from muscle imbalance or paralysis, poor vision, or congenital defect
Because visual axes are not parallel, brain receives two images, and amblyopia can result
Clinical Manifestations
Squints eyelids together or frowns
Has difficulty in focusing from one distance to another
Inaccurate judgment in picking up objects
Unable to see print or moving objects clearly
Closes one eye to see
Tilts head to one side
If combined with refractive errors, may see any of the manifestations listed for refractive errors
Diplopia
Photophobia
Dizziness
Headache
Cross-eye
Treatment
Treatment depends on cause of strabismus
May involve occlusion therapy (patching stronger eye) or surgery to increase visual stimulation to weaker eye
Early diagnosis is essential to prevent vision loss

CATARACTS
Opacity of crystalline lens
Pathophysiology
Prevents light rays from entering eye and refracting on retina

Clinical Manifestations
Gradually less able to see objects clearly
May lose peripheral vision
Nystagmus (with complete blindness)
Gray opacities of lens
Strabismus
Absence of red reflex
Treatment
Requires surgery to remove cloudy lens and replace lens (intraocular lens implant, removable contact lens, prescription glasses)
Must be treated early to prevent blindness from amblyopia

GLAUCOMA
Increased intraocular pressure
Pathophysiology
Congenital type results from defective development of some component related to flow of aqueous humor
Increased pressure on optic nerve causes eventual atrophy and blindness
Clinical Manifestations
Mostly seen in acquired types—loses peripheral vision
May bump into objects not directly in front
Sees halos around objects
May complain of mild pain or discomfort (severe pain, nausea, or vomiting if sudden rise in pressure)
Redness
Excessive tearing (epiphora)
Photophobia
Spasmodic winking (blepharospasm)
Corneal haziness
Enlargement of eyeball (buphthalmos)
Treatment
Requires surgical treatment (goniotomy) to open outflow tracts
May require more than one procedure

Treatment is aimed at preventing further ocular damage and is primarily the responsibility of the ophthalmologist. It involves adequate examination of the injured eye (with the child sedated or anesthetized in severe injuries); appropriate immediate intervention, such as removal of the foreign body or suturing of the laceration; and prevention of complications, such as administration of antibiotics or steroids and complete bed rest to allow the eye to heal and blood to reabsorb (see Emergency Treatment box). The prognosis varies according to the type of injury. It is usually guarded in all cases of penetrating wounds because of the high risk of serious complications.

Infections.   Infections of the adnexa and structures of the eyeball or globe may occur in children. The most common eye infection is *conjunctivitis* (see Chapter 14). Treatment is usually with ophthalmic antibiotics. Severe infections may require systemic antibiotic therapy. Steroids are used cautiously because they exacerbate viral infections such as herpes simplex, increasing the risk of damage to the involved structures.

Nursing Considerations

● *Assessment*

Assessment of children for visual impairment is a critical nursing responsibility. Discovery of a visual impairment as early as possible is essential to prevent social, physical, and psychologic damage to the child. Assessment involves (1) identifying those children who by virtue of their history are at risk, (2) observing for behaviors that indicate a vision loss, and (3) screening all children for visual acuity and signs of other ocular disorders such as strabismus. This discussion focuses on clinical manifestations of various types of visual problems (see Box 19-6). Vision testing is discussed in Chapter 7.

Infancy.   At birth the nurse should observe the neonate's response to visual stimuli, such as following a light or object and cessation of body movement. The infant may vary in the intensity of the response, depending on the state of alertness.

Of special importance in detecting visual impairment during infancy are the parents' concerns regarding visual responsiveness in their child. Their concerns, such as lack of

EMERGENCY TREATMENT

Eye Injuries

FOREIGN OBJECT

Examine eye for presence of a foreign body (evert upper lid to examine upper eye).

Remove a freely movable object with pointed corner of gauze pad lightly moistened with water.

Do not irrigate eye or attempt to remove a penetrating object (see following section).

Caution child against rubbing eye.

CHEMICAL BURNS

Irrigate eye copiously with tap water for 20 minutes.

Evert upper lid to flush thoroughly.

Hold child's head with eye under tap of running lukewarm water.

Take to emergency department.

Have child rest with eyes closed.

Keep room darkened.

ULTRAVIOLET BURNS

If skin is burned, patch both eyes (make sure lids are completely closed); secure dressing with Kling bandages wrapped around head rather than tape.

Have child rest with eyes closed.

Refer to an ophthalmologist.

HEMATOMA ("BLACK EYE")

Use a flashlight to check for gross *hyphema* (hemorrhage into anterior chamber; visible fluid meniscus across iris; more easily seen in light-colored than in brown eyes).

Apply ice for first 24 hours to reduce swelling if no hyphema is present.

Refer to an ophthalmologist immediately if hyphema is present.

Have child rest with eyes closed.

PENETRATING INJURIES

Take child to emergency department.

Never remove an object that has penetrated eye.

Follow strict aseptic technique in examining eye.

Observe for:

Aqueous or vitreous leaks (fluid leaking from point of penetration)

Hyphema

Shape and equality of pupils, reaction to light

Prolapsed iris (not perfectly circular)

Apply a Fox shield if available (not a regular eye patch) and apply patch over unaffected eye to prevent bilateral movement.

Maintain bed rest with child in 30-degree Fowler position.

Caution child against rubbing eye.

---

eye contact from the infant, must be taken seriously. During infancy the child should be tested for strabismus. Lack of binocularity after 4 months of age is considered abnormal and must be treated to prevent amblyopia.

!NURSING ALERT

Suspect blindness if the infant does not react to light and in any-age child if parents express concern.

Childhood. Because the most common visual impairment during childhood is refractive errors, testing for visual acuity is essential. The school nurse usually assumes major responsi-

BOX 19-7 ■ Nursing Diagnoses: The Child With Vision Impairment

Altered family processes related to diagnosis of vision impairment in child

Altered growth and development related to sensory/perceptual alterations (visual)

Risk for injury related to environmental hazards, noncompliance with therapeutic plan

---

bility for vision testing in schoolchildren. Besides refractive errors, the nurse should be aware of signs and symptoms that indicate other ocular problems. If a referral is made to the family requesting further eye testing, the nurse is responsible for follow-up concerning the recommendation.

● *Nursing Diagnoses*

A number of nursing diagnoses are prominent in the nursing care of the child with visual impairment and the child's family (Box 19-7); other diagnoses specific to individual cases become evident.

● *Planning*

The goals of care for the child with visual impairment and family are as follows:

1 Child and family will receive support and education.
2 Parent-child attachment will develop.
3 Child will achieve optimal development.
4 Child will receive appropriate care during hospitalization.

● *Implementation*

Support child and family. The shock of learning that their child is blind or partially sighted is an immense crisis for families. Of all types of disabilities, many people fear loss of sight the most. Vision is involved in almost every activity of daily living. Parents need support during the initial phase of learning about the diagnosis and help to gain a realistic understanding of their child's abilities. The family is encouraged to investigate appropriate stimulation and educational programs for their child as soon as possible. Sources of information include state **Commissions for the Blind,** local schools for the blind, the **American Foundation for the Blind,*** National Federation of the Blind,† National Association for Parents of the Visually Impaired, Inc.,‡ National Association for Visually Handicapped,§ and American Council of the Blind.||

---

*11 Pennsylvania Plaza, Suite 300, New York, NY 10001; (800) 232-5463 or (212) 502-7600; TTY: (212) 502-7662; fax: (212) 502-7777; website: www.afb.org.

†1800 Johnson Street, Baltimore, MD 21230; (410) 659-9314; fax: (410) 685-5653; website: www.nfb.org.

‡PO Box 317, Watertown, MA 02472-0317; (800) 562-6265; fax: (617) 972-74444; website: www.napvi.org.

§22 West 21st Street, 6th Floor, New York, NY 10010; (212) 889-3141; fax: (212) 727-2931; website: www.NAVH.org.

||1155 15th Street NW, Suite 1004, Washington, DC 20005; (800) 424-8666; fax: (202) 467-5085; website: www.acb.org.

¶A source of information in Canada is the **Canadian National Institute for the Blind,** 1929 Bayview Avenue; Toronto, Ontario M4G 3E8, (416) 480-7580; fax: (416) 480-7677; website: www.cnib.ca.

When blindness is not congenital but acquired, newly blind children need much support to help them adjust to the disability. They are usually frightened and confused by the sudden or progressive loss of sight and benefit from an environment that provides security and familiarity.

Promote Parent-Child Attachment.

A crucial time in the life of blind infants is when they and their parents are getting acquainted with each other. Pleasurable patterns of interaction between the infant and parents may be lacking if there is not enough reciprocity. For example, if the parent gazes fondly at the infant's face and seeks eye contact but the infant fails to respond because he or she cannot see the parent, a troubled cycle of responses may occur. The nurse can help parents learn to look for other cues that indicate the infant is responding to them, such as whether the eyelids blink; whether the activity level accelerates or slows; whether respiratory patterns change, such as faster or slower breathing, when the parents come near; and whether the infant makes throaty sounds when they speak to the infant. In time parents learn that the infant has unique ways of relating to them. They are encouraged to show affection using nonvisual methods, such as talking or reading, cuddling, and walking the child.

Promote Child's Optimal Development.

Promoting the child's optimum development requires rehabilitation in a number of important areas. These include learning self-help skills and appropriate communication techniques to become independent. Although nurses may not be directly involved in such programs, they can provide direction and guidance to families regarding the availability of programs and the need to promote these activities in their child.

Development and Independence.

Motor development depends on sight almost as much as verbal communication depends on hearing. From earliest infancy, parents are encouraged to expose the infant to as many visual-motor experiences as possible, such as sitting supported in an infant seat or swing and being given opportunities for holding up the head, sitting unsupported, reaching for objects, and crawling.

Despite visual impairment, the child can become independent in all aspects of self-care. The same principles used for promoting independence in sighted children apply, with additional emphasis on nonvisual cues. For example, the child may need help in dressing, such as special arrangement of clothing for style coordination and braille tags to distinguish colors and prints.

The blind child also must learn to become independent in navigational skills. The two main techniques are the *tapping method* (use of a cane to survey the environment for direction and to avoid obstacles) and *guides,* such as a sighted human guide or a dog guide, such as a Seeing Eye dog. Children who are partially sighted may benefit from ocular aids, such as a monocular telescope.

Play and Socialization.

Blind children do not learn to play automatically. Because they cannot imitate others or actively explore the environment as sighted children do, they depend much more on others to stimulate and teach them how to play. Parents need help in selecting appropriate play material, especially those that encourage fine and gross motor development and stimulate the senses of hearing, touch, and smell. Toys with educational value are especially useful, such as dolls with various clothing closures.

Blind children have the same needs for socialization as sighted children. Because they have little difficulty in learning verbal skills, they are able to communicate with age-mates and participate in suitable activities. The nurse discusses with parents opportunities for socialization outside the home, especially regular preschools. The trend is to include these children with sighted children to help them adjust to the outside world for eventual independence.

To compensate for inadequate stimulation, these children may develop *blindisms* (self-stimulatory activities, such as body rocking, finger flicking, or arm twirling). Such habits restrict the child's social acceptance and are discouraged. Behavior modification is often successful in reducing or eliminating blindisms.

Education.

The main obstacle to learning is the child's total dependence on nonvisual cues. Although the child can learn via verbal lecturing, he or she is unable to read the written word or to write without special education. Therefore the child must rely on *braille,* a system that uses raised dots to represent letters and numbers. The child can then read the braille with the fingers and can write a message using a braille writer. However, unless others read braille, this type of communication is not useful for communicating with others. A more portable system for written communication is the use of a braille slate and stylus or a microcassette tape recorder. A recorder is especially helpful for leaving messages for others and for note taking during classroom lecturing. For mathematic calculations, portable calculators with voice synthesizers are available.*

Records and tapes are significant sources of reading material other than braille books, which are large and cumbersome. The **Library of Congress†** has talking books, braille books, and a special records program, which are available at many local and state libraries and directly from the Library of Congress. The talking book machine and tape player are provided at no cost to families, and there is no postage fee for returning the materials. **Recording for the Blind and Dyslexic‡** also provides texts and tapes of books, which are very helpful for secondary and college students who are blind.

Learning to use a regular typewriter is another form of writing but has the disadvantage of the blind person's being

---

*A catalog of numerous products for people with vision problems is available from the **American Foundation for the Blind** (see previous footnote) and from **Lighthouse International,** 111 East 59th Street, New York, NY 10022-1202; (212) 821-9200; (800) 829-0500; website: www.lighthouse.org.

†**The National Library Service for the Blind and Visually Handicapped,** 1291 Taylor Street NW, Washington, DC 20542; (800) 424-8567; TTD: (202) 707-0744; fax: (202) 707-0712; website: www.loc.gov/nls. (A state-by-state listing of libraries for blind and physically handicapped readers, as well as other reference circulars, is available from this office.)

‡20 Roszel Road, Princeton, NJ 08540; (800) 221-4792; (866) RFBD-585; fax: (609) 987-8116; website: www.rfbd.org.

unable to check the accuracy of the typing. Computers eliminate this drawback; a home computer with a voice synthesizer can be adapted to speak each letter or word that has been typed.

The child with partial sight benefits from specialized visual aids, which produce a magnified retinal image. The basic devices are accommodation (e.g., bringing the object closer), special plus lenses, handheld and stand magnifiers, telescopes, video projection systems, and large print. Special equipment is available to enlarge print. Information about services for the partially sighted is available from the **National Association for Visually Handicapped** and **American Foundation for the Blind.** Children with diminished vision often prefer to do close work without their glasses and compensate by bringing the object very near to their eyes. This should be allowed. The exception is the child with vision in only one eye, who should always wear glasses for protection.

Care for the Child During Hospitalization.

Because nurses are more likely to care for children who are hospitalized for procedures that involve temporary loss of vision than for children who are blind, the following discussion concentrates primarily on the needs of such children. The nursing care objectives in either situation are to (1) reassure the child and family throughout every phase of treatment, (2) orient the child to the surroundings, (3) provide a safe environment, and (4) encourage independence. Whenever possible, the same nurse should care for the child to ensure consistency in the approach. These same principles also apply to a blind child who requires hospitalization.

When sighted children temporarily lose their vision, almost every aspect of the environment becomes bewildering and frightening. They are forced to rely on nonvisual senses for help in adjusting to the blindness without the benefit of any special training. Nurses have a major role in minimizing the effects of temporary loss of vision. They need to talk to the child about everything that is occurring, emphasizing aspects of procedures that are felt or heard. They should approach the child by always identifying themselves as soon as they enter the room. Because unfamiliar sounds are especially frightening, these are explained. Parents are encouraged to room with their child and participate in the care. Familiar objects, such as a teddy bear or doll, should be brought from home to help lessen the strangeness of the hospital. As soon as the child is able to be out of bed, he or she is oriented to the immediate surroundings. If the child is able to see on admission, this opportunity is taken to point out significant aspects of the room. The child is encouraged to practice ambulating with the eyes closed to become accustomed to this experience.

The room is arranged with safety in mind. For example, a stool or chair is placed next to the bed to help the child climb in and out of bed. The furniture is always placed in the same position to prevent collisions. Cleaning personnel are reminded of the need to keep the room in order. If the child has difficulty navigating by feeling the walls, a rope can be attached from the bed to the point of destination, such as the bathroom. Attention to details such as well-fitting slippers or robes that do not drag on the floor is important in preventing tripping. Unlike the child who is blind, these children are not familiar with navigating with a cane.

The child is encouraged to be independent in self-care activities, especially if the visual loss may be prolonged or potentially permanent. For example, during bathing the nurse sets up all the equipment and encourages the child to participate. At mealtime the nurse explains where each food item is on the tray, opens any special containers, prepares cereal or toast, and encourages the child in self-feeding. Favorite finger foods, such as sandwiches, hamburgers, hot dogs, or pizza, may be good selections. The child is praised for efforts at being cooperative and independent. Any improvements made in self-care, no matter how small, are stressed.

Appropriate recreational activities are provided, and if a child-life specialist is available, such planning is done jointly. Because children with temporary blindness have a wide variety of play experiences to draw on, they are encouraged to select activities. For example, if they like to read, they may enjoy being read to. If they prefer manual activity, they may appreciate playing with clay or building blocks or feeling different textures and naming them. If they need an outlet for aggression, activities such as pounding or banging on a drum can be helpful. Simple board and card games can be played with a "seeing partner" or if the opponent helps with the game. They should have familiar toys from home to play with, because familiar items are more easily manipulated than new ones. If parents want to bring presents, they should be objects that stimulate hearing and touch, such as a radio, music box, or stuffed animal.

Occasionally, children who are blind come to the hospital for procedures to restore their vision. Although this is an extremely happy time, it also requires intervention to help them adjust to sight. They need an opportunity to take in all that they see. They should not be bombarded with visual stimuli. They may need to concentrate on people's faces or their own to become accustomed to this experience. They often need to talk about what they see and to compare the visual images with their mental ones. The child may also go through a period of depression, which must be respected and supported. The nurse or parents should refrain from statements such as "How can you be so sad when you can see again?" Instead the child should be encouraged to discuss how it feels to see, especially in terms of seeing himself or herself.

Newly sighted children also need time to adjust to the ability to engage in activities that were impossible before. For example, they may prefer to use braille to read, rather than learning a new "visual approach," because of familiarity with the touch system. Eventually, as they learn to recognize letters and numbers, they will integrate these new skills into reading and writing. However, parents and teachers must be careful not to push them before they are ready. This applies to social relationships and physical activities as well as learning situations.

Assist in Measures to Prevent Visual Impairment.

An essential nursing goal is to prevent visual impairment. This involves many of the same interventions discussed under hearing impairments: (1) prenatal screening for pregnant women at risk, such as those with rubella or syphilis infection and family histories of genetic disorders associated with visual loss; (2) adequate prenatal and perinatal care to prevent prematurity; (3) periodic screening of all children, especially newborns through preschoolers, for congenital blindness and visual impairments caused by refractive errors, strabismus, and other disorders; (4) rubella immunization of all children; and (5) safety counseling regarding the common causes of ocular trauma.

Safety counseling should include safe practices when working with, playing with, or carrying objects such as scissors, knives, and balls.

> ⚠️ **NURSING ALERT**
>
> A helmet with a face mask should be required for children playing football, hockey, or baseball.

After detection of eye problems, the nurse has a responsibility to prevent further ocular damage by ensuring that corrective treatment is used. For the child with strabismus, this often necessitates occlusion patching of the stronger eye. Compliance with the procedure is greatest during the early preschool years. It is more difficult to encourage school-age children to wear the occlusive patch because the poor visual acuity of the uncovered weaker eye interferes with school work and the patch sets them apart from their peers. In school they benefit from being positioned favorably (closer to the chalkboard or other visual media) and allowed extra time to read or complete an assignment. If treatment of the eye disorder requires instillation of ophthalmic medication, the family is taught the correct procedure (see Chapter 22).

For the child with refractive errors, the nurse helps the child adjust to wearing *glasses.* Young children who often pull glasses off benefit from temporal pieces that wrap around the ears or an elastic strap attached to the frames and around the back of the head to hold the glasses on securely. After children appreciate the value of clear vision, they are more likely to wear the corrective lenses.

Glasses should not interfere with any activity. Special protective guards are available during contact sports to prevent accidental injury, and all corrective lenses should be made from safety glass, which is shatterproof. Often, corrective lenses improve visual acuity so dramatically that children are able to compete more effectively in sports. This in itself is a tremendous inducement to continue wearing glasses.

Contact lenses are a popular alternative, especially for adolescents. Several types are available, such as hard lenses, including gas-permeable ones, and soft lenses, which may be designed for daily or extended wear. Contact lenses offer several advantages over glasses, such as greater visual acuity, total corrected field of vision, convenience (especially with the extended-wear type), and optimal cosmetic benefit. Unfortunately, they are usually more expensive and require much more care than glasses, including considerable practice to learn techniques for insertion and removal. If they are prescribed, the nurse can be very helpful in teaching parents or older children how to care for the lenses.

Because trauma is the leading cause of blindness, the nurse has the major responsibility of preventing further eye injury until the specific treatment is instituted. The major principles to follow when caring for an eye injury are outlined in the Emergency Treatment box on p. 612. Because patients with a serious eye injury fear blindness, the nurse should stay with the child and family to provide support and reassurance.

● Evaluation

The effectiveness of nursing interventions is determined by continual reassessment and evaluation of care based on the following observational guidelines and expected outcomes:

1 Interview family regarding their adjustment to the sensory impairment; observe family members' relationship with child; interview child regarding feelings about the sensory impairment and its effect on activities of daily living (especially important if a visual loss).
2 Have parents identify those cues that indicate infant is responding to them; observe nonvisual behaviors of parents as they respond to infant.
3 Observe techniques child uses to read and navigate; inquire if child is enrolled in a visual training program; inquire about socialization opportunities for child (i.e., who are child's friends, what are child's extracurricular activities).
4 Observe preparation of the room and self-care activities that provide for safety and independence during hospitalization.

Expected outcomes

1 Parents express their feelings and concerns regarding loss of sight and demonstrate an understanding of child's disability and its implications.
2 Parents demonstrate attachment behaviors.
3 Infant or child engages in appropriate activities for level of development (specify); child demonstrates an attitude of security in the environment.
4 Child and family receive safe and supportive care during hospitalization.

DEAF-BLIND CHILDREN

The most traumatic sensory impairment is loss of sight and hearing. Obviously, auditory and visual disabilities have profound effects on the child's development. They interfere with the normal sequence of physical, intellectual, and psychosocial growth. Although such children often achieve the usual motor milestones, their rate of development is slower. These children learn communication only with specialized training. *Finger spelling* is one desirable method often taught to these children. Some deaf-blind children, especially those with residual hearing or sight, can learn to speak. Whenever possible, speech is encouraged, because it allows communication with other individuals.

The future prospects for deaf-blind children are, at best, unpredictable. Congenital blindness and/or deafness may be accompanied by other physical or neurologic problems, which further lessen the child's learning potential. The most favorable prognosis is for children who have acquired deafness and blindness and have few, if any, associated disabilities. Their learning capacity is greatly potentiated by their developmental progress before the sensory impairments. Although total independence, including gainful vocational training, is the goal, some deaf-blind children are unable to develop to this level. They may require lifelong parental or residential care. The nurse working with such families helps them deal with future goals for the child, including possible alternatives to home care during the parents' advancing years.

RETINOBLASTOMA

Retinoblastoma, which arises from the retina, is the most common congenital malignant intraocular tumor of childhood. Approximately 11 cases per million occur annually, primarily in children younger than 5 years of age. Retinoblastoma is caused by a mutation in a gene and may occur sporadically or be inherited (Hurwitz and others, 2002). Retinoblastoma develops when the mutated gene is unable to produce the natural signals to stop the growth of retinal cells. Of all cases, the majority are nonhereditary and unilateral, with the remainder divided between hereditary and unilateral, and hereditary and bilateral. Hereditary retinoblastomas are transmitted as an autosomal dominant trait with a 90% penetrance (Hurwitz and others 2002; Lanzkowsky, 2000).

Diagnostic Evaluation

Retinoblastoma has few grossly obvious signs (Box 19-8). Typically it is the parent who first observes a whitish "glow" in the pupil, known as the *cat's eye reflex* (white reflex) or leukokoria. Leukokoria represents visualization of the tumor as the light momentarily falls on the mass (Fig. 19-8).

The first step in diagnosis is carefully listening to and recognizing the significance of reports from family members regarding suspected abnormalities within the eye. Eye abnormalities, including cat's eye reflex, strabismus, decreased vision, and persistent painful erythematous eyes, are referred to an ophthalmologist. Definitive diagnosis is usually based on ophthalmoscopic examination under general anesthesia. Imaging studies, including ultrasonography and computed tomography of the orbit, are done to determine the extent of the disease.

Therapeutic Management

The aim of therapy is to preserve useful vision and eradicate the tumor. Treatment of retinoblastoma depends chiefly on the stage of the tumor at the time of diagnosis. *Reese-Ellsworth (RE) classification* is the commonly used standard for intraocular disease (Box 19-9). Other staging systems such as Grabrowski and Abramson and American Joint Committee on Cancer Systems classify both intraocular and extraocular disease but are not universally used (Hurwitz and others, 2002; Schouten-van Meeteren, 2002).

Recently there has been a shift away from the use of external beam radiation (whole-eye irradiation that damages the cell's DNA) in the treatment of RE groups I, II, and III retinoblastoma toward the use of focal intraocular therapy with or without chemotherapy (De Potter, 2002; Schouten-van Meeteren, 2002). Some of the common focal therapies are (1) plaque brachytherapy (surgical radioactive implant on the sclera until maximum dose has been delivered to the tumor), (2) laser photocoagulation (laser beam to coagulate blood supply to the tumor), (3) cryotherapy (freezing the tumor by destroying the microcirculation to the tumor through microcrystal formation, and (4) thermotherapy (uses microwaves or infrared radiation to deliver heat to the tumor).

Chemotherapy is being used in the early RE groups in an attempt to reduce tumor size to facilitate focal intraocular treatment (chemoreduction). Chemotherapy has been used for several years to prevent metastatic disease in the RE groups IV and V and relapsed patients (chemoprevention or chemoprophylaxis). Chemoreduction and chemoprevention include two to six courses of vincristine, etoposide, and carboplatin with or without cyclophosphamide. Retinoblastoma is chemosensitive but not yet a chemocurable disease (Schouten–van Meeteren, 2002). Chemoreduction and chemoprevention minimize the use of external beam radiation treatment and therefore reduce the risk of radiation-induced malignancies and facial disfigurement.

BOX 19-8 ■ Clinical Manifestations of Retinoblastoma

Cat's eye reflex (most common sign)
Strabismus (second most common sign)
Red, painful eye, often with glaucoma
Blindness (late sign)

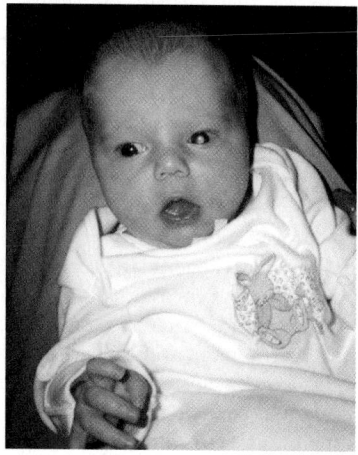

FIG. 19-8 ■ Cat's eye reflex. Whitish appearance of lens is produced as light falls on tumor mass in left eye.

BOX 19-9 ■ Staging of Retinoblastoma

Group I: Very favorable
  Solitary tumor, less than 4 disc diameters (DD), at or behind the equator
  Multiple tumors, none greater than 4 DD, all at or behind the equator
Group II: Favorable
  Solitary tumors, 4 to 10 DD, at or behind the equator
  Multiple tumors, 4 to 10 DD, behind the equator
Group III: Doubtful
  Any lesion anterior to the equator
  Solitary tumors larger than 10 DD, behind the equator
Group IV: Unfavorable
  Multiple tumors, some larger than 10 DD
  Any lesion extending anteriorly to the ora serrata
Group V: Very unfavorable
  Massive tumors involving more than half the retina
  Vitreous seeding

With advanced tumor growth into the optic nerve, choroid, orbit, and anterior chamber or no hope for useful vision, *enucleation* (removal) of the affected eye is the treatment of choice. After enucleation, the orbital implant is placed to provide a more natural cosmetic appearance, minimizes sinking of the prosthesis, and enables motility of the prosthesis.

With bilateral disease, every attempt is made to preserve useful vision in both eyes. Chemotherapy, external beam, radiotherapy, and other treatments (i.e., cryotherapy, laser, plaque brachytherapy, thermotherapy) to both eyes may prevent the need for enucleation.

Trilateral retinoblastoma is a rare, usually fatal syndrome present in 1% to 8% of patients with bilateral retinoblastoma. Trilateral retinoblastoma comprises bilateral retinoblastoma with the involvement of pineal gland tumor or other midline structure (Hurwitz and others, 2002). Trilateral retinoblastoma is treated aggressively with chemotherapy, radiation therapy, adjuvant treatments, and gamma knife therapy with little success. However, a longer survival has been correlated with early tumor diagnosis in the asymptomatic patient and the use of initial chemoreduction at diagnosis (Hurwitz and others, 2002).

Prognosis.   The overall prognosis for retinoblastoma is very favorable, with a survival rate of nearly 90% for both unilateral and bilateral tumors. Retinoblastoma is one of the tumors that may spontaneously regress.

Of major concern in long-term survivors is the development of decreased visual acuity, facial disfiguration, and secondary tumors—especially osteogenic sarcoma, other sarcomas, and melanoma. Children with bilateral disease (hereditary form) are more likely to develop secondary cancers than are children with unilateral disease. It is thought that these individuals are predisposed to developing cancer and that radiation increases their risk.

Chemoprevention and high-dose chemotherapy with autologous stem cell rescue appears to be beneficial for patients with metastatic retinoblastoma (De Potter, 2002). Research studies focused on the use of monoclonal antibodies and gene therapy are being investigated to eradicate metastatic retinoblastoma.

Nursing Considerations

One of the most important nursing goals is to have a high index of suspicion for this rare malignancy. If parents report noticing a strange light in the eye or expression, these concerns must be taken seriously. Families with a history of retinoblastoma require follow-up, and the nurse can be instrumental in reminding parents of appointments.

Because the tumor is usually diagnosed in infants or very young children, most of the preparation for diagnostic tests and treatment involves parents. After indirect ophthalmoscopy, the child may not see very clearly, or the eyes may be sensitive to light because of pupillary dilation. Parents are made aware of these normal reactions before the procedure. Screening tests, such as bone surveys and bone marrow aspiration, are rarely performed unless metastatic disease is suspected.

After the disease is staged, the practitioner confers with the parents regarding treatment. Based on the extent of the disease and the goal of eradicating the tumor and preserving useful vision, an individualized treatment plan is formulated and explained to the parents.

The treatment plan may include focal intraocular therapy with or without chemotherapy, external beam radiation, and, if necessary, enucleation. Enucleation is the treatment of choice if there is extensive disease threatening metastasis or no chance for useful vision. The enucleation procedure and the positive benefits of a prosthesis are explained to the parents. Showing them pictures of another child with an artificial eye may be very helpful in their adjusting to the thought of disfigurement (Fig. 19-9).

After surgery the parents are prepared for the child's facial appearance. An eye patch is in place, and the child's face may be edematous or ecchymotic. Parents often fear seeing the surgical site because they imagine a cavity in the skull. A surgically implanted sphere maintains the shape of the eyeball, and the implant is covered with conjunctiva. When the lids are open, the exposed area resembles the mucosal lining of the mouth. After the child is fitted for a prosthesis, usually within 3 weeks, the facial appearance returns to normal. Initial instructions for care of the prosthesis are given by the ocularist, who fits and manufactures the device.

Care of the socket is minimal and easily accomplished. The wound itself is clean and has little or no drainage. If an antibiotic ointment is prescribed, it is applied in a thin line on the surface of the tissues of the socket. To cleanse the site, an irrigating solution may be ordered and is instilled daily or more frequently, *before* application of the antibiotic ointment. The dressing consists of an eye pad taped over the surgical site and is changed daily. After the socket has healed completely, a dressing is no longer necessary, although it is a preventive measure against infection.

Support Family.   Families with a history of the disorder may feel great guilt for transmitting the defect to their offspring. In families with no history of retinoblastoma, the discovery of the diagnosis is a shock, frequently complicated by guilt and anger for not having found it sooner. The nurse, along with the team—including a pediatric oncologic medical provider, ophthalmologist, radiologist, child psychologist, social workers, genetic counselor, and child-life specialist—

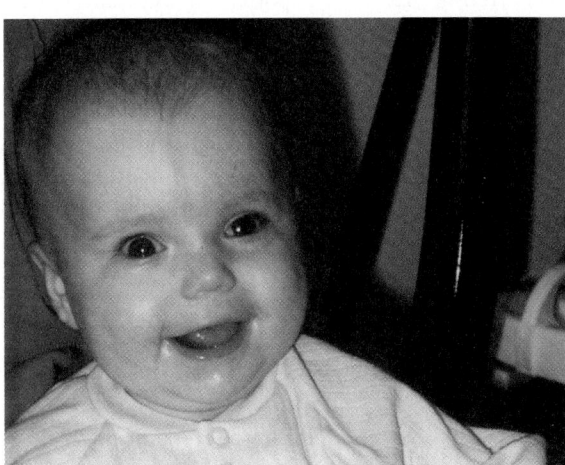

FIG. 19-9 ■ Infant with left prosthetic eye.

support the families dealing with emotional reactions, adjustment, and treatment modalities (see Chapter 18).

See also Nursing Care Plan: The Child With Cancer, Chapter 26.

AUTISM

Autism is a complex developmental disorder of brain function accompanied by a broad range and severity of intellectual and behavioral deficits. It is manifested during early childhood primarily from 24 to 48 months of age. It occurs in 1 in 500 children, is about four times more common in males than in females (although females are more severely affected), and is not related to socioeconomic level, race, or parenting style.

Etiology

The etiology of autism is unknown. However, considerable evidence supports multiple biologic causes. Individuals with autism may have abnormal electroencephalograms, epileptic seizures, delayed development of hand dominance, persistence of primitive reflexes, metabolic abnormalities (elevated blood serotonin), and cerebellar vermal hypoplasia (part of the brain involved in regulating motion and some aspects of memory). Brain overgrowth presenting as a sudden increase in head size between 1-2 months and 6-14 months of age has been observed in children with autism (Courchesne, Carper and Akshoomoff, 2003; Lainhart, 2003).

There is also strong evidence for a genetic basis that in twins is consistent with an autosomal-recessive pattern of inheritance. Twin studies demonstrate a very high concordance (96%) for monozygotic (identical) twins and a 24% concordance for dizygotic (nonidentical) twins. In addition, between 5% and 16% of males with autism are positive for the fragile X chromosome.

There is a 10% to 20% risk of recurrence of autism in families with one affected child (Filipeck and others, 2000). Although several genes have been suggested as possible causative factors in autism, no specific gene for the disorder has been identified (Shao and others, 2003; Tager-Flusberg and Joseph, 2003).

Contrary to previous reports, autism does not appear to be caused by the measles-mumps-rubella (MMR) vaccine (DeStefano and others, 2004; Dales, Hammer, and Smith, 2001). Autism has been reported in association with a number of conditions such as fragile X syndrome, tuberous sclerosis, metabolic disorders, fetal rubella syndrome, *Haemophilus influenzae* meningitis, and structural brain anomalies (Williams, Dalrymple, and Neal, 2000). Recent reports have retrospectively tied autism to perinatal events such as a high incidence of uterine bleeding during pregnancy, a lower incidence of vaginal infections during pregnancy, a decreased maternal use of contraceptives, and a higher incidence of neonatal hyperbilirubinemia (Juul-Dam, Townsend, and Courchesne, 2001). These same researchers, however, urge caution in interpreting these findings.

Clinical Manifestations and Diagnostic Evaluation

Children with autism demonstrate several peculiar and often seemingly bizarre characteristics, primarily in social interactions, communication, and behavior. One hallmark characteristic is the inability to maintain eye contact with another person. Parents of autistic children have noted their infants had difficulties with eye contact and avoidance of body contact at a very early age (Sivberg, 2003). Children with autism also display limited functional play and may interact with toys in an unusual manner (Williams, Dalrymple, and Neal, 2000). Autistic children may have significant gastrointestinal symptoms. Constipation is a common symptom and can be associated with acquired megarectum in children with autism (Afzal and others, 2003). Other clinical manifestations typically seen in children with autism are described in Box 19-10. Studies of these children at play suggest that deficits in social development are a primary feature of the illness. Children with autism do not always have the same manifestations from mild forms, requiring minimal supervision, to severe forms in which self-abusive behavior is common. The majority (50% to 70%) of children with autism have some degree of mental retardation, with scores typically in the moderate to severe range. More females than males tend to have very low intelligence scores. Despite their relatively moderate to severe disability, some children with autism (known as *savants*) excel in particular areas, such as art, music, memory, mathematics, or perceptual skills such as puzzle building.

> **NURSING TIP**
>
> The therapeutic management of autism with the hormone secretin is controversial. One recent study failed to demonstrate significant improvement when autistic children were given one dose of synthetic human secretin (Sandler and others, 1999).*

Speech and language delays are also common in autistic children. The new Practice Parameter Report of the American Academy of Neurology (Filipek and others, 2000) recommends immediate evaluation of any child who does not display such language skills as babbling or gesturing by 12 months, no single word by 16 months, and lack of two-word phrases by 24 months. A sudden deterioration in extant expressive speech is also a red-flag event for further evaluation.

This report emphasizes early recognition, referral, diagnosis, and intensive early intervention to improve outcomes for children with autism. Unfortunately, diagnosis is often not made until 2 to 3 years after symptoms are first recognized. The Academy of Neurology report has a comprehensive set of suggested diagnostic criteria to be used to either rule out or establish the diagnosis of childhood autism (Filipek and others, 2000) (see Box 19-10).

Prognosis

Autism is usually a severely disabling condition. However, some children improve with acquisition of language skills and communication with others (Rapin, 1997). Some ultimately achieve independence, but most require lifelong adult supervision. Aggravation of psychiatric symptoms oc-

---

*Additional information on secretin may be found at www.autism.org/secretin.html; **Autism Society of America,** 7910 Woodmont Avenue, Suite 300, Bethesda, MD 20814-3067; (800) 3AUTISM or (301) 657-0881; website: www.autism-society.org.

BOX 19-10 ■ Diagnostic Criteria for Autistic Disorder

A. A total of six (or more) items from (1), (2), and (3), with at least two from (1), and one each from (2) and (3):
  (1) Qualitative impairment in social interaction, as manifested by at least two of the following:
    (a) Marked impairment in the use of multiple nonverbal behaviors such as eye-to-eye gaze, facial expression, body postures, and gestures to regulate social interaction
    (b) Failure to develop peer relationships appropriate to developmental level
    (c) A lack of spontaneous seeking to share enjoyment, interests, or achievements with other people (e.g., by a lack of showing, bringing, pointing out objects of interest)
    (d) Lack of social or emotional reciprocity
  (2) Qualitative impairments in communication as manifested by at least one of the following:
    (a) Delay in, or total lack of, the development of spoken language (not accompanied by an attempt to compensate through alternative modes of communication such as gestures or mime)
    (b) In individuals with adequate speech, marked impairment in the ability to initiate or sustain a conversation with others
    (c) Stereotyped and repetitive use of language or idiosyncratic language
    (d) Lack of varied, spontaneous make-believe play or social imitative play appropriate to developmental level
  (3) Restricted repetitive and stereotyped patterns of behavior, interests, and activities, as manifested by at least one of the following:
    (a) Encompassing preoccupation with one or more stereotyped and restricted patterns of interest that is abnormal either in intensity or focus
    (b) Apparently inflexible adherence to specific, nonfunctional routines or rituals
    (c) Stereotyped and repetitive motor mannerisms (e.g., hand or finger flapping or twisting, complex whole-body movements)
B. Delays or abnormal functioning in at least one of the following areas, with onset before age 3 years: (1) social interaction, (2) language as used in social communication, or (3) symbolic or imaginative play.
C. The disturbance is not better accounted for by Rett's disorder of childhood disintegrative disorder.

From American Psychiatric Association: *Diagnostic and statistical manual of mental disorders*, ed 4 *(DSM-IV TR)*, Washington, DC, 2000, The Association.

curs in about half of the children during adolescence, with girls having a tendency for continued deterioration.

Early recognition of behaviors associated with autism is critical to implement appropriate interventions and family involvement. The prognosis is most favorable for children with communicative speech development by age 6 years and an intelligence quotient above 50 at the time of diagnosis.

● Nursing Considerations

Therapeutic intervention for the child with autism is a specialized area involving professionals with advanced training. Although there is no cure for autism, numerous therapies have been used. The most promising results have been through highly structured and intensive behavior modification programs. In general the objective in treatment is to promote positive reinforcement, increase social awareness of others, teach verbal communication skills, and decrease unacceptable behavior. Providing a structured routine for the child to follow is a key in the management of autism.

When these children are hospitalized, the parents are essential to planning care and ideally should stay with the child as much as possible. Nurses should recognize that not all children with autism are the same and will require individual assessment and treatment. Decreasing stimulation by using a private room, avoiding extraneous auditory and visual distractions, and encouraging the parents to bring in possessions the child is attached to may lessen the disruptiveness of hospitalization. Because physical contact often upsets these children, minimum holding and eye contact may be necessary to avoid behavioral outbursts. Care must be taken when performing procedures on, administering medicine to, or feeding these children, because they are either fussy eaters who may willfully starve themselves or gag to prevent eating or indiscriminate hoarders, swallowing any available edible or inedible items, such as a thermometer. Eating habits of autistic children may be particularly problematic for families and may involve food refusal, mouthing objects, eating nonedibles, and smelling and throwing food (Williams, Dalrymple, and Neal, 2000).

Children with autism need to be introduced slowly to new situations, with visits with staff caregivers kept short whenever possible. Because these children have difficulty organizing their behavior and redirecting their energy, they need to be told directly what to do. Communication should be at the child's developmental level, brief, and concrete.

Family Support.   Autism, as with so may other chronic conditions, involves the entire family and often becomes "a family disease." Nurses can help alleviate the guilt and shame often associated with this disorder by stressing what is known form a biologic standpoint, as well as how little is known about the cause of autism. It is imperative to help parents understand that they are not the cause of the child's condition.

Parents need expert counseling early in the course of the disorder and should be referred to the **Autism Society of America (ASA).*** ASA provides information about education, treatment programs and techniques, and facilities such as camps and group homes. Other helpful resources for parents of children with autism are the local and state departments of mental health and developmental disabilities; these organizations provide important programs for autistic children and in-school programs throughout the United States.

As much as possible, the family is encouraged to care for the child in the home. With the help of family support programs in many states, families are often able to provide home care and assist with the educational services the child needs. As the child approaches adulthood and parents become older, the family may require assistance in locating a long-term placement facility.

---

*See footnote on opposite page.

KEY POINTS

- The American Association of Mental Retardation defines mental retardation (MR) as significantly subaverage general intellectual functioning existing concurrently with deficits in adaptive behavior and manifested during the developmental period.

- Causes of severe MR are primarily genetic, biochemical, and infectious. Mild MR is associated primarily with familial, social, and environmental causes, whereas severe MR is more likely to be associated with specific syndromes.

- Education of children with cognitive impairment emphasizes sensory and verbal discrimination, improvement of short-term memory, motivation, and technologic support.

- Promoting optimal development may be achieved through family guidance regarding play, communication, discipline, socialization, and sexuality.

- Prevention of MR focused on support for the premature neonate and other high-risk newborns, rubella immunization, genetic counseling, and maternal education regarding the risks of chemical use and the importance of adequate nutrition.

- Down syndrome, a chromosomal abnormality, is characterized by mild to moderate range of retardation (most often), physical characteristics, slowed language development, congenital anomalies, sensory problems, and diminished growth and sexual development.

- Fragile X syndrome is characterized by MR and phenotypic findings in affected males. It is considered the most common hereditary cause and the second leading chromosomal cause of MR after Down syndrome.

- Hearing disorders may be classified according to the location of the defect: conductive, sensorineural, mixed conductive-sensorineural, and central auditory imperception.

- Rehabilitation for hearing loss involves parent education and support, hearing aids, lipreading, sign language, speech therapy, and promotion of socialization.

- Prevention of hearing loss includes treatment of infection, universal newborn screening and child auditory testing, immunization, pregnancy and genetic counseling, and reduction of noise pollution.

- Common visual impairments in childhood include refractive errors, amblyopia, strabismus, cataracts, glaucoma, trauma, and infections.

- Prevention of visual impairment focuses on prenatal screening, prenatal and perinatal care, periodic vision screening, immunization, and safety counseling.

- Nursing goals in visual rehabilitation include helping the family and child adjust to the child's visual impairment, promoting parent-child attachment, fostering optimal development and independence, providing for play and socialization, and being aware of educational facilities.

- For the child undergoing ocular surgery, nursing care is aimed at reassuring the child and family throughout treatment, orienting the child to the surroundings, providing a safe environment, and encouraging independence.

- Retinoblastoma is a rare congenital malignant tumor; its most common clinical manifestations are cat's eye reflex (white pupil) and strabismus.

- Autism is a complex developmental disorder of brain function accompanied by a broad range and severity of intellectual and behavioral deficits.

References

Afzal N and others: Constipation with acquired megarectum in children with autism, *Pediatrics* 112(4):939-942, 2003.

Allegretti CM: The effects of a cochlear implant on the family of a hearing-impaired child, *Pediatr Nurs* 28(6):614-620, 2002.

American Academy of Pediatrics, Committee on Children and Disabilities: Provision of educationally-related services for children and adolescents with chronic diseases and disabling conditions, *Pediatrics* 105(2):448-451, 2000.

American Academy of Pediatrics, Committee on Genetics: Health supervision for children with Down syndrome, *Pediatrics* 107(2):442-449, 2001.

American Academy of Pediatrics, Task Force on Newborn and Infant Hearing: Newborn and infant hearing loss: detection and intervention, *Pediatrics* 103(2):527-530, 1999.

Applebaum E: Detection of hearing loss in children, *Pediatr Ann* 28(6):351-356, 1999.

Berrettini S and others: Progressive sensorineural hearing loss in childhood, *Pediatr Neurol* 20(2):130-136, 1999.

Bosch JJ, Ringdahl J: Functional analysis of problem behavior in children with mental retardation: what is it, and why should pediatric nurses care? *MCN* 26(6):307-311, 2001.

Centers for Disease Control and Prevention: Delayed diagnosis of fragile X syndrome–United States, 1990-1999, *MMWR* 51(33):740-742, 2002.

Cohen W, editor: Health care guidelines for individuals with Down syndrome: 1999 revisions, *Down Syndrome Q* August 1999; available at: www.denison.edu/dsq/health99.shtml.

Crawford DC: FMR1 and the fragile X syndrome, *CDC Fact Sheet*, 2001, available at: http://www.cdc.gov/genomics/hugenet/factsheets/FS_FragileX.htm.

Courchesne E, Carper R, Akshoomoff N: Evidence of brain overgrowth in the first year of life in autism, *JAMA* 290(3):337-344, 2003.

Cunningham M, Cox EO: Committee on Practice and Ambulatory Medicine and the Section on Otolaryngology and Bronchoesophagology: Hearing assessment in infants and children: recommendations beyond neonatal screening, *Pediatrics* 111(2):436-440, 2003.

Daily DK: Identification and evaluation of mental retardation, *Am Fam Physician* 61:1059-1067, 2000.

Dales L, Hammer SJ, Smith NJ: Time trends in autism and in MMR immunization coverage in California, *JAMA* 285(9):1183-1185, 2001.

Davidson PW: Visual impairment and blindness. In Levine MD, Carey WTS, Crocker AC, editors: *Developmental-behavior pediatrics*, ed 3, Philadelphia, 1999, WB Saunders.

De Potter P: Current treatment of retinoblastoma, *Curr Opin Ophthalmol* 13(5):331-336, 2002.

DeStefano F and others: Age at first measles-mumps-rubella vaccination in children with autism and school-matched control subjects: a population-based study in metropolitan Atlanta, *Pediatrics* 113(2):259-266, 2004.

Filipek P and others: Practice parameter: screening and diagnosis of autism: report of the Quality Standards Subcommittee of the American Academy of Neurology and the Child Neurology Society, *Neurology* 55(2 of 2):468-479, 2000.

First MB, McQueen LE, Pincus HA: *DSM-IV coding update*, Washington DC, 1996, American Psychiatric Association.

Fredericks DW, Williams WL: New definition of mental retardation for the American Association of Mental Retardation, *Image J Nurs Sch* 30(1):53-56, 1998.

Grech V: An overview and update regarding medical problems in Down syndrome, *Indian J Pediatr* 68:863-866, 2001.

Greene M: Teaching the mentally retarded parenting skills: international perspectives. In Shaughnessy M and others: *Social and vocational inclusion of persons with mental retardation—an international perspective,* Mahwah, NJ, Lawrence Erlbaum Associates, in press.

Gurrieri F and others: Pervasive developmental disorder and epilepsy due to maternally derived duplication of 15q11-q13, *Neurology* 52(8):1694-1697, 1999.

Hixon M and others: FISH studies of the sperm of fathers of paternally derived cases of trisomy 21: no evidence for an increase in aneuploidy, *Hum Genet* 103(6):654-657, 1998.

Holte L: Early childhood hearing loss: a frequently overlooked cause of speech and language delay, *Pediatr Ann* 32(7):461-465, 2003.

Hurwitz and others: Retinoblastoma. In Pizzo PA, Poplack DG, editors: *Principle and practice of pediatric oncology,* ed 4, Philadelphia, 2002, JB Lippincott.

Juul-Dam N, Townsend J, Courchesne E: Prenatal, perinatal, and neonatal factors in autism, pervasive developmental disorder not otherwise specified, and the general population, *Pediatrics* 107(4):e63, 2001.

Kabra M, Gulati S: Mental retardation, *Indian J Pediatr* 70(2):153-158, 2003.

Lainhart JE: Increased rate of head growth during infancy in autism, *JAMA* 290(3):393-394, 2003.

Lanzkowsky P: *Manual of pediatric hematology and oncology,* San Diego, 2000, Academic Press.

National Down Syndrome Society: *Are any prenatal tests available to detect Down syndrome?* 2003a, available at: http://www.ndss.org.

National Down Syndrome Society: *Down syndrome: myths and truths,* 2003b, available at: http://www.ndss.org.

National Down Syndrome Society: *Questions and answers about Down syndrome,* 2003c, available at: http://www.ndss.org.

National Down Syndrome Society: *What causes Down syndrome?* 2003d, available at: http://www.ndss.org.

National Fragile X Foundation: *Prevalence of fragile X syndrome,* 2002, available at: www.fragilex.org/html/prevalence.htm.

Pueschel SM: The child with Down syndrome. In Levine MD and others, editors: *Developmental-behavioral pediatrics,* ed 3, Philadelphia, 1999, WB Saunders.

Rapin I: Autism, *N Engl J Med* 337(2):97-103, 1997.

Roizen NJ: Etiology of hearing loss in children: nongenetic causes, *Pediatr Clin North Am* 46(1):49-64, 1999.

Sandler AD and others: Lack of benefit of a single dose of synthetic human secretin in the treatment of autism and pervasive developmental disorder, *N Engl J Med* 341(24):1801-1806, 1999.

Schouten–van Meeteren AYN, Moll AC, Imhof SM, and Veerman AJP: Overview chemotherapy for retinoblastoma: an expanding area of clinical research, *Med Pediatr Oncol* 38:428-438, 2002.

Segal S and others: Inner ear damage in children due to noise exposure from toy cap pistols and firecrackers: a retrospective review of 53 cases, *Noise Health* 5(18):13-18, 2003.

Shao Y and others: Fine mapping of autistic disorder to chromosomes 15q11-q13 by phenotypic subtypes, *Am J Hum Genet* 72(3):539-548, 2003.

Sivberg B: Parents' detection of early signs in their children having an autism spectrum disorder, *J Pediatr Nurs* 18(6): 433-440, 2003.

Slattery WH, Fayad, JN: Cochlear implants in children with sensorineural inner ear hearing loss, *Pediatr Ann* 28(6):359-363, 1999.

Tager-Flusberg H, Joseph RM: Identifying neurocognitive phenotypes in autism, *Philos Trans R Soc Lond B Biol Sci* 358(1430):303-314, 2003.

Van Riper M: A change of plans: the birth of a child with Down syndrome doesn't have to be a negative experience, *Am J Nurs* 103(6):71-74, 2003.

Waltzman SB, Roland JT, Cohen NL: Delayed implantation in congenitally deaf children and adults, *Otol Neurotol* 23(3):333-340, 2002.

Welch JL, Williams JK: Fragile X syndrome, *Neonat Netw* 18(6):15-22, 1999.

Williams PG, Dalrymple N, Neal J: Eating habits of children with autism, *Pediatr Nurs* 26(3):259-264, 2000.

Yang YH and others: Prenatal diagnosis of fetal trisomy 21 from maternal peripheral blood, *Yonsei Med J* 44(2):181-186, 2003.

Yoshinaga-Itano C and others: Language of early- and later-identified children with hearing loss, *Pediatrics* 102(5):1161-1171, 1998.

20

Family-Centered Home Care

DAVID WILSON

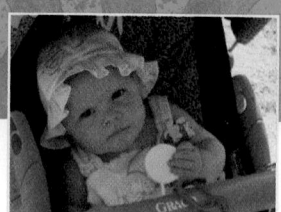

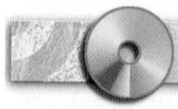 Remember to check out your companion CD-ROM

http://evolve.elsevier.com/Wong/essentials/

CHAPTER OUTLINE

RELATED TOPICS and ADDITIONAL RESOURCES

 IN TEXT

 CD COMPANION

 WEBSITE

GENERAL CONCEPTS OF HOME CARE

Home care nursing is not a new concept in pediatrics. Over time the term has referred to parents caring for mildly ill children at home, to nursing home visits after children are discharged from the hospital, to palliative and hospice care, and, recently, to care at home for children with more serious chronic illness and dependence on medical technology. Home care is one the fastest growing components of the health care industry.

As discussed in this chapter, *home care* refers to care provided in the family's residence for children with complex or simple health care needs; that care also includes the particular needs of the family within the context of the child's health care needs. The purpose of home care services is to promote, maintain, or restore health or to maximize the level of independence while minimizing the effects of disability and illness, including terminal illness. Home care differs from *hospice care,* which is a program of palliative and supportive care that provides physical, psychologic, social, and spiritual care for dying persons, their families, and other loved ones. Hospice services are available both in the home and in inpatient settings. *End-of-life care* and planning should be considered for any child with a terminal diagnosis. Some patients may be admitted for end-of-life home care services before being ready for admission to hospice services. Many hospice programs have admission criteria that do not permit therapies such as intravenous antibiotics, total parenteral nutrition, or enteral feedings that the family may wish to continue. It is therefore important to discuss the type of care the family wishes for the child early in discharge planning to clarify expectations for home care.

HOME CARE TRENDS

The shift toward home-based health care is propelled by numerous factors. Providing quality home health care for children generally requires parental desire and ability, professional assistance, and community preparedness. A natural family environment optimizes growth and development when stress is minimal and support is optimal.

Advances in medical technology have resulted in increased survival for children with congenital and acquired illnesses. Preterm infants or children who are ventilator dependent were once cared for indefinitely in an intensive care unit or long-term care facility. These children are now able to live with their families in their own home.

Children with cancer, kidney disorders, cystic fibrosis, spina bifida, cardiac and respiratory disorders, gastrointestinal disorders, neurodegenerative diseases, and human immunodeficiency virus (HIV) infection may have ongoing health care needs as a result of the disease, its treatment, or side effects of treatment. Parents frequently have ongoing stressors after a child's hospitalization for diagnosis and treatment. Subsequent needs may include reinforcement about the disease process, addressing the physical care needs of the child, emotional support during this change in parental role, and learning in a low-stress environment. Improving the quality of life for both the child and the family is one of the driving forces in the efforts to move technology-dependent children from the hospital to the home setting. The concept of *normalization* describes the process whereby families of children with chronic illness over a period of time begin to perceive the child and their family life as normal (Knafl and Deatrick, 2002). This has important implications for pediatric home care nurses in relation to the assessment of family function and to gain a better understanding of family dynamics. The normalized family tends to be more flexible with treatments and incorporates the child with a disability or illness into the usual routines of daily living (Knafl and Deatrick, 2002).

The *cost of care* is another important factor in the health care delivery system today. Shorter inpatient stays are due in part to the overwhelming cost of lengthy hospitalizations. Children are either not admitted to the hospital at all or are returned home as soon as possible after their acute illness. Shifting the financial burden of health care to home care agencies is an attractive alternative to third-party reimbursers. Likewise, a portion of the financial burden is shifted to the family. The family may be forced to absorb the costs of certain medications, supplies, transportation, shelter, utilities, food, laundry, housekeeping, and a portion of nursing care. Over time chronically ill children can cause a financial burden to the family. Lifetime insurance benefits may be used up quickly, the primary caregiver may be unable to work, and many costs of health care are simply not covered by other means.

Home health care of children, however, is not restricted to children with chronic health care needs. Several short-term intermittent therapies such as phototherapy, apnea monitoring, and intravenous antibiotic administration may be successfully treated in a home setting where the child may remain with the family rather than in an acute care setting.

With the increased demand for nurses in home health and continued pervasive short supply there has been an increased focus on the role of the *family caregiver* in providing home care. A survey by the National Alliance for Caregivers (1997) revealed that 25% of US households have a person being cared for by another family member; this represents care above and beyond the daily routine care of the family household. Legislation for improving resources for family caregivers, including training resources and governmental funding for such training, is currently in progress.

EFFECTIVE HOME CARE

Providing home-based care for children gives the nurse an opportunity to assess and interact with the family in their environment. This assessment can provide the health care team with valuable information about safety, support systems, nutrition, parenting ability, and actual health care practices. This valuable information will determine future decisions for individualized care and realistic outcomes (Thompson, 2000).

There are two distinct areas of implementation of care for the pediatric home care nurse. Nurses who perform *intermittent skilled nursing visits* may see different types and numbers of patients each day. These nurses typically have an assigned patient caseload and accept responsibility for implementing the plan of care. This mode of nursing care is the most often used today as a result of shortage of personnel and decreased reimbursements. Most home visits are now focused on assisting the patient/caregiver in achieving independence with care in the home, including care by therapists, home infusion teaching by nurses, and care management, rather than direct provision of physical care. Nurses who perform *private-duty nursing* or block nursing are usually assigned individual patients, and they remain in the home for a predetermined amount of time (e.g., 8- or 12-hour block of time) providing patient care. The latter model is much less common. The plan of care is implemented over the course of the time in the home, and short-term intermittent plans of care are more common in today's home care. An increasing trend resulting from the nursing shortage and limitations in reimbursement is to have patients receive short-term treatments in non–hospital ambulatory settings (such as ambulatory infusion centers).

A major issue in providing home care in this era is the *nursing shortage.* Agencies and families are facing much more difficulty in staffing required home care services; thus, more and more of the home care provided must be carried out by family members or other caregivers. The lack of pediatric training in some nursing programs, increased acuity of home care patients, and increased pay for nurses working in acute care settings have contributed to a greater than ever nursing shortage in pediatric home health care (Page, 2001). Consideration of the caregiver's willingness, ability, and limitations are of utmost importance when assessing the appropriateness of the plan of care. It is vital to ensure that patients and families have adequate back-up support and access to resources such as social services (Box 20-1). An increasing concern in pediatric home health care is obtaining a managing practitioner for patients in home health. Declining reimbursement and short hospital stays have increased patients moving rapidly through the continuum of care; a patient may be seen in the emergency room or neonatal intensive care unit (ICU), then discharged to home health without ever seeing a primary care physician. It is therefore imperative that the provision of care for home patients involve multidisciplinary cooperation, and communication among health care workers is essential.

BOX 20-1 ■ Services That Support Effective Home Care

Adequate family training and preparation
Primary care physician willing to oversee medical aspects of care
Professional caregivers trained in relevant nursing and communication skills
Developmental intervention (e.g., physical, occupational, and speech therapy; early intervention)
Appropriately designed and well-maintained equipment
Supportive therapies (e.g., respiratory therapy, pharmacy, rehabilitation services, parenteral therapy, physical therapy, durable medical/infusion supplies, nutritional support)
Adequate social and psychologic support services
High-quality respite care
Appropriate home renovation
Telephone service in the home
Appropriate transportation
Appropriate locally available emergency facilities
Competent case management services

Modified from Office of Technology Assessment (OTA), Congress of the United States: *Technology dependent children: hospital v. home care—a technical memorandum* (OTA-TM-H-38), Washington, DC, 1987, US Government Printing Office; Bakewell-Sachs S, Porth S: Discharge planning and home care of the technology-dependent infant, *JOGNN* 24(1):77-83, 1995.

Required nursing skills are determined by patient need, parental ability, complexity of family, and the home environment. In both types of home care, the pediatric nurse is responsible for patient and family assessment and evaluating the appropriateness of the plan of care.

From technology dependence to pain management or failure to thrive, pediatric nurses are appropriate professionals to affect a child's health care needs at home. Quality interdisciplinary care can create a significant, positive impact on family coping and child outcomes (Betz, 2000; Mahony and Murphy, 1999).

DISCHARGE PLANNING

Identifying appropriate local community resources is critical to a successful transfer to home care. The ultimate goal of discharge planning is for the family to become familiar with the child's needs and to be competent in providing that care. A discharge plan should include emergency management and provision of social and emotional support. General guidelines for discharge that allow for family individuality provide for ideal outcomes. The desired attributes of an appropriate home care agency are outlined in Box 20-2.

The American Academy of Pediatrics Committee on Children With Disabilities (1995) states that "the goal for a home health care program for infants, children, or adolescents with chronic conditions is the provision of comprehensive, cost-effective health care with a nurturing home environment that maximizes the capabilities of the individual and minimizes the effects of the disabilities."

> **NURSING TIP**
>
> If home care equipment is different from hospital equipment, deliver portable equipment to be used in the home to the hospital to allow family use before discharge.

Much of the success of home care, particularly for the child who is dependent on medical technology or has com-

BOX 20-2 ■ Quality Pediatric Home Care Agency

Fully trained pediatric staff to provide for all aspects of care (nursing, rehabilitation therapies, pharmacy, dietitian, social worker, home medical equipment)

Prompt responsive staff with 24-hour availability

Family-centered care

Comprehensive continuing education programs

Certification of local, state, and federal regulatory agencies

Accreditation by Joint Commission on Accreditation of Healthcare Organizations (JCAHO) or Community Health Accreditation Program (CHAP)

Data from Dittbrenner H: Pediatric home care as a viable new service, *Caring* 18(2):12-15, 1999; Lovejoy D: *Making the transition to home health nursing: a practical guide,* New York, 1997, Springer.

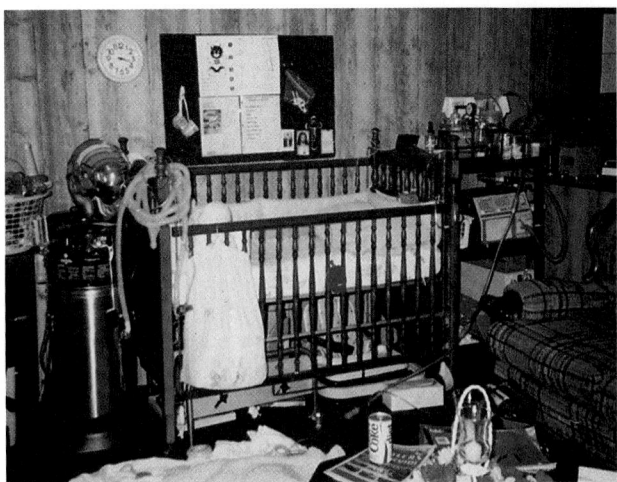

FIG. 20-1 ■ An essential aspect of preparation for home care is arranging equipment and supplies.

BOX 20-3 ■ Critical Home Care Referral Information

Scheduled medications

Durable medical equipment (DME)

Medical supplies

Transportation needs

Adaptive equipment

Rehabilitation therapies (occupational therapy [OT], physical therapy [PT], speech)

Psychologic counseling

Social work referral

Nursing care

Respite plans

Key family members

Demographic information

Reimbursement information

Modified from Townsend JL: Assessment of the child and family. In Votroubek WL, Townsend JL, editors: *Pediatric home care,* ed 2, Gaithersburg, Md, 1997, Aspen.

plex medical problems, depends on careful planning and preparation. Discharge planning must begin early and should be based on child and family readiness, must be a multidisciplinary process and include representatives from inpatient and home care/community settings, and must involve the family. Predischarge assessment and planning should include the following areas:

- The child's medical, nursing, educational, and other therapeutic needs
- Family members' (including siblings') education and training, coping skills, and adjustment needs
- Community readiness in areas such as availability of equipment, appropriate nursing and other personnel, educational and developmental services, respite care, and emergency plans
- Financial arrangements

Creative financial planning, including negotiating arrangements with the insurance company, health maintenance or managed care organization, and public programs, may be required.

Early involvement of the home care agency in the discharge planning process promotes continuity of care and a smooth transition from hospital to home. Before discharge, a general plan, often called an Individualized Home Care Plan (IHCP), should be developed with multidisciplinary input. This plan should address the range of needs identified as part of the comprehensive predischarge assessment.

NURSING TIP

An excellent method of providing home care instructions is with video recordings. After the family masters the procedures, consider video recording their performance. Visual learning may be most helpful for people who cannot read or who are not fluent in English.

The plans for transition from hospital to home should include at least two family members learning and demonstrating all aspects of the child's care in the hospital. An in-hospital trial period during which parents provide total care for the child (such as rooming in) is generally beneficial as well. After a successful trial, the family may benefit from taking the child home on a brief pass before making final discharge plans. (This arrangement may need to be negotiated with the insurance company prior to implementation.) The home care nurse plays an important role in assessing this experience with the family. Whether or not the child is taken home on a pass,

a predischarge home visit offers the home care nurse the opportunity to meet the family, help them assess their preparedness and the preparedness of the home environment, discuss plans for arranging the child's equipment at home (Fig. 20-1), reinforce prior discharge teaching, and implement any additional teaching that may be necessary (Bakewell-Sachs and others, 2000). Additional factors that should be considered in discharge planning include working parents, extended family, and childcare arrangements.

A comprehensive discharge plan includes the IHCP or care map, specific written instructions to facilitate continuity, and detailed information about home care expectations (Box 20-3).

CASE MANAGEMENT

Traditional definitions of *case management* generally focus on cost control, attainment of desired clinical outcomes, and monitoring and evaluation of care provided. However, for optimal home care of the child who is technology dependent, case management—or *care coordination*—should be viewed more broadly (see also Chapter 1).

Care coordination has several purposes. Its primary goal is ensuring continuity for the child and family across hospital, home, educational, therapeutic, and other settings. Other goals involve facilitating timely access to services and enhancing child and family well-being (Lindeke and others, 2002). Care should be coordinated among multiple providers to reduce the complexity of care for the child, reduce fragmentation of care, and decrease the burden of care for the family. Case managers from a number of agencies may be involved in the patient's care, which may add to the parents' confusion; efforts should be made to coordinate all case managers for meetings with the family and a nurse care coordinator to minimize confusion and prevent duplication. Lindeke and others (2002) propose that the ideal situation occurs when the family serves as lead care coordinator within the context of family-centered care. Care coordination should ensure that the medical, nursing, and health maintenance needs of the child, as well as financial issues, psychosocial concerns, and educational needs of the child and family, are addressed (American Academy of Pediatrics, 1999; Dittbrenner, 1999).

Care coordination is most effective if a single person works with the family to accomplish the many tasks and responsibilities involved (Box 20-4).

FYI

The *nurse case manager* should have a minimum of a baccalaureate degree in nursing and 3 years' experience (American Nurses Association, 1998). The nurse case manager should be knowledgeable about community resources, including the following: primary, secondary, and tertiary health care services; speech, language, hearing, and vision resources; respite care services; financial assistance programs; parent groups; advocacy groups; local, state, and federal public officials; transportation services; and private sector individuals with an interest in children with disabilities (Thompson, 2000). With a greater focus on *outcomes of care* in home health care, the nurse case manager is challenged to be resourceful and quite skilled in communication at a number of levels (Rice, 2001). A valuable tool for nurse case managers is the *care path,* which is a multidisciplinary plan of care aimed at measuring quality patient care outcomes derived from standardized patient outcomes; the purpose of a care path is to evaluate the quality of patient care with respect to cost-effectiveness and timeliness (for samples of home care clinical care paths, see Rice, 2001 reference). Care paths may also be used to help nurses and other health care workers learn home care and should be shared with the family members involved in patient care to provide direction and help the family see the eventual goals of care (Rice, 2001).

BOX 20-4 ■ Care Coordination for Children With Special Health Care Needs

Facilitate timely access to services and resources
Promote continuity of care
Provide family support and enhance family well-being
Improve health, developmental, educational, vocational, psychosocial, and functional outcomes
Maximize efficient, effective use of resources

Modified from Presler B: Care coordination for children with special health care needs, *Orthop Nurs* 17(25 suppl):45-51, 1998.

Care coordination should promote the family's role as primary decision maker and enhance the family's capability to meet the special needs of the child and the family as a whole. In 1999 the American Nurses Credentialing Center (ANCC), a subsidiary of the American Nurses Association, began offering specialty certification in case management.

ROLE OF THE NURSE, TRAINING, AND STANDARDS OF CARE

The home care nurse must sometimes share a level of technical expertise with the critical care nurse while being able to adapt equipment, procedures, and the nursing process to the home setting. (See Chapter 22 for specific technical skills that may be required in home care practice.) The need for technical expertise must be matched by knowledge of child development and the ability to work creatively with the child challenged by chronic illness and technology dependence. When caring for patients in the home setting, the nurse must be comfortable making independent nursing judgments, think critically, and solve problems without immediate assistance. At the same time, the nurse must have excellent interpersonal skills, an ability to work with other professionals and the family, and, most important, the ability to respect family autonomy (Box 20-5). Patient outcomes are more readily achievable with a balance of nursing skills that demonstrate clinical excellence, adaptability, accountability, and the ability to develop positive relationships with patients and families.

When working with a home care agency, nurses should expect to receive patient placements appropriate to their expertise. They should also expect to receive orientation to the skills and knowledge base of the home health care nursing specialty and subsequent education to develop as expert practitioners. The minimum initial orientation should include the following areas: the individual patient's care plan and equipment needs; the agency's policies and procedures, including procedures for addressing any problems that may occur when care is provided in the home; documentation procedures; legal liability issues; and emergency procedures.

Reimbursement-driven documentation in home care differs from documentation practices in the hospital setting; increasingly, documentation must be written in specific ways to qualify for reimbursement of services and supplies. Mentoring is an ideal method of orienting a new nurse to home health care.

Nurses in pediatric home health face increasing demands for providing high-quality care with fewer resources to achieve positive patient outcomes. In doing so the nurse often must rely on *delegation* skills to adequately ensure that the patient and family receive the necessary care. Delegation often involves assigning nursing tasks to other health care workers; therefore, the nurse must have good delegation skills as well (Timm, 2003).

BOX 20-5 ■ Qualities of a Pediatric Home Care Nurse

Demonstrates flexibility in skills and case management
Recognizes that the nurse is a guest in the home
Respects family culture and adapts appropriately
Works as an interdisciplinary team member
Demonstrates expertise in pediatric care

Public or private home care agencies that participate in the Medicare or Medicaid programs must be certified by a federally designated, state-certifying body and abide by federal and state regulations. In addition, the **American Nurses Association (ANA)** has developed standards of nursing practice for both community health and home care nurses (see Selected Resources, p. 634). Generalist and clinical specialist certification in both home health and community health is offered by the **ANCC,*** a subsidiary of ANA. The **Hospice Nurses Association** offers certification in hospice nursing. Despite some important differences between pediatric and adult care in the home, as of this writing, no national standards specific to pediatric home care nursing practice have been developed. Nursing practice in pediatric home care should be guided by published guidelines, textbooks, peer-reviewed articles related to pediatric home care, and written standards of care for pediatric patients (see Box 20-6). In addition, professional nursing organizations such as Intravenous Nurses Society (IVS), National Association of Neonatal Nurses (NANN), Society of Pediatric Nurses (SPN), Association of Pediatric Oncology Nurses (APON), National Association of Pediatric Nurse Practitioners (NAPNAP), and others have published standards of care that apply to pediatric home health nursing practice.

A *quality improvement (QI)* program is an important component of an effective home care agency. *Evidence-based practice* is rapidly becoming an important aspect of home health care, as is *benchmarking,* in which the product or practice (in this case, patient outcome) is compared with other agencies' outcomes and practices to determine best practice; this allows agencies to see how they measure in comparison to other similar agencies (Wilson, 2003; Yoder-Wise, 2003). The **OASIS (Outcome and Assessment Information Set),** as part of Medicare, has been established for adults in home health care; however, as of this writing there are no such data for children younger than age 18. As a part of OASIS, home health care quality measures have been established to measure patient care outcomes for Medicare reimbursement purposes. Other certification/licensing organizations that may oversee and regulate practice in home health include Joint Commission on Accreditation of Healthcare Organizations (JCAHO), Centers for Medicare/Medicaid Services (CMS) (formerly HCFA), OSHA (Occupational Safety and Health Administration), and the Community Health Accreditation Program (CHAP). The new HIPAA (Health Insurance Portability and Accountability Act, 1998) guidelines affect the way patient records are handled in home health care to ensure patient confidentiality.

FAMILY-CENTERED HOME CARE

Technology dependence, chronic illness, and complex care requirements cross social, cultural, spiritual, and economic boundaries. Regardless of a family's background, family values must be respected in the provision of home care services. *The home is the family's domain,* and the child is at home because the family's central role is to nurture and raise their child. The ultimate responsibility for managing the child's health, developmental, and emotional needs lies with the family. Roush and Cox (2000) developed a framework for helping the home health care nurse understand the significance of the home to the family. The three central concepts of the model are as follows:

1 Home as familiar—the environment where one is comfortable and at ease because of the familiarity with living arrangements and routines of home
2 Home as protector—the location of everyday experiences related to time, space, and one's social life
3 Home as protector—privacy, safety, and identity may be preserved in the environment of the home (Roush and Cox, 2000).

The nurse must respect the family's central role in the care of the child and must work in collaboration with the family in efforts to care for the child. Family-centered nursing practice is essential in the home setting. Family-centered care has become acknowledged as the standard of care for children with special health care needs (Johnson, 2000).

The philosophic basis for family-centered practice is the recognition that the family is the constant in the child's life, whereas the service systems and personnel within those systems fluctuate. Professionals working with the families of children with complex chronic problems must respect the family's central, caring role; their knowledge; and their particular and unique expertise. Families have the most intimate knowledge of the child's strengths and abilities, the challenges of providing care, and the abilities and needs of other family members. Believing that no one knows the child better than the family is crucial to the success of any health care plan.

DIVERSITY IN HOME CARE

Respect for varied family structures and for racial, ethnic, cultural, spiritual, and socioeconomic diversity among families is essential in home care (see also Chapters 3 and 4). Home care nurses work in close relationship with family members and in the family's own domain. The nurse shares in these relationships, participating in care throughout the course of illness (see Family Focus box). The nurse must assess and respect the family's background and lifestyle choices. Particular attention is given to *communication.* The meaning of the words used and the way in which they are said may affect various cultural groups in different ways. Volume of speech and language style must be taken into consideration as part of a family cultural assessment.

NURSING TIP

Color-coded medication bottles, written schedules, and pillboxes or oral syringes may aid compliance with prescription administration. One should not assume that everyone who speaks English, as a primary or secondary language, is able to adequately read the language. Pictures or special symbols may be helpful when providing instructions for procedures and medication administration.

Families may also differ in their cultural view of children, health care, childrearing practices, and illness—its causes and meaning. The family's health care practices and beliefs may influence the level of investment a family will make in the child's care. The family's *religion* or spirituality is another factor that can have a major influence on a family's

---

*ANCC, c/o ANA, 600 Maryland Avenue SW, Suite 100-W, Washington, DC 20024-2571; (202) 651-7000 or (800) 284-2378; website: www.nursingworld.org/ancc.

FAMILY FOCUS

Developing a Relationship With Culturally Diverse Families

I work in the inner city, and my home care patients come from a variety of racial and ethnic backgrounds. I am Caucasian, from Australia. Often, when I first visit a family, there is an initial coolness or apprehension toward me. This is understandable because I am a stranger, and perhaps families think I'll judge them in one way or another. By the end of the first visit, however, there is usually a smile as I leave; by the second visit they often greet me with a smile at the door; and by the third visit we usually have a friendship, a trust, and an ease of communication.

If I'm working on a case for an extended time, I use a holistic nursing approach. This involves being aware of how the illness of the child affects the entire family. As I listen over many weeks to their fears and questions, and often as I share faith perspectives, a bond begins to form. I find it a privilege to share in their joys and their pain, and I feel rewarded by the trust that they invest in me.

Julie Edgerton, RN
Home Care Nurse
Children's National Medical Center
Washington, DC

response to the child's special health care needs. The family will often look for spiritual meaning and purpose for the illness. Other families may chose to reject past religious ties. In some cultures, religion and beliefs about health care and illness are closely intertwined (McEvoy, 2003), thus it is important that home care nurses assess the relationship between culture, religion, and the family's beliefs about the child's illness (see the spiritual assessment tool BELIEF in Chapter 13).

A variety of cultural assessment tools are available (Giger and Davidhizar, 2002; Spruhan, 1996). The home care nurse, aware that *personal values* drive behavior, needs to learn about the family's culture, ask questions without implying judgment, interpret the mainstream medical culture, and help families design interventions that meet their preferences. When possible, culture-specific teaching materials should be used. Increased emphasis in health care in the United States has been placed on health care workers becoming culturally competent to effectively deliver holistic care to their patients. Home care nurses are challenged to become culturally competent to better understand the patient populations they serve (National Center for Cultural Competence, 2002).

Respect for family diversity and awareness of both family developmental stages (see Chapter 3) and the stages of a family's adjustment to illness in a child (see Chapter 18) will assist the home care nurse in recognizing and promoting family strengths and in respecting varied coping mechanisms. Labels such as "dysfunctional," "difficult," and "noncompliant" can reinforce negative expectations and shape behaviors of both parents and professionals. On the other hand, emphasizing, identifying, and building on family strengths and coping mechanisms are strategies that promote a central goal in nursing care of the child and family: *family empowerment* (see Chapter 1). The home care nurse working with families should remain flexible and open-

minded, because new family strengths may emerge over time and coping mechanisms may wax and wane with the stresses of caring for a child with serious or multiple problems.

PARENT-PROFESSIONAL COLLABORATION

Family-centered nursing practice is built on a foundation of parent-professional collaboration, which represents a shift from the traditional unidirectional relationships between health care providers and families. The *Collaborative Family Health Care Coalition* has developed core competencies for professionals collaborating with families (McDaniel and Campbell, 1996). *Collaborative caring* allows the nurse and family to work together and share outcomes in a deep and meaningful way. This approach, essential in the home care setting, is characterized by the following (Kellett and Mannion, 1999; Gaudet, 1997):

- Encouraging activities to develop self-confidence and self-esteem
- Displaying increased awareness and respect for family caregivers
- Recognizing that families vary in defining their role
- Demonstrating an ability to understand the family's approach to caregiving
- Sharing perspectives, not just tasks and functions
- Supporting family in their primary, irreplaceable role as caregiver
- Exchanging expertise in providing care to the child
- Assisting families in recognizing their contributions as worthwhile
- Identifying strengths and resources of child and family
- Negotiating options, priorities, and preferences
- Assisting coping by allowing families to find meaning in caring

Communication with the family should not be invasive. There is no need to collect information from the family that can be obtained from the child's records. The nurse should explain to the family the reason for questions, particularly those that the family may perceive as intrusive, and should inform families of who will have access to the information. The nurse must also assure families that they have a right to expect confidentiality in regard to the data collected. When working in the home, the nurse must respect the privacy of family members' communications with each other that may be overheard.

! NURSING ALERT

Home care nurses should restrict their communications with other professionals to clinically relevant information about the family.

Home care nurses should respect the family's control of their own environment. The Guidelines box addresses "house rules" that can be negotiated.

Communication with family members should also include sharing with the family, in a supportive manner, complete and unbiased information about all aspects of the child's condition and care. Repeated explanations in simple language may be necessary. Information should be shared with families in a way that will have meaning in their cultural context. Many parents report a preference for interactions with professionals who communicate empathy and concern.

GUIDELINES

Negotiating "House Rules" for Home Care

HOUSE RULES

Parking: Where to park and community regulations.

Access: Where to enter the home. Is knocking preferred or ringing the bell?

Personal belongings: Where does the nurse store own coat, boots, etc.? Does the family prefer slippers to shoes in the home?

Meals: Where may the nurse store own food? NOTE: This is very important given cultural diversity of clients.

Radio and television: Identify preferences regarding usage. Remember, this may help nurses to remain awake at night.

Patient room: The nurse is responsible for the child's immediate environment. Maintaining a clean working area and cleaning up the room at the end of the shift is the nurse's responsibility.

Telephone: Agency policy may dictate that all personal calls be limited to very brief periods and charged to the nurse making them. NOTE: Many nurses do need to check in with home at some interval during the evening.

Visitors: Identify who may enter the home when the parents are away (that is, child's friends or grandparents). A list of names should be available.

Privacy: Describe what parts of the home are off-limits to the nurse and at what times.

CHILD

Routine: Specify times for playtime, bathtime, and bedtime. What does the parent want to participate in regarding these routines?

Mealtime: Specify where the family wants the child fed; if tube fed, specify a preference as to how and where it is done.

Clothing: Identify who picks out the child's clothes. Identify where the laundry is and who is responsible for washing the sick child's clothing.

Discipline: Discuss specific guidelines for discipline.

Homework: Discuss when it should be done and who is responsible for it being completed.

SIBLINGS

Discipline: Establish guidelines regarding how parents should be informed of siblings' conflicts and how discipline should be handled. NOTE: Parents or another caregiver must be in the home when siblings are home.

Patient care: Be specific regarding how children have helped with the child's care. Discuss any concerns regarding behavior that may compromise the child's or siblings' safety.

NURSING

Parental notification: Specify what information the family wishes to be aware of immediately and what can wait until they are home.

Limits of responsibility: Specify duties the nurse may not perform, such as transportation of the child to care facilities.

Environment: Discuss the need to have adequate lighting and a comfortable working area.

Modified from Klug R: Clarifying roles and expectations in home care, *Pediatr Nurs* 19(4):375, 1993.

On occasion, disagreements may arise between parents and nurses over proper procedures for care of the child. Nurses should respect parental preferences in any situation that will not pose danger or risk for the child (see Family Focus box). If parents wish to alter a plan of treatment that is part of medical orders, the nurse should ask that they negotiate the change with the practitioner, because the nurse must follow the written medical orders. If disagreements cannot be resolved, a home care supervisor or case manager should be contacted to assist with problem solving. Increasingly, home care agencies are developing ethics committees and policies for managing difficult situations such as treatment refusal (see Critical Thinking Exercise).

THE NURSING PROCESS

In the home the family is a partner in each step of the nursing process. Assessment should address family strengths and resources (see Family Assessment, Chapter 6). The principles of communication discussed previously guide data collection. The nurse's observations are shared neutrally, without value judgment, and in a way that preserves the family's own role in decision making.

All information gathered as part of the assessment process is shared with the family. The nurse should recognize that the family's perception of their most important need will generally guide their behavior and consume their attention and energy. Family priorities should guide the planning process.

 FAMILY FOCUS

Knowledgeable Parents

It is not unusual for parents, particularly those whose children have chronic illnesses or complex care regimens, to be more knowledgeable about their child's condition than a nurse who is assigned to the child's care. This can be disconcerting for both the parent(s) and the nurse. It is important to remember and reinforce that, regardless of the condition, parents will always know more about their child than the professional caring for the child. The nurse and parents can set goals for care in an atmosphere of mutual respect. If the parents' goal is respite from prolonged caregiving, they are less likely to want to give long explanations about their child's care, and assistance from an experienced peer may be more appropriate for the nurse to seek. If the parents wish to maintain maximum participation in care delivery, the nurse and the parents can negotiate the collaboration.

When teaching parents to perform complex chronic care regimens at home, include teaching them to expect to know more about their child's care than professionals who may come to assist them, whether that be home health, hospital, or outpatient personnel. At the same time, assure them that what various professionals who work with them will have from working with a multitude of families is a scientific knowledge base and a wealth of options for addressing and solving care problems.

Teresa L. Hall, MS, RN
Hathaway Children's Services
Sylmar, Calif

⁇⁇ CRITICAL THINKING EXERCISE ⁇⁇

Family-Centered Home Care and Conflicts

A family wants to begin oral feeding of their 3-year-old daughter, Sarah, who is ventilator dependent, with a tracheostomy, and is being tube fed through a skin-level gastrostomy feeding tube (Mic-Key). The mother, who has assumed the role of being Sarah's primary caretaker, is quite adamant about starting oral feedings so Sarah can be more like other children her age. One day the mother asks you, the nurse case manager overseeing the child's home care, to feed Sarah baby food by mouth to see how she tolerates the feeding. The child is quite alert and sociable yet cannot communicate her wishes except through crying and whining. She does have a seizure disorder and has had several episodes of aspiration pneumonia since birth. Sarah appears to have a considerable amount of tongue thrusting and copious amounts of oral mucus that must be suctioned frequently to prevent aspiration; her cough reflex is compromised and usually only elicited with tracheal suctioning.

QUESTIONS

1. Evidence—Is there sufficient evidence to draw any conclusions about the issue of feeding Sarah at this time?
2. Assumptions—Describe some underlying assumptions about the following:
   a. Sarah's readiness for oral feedings.
   b. Sarah's ability to tolerate oral feedings.
   c. The mother's request for Sarah to start oral feedings.
3. What implications and priorities for nursing care may be drawn at this time?
4. Does the evidence objectively support your argument (conclusion)?
5. Are there alternative perspectives to your arguments? What are they?

ANSWERS

1. Yes, there is sufficient evidence to arrive at some possible conclusions.
2. Assumptions
   a. See text pages 329-331. Sarah demonstrates tongue thrusting, which is common in healthy children from 0 to 4 or 5 months. The extrusion reflex is quite common in children who have little experience with oral feedings and oral stimulation (see Feeding Resistance, p. 237).
   b. Given Sarah's history and assessment data, there are risks involved in starting oral feedings with Sarah, primarily choking and aspiration.
   c. The mother's request is not unusual. Parents want the best for their children despite handicaps that often set them apart from other peers. Although it may seem complicated to engage in communication, negotiation, and consultation over the seemingly simple issue of giving baby food to a 3-year-old, many issues must be considered.
      The family appears to have legitimate reasons for wanting their daughter started on baby foods. The nurse should further explore reasons for wanting the child to be fed orally. They may feel that health care providers have overlooked this aspect of normal development. The implications may be that the family is attempting to assist their daughter in achieving age-appropriate skills and may also want their daughter to participate in family mealtimes. These are legitimate, commendable goals, and the family should be supported in making such choices for their child.
3. A child who is 3 years old and has not been fed orally will benefit from an oral-motor assessment by an occupational therapist/speech therapist (OT/ST) to explore the possibility of starting minimal oral feedings. Specific plans with incremental steps to reduce oral-motor defensiveness and improve the ability to accept foods orally should precede feeding. Nutritional consultation may also be important as feeding plans shift from gastrostomy to oral feedings. The nurse and the family should continue to discuss the issue, plan for consultations and evaluation related to the child's oral-motor progress, and thereby arrange to meet the family's goals of oral feeding in safer incremental steps. Communication between the nurse and the family may also lead to other approaches to normalizing mealtimes for Sarah and her family. After the assessment has been completed by OT/ST specific short- and long-term goals for modified oral feedings may be developed involving the family in such discussions. In addition, the family should be made aware of potential problems with oral feedings, including aspiration pneumonia or airway obstruction with further respiratory compromise.
4. Yes, the evidence supports implementing this plan of care. The nurse should not dismiss the parents' request for oral feedings, yet should not acquiesce to their request without assessing the situation, developing conclusions based on the assessment, and implementing an appropriate plan of care that may be evaluated by the outcomes. It would not be appropriate to begin oral feedings without first consulting OT/ST regarding Sarah's oral-motor abilities.
5. Assessment of the child's status may reveal deficiencies that could preclude attempts at oral feedings altogether. In this case it would be important to involve other health care workers in a discussion with the parents regarding the issue of oral feedings. The home health care nurse must remember, however, that the child is the parent's responsibility and the ultimate decision about oral feedings rests with them. Home care issues that produce conflict about what constitutes the best care for the child between the primary caretaker or parents and the health care team must be handled with utmost care because the parents are ultimately responsible for the child. Such conflicts may lead to mistrust and further alienation if not handled properly. Each case should be handled on an individual basis and all available resources used to make the best care possible available to the child.

Both short-term and long-term goals should be outlined and agreed on by the child, family, and professionals involved. The plan of care should integrate various disciplines that may be involved with the child to minimize duplication and consolidate care requirements. Cross-training of professionals and a transdisciplinary mode of treatment can also be useful when a child has multiple and complex care requirements. For example, certain physical or occupational therapy routines may be incorporated into the child's morning nursing procedures, or speech therapy interventions may be conducted by the parent or nurse around eating times so the entire day is not occupied by procedures. A

FAMILY FOCUS

What I Learned About Home Care

I learned many things as a result of having home care for four children over a period of 8 years. Two of the major areas I learned about were communication and families' rights. It took a long time to learn some of these things.

Initially I tried very hard to be sensitive to the professionals and often put my own feelings and needs aside. It took a while to learn that I could stand up for myself and my family and that my child could continue to receive good care. One area that was important to me was to have nurses withhold judgment on our parenting style, even if they might have parented differently.

Communication needs to be open and two-way. Families and nurses ought to tell each other what is going well. For example, "Thanks for keeping the room so neat while you're here" can help a nurse see a family's appreciation. There was so little I could do as just "Mommy" that it really meant a lot to me when nurses would say, "That's such a cute outfit you picked out for him today." Communicating about little things, even inconsequential topics such as favorite TV shows, makes it easier to communicate about more important things and about problems. Communication has to be open about problems, too.

Jeni Stepanek
Mother
Upper Marlboro, Md

written schedule of daily routines should be developed and followed by all caregivers.

NURSING TIP

At each home visit physically handle and look at all medications. Check them against the medical orders and read the labels. There may be discrepancies, duplications, or changes between hospitalizations. Clarify medication purpose, effect, and dosages for the family.

Goals of care are supported by intervention strategies that reflect normalization (see Chapter 18) and the interests and abilities of the child and family. Nurses can help families explore a range of alternative strategies, services, and resources so that the family can choose the best match for their situation.

Family participation in evaluating a home care plan can occur on several levels. Families and care providers should regularly review the goals of care and then update the care plan as required. The nurse can also ask the family open-ended questions at regular intervals to assess their opinions on the effectiveness of care. As part of the evaluation process, families should be acknowledged for their successes and accomplishments. Finally, families should be given an opportunity to evaluate individual home care nurses, the home care agency, and other service providers periodically. The evaluation should address the nurse's knowledge, skills, and respect for the family's choices. The evaluations should be used by the agency to improve quality of care (see Family Focus box).

Home care nursing encourages a close and rewarding relationship with the family. One of the most important aspects of this relationship is maintaining professional boundaries and a therapeutic role that is supportive but not intrusive. In addi-

tion to maintaining control over their child's care, families need to control their homes and personal lives. Nurses should discuss "house rules" with the family and address issues such as physical environment, private areas in the home, responsibility for maintaining the child's environment, and interactions with siblings and extended family members (see Guidelines box on p. 629 and Critical Thinking Exercise on p. 632).

Technologic trends that influence the nursing process in home care include the use of *laptop computers (notebooks)* to document the home visit; *personal data assistants (PDAs),* or small handheld computers that store large amounts of data including addresses, appointments, patient tracking systems, textbooks, and important data such as pharmacologic databases (Lewis and Sommers, 2003); *Internet and e-mail* services, which increase patient-practitioner accessibility and communication; and *telemedicine or telehealth,* which has various features including electronic systems that can transmit physiologic data directly to the practitioner via the telephone. The American Nurses Association (1999) has established a list of competencies for nurses involved in telehealth technology. *Telephone triage* has become standard in many health care institutions, and standards for triage have been published elsewhere. Concerns with the increase in the use of technology in health care are cost, governmental regulations and patient care standards, liability and malpractice issues, ethics, and confidentiality matters (Rice, 2001). In addition, concerns regarding the nurse-patient relationship (high tech–low touch) and the role of the nurse are raised with the use of any technology.

PROMOTION OF OPTIMAL DEVELOPMENT, SELF-CARE, AND EDUCATION

There is little question that living at home offers most children with complex medical problems great social and emotional advantages over living in the hospital or other institutional setting. However, in infancy and throughout the developmental stages, a child's medical condition(s) and the dependence on medical technology can place constraints on and pose challenges to *normal development.* For example, the child may have lengthy and repeated hospitalizations; developmental regression can occur in response to stress; fatigue may be due to underlying pathology, the flare of an illness, or medication side effects; and equipment requirements may impede mobility, exploration, and independence. The challenge of providing support for normal development in a child who is chronically ill and technology-dependent is to optimize opportunities for developmentally appropriate experiences within the constraints posed by the medical condition and the equipment requirements.

Home care plans are designed to promote optimal child development through initial and periodic assessment, planning, and referrals for further assessment or therapeutic services and by interventions that address normalization issues and self-care. (See Chapter 18 for a discussion of normalization.) General principles for a family-centered assessment and planning process have been addressed earlier in this chapter and are also applied in developmental assessment and planning.

Some parents may not pursue *early developmental intervention* because they do not view their child as needing the

??? CRITICAL THINKING EXERCISE ???

Maintaining Therapeutic Boundaries

As the home care nurse who has been working with a 4-year-old ventilator-dependent child, Derek, weekly for about 5 months, you are aware that the parents have become increasingly argumentative with each other. Most of the arguments are about whether Mr. Jones helps enough with the child's care and the house cleaning. Mr. Jones works full time at one job then supplements the family income by working at a part-time job every weekend. Ms. Jones approaches you to complain about her husband's lack of involvement with the child and his care. Derek requires constant care, and the family has many expenses related to his physical care; the child is severely developmentally impaired and is not expected to improve significantly despite numerous medical interventions. He is the only child, although Ms. Jones stated at one time they wanted to have more children.

QUESTIONS
1. Evidence—Is there sufficient evidence to draw any conclusions about the family situation at this time?
2. Assumptions—Describe some underlying assumptions about the following:
   a. Home care of the child with a chronic, terminal condition (see pp. 623-624, 631)
   b. Impact of the chronic condition, child's prognosis, and required care on the parents
   c. Status of the marriage relationship between Mr. and Ms. Jones
3. What implications and priorities for nursing care may be drawn at this time?
4. Does the evidence objectively support your argument (conclusion)?
5. Are there alternative perspectives to your arguments? What are they?

ANSWERS
1. Yes—there is sufficient evidence to arrive at some conclusions regarding the situation.
2. Assumptions
   a. Home care of any person, especially a child with a chronic debilitating condition, is stressful on any family regardless of their stability and resources. The seeming lack of coping skills and decreased financial resources make the stress worse. It is not unusual for there to be stress and conflict regarding the child's care, especially if one parent seems to be less involved in the daily care. The needs of the primary caretaker, Ms. Jones, in this instance, are not being met, and she is expressing that frustration to the nurse, who perhaps is perceived as an ally in the situation.
   b. The impact of a chronic condition on parents can be devastating and lead to misunderstandings, competition over the care of the child, and neglect of the feelings of the persons involved, which, in this case, are Mr. and Ms. Jones. Because the child's prognosis is poor, this can further exacerbate feelings of frustration, anger, helplessness, fatigue, and conflict among parents. Parents may feel guilty about their feelings toward the child. On one hand, there may be feelings of caring and loving toward the child; on the other hand, the presence of a child with a chronic condition with poor prognosis who requires constant physical care may engender feelings of wanting to see an end to the situation with the child's death. These ambivalent feelings are not unusual in parents, yet it is well-known that there is gender difference in how feelings over such conditions are expressed. Unmet expectations are a source of conflict among parents with a child who is sick; expectations of each other's role in the family setting may have suffered with the loss of the "perfect" child. These feelings may last for months or even years without an appropriate resolution if adequate resources for resolution are not provided.
   c. The status of the marriage appears to be strained at this time; however, there is not sufficient evidence to draw a simple conclusion without further exploration (assessment). This may be the way each parent deals with crisis situations—the mother fusses and complains and the father withdraws by going to work and being less involved. There may be some anticipatory grieving occurring, but this needs to be explored by health care persons who can be objective and properly evaluate the marriage status.
3. The concept of therapeutic boundaries supports the idea that they are not rigid and fixed. The home care nurse must be responsive to the relationship preferred by the family and the style with which the family operates. Individual roles change according to the expectations that person has about her or his role and the context within which that person is living the role. In this situation it would be appropriate for the nurse to mention that home care can be stressful for a family, indicate that referrals for counseling may be provided if desired by the parents, and listen and reflect with Ms. Jones about her feelings. Exploring issues such as an additional home care aide to help take care of Derek might be appropriate; this would enable Ms. Jones to take a break from his care and have time to herself. Additional financial aid may be explored by a qualified case manager or social worker so Mr. Jones would not have to work as much away from home. It is important to explore the couple's feelings regarding Derek's condition and care and their role in providing for him, as well as their relationship to each other. It is not unusual for families in crisis to become so involved in the care of the child that they forget what their marriage and relationship is about within the context of the crisis. If counseling by another professional is not desired by one or both parties, perhaps other avenues such as family support groups could be explored as an option. For any conclusion you may reach, it would be inappropriate to agree with Ms. Jones that her husband is not helping enough with the child's care. Such an action implies a judgment that is not within the nurse's role to make and undermines rather than supports the family system. Families in crisis often require professional assistance in the form of counseling to explore coping skills and help involve appropriate community resources.
4. There is some preliminary evidence to support the argument that professional help is warranted in this situation. In addition, as the feelings of Mr. and Ms. Jones are explored, additional evidence may present which may alter the course of action proposed.
5. Alternative perspectives may arise as more data are obtained during a family interview. It would not be appropriate for the home health care nurse to take sides with Ms. Jones or with Mr. Jones to avoid the main issues, which involve Ms. Jones' sense of isolation in the care of her child.

services. In this case professionals need to explain the child's developmental needs to parents in ways that are meaningful from the parents' own cultural and socioeconomic perspectives. Only then can parents make truly informed decisions. After parents have been fully informed of the child's condition, likely developmental sequelae, and the expected benefits of intervention, developmental goals outlined by the child and family should guide planning and intervention.

Several principles underlie appropriate developmental intervention plans for children with complex medical problems. First, understanding a child's medical condition ensures that the nurse and family can plan to maximize developmental opportunities at times when the child has the most energy and endurance and when stress signals that determine the child's tolerance for type, intensity, and duration of activity will be noted. Second, plans for developmental support should be flexible and tailored to the individual child's abilities, interests, and needs. Third, familiarity with the child's medical equipment facilitates the planning of creative ways to meet the child's developmental needs. For example, the use of lengthy oxygen tubing allows the active toddler freedom of movement during the day (Fig. 20-2); portable equipment of any type facilitates family outings; and mounting a ventilator to a wheelchair allows the adolescent greater independence.

Promoting coping and capability can buffer stress and contribute to mental health and self-esteem in a child with chronic illness. The extent to which a child is involved in his or her own care depends on many factors, including the child's developmental age, level of interest, and physical ability, as well as parental comfort and support. *Self-care,* both in activities of daily living and in regard to the medical condition, is important. The frame of reference for self-care in activities of daily living should be the goal of attaining age-appropriate competence. Some modifications in the environment, the medical equipment, and/or the techniques for daily activities may be required to promote and support self-care. Effective teaching for self-care is focused at the child's own level of conceptual understanding and may be augmented by the use of dolls, other models and diagrams, simple explanations, and repetition.

Educational planning is important for the child who has a chronic medical condition. Federal laws ensure that all children receive a public education. Before age 3, children with developmental delays are eligible for an *early-intervention program.* The child can receive rehabilitation therapies as appropriate (physical therapy/occupational therapy/speech therapy, speech pathology). After age 3, the local school system is responsible for providing this education. Some children may be eligible for special education preschools. The home care nurse should refer the family to local county programs.

Each family is entitled to an *individual family service plan (IFSP)* to help ensure early intervention. All states in the United States provide agencies that develop IFSPs; each state's plan can easily be accessed via the Internet by entering the term *individual family service plan* in an Internet search engine such as Yahoo or Google. The IFSP provides the child with disability from birth to age 3 with a plan for integrating early intervention and rehabilitation, based on the child's and family's needs.

When a child requiring special medical care is to be placed in an educational setting, the parents, child, school health co-

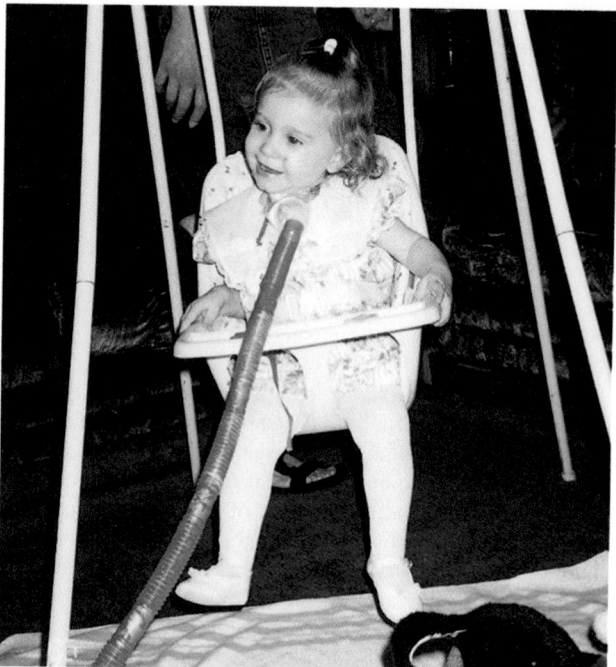

FIG. 20-2 ■ Use of lengthy tubing facilitates a child's freedom of movement.

ordinator, educational evaluation team, and educational and administrative staff should meet to determine safe and appropriate placement and necessary services and personnel to enable the child to attend school in the least restrictive environment. Training of educational staff and caregivers is essential to ensuring the child's safety in the educational setting.* Special assistance can also be beneficial in reintegrating previously schooled children, such as those with cancer, into the school setting. The home care nurse may need to assist parents in developing the skills necessary to advocate effectively for their child in the educational system.

Consultation with a child-life specialist may also be arranged and can be of great assistance to the nurse and family.

SAFETY ISSUES IN THE HOME

Safety is an important consideration in pediatric home care and should be addressed in the home care plan.

> **NURSING TIP**
>
> If the family does not have a telephone, arrangements may be made with the telephone company to supply service. Alternatively, one or two nearby neighbors may agree to let the family use their services. In rural areas a local pharmacy or police or ranger station may be willing to receive messages and relay them to the family. A cell phone may be used in place of a local telephone but it is advisable to check with the local emergency facilities regarding policies for cell phone use and emergency 9-1-1 calls.

*A thorough discussion of training issues, content, and guidelines for care in the school are provided in Porter S, Bierle T, Haynie M, Caldwell TH, Palfrey JS, editors: *Children and youth assisted by medical technology in educational settings: guidelines for care,* ed 2, Baltimore, Md, 1997, Paul H. Brookes; website: www.pbrookes.com.

The telephone and electric companies (if use of medical equipment requires electricity) must be notified that the family needs to be placed on a priority service list so that the family will learn of any anticipated interruptions in service and receive priority in reinstatement of interrupted services. Prior contact with rescue squad and local emergency facility personnel can help ensure prompt and appropriate interventions if required. This is especially important if the family lives in a rural or remote location that may not be familiar to local emergency responders. It is recommended that a map be given to local authorities with key landmarks and intersections for rapid accessibility to the home.

Before hospital discharge, emergency protocols are developed and reviewed with both the parents and the professional caregivers. Cardiopulmonary resuscitation (CPR) guidelines, if appropriate, should be posted near the child's bedside or in another accessible location. A list of emergency telephone numbers can be placed near each home phone and should include those of the rescue squad, emergency room, managing physician(s), nursing agency, and durable medical equipment vendor(s). Additional issues to consider are advance directives and Out of Hospital Do Not Resuscitate (OHDNR) orders (may vary by state), as indicated. If the patient and family desire *advance directives* to be enforced, there are specific guidelines that must be followed and could potentially prevent undesired life-saving measures for children with terminal illnesses.

Another aspect of safety relates to the provision of care by appropriately trained individuals. Family members should receive thorough training in the child's care requirements and have the opportunity to demonstrate knowledge and confidence before hospital discharge. Professional staff caring for the child should have the appropriate background and training for the child's particular care needs. Because of the child's body size, special skill and caution are required both in performing procedures (e.g., gastrostomy feedings, suctioning) and in monitoring the use of equipment (e.g., ventilator settings, intravenous flow rates, total fluid volumes) (see Chapter 22). A tool that might be helpful to the pediatric home care nurse is a 13-item assessment designed to ascertain caregiver stress and subsequently develop appropriate strategies for individual and family coping; this tool is the Caregiver Strain Index (Sullivan, 2003).

The activity level and curiosity of young children raise additional safety considerations in the provision of home care. All medications, needles, syringes, and any contaminated materials are securely stored well out of the reach of curious hands. Arrangements for the disposal of contaminated materials and sharp items can be made with a home health agency or hospital. Special attention is paid to childproofing the control panels for ventilators, pumps, monitors, and other equipment. The use of clear plastic tape, covers, or panels to cover control knobs or buttons reduces the risk of accidental changes in settings. Much of the medical equipment now in use has special lock-out capabilities that may be used to prevent accidentally altering settings. Electrical cords should be kept short and out of reach, and safety covers are used on any open outlets. When not in use, equipment is unplugged, and any wires (e.g., lead wires for an apnea monitor) should be stored out of reach.

BOX 20-6 ■ Selected Resources for Home Care

American Academy of Pediatrics
141 Northwest Point Boulevard
Elk Grove Village, IL 60007-1098
(847) 434-4000
Fax: (847) 434-8000
www.aap.org

Association of Maternal and Child Health Programs
1220 19th Street, NW
Suite 801
Washington, DC 20036
(202) 775-0436
Fax: (202) 775-0061
www.amchp.org

Children's Hospice International
901 N. Pitt Street, Suite 230
Alexandria, VA 22314
(800) 2-4-CHILD
Fax: (703) 684-0226
www.chionline.org

National Association for Home Care
228 Seventh Street SE
Washington, DC 20003
(202) 547-7424
Fax: (202) 547-3540
www.nahc.org
(A special feature on the website is peds@home, an electronic newsletter.)

National Father's Network
16120 NE 8th Street
Bellevue, WA 98008-3937
(206) 747-4404, ext 218
www.fathersnetwork.org

National Information Center for Children and Youth With Disabilities
PO Box 1492
Washington, DC 20013-1492
(202) 884-8200 (voice/TTY) or (800) 695-0285 (voice/TTY)
Fax: (202) 884-8441
www.nichcy.org
Website: www.nichcy.org

Pediatric Home Care Association of America
Division of National Association for Home Care
228 Seventh Street, SE
Washington, DC 20003
(202) 547-7424
Fax: (202) 547-3540
www.nahc.org

Pediatric Nursing.com
Health Resources for Parents
www.pediatricnursing.com/parents/

Sibling Support Project
The Arc of the United States
6512 23rd Avenue NW, Suite 213
Seattle, WA 98117
(206) 297-6368
www.thearc.org/siblingsupport/

Care at night poses other safety concerns. Steps must be taken to prevent accidental strangulation on apnea, pulse oximeter, or cardiac monitor wires or lengthy intravenous tubing during sleep. Parents or other caregivers need to be able to clearly hear monitor, ventilator, or pump alarms at night; an inexpensive intercom system or a baby monitor can be used.

> **NURSING TIP**
>
> Coiling extra tubing and taping it at the exit site, as well as running wires or tubes out the bottoms of pajamas, is a precaution against strangulation.

Safe transportation is a vitally important concern. Wheelchairs and other medical equipment must be properly secured to the vehicle, including vans and buses. Appropriate child restraints must be used at all times. If necessary, an extra adult should be present to monitor the child while in transit. Additional information on car safety and general health supervision is provided in Chapter 18.

FAMILY-TO-FAMILY SUPPORT

Family-to-family support networks can be an important source of emotional and instrumental support and empowerment for families of children with chronic health problems. Family-to-family support does not replace professional sources of support but rather is a unique resource promoting family strengths through shared experience. Families will most likely experience increased emotional stress as a result of living with and caring for a child with special needs. Identifying meaningful sources of support can make a difference in coping abilities (see Box 20-6). The home health nurse can assist the family in increasing their involvement in community social networks. Informal support networks can be extremely beneficial. A link to a family in the same or similar situation allows the sharing of common experiences. Positive outcomes may include understanding, empathy, problem solving, or just talking to someone who will listen. The nurse should remember that the needs of each family member differ. The care plan should acknowledge each family member's needs. Peer support for school-age children and adolescents with complex care needs may be beneficial. These connections can be expanded to include letter writing, e-mails, phone calls, or specialty camping programs (Johnson, Ravert, and Everton, 2001).

Most of the time school-age children and adolescents just want to be accepted by their peers and fit in as a part of the group. Same-age peers may at first be standoffish to children with disabilities, but this is likely out of fear and lack of understanding; helping others see that they have the same dreams, desires, goals, and interests helps promote group cohesiveness and understanding.

KEY POINTS

- Effective home care depends on many factors, including the child's medical stability; the family's/caregiver's willingness, training, and ability to accommodate the child's care requirements; and professional, financial, and community support.

- Comprehensive, multidisciplinary discharge planning should begin early and should include the family and a home care representative in addition to medical personnel.

- Thorough training of the family, including a period of "rooming in" and a predischarge home visit, can ease the transition to home.

- Care coordination ensures continuity of care and reduces fragmentation of services. The family may assume varying degrees of care coordination over time and become the lead care coordinator.

- The home care nurse must share a level of technical expertise with the critical care nurse while being able to adapt equipment, procedures, and the nursing process to the home setting. Education, training, and creativity in care are increasingly important.

- Federal standards apply to agencies that participate in Medicare or Medicaid; standards of practice by the American Nurses Association can guide nurses in the home setting. Specialist and generalist credentialing is available for home care nurses.

- Family-centered nursing practice is the cornerstone of pediatric home health nursing. The family's integrity, privacy, religion, and cultural and personal values are an integral part of the child's life and are respected as such.

- One of the primary goals of pediatric home care is to help the family/caregiver achieve independence in the provision of care for the child and maximize opportunities for the child to be placed in an early learning program or school setting, as the medical condition allows.

- Collaborative relationships are characterized by communication, dialogue, active listening, awareness and acceptance of difference, and negotiation.

- The nursing process is adapted to involve the family in each step and to preserve the family's central role in decision making.

- The current nursing shortage, increased demands on the family for providing for the cost of care, increased regulations for home care nursing, and decreased reimbursements require home care nurses to function as care managers and work closely with the family and other health care providers to maximize family function and care of the child.

- "House rules" agreed on by the nurse and family allow a family to maintain a feeling of control over their own environment when professionals are present.

- Home care plans are designed to promote optimal development of the child and focus on normalization and the impact of the child's medical condition and technologic requirements on development, on self-care, and on educational needs.

- Safety in the provision of home care services involves emergency preparations and protocols, appropriate training of family and home care personnel, and safe use and childproofing of medical equipment.

- Family-to-family support networks can both provide emotional and instrumental support and encourage family empowerment.

References

American Academy of Pediatrics: *The medical home and early intervention*, Elk Grove Village, Il, 1995, The Academy.

American Academy of Pediatrics: *Care coordination: integrating health and related systems of care for children with special health care needs*, Elk Grove Village, Il, 1999, The Academy.

American Nurses Association: *Competencies for telehealth technologies in nursing*, Washington, DC, 1999, The Association.

American Nurses Association: *Standards of community health nursing practice*, Washington, DC, 1986a, The Association.

American Nurses Association: *Standards of home health nursing practice,* Washington, DC, 1986b, The Association.

American Nurses Association: *Nursing case management,* Washington, DC, 1998, The Association.

Bakewell-Sachs S and others: Home care considerations for chronic and vulnerable populations, *Nurse Pract Forum* 11(1):65-72, 2000.

Betz CL: Children and youth in out-of-home placements: nursing care opportunities for pediatric nurses, *J Pediatr Nurs* 15(1):1-2, 2000.

Dittbrenner H: Pediatric home care as a viable new service, *Caring* 18(2):12-15, 1999.

Gaudet L: Stress tolerance. In Votroubek WL, Townsend JL, editors: *Pediatric home care,* ed 2, Gaithersburg, Md, 1997, Aspen.

Giger JN, Davidhizar R: The Giger and Davidhizar Transcultural Assessment Model, *J Transcult Nurs* 13(3):185-188, 2002.

Johnson BH: Family-centered care: facing the new millennium: interview by Elizabeth Ahmann, *Pediatr Nurs* 26(1):87-90, 2000.

Johnson KB, Ravert RD, Everton A: Hopkins Teen Central: assessment of an internet-based support system for children with cystic fibrosis, *Pediatrics* 107(2):e24, 2001.

Kellett UM, Mannion J: Meaning in caring: reconceptualizing the nurse-family carer relationship in community practice, *J Adv Nurs* 29(3):697-703, 1999.

Knafl KA, Deatrick JA: The challenges of normalization for families of children with chronic conditions, *Pediatr Nurs* 28(1):49-53, 56, 2002.

Lewis JA, Sommers CO: Personal data assistants: using new technology to enhance nursing practice, *MCN* 28(2):66-71, 2003.

Lindeke LL and others: Family-centered care coordination for children with special needs across multiple settings, *J Pediatr Health Care* 16(6):290-297, 2002.

Mahony DL, Murphy JM: Neonatal drug exposure: assessing a specific population and services provided by visiting nurses, *Pediatr Nurs* 25(1):27-34, 108, 1999.

McDaniel SH, Campbell TL: Training for collaborative family healthcare, *Fam Systems Health* 14(2):147-150, 1996.

McEvoy M: Culture & spirituality as an integrated concept in pediatric care, *MCN* 28(1):39-43, 2003.

National Alliance of Caregivers: Family caregiving in the U.S.: findings from a national survey, 1997, The Alliance; available at www.caregiving.org.

National Center for Cultural Competence: Developing cultural competence in health care settings, *Pediatr Nurs* 28(2):133-137, 2002.

Page DR: Pediatric home care: nursing the shortage, *Caring* 20(6):46-47, 2001.

Rice R: Case management and leadership strategies for home care nurses. In Rice R, editor, *Home care nursing practice: concepts and application,* ed 3, St Louis, 2001, Mosby.

Roush CV, Cox JE: The meaning of home: how it shapes the practice of home and hospice care, *Home Healthcare Nurse* 18(6):388-394, 2000.

Spruhan JB: Beyond traditional nursing care: cultural awareness and successful home healthcare nursing, *Home Healthcare Nurse* 14(6):445-449, 1996.

Sullivan T: Caregiver Strain Index, *Home Healthcare Nurse* 21(3):197-198, 2003.

Thompson J: Pediatric assessment in the home, *Home Health Nurse* 18(10):639-646, 2000.

Timm S: Effectively delegating nursing activities in home care, *Home Healthcare Nurse* 21(4):260-265, 2003.

Wilson A: Understanding benchmarks, *Home Healthcare Nurse* 21(2):102-107, 2003.

Yoder-Wise P: *Leading and managing in nursing,* ed 3, St Louis, 2003, Mosby.

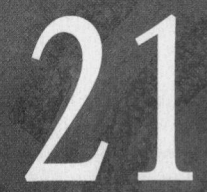

Family-Centered Care of the Child During Illness and Hospitalization

CHRIS ALGREN

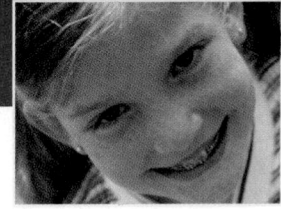

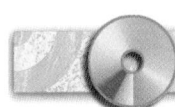
Remember to check out your companion CD-ROM

http://evolve.elsevier.com/Wong/essentials/

CHAPTER OUTLINE

RELATED TOPICS and ADDITIONAL RESOURCES

 IN TEXT

Administration of Medication, *Ch. 22*

Communication and Health Assessment of the Child and Family, *Ch. 6*

Compliance, *Ch. 22*

Cultural/Religious Influences on Health Care, *Ch. 4*

Family-Centered Care, *Ch. 18*

Family-Centered Home Care, *Ch. 20*

Impact of Chronic Illness, Disability, or Death on the Child and Family, *Ch. 18*

Neonatal Pain, *Ch. 9*

Normalization, *Ch. 18*

Nursing Diagnosis, *Ch. 1*

Physical and Developmental Assessment of the Child, *Ch. 7*

Preparation for Procedures, *Ch. 22*

Surgical Procedures, *Ch. 22*

 CD COMPANION

Critical Thinking Exercise—Discharge Planning

Guidelines—Nonpharmacologic Pain Management; Using Buffered Lidocaine; Supporting the Child and Family During Hospital Admission

Clinical Manifestations—Separation Anxiety in Young Children

Nursing Care Plans—The Child in the Hospital; The Family of the Child Who Is Ill or Hospitalized

Drug Dosage Guidelines—Selected Combination of Opioid and Nonopioid Oral Analgesic—Nonaspirin Products; Nonsteroidal Antiinflammatory Drugs Approved for Children; Dosage of Selected Opioids for Children; Selected Analgesics (Equianalgesic)

NCLEX-Style Review Questions

 WEBSITE

WebLinks

NCLEX-Style Review Questions

WONG'S CLINICAL MANUAL OF PEDIATRIC NURSING, 6/E

Community and Home Care Instructions—Applying EMLA and Various Technical Skills such as Giving Oral Medications and Intramuscular Injections

For additional information on pain assessment, please view "Pain Assessment and Management" in *Whaley and Wong's Pediatric Nursing Video Series,* St Louis, 1996, Mosby; (800) 426-4545; website: www.elsevierhealth.com.

LEARNING OBJECTIVES
On completion of this chapter the reader will be able to:

- Identify the stressors of illness and hospitalization for children during each developmental stage.
- List essential priorities of nursing care for a child on admission to the hospital.
- Outline nursing interventions that prevent or minimize the stress of separation during hospitalization.

- Outline nursing interventions that minimize the stress of loss of control during hospitalization.
- Outline nursing interventions that minimize the fear of bodily injury during hospitalization.
- Describe methods of assessing and managing pain in children.

- Outline nursing interventions that support parents, siblings, and family during a child's illness and hospitalization.
- Describe nursing interventions needed when children are admitted to special units such as the emergency department.

STRESSORS OF HOSPITALIZATION AND CHILDREN'S REACTIONS

Often, illness and hospitalization are the first crises children must face. Especially during the early years, children are particularly vulnerable to the crises of illness and hospitalization because (1) stress represents a change from the usual state of health and environmental routine and (2) children have a limited number of coping mechanisms to resolve *stressors* (those events that produce stress). Major stressors of hospitalization include separation, loss of control, bodily injury, and pain. Children's reactions to these crises are influenced by their developmental age; their previous experience with illness, separation, or hospitalization; their innate and acquired coping skills; the seriousness of the diagnosis; and the support system available.

SEPARATION ANXIETY

The major stress from middle infancy throughout the preschool years, especially for children ages 6 to 30 months, is separation anxiety, also called *anaclitic depression.* The principal behavioral responses to this stressor during early childhood are summarized in Box 21-1.

During the phase of *protest,* children react aggressively to the separation from the parent. They cry and scream for their parents, refuse the attention of anyone else, and are inconsolable in their grief (Fig. 21-1). During the phase of *despair,* the crying stops, and depression is evident. The child is much less active, is uninterested in play or food, and withdraws from others (Fig. 21-2).

The third stage is *detachment,* also called *denial.* Superficially it appears that the child has finally adjusted to the

BOX 21-1 ■ Manifestations of Separation Anxiety in Young Children

PHASE OF PROTEST
Observed behaviors during later infancy:
 Cries
 Screams
 Searches for parent with eyes
 Clings to parent
 Avoids and rejects contact with strangers
Additional behaviors observed during toddlerhood:
 Verbally attacks strangers (e.g., "Go away")
 Physically attacks strangers (e.g., kicks, bites, hits, pinches)
 Attempts to escape to find parent
 Attempts to physically force parent to stay
Behaviors may last from hours to days
Protest, such as crying, may be continuous, ceasing only with physical exhaustion
Approach of stranger may precipitate increased protest

PHASE OF DESPAIR
Observed behaviors:
 Inactive
 Withdraws from others
 Depressed, sad
 Uninterested in environment
 Uncommunicative
 Regresses to earlier behavior (e.g., thumb sucking, bed-wetting, use of pacifier, use of bottle)
Behaviors may last for variable length of time
Child's physical condition may deteriorate from refusal to eat, drink, or move

PHASE OF DETACHMENT
Observed behaviors:
 Shows increased interest in surroundings
 Interacts with strangers or familiar caregivers
 Forms new but superficial relationships
 Appears happy
Detachment usually occurs after prolonged separation from parent; rarely seen in hospitalized children
Behaviors represent a superficial adjustment to loss

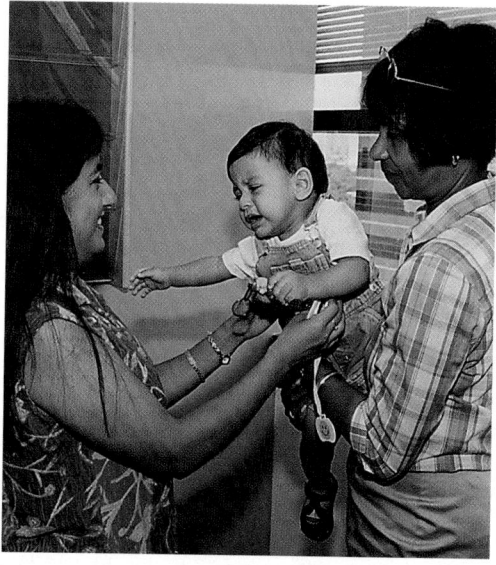

FIG. 21-1 ■ In the protest phase of separation anxiety children cry loudly and are inconsolable in their grief for the parent. (Courtesy James DeLeon, Texas Children's Hospital.)

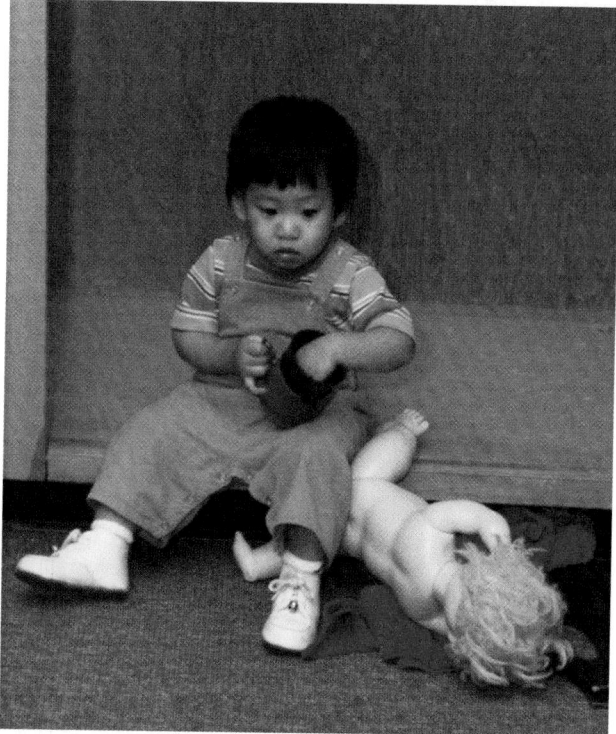

FIG. 21-2 ■ During the despair phase of separation anxiety, children are sad, lonely, and uninterested in food and play.

loss. The child becomes more interested in the surroundings, plays with others, and seems to form new relationships. However, this behavior is the result of resignation and is not a sign of contentment. The child detaches from the parent in an effort to escape the emotional pain of desiring the parent's presence and copes by forming shallow relationships with others, becoming increasingly self-centered, and attaching primary importance to material objects. This is the most serious stage in that reversal of the potential adverse effects is less likely to occur after detachment is established. However, in most situations, the temporary separations imposed by hospitalization do not cause such prolonged parental absences that the child enters into detachment. In addition, considerable evidence suggests that even with stressors such as separation, children are remarkably adaptable and permanent ill effects are rare.

Although progression to the stage of detachment is uncommon, the initial stages are frequently observed even with very brief separations from either parent. Unless health team members understand the meaning of each stage of behavior, they may erroneously label the behaviors as positive or negative. For example, they may see the loud crying of the protest phase as "bad" behavior. Because the protesting increases when a stranger approaches the child, they may interpret that reaction as meaning they should stay away. During the quiet, withdrawn phase of despair, health team members may think that the child is finally "settling in" to the new surroundings, and they may see the detachment behaviors as proof of a "good adjustment." The faster this stage is reached, the more likely it is that the child will be regarded as the "ideal patient."

Because children seem to react "negatively" to visits by their parents, uninformed observers feel justified in restricting parental visiting privileges. For example, during the protest stage, children outwardly do not appear happy to see their parents. In fact, they may even cry louder. If they are depressed, they may reject their parents or begin to protest again. Often they cling to their parents in an effort to ensure their continued presence. Consequently, such reactions may be regarded as "disturbing" the child's adjustment to the new surroundings. If the separation has progressed to the phase of detachment, children will respond no differently to their parents than they would to any other person.

Such reactions are distressing to parents, who are unaware of their meaning. If parents are regarded as intruders, they will see their absence as "beneficial" to the child's adjustment and recovery. They may respond to the child's behavior by staying for only short periods, visiting less frequently, or deceiving the child when it is time to leave. The result is a destructive cycle of misunderstanding and unmet needs.

Early Childhood

Separation anxiety is the greatest stress imposed by hospitalization during early childhood. If separation is avoided, young children have a tremendous capacity to withstand any other stress. During this age period, the typical reactions just described are seen. However, children in the toddler stage demonstrate more goal-directed behaviors. For example, they may plead with the parents to stay and physically try to keep the parents with them or try to find parents who have left. They may demonstrate displeasure on the parents' return or departure by having temper tantrums; refusing to comply with the usual routines of mealtime, bedtime, or toileting; or regressing to more primitive levels of development. However, temper tantrums, bed-wetting, or other behaviors may also be expressions of anger or even a physiologic response to stress.

Because preschoolers are more secure interpersonally than toddlers, they can tolerate brief periods of separation from their parents and are more inclined to develop substitute trust in other significant adults. However, the stress of illness usually renders preschoolers less able to cope with separation; as a result, they manifest many of the stage behaviors of separation anxiety, although in general the protest behaviors are more subtle and passive than those seen in younger children. Preschoolers may demonstrate separation anxiety by refusing to eat, experiencing difficulty in sleeping, crying quietly for their parents, continually asking when the parents will visit, or withdrawing from others. They may express anger indirectly by breaking their toys, hitting other children, or refusing to cooperate during usual self-care activities. Nurses need to be sensitive to these less obvious signs of separation anxiety in order to intervene appropriately.

Later Childhood and Adolescence

Previous research, usually based on adult recollections, indicated that the family does not play as important a role for school-age children as it does during the toddler and preschool years. However, in a recent study that asked children about their fears when hospitalized, children ranked "being away from my family" higher than any other fear associated with hospitalization (Wilson and Yorker, 1997). Although school-age children are better able to cope with separation in general, the stress and often accompanying regression imposed by illness or hospitalization may increase their need for parental security and guidance. This is particularly true for young school-age children who have only recently left the safety of the home and are struggling with the crisis of school adjustment. Middle and late school-age children may react more to the separation from their usual activities and peers than to the absence of their parents. These children have a high level of physical and mental activity that frequently finds no suitable outlets in the hospital environment, and even when they dislike school, they admit to missing its routine and worry that they will not be able to compete or "fit in" with their classmates when they return. Feelings of loneliness, boredom, isolation, and depression are common. Such reactions may occur more as a result of separation than from concern over the illness, treatment, or hospital setting.

School-age children may need and desire parental guidance or support from other adult figures but may be unable or unwilling to ask for it. Because the goal of attaining independence is so important to them, they are reluctant to seek help directly for fear that they will appear weak, childish, or dependent. Cultural expectations to "act like a man" or to "be brave and strong" bear heavily on these children, especially boys, who tend to react to stress with stoicism, withdrawal, or passive acceptance. Often the need to express hostile, angry, or other negative feelings finds outlets in alternate ways, such as irritability and aggression toward parents, withdrawal from hospital personnel, inability to relate to peers, rejection of siblings, or subsequent behavioral problems in school.

For adolescents, separation from home and parents may be a welcomed and appreciated event. However, loss of peer-group contact may pose a severe emotional threat because of loss of group status, inability to exert group control or leadership, and loss of group acceptance. Deviations within peer groups are poorly tolerated, and although group members may express concern for the adolescent's illness or need for hospitalization, they continue their group activities, quickly filling the gap of the absent member. During the temporary separation from their usual group, ill adolescents may benefit from group associations with other hospitalized age-mates.

LOSS OF CONTROL

One of the factors influencing the amount of stress imposed by hospitalization is the amount of control that persons perceive themselves as having. Lack of control increases the perception of threat and can affect children's coping skills. Many hospital situations decrease the amount of control a child feels. Although the usual sensory stimulations are lacking, the additional hospital stimuli of sight, sound, and smell may be overwhelming. Without an insight into the type of environment conducive to children's optimal growth, the hospital experience can at best temporarily slow development and at worst permanently restrict it. Because children's needs vary greatly depending on their age, the major areas of loss of control in terms of physical restriction, altered routine or rituals, and dependency are discussed for each age-group.

Infants

Infants are developing the most important attribute of a healthy personality—trust. Trust is established through consistent, loving care by a nurturing person. Infants attempt to control their environment through emotional expressions, such as crying or smiling. In the hospital setting, cues may be missed or misinterpreted, and routines may be established to meet the hospital staff's needs instead of the infant's needs. Inconsistent care and deviations from the infant's daily routine may lead to mistrust and a decreased sense of control.

Toddlers

Toddlers are striving for autonomy, and this goal is evident in most of their behaviors—motor skills, play, interpersonal relationships, activities of daily living, and communication. When their egocentric pleasures meet with obstacles, toddlers react with negativism, especially temper tantrums. Any restriction or limitation of movement, such as the simple act of making toddlers lie down, can cause forceful resistance and noncompliance.

Loss of control also results from altered routines and rituals. Toddlers rely on the consistency and familiarity of daily rituals to provide a measure of stability and control in their complex world of growing and developing. The experience of hospitalization or illness severely limits their sense of expectation and predictability, since practically every detail of the hospital environment differs from that of the home.

Toddlers' main areas for rituals include eating, sleeping, bathing, toileting, and play. When the routines are disrupted, difficulties can occur in any or all of these areas. The principal reaction to such change is regression. For example, when mealtime and food choices differ from those at home, toddlers often refuse to eat, demand a bottle, or ask others to feed them. Although regression to earlier forms of behavior may seem to increase toddlers' security and comfort, in reality it is very threatening for them to relinquish their most recently acquired achievements.

Enforced dependency is a chief characteristic of the sick role and accounts for the numerous instances of toddler negativism. For example, rigid schedules, different clothes, altered caregiving activities, unfamiliar surroundings, separation from parents, and medical procedures usurp toddlers' control over their world. Although most toddlers initially react negatively and aggressively to such dependency, prolonged loss of autonomy may result in passive withdrawal from interpersonal relationships and regression in all areas of development. Therefore the effects of the sick role are most severe in instances of chronic, long-term illnesses or in those families who foster the sick role despite the child's improved state of health.

Preschoolers

Preschoolers also suffer from loss of control caused by physical restriction, altered routines, and enforced dependency. However, their specific cognitive abilities, which make them feel omnipotent and all-powerful, also make them feel out of control. This loss of control in the context of their sense of self-power is a critical influencing factor in their perception of and reaction to separation, pain, illness, and hospitalization.

Preschoolers' egocentric and magical thinking limits their ability to understand events because they view all experiences from their own self-referenced (egocentric) perspective. Without adequate preparation for unfamiliar settings or experiences, preschoolers' fantasy explanations for such events are usually more exaggerated, bizarre, and frightening than the actual facts. One typical fantasy to explain the reason for illness or hospitalization is that it represents punishment for real or imagined misdeeds. In response to such thinking the child usually feels shame, guilt, and fear.

Preschoolers' preoperational thinking means that explanations are understood only in terms of real events. Purely verbal instructions are often inadequate for them because they are unable to abstract and synthesize beyond what their senses tell them. When combined with their egocentric and magical thinking, this characteristic may lead them to interpret messages according to their particular past experiences. Even with the best preparation for a procedure, they may misconstrue the details.

Transductive reasoning implies that preschoolers deduct from the particular to the particular, rather than from the specific to the general, or vice versa. For example, if preschoolers' concept of nurses is that they inflict pain, preschoolers will think that every nurse (or everyone wearing a similar uniform) will also inflict pain.

School-Age Children

Because of their striving for independence and productivity, school-age children are particularly vulnerable to events that may lessen their feeling of control and power. In particular, altered family roles; physical disability; fears of death, abandonment, or permanent injury; loss of peer acceptance; lack of productivity; and inability to cope with stress according to perceived cultural expectation may result in loss of control.

Because of the nature of the patient role, many routine hospital activities usurp individual power and identity. For school-age children, dependent activities such as enforced bed rest, use of a bedpan, inability to choose a menu, lack of privacy, help with a bed bath, or transport by a wheelchair or stretcher can be a direct threat to their security. Although all of these procedures seem routine and inconsequential, they allow no freedom of choice to children who want to "act grown-up." However, when children are allowed to exert a measure of control, regardless of how limited it may be, they generally respond very well to any procedure. For example, some of the most cooperative, satisfied, and contented patients are school-age children who help make their beds, choose their schedule of activities, assist in procedures, and help the nurses care for younger children. An increased sense of control usually results from a feeling of usefulness and productivity.

In addition to the hospital environment, illness may also cause a feeling of loss of control. One of the most significant problems of children in this age-group centers on boredom.

When physical or enforced limitations curtail their usual abilities to care for themselves or to engage in favorite activities, school-age children generally respond with depression, hostility, or frustration. Keeping a normally active child on bed rest is difficult. However, emphasizing areas of control and capitalizing on quiet activities, particularly hobbies such as building models, promote their adjustment to physical restriction.

Adolescents

Adolescents' struggle for independence, self-assertion, and liberation centers on the quest for personal identity. Anything that interferes with this poses a threat to their sense of identity and results in a loss of control. Illness, which limits one's physical abilities, and hospitalization, which separates one from one's usual support systems, constitute major situational crises.

The patient role fosters dependency and depersonalization. Adolescents may react to dependency with rejection, uncooperativeness, or withdrawal. They may respond to depersonalization with self-assertion, anger, or frustration. Regardless of response, hospital personnel often regard them as difficult, unmanageable patients. Parents may not be a source of help, because these behaviors serve to isolate them further from understanding the adolescent. Although peers may visit, they may not be able to offer the kind of support and guidance needed. Sick adolescents often voluntarily isolate themselves from age-mates until they feel they can compete on an equal basis and meet group expectations. As a result, ill adolescents may be left with virtually no support system.

Loss of control also occurs for many of the reasons discussed for school-age children. However, adolescents are more sensitive to potential instances of loss of control and dependency than are younger children. For example, both groups seek information about their physical status and rely heavily on anticipatory preparation to decrease fear and anxiety. However, adolescents react not only to the kinds of information supplied them, but also to the means by which it is conveyed. They may feel very threatened by others who relate facts in a condescending manner. Adolescents want to know that others can relate to them on their own level. This necessitates a careful assessment of their intellectual abilities, previous knowledge, and present needs. It may also require the nurse's willingness to learn the adolescent's language.

BODILY INJURY AND PAIN

Fears of bodily injury and pain are prevalent among children. The consequences of these fears can be far-reaching; adults who experience more medical fear and pain in childhood are more fearful of pain as adults and tend to avoid medical care (Pate and others, 1996).

In caring for children, nurses must have an appreciation of a child's concerns about bodily harm and the reactions to pain at different developmental periods. Table 21-1 summarizes developmental considerations related to children's understanding of illness and pain. Box 21-2 outlines developmental characteristics of children's reactions to pain.

Infants

Infants' responses to pain after the neonatal period are quite similar to earlier reactions, although there is marked variability in measures of distress, especially the initial cry and heart rate, which may decrease in some infants. The most

TABLE 21-1 ■ Children's Developmental Concepts of Illness and Pain

CONCEPT OF ILLNESS*	CONCEPT OF PAIN†
PREOPERATIONAL THOUGHT (2-7 YEARS)	
Phenomenism: Perceives an external, unrelated, concrete phenomenon as cause of illness (e.g., "being sick because you don't feel well")	Relates to pain primarily as physical, concrete experience
	Thinks in terms of magical disappearance of pain
Contagion: Perceives cause of illness as proximity between two events that occurs by "magic" (e.g., "getting a cold because you are near someone who has a cold")	May view pain as punishment for wrongdoing
	Tends to hold someone accountable for own pain and may strike out at person
CONCRETE OPERATIONAL THOUGHT (7-10 YEARS)	
Contamination: Perceives cause as a person, object, or action external to the child that is "bad" or "harmful" to the body (e.g., "getting a cold because you didn't wear a hat")	Relates to pain physically (e.g., headache, stomach ache)
	Is able to perceive of psychologic pain (e.g., someone dying)
Internalization: Perceives illness as having an external cause but as being located inside the body (e.g., "getting a cold by breathing in air and bacteria")	Fears bodily harm and annihilation (body destruction and death)
	May view pain as punishment for wrongdoing
FORMAL OPERATIONAL THOUGHT (13 YEARS AND OLDER)	
Physiologic: Perceives cause as malfunctioning or nonfunctioning organ or process; can explain illness in sequence of events	Is able to give reason for pain (e.g., fell and hit nerve)
	Perceives several types of psychologic pain
Psychophysiologic: Realizes that psychologic actions and attitudes affect health and illness	Has limited life experiences to cope with pain as adult might cope despite mature understanding of pain
	Fears losing control during painful experience

*From Bibace R, Walsh ME: Development of children's concepts of illness, *Pediatrics* 66(6):912-917, 1980.
†From Hurley A, Whelan EG: Cognitive development and children's perception of pain, *Pediatr Nurs* 14(1):21-24, 1988.

consistent indicator of distress is a facial expression of discomfort (see Fig. 21-3). Infants may express pain by squirming, writhing, jerking, and flailing (Franck, Greenberg, and Stevens, 2000). Some infants may cry loudly after the procedure, whereas others are easily calmed by a gentle hug. It is important to recognize and respect such early signs of individuality and to realize that children who react less intensely may still be experiencing significant discomfort.

Infants younger than 6 months of age seem to have no obvious memory of previous painful experiences and react to a potentially stressful situation with less apprehension and fear than older children. After this time, however, children's response to pain is increasingly influenced by their recall of prior painful experiences and the emotional reaction of parents during the procedure. Older infants react intensely, with physical resistance and uncooperativeness. They may refuse to lie still, attempt to push the person away, or try to escape with whatever motor activity they have achieved. Distraction does little to lessen their immediate reaction to pain, and anticipatory preparation, such as showing them the equipment, can increase their fear and resistance (see Neonatal Pain, Chapter 9).

Toddlers

Toddlers' concept of body image, particularly the definition of body boundaries, is very poorly developed. Intrusive experiences, such as examining the ears or mouth or checking a rectal temperature, are very anxiety producing. Toddlers may react to such painless procedures as intensely as they do to painful ones.

Toddlers' reactions to pain are similar to those seen during infancy, except that the number of variables influencing the individual response is highly complex and varied. Memory, physical restraint, separation from parents, emotional reactions of others, and lack of preparation partially determine the intensity of the behavioral response. In general, children in this age-group continue to react with intense emotional upset and physical resistance to any actual or perceived painful experience. Behaviors indicating pain include grimacing, clenching their teeth or lips, opening their eyes

---

BOX 21-2 ■ Developmental Characteristics of Children's Responses to Pain

YOUNG INFANT
Generalized body response of rigidity or thrashing, possibly with local reflex withdrawal of stimulated area
Loud crying
Facial expression of pain (brows lowered and drawn together, eyes tightly closed, and mouth open and squarish) (Fig. 21-3)
Demonstrates no association between approaching stimulus and subsequent pain

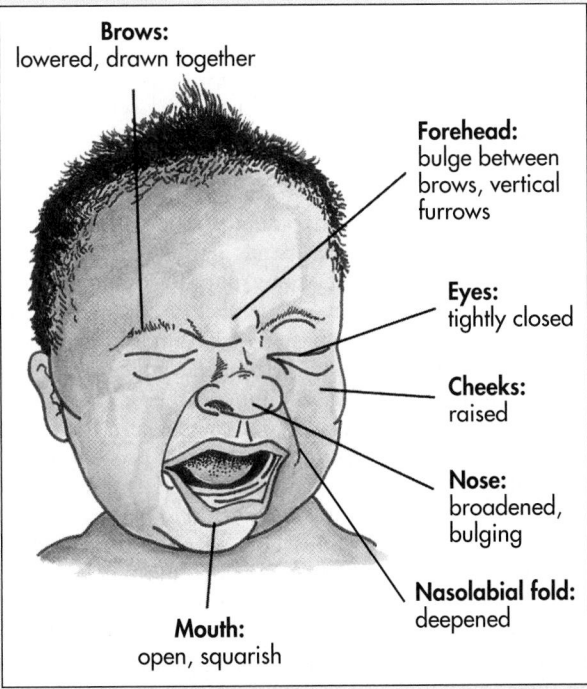

Brows: lowered, drawn together
Forehead: bulge between brows, vertical furrows
Eyes: tightly closed
Cheeks: raised
Nose: broadened, bulging
Nasolabial fold: deepened
Mouth: open, squarish

FIG. 21-3 ■ Facial expression of physical distress is the most consistent behavioral indicator of pain in infants.

OLDER INFANT
Localized body response with deliberate withdrawal of stimulated area
Loud crying
Facial expression of pain or anger (same facial characteristics as pain but eyes are open)
Physical resistance, especially pushing the stimulus away after it is applied

YOUNG CHILD
Loud crying, screaming
Verbal expressions of "Ow," "Ouch," "It hurts"
Thrashing of arms and legs
Attempts to push stimulus away before it is applied
Uncooperative; needs physical restraint
Requests termination of procedure
Clings to parent, nurse, or other significant person
Requests emotional support, such as hugs or other forms of physical comfort
May become restless and irritable with continuing pain
All of these behaviors may be seen in anticipation of actual painful procedure

SCHOOL-AGE CHILD
May see all behaviors of young child, especially during actual painful procedure but less in anticipatory period
Stalling behavior, such as "Wait a minute" or "I'm not ready"
Muscular rigidity, such as clenched fists, white knuckles, gritted teeth, contracted limbs, body stiffness, closed eyes, wrinkled forehead

ADOLESCENT
Less vocal protest
Less motor activity
More verbal expressions, such as "It hurts" or "You're hurting me"
Increased muscle tension and body control

Data from Craig KD and others: Developmental changes in infant pain expression during immunization injections, *Soc Sci Med* 19(12):1331-1337, 1984; Katz ER, Kellerman J, Siegel SE: Behavioral distress in children with cancer undergoing medical procedures: developmental considerations, *J Consult Clin Psychol* 48(3):356-365, 1980.

wide, rocking, rubbing, and acting aggressively, such as biting, kicking, hitting, or running away. Unlike adults, who usually decrease their activity when in pain, young children typically become restless and overly active; frequently, this response is not recognized as a consequence of pain.

By the end of this age period, toddlers usually are able to communicate about their pain. Although they have not developed the ability to describe the type or intensity of the pain, they usually are able to localize it by pointing to a specific area.

Preschoolers

Concepts of illness begin during the preschool period and are influenced by the cognitive abilities of the preoperational stage. Preschoolers differentiate poorly between themselves and the external world. Their thinking is focused on externally perceived events, and causality is based on the proximity of two events. Consequently, children define illness according to what they are told or are given external evidence of, such as "You are sick because you have a fever." The cause of illness is seen as a concrete action the child does or fails to do, such as "Catching a cold because you go out into cold weather"; consequently, it implies a degree of responsibility and self-blame. Another explanation may be based on contagion, that the proximity of two objects or persons causes the illness (e.g., "A person gets a cold when someone else with a cold gets near him").

The psychosexual conflicts of children in this age-group make them very vulnerable to threats of bodily injury. Intrusive procedures, whether painful or painless, are threatening to preschoolers, whose concept of body integrity is still poorly developed. Preschoolers may react to an injection with as much concern for withdrawal of the needle as for the actual pain. They fear that the intrusion or puncture will not reclose and that their "insides" will leak out.

Concerns of mutilation are paramount during this age period. Loss of any body part is threatening, but preschool boys' fears of castration complicate their understanding of surgical or medical procedures associated with the genital area, such as circumcision, repair of hypospadias or epispadias, cystoscopy, or catheterization. Their limited comprehension of body functioning also increases their difficulty in understanding how or why body parts are "fixed." For example, telling preschoolers that their tonsils are to be removed may be interpreted as "taking out their voice" or having the penis "fixed" may be understood as cutting it off. Words such as "dye," "cut off," "take out," or "draw" (e.g., "draw some blood") are understood literally and can lead to confusion and fear (see Communicating With Children, Chapter 6).

Reactions to pain tend to be similar to those seen during toddlerhood, although some differences become apparent. For example, preschoolers respond more favorably than younger children to preparatory interventions, such as explanation and distraction. Physical and verbal aggression are more specific and goal directed. Instead of showing total body resistance, preschoolers may push the offending person away, try to secure the equipment, or attempt to lock themselves in a safe place. Much more thought is evident in their plan of attack or escape.

Verbal expression in particular demonstrates their advanced development in response to stress. They may verbally abuse the nurse by stating, "Get out of here" or "I hate you." They may also use the more cunning approach of trying to persuade the person to give up the intended activity. A common plea is, "Please don't give me a shot; I'll be good." Some statements are not only attempts to avoid the event but also evidence of children's perceptions about the experience.

Preschoolers can locate their pain and can use appropriate pain scales. Children as young as 3 years can use assessment tools that employ facial expressions of pain (see Table 21-2).

School-Age Children

Fears of the physical nature of the illness surface at this time. School-age children may be less concerned with pain than with disability, uncertain recovery, or possible death. Children with chronic illness are more likely to identify intrusive procedures as stressful, whereas children who are acutely ill are more likely to indicate physical symptoms (Boyd and Hunsberger, 1998). Girls tend to express more and stronger fears than boys, and previous hospitalizations may have no effect on the frequency or intensity of these fears. Because of their developing cognitive abilities, school-age children are aware of the significance of different illnesses, the indispensability of certain body parts, potential hazards of treatments, lifelong consequences of permanent injury or loss of function, and the meaning of death. A major concern of school-age children when hospitalized is their fear of being told that something is "wrong" with them. They generally take a very active interest in their health or illness. Even those children who rarely ask questions usually reveal detailed knowledge of their condition by attentively listening to all that is said around them. They request factual information and quickly perceive lies or half-truths. Seeking information tends to be one way of coping or maintaining a sense of control despite the stress and uncertainty of the illness.

School-age children define illness by a set of multiple concrete symptoms, such as signs of a cold, and view the cause as primarily germs or bacteria. The germs have a powerful, almost magical quality, so that in the child's mind, illness can be prevented by avoiding people with the germs. There is also the notion of contamination, which is similar to that seen in the younger age-group; for example, the illness occurs because of physical contact or because the child engaged in a harmful action and became contaminated. Consequently, feelings of self-blame and guilt may be associated with the reason for becoming ill.

School-age children begin to show concern for the potential beneficial and hazardous effects of procedures. Besides wanting to know if a procedure will hurt, they want to know what it is for, how it will make them better, and what injury or harm could result. For example, these children may fear the actual procedure of anesthesia. Unlike preschoolers, who fear the mask and the strange surroundings, school-age children fear what may happen while they are asleep, whether they will wake up, and that they may die. Preadolescents also worry about the procedure itself, particularly if it is one that will result in visible changes in body appearance.

Intrusive procedures of a nonsexual nature, such as routine physical examination of the ears, nose, mouth, and throat, are generally well-tolerated. However, concerns for privacy become evident and increasingly significant. Although school-age children may cooperate during examination of, or procedures performed on, the genital area, it is usually very stressful for them, especially in the case of preadolescents who are beginning pubertal changes. Nurses who respect children's need for privacy can provide them with much assurance and support.

By age 9 or 10, most school-age children show less fright or overt resistance to pain than younger children. They generally have learned coping methods of dealing with discomfort, such as holding rigidly still, clenching their fists or teeth, or trying to act brave through the "grin-and-bear-it" routine. If they do display signs of overt resistance, such as biting, kicking, pulling away, trying to escape, crying, or plea bargaining, they may deny such reactions later, especially to their peers for fear of embarrassment.

School-age children verbally communicate about their pain in respect to its location, intensity, and description. Unlike younger children, who may have difficulty choosing words to describe pain, children 8 years and older use a wide variety of words and phrases, such as "hurting," "sore," "burning," "stinging," "aching," and "like a sharp knife" (Franck, Greenberg, and Stevens, 2000).

School-age children also use words as a means of controlling their reactions to pain. For example, these children may ask the nurse to talk to them during a procedure. Some prefer to participate in a procedure, whereas others choose to distance themselves by not looking at what is happening. Most appreciate an explanation of the procedure and seem less fearful when they know what to expect. Others try to gain control by attempting to postpone the event or bargain their way out of it. A typical request is, "Start the IV when I am finished with this." Although the ability to make decisions does increase their sense of control, unlimited procrastination results in heightened anxiety. When choices are allowed, such as selection of the intravenous (IV) site, it is best to structure the number of possible sites and to limit the number of "procrastination" techniques.

Similar to their more passive acceptance of pain is their nondirective request for support or help. School-age children will rarely initiate a conversation about their feelings or request someone to stay with them during a lonely or stressful period. Their visible composure, calmness, and acceptance often mask their inner longing for support. It is especially important to be aware of nonverbal clues, such as a serious facial expression, a half-hearted reply of "I am fine," silence, lack of activity, or social isolation, as signs of the need for help. Usually when someone identifies the unspoken messages and offers support, they readily accept it.

NURSING ALERT

If children's behaviors appear to differ from their rating of pain, believe their pain rating.

Adolescents

Although the development of body image begins at birth, its relevance is paramount during adolescence. Injury, pain, disability, and death are viewed primarily in terms of how each affects adolescents' views of themselves in the present. Any change that differentiates the adolescent from peers is

regarded as a major tragedy. For example, diseases such as diabetes mellitus often present a more difficult adjustment period for children in this age-group than for younger children because of the necessary changes in the adolescent's lifestyle. Conversely, serious, even life-threatening illnesses that entail no visible body changes or physical restrictions may have less immediate significance for the adolescent. Therefore the nature of bodily injury may be more important in terms of adolescents' perception of the illness than its actual degree of severity.

Adolescents' rapidly changing body image during pubertal development often makes them feel insecure about their bodies. Illness, medical or surgical intervention, and hospitalization increase their existing concerns for normalcy. They may respond to such events by asking numerous questions, withdrawing, rejecting others, or questioning the adequacy of care. Frequently their fear of loss of control and body-image change is demonstrated as overconfidence.

Because of the development of secondary sex characteristics, adolescents are very concerned about privacy. Lack of respect for this need can cause greater stress than physical pain. In addition, adolescents look for signs that indicate they are developing normally and according to acceptable standards. When illness occurs, they fear that growth may be retarded, leaving them behind their peers. Although they may not voice this concern, they may demonstrate it by carefully observing others' reactions to them.

Adolescents typically react to pain with much self-control. Physical resistance and aggression are less likely at this age unless the adolescent is totally unprepared for a procedure. As with older school-age children, adolescents are very concerned with remaining composed and feel embarrassed and ashamed of losing control. They are able to describe their pain experience and to use any of the pain assessment tools developed for adults. However, they may be reluctant to disclose their pain, requiring the nurse to listen closely and observe physical indications, such as limited movement, excessive quiet, or irritability. Adolescents may also believe that the nurse knows how they feel; thus they may see no need to ask for analgesia.

EFFECTS OF HOSPITALIZATION ON THE CHILD

Children may react to the stresses of hospitalization before admission, during hospitalization, and after discharge. A child's conception of illness is even more important than age and intellectual maturity in predicting the level of anxiety before hospitalization (Clatworthy, Simon, and Tiedeman, 1999). This may or may not be affected by the duration of the condition or prior hospitalizations; therefore, nurses should avoid overestimating the illness concepts of children with prior medical experience (Box 21-3).

Individual Risk Factors

A number of risk factors make certain children more vulnerable than others to the stresses of hospitalization (Box 21-4). It has also been noted that rural children exhibit significantly greater degrees of psychologic upset than urban children, possibly because urban children have opportunities to become familiar with a local hospital. Because separation is such an important issue surrounding hospitalization for young children, children who are active and strong-willed tend to

BOX 21-3 ■ Posthospital Behaviors in Children

YOUNG CHILDREN

Initial aloofness toward parents; may last from a few minutes (most common) to a few days

Frequently followed by dependency behaviors:

Tendency to cling to parents

Demand parents' attention

Vigorously oppose any separation (e.g., staying at preschool or with a baby-sitter)

Other negative behaviors include the following:

New fears (e.g., nightmares)

Resistance to going to bed, night waking

Withdrawal and shyness

Hyperactivity

Temper tantrums

Food finickiness

Attachment to blanket or toy

Regression in newly learned skills (e.g., self-toileting)

OLDER CHILDREN

Negative behaviors include the following:

Emotional coldness, followed by intense, demanding dependence on parents

Anger toward parents

Jealousy toward others (e.g., siblings)

BOX 21-4 ■ Risk Factors That Increase Children's Vulnerability to the Stresses of Hospitalization

"Difficult" temperament

Lack of fit between child and parent

Age (especially between 6 months and 5 years)

Male gender

Below-average intelligence

Multiple and continuing stresses (e.g., frequent hospitalizations)

fare better when hospitalized than youngsters who are passive. Consequently, nurses should be alert to children who passively accept all changes and requests; these children may need more support than the "oppositional" child.

The stressors of hospitalization may cause young children to experience short- and long-term negative outcomes. Adverse outcomes may be related to the length and number of admissions, multiple invasive procedures, and the anxiety of parents. Common responses include regression, separation anxiety, apathy, fears, and sleeping disturbances, especially for children younger than 7 years of age (Melnyk, 2000). Supportive practices, such as family-centered care and frequent family visiting, may lessen the detrimental effects of such admissions. Research also indicates that a child's pain experience determines how the overall hospitalization is experienced (Woodgate and Kristjanson, 1996).

Changes in the Pediatric Population. The pediatric population in hospitals today has changed dramatically over the last two decades. Although there is a growing trend toward shortened hospital stays and outpatient surgery, a greater percentage of the children hospitalized today have more serious and complex problems than those hospitalized in the past. Many of these children are fragile newborns and children with severe injuries or disabilities who have survived because of major technologic advances, yet have been left with chronic or disabling conditions that require often frequent and lengthy hospital stays. The nature of their conditions increases the likelihood that they will experience more invasive and traumatic procedures while they are hospitalized. These factors make them more vulnerable to the emotional consequences of hospitalization and result in their needs being significantly different from those of the short-term patients of the past (see Chapter 18 for further discussion on children with special needs). The majority of these children are infants and toddlers, the age-group most vulnerable to the effects of hospitalization.

Concern in recent years has focused on the increasing length of hospitalization because of complex medical and nursing care, elusive diagnoses, and complicated psychosocial issues. Without special attention devoted to meeting the child's psychosocial and developmental needs in the "artificial" hospital environment, the detrimental consequences of prolonged hospitalization may be severe.

Beneficial Effects of Hospitalization

Although hospitalization can be and usually is stressful for children, it can also be beneficial. The most obvious benefit is the recovery from illness, but hospitalization also can present an opportunity for children to master stress and feel competent in their coping abilities. The hospital environment can provide children with new socialization experiences that can broaden their interpersonal relationships. The psychologic benefits need to be considered and maximized during hospitalization. Appropriate nursing strategies to achieve this goal are presented on p. 686.

STRESSORS AND REACTIONS OF THE FAMILY OF THE CHILD WHO IS HOSPITALIZED

PARENTAL REACTIONS

The crisis of childhood illness and hospitalization affects every member of the nuclear family. Parents' reactions to illness in their child depend on a variety of influencing factors. Although one cannot predict which factors are most likely to influence their response, a number of variables have been identified (Box 21-5). (See also Chapter 18.)

Almost all parents respond to their child's illness and hospitalization with remarkably consistent reactions. Initially parents may react with *disbelief*, especially if the illness is sudden and serious. Following the realization of illness, parents react with *anger* or *guilt* or both. They may blame themselves for the child's illness or become angry at others for some wrongdoing. Even in the mildest of illnesses, parents question their adequacy as caregivers and review any actions or omissions that could have prevented or caused the illness. When hospitalization is indicated, parental guilt is intensified because the parents feel helpless in alleviating the child's physical and emotional pain.

BOX 21-5 ■ Factors Affecting Parents' Reactions to Their Child's Illness

Seriousness of the threat to the child
Previous experience with illness or hospitalization
Medical procedures involved in diagnosis and treatment
Available support systems
Personal ego strengths
Previous coping abilities
Additional stresses on the family system
Cultural and religious beliefs
Communication patterns among family members

Fear, anxiety, and *frustration* are common feelings expressed by parents. Fear and anxiety may be related to the seriousness of the illness and the type of medical procedures involved. Often great anxiety is related to the trauma and pain inflicted on the child. Feelings of frustration are often related to lack of information about procedures and treatments, unfamiliarity with hospital rules and regulations, unfriendly staff, or fear of asking questions. Much frustration can be alleviated in a pediatric unit when parents are aware of what to expect and what is expected of them, are encouraged to participate in their child's care, and are regarded as the most significant contributors to the child's total health.

Parents eventually may react with some degree of *depression.* Mothers often comment on their feeling of physical and mental exhaustion after all of the other family members have adapted to the crisis. Parents may also worry about and miss their other children, who may be left in the care of family, friends, or neighbors. Other reasons for anxiety and depression are related to concerns for the child's future well-being, including negative effects produced by the hospitalization and any financial burden incurred from the hospitalization.

SIBLING REACTIONS

Siblings' reactions to a sister's or brother's illness or hospitalization are discussed in Chapter 18 and differ little when a child becomes temporarily ill. Siblings experience loneliness, fear, and worry, as well as anger, resentment, jealousy, and guilt. Various factors have been identified that influence the effects of the child's hospitalization on siblings. Although these factors are similar to those seen when a child has a chronic illness, Craft (1993) reported that the following factors regarding siblings are related specifically to the hospital experience and have been found to increase the effects on the sibling:

- Younger and experiencing many changes
- Cared for outside the home by care providers who are not relatives
- Received little information about their ill brother or sister
- Perceived their parents to be treating them differently compared with before their sibling's hospitalization

Simon (1993) interviewed 45 siblings of children who were hospitalized and asked about their perceptions of the stress of the hospitalization of a brother or sister. The siblings' perceptions of the stress they experienced were equal to the level of stress of hospitalized children.

Parents are often unaware of the number of effects that siblings experience during the sick child's hospitalization and the benefit of simple interventions to minimize such effects, such as explicit explanations about the illness and provisions for the siblings to remain at home. Sibling visitation is usually beneficial to the patient, sibling, and parent but should be evaluated on an individual basis.

ALTERED FAMILY ROLES

In addition to the effects of separation on family roles, loss of parenting, sibling, and offspring roles may affect each family member differently. One of the most common reactions of parents is specialized and intensified attention toward the sick child. The other siblings may regard this as unfair and interpret the parents' attitude toward them as rejection. Although such responses are usually unconscious and unintended, they place unique burdens on ill children. For example, the ill child may feel obligated to play the sick role to meet parents' expectations, especially those children who have had limited physical ability and regain normal health status, such as after corrective heart surgery. Parents may be unable to perceive the child's recovery and therefore continue the pattern of overprotection and indulgent attention.

Ill children may also feel jealousy and resentment from other siblings. Because of their singular position in the family, they may be denied the companionship of their brothers and sisters. Rivalry between siblings tends to be greatest in the sibling who is nearest in age to the ill child. Without an understanding of the interpersonal dynamics between siblings, parents are likely to blame the well children for antisocial behavior. Illness may also result in children's loss of status within either their family or social group. For example, illness in the oldest child may temporarily terminate special privileges as "big" brother or sister.

NURSING CARE OF THE CHILD WHO IS HOSPITALIZED

PREPARATION FOR HOSPITALIZATION

The rationale for preparing children for the hospital experience and related procedures is based on the principle that fear of the unknown (fantasy) exceeds fear of the known. Therefore decreasing the elements of the unknown results in less fear. When children do not have paralyzing fear to cope with, they are able to direct their energies toward dealing with the other, unavoidable stresses of hospitalization and to benefit optimally from the growth potential of the experience.

Although preparation for hospitalization is a common practice, there is no universal standard or program that is advocated for all settings. The preparation process may be elaborate with tours, puppet shows, and playtime with miniature hospital equipment; it may involve the use of books, videos, or films; or it may be limited to a brief description of the major aspects of any hospital stay (Stewart, Algren, and Arnold, 1994). No firm consensus exists on the timing of the event. Some authorities recommend preparing children 4 to 7 years of age about 1 week in advance so that they can assimilate the information and ask questions. For older children the time may be longer. However, for young children, who may begin to fantasize about what they observed, 1 or 2 days before admission is sufficient time for anticipatory preparation. The length of the session should be suited to the children's attention span—the younger the child, the shorter the program. The optimal approach is one that is individualized for each child and family. Regardless of the specific type of program, all children, even those who have been hospitalized before, benefit from an introduction to the environment and routine of the unit.

FYI

In many hospitals, child-life specialists, health care professionals with extensive knowledge of child growth and development and of the special psychosocial needs of children who are hospitalized and their families, help prepare children for hospitalization, surgery, and procedures. A collaborative effort between the nurse, child-life specialist, and other members of the child's health care team helps ensure the best possible hospital experience for the child and family.

Assessment

Assessment is the first step in identifying nursing diagnoses and planning care for an individual child. In some instances, such as with elective admission, assessment begins even before the child is hospitalized so that appropriate preadmission preparation can be instituted. At other times, assessment occurs at the time of admission and should be integrated into other admission procedures so that the child's specific needs are recognized *early* in the hospitalization. One critical area is assessment of pain for implementing appropriate relief of discomfort (see p. 656). Although assessment is discussed under nursing care of the child who is hospitalized, a comprehensive approach must involve the child's parents or other caregivers.

The nurse's primary intent is to provide *atraumatic care* (see Chapter 1). Therefore patient assessment should be individualized and include an evaluation of the child's growth and development, psychosocial needs, educational needs, cultural background, and the effects of the illness on the child's family or guardian.

Admission Assessment

The nursing admission history refers to a systematic collection of data about the child and family that allows the nurse to plan individualized care. The nursing admission history presented in Box 21-6 is organized according to the Functional Health Patterns outlined by Gordon (1994, 2002) (see Nursing Diagnosis, Chapter 1). This assessment framework is a guideline for formulating nursing diagnoses. One of the main purposes of the history is to assess the child's usual health habits at home to promote a more normal environment in the hospital. Therefore questions related to activities of daily living in the nutritional-metabolic, elimination, sleep-rest, and activity-exercise patterns are a major part of the assessment. The questions found under the health perception–health management pattern are directed toward evaluation of the child's preparation for hospitalization and are key factors in determining if additional preparation is needed. The questions included in the self-perception–self-concept and role-relationship patterns

offer insight into the child's potential reaction to hospitalization, especially in terms of separation.

The nurse should also inquire about the use of any complementary medicine practices (Box 21-7). In a study of children with cancer, 42% had used alternative or complementary therapies simultaneously with or after conventional treatments (Fernandez, Pyesmany, and Stutzer, 1999). Widespread use of complementary medicine is often explored, however, without discussion with the primary care physician or nurse (Moenkhoff and others, 1999; Spiegel, Stroud, and Fyfe, 1998). It is important that the use of any herbal or complementary therapy be noted in a preoperative assessment because of possible anesthesia or surgical complications related to herbal products (Flanagan, 2001) (see Critical Thinking Exercise on p. 651).

After the data are collected, the information must be applied to the nursing process and communicated to other staff. It makes little sense to assess a child's home routine if none of this knowledge is integrated into the plan of care. Most nursing units have provisions for care plans in which specific information about the child's habits and needs are recorded.

As with any history form, the questions are only guidelines: for maximum communication, nurses should ask these questions as a part of conversation, not as a direct questionnaire. Answers to questions that are broad and nonspecific, such as "What does your child know about this hospitalization?" need to be followed by more specific questions such as "Tell me what you told him." Children may respond to questions regarding their knowledge of hospitalization with statements such as "I don't know why I am here." Although this may be correct, they have often been given some explanation concerning the reason for hospitalization. Such an answer may mean that the explanation was inadequate, their anxiety blocked the recall, or they are testing the explanation by prompting the nurse to supply additional information.

Besides taking the nursing admission history, nurses should also perform a physical assessment (see Chapter 7) or obtain the information from the medical examination before planning care. At the very least, the nurse's physical assessment of the child should include observation of the body for any bruises, rashes, signs of neglect, deformities, or physical limitations. The nurse should also listen to the heart and lungs to assess overall physical status. For example, it is impossible to evaluate improvement in respiratory function in a child admitted with pulmonary disease unless there are baseline data with which to compare subsequent findings.

Nursing Diagnoses

A number of nursing diagnoses are prominent in the nursing care of children who are ill or hospitalized. Other nursing diagnoses specific to individual cases may become evident in addition to those outlined in the Nursing Care Plan on pp. 686-690.

Planning

An effective plan of care for the child who is hospitalized is based on patient- and family-identified needs, as well as those identified by the nurse. Family members and the child should play active roles in developing the plan whenever possible.

BOX 21-6 ■ Nursing Admission History According to Functional Health Patterns*

HEALTH PERCEPTION–HEALTH MANAGEMENT PATTERN

Why has your child been admitted?

How has your child's general health been?

What does your child know about this hospitalization?

Ask the child why he or she came to the hospital.

If the answer is "For an operation or for tests," ask the child to tell you about what will happen before, during, and after the operation or tests.

Has your child ever been in the hospital before?

How was that hospital experience?

What things were important to you and your child during that hospitalization? How can we be most helpful now?

What medications does your child take at home?

Why are they given?

When are they given?

How are they given (if a liquid, with a spoon; if a tablet, swallowed with water; or other)?

Does your child have any trouble taking medication? If so, what helps?

Is your child allergic to any medications?

What, if any, forms of complementary medicine practices are being used?

NUTRITION-METABOLIC PATTERN

What are the family's usual mealtimes?

Do family members eat together or at separate times?

What are your child's favorite foods, beverages, and snacks?

Average amounts consumed or usual size of portions

Special cultural practices, such as family eats only ethnic food

What foods and beverages does your child dislike?

What are your child's feeding habits (bottle, cup, spoon, eats by self, needs assistance, any special devices)?

How does your child like the food served (warmed, cold, one item at a time)?

How would you describe your child's usual appetite (hearty eater, picky eater)?

Has being sick affected your child's appetite? In what ways?

Are there any known or suspected food allergies?

Is your child on a special diet?

Are there any feeding problems (excessive fussiness, spitting up, colic); any dental or gum problems that affect feeding?

What do you do for these problems?

ELIMINATION PATTERN

What are your child's toilet habits (diaper, toilet trained—day only or day and night, use of word to communicate urination or defecation, potty chair, regular toilet, other routines)?

What is your child's usual pattern of elimination (bowel movements)?

Do you have any concerns about elimination (bed-wetting, constipation, diarrhea)?

What do you do for these problems?

Have you ever noticed that your child sweats a lot?

SLEEP-REST PATTERN

What is your child's usual hour of sleep and awakening?

What is your child's schedule for naps; length of naps?

Is there a special routine before sleeping (bottle, drink of water, bedtime story, night-light, favorite blanket or toy, prayers)?

Is there a special routine during sleep time, such as waking to go to the bathroom?

What type of bed does your child sleep in?

Does your child have a separate room or share a room; if shares, with whom?

What are the home sleeping arrangements (alone or with others, e.g., sibling, parent, other person)?

What is your child's favorite sleeping position?

Are there any sleeping problems (falling asleep, waking during night, nightmares, sleep walking)?

Are there any problems in awakening and getting ready in the morning?

What do you do for these problems?

ACTIVITY-EXERCISE PATTERN

What is your child's schedule during the day (preschool, day care center, regular school, extracurricular activities)?

What are your child's favorite activities or toys (both active and quiet interests)?

What is your child's usual television-viewing schedule at home?

What are your child's favorite programs?

Are there any television restrictions?

Does your child have any illness or disabilities that limit activity? If so, how?

What are your child's usual habits and schedule for bathing (bath in tub or shower, sponge bath, shampoo)?

What are your child's dental habits (brushing, flossing, fluoride supplements or rinses, favorite toothpaste); schedule of daily dental care?

Does your child need help with dressing or grooming, such as hair combing?

Are there any problems with these patterns (dislike of or refusal to bathe, shampoo hair, or brush teeth)?

What do you do for these problems?

Are there special devices that your child requires help in managing (eyeglasses, contact lenses, hearing aid, orthodontic appliances, artificial elimination appliances, orthopedic devices)?

NOTE: Use the following code to assess functional self-care level for feeding, bathing/hygiene, dressing/grooming, toileting:

O: Full self-care

I: Requires use of equipment or device

II: Requires assistance or supervision from another person

III: Requires assistance or supervision from another person and equipment or device

IV: Is totally dependent and does not participate

COGNITIVE-PERCEPTUAL PATTERN

Does your child have any hearing difficulty?

Does the child use a hearing aid?

Have "tubes" been placed in your child's ears?

Does your child have any vision problems?

Does the child wear glasses or contact lenses?

Does your child have any learning difficulties?

What is the child's grade in school?

For information on pain, see Box 21-12.

*The focus of the admission history is the child's psychosocial environment. Most of the questions are worded in terms of parental responses. Depending on the child's age, they should be addressed directly to the child when appropriate.

Continued

BOX 21-6 ■ Nursing Admission History According to Functional Health Patterns—*cont'd*

SELF-PERCEPTION–SELF-CONCEPT PATTERN

How would you describe your child (e.g., takes time to adjust, settles in easily, shy, friendly, quiet, talkative, serious, playful, stubborn, easygoing)?

What makes your child angry, annoyed, anxious, or sad? What helps?

How does your child act when annoyed or upset?

What have been your child's experiences with and reactions to temporary separation from you (parent)?

Does your child have any fears (places, objects, animals, people, situations)? How do you handle them?

Do you think your child's illness has changed the way he or she thinks about self (e.g., more shy, embarrassed about appearance, less competitive with friends, stays at home more)?

ROLE-RELATIONSHIP PATTERN

Does your child have a favorite nickname?

What are the names of other family members or others who live in the home (relatives, friends, pets)?

Who usually takes care of your child during the day/night (especially if other than parent, such as baby-sitter, relative)?

What are the parents' occupations and work schedules?

Are there any special family considerations (adoption, foster child, stepparent, divorce, single parent)?

Have any major changes in the family occurred lately (death, divorce, separation, birth of a sibling, loss of a job, financial strain, mother beginning a career, other)? Describe child's reaction.

Who are your child's play companions or social groups (peers, younger or older children, adults, prefers to be alone)?

Do things generally go well for your child in school or with friends?

Does your child have "security" objects at home (pacifier, bottle, blanket, stuffed animal or doll)? Did you bring any of these to the hospital?

How do you handle discipline problems at home? Are these methods always effective?

Does your child have any condition that interferes with communication? If so, what are your suggestions for communicating with your child?

Will your child's hospitalization affect the family's financial support or care of other family members (e.g., other children)?

What concerns do you have about your child's illness and hospitalization?

Who will be staying with your child while hospitalized?

How can we contact you or another close family member outside of the hospital?

SEXUALITY-REPRODUCTIVE PATTERN

(Answer questions that apply to your child's age-group.)

Has your child begun puberty (developing physical sexual characteristics, menstruation)? Have you or your child had any concerns?

Does your daughter know how to do breast self-examination?

Does your son know how to do testicular self-examination?

How have you approached topics of sexuality with your child?

Do you feel you might need some help with some topics?

Has your child's illness affected the way he or she feels about being a boy or a girl? If so, how?

Do you have any concerns with behaviors in your child, such as masturbation, asking many questions or talking about sex, not respecting others' privacy, or wanting too much privacy?

Initiate a conversation about an adolescent's sexual concerns with open-ended to more direct questions and using the terms "friends" or "partners" rather than "girlfriend" or "boyfriend:"
Tell me about your social life.

Who are your closest friends? (If one friend is identified, could ask more about that relationship, such as how much time they spend together, how serious they are about each other, if the relationship is going the way the teenager hoped.)

Might ask about dating and sexual issues, such as the teenager's views on sexuality education, "going steady," "living together," or premarital sex.

Which friends would you like to have visit in the hospital?

COPING-STRESS TOLERANCE PATTERN

(Answer questions that apply to your child's age-group.)

What does your child do when tired or upset?
If upset, does your child want a special person or object?
If so, explain.

If your child has temper tantrums, what causes them and how do you handle them?

Whom does your child talk to when worried about something?

How does your child usually handle problems or disappointments?

Have there been any big changes or problems in your family recently? If so, how have you handled them?

Has your child ever had a problem with drugs or alcohol or tried to commit suicide?

Do you think your child is "accident prone"? If so, explain.

VALUE-BELIEF PATTERN

What is your religion?

How is religion or faith important in your child's life?

What religious practices would you like continued in the hospital (e.g., prayers before meals/bedtime; visit by minister, priest, or rabbi; prayer group)?

BOX 21-7 ■ Complementary Medicine Practices and Examples

Nutrition, diet, and lifestyle/behavioral health changes—Macrobiotics, megavitamins, diets, lifestyle modification, health risk reduction/health education, wellness

Mind/body control therapies—Biofeedback, relaxation, prayer therapy, guided imagery, hypnotherapy, music/sound therapy, massage, aromatherapy, education therapy

Traditional and ethnomedicine therapies—Acupuncture, ayurvedic medicine, herbal medicine, homeopathic medicine, Native American medicine, natural products, traditional Asian medicine

Structural manipulation and energetic therapies—Acupressure, chiropractic medicine, massage, reflexology, rolfing, therapeutic touch, Qi Gong

Pharmacologic and biologic therapies—Antioxidants, cell treatment, chelation therapy, metabolic therapy, oxidizing agents

Bioelectromagnetic therapies—Diagnostic and therapeutic application of electromagnetic fields (e.g., transcranial electrostimulation, neuromagnetic stimulation, electroacupuncture)

?? CRITICAL THINKING EXERCISE

Complementary/Alternative Medicine

Maria, a 10-year-old Hispanic girl, has had severe nosebleeds. She is admitted to the hospital for a complete workup in an attempt to determine the cause. Her parents and grandparents have gathered around her bed. When you enter her room to begin admitting procedures, you notice an unusual scent. Maria's mother is rubbing the contents from an unfamiliar bottle of liquid on Maria. Meanwhile, the grandmother is rubbing Maria's head. She is startled at your entry and drops something on the floor near your feet. You bend over to pick it up and discover that it is a penny.

QUESTIONS

1. Evidence—Is there sufficient evidence to draw any conclusions?
2. Assumptions—What are some underlying assumptions that may be drawn from the data about the following:
    a. Complementary or alternative medical remedies
    b. The role of ethnic or folk remedies in modern health care practice
    c. The nurse's role in cases where alternative medicine is practiced (versus traditional medicine)
3. What implications and priorities for nursing care can be drawn at this time?
4. Does the evidence objectively support your argument (conclusion)?
5. Are there alternative perspectives to your arguments? If so, what are they?

ANSWERS

1. There is limited evidence to draw certain conclusions without obtaining more data from the parents. It would be appropriate to gather more information before jumping to any major conclusions at this time.
2. Assumptions:
    a. Complementary and alternative medicine (CAM) is more common in US households than previously reported. Much of the concern surrounding complementary therapies, especially in children, is the lack of sufficient data regarding their effectiveness, benefit, and the potential harm that may occur as a result of such treatments. In some cases CAM therapies may counteract certain medications or the effects of prescribed therapies. It has become more common for practitioners in emergency medicine to encounter patients who are taking CAM therapy in addition to prescription medications/treatments for conditions such as eczema, asthma, colds, and upper respiratory problems.
    b. Folk remedies are quite common among certain ethnic groups and subgroups within the United States. Many are based on traditional family remedies that have neither been proven to be effective or entirely harmful in most cases. However there remain a few remedies that could be potentially harmful, especially to children, if these remedies counteract the effects of prescribed treatments that are known to be effective.
    c. The nurse's role in such cases is to gather sufficient data from the family about the practice, discuss the treatment (CAM) in a nonjudgmental manner, and be cognizant of the effects of the treatment on the child's current health status and potential effects on other medical treatment regimens.
3. Give the family their penny and open a dialog about the traditional practice they are using. Additional information should be gathered in a nonjudgmental manner, and the discussion should center on the family's traditional beliefs regarding the practices, the prescribed medical regimen, and whether there is conflict or potential for harm. There is no need to stop the treatment unless potential harm to the child may occur. A discussion with the primary practitioner regarding the use of CAM for Maria should ensue, followed by a discussion with the entire family, if necessary.
   The contents of the bottle will more than likely be revealed during the discussion with the family. It is important to respect the family's wishes regarding traditional folk or CAM rituals, yet remain mindful of potential harmful effects on the child. It is not likely that telling the family to stop the ritual will be successful because these beliefs are deeply ingrained into cultural, religious, and medical practice; the family is more likely to continue the ritual at home on discharge and further disregard other instructions for care should a confrontational approach be adopted by the nursing and medical staff. The important concept for the staff and family to focus upon is the ultimate well-being of the child. What you have probably observed is Santeria, the African-Caribbean religion that was brought to the New World by slaves from West Africa. It is common among immigrants from Cuba, Puerto Rico, Brazil, and Santo Domingo, and it is believed that a majority of Latin immigrants will have contact with Santeria sometime in their lives.
4. As yet, there is insufficient evidence to indicate that harm is being done by the CAM ritual. Further data need to be gathered, and then a decision about further discussion of the CAM practice may occur.
5. There are no alternative views other than the notion that if the nursing and medical staff is confrontational and judgmental with the family, there is less likely to be a sense of trust of the staff by the family, thereby negating any treatments and discharge instructions for the care of the child.

The main goals for the child who is ill or hospitalized are as follows:

1. Child will be prepared for hospitalization.
2. Child will experience little or no separation.
3. Child will maintain a sense of control.
4. Child will exhibit decreased fear of bodily injury.
5. Child will experience a reduction of pain that is acceptable to child.
6. Child will have opportunities to participate in developmentally appropriate diversional activities.
7. Child will experience maximum benefits from hospitalization.

Implementation

Preparing Child for Admission

The preparation that children require on the day of admission depends on the kind of prehospital counseling they have received. If they have been prepared in a formalized program, they will usually know what to expect in terms of

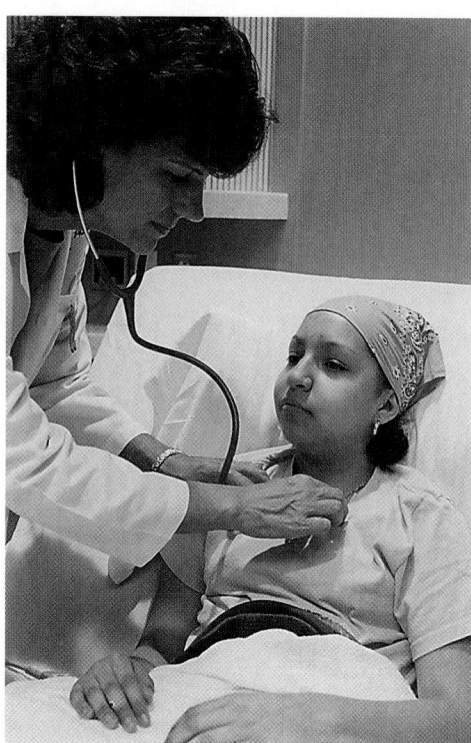

FIG. 21-4 ■ The initial admission procedures give the nurse an opportunity to get to know the child and to assess the child's understanding of the hospital experience.

BOX 21-8 ■ Guidelines for Admission

PREADMISSION

Assign a room based on developmental age, seriousness of diagnosis, communicability of illness, and projected length of stay.

Prepare roommate(s) for the arrival of a new patient; when children are too young to benefit from this consideration, prepare parents.

Prepare room for child and family, with admission forms and equipment nearby to eliminate need to leave child.

ADMISSION

Introduce primary nurse to child and family.

Orient child and family to inpatient facilities, especially to assigned room and unit; emphasize positive areas of pediatric unit.

Room: Explain call light, bed controls, television, bathroom, telephone, etc.

Unit: Direct to playroom, desk, dining area, or other areas.

Introduce family to roommate and his or her parents.

Apply identification band to child's wrist, ankle, or both (if not done).

Explain hospital regulations and schedules (e.g., visiting hours, mealtimes, bedtime, limitations [give written information if available]).

Perform nursing admission history (see Box 21-6).

Take vital signs, blood pressure, height, and weight.

Obtain specimens as needed and order needed laboratory work.

Support child and assist practitioner with physical examination (for purposes of nursing assessment).

---

initial medical procedures, inpatient facilities, and nursing staff. However, prehospital counseling does not preclude the need for support during procedures such as obtaining blood specimens, x-ray tests, or physical examination. For example, undressing young children before they feel comfortable in their new surroundings can be very upsetting. Causing needless anxiety and fear during admission may adversely affect the nurse's establishment of trust with these children. Therefore nursing assistance during the admission procedure is vital, regardless of how well-prepared any child is for the experience of hospitalization. In addition, spending this time with the child gives the nurse an opportunity to evaluate the child's understanding of subsequent procedures (Fig. 21-4). Ideally, a primary nurse is assigned whenever possible to allow for individualized care and to provide a substitute support person for the child.

When a child is admitted, nurses follow several fairly universal admission procedures, which are outlined in Box 21-8. One particularly important decision is room assignment. The minimum considerations for room assignment are age, sex, and nature of the illness. Ideally, however, room selection should be based on a variety of developmental and psychobiologic needs. Determining compatible roommates, both for the children and for rooming-in parents, greatly influences the growth potential from the hospital experience.

No absolute rules govern room selection, but in general, placing children of the same age-group and with similar types of illness in the same room is both psychologically and medically advantageous. However, there are many exceptions. For example, a school-age child may thrive on the responsibility of caring for a younger child. A child in traction may be very therapeutic for another child confined to bed because of a serious illness. A child who is very independent despite physical disabilities may help another child with similar or different limitations, and the parents of the child with disabilities may achieve deeper insight and acceptance of their child's disorder.

Age-grouping is especially important for adolescents. Many hospitals make an effort to place teenagers on their own unit or in a separate, designated section of the pediatric or general unit whenever possible.

Preventing or Minimizing Separation

A primary nursing goal is to prevent separation, particularly in children younger than 5 years of age. Changes in hospitals' policies over recent years reflect a changed attitude toward parents; many hospitals no longer consider parents "visitors" and welcome their presence at all times throughout the child's hospitalization. Many hospitals have developed a system of *family-centered care.* This philosophy of care recognizes the integral role of the family in a child's life and acknowledges the family as an essential part of the child's care and illness experience. The family is considered to be partners in the care of the child (Smith and Conant Rees, 2000) (see Chapter 1).

At the least, most hospitals welcome parents at any time. Many provide facilities such as a chair or bed for at least one person per child, unit kitchen privileges, and other amenities that create a welcoming atmosphere for parents. However, not all hospitals provide such amenities, and parents' own schedules may prevent rooming-in. In such instances, strategies to minimize the effects of separation must be implemented.

A thorough, detailed nursing history specifically identifies the child's established daily routine. Usual daily activities, such as food preparation and method of feeding, help establish a complementary schedule of caregiving practices. Incorporating these normal activities also helps the parents feel that they are participating in the child's care, even if through another person. A consistent staff member can be designated to keep the family informed of the child's condition and to support the family's concerns and priorities without being judgmental (Kauffmann and others, 1998).

Nurses must have an appreciation of the child's separation behaviors. As discussed earlier, the phases of protest and despair are normal. The child is allowed to cry. Even if the child rejects strangers, the nurse provides support through physical presence. *Presence* is defined as spending time being physically close to the child while using a quiet tone of voice, appropriate choice of words, eye contact, and touch in ways that establish rapport and communicate empathy. If behaviors of detachment are evident, the nurse maintains the child's contact with the parents by frequently talking about them, encouraging the child to remember them, and stressing the significance of their visits, telephone calls, or letters.

Separation may be equally as difficult for parents, especially when they do not understand the behaviors of separation anxiety. To avoid the immediate protest, parents may sneak out or lie to the child about leaving. As a result, the child does not learn that absence is associated with a guaranteed return, but that absence means loss of parents. Helping parents recognize that separation behaviors are normal and expected can decrease the parents' anxiety and may ease their fears about leaving without telling the child. Explaining to parents how the child reacts after they leave may also be helpful. Many parents imagine that the child cries for hours after they leave, whereas in reality the child may cry for a few minutes but settle down when comforted by someone else.

Toddlers and preschoolers have a very limited concept of time. The young child's question, "Will my mommy come yesterday?" symbolizes a lack of understanding for usual measurements of time, such as days, hours, and weeks. Time is measured in associations, such as eating dinner "when Daddy comes home." Therefore, when helping parents with their fears of separation, nurses need to suggest ways of explaining leaving and returning. For example, if parents must leave to go to work or to make meals for the other family members, they should tell the child the reason for leaving. They also need to convey the expected time of return in terms of anticipated events. For example, if the parents will return in the morning, they can say to the child, "We'll see you after the sun comes up" or "We'll come back when (a favorite program) is on television."

The young child's ability to tolerate parental absence is very limited. Therefore parental visits should be frequent (e.g., visiting three times a day for short periods rather than once a day for an extended time). This may necessitate that each parent visit at different times to lessen the length of separation. When parents cannot visit, the presence of other significant people can be most comforting for the child (Fig. 21-5).

If parents leave after the child is asleep, they still need to communicate their absence. The parents of a 5-year-old boy solved this problem by devising a sign; on one side they

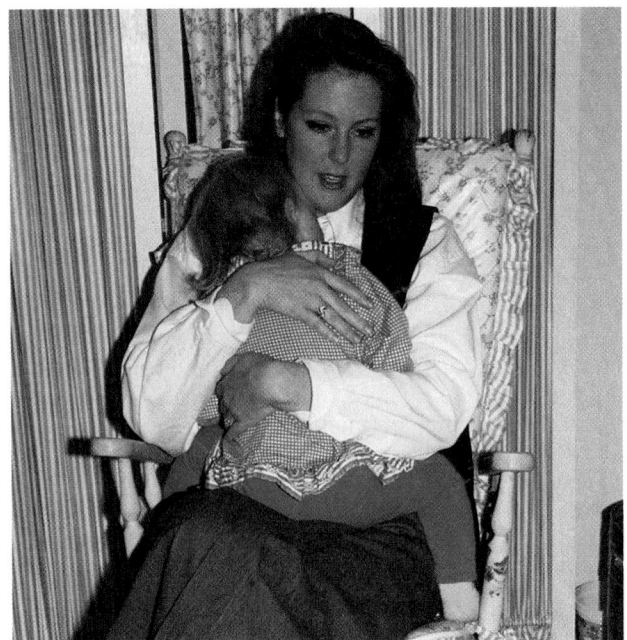

FIG. 21-5 ■ When parents cannot visit, other significant persons can provide comfort to the hospitalized child.

drew a picture of a telephone, and on the other they drew a hamburger. Before they left, they turned the sign to the appropriate side to tell the child when he awoke that they were out using the telephone or eating.

Older children who know how to tell time may find it helpful to have a clock or watch. However, these children have the same need for honesty from their parents regarding visiting schedules. Because their peer groups are important, adolescents often appreciate planning visiting hours with their parents to ensure that the patient has some private time for friends.

Familiar surroundings also increase the child's adjustment to separation. If parents cannot room-in, they should leave favorite articles from home with the child, such as a blanket, toy, bottle, feeding utensil, or article of clothing. Because young children associate such inanimate objects with significant people, they gain comfort and reassurance from these possessions. They make the association that if the parents left this, the parents will surely return. Placing an identification band on the toy lessens the chances of its being misplaced and provides a symbol that the toy is experiencing the same needs as the child. Other mementos of home include photographs and audiotape or videocassette recordings of family members reading a story, singing a song, saying prayers before bedtime, relating events at home, or taking a "talking walk" through the home. The tapes can be played at lonely times, such as on awakening or before sleeping. Some units allow pets to visit, which can have therapeutic benefits for a child. Animals should be carefully screened for medical or behavioral problems, and patients should be screened for allergies.

Older children also appreciate familiar articles from home, particularly photographs, a radio, a favorite toy or game, and the usual pajamas. Often the importance of treasured objects to school-age children is overlooked or criticized. However, many school-age children have a special object to which they formed an attachment in early childhood. Therefore such treasured or transitional objects can help even older children feel more comfortable in a strange environment.

The strange sights, smells, and sounds in the hospital that are commonplace for the nurse can be frightening and confusing for children. It is important for the nurse to try to evaluate stimuli in the environment from the child's point of view (considering also what the child may see or hear happening to other patients) and to make every effort to protect the child from frightening and unfamiliar sights, sounds, and equipment. The nurse should offer explanations or prepare the child for those experiences that are unavoidable. Combining familiar or comforting sights with the unfamiliar can relieve much of the harshness of medical equipment.

"Soften" medical equipment (e.g., clip a bear or other animal to a stethoscope; use paper, fabric, or stickers to transform an IV pump into a friendly animal) to create a pleasant and more familiar environment for children.

Helping children maintain their usual nonhome contacts also minimizes the effects of separation imposed by hospitalization. This includes continuing school lessons during the illness and confinement, visiting with friends either directly or through letter writing or telephone calls, and participating in stimulating projects whenever possible (Fig. 21-6). For extended hospitalizations, youngsters enjoy personalizing the hospital room to make it "home" by decorating the walls with posters and cards, rearranging the furniture (when possible), and displaying a collection or hobby.

Minimizing Loss of Control

Feelings of loss of control result from separation, physical restriction, changed routines, enforced dependency, and magical thinking. Although some of these cannot be prevented, most can be minimized through individualized planning of nursing care.

Promoting Freedom of Movement. Younger children react most strenuously to any type of physical restriction or immobilization. Although temporary immobilization may be necessary for some interventions such as maintaining an IV line, most physical restriction can be prevented if the nurse gains the child's cooperation.

For young children, particularly infants and toddlers, preserving parent-child contact is the best means of decreasing the need for or stress of restraint. For example, almost the entire physical examination can be done in a parent's lap, with the parent hugging the child for procedures such as otoscopy. For painful procedures the parents' preferences for assisting, observing, or waiting outside the room are evaluated.

Environmental factors may also restrict movement. Keeping children in cribs or playpens may not represent immobilization in a concrete sense, but it certainly limits sensory stimulation. Increasing mobility by transporting children in carriages, wheelchairs, carts, wagons, or on stretchers or beds provides them with mechanical freedom.

Maintaining Child's Routine. Altered daily schedules and loss of rituals are particularly stressful for toddlers and early preschoolers and may increase the stress of separation. The nursing admission history provides a baseline for planning care around the child's usual home activities.

A frequently neglected aspect of altered routines is the change in the child's daily activities. A nonhospitalized child's day, especially during the school years, is structured with specific times for eating, dressing, going to school, playing, and sleeping. However, this time structure vanishes when the child is hospitalized. Although nurses have a set schedule, the child is frequently unaware of it; new schedules are imposed that may be rigid or flexible. For example, some units have uniform nap times and bedtimes for all children, whereas others allow children to stay up late at night. Many children obtain significantly less sleep in the hospital than at home; the primary causes are delay in sleep onset and early termination of sleep because of hospital routines. Not only are hours of sleep disrupted, but waking hours are spent in passive activities. For example, few institutions impose any regulation on the amount of time the child spends watching television.

One technique that can minimize the disruption in the child's routine is ***time structuring***. This approach is most suitable for the non–critically ill school-age or adolescent child who has mastered the concept of time. It involves scheduling the child's day to include all those activities that are important to the child and nurse, such as treatment procedures, schoolwork, exercise, television, playroom, and hobbies. Together, the nurse, parent, and child then plan a daily schedule with times and activities written down (Fig. 21-7). This is left in the child's room, and a clock or watch is available for the child's use. Whenever possible, a calendar is also constructed with special events marked, such as favorite television programs, visits by friends or relatives, events in the playroom, and holidays or birthdays. If specific changes in treatment are expected (e.g., "beginning physical therapy in 2 days"), these are added.

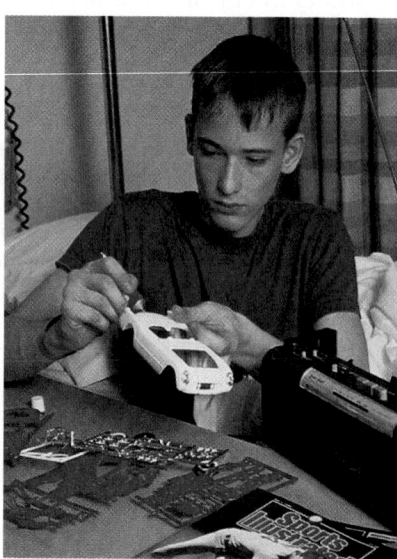

FIG. 21-6 ■ For extended hospitalizations children enjoy having projects to occupy time. (Courtesy St. Louis Children's Hospital.)

NURSING TIP

Ask the young child to select or draw pictures or symbols to represent daily or weekly fun activities (e.g., favorite television programs, family visits, playroom times). Draw a clock face with the hands of the clock depicting the time each event will occur next to the child's representation. Have the child compare the clock on the schedule with a clock or watch in the room. When the two match, the child knows that it is time for a favorite activity and exactly what that activity is.

Encouraging Independence. The dependent role of the hospitalized patient imposes tremendous feelings of loss on older children. Principal interventions should focus on respect for individuality and the opportunity for decision making. Although these sound simple, their efficacy lies with nurses who are flexible, tolerant, and personally secure. The last is particularly important because, when decision making is geared toward the patient, nurses can feel threatened by a sense of lessened control.

Promoting children's control involves maintaining independence, and the concept of self-care can be most beneficial. ***Self-care*** refers to the practice of activities that individuals personally initiate and perform on their own behalf in maintaining life, health, and well-being (Orem, 1995). Although self-care is limited by the child's age and physical condition, most children beyond infancy can perform some activities with little or no help. Whenever possible, these activities are encouraged in the hospital. Other approaches include jointly planning care, time structuring, wearing street clothes, making choices in food selections and bedtime, continuing school activities, and rooming with an appropriate age-mate.

Promoting Understanding. Loss of control can occur from feelings of having too little influence on one's destiny, as well as from sensing overwhelming control or power over fate. Although preschoolers' cognitive abilities predispose them most to magical thinking and self-power, all children are vulnerable to misinterpreting causes for stresses such as illness and hospitalization.

ERIC'S DAILY SCHEDULE:

7:00 AM	– Breakfast, Watch TV, Brush Teeth, Wash up	3:00 PM	– Tutor (M, W, F) Study Time (T, Th)
9:00	– Tub Room, Dressing Change	4:00	– Physical Therapy
		5:00	– Dinner
10:00	– Rest, TV, Snack	6:30	– Dressing Change
11:00	– Physical Therapy	7:00 to 9:00	– TV, Reading, Snack, Friends Visit
12:00 PM	– Lunch		
1:00	– Playroom, Quiet Play, Rest, Friends Visit	9:00	– Brush Teeth, Wash up
		9:15	– Bedtime

FIG. 21-7 ■ Time structuring is an effective strategy for normalizing the hospital environment and increasing the child's sense of control.

Most children feel more in control when they know what to expect, because the element of fear is reduced. Anticipatory preparation and providing information help greatly to lessen stress and prevent lack of understanding (see Preparation for Procedures, Chapter 22).

Informing children of their rights while hospitalized fosters greater understanding and may relieve some of the feelings of powerlessness they typically experience. Hospitals providing services to children should have a hospital-wide policy on the rights and responsibilities of these patients and of their parents or guardians (Joint Commission on Accreditation of Healthcare Organizations, 1999). An increasing number of hospitals and organizations have developed a patient "Bill of Rights" that is prominently displayed throughout the hospital or is presented to children and their families on admission (Box 21-9).

Preventing or Minimizing Fear of Bodily Injury

Beyond early infancy all children fear bodily injury either from mutilation, bodily intrusion, body-image change, disability, or death. In general, preparation of children for painful procedures decreases their fears. Manipulating procedural techniques for children in each age-group also minimizes fear of bodily injury. For example, because toddlers and young preschoolers are traumatized by insertion of a rectal thermometer, axillary temperatures or temperatures taken with electronic or tympanic membrane devices can effectively be substituted. Whenever procedures are performed on young children, the most supportive intervention is to do the procedure as quickly as possible while maintaining parent-child contact.

Because of young children's poorly defined body boundaries, the use of bandages may be particularly helpful. For example, telling children that the bleeding will stop after the needle is removed does little to relieve their fears, whereas applying a small Band-Aid usually provides much reassurance. The size of bandages is also significant to children in this age-group; the larger the bandage, the more importance is attached to the wound. Watching their surgical dressings become successively smaller is one way young children can measure healing and improvement. Prematurely removing a dressing may cause these children considerable concern for their well-being.

For children who fear mutilation of body parts, it is essential that the nurse repeatedly stress the reason for a procedure and evaluate the child's understanding. For example,

BOX 21-9 ■ Bill of Rights for Children and Teens

In this hospital you and your family have the right to:
- Respect and personal dignity
- Care that supports you and your family
- Information you can understand
- Quality health care
- Emotional support
- Care that respects your need to grow, play, and learn
- Make choices and decisions

From Association for the Care of Children's Health: *A pediatric bill of rights,* Bethesda, Md, 1991, The Association.

explaining cast removal to preschoolers may seem simple enough, but children's comprehension of the details may vary considerably from the explanation. Asking them to draw a picture of what they think will happen presents substantial evidence of the perceived events.

Children may fear bodily injury from a great variety of sources. X-ray machines, use of strange equipment for examination, unfamiliar rooms, or awkward positions can be perceived as potentially hazardous. In addition, thoughts and actions can be imagined sources of bodily damage. For older children, masturbation or sex play may be perceived as powerful weapons of potential destruction. Therefore it is important to investigate imagined reasons, particularly of a sexual nature, for illness. Because children may fear revealing such thoughts, using projective techniques such as drawing or doll play may elicit previously undisclosed misconceptions.

Older children fear bodily injury of both internal and external origins. For example, school-age children are aware of the significance of the heart and may fear the actual operation as much as the pain, the stitches, and the possible scar. Adolescents may express concern about the actual procedure but be much more anxious over the resulting scar. An appreciation of each child's special concerns helps nurses focus on critical areas during preparation for procedures or when giving explanations of the disease processes.

Children can grasp information only if it is presented on or close to their level of cognitive development. This necessitates an awareness of the words used to describe events or processes. For example, young children told that they are going to have a CAT (i.e., CT, computed tomography) scan may wonder, "Will there be cats? Or something that scratches?" It is clearer to describe the procedure in simple terms and explain what the letters of the common name stand for.

When children are upset about their illness, their perception can be changed by (1) providing a somewhat different and less negative account of the disease or (2) offering an explanation that is characteristic of the next stage of cognitive development. An example of the first strategy is reassuring a preschooler who fears that after a tonsillectomy, another sore throat means a second operation. Explaining that after tonsils are "fixed" they do not need fixing again can help relieve the fear. An example of the latter strategy is to explain that germs made the tonsils sick and even though germs can cause another sore throat, they cannot cause the tonsils to ever be sick again. This higher-level explanation is based on the school-age child's concept of germs as a cause of disease.

Pain Assessment

Pain assessment is a critical component in managing pain. Pain is multifactorial and includes sensory, affective, behavioral, cognitive, sociocultural, and physiologic components. All of these require assessment (Broome and Huth, 2003). Unfortunately, health professionals, including nurses, continue to underestimate and sporadically manage pain in infants and children (Vincent and Denyes, 2004; Ellis and others, 2002; Broome and others, 1996) (see Evidence-Based Practice box). One of the reasons for inadequate management of pain is a lack of understanding of what pain

is—a personal phenomenon that *cannot* be experienced by any other individual. Therefore defining pain in terms of another's perceptions is inappropriate and inaccurate. An operational definition that is useful in clinical practice follows: *pain is whatever the experiencing person says it is, existing whenever the person says it does* (McCaffery and Pasero, 1999). This definition implies a very important attitude toward patients—*that they are believed.* It includes both verbal and nonverbal expressions of pain.

Fallacies and Facts

Children are undertreated for pain for a number of complex and interrelated reasons, including professionals' misconceptions about pain; the complexities of pain assessment, particularly in nonverbal children; and the lack of information regarding currently available pain reduction techniques. A number of fallacies continue to flourish because of incorrect knowledge about pain in infants and children, despite these fallacies having been disproved by current research on pediatric pain (Box 21-11).

Fear of Addiction. A major concern that prevents health professionals from adequately using opioids* to relieve pain is an unwarranted fear of addiction. Studies on addiction rates in patients treated with opioids have found an incidence of less than 1% (McCaffery and Pasero, 1999). One of the reasons for the unfounded and prevalent fear regarding addiction is confusion among the three terms: physical dependence, tolerance, and addiction. The American Society of Addiction Medicine (2001) has defined physical dependence, tolerance, and addiction, and these definitions are found in the Community Focus box.

Fear of Respiratory Depression. Although respiratory depression is the most serious side effect of opioids, it is a rare occurrence in children. Evidence suggests that in children older than 3 months of age, opioids cause no greater respiratory depression than in adults (Kart, Christrup, and Rasmussen, 1997). Respiratory depression is most likely to occur when the opioid is administered with other sedating drugs, such as hydroxyzine (Vistaril), promethazine (Phenergan), chlorpromazine (Thorazine), midazolam (Versed), or diazepam (Valium). Unlike many sedatives, opioids have the advantage of the antidote naloxone (Narcan), which rapidly reverses the respiratory depressant effect. Fortunately, the benzodiazepines, such as diazepam and midazolam, have the drug flumazenil (Romazicon) to treat respiratory depression (see Guidelines box, p. 681).

In addition, as tolerance to the analgesic effect of opioids occurs, tolerance to the respiratory depressant effect also occurs. Pain acts as a natural antagonist to the respiratory depressant effect of opioids. With increased pain, a patient can receive increased doses of opioids without necessarily

Text continued on p. 661.

---

*The term *opioid* refers to natural or synthetic analgesics with morphine-like actions. It is preferred to the term *narcotic,* which in a legal context refers to any substance that causes psychologic dependence, such as cocaine, which is not an opioid. The word "narcotic" also engenders fears of addiction in older children and parents that are unwarranted when opioids are used for pain control.

EVIDENCE-BASED PRACTICE

Undermedication of Pain in Children

Several studies have examined the pattern of pain medication for children as compared with adults and have found remarkably consistent findings—that children have been undermedicated for pain. Eland and Anderson (1977) investigated the incidence of administration of analgesics to 25 hospitalized children for postoperative pain. Twelve of the children received a total of 24 doses of analgesics; the remaining 13 children were never given any medication for pain relief. In contrast, 18 adults with identical diagnoses received 372 opioid analgesic doses and 299 nonopioid analgesic doses for a total of 671 doses. One of the saddest findings was that more than twice as many children had pain medication ordered as received it. This lack of response to the need for pain medication directly relates to the nurses who failed to administer the analgesic.

Another study investigating analgesic prescriptions given to children and adults after open heart surgery found that all of the adults received medication, for a total of 564 doses, but only three fourths of the children were given medication, for a total of 237 doses during the first 3 postoperative days. This difference was even greater on the fifth postoperative day, when 83% of the adults continued to receive analgesics (a total of 136 doses) but only 12% of the children were medicated (a total of 10 doses) (Beyer and others, 1983).

Another study on postoperative pain found that 75% of the children reported pain on the day of surgery, and if orders for opioid or nonopioid analgesics were written, the nonopioid was given exclusively. In addition, the doses ordered were usually too small or too infrequent to be maximally effective. Most orders were written "PRN," which was often interpreted by nursing staff to mean "as little as possible" (Mather and Mackie, 1983).

A review of analgesic use in the emergency department reported significantly low use in children with mild to moderate trauma, including children with painful fractures. Head injury was associated with especially low use of analgesics (Friedland and Kulick, 1994).

Johnston and others (1992) studied 150 randomly selected hospitalized children and found that 87% reported pain, with 19% stating that their pain was severe. Of the 150 children, only 38% had received analgesics during the previous 24 hours.

An even sadder and more disappointing finding is that two decades after Eland's seminal research, some nurses may neither have knowledge about appropriate analgesic medications for children nor appreciate the consequences of undermedication. In Boughton and others' study (1998), 25% of 36 patients were given no pain medication, and 25% of the patients stated that their pain intervention was only partially effective. All patients had PRN orders for analgesics. Clearly, the responsibility for inadequate pain control rested with the nurses. Vincent and Denyes (2004) recently studied 67 nurses' ability to appropriately manage pain in a group of 132 hospitalized children. In this study, there was a positive relationship between nurses' analgesic administration and children's pain. However, of the 117 children who reported pain, only 74% received analgesia. For those children who received pain medication, 51% reported moderate to high levels of pain.

The situation is even more serious with infants. One analysis of anesthetic practices with newborns undergoing surgical ligation of patent ductus arteriosus found that 76% of the infants received only nitrous oxide and a paralyzing agent. These infants could not move during surgery but could feel all the pain of a thoracotomy (Anand and Aynsley-Green, 1985). In a survey of nurses working in neonatal intensive care units, 79% believed that infants were undermedicated for pain. The same study found that more than half of the medications used for pain relief had no analgesic properties (Franck, 1987). A study comparing premedication for procedures such as arterial line or chest tube placement found that infants in neonatal intensive care units received no premedication much more often than children in pediatric intensive care units (Bauchner, May, and Coates, 1992). In the United States the use of analgesia and anesthesia for newborn circumcision is not routine. A survey of pediatric, obstetric, and family practice residents showed that training in the use of pain reducers during this painful procedure was inadequate (Howard and others, 1998). Unfortunately, the amount of content on pain in nursing curricula also is inadequate, and some of the textbooks contain inaccurate information (Davis, 1998; Ferrell, McCaffery, and Rhiner, 1992).

Much research has been done examining the stress response in premature infants, and the results support the belief that unrelieved pain has detrimental physiologic, anatomic, and behavioral effects (see also Neonatal Pain, Chapter 9). Much less research has been done on the long-term effects of pain on children, from both a psychologic and a physiologic point of view. Stuber and others (1997) examined the psychologic effects on survivors of childhood cancer. Many children reported long-term sequelae that resembled posttraumatic stress syndrome (see Chapter 17). Children's fears were related to their perception of the intensity of treatment, not the illness itself. Symptoms included stomach aches and bad dreams. Another study found that memory of a painful experience may cause anxiety about subsequent procedures. Weisman, Bernstein, and Schechter (1998) showed that children who had a placebo, rather than oral transmucosal fentanyl, before a painful procedure were more anxious than the medicated group for the subsequent procedure even when the analgesic was given. Based on their results, the authors argue strongly for aggressive pain control beginning with the first noxious procedure.

On a positive note, Schechter (1997) outlines the growth in research and published literature (33 articles in 1974 to 2966 articles between 1980 and 1991) in pediatric pain management that comprises many topics such as oncology, sickle cell disease, acute pain, and chronic pain. One outcome of the large number of research studies has been the development of pain teams or pain specialists. Unfortunately, when these services exist, other health care professionals may abandon any responsibility for pain control to the pain experts or neglect to consult the pain team. Although pain teams play a very important role in treating pain adequately (Ferrell and others, 1994), in a survey of 35 pediatric pain services only 17% had written guidelines (Tyc and others, 1998).

Guidelines are available to help practitioners assess and manage pain using methods based on the published scientific literature. In the United States the **Agency for Healthcare Research and Quality (AHRQ)** has published guidelines developed by pain experts that focus on the issues of postoperative, procedure-related or trauma, and cancer pain. Other national and international organizations, including the Joint Commission for the Accreditation of Health Care Organizations, have also contributed research-based recommendations that nurses can use to improve pain control (Box 21-10).

If these references are not readily available to staff, order them, especially the AHRQ publications, and distribute them, stressing that they provide state-of-the-art information. As you practice, carry your copy of the guidelines; mark sections, such as those discussing addiction and listing drug dosages, for quick reference. Compare your pain assessment and management interventions with those in the published guidelines, and make a commitment to increase your knowledge. Remember: to relieve pain effectively, its management must be based on scientific research, not personal opinion or belief.

BOX 21-10 ■ Selected Resources on Pain

FEDERAL GUIDELINES ON PAIN

Acute pain management: operative or medical procedures and trauma (1992)

Quick reference guide for clinicians: acute pain management in adults: operative procedures

Quick reference guide for clinicians: acute pain management in infants, children and adolescents: operative and medical procedures

Pain control after surgery: a patient's guide

Management of cancer pain

Quick reference guide for clinicians: management of cancer pain: adults (1994)

Managing cancer pain: patient guide*

Management of cancer pain: infants, children, and adolescents

Not published. (For excerpts see *J Pharm Care Pain Symptom Control* 2[1]:75-103, 1994.) Resources contain federal medical practice guidelines written by a panel of experts. Available at no charge from the Agency for Healthcare Research and Quality [AHRQ]) Publications, PO Box 8527, Silver Spring, MD 20907; (800) 358-9295; website: www.ahrq.gov

OTHER PROFESSIONAL ORGANIZATIONS' GUIDELINES

AHRQ guidelines on pain: nursing implications. Booklet and two audiotapes describing the development and clinical applications of the guidelines. (From American Pain Society [see below]).

Definitions related to the use of opioids for the treatment of pain. A consensus statement from the American Academy of Pain Medicine, the American Pain Society, and the American Society of Addiction Medicine (2001); www.asam.org/pp01/paindef.htm.

Principles of analgesic use in the treatment of acute pain and cancer pain, ed 4, 1999. Booklet describing consensus guidelines for treating pain. (From American Pain Society, 4700 W Lake Avenue, Glenview, IL 60025-1485; (847) 375-4715; fax: 877-734-8758; website: www.ampainsoc.org).

Management of acute pain: a practical guide. Book describing effective pain management strategies. (Available from the International Association for the Study of Pain [IASP], 909 NE 43rd Street, Suite 306, Seattle, WA 98105-6020; (206) 547-6409; e-mail: iaspdesk@juno.com; website: www.iasppain.org).

Cancer pain relief and palliative care in children (in English, French, Spanish Russian, and Chinese in preparation). World Health Organization in conjunction with IASP, 1998, ISBN 92-4-154512-7, 76 pp. Order from WHO Distribution & Sales, 1211 Geneva 27, Switzerland; price, CHF 18.00, US$16.20, $5 shipping and handling. Order no. 1150459, website: www.who.org.

Joint Commission on Accreditation of Healthcare Organizations (JCAHO) has established pain assessment and management standards and a toll-free hotline: (800) 994-6610 to encourage patients, their families, caregivers, and others to share concerns regarding quality of care issues at accredited health care organizations. Complaints (may be anonymous) may be sent by e-mail to complaint@jcaho.org; faxes to the office of Quality Monitoring at (630) 792-5636; mail to the Office of Quality Monitoring, Joint Commission, One Renaissance Boulevard, Oakbrook Terrace, IL 60181. The pain standards are available from www.jcaho.org/standard/pm_hap.html. A reference book, *Pain assessment and management: an organizational approach,* and an in-

teractive CD-ROM for clinical staff development, *Pain management,* are also available from the Joint Commission.

Guideline for the management of pain in osteoarthritis, rheumatoid arthritis, and juvenile chronic arthritis (2002). Book reviews types, assessment, and treatment of pain in children and adults with arthritis, including use of opioids for chronic pain. (Available from American Pain Society, website: www.ampainsociety.org).

Guideline for the management of acute and chronic pain in sickle-cell disease (1999). Book reviews types, assessment, and treatment of pain in children and adults with SCD. (Available from American Pain Society, website: www.ampainsociety.org).

The use of opioids for the treatment of chronic pain. A consensus statement from the American Academy of Pain Medicine and the American Pain Society. (From *Clin J Pain* 13[1]:6-8, 1997.) (Also Wilson PR: Opioids and chronic pain [editorial], *Clin J Pain* 13[1]:1-2, 1997).

LEGAL IMPLICATIONS AND STATE/FEDERAL REGULATIONS

Pain management on trial. Cushing M, *Am J Nurs* 92(2):21-22, 1992; website: www.nursingcenter.com.

Must we make the courts our last resort? (editorial), Lipman AG, *J Pharm Care Pain Symptom Control* 5(1):1-3, 1997.

Pain management: legal risks and ethical responsibilities. Rich BA, *J Pharm Care Pain Symptom Control* 5(1):5-20, 1997.

The undertreatment of pain: are providers accountable for it? Pasero CL, *Am J Nurs* 101(11):62-63, 2001; website: www.nursingcenter.com.

2001 Annual review of state pain policies: a question of balance.* Joranson DE and others, Pain & Policy Studies Group, University of Wisconsin Comprehensive Cancer Center, Madison, February 2002; website: www.medsch.wisc.edu/painpolicy/publicat/01annrev.

Achieving balance in federal and state pain policy: a guide to evaluation.* Joranson DE and others, Pain & Policy Studies Group, University of Wisconsin Comprehensive Care Center, Madison, July 2000; website: www.medsch.wisc.edu/painpolicy/2003_balance/.

Model guidelines for the use of controlled substances for the treatment of pain (May 1998).* Federation of State Medical Boards of the United States, Inc; website: www.medsch.wisc.edu/painpolicy/domestic/model.htm

Position of the Federation of State Medical Boards in Support of Adoption of Pain Management Guidelines (February 2000).* Federation of State Medical Boards of the United States, Inc; website: www.medsch.wisc.edu/painpolicy/domestic/FSMBwp.htm.

Promoting pain relief and preventing abuse of pain medications; a critical balancing act.* Last Acts, Drug Enforcement Administration, Pain & Policy Studies Group, and others: A joint statement from 21 health organizations and the Drug Enforcement Administration (Oct 2001); website: www.deadiversion.usdoj.gov/pubs/pressrel/consensus.pdf or www.medsch.wisc.edu/painpolicy/dea01.htm.

Resource guide: information about regulatory issues in pain management.* Pain & Policy Studies Group, University of Wisconsin Comprehensive Cancer Center, Madison, 1998; website: www.medsch.wisc.edu/painpolicy/domestic/resource.htm.

*Links may change subsequent to printing. The reader is directed to http://www.medsch.wisc.edu/painpolicy/, the home page of the Pain & Policy Studies Group, to locate appropriate links in case of change.

BOX 21-10 ■ Selected Resources on Pain—*cont'd*

SELECTED RESOURCES ON PEDIATRIC/ADULT PAIN

A child in pain: how to help, what to do. Leora Kuttner (1996). Book written for consumers that focuses on the effects, assessment, and treatment of pain in children. From Hartley & Marks, PO Box 147, Pt Roberts, WA 98281; (800) 277-5887; fax: (800) 707-5887.

Adolescent Pediatric Pain Tool (APPT). Assessment includes use of human figure drawing, Word-Graphic Rating Scale, and choice of descriptive words. From Pediatric Pain Study, UCFS School of 0606; website: www.savedra@linex.com.

American Cancer Society's guide to pain control. Book written for consumers that focuses on numerous aspects of management of cancer pain but would be valuable for any person with pain. Available from American Cancer Society, Health Content Products, 1599 Clifton Road NE, Atlanta, GA 30329; (800) ACS-2345; website: www.cancer.org.

Building an institutional commitment to pain management: the Wisconsin resource manual, ed 2 (2000). An excellent compilation of resource material to promote institutional support of pain management; all of the sample resource tools are available on a disk. Available from American Alliance of Cancer Pain Initiatives, 1300 University Avenue, Madison, WI 53706; (608) 265-4013; fax: (608) 265-4014; e-mail: aacpi@aacpi.org; website: www.aacpi.org

Children's cancer pain can be relieved: a guide for parents and families and Jeff asks about cancer pain. Booklets provide parents and older children with facts about pain and its management in pediatric cancer. Available from American Alliance of Cancer Pain Initiatives, 1300 University Avenue, Madison, WI 53706; (608) 265-4013; fax: (608) 265-4014; e-mail: aacpi@aacpi.org; website: www.aacpi.org.

Circumcision: information for parents. Pamphlet describes the benefits and risks of the procedure and the importance of providing analgesia for the infants. Available from the American Academy of Pediatrics, Division of Pediatrics, 141 Northwest Point Boulevard, PO Box 747, Elk Grove Village, IL 60009-0747; (800) 433-9016; fax: (847) 228-1281; website: www.aap.org.

Circumcision policy statement. Task Force on Circumcision of the American Academy of Pediatrics, *Pediatrics* 103(3):686-693, 1999; www.aap.org.

City of Hope Pain/Palliative Care Resource Center. Serves as a clearinghouse to disseminate information and resources to improve the quality of pain management. (From City of Hope Pain/Palliative Care Resource Center, 1500 East Duarte Road, Duarte, CA 91010; (626) 359-8111, ext 3829; fax: (626) 301-8941; e-mail: mayday_pain@smtplink.coh.org; website: http://mayday.coh.org.

Clinical reference guide for health care providers; sickle cell related pain: assessment and management conference proceedings; sickle cell related pain: assessment and management—a guide for patients and parents. An excellent compilation of resource material to promote pain management in people with SCD. Available from the New England Regional Genetics Groups [NERGG], #28 Clarendon Street, Newton, MA 02460, or Mary Aten (617) 243-3033; e-mail: maryaten@mediaone.net; website: www.acadia.net/NERGG.

Compounding specialist. For information about specially compounded medications, such as Tetracaine 1% Sucker (80 mg), contact Deril J. Lees, RPh, The Apothecary Shoppe, 3707 East 51st Street, Tulsa, OK 74135, (800) 610-2003 in United States or (918) 665-2003; fax: (918) 665-8283. See also Professional Compounding Centers of America (PCCA), 9901 S Wilcrest Drive, Houston, TX 77099; (800) 331-2498; fax: (800) 874-5760; www.pccarx.com.

Consensus statement for the prevention and management of pain in the newborn. Anand KJS and International Evidence-Based Group for Neonatal Pain: *Arch Pediatr Adolesc Med* 155(2):173-180, 2001.

End-of-life care for children, by Texas Children's Cancer Center, Texas Children's Hospital, Houston. Published by the Texas Cancer Council, Austin, 2000. Book provides guidelines for care of children and their families during the transition from aggressive treatment to quality palliative care at the end of life. For additional booklets or information, see www.childendoflifecare.org.

Epidural analgesia for acute pain management: a self-directed learning program and pre- and posttests/answers and explanations, by Chris Pasero, MS, RN. The objectives for the program are to identify the nurse's role in assessing and managing acute pain of adult patients and to identify how to care for adult patients who are receiving epidural analgesia. Available from American Society of Pain Management Nurses [ASPMN], 7794 Grow Drive, Pensacola, FL 32514-7072; (888) 34ASPMN or (888) 342-7766; fax (805) 484-7862; e-mail: aspmn@puetzamc.com; website: www.aspmn.org.

Guidelines for treatment of cancer pain: the pocket edition of the final report of the Texas Cancer Council's Workgroup on Pain Control in Cancer Patients by C. Stratton Hill, Jr, MD (1997). Available free from Texas Cancer Council, PO Box 12097, Austin, TX 78711; (512) 463-3190; fax: (512) 475-2563; website: www.tcc.state.tx.us.

Managing pain before it manages you. Margaret A. Caudill, MD, PhD (1995). Available from The Guilford Press, A Division of Guilford Publications, Inc, 72 Spring Street, New York, NY 10012.

McCaffery: Contemporary issues in pain management. Four videotapes focus on pain management in the elderly; improving the quality of pain management; epidural analgesia for chronic pain; and preventing and managing opioid-induced respiratory depression. **McCaffery on pain: nursing assessment and pharmacological intervention in adults.** Four videotapes focus on nursing assessment of the patient with pain; the three analgesic groups: practical considerations; use of opioid analgesic; and undertreatment of pain. A resource manual also accompanies the videotapes. (Available for purchase from Lippincott Williams & Wilkins; (800) 527-5597; www.lww.com).

No fears, no tears: children with cancer coping with pain. Videotape demonstrates the use of distraction and imagery to reduce distress from various procedures. Available from Canadian Cancer Society; (604) 872-4400; fax: (604) 879-4533. For information on **No fears, no tears—13 years later,** contact Leora Kuttner, PhD; work (604) 736-8801; fax: (604) 294-9986; e-mail: leora_kuttner@sfu.ca (Vancouver, Canada) or order directly from www.burnessc.com/nofears.

No more crying: reducing distress during venipuncture. Videotape describes distraction, limit setting, and positive reinforcement to reduce the distress associated with procedures. Rental or purchase from www.leomedia.net; (217) 337-0700.

Nurse's guide to breakthrough cancer pain. Betty Ferrell, RN, PhD, FAAN with contributions by Michelle Rhiner, RN, MSN, NP (2001). Book provides guidelines for treating breakthrough cancer pain. Available free from Triplei, 295 North Street, Teterboro, NJ 07608; (201) 727-9300; fax: (201) 727-0099.

*Links may change subsequent to printing. The reader is directed to http://www.medsch.wisc.edu/painpolicy/, the home page of the Pain & Policy Studies Group, to locate appropriate links in case of change.

Continued

BOX 21-10 ■ Selected Resources on Pain—*cont'd*

SELECTED RESOURCES ON PEDIATRIC/ADULT PAIN—*cont'd*

Pain management in children with cancer. Marilyn Hockenberry-Eaton, PhD, RN-CS, PNP, CPON, FAAN, and others, published by Texas Cancer Council (1999). Book provides information on treating pain in children with cancer but provides guidelines that apply generally to acute pain management as well. For additional information, see www.childcancerpain.org.

Pain relief electro membrane (PREM) is a high-technology electron reservoir membrane that on contact with skin releases the electrons in the form of microcurrent impulses. PREM relieves acute or chronic musculoskeletal pain, including soft tissue injuries, sports injuries, arthritis, back pain, fibromyalgia, neurogenic pain, and myofascial pain. Available from Helio Medical Supplies, Inc, 606 Charcot Avenue, San Jose, CA 95131; (888) PAINTEM; fax: (408) 433-5566; e-mail: eileen@heliomed.com

Pain relief: how to say no to acute, chronic, & cancer pain! Jane Cowles (1997). Book written for consumers that focuses on the prevention, assessment, and individualized treatment of pain in children and adults. From MasterMedia Publishing, PO Box 1117, Sandy, OR 97055; (800) 334-8232; fax: (503) 668-0494.

Palliative care for children. Committee on Bioethics and Committee on Hospital Care of the American Academy of Pediatrics, *Pediatrics* 106(2):351-356, 2000; website: www.aap.org.

Pediatric Pain Letter by Patrick J. McGrath, PhD, and G. Allen Finley, MD, FRCPC. The Pediatric Pain Letter is a quarterly review of the literature on pain in infants, children, and adolescents that presents series of structured abstracts accompanied by critical commentaries. Questions and subscriptions may be addressed to Julie Goodman, Managing Editor, Pediatric Pain Letter, Psychology Department, Dalhousie University, Halifax, Nova Scotia, B3H 4J1; e-mail: jgoodman@is2.dal.ca.

Perioperative analgesia approaching the 21st century. Study guide and audiocassette reviews current and emerging approaches, such as preemptive analgesia, for surgery. From American Pain Society, 4700 W Lake Drive, Glenview, IL 60025; (847) 375-4715; fax: (847) 375-6315; e-mail: info@ampainsoc.org; website: www.ampainsoc.org/.

Prevention and management of pain and stress in the neonate. American Academy of Pediatrics Committee on Drugs, Section on Anesthesiology, and Section on Surgery; and Canadian Paediatric Society Fetus and Newborn Committee. This statement is intended for health care professionals caring for neonates (preterm to 1 month of age). *Pediatrics* 105(2):454-461, 2000; website: www.aap.org.

Quality of mercy: a case for better pain management. Videotape highlights problems in infant pain control and cancer and burn pain. Rental or purchase from Filmmakers Library, 124 East 40th Street, New York, 10016; (212) 808-4980; fax: (212) 808-4983; e-mail: info@filmakers.com; website: www.filmakers.com.

Reducing the anxiety and pain of injections (1998) is a guide based on a composite of research data, clinical studies, and expert opinion. Available from Becton Dickinson Media Center, 800 ALL MEDIA; fax: (201) 847-4862; website: www.bd.com (reorder number BDM#01). Another excellent article is Reis EC and others: **Taking the sting out of shots: control of vaccination-associated pain and adverse reactions,** *Pediatr Ann* 27(6):376-386, 1998.

Whaley and Wong's Pediatric Pain Assessment and Management. Donna Wong, PhD, RN. Videotape focuses on process of QUESTT for pain assessment and Six Rights for Pharmacologic Pain Relief. Available from Mosby, 11830 Westline Industrial Drive, St. Louis, MO 63146; (800) 426-4545; fax: (800) 535-9935; website: www.mosby.com.

Wong D, Baker C: Reference manual for the Wong-Baker FACES Pain Rating Scale **(2004)** describing development and research of the scale is available from the City of Hope National Medical Center, Pain/Palliative Care Resource Center, 1500 East Duarte Road, Duarte, CA 91010; (626) 359-8111, ext 3829; fax: (626) 301-8941; e-mail: mayday_pain@smtplink.coh.org. To obtain permission to use the scale, contact Elsevier Health Sciences Center, The Curtis Center, 625 Walnut Street, Philadelphia, PA 19106; (800) 523-1649; fax: (215) 238-2239; website: www.mosby.com/WOW/.

Wong-Baker FACES pain rating scale pins. The cost for 1-99 pins is US$5 each. U.S. postage and handling for up to 50 pins is $5; postage for 51-99 pins is $8. The cost for orders of 100 or more is $4 each. Postage and handling are $10 for 100 pins and, for each additional set of 50, $5. Pins may be purchased in gold, red, or blue and with coding of 0-5 for all colors and 0-10 for red only. Please specify color and coding, or one will be chosen. Orders can be sent to Linda Toth, PO Box 2984, Sanford, NC 27331; (919) 498-1158; fax: (919) 498-3993. Make check payable to Linda Toth.

BOX 21-11 ■ Fallacies and Facts About Children and Pain

Fallacy: Infants do not feel pain.

Fact: Infants demonstrate behavioral, especially facial, and physiologic, including hormonal, indicators of pain. Neonates have the neural mechanisms to transmit noxious stimuli by 20 weeks of gestation (Stevens, Johnston, and Horton, 1993; Shapiro, 1989; Anand and Hickey, 1987; Marshall, 1989). (See also Neonatal Pain, Chapter 9.)

Fallacy: Children tolerate pain better than adults.

Fact: Children's tolerance for pain actually increases with age (Lander and Fowler-Kerry, 1991; Haslam, 1969). Younger children tend to rate procedure-related pain higher than older children (Humphrey and others, 1992; Wong and Baker, 1988).

Fallacy: Children cannot tell you where they hurt.

Fact: By 4 years of age, children can accurately point to the body area or mark the painful site on a drawing (Savedra and others, 1993, 1989; Van Cleve and Savedra, 1993); children as young as 3 years old can use pain scales, such as faces (Beyer, Denyes, and Villarruel, 1992; Wong and Baker, 1988).

Fallacy: Children always tell the truth about pain.

Fact: Children may not admit having pain to avoid an injection; because of constant pain, they may not realize how much they are hurting; children may believe that others know how they are feeling and not ask for analgesia (Favaloro and Touzel, 1990; Hester, 1989).

Fallacy: Children become accustomed to pain or painful procedures.

Fact: Children often demonstrate increased behavioral signs of discomfort with repeated painful procedures (Lander and Fowler-Kerry, 1991; Dolgin and others, 1989; Fitzgerald, Millard, and MacIntosh, 1988; Katz, Kellerman, and Siegel, 1980).

Fallacy: Behavioral manifestations reflect pain intensity.

Fact: Children's developmental level, coping abilities, and temperament, such as activity level and intensity of reaction to pain, influence pain behavior (Beyer, McGrath, and Berde, 1990; Wallace, 1989; Young and Fu, 1988). Children with more active, resisting behaviors may rate pain lower than children with passive, accepting behaviors (Broome and others, 1990).

Fallacy: Narcotics are more dangerous for children than they are for adults.

Fact: Narcotics (opioids) are no more dangerous for children than they are for adults. Addiction to opioids used to treat pain is extremely rare in children (Morrison, 1991; Rogers, 1990; Rodgers and others, 1988; Rogers, 1990). Reports of respiratory depression in children are also uncommon (Berde and others, 1991; Billmire, Neale, and Gregory 1985; Dilworth and MacKellar, 1987). By 3 to 6 months of age, healthy infants can metabolize opioids similarly to other children (Hertzka and others, 1989; Koren and others, 1985).

COMMUNITY FOCUS

Fear of Opioid Addiction

One of the reasons for the unfounded but prevalent fear of addiction from opioids used to relieve pain is a misunderstanding of the differences between physical dependence, tolerance, and addiction. Health professionals and the community often confuse addiction with the physiologic effects of opioids, when in reality these three events are unrelated.

The American Society of Addiction Medicine (2001) defines these three terms as follows:

Physical dependence on an opioid is a physiologic state in which abrupt cessation of the opioid, or administration of an opioid antagonist, results in a withdrawal syndrome. Physical dependency on opioids is an expected occurrence in all individuals in the presence of continuous use of opioids for therapeutic or for nontherapeutic purposes. It does not, in and of itself, imply addiction.

Tolerance is a form of neuroadaptation to the effects of chronically administered opioids (or other medications) that is indicated by the need for increasing or more frequent doses of the medication to achieve the initial effects of the drug. Tolerance may occur both to the analgesic effects of opioids and to some of the unwanted side effects, such as respiratory depression, sedation, or nausea. The occurrence of tolerance is variable in occurrence, but it does not, in and of itself, imply addiction.

Addiction in the context of pain treatment with opioids is characterized by a persistent pattern of dysfunctional opioid use that may involve any or all of the following:

■ Adverse consequences associated with the use of opioids
■ Loss of control over the use of opioids
■ Preoccupation with obtaining opioids, despite the presence of adequate analgesia

Unfortunately, individuals who have severe, unrelieved pain may become intensely focused on finding relief for their pain. Sometimes behaviors such as "clock watching" make patients appear to others to be preoccupied with obtaining opioids. However, this preoccupation focuses on finding relief of pain, not on using opioids for reasons other than pain control. This phenomenon has been termed *pseudoaddiction* and must not be confused with real addiction.

Nurses must educate older children, parents, and health professionals about the extremely low risk of real addiction (less than 1%) from the use of opioids to treat pain. Infants, young children, and comatose or terminally ill children simply cannot become addicted, because they are incapable of a consistent pattern of drug-seeking behavior, such as stealing, drug-dealing, prostitution, and use of family income, to obtain opioids for nonanalgesic reasons.

Data from American Society of Addiction Medicine: *Public policy statement on definitions related to the use of opioids for pain treatment,* February, 2001; website: www.asam.org.

BOX 21-12 ■ Pain Experience Inventory

QUESTIONS FOR PARENTS

Describe any pain your child has had before.
How does your child usually react to pain?
Does your child tell you or others when he or she is hurting?
How do you know when your child is in pain?
What do you do to ease discomfort for your child when your child is hurting?
What does your child do to get relief when hurting?
Which of these actions work best to decrease or take away your child's pain?
Is there anything special that you would like me to know about your child and pain? (If yes, have parent[s] describe.)

QUESTIONS FOR CHILD

Tell me what pain is.
Tell me about the hurt you have had before.
What do you do when you hurt?
Do you tell others when you hurt?
What do you want others to do for you when you hurt?
What don't you want others to do for you when you hurt?
What helps the most to take away your hurt?
Is there anything special that you want me to know about you when you hurt? (If yes, have child describe.)

From Hester N, Barcus C: Assessment and management of pain in children, *Pediatr Nurs Update* 1(14):3, 1986.

ment is to assess patients for pain every time the nurse checks for pulse, blood pressure, temperature, and respiratory rate (Federwisch, 1999). Because pain is both a sensory and an emotional experience, several assessment strategies should be used to gather information about pain. One approach to pain assessment in children is QUESTT (Baker and Wong, 1987):

Question the child.
Use a pain rating scale.
Evaluate behavioral and physiologic changes.
Secure parents' involvement.
Take the cause of pain into account.
Take action and evaluate results.

Question the Child. Children's verbal statements and descriptions of pain are the *most* important factors in assessing pain. However, young children may not know what the word "pain" means and may need help in describing it using familiar language. Using a variety of words to describe pain, such as "owie," "boo-boo," "feel funny," or "hurt," is necessary. The nurse should also use appropriate foreign language words; for example, in Spanish, "pain" may be described as "le le," "duele," "dolor," or "ai ai" (see Guide for Spanish words and phrases). Older children benefit from using simple words to describe pain. Questions for obtaining information about children's experiences with pain are presented in Box 21-12. Asking children to locate the pain is also helpful, and play can provide other means for helping children to reveal discomfort.

experiencing clinically significant respiratory depression. Respiratory depression is rare in children receiving long-term opioid therapy, because tolerance to the respiratory depression develops (Collins, 1997).

Principles of Pain Assessment in Children. The American Pain Society* (1999) created the phrase "pain: the fifth vital sign" to increase awareness of pain assessment among health care professionals. The rationale is that if pain were assessed seriousness as other vital signs, it would more likely be treated properly. This one principle of pain assess-

---

*A number of resources on pain management are available from **American Pain Society,** 4700 West Lake Avenue, Glenview, IL 60025-1485; (847) 375-4715; website: www.ampainsoc.org.

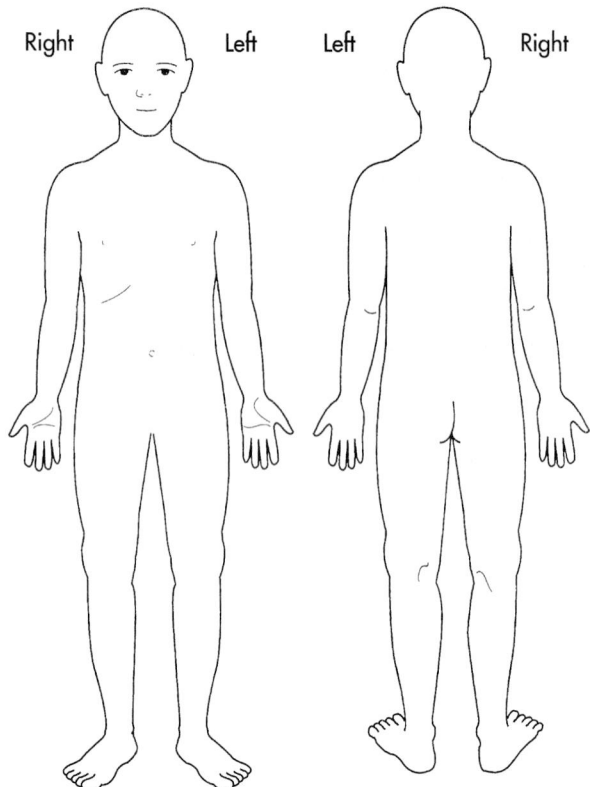

Right   Left   Left   Right

FIG. 21-8 ■ Adolescent pediatric pain tool (APPT): body outlines for pain assessment. Instructions: "Color in the areas on these drawings to show where you have pain. Make the marks as big or as small as the place where the pain is." (From Savedra MC, Tesler MD, Holzemer WL, Ward JA, School of Nursing, University of California–San Francisco; copyright 1989, 1992.)

NURSING TIP

Ask child to point to where it hurts; have child mark or color the painful area on a drawing of a human figure (Fig. 21-8); ask child to tell how a puppet, doll, or stuffed animal is feeling or to point out areas on these models that "hurt" or "don't feel good."

When asking children about pain, the nurse must remember that they may deny pain because they fear receiving an injectable analgesic or because they believe they deserve to suffer as punishment for some misdeed. They may also deny pain to a stranger but readily admit it to a parent. This behavior should not be interpreted as seeking attention from the parent, but as a valid indication of pain.

Use a Pain Rating Scale.   Pain rating scales provide a quantitative self-reporting measure of pain. Although various pain scales exist (Table 21-2), not all of them are appropriate for young children. For the most valid and reliable pain intensity rating, a scale is selected that is suitable to the child's age, abilities, and preference. Scales using facial expressions are readily accepted by children and can be used by children as young as 3 years of age. Evidence indicates that children may prefer a faces scale to other tools (Luffy and Grove, 2003; Keck and others, 1996; Wong and Baker, 1988).

It is best to use the same scale with children to avoid confusing them with different instructions and to use the pain measurement scale for pain only. Multiple uses of the scale (e.g., as a general measure of the child's feelings) can cause the child to lose interest in the scale. Ideally, children should be taught to use the scale before pain is expected, such as preoperatively. Familiarizing children with the scale facilitates its use when children are actually in pain.

Evaluate Behavioral and Physiologic Changes.   Behavioral changes are common indicators of pain and are especially valuable in assessing pain in nonverbal children. Children's behavioral responses to pain change with age and follow a developmental trend (see Box 21-2). However, children vary widely in their responses and may exhibit behaviors at one age that are more typically seen at a different age. Children with more positive moods may appear to be in less pain than they actually are. Children who use passive coping behaviors (offering no resistance, cooperating) may rate pain as more intense than children who use active coping behaviors (resisting, attacking). Recent evidence, however, indicates that temperament does not seem to be a useful predictor of response to pain (Broome, Rehwaldt, and Fogg, 1998). Cultural background may also play a role in children's pain responses (Lipson, Dibble, and Minarik, 1996). In addition, cultural and linguistic differences may hinder assessment. Unfortunately, making judgments about pain based solely on behavior may lead to underestimation of its severity and inadequate pain management (McCaffery and Pasero, 1999; Tesler, Holzemer, and Savedra, 1998).

Depending on the characteristics of pain, children may display behaviors that indicate local body pain, such as pulling the ears for ear pain, rolling the head from side to side for head and ear pain, lying on the side with legs flexed for abdominal pain, limping for leg or foot pain, and refusing to move a body part. Children who experience chronic or repeated pain often develop effective behavioral coping strategies, such as squeezing a hand, talking, counting, relaxing, or thinking about pleasant events. After these coping skills are identified, the child is encouraged to use them in future experiences with pain.

Physiologic responses indicating pain include flushing of the skin; increases in sweating, blood pressure, pulse, and respiration; restlessness; and dilation of the pupils. However, these signs vary considerably—for example, heart rate may actually decrease—and they may be produced by emotions such as fear, anger, or anxiety. They occur primarily in acute pain from stimulation of the sympathetic nervous system. If pain persists, the body begins to adapt and these responses decrease or stabilize. Consequently, if nurses rely primarily on observing these physiologic indications or expecting "pain" behaviors before believing that pain exists, many instances of pain will go unrecognized (Van Cleve, Johnson, and Pothier, 1996).

Several scales have been developed that use changes in behavioral and physiologic parameters to measure pain in young, nonverbal children (Table 21-3). The most common cues assessed in these instruments are facial expression, cry, activity, heart rate, or oxygen saturation, and body movements. One example of such a tool is the **FLACC Postoperative Pain Scale** (Merkel and others, 2002) (see

Text continued on p. 665.

TABLE 21-2 ■ Pain Rating Scales for Children

PAIN SCALE/DESCRIPTION	INSTRUCTIONS	RECOMMENDED AGE/COMMENTS
FACES Pain Rating Scale* Consists of six cartoon faces ranging from smiling face for "no pain" to tearful face for "worst pain"	*Original instructions:* Explain to child that each face is for a person who feels happy because there is no pain (hurt) or sad because there is some or a lot of pain. FACE 0 is very happy because there is no hurt. FACE 1 hurts just a little bit. FACE 2 hurts a little more. FACE 3 hurts even more. FACE 4 hurts a whole lot, but FACE 5 hurts as much as you can imagine, although you don't have to be crying to feel this bad. Ask child to choose face that best describes own pain. Record the number under chosen face on pain assessment record. *Brief word instructions:* Point to each face using the words to describe the pain intensity. Ask the child to choose face that best describes own pain, and record the appropriate number.	For children as young as 3 years. Using original instructions without affect words, such as *happy* or *sad,* or brief words resulted in same ranging pain rating, probably reflecting child's rating of pain intensity. For coding purposes, numbers 0, 2, 4, 6, 8, 10 can be substituted for 0-5 system to accommodate 0-10 system. The FACES provides three scales in one: facial expressions, numbers, and words Research supports cultural sensitivity of FACES for white, black, Hispanic, Thai, Chinese, and Japanese children.

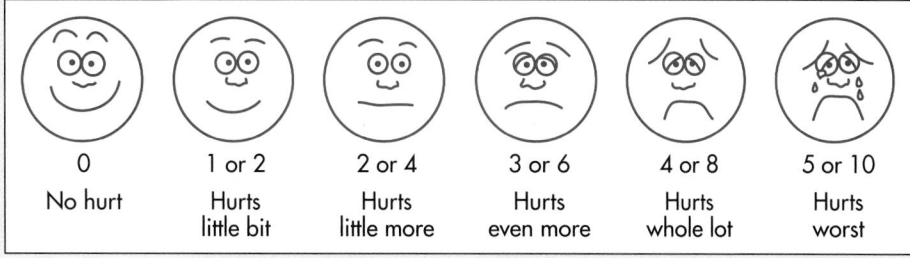

0 No hurt	1 or 2 Hurts little bit	2 or 4 Hurts little more	3 or 6 Hurts even more	4 or 8 Hurts whole lot	5 or 10 Hurts worst

Oucher (Beyer, Denyes, and Villarruel, 1992): Consists of six photographs of white child's face representing "no hurt" to "biggest hurt you could ever have"; also includes a vertical scale with numbers from 0 to 100; scales for black and Hispanic children have been developed (Villarruel and Denyes, 1991)	**Numeric scale** Point to each section of scale to explain variations in pain intensity: "O means no hurt." "This means little hurts" (pointing to lower part of scale, 1 to 29). "This means middle hurts" (pointing to middle part of scale, 30 to 69). "This means big hurts" (pointing to upper part of scale, 70 to 99). "100 means the biggest hurt you could ever have." Score is the actual number stated by child. **Photographic scale** Point to each photograph on Oucher and explain variations in pain intensity using following language: first picture from the bottom is "no hurt," second is "a little hurt," third is "a little more hurt," fourth is "even more hurt than that," fifth is "pretty much or a lot of hurt," and the sixth is the "biggest hurt you could ever have." Score pictures from 0 to 5, with the bottom picture scored as 0. **General** Practice using Oucher by recalling and rating previous pain experiences (e.g., falling off a bike). Child points to number or photograph that describes pain intensity associated with experience. Obtain current pain score from child by asking, "How much hurt do you have right now?"	Children 3-13 years Use numeric scale if child can count to 100 by ones and identify larger of any two numbers, or by tens (Jordan-Marsh and others, 1994). Determine whether child has cognitive ability to use photographic scale; child should be able to rate six geometric shapes from largest to smallest. Determine which ethnic version of Oucher to use. Allow the child elect a version of Oucher, or use version that most closely matches physical characteristics of child. NOTE: Ethnically similar scale may not be preferred by child when given choice of ethnically neutral cartoon scale (Luffy and Grove, 2003).

*Wong-Baker FACES Pain Rating Scale reference manual describing development and research of the scale is available from the Pain/Palliative Care Resource Center, City of Hope National Medical Center, 1500 East Duarte Road, Duarte, CA 91010; (626) 359-8111, ext. 3829; fax: (626) 301-8941; website: www.elsevierhealth.com/WOW/. The use of FACES with children is demonstrated in *Whaley and Wong's Pediatric Nursing Video Series,* "Pain Assessment and Management," narrated by Donna Wong, PhD, RN. Available from Mosby, 11830 Westline Industrial Drive, St Louis, MO 63146; (800) 426-4545; fax: (800) 535-9935; website: www.elsevierhealth.com.   *Continued*

TABLE 21-2 ■ Pain Rating Scales for Children—*cont'd*

PAIN SCALE/DESCRIPTION	INSTRUCTIONS	RECOMMENDED AGE/COMMENTS
Poker Chip Tool† (Hester and others, 1998): Uses four red poker chips placed horizontally in front of child	Say to the child: "I want to talk with you about the hurt you may be having right now." Align the chips horizontally in front of the child on the bedside table, a clipboard, or other firm surface. Tell the child, "These are pieces of hurt." Beginning at the chip nearest the child's left side and ending at the one nearest the right side, point to the chips and say, "This (first chip) is a little bit of hurt and this (fourth chip) is the most hurt you could ever have." For a young child or for any child who may not fully comprehend the instructions, clarify by saying, "That means this (one) is just a little hurt, this (two) is a little more hurt, this (three) is more yet, and this (four) is the most hurt you could ever have." Do not give children an option for zero hurt. Research with the Poker Chip Tool has verified that children without pain, will so indicate by responses such as "I don't have any." Ask the child, "How many pieces of hurt do you have right now?" After initial use of the Poker Chip Tool, some children internalize the concept "pieces of hurt." If a child gives a response such as "I have one right now," before you ask or before you lay out the poker chips, record the number of chips on the Pain Flow Sheet. Clarify the child's answer by statements such as "Oh, you have a little hurt? Tell me about the hurt."	Children as young as 4 years Determine whether child has cognitive ability to use numbers by identifying larger of any two numbers
Word-Graphic Rating Scale‡ (Tesler and others, 1991): Uses descriptive words (may vary in other scales) to denote varying intensities of pain	Explain to child, "This is a line with words to describe how much pain you may have. This side of the line means no pain, and over here the line means worst possible pain." (Point with your finger where "no pain" is, and run your finger along the line to "worst possible pain," as you say it.) "If you have no pain, you would mark like this." (Show example.) "If you have some pain, you would mark somewhere along the line, depending on how much pain you have." (Show example.) The more pain you have, the closer to worst pain you would mark. The worst pain possible is marked like this." (Show example.) "Show me how much pain you have right now by marking with a straight, up-and-down line anywhere along the line to show how much pain you have right now." With a millimeter rule, measure from the "no pain" end to the mark and record this measurement as the pain score.	Children 4-17 years

No pain	Little pain	Medium pain	Large pain	Worst possible pain

†Developed in 1975 by N.O. Hester, University of Colorado Health Sciences Center, School of Nursing, Denver, CO 80262. Also available in Spanish and French.
‡Instructions for Word-Graphic Rating Scale from Acute Pain Management Guideline Panel: *Acute pain management in infants, children, and adolescents: operative and medical procedures; quick reference guide for clinicians,* ACHPR Pub No 92-0020, Rockville, Md, 1992, Agency for Health Care Research and Quality, US Department of Health and Human Services. Word-Graphic Rating Scale is part of the Adolescent Pediatric Pain Tool and is available from Pediatric Pain Study, University of California, School of Nursing, Department of Family Health Care Nursing, San Francisco, CA 94143-0606; (415) 476-4040.

TABLE 21-2 ■ Pain Rating Scales for Children—*cont'd*

PAIN SCALE/DESCRIPTION	INSTRUCTIONS	RECOMMENDED AGE/COMMENTS
Numeric Scale Uses straight line with end points identified as "no pain" and "worst pain" and sometimes "medium pain" in the middle; divisions along line are marked in units from 0 to 10 (high number may vary)	Explain to child that at one end of the line is a 0, which means that a person feels no pain (hurt). At the other end is usually a 5 or a 10, which means the person feels the worst pain imaginable. The numbers 1 to 5 or 10 are for a very little pain to a whole lot of pain. Ask child to choose a number that best describes own pain.	Children as young as 5 years, as long as they can count and have some concept of numbers and their values in relation to other numbers Scale may be used horizontally or vertically. Number coding should be same as other scales used in a facility.

```
No pain                                          Worst pain
  |___|___|___|___|___|___|___|___|___|___|
  0   1   2   3   4   5   6   7   8   9   10
```

Visual Analogue Scale (VAS) (Cline and others, 1992): Defined as a vertical or horizontal line that is drawn to a certain length, such as 10 cm, and anchored by items that represent the extremes of the subjective phenomenon, such as pain, that is measured	Ask child to place a mark on line that best describes amount of own pain. With a centimeter ruler, measure from the "no pain" end to the mark, and record this measurement as the pain score.	Children as young as 4.5 years, preferable 7 years Vertical or horizontal scale may be used Research supports that children ages 3-18 years least prefer VAS to other scales (Luffy and Grove, 2003; Wong and Baker, 1988).

```
No pain                    Worst pain
  |___|___|___|___|___|
```

Color Tool (Eland and Banner, 1999): Uses markers for child to construct own scale that is used with body outline	Present eight markers to child in a random order. Ask child, "Of these colors, which color is like . . . ?" (the event identified by the child as having hurt the most). Place the marker (represents severe pain) away from the other markers. Ask child, "Which color is like a hurt, but not quite as much as . . . ?" (the event identified by the child as having hurt the most). Place the marker with the marker chosen to represent severe pain. Ask child, "Which color is like something that hurts just a little?" Place the marker with the other colors. Ask child, "Which color is like no hurt at all?" Show the four marker choices to the child in order from the worst to the no-hurt color. Ask child to show on the body outlines where they hurt, using the markers chosen. After child has colored the hurts, ask if they are current hurts or hurts from the past. Ask if child knows why the area hurts if it is not clear to you why it does.	Children as young as 4 years, provided they know their colors, are not color blind, and are able to construct the scale if in pain

Table 21-3). Unfortunately, many of these cues can be affected by events other than pain (e.g., anxiety and fear) and may be open to misinterpretation. For a discussion of pain scales for newborns, see Neonatal Pain, Chapter 9.

The issue of assessing pain in children with developmental or physical disabilities or children in a coma, on a ventilator, pharmacologically paralyzed, or heavily sedated remains challenging and, for the most part, unexplored. Researchers are investigating parents' descriptions of recognizing pain in the child with serious cognitive and physical impairment (Fanurik and others, 1999; Oberlander, O'Donnell, and Montgomery, 1999).

One of the most valuable clues to pain is a change in behavior and vital signs after administration of an analgesic. Behaviors such as less irritability or cessation of crying and decreased pulse, respirations, and blood pressure provide important evidence for pain existing before treatment. Often the change in vital signs is attributed to the depressant effect of opioids, when in reality the return to more normal physiologic functioning is due to pain relief.

Encourage Parents' Involvement.   Parents are often the primary source of information about how their child exhibits pain and should play a key role in the assessment

TABLE 21-3 ■ Summary of Selected Behavioral Pain Assessment Scales for Young Children

TOOLS AND AUTHORS/ AGES OF USE	RELIABILITY AND VALIDITY	VARIABLES AND SCORING RANGE
Objective Pain Score (OPS) (Hannallah and others, 1987) *Ages of use:* 4 months-18 years	No testing in original publication Later tested by original authors 1988: concurrent validity with Linear Analog Pain Scale, Spearman's $r = 0.721$ with scores ≥ 6 and 0.419 with scores < 6 1991: interrater agreement, coefficient alpha = 0.986 for one rater and 0.983 for the other 1991: concurrent validity with CHEOPS, Pearson correlation coefficient = 0.88 and 0.94	Blood pressure (0-2) Crying (0-2) Moving (0-2) Agitation (0-2) Verbal evaluation/body language (0-2) *Scoring range:* 0 = no pain; 10 = worst pain
Children's Hospital of Eastern Ontario Pain Scale (CHEOPS) (McGrath and others, 1985) *Ages of use:* 1-5 years	Interrater reliability = 90%-99.5%; internal correlation = significant correlations between pairs of items; concurrent validity between CHEOPS and VAS = 0.91; between individual and total scores of CHEOPS and VAS = 0.50-0.86; construct validity with preanalgesia and postanalgesia scores = 9.9-6.3	Cry (1-3) Facial (0-2) Child verbal (0-2) Torso (1-2) Touch (1-2) Legs (1-2) *Scoring range:* 4 = no pain; 13 = worst pain
Nurses Assessment of Pain Inventory (NAPI) (Stevens, 1990) *Ages of use:* newborn-16 years	Not tested by original author. Later tested by Joyce and others (1994); interrater agreement: weighted kappa 0.37-0.80 Discriminant validity: statistically significant differences between preanalgesia and postanalgesia scores ($p < 0.0001$) Reliability: Cronbach's alpha = 0.35-0.69	Body movement (0-2) Facial (0-3) Touching (0-2) *Scoring range:* 0 = no pain; 7 = worst pain
Behavioral Pain Score (BPS) (Robieux and others, 1991) *Ages of use:* 3-36 months	Original article stated, "reliability of the VAS and BPS scores was tested by a k test"; no further testing of reliability or validity was mentioned	Facial expression (0-2) Cry (0-3) Movements (0-3) *Scoring range:* 0 = no pain; 8 = worst pain
Modified Behavioral Pain Scale (MBPS) (Taddio and others, 1995) *Ages of use:* 4-6 months	Concurrent validity between MBPS and VAS scores = correlation coefficient 0.68 ($p < 0.001$) and 0.74 ($p < 0.001$) Construct validity using prevaccination and postvaccination scores with EMLA versus placebo: significantly lower scores with EMLA ($p < 0.01$) Internal consistency of items = significant correlations between items Interrater agreement: ICC = 0.95, $p < 0.001$ Test-retest reliability: 0.95, $p < 0.001$	Facial expression (0-3) Cry (0-4) Movements (0, 2, 3) *Scoring range:* 0 = no pain; 10 = worst pain
Riley Infant Pain Scale (RIPS) (Schade and others, 1996) *Ages of use:* < 36 months and children with cerebral palsy	Interrater agreement using intraclass correlation coefficient = 0.53-0.83, $p < 0.0001$ Discriminant validity using Mann-Whitney U test with preanalgesia and postanalgesia scores = statistically significant ($p < 0.001$) Sensitivity = 0.31-0.23 Specificity = 0.86-0.90 Interrater reliability using two-way cross tabulations and kappa statistics ($r[87] = 0.94$; $p < 0.001$) and kappa values above 0.50 for each category	0: Neutral face/smiling, calm, sleeping quietly, no cry, consolable, moves easily 1: Frowning/grimace, restless body movements, restless sleep, whimpering, winces with touch 2: Clenched teeth, moderate agitation, sleeps intermittently, pain crying, difficult to console, cries with touch 3: Full cry expression, thrashing/flailing, sleeping prolonged periods interrupted by jerking or no sleep, screaming/high-pitched cry, inconsolable, screams when touched/moved *Scoring range:* 0 = no pain; 3 = worst pain

TABLE 21-3 ■ Summary of Selected Behavioral Pain Assessment Scales for Young Children—*cont'd*

TOOLS AND AUTHORS/ AGES OF USE	RELIABILITY AND VALIDITY	VARIABLES AND SCORING RANGE
FLACC Postoperative Pain Tool (Merkel and others, 1997) *Ages of use:* 2 months-7 years	Validity using analysis of variance for repeated measures to compare FLACC scores before and after analgesia; pre-analgesia FLACC scores were significantly higher than postanalgesia scores at 10, 30, and 60 minutes ($p < 0.001$ for each time) Correlation coefficients used to compare FLACC pain scores and OPS pain scores; significant positive correlation between FLACC and OPS scores ($r = 0.80$; $p < 0.001$); positive correlation also found between FLACC scores and nurses' global ratings of pain ($r[47] = 0.41$; $p < 0.005$)	Face (0-2) Legs (0-2) Activity (0-2) Cry (0-2) Consolability (0-2) ***Scoring range:*** 0 = no pain; 10 = worst pain

FLACC SCALE*

	0	1	2
Face	No particular expression or smile	Occasional grimace or frown, withdrawn, disinterested	Frequent to constant frown, clenched jaw, quivering chin
Legs	Normal position or relaxed	Uneasy, restless, tense	Kicking, or legs drawn up
Activity	Lying quietly, normal position, moves easily	Squirming, shifting back and forth, tense	Arched, rigid, or jerking
Cry	No cry (awake or asleep)	Moans or whimpers, occasional complaint	Crying steadily, screams or sobs, frequent complaints
Consolability	Content, relaxed	Reassured by occasional touching, hugging, or talking to; distractible	Difficult to console or comfort

*From Merkel S and others: The FLACC: a behavioral scale for scoring postoperative pain in young children, *Pediatr Nurs* 23(3):293-297, 1997. Used with permission of Jannetti Publications, Inc., and the University of Michigan Health System. Can be reproduced for clinical and research use.

of their child's pain. They are sensitive to changes in their child's behavior and typically want to be involved in their child's pain relief. Parents' ability to recognize pain in their children varies. Some parents may never have seen their child in severe pain and may not equate certain responses, such as irritability or withdrawal, with discomfort. Others are aware that certain behaviors signal pain because the child has acted similarly during previous painful events. Parents usually know what comforts their child, such as rocking, stroking, or talking. They are the persons most consistently caring for the child. Encouraging their participation gives them control and a sense of helping.

To better assess the child's pain, the nurse can interview the parents about their child's previous pain experiences (see Box 21-12). Ideally, this questioning should occur before the child is in pain, such as on admission to the hospital. Parents need to realize that their knowledge of their child is important in providing care. Parents sometimes leave the assessment of pain up to the nurse because "nurses are more experienced," and they expect the nurse to know when their child is in pain (Woodgate and Kristjanson, 1996). Consequently, parents do not report pain. Parents need to be taught nonverbal pain behaviors in children and encouraged to inform the staff when they think their child is in pain.

Take the Cause of Pain Into Account. When children exhibit behaviors or other clues that suggest pain, reasons for discomfort should be investigated. The pathologic condition may give clues to the expected intensity and type of pain. For example, pain associated with vaso-occlusive crises in sickle cell disease is severe. Pain caused by bone marrow puncture is typically greater than the discomfort associated with a venipuncture. However, it is a mistake to assume that certain conditions or procedures always produce a standard amount of pain. For example, sore throat pain may be mild or severe—only the child knows the intensity.

> **❗NURSING ALERT**
>
> A golden rule to follow in pain assessment is this: Whatever is painful to an adult is painful to an infant or child, until proved otherwise. Be aware that temperament affects coping style, and children with more positive moods may appear to be in less pain than they actually are. Children who use passive coping behaviors (offering no resistance, cooperating) may rate pain as more intense than children who use active coping behaviors (resisting, attacking). If children's behaviors appear to differ from their rating of pain, believe their pain rating, unless they appear to be in pain. In this case, inquire about possible reasons for denying pain (i.e., children with burns may deny pain because they believe they should suffer for setting the fire).

Take Action and Evaluate Results. The reason for assessing pain is to relieve it (p. 669). Complete pain relief, with the combined use of pharmacologic and nonpharmacologic interventions, should be the goal. However, complete relief may not be possible.

Pain Assessment Record

Directions for each column:
1. Record date and time of assessment and analgesic administration; assess analgesic effect _____ minutes later and then _____
2. Use a pain rating scale if child understands its use. Name of scale: _____

   Ratings: No pain = _____ Worst pain = _____ Comfort/function goals* _____
3. Record analgesic, dose, and route
4. Record possible indications or effects of pain, such as shallow breathing due to incisional pain, parental request for pain relief; record indications or effects of pain relief, such as "moves easily, playing"
5. Record any other side effects (e.g., nausea, itching)
6. Record LOS (see inset) R (respiratory function); record breaths per minute and/or other observations of respiratory status (e.g., depth of respiration, change in color of skin)
7. Signature or initials of person recording information

> **Level of Sedation (LOS) Scale†**
>
> S = Sleeping, easily aroused
>   Requires no action
> 1 = Awake and alert
>   Requires no action
> 2 = Occasionally drowsy, easy to arouse
>   Requires no action
> 3 = Frequently drowsy, arousable, drifts off to sleep during conversation
>   Notify practitioner and decrease dose
> 4 = Somnolent, minimal or no response to stimuli
>   Notify practitioner and stop opioid

1 Date/time	2 Pain rating	3 Analgesic	4 Possible effects/indications of pain or relief of pain	5 Side effects	6 LOS/R	7 Signature

*Ask the child what pain rating would be acceptable in terms of usual function (e.g., activities of daily living, playing, attending school, and so on). From McCaffery M, Pasero C, editors: *Pain: a clinical manual,* ed 2, St Louis, 1999, Mosby.

†From Pasero C, McCaffery M: Providing epidural analgesia: how to maintain a delicate balance, *Nurs99* 29(8):34-39, 1999.

FIG. 21-9 ■ Pain assessment record.

Regardless of the type of pain intervention, *evaluation of the results is essential*. No one pain reduction technique is effective for all children. Therefore a pain assessment record is used to monitor the effectiveness of the interventions (Fig. 21-9). With nonverbal children, behavioral and physiologic signs are evaluated for evidence of pain relief. With verbal children, their statements about pain relief and pain ratings are also recorded. Changes in the medication regimen are made as needed to provide the maximum pain relief with minimal side effects. Family members are often excellent partners for keeping a pain assessment record for the nurse.

NURSING ALERT

Presenting practitioners with objective documentation of pain, rather than opinion, is more likely to lead to a favorable change in analgesic orders (Walker and Wong, 1991).

Pain Management

Relief of pain is a basic need and right of all children. Effective pain management requires that health professionals be willing to try a number of interventions to achieve optimal results. Basically, pain-reducing methods can be grouped into two categories: nonpharmacologic and pharmacologic. Whenever possible, both should be used; however, nonpharmacologic measures are not substitutes for analgesics.

Nonpharmacologic Management.   Pain is often associated with fears, anxiety, and stress. A number of nonpharmacologic techniques, such as distraction, relaxation, guided imagery, and cutaneous stimulation (see Guidelines box), provide coping strategies that may help reduce pain perception, make pain more tolerable, decrease anxiety, and enhance the effectiveness of analgesics (Kachoyeanos and Friedhoff, 1993). Although there is inconclusive research on the effectiveness of many of these interventions, the strategies are safe, noninvasive, and inexpensive, and most are independent nursing functions. Experimentation with several strategies that are appropriate for the child's age, pain intensity, interest, and abilities is often necessary to determine the most effective approach.

NURSING ALERT

Most specific nonpharmacologic strategies require children's understanding and cooperation; therefore, try to match the strategy with the pain severity. Children in severe pain may not be able to expend the effort necessary to learn the technique, and those with very mild symptoms may not be motivated to learn. As a result, these strategies may be most useful with midrange pain.

In the selection of a nonpharmacologic intervention, it is best to use a technique familiar to the child or to describe several strategies and let the child select the most appealing one. Parents should be involved in the selection process; they may be familiar with the child's usual coping skills and can help identify potentially successful strategies. Involving parents also encourages their participation in learning the skill with the child and acting as coach. If the parent cannot assist the child, other appropriate persons may include a grandparent, older sibling, nurse, or child-life specialist.

Children should learn a specific strategy *before* pain occurs or before it becomes severe. To reduce the child's effort, instructions for a strategy, such as distraction or relaxation, can be audiotaped and played during a period of discomfort.

Pharmacologic Management.   Using pharmacologic methods to control pain requires attention to four "rights:" right drug, right dose, right route, and right time. In addition, observing for side effects is an essential nursing intervention. Although nurses may not prescribe the medication, knowledge of these essential principles assists in optimally implementing analgesic orders and discussing with other practitioners possible strategies to improve pain control. In addition, observing for side effects of the drug and using supportive approaches with children when administering the drug are important nursing interventions.

Right   Drug.   Nonopioids, including acetaminophen (Tylenol, paracetamol) and nonsteroidal antiinflammatory drugs (NSAIDs), are suitable for mild to moderate pain; *opioids* are needed for moderate to severe pain. A combination of the two analgesics attacks pain on two levels: nonopioids primarily at the peripheral nervous system and opioids primarily at the central nervous system (CNS). This approach provides increased analgesia without increased side effects. Several commercially available combinations, such as Tylenol with Codeine, may have increasing doses of the opioid but a constant dose of the nonopioid (Box 21-13). Therefore, before increasing the opioid, it may be preferable to increase the nonopioid component (e.g., adding 300 mg of plain Tylenol to Tylenol with Codeine No. 3 before advancing to Tylenol with Codeine No. 4). However, if this approach is not successful, the pain most likely requires a stronger opioid.

Actions of various opioids differ. Morphine is considered the gold standard for the management of severe pain. When morphine is not a suitable opioid, drugs such as oxycodone, hydromorphone (Dilaudid), and fentanyl (Sublimaze) are effective substitutes. Although fentanyl is used as an anesthetic in the operating room, it is classified as an analgesic. It can be safely administered by nurses as a continuous infusion (Algren and Algren, 1998). Although methadone is usually thought of as a drug used to treat opioid-dependent patients, it is increasingly being used for postoperative analgesia or intractable pain. When administered orally or intravenously, a single dose of methadone may provide up to 36 hours of pain relief (Yaster, Kost-Byerly, and Maxwell, 2003).

Meperidine (Demerol, pethidine) is not recommended as a first-line opioid analgesic for the management of any kind of pain (American Pain Society, 1999; McCaffery and Pasero, 1999). A major drawback in the use of meperidine is its metabolite, normeperidine. Normeperidine is a CNS stimulant that can produce restlessness, irritability, twitching, jerking, agitation, tremors, and seizures. The CNS side effects caused by normeperidine are not reversed with naloxone. Another disadvantage of meperidine is the long half-life of its metabolite. Normeperidine has a half life of 15 to 20 hours, compared with meperidine's half-life of 3 hours (Tobias, 2003).

GUIDELINES

Nonpharmacologic Strategies for Pain Management

GENERAL STRATEGIES

Use nonpharmacologic interventions to supplement, not replace, pharmacologic interventions and use for mild pain and pain that is reasonably well-controlled with analgesics.

Form a trusting relationship with child and family.

Express concern regarding their reports of pain and intervene appropriately.

Take an active role in seeking effective pain management strategies.

Use general guidelines to prepare child for procedure (see Chapter 22).

Prepare child before potentially painful procedures but avoid "planting" the idea of pain. For example, instead of saying, "This is going to (or may) hurt," say, "Sometimes this feels like pushing, sticking, or pinching, and sometimes it doesn't bother people. Tell me what it feels like to you."

Use "nonpain" descriptors when possible (e.g., "It feels like heat" rather than "It's a burning pain"). This allows for variation in sensory perception, avoids suggesting pain, and gives child control in describing reactions.

Avoid evaluative statements or descriptions (e.g., "This is a terrible procedure" or "It really will hurt a lot").

Stay with child during a painful procedure.

Allow parents to stay with child if child and parent desire; encourage parent to talk softly to child and to remain near child's head.

Involve parents in learning specific nonpharmacologic strategies and in assisting child with their use.

Educate child about the pain, especially when explanation may lessen anxiety (e.g., that pain may occur after surgery and does not indicate something is wrong); reassure that child is not responsible for the pain.

For long-term pain control, give child a doll, which represents "the patient," and allow child to do everything to the doll that is done to the child; pain control can be emphasized through the doll by stating, "Dolly feels better after the medicine."

Teach procedures to child and family for later use.

SPECIFIC STRATEGIES

Distraction

Involve parent and child in identifying strong distractors.

Involve child in play; use radio, tape recorder, CD player, or computer game; have child sing or use rhythmic breathing.

Have child take a deep breath and blow it out until told to stop (French, Painter, and Coury, 1994).

Have child blow bubbles to "blow the hurt away."

Have child concentrate on yelling or saying "ouch" by focusing on "yelling as loud or soft as you feel it hurt: that way I know what's happening."

Have child look through kaleidoscope (type with glitter suspended in fluid-filled tube) and encourage to concentrate by asking, "Do you see the different designs?" (Vessey, Carlson, and McGill, 1994).

Use humor, such as watching cartoons, telling jokes or funny stories, or acting silly with child.

Have child read, play games, or visit with friends.

Relaxation

With an infant or young child:

Hold in a comfortable, well-supported position, such as vertically against the chest and shoulder.

Rock in a wide, rhythmic arc in a rocking chair or sway back and forth, rather than bouncing child.

Repeat one or two words softly, such as "Mommy's here."

With a slightly older child:

Ask child to take a deep breath and "go limp as a rag doll" while exhaling slowly; then ask child to yawn (demonstrate if needed).

Help child assume a comfortable position (e.g., pillow under neck and knees).

Begin progressive relaxation: starting with the toes, systematically instruct child to let each body part "go limp" or "feel heavy"; if child has difficulty with relaxing, instruct child to tense or tighten each body part and then relax it.

Allow child to keep eyes open, since children may respond better if eyes are open rather than closed during relaxation.

Guided Imagery

Have child identify some highly pleasurable real or imaginary experience.

Have child describe details of the event, including as many senses as possible (e.g., "feel the cool breezes," "see the beautiful colors," "hear the pleasant music").

Have child write down or tape record script.

Encourage child to concentrate only on the pleasurable event during the painful time; enhance the image by recalling specific details through reading the script or playing the tape.

Combine with relaxation and rhythmic breathing.

Positive Self-Talk

Teach child positive statements to say when in pain (e.g., "I will be feeling better soon," "When I go home, I will feel better, and we will eat ice cream").

Thought Stopping

Identify positive facts about the painful event (e.g., "It does not last long").

Identify reassuring information (e.g., "If I think about something else, it does not hurt as much").

Condense positive and reassuring facts into a set of brief statements and have child memorize them (e.g., "Short procedure, good veins, little hurt, nice nurse, go home").

Have child repeat the memorized statements whenever thinking about or experiencing the painful event.

Cutaneous Stimulation

Includes simple rhythmic rubbing; use of pressure or electric vibrator; massage with hand lotion, powder, or menthol cream; application of heat or cold, such as vapocoolant spray on the site before giving injection or application of ice to the site opposite the painful area (e.g., if right knee hurts, place ice on left knee).

A more sophisticated method is *transcutaneous electrical nerve stimulation (TENS)* (use of controlled low-voltage electricity to the body via electrodes placed on the skin).

Another method is the use of *Pain Relief Therapeutic Electro-Membrane (P.R.E.M.),* a high-technology membrane electron reservoir fabricated from a nonwoven, nonallergenic dressing that when placed in contact with the skin, releases the stored electrons in the form of microcurrent impulses.*

*For more information contact **Helio Medical Supplies, Inc.,** 606 Charcot Avenue, San Jose, CA 95131; (888)-PAINTEM (724 6836); e-mail: eileen@heliomed.com.

GUIDELINES

Behavioral Contracting

Informal—May be used with children as young as 4 or 5 years of age:

Use stars, tokens, or cartoon character stickers as rewards.

Give uncooperative or procrastinating children (during a procedure) a limited time (measured by a visible timer) to complete the procedure.

Proceed as needed if child is unable to comply.

Reinforce cooperation with a reward if the procedure is accomplished within specified time.

Formal—Use written contract, which includes:

Realistic (seems possible) goal or desired behavior

Measurable behavior (e.g., agrees not to hit anyone during procedures)

Contract written, dated, and signed by all persons involved in any of the agreements

Identified rewards or consequences that are reinforcing

Goals that can be evaluated

Commitment and compromise requirements for both parties (e.g., while timer is used, nurse will not nag or prod child to complete procedure)

BOX 21-13 ■ Selected Combination Opioid and Nonopioid Oral Analgesics—Nonaspirin Products*

Fioricet with codeine	30 mg codeine 325 mg acetaminophen 50 mg butalbital 40 mg caffeine	Percocet 10/650	10 mg oxycodone 650 mg acetaminophen
Hydrocet	5 mg hydrocodone 500 mg acetaminophen	Tylenol with codeine No. 1	7.5 mg codeine 300 mg acetaminophen
Lorcet-HD	5 mg hydrocodone 500 mg acetaminophen	Tylenol with codeine No. 2	15 mg codeine 300 mg acetaminophen
Lorcet Plus	7.5 mg hydrocodone 650 mg acetaminophen	Tylenol with codeine No. 3	30 mg codeine 300 mg acetaminophen
Lorcet 10/650	10 mg hydrocodone 650 mg acetaminophen	Tylenol with codeine No. 4	60 mg codeine 300 mg acetaminophen
Lortab 2.5/500	2.5 mg hydrocodone 500 mg acetaminophen	Tylenol and codeine elixir (each 5 mL)	12 mg codeine 120 mg acetaminophen 7% alcohol
Lortab 5/500	5 mg hydrocodone 500 mg acetaminophen	Tylox†	5 mg oxycodone HCl 500 mg acetaminophen
Lortab 10/500	10 mg hydrocodone 500 mg acetaminophen	Vicodin	5 mg hydrocodone 500 mg acetaminophen
Lortab Elixir (each 15 mL)	7.5 mg hydrocodone 500 mg acetaminophen	Vicodin ES	7.5 mg hydrocodone 750 mg acetaminophen
Percocet 2.5/325†	2.5 mg oxycodone 325 mg acetaminophen	Vicodin HP	10 mg hydrocodone 650 mg acetaminophen
Percocet-5/325	5 mg oxycodone HCl 325 mg acetaminophen	Vicoprofin	7.5 mg hydrocodone 200 mg ibuprofen
Percocet 7.5/500	7.5 mg oxycodone 500 mg acetaminophen		

*Aspirin is not recommended for children, because of its possible association with Reye syndrome. Analgesic compounds with aspirin include Darvon Compound, Darvon with A.S.A., Percodan, and Percodan-Demi, Darvon, or Darvocet (propoxyphene) is not recommended; its analgesic effect is no greater than that from aspirin, acetaminophen, or other nonsteroidal antiinflammatory drugs. Propoxyphene, an opioid, can depress respirations, and its major metabolite is cardiotoxic and is a central nervous system stimulant that can produce seizures (Dahl, 1998).

†All medications require a prescription, but these are classified as schedule II drugs (such as morphine), and each filling requires a written prescription that includes the patient's name and address, the practitioner's DEA (Drug Enforcement Agency) number, and the date. In case of emergency, verbal prescriptions for schedule II substances may be filled; however, the practitioner must provide a signed prescription within 72 hours. Schedule II prescriptions cannot be refilled but require a new prescription.

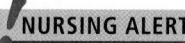 NURSING ALERT

By any route of administration, the use of meperidine for any type of pain management in children should be questioned, because there are other, less toxic, more effective opioid drugs available. Meperidine should be used only for short-term (48 hours) pain management in healthy patients who have demonstrated an unusual reaction or allergic response during treatment with other opioids. When meperidine is administered, assess the child frequently for signs of toxicity such as tremors of the outstretched hands, twitching or jerk-ing, or increased agitation. If toxicity is suspected, discontinue the meperidine, maintain the IV infusion, and notify the practitioner immediately. An adverse drug reaction should also be reported.*

---

*The **FDA Medical Products Reporting Program,** Food and Drug Administration, 5600 Fishers Lane, Rockville, MD 20852-9787; (800) FDA-1088; fax: (800) FDA-0178; website: www.fda.gov/medwatch.

Opioids are frequently combined with other drugs that are considered "potentiators." However, little evidence indicates that any drug potentiates the analgesic effect of opioids; rather, drugs that produce sedation are erroneously equated with producing analgesia. One common drug combination—*meperidine (pethidine [Demerol]), promethazine (Phenergan),* and *chlorpromazine (Thorazine),* known as *DPT* or *lytic cocktail*—has commonly been used to sedate children for procedures (see Preoperative Care, Chapter 22). Meperidine, a short-acting analgesic, provides pain relief for 2 to 3 hours but is irritating to the tissues when given intramuscularly. Promethazine has antianalgesic properties, produces excessive sedation, and can cause extrapyramidal reactions (spasms of neck, face, and back; shuffling gait; drooling; speech impairment; restlessness). Besides producing prolonged deep sedation, all of these drugs can cause respiratory depression and lower the seizure threshold, a particular risk to those with a seizure disorder. In addition, the "cocktail" is usually administered intramuscularly, causing additional pain. **For these reasons, DPT is not recommended for general use** (Yaster, Kost-Byerly, and Maxwell, 2003). Appropriate drugs for sedation are listed in Table 21-4.

Several drugs, known as *adjuvant analgesics* or *coanalgesics,* may be used alone or with opioids to control pain symptoms. Frequently used drugs to relieve anxiety, cause sedation, and provide amnesia are diazepam (Valium) and midazolam (Versed); however, they are not analgesics. Other adjuvants include tricyclic antidepressants (i.e., amitriptyline, imipramine) and antiepileptics for neuropathic pain (brief, lancinating pain); steroids for inflammation and bone pain; and dextroamphetamine and caffeine for increased analgesia and decreased sedation (McCaffery and Pasero, 1999).

At times, health professionals question whether pain really exists and administer *placebos* to "see if the pain is real." This practice is unjustified and unethical; a positive response to a placebo, such as a saline injection, is common in patients who have a documented organic basis for pain. Therefore the deceptive use of placebos does not provide

TABLE 21-4 ■ Suggested Medications for Sedation

DRUG	DOSING	SIDE EFFECTS	REVERSAL AGENTS
CONSCIOUS SEDATION			
Midazolam A benzodiazepine (short acting), CNS depressant *Onset:* 1-5 minutes *Peak effect:* 3-5 minutes (IV) *Half-life:* 1.5-2 hours	Oral: 0.2-1 mg/kg; 30-45 minutes before procedure; maximum: 20 mg IV: 0.05 mg/kg 3 minutes before procedure (may repeat dose × 2); maximum: 2 mg/dose	Respiratory distress, depression, apnea, PVCs, amnesia, blurred vision, or hyperexcitability	Flumazenil: 0.2 mg/dose every 1 minute; maximum cumulative = 1 mg
Fentanyl A narcotic analgesic *Onset:* 1-5 minutes *Peak effect:* no data available *Half-life:* 1.5-6 hours	IV: 0.5-3 μg/kg/dose; may repeat after 30-60 minutes; maximum: 50 μg/dose Use lower doses (0.5-1 μg/kg/dose) when used in combination with other agents, such as midazolam	Respiratory distress or depression, apnea, seizures, shock, chest wall rigidity (with rapid infusion or high doses)	Naloxone: 5-10 μg/kg/dose; single dose should not exceed maximum likely to occur with recommended adult dose of 0.2 mg
Morphine A narcotic analgesic *Onset:* 15-60 minutes *Peak effect:* 30-40 minutes *Half life:* 1.5-2 hours	IV: 0.05-0.1 mg/kg 5 minutes before procedure; maximum: 15 mg/dose	Sedation, somnolence, respiratory distress or depression, pruritus	Naloxone: 5-10 μg/kg/dose; single dose should not exceed maximum recommended adult dose of 0.2 mg
UNCONSCIOUS SEDATION			
Propofol A general anesthetic *Onset:* within 30 seconds *Peak effect:* 3-10 minutes *Half life:* three-compartment model Initial: 2-8 minutes second distribution: 40 minutes Terminal: 200 minutes	IV: 1-2 mg/kg followed by 75-100 μg/kg/min **(only with qualified anesthesia personnel available)**	Pain on injection, involuntary movements, hypotension, apnea	None
Ketamine A general anesthetic *Onset:* 30 seconds with IV administration; PO 20-45 minutes *Peak effect:* 5 minutes *Half-life:* unknown	Oral: 6-10 mg/kg given 30 minutes before procedure IV: 0.25-0.75 mg/kg **(only with anesthesia personnel available)**	Laryngospasm, severe hypotension/hypertension, respiratory depression, apnea, excessive salivation	None

useful information about the presence or severity of pain. In addition, the use of placebos can cause side effects similar to those of opioids, can destroy the client's trust in the health care staff, and raises serious ethical and legal questions (Pasero, 1995). The position of the American Society of Pain Management Nurses (1998) is that placebos should not be used by any route in the assessment or management of pain in any patient regardless of age or diagnosis.

Right Dosage.   The optimal dosage is one that controls pain without causing severe side effects. This usually requires *titration,* the gradual adjustment of drug dosage (usually by increasing or decreasing the dose) until optimal pain relief without excessive sedation is achieved. Dosage recommendations, such as those in Tables 21-5 and 21-6, are only safe initial dosages, not optimal dosages. Children (except infants younger than about 3 to 6 months of age) metabolize drugs more rapidly than adults; younger children may require higher doses of opioids to achieve the same analgesic effect. Therefore the therapeutic effect and duration of analgesia vary. Children's dosages are usually calculated according to body weight, except in children who weigh 50 kg (110 pounds) or more, when the weight formula may exceed the average adult dose. In this case the adult dose is used.

A reasonable starting dose of opioid for infants younger than 6 months of age who are not mechanically ventilated is one fourth to one third of the recommended starting dose for older children. The infant is monitored very closely for signs of pain relief and respiratory depression. The dose is titrated to response. Because tolerance can develop rapidly, very large opioid doses may be needed for continued severe pain (American Pain Society, 1999).

If pain relief is inadequate, the initial dosage is increased (usually by 25% to 50% and sometimes more to provide greater analgesic effectiveness). Decreasing the interval between doses may also provide more continuous pain relief. A major difference between opioids and nonopioids is that nonopioids have a *ceiling effect,* which means that doses higher than the recommended dose will not produce greater pain relief. Opioids do not have a ceiling effect other than that imposed by side effects; therefore larger dosages can be given safely for increasing severity of pain.

> **!NURSING ALERT**
>
> A frequent error in attempts to improve pain control is to change to another analgesic. If an opioid, such as morphine, hydromorphone, or fentanyl, is used, rarely is the problem one of drug choice. Rather, the problem is usually one of inadequate dosage. If changing to another analgesic is warranted because of adverse side effects, the new drug should be slightly less or equal in potency to the original analgesic.

TABLE 21-5 ■ Nonsteroidal Antiinflammatory Drugs (NSAIDs) Approved for Children*

DRUG (TRADE NAME)	DOSE	COMMENTS
Acetaminophen (Tylenol and other brands)†	10-15 mg/kg/dose every 4-6 hours not to exceed five doses in 24 hours or 75 mg/kg/day, orally	Available in numerous preparations Nonprescription Higher dosage range may provide increased analgesia
Choline magnesium trisalicylate (Trilisate)†	Children <37 kg: 50 mg/kg/day divided into two doses Children >37 kg: 2250 mg/day divided into two doses	Available in suspension, 500 mg/5 mL Prescription

Ibuprofen‡
  Children's Motrin
  Children's Advil
	Children <6 months: 5-10 mg/kg/dose every 6-8 hours not to exceed 40 mg/kg/day	Available in numerous preparations
		Available in suspension, 100 mg/5 mL, and drops, 100 mg/2.5 mL
		Nonprescription

Naproxen (Naprosyn)	Children >2 years: 10 mg/kg/day divided into two doses	Available in suspension, 125 mg/5 mL, and several different dosages for tablets Prescription
Tolmetin (Tolectin)	Children >2 years: 20 g/kg/day divided into three or four doses	Available in 200-mg, 400-mg, and 600-mg tablets Prescription

Data from Olin BR and others: *Drug facts and comparisons,* St Louis, 2002, Facts and Comparisons.
NOTE: Newer formulations of NSAIDs, such as celecoxib (Celebrex), rofecoxib (Vioxx), or valdecoxib (Bextra), selectively inhibit one of the enzymes of cyclooxygenase (COX-2, which is responsible for pain transmission) but do not inhibit the other (COX-1). Inhibition of COX-1 decreases prostaglandin production, which is necessary for normal organ function. For example, prostaglandins help maintain gastric mucosal blood flow and barrier protection, regulate blood flow to the liver and kidneys, and facilitate platelet aggregation and clot formation. Theoretically, the COX-2 NSAIDs provide similar analgesic and antiinflammatory benefits with fewer gastric and platelet side effects than the nonselective agents. COX-2 NSAIDs are approved for use in patients older than 18 years of age.
*All NSAIDs in this table (except acetaminophen) have significant antiinflammatory, antipyretic, and analgesic actions. Acetaminophen has a weak antiinflammatory action, and its classification as an NSAID is controversial. Patients respond differently to various NSAIDs; therefore, changing from one drug to another may be necessary for maximum benefit. Acetylsalicylic acid (aspirin) is also an NSAID but is not recommended for children because of its possible association with Reye syndrome. The NSAIDs in this table have no known association with Reye syndrome. However, caution should be exercised in prescribing any salicylate-containing drug (e.g., Trilisate) for children with known or suspected viral infection.
†Acetaminophen and choline magnesium trisalicylate are well-tolerated in the gastrointestinal tract and do not interfere with platelet function. NSAIDs (except acetaminophen) should not be given to patients with allergic reactions to salicylates. All the NSAIDs should be used cautiously in patients with renal impairment.
‡Side effects of ibuprofen, naproxen, and tolmetin include nausea, vomiting, diarrhea, constipation, gastric ulceration, bleeding nephritis, and fluid retention.

TABLE 21-6 ■ Dosage of Selected Opioids for Children

DRUG	APPROPRIATE EQUIANALGESIC	APPROXIMATE EQUIANALGESIC PARENTERAL DOSE	RECOMMENDED STARTING DOSE (children less than 50-kg body weight)*	
			ORAL	PARENTERAL
Morphine‖	30 mg every 3-4 hours	10 mg every 3-4 hours	0.2-0.4 mg/kg every 3-4 hours 0.3-0.6 mg/kg time released every 12 hours	0.1-0.2 mg/kg intramuscularly (IM) every 3-4 hours 0.02-0.1 mg/kg intravenously (IV) bolus every 2 hours 0.015 mg/kg every 8 minutes for patient-controlled analgesia 0.01-0.02 mg/kg/hr IV infusion (neonates) 0.01-0.06 mg/kg/hr IV infusion (child)
Fentanyl (Sublimaze) (oral mucosal form—Actiq)§	Not available	0.1 mg IV	5-15 μg/kg; maximum dose 400 μg	0.5-1.5 μg/kg IV bolus every half hour 1-2 μg/hr IV infusion
Codeine‡	200 mg every 3-4 hours	130 mg every 3-4 hours	1 mg/kg every 3-4 hours	Not recommended
Hydromorphone‖ (Dilaudid)	7.5 mg every 3-4 hours	1.5 mg every 3-4 hours	0.04-0.1 mg/kg every 3-4 hours	0.02-0.1 mg/kg every 3-4 hours 0.005-0.2 mg/kg IV bolus every 2 hours Not available
Hydrocodone (in Lorcet, Lortab, Vicodin, others)	30 mg every 3-4 hours	Not available	0.2 mg/kg every 3-4 hours	0.02 mg/kg every 6-8 hours
Levorphanol (Levo- Dromoran)	4 mg every 6-8 hours	2 mg every 6-8 hours	0.04 mg/kg every 6-8 hours	0.75 mg/kg every 2-3 hours
Meperidine (Demerol)#	300 mg every 2-3 hours	100 mg every 3 hours	Not recommended	0.1 mg/kg every 6-8 hours
Methadone (Dolophine, others)**	20 mg every 6-8 hours	10 mg every 6-8 hours	0.2 mg/kg every 6-8 hours	Not available
Oxycodone (Roxicodone, OxyContin; also in Percocet, Percodan, Tylox, others)	20 mg every 3-4 hours	Not available	2 mg/kg every 3-4 hours¶	

Data from Acute Pain Management Guideline Panel: *Acute pain management: operative or medical procedures and trauma: clinical practice guideline,* AHCPR Pub No 92-0032, Rockville, Md, 1992, Agency for Health Care Policy and Research, Public Health Service, US Department of Health and Human Services; Berde C and others: Report of the subcommittee on disease-related pain in childhood cancer, *Pediatrics* 86(5 pt 2):820, 1990.
ATC, Around the clock; *IM,* intramuscular; *IV,* intravenous; *PCA,* patient-controlled analgesia.
NOTE: Published tables vary in the suggested doses that are equianalgesic to morphine. Clinical response is the criterion that must be applied for each patient; titration to clinical response is necessary. Because there is not complete cross-tolerance among these drugs, it is usually necessary to use a lower than equianalgesic dose when changing drugs and to retitrate to response. **CAUTION:** Recommended doses do not apply to patients with renal or hepatic insufficiency or other conditions affecting drug metabolism and kinetics.
*CAUTION: Doses listed for patients with body weight less than 50 kg cannot be used as initial starting doses in infants less than 6 months of age. For nonventilated infants younger than 6 months of age, the initial opioid dose should be about one fourth to one third of the dose recommended for older infants and children. For example, morphine could be used at a dose of 0.03 mg/kg instead of the traditional 0.1 mg/kg.
‡CAUTION: Codeine doses above 65 mg often are not appropriate because of diminishing incremental analgesia with increasing doses but continually increasing constipation and other side effects. Dosages are from McCaffery M, Pasero C: *Pain: a clinical manual,* ed 2, St Louis, 1999, Mosby.
‖For morphine, hydromorphone, and oxymorphone, rectal administration is an alternate route for patients unable to take oral medications, but equianalgesic doses may differ from oral and parenteral doses because of pharmacokinetic differences.
§Actiq is indicated only for management of breakthrough cancer pain in patients with malignancies who are already receiving and are tolerant to opioid therapy but can be used for preoperative or preprocedural sedation/analgesia.
#Meperidine is not recommended for continuous pain control (i.e., postoperatively) because of risk of normeperidine toxicity.
¶CAUTION: Doses of aspirin and acetaminophen in combination with opioid/NSAID preparations must also be adjusted to patient's body weight. Daily dose of acetaminophen should not exceed 75 mg/kg or 4000 mg.
**Initial dose is 10%-25% of equianalgesic morphine dose. Parenteral Dolophine is no longer available in the United States.

TABLE 21-7 ■ Selected Analgesics (Equianalgesia)

DRUG*	EQUAL TO ORAL MORPHINE (mg)	EQUAL TO INTRAMUSCULAR/ INTRAVENOUS MORPHINE (mg)
Hydromorphone (Dilaudid), 1 mg	4	1.3
Codeine, 30 mg	4.5	1.5
Meperidine (Demerol), 50 mg	4.8	1.6
Codeine, 30 mg; acetaminophen, 300 mg (Tylenol No. 3)	7.2	2.4
Oxycodone, 5 mg; acetaminophen, 325 mg (Percocet)	7.2	2.4
Oxycodone, 5 mg; aspirin, 325 mg (Percodan)	7.2	2.4
Hydrocodone, 5 mg; acetaminophen, 500 mg (Vicodin, Lortab)	9	3
Oxycodone, 5 mg; acetaminophen, 500 mg (Tylox)	9	3
Dolophine (Methadone), 10 mg	15	7.5
Acetaminophen (Tylenol), 325 mg	2.7	0.9
Aspirin, 325 mg	2.7	0.9
Acetaminophen (Tylenol Extra Strength), 500 mg	4	1.3
Codeine, 60 mg; acetaminophen, 300 mg (Tylenol No. 4)	11.7	3.9
Transdermal fentanyl patch (Duragesic) (based on 25 μg/hr patch applied every 3 days = 50 mg oral morphine every 24 hours or divided into six doses = 8.3 mg)	8.3	2.77

or use:

RECOMMENDED INITIAL DURAGESIC DOSE BASED ON DAILY ORAL MORPHINE DOSE†

ORAL 24-HOUR MORPHINE (mg/day)	DURAGESIC DOSE (mg/hr)
45-134	25
135-224	50
225-314	75
315-404	100
405-494	125
495-584	150
585-674	175
675-764	200
765-854	225
855-944	250
945-1034	275
1035-1124	300

Courtesy of Betty R. Ferrell, PhD, FAAN, 1999. Used with permission.

NOTE: When converting to oral oxycodone from oral morphine, an appropriate conservative estimate is 15-20 mg of oxycodone per 30 mg of morphine; however, when converting to oral morphine from oral oxycodone, an appropriate conservative estimate is 30 mg of morphine per 30 mg of oxycodone (McCaffery M, Pasero C: *Pain: a clinical manual*, ed 2, St Louis, 1999, Mosby, p 198).

*Oral medication with exception of fentanyl.

†Data from Duragesic package insert, Janssen, Pharmaceutical Products, Titusville, NJ, 2001.

Parenteral and oral dosages of opioids are not the same. Because of the *first-pass effect*, an oral opioid is rapidly absorbed from the gastrointestinal tract and enters the portal circulation, where it is partially metabolized before reaching the central circulation. Therefore oral dosages must be larger to compensate for the partial loss of analgesic potency to achieve *equianalgesia* (equal analgesic effect). Conversion factors for selected opioids, when a change is made from intramuscular (IM) or IV to oral, are listed in Tables 21-6 and 21-7. Immediate conversion from IM or IV to the suggested equianalgesic oral dose may result in a substantial error in the individual child. For example, the dose may be significantly more or less than what the child requires. Small changes ensure small errors.

Right Route. Several routes of analgesic administration exist (Box 21-14). Children should not have to endure pain, such as from IM injections, to achieve pain relief.

Therefore the most effective and least traumatic route of administration should be selected.

A significant advance in the administration of IV, epidural, or subcutaneous (SC) analgesics is the use of *patient-controlled analgesia (PCA)*. As the name implies, the patient controls the amount and frequency of the analgesic, which is typically delivered through a special infusion device. Successfully using a PCA pump requires a patient to have enough intelligence, manual dexterity, and strength to push the button to operate the pump. Children who are able to play a video or computer game (5 to 6 years of age) often can successfully use PCA. Contraindications to using PCA include inability to understand how to use the button, inability to push the button because of limitations of mobility (weakness, presence of a cast, or traction), or an unwillingness to use the pump. Although it is controversial, parents and nurses have used the PCA system for the child. When used as "nurse"- or "parent"-controlled analgesia, the concept of patient control is negated,

BOX 21-14 ■ Routes and Methods of Analgesic Drug Administration

ORAL

Preferred because of convenience, cost, and relatively steady blood levels

Higher dosages of oral form of opioids required for equivalent parenteral analgesia

Peak drug effect occurs after 1-2 hours for most analgesics
Delay in onset is disadvantage when rapid control of severe pain or of fluctuating pain is desired

SUBLINGUAL/BUCCAL/TRANSMUCOSAL

Tablet or liquid placed between cheek and gum (buccal) or under tongue (sublingual)

Highly desirable because more rapid onset than with oral route
Less first-pass effect through liver than oral route, which normally reduces analgesia from oral opioids (unless sublingual/buccal form swallowed, which occurs often in children)

Few drugs commercially available in this form
Many drugs can be compounded into a sublingual troche or lozenge*

Actiq—Oral transmucosal fentanyl citrate in hard confection base on a plastic holder; indicated only for management of breakthrough cancer pain in patients with malignancies who are already receiving and are tolerant to opioid therapy but can be used for preoperative or preprocedural sedation/analgesia

INTRAVENOUS (IV) (BOLUS)

Preferred for rapid control of severe pain

Provides most rapid onset of effect, usually in about 5 minutes
Advantage for acute pain, procedural pain, and breakthrough pain

Needs to be repeated hourly for continuous pain control
Drugs with short half-life (morphine, fentanyl, hydromorphone) are preferred, to avoid toxic accumulation of drug

INTRAVENOUS (CONTINUOUS)

Preferred over bolus and intramuscular injection for maintaining control of pain

Provides steady blood levels

Easy to titrate dosage

SUBCUTANEOUS (SC) (CONTINUOUS)

Used when oral and IV routes not available

Provides equivalent blood levels to continuous IV infusion

Suggested initial bolus dose to equal 2-hour IV dose; total 24-hour dose usually requires concentrated opioid solution to minimize infused volume. Use smallest gauge needle that accommodates infusion rate

PATIENT-CONTROLLED ANALGESIA (PCA)

Generally refers to self-administration of drugs, regardless of route

Typically uses programmable infusion pump (IV, epidural, SC) that permits self-administration of boluses of medication at preset dose and time interval (lockout interval is time between doses)

PCA bolus administration may be combined with initial bolus and continuous (basal or background) infusion of opioid

Optimal lockout interval not known but must be at least as long as time needed for onset of drug
Should effectively control pain during movement or procedures
Longer lockout provides larger dose

FAMILY-CONTROLLED ANALGESIA

One family member (usually a parent) or other caregiver is designated child's primary pain manager and has responsibility of pressing PCA button

Guidelines for selecting a primary pain manager for family-controlled analgesia
Spends a significant amount of time with the patient
Is willing to assume responsibility of being primary pain manager
Is willing to accept and respect patient's reports of pain (if able to provide) as best indicator of how much pain the patient is experiencing; knows how to use and interpret a pain rating scale
Understands the purpose and goals of patient's pain management plan
Understands concept of maintaining a steady analgesic blood level
Recognizes signs of pain and side effects and adverse reactions to opioid

NURSE-ACTIVATED ANALGESIA

Child's primary nurse is designated primary pain manager and is only person who presses PCA button during that nurse's shift

Guidelines for selecting primary pain manager for family-controlled analgesia apply to nurse-activated analgesia

May be used in addition to a basal rate to treat breakthrough pain with bolus doses; patients are assessed every 30 minutes for the need for a bolus dose

May be used without a basal rate as a means of maintaining analgesia with ATC bolus doses

INTRAMUSCULAR

NOT RECOMMENDED FOR PAIN CONTROL; NOT CURRENT STANDARD OF CARE

Painful administration (hated by children)

Some drugs (e.g., meperidine) can cause tissue and nerve damage

Wide fluctuation in absorption of drug from muscle

Faster absorption from deltoid than from gluteal sites

Shorter duration and more expensive than oral drugs

Time consuming for staff and unnecessary delay for child

INTRANASAL

Available commercially as Stadol NS (butorphanol); approved for those older than 18 years of age; should not be used in patient receiving morphine-like drugs because butorphanol is partial antagonist that will reduce analgesia and may cause withdrawal

INTRADERMAL

Used primarily for skin anesthesia (e.g., before lumbar puncture, bone marrow aspiration, arterial puncture, skin biopsy)

Local anesthetics (e.g., lidocaine) cause stinging, burning sensation
Duration of stinging may depend on type of "caine" used

To avoid stinging sensation associated with lidocaine:
Buffer the solution by adding 1 part sodium bicarbonate (1 mEq/mL) to 9 to 10 parts 1% or 2% lidocaine with or without epinephrine (see Guidelines box on p. 680)

Normal saline with preservative, benzyl alcohol (except neonates), anesthetizes venipuncture site

Use same dose as for buffered lidocaine (see Guidelines box on p. 680).

Data primarily from American Pain Society: *Principles of analgesic use in the treatment of acute pain and chronic cancer pain,* ed 4, Skokie, Il, 1999, The Society; McCaffery M, Pasero C: *Pain: a clinical manual,* ed 2, St Louis, 1999, Mosby.

*For further information about compounding drugs in troche or suppository form, contact: **Professional Compounding Centers of America (PCCA), Inc,** 9901 South Wilcrest Drive, Houston, TX 77009; (800) 331-2498; website: www.pccarx.com

BOX 21-14 ■ Routes and Methods of Analgesic Drug Administration—*cont'd*

TOPICAL/TRANSDERMAL

EMLA (eutectic mixture of local anesthetics [lidocaine/ prilocaine]) cream and Anesthetic Disc or LMX4 (4% lidocaine cream)

Eliminates or reduces pain from most procedures involving skin puncture

Must be placed on intact skin over puncture site and covered by occlusive dressing or applied as anesthetic disk for 1 hour or more before procedure (see Guidelines box on p. 679)

LAT (lidocaine/adrenaline/tetracaine) or tetracaine/ phenylephrine (tetraphen)

Provides skin anesthesia about 15 minutes after application on nonintact skin

Gel (preferable) or liquid placed on wounds for suturing

Adrenaline must not be used on end arterioles (fingers, toes, tip of nose, penis, earlobes) because of vasoconstriction

Numby Stuff

Uses iontophoresis to transport lidocaine 2% and epinephrine 1:100,000 (Iontocaine) into the skin

A small battery-powered device delivers current via an electrode with Iontocaine and a ground electrode

Produces local dermal anesthesia in about 10 minutes to a depth of approximately 10 mm at maximum setting

May be frightening to young children when they see the device and feel the current

Child should be observed during iontophoresis, and all metal, such as jewelry, is removed from application site to prevent burns

Transdermal fentanyl (Duragesic)

Available as patch for continuous pain control

Safety and efficacy not established in children younger than 12 years of age

Not appropriate for initial relief of acute pain because of long interval to peak effect (12-24 hours); for rapid onset of pain relief, an immediate release opioid must be given

Orders for "rescue doses" of an immediate release opioid should be available for breakthrough pain, a flare of severe pain that breaks through the medication being administered at regular intervals for persistent pain

Has duration of up to 72 hours for prolonged pain relief

If respiratory depression occurs, several doses of naloxone may be needed

Vapocoolant

Use of prescription spray coolant, such as Fluori-Methane or ethyl chloride (Pain-Ease); applied to the skin for 10-15 seconds immediately before the needle puncture; anesthesia lasts about 15 seconds

Some children dislike the cold; spraying the coolant on a cotton ball and then applying this to the skin may be less uncomfortable

Application of ice to the skin for 30 seconds has been found to be ineffective

RECTAL

Alternative to oral or parenteral routes

Variable absorption rate

Generally disliked by children

Many drugs can be compounded into rectal suppositories*

REGIONAL NERVE BLOCK

Use of long-acting local anesthetic (bupivacaine or ropivacaine) injected into nerves to block pain at site

Provides prolonged analgesia postoperatively, such as after inguinal herniorrhaphy

May be used to provide local anesthesia for surgery, such as dorsal penile nerve block for circumcision or for reduction of fractures

INHALATION

Use of anesthetics, such as nitrous oxide, to produce partial or complete analgesia for painful procedures

Occupational exposure to high levels of nitrous oxide may cause side effects (e.g., headache)

EPIDURAL/INTRATHECAL

Involves catheter placed into epidural, caudal, or intrathecal space for continuous infusion or single or intermittent administration of opioid with or without a long-acting local anesthetic (e.g., bupivacaine, ropivacaine)

Analgesia primarily from drug's direct effect on opioid receptors in spinal cord

Respiratory depression is rare but may have slow and delayed onset; can be prevented by checking level of sedation and respiratory rate and depth hourly for initial 24 hours and decreasing dose when excessive sedation is detected

Nausea, itching, and urinary retention are common dose-related side effects from the epidural opioid

Mild hypotension, urinary retention, and temporary motor or sensory deficits are common unwanted effects of epidural local anesthetic

Catheter for urinary retention should be inserted during surgery to decrease trauma to child; if inserted when child is awake, anesthetize urethra with lidocaine

*For further information about compounding drugs in troche or suppository form, contact: **Professional Compounding Centers of America (PCCA), Inc,** 9901 South Wilcrest Drive, Houston, TX 77009; (800) 331-2498; website: www.pccarx.com.

however, and the inherent safety of PCA may be compromised. Nevertheless, recent research reported safe and effective analgesia in children when the PCA was controlled by patient, parent, or nurse (Yaster, Kost-Byerly, and Maxwell, 2003; Algren and others, 1998).

PCA infusion devices typically allow for the following three methods or modes of drug administration to be used alone or in combination:

1 **Patient-administered boluses** that can only be infused according to the preset amount and lockout interval (time between doses); more frequent "pushing of the button" means no drug is delivered, but the patient may need the dose or time adjusted for better pain control

2 **Nurse-administered boluses** that are typically used to give an initial loading dose to increase blood levels rapidly and to relieve **breakthrough pain** (pain not relieved with the usual programmed dose)

3 **Continuous basal** or **background infusion** that delivers a constant amount of analgesic and prevents

TABLE 21-8 ■ **Suggested Intravenous Patient-Controlled Analgesia Opioid Infusion Orders**

DRUG	BASAL RATE (μg/kg/hr)	BOLUS RATE (μg/kg/dose)	LOCKOUT PERIOD (min)	MAXIMUM DOSE/ HOUR (mg/kg)
Morphine	10-30	10-30	6-10	0.1-0.15
Hydromorphone	3-5	6-10	0.015-0.02	3-5
Fentanyl	0.5-1.00	0.5-1.0	6-10	0.002-0.004

From Yaster M and others: *Pediatric pain management and sedation handbook*, St Louis, 1997, Mosby.

pain from returning during those times, such as sleep, when the patient cannot control the infusion; may decrease safety of PCA

The optimal use of these three modes continues to be investigated. However, as with any type of analgesic management plan, continued assessment of the child's pain relief is essential for the greatest benefit from PCA. Typical uses of PCA are for controlling perioperative pain, sickle cell crisis, trauma, and cancer.

The most commonly prescribed opioids for intravenous PCA are morphine, hydromorphone, and fentanyl. (See Table 21-8.) Because PCA is typically used for continuous and extended pain control, meperidine should not be administered (p. 669). Another risk of using meperidine is confusion between its concentration (10 mg/mL) and that of morphine when the PCA pump is programmed, which can result in undermedication or overmedication.

Epidural analgesia, primarily used postoperatively or in selected cases of terminal care, can be achieved by placing a catheter in the epidural space of the spinal column. An opioid (usually fentanyl, hydromorphone, or preservative-free morphine), often with a long-acting local anesthetic (usually bupivacaine or ropivacaine), is administered via single or intermittent bolus, continuous infusion, or patient-controlled epidural analgesia (PCEA). Analgesia results from the opioid's direct effect on receptors in the dorsal horn of the spinal cord, which block transmission of pain impulses to the brain (Rasmussen, 1996). Respiratory depression is rare, but if it occurs, it develops slowly and is evident several hours after the infusion begins. It is important to examine the epidural insertion site daily for evidence of infection and to ensure the occlusive dressing is intact. A mild erythema is not uncommon when catheters have been in place for several days. Catheters should be removed, however, if there is a fever of unknown origin or purulent drainage is present. Occasionally, when the nurse is examining the insertion site, a collection of fluid is seen between the skin and the clear occlusive dressing. Usually this edema is the result of fluid leaking through the insertion site hole and is not cerebrospinal fluid. It does not require any special treatment. The dressing should be changed or reinforced.

NURSING ALERT

When the epidural route is used, check the child's level of sedation and respiratory rate and depth hourly for the first 24 hours to detect delayed-onset respiratory depression (Pasero, 1999).

Although opioids are usually administered parenterally, spinally, or orally, new routes such as *oral transmucosal* and *transdermal* have recently been developed. Fentanyl is readily absorbed through the skin. However, because of its long onset, an inability to adjust drug delivery, and a long elimination half-life, transdermal fentanyl is contraindicated for acute pain management. A transdermal patch (Duragesic), however, may be used in older children and adolescents who have chronic cancer pain.

Conversely, the transmucosal route of fentanyl (Fentanyl Actiq) provides atraumatic preoperative and procedural sedation and analgesia. It is also useful in the treatment of cancer pain. As with all opioid administration, using these routes requires vigilant patient monitoring (Yaster, Kost-Byerly, and Maxwell, 2003).

One of the most significant improvements in the ability to provide atraumatic care to children is the anesthetic cream *EMLA,* a eutectic mixture of local anesthetics (lidocaine 2.5% and prilocaine 2.5%). The eutectic mixture, whose melting point is lower than that of the two anesthetics alone, permits effective concentrations of the drug to penetrate *intact* skin. A thick layer of cream under an occlusive transparent dressing or a "peel-and-stick" Anesthetic Disc is applied for 1 hour or more before procedures such as lumbar, venous, arterial, finger, heel, or earlobe punctures; implanted port access; insertion of peripherally inserted central catheter (PICC) lines; superficial biopsy; skin graft; laser treatment of port-wine stains; removal of epicardial (pacing) wires, chest tubes, or hair (electrolysis); bone marrow examination; allergy testing; and IM or SC injections. For deeper pain, such as IM injections, the application time should be extended up to 3 hours (see Guidelines box). The duration of anesthesia is 1 to 2 hours after removal (Wong, 2003). A recent review of the literature comparing EMLA with placebo, iontophoresis, and amethocaine cream found EMLA to be an effective local anesthetic for venipuncture pain from intravenous cannulation and phlebotomy (Rogers and Ostrow, 2004).

EMLA is approved for children 37 weeks of gestational age and older. It should be used cautiously on infants between ages 1 and 12 months who are receiving treatment with methemoglobin-inducing agents, such as sulfonamides, phenytoin (Dilantin), and acetaminophen (Tylenol). However, the use of these drugs is not a contraindication for applying EMLA, and there are no published reports of methemoglobinemia caused by EMLA when an infant received acetaminophen. Because of their diminished levels of erythrocyte-methemoglobin reductase, infants younger than 3 months old are more susceptible to prilocaine-induced

GUIDELINES

Using EMLA (Eutectic Mixture of Local Anesthetics—Lidocaine 2.5% and Prilocaine 2.5%)

Explain to child that EMLA is a "cream that takes hurt away." Tap or lightly scratch site of procedure to show child that "skin is now awake."

Apply the "peel-and-stick" Anesthetic Disc or a thick layer (dollop) of EMLA cream over normal intact skin to anesthetize site (about one half of a 5-g tube; can use one third of tube if puncture site is localized and superficial (e.g., intradermal injection or heel/finger puncture).

For venous access, apply to two sites; place enough cream on antecubital fossa to cover medial and lateral veins. Do not rub the cream.

If using the cream, place transparent adhesive dressing (e.g., Tegaderm) over EMLA. Make sure cream remains in a dollop or mound. A piece of plastic film (e.g., Saran Wrap) can be used, with tape to seal the edges. Use only as much adhesive as needed to prevent leakage.

To make the dressing less accessible, cover it loosely with a self-adhering Ace-type bandage (such as Coban) or an IV protector (such as I.V. House*). Label the dressing with "EMLA applied" and the date and time to distinguish it from other types of dressings. Instruct older children not to disturb the dressing. (Covering the dressing with an opaque material may reduce the attraction and discourage "fingering.") Supervise younger or cognitively compromised children throughout the application time.

Leave EMLA on skin for at least 60 minutes for superficial puncture and 2.5 hours for deep penetration (e.g., IM injection, biopsy). EMLA may be applied at home and may need to be kept on longer in persons with dark or thicker skin. Anesthesia may last up to 4 hours after EMLA is removed.

Remove Anesthetic Disc or dressing before procedure and wipe cream from skin. For transparent dressing, grasp opposite sides, and while holding dressing parallel to skin, pull sides away from each other to stretch and loosen. An adhesive remover may be used.

Observe skin reaction (e.g., either blanched or reddened). If there is no obvious skin reaction, EMLA may not have penetrated adequately. Test skin sensitivity and reapply if needed.

Repeat tapping or lightly scratching on skin to show child that "skin is asleep" and that it cannot feel a needle.

After procedure, assess behavioral response. If child was upset, use pain scale (e.g., FACES) to help child distinguish between pain and fear. (See FACES Pain Rating Scale in Table 21-2.)

In the United States, EMLA is approved for use in infants born at 37 weeks of gestation and older. It should not be used in those rare patients with congenital or idiopathic methemoglobinemia or in infants under the age of 12 months who are receiving treatment with methemoglobin-inducing agents such as sulfonamides, phenytoin (Dilantin), phenobarbital, and acetaminophen (Tylenol). Methemoglobin, a dysfunctional form of hemoglobin, reduces the blood's oxygen-carrying capacity, causing cyanosis and hypoxemia. The use of IV methylene blue promptly eliminates the methemoglobinemia.

NOTE: Although the package insert lists under "Warnings" that patients taking drugs associated with drug-induced methemoglobinemia, such as acetaminophen, are at greater risk for developing methemoglobinemia, there have been no reported cases of this complication occurring in children taking acetaminophen and using EMLA.

Follow the manufacturer's guidelines for MAXIMUM RECOMMENDED APPLICATION AREA TO INTACT SKIN FOR INFANTS AND CHILDREN:

Age and body weight requirements	Maximum total dose of EMLA	Maximum application area
0 to 3 months or <5 kg	1 g	10 cm² (1.25 × 1.25 in)
3 to 12 months and >5 kg	2 g	20 cm² (1.75 × 1.75 in)
1 to 6 years and >10 kg	10 g	100 cm² (4 × 4 in)
7 to 12 years and >20 kg	20 g	200 cm² (5.5 × 5.5 in)

NOTE: If a patient over 3 months old does not meet the minimum weight requirement, the maximum total dose of EMLA should be restricted to that which corresponds to the patient's weight.

*For more information, contact **I.V. House,** 7400 Foxmont Drive, Hazelwood, MO 63042-2198; (800) 530-0400; fax: (314) 831-3683; e-mail: ivhouse@ivhouse.com; website: www.ivhouse.com.

---

methemoglobinemia, a very rare and reversible side effect. *Methemoglobin* is a dysfunctional form of hemoglobin that reduces the oxygen-carrying capacity of the blood, causing cyanosis and hypoxemia. The use of IV methylene blue promptly eliminates the methemoglobinemia (McCaffery and Pasero, 1999). Other side effects are very mild and include pallor, erythema, or edema at the application site.

LMX4 (formerly Ela-Max) is a new over-the-counter topical anesthetic that produces dermal anesthesia in 15 to 30 minutes. Researchers concluded that a 30-minute application was as effective as a 60-minute application of EMLA in reducing pain associated with intravenous cannulation in the hands of a child. Although an occlusive dressing was used in this study, an occlusive dressing is not required when using LMX4 (Kleiber and others, 2002); however, a dressing may be used to prevent accidental ingestion by small children.

Another topical option is *Numby Stuff,* which uses iontophoresis (mild electrical current) to actively push the drug

into the skin. This preparation of Iontocaine (lidocaine HCl 2% with epinephrine 1:100,000 topical solution) provides dermal anesthesia to a depth of 10 mm in approximately 10 minutes without causing vasoconstriction. This painless needle-free process is noninvasive, minimizes trauma, and reduces risk of infection. It can be used for IV placement, insertion of PICC lines, lumbar punctures, implantable port needle insertion, and pulsed dye laser therapy (IOMED, 1996). In one study of children ages 5 to 12 years, iontophoresis was more effective than EMLA at reducing the pain of intravenous cannulation (Squire, Kirchoff, and Hissong, 2000). It is important to provide explanations and let the child become familiar with the equipment. Some children may be frightened by a warm or tingling sensation under the patches. This decreases after a few minutes (McCaffery and Pasero, 1999).

In some situations where there is not ample time for preparations like EMLA to take effect, refrigerant sprays such as ethyl chloride and fluori-methane (vapocoolant or skin refrigerant spray) can be used. When sprayed on the skin, these sprays vaporize, rapidly cool the area, and provide superficial anesthesia. Ethyl chloride wears off in about 2 minutes, and there are virtually no side effects (New Products, 2002).

The *intradermal route* is often used to inject a local anesthetic, typically lidocaine (Xylocaine), into the skin to reduce the pain from a lumbar puncture, bone marrow aspiration, or venous or arterial access. One problem with the use of lidocaine is the stinging and burning that initially occur. However, the use of *buffered lidocaine* reduces the stinging sensation (Wong and Pasero, 1997) (see Guidelines box). Warming the lidocaine to 37° C (98.6° F) may also accomplish the same effect (Mader, Playe, and Garb, 1994).

Right Time. The right timing for administering analgesics depends on the type of pain. For continuous pain control, such as for postoperative or cancer pain, a preventive schedule of medication *around the clock (ATC)* is effective. The ATC schedule avoids low plasma concentrations that permit breakthrough pain. If analgesics are administered only when pain returns (a typical use of the PRN, or "as needed," order), pain relief may take several hours. This may require higher doses, leading to a cycle of undermedication of pain alternating with periods of overmedication and drug toxicity. This cycle of erratic pain control also promotes "clock watching," which may be erroneously equated with "addiction." Nurses can effectively use PRN orders by giving the drug at regular intervals, because "as needed" can be interpreted to mean "as needed to prevent return of pain."

Preventive pain control is best provided through continuous IV infusion rather than intermittent boluses. If intermittent boluses are given, the intervals between doses should not exceed the drug's expected duration of effectiveness. For extended pain control with fewer administration times, drugs that provide longer duration of action (e.g., some NSAIDs, time-released morphine or oxycodone, methadone, levorphanol) can be used.

> **⚠ NURSING ALERT**
>
> Because breakthrough pain can occur even with optimal ATC scheduling, there should be an order for PRN "rescue" doses of an analgesic.

Continuous analgesia is not always appropriate, because not all pain is continuous. Frequently, temporary pain control is needed to provide analgesia before a scheduled procedure. When pain can be predicted, the drug's peak effect should be timed to coincide with the painful event. For example, with opioids the peak effect is only a few minutes for the IV route; with nonopioids, the peak effect occurs about 2 hours after oral administration. For rapid onset and peak of action, opioids that quickly penetrate the blood-brain barrier (e.g., IV fentanyl) provide excellent pain control.

Observe for Side Effects.   Both NSAIDs and opioids have side effects, although the major concern is with those from opioids (Box 21-15). Respiratory depression is the most serious complication and is most likely to occur in sedated patients. The respiratory rate may decrease gradually or may cease abruptly; lower limits of normal are not established for children, but any significant change from a previous rate calls for increased vigilance. A slower respiratory rate does not necessarily reflect decreased arterial oxygenation; an increased depth of ventilation may compensate for the altered rate (McCaffery and Pasero, 1999). If respiratory depression or arrest occurs, the nurse must be prepared to intervene quickly (see Guidelines box).

Although respiratory depression is the most feared side effect, constipation is a common and sometimes serious side effect of opioids, which decrease peristaltic activity and increase anal sphincter tone. Prevention with stool softeners and laxatives is more effective than treatment after constipation occurs. Dietary treatment, such as increased fiber, is usually not sufficient to promote regular bowel evacuation.

〰 GUIDELINES

Using Buffered Lidocaine

SUPPLIES

8.4% sodium bicarbonate (1 mEq/mL), 1% to 2% lidocaine with or without epinephrine, syringe with removable needle, and a 30-gauge needle

INSTRUCTIONS

Use 1 part sodium bicarbonate to 10 parts lidocaine (e.g., draw up 1 mL lidocaine and 0.1 mL sodium bicarbonate).

Change needle used to withdraw buffered lidocaine (BL) to 30-gauge needle for intradermal injection.

For venipuncture or port access, inject 0.1 mL or less BL intradermally directly over intended puncture site; anesthesia occurs almost immediately.

Suggested maximum dose of lidocaine for local anesthesia is 4.5 mg/kg.

If buffering lidocaine vial (e.g., 20 mL lidocaine with 2 mL sodium bicarbonate), solution may be used for 7 days if unrefrigerated or 14 days if refrigerated.

BOX 21-15 ■ Side Effects of Opioids

GENERAL	SIGNS OF WITHDRAWAL
Constipation (possibly severe)	SYNDROME IN PATIENTS
Respiratory depression	WITH PHYSICAL
Sedation	DEPENDENCE
Nausea and vomiting	Initial signs of withdrawal:
Agitation, euphoria	Lacrimation
Mental clouding	Rhinorrhea
Hallucinations	Yawning
Orthostatic hypotension	Sweating
Pruritus	Later signs:
Urticaria	Restlessness
Sweating	Irritability
Miosis (may be sign of toxicity)	Tremors
Anaphylaxis (rare)	Anorexia
	Dilated pupils
SIGNS OF TOLERANCE	Gooseflesh
Decreasing pain relief	Nausea/vomiting
Decreasing duration of pain relief	

However, dietary measures, such as increased fluid, fruit, and bran intake, and especially activity, are encouraged.

Pruritus from epidural or IV infusion can be treated with low doses of naloxone infused slowly or with IV nalbuphine. Pruritus from IV infusion usually responds to oral antihistamines. Nausea, vomiting, and sedation usually subside after 2 days of opioid administration, although intravenous, oral, or rectal antiemetics may be necessary.

Both tolerance and physical dependence can occur with prolonged use of opioids. Treatment of tolerance involves increasing the dose or decreasing the duration between doses. Treatment of physical dependence involves gradually reducing the dose over several days to prevent occurrence of withdrawal symptoms (similar to tapering of steroid dosages after chronic steroid therapy). The following are suggested guidelines for treating physical dependence (American Pain Society, 1999):

- Gradually reduce dose (similar to tapering of steroids): Give one half of previous daily dose in every-6-hour doses for first 2 days, then reduce dose by 25% every 2 days.
- Continue this schedule until total daily dose of 0.6 mg/kg/day of morphine (or equivalent) is reached.
- After 2 days on this dose, discontinue opioid.
- May also switch to oral methadone, using one fourth of equianalgesic dose as initial weaning dose and proceeding as described above.

Use supportive statements when administering analgesics. The effectiveness of analgesics can be enhanced by a supportive attitude toward the child. By reinforcing the cause and effect of the medication and analgesia, the nurse can

GUIDELINES

Managing Opioid-Induced Respiratory Depression

IF RESPIRATIONS ARE DEPRESSED:

Assess sedation level (see Fig. 21-9 for sedation scale)

Reduce infusion by 25% when possible.

Stimulate patient (shake shoulder gently, call by name, ask to breathe).

IF PATIENT CANNOT BE AROUSED OR IS APNEIC (AMERICAN PAIN SOCIETY, 1999):

Administer naloxone (Narcan):

For children weighing less than 40 kg, dilute 0.1 mg naloxone in 10 mL sterile saline to make 10 µg/mL solution and give 0.5 µg/kg.

For children weighing more than 40 kg, dilute 0.4-mg ampule in 10 mL sterile saline and give 0.5 mL.

Administer bolus slow IV push every 2 minutes until effect is obtained.

Closely monitor patient. Naloxone's duration of antagonist action may be shorter than that of opioid, requiring repeated doses of naloxone

NOTE: Respiratory depression caused by benzodiazepines (e.g., diazepam [Valium] or midazolam [Versed]) can be reversed with flumazenil (Romazicon). Pediatric dosing experience suggests 0.01 mg/kg (0.1 mL/kg); if no (or inadequate) response after 1 to 2 minutes, administer same dose and repeat as needed at 60-second intervals for maximum dose of 1 mg (10 mL) (Yaster and others, 1997).

condition the child to expect pain relief, provided that the regimen is likely to be effective. Although IM injections should *not* be given, when they are, children need to understand that the "little hurt from the needle will take away the bigger hurt for a long time."

Parents and older children may have concerns about the use of opioids because of fear of addiction. These concerns should be addressed with assurance that any such risk is extremely low. It may be helpful to ask the question, "If you did not have this pain, would you want to take this medicine?" The answer is invariably no, which reinforces the solely therapeutic nature of the drug. It is also important to avoid making statements to the family such as "We don't want you to get used to this medicine" or "By now you shouldn't need this medicine," which may reinforce the fear of becoming addicted.

Providing Developmentally Appropriate Activities

A primary goal of nursing care for the child who is hospitalized is to minimize threats to the child's development. Many strategies (e.g., minimizing separation) have been discussed and may be all that the short-term patient requires. However, children who experience prolonged or repeated hospitalization are at greater risk for developmental delays or regression. The nurse who provides opportunities for the child to participate in developmentally appropriate activities further normalizes the child's environment and helps reduce interference with the child's ongoing development (see Normalization, Chapter 18).

Play is the "work" of children of all ages and assumes a critical role in their development. Because of its other important purposes in the hospital setting, play is the focus of a separate discussion.

Interference with normal development may have long-term implications for the developing infant and toddler. The nurse plays a primary role in identifying children at risk and helping to plan, implement, and evaluate developmental intervention (see Chapters 10 and 12).

School is an integral part of the school-age child's and adolescent's development. Accreditation standards for hospitals serving children consider access to appropriate educational services a key factor in the accreditation decision process when a child's treatment requires a significant absence from school (Joint Commission on Accreditation for Healthcare Organizations, 1999). The nurse can encourage children to resume schoolwork as quickly as their condition permits, help them schedule and protect a selected time for studies, and help the family coordinate hospital educational services with their children's schools. Children should have the opportunity to "keep up" with art and music classes, as well as their academic subjects.

To meet the unique developmental needs of adolescents, special units have been developed that provide privacy, increased socialization, and appropriate activities for these young people. Typically these units are set apart from the general pediatric facility so that the teenagers do not share space with younger children, who are often perceived as a threat to their maturity.

These units often provide flexible routines and activities, such as more group activity, wearing of street clothes, and access to the items so critical to adolescents—telephones, compact disc players, DVD players, videocassette recorders (VCRs), computers, email, and televisions. Because adolescents' food habits are rarely limited to the three traditional meals a day, a ready supply of snacks should be available. However, the most important benefit of these units is increased socialization with peers. In addition, staff members usually enjoy working with this age-group and are well-suited to establishing the trust so essential for communication.

> **NURSING TIP**
>
> When adolescents must share a common activity room with younger patients, referring to the area as the "activity" room rather than the "playroom" may entice them to visit the room and participate in activities.

Although regression is expected and normal, nurses have the responsibility of fostering the child's growth and development. Hospitalization can become a significant opportunity for learning and advancing. Extended hospitalizations for long-term chronic illness or situations of failure to thrive, abuse, or neglect represent instances in which regression must be seen as an adjustment period, to be followed by plans for promoting appropriate developmental skills.

Providing Opportunities for Play and Expressive Activities

Play is one of the most important aspects of a child's life and one of the most effective tools for managing stress. Because illness and hospitalization constitute crises in a child's life and often involve overwhelming stresses, children need to act out their fears and anxieties as a means of coping with these stresses. Play is essential to children's mental, emotional, and social well-being. As with their developmental needs, the need for play does not stop when children are ill or in the hospital. On the contrary, play in the hospital serves many functions (Box 21-16).

Engaging in such activities gives children a sense of control. In the hospital environment, most decisions are made for the child; play and other expressive activities offer the child much-needed opportunities to make choices. Even if a child chooses not to participate in a particular activity, the nurse has offered the child a choice, perhaps one of but a few real choices the child has had that day.

Of all hospital facilities, probably no room does more to alleviate the stressors of hospitalization than the playroom or activity room. In this nonthreatening environment children temporarily distance themselves from the fears of separation, loss of control, and bodily injury. Time spent in this area should be protected. No treatments or intrusive or painful procedures should be allowed (see Critical Thinking Exercise).

Diversional Activities.   Almost any form of play can be used for diversion and recreation, but the activity should be selected on the basis of the child's age, interests, and limitations (Fig. 21-10). Children do not necessarily need special direction for using play materials. All they require is the raw materials with which to work and adult approval and supervision to help keep their natural enthusiasm or expression of feelings from getting out of control. Small children enjoy a variety of small, colorful toys that they can play with in bed or in their room, or more elaborate play equipment, such as playhouses, sandboxes, rhythm instruments, or large boxes and blocks, that may be a part of the hospital playroom.

Games that can be played alone or with another child or an adult are popular with older children, as are puzzles; reading material; quiet, individual activities, such as sewing, stringing beads, and weaving; and Lego blocks and other building materials. Assembling models is an excellent pastime, but one should make certain that all pieces and necessary materials are included in the package so that the child is not disappointed and frustrated.

Well-selected books are of infinite value to the child. Children never tire of stories; having someone read aloud gives them endless hours of pleasure and is of special value to the child who has limited energy to expend in play. A radio, VCR, electronic games, and television, included among most hospital room equipment, are useful tools for entertaining a child. Computers with access to the Internet can provide diversion, educational opportunities, and online support groups.

When supervising play for ill or convalescent children, it is best to select activities that are simpler than would normally be chosen according to the specific developmental level of the child. These children usually do not have the energy to cope with more challenging activities. Other limitations also influence the type of activities. Special consideration must be given to the child who is confined in terms of movement, has a restricted extremity, or is isolated. Toys for isolated children may need to be disinfected before or after use.

Toys.   Parents of hospitalized children often ask nurses about the types of toys that would be best to bring for their child. Although parents often want to buy new toys for the hospitalized child, it is often better to wait awhile to bring new things, especially in the case of younger children. Small children need the comfort and reassurance of familiar things, such as the stuffed animal the child hugs for comfort and takes to bed at night. These familiar items are a link with home and the world outside the hospital.

Large numbers of toys often confuse and frustrate a small child. A few small, well-chosen toys are usually preferred to one large, expensive one. Children who are hospitalized for an extended time benefit from changes. Rather than a confusing accumulation of toys, older toys should be replaced periodically as interest wanes.

BOX 21-16 ■ Functions of Play in the Hospital

Provides diversion and brings about relaxation
Helps the child feel more secure in a strange environment
Helps to lessen the stress of separation and the feeling of homesickness
Provides a means for release of tension and expression of feelings
Encourages interaction and development of positive attitudes toward others
Provides an expressive outlet for creative ideas and interests
Provides a means for accomplishing therapeutic goals (see Use of Play in Procedures, Chapter 22)
Places child in active role and provides opportunity to make choices and be in control

?? CRITICAL THINKING EXERCISE

Playroom and Hospital Procedures

Hannah, a 7-year-old with cystic fibrosis, has been hospitalized numerous times with complications from the condition. She is playing Candyland with her brother, sister, and several other children in the playroom on the pediatric unit. A pediatric phlebotomist enters the playroom and says, "Hannah, I need to take some blood. I can see that you are playing a game, so I'll just do it while you play. It will just take a minute." Hannah nods her head indicating that she agrees to let the phlebotomist draw the blood at this time. The playroom is usually off-limits for invasive procedures. As Hannah's nurse, you are aware that Dr. Lung wants the results of the laboratory studies as soon as possible to make a decision about her course of therapy.

QUESTIONS

1. Evidence—Is there sufficient evidence to draw any conclusions about this situation at this time?
2. Assumptions—What are some underlying assumptions about the following:
   a. Children and painful procedures such as venipunctures
   b. The function of play in a hospitalized child.
   c. The priority in performing the procedure
   d. Implications of performing the procedure in the playroom
3. What implications and priorities for nursing care can be drawn at this time (i.e., what will you do)?
4. Does the evidence objectively support your argument (conclusion)?
5. Are there alternative perspectives to your conclusions? If so, what are they?

ANSWERS

1. There is sufficient evidence regarding this incident to draw some conclusions.
2. Assumptions:
   a. Regardless of how minor a procedure such as a venipuncture may seem to an adult health care worker, it represents a major threat to a child. One must consider the child's age, illness, developmental level, and previous experiences with venipunctures.
   b. Play is an important function of childhood whether the child is sick or well. Through play children may act out fears, concerns, anger, and other behaviors they may not feel comfortable expressing to adults in a confrontational manner. Play is an important part of the hospitalized child's life, and it is a vehicle for promoting optimal development.
   c. It is important to have the blood drawn so Dr. Lung may plan a therapeutic regimen; however, one must consider another issue and that is that there appears to have been no advance preparation of the child's skin to minimize or prevent pain from the procedure. Regardless of the phlebotomist's skill in performing the procedure, it is also important to consider the fact that the negative repercussions for performing the procedure at this point may outweigh the positive benefits.
   d. All staff on the pediatric floor must be in agreement about respecting the child's personal space in the playroom and in adhering to unit policies or rules so that respect is maintained. Failure to respect the child's space may engender further fear by other children who perceive that the playroom is not a safe place after all, when certain procedures need to be done. The fear of having other procedures performed in the playroom may prevent children from going there to participate in therapeutic and interactive play.
3. It is important to maintain a fair balance between what constitutes therapeutic management of illness and childhood recreation. It would be appropriate in this situation to intervene and ask the phlebotomist to return in 30 minutes to an hour and indicate that the child will be ready for the venipuncture in the treatment room at that time. It is important to stress that the playroom is off-limits for procedures. It would be appropriate to discuss this plan with Hannah, indicating that the procedure will be performed at the designated time. It is also important to explore pain management issues with Hannah—does she usually use EMLA or other topical remedy to prevent pain at the site? If so, it will be necessary to make such arrangements in advance, possibly now, so her pain is managed appropriately. As the nurse, it is appropriate to discuss a delay in obtaining the lab results with Dr. Lung and the reasons for the delay. As workers on the pediatric floor it is important for medical and nursing staff to communicate effectively. Should this arrangement not suit Dr. Lung's time frame for accomplishing certain tasks, one might suggest a trade-off. The nurse may draw the blood in the treatment room after preparations are made and a time is agreed on by Hannah. Remember however that school-age children are prone to "bargain" for more time to delay or prevent the event because it is painful. One must be gently firm about the agreed-on time of the procedure and not allow further delays to accommodate the child who just does not want the procedure performed—ever, in most cases.

   Even if one accepts the conclusion that it is "okay" with Hannah, it is important to consider the possible negative implications for the other children in the room, who may be confused about even a simple procedure (e.g., checking blood pressure) or the sanctuary status of the playroom for themselves.

   To proceed with the blood draw in the playroom would violate the child's trust about what adult health care workers say regarding the purpose of the playroom as a sanctuary from painful procedures. Such action would likely result in less cooperation from the children who are present and may also make other parents present (or who obtain knowledge of the incident) wonder about the sincerity of the staff. Interrupting the children's game is not necessary because this does not represent a life-threatening condition at this time.
4. Yes, there is sufficient evidence to support these decisions and the plan of action.
5. An exception is sometimes made when all of the children present are older and the procedure is a quick, painless one (e.g., checking blood pressure, giving oral medication) that all the children present have experienced. In such cases the patient and the other children are asked if it is okay and give permission before the procedure is undertaken.

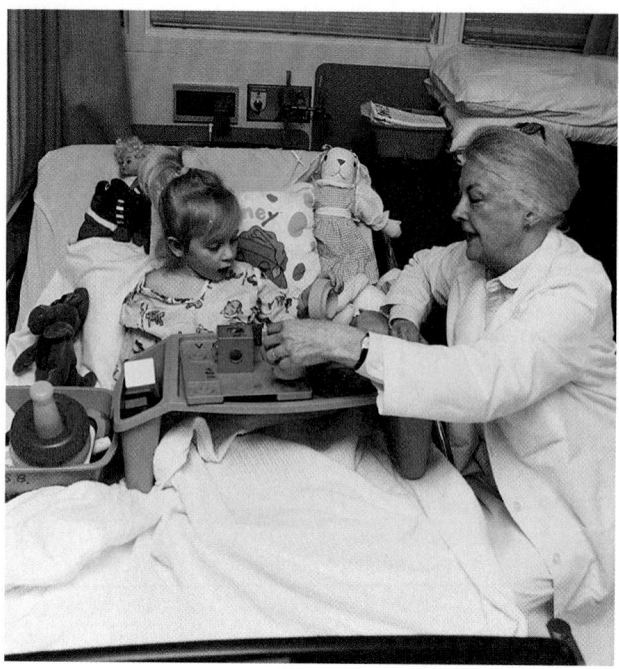

FIG. 21-10 ■ Play materials for children in the hospital need to be appropriate for their age, interests, and limitations.

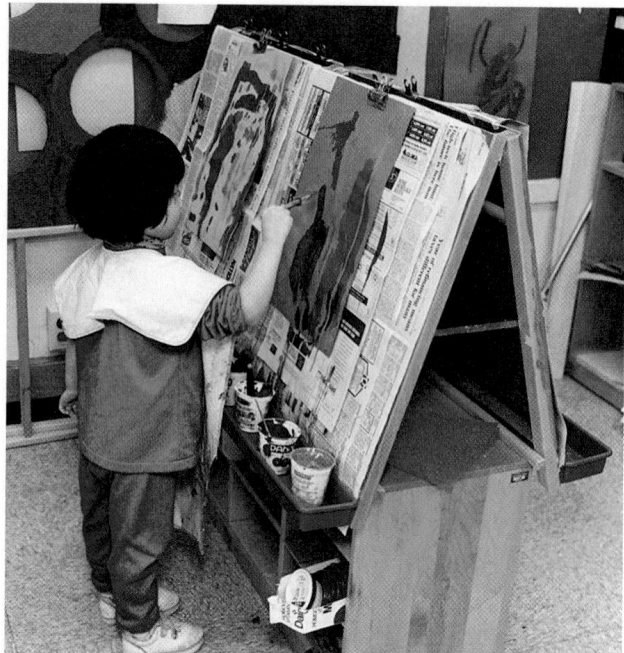

FIG. 21-11 ■ Drawing and painting are excellent media for expression.

Have parents provide the child with a shoe box, a child's small suitcase, or a backpack to attach to the bed for an easy storage receptacle to prevent small items from becoming lost in the sheets or under the bed.

A highly successful diversion for a child who is hospitalized for a length of time and whose parents are unable to visit frequently is having the parents bring a box with several small, inexpensive, brightly wrapped items with a different day of the week printed on the outside of each package. The child will eagerly anticipate the time for opening each one. When the parents know when their next visit will be, they can provide the number of packages that corresponds to the time between visits. In this way the child knows that the diminishing packages also represent the anticipated visit from the parent.

Expressive Activities. Play and other expressive activities provide one of the best opportunities for encouraging emotional expression, including the safe release of anger and hostility. Nondirective play that allows children freedom for expression can be tremendously therapeutic. Therapeutic play, however, should not be confused with ***play therapy,*** a psychologic technique reserved for use by trained and qualified therapists as an interpretative method with emotionally disturbed children. ***Therapeutic play,*** on the other hand, is a very effective, nondirective modality for helping children deal with their concerns and fears, and at the same time it often helps the nurse to gain insights into children's needs and feelings.

Tension release can be facilitated through almost any activity, and with younger ambulatory children, large-muscle activity such as use of tricycles and wagons is especially beneficial. Much aggression can be safely directed into pounding and throwing games and activities. Beanbags are often thrown at a target or open receptacle with surprising vigor and hostility. A pounding board is employed with enthusiasm by young children; clay and Play Doh are marvelous media for use at any age.

Creative Expression. Although all children derive physical, social, emotional, and cognitive benefits from engaging in art or other creative activities, children's need for such activities is intensified when they are hospitalized. Children are more at ease expressing their thoughts and feelings through art, because humans think first in images and later learn to translate these images into words. A child's drawing before surgery, for example, will often reveal unvoiced concerns about mutilation, body changes, and loss of self-control (Clatworthy, Simon, and Tiedeman, 1999). Drawing and painting are excellent media for expression. The child needs only to be supplied with the raw materials, such as crayons and paper; large brushes, and an ample supply of newsprint supported on easels; or materials for finger painting (Fig. 21-11). Children can work individually or collaborate on a group project, such as a mural painted on a long piece of paper.

Although interpretation of children's drawing requires special training, observing changes in a series of the child's drawings over time can be helpful in assessing psychosocial adjustment and coping (Clatworthy, Simon, and Tiedeman, 1999). The nurse can use children's drawings, stories, poetry, and other products of creative expression as a springboard for discussion of thoughts, fears, and understanding of concepts or events (see Communication Techniques, Chapter 6).

Nurses can incorporate opportunities for musical expression into routine nursing care. For example, simple musical instruments, such as bracelets with bells, can be placed on infants' legs for them to shake to accompany mealtime music, or dressing changes. Dance and movement suggestions may encourage a child to ambulate.

Holidays provide stimulus and direction for unlimited creative projects. Children can participate in decorating the pediatric unit, and making pictures and decorations for their rooms gives the children a sense of pride and accomplishment. This is especially beneficial for children who are immobilized and isolated. Making gifts for someone at home helps to maintain interpersonal ties.

Dramatic Play.   Dramatic play is a well-recognized technique for emotional release, allowing children to reenact frightening or puzzling hospital experiences. Through use of puppets, replicas of hospital equipment, or some actual hospital equipment, children can play out the situations that are a part of their hospital experience. Dramatic play enables children to learn about procedures and events that will concern them and to assume the roles of the adults in the hospital environment.

Puppets are universally effective for communicating with children. Most children see them as peers and readily communicate with them. Children will relate to the puppet feelings that they hesitate to express to adults. Puppets can share children's own experiences and help them to find solutions to their problems. Puppets dressed to represent figures in the child's environment—for example, a physician, nurse, child patient, therapist, and members of the child's own family—are especially useful (Fig. 21-12). Small, appropriately attired dolls are equally effective in encouraging the child to play out situations, although puppets are usually best for direct conversation.

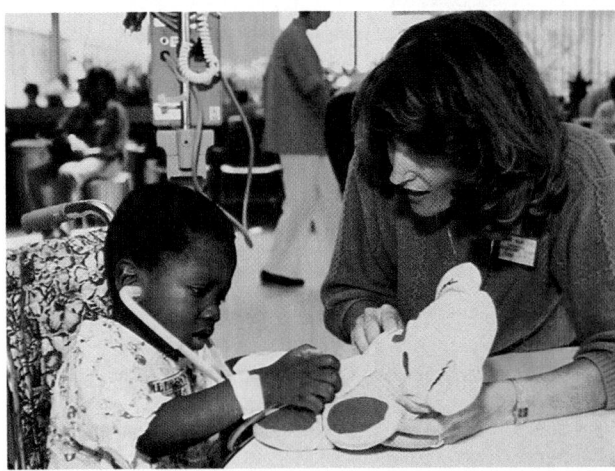

FIG. 21-12 ■ Playing with stuffed animals allows children to safely explore feelings and concerns. (Courtesy St. Louis Children's Hospital.)

Make a simple puppet using a large handkerchief. Place some cotton balls in the center of the cloth and wrap a rubber band over the handkerchief and cotton balls to form a "head." Place the head over the index finger so that the rubber band secures it to the finger. Let the cloth drape over the front and back of the hand. The cloth forms four parts of the puppet: the index finger is the head, the thumb and other fingers are the arms, and the draped cloth is the body. Decorate the head by drawing features on it.

Play must consider medical needs, but at times a procedure can be postponed for a short time to allow the child to complete a special activity (see Critical Thinking Exercise on p. 683). Play must consider any limitations imposed by the child's condition. For example, small children may eat paste and other creative media; therefore, a child who is allergic to wheat should not be given finger paint made from wallpaper paste or modeling dough made with flour. A child on a restricted salt intake should not play with modeling dough, because salt is one of its major constituents. At home the play program can be planned around the therapy regimen. However, play can be satisfactorily incorporated into the child's care if the nurse and others involved allow some flexibility and use creativity in planning for play.

Maximizing Potential Benefits of Hospitalization

Although hospitalization generally represents a stressful time for children and families, it also represents an opportunity for facilitating positive change within the child and among family members. For some families the stress of a child's illness, hospitalization, or both can lead to strengthening of family coping behaviors and the emergence of new coping strategies (Kirby and Whelan, 1996). Therefore nursing interventions must also focus on maximizing the potential benefits of the experience.

Fostering Parent-Child Relationships.   The crisis of illness or hospitalization can mobilize parents into more acute awareness of the needs of their children. For example, hospitalization provides opportunities for parents to learn more about their children's growth and development. When parents are helped to understand children's usual reactions to stress, such as regression or aggression, they are not only better able to support the child through the hospital experience, but also may extend their insights into childrearing practices after discharge.

Difficulties in parent-child relationships that may result in feeding problems, negative behavior, and sleep disturbances may decrease during hospitalization. The temporary cessation of such problems sometimes alerts parents to the role they may be playing in propagating the negative behavior. With assistance from health professionals, parents can restructure ways of relating to their children to foster more positive behavior.

Hospitalization may also represent a temporary reprieve or refuge from a disturbed home. Typically, abused or neglected children's dramatic physical and social improvement during hospitalization is proof of the growth potential of this experience. Hospitalized children temporarily are able to seek support, reassurance, and security from new relationships, particularly with nurses and hospitalized peers.

Providing Educational Opportunities.   Illness and hospitalization represent excellent opportunities for children and other family members to learn more about their bodies, each other, and the health professions. For example, during a hospital admission for a diabetic crisis, the child may learn about the disease; the parents may learn about the child's needs for independence, normalcy, and appropriate limits; and each of them may find a new support system in the hospital staff.

Text continued on p. 690.

NURSING DIAGNOSIS ■ Anxiety/fear related to separation from accustomed routine and support system; unfamiliar surroundings

PATIENT GOAL 1: Will experience minimized separation

NURSING INTERVENTIONS/*RATIONALES*

Assign same nursing personnel as much as possible and a primary nurse *to provide the consistency that builds trust*

Arrange workload and schedule to allow personal contact with child

Encourage parents to be present whenever possible *to prevent separation*

Provide an atmosphere of warmth and acceptance for both child and parents

Encourage parents and others to demonstrate affection for child

Recognize child's separation behaviors as normal

    Allow child to cry *because this is a normal response to separation*

    Provide support through physical presence

Maintain child's contact with parents and siblings and home

    Talk about child's parents frequently

    Encourage child to talk about and remember family members, pets

    Stress significance of parents' and siblings' visits, telephone calls, or letters

Help parents understand the behaviors of separation anxiety and suggest ways of supporting the child

    Explain to child when parents leave and when they will return

    Tell hospitalized child the reason for leaving

    Convey the expected time of return in terms of anticipated events; for example, if the parents will return in the morning, they can say they will see the child "After the sun comes up" or "When (a favorite program) is on television"

    Use a clock or calendar for an older child *so child can anticipate next family visit*

    Visit for short but frequent times rather than one long time; encourage parents and relatives to take turns visiting

    Encourage siblings, grandparents, and other significant persons in child's life to visit

    Leave favorite articles from home, such as a blanket, toy, bottle, feeding utensil, or article of clothing, with child *because this helps child tolerate separation*

    Respect treasured objects of older children, such as a stuffed animal

    Encourage family to provide photographs of family members and recordings of the parents' voices (e.g., reading a story, singing a song, saying prayers before bedtime, relating events at home) *to familiarize the unfamiliar environment and to provide comfort during times of separation*

Play family recordings at lonely times, such as before sleep

Suggest that the family leave small gifts for the child to open each day: if the parents know when their next visit will be, have them leave the number of packages that correspond to the time between visits

Assign a "foster grandparent" or consistent volunteer to be with child if available

EXPECTED OUTCOMES

Child has consistent caregivers

Parents visit as much as possible

Parents cooperate in care (specify)

Child accepts and responds positively to comforting measures

Child discusses the family, including pets

Parents demonstrate an understanding of separation behaviors

Siblings, grandparents, and other significant persons visit as much as possible

Family provides child with familiar or cherished articles from home

Assigned person spends time with child (specify amount)

PATIENT GOAL 2: Will express feelings

NURSING INTERVENTIONS/*RATIONALES*

Accept expression of feelings *so that child continues these expressions*

Provide an atmosphere that encourages free expression of feelings

Provide opportunities for the child to verbalize, "play out," or otherwise express feelings without fear of punishment

Encourage drawing and other expressive activities *because children often find it easier to express themselves in images instead of words*

Encourage keeping a journal or diary *to allow child to review progress and changes in feelings*

EXPECTED OUTCOME

Child verbalizes or plays out feelings or concerns

PATIENT GOAL 3: Will remain calm

NURSING INTERVENTIONS/*RATIONALES*

Maintain a calm, relaxed, and reassuring manner

Spend time with child and family *to establish rapport*

Give competent, consistent nursing care *to instill confidence in both parents and child*

Explain intrusive procedures in a developmentally appropriate manner

EXPECTED OUTCOMES

Child exhibits no signs of apprehension

Child rests quietly and calmly

PATIENT GOAL 4: Will exhibit trusting behaviors

NURSING INTERVENTIONS/*RATIONALES*

Be positive in approach to child

Be honest with child *to encourage child to trust*

Convey to child the behaviors expected

Be consistent in expectations and relationships with child *because consistency is an important component of the development of trust*

Treat child fairly

Encourage parents to maintain a truthful relationship with the child

Make certain child has call light or other signal device within reach

EXPECTED OUTCOMES

Child develops rapport with nurse

Child maintains trust of family

PATIENT GOAL 5: Will experience feelings of security

NURSING INTERVENTIONS/*RATIONALES*

Maintain child's identity

    Address child by name or usual nickname

    Avoid assigning a nickname to child or converting a given name to its counterpart in another language (e.g., using Joe instead of José)

Avoid communicating any signals of rejection, distaste, or other negative feelings to child

When necessary communicate disapproval of unacceptable *behavior,* not disapproval of the *child*

Communicate, verbally and nonverbally, that the child is a valued person

Discourage treatments or procedures in the child's room or playroom *to maintain these areas as "safe places"*

EXPECTED OUTCOMES

Child interacts with staff

*Staff demonstrates respect for child

*Nursing outcome.

NURSING CARE PLAN   The Child in the Hospital—*cont'd*

PATIENT GOAL 6: Will experience reduction of or no fear

NURSING INTERVENTIONS/*RATIONALES*

Explain routines, items, procedures, and events in a language and method appropriate to the child's developmental level; use simple language, drawings, and play *to facilitate understanding and mastery*

Reassure child and repeat reassurance as necessary

Ask child to explain reason for hospitalization and correct if necessary *to help absolve child from any guilt about being hospitalized*

Encourage parent(s) to participate in child's care

Encourage child to handle items that may seem strange or threatening *to reduce fear of the unknown*

Give encouragement and positive feedback for cooperation in care

EXPECTED OUTCOMES

Child exhibits understanding of information presented (specify information and means of demonstration)

Child discusses procedures and activities without evidence of anxiety

PATIENT GOAL 7: Will be allowed to express regressive behavior

NURSING INTERVENTIONS/*RATIONALES*

Inform parents that regressive behavior is a feature of illness *so that it is not viewed as abnormal*

Accept regressive behavior and help child with dependency

Assist child in reconquering the negative counterpart of the psychosocial stage to which child has regressed (e.g., overcome mistrust; facilitate development of trust)

EXPECTED OUTCOME

*Staff and parents exhibit an attitude of acceptance of regressive behaviors

PATIENT GOAL 8: Will experience adequate comfort level

NURSING INTERVENTIONS/*RATIONALES*

Provide pacifier, if appropriate, *to meet oral needs and to provide comfort*

Hold infant or young child when this does not interfere with therapy

Touch, talk, and otherwise comfort child who cannot be held

Provide sensory stimulation and diversion appropriate to child's level of development and need for rest

Encourage family members to visit and allow them to comfort and care for child to the extent possible

EXPECTED OUTCOMES

Infant or young child engages in nonnutritive sucking

Child exhibits no signs of distress

Family is involved in care

NURSING DIAGNOSIS ▪ **Anxiety/fear related to distressing procedures, events**

PATIENT GOAL 1: Will be prepared for hospitalization

NURSING INTERVENTIONS/*RATIONALES*

Prepare child as needed *to reduce fear of the unknown and to promote cooperation*

Select appropriate preparatory materials

Involve parents *to enable them to serve as effective resources for their child*

Modify preparation in special situations (e.g., ambulatory/outpatient setting, emergency admission, intensive care unit) (see pp. 698 to 702)

EXPECTED OUTCOME

Child is prepared for hospital experience

PATIENT GOAL 2: Will exhibit decreased fear of bodily injury

NURSING INTERVENTIONS/*RATIONALES*

Recognize developmental fears associated with illness and procedures *to ensure appropriate intervention*

Provide age-appropriate explanations for procedures, especially those that are intrusive or involve the genitals, and include information about what body parts will not be affected, as well as those that will

Provide age-appropriate explanations for procedures the child may see or hear performed on other patients *to decrease child's fears*

Reassure child that certain body parts can be removed without producing harm (e.g., blood, tonsils, appendix)

Provide privacy for any procedure that exposes the body

Use interventions that preserve child's concept of body integrity (e.g., bandages over puncture sites)

EXPECTED OUTCOME

Child displays minimal fear of bodily injury

PATIENT GOAL 3: Will receive support during tests and procedures

NURSING INTERVENTIONS/*RATIONALES*

Prepare child for procedures according to age and level of understanding, including strategies for coping

Remain with child *to provide support by physical presence*

Prepare child and family for surgery if appropriate

Answer questions and explain purposes of activities

Keep child (and family) informed of progress

EXPECTED OUTCOME

Child remains calm and cooperative during procedures

Child feels supported during procedures

NURSING DIAGNOSIS ▪ **Pain related to (specify)**

PATIENT GOAL 1: Will perceive less pain by using appropriate strategies

NURSING INTERVENTIONS/*RATIONALES*

Employ nonpharmacologic strategies to help child manage pain *because techniques such as relaxation, rhythmic breathing, and distraction can make pain more tolerable*

Use nonpharmacologic strategy that is familiar to child or describe several strategies and let child select one (see Guidelines box, p. 670) *to facilitate child's learning and use of strategy*

Involve parent in selection of strategy *because parent knows child best*

Select appropriate person(s), usually parent, to assist child with strategy

Teach child to use specific nonpharmacologic strategies before pain occurs or before it becomes severe *because these approaches appear to be most effective for mild pain*

Assist or have parent assist child with using strategy during actual pain *because coaching may be needed to help child focus on required actions*

*Nursing outcome.

Continued

EXPECTED OUTCOMES

Child exhibits acceptable pain level

Child learns and implements effective coping strategies

Parent learns coping skills and is effective in assisting child to cope

PATIENT GOAL 2: Will experience no pain or reduction of pain to level acceptable to child when receiving analgesics

NURSING INTERVENTIONS/*RATIONALES*

Plan to administer prescribed analgesic before procedure *so that its peak effect coincides with painful event*

Plan preventive schedule of medication around the clock (ATC) or "PRN as needed to prevent pain" when pain is continuous and predictable (e.g., postoperatively) *to maintain steady blood levels of analgesic*

Administer analgesia by least traumatic route whenever possible *to avoid causing additional pain;* avoid intramuscular or subcutaneous injections (see Box 21-14)

Prepare child for administration of analgesia by using supportive statements (e.g., "This medicine I am putting in the IV will make you feel better in a few minutes")

Reinforce effect of analgesic by saying that child will begin to feel better in (fill in appropriate amount of time, according to drug use); use clock or timer to measure onset of relief with child; reinforce cause and effect of pain and analgesic *so that child becomes conditioned to expecting relief*

If injection must be given, provide an age-appropriate explanation

Avoid statements such as "By now you shouldn't need so much pain medicine" *because they convey a judgmental and belittling attitude*

Give child control whenever possible (e.g., using patient-controlled analgesia, choosing which arm for a venipuncture, taking bandages off, holding tape or other equipment)

*Administer prescribed analgesic; nonopioids, including acetaminophen (Tylenol, paracetamol) and nonsteroidal antiinflammatory drugs (NSAIDs), are suitable for mild to moderate pain (Table 21-5); opioids are needed for moderate to severe pain (Table 21-6); combination of the two analgesics (see Table 21-7) attacks pain at peripheral nervous system and at central nervous system and provides increased analgesia without increased side effects

Titrate (adjust) dosage for maximum pain relief

If using parenteral route, change to oral route as soon as possible using equianalgesic dosages (see Tables 21-6 and 21-7) *because of first-pass effect (oral opioid is rapidly absorbed from gastrointestinal tract and enters portal circulation, where it is partially metabolized before reaching central circulation; therefore, oral dosages must be larger)*

*Avoid combining opioids with so-called "potentiators" *because combining drugs such as promethazine (Phenergan) and chlorpromazine (Thorazine) adds risk of sedation and respiratory depression without increasing analgesia*

Do not use placebos in the assessment or treatment of pain *because deceptive use of placebos does not provide useful information about presence or severity of pain, can cause side effects similar to those of opioids, can destroy child's and family's trust in health care staff, and raises serious ethical and legal questions*

EXPECTED OUTCOMES

Child exhibits absence or minimal evidence of pain

Child accepts administration of analgesia with minimal distress

---

NURSING DIAGNOSIS ■ **Risk for poisoning or injury related to sensitivity, excessive dose, decreased gastrointestinal motility**

PATIENT GOAL 1: Will exhibit normal respiratory function

NURSING INTERVENTIONS/*RATIONALES*

Monitor rate and depth of respirations and level of sedation

Have emergency drugs and equipment in case of respiratory depression from opioids (see Guidelines box, p. 681) *to begin therapy as soon as needed*

EXPECTED OUTCOME

Child's respirations and sedation level remain within acceptable limits (see inside back cover for normal variations)

PATIENT GOAL 2: Will not develop constipation and will receive treatment for other opioid-related side effects

NURSING INTERVENTIONS/*RATIONALES*

*Administer stool softener or laxative *to prevent constipation*

*Stop or decrease medication if evidence of rash

*Administer antipruritic *for itching*

*Administer antiemetic for nausea and vomiting

Encourage child to lie quietly *because movement increases nausea and vomiting*

Recognize signs of tolerance: decreasing pain relief, decreasing duration of pain relief

Recognize signs of withdrawal after discontinuation of drug (physical dependence) (see Box 21-16)

†Help treat tolerance and physical dependence appropriately *because these are involuntary, physiologic responses that occur from prolonged use of opioids*

Never refer to child who is tolerant or physically dependent as "addicted"

EXPECTED OUTCOMES

Child has regular bowel movements

Child exhibits no evidence of rash or itching

Child receives appropriate therapy for tolerance or dependency

See also Preparation for Procedures, Chapter 22

See also Administration of Medications, Chapter 22

NURSING DIAGNOSIS ■ **Powerlessness related to the health care environment**

PATIENT GOAL 1: Will experience "homelike" atmosphere in the hospital environment

NURSING INTERVENTIONS/*RATIONALES*

Determine child's customary routine and usual manner of handling child from parents or other caregiver (see Box 21-6)

Maintain a routine similar to one that child is accustomed to at home

Minimize a hospital-like environment as much as possible; allow child to sit at table to eat and wear own pajamas or street clothes

Use terms familiar to child, such as those for body functions

Encourage patients with extended hospitalizations to decorate room (e.g., pictures, bedspread from home) *to make it more "homelike"*

Encourage sibling visitation

Explore possibility of pet visitation for children with extended hospitalizations

EXPECTED OUTCOME

Child's routines and environment are similar to those at home (specify)

---

*Dependent nursing action.

†Nursing outcome.

PATIENT GOAL 2: Will experience opportunities to exert control

NURSING INTERVENTIONS/*RATIONALES*

Allow child choices whenever possible, such as food selection, clothing, options for time of basic care (bath, play, bedtime), selection of television channels, and choice of activities, *to give child some measure of control*

Use time structuring with an older child (a jointly planned and written schedule of daily activities)

Permit freedom on the unit within defined and enforced limitations

Explain reason for physically restraining a child to both child and parents

Encourage self-care according to child's abilities

Assign tasks to an older child, especially in extended hospitalization (e.g., making the bed, supervising younger children, distributing menus, collating charts)

Respect child's need for privacy

EXPECTED OUTCOMES

Child participates in planning care (specify)

Child moves about the unit but respects limits

Child participates in care activities (specify activities)

Child assumes responsibility for tasks (specify)

†Child's need for privacy is maintained

NURSING DIAGNOSIS ▪ **Diversional activity deficit related to impaired mobility, musculoskeletal impairment, confinement to hospital or home, effects of illness**

PATIENT GOAL 1: Will have opportunity to participate in activities

NURSING INTERVENTIONS/*RATIONALES*

Schedule therapies and periods of rest to allow for activities

Involve child in planning care to the extent of capabilities

Arrange for and encourage interaction with others as feasible

Encourage visits from family and friends

Provide opportunity to socialize with noninfectious children

EXPECTED OUTCOMES

Child helps plan care and schedule

Child interacts with family and other children

PATIENT GOAL 2: Will have opportunity to participate in diversional activities

NURSING INTERVENTIONS/*RATIONALES*

Spend time with child

Query child and parents regarding child's favorite diversional activities

Change position of bed in room periodically *to alter sensory stimuli* if child is confined to bed

Provide activities appropriate to child's condition, physical limitations, and developmental level

Encourage family to caress and hold infant or child

Maintain accustomed home routine of diversional activities, when possible

Consult with a child-life specialist *to provide diversional activities*

Encourage interaction with other children

Choose a roommate compatible in age, sex, and physical abilities

Monitor time spent watching television or playing electronic games versus interactive or creative activities

Allow ample time for play

Make play, art, music, and other expressive materials available to child

Encourage play activities and diversions appropriate to child's age, condition, and capabilities

Help facilitate an activity by acting under child's instructions to perform tasks child is unable to do

Use play as a teaching strategy and an anxiety-reducing technique

Promote the use of a separate activity room or area for adolescents

EXPECTED OUTCOMES

Child engages in activities appropriate for age, interests, and physical limitations (specify activities)

Child receives attention and comfort

Child engages in age-appropriate play (specify)

NURSING DIAGNOSIS ▪ **Activity intolerance related to generalized weakness, fatigue, imbalance between oxygen supply and demand**

PATIENT GOAL 1: Will maintain adequate energy levels

NURSING INTERVENTIONS/*RATIONALES*

Assess child's level of physical tolerance

Anticipate child's need for rest, as evidenced by irritability, short attention span, and fretfulness; assist child in those activities of daily living that may be beyond tolerance

Provide entertainment and quiet diversional activities appropriate to child's age and interest *to conserve energy*

Provide diversional play activities *that promote rest and quiet but prevent boredom and withdrawal*

Instruct child to rest when feeling tired

Balance rest and activity when ambulatory

EXPECTED OUTCOMES

Child plays and rests quietly and engages in activities appropriate to age and capabilities (specify)

Child tolerates increasingly more activity

PATIENT GOAL 2: Will receive optimal rest

NURSING INTERVENTIONS/*RATIONALES*

Provide quiet environment *to promote rest*

Organize activities for maximum sleep time

Schedule visiting to allow for sufficient rest

Keep visiting periods with friends and family short

Encourage parents to remain with child *to decrease separation and anxiety*

*Administer sedatives and analgesics as indicated, if ordered, *for restlessness and pain*

Encourage frequent rest periods

Enforce regular sleep times

Follow child's usual routine for bedtime, nap time

Implement measures to ensure sleep, such as quiet, darkened room

Be alert to signs that child is tired or overstimulated *to allow flexibility in scheduling or enforcing rest and sleep periods*

EXPECTED OUTCOMES

Child remains calm, quiet, and relaxed

Child has sufficient amount of rest (specify)

†Nursing outcome.
*Dependent nursing action.

Continued

NURSING CARE PLAN   The Child in the Hospital—*cont'd*

NURSING DIAGNOSIS ■ **Risk for injury/trauma related to unfamiliar environment, therapies, hazardous equipment**

PATIENT GOAL 1: Will experience no injury

NURSING INTERVENTIONS/*RATIONALES*

Employ environmental safety measures

Report any potential hazards (e.g., slippery floors, poor illumination, electrical hazards, damaged or malfunctioning furniture or equipment, unprotected windows, stairwells)

Dispose of breakable items appropriately (syringe caps, thermometers, bottles) to prevent aspiration or laceration

Keep potentially hazardous articles out of child's reach

Check bathwater for temperature before bathing infant or child *to prevent burns*

Do not leave children unsupervised in bath or shower

Keep crib sides up and securely fastened; use siderails for children who may fall out of bed

Use safety restraints only when absolutely necessary (Follow hospital policies)

   Remove as often as possible

   Discontinue as soon as possible

   Check regularly for adequate circulation to restrained area and any pressure points and that restraint is applied properly

Maintain hand contact while caring for a child in a crib with siderails down *to prevent falls*

Transport infants and children appropriately

   Hold with proper support

   Fasten safety belt on gurney, wheelchair

Alert parents and ancillary hospital personnel regarding child's physical tolerance and need for assistance during activity

Fasten safety belts in high chairs, swings

EXPECTED OUTCOME

Child remains free of injury

NURSING DIAGNOSIS ■ **Bathing/hygiene and dressing/grooming self-care deficit related to physical or cognitive disability, mechanical restrictions**

PATIENT GOAL 1: Will engage in self-help activities

NURSING INTERVENTIONS/*RATIONALES*

Allow child to help plan own daily routine and choose from alternatives when appropriate *to promote sense of control*

Encourage participation in self-care activities according to developmental level and capabilities *to promote mastery and decrease regression*

Provide devices, equipment, and methods to assist child in self-care

Advocate for child-sized features *that foster independence* (e.g., bathroom door handles low enough for children to reach)

Assist with dressing, grooming, bathing as indicated

EXPECTED OUTCOME

Child engages in self-help activities to maximum capabilities

NURSING DIAGNOSIS ■ **Toileting self-care deficit related to physical or cognitive disability, mechanical restrictions**

PATIENT GOAL 1: Will exhibit normal elimination patterns

NURSING INTERVENTIONS/RATIONALES

Solicit information from child and parents regarding child's normal patterns and procedures of elimination

Sit child in upright position when possible *to encourage elimination*

Employ special devices when appropriate (e.g., fracture pan, commode, elevated toilet seat)

Carry out bowel-training program with hydration, high-fiber diet, stool softeners, and mild laxatives if needed

Provide privacy

EXPECTED OUTCOME

Child has regular bowel movement

NURSING DIAGNOSIS ■ **Altered patterns of urinary elimination related to discomfort, positioning**

PATIENT GOAL 1: Will exhibit normal voiding

NURSING INTERVENTIONS/*RATIONALES*

Solicit information from child and parents regarding child's normal patterns and procedures of elimination

Position child as upright as possible to void

Hydrate child *to ensure adequate urine output for age*

Stimulate bladder emptying with running water

Catheterize as needed

EXPECTED OUTCOME

Child exhibits no urinary retention

See also:

   Nursing Care Plan: The Child Undergoing Surgery, Chapter 22

   Nursing Care Plan: The Child Who Is Terminally Ill or Dying, Chapter 18

Illness or hospitalization can also help older children in choosing a vocation. Frequently, children have impressions of physicians or nurses that are disproportionately glorified or horrified. Actual experience with different health professionals can influence their attitude about health professionals and even a decision regarding a health career.

Promoting Self-Mastery.   The experience of facing a crisis such as illness or hospitalization, coping successfully with it, and maturing as a result of it constitutes an opportunity for self-mastery. Younger children have the chance to test fantasy versus reality fears. They realize that they were not abandoned, mutilated, castrated, or punished. In fact, they were loved, cared for, and treated with respect for their individual concerns. It is not unusual for children who have undergone hospitalization or surgery to tell others that "it was nothing" or to display proudly their scars or bandages. For older children, hospitalization may represent an opportunity for decision making, independence, and self-reliance. They are proud of having survived the experience and may feel a genuine self-respect for their achievements. Nurses can facilitate such feelings of self-mastery by emphasizing aspects of personal competence in the child and not focusing on uncooperative or negative behavior.

Providing Socialization.   Hospitalization may offer children a special opportunity for social acceptance. Lonely, asocial, sometimes delinquent children find a sympathetic environment in the hospital. Children who have a physical handicap or are in some other way "different" from their age-mates may find an accepting social peer group (Fig. 21-13). Although this does not always spontaneously occur, nurses can structure the environment to foster a supportive child group. For example, selection of a compatible roommate can help children gain a new friend and learn more about themselves. Forming relationships with significant members of the health care team, such as the physician, nurse, child-life specialist, or minister, can greatly enhance children's adjustment in many areas of life.

Parents may also encounter a new social group in other parents who have similar problems. The waiting room or hallway "self-help" groups are inherent to every institution. Nurses can capitalize on this informal gathering by encouraging parents to discuss collectively their concerns and feelings. Nurses can also refer parents to organized parent groups or can use the help and support of recovered hospitalized patients.

Evaluation

The effectiveness of nursing interventions is determined by continual reassessment and evaluation of care based on the following observational guidelines:

1 Interview child and parents regarding the type of preparation for hospitalization the child received.
2 Review the medical record for evidence of parental visitation; interview parents and child regarding strategies used to minimize separation.
3 Compare child's hospital schedule with the schedule the child typically follows at home; interview child and family for examples of when they were allowed choices in the child's care.
4 Review the medical record for evidence of pain assessment and administration of analgesics or nonpharmacologic pain reducers. Compare child's behavior and pain scores before and after administration of pain reducers for evidence of pain relief.
5 Interview child regarding the types of play and other activities that were introduced by the nurses or child-life specialist and the times the child visited the playroom. For preverbal child, observe child's use of play materials.
6 Interview child and parents regarding their perception of any beneficial aspects of the hospitalization. Observe behaviors that indicate benefits, such as the formation of new friendships.

The *expected outcomes* are described in the Nursing Care Plan on pp. 686 to 690.

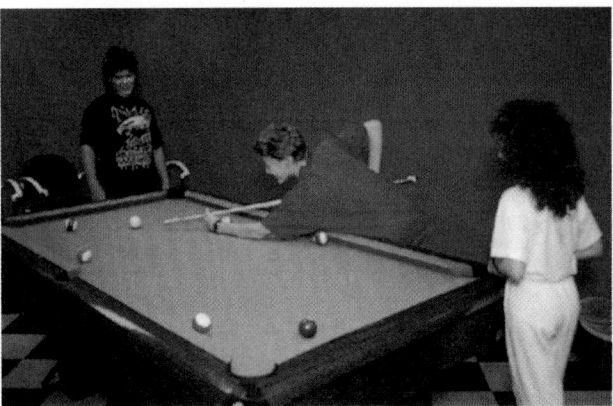

FIG. 21-13 ■ The hospital environment can present an opportunity for forming new friendships and an accepting peer group for children.

NURSING CARE OF THE FAMILY

Assessment

Assessment involves those factors that are most likely to influence the family's responses to the child's illness or hospitalization. Although it is not possible to predict exactly which factors are most likely to have an effect on the family's reactions, the areas discussed in Table 18-2 should be included in the assessment process. Other important variables are (1) the seriousness of the child's illness, (2) the family's previous experience with hospitalization, and (3) the medical procedures involved in the diagnosis and treatment. Important information is also obtained in the nursing admission history (see Box 21-6).

Discharge Assessment

Throughout the hospitalization the nurse should be aware of the need for discharge planning and those assessment factors that affect the family's ability to provide home care. Discharge planning must begin early in the hospital admission to permit sufficient time to assess the family's ability to perform care at home and to institute needed teaching. With the current concern for cost containment and recognition of children's emotional needs, home care for children with technologically complex care, such as children requiring mechanical ventilation, has become increasingly common. The current nursing shortage has placed more of the burden for caring for children in the home on the parents, who often become the child's *caregiver,* supervised by the nurse who acts as *case manager* (see Home Care in Chapter 20).

In terms of home care for children with complex care, a thorough assessment of the family and home environment should be performed to ensure that the family's emotional and physical resources are sufficient to manage the tasks of home care. (For a discussion of family and home assessment strategies, see Chapter 6.) In addition to adequate family resources, an investigation of community services, including respite care, is needed to ensure that appropriate support agencies are available, such as emergency facilities, home health agencies, and equipment vendors. Financial resources are also a consideration. To coordinate the immense task of assessment and to plan implementation, a care coordinator or manager should be appointed early in the discharge program.

Discharge planning is also concerned with those treatments that parents or children are expected to continue at home. Assessment for planning appropriate teaching includes knowledge of (1) the actual and perceived complexity of the skill, (2) the parents' or child's ability to learn the skill, and (3) the parents' or child's previous or present experience with such procedures.

● Nursing Diagnoses

A number of nursing diagnoses are prominent in the nursing care of the family of the hospitalized child, and others specific to individual cases become evident. The most common nursing diagnoses are outlined in the Nursing Care Plan on pp. 695 to 697.

● Planning

The main goals for the family are as follows:
1 Family will participate in child's care to the extent they desire.
2 Family will receive support.
3 Family will be informed of child's care.
4 Family will be prepared for discharge and home care.

● Implementation

Encouraging Parent Participation

Preventing or minimizing separation is a key nursing goal with the child who is hospitalized, but maintaining parent-child contact is also beneficial for the family. One of the best approaches is encouraging parents to stay with their child and to participate in the care whenever possible. Although some health facilities provide special accommodations for parents, the concept of "rooming-in" can be instituted anywhere. The first requirement is the staff's positive attitude toward parents. A negative attitude toward parent participation can create barriers to collaborative working relationships (Johnson and Lindschau, 1996). Although nurses often express explicit support for the concept of family-centered care, some of their practices and beliefs suggest otherwise (Bruce and Ritchie, 1997).

When hospital staff genuinely appreciate the importance of continued parent-child attachment, they foster an environment that encourages parents to stay. When parents are included in the care planning and understand that they are a contributing factor to the child's recovery, they are more inclined to remain with their child and have more emotional reserves to support themselves and the child through the crisis. An empowerment model of helping allows the nurse to focus on parents' strengths and seek ways to promote growth and family functioning so that the parents become empowered in caring for their child (Fig. 21-14).

Because the mother tends to be the usual family caregiver, she usually spends more time in the hospital than the father. However, not all mothers (or fathers) feel equally comfortable in assuming responsibility for their child's care. Some may be under such great emotional stress that they need a temporary reprieve from total participation in care-

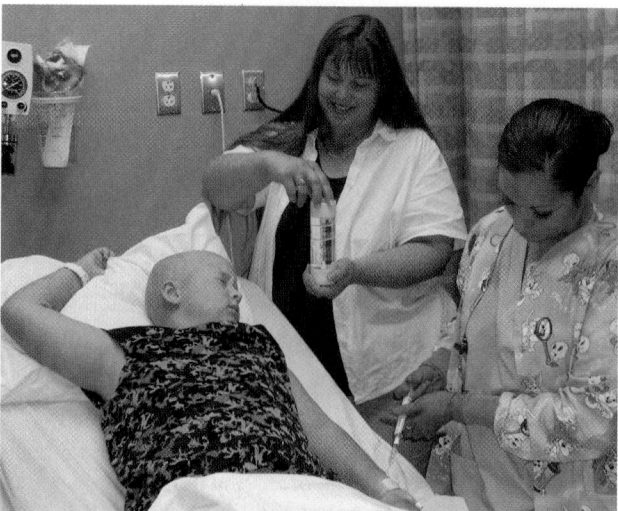

FIG. 21-14 ■ Parental presence during hospitalization provides emotional support for the child and increases the parent's sense of empowerment in the caregiver role. (Courtesy Texas Children's Hospital).

giving activities (Remmel, 1997). (See Ethical Case Study.) Others may feel insecure in participating in specialized areas of care, such as bathing the child after surgery. On the other hand, some mothers may feel a great need to have control of their child's care. This seems particularly true of young mothers, who have more recently established their role as a parent; mothers of children too young to verbalize their needs; and ethnic minority mothers when the hospital setting is predominantly staffed by nonminority personnel. Individual assessment of each parent's preferred involvement is necessary to prevent the effects of separation while supporting parents in their needs as well.

With lifestyles and gender roles changing, fathers may assume all or some of the usual "mothering" roles in the household. In this case it may be the father-child relationship that requires preservation. Fathers need to be included in the plan of care and respected for their parental role. For some fathers the child's hospitalization may represent an opportunity to alter their usual caregiving role and increase their involvement. In single-parent families the caregiver may not be a parent but an extended family member, such as a grandparent or aunt.

One of the potential problems with continuous parent involvement is neglect of the parent's need for sleep, nutrition, and relaxation (see Family Focus box). Often the sleeping accommodations are limited to a chair, and sleep is disrupted by nursing procedures. Encouraging the parents to leave for brief periods, arranging for sleeping quarters on the unit but outside the child's room, and planning a schedule of alternating visiting with another family member can minimize the stresses for the parent.

NURSING TIP

If parents are reluctant to leave the hospital (usually for fear of not being there when the child awakens or the practitioner visits), arrange for them to have a remote "beeper" that can provide immediate communication regardless of their location (Ashenberg and others, 1996).

✕ ETHICAL CASE STUDY

Ethical Decision Making Model	Carrie is a 3-month-old infant who has been admitted to the hospital for bronchiolitis and respiratory syncytial virus (RSV). She also is diagnosed with failure to thrive. Carrie's mother is 18 years of age and has a history of drug addiction. On arrival at the hospital, Carrie's mother informs the nurse that she cannot stay with Carrie because she has to go to work. She leaves shortly after the nurse completes the admission history and has not returned to the hospital for 2 days. No other family members are listed in the chart, and no one has visited Carrie since her mother left.
Evaluate the issue	The first priority is Carrie's recovery from bronchiolitis and RSV. The hospital policies for supervision of a young infant without family presence should be followed. Social services should be involved, and an investigation of the mother should occur prior to Carrie's discharge. A review of any past hospital or emergency department visits could be helpful in trying to locate a family member as well as provide additional information on Carrie's health.
Treat all involved with respect	It is difficult for nursing staff not to judge a mother who has left her young child in a hospital for 2 days without visiting. Nurses who realize the difficulties facing this drug-addicted mother can provide support and serve as resources for helping the mother receive care.
Hear all sides	Assumptions are easily made in this case because the mother is young and has a history of drug addiction. It is important for the nursing staff to remember to be objective during the investigation of the mother and to provide professional support for needed referrals for counseling and guidance.
Initiate action	Carrie's situation warrants immediate action to begin plans for Carrie's care outside the hospital. If the mother cannot be found, social services must begin working with outside resources to place Carrie in a foster home. While investigation of Carrie's mother continues, comfort and support for Carrie should be provided by child-life specialists, volunteers, and the nursing staff.
Consider the outcome	There are a number of outcomes to be considered that could positively affect Carrie's well-being. One is that the mother would receive the appropriate counseling needed to cope with life and its problems without depending on substances or drugs that may affect her and her daughter. If the mother demonstrates the capacity to adequately care for Carrie at home, it would be best if the child remains in the home setting with her mother. Carrie's failure to thrive must be adequately addressed before such actions take place. The second scenario would entail Carrie recovering from the bronchiolitis and RSV and going into a temporary foster home while her mother receives appropriate assistance for substance abuse. Carrie needs a constant, stable primary caretaker and home environment in order to be able to grow and develop appropriately. The issue of the failure to thrive must be investigated to ensure that organic problems are not a contributing factor. If the lack of an appropriate and consistent home environment is the cause of her failure to thrive, this must be addressed by the nursing staff and social services.

 FAMILY FOCUS

Parents' Reluctance to Leave Their Children Unattended

Parents are often very reluctant to leave their children or to ask the nurse to watch their children while they take a break. In his research on the experiences of nurses and parents when parents room-in, Darbyshire (1994) found that many parents did not eat properly or, in some cases, at all. The following are two mothers' experiences:

I just about starved to death the first couple of days . . . just . . . I mean, it was my own fault really, 'cos I wouldn't leave the wee one. There was always going to be something else happening and I thought . . . if he gets upset I'd better be there when it finishes.

There was one day I couldn't get any of the visitors to look after the wee chap so I could go for something to eat and it was about six o'clock at night and nurse said, "You look awful, are you OK?" and I said, "No, actually I feel awful and I think I'm going to pass out," and she said, "Oh, you've just gone a funny colour," and I said, "What time is it?" and I said, "It's OK, it's just because I haven't eaten all day"—because none of my family had come to take the child from me, and I didn't think to say to a nurse, "Could you watch him till I go for something to eat?"

Data from Darbyshire P: *Living with a sick child in hospital,* London, 1994, Chapman & Hall.

All too often, nurses respond to parent participation by abandoning their patient responsibilities. Nurses need to restructure their roles to complement and augment the caregiving functions of parents. Even in units structured to provide care by parents, parents frequently feel anxiety in their caregiving responsibilities; those more involved in direct care may feel more anxiety than those less involved in direct care. Therefore 24-hour responsibility may be too much for some parents. Assistance and relief by nursing personnel should always be available to these families, and nurses must often work diligently to establish the strong bond of trust some parents need to take advantage of these opportunities.

Supporting Family Members

Support involves the willingness to stay and listen to parents' verbal and nonverbal messages. Sometimes the nurse does not give this support directly. For example, the nurse may offer to stay with the child to allow the parents time alone or may discuss with other family members the parents' need for extra relief. Often relatives and friends want to help but do not know how. Suggesting ways, such as baby-sitting, preparing meals, tending the garden or home, doing laundry, or transporting the siblings to school, can prompt others to help lessen the responsibilities that burden parents. An ongoing parent support group held on the pediatric unit during the children's traditional nap time has also proved effective in helping parents share emotions and concerns related to hospitalization (Bracht and others, 1998; Santelli, Turnbull, and Higgins, 1997).

Support may also be provided through the clergy. Parents with deep religious beliefs may appreciate the counsel of a clergy member, but because of their stress they may not have sufficient energy to initiate the contact. Nurses can be supportive by arranging for clergy to visit, upholding parents' religious beliefs, and respecting the individual meaning and significance of those beliefs.

Support involves an acceptance of cultural, socioeconomic, and ethnic values. For example, health and illness are defined differently by various ethnic groups. For some, a disorder that has few outward manifestations of illness, such as diabetes, hypertension, or cardiac problems, is not a sickness. Consequently, following a prescribed treatment may be seen as unnecessary. Nurses who appreciate the influences of culture are more likely to intervene therapeutically. (See also Chapter 4 for an extensive discussion of cultural and religious influences on health care.)

Parents need help in accepting their own feelings toward the ill child. If given the opportunity, parents often disclose their feelings of loss of control, anger, and guilt. They often resist admitting to such feelings because they expect others to disapprove of behavior that is less than perfect. Unfortunately, health personnel, including nurses, sometimes do exercise little tolerance for deviation from the expected norm. This only increases the psychologic impact of a child's illness on family members. Helping parents identify the specific reason for such feelings and emphasizing that each is a normal, expected, and healthy response to stress provides the parents with an opportunity to lessen their emotional burden.

Family-centered care also addresses the needs of siblings. Support may involve preparing siblings for hospital visits, assessing their adjustment, and providing appropriate interventions or referrals when needed. The Family Home Care box suggests ways that parents can support siblings during hospitalization.

Providing Information

One of the most important nursing interventions is providing information about (1) the disease, its treatment, prognosis, and home care; (2) the child's emotional, as well as physical, reaction to illness and hospitalization; and (3) the probable emotional reactions of family members to the crisis.

For many families the child's illness is the first contact they have with the hospital experience. Often parents are not prepared for the child's behavioral reactions to hospitalization, such as separation behaviors, regression, aggression, and hostility. Providing the parents with information about these normal and expected behavioral responses can lessen the parents' anxiety during the hospital admission. The family is equally unfamiliar with hospital rules, which often adds to feelings of confusion and anxiety. Therefore the family needs clear explanations about what to expect and what is expected of them.

Parents also need to be aware of the effects of illness on the family and strategies that prevent negative changes. Specifi-

---

FAMILY HOME CARE

Supporting Siblings During Hospitalization

Trade off staying at the hospital with spouse or have a parent surrogate who knows the siblings well stay in the home.

Offer information about the child's condition to young siblings as well as older siblings; respect the sibling who avoids information as a means of coping with the situation.

Arrange for children to visit their brother or sister in the hospital if possible.

Encourage phone visits and mail between brothers and sisters; provide children with phone numbers, writing supplies, and stamps.

Help each sibling identify an extended family member or friend to be their support person and provide extra attention during parental absence.

Make or buy inexpensive toys or trinkets for siblings, one gift for each day the child will be hospitalized.

Wrap each gift separately and place in a basket, box, or other container at each child's bedside.

Instruct siblings to open one gift each night at bedtime and to remember that he or she is in the parent's thoughts.

If the child's condition is stable and distance is not prohibitive, plan a special time at home with the siblings or have spouse or another relative or friend bring the children to meet parent(s) at a restaurant or other location near the hospital.

Have extended family members or friends schedule a visit to the child in the hospital during parental absence.

Arrange a pass for the child to leave the hospital to join the family if the child's condition permits.

Modified from Craft M, Craft J: Perceived changes in siblings of hospitalized children: a comparison of sibling and parent reports, *Child Health Care* 18(1):42-48, 1989; Rollins J: *Brothers and sisters: a discussion guide for families*, Landover, Md, 1992, Epilepsy Foundation of America.

---

cally, parents should keep the family well-informed and communicating as much as possible. They should treat all of the children equally and as normally as before the illness occurred. Discipline, which initially may be lessened for the ill child, should be continued to provide a measure of security and predictability. When ill children know that their parents expect certain standards of conduct from them, they feel certain that they will recover. Conversely, when all limits are removed, they fear that something catastrophic will happen.

Nurses should help parents understand and accept the meaning of posthospitalization behaviors so that the parents can tolerate and support such behaviors. Consequently, parents should be forewarned of the usual continuance of such reactions after discharge (see Box 21-3). Parents who do not expect such reactions may misinterpret them as evidence of the child's "being spoiled" and demand perfect behavior at a time when the child is still reacting to the stress of illness and hospitalization. If the behaviors, especially the demand for attention, are dealt with in a supportive manner, most children are able to relinquish them and assume precrisis levels of functioning.

Nurses should also forewarn parents of the reactions of siblings, particularly anger, jealousy, and resentment. Older siblings may deny such reactions because they provoke feelings of guilt. However, everyone needs outlets for emo-

Text continued on p. 698.

NURSING CARE PLAN   The Family of the Ill or Hospitalized Child

NURSING DIAGNOSIS ▪ Anxiety/fear related to situational crisis, threat to role functioning, change in environment

FAMILY GOAL 1: Will adjust to hospital environment

NURSING INTERVENTIONS/RATIONALES

Introduce family to significant staff members

Describe hospital routine that affects child

Acclimate family to the new and strange surroundings (e.g., physical layout of unit, including playroom, unit kitchen, toilet, and telephone)

Direct family to areas they may need to use outside the unit (e.g., dining room, chapel, laundry facilities)

Provide an atmosphere that promotes questioning, expression of doubts and feelings

Be available to family for questions or concerns

Be alert to signs of tension in family members

Provide for privacy

EXPECTED OUTCOMES

Family demonstrates familiarity with hospital environment

Family members ask questions pertinent to hospitalization and care

FAMILY GOAL 2: Will continue to be child's primary caregivers

NURSING INTERVENTIONS/RATIONALES

Employ a polite approach and demeanor toward family

Recognize that family knows child's non–health care needs better than staff (favorite food, activity, diversions)

Greet family by name when they arrive on the unit

Encourage family's presence

Include family in planning patient care

Encourage family to select and assume specific roles in child's care

Offer encouragement for their efforts

Ask family to share with staff what they know about child's care and needs

Convey an attitude of collegiality with family, not competition

EXPECTED OUTCOME

Family is involved in planning and caring for the child

FAMILY GOAL 3: Will experience reduced apprehension

NURSING INTERVENTIONS/RATIONALES

Allow for expression of feelings about child's hospitalization and illness

Provide needed information *to alleviate fear of the unknown*

Prepare family for what to expect (e.g., procedures, behaviors)

Explore family's expectations

Explore family's concerns and feelings of irritation, guilt, anger, disappointment, inadequacy

Explore family's fears and anxieties regarding child's status and expectations of results of procedures or therapy

Introduce parents to other families who have a child in the hospital, especially a child who is similarly affected, *to facilitate family-to-family support*

Provide something constructive and meaningful for family to focus on (e.g., keeping record of intake and output, pain relief record, ensuring a specified amount of fluid intake, collecting a specimen)

EXPECTED OUTCOMES

Family members verbalize feelings and concerns

Family demonstrates an understanding of procedures and behaviors (specify manner of demonstration and learning)

Family interacts with other families, as desired

FAMILY GOAL 4: Will be prepared for special procedures (e.g., radiology, diagnostic tests, surgery)

NURSING INTERVENTIONS

Assess family's understanding of the procedure and its purpose

Provide needed information; clarify misconceptions

Explain special preparation needed (e.g., nothing by mouth [NPO], shaving, preprocedural medication or equipment)

Describe:

Where child will be during the procedure

Whether family can be with child

Where family can wait

Approximate length of time procedure requires

Reassure family that they will be notified regarding progress of the procedure

EXPECTED OUTCOME

Family demonstrates an understanding of procedures and tests (specify)

FAMILY GOAL 5: Will receive support during child's absence

NURSING INTERVENTIONS/RATIONALES

Provide a comfortable place for family to wait

Suggest activities to help reduce anxiety (e.g., go to the coffee shop or dining room, take a short walk [specify activity])

Be available to family *for support*

Make contact with family at frequent intervals *to relay information, provide comfort*

EXPECTED OUTCOME

Family feels a sense of support

FAMILY GOAL 6: Will adjust to child's appearance and behavior after procedure(s) or in special care unit

NURSING INTERVENTIONS/RATIONALES

Remain calm *to decrease family's anxiety*

Describe the environment, as appropriate (e.g., intensive care unit)

Apply principles of learning to explanations

Begin with small amounts of information

Begin with very general information

Allow ample time for family to absorb information and to ask questions

Use age-appropriate explanations and techniques for siblings

Explain how child will look and the reasons for the child's appearance and equipment

Explain what child may be experiencing

Prepare child and surrounding *to lessen impact of the first impression*

Keep the bed clean and neat

Personalize the bed and bedside with a toy or other item(s)

Provide chairs for family

Be prepared for possible adverse reaction (e.g., fainting)

Convey an attitude of caring *about*, as well as *for*, the child

Accompany the family to the child's bedside

Allow time for follow-up discussion of questions and concerns

EXPECTED OUTCOME

Family feels prepared before coming to child's bedside

Continued

FAMILY GOAL 7: Will experience reduction or absence of fear

NURSING INTERVENTIONS

Help family distinguish between realistic and unfounded fears
Help eliminate unfounded fears
Discuss with family their fears regarding:
    Child's signs and symptoms
    Child's anxiety
    Consequences of disease or therapy
    Deterioration of child's condition
    Tests and procedures
    Death
Answer questions honestly and compassionately

EXPECTED OUTCOME

Family members verbalize fears and explore nature and ramifications of these fears

NURSING DIAGNOSIS ▪ **Powerlessness related to health care environment**

FAMILY GOAL 1: Will experience a sense of control

NURSING INTERVENTIONS/*RATIONALES*

Encourage family's presence at times convenient for them; consider variations (e.g., cultural, occupational) in visiting
Encourage expression of concerns regarding child's care and progress
Explore family's feelings regarding prescribed therapies
Encourage family to assume as much control as possible in child's management
    Encourage participation in child's care
    Include family in setting goals for care
    Involve family in scheduling and other aspects of care
    Explain what family can do for child and how to handle child to maintain therapy (e.g., how to pick up the child who has an intravenous line)
    Employ family's suggestions regarding child's care whenever possible

EXPECTED OUTCOMES

Family schedules time to be with child
Family readily discusses feelings and concerns
Family contributes to care and management of child
*Family's suggestions are incorporated into plan of care

NURSING DIAGNOSIS ▪ **Altered family processes related to situational crisis (threat to role functioning, hospitalization of a child)**

FAMILY GOAL 1: Will demonstrate knowledge of child's illness

NURSING INTERVENTIONS/*RATIONALES*

Recognize family's concern and need for information, support
Assess family's understanding of diagnosis and plan of care
Reinforce and clarify health professional's explanation of child's condition, suggested procedures and therapies, and prognosis
Use every opportunity to increase family's understanding of the disease and its therapies
Repeat information as often as necessary *to facilitate understanding*
Interpret technical information *because family may not understand*
Help family interpret infant's or child's behaviors and responses
Set and keep appointed time for patient/family education

EXPECTED OUTCOME

Family demonstrates an understanding of the disease and its therapies (specify knowledge)

FAMILY GOAL 2: Will experience reduction of or no guilt feelings

NURSING INTERVENTIONS

Acknowledge feelings of guilt
Provide accurate and specific information regarding the cause of the illness
Clarify misconceptions and false assumptions

EXPECTED OUTCOME

Family verbalizes their understanding of the cause of the illness (specify)

FAMILY GOAL 3: Will receive adequate support

NURSING INTERVENTIONS/*RATIONALES*

Respect parental rights
Convey an attitude of respectful caring for both child and family
Support and emphasize family's strengths and abilities
Provide feedback and praise
Refer to other professionals *for additional interpersonal and concrete support* (e.g., social service, clergy)

EXPECTED OUTCOMES

Family exhibits behaviors that indicate a feeling of self-respect
Family uses supportive services

FAMILY GOAL 4: Will demonstrate positive coping behaviors toward child

NURSING INTERVENTIONS

Determine family's understanding of the normal childhood responses to the stress of illness and hospitalization
Explain child's regression, magical thinking, egocentricity, separation anxiety, fears
Explain behavioral reactions generally expected of child (specify according to age and developmental level)
Explain what child is (family are) permitted to do in coping with child's behavior
Reinforce family's endeavors

EXPECTED OUTCOME

Family demonstrates an understanding of child's unfamiliar behaviors (specify manner of demonstration: verbalization, physical attitude, behaviors with child)

FAMILY GOAL 5: Will assist child in coping effectively with hospitalization

NURSING INTERVENTIONS

Help parents determine the best way to prepare child for hospitalization, procedures
Provide family with precise information about what will take place so that they know what child is likely to experience
Encourage family to trust child's capacity to cope
Impress on family the need for honesty in relating to child
Encourage family to use play as a coping strategy
Suggest appropriate items to bring to child (e.g., pajamas, favorite toys)
See also Nursing Care Plan: The Child in the Hospital, pp. 686 to 690

*Nursing outcome.

NURSING CARE PLAN   The Family of the Ill or Hospitalized Child—*cont'd*

EXPECTED OUTCOMES

Family helps in planning strategies

Family is honest with child and staff

Family uses play as a tool for relating with child

FAMILY GOAL 6: Will experience positive relationships

NURSING INTERVENTIONS/*RATIONALES*

Recognize that family members know child best and are "cued in" to child's needs

Welcome unlimited family presence *to promote family relationships*

Encourage family to bring other significant family members to visit (e.g., siblings, grandparents, and, where permitted, pets)

Encourage family to provide child with significant, but manageable, items from home *to provide security*

Arrange for family members to have a meal together

EXPECTED OUTCOMES

Child and family exhibit behaviors that indicate positive coping

Family is with child at appropriate times and in appropriate numbers

Child demonstrates an attitude of security with familiar persons and things

---

FAMILY GOAL 7: Will exhibit evidence of optimal health

NURSING INTERVENTIONS/*RATIONALES*

Stress importance of maintaining family members' health during child's illness and hospitalization

Encourage adequate rest *to promote health of family*

　Provide sleeping facilities where possible

　Encourage members to alternate visiting with child *to allow some time at home*

Explore means for respite care of dependent family members

Assure family that child will receive optimal care in their absence

Provide relief for family from direct care of child as needed

Promote adequate nutrition

Provide meals for parents if possible

Direct family to nutritious resources for meals

Encourage regular mealtimes away from unit

Provide access to unit kitchen to store and prepare snacks

EXPECTED OUTCOMES

Family shows no evidence of illness

Family members appear well-rested

Family members eat regularly

FAMILY GOAL 8: Will experience smooth transition from hospital to home

NURSING INTERVENTIONS

Assess family's learning needs

Outline and carry out a teaching plan

Determine services needed and make necessary referrals

Include family in planning and problem solving

Maintain open communication between family and health care providers

EXPECTED OUTCOME

Child and family demonstrate ability to provide needed care in the home

---

FAMILY GOAL 9: Will demonstrate knowledge of home care

NURSING INTERVENTIONS/*RATIONALES*

Assess family's knowledge *to facilitate planning*

Teach family the skills needed to carry out the therapeutic program (specify)

　Allow ample time for preparation

　Teach necessary techniques and observations

　Help family by demonstration

　Distribute appropriate home care instructions or other educational materials

　Encourage questions and expression of feelings and concerns

　Allow sufficient time for family to perform procedures under supervision

Inform parents of:

　Signs of progress to observe for

　Any unfavorable signs to be alert for

　Problems that can be anticipated (e.g., care of equipment or devices)

　Behaviors that indicate special needs (e.g., pain medication, imminent seizures)

　A course of action to follow (e.g., seizure care)

　Make certain family knows how to contact appropriate persons if or when needed

Prepare family for possible posthospital behaviors of the child (see Box 21-3)

Ensure family's comprehension of child's needs before discharge

EXPECTED OUTCOMES

Family demonstrates procedures needed to care for child in the home (specify learning and method of demonstration)

Family is aware of how to seek help

FAMILY GOAL 10: Will demonstrate understanding of continuity of care

NURSING INTERVENTIONS

Inform family of community resources available

Refer to agencies as appropriate (specify)

Help identify support group(s) for family

Be available to family by telephone or other means

Schedule follow-up appointments as needed

EXPECTED OUTCOMES

Family seeks appropriate assistance

Family keeps appointments

See also:

　Nursing Care Plan: The Child in the Hospital, pp. 686 to 690.

　Nursing Care Plan: The Child Who Is Terminally Ill or Dying, Chapter 18

tions, and the repressed feelings may surface as problems in school, with age-mates, as psychosomatic illnesses, or in delinquent behavior.

Probably one of the most neglected areas involves giving information to siblings. Frequently, age becomes the only factor that leads to an awareness of this problem, because older children may begin to ask questions or request explanations. Even in this situation, however, the information may be seriously inadequate. Children in every age-group deserve some explanation of the sibling's illness or hospitalization. Although the exact wording may differ, the explanation should focus on the following concerns: (1) "Will I get sick and have to go to the hospital?" (2) "Did I cause the illness?" (for actual or imagined reasons), and (3) "Will my parents abandon me if my brother or sister doesn't recover?" If parents or nurses address the explanations to these three questions, the siblings' own fears of illness, guilt, and abandonment are minimized (Melnyk and Alpert-Gillis, 1998).

Preparing for Discharge and Home Care

Most hospitalizations necessitate some type of discharge preparation. Often this involves education of the family for continued care and follow-up in the home. Depending on the diagnosis, this may be relatively simple or highly complex. Preparing the family for home care demands a high degree of competence in planning and implementing discharge instructions. This usually is best accomplished using an *interdisciplinary team approach,* which requires a shift from the *multidisciplinary team approach* used during an acute phase of a child's illness (Hornick, 1996).

Nurses are the ones responsible for all or some of the discharge teaching, which may be further carried out by the parent as the home caregiver, with a nurse acting as resource case manager. The teaching plan incorporates levels of learning, such as observing, participating with assistance, and finally, acting without help or guidance. The skill is divided into discrete steps, and each step is taught to the family member until it is learned. Return demonstration of the skill is requested before new skills are introduced. A record of teaching and performance provides an efficient checklist for evaluation. All families need to receive detailed *written* instructions about home care, with telephone numbers for assistance, before they leave the hospital. Communication between the nurse performing discharge planning and home health care is essential for ensuring a smooth transition for the child and family.

Videocassette recordings offer another excellent vehicle for home teaching. The actual teaching session in the hospital can be recorded and played for the family as often as needed. If the family has a VCR at home, the filmed instructions serve as a refresher when parents have questions about the procedure.

After the family is competent in performing the skill, they are given responsibility for the care. When possible, the family should have a transition or trial period to assume care with minimal health care supervision. This may be arranged on the unit, during a home pass, or in a facility, such as a motel, near the hospital. Such transitions provide a safe practice period for the family, with assistance readily available when needed, and are especially valuable when the family lives at a distance from the treating center.

In many instances parents need only simple instructions and understanding of follow-up care. However, the often overwhelming care assumed by some families, coupled with other stressors they may be experiencing, necessitates continued professional support after discharge. A follow-up home visit or telephone call gives the nurse a better opportunity to individualize care and provide information in perhaps a less stressful learning environment than the hospital (Snowdon and Kane, 1995). Appropriate referrals and resources may include visiting nurse or home health agencies, private nurse services, the school system, a physical therapist, a mental health counselor, a social worker, and any number of community agencies. Sharing the important issues surrounding the child's and family's needs is essential. Referral summaries should be concise, specific, and factual. When numerous support services are involved, periodic collaboration among the professionals involved and the family is an excellent strategy to ensure efficient usage and comprehensive delivery of services.

● *Evaluation*

The effectiveness of nursing interventions is determined by continual reassessment and evaluation of care based on the following observational guidelines:

1 Observe schedule of parental presence and amount of participation in child's care; observe parents' willingness and ability to take care of their own needs, such as regular breaks to eat, sleep, and care for the family's needs at home.

2 Interview family regarding their concerns; observe support offered by others, such as relatives, friends, and clergy; observe if special cultural practices (if applicable) are respected in the hospital.

3 Interview family regarding their knowledge of child's illness, child's expected reactions to the hospitalization experience, and the emotional needs of the other family members, especially siblings. Observe frequency of siblings' visits and interview siblings regarding their understanding of the ill child's condition.

4 Observe family's performance of skills and determine their understanding of other aspects of home care before discharge; interview family or resource persons regarding the family's use of appropriate referral services.

The *expected outcomes* are described in the Nursing Care Plan on pp. 695 to 697.

CARE OF THE CHILD AND FAMILY IN SPECIAL HOSPITAL SITUATIONS

In addition to a general pediatric unit, children may be admitted to special facilities such as an ambulatory/outpatient setting, an isolation room, or intensive care.

AMBULATORY/OUTPATIENT SETTING

The ambulatory or outpatient setting provides needed medical services for the child while eliminating the necessity of overnight admission. Among the benefits of ambulatory care are (1) minimization of the stressors of hospitalization, especially separation from the family; (2) reduced chance of infection; and (3) cost savings. Admission to the ambulatory or outpatient hospital setting usually is for surgical or diagnostic procedures, such as insertion of tympanostomy tubes, hernia repair, adenoidectomy, tonsillectomy, cystoscopy, or bronchoscopy.

In the ambulatory/outpatient setting, adequate preparation is particularly challenging (Stewart, Algren, and Arnold, 1994). Ideally, the child and parents should receive preadmission preparation, including a tour of the facility and a review of the day's events (Brewer and Lambert, 1997). Parents need information in advance to help prepare the child and themselves for surgery and enable them to care for the child at home after the procedure. Parents also appreciate suggestions for items to bring to the hospital, such as blankets or stuffed animals. When preadmission preparation is not possible, time should be allowed on the day of the procedure for children to become acquainted with their surroundings and for nurses to assess, plan, and implement appropriate teaching.

Waiting is usually inevitable in ambulatory settings. Families frequently report waiting to be the most stressful part of the experience. Providing a pager is one way to allow the family (and at times the child) to leave the area and then be paged to return when needed (Ashenberg and others, 1996).

Explicit discharge instructions are important after outpatient surgery (see Family Home Care box below and Preparing for Discharge and Home Care, p. 698). Parents need guidelines on when to call their practitioner regarding a change in the child's condition. A follow-up telephone call system allows for nurses to check on the child's progress within 48 to 72 hours after discharge. It also provides an opportunity for the nurse to review discharge information and answer questions.

NURSING TIP

Help the family prepare for the transportation home by offering these suggestions:
- Have a blanket and pillow in the car. (Always use the car safety restraint system.)
- Take a basin or plastic bag in case of vomiting.
- Use a cup with a cap and straw for the child to drink fluids (except in cases of orofacial surgery where a straw may be contraindicated).
- Give any prescribed pain medication before leaving facility.
- Provide parents verbal and written information regarding potential side effects of pain medication for which they should be vigilant after discharge.

 FAMILY HOME CARE

Discharge From Ambulatory Settings

Before beginning, explain that all instructions will also be presented in writing for the family to refer to later.

Provide an overview of the typical trajectory (expected pattern) of recovery.

Discuss expected progression of the child's activity level during the postdischarge period (e.g., "Mary will probably sleep for the rest of the day, feel kind of tired most of tomorrow, but be back to her usual activities the next day.").

Explain which activities the child is allowed and what is not permitted (e.g., bed rest, bathing).

Discuss dietary restrictions, being very specific and giving examples of "clear fluids" or what is meant by a "full liquid diet."

Discuss nausea and vomiting, if applicable, explaining how much is "normal" and what to do if more occurs (e.g., "Juan may be sick to his stomach and vomit. This is normal. However, if he vomits more than three times, please call us at this number right away.").

Discuss fever and appropriate comfort measures, explaining how much fever is considered "normal," and specifically what to do if the child goes beyond the range.

Explain the amount, location, and kind of pain or discomfort the child may experience.

   Give any prescribed medication before leaving the facility.

   Send a pain scale home with the family.

   Explain how much pain and discomfort is "normal" and what to do if the child surpasses that level or if pain management interventions are unsuccessful.

Discuss pain management, including dosage for pain medications and details on how to administer them.

Describe appropriate nonpharmacologic comfort measures, such as holding, rocking, or swaddling.

Provide information about each medication that the child will be taking at home.

   Review the details, including dose and route.

   Demonstrate how to administer medications, if necessary (e.g., how to take wrapping off suppositories, how to insert).

   Discuss guidelines for requesting other medications.

   Request that all prescriptions be filled and with the family before discharge.

Make certain the family has all of the equipment and supplies (e.g., gauze and tape for dressing changes) they will need at home.

Discuss complications that may occur and the steps to take if they do.

Ensure that appropriate measures are in place for safe transport home.

   Remind family to use a seat belt or car seat for the child.

   Determine if there will be one person whose sole responsibility is helping ensure the child's safety and comfort during transport.

   Discuss measures the driver may need to take if this is impossible (e.g., be certain a basin is within the child's reach should vomiting occur; take a route that permits slower traffic and has places along the roadside to stop if necessary).

   Determine the availability of a blanket, pillow, and cup with a cap and straw for the child's use in the car.

   Provide a basin or plastic bag in case of vomiting.

Provide emergency phone numbers for the family to call with any concerns.

Explain that the family will be contacted (giving an approximate time) to follow-up on the child but that they should not hesitate to call if concerns arise before then.

Ask the family and child, if appropriate, if they have any questions, and problem solve with family members to meet their unique needs.

ISOLATION

Admission to an isolation room increases all of the stressors typically associated with hospitalization. There is further separation from familiar persons, additional loss of control, and added environmental changes, such as sensory deprivation and the strange appearance of visitors. Orientation to time and place is affected. These stressors are compounded by children's limited understanding of isolation. Preschool children have difficulty understanding the rationale for isolation because they cannot comprehend the cause-and-effect relationship between germs and illness. They are likely to view isolation as punishment. Older children understand the causality better but still require information to decrease fantasizing or misinterpretation.

When a child is placed in isolation, preparation is essential for the child to feel in control. With young children the best approach is a simple explanation, such as "You need to be in this room to help you get better. This is a special place to make all the germs go away. The germs made you sick, and you could not help that."

All children, but especially younger ones, need preparation in terms of what they will see, hear, or feel in isolation. Therefore they are shown the mask, gloves, and gown and are encouraged to "dress up" in them. Playing with the strange apparel lessens the fear of seeing "ghostlike" people walk into the room. Before entering the room, nurses and other health personnel should introduce themselves and let the child see their face before donning a mask. In this way the child associates them with significant experiences and gains a sense of familiarity in an otherwise strange and lonely environment.

When the child's condition improves, appropriate play activities are provided to minimize boredom, stimulate the senses, provide a real or perceived sense of movement, orient the child to time and place, provide social interaction, and reduce depersonalization. For example, the environment can be manipulated to increase sensory freedom by moving the bed toward the door or window. Opening window shades; providing musical, visual, or tactile toys; and increasing interpersonal contact can substitute mental mobility for the limitations of physical movement. Rather than dwelling on the negative aspects of isolation, the child can be encouraged to view this experience as challenging and positive. For example, the nurse can help the child look at isolation as a method of keeping others out and letting only special people in. Children often think of intriguing signs for their doors, such as "Enter at your own risk." These signs also encourage people "on the outside" to talk with the child about the ominous greeting.

> **NURSING TIP**
>
> Have the child select a place he or she would like to visit. Help the child decorate the bed and equipment to suit the theme (e.g., truck, circus tent, spaceship, sky). At a set time each day pretend to go with the child to the special place. Consider including props such as a suitcase or picnic basket.

EMERGENCY ADMISSION

One of the most traumatic hospital experiences for the child and parents is an emergency admission. The sudden onset of an illness or the occurrence of an injury leaves little time for preparation and explanation. Sometimes the emergency admission is compounded by admission to an intensive care unit or the need for immediate surgery. However, even in those instances requiring only outpatient treatment, the child is exposed to a strange, frightening environment and to experiences that may elicit fear or cause pain. Thus every medical emergency requires psychologic intervention to reduce the fear and anxiety frequently associated with the experience. Although underused, child-life specialists may provide teaching and support (Krebel, Clayton, and Graham, 1996).

There is a wide discrepancy between what constitutes a medically defined emergency and a client-defined emergency. A growing concern is the use of major emergency departments for routine primary care health visits. To offset overcrowding in emergency departments many facilities have minor emergency units or pediatric minor emergency units for after-hours health care. Telephone triage for minor illnesses for patients is also emerging as a health care delivery mode to triage illnesses such as a common cold from true life-threatening conditions that require immediate practitioner attention and intervention. Other factors contributing to the overuse of emergency departments (as opposed to the primary practitioner's office) include the increasing number of noninsured persons and households where both parents work full time and cannot afford to take off during the daytime to take the sick child to a practitioner.

In pediatric populations most visits are for respiratory infections, with skin conditions, gastrointestinal disorders, and trauma such as poisoning accounting for the remainder of cases. The most common reason parents give for bringing the child to the emergency department is concern about the illness worsening. However, practitioners may not consider the progressive symptoms as necessitating immediate or emergency care. One of the nurse's primary goals is to assess the parents' perception of the event and their reasons for considering it serious or life-threatening.

Lengthy preparatory admission procedures are often inappropriate for emergency situations. In such instances, nurses must focus their nursing interventions on the essential components of admission counseling (Box 21-17) and complete the process as soon as the child's condition is stabilized.

Unless an emergency is life-threatening, children need to participate in their care to maintain a sense of control. Because emergency departments are frequently hectic, there is a tendency to rush through procedures to save time. However, the extra few minutes needed to allow children to participate may save many more minutes of useless resistance and uncooperativeness during subsequent procedures. Other supportive measures include ensuring privacy, accepting various emotional responses to fear or pain, preserving parent-child contact, explaining all events before or as they occur, and personally remaining calm.

At times, because of the child's physical condition, little or no preparatory counseling for emergency hospitalization can be done. In such situations the implementation of *postvention,* or counseling subsequent to the event, has therapeutic value. The process of postvention involves evaluating children's thoughts regarding admission and related procedures. It is similar to precounseling techniques; however, instead of supplying information, the nurse listens to

BOX 21-17 ■ Guidelines for Special Hospital Admission*

EMERGENCY ADMISSION

Lengthy preparatory admission procedures are often impossible and inappropriate for emergency situations.

Focus assessment on airway, breathing, and circulation; weigh child whenever possible for calculation of drug dosages.

Unless an emergency is life-threatening, children need to participate in their care to maintain a sense of control.

Focus on essential components of admission counseling, including:
Appropriate introduction to the family
Use of child's name, not terms such as "honey" or "dear"
Determination of child's age and some judgment about developmental age (if the child is of school age, asking about the grade level will offer some evidence for concurrent intellectual ability)
Information about child's general state of health, any problems that may interfere with medical treatment (e.g., allergies), and previous experience with hospital facilities
Information about the chief complaint from both the parents and the child

ADMISSION TO INTENSIVE CARE UNIT (ICU)

Prepare child and parents for elective ICU admission, such as for postoperative care after cardiac surgery.

Prepare child and parents for unanticipated ICU admission by focusing primarily on the sensory aspects of the experience and on usual family concerns (e.g., persons in charge of child's care, schedule for visiting, area where family can stay).

Prepare parents regarding child's appearance and behavior when they first visit child in ICU.

Accompany family to bedside to provide emotional support and answer questions.

Prepare siblings for their visit; plan length of time for sibling visitation; monitor siblings' reactions during visit to prevent them from becoming overwhelmed.

Encourage parents to stay with their child:
If visiting hours are limited, allow flexibility in schedule to accommodate parental needs.
Give family members a written schedule of visiting times.
If visiting hours are liberal, be aware of family members' needs and suggest periodic respites.
Assure family they can call the unit at any time.

Prepare parents for expected role changes and identify ways for parents to participate in child's care without overwhelming them with responsibilities:
Help with bath or feeding.
Touch and talk to child.
Help with procedures.
Provide information about child's condition in understandable language:
Repeat information often.
Seek clarification of understanding.
During bedside conferences, interpret information for family members and child or, if appropriate, conduct report outside room.
Prepare child for procedures, even if this involves explanation while procedure is performed.
Assess and manage pain; recognize that a child who cannot talk, such as an infant or child in a coma or on mechanical ventilation, can be in pain.
Establish a routine that maintains some similarity to daily events in child's life whenever possible:
Organize care during normal waking hours.
Keep regular bedtime schedules, including quiet times when television or radio is lowered or turned off.
Provide uninterrupted sleep cycles (60 minutes for infant, 90 minutes for older child).
Close and open drapes and dim lights to allow for day/night.
Place curtain around bed for privacy.
Orient child to day and time; have clocks or calendars in easy view for older children.
Schedule a time when child is left undisturbed (e.g., during naps, visit with family, playtime, or favorite program).
Provide opportunities for play.
Reduce stimulation in environment:
Refrain from loud talking or laughing.
Keep equipment noise to a minimum:
Turn alarms as low as safely possible.
Perform treatments requiring equipment at one time.
Turn off bedside equipment that is not in use, such as suction and oxygen.
Avoid loud, abrupt noises.

*See also Box 21-8.

---

the explanations offered by the child. Projective techniques such as drawing, doll play, or storytelling are especially effective. The nurse then bases additional information on what has already been revealed.

INTENSIVE CARE UNIT

Parents who have a child in an intensive care unit (ICU) are stressed (Fig. 21-15). The nature and severity of the illness and the circumstances surrounding the admission are major factors, especially for parents. Parents experience significantly more stress when the admission is unexpected rather than expected. A recent study found that parental anxiety levels reached near panic levels initially (Huckabay and Tilem-Kessler, 1999). Stressors for the child and parent are described in Box 21-18. Although several studies have described what parents perceive as most stressful, the most effective strategy may be to simply ask parents what is stress-

ful and implement interventions that will enhance coping outcomes (Board and Ryan-Wenger, 2003; Melnyk and Alpert-Gillis, 1998). Assessment should be repeated periodically to account for changes in perceptions over time.

The emotional needs of the family are paramount when a child is admitted to an ICU. Although the same interventions discussed earlier for the stressors of separation, loss of control, and bodily injury and pain apply here, additional interventions may also benefit the family and child (see Box 21-18 and Family Focus box). Critical care must be centered on the family. Visiting hours should be liberal and flexible enough to accommodate parental needs (Hazinski, 1999).

Critically ill children become the focus of the parents' lives, and parents' most pressing need is for information (Scott, 1998). They want to know if their child will live, and, if so, whether the child will be the same as before. They need to know why various interventions are being

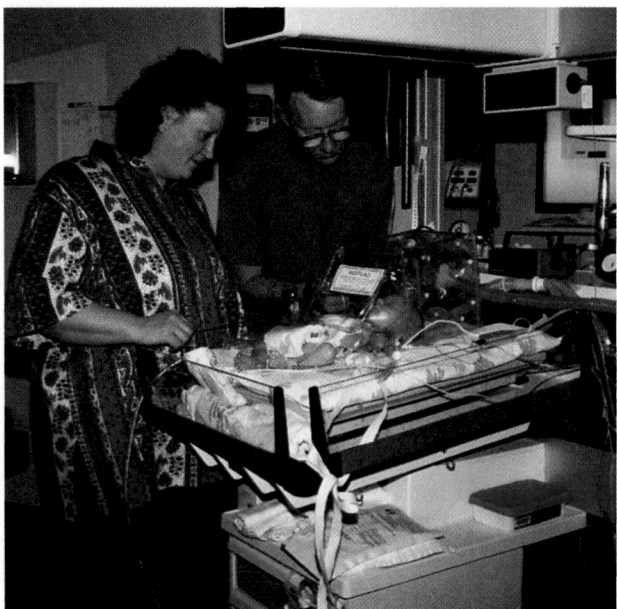

FIG. 21-15 ■ Parents can be overwhelmed when their child is critically ill and requires care in an ICU.

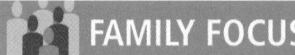

FAMILY FOCUS

Artists as Partners in Care

A teenage boy with a rare genetic disorder, having made steady progress after awakening from a coma, relapsed and seemed very depressed. When told that a musician was visiting the pediatric intensive care unit (PICU), he immediately perked up and asked to have his room lights turned on. He whispered endless song requests to the musician. Family members and staff were treated to some of his first smiles in days; his biggest came when the musician held his hand and guided it across the guitar strings while they sang "Born to Be Wild" together at the boy's request. His dad was misty-eyed as he thanked the musician for the visit.

A few weeks later the boy's condition worsened and he again lapsed into a coma. There was nothing more to be done. His parents began the necessary preparations to take their son home to die.

We continued to visit our friend and his family, offering a song, a story, or just simply to say hello. I hold a vivid picture of our final visit. We stood around the boy's bed with his parents singing together songs they remembered from their youth, from more carefree times. Song and laughter filled the boy's room.

Perhaps the boy heard his parents' laughter and knew then that they would be okay. He died a few days later on the morning he was to have been discharged.

Judy Rollins, MS, RN
Washington, DC

Modified from Rollins J: *Placed in our keeping,* 1995, Unpublished.

BOX 21-18 ■ Neonatal/Pediatric Intensive Care Unit Stressors for the Child and Family

PHYSICAL STRESSORS
Pain and discomfort (e.g., injections, intubation, suctioning, dressing changes, other invasive procedures)
Immobility (e.g., use of restraints, bed rest)
Sleep deprivation
Inability to eat or drink
Changes in elimination habits

ENVIRONMENTAL STRESSORS
Unfamiliar surroundings (e.g., crowding)
Unfamiliar sounds
   Equipment noise (e.g., monitors, telephone, suctioning, computer printout)
   Human sounds (e.g., talking, laughing, crying, coughing, moaning, retching, walking)
Unfamiliar people (e.g., health care professionals, patients, visitors)
Unfamiliar and unpleasant smells (e.g., alcohol, adhesive remover, body odors)

Constant lights (disturb day/night rhythms)
Activity related to other patients
Sense of urgency among staff
Unkind or thoughtless comments from staff

PSYCHOLOGIC STRESSORS
Lack of privacy
Inability to communicate (if intubated)
Inadequate knowledge and understanding of situation
Severity of illness
Parental behavior (expression of concern)

SOCIAL STRESSORS
Disrupted relationships (especially with family and friends)
Concern with missing school or work
Play deprivation

Data primarily from Tichy AM and others: Stressors in pediatric intensive care units, *Pediatr Nurs* 14(1):40-42, 1988.

done for the child, that the child is being treated for pain or is comfortable, and that the child may be able to hear them even though not awake.

Despite the stresses normally associated with ICU admission, a special security develops from being carefully monitored and receiving individualized care. Therefore planning for transition to the regular unit is essential and should include (1) assignment of a primary nurse on the regular unit who visits before the transfer; (2) continued visits by the ICU staff to assess the child's and parents' adjustment and to act as a temporary liaison with the nursing staff; (3) explanation of the differences between the two units and the rationale for the change to less intense monitoring of the child's physical condition; and (4) selection of an appropriate room, such as one that is close to the nursing station, and a compatible roommate.

- Children are particularly vulnerable to the stressors of illness and hospitalization because stress represents a change from the usual state of health and routine and because they possess limited coping mechanisms.

- The three phases of separation anxiety are protest, despair, and detachment.

- Feelings of loss of control are caused by unfamiliar environmental stimuli, physical restriction, altered routine, and dependency.

- Fear of bodily pain may be manifested in the following ways: infants—facial expressions, body movements; toddlers—intense emotional upset, physical resistance; preschoolers—aggression, verbal expression, dependency; school-age children—precise verbalization of pain, passive requests for support or help, procrastination technique; adolescents—self-control, limited movement.

- Because of their separation from significant people, children who are hospitalized may lack the opportunity to form new attachments in the strange environment of the hospital and exhibit negative behaviors after discharge.

- Nursing care of the child in the hospital is aimed at preventing or minimizing separation, decreasing loss of control, minimizing fear of bodily injury, assessing and managing pain, promoting normal development, using play/expressive activities to lessen stress, and maximizing the potential benefits of hospitalization.

- Pain assessment includes questioning the child, using pain rating scales, evaluating behavior, securing parents' involvement, taking the cause of the pain into account, and taking action. Pain management should incorporate both pharmacologic and nonpharmacologic methods.

- The nurse can maximize potential benefits of hospitalization by fostering parent-child relations, providing educational opportunities, promoting self-mastery, and encouraging socialization.

- Family reactions are influenced by the seriousness of the illness; experience with illness or hospitalization and diagnostic or therapeutic procedures; available support systems; personal ego strengths; coping abilities; presence of additional stressors; cultural and religious beliefs; and family communication patterns.

- Fear of contracting illness, their younger age, a close relationship with the ill sibling, substitute child care, minimal explanation of the illness, and perceived changes in parenting all increase the deleterious effects of a brother's or sister's illness and hospitalization on siblings.

- Nursing care of the family involves listening to parents' verbal and nonverbal messages; providing clergy support; accepting cultural, socioeconomic, and ethnic values; giving information to families and siblings; and preparing for discharge and home care.

- Admission to an outpatient setting, emergency department, isolation room, or intensive care unit requires additional intervention strategies to meet the child's and family's needs.

References

Algren JT, Algren CL: Management of procedural and perioperative pain in children. In Weiner R, editor: *Pain management: a practical guide for clinicians,* Boca Raton, Fla, 1998, St Lucie Press.

Algren JT and others: Efficacy and safety of morphine administered by patient-, parent-, or nurse-controlled analgesia in children, *Anesthesiology* 89:A1003, 1998 (abstract).

American Pain Society: *Principles of analgesic use in the treatment of acute pain and chronic cancer pain,* ed 4, Glenview, IL, 1999, The Society.

American Society of Addiction Medicine: *Public policy statement on definitions related to the use of opioids for pain treatment,* February 2001.

American Society of Pain Management Nurses: ASPMN position statement: use of placebos for pain management, *Ostomy Wound Manage* 44(2):56-57, 1998.

Anand K, Aynsley-Green A: Metabolic and endocrine effects of surgical ligation of patent ductus arteriosus in the human preterm neonate: are there implications for further improvement of postoperative outcome? *Mod Probl Paediatr* 23:143-157, 1985.

Anand KJS, Hickey P: Pain and its effects in the human neonate and fetus, *N Engl J Med* 317(21):1321-1329, 1987.

Ashenberg MD and others: Easing the wait: development of a pager program for families, *Pediatr Nurs* 22(2):103-107, 1996.

Baker C, Wong D: Q.U.E.S.T.: a process of pain assessment in children, *Orthop Nurs* 6(1):11-21, 1987.

Bauchner H, May A, Coates E: Use of analgesic agents for invasive medical procedures in pediatric and neonatal intensive care units, *J Pediatr* 121(4):647-649, 1992.

Berde C and others: Patient-controlled analgesia in children and adolescents: a randomized, prospective comparison with intramuscular administration of morphine for postoperative analgesia, *J Pediatr* 118(3):460-466, 1991.

Beyer JE, Denyes MJ, Villarruel AM: The creation, validation and continuing development of the Oucher: a measure of pain intensity in children, *J Pediatr Nurs* 7(5):335-346, 1992; www.oucher.org.

Beyer JE, McGrath PJ, Berde CB: Discordance between self-report and behavioral pain measures in children aged 3-7 years after surgery, *J Pain Symptom Manage* 5(6):350-356, 1990.

Beyer J and others: Patterns of postoperative analgesic use with adults and children following cardiac surgery, *Pain* 17:71-81, 1983.

Billmire DA, Neale HW, Gregory RO: Use of IV fentanyl in the outpatient treatment of pediatric facial trauma, *J Trauma* 25(11):1079-1080, 1985.

Board R, Ryan-Wenger N: Stressors and symptoms of mothers with children in the PICU, *J Pediatr Nurs* 18(3):195-201, 2003.

Boughton K and others: Impact of research on pediatric pain assessment and outcomes, *Pediatr Nurs* 24(1):31-35, 62, 1998.

Boyd, J, Hunsberger M: Chronically ill children coping with repeated hospitalizations: their perceptions and suggested interventions, *J Pediatr Nurs* 13(6):330-342, 1998.

Bracht M and others: Initiation and maintenance of a hospital-based parent group for parents of premature infants: key factors for success, *Neonatal Network* 17(3):33-37, 1998.

Brewer S, Lambert C: Preparing children for same day surgery: innovative approaches, *J Pediatr Nurs* 12(4):257-259, 1997.

Broome ME, Huth MM: Nursing management of the child in pain. In Schechter NL, Berde CB, Yaster M, editors: *Pain in infants, children, and adolescents,* ed 2, Philadelphia, 2003, Lippincott Williams & Wilkins.

Broome M, Rehwaldt M, Fogg L: Relationships between cognitive behavioral techniques, temperament, observed distress, and pain reports in children and adolescents during lumbar puncture, *J Pediatr Nurs* 13:48-54, 1998.

Broome M and others: Pediatric pain practices: a national survey of health professionals, *J Pain Symptom Manage* 11(5):312-320, 1996.

Broome M and others: Children's medical fears, coping behaviors, and pain perceptions during a lumbar puncture, *Oncol Nurs Forum* 17(3):361-367, 1990.

Brozovic M and others: Pain relief in sickle cell crises, *Lancet* 2(8507):624-625, 1986.

Bruce B, Ritchie J: Nurses' practices and perceptions of family centered care, *J Pediatr Nurs* 12(4):214-222, 1997.

Clatworthy S, Simon K, Tiedeman ME: Child drawing: hospital—an instrument designed to measure the emotional status of hospitalized school-aged children, *J Pediatr Nurs* 14(1):2-9, 1999.

Cline ME and others: Standardization of the visual analogue scale, *Nurs Res* 41(6):378-380, 1992.

Collins J: Intractable cancer pain in children, *Child Adolesc Psychiatr Clin* 6(4):879-888, 1997.

Craft MJ: Siblings of hospitalized children: assessment and intervention, *J Pediatr Nurs* 8(5):289-297, 1993.

Dahl JL: Darron: a drug with dubious distinction, *Cancer Pain Update* 48:3, 6, Summer 1998.

Davis GC: Nursing's role in pain management across the health care continuum, *Nurs Outlook* 46(1):19-23, 1998.

Dilworth NM, MacKellar A: Pain relief for the pediatric surgical patient, *J Pediatr Surg* 22:264-266, 1987.

Dolgin M and others: Behavioral distress in pediatric patients with cancer receiving chemotherapy, *Pediatrics* 84(1):103-110, 1989.

Eland JM, Anderson JE: The experience of pain in children. In Jacox A, editor: *Pain: a source book for nurses and other health professionals,* Boston, 1977, Little, Brown.

Eland JA, Banner W: Analgesia, sedation, and neuromuscular blockage in pediatric critical care. In Hazinski ME, editor: *Manual of pediatric critical care,* St Louis, 1999, Mosby.

Ellis JA and others: Pain in hospitalized pediatric patients: how are we doing? *Clin J Pain* 18(4):262-269, 2002.

Fanurik D and others: Children with cognitive impairment: parent report of pain and coping, *J Dev Behav Pediatr* 20(4):228-234, 1999.

Favaloro R, Touzel B: A comparison of adolescents' and nurses' postoperative pain ratings and perceptions, *Pediatr Nurs* 16(4):414-417, 424, 1990.

Federwisch A: Complete assessment: making pain the fifth vital sign, *Health Week* 4(14):18, 1999.

Fernandez C, Pyesmany A, Stutzer C: Alternative therapies in childhood cancer, *N Engl J Med* 340(7):569-570, 1999.

Ferrell BR, McCaffery M, Rhiner M: Pain and addiction: an urgent need for change in nursing education, *J Pain Symptom Manage* 7: 48-55, 1992.

Ferrell BR and others: The experience of pediatric cancer pain. I. Impact of pain on the family, *J Pediatr Nurs* 9(6):368-379, 1994.

Fitzgerald M, Millard C, MacIntosh N: Hyperalgesia in premature infants, *Lancet* 6(8580):292, 1988.

Flanagan K: Preoperative assessment: safety considerations for patients taking herbal products, *J Perianesth Nurs* 16(1):19-26, 2001.

Fradet C and others: A prospective survey of reactions to blood tests by children and adolescents, *Pain* 40(1):53-60, 1990.

Franck L: A national survey of the assessment and treatment of pain and agitation in the neonatal intensive care unit, *JOGNN* 16: 387-395, 1987.

Franck LS, Greenberg CS, Stevens B: Pain assessment in infants and children, *Pediatr Clin North Am* 47(3):487-512, 2000.

French GM, Painter EC, Coury DL: Blowing away shot pain: a technique for pain management during immunization, *Pediatrics* 93(3):384-388, 1994.

Friedland LR, Kulick RM: Emergency department analgesic use in pediatric trauma victims with fractures, *Ann Emerg Med* 23(2):203-207, 1994.

Gordon M: *Nursing diagnosis: process and application,* ed 3, St Louis, 1994, Mosby.

Gordon M: *Manual of nursing diagnosis,* ed 10, St Louis, 2002, Mosby.

Hannallah RS and others: Comparison of caudal and ilioinguinal/ iliohypogastric nerve blocks for control of post-orchiopexy pain in pediatric ambulatory surgery, *Anesthesiology* 66:832-834, 1987.

Haslam DR: Age and the perception of pain, *Psychosom Sci* 15:86, 1969.

Hazinski MF: *Manual of pediatric critical care,* St Louis, 1999, Mosby.

Hertzka R and others: Fentanyl-induced ventilatory depression: effects of age, *Anesthesiology* 70:213-218, 1989.

Hester NO: Comforting the child in pain. In Funk SG and others, editors: *Key aspects of comfort,* New York, 1989, Springer.

Hester NO and others: Putting pain measurement into clinical practice. In Finley GA, McGrath PJ, editors: *Measurement of pain in infants and children,* vol 10, Seattle, 1998, International Association for the Study of Pain Press.

Hornick R: Discharge teams. In Gunter K, Manago R, editors: *Beyond discharge: interdisciplinary perspectives for transitioning children with complex medical needs from hospital to home,* Bethesda, Md, 1996, Association for the Care of Children's Health.

Howard CR and others: Neonatal circumcision and pain relief: current training practices, *Pediatrics* 101(3):423-428, 1998.

Huckabay LMD, Tilem-Kessler D: Patterns of parental stress in PICU emergency admission, *Dimens Crit Care Nurs* 18(2):36-42, 1999.

Humphrey BG and others: The occurrence of high levels of acute behavioral distress in children and adolescents undergoing routine venipunctures, *Pediatrics* 90(1):87-91, 1992.

IOMED, Inc: Iontocaine package insert, Salt Lake City, Utah, 1996, IOMED, Inc.

Johnson A, Lindschau A: Staff attitudes toward parent participation in the care of children who are hospitalized, *Pediatr Nurs* 22(2):99-102, 1996.

Johnston CC and others: A survey of pain in hospitalized patients aged 4-14 years, *Clin J Pain* 8(2):154-163, 1992.

Joint Commission on Accreditation of Healthcare Organizations: *AMH92 accreditation manual for hospitals,* Chicago, 1999, The Commission.

Jordan-Marsh M and others: Alternate Oucher form testing gender ethnicity and age variations, *Res Nurs Health* 17:111-118, 1994.

Joyce BA and others: Reliability and validity of preverbal pain assessment tools, *Issues Comp Pediatr Nurs* 17:121-135, 1994.

Kachoyeanos MK, Friedhoff M: Cognitive and behavioral strategies to reduce children's pain, *MCN* 18(1):14-19, 1993.

Kart T, Christrup LL, Rasmussen M: Recommended use of morphine in neonates, infants and children based on a literature review. I. Pharmacokinetics, *Paediatr Anaesth* 7(1):5-11, 1997.

Katz E, Kellerman J, Siegel S: Behavioral distress in children with cancer undergoing medical procedures: developmental considerations, *J Consult Clin Psychol* 48(3):356-365, 1980.

Kauffmann E and others: Stress-point intervention for parents of children hospitalized with chronic conditions, *Pediatr Nurs* 24(4): 362-366, 1998.

Keck J and others: Reliability and validity of the FACES and Word Descriptor scales to measure procedural pain, *J Pediatr Nurs* 11(6): 368-374, 1996.

Kirby R, Whelan T: The effects of hospitalization and medical procedures on children and their families, *J Fam Stud* 2(1):65-77, 1996.

Kleiber C and others: Topical anesthetics for intravenous insertion in children: a random equivalency study, *Pediatr* 110(4):758-761, 2002.

Koren G and others: Postoperative morphine infusion in newborn infants: assessment of disposition characteristics and safety, *J Pediatr* 107(6):963-967, 1985.

Krebel MS, Clayton C, Graham C: Child life programs in the pediatric emergency department, *Pediatr Emerg Care* 12(1):13-15, 1996.

Lander J, Fowler-Kerry S: Assessment of sex differences in children's and adolescents' self-reported pain from venipuncture, *J Pediatr Psychol* 16(6):783-793, 1991.

Lipson J, Dibble S, Minarik P: *Culture and nursing care: a pocket guide,* San Francisco, 1996, UCSF Nursing Press.

Luffy R, Grove SK: Examining the validity, reliability, and preference of three pediatric pain measurement tools in African-American children, *Pediatr Nurs* 29(1):54-60, 2003.

Mader TJ, Playe SJ, Garb JL: Reducing the pain of local anesthetic infiltration: warming and buffering have a synergistic effect, *Ann Emerg Med* 23(3):550-554, 1994.

Marshall RE: Neonatal pain associated with caregiving procedures, *Pediatr Clin North Am* 36(4):885-903, 1989.

Mather L, Mackie J: The incidence of postoperative pain in children, *Pain* 15:271-282, 1983.

McCaffery M, Pasero C: *Pain: a clinical manual,* ed 2, St Louis, 1999, Mosby.

McGrath PJ and others: The Children's Hospital of Eastern Ontario Pain Scale (CHEOPS): a behavioral scale for rating post-operative pain in children. In Fields HL, Dubner R, Cervero F, editors: *Advances in pain research and therapy,* New York, 1985, Raven Press.

Melnyk B, Alpert-Gillis L: The COPE Program: a strategy to improve outcomes of critically ill young children and their parents, *Pediatr Nurs* 24(6):521-527, 1998.

Melnyk BM: Intervention studies involving parents of hospitalized young children: an analysis of the past and future recommendations, *J Pediatr Nurs* 15(1):4-13, 2000.

Merkel S and others: Pain assessment in infants and young children: the FLACC scale, *Am J Nurs* 102(10):55-57, 2002.

Moenkhoff M and others: Parental attitude towards alternative medicine in the paediatric intensive care unit, *Eur J Pediatr* 158(1):12-17, 1999.

Morrison R: Update on sickle cell disease: incidence of addiction and choice of opioid in pain management, *Pediatr Nurs* 17(6):503, 1991.

New Products: Gebauer's ethyl chloride topical refrigerant eases anxiety for patients and parents, *Pediatr Nurs* 28(6):636, 644, 2002.

Oberlander TF, O'Donnell ME, Montgomery CJ: Pain in children with neurological impairment, *J Dev Behav Pediatr* 20(4):234-243, 1999.

Orem D: *Nursing: concepts of practice,* ed 5, New York, 1995, Mosby.

Pasero C: Pain control: reality check on placebos, *Am J Nurs* 95(8):20, 1995.

Pasero C: Pain control, epidural analgesia in children, *Am J Nurs* 99(5):20, 1999.

Pate J and others: Childhood medical experience and temperament as predictors of adult functioning in medical situations, *Child Health Care* 25(4):281-298, 1996.

Rasmussen G: Epidural and spinal anesthesia and analgesia. In Deshpande J, Tobias J, editors: *Pediatric pain handbook,* St Louis, 1996, Mosby.

Remmel M: Don't assume all parents want to be involved, *RN* 60(9):9, 1997 (letter).

Robieux I and others: Assessing pain and analgesia with a lidocaine-prilocaine emulsion in infants and toddlers during venipuncture, *J Pediatr* 118(6):971-973, 1991.

Rodgers BM and others: Patient-controlled analgesia in pediatric surgery, *J Pediatr Surg* 23(3):259-262, 1988.

Rogers A: The ABC of pediatric pain, *Prim Care Cancer* 10:7-8, 1990.

Rogers TA, Ostrow CL: The use of EMLA cream to decrease venipuncture pain in children, *J Pediatr Nurs* 19(1):33-39, 2004.

Santelli B, Turnbull A, Higgins C: Parent to parent support and health care, *Pediatr Nurs* 23(3):303-306, 1997.

Savedra M and others: Pain location: validity and reliability of body outline markings by hospitalized children and adolescents, *Res Nurs Health* 12:307-314, 1989.

Savedra MC and others: Assessment of postoperative pain in children and adolescents using the Adolescent Pediatric Pain Tool, *Nurs Res* 42(1):5-9, 1993.

Schade JG and others: Comparison of three preverbal scales for postoperative pain assessment in a diverse pediatric sample, *J Pain Symptom Manage* 12(6):348-359, 1996.

Schechter NL: The need for premedication for painful procedures in children, *Am J Anesthesiol* 24(1 suppl):10-12, 1997.

Scott LD: Perceived needs of parents of critically ill children, *J Soc Pediatr Nurses* 3(1):4-12, 1998.

Shapiro C: Pain in the neonate: assessment and intervention, *Neonatal Network* 8(1):7-21, 1989.

Simon K: Perceived stress of nonhospitalized children during the hospitalization of a sibling, *J Pediatr Nurs* 8(5):298-304, 1993.

Smith T, Conant Rees HL: Making family-centered care a reality, *Semin Nurs Manage* 8(3):136-142, 2000.

Snowdon A, Kane D: Parental needs following the discharge of a hospitalized child, *Pediatr Nurs* 21(5):425-428, 1995.

Spiegel D, Stroud P, Fyfe A: Complementary medicine, *West J Med* 168(4):241-247, 1998.

Squire SJ, Kirchoff KT, Hissong K: Comparing two methods of topical anesthesia used before intravenous cannulation in pediatric patients, *J Pediatr Health Care* 14(2):68-72, 2000.

Stevens B: Development and testing of a pediatric pain management sheet, *Pediatr Nurs* 16(6):543-548, 1990.

Stevens BJ, Johnston CC, Horton L: Multidimensional pain assessment in premature neonates: a pilot study, *JOGNN* 26(5):531-541, 1993.

Stewart E, Algren C, Arnold S: Preparing children for a surgical experience, *Today's OR Nurse* 16(2):9-14, 1994.

Stuber M and others: Predictors of posttraumatic stress symptoms in childhood cancer survivors, *Pediatrics* 100(6):958-964, 1997.

Taddio A and others: A revised measure of acute pain in infants, *J Pain Symptom Manage* 10(6):456-463, 1995.

Tesler M, Holzemer W, Savedra M: Pain behaviors: postsurgical responses of children and adolescents, *J Pediatr Nurs* 13(1):41-47, 1998.

Tesler M and others: The word-graphic rating scale as a measure of childrens' and adolescents' pain intensity, *Res Nurs Health* 14:361-371, 1991.

Tobias JD: Pain management for the critically ill child in the pediatric intensive care unit. In Schechter NL, Berde CB, Yaster M, editors: *Pain in infants, children and adolescents,* ed 2, Philadelphia, 2003, Lippincott Williams & Wilkins.

Tyc V and others: A survey of pain services for pediatric oncology patients: their composition and function, *Pediatr Oncol Nurs* 15(4):207-215, 1998.

Van Cleve L, Johnson L, Pothier P: Pain responses of hospitalized infants and children to venipuncture and intravenous cannulation, *J Pediatr Nurs* 11:161-168, 1996.

Van Cleve L, Savedra M: Pain location: validity and reliability of body outline markings for 4- to 7-year-old children who are hospitalized, *Pediatr Nurs* 19(3):217-220, 1993.

Vessey JA, Carlson KL, McGill J: Use of distraction with children during an acute pain experience, *Nurs Res* 43(6):369-372, 1994.

Villaruel AM, Denyes MJ: Pain assessment in children: theoretical and empirical validity, *Adv Nurs Sci* 14(2):32-41, 1991.

Vincent CVH, Denyes MJ: Relieving children's pain: nurses' abilities and analgesic administration practices, *J Pediatr Nurs* 19(1):40-50, 2004.

Walker M, Wong DL: A battle plan for patients in pain, *Am J Nurs* 91(5):32-36, 1991.

Wallace M: Temperament: a variable in children's pain management, *Pediatr Nurs* 15(2):118-121, 1989.

Weisman SJ, Bernstein B, Schechter NL: Consequences of inadequate analgesia during painful procedures in children, *Arch Pediatr Adolesc Med* 132(2):147-149, 1998.

Wilson A, Yorker B: Fears of medical events among school-age children with emotional disorders, parents and health care providers, *Issues Ment Health Nurs* 18:57-71, 1997.

Wong D: Topical anesthetics: two products for pain relief during minor procedures, *Am J Nurs* 103(6):42-45, 2003.

Wong DL, Baker C: Pain in children: comparison of assessment scales, *Pediatr Nurs* 14(1):9-17, 1988.

Wong DL, Pasero CL: Pain control: reducing the pain of lidocaine, *Am J Nurs* 97(1):17-18, 1997.

Woodgate R, Kristjanson L: "Getting better from my hurts": toward a model of the young child's pain experience, *J Pediatr Nurs* 11(4):233-242, 1996.

Yaster M and others: *Pediatric pain management and sedation handbook,* St Louis, 1997, Mosby.

Yaster M, Kost-Byerly S, Maxwell LG: Opioid agonists and antagonists. In Schechter NL, Berde CB, Yaster M, editors: *Pain in infants, children, and adolescents,* ed 2, Philadelphia, 2003, Lippincott Williams & Wilkins.

Young M, Fu V: Influence of play and temperament on the young child's response to pain, *Child Health Care* 16(3):209-215, 1988.

22

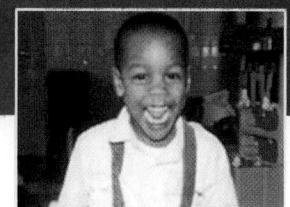

Pediatric Variations of Nursing Interventions

CHRIS ALGREN and DEBRA ARNOW

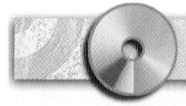

Remember to check out your companion CD-ROM

http://evolve.elsevier.com/Wong/essentials/

CHAPTER OUTLINE

RELATED TOPICS and ADDITIONAL RESOURCES

LEARNING OBJECTIVES
On completion of this chapter the reader will be able to:

- Identify those instances in which informed consent is required and in which minors may be considered emancipated.
- Formulate general guidelines for preparing children for procedures, including surgery.
- Implement play in therapeutic procedures.
- List general strategies for enhancing compliance in children and families.

- Outline general hygiene and care procedures for hospitalized children.
- Implement feeding techniques that encourage food and fluid intake.
- Describe methods of reducing temperature of child with fever or hyperthermia.
- Describe systems that can be used for infection control.
- Describe safe methods of administering oral, parenteral, rectal, optic, otic, and nasal medications to children.

- Identify nursing responsibilities in maintaining fluid balance.
- Demonstrate correct procedures for postural drainage and tracheostomy care.
- Describe the procedures involved in providing nutrition via gavage, gastrostomy, and parenteral routes.
- Describe the procedures involved in administering an enema and ostomy care to children.

GENERAL CONCEPTS RELATED TO PEDIATRIC PROCEDURES

INFORMED CONSENT

Before undergoing any invasive procedure, including a surgical procedure, the patient or the patient's legal surrogate must receive sufficient information on which to make an informed decision. *Informed consent* refers to the legal and ethical requirement that the patient clearly, fully, and completely understands the proposed procedure or treatment to be performed. This information must include the nature of the procedure, the risks associated with the procedure, the alternatives to the procedure, and the benefits of the proce-

dure. To obtain valid informed consent, the following three conditions must be met:

1 The person must be capable of giving consent; he or she must be over the age of majority (usually age 18) and must be considered competent (i.e., possess the mental capacity to make choices and understand their consequences).
2 The person must receive the information needed to make an intelligent decision.
3 The person must act voluntarily when exercising freedom of choice without force, fraud, deceit, duress, or other forms of constraint or coercion.

The patient has the right to accept or refuse any health care. If treated without consent, the hospital or health care provider may be charged with assault and held liable for damages.

Requirements for Obtaining Informed Consent

Written informed consent of the parent or legal guardian is usually required for medical or surgical treatment, including many diagnostic procedures. One blanket consent is not sufficient. Separate informed permissions must be obtained for each surgical or diagnostic procedure, including:

- Major surgery
- Minor surgery (e.g., cutdown, biopsy, dental extraction, suturing a laceration)
- Diagnostic tests with an element of risk
- Medical treatments with an element of risk (e.g., blood transfusion, thoracentesis or paracentesis, radiation therapy, shock therapies)

Other situations that require parental consent include:

- Taking photographs for medical, educational, or other public use
- Removal of the child from the health care institution against medical advice
- Postmortem examinations, except in unexplained deaths, such as sudden infant death, violent death, or suspected suicide
- Release of medical information (See Evidence-Based Practice box)

Decision-making involving the care of older children and adolescents should include, to the extent feasible, the *assent* of the patient as well as the parents and the physician. Assent means the child/adolescent has been informed about what will happen during the treatment or procedure and is willing to permit a health care provider to perform it. *Assent* should include the following elements:

- Helping the patient achieve a developmentally appropriate awareness of the nature of his or her condition.
- Telling the patient what he or she can expect.

EVIDENCE-BASED PRACTICE

Informed Consent and Parental Right to the Child's Medical Chart

Does the right to certain types of information before giving valid informed consent include the right to review medical records? Because the process of consent continues throughout the patient's treatment, is there an ongoing right of parents to see their children's medical charts?

The answer to these questions varies depending on state law. Some state statutes give parents the unrestricted right to a copy of children's medical records. Other states have no statutes that address this point. In these states the best practice is to allow parents to review or have a copy of minors' charts under reasonable circumstances. That is, records should be available in a reasonable time. In addition, practitioners should avoid restrictive requirements such as review permitted only in the presence of a clinician. Rather, an appropriate practitioner should be available to answer any questions that parents may have during their reviews.

- Making a clinical assessment of the patient's understanding.
- Soliciting an expression of the patient's willingness to accept the proposed procedure of care. (American Academy of Pediatrics, 1995). Assent may minimize the trauma to the child and maximize the success of the procedure.

Multiple methods should be used to explain the study, including age-appropriate methods (e.g., videotapes, peer discussion, diagrams, written materials). An assent form should be provided to each child to sign, and the child should keep a copy (Broome, 1999). By including children in the decision-making process and gaining their acceptance, children are treated with respect. Assent is not a legal requirement but an ethical one to protect the rights of children. The nurse, whether acting as a researcher, assisting in research, or caring for the child, must ultimately have the best interest of the child in mind (Algren and Schwartz, 1998).

Eligibility for Giving Informed Consent

Informed Consent of Parents or Legal Guardians. Parents have full responsibility for the care and rearing of their minor children, including legal control over them. Therefore, as long as children are minors, their parents or legal guardians are required to give informed consent before medical treatment is rendered or any procedure is performed on them. Parents also have a right to withdraw consent later. If the parents are divorced, responsibility for informed consent rests with the parent who has legal custody.

Evidence of Consent. Obtaining informed consent varies from state to state and policies differ at each health care facility. It is the physician's responsibility to explain the procedure, risks, benefits, and alternatives. The nurse witnesses the patient or legal surrogate's signature on the consent form and may reinforce what the patient has been told. A signed consent form is the legal document that signifies that the process of informed consent has occurred. If parents are unavailable to sign consent forms, verbal consent may be obtained via the telephone in the presence of two witnesses. Both witnesses record that informed consent was given and by whom. Their signatures indicate that they witnessed the verbal consent.

Informed Consent of Mature and Emancipated Minors. State laws differ with regard to the so-called *age of majority,* the age at which a person is considered to have all the legal rights and responsibilities of an adult. Although some variation still exists, children become adults on their eighteenth birthday in most states. Competent adults can give informed consent on their own behalf. Nonetheless, some courts have permitted minors to consent to their treatment based on the *mature minors' doctrine,* which permits minors to give consent even though they are not technically adults as long as they demonstrate the maturity to understand the risks and benefits of the treatment or procedure (Moskop, 1999; Guertler, 1997). For example, statutes in many states permit minors to give consent on their own behalf to certain treatments, such as for sexually transmitted diseases, contraceptive services, pregnancy, or drug or alcohol abuse.

An *emancipated minor* is one who is legally under the age of majority but is recognized as having the legal capacity of an adult under circumstances prescribed by state law, such as pregnancy, marriage, high school graduation, living independently, or military service.

Treatment Without Parental Consent.   Exceptions to requiring parental consent before treating minor children occur in situations in which children need prompt medical or surgical treatment and a parent is not readily available to give consent or refuses to give consent. For example, a child may be brought to an emergency department accompanied by a grandparent, child care provider, teacher, older sibling, or others. In the absence of parents or legal guardians, some providers permit persons in charge of the child to give informed consent for treatment. Appropriate care for urgent or emergent problems should not be withheld or delayed because of problems obtaining consent. Efforts made to obtain consent should be documented (American Academy of Pediatrics, 2003). Emergencies include danger to life or the possibility of permanent injury.

With the growing number of single-parent households and a significant percentage of children living with someone other than a biologic parent, the need for consent by proxy for nonurgent care is becoming more common. Clinicians and nurses need to be aware of state and federal laws as well as institutional guidelines regarding consent by proxy. The American Academy of Pediatrics Committee on Medical Liability has put forth suggested guidelines for nurses and clinicians on consent by proxy (Berger and Committee on Medical Liability, 2003).

Refusal to give consent can occur when the treatment, such as blood transfusions, conflicts with the parents' religious beliefs. All states recognize such exceptions and have statutory procedures to permit treatment if the life or health of such a minor is in jeopardy or if delayed treatment would create a risk to the minor's health. The state is also able to intervene in situations that jeopardize the health and welfare of children, as in cases in which parents neglect or impose excessive or improper punishment on a child. Most communities have procedures by which custody of the child can be transferred to a governmental or a private agency when parental neglect or abuse can be proved.

PREPARATION FOR DIAGNOSTIC AND THERAPEUTIC PROCEDURES

Technologic advances and changes in health care have resulted in more pediatric procedures being performed in a variety of settings. Many procedures are both stressful and painful experiences for children and their parents. For most procedures, the focus of care is psychologic preparation of the child and family. Some procedures, however, require some physical preparation and the administration of sedatives/analgesics.

Psychologic Preparation

Preparing children for procedures decreases their anxiety, promotes their cooperation, supports their coping skills and may teach them new ones, and facilitates a feeling of mastery in experiencing a potentially stressful event. Many institutions have developed preadmission teaching programs designed to educate the pediatric patient and family about hospitalization and various procedures by offering hands-on experience with hospital equipment, information about the procedure to be

preformed, and departments they may visit (Algren, Ireland, and Stewart, 1998). Preparatory methods may be formal, such as group preparation for hospitalization. Most preparation strategies used by nurses are informal, focus on providing information about the experience, and are directed at stressful or painful procedures. Especially for painful procedures, the most effective preparation includes the provision of sensory-procedural information and helping the child develop coping skills, such as imagery, distraction, or relaxation (Broome, Rehwaldt, and Fogg, 1998).

General guidelines for preparing children for procedures are described in Box 22-1, and age-specific guidelines that consider children's developmental needs and cognitive abilities are presented in Box 22-2. In addition to these suggestions, nurses should consider the child's temperament,

BOX 22-1 ■ General Guidelines for Preparing Children for Procedures

Determine details of exact procedure to be performed.
Review parents' and child's present level of understanding.
Plan actual teaching based on child's developmental age and existing level of knowledge.
Incorporate parents in the teaching if they desire, especially if they plan to participate in care.
Inform parents of their role during procedure, such as standing near child's head or in child's line of vision and talking softly to child.
While preparing child and family, allow for ample discussion to prevent information overload and ensure adequate feedback.
Use concrete, not abstract, terms and visual aids to describe procedure. For example, use a simple line drawing of a boy or girl (Fig. 22-1), and mark the body part that will be involved in the procedure. Use nonthreatening but realistic models.*
Emphasize that no other body part will be involved.
If the body part is associated with a specific function, stress the change or noninvolvement of that ability (e.g., after tonsillectomy, child can still speak).
Use words appropriate to child's level of understanding (a rule of thumb for number of words is age in years plus 1).
Avoid words and phrases with dual meanings (see Guidelines box, p. 713) unless child understands such words.
Clarify all unfamiliar words (e.g., "Anesthesia is a *special* sleep").
Emphasize sensory aspects of procedure—what child will feel, see, smell, and touch and what child can do during procedure (e.g., lie still, count out loud, squeeze a hand, hug a doll).
Allow child to practice those procedures that will require cooperation (e.g., turning, deep breathing, using an incentive spirometer or mask).
Introduce anxiety-laden information last (e.g., starting an intravenous line).
Be honest with child about unpleasant aspects of a procedure but avoid creating undue concern. When discussing that a procedure may be uncomfortable, state that it feels differently to different people and have child describe how it felt.
Emphasize end of procedure and any pleasurable events afterward (e.g., going home, seeing parents).
Stress positive benefits of procedure (e.g., "After your tonsils are fixed, you won't have as many sore throats").

*Soft-sculptured dolls and customized adapters and overlays for preparing children and families about procedures and as teaching models for technical care are available from **Legacy Products, Inc.**, PO Box 267, Cambridge City, IN 47327; (800) 238-7951; e-mail: legacyez2b@aol.com; website: www.legacyproductsinc.com.

BOX 22-2 ■ Age-Specific Guidelines for Preparing Children for Procedures Based on Developmental Characteristics

INFANT: DEVELOPING A SENSE OF TRUST AND SENSORIMOTOR THOUGHT

Attachment to Parent

*Involve parent in procedure if desired.

Keep parent in infant's line of vision.

If parent is unable to be with infant, place familiar object with infant (e.g., stuffed toy).

Stranger Anxiety

*Have usual caregivers perform or assist with procedure.

Make advances slowly and in nonthreatening manner.

*Limit number of strangers entering room during procedure.

Sensorimotor Phase of Learning

During procedure use sensory soothing measures (e.g., stroking skin, talking softly, giving pacifier).

*Use analgesics (e.g., local anesthetic, intravenous opioid) to control discomfort.

Cuddle and hug child after stressful procedure; encourage parent to comfort child.

Increased Muscle Control

Expect older infants to resist.

Restrain adequately.

Keep harmful objects out of reach.

Memory for Past Experiences

Realize that older infants may associate objects, places, or persons with prior painful experiences and will cry and resist at the sight of them.

*Keep frightening objects out of view.

*Perform painful procedures in a separate room, not in crib (or bed).

*Use nonintrusive procedures whenever possible (e.g., axillary or tympanic temperatures, oral medications).

Imitation of Gestures

Model desired behavior (e.g., opening mouth).

TODDLER: DEVELOPING A SENSE OF AUTONOMY AND SENSORIMOTOR TO PREOPERATIONAL THOUGHT

Use same approaches as for infant in addition to the following:

Egocentric Thought

Explain procedure in relation to what child will see, hear, taste, smell, and feel.

Emphasize those aspects of procedure that require cooperation (e.g., lying still).

Tell child it's okay to cry, yell, or use other means to express discomfort verbally.

Negative Behavior

Expect treatments to be resisted; child may try to run away.

Use firm, direct approach.

Ignore temper tantrums.

Use distraction techniques (e.g., singing a song *with* a child).

Restrain adequately.

Animism

Keep frightening objects out of view (young children believe objects have lifelike qualities and can harm them).

Limited Language Skills

Communicate using behaviors.

Use a few, simple terms familiar to child.

Give one direction at a time (e.g., "Lie down," then "Hold my hand").

Use small replicas of equipment; allow child to handle equipment.

Use play; demonstrate on doll but avoid child's favorite doll, because child may think doll is really "feeling" procedure.

Prepare parents separately to avoid child's misinterpreting words.

Limited Concept of Time

Prepare child shortly or immediately before procedure.

Keep teaching sessions short (about 5 to 10 minutes).

Have preparations completed before involving child in procedure.

Have extra equipment nearby (e.g., alcohol swabs, new needle, adhesive bandages) to avoid delays.

Tell child when procedure is completed.

Striving for Independence

Allow choices whenever possible but realize that child may still be resistant and negative.

Allow child to participate in care and to help whenever possible (e.g., drink medicine from a cup, hold a dressing).

PRESCHOOLER: DEVELOPING A SENSE OF INITIATIVE AND PREOPERATIONAL THOUGHT

Egocentric

Explain procedure in simple terms and in relation to how it affects child (as with toddler, stress sensory aspects).

Demonstrate use of equipment.

Allow child to play with miniature or actual equipment.

Encourage "playing out" experience on a doll both before and after procedure to clarify misconceptions.

Use neutral words to describe the procedure (see Guidelines box, p. 713).

Increased Language Skills

Use verbal explanation but avoid overestimating child's comprehension of words.

Encourage child to verbalize ideas and feelings.

Concept of Time and Frustration

Tolerance Still Limited

Implement same approaches as for toddler but may plan longer teaching session (10 to 15 minutes); may divide information into more than one session.

Illness and Hospitalization May Be Viewed as Punishment

Clarify why each procedure is performed; a child will find it difficult to understand how medicine can make him or her feel better and can taste bad at the same time.

Ask child thoughts regarding why a procedure is performed.

State directly that procedures are never a form of punishment.

Animism

Keep equipment out of sight, except when shown to or used on child.

*Applies to any age.

BOX 22-2 ■ Age-Specific Guidelines for Preparing Children for Procedures Based on Developmental Characteristics—*cont'd*

Fears of Bodily Harm, Intrusion, and Castration

Point out on drawing, doll, or child where procedure is performed.

Emphasize that no other body part will be involved.

Use nonintrusive procedures whenever possible (e.g., axillary temperatures, oral medication).

Apply an adhesive bandage over puncture site.

Encourage parental presence.

Realize that procedures involving genitals provoke anxiety.

Allow child to wear underpants with gown.

Explain unfamiliar situations, especially noises or lights.

Striving for Initiative

Involve child in care whenever possible (e.g., hold equipment, remove dressing).

Give choices whenever possible but avoid excessive delays.

Praise child for helping and attempting to cooperate; never shame child for lack of cooperation.

SCHOOL-AGE CHILD: DEVELOPING A SENSE OF INDUSTRY AND CONCRETE THOUGHT

Increased Language Skills; Interest in Acquiring Knowledge

Explain procedures using correct scientific/medical terminology.

Explain reason for procedure using simple diagrams of anatomy and physiology.

Explain function and operation of equipment in concrete terms.

Allow child to manipulate equipment; use doll or another person as model to practice using equipment whenever possible (doll play may be considered "childish" by older school-age child).

Allow time before and after procedure for questions and discussion.

Improved Concept of Time

Plan for longer teaching sessions (about 20 minutes).

Prepare in advance of procedure.

Increased Self-Control

Gain child's cooperation.

Tell child what is expected.

Suggest ways of maintaining control (e.g., deep breathing, relaxation, counting).

Striving for Industry

Allow responsibility for simple tasks (e.g., collecting specimens).

Include child in decision making (e.g., time of day to perform procedure, preferred site).

Encourage active participation (e.g., removing dressings, handling equipment, opening packages).

Developing Relationships With Peers

May prepare two or more children for same procedure or encourage one to help prepare another peer.

Provide privacy from peers during procedure to maintain self-esteem.

ADOLESCENT: DEVELOPING A SENSE OF IDENTITY AND ABSTRACT THOUGHT

Increasingly Capable of Abstract Thought and Reasoning

Supplement explanations with reasons why procedure is necessary or beneficial.

Explain long-term consequences of procedures.

Realize that adolescent may fear death, disability, or other potential risks.

Encourage questioning regarding fears, options, and alternatives.

Conscious of Appearance

Provide privacy.

Discuss how procedure may affect appearance (e.g., scar) and what can be done to minimize it.

Emphasize any physical benefits of procedure.

Concerned More With Present Than With Future

Realize that immediate effects of procedure are more significant than future benefits.

Striving for Independence

Involve in decision making and planning (e.g., choice of time; place; individuals present during procedure, such as parents; clothing to wear).

Impose as few restrictions as possible.

Suggest methods of maintaining control.

Accept regression to more childish methods of coping.

Realize that adolescent may have difficulty in accepting new authority figures and may resist complying with procedures.

Developing Peer Relationships and Group Identity

Same as for school-age child but assumes even greater significance.

Allow adolescents to talk with other adolescents who have had the same procedure.

existing coping strategies, and previous experiences in individualizing the preparatory process. Children who are distractible and highly active, as well as those who are "slow to warm up," may need individualized sessions that are shorter for the active child but more slowly paced for the shy child. Youngsters who tend to cope well may need more emphasis on using their present skills, whereas those who appear to cope less adequately can benefit from more time devoted to simple coping strategies, such as relaxing, breathing, counting, squeezing a hand, or singing.

NURSING TIP

Prepare a basket (toy or treasure chest or cart) to keep near the treatment area. Items ideal for the basket are a Slinky; a sparkling "magic" wand (clear, acrylic tube sealed on both ends and partially filled with liquid in which is suspended metallic confetti); a soft foam ball; bubble solution; party blowers; pop-up books with foldout, three-dimensional scenes; real medical equipment, such as a syringe, adhesive bandages, and alcohol packets; toy medical supplies or a toy medical kit; marking pens; a notepad; and stickers. Have the child choose an item to use during a procedure, such as a party blower, to help distract and relax the youngster. After the procedure, allow the child to choose a small gift, such as a sticker, or to play with items from the basket, such as the medical equipment (Heiney, 1991).

Children differ in their "information-seeking dimension." Some actively solicit information about the intended procedure, whereas others characteristically avoid information. Parents can often guide nurses in deciding how much information is enough for the child, because parents know whether the child is typically inquisitive or satisfied with short answers. Drawings may also be helpful in preparing children for procedures (Fig 22-1).

The exact timing of the preparation for a procedure varies with the child's age and the type of procedure. There are no exact guidelines to govern timing, but in general the younger the child, the closer the explanation should be to the actual procedure to prevent undue fantasizing and worrying. With complex procedures, more time may be needed for assimilation of information, especially with older children. For example, the explanation for an x-ray can immediately precede the procedure for all ages, but preparation for surgery may begin the day before for young children.

Establish Trust and Provide Support. The nurse who has spent time with and who has established a positive relationship with a child will usually find it easier to gain the child's cooperation. If the relationship is based on trust, the child will associate the nurse with caregiving activities that give comfort and pleasure most of the time and not regard the nurse as someone who brings discomfort and stress. If the nurse does not know the child, it is best that the nurse be introduced by another staff person whom the child trusts. The first visit with the child should not include any painful procedure and ideally should focus on the child first, then on the explanation of the procedure. When talking with the child, the nurse uses the same guidelines for communicating with children that are discussed in Chapter 6.

Parental Presence and Support. Children need support during procedures, and for young children the greatest source of comfort is the parents. They represent security, safety, and comfort. However, controversy exists regarding the role parents should assume during the procedure, especially if discomfort is involved. Nurses need to consider the issues in deciding whether parental presence is beneficial. The parents' preferences for assisting, observing, or waiting outside the room should be assessed, as well as the child's preference for parental presence. The child's choice should be respected. Parents who want to stay should be educated, because they do not automatically know what to do, where

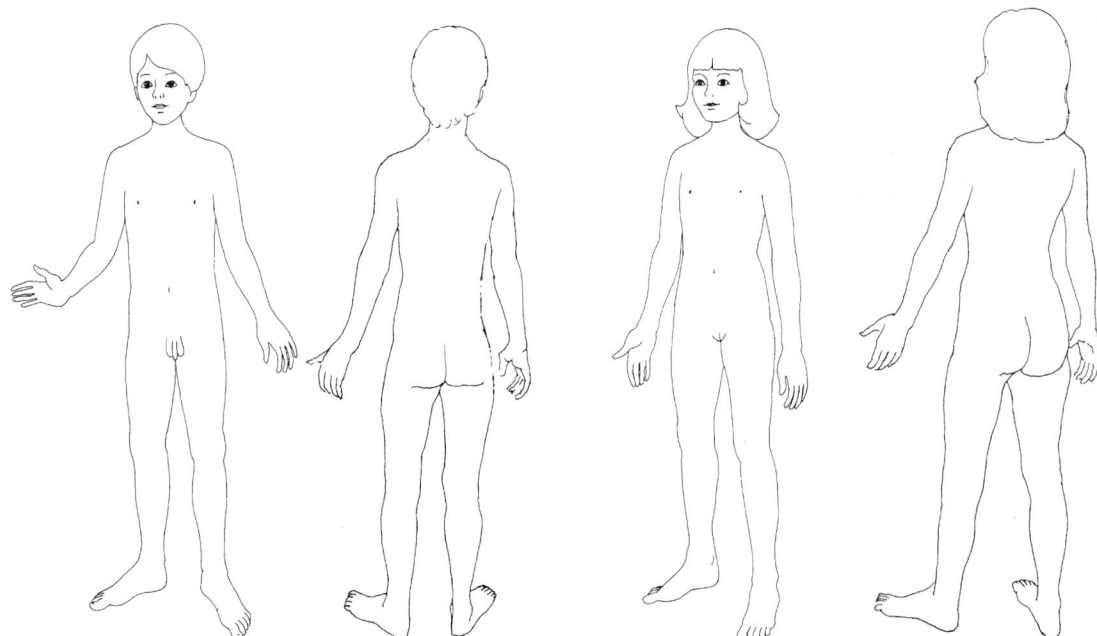

FIG. 22-1 ■ Examples of line drawings to be used in preparing child for procedures.

to be, and what to say to help their child through the procedure. Simple instructions such as clarifying where parents can stand or sit in the room and positioning them where they have eye contact with the child provide support and lessen anxiety. Parents who do not want to be present or participate are supported in their decision and encouraged to remain close by so that they can be available to console the child immediately after the procedure (see Evidence-Based Practice box). Parents should also know that someone will be with their child to provide support. Ideally, this person should inform the parents after the procedure about how the child did.

Provide an Explanation.

Children need an explanation for anything that involves them directly. Before performing a procedure, the nurse explains to children what is to be done and what is expected of them. The explanation should be short, simple, and appropriate to the child's level of comprehension. Long explanations are not necessary and may only increase anxiety in a small child. This is especially true regarding painful procedures. When explaining the procedure to parents with the child present, the nurse uses language appropriate to the child because unfamiliar words can be misunderstood (see Guidelines box). If the parents need additional preparation, this is done in an area away from the child. Teaching sessions are planned at times most conducive to the child's learning (e.g., after a rest period) and for the usual span of attention.

Special equipment is not necessary for preparing a child, but for young children who cannot yet think in concepts, using objects to supplement verbal explanation is important. Allowing children to handle actual items that will be used in their care, such as a stethoscope, sphygmomanometer, or oxygen mask, helps them to develop familiarity with these items and to reduce the threat often associated with their use. Miniature versions of hospital items such as gurneys and x-ray and intravenous equipment can be used to explain what the children can expect and permit them to safely experience situations that are unfamiliar and potentially frightening. Written and illustrated materials are also valuable aids to preparation.*

*Sources of preparatory materials include *Going to the Hospital* and *Going to the Doctor,* available from **Family Communications, Inc.,** 4802 Fifth Avenue, Pittsburgh, PA 15213; (412) 687-2990; *Hospital Friends,* available from the **Centering Corporation,** 1531 North Saddle Creek Road, Omaha, NE 68104; (402) 553-1200; and *Health, Illness, and Disability: A Guide to Books for Children and Young Adults,* available from **Pediatric Projects, Inc.,** PO Box 571555, Tarzana, CA 91357-1555; (800) 947-0947. Other resources include *Berenstein Bears Go to the Doctor* and *Berenstein Bears Visit the Dentist* (Random House), available in most bookstores.

NURSING TIP

Use photographs of children in different areas of the hospital (e.g., radiology department, operating room) to give children a more realistic idea of equipment they may encounter.

Physical Preparation.

For many diagnostic and therapeutic procedures, no special physical preparation is needed. However, some do require physical preparation. One area of special concern is the administration of appropriate sedation and analgesia before stressful procedures. The drug should be given at an interval before the procedure to allow time for the medication to reach its peak effect (Box 22-3).

Often children younger than age 6 years and those with developmental delays require deep levels of sedation to gain their cooperation. The safety of sedated children can be facilitated by performing a detailed presedation assessment, carefully selecting patients for sedation, and using drugs with a wide margin of safety. After sedatives are adminis-

---

EVIDENCE-BASED PRACTICE

Parental Presence During Their Child's Stressful Procedure

Many institutions permit parents and children to be together during painful or stressful situations. However, allowing parents to stay with the child during induction of anesthesia (see p. 717), recovery from anesthesia, and cardiopulmonary resuscitation during an arrest tends to remain restricted. When parents and children are asked their preference regarding visiting during these times, however, the results favor offering the family a choice. For example, 98% of parents thought that they and their child benefited from the parents' presence in recovery. When given the choice, 100% of parents came to recovery (Turner, 1997). (See also Parental Support.) When one hospital considered a policy of allowing parents in the operating room if the child was dying, the parent advisory committee simply asked, "What right has Children's Hospital to dictate to families how they should experience the death of a child or how they should grieve?" (Fina, 1994). Shouldn't this question apply to all "visiting" policies?

GUIDELINES

Selecting Nonthreatening Words or Phrases

WORDS/PHRASES TO AVOID	SUGGESTED SUBSTITUTIONS
Shot, bee sting, stick	Medicine under the skin
Organ	Special place in body
Test	See how (specify body part) is working
Incision	Special opening
Edema	Puffiness
Stretcher, gurney	Rolling bed
Stool	Child's usual term
Dye	Special medicine
Pain	Hurt, discomfort, "owie," "boo-boo"
Deaden	Numb, make sleepy
Cut, fix	Make better
Take (as in "take your temperature")	See how warm you are
Take (as in "take your blood pressure")	Check your pressure; hug your arm
Put to sleep, anesthesia	Special sleep
Catheter	Tube
Monitor	Television screen
Electrodes	Stickers, ticklers
Specimen	Sample

BOX 22-3 ■ Commonly Used Sedation Medications

OPIOIDS*

Morphine sulfate, 0.05 to 0.10 mg/kg IV over 1 to 2 minutes given 5 minutes before procedure

Fentanyl, 1 to 2 μg/kg (0.001 to 0.002 mg/kg) IV 3 minutes before procedure

Fentanyl Oralet, 5 to 15 μg/kg, to maximum of 400 μg, orally 20 to 40 minutes before procedure†

Hydromorphone (Dilaudid), 0.015 to 0.02 mg/kg IV over 1 to 2 minutes given 5 minutes before procedure

Meperidine (if morphine sulfate or fentanyl is not available), 0.5 to 1 mg/kg IV over 1 to 2 minutes given 2 to 5 minutes before procedure or 1.5 mg/kg orally 45 to 60 minutes before procedure

SEDATIVES‡

Midazolam (Versed), 0.25 to 0.5 mg/kg (children 6 months to less than 6 years of age and less cooperative children may require a higher dose of up to 1 mg/kg), to maximum of 20 mg, using oral preparation, 10 to 20 minutes, or 0.05 mg/kg IV 3 minutes before procedure

Diazepam (Valium), 0.2 to 0.3 mg/kg, to maximum of 10 mg, orally 45 to 60 minutes before procedure

Pentobarbital (Nembutal), 1 to 3 mg/kg IV boluses to maximum of 100 mg until asleep

Chloral hydrate, 50 to 75 mg/kg, to maximum of 100 mg/kg or 2.5 g; orally or rectally 60 minutes before procedure

Modified from Zeltzer LK and others: Report of the subcommittee on the management of pain associated with procedures in children with cancer, *Pediatrics* 86(suppl):826-831, 1990; Yaster M and others: *Pediatric pain management and sedation handbook,* St Louis, 1997, Mosby.
*Provide analgesia and sedation.
†Not recommended for children weighing less than 15 kg. Lozenge should be sucked, not chewed and swallowed. If chewed, drug is less effective because part of it is metabolized by liver before entering bloodstream. Swallowing drug rapidly does not increase risk of respiratory depression during first 15 to 30 minutes, period of greatest risk for decreased respiration.
‡Provide sedation but no analgesia.

tered, stringent monitoring will permit early recognition of any untoward effects. The use of sedatives for procedures has serious associated risks, such as hypoventilation, apnea, airway obstruction, and cardiopulmonary impairment. In a recent study, adverse events were associated with all routes and all classes of drugs, even those thought to have minimal effect on respiration (Coté and others, 2000).

Regardless of the intended level of sedation or the route of administration of sedatives, sedation should be viewed as a continuum, ranging from minimal sedation to general anesthesia. *Minimal sedation (anxiolysis)* is a drug-induced state during which patients respond normally to verbal commands. Although cognitive function and coordination may be impaired, ventilatory and cardiovascular functions are unaffected. This level of sedation is difficult, if not impossible, to achieve in the pediatric patient undergoing diagnostic or therapeutic procedures. *Moderate sedation* (previously known as *"conscious sedation"*) is a drug-induced depression of consciousness during which patients respond purposefully to verbal commands, either alone or accompanied by light tactile stimulation. No interventions are required to maintain a patient airway, and spontaneous ventilation is adequate. Cardiovascular function is usually maintained. *Deep sedation/analgesia* is a drug-induced depression of consciousness during

which patients cannot be easily aroused, but respond purposefully after repeated or painful stimulation. The ability to independently maintain ventilatory function may be impaired. Patients may require assistance in maintaining a patent airway and spontaneous ventilation may be inadequate. Cardiovascular function is usually maintained (American Society of Anesthesiologists, 2002).

Reports of adverse events have led to the development of guidelines and standards of care to ensure the safety of sedated children. The American Society of Anesthesiologists (2002) and the American Academy of Pediatrics (2002) have developed policies and guidelines for sedation. These guidelines emphasize provision of emergency equipment, such as a positive-pressure oxygen delivery system, airway management and breathing equipment, and an emergency cart. The patient's level of consciousness and responsiveness, heart rate, blood pressure, respiratory rate, and oxygen saturation must be monitored during and after the procedure by an individual who has no other responsibilities. In all cases the patient's condition after the procedure is also documented. Specific discharge criteria must be used.

Nitrous oxide, a mixture of 50% or less of nitrous oxide with the balance as oxygen, without any other sedative, opioid, or other depressant, can be administered for sedation. Although pulse oximetry monitoring is not required, it is strongly recommended. The patient is able to maintain verbal communication throughout, and a second individual whose responsibility is to monitor the patient may also assist with the procedure. The patient's condition after the procedure is also documented.

Performance of the Procedure

Supportive care continues during the procedure and can be a major factor in a child's ability to cooperate and achieve mastery. Before the procedure is begun, all equipment is assembled and the room is readied to prevent unnecessary delays and interruptions that only serve to increase the child's anxiety.

NURSING TIP

To avoid a delay during a procedure, have extra supplies handy. For example, have tape, bandages, alcohol swabs, and an extra needle in your pocket when giving an injection or performing a venipuncture.

If at all possible, procedures are performed in a special treatment room rather than the child's hospital room. Traumatic procedures should never be performed in "safe" areas, such as the playroom. If the procedure is lengthy, conversation that could be misinterpreted by the child is avoided. As the procedure is nearing completion, the nurse should inform the child that it is almost over in language that the child understands.

Expect Success. Nurses who approach children with confidence and who convey the impression that they expect to be successful are less likely to encounter difficulty. It is best to approach children as though cooperation is expected. Children sense anxiety in another and may respond to a perceived threat by striking out or with active resistance. Although it is not possible to eliminate such behavior in every child, a firm approach with a positive attitude by the nurse tends to convey a feeling of security to most children.

Involve the Child.   As in any other aspect of care, involving children helps to gain their cooperation. Permitting them to make choices gives them some measure of control. However, a choice is given only in situations in which one is available. Asking children, "Do you want to take your medicine now?" leads them to believe that there is an option and provides them with the opportunity to legitimately refuse or delay the medication. This places the nurse in an awkward, if not impossible, position. It is much better to state firmly, "It's time to take your medicine now." Children usually like to make choices, but the choice must be one that they may have (e.g., "It's time for your medicine. Do you want to drink it plain or with a little water?").

Many children respond to tactics that appeal to their maturity or courage. This approach also gives them a sense of participation and achievement. For example, preschool children will be proud that they can hold the dressing during the procedure or remove the tape. The same is true for the school-age child, who often cooperates with minimal resistance.

Provide Distraction.   When children are occupied with an activity that interests them, they are less likely to focus on the procedure. The acute pain of procedures can be made more bearable when the patient is distracted during the process. Reading, watching television, or listening to music are a few potential activities. Other strategies for diverting attention are to have the child tightly squeeze the hands of a parent or an assistant, count aloud, sing a familiar song such as a nursery rhyme, or verbally express discomfort.

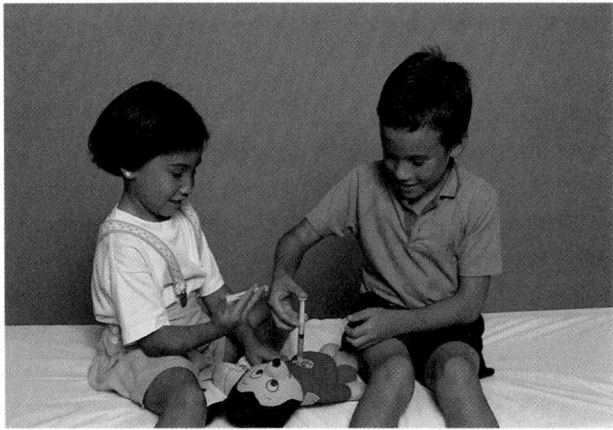

FIG. 22-2 ■ Playing with syringes provides children with the opportunity to play out fears and concerns.

> **NURSING TIP**
>
> Help the child to select and practice a coping technique before the procedure. Consider having the parent or some other supportive person, such as a child-life specialist, "coach" the child in learning and using the coping skill.

For other nonpharmacologic interventions that may lessen discomfort, see Pain Management, Chapter 21.

Allow Expression of Feelings.   The child should be allowed to express feelings of anger, anxiety, fear, frustration, or any other emotion. It is natural for children to strike out in frustration or to try to avoid stress-provoking situations. The child needs to know that it is all right to cry. Behavior is children's primary means of communication and coping and should be permitted unless it inflicts harm on them or those caring for them.

Postprocedural Support

After the procedure the child continues to need reassurance that he or she performed well and is accepted and loved. If the parents did not participate, the child is united with them as soon as possible so that they can provide comfort.

Encourage Expression of Feelings.   Planned activity after the procedure is helpful in encouraging constructive expression of feelings. For verbal children, reviewing the details of the procedure can help clarify misconceptions and provide feedback for improving the nurse's preparatory strategies. Play is an excellent activity for all children. Infants and young children are given the opportunity for gross motor movement. Even older children can vent their anger and frustration in acceptable pounding or throwing activities. Play-Doh is a remarkably versatile medium for pounding and shaping. Dramatic play provides an outlet for anger and places the child in a position of control, in contrast to the position of helplessness in the real situation. Puppets may also be used to allow the child to communicate in a nonthreatening way. One of the most effective interventions is *therapeutic play,* which includes activities such as permitting the child to give an injection to a doll or stuffed toy to reduce the stress of injections (Fig. 22-2).

Provide Positive Reinforcement.   Children need to hear from adults that they know the youngsters did the best they could in the situation, no matter how they behaved. It is important for children to know that their worth is not being judged on the basis of their behavior in a stressful situation. Reward systems, such as earning stars, stickers, or a badge of courage, are appealing to children.

Returning to the child a short while after the procedure helps the nurse to strengthen a supportive relationship. Relating with the child during a relaxed and nonstressful period allows him or her to see the nurse not only as someone associated with stressful situations but also as someone with whom to share pleasurable experiences.

Use of Play in Procedures

The use of play is an integral part of relationships with children. As such, its value in specific situations is discussed throughout this book, such as in Chapter 21, in relation to hospitalization. Nurses can easily include play activities as part of nursing care. Play can be used to teach, for expression of feelings, or as a method to achieve a therapeutic goal. Consequently, it should be included in preparing children for and encouraging their cooperation during procedures. Play sessions after procedures can be structured, such as directed toward playing with syringes, or general, with a wide variety of equipment available for children to play with. Suggestions for incorporating play into nursing procedures and activities for the hospitalized child that facilitate learning and adjustment to a new situation are described in Box 22-4.

BOX 22-4 ■ Play Activities for Specific Procedures*

FLUID INTAKE

Make ice pops using child's favorite juice.

Cut gelatin into fun shapes.

Make a game out of taking a sip when turning page of a book or in games such as Simon Says.

Use small medicine cups; decorate the cups.

Color water with food coloring or powdered drink mix.

Have a tea party; pour at a small table.

Let child fill a syringe and squirt it into mouth or use it to fill small decorated cups.

Cut straws in half and place in a small container (much easier for child to suck liquid).

Decorate a straw: cut out small design with two holes and pass straw through; place small sticker on straw.

Use a "crazy" straw.

Make a "progress poster"; give rewards for drinking a predetermined quantity.

DEEP BREATHING

Blow bubbles with a bubble blower.

Blow bubbles with a straw (no soap).

Blow on a pinwheel, feather, whistle, harmonica, balloon, toy horn, party blower.

Practice band instruments.

Have blowing contest using balloons,* boats, cotton balls, feathers, marbles, Ping-Pong balls, pieces of paper; blow such objects on a table top over a goal line, over water, through an obstacle course, up in the air, against an opponent, or up and down a string.

Suck paper or cloth from one container to another using a straw.

Use blow bottles with colored water to transfer water from one side to the other.

Dramatize stories such as "I'll huff and puff and blow your house down" from the Three Little Pigs.

Do straw-blowing painting.

Take a deep breath and "blow out the candles" on a birthday cake.

Use a little paint brush to "paint" nails with water and blow nails dry.

RANGE OF MOTION AND USE OF EXTREMITIES

Throw beanbags at a fixed or movable target or throw wadded-up paper into a wastebasket.

Touch or kick Mylar balloons held or hung in different positions (if child is in traction, hang balloon from a trapeze).

Play "tickle toes"; wiggle them on request.

Play Twister game or Simon Says.

Play pretend and guess games (e.g., imitate a bird, butterfly, horse).

Have tricycle or wheelchair races in safe area.

Play kickball or throw ball with a soft foam ball in a safe area.

Position bed so that child must turn to view television or doorway.

Climb wall like a "spider."

Pretend to teach "aerobic" dancing or exercises; encourage parents to participate.

Encourage swimming if feasible.

Play video games or pinball (fine motor movement).

Play "hide and seek": hide toy somewhere in bed (or room if ambulatory) and have child find it using specified hand or foot.

Provide clay to mold with fingers.

Paint or draw on large sheets of paper placed on floor or wall.

Encourage combing own hair; play "beauty shop" with "customer" in different positions.

SOAKS

Play with small toys or objects (cups, syringes, soap dishes) in water.

Wash dolls or toys.

Bubbles may be added to bathwater if permissible; move bubbles to create shapes or "monsters."

Pick up marbles or pennies* from bottom of bath container.

Make designs with coins on bottom of container.

Pretend a boat is a submarine by keeping it immersed.

Read to child during soaks, sing with child, or play game, such as cards, checkers, or other board game (if both hands are immersed, move board pieces for child).

Sitz bath: give child something to listen to (music, stories) or look at (View-Master, book).

Punch holes in bottom of plastic cup, fill with water, and let it "rain" on child.

INJECTIONS

Let child handle syringe, vial, and alcohol swab, and give an injection to doll or stuffed animal.

Use syringes to decorate cookies with frosting, squirt paint, or target shoot into a container.

Draw a "magic circle" on area before injection; draw smiling face in circle after injection, but avoid drawing on puncture site.

Allow child to have a "collection" of syringes (without needles); make "wild" creative objects with syringes.

If multiple injections or venipunctures, make a "progress poster"; give rewards for predetermined number of injections.

Have child count to 10 or 15 during injection.

AMBULATION

Give child something to push.

Toddler: push-pull toy

School-age child: wagon or decorated IV stand

Adolescent: a baby in a stroller or wheelchair

Have a parade; make hats, drums, etc.

EXTENDING ENVIRONMENT (FOR EXAMPLE, FOR PATIENTS IN TRACTION)

Make bed into a pirate ship or airplane with decorations.

Put up mirrors so patient can see around room.

Move patient's bed frequently, especially to playroom, hallway, or outside.

*Small objects such as marbles or coins, as well as gloves or balloons, are unsafe for young children because of possible aspiration. Latex products also carry the risk of an allergic reaction.

NURSING TIP

Play can also be spontaneous at the bedside and does not always require many supplies or much nursing time. Small items such as finger puppets or a small bottle of bubbles can be kept in the nurse's pocket for immediate use.

SURGICAL PROCEDURES
Preoperative Care

Children undergoing surgical procedures require both psychologic and physical preparation. In general, psychologic preparation is similar to that previously discussed for a pro-

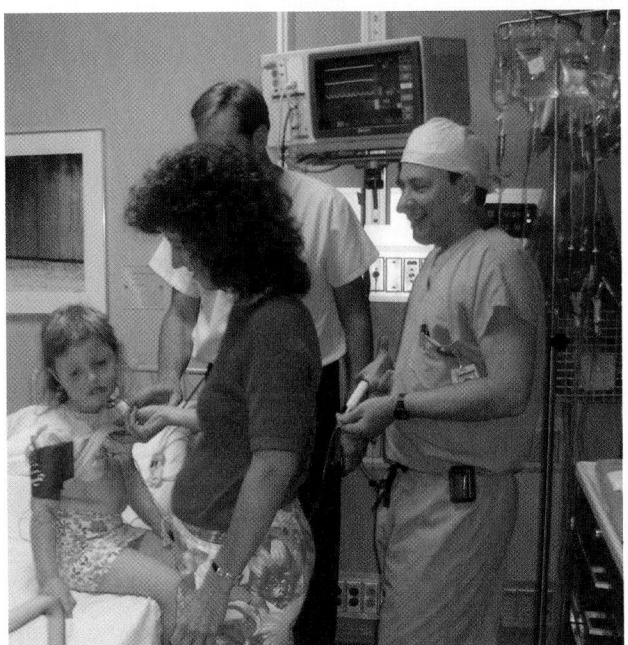

FIG. 22-3 ■ Parental presence during induction of anesthesia can minimize child's and parents' anxiety during the preoperative period.

BOX 22-5 ■ Summary of Fasting Recommendations to Reduce the Risk of Pulmonary Aspiration*

INGESTED MATERIAL	MINIMUM FASTING PERIOD (hours)†
Clear liquids‡	2
Breast milk	4
Infant formula	6
Nonhuman milk§	6
Light meal‖	6

From American Society of Anesthesiologists: Practice guidelines for preoperative fasting and the use of pharmacologic agents to reduce the risk of pulmonary aspiration: application to healthy patients undergoing elective procedures, *Anesthesiology* 90(3):896-905, 1999 (www.ASAhq.org/practice/NPO/NPOguide.html).

*These recommendations apply to healthy patients who are undergoing elective procedures. They are not intended for women in labor. Following the guidelines does not guarantee a complete gastric emptying has occurred.

†The fasting periods noted in the chart apply to all ages.

‡Examples of clear liquids include water, fruit juices without pulp, carbonated beverages, clear tea, and black coffee.

§Because nonhuman milk is similar to solids in gastric emptying time, the amount ingested must be considered when determining an appropriate fasting period.

‖A light meal typically consists of toast and clear liquids. Meals that include fried or fatty foods or meat may prolong gastric emptying time. Both the amount and type of foods ingested must be considered when determining an appropriate fasting period.

cedure and employs many of the same techniques used in preparing a child for hospitalization, such as films, books, play, and tours. However, some important differences exist. Even though children are anesthetized for the actual surgical intervention, they may be subjected to numerous preoperative and postoperative procedures. Stress points before and after surgery include the admission process, blood tests, administration of preoperative medications (if prescribed), the period before and during transport to the operating room, and the return from the postanesthesia care unit (PACU).

Psychologic intervention consisting of systematic preparation, rehearsal of the forthcoming events, and supportive care during times of stress has been shown to be more effective than a single-session preparation or consistent supportive care without systematic preparation and rehearsal. Play is always an effective strategy in preparing children, and increased familiarity with medical procedures decreases anxiety.

Parental presence during induction of anesthesia (PPIA) is allowed in some institutions (Fig 22-3). Potential benefits include minimizing the need for premedication and avoiding an upsetting separation of the child from the parents. Other benefits are controversial but may include decreasing the child's anxiety during induction and decreasing the long term behavioral effects of surgery (Kain, Caldwell-Andrews, and Wang, 2002). Based on the parents' favorable response to the practice and most children's desire to have parents with them during any stressful procedure, a policy of offering parents the option of attending the induction, combined with a program that prepares them for what to expect and what is expected of them, is recommended. When parents choose not to or are not allowed to attend this induction, leaving a favorite possession with the child and uniting the child and parents as soon as possible after surgery

(preferably in the PACU) are important interventions. During surgery the family should have a designated place to wait and needs to be kept informed of the child's progress. Family members also should know where and when they can visit the child after surgery.

Aside from possibly being separated from the parents before and after surgery, children may be cared for by a number of unfamiliar practitioners. Although the same supportive nurse should remain with the child through as many of the procedures as possible, the child may have several nurses. Many hospitals have surgical tours for children and parents to familiarize them with the strange environment and to introduce them to other individuals who will be involved in their care.

Besides psychologic preparation, children usually require various types of physical care before surgery, such as those listed in the Nursing Care Plan on pp. 718 to 720 and in the preoperative checklist (see Guidelines box). An important concern is restriction of food and fluids before surgery to avoid aspiration during anesthesia. Before fluids are restricted, children are encouraged to drink to promote hydration and minimize the dryness and thirst they experience. Infants require special attention to fluid needs. They should not be without oral fluids for an extended period preoperatively to avoid glycogen depletion and dehydration. Current preoperative fasting guidelines are found in Box 22-5.

Although most preoperative care procedures are routine, nurses should keep in mind that they can be anxiety-provoking for children and parents. For example, for young children, having to wear a loose-fitting hospital gown without the security of underpants or pajama bottoms can be traumatic. Therefore these articles of clothing should be allowed to be worn to the operating room. They can be removed after induction of anesthesia.

Text continued on p. 722.

PREOPERATIVE CARE

NURSING DIAGNOSIS ■ Risk for injury related to surgical procedure, anesthesia

PATIENT GOAL 1: Will give fully informed consent and sign appropriate documents

NURSING INTERVENTIONS/*RATIONALES*

Inquire whether parents have any questions about procedure *to determine their level of understanding and to provide for additional information (from nurse or other professional)*

Confirm that all required consent forms are fully completed, with dates, specific procedure, and signatures; *informed consent is physician's responsibility*

Obtain or witness signature if not obtained earlier

EXPECTED OUTCOMES

Family gives fully informed consent
Family signs appropriate documents

PATIENT GOAL 2: Will receive proper hygiene measures

NURSING INTERVENTIONS/*RATIONALES*

Bathe child, groom hair
Provide mouth care *to promote comfort while NPO*
Cleanse operative site according to prescribed method, if ordered, *to minimize risk of infection*
Remove nail polish from fingers and toes

EXPECTED OUTCOME

Child is cleansed and prepared appropriately (specify)

PATIENT GOAL 3: Will receive proper preparation

NURSING INTERVENTIONS/*RATIONALES*

Perform special procedures
Order or assist with special tests, such as x-ray films
Consult with practitioner for appropriate change in schedule or route of administration of any medication child ordinarily receives
Attire child appropriately
    Allow child to wear underwear or pajama bottoms *to provide privacy*
    Label personal articles and clothing
Document height and weight
Remove jewelry, contact lenses, or prosthetic devices (e.g., orthodontic appliances and body piercings) *because they may be lost or interfere with anesthesia and surgery*
Check for loose teeth
Inform anesthesiologist, if detected, *to prevent aspiration of teeth during anesthesia*

EXPECTED OUTCOME

Child is prepared appropriately (specify)

PATIENT GOAL 4: Will experience no complications

NURSING INTERVENTIONS/*RATIONALES*

Keep child NPO (nothing by mouth) as ordered *to prevent aspiration during anesthesia*
Be sure child is well-hydrated before NPO status begins, especially infants, *who are more at risk for dehydration*
Take and record vital signs
    Report any deviations from admission readings, especially elevated temperature, *which may indicate infection*
Encourage child to void before preoperative medication is administered *to prevent bladder distention or incontinence during anesthesia*
    Record time of last voiding if unable to void

Be certain allergies are clearly indicated on chart *to decrease risk of adverse reaction*
Elicit any family history of reaction to anesthesia, which indicates risk of malignant hyperthermia
Check laboratory values for any sign of systemic abnormality, such as infection (increased white blood cells), anemia (decreased hemoglobin or hematocrit), or bleeding tendencies (reduced platelets or prolonged bleeding or clotting time)
Keep small infants warm during transport and waiting time
*Administer antibiotics as ordered, observing for side effects

EXPECTED OUTCOMES

Child is NPO for designated time preoperatively
Child voids
Pertinent information about child is visible

PATIENT GOAL 5: Will experience no injury

NURSING INTERVENTIONS/*RATIONALES*

Check that identification band is securely fastened
Follow institutional policies for accurate identification and verification of the correct patient, procedure, site, and side
Fasten siderails of bed or crib *to prevent falls*
Use restraints during transport by stretcher (or other conveyance) *to prevent falls*
Do not leave child unattended

EXPECTED OUTCOMES

Child is safe from immediate harm
Child, procedure, and site are clearly and correctly identified

NURSING DIAGNOSIS ■ Anxiety/fear related to separation from support system, unfamiliar environment, knowledge deficit

PATIENT GOAL 1: Will demonstrate optimal sense of security

NURSING INTERVENTIONS/*RATIONALES*

Institute preoperative teaching *to reduce anxiety/fear*
Orient child to strange surroundings
Explain where parents will be while child is in operating room
Have someone stay with child *to provide increased sense of security*

EXPECTED OUTCOME

Child demonstrates minimum insecurity or anxiety

PATIENT/FAMILY GOAL 2: Will demonstrate understanding of surgery and postoperative care

NURSING INTERVENTIONS/*RATIONALES*

Prepare for postoperative procedures, as indicated (e.g., nasogastric tube, intravenous [IV] fluids, nothing by mouth, dressing changes, wound drains if necessary)
Explain reason for surgery; if special operative procedure is to be performed, explain basic principles and briefly outline care, if needed, *to reinforce information given by practitioner*
Explain all preoperative procedures (e.g., blood work, other laboratory tests)
In emergency situation, explain most essential components of surgery (e.g., where child will be before and after surgery, anesthesia, dressing)
Accept behavioral reactions of parents and child *because these can vary greatly*

EXPECTED OUTCOMES

Child and family demonstrate an understanding of forthcoming events (specify methods of learning and evaluation)
*Family's behavioral reactions are accepted and supported

*Dependent nursing action.

PATIENT GOAL 3: Will exhibit signs of optimal relaxation, sedation, and support before arriving in operating room

NURSING INTERVENTIONS/*RATIONALES*

†Administer preoperative sedation (preferably oral), if ordered, *to promote relaxation and sleep*

Place unfamiliar equipment out of child's view *to decrease anxiety/fear*

Place child in quiet environment with minimum distraction *to promote relaxation and encourage sleep*

Do not leave child unattended

Explain what is happening, unless child is asleep

Encourage parents to stay with child as long as permitted and according to their wishes

Permit parent to hold child until child falls asleep, if desired

Encourage parents to remain with child as long as possible, preferably through induction of anesthesia if allowed

Allow significant objects to accompany child (e.g., a favorite toy, blanket) *to provide comfort and sense of security*

EXPECTED OUTCOMES

Child falls asleep or lies quietly

Child is not left alone

NURSING DIAGNOSIS ■ **Altered family processes related to a surgical procedure**

PATIENT (FAMILY) GOAL 1: Will receive adequate support and reassurance

NURSING INTERVENTIONS/RATIONALES

Reinforce and clarify information given by practitioner

Explain associated diagnostic tests and procedures (e.g., x-ray examinations)

Explain child's schedule

    When child will receive premedication

    Time child will leave for surgery

    Where parents can wait for child to return

    Room to which child will return

    Postprocedural care and routines

Explore family's feelings regarding the procedure and its implications *to assess need for further intervention*

Include parents in preparation of child

Be available to family *to provide support and reassurance as needed*

See also Nursing Care Plan: The Family of the Ill or Hospitalized Child, Chapter 21

EXPECTED OUTCOMES

Family demonstrates an understanding of procedure (specify demonstration) and related information (specify)

Family complies with directives (specify)

POSTOPERATIVE CARE

NURSING DIAGNOSIS ■ **Risk for injury related to surgical procedure, anesthesia, and hypothermia**

IMMEDIATE POSTANESTHESIA CARE:

NURSE GOAL 1: Assist a noncomplicated return to safe physiologic function after emergence from anesthesia

NURSING INTERVENTIONS/RATIONALES

Transfer to recovery stretcher using techniques appropriate to type of surgery to prevent injury

Position the child to ensure airway patency

Receive report from anesthesia/OR team

Hang IV fluids as ordered

Closely monitor all vital physiologic functions and oxygen saturation until effects of anesthetic agents are diminished

Stay at bedside until gag reflex returns

Monitor oxygen saturation; administer oxygen as ordered

Have suction immediately available

Assess temperature for hypothermia and apply warm blankets

Manage drainage tubes

Promote comfort by administration of analgesics and antiemetics

EXPECTED OUTCOME

Child is discharged from postanesthesia care unit (PACU) without injury or complications

POSTOPERATIVE CARE (AFTER PACU)

PATIENT GOAL 2: Will exhibit signs of wound healing without evidence of infection

NURSING INTERVENTIONS/*RATIONALES*

Use proper handwashing techniques and other standard precautions, especially if drainage is present

Practice careful surgical incision care *to minimize risk of infection*

    Check incision regularly for bleeding

    Keep dressing intact

    Apply dressing that promote moist wound healing

    Change dressing as needed; carefully dispose of soiled dressing

    Carry out special wound care, such as drain care

    Cleanse with prescribed preparation (if ordered)

    Apply antibacterial solutions or ointments as ordered *to prevent infection*

    Report any unusual appearance or drainage for early detection of infection

Maintain skin integrity by repositioning every two hours and keeping linens clean and dry

Monitor vital signs for any signs of infection

Monitor IV site for any signs of infection

When child begins oral feedings, provide nutritious diet as ordered *to promote wound healing*

EXPECTED OUTCOMES

Child exhibits no evidence of wound infection

PATIENT GOAL 3: Will exhibit no evidence of complications

NURSING INTERVENTIONS/*RATIONALES*

Ambulate as prescribed to *decrease complications associated with immobility*

Maintain child NPO until fully awake to *prevent aspiration*

Encourage to void when awake

    Offer bedpan

    Boys may be allowed to stand at bedside

Notify practitioner if child is unable to void *to ensure appropriate intervention*

Maintain abdominal decompression, chest tubes, or other equipment, if prescribed

Provide diet as prescribed; advance as appropriate

EXPECTED OUTCOME

Child exhibits no evidence of complications

*Dependent nursing action.

Continued

NURSING DIAGNOSIS ■ **Anxiety/fear related to surgery, unfamiliar environment, separation from support systems, discomfort**

PATIENT GOAL 1: Will experience reduced anxiety

NURSING INTERVENTIONS/RATIONALES
Maintain calm, reassuring manner
Encourage expression of feelings *to facilitate coping*
Explain procedures and other activities before initiating
Answer questions and explain purposes of activities
Keep informed of progress
Remain with child as much as possible
Give encouragement and positive feedback for cooperation in care
Encourage parental presence as soon as permitted *to decrease stress of separation*
If emergency procedure, review child's memory of previous events *so that misconceptions can be clarified*

EXPECTED OUTCOMES
Child rests quietly and calmly
Child discusses procedures and activities without evidence of anxiety

NURSING DIAGNOSIS ■ **Pain related to surgical procedure**

PATIENT GOAL 1: Will experience adequate comfort level and reduction of pain

NURSING INTERVENTIONS/RATIONALES
Assess level of pain using appropriate pain scale
Administer analgesics as ordered
Monitor effectiveness of analgesics by reassessing child after administration
Use age-appropriate nonpharmacologic strategies as adjuncts to analgesics (e.g., distraction, positioning)
Avoid palpating operative area unless necessary
Encourage child to void *to prevent bladder distention*
Administer mouth care *to provide comfort*
Lubricate nostril *to decrease irritation from nasogastric tube, if present*
Allow child position of comfort if not contraindicated
Perform nursing activities and procedures after analgesia
Administer antiemetics as ordered for nausea and vomiting

EXPECTED OUTCOME
Child's pain is adequately controlled as demonstrated by a lower number on pain scale

NURSING DIAGNOSIS ■ **Risk for fluid volume deficit related to NPO status before or after surgery, loss of appetite, vomiting**

PATIENT GOAL 1: Will receive adequate hydration

NURSING INTERVENTIONS/RATIONALES
Monitor IV infusion at prescribed rate *to ensure adequate hydration*
  Attach pediatric IV apparatus if not done in operating room
Offer fluids as soon as ordered or child tolerates them
  Start with small sips of water and advance as tolerated or ordered
Encourage to drink
  Tempt with favorite fluids, ice chips, or flavored ice pops
  Closely monitor intake and output

EXPECTED OUTCOMES
Child exhibits no evidence of dehydration
Child takes and retains fluid when allowed (specify)

NURSING DIAGNOSIS ■ **Risk for infection related to surgical procedure and IV line**

PATIENT GOAL 1: Will maintain normal respiratory function

NURSING INTERVENTIONS/RATIONALES
Assess respirations and auscultate lungs every 2 hours
Assess need for pain medication before respiratory therapy, ambulation, or any activity
Encourage to turn and deep breathe every 2 hours
  Splint operative site with hand or pillow, if possible, before coughing (if coughing prescribed) *to minimize pain*
Assist with use of incentive spirometer, blow bottle, or pinwheels
Perform percussion and vibration if indicated
Suction secretions if needed
Reposition or encourage ambulation every 2 hours

EXPECTED OUTCOME
Child remains free of respiratory complications

NURSING DIAGNOSIS ■ **Altered family processes related to situational crisis (emergency hospitalization of child), knowledge deficit**

PATIENT/FAMILY GOAL 1: Will receive adequate support and reassurance related to postoperative care and outcome

NURSING INTERVENTIONS/RATIONALES
Reassure child and family that anxiety about surgery is normal
Explain all procedures *to reduce anxiety/fear*
Keep family informed of child's progress
Encourage expression of feelings *to facilitate coping*
Refer to home health care agency, if indicated, *for follow-up care*
Refer to appropriate agency or persons for specific help (e.g., social service, clergy)
See also Nursing Care Plan: The Child in the Hospital, Chapter 21
See also Nursing Care Plan: The Family of the Ill or Hospitalized Child, Chapter 21

EXPECTED OUTCOMES
Family discusses child's condition and therapies comfortably
Family demonstrates an awareness of child's progress (specify method of evaluation)
Family members avail themselves of appropriate assistance

PATIENT (FAMILY) GOAL 2: Will demonstrate understanding of home care

NURSING INTERVENTIONS/*RATIONALES*
If dressing changes are required at home, teach parents sterile or aseptic procedures; provide written list of necessary equipment and instructions *for referral at home*
Instruct parents regarding administration of medications, if ordered, including possible side effects and untoward reactions, *to ensure adequate home care*
Instruct parents in care and management of special procedures (e.g., ostomy care, irrigations) *to ensure adequate home care*
Provide written home care instructions regarding wound care, activity level, medications, diet, and follow-up care

EXPECTED OUTCOME
Family demonstrates an understanding of instructions (specify methods of learning and evaluation)

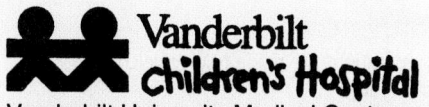

Vanderbilt Children's Hospital
Vanderbilt University Medical Center

PRE-PROCEDURE CHECKLIST

Weight:_____

Location of Patient's Family During Procedure:

_____

Date:_____

NPO Status Maintained Since:_____

PATIENT IDENTIFICATION (Indicate two identifiers):
☐ Patient Name   ☐ Date of Birth   ☐ Medical Record Number   ☐ Social Security Number   ☐ Photo ID

Source: ☐ Patient Statement   ☐ Parent   ☐ Guardian   ☐ Spouse   ☐ Domestic Partner
☐ Adult Sibling (18y or older)   ☐ Adult Child   ☐ Transferring Facility Representative/Documents
☐ **Identification Band On / Name, Numbers Match Patient's Statement &/or Permanent Medical Record Document**

PROCEDURE (Patient's or Other Identifying Source's Statement): _____

_____

Procedure Statement Consistent With: (Check ALL that apply)
☐ **Procedure Consent**   ☐ **History & Physical**   ☐ Physician orders/notes   ☐ Procedure Schedule   ☐ Diagnostic x-rays / reports

SITE / SIDE IDENTIFICATION: ☐ Site Not Applicable (Procedure performed through a natural body orifice)

Patient's / Other Source's Statement – SITE:_____

SIDE:_____

Site / Side Statement Consistent With: (Check ALL that apply)
☐ **Procedure Consent**   ☐ **History & Physical**   ☐ Physician orders / notes   ☐ Procedure Schedule   ☐ Diagnostic x-rays / reports

Procedure / Site / Side Identified By: ☐ Patient Statement   ☐ Parent   ☐ Guardian   ☐ Spouse
☐ Domestic Partner   ☐ Adult Sibling (18y or older)   ☐ Adult Child   ☐ Transferring Facility Representative / Documents

---

PRE-PROCEDURE PREPARATION				
	Staff Initials			**Staff Initials**
Procedure Consent Completed	_____	Lab Work Obtained & Results Acceptable to Proceed		_____ ☐ N/A
History & Physical Completed	_____	Radiology / Cardiology / Other Studies Completed		_____ ☐ N/A
Anesthesia History & Physical Completed	_____ ☐ N/A	Pre-Procedure Scrub / Site Prep Completed		_____ ☐ N/A
Anesthesia Day of Surgery Evaluation Completed	_____ ☐ N/A	Patient Voided / Catheterized		_____ ☐ N/A
Patient ID Card in Chart (Inpatient Only)	_____ ☐ N/A	Dentures / Prostheses Removed *		_____ ☐ N/A
Current Chart(s) Available	_____ ☐ N/A	Eye Glasses / Contact Lenses Removed *		_____ ☐ N/A
"Old" Chart(s) Available	_____ ☐ N/A	Jewelry Removed *		_____ ☐ N/A
Pre-Procedure Medications Administered/Documented	_____ ☐ N/A	Other Valuables:*_____		_____ ☐ N/A
IV Patent	_____ ☐ N/A	* ☐ Given to Family ☐ Stored:_____		

SYNTHETIC / TISSUE IMPLANTS (If Applicable):   ☐ Available in procedure suite   ☐ Identification matches procedure request
SITE MARKING: **Site Initialed By:** ☐ Physician   ☐ Non-Physician Proceduralist   ☐ Site Marking Not Indicated   ☐ See OR documentation
All Team Members Concur With Site Identification and Marking: ☐ YES   ☐ Not Indicated
Site Marking Visible After Draping: ☐ YES   ☐ Not Indicated   ☐ See OR documentation

---

Comments:

_____

_____

_____

_____

Staff Confirming Patient, Procedure, Site, & Side Identification: Initials_____   Signature/Title_____

Initials_____   Signature/Title_____   Initials_____   Signature/Title_____

Initials_____   Signature/Title_____   Initials_____   Signature/Title_____

MC 0014 (04/2003)

Historically the most upsetting event for children has been the preoperative injection. Unfortunately, little research has been done on the value of this practice. If children have no preoperative pain, are well-prepared psychologically for surgery, and have their parents nearby, preanesthetic medication may be unnecessary. When drugs are used, they should be "atraumatic" by using oral or existing intravenous (IV) route.

Numerous preanesthetic drug regimens are used with children, and no consensus exists on the optimal method. Drugs used should achieve five goals (American Academy of Pediatrics, 1992): (1) guard the patient's safety and welfare; (2) minimize physical discomfort or pain; (3) minimize negative psychologic responses to treatment by providing analgesia, and maximize the potential for amnesia; (4) control behavior; and (5) return the patient to a state in which safe discharge, as determined by recognized criteria, is possible.

Midazolam (Versed) provides excellent preoperative anxiety reduction, amnesia, and sedation. It is popular because of its short duration, predictable onset, and rare occurrence of respiratory depression. Oral transmucosal fentanyl (OTFC), or Fentanyl Oralet, is available as a sweetened lozenge on a plastic stick. When first approved, this appeared to be an excellent, atraumatic route of administration. However, associated nausea and vomiting, respiratory depression, and the need for more intensive monitoring and observation than with other oral sedatives have limited its popularity to date (Cravero, Manzi, and Rice, 1998).

Children may also fear induction of anesthesia by mask. Practices that can minimize anxiety related to inhalation anesthesia include (1) disguising the unpleasant odor of anesthetic gases by applying a pleasant-smelling substance on the mask; (2) using a transparent plastic mask rather than an opaque black mask and gradually bringing it toward the face; (3) directing a stream of gas toward the child's face from the bare tube until the child becomes drowsy, then using the mask; (4) allowing the child to sit up rather than lie down for anesthesia induction; and (5) allowing preoperative play with a mask and a doll or manikin.

> ⚠️ **NURSING ALERT**
>
> When taking the preoperative history, ask the family if any relatives have had anesthetic difficulties suggesting malignant hyperthermia; report findings immediately.

Postoperative Care

After surgical procedures, psychologic and physical observations and interventions are required to prevent or minimize possible untoward effects from anesthesia and the surgical procedure (see Nursing Care Plan, pp. 718 to 720, and Guidelines box). Although most of these interventions are prescribed by physicians, it is the nurse's responsibility to exercise judgment in their implementation. For example, vital signs are taken as frequently as necessary until they are stable. Simply recording temperature, pulse, respiration, and blood pressure without comparing the present readings with previous ones is a useless technical function. Each vital sign is evaluated in terms of side effects from anesthesia and signs of impending shock, respiratory compromise, or pain (Table 22-1). The nurse should also be alert for the development of *malignant hyperthermia*, a potentially lethal ge-

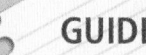

GUIDELINES

Postoperative Care

Ensure that preparations are made to receive child.
  Bed or crib is ready.
  Intravenous equipment, such as pumps, and any other relevant equipment, such as suction apparatus, oxygen flow meter, or Gomco suction, is at bedside.
Obtain baseline information:
  Take vital signs, including blood pressure (BP); keep BP cuff in place and deflated to lessen amount of disturbance to child.
  Take and record vital signs more frequently if any value fluctuates.
  Inspect operative area.
  Check dressing if present.
    Outline any bleeding area on dressing or cast with pen.
    Reinforce, but do not remove, loose dressing.
    Observe areas below surgical site for blood that may have drained toward bed.
    Assess for bleeding and other symptoms in areas not covered with a dressing, such as throat after tonsillectomy.
  Assess skin color and characteristics.
  Assess level of consciousness and activity.
Notify physician of any irregularities in child's condition.
Assess for evidence of pain (see Pain Assessment, Chapter 21).
Review surgeon's orders after completing initial assessment, and check that any preoperative orders, such as seizure or cardiac medications, have been reordered and can be given by available routes (oral preparations may be contraindicated).
Monitor vital signs as ordered and more often if indicated.
Check dressings for bleeding or other abnormalities.
Check bowel sounds.
Observe for signs of shock, abdominal distention, and bleeding.
Assess for bladder distention.
Observe for signs of dehydration.
Detect presence of infection:
  Take vital signs every 2 to 4 hours, as ordered.
  Collect or request needed specimens.
  Inspect wound for signs of infection—redness, swelling, heat, pain, and purulent drainage.

netic myopathy. In susceptible children, certain anesthetic agents such as succinylcholine and halothane trigger the disorder, producing elevated temperature, muscle rigidity, hypermetabolism, and muscle cell destruction. The symptoms may or may not occur during surgery; therefore, alert observation in the PACU and regular care unit is essential. Early signs of the disorder include tachycardia, rising blood pressure, tachypnea, mottled skin, and muscle rigidity. An elevated temperature is considered by many to be a late sign of the disorder (Dunn, 1997).

Managing pain is a major nursing responsibility after surgery. Pain is assessed, and analgesics are administered to provide comfort and to facilitate the child's cooperation with postoperative procedures such as ambulating and deep breathing. Opioids are the most commonly used analgesics for this purpose. Routinely scheduled IV analgesics, patient-controlled analgesia (PCA), and epidural infusions, rather than as needed (PRN) orders, provide excellent analgesia in postoperative pediatric patients.

Because respiratory infections are a potential complication, every effort is taken to aerate the lungs and remove se-

TABLE 22-1 ■ Potential Causes of Postoperative Vital Sign Alterations in Children

ALTERATION	POTENTIAL CAUSE	COMMENTS
HEART RATE		
Increase	Decreased profusion (shock) Elevated temperature Pain Respiratory distress (early) Medications (atropine, morphine, epinephrine)	Heart rate may increase to maintain cardiac output
Decrease	Hypoxia Vagal stimulation Increased intracranial pressure Respiratory distress (late) Medications (prostigmine)	Bradycardia is of more concern in the young child than tachycardia
RESPIRATORY RATE		
Increase	Respiratory distress Fluid volume excess Hypothermia Elevated temperature Pain	Body responds to respiratory distress primarily by increasing rate
Decrease	Anesthetics, opioids Pain	Decreased respiratory rate from opioids may be compensated for by increase depth of respiration
BLOOD PRESSURE		
Increase	Excess intravascular volume Increased intracranial pressure Carbon dioxide retention Pain Medication (ketamine, epinephrine)	Serious in premature infants because it increases risk of intraventricular hemorrhage
Decrease	Vasodilating anesthetic agents (halothane, isoflurane, enflurane) Opioids (e.g., morphine)	Decrease in blood pressure is late sign of shock because of elasticity and constriction of vessels to maintain cardiac output
TEMPERATURE		
Increase	Shock (late sign) Infection Environmental causes (warm room, excess coverings) Malignant hyperthermia	Fever associated with infection usually occurs later than fever of noninfection origin Absence of fever does not rule out infection, especially in infants
Decrease	Vasodilating anesthetic agents (halothane, isoflurane, enflurane) Muscle relaxants Environmental causes (cool room) Infusion of cool fluids/blood	Malignant hyperthermia requires immediate treatment Neonates are especially susceptible to hypothermia, with serious or fatal consequences

From Smith DP and others, editors: *Comprehensive child and family nursing skills*, St. Louis, 1991, Mosby.

cretions. The lungs are auscultated regularly to identify abnormal sounds or any areas of diminished or absent breath sounds. To prevent hypostatic pneumonia, respiratory movement can be encouraged with incentive spirometers or other motivating activities (see Box 22-4). If these measures are presented as games, the child is more likely to comply. The child's position is changed every 2 hours, and deep breathing is encouraged.

NURSING TIP

Because deep breathing is usually painful after surgery, administer analgesics before asking the child to take deep breaths. Have the child splint the operative site (depending on its location) by hugging a small pillow or a favorite stuffed animal.

❗NURSING ALERT

Early signs of respiratory involvement are abnormal rate, shallow depth, and cough. Report these findings immediately.

During the recovery period, some time should be spent with children to assess their perception of surgery. Play, drawing, and storytelling are excellent methods of discovering their thoughts. With such information the nurse can support or correct their perceptions and assist children in feeling a sense of mastery for having gone through a stressful procedure.

COMPLIANCE

Compliance, also termed *adherence*, refers to the extent to which the patient's behavior in terms of taking medication, following diets, or executing other lifestyle changes coincides with the prescribed regimen. Because nurses are frequently responsible for teaching families about treatment protocols, they must have knowledge of factors that influence compliance, methods to measure compliance, and strategies to enhance adherence to prescribed treatment.

Assessment of Compliance

In developing strategies to provide compliance, the nurse must first assess factors that influence compliance in the patient. Because many children are too young to assume partial or total responsibility for their care, parents are usually the primary caregivers at home. Consequently, the nurse needs to assess their ability to carry out instructions. The first approach to assessment is knowledge of those factors that influence compliance. The second is to apply methods to objectively assess the child's and parent's levels of compliance.

Several factors influence compliance (Box 22-6), although no typical characteristics of noncompliers exist, and even education is not correlated with compliance (Rosenstock, 1988). Basically, any aspect of the health care environment that increases the family's satisfaction with the care they are receiving positively influences adherence to the treatment regimen. However, the more complex, expensive, inconvenient, and disruptive the treatment protocol, the less likely the family is to comply. During long-term conditions that involve multiple treatments and considerable rearrangement of lifestyle, compliance is severely affected.

Although it is helpful to know those factors that influence compliance, assessment must include more direct measurement techniques. A number of methods exist, each with advantages and disadvantages. The most successful approach includes a combination of at least two of the following methods:

Clinical judgment. The nurse judges family compliance. This is a very poor method that is subject to bias and inaccuracy

BOX 22-6 ■ Factors That Positively Influence Compliance

INDIVIDUAL/FAMILY FACTORS
High self-esteem
Positive body image
High degree of autonomy (increased locus of control)
Supportive and well-adjusted family
Effective family communication
Family expectation for successful completion of therapy

CARE-SETTING FACTORS
Perceived satisfaction with care
Positive interactions with practitioners
Continuity of care
Individualized care
Minimum waiting time for appointments
Convenient care setting

TREATMENT FACTORS
Simple regimen
Minimum disruption in usual lifestyle
Short duration
Inexpensive
Visible benefits
Tolerable side effects

unless the nurse carefully evaluates the criteria used in evaluation.

Self-reporting. The family is asked about their ability to carry out the prescribed treatments, although most people overestimate their compliance by about 20% even when they admit to lapses in treatment.

Direct observation. The nurse directly observes the patient or family performing the treatment. This method is difficult to employ outside the health care setting, and the family's awareness of being observed frequently affects their performance.

Monitoring appointments. The family's attendance at scheduled appointments is recorded, although this method only indirectly indicates compliance with the prescribed care.

Monitoring therapeutic response. The child's response in terms of benefit from treatment is monitored and preferably recorded on a graph or chart. Unfortunately, few treatments yield directly measurable results (e.g., decreased blood pressure, weight loss).

Pill counts. The nurse counts the number of pills remaining in the original container and compares the amount missing with the number of days the medication should have been taken. Although this is a simple method, families may forget to bring the container or deliberately alter the number of pills to avoid detection. This method is also poorly suited to liquid medication, which is often prescribed in pediatrics. Another strategy is to call the pharmacy and check on the number of refills for long-term prescriptions.

Chemical assay. For certain drugs, such as digoxin and phenytoin, measurement of plasma drug levels provides information on the amount of drug recently ingested. However, this method is expensive, indicates only short-term compliance, and requires precise timing of the assay for accurate results.

Strategies to Enhance Compliance

Strategies to improve compliance are concerned with those interventions that encourage families to follow the prescribed treatment regimen. No one approach is always successful, and the best results occur when at least two strategies are used.

Organizational strategies refer to those interventions that involve the care setting and the therapeutic plan. They include employing the factors listed in Box 22-6, which are known to positively affect compliance. Depending on the individual situation, this may involve increasing the frequency of appointments, designating a primary practitioner, reducing the cost of medication by purchasing generic brands, reducing the treatment's disruption of the family's lifestyle, and using "cues" to minimize forgetting. Numerous devices are available commercially or can be improvised for cueing, such as pill dispensers; watches with alarms; charts to record completed therapy; reminders, such as messages on the refrigerator or morning coffee pot; and treatment schedules that incorporate the treatment plan into the daily routine, such as physical therapy after the evening bath.

Educational strategies are concerned with instructing the family about the treatment plan. Although education is an important component in enhancing compliance and patients who are more knowledgeable about their condition are more likely to comply, education alone does not ensure compliant behavior. Also, for education to be effective, it must incorporate teaching principles known to enhance understanding and retention of material (see Guidelines box). Written materials are essential, especially in any regimen requiring multiple or complex treatments, and need to be understandable to the average individual, who reads at about the fourth-grade level. Involvement of the immediate and extended family (e.g., grandparents) in education sessions may enhance compliance (Liptak, 1996).

Treatment strategies are related to the child's refusal or inability to take the prescribed medication. The family may also have difficulty following a prescribed treatment regimen. They may remember and understand the instructions but may not be able to give the medicine as prescribed. It is essential to assess the reason for refusal. For example, the child may not be able to swallow pills. In this case, perhaps the pills can be crushed or a liquid medication substituted (always review medication to make sure that crushing is acceptable before giving this instruction). The opposite also may occur; the child may have difficulty drinking a liquid medication but is able to swallow pills.

Also assess the treatment and medication schedule to determine if it is reasonable for a home situation. Although an every-6-hour or every-8-hour schedule is reasonable for hospitals, a parent would have difficulty awakening one or two times at night when a medication could be given during the day at times that would be easy to remember.

Behavioral strategies encompass those interventions designed to modify behavior directly. Several strategies exist that are effective in encouraging the desired behavior and are very useful with children. Also, positive reinforcement may be employed to strengthen the behavior; this may consist of earning stars or tokens, which gains the child a special privilege or gift. At times, however, techniques such as time-out for young children or withholding privileges for

---

GUIDELINES

Effective Teaching of Family Members

Establish rapport; reduce anxiety and fear.

Assess what family members know and expect to learn, especially if they have concerns, and address their concerns before beginning teaching.

Assess family's learning style; ask if they prefer to have everything explained in detail or if they prefer knowing only the major facts.

Use a variety of teaching materials (lecture, demonstration, video or slide presentation, written material).

Speak family's language, avoid jargon, and clarify all terms.

Be specific when giving information.

Divide the information into small steps.

Keep information short, simple, and concrete.

Introduce most important information first.

Use "verbal" headings to organize information, such as "There are two things you need to learn: how to give the medicine and what side effects to look for. First, how to give. . . . Second, what side effects. . . ."

Stress how important the instructions are and the expected benefits; explain the detrimental effects of inadequate treatment but avoid fear tactics.

Evaluate the teaching by eliciting feedback to ensure that family members understand the information.

Repeat information as needed.

Reward family for learning through verbal praise.

Use "teachable moments"—times when family members are most likely to accept new information (e.g., when a member asks a question or when symptoms are present).

Use "hands on" demonstration and return demonstration to encourage mastery of skills and retention of information.

---

older children may be needed to reduce noncompliance (see Limit Setting and Discipline, Chapter 3).

NURSING TIP

To encourage a child to perform a treatment for a certain time frame (e.g., soaking a foot), ask the child to soak during a favorite television show, including commercials. This technique also helps evaluate compliance by asking the child what show was watched (Woolverton, 1991).

GENERAL HYGIENE AND CARE

MAINTAINING HEALTHY SKIN*

Skin, the largest organ of the body, is not merely a covering but also a complex structure that serves many functions, the most important of which is to protect the tissues that it encloses and to protect itself. Many routine nursing activities—maintaining an IV line, removing a dressing, positioning a child in bed, changing a diaper, using electrode patches, or maintaining restraints—have the potential to contribute to skin injury. Skin care must go beyond the daily bath and become a part of each nursing intervention. General guidelines for skin care are listed in the Guidelines box on p. 726. Specific guidelines for skin care of neonates are provided in Chapter 9 under Skin Care.

Assessment of the skin is most easily accomplished during the bath, but often the nurse is not the one who bathes the child. In this case the nurse needs to plan a time to observe the child's skin and to request feedback from the caregiver. The skin is examined for any early signs of injury, especially for the child who is at risk. Risk factors include impaired mobility, protein malnutrition, edema, incontinence, sensory loss, anemia, and infection. Other risk factors include not turning the patient, intubation, patients ventilated with high positive end-expiratory pressure (PEEP), patients on low–air-loss beds, edema, and weight loss. Critically ill children often are at higher risk of pressure ulcers and skin breakdown, as they often have several risk factors in combination. Identification of risk factors helps to determine those children who need a more thorough skin assessment. Assessment should occur within 24 hours of admission so that pressure ulcers and wounds that occurred before admission can be identified (Ratcliff and Rodheaver, 1999; Quigley & Curley, 1996).

When capillary blood flow is interrupted by pressure, the blood flows back into the tissue when the pressure is relieved. As the body attempts to reoxygenate the area, a bright red flush appears. This *reactive hyperemia,* or flush, is the earliest sign of tissue compromise and pressure-related ischemia. If pressure is prolonged, reactive hyperemia will not be sufficient to revitalize ischemic tissue (Calianno, 1999).

NURSING ALERT

The tissue in the wound must be visible to be staged (Box 22-7). Wounds covered with necrotic tissue or a scab should not be staged. Reverse staging should not be used to describe wounds as they heal. Accurate documentation of redness or obvious skin breakdown is essential. Color, size (height × width × depth), location, presence of sinus tracts, odor, exudate, eschar, and response to treatment are observed and recorded at least daily.

---

*This section was revised by Shannon McCord, MSN, RN, CPNP.

GUIDELINES

Skin Care

Cleanse skin with mild nonalkaline soap or soap-free cleaning agents for routine bathing.

Provide daily cleansing of eyes, oral and diaper or perianal areas, and any areas of skin breakdown.

Apply moisturizing agents after cleansing to retain moisture and rehydrate skin; however, cleanse skin of any old cream before adding a new layer. Commonly used agents include lactic acid, glycolic acid, mineral oil, glycerin, and petrolatum. Moisturizing agents are more effective when applied during or immediately after bathing.

Use minimum amount of tape or adhesive. On very sensitive skin, use a protective, pectin-based or hydrocolloid skin barrier between skin and tape or adhesives.

Use water or possibly adhesive remover (if skin is not fragile) when removing tape or adhesives.

Place pectin-based or hydrocolloid skin barriers directly over excoriated skin. Leave barrier undisturbed until it begins to peel off, or for 5 to 7 days. With wet, oozing excoriations, place a small amount of stoma powder (as used in ostomy care) on site, remove excess powder, and apply skin barrier. Hold barrier in place for several minutes to allow barrier to soften and mold to skin surface.

Alternate electrode placement and thoroughly assess skin underneath electrodes at least every 24 to 72 hours. Alcohol free skin sealant under leads may protect the skin from epidermal stripping with changes.

Be certain fingers or toes are visible whenever extremity is used for intravenous (IV) or arterial line.

Reduce friction by keeping skin dry (may apply absorbent powder, for example, cornstarch) and using soft, smooth bed linen and clothes.

Use a draw sheet to move a child in bed or onto a gurney to reduce friction and shearing injuries; do not drag the child from under the arms.

Identify children who are at risk for skin breakdown before it occurs. Employ measures, such as pressure-reducing or pressure-relieving devices (e.g., mattress overlays, low–air-loss bed, gel pillows) to prevent breakdown.

Do not massage reddened bony prominences because it can cause deep tissue damage; provide pressure relief to those areas instead.

Keep skin free of excess moisture (i.e., urine or fecal incontinence, wound drainage, excessive perspiration).

Routinely assess the child's nutritional status. A child who is NPO (nothing by mouth) for several days and is only receiving IV fluid is nutritionally at risk, which can also affect the skin's ability to maintain its integrity. Parenteral nutrition should be considered for these children before they are at risk.

Staging of pressure ulcers is used to classify the amount of tissue damage that has occurred. The tissue in the wound must be visible to be staged; it is difficult to assess a wound that is covered with necrotic tissue or a scab (Box 22-7). Accurate documentation of redness or obvious skin breakdown is essential. Color, size (diameter and depth), location, presence of sinus tracts, odor, exudate, and response to treatment are observed and recorded at least daily. (For treatment of wounds, see Chapter 30).

The nurse must also have an understanding of the types of mechanical damage that can occur, such as pressure, friction, shearing, and epidermal stripping. When a combination of risk factors and mechanical injury is present, skin breakdown can occur (Hagelgans, 1993).

When a child is identified as being at risk for skin breakdown, nursing interventions are directed toward prevention of mechanical injury. Wounds caused by pressure can be prevented by using current technology and resources. *Pressure ulcers* can develop when the pressure on the skin and underlying tissues is greater than the capillary closing pressure, causing capillary occlusion. If the pressure remains unrelieved, vessels can collapse, resulting in tissue anoxia and cellular death. Pressure ulcers most often occur over bony prominences. These lesions are usually very deep (stage IV), extending into subcutaneous tissue or even deeper into muscle, tendon, or bone. Prevention of pressure ulcers includes measures that reduce or relieve pressure (Laurent, 1999).

A *pressure-reduction device* (e.g., gel pillows, foam mattress overlays) reduces pressure by redistributing the pressure. These products do not prevent pressure from causing capillary closing; therefore, turning and repositioning are always included when using these devices. Most of these items are overlays that are placed on top of the regular mattress. A *pressure-relief device* maintains pressure below that which would cause capillary closing. These devices are usually high-technology beds (e.g., low–air-loss beds) that are used for patients who have multiple pressure ulcer risk factors and cannot be turned effectively. Manufacturers of these beds recommend turning patients on low–air-loss beds when it can be clinically tolerated because the beds do not alleviate all interface pressure. Low–air-loss beds do not take the place of manually turning and have not been proven to relieve pressure in pediatric patients (McLane and others, 2002). Some bed manufacturers do not recommend placing patients weighing less than 22.7 kg on a low–air-loss bed. If the bed is in the turning mode, patients may continue to pivot on one area (i.e., occiput), potentially causing friction and skin breakdown in that area.

> **NURSING ALERT**
>
> Pressure-reducing devices on the bed for at-risk patients: on a bed, the device can be placed on top of a standard mattress or used as a mattress-replacement system; or a pressure-reducing bed can be used (Calianno, 1999).

Friction and shear both contribute to pressure ulcers. *Friction* occurs when the surface of the skin rubs against another surface, such as the sheets on the bed. The skin may have the appearance of an abrasion. The skin damage is usually limited to the epidermal and upper layers. It most often occurs over the elbows, heels, or occiput. Prevention of friction injury includes the use of protective sheepskin over the elbows or heels, moisturizing agents, transparent dressings over susceptible areas, and soft, smooth bed linen and clothing. Friction alone does not cause tissue necrosis, but when it acts with gravity, it results in shear injury.

Shear is the result of the force of gravity pushing down on the body and friction of the body against a surface, such as the bed or chair. For example, when a patient is in the semi-Fowler position and begins to slide to the foot of the

BOX 22-7 ■ **Staging of Pressure Ulcers**

STAGE I

An observable pressure-related alteration of intact skin whose indicators as compared with the adjacent or opposite area on the body may include changes in one or more of the following: skin temperature (warmth or coolness), tissue consistency (firm or boggy feel), or sensation (pain, itching). The ulcer appears as a defined area of persistent redness in lightly pigmented skin, whereas in darker skin tones, the ulcer may appear with persistent red, blue, or purple hues.

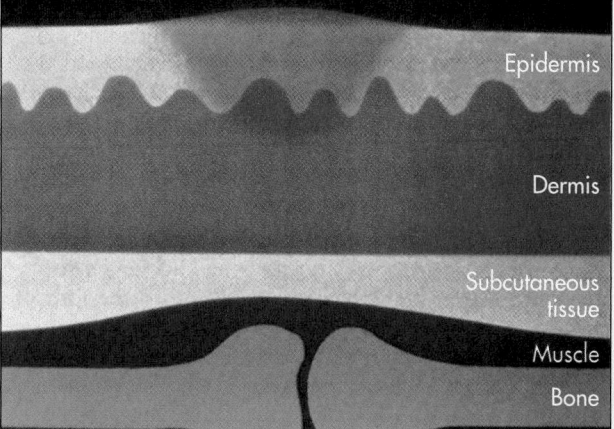

STAGE II

Partial-thickness skin loss involving epidermis, dermis, or both. The ulcer is superficial and presents clinically as an abrasion, blister, or shallow crater.

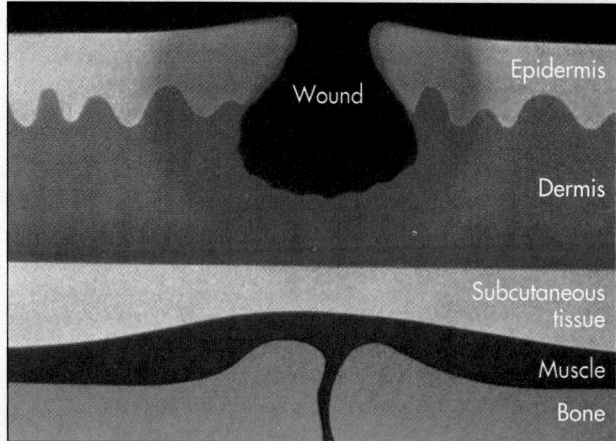

STAGE III

Full-thickness skin loss involving damage to or necrosis of subcutaneous tissue that may extend down to, but not through, underlying fascia. The ulcer presents clinically as a deep crater with or without undermining of adjacent tissue.

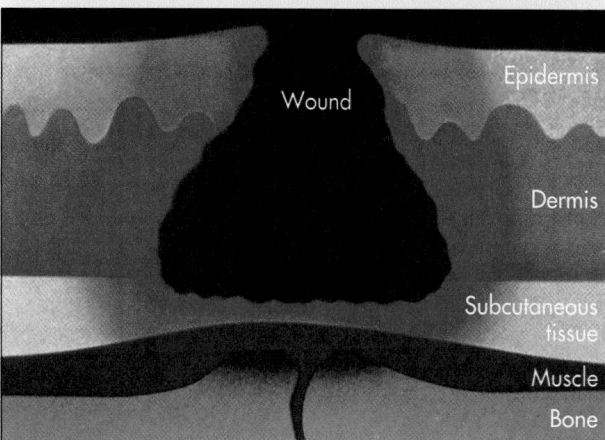

STAGE IV

Full-thickness skin loss with extensive destruction, tissue necrosis, or damage to muscle, bone, or supporting structures (e.g., tendon, joint capsule). NOTE: Undermining and sinus tracts may also be associated with stage IV pressure ulcers.

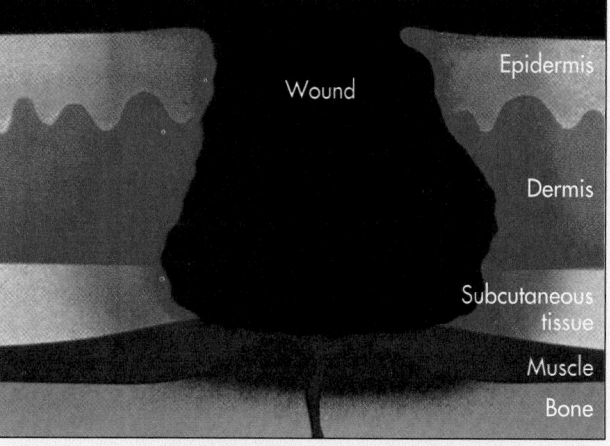

From National Pressure Ulcer Advisory Panel, 11250 Roger Bacon Drive, Suite 8, Reston, VA 20190-5202; www.nuap.org (original source); adapted and printed in table form by the Wound Ostomy and Continence Nurse Society: *Guideline For Prevention and Management of Pressure Ulcers* (2003), 4700 West Lake Avenue, Glenview, IL 60025-1485; www.wocn.org.

bed, the skin over the sacral area remains in the same place because of the resistance of the bed surface. The blood vessels in the area are stretched and may cause small-vessel thrombosis and tissue death (Bryant and Doughty, 2000). The same type of damage can occur when a patient is pulled up in the bed if the skin does not move with the patient. Prevention of shear injury includes using "lift sheets" when repositioning a patient, elevating the bed no more than 30 degrees for short periods, and using the knee gatch to interrupt the pull of gravity on the body toward the foot of the bed.

Epidermal stripping results when the epidermis is unintentionally removed with tape removal. These lesions are usually shallow and irregularly shaped; they may blister or weep after the epidermal injury. Babies are at increased risk for epidermal injury, as their epidermal bond is only 40% to 60% of that of adults. Prevention of epidermal stripping includes using no tape when possible, securing dressings with laced binders (Montgomery straps) or stretchy netting (Spandage or stockinette). Use of porous or low-tack tapes (e.g., Medipore, paper, hydrogel), alcohol-free skin sealants (No Sting Barrier), and picture framing wounds with hydrocolloid or wafer barriers (e.g., Duoderm, Coloplast, Stomahesive) and then taping on top of the barrier also will reduce epidermal stripping.

Tape is placed so that there is no tension, traction, or wrinkles on the skin. To remove tape, the nurse slowly peels the tape away while stabilizing the underlying skin. Adhesive remover may be used to break the adhesive bond but may be drying to the skin; adhesive removers should be avoided in preterm neonates, because absorption rates vary and toxicity may occur. The adhesive is removed with water to prevent absorption and irritation. Wetting the tape with water may facilitate removal.

Chemical factors can also lead to skin damage. Fecal incontinence, especially when mixed with urine; wound drainage; or gastric drainage around gastrostomy tubes can erode epidermis. The skin can very quickly progress from redness to denudement if exposure continues. Moisture barriers, gentle cleansing as soon after exposure as possible, and skin barriers can be used to prevent damage caused by chemical factors (see also Diaper Dermatitis, Chapter 30). In addition, foam dressings that wick moisture away from the skin are helpful around gastrostomy tubes and tracheostomy sites.

BATHING

Gentle, pH-balanced soaps should be used (e.g., Dove, Neutrogena, Lever 2000). Be careful of cleansers that are not pH-balanced and contain artificial color, alcohol, and lanolin because patients may have sensitivity to these cleansers. A moisturizer, if needed, is most effective when applied within minutes after the bath, after the skin has been patted dry and is still warm and moist.

Unless contraindicated, most infants and children can be bathed in a tub at the bedside, on the bed, or in a standard bathtub or shower located on the unit, which is often conveniently adapted for pediatric use. For infants and young children confined to bed, the towel method can be used. Two towels are immersed in a diluted soap solution and wrung damp. With the child lying supine on a dry towel, one damp towel is placed on top of the child and used to gently clean the body. This towel is discarded, and the child is dried and turned prone. The procedure is repeated using the second damp towel.

Infants and small children are *never* left unattended in a bathtub, and infants who are unable to sit alone are securely held with one hand during the bath. The infant's head is supported securely with one hand, or the farther arm is firmly grasped in the nurse's hand while the head rests comfortably on the nurse's wrist or arm. This hold provides secure control of the infant while the other hand is free to wash the infant's body (Fig. 22-4). Infants or children who are able to sit without assistance need only close supervision and a pad placed in the bottom of the tub to prevent slipping and loss of balance, which could result in a bumped head or submersion of the face.

Recent literature has challenged the practice of the daily bath, suggesting that it may be more harmful than helpful by stripping the skin of essential oils, disturbing pH balance and normal bacterial flora, and overdrying the skin. In hospitalized patients bathing regimens should be decided on an individual basis. Most children who feel well require little encouragement to participate in their daily care. Nurses need to use judgment regarding the amount of supervision the child requires. Some can be trusted to assume this responsibility unaided, whereas others will need someone in constant attendance. Children with mental or physical limitations and suicidal or psychotic children (who may commit bodily harm) require close supervision.

Areas that require special attention during bed baths and for children performing their own care are the ears, between skinfolds, the neck, the back, and the genital area. The genital area should be carefully cleansed and dried with particular care to skinfolds, and in uncircumcised boys, usually those older than 3 years of age, the foreskin should be gently retracted and the exposed surfaces cleansed and then the foreskin replaced. Do not attempt to retract the foreskin in newborns. If the condition of the glans indicates inadequate cleaning, such as accumulated smegma, inflammation, phimosis, or foreskin adhesions, teaching proper hygiene is indicated. In the Vietnamese and Cambodian cultures the foreskin is traditionally not retracted until adulthood (Krueger and Osborn, 1986). Older children have the tendency to avoid these areas; therefore, they may need a gentle reminder.

Children who are ill or debilitated need more extensive assistance with bathing and other aspects of hygienic care, but they should be encouraged to perform as much as they can without overtaxing their energies. Increasing involvement can be expected with improved strength and endurance. Children with limited capacity for self-care but no other contraindications benefit greatly from tub baths. They can be transported to the tub and, with the aid of lifting devices or an appropriate number of persons to assist, gain the advantages of a tub bath.

ORAL HYGIENE

Mouth care is an integral part of daily hygiene and should be continued in the hospital. Infants and debilitated children require the nurse or a family member to perform mouth care. Although young children can manage a toothbrush and should be encouraged to use it, most will need

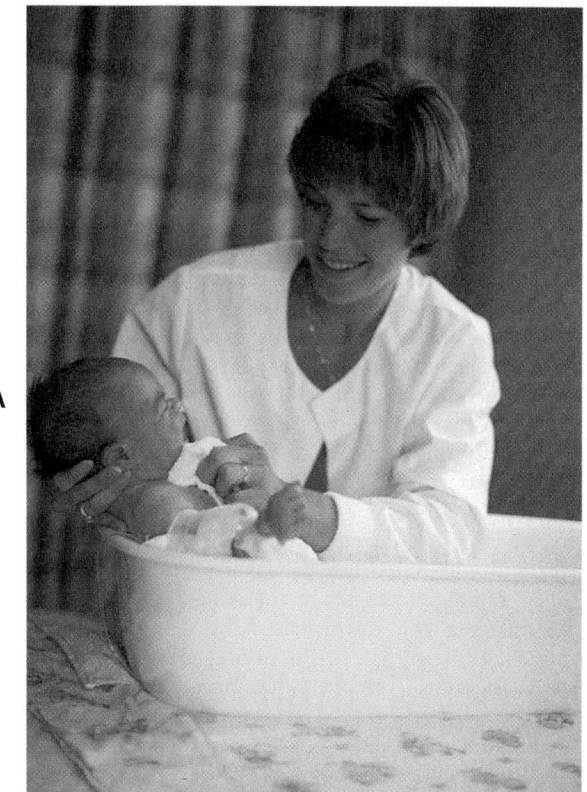
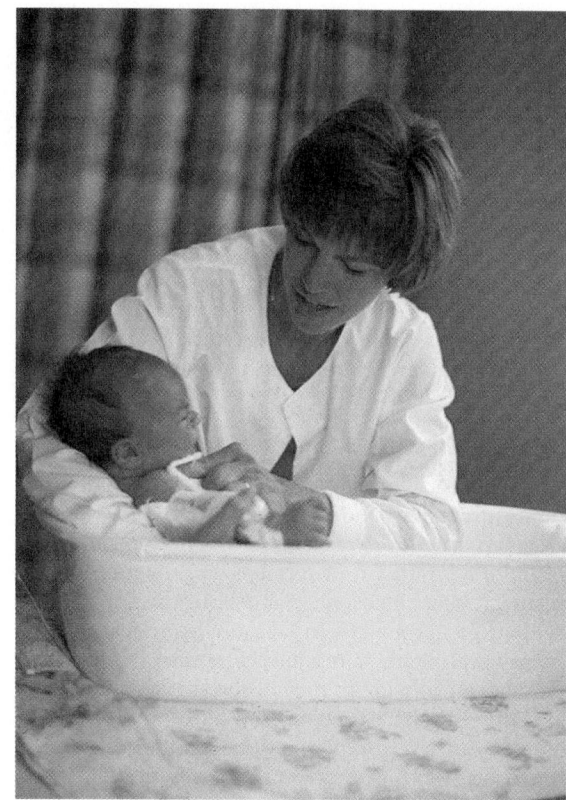

FIG. 22-4 ■ Two methods of supporting infant during tub bath. **A,** Using hand to support neck and head. **B,** Using arm to support neck and head.

assistance to perform a satisfactory job. Older children, although capable of brushing and flossing without assistance, sometimes need to be reminded that this is a part of their hygienic care. Most hospitals have equipment available for those children who do not have a toothbrush or toothpaste of their own. (See Dental Health, Chapters 10 and 12, for specific oral hygiene techniques; mouth care of children with mucosal ulcers is discussed under nursing care of the child with leukemia in Chapter 26.)

HAIR CARE

Brushing and combing hair are a part of the daily care for all persons in the hospital, including infants and children. If the child does not have a brush or comb, many hospitals provide one as part of the usual admission kit. If not, the parents should be asked to bring hair care equipment for the child's use. Both boys and girls should be helped to comb or brush their hair, or it should be done for them, at least once daily. The hair is styled for comfort and in a manner pleasing to the child and parents. A satisfactory style for girls with longer hair is French braiding, which is done by starting with three equal portions of hair from the top of the scalp; as the hair is braided, segments of hair are added at successive intervals until all the hair has been incorporated into one or more neat, head-hugging braids. The ends are firmly anchored with a coated elastic band or barrette. The hair should not be cut without parental permission, although shaving hair to provide access to a scalp vein for IV needle insertion may be necessary.

If children are hospitalized for more than a few days, the hair may need shampooing. With infants the hair may be washed during the daily bath or less frequently. For most children washing the hair and scalp once or twice weekly is sufficient unless there is an indication to wash it more frequently, such as following a high fever and profuse sweating. Some hospitals have shampoo basins, but almost any child can be conveniently transported by a gurney to an accessible sink or washbasin for shampooing. Those who are unable to be transported can receive a shampoo in their beds with adequate protection or specially adapted equipment or positioning. A convenient method involves positioning the child near the edge of the bed, placing towels under the shoulders, and draping a large plastic garbage bag at the edge of the bed with one open side under the shoulders and the other side opened away from the head so that the hair is placed inside the opening. Water can be transported in a basin or placed in a clean enema bag. The nurse should fill a clean enema bag with warm water, hang the bag from an IV pole, and use the clamp on the bag's tubing to adjust the flow of water.

Teenagers, with their normally increased oily sebaceous secretions, are particularly in need of frequent hair care and usually require more frequent shampoos. Commercial no-rinse products also may prove useful on a short-term basis.

African-American children require special hair care, and this need is frequently neglected or inadequately managed. Most standard combs are inadequate and may cause hair breakage and discomfort to the child. If a special comb with widely spaced teeth is not available on the unit, the parent can be reminded to bring a comb, if possible, for the child's use. It is also much easier to comb the hair after shampooing when it is wet. This type of hair also requires a special hair dressing or pomade, which usually has a coconut oil base. The preparation is rubbed on the hands and then transferred to the hair to make it more pliable and manageable. The child's parents should be consulted regarding the preparation they want to be used on their child's hair, and they should be asked if they can provide some for use during the child's hospitalization. Petroleum jelly should *not* be used. If braiding or plaiting the hair is desired, the hair should be damp and loosely woven. The hair tightens as it dries, which could result in tension folliculitis (Jackson, 1998).

FEEDING THE SICK CHILD

Loss of appetite is a symptom common to most childhood illnesses and is frequently the initial evidence of illness, preceding fever and other overt signs of infection. In most cases children can be permitted to determine their own need for food. Because an acute illness is usually short, the nutritional state is seldom compromised. In fact, urging foods on the sick child may precipitate nausea and vomiting and in some cases even cause an aversion to the feeding situation that can extend into the convalescent period and beyond.

Refusing to eat may also be one way children can exert power and control in an otherwise helpless situation. For young children, loss of appetite may be related to the depression of separation from their parents and their natural tendency toward negativism. Parents' concern with eating can intensify the problem. Forcing a child to eat only meets with rebellion and reinforces the behavior as a control mechanism. Parents are encouraged to relax any pressure during the period of acute illness. Although it is best to encourage high-quality nutritious foods, the child may desire foods and liquids that contain mostly empty or nonnutritional calories. Some well-tolerated foods include gelatin, clear soups, carbonated drinks, flavored ice pops, dry toast, crackers, and hard candy. Even though these substances are not nutritious, they can provide necessary fluid and calories.

Dehydration is always a hazard when children are febrile or anorexic, especially when this is accompanied by vomiting or diarrhea. An adequate fluid intake is encouraged by offering small amounts of favored fluids at frequent intervals and by offering salty foods (that increase thirst) if allowed. If diarrhea is present, high-carbohydrate liquids (e.g., carbonated beverages, gelatin, flavored ice pops) are avoided because they may aggravate the diarrhea by an osmotic effect. Also, replacing abnormal losses with plain water or undiluted broth may worsen the electrolyte imbalance. Fluids should not be forced, and the child should not be wakened from rest to take fluids. Forcing fluids may create the same difficulties as urging unwanted food. Gentle persuasion with preferred beverages will usually meet with success. Using play techniques can also be very effective (see Guidelines box).

When children are placed on special diets, such as clear liquids after surgery or during episodes of diarrhea, assessment of their intake and readiness to advance to more complex foods is essential.

GUIDELINES

Feeding the Sick Child

Take a dietary history (see Chapter 6) and use information to make eating time as much like home as possible.

Encourage parents or other family members to feed child or to be present at mealtimes.

Make mealtimes pleasant; avoid any procedures immediately before or after eating; make sure child is rested and pain free.

Serve small, frequent meals rather than three large meals or serve three meals and nutritious between-meal snacks.

Provide finger foods for young children.

Involve children in food selection and preparation whenever possible.

Serve small portions, and serve each course separately, such as soup first; followed by meat, potatoes, and vegetables; and ending with dessert. With young children, camouflage size of food by cutting meat thicker so that less appears on plate or by folding a cheese slice in half. Offer second helpings. Ensure a variety of foods, textures, and colors.

Provide food selections that are favorites of most children, such as peanut butter–and-jelly sandwiches, hot dogs, hamburgers, macaroni and cheese, pizza, spaghetti, tacos, fried chicken, corn on the cob, and fruit yogurt.

Avoid foods that are highly seasoned, have strong odors, are served hot, or are all mixed together, unless typical of cultural practices.

Provide fluid selections that are favorites of most children, such as fruit punch, cola, ginger ale, sweetened tea, flavored ice pops, sherbet, ice cream, milk and milkshakes, eggnog, pudding, gelatin, clear broth, or creamed soups.

Offer nutritious snacks, such as frozen yogurt or pudding, ice cream, oatmeal or peanut butter cookies, hot cocoa, cheese slices, pieces of raw vegetable or fruit, and dried fruit or cereal.

Make food attractive and different; for example:
Serve a "picnic lunch" in a paper bag.
Pack food in a Chinese-food container; decorate container.
Put a "face" or a "flower" on a hamburger or sandwich with pieces of vegetable.
Use a cookie cutter to shape a sandwich.
Serve pudding, yogurt, or juice frozen as an ice pop.
Make Slurpies or snow cones by pouring flavored syrup on crushed ice.
Add food coloring to water or milk.
Serve fluids through brightly colored or unusually shaped straws.
Make "bowtie" sandwiches by cutting them in triangles and placing two points together.
Slice sandwiches into "fingers."
Grate mounds of cheese.
Cut apples horizontally to make circles.
Put a banana on a hot dog bun and spread with peanut butter.
Break uncooked spaghetti into toothpick lengths and skewer cheese, cold meat, vegetables, or fruit chunks.

Praise children for what they do eat.

Do not punish children for not eating by removing their dessert or putting them to bed.

Once the child is feeling better, the appetite usually begins to improve. It is best to take advantage of any hungry period by serving high-quality foods and snacks. If the child still refuses to eat, nutritious fluids, such as prepared breakfast drinks, should be encouraged.

The admission nutritional assessment provides information pertinent to the patient's dietary preferences and cultural or religious preference. It is more advantageous to work with preferred food choices than with selections that children rarely eat. A number of creative approaches to food preparation can increase the child's interest in eating (see Guidelines box).

Regardless of the type of diet, charting of the amount consumed is an important nursing responsibility. Descriptions need to be detailed and accurate, such as "4 ounces of orange juice, one pancake, no bacon, and 8 ounces of milk." Comments such as "ate well" or "ate poorly" are inadequate. Charting the percentage of the meal eaten is also inadequate unless food is measured before serving.

If parents are involved in the child's care, they are encouraged to keep a list of everything eaten. Using a premeasured cup for fluids ensures a more accurate estimate of intake. A comparison of the intake at each meal can isolate food deficiencies, such as insufficient intake of meat or vegetables. Behaviors associated with mealtime also identify possible factors influencing appetite. For example, the observation that "Child eats well when with other children but plays with food if left alone in room" helps the nurse plan mealtime activities that stimulate the appetite.

CONTROLLING ELEVATED TEMPERATURES

An elevated temperature, most frequently from fever but occasionally caused by hyperthermia, is one of the most common symptoms of illness in children. This manifestation is frequently misunderstood and of great, but often unnecessary, concern to parents. To facilitate an understanding of fever, the following terms are defined:

Set point—The temperature around which body temperature is regulated by a thermostat-like mechanism in the hypothalamus

Fever—An elevation in set point such that body temperature is regulated at a higher level; may be arbitrarily defined as temperature higher than 38° C (100° F)

Hyperthermia—A situation in which body temperature exceeds the set point, which usually results from the body or external conditions creating more heat than the body can eliminate, such as in heatstroke, aspirin toxicity, seizures, or hyperthyroidism

Body temperature is regulated by a thermostat-like mechanism in the hypothalamus. This mechanism receives input from centrally and peripherally located receptors. When temperature changes occur, these receptors relay the information to the thermostat, which either increases or decreases heat production to maintain a constant set point temperature. During an infection, however, pyrogenic substances cause an increase in the body's normal set point, a process that is mediated by prostaglandins. Consequently, the hypothalamus increases heat production until the core (internal) temperature reaches the new set point (Connell, 1997).

Most fevers are of brief duration with limited consequences and are viral in nature. When fever is caused by bacteria, endotoxins are produced that activate the inflammatory process and produce fever (Rote, Huether, and McCance, 2000). In addition, fever probably plays a role in enhancing the development of both specific and nonspecific immunity and in aiding recovery and survival from infection. Contrary to popular belief, neither the rise in temperature nor its response to antipyretics indicates the severity or etiology of infection, which casts doubt on the value of using fever as a diagnostic or prognostic indicator.

Measures to Reduce Elevated Temperature

Treatment of elevated temperature depends on whether it is caused by a fever or hyperthermia. Because the set point is normal in hyperthermia but increased in fever, different approaches must be used to lower body temperature successfully.

Fever.   The principal reason for treating fever is the relief of discomfort; there is no specific degree of fever that requires treatment. Relief measures include pharmacologic or environmental intervention. The most effective intervention is the use of antipyretics to lower the set point.

Antipyretic drugs include acetaminophen, aspirin, and nonsteroidal antiinflammatory drugs (NSAIDs). Acetaminophen is the preferred drug; aspirin should *not* be given to children because of the association between aspirin use in children with influenza virus or chickenpox and Reye syndrome. One nonprescription NSAID, ibuprofen, is approved for fever reduction in children as young as 6 months of age (Table 22-2). Dosage is based on the initial temperature level: 5 mg/kg of body weight for temperatures less than 39.1° C (102.5° F) or 10 mg/kg for temperatures greater than 39.1° C. The recommended dosage for pain is 10 mg/kg every 6 to 8 hours, and the recommended maximum daily dose for pain and fever is 40 mg/kg. The duration of fever reduction is generally 6 to 8 hours and is longer with the higher dose. Table 22-3 lists the recommended dosages of acetaminophen. It may be given every 4 hours but no more than five times in 24 hours. Because body temperature normally decreases at night, three to four doses in 24 hours are usually sufficient to control most fevers. The temperature is usually retaken 30 minutes after the antipyretic is given to assess its effect but should not be

TABLE 22-2 ■ Dosage Recommendations for Ibuprofen* (Children's Motrin)

WEIGHT						
(pounds)	(kilograms)	AGE	ORAL DROPS (50 mg/1.25 mL)	SUSPENSION (100 mg/5 mL)	CHEWABLE TABLETS (50 mg†)	CAPLETS (100 mg)
12-17	5.4-7.7	6-11 months	1 dropper	0.25 tsp		
18-23	8.2-10.4	12-23 months	1.5 droppers	0.5 tsp		
24-35	10.9-15.9	2-3 years		1 tsp	2	1
36-47	16.3-21.3	4-5 years		1.5 tsp	3	1.5
48-59	21.8-26.8	6-8 years		2 tsp	4	2
60-71	27.2-32.2	9-10 years		2.5 tsp	5	2.5
72-95	32.7-43.1	11 years		3 tsp	6	3

Modified from *Physician's desk reference*, Monvale, NJ, 2001, Medical Economics.
*Dosages based on fever <39.2° C using 5 mg/kg. For fever = 39.2° C may use 10 mg/kg.
Doses administered every 6 to 8 hours. Another nonprescription ibuprofen is Children's Advil.
†Also available in 100-mg tablets.

TABLE 22-3 ■ Dosage Recommendations for Acetaminophen (Tylenol)*

AGE	WEIGHT (pounds)	DOSE (mg)
Less than 3 months	6-11	40
4-11 months	12-17	80
12-23 months	18-23	120
2-3 years	24-35	160
4-5 years	36-47	240
6-8 years	48-59	320
9-10 years	60-71	400
11 years	72-95	480
12 years and above	96+	640

*Doses should be administered four or five times daily but should not exceed five doses in 24 hours.

repeatedly measured; the child's level of discomfort is the best indication for continued treatment.

> **NURSING ALERT**
>
> Acetaminophen is an effective antipyretic and analgesic when administered as recommended. However, it is important to recognize its full toxic potential in both acute overdose and excessive therapeutic administration. Several cases of acetaminophen hepatotoxicity in children who received overdoses of the drug as part of therapeutic administration have been reported (Kearns, Leeder, and Wasserman, 1998).

Environmental measures to reduce fever may be used if tolerated by the child and if they do not induce shivering. Shivering is the body's way of maintaining the elevated set point by producing heat. Compensatory shivering greatly increases metabolic requirements above those already caused by the fever.

> **NURSING ALERT**
>
> Treatment of shivering is directed at modifying or interfering with the rate of heat loss by warming the body, especially on extremities.

Traditional cooling measures, such as wearing minimum clothing, exposing the skin to the air, reducing room temperature, increasing air circulation, and applying cool, moist compresses to the skin (e.g., the forehead), are effective if employed approximately 1 hour *after* an antipyretic is given so that the set point is lowered. Cooling procedures such as sponging or tepid baths are ineffective in treating febrile children either when used alone or in combination with antipyretics, and they cause considerable discomfort (Sharber, 1997). These measures are used for hyperthermia.

Seizures associated with a fever occur in 3% to 4% of all children, usually those 3 months to 5 years of age. Although most children never have febrile seizures after the first occurrence, a younger age at onset and a family history of febrile seizures are associated with recurring episodes. For children who have febrile seizures, administration of antipyretics does not prevent recurrences (El-Radhi and Barry, 2003; Shinnar and others, 2001). There is little evidence to support the use of antipyretic drugs to prevent febrile seizures; nursing interventions should focus on ways in which care and comfort can be provided during a febrile illness (Purssell, 2000).

Hyperthermia. Unlike with fever, antipyretics are of no value in hyperthermia, because the set point is already normal. Consequently, cooling measures are used. Cool applications to the skin help to reduce the core temperature. Cooled blood from the skin surface is conducted to inner organs and tissues, and warm blood is circulated to the surface, where it is cooled and recirculated. The surface blood vessels dilate as the body attempts to dissipate heat to the environment and facilitate this cooling process.

Commercial cooling devices, such as cooling blankets or mattresses, are available to reduce body temperature. They are placed on the bed and covered with a sheet or lightweight blanket. Frequent temperature monitoring is essential to prevent excessive cooling of the body.

Traditionally, cool compresses have been used to decrease high temperature. However, no particular temperature of water is agreed on as optimal. For tepid tub baths it is usually best to start with warm water and gradually add cool water until the desired water temperature of 37° C

(98.6° F) is reached to accustom the child to the lower water temperature. Generally, the temperature of the water only has to be 1° to 2° (usually a warm temperature) less than the child's temperature to be effective (Kinmonth, Fulton, and Campbell, 1992). The child is placed directly in the tub of tepid water for 20 to 30 minutes while water is gently squeezed from a washcloth over the back and chest or gently sprayed over the body from a sprayer. In the bed or crib, cool washcloths or towels are used, exposing only one area of the body at a time. The sponging is continued for approximately 30 minutes.

After the tub or sponge bath, the child is dried and dressed in lightweight pajamas, a nightgown, or a diaper and placed in a dry bed. The temperature is retaken 30 minutes after the tub bath or sponge bath. The child is dried by gently rubbing the skin surface with a towel to stimulate circulation. The tub or sponge bath should not be continued or restarted until the skin surface is warm or if the child feels chilled. Chilling causes vasoconstriction, which defeats the purpose of the cool applications. In this condition, little blood is carried to the skin surface; the blood remains primarily in the viscera to become heated.

Whether a temperature elevation in the critically ill child is caused by fever or hyperthermia, it should be treated more aggressively. The metabolic rate increases 10% for every 1° C increase in temperature and three to five times during shivering, increasing oxygen, fluid, and caloric requirements. If the child's cardiovascular or neurologic system is already compromised, these increased needs are especially hazardous. In all children with elevated temperature, attention to adequate hydration is essential. Most children's needs can be met through additional oral fluids.

FAMILY TEACHING AND HOME CARE

Nurses have a unique opportunity for teaching the family about health care practices while the child is hospitalized. Although most children have learned self-care and hygiene in the home or at school, many have not. For some young children, this is their first introduction to the use of a toothbrush. Much health teaching can be accomplished even when the child is hospitalized for only a short time. The daily bath, handwashing before meals and after bowel and bladder evacuation, and conscientious dental hygiene are taught by example during routine care. Clean hair, nails, and clothing, as well as good grooming, are emphasized as being essential to a pleasing appearance. Positive reinforcement of good hygiene practices helps to create a positive body image, promote the development of self-esteem, and prevent health problems (e.g., teaching girls to wipe the genital area from front to back after toileting).

Although sick children's appetites may be poor and not characteristic of their home eating habits, the hospital stay provides numerous opportunities for nurses to assess the family's knowledge of good nutrition and to implement teaching as needed to improve nutritional intake.

Fever is one of the most common problems in pediatrics for which parents seek health care. Parental anxiety levels are increased with temperature elevation and its management (Liebman and Barnsteiner, 2001). Parents also need to know that sponging is indicated for elevated temperatures from hyperthermia rather than fever and that ice water and alcohol are inappropriate, potentially dangerous, solutions (Axelrod, 2000). Parents should know how to take the child's temperature and read the thermometer accurately, and should have guidelines for seeking professional care (see Family Home Care box). Some of the newer temperature-measuring devices, such as tympanic membrane sensors, plastic strips, or digital thermometers, may be better suited for home use, because many parents are unable to read a mercury thermometer or calculate the correct decimal point (see Temperature, Chapter 7).

If the use of acetaminophen and ibuprofen is indicated, the parents need instruction in administering the drug. It is important to emphasize accuracy in both the amount of drug given and the time intervals at which the drug is administered. Because many forms of acetaminophen are available, the nurse must be certain of the type being used in the home when discussing dosage. For example, the chewable tablets come in *two* strengths (80 and 160 mg), and the specially coated, swallowable tablets for older children are 160 mg only. The nurse should alert the parents to this because the tablets for older children may contain *twice* the amount of drug as the lower-dose chewable ones. If parents switch from the infant drops to the elixir, they are cautioned against using the dropper to measure the elixir, which is much less concentrated than the drops. Also, as children grow, their dosage needs to be recalculated.

SAFETY

Safety is an essential component of any patient's care, but children have special characteristics that require an even greater concern for safety. Because small children are separated from their usual environment and do not possess the capacity for abstract thinking and reasoning, it is the responsibility of everyone who comes in contact with them to maintain protective measures throughout their hospital stay. Nurses need to understand the age level at which each child is operating and plan for safety accordingly.

FAMILY HOME CARE

The Child With Fever

CALL THE OFFICE IMMEDIATEILY IF:
Your child is younger than 3 months old.
The fever is over 40.6° C (105° F).
Your child looks or acts very sick.

CALL WITHIN 24 HOURS IF:
Your child is 3 to 6 months old (unless the fever is due to a diphtheria-pertussis-tetanus [DPT] shot).
The fever is between 40° and 40.6° C (104° and 105° F), especially if your child is younger than 2 years old.
Your child has had a fever for more than 24 hours without an obvious cause or location of infection.
Your child has had a fever for more than 3 days.
The fever went away for more than 24 hours and then returned.
You have other concerns or questions.

Modified from Schmitt BD: *Instructions for pediatric patients,* ed 2, Philadelphia, 1999, WB Saunders.

Name bands, a part of hospital safety practices, are particularly important for the pediatric age-group. Infants and unconscious patients are unable to tell or respond to their names. Toddlers may answer to any name or to a nickname only. Older children may exchange places, give an erroneous name, or choose not to respond to their own names as a form of joke, unaware of the hazards of such practices.

INFECTION CONTROL

The use of medical asepsis and appropriate barrier precautions to reduce the risk of *nosocomial* (hospital-acquired) infections is essential in caring for children. Children are infected frequently with organisms, such as varicella (chickenpox), that are transmissible and may be dangerous to others, especially immunocompromised patients. In addition, children may not have developed good hygiene habits, such as handwashing after toileting. Young children are especially at risk for infection because of their high oral activity. Children in diapers present infection risks if caregivers do not practice meticulous cleaning and disposal techniques.

To assist hospitals in maintaining up-to-date isolation practices, the **Centers for Disease Control and Prevention (CDC)** and the **Hospital Infection Control Practices Advisory Committee (HICPAC)** have revised the "CDC Guideline for Isolation Precautions in Hospitals," which was published in 1983. The guideline was revised to meet the following objectives: (1) to be epidemiologically sound; (2) to recognize the importance of all body fluids, secretions, and excretions in the transmission of nosocomial pathogens; (3) to contain adequate precautions for infections transmitted by the airborne, droplet, and contact routes of transmission; (4) to be as simple and user friendly as possible; and (5) to use new terms to avoid confusion with existing infection control and isolation systems.*

The revised guideline contains two levels of precautions. In the first, and most important, level are those precautions designed for the care of all patients in hospitals regardless of their diagnosis or presumed infection status. Implementation of these "standard precautions" is the primary strategy for successful nosocomial infection control. In the second level are precautions designed only for the care of specified patients. These additional "transmission-based precautions" are used for patients known or suspected to be infected or colonized with epidemiologically important pathogens that can be transmitted by airborne or droplet transmission or by contact with dry skin or contaminated surfaces.

Standard precautions synthesize the major features of universal (blood and body fluid) precautions (UP) (designed to reduce the risk of transmission of blood-borne pathogens) and body substance isolation (BSI) (designed to reduce the risk of transmission of pathogens from moist body substances). Standard precautions involve the use of *barrier protection,* such as gloves, goggles, gown, or mask, to prevent contamination from (1) blood; (2) all body fluids, secretions, and excretions *except sweat,* regardless of whether or not they contain visible blood; (3) nonintact

skin; and (4) mucous membranes. Standard precautions are designed to reduce the risk of transmission of microorganisms from both recognized and unrecognized sources of infection in hospitals.

Transmission-based precautions are designed for patients documented or suspected to be infected or colonized with highly transmissible or epidemiologically important pathogens for which additional precautions beyond standard precautions are needed to interrupt transmission in hospitals. There are three types of transmission-based precautions: airborne precautions, droplet precautions, and contact precautions. They may be combined for diseases that have multiple routes of transmission (Box 22-8). When used either singularly or in combination, they are to be used in addition to standard precautions.

Airborne precautions are designed to reduce the risk of airborne transmission of infectious agents. Airborne transmission occurs by dissemination of either airborne droplet nuclei (small-particle residue [5 μm or smaller in size] of evaporated droplets that may remain suspended in the air for long periods) or dust particles containing the infectious agent. Microorganisms carried in this manner can be dispersed widely by air currents and may become inhaled by or deposited on a susceptible host within the same room or over a longer distance from the source patient, depending on environmental factors; therefore, *special air handling* and *ventilation* are required to prevent airborne transmission. Airborne precautions apply to patients known or suspected to be infected with epidemiologically important pathogens that can be transmitted by the airborne route. Examples of such illnesses include measles, varicella (chickenpox), and tuberculosis.

Droplet precautions are designed to reduce the risk of droplet transmission of infectious agents. Droplet transmission involves contact of the conjunctivae or the mucous membranes of the nose or mouth of a susceptible person with large-particle droplets (larger than 5 μm in size) containing microorganisms generated from a person who has a clinical disease or who is a carrier of the microorganism. Droplets are generated from the source person primarily during coughing, sneezing, or talking and during the performance of certain procedures such as suctioning and bronchoscopy. Transmission via large-particle droplets requires close contact between source and recipient persons, because droplets do not remain suspended in the air and generally travel only short distances, usually 3 feet or less, through the air. Special air handling and ventilation are not required to prevent droplet transmission. Droplet precautions apply to any patient known or suspected to be infected with epidemiologically important pathogens that can be transmitted by infectious droplets (see Box 22-8).

Contact precautions are designed to reduce the risk of transmission of epidemiologically important microorganisms by direct or indirect contact. *Direct-contact transmission* involves a direct body surface–to–body surface contact and physical transfer of microorganisms to a susceptible host from an infected or colonized person, such as occurs when personnel turn patients, bathe patients, or perform other patient care activities that require physical contact. Direct-contact transmission also can occur between two patients (e.g., by hand contact), with one serving as the source

---

*This section is modified from Garner JS: What's in a name? The evolution of universal precautions to standard precautions: A guide to the latest recommendations in isolation practices, *Today's Surg Nurse* 19(1):14-21, 1997.

BOX 22-8 ■ Summary of Types of Precautions and Patients Requiring Them

STANDARD PRECAUTIONS
Use standard precautions for the care of all patients.

AIRBORNE PRECAUTIONS
In addition to standard precautions, use airborne precautions for patients known or suspected to have serious illnesses transmitted by airborne droplet nuclei. Examples of such illnesses include measles, varicella (including disseminated zoster), and tuberculosis.

DROPLET PRECAUTIONS
In addition to standard precautions, use droplet precautions for patients known or suspected to have serious illnesses transmitted by large-particle droplets. Examples of such illnesses include the following:
Invasive *Haemophilus influenzae* type b disease, including meningitis, pneumonia, epiglottitis, and sepsis
Invasive *Neisseria meningitidis* disease, including meningitis, pneumonia, and sepsis
Other serious bacterial respiratory infections spread by droplet transmission, including diphtheria (pharyngeal), mycoplasmal pneumonia, pertussis, pneumonic plague, streptococcal pharyngitis, pneumonia, or scarlet fever in infants and young children
Serious viral infections spread by droplet transmission including adenovirus, influenza, mumps, parvovirus B19, rubella

CONTACT PRECAUTIONS
In addition to standard precautions, use contact precautions for patients known or suspected to have serious illnesses easily transmitted by direct patient contact or by contact with items in the patient's environment. Examples of such illnesses include the following:
Gastrointestinal, respiratory, skin, or wound infections or colonization with multidrug-resistant bacteria judged by the infection control program, based on current state, regional, or national recommendations, to be of special clinical and epidemiologic significance
Enteric infections with a low infectious dose or prolonged environmental survival, including *Clostridium difficile*. For diapered or incontinent patients: enterohemorrhagic *Escherichia coli* O157:H7, *Shigella* sp., hepatitis A, or rotavirus
Respiratory syncytial virus, parainfluenza virus, or enteroviral infections in infants and young children
Skin infections that are highly contagious or that may occur on dry skin, including diphtheria (cutaneous), herpes simplex virus (neonatal or mucocutaneous), impetigo, major (noncontained) abscesses, cellulitis or decubiti, pediculosis, scabies, staphylococcal furunculosis in infants and young children, zoster (disseminated or in the immunocompromised host)
Viral/hemorrhagic conjunctivitis
Viral hemorrhagic infections (Ebola, Lassa, or Marburg)

From Garner JS: Guidelines for isolation precautions in hospitals, *Infect Control Hosp Epidemiol* 17(1):66, 1996.

of infectious microorganisms and the other as a susceptible host. *Indirect-contact transmission* involves contact of a susceptible host with a contaminated intermediate object, usually inanimate, in the patient's environment (e.g., a contaminated instrument or contaminated hands that are not washed and gloves that are not changed between patients). Contact precautions apply to specified patients known or

suspected to be infected or colonized (presence of microorganism in or on the patient but without clinical signs and symptoms of infection) with epidemiologically important microorganisms that can be transmitted by direct or indirect contact.

> **!NURSING ALERT**
>
> **The most common piece of medical equipment, the stethoscope, can be a potent source of harmful microorganisms and nosocomial infections. One study found that 80% of 200 stethoscopes were contaminated with at least one microbe (Eckler, 1997).**

Nurses caring for young children are frequently in contact with body substances, especially urine, feces, and vomitus. Nurses need to exercise judgment for those situations when gloves, gowns, or masks are necessary. For example, gloves and possibly gowns should be worn for changing diapers when there are loose or explosive stools. Otherwise, the plastic lining of disposable diapers provides a sufficient barrier between the hands and body substances. The type of diaper may be an important aspect of infection control. Superabsorbent disposable diapers with elastic legs contain urine and feces better than cloth diapering systems, and their use can reduce fecal contamination in the environment (Kubiak and others, 1993).

Antimicrobial-resistant organisms are causing increasing numbers of nonsocial infections. Nearly 70% of nonsocial infections can be attributed to seven pathogens: *Staphylococcus aureus*, coagulase-negative staphylococci, and enterococci; and the gram-negative organisms *Escherichia coli*, *Pseudomonas aerations*, *Enterobacter*, and *Klebsiella pneumoniae*. The main mode of transmission is patient to patient via the health care provider (Russell, 1999).

> **!NURSING ALERT**
>
> **Handwashing is the most critical infection-control practice.**

During feedings, gowns should be worn if the child is likely to vomit or spit up, which often occurs during burping. When gloves are worn, the hands are washed thoroughly after removing the gloves, because both latex and vinyl gloves fail to provide complete protection.

Another essential practice of infection control is that all needles (uncapped and unbroken) are disposed of in a rigid, puncture-resistant container located near the site of use. Consequently, these containers are installed in patients' rooms. Because children are naturally curious, extra attention is needed in selecting a suitable type of container and a location that discourages access to the disposed needles (Fig. 22-5). The use of needleless systems allow secure syringe or IV tubing attachment to vascular access devices without the risk of needle-stick injury to the child or nurse. These devices also help maintain IV line integrity (see p. 765).

ENVIRONMENTAL FACTORS

All of the environmental safety measures in operation for the protection of adults apply to children as well and include good illumination, floors clear of fluid or objects that might contribute to falls, and nonskid surfaces in showers and tubs. Electrical equipment, which is maintained in good working order,

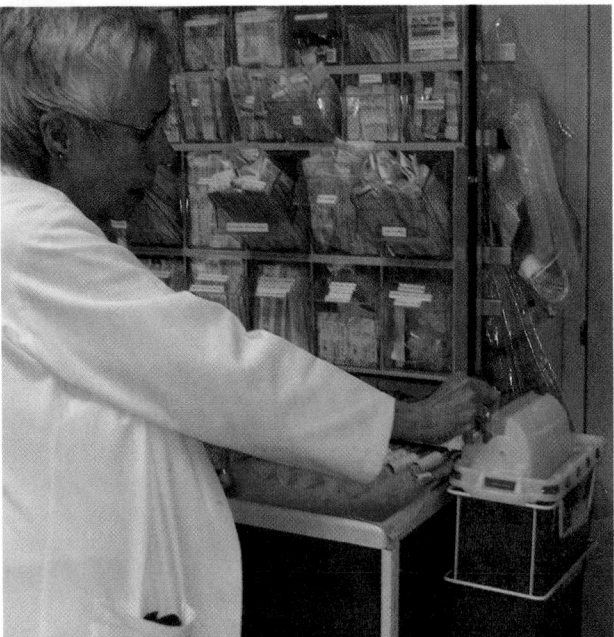

FIG. 22-5 ■ To prevent needle-stick injuries, used needles (and other sharp instruments) are not capped or broken and are disposed of in a rigid, puncture-resistant container located near the site of use. Note placement of the container to prevent children's access to the contents.

is operated only by personnel familiar with its use and is not in contact with moisture or near tubs, where it could prove to be a shock hazard. Beds of ambulatory patients are locked in place and at a height that allows easy access to the floor. A special hazard for children is the danger of entrapment under an electronically controlled bed when it is activated to descend. Staff members should practice proper care and disposal of breakable items such as thermometers and bottles and small items such as syringe caps or needle covers. All staff members should be familiar with the area-specific fire plan.

All windows should be securely screened, and elevators and stairways made safe. Ideally, electrical outlets should be provided with covers to prevent burns in small children, whose exploratory activities may extend to inserting objects into the small openings. Bathwater is carefully checked before placing the child in it, and children must never be left alone in a bathtub. Infants are helpless in water, and small children (and some older ones) may turn on the hot water faucet and be severely burned.

Furniture is safest when it is scaled to the child's proportions, is sturdy, and is well-balanced to prevent its being easily tipped over. Infants and small children must be securely strapped into infant seats, feeding chairs, and strollers. Baby walkers should be discouraged because they provide access to hazards, resulting in burns, falls, and poisonings. Infants, young children, and those who are weak, paralyzed, agitated, confused, sedated, or cognitively impaired are never left unattended on treatment tables, on scales, or in treatment areas. Even premature infants are capable of surprising mobility; therefore, portholes in incubators must be securely fastened when not in use. Beds of ambulatory patients should remain locked in place and at a height that allows easy access to the floor.

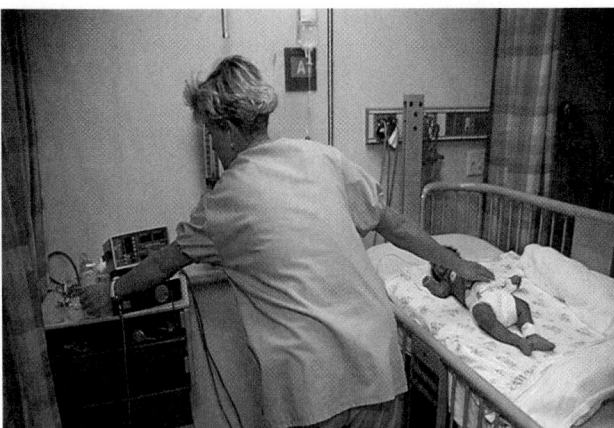

FIG. 22-6 ■ Nurse maintains hand contact when back is turned.

Crib sides should be elevated and fastened securely unless an adult is at the bedside. It is safer to leave crib sides up, regardless of the child's ability to get out and even when the crib is unoccupied, to remove the child's temptation to climb in. Anyone attending an infant or small child in a crib with the sides down should never turn away without maintaining hand contact with the child; that is, one hand should be kept on the child's back or abdomen to prevent the child from rolling, crawling, or jumping from the open crib (Fig. 22-6). A child who is apt to or has demonstrated the inclination to climb over the sides of the crib is safest when placed in a specially constructed crib with a cover. Cribs are not placed within reach of heating units, appliances, dangling cords, or other objects that can be grabbed by curious hands, and toys are not tied to or across crib rails once children are old enough to reach them.

Toys. Toys play a vital role in the everyday life of children, and they are no less important in the hospital setting. However, nurses are responsible for assessing the safety of toys brought to the hospital by well-meaning parents and friends. Toys and gifts should be appropriate to the child's age, condition, and treatment. For example, if the child is in an oxygen tent, electrical or friction toys cannot be placed in the tent. Toys are inspected to make certain that they are nonallergenic, washable, and unbreakable and that they have no small, removable parts that can be aspirated or swallowed or that can in other ways inflict injury to a child. Latex balloons pose a serious threat to children of all ages. If the balloon breaks, a child may put a piece of the latex in his or her mouth. If it is aspirated or swallowed, the latex piece is difficult to remove, resulting in choking. Latex balloons should *never* be permitted in the hospital setting.

> **! NURSING ALERT**
>
> Plants and flowers harbor gram-negative bacteria and molds that may be a risk to the immunocompromised child. These items may also pose the danger of poisoning to curious toddlers.

LIMIT SETTING

Setting limits is essential to a child's safety. Children must understand where they are permitted to go and what they are permitted to do in the hospital. These limitations should

A   **B**   **C**

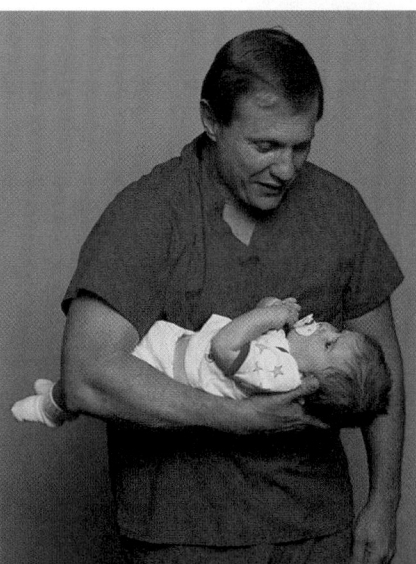 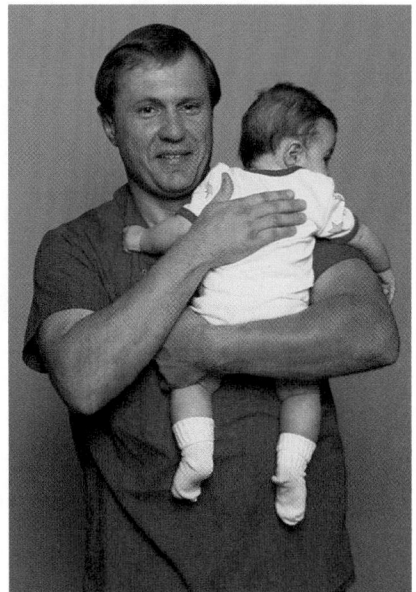

FIG. 22-7 ■ Transporting infants, **A,** Infant's thigh firmly grasped in nurse's hand. **B,** Football hold. **C,** Back supported.

be made clear to them, consistently enforced, and repeated as frequently as necessary to make certain that they are understood. The nurse is responsible for a child's whereabouts at all times. Children can easily wander off unnoticed, and their access to tubs, laundry chutes, medication rooms and carts, and elevators must be prevented. Normally active older children often become restless when their activity is restricted and may resort to pillow fights, water fights, and other rough play that might endanger the safety of the involved children or other children, staff, or visitors. Children in the hospital require supervision, and appropriate tension-reducing activities can be planned and supervised by nurses or by the child-life therapist. A useful discipline technique is time-out (see Limit Setting and Discipline, Chapter 3).

TRANSPORTING INFANTS AND CHILDREN

In the course of a hospital stay, infants and children usually need to be transported within the unit and to areas outside the pediatric unit. Infants and small children can be carried for short distances within the unit, but for more extended trips the child should be securely transported in a suitable conveyance.

Small infants can be held or carried in the horizontal position with the back supported and the thigh grasped firmly by the carrying arm (Fig. 22-7, *A*). In the football hold, the infant is carried on the nurse's arm with the head supported by the hand and the body held securely between the nurse's body and elbow (Fig. 22-7, *B*). Both of these holds leave the nurse's other arm free for activity. The infant can be held in the upright position with the buttocks on the nurse's forearm and the front of the body resting against the nurse's chest. The infant's head and shoulders are supported by the nurse's other arm to allow for any sudden movement by the infant (Fig. 22-7, *C*). Older infants are able to hold their heads erect but can still make sudden movements.

Infants can be transported to other areas, such as the radiography department, in their bassinets or cribs. Baby car-

riages are sometimes used for infants who are not likely to stand up. Strollers and wheeled feeding chairs or tables are also convenient transporters in some situations, such as trips to the playroom or nurse's station.

The method of transporting children is determined by their age, condition, and destination. Most older children are safe in wheelchairs or on stretchers. A younger child can be transported in a crib, on a stretcher, in a wagon with raised sides, or in a wheelchair with a safety belt. Stretchers should be equipped with high sides and a safety belt, both of which are secured during transport.

RESTRAINING METHODS AND THERAPEUTIC HUGGING

Sometimes restraining methods and therapeutic hugging are common practices in nursing to ensure a child's safety or comfort, facilitate examination, and aid in performing diagnostic tests and therapeutic procedures. *Therapeutic hugging* is the use of a secure, comfortable, temporary holding position that provides close physical contact with the parent or caregiver (see Fig. 22-8).

Nurses need to assess whether or not restraints are needed. Restraints can often be avoided with adequate preparation of the child, parental or staff supervision of the child, and adequate protection of a vulnerable site, such as an infusion device. The nurse needs to take into account the child's development, mental status, potential threat to others or self, and safety. The Joint Commission on Accreditation of Healthcare Organizations (JCAHO) points to the need for a physician's order before application of restraint. However, alternative approaches to restraint must be attempted before seeking a physician's order for restraint (Selekman and Snyder, 1996). Therefore alternative measures to using restraints should be a careful consideration of the nurse. Creative approaches may make physical restraint unnecessary. For example, a young child might be brought

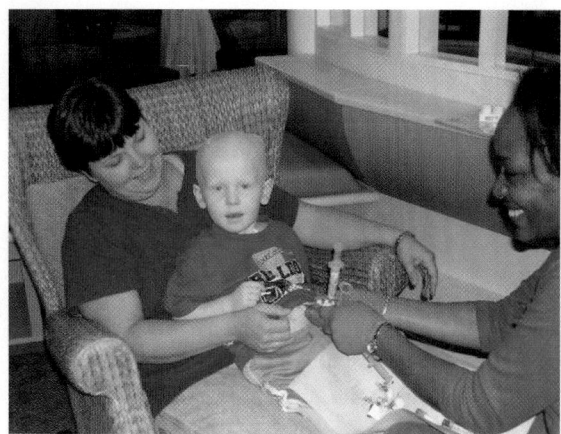

FIG. 22-8 ■ Therapeutic hugging by a parent.

to the nurses' station for observation and stimulation when parents are not present.

When a child must be restrained, it is important to explain to the child the reason for the restraint. This information should be repeated as often as needed to gain cooperation. Have the child verbalize understanding of the need for restraint. Explain how the child can help (i.e., "Your job is to keep your arm as still as a tree"). Most important, reassure the child that the restraint is not a punishment.

Parents need to know the purpose of restraints, how to remove and reapply them, and the signs of complications from their use. Document parental consent for restraints. Sometime parents are upset when their child must be restrained and need to understand how they can help. Explain ways in which they can help to ensure maximal benefit and minimal stress (i.e., have the parent emotionally support the child by staying near the child). Position the parent at the head of the bed (provide a chair for the parent) so that the parent can soothe or calm the child by talking softly, singing, or stroking the child's skin.

After the decision is made that some restraint is necessary, it must be determined what type of restraint should be applied. For example, arm boards are less restrictive than four-point extremity restraints. Using less restrictive restraints is often possible by gaining the cooperation of the child and parents. It is the nurse's responsibility to select the most appropriate and least restrictive type of restraint.

Restraining devices are not without risk and must be checked and documented every 1 to 2 hours to ensure that they are accomplishing their purpose; that they are applied correctly; and that they do not impair circulation, sensation, or skin integrity. Restraints with ties must be secured to the bed or crib frame, not the siderails.

Selekman and Snyder (1997) recommend appropriate nursing interventions for the child who is restrained. Parental participation is always encouraged. These include, but are not limited to, the following:

- Remove and reapply restraints periodically.
- Offer comfort measures; use "therapeutic hugging" rather than mechanical restraint.
- Raise head of bed 30 degrees unless contraindicated.
- Provide range of motion as appropriate.
- Offer food, fluids, and toileting as appropriate; give pacifier.
- Discuss criteria for removal of restraint.
- Administer analgesics and sedatives if ordered or request whether needed.
- Avoid psychologic upset to other patients.
- Provide distraction (read a book) and touch.
- Maintain child's dignity.
- Provide ongoing nursing assessment.
- Document use of restraints.

Nurses play an important role in the practice of using physical restraints on children. Until more research is available, nurses need to carefully assess the children in their care and apply the nursing process in the use of restraints.

Jacket Restraint

A jacket restraint is sometimes used to keep the child safe in various chairs. The jacket is put on the child with the ties in back so that the child is unable to manipulate them. The long tapes, secured to the understructure of the crib, keep the child inside the crib. The jacket restraint is also useful as a means of maintaining the child in a desired horizontal position.

Mummy Restraint or Swaddle

When an infant or small child requires short-term restraint for examination or treatment that involves the head and neck, such as venipuncture, throat examination, and gavage feeding, the mummy device effectively controls the child's movements. A blanket or sheet is opened on the bed or crib with one corner folded to the center. The infant is placed on the blanket with shoulders at the fold and feet toward the opposite corner (Fig. 22-9, A). With the infant's right arm straight down against the body, the right side of the blanket is pulled firmly across the infant's right shoulder and chest and secured beneath the left side of the body (Fig. 22-9, B). The left arm is placed straight against the child's side, and the left side of the blanket is brought across the shoulder and chest and locked beneath the child's body on the right side. The lower corner is folded and brought over the body and tucked or fastened securely with safety pins (Fig. 22-9, C). Safety pins can be used to fasten the blanket in place at any step in the process.

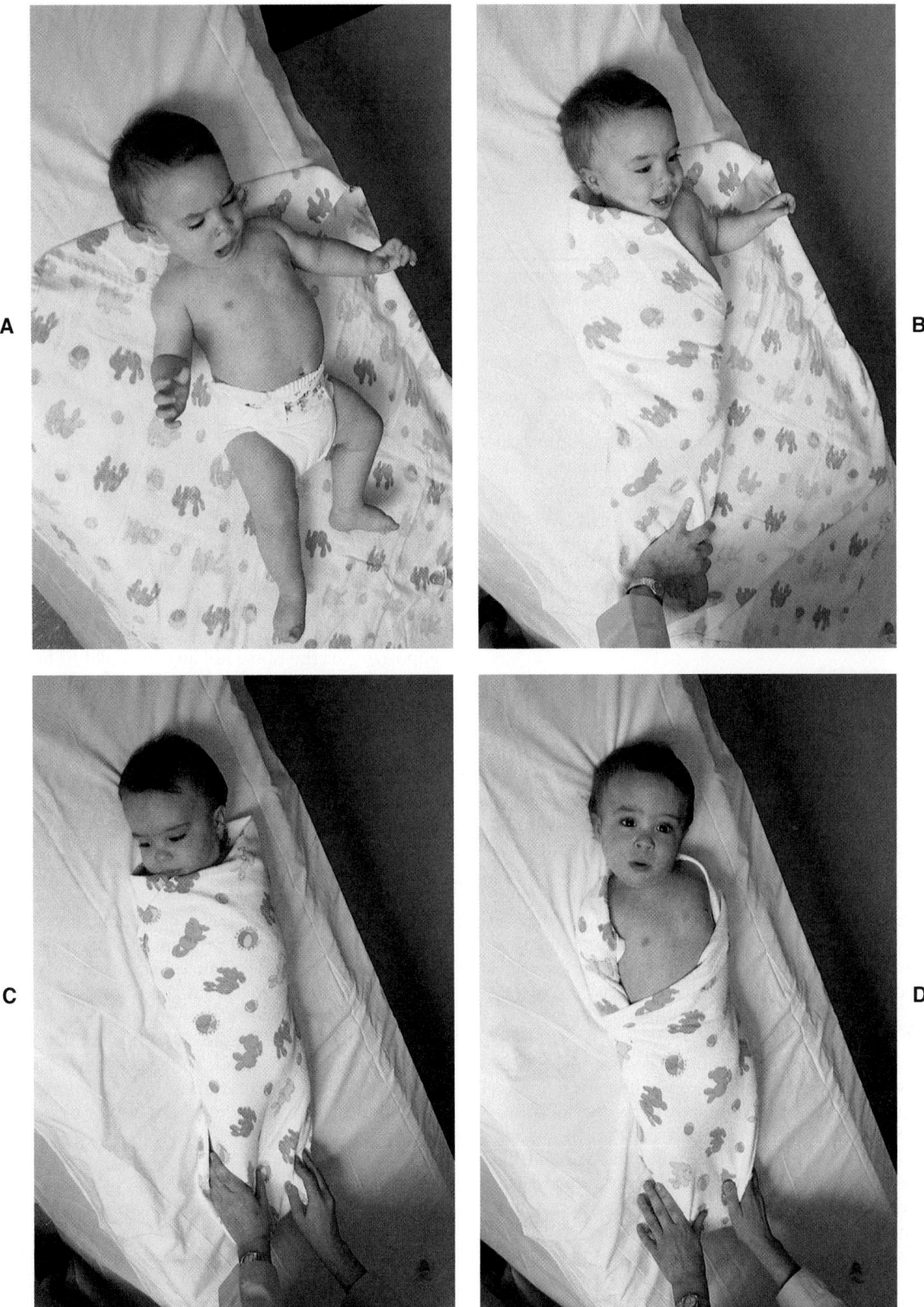

FIG. 22-9 ■ Application of mummy restraint. **A,** Infant placed on folded corner of blanket. **B,** One corner of blanket brought across body and secured beneath body. **C,** Second corner brought across body and secured, and lower corner folded and tucked or pinned in place. **D,** Modified mummy restraint with chest uncovered.

To modify the mummy restraint for chest examination, the folded edge of the blanket is brought over each arm and under the back, after which the loose edge is folded over and secured at a point below the chest to allow visualization and access to the chest (Fig. 22-9, *D*).

The papoose board has the same function as the mummy restraint. It is a solid board with straps attached that secure the infant or small child to the board, similar to a mummy restraint. For maximum comfort the board should be padded.

> **!NURSING ALERT**
>
> Papoose boards or mummy wraps are not substitutes for use of sedation and analgesia during painful procedures. They should be used only when no other options exist.

Arm and Leg Restraints

Arm and leg restraints are sometimes used to immobilize one or more extremities for treatment or procedures or to facilitate healing. Several commercial restraining devices are available, including disposable wrist and ankle restraints. When this type of restraint is used, it must be appropriate to the size of the child; it must be padded to prevent undue pressure, constriction, or tissue injury; and the extremity must be observed frequently for signs of irritation or impairment of circulation. The ends of the restraints are never tied to the crib rails, because lowering the rail will disturb the extremity, frequently with a jerk that may hurt or injure the child.

Elbow Restraint

Sometimes it is important to prevent the child from bending an elbow or reaching the head or face (e.g., after lip surgery, when a scalp vein infusion is in place, to prevent scratching in skin disorders). For this purpose, elbow restraints fashioned from a variety of materials function very well. The most common form of elbow restraints consists of a piece of muslin long enough to reach comfortably from just below the axilla to the wrist with a number of vertical pockets into which tongue depressors are inserted. The restraint is wrapped around the arm and secured with tapes or pins. It may be necessary to pin the top of the restraint to the undershirt sleeve to prevent the restraint from slipping. Similar restraints can be made from commonly available products.

POSITIONING FOR PROCEDURES

Infants and small children are unable to cooperate for many procedures; therefore, the nurse is responsible for minimizing their movement and discomfort with proper positioning. Older children usually need only minimal, if any, restraint. Careful explanation and preparation beforehand and support and simple guidance during the procedure are usually sufficient. Encourage parental participation to ease anxiety. For painful procedures the child should receive adequate analgesia and sedation to minimize pain and the need for excessive restraint. For local anesthesia, use buffered lidocaine to reduce the stinging sensation of infiltration, or use the topical anesthetic EMLA or Numby Stuff (see Pain Management, Chapter 21).

Jugular Venipuncture

The large, superficial external jugular vein may be used to obtain blood specimens from infants and young children. For easy access to the vein, the child is first placed in a

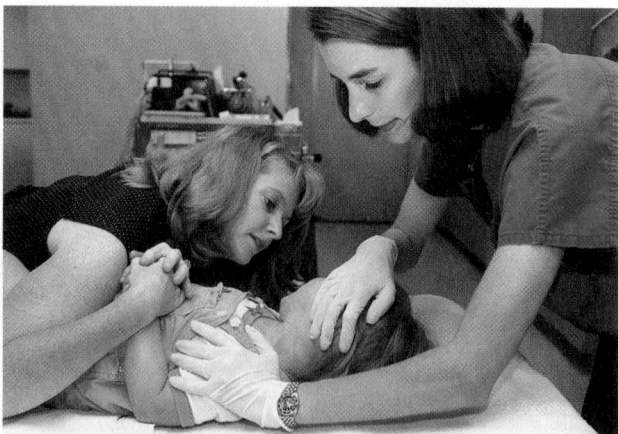

FIG. 22-10 ■ Therapeutic hugging of child for jugular vein puncture with parental assistance.

mummy restraint in which the top edge of the restraint is low enough to permit access to the vein. The child is placed so that the head and shoulders extend over the edge of a table or a small pillow, with the neck extended and the head turned sharply to the side. One alternate method (therapeutic hugging) for restraining arms and legs is with the parent holding the child's arms and legs at the same time that the child's head is restrained and positioned (Fig. 22-10). It is important for the nurse holding the child to maintain control of the child's head without interfering with the practitioner's approach to the vein. The child's crying during the procedure increases IV pressure, which facilitates visualization of the vein. After venipuncture, digital pressure is applied to the site with a dry gauze square for 3 to 5 minutes or until bleeding stops. Care must be taken not to apply excessive pressure that might compromise circulation or breathing during or after the procedure.

Femoral Venipuncture

Other frequently used sites for venipuncture are the large femoral veins. The nurse restrains the infant by placing the child supine with the legs in a frog position to provide extensive exposure of the groin area. Both the arms and the legs of the infant can be effectively controlled by the nurse's forearms and hands (Fig. 22-11). Only the side used for the venipuncture is uncovered, so the practitioner is protected should the child urinate during the procedure. Pressure is applied to the site after the withdrawal of blood to prevent oozing from the site.

Extremity Venipuncture

The most common sites of venipuncture are the veins of the extremities, especially the arm and hand. A convenient position is to place the child in the parent's (or assistant's) lap, with the child facing the parent and in the straddle position. Next, place the child's arm for venipuncture on a firm surface, such as a treatment table, for support and on top of a soft cloth or towel. Have an assistant immobilize the arm for venipuncture, or have the parent do this if an assistant is not available. Then have the parent hug the child around the body to hold the child's free arm, and place the child's legs between the parent's legs (Fig. 22-12). If the child must remain supine, have the parent (or assistant) on one

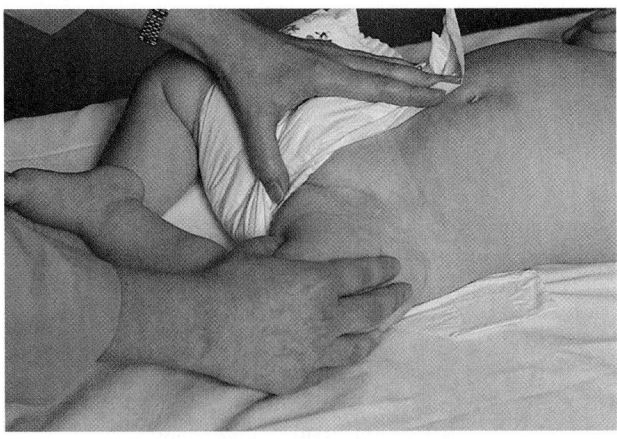

FIG. 22-11 ■ Restraining infant for femoral vein puncture.

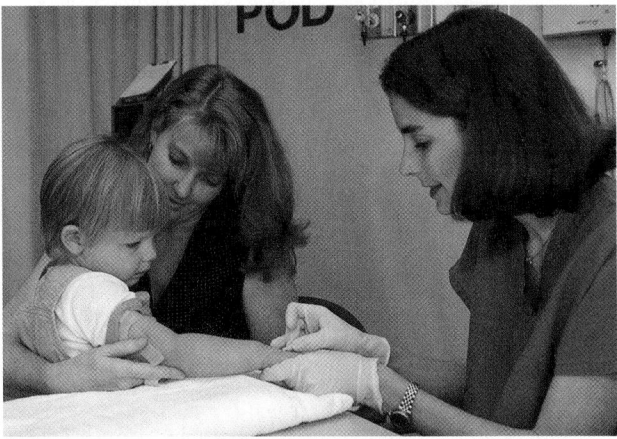

FIG. 22-12 ■ Therapeutic hugging of child for extremity vein puncture with parental assistance.

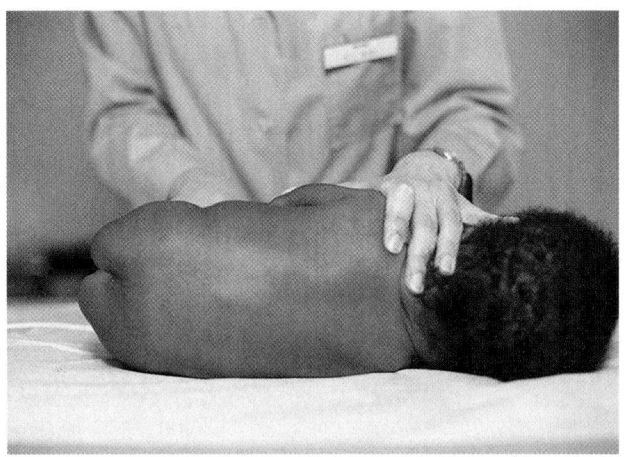

A

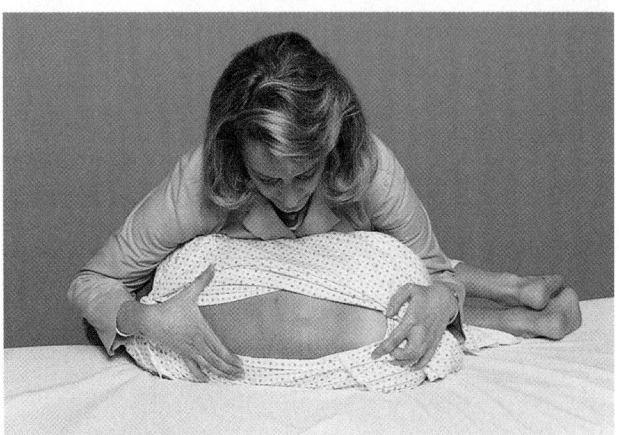

B

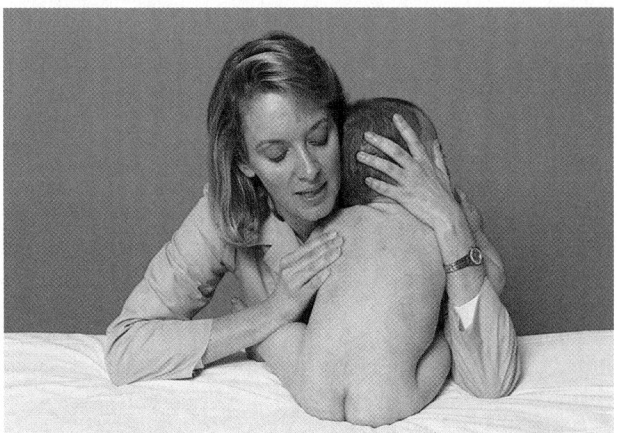

C

FIG. 22-13 ■ **A,** Modified side-lying position for lumbar puncture. **B,** Older child in side-lying position. **C,** Infant's sitting position allows for flexion of lumbar spine.

side of the bed and lean over the child's upper body to apply restraint, using the hand to hold the arm for the venipuncture. Have the operator stand on the other side of the bed for access to the arm for venipuncture.

Lumbar Puncture

The technique for lumbar puncture (LP) in infants and children is similar to that in the adult, although modifications are suggested in neonates, who have less distress in a side-lying position with modified neck extension than in flexion or a sitting position (Fig. 22-13, *A*). Neonates tend to have more cardiorespiratory changes during an LP than older infants regardless of positioning; therefore, oximetry and heart rate monitoring are advisable (Lehmann and others, 1990). Pediatric LP sets contain smaller spinal needles, but sometimes the practitioner will specify a particular size or type of needle that the nurse should make certain is placed on the tray.

Children should receive adequate analgesia or anesthesia to relieve pain. EMLA, a mixture of a local and topical anesthetic in a cream form, should be applied before the LP (see Atraumatic Care box).

Children are usually controlled best in the side-lying position, with the head flexed and the knees drawn up toward the chest. Even cooperative children need to be restrained to prevent possible trauma from unexpected, involuntary

movement. They can be reassured that although they are trusted, the holding will serve as a reminder to maintain the desired position. It also provides a measure of support and reassurance to them.

The child is placed on the side with the back close to the edge of the examining table on the side from which the practitioner is working. The nurse maintains the child's spine in a flexed position by holding the child with one arm behind the neck and the other behind the thighs (Fig. 22-13, *B*). The flexed position enlarges the spaces between the lumbar

ATRAUMATIC CARE

Lumbar Puncture and Bone Marrow Test

Apply EMLA to the puncture site at least 60 minutes before the procedure or apply LMX cream to the site. To identify the lumbar puncture (LP) site, draw an imaginary line from the posterior iliac crest across the spine to the opposite iliac crest. The puncture site is intersected by the line at approximately L4 (Fig. 22-14). For additional anesthesia, buffered lidocaine with a 30-gauge needle can be used. *Unconscious sedation* with agents such as propofol (Diprivan) or ketamine is recommended for bone marrow biopsy and aspiration. Conscious or unconscious sedation is recommended for LP.

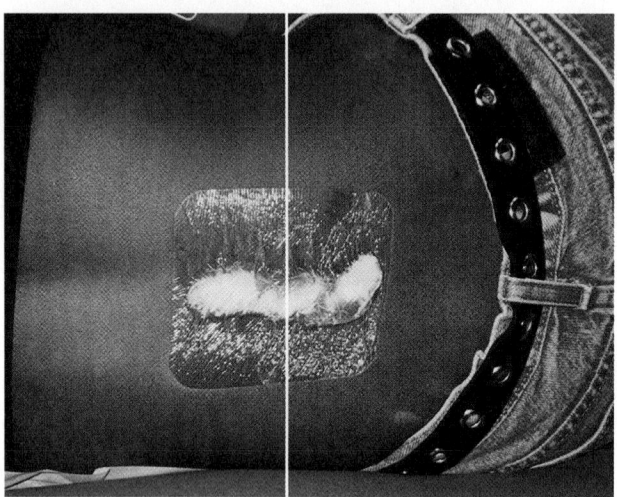

FIG. 22-14 ■ EMLA, a local anesthetic cream, is placed under an occlusive dressing to decrease pain caused by lumbar puncture. The site is located by drawing an imaginary line from the top of the iliac crest that crosses the spine at the approximate needle insertion site.

vertebral spines, which facilitates access to the spinal fluid space. It is helpful to wrap the legs before positioning to decrease leg movement.

An alternate position used with small infants and some older children is the sitting position. The child is placed with the buttocks at the edge of the table and with the neck flexed so that the chin rests on the chest or the nurse's arm. The infant's arms and legs are immobilized by the nurse's hands (Fig. 22-13, *C*).

! NURSING ALERT

The sitting position may interfere with chest expansion and diaphragm excursion, and in infants the soft, pliable trachea may collapse. Therefore observe the child for difficulty with breathing.

Another position that employs close and comforting contact for the child involves holding the child upright against the nurse's (or parent's) chest with the child's legs wrapped around the adult's waist. The adult's arms are used to hug and restrain the child. For ease of the examiner, the adult should be standing. A small pillow is placed between the child's abdomen and the adult to help arch the child's back. If the pillow proves unsuccessful, a third person can place an arm in this space to achieve the desired position. Care should be taken that excessive pressure does not compromise circulation or breathing and that the nose and mouth are not covered by the restrainer's body.

Specimens and spinal fluid pressure are obtained, measured, and sent for analysis in the same manner as for the adult patient. Vital signs are taken as ordered, and the child is observed for any changes in level of consciousness, motor activity, or other neurologic signs. Post-LP headache may occur and is related to postural changes; this is less severe when the child lies flat. Headache is seen much less frequently in young children than in adolescents.

Bone Marrow Aspiration or Biopsy

Positioning for a bone marrow aspiration or biopsy depends on the location of the chosen site. In children the posterior or anterior iliac crest is most frequently used, although in infants the tibia may be selected because of easy access to the site and holding of the child.

If the posterior iliac crest is used, the child is positioned prone. Sometimes a small pillow or folded blanket is placed under the hips to facilitate obtaining the bone marrow specimen. Children should receive adequate analgesia or anesthesia to relieve pain. If the child awakens, holding may be needed, and is best done with two people—one person to immobilize the upper body and a second person to immobilize the lower extremities (see Atraumatic Care box).

Other Procedures

For subdural puncture through a fontanel or burr hole, the infant is wrapped in a mummy restraint and placed in the supine position with the head accessible to the examiner. To control the head, the nurse uses a firm hold on each side of it. Procedures for immobilizing the head for examining the ears, nose, or throat are discussed in Chapter 7.

COLLECTION OF SPECIMENS

URINE SPECIMENS

When children are admitted to the hospital or are seen in a clinic or office, a urine specimen may be needed. Older children and adolescents can use a bedpan or urinal or can be trusted to follow directions for collection in the bathroom. However, attention to their special needs and concerns is warranted. School-age children are cooperative but curious. They are likely to ask questions regarding the disposition of their specimen and what one expects to discover from it. Self-conscious adolescents may be reluctant to carry a specimen bottle through a hallway or waiting room and appreciate a paper bag or other means for disguising the container. The presence of menses is sometimes an embarrassment or a concern to teenage girls; therefore, it is a good idea to ask if they are menstruating and to make adjustments as necessary. The specimen can be delayed, or a notation made on the laboratory slip to explain the presence of red blood cells.

Preschoolers and toddlers are usually unable to void on request. It is often best to offer them water or other liquids

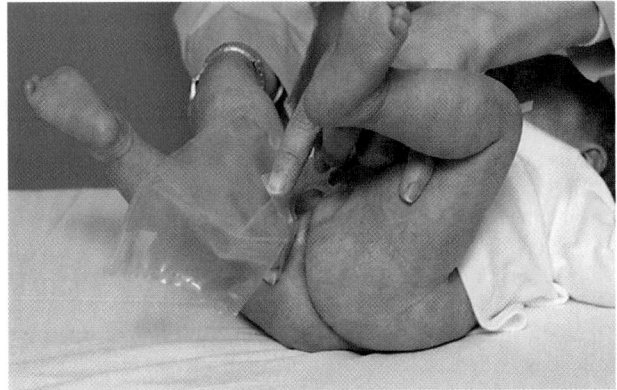
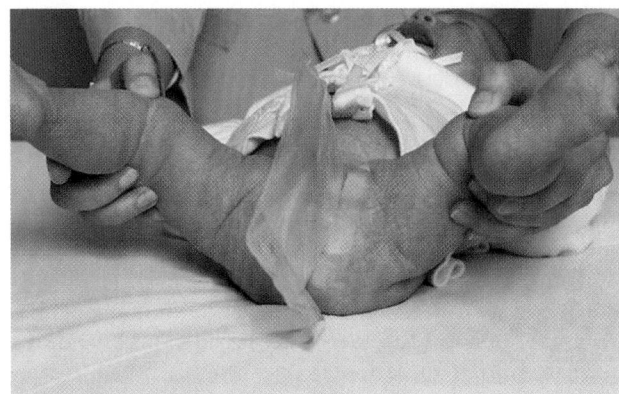

FIG. 22-15 ■ Application of urine collection bag. **A,** On female infants, adhesive portion is applied to exposed and dried perineum first. **B,** Bag adheres firmly around perineal area to prevent urine leakage

that they enjoy and wait about 30 minutes until they are ready to void voluntarily or to set a timer to alert them that they need to void shortly. The child will better understand what is expected if the nurse uses familiar terms, such as "pee-pee," "wee-wee," "tee-tee," or "tinkle." Some children will have difficulty voiding in an unfamiliar receptacle. Potty chairs or a potty hat placed on the toilet will usually prove satisfactory. Toddlers who have recently acquired bladder control may be especially reluctant, because they undoubtedly have been admonished for "going" in places other than those approved by parents. A useful approach is to enlist the help of parents; they are likely to be successful, and this helps them feel a part of the child's care.

For infants and toddlers who are not toilet trained, special urine collection devices may be used. These devices are clear, plastic, single-use bags with self-adhering material around the opening at the point of attachment. To prepare the infant, the genitalia, perineum, and surrounding skin are washed and dried thoroughly, because the adhesive will not stick to a moist, powdered, or oily skin surface. The collection bag is easiest to apply if attached first to the perineum, progressing to the symphysis (Fig. 22-15). With little girls the perineum is stretched taut during application to that area to ensure a leakproof fit. With small boys the penis and scrotum are placed inside the bag. The adhesive portion of the bag must be firmly applied to the skin all around the genital area to avoid possible leakage. For low-birth-weight infants, small bags with adhesive that is gentle to the skin are available.* Anatomically correct urine collection bags are also available.†

The diaper is carefully replaced. The bag is checked frequently and removed as soon as the specimen is available, because the moist bag may become loosened on an active child. When urine is collected for culture, the bag is removed immediately. If the urine is not tested within 30 minutes, the specimen is refrigerated or placed in a sterile container with a preservative.

_____
*Available from **Hollister, Inc.,** 2000 Hollister Drive, Libertyville, IL 60048; (800) 323-4060; website: www.hollister.com.
†Available from **ConvaTec,** CN 5254, Princeton, NJ 08543-5254; (800) 422-8811; website: www.convatec.com.

Urine obtained from disposable diapers can be tested accurately for glucose, ketones, protein, blood, bilirubin, urobilinogen, nitrates, potassium, creatinine, and urea. In one study, urine obtained from a disposable diaper provided a valid sample for diagnosing urinary tract infections (Cohen and others, 1997). Erythrocyte and leukocyte counts may be low. Superabsorbent disposable diapers may produce a false crystalluria. Specific gravity measurements are accurate for up to 4 hours provided that the disposable diapers are kept folded. The accuracy of these tests performed on urine obtained from cloth diapers is unknown. Urine samples collected by the cotton ball method were accurate for pH and specific gravity and were atraumatic to the skin of newborns (Burke, 1995). Traditionally, specific gravity refractometers have been used on nursing units to measure specific gravity. One study showed strong agreement between the use of a refractometer and reagent strip to test urine-specific gravity (Barton and Holmes, 1998). However, current regulations have limited the refractometer's use to the laboratory. Urine dipsticks can be used on the nursing unit with reasonable accuracy.

NURSING TIPS

• When using a urine collection bag, cut a small slit in the diaper and pull the bag through to allow room for urine to collect and to facilitate checking on the contents.
• To obtain small amounts of urine, use a syringe without a needle to aspirate urine directly from the diaper; if diapers with absorbent gelling material that trap urine are used, place a small gauze dressing, some cotton balls, or a urine collection device* inside the diaper to collect urine and aspirate the urine with a syringe.

At times parents may be requested to bring a urine sample to a health care facility for examination, especially when infants are unable to void during an outpatient visit. In this instance parents need instruction on applying the collection

_____
*The Bard Sure Catch is available from Bard Urological Division, **C.R. Bard, Inc.,** 8195 Industrial Boulevard, Covington, GA 30209; (770) 786-9051; website: www.crbard.com.

device and storage of the specimen. Ideally, the specimen should be brought to the designated place as soon as possible; if there is a delay, the sample is refrigerated and the lapsed time reported to the examiner.

Clean-Catch Specimens

The term *clean-catch specimen* traditionally refers to a urine sample obtained for culture after the urethral meatus is cleaned and the first few milliliters of urine are voided before the urine is collected *(midstream specimen)*. The procedure consists of cleaning the perineum or tip of the penis with a soap- or antiseptic-soaked sterile pad in males and of wiping from front to back only once with each pad in females. This is repeated at least two times. The area may be wiped with sterile water to prevent accidental contamination of the urine with a solution that may destroy the pathogens, although minute amounts of antiseptic such as iodine do not alter bacterial counts.

FYI

Although this traditional cleansing procedure is often practiced, studies have found that it does not significantly reduce contamination rates in infants, circumcised or uncircumcised males, or toilet-trained prepubertal children. Also, midstream collection does not significantly reduce contamination rates over non-midstream specimens (Prandoni and others, 1996).

⬤❗NURSING ALERT

Use a urinary catheter of appropriate length to prevent knotting of the catheter in the bladder and urethral trauma. Feeding tubes for intermittent catheterization have been associated with a high incidence of catheter knotting in the bladder. The catheter's extra length coils around its end as bladder decompression occurs, causing subsequent catheter knotting. Surgical removal of a knotted catheter may be required (Carlson and Mowery, 1997).

Twenty-Four-Hour Collection

Collection of urine voided over a 24-hour period creates a special challenge in infants and children. Collection bags are required to collect specimens from infants and small children. Older children require special instruction about notifying someone when they need to void or have a bowel movement so that urine can be collected separately and not discarded. Some older school-age children and adolescents can be trusted to take responsibility for collection of their own 24-hour specimens. They can keep output records and transfer each voiding to the 24-hour collection container if this is permitted.

As in any 24-hour urine collection, the collection period always starts and ends with an empty bladder. At the time the collection begins, the child is instructed to void and the specimen is discarded. All urine voided in the subsequent 24 hours is saved in a container with a preservative or is refrigerated or placed on ice. Twenty-four hours from the time the precollection specimen was discarded, the child is again instructed to void, the specimen is added to the container, and the entire collection is taken to the laboratory for examination.

Infants and small children who need a 24-hour urine collection require a special collection bag; frequent removal and replacement of adhesive collection devices can produce skin irritation. A thin coating of sealant, such as Skin-Prep, applied to the skin helps to protect it and aids adhesion, unless its use is contraindicated, such as in a premature infant or a child with irritated skin. Plastic collection bags with collection tubes attached are ideal when the container must be left in place for a time. These can be connected to a collecting device or emptied periodically by aspiration with a syringe. When such devices are not available, a regular bag with a feeding tube inserted through a puncture hole at the top of the bag serves as a satisfactory substitute. However, care must be taken to empty the bag as soon as the infant urinates to prevent leakage and loss of contents. An indwelling catheter may also be placed for the collection period.

Bladder Catheterization and Other Techniques

Bladder catheterization or *suprapubic aspiration* is employed when a specimen is urgently needed or when the child is unable to void or otherwise provide an adequate specimen. Catheterization is used to obtain a sterile urine specimen and when urethral obstruction or anuria caused by renal failure is believed to be the cause of the child's failure to void. Suprapubic aspiration is useful in clarifying the diagnosis of suspected urinary tract infection in acutely ill infants.

The anxiety, fear, and discomfort experienced during catheterization can be significantly alleviated by adequate preparation of the child and parents, by selection of the correct catheter, and by the appropriate technique of insertion. Specifically, generous lubrication of the urethra before catheterization and use of a lubricant containing 2% lidocaine (Xylocaine) may significantly reduce or eliminate the burning and discomfort frequently associated with this invasive procedure.

Preparation for catheterization includes instruction on pelvic muscle relaxation whenever possible. The toddler, preschooler, or younger child is taught to blow a pinwheel and to press the hips against the bed or procedure table during catheterization to relax the pelvic and periurethral muscles. The location and function of the pelvic muscles are described briefly to the older child or adolescent. The patient is then taught to contract and relax the pelvic muscles, and the relaxation procedure is repeated during catheter insertion. If the patient vigorously contracts the pelvic muscles when the catheter reaches the striated sphincter (proximal urethra in boys and midurethra in girls), catheter insertion is temporarily stopped. The catheter is neither removed nor advanced; instead, the child is helped to press the hips against the bed or examining table and relax the pelvic muscles. The catheter is then gently advanced into the bladder.

Catheterization is a sterile procedure, and standard precautions for body substance protection should be followed. When placing a catheter for a sterile urine specimen or to check for residual urine, a sterile feeding tube may be used. If the catheter is to remain in place, a Foley catheter is used. Table 22-4 gives guidelines for choosing an appropriate catheter size and length of insertion. The supplies needed for this procedure include sterile gloves, sterile lubricant anesthetic, an appropriately sized catheter, povidone-iodine (Betadine) swabs or an alternative cleansing agent and 4 × 4

TABLE 22-4 ■ Straight Catheter or Foley Catheter*

	SIZE (LENGTH OF INSERTION [cm]) FOR GIRLS	SIZE (LENGTH OF INSERTION [cm]) FOR BOYS
Term neonate	5-6 (5)	5-6 (6)
Infant to 3 years	5-8 (5)	5-8 (6)
4-8 years	8 (5-6)	8 (6-9)
8 years to prepubertal	10-12 (6-8)	8-10 (10-15)
Pubertal	12-14 (6-8)	12-14 (13-18)

*Foley catheters are approximately 1 French size larger because of the circumference of the balloon. Example: 10 French Foley = approximately 12 French calibration.

inch gauze squares, a sterile drape, and a syringe with sterile water if a Foley catheter is being used. Test the balloon of the Foley catheter by injecting sterile water before catheter insertion. Place a sterile drape under the buttocks of the female patient.

NURSING ALERT

Identify patients who have allergies to povidone-iodine or latex before using these items in catheterization.

Adolescent boys and children with a history of urethral surgery may be catheterized with a coudé-tipped catheter. The child with myelodysplasia or one who has been identified as being sensitive or allergic to latex is catheterized with a catheter or feeding tube manufactured of an alternative material. When an indwelling catheter is indicated for urinary drainage, a lubricious or silicone catheter is selected because these materials produce less irritation of the urethral mucosa as compared with a Silastic or latex catheter when the catheter is left in place for more than 72 hours.

A 2% lidocaine lubricant with applicator is assembled according to the manufacturer's instructions,* and several drops of the lubricant are placed at the meatus. The child is advised that the lubricant is used to reduce any discomfort associated with inserting the catheter and that introduction of the lubricant into the urethra will produce a sensation of pressure and a desire to urinate (Gray, 1996).

In male patients the tip of the applicator is gently introduced into the urethra 1 to 2 cm so that the lubricant flows only into the urethra; 5 to 10 mL 2% lidocaine lubricant is slowly inserted into the urethra and held in place for 2 to 3 minutes by gently squeezing the distal penis. This maneuver allows the mucosa to absorb the active ingredient. Additional lubricant is placed on the catheter tip, which is inserted into the urethra without allowing the intraurethral lubricant to exit the urethral meatus. Using this technique of retaining the lubricant as the catheter is inserted provides lubrication of the urethra and promotes opening of the sphincter mechanism.

---

*Lidocaine hydrochloride 2% jelly is available in 5-, 10-, and 20-mL (20 mg/mL) glass prefilled sterile syringes from **International Medication Systems, Ltd. (IMS)**, South El Monte, CA 91733; (818) 913-4660. Lidocaine hydrochloride 2% jelly is available in 10- and 20-mL (20 mg/mL) plastic prefilled sterile syringes from **AstraZeneca**, 725 Chesterbrook Boulevard, Wayne, PA 19087; (800) 237-8898.

In female patients, 1 to 2 mL 2% lidocaine lubricant is placed on the periurethral mucosa, and 1 to 2 mL is inserted into the urethral meatus. Catheterization is delayed for 2 to 3 minutes to maximize absorption of the anesthetic into the periurethral and intraurethral mucosa. Additional lubricant is added to the catheter, which is gently inserted into the urethra until urine returns. This additional lubrication, combined with the mild anesthetic effects of the 2% lidocaine lubricant, greatly reduces the discomfort frequently associated with insertion of a catheter.

Because the use of lidocaine jelly can increase the volume of intraurethral lubricant, urine return may not be as rapid as when minimum lubrication is used. However, with patience, a urine return will occur, and the discomfort and anxiety commonly associated with catheterization will be avoided.

Suprapubic aspiration is mainly used when the bladder cannot be accessed through the urethra (such as with some congenital urologic birth defects) or to reduce the risk of contamination that may be present when passing a catheter. In general, with the advent of small-sized catheters (5 and 6 French straight catheters), the need for suprapubic aspiration has decreased. Access to the bladder via the urethra has a much higher success rate than suprapubic aspiration, where success depends on the practitioner's skill at assessing the location of the bladder and the amount of urine in the bladder.

Suprapubic aspiration, which is performed by a practitioner skilled in the procedure, involves aspirating bladder contents by inserting a 20- or 21-gauge needle in the midline approximately 1 cm above the symphysis pubis and directed vertically downward. The skin is prepared as for any needle insertion, and the bladder should contain an adequate volume of urine. This can be assumed if the infant has not voided for at least 1 hour or the bladder can be palpated above the symphysis pubis. This technique is useful for obtaining sterile specimens from young infants, because the bladder is an abdominal organ and is easily accessed. Suprapubic aspiration is painful, and therefore pain management during the procedure is important (see Atraumatic Care box; see also Cultural Awareness box).

ATRAUMATIC CARE

Bladder Catheterization or Suprapubic Aspiration

Use distraction to help the child relax (blowing bubbles, deep breathing, singing a song).

Use lidocaine jelly to anesthetize the area before insertion of catheter (see text above). EMLA cream or LMX cream may lessen an infant's discomfort as the needle passes through the skin for suprapubic aspiration, but care should be taken that the site is thoroughly cleaned and prepped before the procedure.

Have the parent sit in a chair or on an examining table with a back support. Next, place the child leaning back in the parent's lap with the parent's arms hugging the child's upper body. Then place the child's legs in the frog position with the parent's legs over the child's to stabilize them. In this comfortable position the perineum or lower abdomen is exposed for the procedure.

Children often become agitated at being restrained for either procedure. Use comfort measures through touch and voice, both during and after the procedure, to help reduce the child's distress.

CULTURAL AWARENESS

Bladder Catheterization

Parents may be upset when their child is catheterized. Aside from the trauma the child experiences, some parents, especially those from different cultures, may fear that the procedure affects the daughter's virginity. To correct this misconception, the family may benefit from a detailed explanation of the genitourinary anatomy, preferably with a model that shows the separate vaginal and urethral openings. The nurse can also indicate that catheterization has no effect on virginity.

STOOL SPECIMENS

Stool specimens are frequently collected in children to identify parasites and other organisms that cause diarrhea, to assess gastrointestinal function, and to check for occult (hidden) blood. Ideally, stool should be collected without contamination with urine, but in children wearing diapers this is difficult unless a urine bag is applied. Children who are toilet trained should urinate first, flush the toilet, then defecate in the toilet, a bedpan (preferably one that is placed on the toilet to avoid embarrassment), or a commercial potty hat.

NURSING TIP

To obtain a stool specimen, place plastic wrap over the toilet bowl to collect the stool. Use a tongue depressor or disposable spoon or knife to collect the stool and place the specimen in a covered cup or plastic bag.

Stool specimens should be large enough to obtain an ample sampling, not merely a fecal fragment. Specimens are placed in an appropriate container, which is covered and labeled. If several specimens are needed, the containers are marked with the date and time and kept in a specimen refrigerator. Special care is exercised in handling the specimen because of the risk of contamination.

BLOOD SPECIMENS

Although most blood specimens are obtained by the laboratory staff, nurses are increasingly responsible for specimen collection, especially if the child has an arterial or venous device. However, whether the specimen is collected by the nurse or others, the nurse is responsible for making certain that specimens, such as serial examinations and fasting specimens, are collected on time and that the proper equipment is available, such as correct collection tubes and ice for blood gas samples. Collecting, transporting, and storing of specimens can have a major impact on laboratory results (Frizzell, 1998).

Venous blood samples can be obtained by venipuncture or by aspiration from a peripheral or central access device. Withdrawing blood specimens through peripheral lock devices in small peripheral veins has met with varying degrees of success. Although it avoids an additional venipuncture for the child, attempting to aspirate blood from the peripheral lock may shorten the life of the device. When using an IV infusion site for specimen collection, it is important to consider the type of fluid being infused. For example, a specimen collected for glucose determination would be inaccurate if removed from a catheter through which glucose-containing solution were being administered.

NURSING TIPS

- To obtain a blood specimen from a central venous line or peripheral lock when the infusion solution may interfere with tests results, first aspirate a quantity of blood equal to the volume of fluid in the catheter and discard; then aspirate the blood sample.
- For a blood culture, use the first sample of blood, because organisms are most likely to collect within the catheter itself.

NURSING ALERT

On small or anemic children, keep track of the amount drawn and discarded over time. Frequent taking of blood specimens can rapidly decrease a child's blood volume. Coordinate blood samples and ask the laboratory to save blood as much as possible to reduce the frequency.

Arterial blood samples are sometimes needed for blood gas measurement, although noninvasive techniques, such as transcutaneous oxygen/carbon dioxide monitoring and pulse oximetry, are used frequently. Arterial samples may be obtained by arteriopuncture using the radial, brachial, or femoral arteries; by deep heel puncture; or from indwelling arterial catheters). Adequate circulation should be assessed before arterial puncture by observing capillary refill or performing the *Allen test,* a procedure that assesses the circulation of the radial, ulnar, or brachial arteries. Because unclotted blood is required, only heparinized collection tubes are used. In addition, no air bubbles should enter the tube, because they can alter blood gas concentration. Crying, fear, and agitation also affect blood gas values; therefore, every effort is made to comfort the child. The blood samples are packed in ice to reduce blood cell metabolism and are taken to the laboratory for immediate analysis.

Capillary blood samples are taken from children by a finger or earlobe stick, just as in the adult patient. A common method for taking peripheral blood samples from infants is by a heel stick. Before the blood sample is taken, the heel is warmed with warm, moist compresses for 5 to 10 minutes to dilate the vessels in the area. Although this is a well-accepted practice, one study questioned its effectiveness. In a study of healthy full-term infants, warming the heel with a warm gel pack (40° C [104° F] for 10 minutes before capillary blood sampling with an automated device (Autolet) did not significantly decrease the sampling time required (Barker and others, 1996).

The area is cleansed with alcohol, and with the infant's foot firmly restrained with the free hand, the heel is punctured with a blade or an automatic lancet device. An automatic device, such as Tenderfoot* or Autolet, delivers a more precise puncture depth and is a less painful puncture than that achieved with a blade or lance (Vertanen and others, 2001; McIntosh, van Veen, and Brameyer, 1994). Although obtaining capillary blood gases is a common prac-

*Available from **International Technidyne Corporation,** 8 Olsen Avenue, Edison, NJ 08820; (732) 548-5700 or (800) 631-5945; website: www.itemed.com.

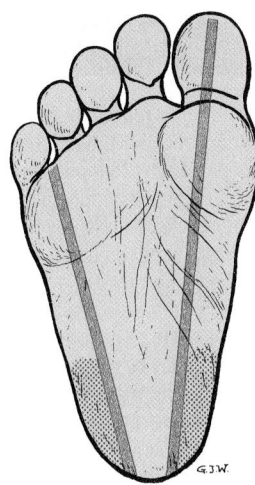

FIG. 22-16 ■ Puncture site (colored stippled area) on sole of infant's foot.

tice, some practitioners believe that these measures may not accurately reflect arterial values.

The most serious complication of infant heel puncture is necrotizing osteochondritis from lancet penetration of the underlying calcaneus bone. To avoid this, the puncture should be no deeper than 2.4 mm and should be made at the outer aspect of the heel. The boundaries of the calcaneus can be marked by an imaginary line extending posteriorly from a point between the fourth and fifth toes and running parallel to the lateral aspect of the heel and another line extending posteriorly from the middle of the great toe and running parallel to the medial aspect of the heel (Fig. 22-16).

The needed specimens are collected quickly, and then pressure is applied to the puncture site with a dry gauze square until bleeding stops. The arm is kept extended, not flexed, while pressure is applied for a few minutes after venipuncture in the antecubital fossa to reduce bruising. The site is then covered with an adhesive bandage. In young children, adhesive bandages pose an aspiration hazard; their use should be avoided or the adhesive bandage should be removed as soon as the bleeding stops. Applying warm compresses to ecchymotic areas increases circulation, helps remove extravasated blood, and decreases pain.

No matter how or by whom the specimen is collected, children, even some older ones, fear the loss of their blood. This is particularly true for children whose condition requires frequent blood specimens. They mistakenly believe that blood removed from their bodies is a threat to their lives. Explaining to them that their blood is continually being produced by their bodies provides them with a measure of reassurance regarding this aspect of the stress-provoking procedure. When the blood is drawn, a simple comment, such as "Just look how red it is. You're really making a lot of nice red blood," confirms this information and affords them an opportunity to express their concern. Covering the puncture site with an adhesive bandage strip gives them added assurance that the vital fluids will not leak out.

Children also dislike the discomfort associated with venous, arterial, or capillary punctures. In fact, children have identified these procedures as the ones most frequently causing pain during hospitalization and arterial punctures as being one of the most painful of all procedures experienced (Wong and Baker, 1988). Consequently, nurses need to institute pain reduction techniques to lessen the discomfort of these procedures (see Atraumatic Care box). Younger children are more distressed by venipuncture than are older children.

RESPIRATORY SECRETION AND THROAT SPECIMENS

Collection of sputum or nasal discharge is sometimes required for diagnosis of respiratory infections, especially tuberculosis and respiratory syncytial virus (RSV). Older children and adolescents are able to cough as directed and supply sputum specimens when given proper directions. It must be made clear to them that a coughed specimen is needed, not mucus that is cleared from the throat. It is helpful to demonstrate a deep cough so that communication is clear. Infants and small children are unable to follow directions to cough and will swallow any sputum produced; therefore, *gastric washings (lavage)* may be used to collect a sputum specimen. Sometimes it is possible to obtain a satisfactory specimen by using a suction device such as a mucus trap if the catheter is inserted into the trachea and the cough reflex is elicited. A catheter that is inserted into the back of the throat is not sufficient. For children with a tracheostomy, a specimen is easily aspirated from the trachea or major bronchi by attaching a collecting device to the suction apparatus.

Nasal washings are usually obtained to diagnose an infection of RSV. The child is placed supine, and 1 to 3 mL sterile normal saline is instilled with a sterile syringe (without needle) into one nostril. The contents are aspirated using a small, sterile bulb syringe and are placed in a sterile container. To prevent any additional discomfort to the child, all of the equipment should be ready before the procedure is begun.

Other respiratory secretion collection methods include nasopharyngeal swabs to diagnose *Bordetella pertussis* and throat cultures. The nurse swabs both the tonsils and the posterior pharynx when obtaining a throat culture. The swab stick is inserted into the culture tube. Some culture kits require squeezing an ampule to release the culture medium.

> **⚠ NURSING ALERT**
>
> Do not attempt to obtain a throat culture if acute epiglottitis is suspected. The trauma from the swab may increase edema, possibly occluding the airway.

ADMINISTRATION OF MEDICATION

PREPARATION FOR SAFE ADMINISTRATION

The safe administration of medication to children presents a number of problems that are not encountered when giving medication to adult patients. Children vary widely in age, weight, body surface area, and the ability to absorb, metabolize, and excrete medications. Nurses must be particularly alert when computing and administering drugs to infants and children.

Determination of Drug Dosage

It is the physician's responsibility to prescribe drugs in the correct dosage to achieve the desired effect without endangering the health of the child. However, nurses must have an understanding of the safe dosage of medications they

ATRAUMATIC CARE

Guidelines for Skin/Vessel Punctures

To reduce the pain associated with heel, finger, venous, or arterial punctures:

Apply EMLA topically over the site if time permits (at least 60 minutes). LMX cream also may be used and requires a shorter application time (30 minutes). To remove the Tegaderm dressing atraumatically, grasp opposite sides of the film and pull the sides away from each other to stretch and loosen the film. After the film begins to loosen, grasp the other two sides of the film and pull. Use iontophoresis (Numby Stuff) over the site if time permits (8 to 20 minutes, depending on the amount of current), a vapocoolant spray, or buffered lidocaine (injected intradermally near the vein with a 30-gauge needle) to numb the skin.

Use nonpharmacologic methods of pain and anxiety control (e.g., ask child to take a deep breath when the needle is inserted and again when the needle is withdrawn; have child exhale a large breath or blow bubbles to "blow hurt away"; ask child to count slowly and then faster and louder if pain is felt).

Keep all equipment out of sight until used.

Enlist parents' presence or assistance if they wish to participate.

Restrain child *only as needed* to perform the procedure safely; use therapeutic hugging (p. 737).

Allow the skin preparation to dry completely before penetrating the skin.

Use the smallest-gauge needle (e.g., 25 gauge) that permits free flow of blood; a 27-gauge needle can be used for obtaining 1 to 1.5 mL blood and for prominent veins (needle length is only 0.5 inches).

Avoid putting an intravenous (IV) line in the dominant hand or the hand the child uses to suck the thumb.

Use an automatic lancet device for precise puncture depth of the finger or heel; press the device lightly against the skin and avoid steadying the finger against a hard surface.

Emphasize that blood entering the syringe or tube does not hurt and reassure young children that you did not "take their blood" away and that they have a lot more inside.

Place a small bandage over the puncture site to make removal easy and less painful and to reassure young children that "their blood will not leak out."*

Have a "two-try" only policy to reduce excessive insertion attempts—two operators each have two insertion attempts; if insertion is not successful after four punctures, consider alternative venous access, such as a peripherally inserted central catheter (PICC); have a policy for identifying children with difficult access and appropriate interventions (e.g., most experienced operator for the first attempt).†

FOR MULTIPLE BLOOD SAMPLES

Use an intermittent infusion device ("saline or heparin lock") to collect additional samples from an existing IV line; consider PICC lines early, not as a last resort. Preferably, use a saline flush for a catheter larger than 24 gauge (less painful, compatible with drugs, and less costly).

Coordinate care to allow several tests to be performed on one blood sample using micromethods of testing.

Anticipate tests (e.g., drug levels, chemistry, immunoglobulin levels) and ask the laboratory to save blood for additional testing.

FOR HEEL LANCING IN NEWBORNS

Heel lancing has been shown to be more painful than venipuncture (Larsson and others, 1998); consider venipuncture when the amount of blood from the heel would require much squeezing (e.g., genetic screening tests).

The effectiveness of EMLA is controversial, although application of 0.5 g for 30 minutes four times a day in preterm infants was found to be safe (Essink-Tebbes and others, 1999).

Place diapered newborn against mother's bare chest in skin-to-skin contact 10 to 15 minutes before and during heel lance (Gray, Watt, and Blass, 2000).

During the procedure, allow newborn to suck a pacifier coated with a slurry of sugar and water: to make an approximate 24% sucrose solution, add 1 teaspoon of table sugar to 4 teaspoons of sterile water. Use this solution to coat the pacifier or administer 2 mL to the tongue 2 minutes before the procedure (Blass and Watt, 1999).

*Contrary to popular belief, a study of children ages 3 to 6 years found that asking them not to look at the finger stick to avoid the sight of blood or applying a decorated bandage did not lessen their rating of pain intensity (Johnston, Stevens, and Arbess, 1993).

†For an example of one hospital's guidelines for reducing excessive IV insertion attempts, see Catudal (1999).

---

administer to children, as well as the expected action, possible side effects, and signs of toxicity (Kennedy, 1996). Unlike with adult medications, there are few standardized pediatric dosage ranges, and with a few exceptions, drugs are prepared and packaged in average adult-dosage strengths.

Factors related to growth and maturation significantly alter an individual's capacity to metabolize and excrete drugs, and deficiencies associated with immaturity become more important with decreasing age. Immaturity or defects in any or all of the important processes of absorption, distribution, biotransformation, or excretion can significantly alter the effects of a drug. Newborn and premature infants with immature enzyme systems in the liver (where most drugs are broken down and detoxified), lower plasma concentrations of protein for binding with drugs, and immaturely functioning kidneys (where most drugs are excreted) are particularly vulnerable to the harmful effects of drugs. Beyond the newborn period, many drugs are metabolized more rapidly by the liver, necessitating larger doses or more frequent administration. This is particularly important in pain control, when the dosage may need to be increased or the interval between administering analgesics may need to be decreased.

Various formulas involving age, weight, and body surface area as the basis for calculations have been devised to determine children's drug dosage from a standard adult dose. Because the administration of medication is a nursing responsibility, nurses need not only a knowledge of drug action and patient responses, but also some resources for estimating safe dosages for children. The method most often used to determine children's dosage is based on a specific dose per kilogram of body weight, such as 0.1 mg/kg.

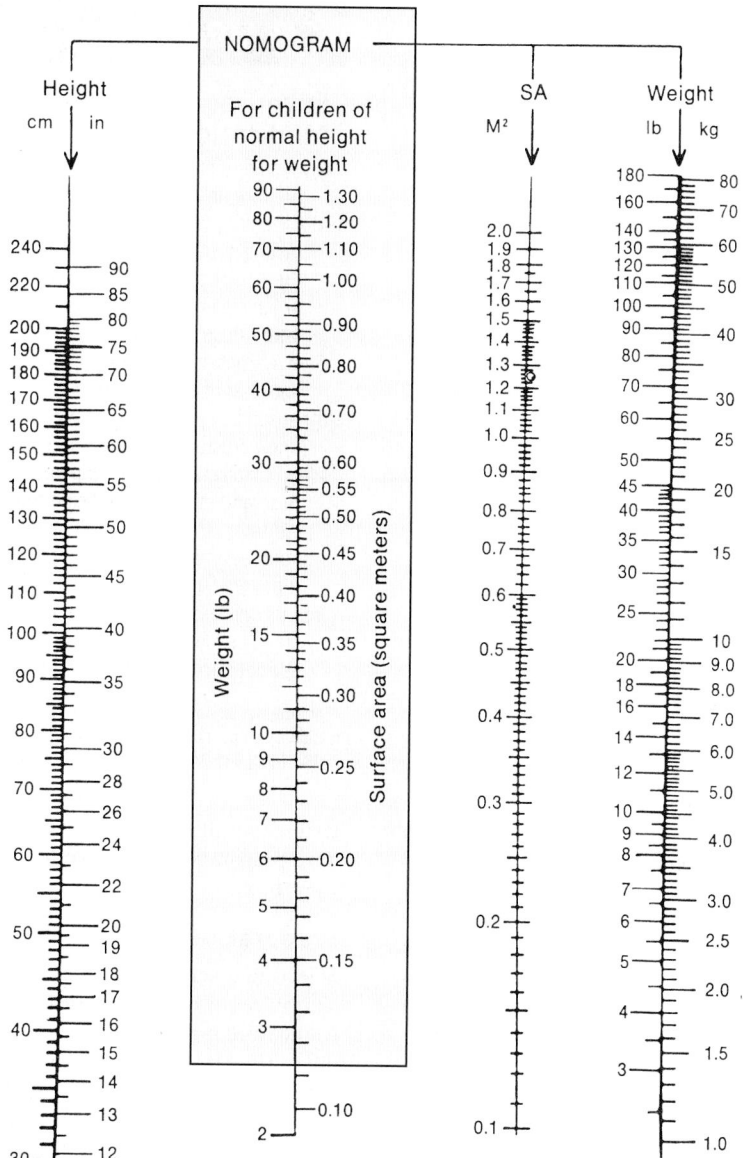

FIG. 22-17 ■ West nomogram for estimation of surface areas. Surface area is indicated where a straight line connecting height and weight intersects surface area (SA) column or, if patient is approximately of normal proportion, from weight alone (yellow area). (Nomogram modified from data of E. Boyd by C.D. West; from Behrman RE, Kleigman RM, Jenson HB, editors: *Nelson textbook of pediatrics,* ed 17, Philadelphia, 2000, WB Saunders.)

The most reliable method for determining children's dosage is to calculate the proportional amount of *body surface area (BSA)* to body weight. The ratio of BSA to weight varies inversely with length; therefore, the infant who is shorter and weighs less than an older child or adult has relatively more surface area than would be expected from the weight. The usual determination of BSA requires the use of the *West nomogram* (Fig. 22-17). The BSA is estimated from the height and weight of the child.

Checking Dosage. Administering the correct dosage of a drug is a shared responsibility between the practitioner who orders the drug and the nurse who carries out that order. Children react with unexpected severity to some drugs,

and ill children are especially sensitive to drugs. Therefore checking the dose if any doubt exists about its accuracy is a professional duty. When a dose is ordered that is outside the usual range or if there is some question regarding the preparation or the route of administration, the nurse should always check with the prescribing practitioner before proceeding with the administration, because the nurse is legally liable for any drug administered.

Administering some medications requires added safeguards. Even when it has been determined that the dosage is correct for a particular child, many drugs are potentially hazardous or lethal. Most hospital units or other facilities where medications are given to children have regulations requiring that specified drugs be double-checked by another nurse before they are given to the child. Among drugs that require such safeguards are digoxin, heparin, chemotherapeutic agents, and insulin. Others frequently included are epinephrine, opioids, and sedatives. Even if this precaution is not mandatory, nurses are wise to take such precautions for their own sense of security. Errors in decimal point placement may easily occur and may result in a tenfold or more dosage error.

Identification

Before the administration of any medication, the child must be correctly identified, because children are not totally reliable in giving correct names on request. Infants are unable to give their name, a toddler or preschooler may admit to any name, and school-age children may deny their identity in an attempt to avoid the medication. Children sometimes exchange beds during play. Parents may be present to identify their child, but the only safe method for identifying children is to check their hospital identification band with the labeled medication or medication card. Two identifiers are required before medication administration. An example of identifiers include name, medical record number, and birth date.

Family Aspects

Parents can be useful sources of information regarding the child and his or her capabilities. Nearly all parents have given some kind of medication to their child and can describe approaches that they have found to be successful. In some cases it is less traumatic for the child if a parent gives the medication, provided that the nurse prepares the medication and supervises its administration and the practice is consistent with hospital or unit policy. Children being given daily medications at home are accustomed to the parent's functioning in this capacity and are less apt to object than they would if the medication were administered by a stranger.

Every child requires psychologic preparation for parenteral administration of medication and supportive care during the procedure (p. 709). Even if children have received several injections, they rarely become accustomed to the discomfort and have as much right as any other child to understanding and patience from those involved in giving the injection. Safe administration of any drug requires meticulous attention to the safeguards discussed here.

ORAL ADMINISTRATION

The oral route is preferred for administering medications to children whenever possible. Because of the ease of administration of oral medications, most are dissolved or suspended in liquid preparations. Although some children are able to swallow or chew solid medications at an early age, solid preparations are not recommended for young children because of the danger of aspiration.

Most pediatric medications come in palatable and colorful preparations for added ease of administration. Some have a slightly unpleasant aftertaste, but most children will swallow these liquids with little if any resistance. The nurse should taste a minute amount of an oral preparation to ascertain if it is palatable or bitter. In this way legitimate complaints of dislike from the child can be accepted and the

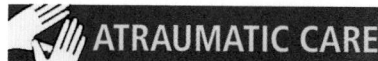

ATRAUMATIC CARE

Encouraging a Child's Acceptance of Oral Medication

Give child a flavored ice pop or small ice cube to suck to numb the tongue before giving the drug.

Mix the drug with a small amount (about 1 teaspoon) of sweet-tasting substance, such as honey (except in infants because of the risk of botulism), flavored syrups, jam, fruit purees, sherbet, or ice cream; avoid essential food items, because the child may later refuse to eat them.

Give a "chaser" of water, juice, soft drink, or ice pop or frozen juice bar after the drug.

If nausea is a problem, give a carbonated beverage poured over finely crushed ice before or immediately after the medication.

When medication has an unpleasant taste, have child pinch the nose and drink the medicine through a straw. Much of what we taste is associated with smell.

Another alternative is to have the pharmacist prepare the drug in a flavored, chewable troche or lozenge.*

Infants will suck medicine from a needleless syringe or dropper in small increments (0.25 to 0.50 mL) at a time. Use a nipple or special pacifier with a reservoir for the drug.

*For information about compounding drugs in troches, contact Technical Staff, Professional Compounding Centers of America (PCCA), PO Box 368, Sugarland, TX 77487; (800) 331-2498; website: www.thecompounders.com.

taste camouflaged whenever possible. Most pediatric units have preparations available for this purpose (see Atraumatic Care box).

Preparation

Selecting a vehicle for measuring and administering a medication requires careful consideration. The devices available to measure medicines are not always sufficiently accurate for measuring the small amounts needed in pediatric nursing practice (Fig. 22-18). Disposable plastic calibrated cups offer reasonable accuracy in measuring moderate doses of liquids (paper cups are likely to have irregularly shaped or crumpled bottoms). However, the personal interpretation of a given measure is highly variable, and considerable amounts of thick medication may remain in the cup. Measures of less than a teaspoon are impossible to determine accurately with a cup.

Many liquid preparations are prescribed in measurements of teaspoons. However, the teaspoon is an inaccurate measuring device and is subject to error from a number of variables. For example, household teaspoons vary greatly in capacity, and different persons using the same spoon will pour different amounts. Therefore a drug ordered in teaspoons should be measured in milliliters; the established standard is 5 mL per teaspoon. A convenient hollow-handled medicine spoon is available to accurately measure and administer the drug (see Fig. 22-18). Household *measuring* spoons can also be used when other devices are not available.

Another unreliable device for measuring liquids is the dropper, which varies to a greater extent than the teaspoon or measuring cup. Droppers are available in numerous sizes, but even with the standard USP dropper, the volume of a drop will vary according to the viscosity of the liquid measured; viscid fluids produce much larger drops than thin liquids. Many medications are supplied with caps or droppers designed for measuring each specific preparation. These are accurate when used to measure that specific medication but are not reliable for measuring other liquids. Emptying dropper contents into a medicine cup invites additional error. Because some of the liquid clings to the sides of the cup, a significant amount of the drug can be lost.

NURSING ALERT

Many pediatric medications are given by drops or dropper. A misunderstanding of these terms by parents can result in a potential overdose. In addition, many droppers that come with medications are marked in tenths of cubic centimeters. If a parent were to use a syringe instead of the dropper, 0.4 cc may be thought to be the same as 4 cc. Provide education to parents on correct methods for giving medication. Demonstrate the technique.

The most accurate means for measuring small amounts of medication is the plastic disposable (never glass) syringe, especially the tuberculin syringe for volumes less than 1 mL. Not only does the syringe provide a reliable measure, but it also serves as a convenient means for transporting and administering the medication. The medication can be placed directly into the child's mouth from the syringe. For added safety, a short length of flexible tubing can be placed on the tip of the syringe to prevent injury to the mouth, although the tubing must be completely emptied of medication.

Young children and some older children as well have difficulty swallowing tablets or pills. Because a number of drugs are not available in pediatric preparations, the tablet needs to be crushed before it can be given to these children. Commercial devices* are available, or simple methods can be employed for crushing tablets. Not all drugs can be crushed (e.g., medication with an enteric or protective coating or formulated for slow release).

NURSING TIP

To minimize loss of the drug, crush the tablet between two spoons or place the tablet in either a medicine cup or between two small paper soufflé cups and use a pestle for crushing; collect the bits of pulverized medication that tend to cling to the sides of the cup or spoon and mix the crushed tablet with a palatable substance.

Children who must take oral medication for an extended period can be taught to swallow tablets or capsules. Training sessions include using verbal instruction, demonstration, reinforcement of swallowing progressively larger candy/capsules, no attention for inappropriate behavior, and gradual withdrawal of guidance once children can swallow their medication.

Because pediatric doses often require dividing adult preparations of medication, the nurse may be faced with the

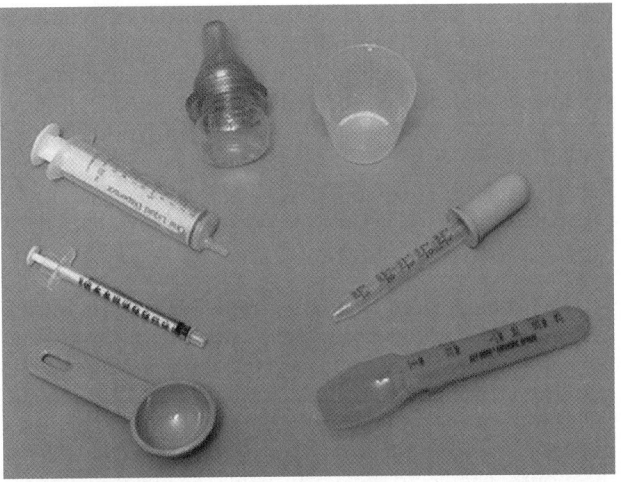

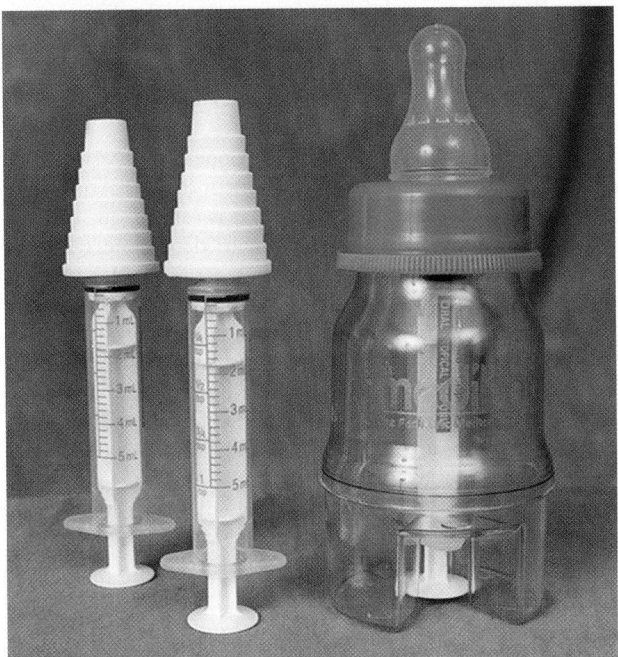

FIG. 22-18 ■ **A,** Acceptable devices for measuring and administering oral medication to children (clockwise): measuring spoon, plastic syringes, calibrated nipple, plastic medicine cup, calibrated dropper, hollow-handled medicine spoon. **B,** Medi-bottle used to deliver oral medication via a syringe. **(B,** Photo by Paul Vincent Kuntz, Texas Children's Hospital.)

dilemma of accurate dosage. With tablets, only those that are scored can be halved or quartered accurately. If the medication is soluble, the tablet or contents of a capsule can be mixed in a small, premeasured amount of liquid and the appropriate portion given. If half a dose is required, the tablet is dissolved in 5 mL water or flavored liquid and 2.5 mL is given.

Administration

Although administering liquids to infants is relatively easy, the nurse must be careful to prevent aspiration. With the infant held in a semireclining position, the medication is placed in the mouth from a spoon, plastic cup, plastic dropper, or

---

*__Trademark Medical__ manufactures a pill crusher and has compiled a list of more than 190 medications that should not be crushed or chewed. Both are available from Trademark Medical, 1053 Headquarters Park, Fenton, MO 63026-2033; (800) 325-9044; website: www.trademarkmedical.com.

plastic syringe (without needle). The dropper or syringe is best placed along the side of the infant's tongue, with the contents administered slowly in small amounts, allowing the child to swallow between deposits.

In infants up to 11 months of age and children with neurologic impairments, blowing a small puff of air in the face frequently elicits a swallow reflex.

Medicine cups can be used effectively for older infants who are able to drink from a cup. Because of the natural outward tongue thrust in infancy, medications may need to be retrieved from the lips or chin and refed. Allowing the infant to suck medication that has been placed in an empty nipple or inserting the syringe or dropper into the side of the mouth, parallel to the nipple, while the infant nurses are other convenient methods for giving liquid medications to infants. Medication is not added to the infant's formula feeding. Dispose of any plastic covers that may be on the ends of syringes. These covers are small enough to be aspirated by young children.

The young child who refuses to cooperate or resists consistently despite explanation and encouragement may require mild physical coercion. If so, it is carried out quickly and carefully. Every effort is made to determine why the child resists, and the reasons for the coercion are explained to the child in such a way that the child will know that it is being carried out for his or her well-being and is not a form of punishment. There is always a risk in using even mild forceful techniques. A crying child can aspirate a medication, particularly when lying on the back. If the nurse holds the child in the lap with the child's right arm behind the nurse, the left hand firmly grasped by the nurse's left hand, and the head securely restrained between the nurse's arm and body, the medication can be slowly poured into the mouth (Fig. 22-19).

INTRAMUSCULAR ADMINISTRATION
Selecting the Syringe and Needle

The volume of medication prescribed for small children and the small amount of tissue for injection require that a syringe be selected that can measure very small amounts of solution. For volumes of less than 1 mL, the tuberculin syringe, calibrated in one-hundredth increments, is appropriate. Very minute doses may require the use of a 0.5-mL, low-dose syringe. These syringes with specially constructed needles minimize the possibility of inadvertently administering incorrect amounts of a drug because of *dead space*, which allows fluid to remain in the syringe and needle after the plunger is pushed completely forward. A minimum of 0.2 mL solution remains in a standard needle hub; therefore, when very small amounts of two drugs are combined in the syringe, such as mixtures of insulin, the ratio of the two drugs can be altered significantly. Measures that minimize the effect of dead space follow: (1) when two drugs are combined in the syringe, always draw them up in the same order to maintain a consistent ratio between the drugs; (2) use the same brand of syringe (dead space may vary between brands); and (3) use one-piece syringe units (needle permanently attached to the syringe).

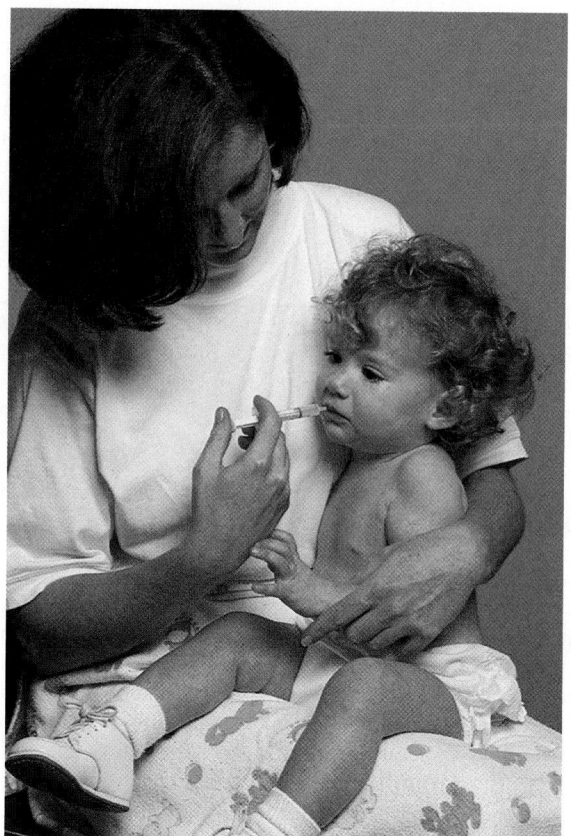

FIG. 22-19 ■ Nurse partially restrains child for easy and comfortable administration of oral medication.

Dead space is also an important factor to consider when injecting medication, because flushing the syringe with an air bubble or parenteral fluid adds an additional amount of medication to the prescribed dose. This can be hazardous when very small amounts of a drug are given. For example, a tuberculin syringe filled to the 0.05-mL mark can deliver *more than twice* the calculated dose of medication when it is flushed with parenteral fluid from an IV line. Consequently, flushing is not advisable, especially when less than 1 mL of medication is given. Syringes are calibrated to deliver a prescribed drug dose, and the amount of medication left in the hub and needle is not part of the syringe barrel calibrations. However, the air-bubble technique (drawing up about 0.2 mL of air into the syringe after withdrawing the medication) may be beneficial with certain drugs, such as iron dextran and diphtheria and tetanus toxoid, to avoid tracking the drug through the tissue. Other techniques to minimize tracking include changing the needle after withdrawing the fluid from the vial (not always effective) and using the Z-track method.

The *needle length* must be sufficient to penetrate the subcutaneous tissue and deposit the medication in the body of the muscle. The needle gauge should be as small as possible to deliver fluid safely. Smaller-diameter (25- to 30-gauge) needles cause the least discomfort, but larger diameters are needed for viscous medication and prevention of accidental bending of longer needles (Table 22-5).

Based on ultrasonography, two injection techniques have been studied to determine the best needle length for the

TABLE 22-5 ■ Intramuscular Injection Sites in Children

SITE	DISCUSSION
VASTUS LATERALIS 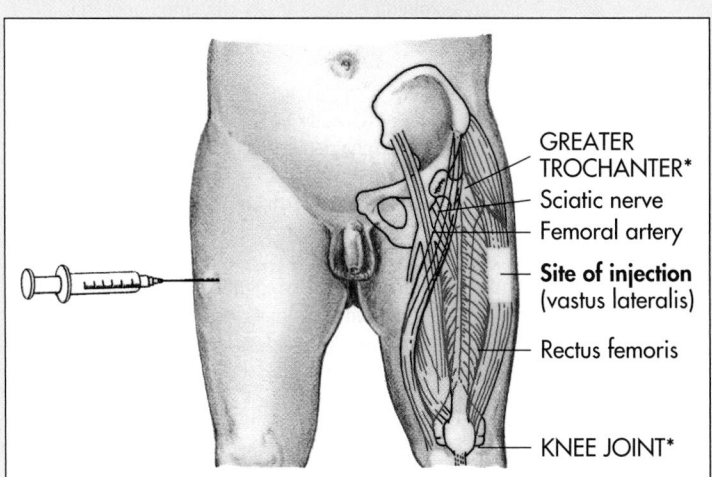 GREATER TROCHANTER* Sciatic nerve Femoral artery **Site of injection** (vastus lateralis) Rectus femoris KNEE JOINT*	**LOCATION*** Palpate to find greater trochanter and knee joints; divide vertical distance between these two landmarks into thirds; inject into middle third **NEEDLE INSERTION AND SIZE** Insert needle perpendicular to knee in infants and young children or perpendicular to thigh or slightly angled toward anterior thigh 22 to 25 gauge, 0.625 to 1 inch† **ADVANTAGES** Large, well-developed muscle that can tolerate larger quantities of fluid (0.5 mL [infant] to 2.0 mL [child]) Easily accessible if child is supine, side-lying, or sitting **DISADVANTAGES** Thrombosis of femoral artery from injection in midthigh area Sciatic nerve damage from long needle injected posteriorly and medially into small extremity More painful than deltoid or gluteal sites
VENTROGLUTEAL 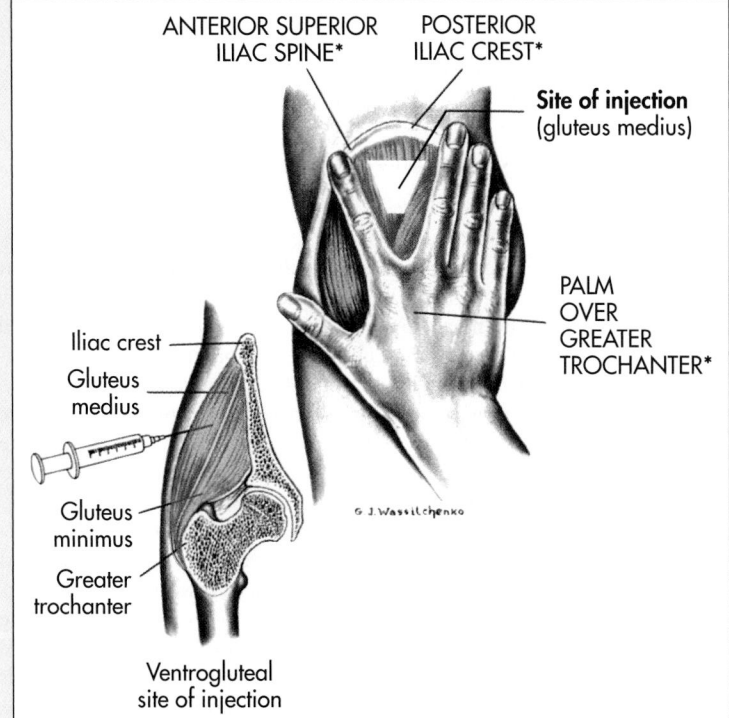 ANTERIOR SUPERIOR ILIAC SPINE* POSTERIOR ILIAC CREST* **Site of injection** (gluteus medius) Iliac crest Gluteus medius PALM OVER GREATER TROCHANTER* Gluteus minimus Greater trochanter G. J. Wassilchenko Ventrogluteal site of injection	**LOCATION*** Palpate to locate greater trochanter, anterior superior iliac tubercle (found by flexing thigh at hip and measuring up to 1 to 2 cm above crease formed in groin), and posterior iliac crest; place palm of hand over greater trochanter, index finger over anterior superior iliac tubercle, and middle finger along crest of ilium posteriorly as far as possible; inject into center of V formed by fingers **NEEDLE INSERTION AND SIZE** Insert needle perpendicular to site but angled slightly toward iliac crest 22 to 25 gauge, 0.625 to 1 inch‡ **ADVANTAGES** Free of important nerves and vascular structures Easily identified by prominent bony landmarks Thinner layer of subcutaneous tissue than in dorsogluteal site, thus less chance of depositing drug subcutaneously rather than intramuscularly Can accommodate larger quantities of fluid (0.5 mL [infant] to 2.0 mL [child]) Easily accessible if child is supine, prone, or side-lying Less painful than vastus lateralis **DISADVANTAGES** Health professionals' unfamiliarity with site

*Locations are indicated by asterisks on illustrations.
†Research has shown that a 1-inch needle is needed for adequate muscle penetration in infants 4 months old and possibly in infants as young as 2 months (Hicks and others, 1989).
‡*A Guide for Managing the Pediatric Patient, Reducing the Anxiety and Pain of Injections* (1998) is available from Becton Dickinson & Co., 1 Becton Drive, Franklin Lakes, NJ 07417; (888) 237-2762; fax: (201) 847-4682; website: www.bd.com. In Canada: Becton Dickinson Canada, Inc., 2464 South Sheridan Way, Mississauga, Ontario L5J 2M8; (800) 268-5430 (Ontario and Quebec) or (800) 268-5450 (other areas).

Continued

TABLE 22-5 ■ **Intramuscular Injection Sites in Children—*cont'd***

SITE	DISCUSSION
DELTOID Clavicle ACROMION PROCESS* Site of injection (deltoid) AXILLA Brachial artery Humerus Radial nerve G.J.Wassilchenko	**LOCATION*** Locate acromion process; inject only into upper third of muscle that begins about 2 fingerbreadths below acromion **NEEDLE INSERTION AND SIZE** Insert needle perpendicular to site but angled slightly toward shoulder 22 to 25 gauge, 0.625 to 1 inch **ADVANTAGES** Faster absorption rates than gluteal sites Easily accessible with minimal removal of clothing Less pain and fewer local side effects from vaccines as compared with vastus lateralis **DISADVANTAGES** Small muscle mass; only limited amounts of drug can be injected (0.5 to 1.0 mL) Small margins of safety with possible damage to radial nerve and axillary nerve (not shown, lies under deltoid at head of humerus)

*Locations are indicated by asterisks on illustrations.

deltoid and vastus lateralis sites. If the muscle is grasped or bunched, a needle length of 25 mm (1 inch) is recommended. If the muscle is stretched or flattened, a needle length of 16 mm (0.625 inch) is adequate (Groswasser and others, 1997). Unfortunately, the conclusions of the study fail to address whether these lengths apply to both muscles. From the data, it appears more likely that the recommendations apply to the thigh muscle only. Other recommendations for needle size and volume of fluid are based on traditional practice and have not been verified by research.

Determining the Site

Factors that are considered when selecting a site for an intramuscular (IM) injection on an infant or child include:

- The amount and character of the medication to be injected
- The amount and general condition of the muscle mass
- The frequency or number of injections to be given during the course of treatment
- The type of medication being given
- Factors that may impede access to or cause contamination of the site
- The child's ability to assume the required position safely

Older children and adolescents usually pose few problems in selecting a suitable site for IM injections, but infants, with their small and underdeveloped muscles, have fewer

available sites. It is sometimes difficult to assess the amount of fluid that can be safely injected into a single site. Usually 1 mL is the maximum volume that should be administered in a single site to small children and older infants. The muscles of small infants may not tolerate more than 0.5 mL. As the child approaches adult size, volumes approaching those given to adults may be used. However, the larger the amount of solution, the larger the muscle must be into which it is injected.

Injections must be placed in muscles large enough to accommodate the medication; however, major nerves and blood vessels must be avoided. There is no universal agreement regarding the best IM injection site for children. The preferred site for infants is the vastus lateralis (the rectus femoris is not an acceptable site). The ventrogluteal site is relatively free of major nerves and blood vessels, is a relatively large muscle with less subcutaneous tissue than the dorsal site, has well-defined landmarks for safe site location, is less painful than the vastus lateralis, and is easily accessible in several positions. These advantages make it a preferred site over the dorsogluteal muscle and challenge the recommendation that the ventrogluteal site not be used until children have been walking. Although there are published recommendations regarding age, in clinical practice the ventrogluteal site has been used in children as young as newborns. The dorsogluteal site is not recommended in infants and young children because of the close proximity to the sciatic nerve and superior gluteal artery. Other sites discussed previously provide better choices for IM injections in children. Table 22-5 summarizes the major injection sites and illustrates the location of the preferred IM injection sites for children.

Administration

Although injections that are executed with care seldom cause trauma to the child, there have been reports of serious disability related to IM injections in children. Repeated use of a single site has been associated with fibrosis of the muscle with subsequent muscle contracture. Injections close to large nerves, such as the sciatic nerve, have been responsible for permanent disability, especially when potentially neurotoxic drugs are administered. There are several reports of tissue damage from penicillin. One of the difficulties in administering the opaque preparations, such as Bicillin, is that aspirated blood cannot be detected at the bottom of the syringe, thus increasing the risk of injecting into a blood vessel. When such drugs are injected, great care must be used in locating the correct site. When aspirating, the nurse should look for blood at the *top* of the syringe near the plunger, because blood may be drawn up through the column of penicillin. One study of IM injection techniques revealed that the straighter the path of needle insertion (e.g., 90-degree angle), the less displacement there is, causing less discomfort (Katsma and Smith, 1997).

A reported potential hazard with medication in glass ampules is the presence of glass particles in the ampule after the container is broken. When the medication is withdrawn into the syringe, the glass particles may also be withdrawn and subsequently injected into the patient. As a precaution, medication from glass ampules should be drawn up only through a needle with a filter or injected intravenously through a site in the tubing that is distal to an IV filter. Other precautions related to needle use and disposal are on p. 735.

Children may be unpredictable and cannot be expected to cooperate totally when receiving an injection. Even children who appear to be relaxed and constrained can lose control under the stress of the procedure. It is advisable to have someone available to help hold the child if needed. Because children often jerk or pull away unexpectedly, the nurse should carry an extra needle to exchange for a contaminated one so that the delay is minimal. The child, even a small one, is told that he or she is receiving an injection (preferably using a phrase such as "putting medicine under the skin"), and then the procedure is carried out as quickly and skillfully as possible to avoid prolonging the stressful experience. Delay caused by lengthy explanations, attempts to hide the syringe from sight, or efforts to soothe the child only increase the anxiety. It must be kept in mind that intrusive procedures such as injections are especially anxiety provoking in preschool children and that small children usually associate any assault to the "behind" area with punishment. Most children hate intramuscular injections; studies show that getting an injection is one of the most feared procedures (Huth, 1999). Because injections are painful, the nurse should employ excellent injection technique and effective pain reduction measures to reduce discomfort (see Guidelines box).

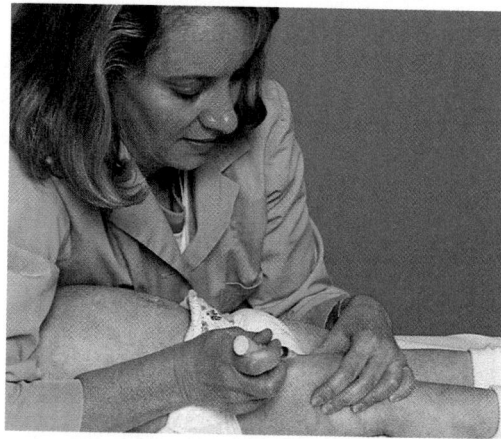

FIG. 22-20 ■ Holding small child for intramuscular injection. Note how nurse isolates and stabilizes muscle.

Small infants offer little resistance to injections. Although they squirm and may be difficult to hold in position, they can usually be restrained without assistance. The body of a larger infant can be securely held between the nurse's arm and body (Fig. 22-20). To inject into the body of the muscle, the muscle mass is firmly grasped between the thumb and fingers to isolate and stabilize the site. In obese children, however, it is preferable first to spread the skin with the thumb and index finger to displace subcutaneous tissue and then grasp the muscle deeply on each side. For an injection into the arm, place the child in the parent's (or assistant's) lap, with the child facing sideward. Next, place the child's arm that is closest to the parent under the parent's arm and wrap toward the back. Then have the parent hold the arm for the injection against the child's body.

If the medication is given around the clock, the nurse should not try to administer an injection to a sleeping child, even though it may seem to be easier than waking the youngster. This practice can cause the child to fear going to sleep. When awakened first, the child knows that nothing will be done unless he or she is forewarned.

A needless injection system delivers IM or subcutaneous injections without the use of a needle and eliminates the risk of accidental needle puncture. This needle-free injection system is powered by a carbon dioxide cartridge that provides the power to deliver the medication through the skin. Although it is not painless, it may reduce pain and also the anxiety of seeing the needle (Polillio and Killy, 1997).

SUBCUTANEOUS AND INTRADERMAL ADMINISTRATION

Subcutaneous and intradermal injections are frequently administered to children, but the technique differs little from the method used with adults. Examples of *subcutaneous injections* include insulin, hormone replacement, allergy desensitization, and some vaccines. Tuberculin (TB) testing, local anesthesia, and allergy testing are examples of frequently administered *intradermal injections.*

Techniques to minimize the pain associated with these injections include changing the needle if it pierced a rubber stopper on a vial, using 26- to 30-gauge needles (only to inject the solution), and injecting small volumes (up to 0.5 mL).

GUIDELINES

Intramuscular Administration of Medication

Use safety precautions in administering medication (e.g., check child's identification).

Apply EMLA topically over site if time permits (at least 60 minutes, preferably 2 to 2.5 hours for (intramuscular [IM] injection). LMX cream may be applied for a shorter interval (see Pain Management, Chapter 21).

Prepare medication.

Select needle and syringe appropriate to the following:

Amount of fluid to be administered (syringe size)

Viscosity of fluid to be administered (needle gauge)

Amount of tissue to be penetrated (needle length)

Maximum volume to be administered in a single site is 1 mL for older infants and small children.

Determine site of injection (see Table 22-5), make certain that muscle is large enough to accommodate volume and type of medication.

Following are acceptable sites for infants and small or debilitated children:

Vastus lateralis muscle

Ventrogluteal muscle

Dorsogluteal muscle is insufficiently developed to be a safe site for infants and small children.

Administer medication.

Provide for sufficient help in restraining child; children are often uncooperative, and their behavior is usually unpredictable.

Explain briefly what is to be done and, if appropriate, what child can do to help.

Expose injection area for unobstructed view of landmarks.

Select a site where skin is free of irritation and danger of infection; palpate for and avoid sensitive or hardened areas.

With multiple injections, rotate sites.

Place child in a lying or sitting position; child is not allowed to stand because:

Landmarks are more difficult to assess.

Restraint is more difficult.

Child may faint and fall.

Use a new, sharp needle with smallest diameter that permits free flow of the medication.

Grasp muscle firmly between thumb and fingers to isolate and stabilize muscle for deposition of drug in its deepest part; in obese children, spread skin with thumb and index finger to displace subcutaneous tissue and grasp muscle deeply on each side.

Allow skin preparation to dry completely before skin is penetrated.

Have medication at room temperature.

Decrease perception of pain.

Distract child with conversation.

Give child something on which to concentrate (e.g., squeezing a hand or side rail, pinching own nose, humming, counting, yelling "Ouch!").

Spray vapocoolant (e.g., ethyl chloride or fluori-methane) on site 11 to 15 seconds before injection or place a cold compress or wrapped ice cube on site about a minute before injection, or apply cold to contralateral site.

Say to child, "If you feel this, tell me to take it out, please."

Have child hold a small adhesive bandage and place it on puncture site after IM injection is given.

Insert needle quickly, using a dartlike motion at a 90-degree angle unless contraindicated.

Use new needle, not one that has pierced rubber stopper on vial.

Avoid tracking any medication through superficial tissues:

Replace needle after withdrawing medication, or wipe medication from needle with sterile gauze.

If withdrawing medication from an ampule, use a needle equipped with a filter that removes glass particles; then use a new, nonfilter needle for injection.

Use the Z-track or air-bubble technique as indicated.

Avoid any depression of the plunger during insertion of the needle.

Aspirate for blood.

If blood is found, remove syringe from site, change needle, and reinsert into new location.

If no blood is found, inject into a relaxed muscle:

Ventrogluteal—Place child on side with upper leg flexed and placed in front of lower leg.

Vastus Lateralis—Child can be supine, lying on the side, or sitting.

Inject medication slowly.

Remove needle quickly; hold gauze sponge firmly against skin near needle when removing it to avoid pulling on tissue.

Apply firm pressure to site after injection; massage site to hasten absorption unless contraindicated, as with irritating drugs.

Place a small adhesive bandage on puncture site; with young children decorate it by drawing a smiling face or other symbol of acceptance.

Hold and cuddle young child and encourage parents to comfort child; praise older child.

Allow expression of feelings.

Discard syringe and uncapped, uncut needle in puncture-resistant container located near site of use.

Record time of injection, drug, dose, and injection site.

The angle of the needle for the subcutaneous injection is typically 90 degrees. In children with little subcutaneous tissue, some practitioners insert the needle at a 45-degree angle. However, the benefit of using the 45-degree angle rather than the 90-degree angle remains controversial.

Although subcutaneous injections can be given anywhere there is subcutaneous tissue, common sites include the center third of the lateral aspect of the upper arm, the abdomen, and the center third of the anterior thigh. Some practitioners believe it is not necessary to aspirate before injecting subcutaneously. For example, not aspirating is an ac-

cepted practice in the administration of insulin. Automatic injector devices do not aspirate before injecting.

When giving an intradermal injection into the volar surface of the forearm, the nurse should avoid the medial side of the arm, where the skin is more sensitive.

NURSING TIP

Families often need to learn subcutaneous injection techniques to administer medications, such as insulin, at home. Begin teaching as early as possible to allow the family the maximum amount of practice time possible.

INTRAVENOUS ADMINISTRATION

The IV route for administering medications is frequently used in pediatric therapy. For some important drugs it is the only effective route of administration. This method is used for giving drugs to children who have poor absorption as a result of diarrhea, dehydration, or peripheral vascular collapse; children who need a high serum concentration of a drug; children who have resistant infections that require parenteral medication over an extended time; children who need continuous pain relief; and children who require emergency treatment.

Insertion sites and observation of the IV infusion are discussed on p. 764. However, several factors need to be considered in relation to IV medication. When a drug is administered intravenously, the effect is almost instantaneous and further control is limited. Most drugs for IV administration require a specified minimum dilution and/or rate of flow, and many are highly irritating or toxic to tissues outside the vascular system. In addition to the precautions and nursing observations related to IV therapy, factors to consider when preparing and administering drugs to infants and children by the IV route include the following:

- Amount of drug to be administered
- Minimum dilution of drug and if child is fluid-restricted
- Type of solution in which drug can be diluted
- Length of time over which drug can be safely administered
- Rate of infusion that child and vessels can tolerate safely
- IV tubing volume capacity
- Time that this or another drug is to be administered
- Compatibility of all drugs that child is receiving intravenously

Before any IV infusion, the site of insertion is checked for patency. Medications are never administered with blood products. Only one antibiotic should be administered at a time.

IV infusion is suitable for children who can tolerate the necessary infusion rate and the extra fluid needed to administer the medication. For the very small infant or fluid-restricted child who is not able to tolerate the increased rate of fluids, special delivery systems, such as syringe pumps, are used. Regardless of the technique used, the nurse must know the minimum dilutions for safe administration of IV medications to infants and children. The package insert often includes this information, but if there is any doubt regarding the amount of dilution, the pharmacist should be contacted.

Peripheral Venous Access Devices

The *peripheral lock,* also known as an *intermittent infusion device* or *saline* or *heparin lock,* is used as an alternative for a keep-open infusion when extended access to a vein is required without the need for continuous fluid. It is most frequently employed for intermittent infusion of medication into a peripheral venous route. A short, flexible catheter is used as the lock device, and a site is selected where there will be minimal movement, such as the forearm. The catheter device is inserted and secured in the same manner as for any IV infusion device, but the hub is occluded with a stopper.

The type of device used may vary, and the care and use of the peripheral intermittent infusion device (PIID) are carried out according to the specific protocol of the institution or unit. However, the general concept is the same. The catheter remains in place and is flushed with saline after infusion of the medication. Many studies have shown that normal saline alone is as effective as heparin in maintaining IV patency, especially in catheters larger than 24 gauge (Heilskov and others, 1998; Beecroft and others, 1997; Paisley and others, 1997; Kotter, 1996). Two factors that may account for the difference in small-gauge catheters is frequency of flush and use of the positive-pressure technique. This technique involves instilling the final flush solution as the clamp is closed. Theoretically the procedure is thought to prevent backflow of blood into the catheter, preventing a small clot from forming.

Children may be discharged with a PIID in place to continue receiving medications without hospitalization; this is usually reserved for children who require medications on a short-term basis and are referred to a home-based infusion company. Those with chronic illnesses who require repeated blood sampling or medications, long-term chemotherapy, or frequent hyperalimentation or antibiotic therapy are best managed with a central venous catheter or a peripherally inserted central catheter.

Central Venous Access Devices

Central venous access devices (VADs) have several different characteristics. The practitioner has to consider the best type of catheter for the individual patient's needs. Factors that can influence the decision include the reason for placement of the catheter (diagnosis), length of therapy, risk to the patient in placement of the catheter, and availability of resources to assist the family in maintaining the catheter.

Short-term or *nontunneled catheters* are used in acute care, emergency, and intensive care units. These catheters are made of polyurethane and are placed in large veins such as the subclavian, femoral, or jugular. Insertion is by surgical incision or large percutaneous threading. A chest x-ray film should be taken to verify placement of the catheter tip before administration of fluids or medications.

Peripherally inserted central catheters (PICCs) can be used for short-term to moderate-length therapy. Researchers have shown catheter longevity ranging to more than 200 days (Donaldson and others, 1995; Frey, 1995). These catheters consist of silicone or polymer material and are placed by specially trained nurses, physicians, or interventional radiologists (Chung and Ziegler, 1998). The most common insertion site is above the antecubital area using the median, cephalic, or basilic vein. The catheter is threaded either with or without a guidewire into the superior vena cava. PICCs can be trimmed before insertion, and the decision can be made to insert the catheter "midline," which is considered between the insertion site and the head of the clavicle. If the catheter is threaded midline, total parenteral nutrition (TPN) or any other drug known to irritate a peripheral vein (e.g., chemotherapy drugs) should not be administered. The high concentration of glucose in TPN makes it irritating to the vessel; thus it should be infused through a central catheter.

The decision to insert a PICC needs to be made *before* there are several unsuccessful attempts at IV lines or blood sampling by phlebotomy. After the antecubital veins have been punctured repeatedly, they are not considered to be a candidate for this type of catheter. Because this catheter is the least costly and has less chance of complications than other central VADs, it is an excellent choice for many pediatric patients. This catheter is also usually inserted either at the child's bedside or, more appropriately when available, in the unit's treatment room.

! NURSING ALERT

Most PICC lines are not sutured into place, so care needs to be maintained when changing the dressing.

Long-term central VADs include tunneled and implanted infusion ports (Table 22-6). They may have single, double, or triple lumens. Several lumens (multilumen catheters) allow more than one therapy to be administered at the same time. Reasons to use multilumen catheters include repeated blood sampling, TPN, administration of blood products or infusion of large quantities and/or concentrations of fluids, ability to administer incompatible drugs or fluids at the same time (through different lumens), and central venous pressure (CVP) monitoring.

With any of the central venous catheters, instilling medication through the injection cap is easily accomplished. With the implanted device the port must be palpated for placement and stabilized, the overlying skin cleansed, and only special noncoring Huber needles used to pierce the port's diaphragm on the top or side, depending on the

TABLE 22-6 ■ Comparison of Long-Term Central Venous Access Devices

DESCRIPTION	BENEFITS	CARE CONSIDERATIONS
TUNNELED CATHETER (SUCH AS HICKMAN/BROVIAC CATHETER)		
Silicone, radiopaque, flexible catheter with open ends	Reduced risk of bacterial migration after tissue adheres to Dacron cuff or VitaCuff	Requires daily heparin flushes
One or two Dacron cuffs or VitaCuffs (biosynthetic material impregnated with silver ions) on catheter(s) enhances tissue ingrowth	Easy to use for self-administered infusions	Must be clamped or have clamp nearby at all times
May have more than one lumen	Removal requires pulling catheter from site (nonsurgical procedure)	Must keep exit site dry
		Heavy activity restricted until tissue adheres to cuff
		Water sports may be restricted (risk of infection)
		Risk of infection still present
		Protrudes outside body; susceptible to damage from sharp instruments and may be pulled out; may affect body image
		More difficult to repair
		Patient/family must learn catheter care
GROSHONG CATHETER		
Clear, flexible, silicone, radiopaque catheter with closed tip and two-way valve at proximal end	Reduced time and cost for maintenance care; no heparin flushes needed	Requires weekly irrigation with normal saline
Dacron cuff or VitaCuff on catheter enhances tissue ingrowth	Reduced catheter damage; no clamping needed because of two-way valve	Must keep exit site dry
May have more than one lumen	Increased patient safety because of minimal potential for blood backflow or air embolism	Heavy activity restricted until tissue adheres to cuff
	Reduced risk of bacterial migration after tissue adheres to Dacron cuff or VitaCuff	Water sports may be restricted (risk of infection)
	Easily repaired	Risk of infection still present
	Easy to use for self-administered intravenous infusions	Protrudes outside body; susceptible to damage from sharp instruments and may be pulled out; can affect body image
		Patient/family must learn catheter care
IMPLANTED PORTS (PORT-A-CATH, INFUS-A-PORT, MEDIPORT, NORPORT, GROSHONG PORT)		
Totally implantable metal or plastic device that consists of self-sealing injection port with top or side access with preconnected or attachable silicon catheter that is placed in large blood vessel	Reduced risk of infection	Must pierce skin for access; pain with insertion of needle; can use local anesthetic (EMLA, LMX) or intradermal buffered lidocaine before accessing port
	Placed completely under the skin; therefore, much less likely to be pulled out or damaged	Special noncoring needle (Huber) with straight or angled design must be used to inject into port
	No maintenance care and reduced cost for family	Skin preparation needed before injection
	Heparinized monthly and after each infusion to maintain patency (Groshong port only requires saline)	Difficult to manipulate for self-administered infusions
	No limitations on regular physical activity, including swimming	Catheter may dislodge from port, especially if child "plays" with port site (twiddler syndrome)
	Dressing only needed when port accessed with Huber needle that is not removed	Vigorous contact sports generally not allowed
	No or only slight change in body appearance (slight bulge on chest)	Removal requires surgical procedure

style. To avoid repeated skin punctures, a special infusion set with a Huber needle and extension tubing with a Luer connection can be used (Fig. 22-21). With this attached, the injection procedure is the same as for an intermittent infusion device or a central venous catheter. To prevent infection, meticulous aseptic technique must be used any time the devices are entered, including instillation of heparin or saline to prevent clotting (Long and others, 1996). There should be a protocol stating that the Huber needle needs to be charged at established intervals, usually 5 to 7 days.

The children and parents are taught the procedure for care of the VAD before discharge from the hospital, including preparation and injection of the prescribed medication, the flush, and dressing changes. A protective device may be recommended for some active children to prevent their accidentally dislodging the needle. Many children take responsibility for preparing and administering medications. Both verbal and written step-by-step instructions are provided for the learners (Table 22-7).

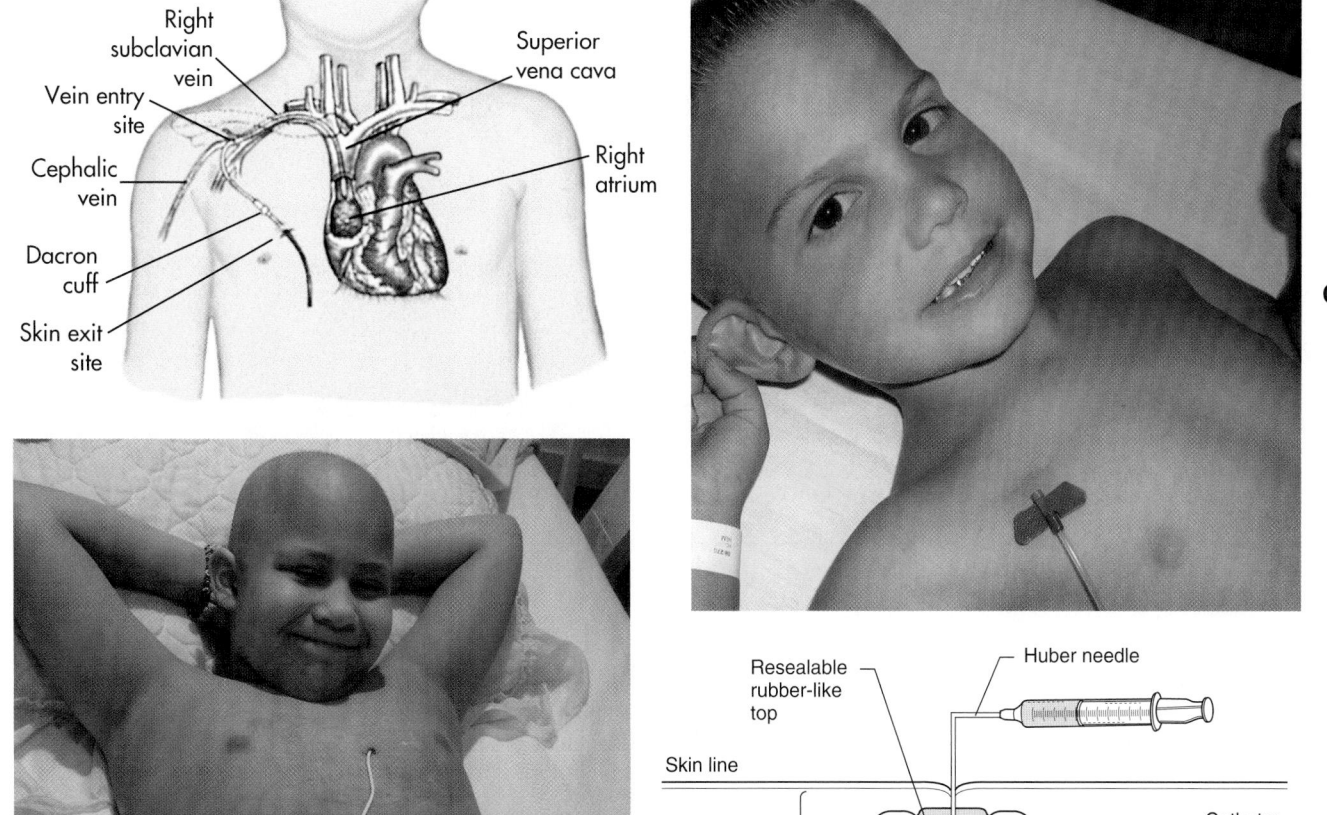

FIG. 22-21 ■ Venous access devices. **A,** External central venous catheter insertion and exit site. **B,** Child with external central venous catheter. **C,** Child with implanted port with Huber needle in place. **D,** Side view of implanted port.

TABLE 22-7 ■ Heparin Flush Guidelines

	INTERMITTENT		DORMANT	
CHILDREN	≤2 years or ≤24-g catheter	>2 years	≤2 years or ≤24-g catheter	>2 years
Peripheral lines (Heplock)	10 units/mL; 1 mL heparin after meds or every 8 hours	5 mL normal saline after meds or every 8 hours	10 units/mL; 1 mL heparin every 8 hours	5 mL normal saline every 8 hours
External central line (nonimplanted, tunneled, or peripherally inserted central catheter [PICC])	10 units/mL; 3 mL heparin after meds		10 units/mL; 3 mL heparin every day	100 units/mL; 3 mL heparin every day
Totally implanted central line	10 units/mL; 5 mL heparin after meds		100 units/mL; 5 mL every month; or 10 units/mL, 5 mL every day if accessed	100 units/mL; 5 mL heparin every month or every day if accessed
Midline	10 units/mL; 3 mL heparin in a 5-mL syringe after meds or every 8 hours		10 units/mL; 3 mL heparin in a 5-mL syringe every 8 hours	
Arterial and central venous pressure continuous monitored lines	Heparin, 2 units/mL, in 55-mL syringes run at 1 mL/hr		N/A	
NEONATES/INFANTS				
Peripheral lines (Heplock)	2 units/mL; 2 mL heparin to check for line patency and between meds or TPN known to be incompatible		2 units/mL; 2 mL heparin every 8 hours	
Percutaneous central catheter	2 units/mL in 20-mL syringe run at 0.2 mL/hr		N/A	
Surgically placed central venous catheter (CVC) ≤5 French	2 units/mL; 2 mL heparin to check for line patency and between meds or TPN known to be compatible		2 units/mL; 2 mL heparin every 8 hours	
Surgically placed CVC (central venous catheter) >5 French	2 units/mL; 3 mL heparin to check for line patency and between meds or TPN known to be compatible		2 units/mL; 3 mL heparin every 8 hours	

Modified from Texas Children's Hospital, Houston, Tex, 2002.
N/A, Not applicable; *TPN,* total parenteral nutrition.

- A pocket sewn on the inside of a T-shirt provides a place in which to coil the catheter line while the child is at play if a dressing is not used. A commercial elastic vest is also available.*

---

*Available from **Advanced Patient Devices**, 3564 Sabaka Trail, Verona, WI 53593; (800) 547-6412; fax: (608) 833-6694.

Infection and an occluded catheter are two of the most common complications of central venous catheters. Although neither is an emergency, they require treatment with antibiotics for infection and a fibrinolytic agent, such as alteplase, for clots (Reed and Phillip, 1996). Uncapping can be prevented by taping the cap securely to the catheter and the clamped line to the dressing. Leaks can be prevented by using a smooth-edged clamp only. Parents are cautioned to keep scissors away from the child to prevent accidental cutting of the catheter. If the catheter leaks, they are instructed to tape it above the leak and then clamp the catheter at the taped site. The child should be taken to the practitioner as soon as possible to prevent infection or clotting after a catheter leak.

! NURSING ALERT

If a central venous catheter is accidentally removed, apply pressure to the entry site to the vein, not the exit site on the skin.

NASOGASTRIC, OROGASTRIC, OR GASTROSTOMY ADMINISTRATION

When a child has an indwelling feeding tube or a gastrostomy, oral medications are usually given via that route. An advantage of this method is the ability to administer oral medications around the clock without disturbing the child. A disadvantage is the risk of occluding or "clogging" the tube, especially when giving viscous solutions through small-bore feeding tubes. The most important preventive measure is adequate flushing after the medication is instilled. Guidelines for administration are presented in the Guidelines box.

> ### ❗ NURSING ALERT
>
> Sprinkle-type medication should be avoided. However, if there is no other option and the tube is large gauge (18 French or greater), but usually not a Foley catheter, it may be given by mixing the sprinkles with a small amount of pureed fruit and thinning with water. The fruit keeps the sprinkles suspended so that they do not float to the top. Flush well. This procedure is not recommended for skin-level gastrostomy devices.

RECTAL ADMINISTRATION

The rectal route for administration is less reliable but is sometimes used when the oral route is difficult or contraindicated. Some of the drugs available in suppository

---

⌇ GUIDELINES

Nasogastric, Orogastric, or Gastrostomy Medication Administration in Children

Use elixir or suspension (rather than tablet) preparations of medication whenever possible.

Dilute viscous medication or syrup with a small amount of water if possible.

If administering tablets, crush tablet to a very fine powder and dissolve drug in a small amount of warm water.

Never crush enteric-coated or sustained-release tablets or capsules.

Avoid oily medications because they tend to cling to side of tube.

Do not mix medication with enteral formula unless fluid is restricted. If adding a drug:
  Check with pharmacist for compatibility.
  Shake formula well and observe for any physical reaction (e.g., separation, precipitation).
  Label formula container with name of medication, dosage, date, and time infusion started.

Have medication at room temperature.

Measure medication in a calibrated cup or syringe.

Check for correct placement of nasogastric or orogastric tube (see Guidelines box, p. 779).

Attach syringe (with adaptable tip but without plunger) to tube.

Pour medication into syringe.

Unclamp tube and allow medication to flow by gravity.

Adjust height of container to achieve desired flow rate (e.g., increase height for faster flow).

As soon as syringe is empty, pour in water to flush tubing.

Amount of water depends on length and gauge of tubing.

Determine amount before administering any medication by using a syringe to fill completely an unused nasogastric or orogastric tube with water. Amount of flush solution is usually 1.5 times this volume.

With certain drug preparations (e.g., suspensions) more fluid may be needed.

If administering more than one drug at the same time, flush tube between each medication with clear water.

Clamp tube after flushing, unless tube is left open.

---

form are acetaminophen, sedatives, analgesics (morphine), and antiemetics. The difficulty in using the rectal route is that unless the rectum is empty at the time of insertion, the absorption of the drug may be delayed, diminished, or prevented by the presence of feces. Sometimes the drug is later evacuated, securely surrounded by stool. However, the rectal route is used most frequently in children who are unable to take anything by mouth and are unlikely to have large amounts of stool. It is also used when oral preparations are unsuitable for controlling vomiting.

To insert a suppository, the wrapper is removed and the suppository lubricated with water-soluble jelly or warm water. A gloved finger is used to quickly but gently insert the suppository into the rectum, beyond both of the rectal sphincters. The buttocks are then held together firmly to relieve pressure on the anal sphincter until the urge to expel the suppository has passed—5 to 10 minutes. Sometimes the amount of drug ordered is less than the dosage available. The irregular shape of most suppositories makes the process of dividing them into a desired dose difficult if not dangerous. If the suppository must be halved, it should be cut lengthwise. However, there is no guarantee that the drug is evenly dispersed throughout the petrolatum base.

Rectal suppositories are usually inserted with the apex (pointed end) foremost. One study demonstrated easier insertion and a lower expulsion rate when the suppository was inserted with the base (blunt end) first. Reverse contractions or the pressure gradient of the anal canal may help the suppository to slip higher into the canal (Moppett and Parker, 1999).

If medication is administered via a retention enema, the same procedure is used. Drugs given by enema are diluted in the smallest amount of solution possible to minimize the likelihood of being evacuated.

OPTIC, OTIC, AND NASAL ADMINISTRATION

There are few differences in administering eye, ear, and nose medication to children or to adults. The major difficulty is in gaining children's cooperation. The infant's or young child's head is immobilized in the same manner as described in Fig. 7-17, *B*. Older children need only explanation and direction. Although the administration of optic, otic, and nasal medication is not painful, these drugs can cause unpleasant sensations that can be eliminated with various techniques. Parental involvement is an important component during administration. A parent's presence can decrease levels of anxiety in the child.

> ### NURSING TIPS
>
> To reduce unpleasant sensations, perform the following:
> - **Eye.** Apply finger pressure to the lacrimal punctum at the inner aspect of the lid for 1 minute to prevent drainage of medication to the nasopharynx and the unpleasant "tasting" of the drug.
> - **Ear.** Allow medications stored in the refrigerator to warm to room temperature before instillation.
> - **Nose.** Position the child with the head hyperextended to prevent strangling sensations caused by medication trickling into the throat rather than up into the nasal passages.

To instill eye medication, the child is placed supine or sitting with the head extended, and the child is asked to look

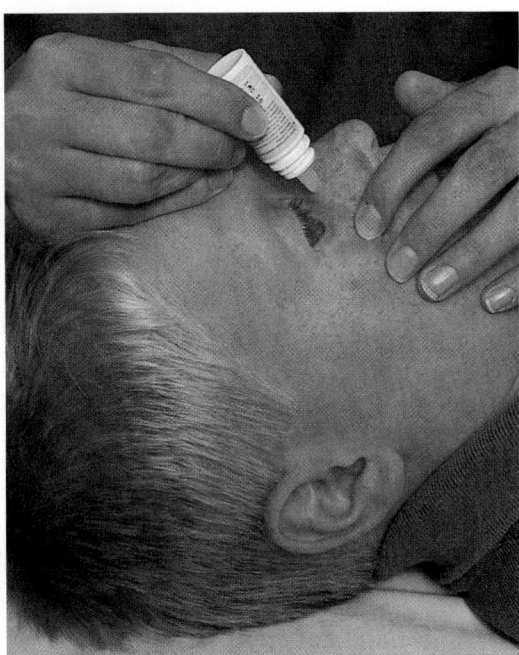

FIG. 22-22 ■ Administering eye drops.

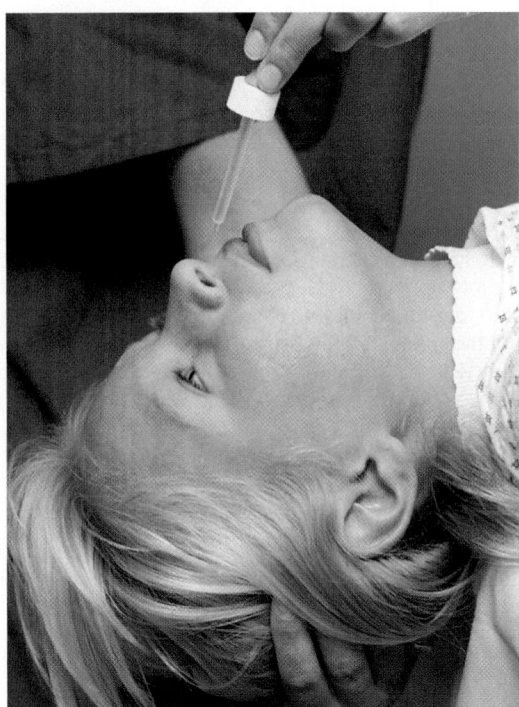

FIG. 22-23 ■ Proper position for instilling nose drops.

up. One hand is used to pull the lower lid downward; the hand that holds the dropper rests on the head so that it may move synchronously with the child's head, thus reducing the possibility of trauma to a struggling child or of dropping medication on the face (Fig. 22-22). As the lower lid is pulled down, a small conjunctival sac is formed; the solution or ointment is applied to this area, never directly on the eyeball. Another effective technique is to pull the lower lid down and out to form a cup, into which the medication is dropped. The lids are gently closed to prevent expression of the medication, and the child is asked to look in all directions to enhance even distribution of the preparation. Excess medication is wiped from the inner canthus outward to prevent contamination to the contralateral eye.

Instilling eye drops in infants can be most difficult, because they often clench the lids tightly closed. One approach is to place the drops in the nasal corner where the lids meet. The medication pools in this area, and when the child opens the lids, the medication flows onto the conjunctiva. For young children, playing a game can be helpful, such as instructing the child to keep the eyes closed until the count of 3 and then open them, at which time the drops are quickly instilled. Ointment can be applied by gently pulling down the lower lid and placing the ointment in the lower conjunctival sac.

> **! NURSING ALERT**
>
> If both eye ointment and drops are ordered, give drops first, wait 3 minutes, and then apply the ointment to allow each drug to work. When possible, administer eye ointments before bedtime or naptime, because the child's vision will be blurred temporarily.

Ear drops are instilled with the child in the prone or supine position and the head turned to the appropriate side. For children younger than 3 years of age, the external auditory canal is straightened by gently pulling the pinna down-

ward and straight back. The pinna is pulled upward and back in children older than 3 years of age (see Fig. 7-20). To place the drops deep in the ear canal without contaminating the tip of the dropper, place a disposable ear speculum in the canal and administer the drops through the speculum. After instillation, the child should remain lying on the unaffected side for a few minutes. Gentle massage of the area immediately anterior to the ear facilitates the entry of drops into the ear canal. The use of cotton pledgets prevents medication from flowing out of the external canal. However, the pledgets should be loose enough to allow any discharge to exit from the ear. Premoistening the cotton with a few drops of medication prevents the wicking action from absorbing the medication instilled in the ear.

Nose drops are instilled in the same manner as in the adult patient. Unpleasant sensations associated with medicated nose drops are minimized when care is taken to position the child with the head extended well over the edge of the bed or a pillow (Fig. 22-23). Depending on size, the infant can be positioned in the football hold (see Fig. 22-7, *B*); in the nurse's arm with the head extended and stabilized between the nurse's body and elbow, and the arms and hands immobilized with the nurse's hands; or as in Fig. 22-23. After instillation of the drops, the child should remain in position for 1 minute to allow the drops to come in contact with the nasal surfaces.

Nasal spray dispensers are inserted into the naris vertically and then angled nasally to avoid trauma to the septum and to direct medication toward the inferior turbinate.

FAMILY TEACHING AND HOME CARE

The nurse usually assumes the responsibility for preparing families to administer medications at home. The family should have an understanding of why the child is receiving the medication and the effects that might be expected, as well as the amount, frequency, and length of time the drug is to be administered. Instruction should be carried out in an unhurried, relaxed manner, preferably in an area away from busy ward or office routine, following the same guidelines for teaching as outlined in the Guidelines box on p. 725.

The caregiver is carefully instructed regarding the correct dosage, and the nurse is responsible for preparing parents for the specifics of the task. Some persons have difficulty understanding or interpreting terminology from the pharmacy, and just because they nod or otherwise indicate an understanding, it cannot be assumed that the message is clear. It is important to ascertain their interpretation of a teaspoon, for example, and to be certain they have acceptable devices for measuring the drug. If the drug is packaged with a dropper, syringe, or plastic cup, the nurse should show or mark the point on the device that indicates the prescribed dose and demonstrate how the dose is drawn up into a dropper or syringe and measured, and how any bubbles are eliminated. Also, the nurse must be certain that families understand that a prescription ordered in drops means single drops, not dropperfuls, a potential source of administration error (see Nursing Alert, p. 751). If the nurse has any doubts about the parent's ability to administer the correct dose, the parent should be asked to give a return demonstration. This verification is especially important when the drug has potentially serious consequences from incorrect dosage, such as insulin or digoxin, or when more complex administration is required, such as parenteral injections. When teaching a parent to give an injection, adequate time for instruction and practice must be allotted.

Home modifications are often necessary because the availability of equipment or assistance can differ from that of the hospital setting. For example, the parent may need guidance in devising methods that allow for one person to hold the child and safely give the drug.

> **NURSING TIP**
>
> To administer oral, nasal, or optic medication when only one person is available to hold the child, use the following procedure:
> - Place child supine on flat surface (bed, couch, floor).
> - Sit facing child so that his or her head is between operator's thighs and his or her arms are under operator's legs.
> - Place lower legs over child's legs to restrain lower body, if necessary.
> - To administer oral medication, place small pillow under child's head to reduce risk of aspiration.
> - To administer nasal medication, place small pillow under child's shoulders to aid flow of liquid through nasal passages.

The time that the drug is to be administered is clarified with the parent. For instance, when a drug is prescribed in association with meals, the number of meals that the family is accustomed to eating influences the amount of drug the child receives. Does the child have meals twice a day or five times a day? When a drug is to be given several times during the day, together the nurse and parents can work out a schedule that accommodates the family's routine. This is particularly significant if the drug must be given at equal intervals throughout a 24-hour period. For example, telling parents that the child needs 1 teaspoon of medicine four times a day is subject to misinterpretation, because parents may routinely schedule the doses at incorrect times. Instead, a preplanned schedule based on 6-hour intervals should be set up with the number of days required for therapeutic dosage listed. Modification should also be made to accommodate sleep schedules. For example, at nighttime a 6-hour interval may be extended to 8 hours (e.g., 11 PM, 7 AM, noon, and 6 PM. Written instruction should accompany all drug prescriptions.

> **NURSING TIP**
>
> If parents have difficulty reading or understanding English, use colors to convey instructions. For example, mark each drug with a color and place the appropriate color on a calendar chart or on a drawing of a clock to identify when the drug needs to be given. If a liquid medication and syringe are used, also mark the syringe at the place the plunger needs to be with color-coded tape.

PROCEDURES RELATED TO MAINTAINING FLUID BALANCE

MEASUREMENT OF INTAKE AND OUTPUT

One of the most important roles of the nurse in maintaining fluid balance is accurate measurement of fluid intake and output (I&O). Accurate measurements are essential to the assessment of fluid balance. Measurements from all sources—including both gastrointestinal and parenteral I&O from urine, stools, vomitus, fistulas, nasogastric suction, sweat, and drainage from wounds—must be taken and considered. Although the practitioner usually indicates when I&O measurements are to be recorded, it is a nursing responsibility to keep an accurate I&O record on patients in the following situations:

- After major surgery
- IV, diuretic, or corticosteroid therapy
- Severe thermal burns or injuries
- Renal disease or damage
- Congestive heart failure
- Dehydration (vomiting and diarrhea)
- Diabetes mellitus
- Oliguria
- Two years of age or younger
- Respiratory distress

Infants or small children who are unable to use a bedpan or those who have bowel movements with every voiding require the application of a collecting device (p. 742). If collecting bags are not used, wet diapers or pads are carefully weighed to ascertain the amount of fluid lost. This includes liquid stool, vomitus, and other losses. The volume of fluid in milliliters is equivalent to the weight of the fluid measured in grams. The specific gravity as a measure of osmolality is determined with a refractometer or urine dipsticks and assists in assessing the degree of hydration (see FYI on p. 743).

> **NURSING TIP**
>
> 1 g of wet diaper weight = 1 mL urine.

The weighed-diaper method of fluid measurement has disadvantages, including (1) inability to differentiate one type of loss from another because of admixture, (2) loss of urine or liquid stool from leakage or evaporation (especially if the infant is under a radiant warmer), and (3) additional fluid in the diaper (superabsorbent disposable type) from absorption of atmospheric moisture (from high-humidity incubators). However, when several types of diapers, including cloth, conventional disposable, and superabsorbent disposable, were compared for accuracy in terms of evaporative effects, closed superabsorbent disposable diapers followed by open superabsorbent disposable diapers were affected the least (Fox, 1992). To avoid the problem of evaporative losses and leakage of excreta, diapers should be weighed as soon as possible after becoming soiled.

Special Needs When the Child Is NPO

Infants or children who are unable or not permitted to take fluids by mouth (NPO) have special needs. To ensure that they do not receive fluids, a sign can be placed in some obvious place, such as over their beds or on their shirts, to alert others to the NPO status. To prevent the temptation to drink, fluids should not be left at the bedside.

Oral hygiene, a part of routine hygienic care, is especially important when fluids are restricted or withheld (p. 728). For the young child who cannot brush the teeth or rinse the mouth without swallowing fluid, the nurse can institute oral hygiene by wiping the teeth, gums, and tongue with a cloth moistened with saline.

> **NURSING TIP**
>
> To keep the mouth feeling moist when the child is NPO, give ice chips (if this is permitted by the practitioner) or spray the mouth with a fine mist of cool water (a clean perfume atomizer works well).

To keep the lips moist and prevent cracking, petrolatum (Vaseline) or some other commercial lip aid is applied. Lemon-glycerin swabs are avoided because they dry the skin, irritate open lesions, and can decay the teeth. To meet the need to suck, the infant is provided with a safe commercial pacifier.

The child who is fluid-restricted presents an equal challenge. Limiting fluids is often more difficult for the child than NPO, especially when IV fluids are also eliminated. To make certain the child does not drink the entire amount allowed early in the day, the daily allotment is calculated to provide fluids at periodic intervals throughout the child's waking hours. Serving the fluids in small containers gives the illusion of larger servings. No extra liquid is left at the bedside if compliance is a problem.

PARENTERAL FLUID THERAPY
Site and Equipment

The site selected for IV infusion depends on accessibility and convenience. Although it is possible to use any accessible vein in older children, attention must be directed toward the child's developmental, cognitive, and mobility needs when selecting a site. Ideally in older children, the superficial veins of the forearm should be used, leaving the hands free. An older child can help select the site and thereby maintain some measure of control. For veins in the extremities it is best to start with the most distal site and avoid the child's favored hand to reduce the disability related to the procedure. A site is chosen that restricts the child's movements as little

as possible—a site over a joint in an extremity, such as the antecubital space, is avoided. In small infants a superficial vein of the hand, wrist, forearm, foot, or ankle is usually most convenient and most easily stabilized (Fig. 22-24). Foot veins should be avoided in children learning to walk and in children already walking. Superficial veins of the scalp have no valves, insertion is easy, and they can be used in infants up to about 9 months of age, but they should be used only when other site attempts have failed.

Selection of a scalp vein as the venipuncture site requires shaving the area around the site to visualize the vein better and to provide a smooth surface on which to tape the catheter hub and tubing. A rubber band slipped onto the head from brow to occiput will usually suffice as a tourniquet. Shaving off a portion of the infant's hair is very upsetting to parents; therefore, they should be told what to expect and reassured that the hair will grow in again rapidly (save the hair because parents often wish to keep it). Remove as little as possible, directly over the insertion site and taping surface.

> **NURSING TIP**
>
> A tab of tape should be placed on the rubber band to help grasp it when removing it from the infant's head. The rubber band should be cut to avoid accidentally dislodging the catheter when moving the rubber band over the IV insertion site. The tape tab will lift the rubber band and allow it to be cut. Hold the rubber band in two places and cut between these areas to prevent the rubber band from snapping on the head.

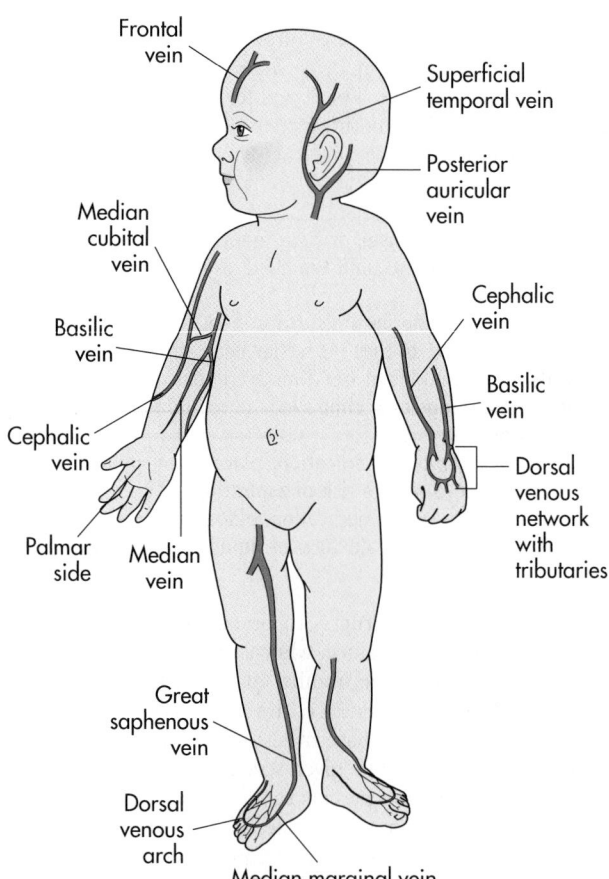

FIG. 22-24 ■ Preferred sites for venous access in infants.

Situations may occur in which rapid establishment of a systemic access is vital, and venous access may be hampered by peripheral circulatory collapse, hypovolemic shock (secondary to vomiting or diarrhea, burns, or trauma), cardiopulmonary arrest, or other conditions (Banerjee and others, 1994). *Intraosseous infusion* provides a rapid, safe and lifesaving alternate route for administration of fluids and medications until intravascular access can be attained, especially in children who are 6 years of age and younger.

A large-bore needle, such as a bone marrow aspiration needle (e.g., Jamshidi) or an intraosseous needle (e.g., Cook), is inserted into the medullary cavity of a long bone, most often the proximal tibia. This procedure is usually reserved for children who are unconscious or for those who are receiving analgesia, because the procedure is painful. Local anesthesia should be used for a semiconscious patient.

In situations in which fluids are urgently needed and there is difficulty in entering a vein, a polyethelene catheter inserted by the *surgical cutdown procedure* may be necessary, but this procedure is time-consuming. The vessel of choice is the internal saphenous vein located just anterior to the medial malleolus of the tibia. For long-term IV therapy a number of other devices may be used (p. 757).

For most IV infusions in children, an over-the-needle 22- to 24-gauge catheter may be used if therapy is expected to last less than 5 days. The smallest-gauge and shortest-length catheter that will accommodate the prescribed therapy should be chosen when evaluating the placement of a peripheral IV line. The length of the catheter may be directly related to infection and/or embolus formation—the shorter the catheter, the fewer the complications (Maki, 1994). The gauge of the catheter should maintain adequate flow of the infusate into the cannulated vein while allowing adequate blood flow around the catheter walls to promote proper hemodilution of the infusate. Because stainless steel needles tend to dislodge and infiltrate more frequently than catheters, the use of these should be limited to short-term or single-dose administration (Intravenous Nurses Society, 1998).

The goal of IV therapy is to deliver the prescribed fluids or medications without complications. Determining the best catheter for the patient early in the therapy provides the best chance of avoiding catheter-related complications (Moureau, 1999). As the length of therapy increases, decisions regarding the type of infusion device (short peripheral, midline, peripherally inserted central catheter, or central venous catheter) should be explored. Guidelines such as flow charts or algorithms are available to help in these decisions (Catudal, 1999).

Safety Catheters and Needleless Systems

One of the main causes for change in IV therapy is the concern of needle-stick injuries. To provide safer care for the patient and health care worker, manufacturers have developed safety catheters and needleless IV systems.

Over-the-needle IV catheters with hollow-bore needles carry a high risk for transmission of blood-borne pathogens from needle-stick injuries. Safety catheters prevent accidental needle sticks with the use of over-the-needle IV catheters.

Needleless IV systems, which are designed to prevent needle-stick injuries during administration of IV push medications and IV piggyback medications, may vary from manufacturer to manufacturer, but the concept is essentially the same. Some needleless systems are universal, whereas others require complete use of the entire IV delivery system for compatibility. Needleless IV systems rely on prepierced septa that are accessed by blunted plastic cannulas or systems that use valves that open and close a fluid path when activated by insertion of a syringe.

Blunt plastic cannulas and preslit injection port sites (Fig. 22-25) eliminate the need for steel needles and conventional injection port sites but remain accessible via hypodermic needles, a drawback except in emergent situations. Systems that do not permit needled access enhance safety by preventing health care workers from attempting to use needles; however, such systems are limited by the lack of needled access, especially in emergency situations (Orenstein, 1999). A syringe with a blue spike is available to access a single-dose vial (Fig. 22-25, *A*). The preslit injection port sites are identified by a white ring surrounding the port; this ring alerts users that the system is needleless (Fig. 22-25, *B*). Syringes are available with the blunt plastic cannula for accessing these sites (Fig. 22-25, *C*). A lever lock (Fig. 22-25, *D*) or threaded lock cannula (Fig. 22-25, *E*) attaches to an IV line, IV Y site, or peripheral intermittent infusion device. A preslit universal vial adapter (not pictured) provides access to standard multiple-dose vials, and syringe cannulas are then used to access the adapter.

Infusion Pumps

A variety of infusion pumps are available, refillable from the bag or bottle above or contained in a syringe pump to minimize the possibility of overloading the circulation. Infusion devices are almost always used in pediatrics because they can accurately infuse fluids (especially the syringe pumps, which infuse very small amounts of fluid), as well as accurately provide the prescribed amount of IV solution. It is an important nursing responsibility to calculate the amount to be infused in a given length of time, set the infusion rate, and monitor the apparatus frequently (at least every 1 to 2

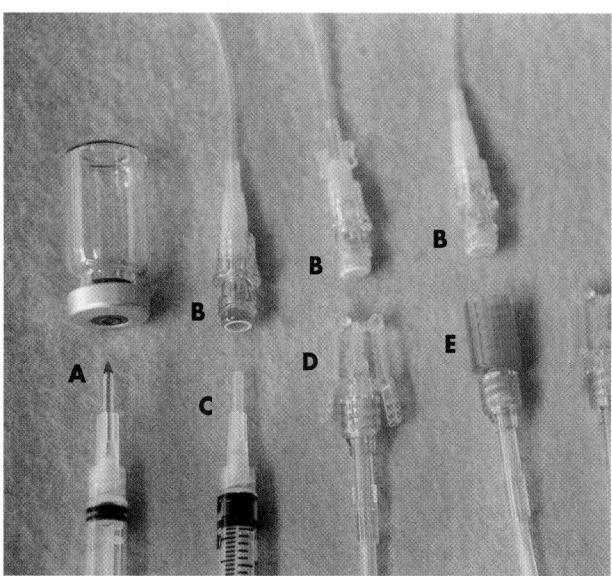

FIG. 22-25 ■ Interlink IV access systems: **A,** blue spike syringe; **B,** preslit injection port (needleless); **C,** blunt plastic cannula syringe; **D,** lever lock cannula; **E,** threaded lock cannula.

hours) to make certain that the desired rate is maintained, the integrity of the system remains intact, the site remains intact (free of redness, edema, infiltration, or irritation), and the infusion does not stop.

Continuous infusion pumps, although convenient and efficient, are not without risks. Overreliance on the accuracy of the machine can cause either too much or too little fluid to be infused; therefore, its use does not eliminate careful periodic assessment by the nurse. Excess pressure can build up if the machine is set at a rate faster than the vein is able to accommodate (or continues to pump when the needle is out of the lumen). This is especially true in very small infants. No matter what device is used, a thorough understanding of the apparatus is essential for safe fluid administration.

Securement of a Peripheral Intravenous Line

To maintain the integrity of the IV line, adequate protection of the site is required. The catheter hub is firmly secured at the puncture site with a transparent dressing or clear, nonallergenic tape. Transparent dressings are ideal because the insertion site is easily observed. Minimal tape should be used at the puncture site and on about 1 to 2 inches of skin beyond the site to avoid obscuring the insertion site for early detection of infiltration.

A protective cover is applied directly over the catheter insertion site to protect the infusion site. Easy access to the IV site for frequent (1- to 2-hour) assessments must be considered. Improvised plastic cups that are cut in half with the ridged edges covered with tape should not be used, because they have caused injury to patients. A commercial site protector, *I.V. House,** is available in different sizes (Fig. 22-26). Its ventilation holes prevent moisture from accumulating under the dome (Lee and Vallino, 1996). This device is designed to protect the IV site; allow for visibility of the site; minimize use of padded boards, splints, or other restraints and tape; and maintain skin integrity. The connector tubing or extension tubing can be looped to make it small enough to fit under the protective cover to prevent accidental snagging of the catheter. It is important to safely secure the IV tubing to prevent infants and children from becoming entangled in the tubing or from accidentally pulling the catheter or needle out. Securing the tubing in this manner also eliminates movement of the catheter hub at the insertion site (mechanical manipulation). A colorful and interesting sticker can be applied to the protecting device to add a positive note to the procedure.

> **NURSING TIP**
>
> I.V. House may be used to protect surgical insertion sites, such as jugular, femoral, or subclavian lines; implanted ports; or peripherally inserted central catheter lines; and for the application of EMLA or LMX.

Finger or toe areas are left unoccluded by dressings or tape to allow for assessment of circulation. The thumb is never immobilized because of the danger of contractures with limited movement later on. An extremity should never

*Available from **I.V. House,** 7400 Foxmont Drive, Hazelwood, MO 63042; (800) 530-0400; fax: (314) 831-3863; website: www.ivhouse.com.

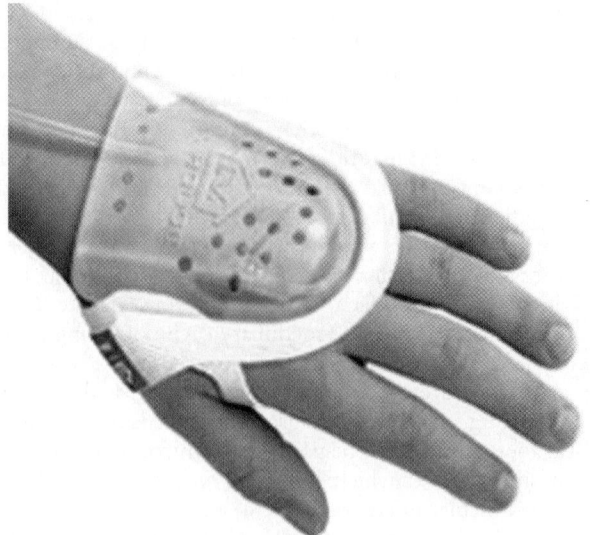

FIG. 22-26 ■ I.V. House.

be encircled with tape. The use of roll gauze, self-adhering stretch bandages (Coban), and Ace bandages can cause the same constriction and hide signs of infiltration (Intravenous Nurses Society, 1998).

> **NURSING ALERT**
>
> Opaque covering should be avoided; however, if any type of opaque covering is used to secure the IV line, the insertion site and extremity distal to the site should be visible to detect an infiltration. If these sites are not visible, they must be checked frequently to detect problems early.

Traditionally, padded boards or splints have been used to partially immobilize the IV site. Some institutions have even used rigid elbow restraints that do not allow the arm to bend at all. Padded boards or splints and restraints were appropriate when metal needles were inserted into the vein to prevent the sharp end from puncturing the vessel, especially at a joint. With the more recent use of soft, pliable catheters, arm or leg boards may not be necessary and have several disadvantages. They obscure the IV site, can constrict the extremity, may excoriate the underlying tissue and promote infection, can cause a contracture of a joint, restrict useful movement of the extremity, and are uncomfortable. Unfortunately, no research has been conducted to demonstrate their proposed benefit of increasing dwell time (patency of the IV line). Adequate taping and protection with a commercial device should eliminate the need for padded boards in most circumstances. Older children who are alert and cooperative can usually be trusted to protect the IV site.

Removal of a Peripheral Intravenous Line

When it comes time to discontinue an IV infusion, many children are distressed by the thought of catheter removal. Therefore they need a careful explanation of the process and suggestions for helping. Encouraging children to remove or help remove the tape from the site provides them with a measure of control and often encourages their cooperation.

The procedure consists of turning off any pump apparatus, occluding the IV tubing, removing the tape, pulling the catheter out of the vessel in the opposite direction of insertion, and exerting firm pressure at the site. A dry dressing (adhesive bandage strip) is placed over the puncture site. The use of adhesive-removal pads can decrease the pain of tape removal, but the skin should be washed after use because it can become irritated. To remove transparent dressings (e.g., Opsite, Tegaderm), pull the opposing edges parallel to the skin to loosen the bond. If a catheter was used for the IV infusion, the tip is inspected to make certain that the catheter is intact and that no portion remains in the vein.

> **❗ NURSING ALERT**
>
> Removal of the IV line, especially the tape, is another painful and frightening experience for the child. Consider the child's age, development, and neurologic status, as well as the predictability of the child (how does the child respond to painful treatments), when determining the need for assistance to maintain safety with this procedure. Manual removal of tape is the preferred method. Only if absolutely necessary should a small cut be made in the tape, using bandage scissors, to facilitate its removal. Before cutting the tape:
> - Ensure that all digits are visible.
> - Remove any barrier that hinders visibility, such as a protective covering.
> - Protect the child's skin and digits by sliding own finger(s) between the tape and the child's skin so that the scissors do not touch the patient.
> - Place a cut on the tape located on the medial aspect (thumb side) of the extremity.

Complications

The same precautions regarding maintenance of asepsis, prevention of infection, and observation for infiltration are carried out with patients of any age. However, infiltration is more difficult to detect in infants and small children than in adults. The increased amount of subcutaneous fat and the amount of tape used to secure the needle often obscure the signs of early infiltration. When the fluid appears to be infusing too slowly or ceases, the usual assessment for obstruction within the apparatus—kinks, screw clamps, shutoff valve, and positioning interference (e.g., a bent elbow)—often locates the difficulty. When these actions fail to detect the problem, it may be necessary to carefully remove some of the tape and other material that obscure a clear view of the venipuncture site. Dependent areas, such as the palm and undersides of the extremity or the occiput and behind the ears, are examined.

Whenever possible, the IV infusion should be placed in an extremity to which the identification band (or bracelet) is not attached. Serious circulatory impairment can result from infiltrated solution distal to the band, which acts as a tourniquet, preventing adequate venous return. To check for return blood flow through the catheter, the tubing is removed from the infusion pump, and the bag is lowered below the level of the infusion site. If the tubing is connected to an infusion pump, it must be removed from the pump before lowering. A good blood return, or lack thereof, is not always an indicator of infiltration in small infants. Flush-

ing the catheter/needle and observing for edema, redness, or streaking along the vein is an appropriate assessment of IV. Resistance during flushing or aspiration for blood return also indicates that the IV infusion may have infiltrated surrounding tissue.

IV therapy in pediatrics tends to be difficult to maintain because of mechanical factors that may predispose the IV infusion to shortened dwell times (number of days the catheter has been in place). Such factors include vascular trauma resulting from a peripheral intravenous (PIV) device selection (gauge and length of the catheter), the insertion site, the length of catheter dwell, the size of vessel, vessel fragility, the activity level of the patient, operator skill and insertion technique, forceful administration of boluses of fluid, and infusion of irritants or vesicants through a small vessel (Pettit and Hughes, 1999). These factors cause infiltration and extravasation injuries, which are reported with relative frequency. *Infiltration* is defined as inadvertent administration of a nonvesicant solution/medication into surrounding tissue. *Extravasation* is defined as inadvertent administration of vesicant solution/medication into surrounding tissue (Intravenous Nurses Society, 1998). A *vesicant* or *sclerosing agent* causes varying degrees of cellular damage when even minute amounts escape into surrounding tissue. Guidelines for determining the severity of tissue injury by staging characteristics, such as the amount of redness, blanching, the amount of swelling, pain, the quality of pulses below infiltration, capillary refill, and warmth or coolness of the area, are available (Montgomery and others, 1999; Intravenous Nurses Society, 1998).*

Treatment of an infiltration/extravasation varies according to the type of vesicant. Guidelines are available outlining the sequence of interventions and specific treatment of infiltration/extravasation with antidotes (Oncology Nursing Society, 1998; Montgomery and others, 1999).†

> **❗ NURSING ALERT**
>
> When an infiltration/extravasation is observed (signs may include erythema, pain, edema, blanching, streaking on the skin along the vein, and darkened area at the insertion site), immediately stop the infusion, elevate the extremity, notify the practitioner, and initiate the ordered treatment as soon as possible. Dry heat may be applied, except if the infused solution is sclerosing. Remove the IV line when it is no longer needed (e.g., after infusing an antidote).

PIV catheters are the most commonly used intravascular device. Heavy cutaneous colonization of the insertion site is the single most important predictor of catheter-related infection with all types of short-term, percutaneously inserted catheters. Phlebitis, largely a mechanical rather than infectious process, remains the most important

---

*Guidelines for determining tissue injury severity are available from the **Intravenous Nurses Society,** Fresh Pond Square, 10 Fawcet Street, Cambridge, MA 02138; (617) 441-3008; fax: (617) 441-3009; website: www.ins1.org.
†Guidelines on interventions for infiltration/extravasation are available from the **Oncology Nursing Society,** 501 Holiday Drive, Pittsburgh, PA 15220-2749; (412) 921-7373; fax: (412) 921-2131; website: www.ons.org.

complication associated with the use of peripheral venous catheters.*

Proper education of the patient and family regarding signs and symptoms of an infected site can help prevent infections from going unnoticed. When an IV infusion continues for several days, the tubing and solution are changed at regular intervals according to hospital policy, most often every 72 hours (Pearson, 1995). The dressing, whether transparent dressing or sterile gauze and tape, can be left in place for the duration of the IV infusion (Maki, 1994) unless the integrity has been compromised. To ensure that the equipment is changed regularly, it is labeled with the date and time that the new bag and tubing are attached. Any signs of inflammation, such as redness or pain, are reported immediately. This usually requires removal of the infusion and restarting it at another site or administering the medication by another route.

PROCEDURES FOR MAINTAINING RESPIRATORY FUNCTION

INHALATION THERAPY

The term ***inhalation therapy*** is an all-inclusive term that encompasses a variety of therapies that involve changing the composition, volume, or pressure of inspired gases. These therapies include primarily increasing the oxygen concentration of inspired gas (oxygen therapy), increasing the water vapor content of inspired gas (humidification), adding airborne particles with beneficial properties (aerosol therapy), and employing various means for controlling or assisting respiration (artificial ventilation, continuous positive airway pressure).

Oxygen Therapy

Oxygen (O_2) therapy is primarily carried out in the hospital, although increasing numbers of children are receiving O_2 in the home. O_2 delivered to the infant via the incubator is satisfactory when lower levels are adequate to prevent cyanosis, but the highest concentration (almost 100%) is supplied by way of a ***plastic hood*** (Fig. 22-27). The humidified O_2 should not be blown directly into the infant's face,

---

*Guidelines for prevention of intravascular device-related infections are available from the **Centers for Disease Control and Prevention,** 1600 Clifton Road NE, Atlanta, GA 30333; (404) 639-3311; website: www.cdc.gov/ncidod/hip/iv/iv.htm.

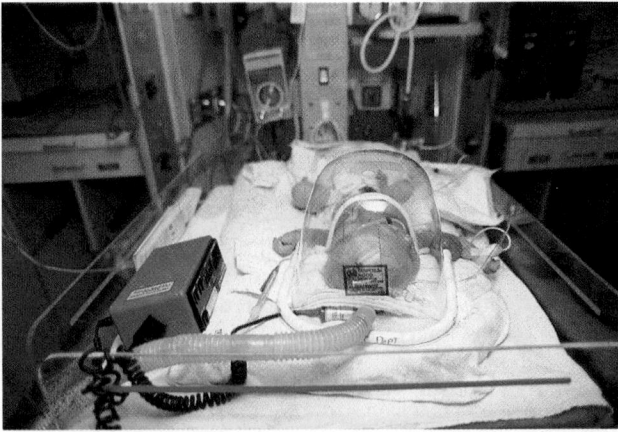

FIG. 22-27 ■ Oxygen administered to infant by means of a plastic hood. Note oxygen analyzer (*blue machine*).

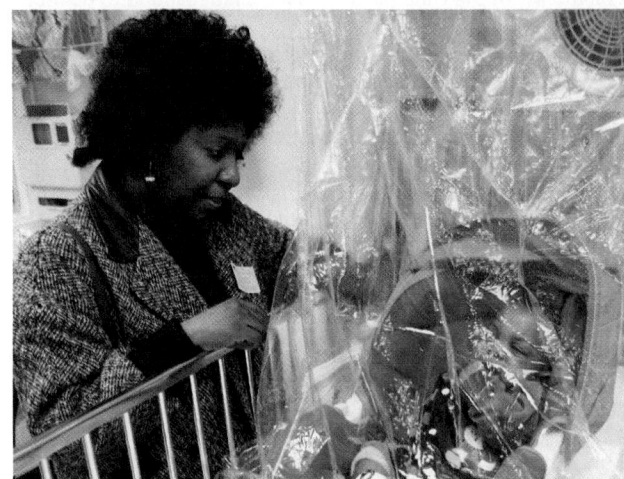

FIG. 22-28 ■ The tent provides a comfortable method for oxygen administration. (From Wilson SF, Thompson JM: *Respiratory disorders,* St Louis, 1990, Mosby.)

and the hood should not rub against the infant's neck, chin, or shoulder. Older, cooperative infants and children can use a ***nasal cannula*** or ***prongs,*** which can supply a concentration of O_2 of about 50%. A ***mask*** is not well-tolerated by children.

For children beyond early infancy, the ***oxygen tent*** is a satisfactory means for administration of O_2 (Fig. 22-28). A tent does not require any device to come into direct contact with the face, but the concentration of O_2 within the tent is difficult to control and to maintain above 30% to 50%. A major difficulty with the use of the tent is keeping the tent closed so that the O_2 concentration is maintained.

To reduce O_2 loss, nursing care is planned carefully so that the tent is opened as little as possible. Because O_2 is heavier than air, loss will be greater at the bottom of the tent; therefore, the tent is tucked in snugly without open edges. The bottom of the tent should be examined more often when the child is restless and fussy and liable to pull the covers loose. Some tents are even open at the top. Because of the rapid diffusing qualities of carbon dioxide (CO_2), the levels of the gas do not build up within these enclosures.

After the tent has been opened for an extended period, it is flushed with O_2 by increasing the flow meter for a few minutes to quickly raise the O_2 and mist concentration. The flow meter is then reset to the prescribed number of liters.

The enclosed tent becomes very warm; therefore, some type of cooling mechanism is provided. The temperature inside the tent must be checked periodically to be certain that it is maintained at the desired level. Although the cool environment can reduce fever and airway inflammation, it can also produce hypothermia and cold stress. It is important to make certain that the child is kept warm and dry. Because O_2 is drying to the tissues, the gas is humidified, which causes moisture to condense on the tent walls.

> **NURSING ALERT**
>
> Keep the child warm and dry by checking the temperature inside the tent and the child's bedding and clothing frequently. Adjust the temperature and change clothing as often as needed.

The reactions of children to the O_2 tent are variable. Some, especially older children, feel comfortable in the tent and like the cozy, close privacy it affords. Others, more often younger children, may be frightened by the forced enclosure. The plastic walls distort their view of the world and constitute a barrier between them and their source of comfort, their parent. Their distress can be minimized if they are able to see someone nearby and are reassured that they will not be left alone. A favorite toy or object can accompany the child inside the tent. However, all toys should be inspected for safety and suitability. Other familiar items can be placed at the foot of the bed or otherwise in view.

> **NURSING ALERT**
>
> Inspect all toys for safety and suitability (e.g., vinyl or plastic, not stuffed items that absorb moisture and are difficult to keep dry). The high-level O_2 environment makes any source of sparks (e.g., mechanical or electrical toys) a potential fire hazard.

In most instances the child can be removed from the O_2 tent for activities such as feeding and bathing, whereas in other cases the child is placed in the tent only during periods of rest. Still other children may require O_2 continuously and can be removed from the tent or incubator only if an O_2 source is held close to the child's face. Any change in color, increased respiratory effort, or restlessness is an indication to return the child to the O_2 tent.

Oxygen Toxicity. O_2 is essential to life and a valuable therapeutic aid. However, prolonged exposure to high O_2 tensions can be damaging to some body tissues and functions. The organs most vulnerable to the adverse effects of excessive oxygenation are the retina of the premature infant and the lungs of persons at any age.

Oxygen-induced carbon dioxide (CO_2) narcosis is a physiologic hazard of O_2 therapy that may occur in persons with chronic pulmonary disease, such as cystic fibrosis. These children have chronic alveolar hypoventilation with a concomitant chronic CO_2 retention and hypoxemia. In these patients the respiratory center has adapted to the con-

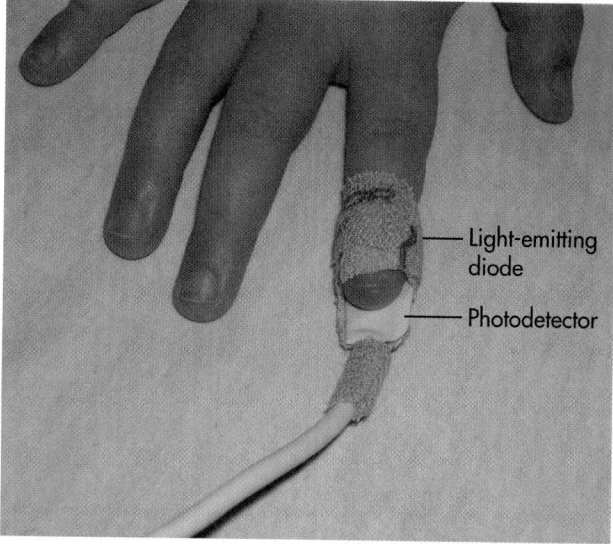

FIG. 22-29 ■ Oximeter sensor on right second finger. Note that sensor is positioned with light-emitting diode opposite photodetector.

tinuously higher arterial carbon dioxide tension ($PaCO_2$) levels, and therefore hypoxia becomes the more powerful stimulus for respiration. When the arterial oxygen tension (PaO_2) level is elevated during O_2 administration, the hypoxic drive is removed, causing progressive hypoventilation and increased $PaCO_2$ levels, and the child rapidly becomes unconscious. CO_2 narcosis can also be induced by the administration of sedation in these patients.

Monitoring Oxygen Therapy

Pulse oximetry is a simple, continuous, noninvasive method of determining oxygen saturation (SaO_2) to guide O_2 therapy. A sensor comprising a light-emitting diode (LED) and a photodetector is placed in opposition around a foot, hand, finger, toe, or earlobe, with the LED placed on top of the nail when digits are used (Fig. 22-29). The LED emits red and infrared lights that pass through the skin to the photodetector. The photodetector measures the amount of each type of light absorbed by functional hemoglobins. Hemoglobin saturated with O_2 (oxyhemoglobin) absorbs more infrared light than does hemoglobin not saturated with O_2 (deoxyhemoglobin). Therefore pulsatile blood flow is the primary physiologic factor that influences accuracy of the pulse oximeter.

Another noninvasive method is *transcutaneous monitoring (TCM)*, which provides continual monitoring of transcutaneous partial pressure of oxygen in arterial blood ($tcPaO_2$) and, with some devices, of carbon dioxide in arterial blood ($tcPaCO_2$). An electrode is attached to the warmed skin to facilitate arterialization of cutaneous capillaries. The site of the electrode must be changed every 3 to 4 hours to prevent burning the skin, and the machine must be calibrated with every site change. TCM is used frequently in neonatal intensive care units, but it may not reflect PaO_2 in infants with impaired local circulation or in older infants whose skin is thicker.

The PaO_2 can be correlated with the SaO_2 by means of the *oxyhemoglobin dissociation curve* (Fig. 22-30). Most

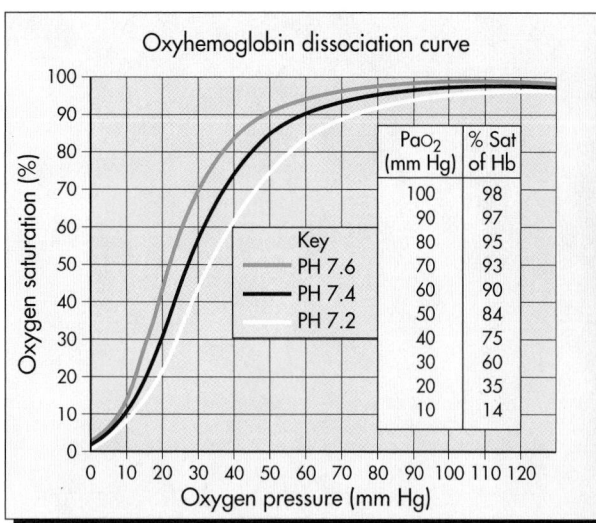

FIG. 22-30 ■ Oxyhemoglobin dissociation curve. Changes in affinity of hemoglobin for oxygen shift position of curve. Shift to left (*colored line*) indicates increased affinity of hemoglobin for oxygen. Shift to right (*white line*) indicates decreased affinity of hemoglobin for oxygen.

important, changes in PaO_2 do not cause identical changes in SaO_2. Rather, in the steep portion of the curve, small changes in PaO_2 result in large changes in SaO_2. In the flat portion of the curve, large changes in PaO_2 result in only small changes in SaO_2.

A quick formula for calculating the correlation of PaO_2 with SaO_2 is the 30-60, 60-90 rule. Assuming a normal pH, $PaCO_2$, and body temperature, this rule can apply: when PaO_2 = 30 mm Hg, SaO_2 = 60%; when PaO_2 = 60 mm, SaO_2 = 90%.

Also, oximetry is insensitive to hyperoxia because hemoglobin approaches 100% saturation for all PaO_2 readings greater than approximately 100 mm Hg, which is a dangerous situation for the premature infant at risk for developing retinopathy of prematurity (see Chapter 9). Therefore the premature infant being monitored with oximetry should have upper limits identified, such as 90% to 95%, and a protocol established for decreasing O_2 when saturations are high.

The degree to which O_2 combines with hemoglobin is affected by several factors. A shift of the curve to the left causes an increased affinity of hemoglobin for O_2, but the O_2 is not easily released to the tissues. This represents an increase in the SaO_2 if it is measured against the same PaO_2 of the normal oxyhemoglobin dissociation curve. This left shift can be caused by an increase in blood pH or a decrease in $PaCO_2$, body temperature, or 2,3-diphosphoglycerate (2,3-DPG), a substance in the red blood cells.

A shift of the curve to the right causes a decreased affinity of hemoglobin for O_2, but improved O_2 release to the tissues. This represents a lower SaO_2 if measured against the same PaO_2 of the normal oxyhemoglobin dissociation curve. This right shift can be caused by a decrease in blood pH or an increase in $PaCO_2$, body temperature, or 2,3-DPG.

Oximetry offers several advantages over TCM. Oximetry (1) does not require heating the skin, thus reducing the risk

of burns; (2) eliminates a delay period for transducer equilibration; and (3) maintains an accurate measurement regardless of the patient's age or skin characteristics or the presence of lung disease.

! NURSING ALERT

It is important to make certain that sensor connectors and oximeters are compatible. Wiring that is incompatible can generate considerable heat at the tip of the sensor, causing second- and third-degree burns under the sensors. Pressure necrosis can also occur from sensors attached too tightly. Therefore inspect the skin under the sensor frequently.

Applying the sensor correctly is essential for accurate SaO_2 measurements. Because the sensor must identify every pulse beat to calculate the SaO_2, movement can interfere with sensing. Some devices synchronize the SaO_2 reading with the heartbeat, thereby reducing the interference caused by motion. Sensors are not placed on extremities used for blood pressure monitoring or with indwelling arterial catheters, because pulsatile blood flow can be affected.

NURSING TIPS

- **Infant.** Tape the sensor securely to the great toe and tape the wire to the sole of the foot (or use a commercial holder that fastens with a self-adhering closure). Place a snugly fitting sock over the foot.
- **Child.** Tape the sensor securely to the index finger and tape the wire to the back of the hand. Use self-adhering Ace-type wrap (e.g., Coban) around the finger or hand to further secure the sensor and wire.

Ambient light from ceiling lights and phototherapy, as well as high-intensity heat and light from radiant warmers, can interfere with readings. Therefore the sensor should be covered to block these light sources. IV dyes; green, purple, or black nail polish; nonopaque synthetic nails; and possibly ink used for footprinting can also cause inaccurate SaO_2 measurements. The dyes should be removed or, in the case of porcelain nails, a different area used for the sensor. Skin color, thickness, and edema do not affect the readings.

Aerosol Therapy

Aerosol therapy can be effective in depositing medication directly into the airway. The value of aerosolized water, or "mist therapy," is controversial (see Evidence-Based Practice box). This route of administration can be useful in avoiding the systemic side effects of certain drugs and in reducing the amount of drug necessary to achieve the desired effect. Bronchodilators, steroids, and antibiotics can be suspended in particulate form and then inhaled so that the medication reaches the small airways. The use of aerosol therapy is particularly challenging in children who are too young to cooperate with controlling the rate and depth of breathing. Administration of this therapy requires skill, patience, and creativity.

Medications can be aerosolized or nebulized with air or with O_2-enriched gas. **Handheld nebulizers** are the most frequently used equipment. The medicated "mist" is discharged into a small plastic mask, which the child holds over the nose and mouth. To avoid particle deposition in the nose and pharynx, the child is instructed to take slow, deep

EVIDENCE-BASED PRACTICE

Mist Therapy

Continuous administration of mist, or aerosolized water, often viewed as a traditional and helpful remedy, is not a treatment of choice for most inflammatory conditions of the airways. The exception is the child with mild viral croup, who might be helped by cool-mist therapy, including a walk outside in the cool, humid, night air. The beneficial effect of cool mist may include moistening of airway secretions, a reflex reaction to the cool air that slows rapid respiration, and a feeling of reassurance from holding the child near the mist that may help lessen the anxiety for both the child and the parent (Kaditis and Wald, 1999). Mist therapy may not help the child with reactive airway disease and croup, because humidity may worsen the bronchospasm.

The notion that inhaled mist can influence the viscosity of mucus in dehydrated children is erroneous. If dehydration is evident, oral or parenteral rehydration will normalize the water content of respiratory mucus.

breaths through an open mouth during the treatment. For home use an air compressor is necessary to force air through the liquid medication to form the aerosol. Fairly compact, portable units can be rented from health equipment companies. The *metered-dose inhaler (MDI)* is a self-contained, handheld device that allows for intermittent delivery of a specified amount of medication. Many bronchodilators are available in this form and are successfully used by children with asthma. For children under the age of 5 or 6 years, a *spacer device* attached to the MDI can help with coordination of breathing and aerosol delivery. It allows the aerosolized particles to remain in suspension longer. (See also Asthma, Chapter 23.)

A major nursing responsibility during aerosol therapy is to assess the effectiveness of the treatment and the patient's tolerance of the procedure. Assessments of breath sounds and work of breathing should be done before and after treatments. Small children who become upset with having a mask held close to the face may become fatigued with fighting the procedure and may actually appear worse during and immediately after the therapy. Careful assessment is required by the nurse and practitioner to determine if the treatment is worthwhile. It may be necessary to spend a few minutes calming the child after the procedure, and allowing the vital signs to return to baseline to accurately assess changes in breath sounds and work of breathing.

BRONCHIAL (POSTURAL) DRAINAGE

Bronchial drainage is indicated whenever excessive fluid or mucus in the bronchi is not being removed by normal ciliary activity and cough. Positioning the child to take maximum advantage of gravity facilitates removal of secretions. The effect is sometimes dramatic in children with chronic lung disease characterized by thick mucus, such as asthma or cystic fibrosis.

Postural drainage is carried out three to four times daily and is more effective when it follows other respiratory therapy, such as bronchodilator or nebulization medication. Bronchial drainage is generally performed before meals (or 1 to 1.5 hours after meals) to minimize the chance of vom-

iting and is repeated at bedtime. The length and duration of treatment depend on the child's condition and tolerance level, usually 20 to 30 minutes. There are positions to facilitate drainage from all major lung segments (Fig. 22-31), but all positions are not employed at each session. Children will usually cooperate for four to six positions, but more than six tend to exceed their limits of tolerance. Older children can be expected to tolerate longer periods.

In the hospital an older child can be positioned over an elevated knee rest. Small children and infants can be positioned with pillows or on the therapist's lap and legs (Fig. 22-32). Infants should not be placed in the Trendelenburg position because they do not have an autonomic regulation of blood flow to the head. Special modifications of the techniques are required in children whose conditions contraindicate the standard positioning, such as head injuries, some types of surgical incisions or burns, and casts or traction. At home small children can be positioned on a padded ironing board. Children who require postural drainage over months or years may benefit from specially constructed tables padded and adjusted to their individual needs. The position used and the frequency and duration of treatment are individualized.

CHEST PHYSIOTHERAPY

Chest physiotherapy (CPT) usually refers to the use of postural drainage in combination with adjunctive techniques that are thought to enhance the clearance of mucus from the airway. These techniques include manual percussion, vibration, and squeezing of the chest; cough; forceful expiration; and breathing exercises. The efficacies of these techniques, both individually and combined, are controversial, however. Postural drainage in combination with forced expiration has been shown to be beneficial, but the benefit of the other techniques has yet to be demonstrated. The results of a study evaluating the effects of noninvasive inspiratory nasal pressure–support ventilation (PSV) during CPT showed a significant improvement in respiratory muscle performance and a reduction in O_2 desaturation when used in combination (Fauroux and others, 1999).

The most common technique used in association with postural drainage is manual percussion of the chest wall. Nurses are often responsible for this maneuver if a respiratory therapist is not available, so they should be skilled in the technique. The patient is dressed in a lightweight shirt and placed in a postural drainage position; then the nurse gently but firmly strikes the chest wall with a cupped hand (Fig. 22-33, *A*). For infants, special devices are available for percussing small areas (Fig. 22-33, *B*). A "popping," hollow sound should be the result, not a slapping sound. The procedure should be done over the rib cage only and should be painless. Percussion can be performed with a soft circular mask (adapted to maintain air trapping) or a percussion cup marketed especially for the purpose of aiding the loosening of secretions.

CPT is contraindicated when patients have pulmonary hemorrhage, pulmonary embolism, end-stage renal disease, increased intracranial pressure, osteogenesis imperfecta, or minimal cardiac reserves.

CPT should be used for patients who have increased sputum production. It is probably of no value to the uncom-

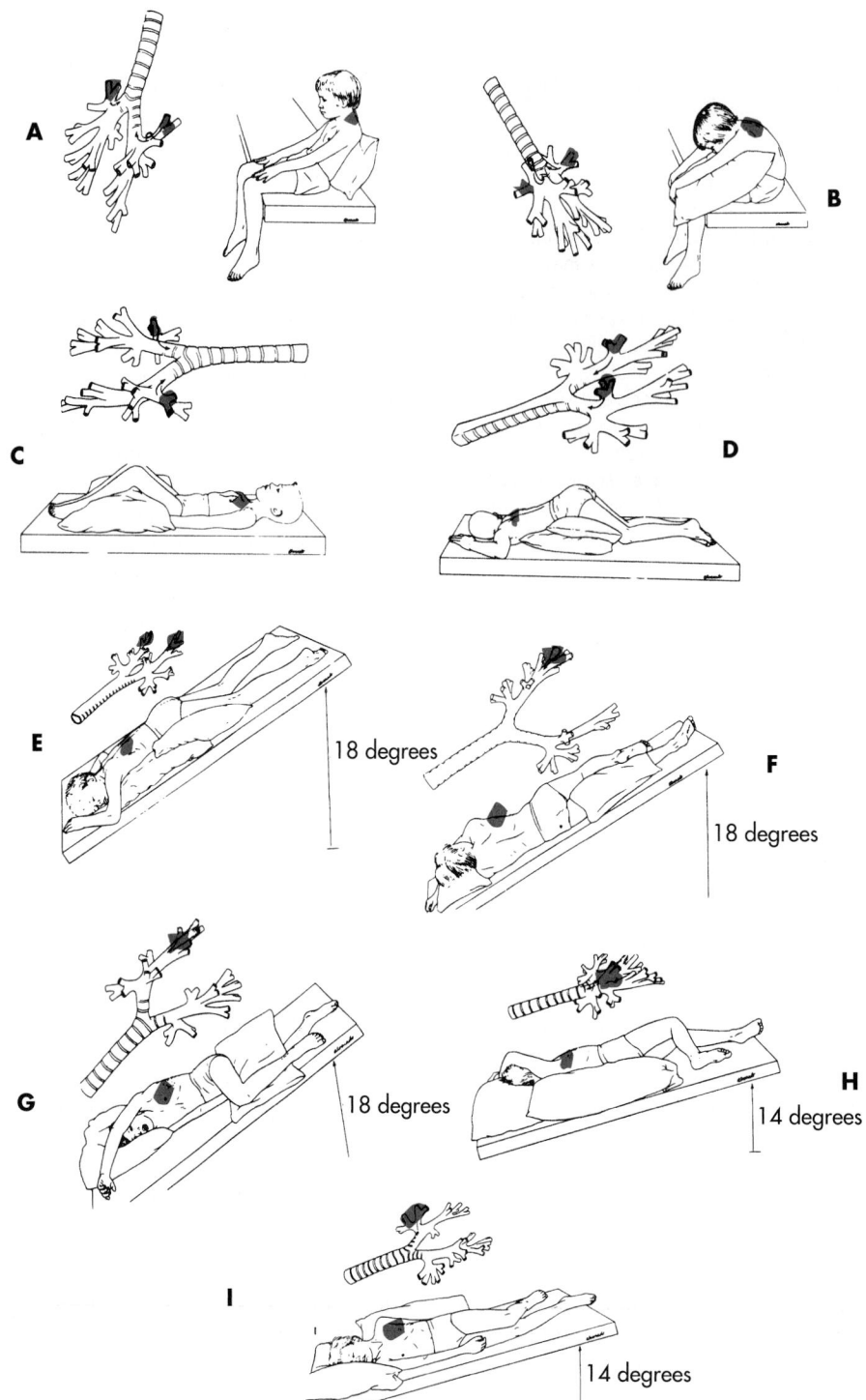

FIG. 22-31 ■ Bronchial drainage positions for all major segments of child. For each position, model of tracheobronchial tree is projected beside child to show segmental bronchus (*red*) being drained and pathway of secretions out of bronchus. Drainage platform is horizontal unless otherwise noted. Red area on child's chest indicates area to be cupped or vibrated by therapist. **A,** Apical segment of right upper lobe and apical subsegment of apical-posterior segment of left upper lobe. **B,** Posterior segment of right upper lobe and posterior subsegment of apical-posterior segment of left upper lobe. **C,** Anterior segments of both upper lobes; child should be rotated slightly away from side being drained. **D,** Superior segments of both lower lobes. **E,** Posterior basal segments of both lower lobes. **F,** Lateral basal segments of right lower lobe; left lateral basal segment would be drained by mirror image of this position (right side down). **G,** Anterior basal segment of left lower lobe; right anterior basal segment would be drained by mirror image of this position (left side down). **H,** Medial and lateral segments of right middle lobe. **I,** Lingular segments (superior and inferior) of left upper lobe (homologue of right middle lobe). (From Chernick V, editor: *Kendig's disorders of the respiratory tract of children,* ed 6, Philadelphia, 1998, WB Saunders.)

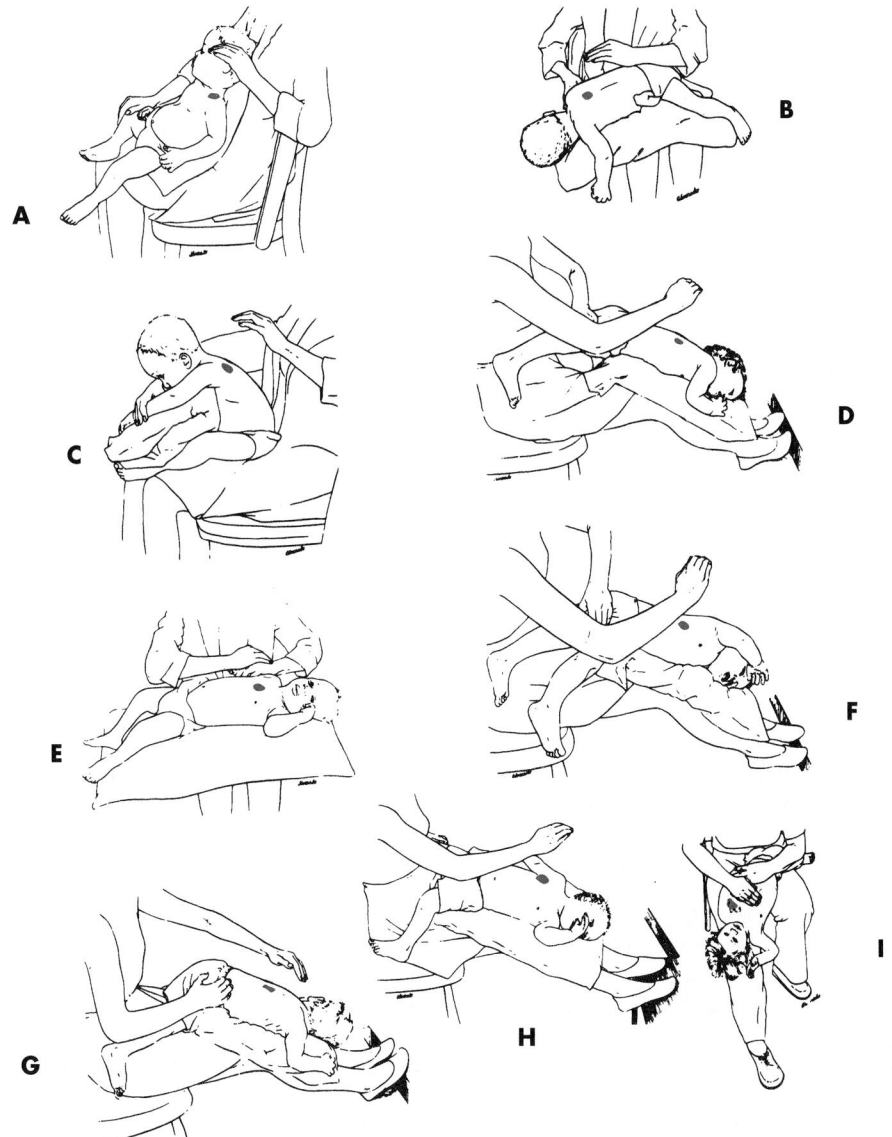

FIG. 22-32 ■ Bronchial drainage positions for major segments of all lobes in infant. Procedure is most easily carried out in therapist's lap. Therapist's hand on chest indicates area (red) to be cupped or vibrated. **A,** Apical segment of left upper lobe. **B,** Posterior segment of left upper lobe. **C,** Anterior segment of left upper lobe. **D,** Superior segment of right lower lobe. **E,** Posterior basal segment of right lower lobe. **F,** Lateral basal segment of right lower lobe. **G,** Anterior basal segment of right lower lobe. **H,** Medial and lateral segments of right middle lobe. **I,** Lingular segments (superior and inferior) of left upper lobe. (Modified from Cystic Fibrosis Foundation: *Infant segmental bronchial drainage,* Rockville, Md, The Foundation.)

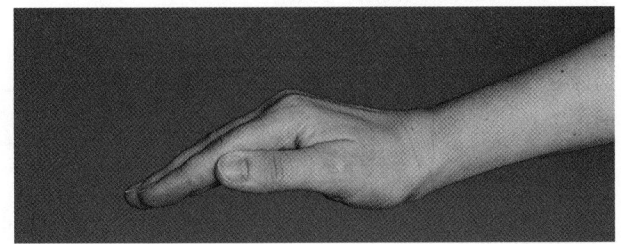

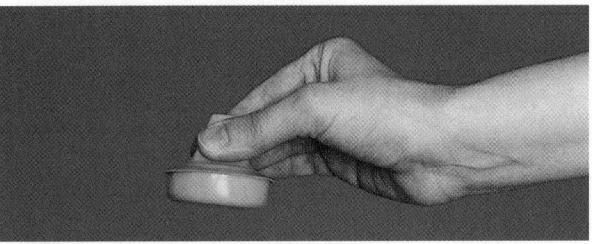

FIG. 22-33 ■ **A,** Cupped hand position for percussion. **B,** Device for infant percussion.

plicated postoperative patient or the patient with pneumonia. Forced expiration combined with postural drainage is more effective than cough alone, but percussion and vibration have no proven value. Appropriate use of nebulized bronchodilators before CPT therapy will enhance mucus clearance.

ARTIFICIAL VENTILATION
Artificial Airways

An artificial airway is usually used in association with artificial ventilation and in children with upper airway obstruction. Endotracheal intubation can be accomplished by the nasal (nasotracheal), oral (orotracheal), or direct tracheal (tracheostomy) routes. Although it is more difficult to place, nasotracheal intubation is preferred to orotracheal intubation because it facilitates oral hygiene and provides more stable fixation, which reduces the complication of tracheal erosion and the danger of accidental extubation. Only uncuffed endotracheal (ET) tubes should be used in children younger than 8 years of age (Hazinski, 1996). Cuffed tubes may be used with adolescents to help provide an airtight seal. Air or gas delivered directly to the trachea must be humidified as in tracheostomy.

Tracheostomy

A tracheostomy is a surgical opening in the trachea; the procedure may be done on an emergency basis or may be an elective one, and it may be combined with mechanical ventilation.

Pediatric tracheostomy tubes are usually made of plastic or Silastic (Fig. 22-34). The most common types are the Hollinger, Jackson, Aberdeen, and Shiley tubes. These tubes are constructed with a more acute angle than adult tubes, and they soften at body temperature, conforming to the contours of the trachea. Because these materials resist the formation of crusted respiratory secretions, they are made without an inner cannula. Some children require a metal tracheostomy tube (usually made of sterling silver or stainless steel), which contains an inner cannula. The principal advantage of metal tubes is their nonreactivity and decreased chance of causing an allergic reaction.

Children who have undergone a tracheostomy require a hospital stay. During this time the child is closely monitored for the development of complications such as hemorrhage, edema, aspiration, accidental decannulation, tube obstruc-

tion, or the entrance of free air into the pleural cavity. The focus of postoperative nursing care is maintaining a patent airway, facilitating the removal of pulmonary secretions, providing humidified air or O_2, cleansing the stoma, monitoring the child's ability to swallow, and teaching while simultaneously preventing complications. The most dangerous complication is related to accidental decannulation and tube obstruction. Because the child may be unable to signal for help, direct observation and use of respiratory and cardiac monitors is essential. Respiratory assessments include breath sounds and work of breathing, vital signs, tightness of the tracheostomy ties, and the type and amount of secretions. Large amounts of bloody secretions are uncommon and should be considered a sign of hemorrhage. The practitioner should be notified immediately if this occurs.

The child is positioned with the head of the bed raised or in the position most comfortable to the child, with the call light easily available. Suction catheters, suction source, gloves, sterile saline, sterile gauze for wiping away secretions, scissors, an extra tracheostomy tube of the same size with ties already attached, another tracheostomy tube one size smaller, and the obturator are kept at the bedside. A source of humidification is provided, because the normal humidification and filtering functions of the airway have been bypassed. IV fluids ensure adequate hydration until the child is able to swallow sufficient amounts of fluids.

Suctioning. The airway must remain patent and requires frequent suctioning during the first few hours after a tracheostomy to remove mucous plugs and excessive secretions. Proper vacuum pressure and suction catheter size are important to prevent atelectasis and decrease hypoxia from the suctioning procedure. Vacuum pressure should range from 60 to 100 mm Hg for infants and children and from 40 to 60 mm Hg for premature infants. Unless secretions are thick and tenacious, the lower range of negative pressure is recommended. Tracheal suction catheters are available in a variety of sizes. The catheter selected should have a diameter one-half the diameter of the tracheostomy tube. If the catheter is too large, it can block the airway. The catheter is constructed with a side port so that the catheter is introduced without suction and removed while simultaneous intermittent suction is applied by covering the port with the thumb (Fig. 22-35). The catheter is inserted to 0.5 cm beyond or just to the end of the tracheostomy tube. The practice of instilling sterile saline in the tracheostomy tube before suctioning is not supported by research and is no longer recommended. (See Evidence-Based Practice box.)

> **NURSING ALERT**
>
> Suctioning should require no more than 5 seconds. Counting 1—one thousand, 2—one thousand, 3—one thousand, and so on, while suctioning is a simple means for monitoring the time. Without a safeguard, the airway may be obstructed for too long a period. Hyperventilating the child with 100% O_2 before and after suctioning (using a bag-valve-mask or increasing the fraction of inspired oxygen concentration [Fio$_2$] ventilator setting) is also performed to prevent hypoxia. Closed tracheal suctioning systems that allow for uninterrupted O_2 delivery may also be used.

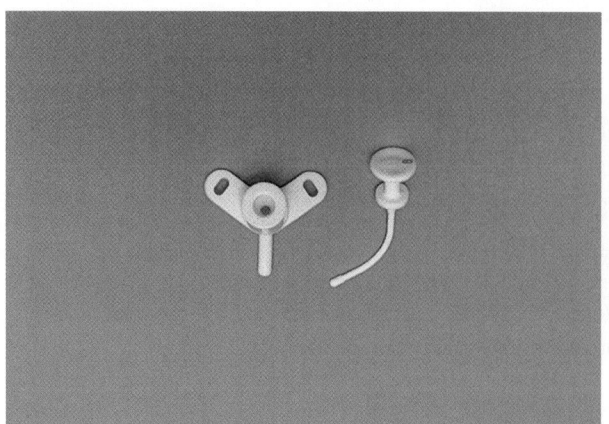

FIG. 22-34 ■ Silastic pediatric tracheostomy tube and obturator.

FYI

In a closed suction system, a suction catheter is directly attached to the ventilator tubing. This system has several advantages. First, there is no need to disconnect the patient from the ventilator, which allows for better oxygenation. Second, the suction catheter is enclosed in a plastic sheath, which reduces the risk of exposure to the patient's secretions (Carroll, 1998).

The child is allowed to rest for 30 to 60 seconds after each aspiration to allow O_2 tension to return to normal; then the process is repeated until the trachea is clear. Suctioning should be limited to about three aspirations in one period. Oximetry is used to monitor suctioning and prevent hypoxia.

NURSING ALERT

Suctioning is carried out *only as often as needed* to keep the tube patent. Signs of mucus partially occluding the airway include an increased heart rate, a rise in respiratory effort, a drop in Sao_2, cyanosis, and an increase in the positive inspiratory pressure (PIP) on the ventilator.

In the acute care setting, aseptic technique is used during care of the tracheostomy. Secondary infection is a major concern, because the air entering the lower airway bypasses the natural defenses of the upper airway. Gloves are worn during the aspiration procedure, although a sterile glove is needed only on the hand touching the catheter. A new tube, gloves, and sterile saline solution are used each time (see Critical Thinking Exercise).

Routine Care.   The tracheostomy stoma requires daily care. Assessments of the stoma area include observations for signs of infection and breakdown of the skin. The skin is kept clean and dry, and secretions around the stoma may be gently removed with half-strength hydrogen peroxide. Hydrogen peroxide should not be used with sterling silver tracheostomy tubes because it tends to pit and stain the silver surface. The nurse should be aware of wet tracheostomy dressings, which can predispose the peristomal area to skin breakdown. Several products are available to prevent or treat excoriation. The Allevyn tracheostomy dressing is a hydrophilic sponge with a polyurethane back that is highly absorptive. Other possible barriers to help maintain skin integrity include the use of hydrocolloid wafers (e.g., Duoderm CGF, Hollister Restore) under the tracheostomy flanges, as well as use of extra-thin hydrocolloid wafers under the chin.

The tracheostomy tube is held in place with tracheostomy ties made of a durable, nonfraying material. The ties are changed daily and when soiled. New ties are looped through the flanges and tied snugly in a triple knot at the side of the neck *before* the soiled ties are cut and removed. Some nurses have found that threading the ties through a piece of 0.25-inch surgical tubing cushions the ties; others have found the tubing to be irritating to the skin. The ties should be tight enough to allow just a fingertip to be inserted between the ties and the neck (Fig. 22-36). It is easier to ensure a snug fit if the child's head is flexed rather than extended while the ties are being secured. Ties fastened with self-adhering closures are also available. These devices, such as the Dale tracheostomy tube holder, are made of a soft, cushioning, and slightly stretchy material that is very comfortable. They are becoming increasingly popular because of their ease of use and ability to maintain better skin integrity. However, nurses and family members

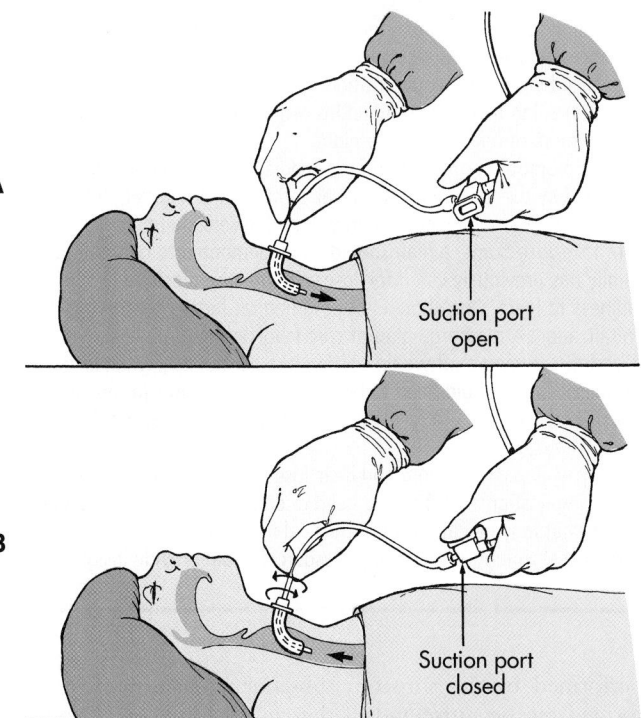

FIG. 22-35 ■ Tracheostomy suctioning. **A,** Insertion, port open. **B,** Withdrawal, port occluded. Note that catheter is inserted just slightly beyond end of tracheostomy tube.

EVIDENCE-BASED PRACTICE

Suctioning, Catheter Length, and Saline

Traditional technique for suctioning endotracheal (ET) or tracheostomy tubes recommends advancing a suction catheter into the tube until it meets resistance, then withdrawing it slightly and applying suction. However, studies indicate that this approach causes trauma to the tracheobronchial wall. This trauma can be avoided by inserting the catheter and advancing it to the premeasured depth of just to the tip (especially in infants) or no more than 0.5 cm beyond the tube (Kleiber, Krutzfield, and Rose, 1988).

Calibrated catheters are easier to use for premeasured suctioning technique, but unmarked catheters can also be used. To measure the length for catheter insertion, place the catheter near a sample ET or tracheostomy tube (the same size as the child's tube) with the end of the catheter at the correct position. Grasp the catheter with a sterile-gloved hand to mark the length, and insert the catheter until the hand reaches the stoma.

It has been common practice to instill a bolus of normal saline into the tube before suctioning. However, this technique may contribute to lower airway colonization and nosocomial pneumonia through repeated washing of organisms from the tube's surface into the lower airway. Also, the use of saline has been shown to have an adverse effect on oxygen saturation (Sao_2) and should not be used routinely in patients receiving mechanical ventilation who have a pulmonary infection (Ackerman, 1998). Although the pediatric research is scarce, routine use of normal saline with ET tube suctioning should be avoided (Curley and Moloney-Harmon, 2001; Blackwood, 1999).

?? CRITICAL THINKING EXERCISE

Planning for Home Tracheostomy Care

Jose Munoz, 18 months old, has a tracheostomy and has been ventilator-dependent since birth. He is hospitalized with pneumonia that has responded well to systemic antibiotic therapy. You are discussing plans for discharge and home care with the family. Jose lives with his mother, Gabriela, and her parents. None of the family members have previous health care experience. Home nursing support for Jose is available only during the day, and the family verbalizes concerns about taking the child home because he requires frequent suctioning at night.

QUESTIONS

1. Evidence—Is there sufficient evidence to draw conclusions about the family's concerns?
2. Assumptions—Describe an underlying assumption about each of the following:
   a. Ventilator use in the home
   b. Tracheostomy suctioning
   c. Need for nursing support
   d. Needs of a ventilator-dependent child
3. What priorities for nursing care should be established for Jose and his family?
4. Does the evidence support your nursing intervention?
5. What alternative perspectives might you have?

ANSWERS

1. Further evidence needs to be explored before implementing a plan for discussing home care. One item that needs clarification relates to how Jose's family managed with daytime nursing assistance before this hospitalization. Perhaps there is miscommunication between the family and nursing staff regarding the continued need for frequent nighttime suctioning. It is important to discuss with the family whether Jose's status has changed with this hospitalization. The family may need further teaching regarding home care, yet these issues must be carefully explored with the family. More information is needed regarding the family's understanding and knowledge of Jose's status.
2. a. Ventilator use in the home. Because Jose has required mechanical ventilation since birth, the family is knowledgeable about his respiratory care needs and seems to be comfortable with his care. Care of a child on mechanical ventilation is a complex skill for persons without health care experience, yet in most cases families who receive adequate training, resources, and support manage the child effectively in the home environment and adapt quite successfully to such care.
   b. Tracheostomy (tracheal) suctioning. Tracheal suctioning should not be performed on a set schedule, but only as needed to clear secretions that may accumulate and block the airway. Tracheal suctioning is not without inherent complications, including hypoxia and tracheal irritation. Suctioning should take place over a time frame of 10 to 25 seconds to prevent hypoxia, and the child should be adequately oxygenated before performing the procedure. Irritation of the tracheal tissues may lead to permanent damage if the suction catheter is advanced past the cannula; therefore, the suction catheter is premeasured to the length of the cannula to avoid deep suctioning. Equipment needed for tracheal suctioning, such as suction catheters, manual insufflation bag, and gloves, should always be gathered before the procedure and made readily available in case of an emergency. In the event of an illness such as pneumonia the amount of pulmonary secretions may be increased as a result of the illness; the amount usually decreases once the illness has resolved.
   c. Need for nursing support. The family managed with daytime nursing assistance before this hospitalization. After the pneumonia has resolved, frequent suctioning should not be required unless there are other intervening factors that affect his respiratory status. As noted in this case, changing the suctioning regimen decreased the frequency to a minimum of once or twice a night.
   d. Jose should be discharged as soon as possible to avoid nosocomial infection, promote normalization for a toddler, and contain health care costs. The child's needs for normal growth and development are not minimized by the fact that mechanical ventilation is required. It is important that the child be involved in early developmental assessment and care to promote adequate growth and development.
3. After adequate data have been gathered regarding the family's reluctance to take Jose home, a plan should be implemented to help the family cope with the care of a child on mechanical ventilation. Although the family has previously cared for Jose at home, the teaching should proceed in accordance to their level of understanding, willingness, and readiness to learn. One should not assume that further teaching is not required because the family has successfully cared for him before this hospitalization. A discharge plan of care involving the family should take place to provide effective home care for Jose. While Jose was hospitalized the nursing staff would suction him periodically when in the room, leading the family to believe that the frequency of suctioning seen in the hospital would need to be maintained at home. In this particular case the suctioning regimen gradually decreased to a minimum of once or twice a night—a level of care the family felt they would be able to manage.
4. Yes. In talking with the night staff, you find that the nurses suction any time they walk past the room and hear Jose "gurgling." Also, if you accept the conclusion that they do not use premeasured suctioning technique, the implications are that you need to discuss with them a program of premeasured suctioning only as needed to reduce the production of secretion that may be caused from tracheal irritation.
5. Further exploration of the family's concerns and worries is warranted. A detailed assessment of the family's resources could provide insight into issues that might not be related to Jose's respiratory care.

must consider the safety factor and use them only on a child who will not pull and undo the fastener.

Routine tracheostomy tube changes are usually carried out weekly after a tract has been formed to minimize the formation of granulation tissue. The first change is usually performed by the surgeon; subsequent changes are performed by the nurse and, if the child is discharged home with the tracheostomy, by either a parent or a visiting nurse. Ideally, two caregivers participate in the procedure to assist with positioning the child.

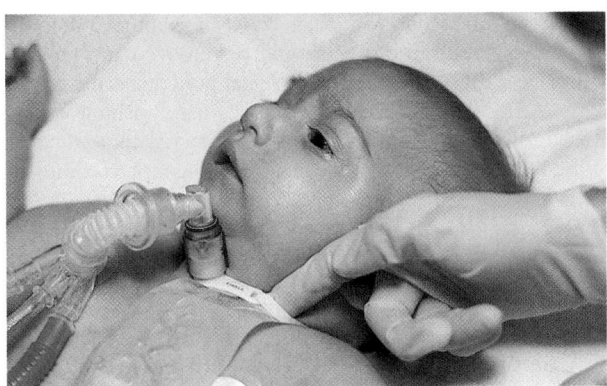

FIG. 22-36 ■ Tracheostomy ties are snug but allow one finger to be inserted.

Changing the tracheostomy tube is accomplished using sterile technique. The new, sterile tube is prepared by inserting the obturator and attaching new ties. The child is suctioned before the procedure to minimize secretions, then restrained and positioned with the neck slightly extended. One caregiver cuts the old ties and removes the tube from the stoma. The new tube is inserted gently into the stoma (using a downward and forward motion that follows the curve of the trachea), the obturator is removed, and the ties are secured. The adequacy of ventilation must be assessed after a tube change because the tube can be inserted into the soft tissue surrounding the trachea; therefore, breath sounds and respiratory effort are carefully monitored.

Supplemental O_2 is always delivered with a humidification system to prevent drying of the respiratory mucosa. Humidification of room air for an established tracheostomy can be intermittent if secretions remain thin enough to be coughed or suctioned from the tracheostomy. Direct humidification via a tracheostomy mask can be provided during naps and at night so that the child is able to be up and around unencumbered during much of the day. Room humidifiers are also used successfully.

The inner cannula, if used, should be removed with each suctioning, cleaned with sterile saline and pipe cleaners to remove crusted material, dried thoroughly, and reinserted.

Emergency Care: Tube Occlusion and Accidental Decannulation.   Occlusion of the tracheostomy tube is life-threatening, and infants and children are at greater risk than adults because of the smaller diameter of the tube. Maintaining patency of the tube is accomplished with suctioning and routine tube changes to prevent the formation of crusts that can occlude the tube.

> **NURSING ALERT**
>
> Life-threatening occlusion is apparent when the child displays signs of respiratory distress and a suction catheter cannot be passed to the end of the tube despite several attempts and instillation of saline. This situation requires an immediate tube change.

Accidental decannulation also requires immediate tube replacement. Some children have a fairly rigid trachea, so the airway remains partially open when the tube is removed. However, others have malformed or flexible tracheal cartilage, which causes the airway to collapse when the tube is removed or dislodged. Because many infants and children with upper airway problems have little airway reserve, if replacement of the dislodged tube is impossible, a smaller-sized tube should be inserted. If the stoma cannot be cannulated with another tracheostomy tube, oral intubation should be performed.

FAMILY TEACHING AND HOME CARE

Some of the treatments families need to continue at home are often related to respiratory procedures. Some of these treatments, such as postural drainage, require less preparation than others, such as tracheostomy care. Regardless of the home therapy, the family needs ample time to learn the skills and demonstrate them before discharge; therefore, instruction should begin as soon as it is identified that the child will go home with a tracheostomy. The more comfortable they are with all the aspects of care, the more confident and less anxious the family will be when faced with total care of the child at home. For example, the family may require many practice sessions before they feel comfortable with suctioning, cleaning, and changing a tracheostomy tube and performing cardiopulmonary resuscitation (CPR) in case of an emergency. Teaching sessions should be short, and written material must accompany instructions to reinforce what is being taught. To facilitate the family's adjustment, supplies identical to the ones to which they are accustomed should be available in the home. In the event of substitution, parents need to be reassured that the unfamiliar equipment is safe to use on their child. The home should be properly equipped with all supplies and equipment needed before the child arrives.

A nurse from the public health department or other home care service should be available to the family and should periodically assess the family's ability to carry out the activities needed in care of the child. The parents may find it helpful to talk with other parents of children with similar needs. They also need to know whom to call and where they can get help and support in times of uncertainty or in an emergency.

To prepare for any emergency, the family must be taught infant or child CPR. The local utilities company and local emergency medical services (EMS) should be notified of the child's condition and the equipment used in the home. Prior notification allows for a quicker response if help is needed.

When a child has a tracheostomy, parents are encouraged to provide as normal a life as possible for their child and other family members. Vocalization for the child with a tracheostomy has recently become a reality. Several tracheostomy speaking valves have been created to aid in the development of uninterrupted speech without the necessity of finger occlusion. One valve of several available on the market is the *Passy Muir* valve.* It is a one-way valve that attaches to the hub of all types and sizes of tracheostomies. It can be used in infants and in children who are ventilator-assisted (Engleman and Turnage-Carrier, 1997).

The child who is physically able (e.g., a child with a tracheostomy without respiratory disability such as recurrent laryngeal polyps) can usually be allowed to engage in most

---

*Further information can be obtained from **Passy & Passy, Inc.,** 4521 Campus Drive, Suite 273, Irvine, CA 92612; (800) 634-5397; fax: (949) 833-8299; website: www.passy-muir.com.

activities that are appropriate for the child's age. The child may play outdoors with a scarf or other protection to loosely cover the tracheostomy stoma. Both child and parents must be cautioned regarding play near any body of water, such as a swimming pool or stream, and informed about safety precautions in the bathtub. The child should not be exposed to noxious fumes (e.g., paint, varnish, hair spray) or talc (baby powder). Young children who may spill food near the stoma should wear a fabric bib (without plastic lining) or other device to prevent dribbled food or crumbs from being aspirated. The family should have a bag with routine and emergency supplies to take with the child at all times.

PROCEDURES RELATED TO ALTERNATIVE FEEDING TECHNIQUES

Some children are unable to take nourishment by mouth because of conditions such as anomalies of the throat, esophagus, or bowel; impaired swallowing capacity; severe debilitation; respiratory distress; or unconsciousness. These children are frequently fed by way of a tube inserted orally or nasally into the stomach *(orogastric* or *nasogastric gavage)* or duodenum/jejunum *(enteral gavage),* or by a tube inserted directly into the stomach *(gastrostomy)* or jejunum *(jejunostomy).* Such feedings may be intermittent or by continuous drip. At times the entire alimentary tract must be bypassed, using IV feeding called total parenteral nutrition (TPN). Because enteral feedings are used less often than gastric or IV feedings, the following discussion is limited to gastric gavage, gastrostomy, and TPN.

Feeding resistance, a problem that may result from any long-term feeding method that bypasses the mouth, is discussed in Chapter 9. During gavage or gastrostomy (nonoral) feedings, infants are given a pacifier. Nonnutritive sucking has several advantages, such as increased weight gain and decreased crying. However, to prevent the possibility of aspiration, only pacifiers with a safe design may be used. Using improvised pacifiers made from bottle nipples is not a safe practice. (See Injury Prevention: Aspiration in Chapter 10.)

! NURSING ALERT

When a child is concurrently receiving continuous-drip gastric or enteral feedings and parenteral (IV) therapy, the potential exists for inadvertent administration of the enteral formula through the circulatory system, especially when the parenteral solution is a fat emulsion, which looks milky. Safeguards to prevent this potentially serious error include:

Use a separate, specifically designed enteral feeding pump mounted on a separate pole for continuous-feeding solutions.

Label all tubing for continuous enteral feeding with brightly colored tape or labels.

Use specifically designed continuous-feeding bags to contain the solutions instead of parenteral equipment, such as a burette.

GAVAGE FEEDING

Infants and children can be fed simply and safely by a tube passed into the stomach through either the nares or the mouth. The tube can be left in place or inserted and removed with each feeding. In older children it is usually less traumatic

to tape the tube securely in place between feedings. When this alternative is used, the tube should be removed and replaced with a new tube according to hospital policy, specific orders, and the type of tube used. Meticulous handwashing is practiced during the procedure to prevent bacterial contamination of the feeding, especially during continuous-drip feedings.

Preparation

The equipment needed for gavage feeding includes:

- A suitable tube selected according to the size of the child and the viscosity of the solution being fed. Feeding tubes are available in silicone rubber, polyurethane, polyethylene, or polyvinylchloride. Polyurethane and silicone rubber tubes are smaller in diameter and more flexible than the others and are often referred to as small-bore tubes.
- A receptacle for the fluid; for small amounts a 10- to 30-mL syringe barrel or Asepto syringe is satisfactory; for larger amounts a 50-mL syringe with a catheter tip is more convenient.
- A syringe to aspirate stomach contents and/or to inject air after the tube has been placed.
- Water or water-soluble lubricant to lubricate the tube; sterile water is used for infants.
- Paper or nonallergenic tape to mark the tube and to attach the tube to the infant's or child's cheek (and nose, if placed through the nares).
- A stethoscope to determine the correct placement in the stomach.
- The solution for feeding.

Not all feeding tubes are the same. Polyethylene and polyvinylchloride types lose their flexibility and need to be replaced frequently, usually every 3 to 4 days. The polyurethane and silicone rubber tubes are indwelling and remain flexible; thus, they can remain in place longer and afford more patient comfort. Use of these small-bore tubes for continuous feeding has greatly reduced the incidence of complications such as pharyngitis, otitis media, and incompetence of the lower esophageal sphincter. Although the increased softness and flexibility of the tubes are advantages, they also result in problems such as difficult insertion (may require a stylet or metal guidewire), collapse of the tube during aspiration of gastric contents when testing for correct placement, dislodgment during forceful coughing, and unsuitability for thick feedings. Traditional methods for verifying placement are less reliable with the small-bore tubes.

Procedure

Even tiny infants with random movements can grasp and dislodge the tube. Premature infants do not ordinarily require restraint, but if they do, a small towel folded across the chest and secured beneath the shoulders is usually sufficient. Care must be taken so that breathing is not compromised.

Whenever possible, the infant should be held during the procedure to associate the comfort of physical contact with the feeding. When this is not possible, gavage feeding is carried out with the infant or child on the back or toward the right side and the head and chest elevated. Feeding the child in a sitting position helps maintain the placement of the tube in the lowest position, thus increasing the likelihood of correct placement in the stomach.

The feeding tube can be passed through either the nose (nasogastric) or the mouth (orogastric). Because most young infants are obligatory nose breathers, insertion through the mouth causes less distress and helps to stimulate sucking. A tube passed through one of the nares in older infants and children is satisfactory once the tube is in place. An indwelling tube is almost always placed through the nose; the tube is alternated between nares with each insertion to minimize irritation, chance of infection, and possible breakdown of mucous membranes from pressure that occurs over time (see Atraumatic Care box). The procedure for gavage feeding is described in the Guidelines box.

ATRAUMATIC CARE

Reducing the Distress of Nasogastric Tube Insertion

Numerous strategies can be used to decrease discomfort during nasogastric (NG) tube insertion. Most important, the nurse performing the procedure should be competent in NG tube placement. The procedure should be discussed with the child in a developmentally appropriate way, and family members should be given the details of what to expect during the procedure. Administration of sedation and analgesia should be considered before NG insertion. The use of topical lidocaine and phenylephrine for the nose and tetracaine and benzocaine spray for the throat before NG insertion has been found to reduce pain and discomfort in a group of adult patients (Singer and Konia, 1999). A smaller-caliber, soft, flexible tube should be used. To prevent the trauma of reinsertion, make sure the NG tube is well secured following placement.

Data from Maglinte C: Strategies for reducing the pain and discomfort of nasogastric intubation, *Acad Emerg Med* 6(3):166-168, 1999.

GUIDELINES

Nasogastric Tube Feedings in Children

Place child supine with head slightly hyperflexed or in a sniffing position (nose pointed toward ceiling).

Measure the tube for approximate length of insertion and mark the point with a small piece of tape.

Insert the tube that has been lubricated with sterile water or water-soluble lubricant through either the mouth or one of the nares to the predetermined mark. Because most young infants are obligatory nose breathers, insertion through the mouth causes less distress and helps to stimulate sucking. In older infants and children the tube is passed through the nose and alternated between nostrils. An indwelling tube is almost always placed through the nose.

When using the nose, slip the tube along the base of the nose and direct it straight back toward the occiput.

When entering through the mouth, direct the tube toward the back of the throat (Fig. 22-37, *B*).

If the child is able to swallow on command, synchronize passing the tube with swallowing.

Check the position of the tube by doing *both* of the following:

Attach the syringe to the feeding tube and apply negative pressure. Aspiration of stomach contents indicates proper placement, but aspiration of respiratory secretions may be mistaken for stomach contents. However, absence of fluid is not necessarily evidence of improper placement. The stomach may be empty, the tube may not be in contact with stomach contents, or a small-bore flexible tube may collapse. Note the amount and character of any fluid aspirated and return the fluid to the stomach.

With the syringe, inject a small amount of air (0.5 to 1 mL in premature or very small infants to 5 mL in larger children) into the tube while simultaneously listening with a stethoscope over the stomach area. Sounds of gurgling or growling will be heard if the tube is properly situated in the stomach, although it is possible to hear the air entering the stomach even when the tube is positioned above the gastroesophageal sphincter.

Stabilize the tube by holding or taping it to the cheek, not to the forehead, because of possible damage to the nostril. To maintain correct placement, measure and record the amount of tubing extending from the nose or mouth to the distal port when the tube is first positioned. Recheck this measurement before each feeding.

Warm the formula to room temperature. Do not microwave! Pour formula into the barrel of the syringe attached to the feeding tube. To start the flow, give a gentle push with the plunger, but then remove the plunger and allow the fluid to flow into the stomach by gravity. The rate of flow should not exceed 5 mL every 5 to 10 minutes in premature and very small infants and 10 mL/min in older infants and children to prevent nausea and regurgitation. The rate is determined by the diameter of the tubing and the height of the reservoir containing the feeding and is regulated by adjusting the height of the syringe. A usual feeding may take from 15 to 30 minutes to complete.

Flush the tube with sterile water (1 or 2 mL for small tubes to 5 to 15 mL or more for large ones), or see discussion of flushing for administering medication through nasogastric tubes in the Guidelines box on p. 761 to clear it of formula.

Cap or clamp indwelling tubes to prevent loss of feeding.

If the tube is to be removed, first pinch it firmly to prevent escape of fluid as the tube is withdrawn. Withdraw the tube quickly.

Position the child with the head elevated about 30 degrees and on the right side or abdomen for at least 1 hour in the same manner as after any infant feeding to minimize the possibility of regurgitation and aspiration. If the child's condition permits, bubble the youngster after the feeding.

Record the feeding, including the type and amount of residual, the type and amount of formula, and how it was tolerated. For most infant feedings, any amount of residual fluid aspirated from the stomach is refed to prevent electrolyte imbalance, and the amount is subtracted from the prescribed amount of feeding. For example, if the infant is to receive 30 mL and 10 mL is aspirated from the stomach before the feeding, the 10 mL of aspirated stomach contents is refed along with 20 mL of feeding. Another method can be used in children. If residual fluid is more than one fourth of the last feeding, return the aspirate and recheck in 30 to 60 minutes. When residual fluid is less than one fourth of the last feeding, give the scheduled feeding. If large amounts of aspirated fluid persist and the child is due for another feeding, notify the practitioner.

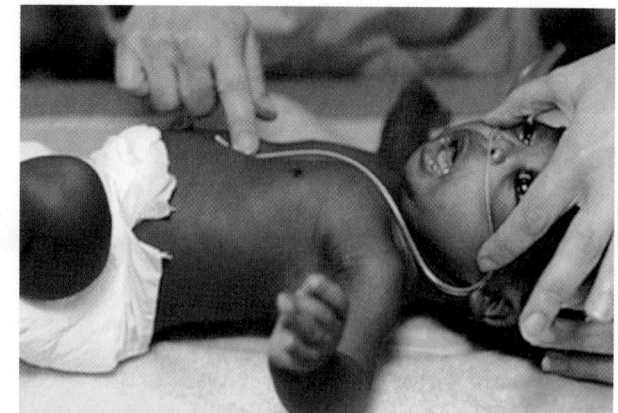 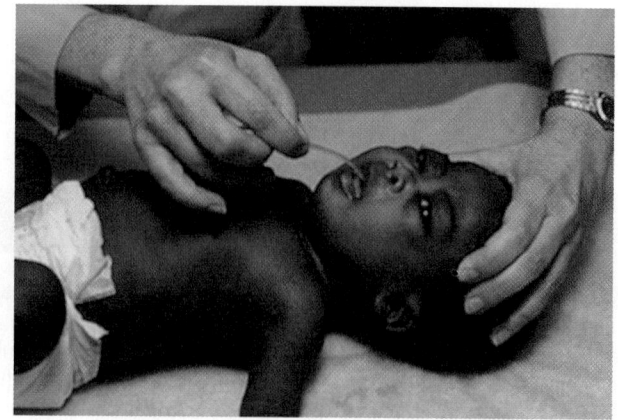

FIG. 22-37 ■ Gavage feeding. **A,** Measuring tube for orogastric feeding from tip of nose to earlobe and to midpoint between end of xiphoid process and umbilicus. **B,** Inserting tube.

TABLE 22-8 ■ **Recommended Minimum Insertion Lengths for Orogastric Tubes in Very-Low-Birth-Weight Infants**

	DAILY WEIGHT (g)			
	<750	750-999	1000-1249	1250-1499
Insertion length (cm)	13	15	16	17

From Gallaher KJ and others: Orogastric tube insertion length in very-low-birth-weight infants (<1500 grams), *J Perinatol* 13(2):128-131, 1993.

Two standard methods of measuring tube length for insertion are (1) measuring from the nose to the bottom of the earlobe and then to the end of the xiphoid process or (2) measuring from the nose to the earlobe and then to a point midway between the xiphoid process and the umbilicus (Fig. 22-37, *A*). Ellett (1998) found significant tube placement errors (43.5%) in a study of 39 hospitalized children. For very-low-birth-weight infants, daily weight can be used to predict insertion length (Table 22-8).

Unfortunately, "bedside" methods used to verify the placement of the tube have serious shortcomings (see Guidelines box). The most accurate method for testing tube placement is radiography, but this practice is not feasible before each feeding. One method that appears promising is the consideration of aspirate color and pH to determine placement, because respiratory, gastric, and intestinal fluids have a different pH and color. Metheny and others (1998) found that acidic pH values of 4 or less were reasonable indicators of gastric tube placement, whereas respiratory fluid had pH values greater then 6. The color of the gastric fluid aspirated was found to be most often grassy green, off-white to tan, bloody, or brown, whereas the color of pleural fluid was off-white and tinged with mucus and blood. These authors suggest that an aspirate's pH and color can help determine tube placement. Until pH is studied further, especially in children, nurses need to use the traditional methods with an awareness of their limitations. If doubt exists regarding correct placement, the practitioner should be consulted.

NURSING ALERT

Nurses need to take precaution when assessing tube placement. One study reported that out of 201 children, 32 had nasogastric (NG) tube placement errors as viewed by radiography (Ellett, 1998).

GASTROSTOMY FEEDING

Feeding by way of a gastrostomy tube is a variation of tube feeding that is often used for children in whom passage of a tube through the mouth, pharynx, esophagus, and cardiac sphincter of the stomach is contraindicated or impossible. It is also used to avoid the constant irritation of a gastric tube in children who require tube feeding over an extended period. Placement of a gastrostomy tube may be performed with the patient under general anesthesia or percutaneously using an endoscope with the patient sedated and under local anesthesia (percutaneous endoscopic gastrostomy [PEG]). The tube is inserted through the abdominal wall into the stomach about midway along the greater curvature and when surgically placed is secured by a purse-string suture. The stomach is anchored to the peritoneum at the operative site. The tube used can be a Foley, wing-tip, or mushroom catheter.

Immediately after surgery the catheter is left open and attached to gravity drainage for 24 hours or more. Postoperative care of the wound site is directed toward prevention of infection and irritation. The area is cleansed with a mild, pH-balanced cleanser such as normal saline. A cotton-tipped applicator is used to remove drainage close to the tube site (O'Brien and others, 1999). After healing takes place, meticulous care is needed to keep the area surrounding the tube clean and dry to prevent excoriation and infection. Daily applications of antibiotic ointment or other preparations may be prescribed to aid in healing and prevention of irritation. Care is exercised to prevent excessive pull on the catheter that might cause widening of the opening and subsequent leakage of highly irritating gastric juices.

For children receiving long-term gastrostomy feeding, a *skin-level device* (e.g., MIC-KEY, Bard Button, Gastroport) offers several advantages. The small, flexible silicone device protrudes slightly from the abdomen, is cosmetically pleasing in appearance, affords increased comfort and mo-

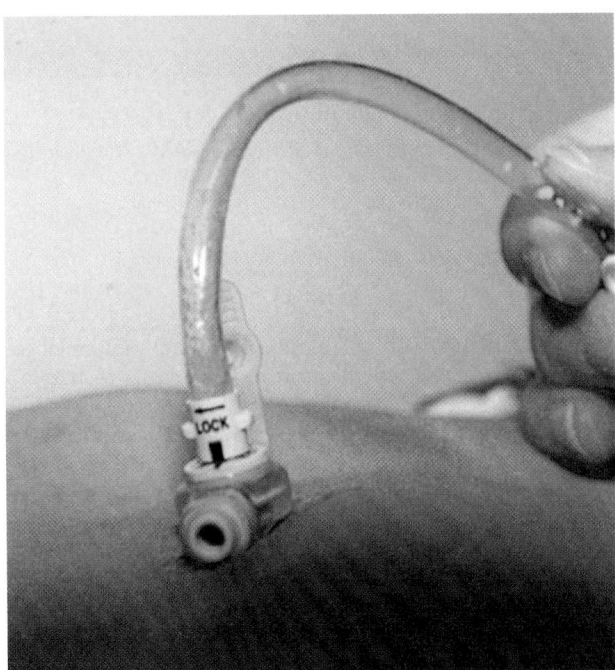

FIG. 22-38 ■ Child with skin-level gastrostomy device (MIC-KEY), which provides for secure attachment of extension tubing to gastrostomy opening.

bility to the child, is easy to care for, and is fully immersible in water. The one-way valve at the proximal end minimizes reflux and eliminates the need for clamping. However, the button requires a well-established gastrostomy site and is more expensive than the conventional tube. In addition, the valve may become clogged. When functioning, the valve prevents air from escaping; therefore, the child may require frequent bubbling. With some devices, during feedings the child must remain fairly still, because the tubing easily disconnects from the opening if the child moves. With other devices, extension tubing can be securely attached to the opening (Fig. 22-38). The feeding is instilled at the other end of the tubing in a manner similar to that for a regular gastrostomy. The extension tubing may also have a separate medication port. Both the feeding and the medication ports have plugs attached. Some skin-level devices require a special tube to decompress the stomach (to check residual or release air).

Feeding of water, formula, or pureed foods is carried out in the same manner and rate as in gavage feeding. A mechanical pump may be used to regulate the volume and rate of feeding. After feedings, in an effort to encourage gastric emptying and reduce potential aspiration, the child is positioned to sleep at a 30-degree angle in bed. Older children are propped up on pillows, whereas the infant can have a small wedge or pillow placed under the head end of the mattress (Holden and others, 1997). It is also recommended that the infant or child be positioned on the right side. The tube may be clamped, left open, or suspended between feedings, depending on the child's condition. A clamped tube allows more mobility but is appropriate only if the child can tolerate intermittent feedings without vomiting or prolonged backup of feeding into the tube. Some-

times a Y tube is used to allow for simultaneous decompression during feeding. If a Foley catheter is used as the gastrostomy tube, very slight tension is applied. The tube is securely taped to maintain the balloon at the gastrostomy opening to prevent leakage of gastric contents and to prevent the tube's progression toward the pyloric sphincter, where it may occlude the stomach outlet. As a precaution, the length of the tube should be measured postoperatively and then remeasured each shift to be sure it has not slipped. A mark can be made above the skin level to further ensure its placement. When the gastrostomy tube is no longer needed, it is removed; the skin opening usually closes spontaneously by contracture.

TOTAL PARENTERAL NUTRITION

TPN provides for the total nutritional needs of infants or children whose lives are threatened because feeding by way of the gastrointestinal tract is impossible, inadequate, or hazardous.

TPN therapy involves IV infusion of highly concentrated solutions of protein, glucose, and other nutrients. The solution is infused through conventional tubing with a special filter attached to remove particulate matter or microorganisms that may have contaminated the solution. The highly concentrated solutions require infusion into a vessel with sufficient volume and turbulence to allow for rapid dilution. The wide-diameter vessels selected are the superior vena cava and innominate or intrathoracic subclavian veins approached by way of the external or internal jugular veins. The highly irritating nature of concentrated glucose precludes the use of the small peripheral veins in most instances. However, dilute glucose-protein hydrolysates that are appropriate for infusing into peripheral veins are being used with increasing frequency. When peripheral veins are used, intralipid becomes the major calorie source. For long-term alimentation, VADs are usually used (see p. 757).

The major nursing responsibilities are the same as for any IV therapy: control of sepsis, monitoring of the infusion rate, and assessment of the patient. The TPN solution must be prepared under rigid aseptic conditions best accomplished by specially trained technicians. The solution and tubing are changed and the infusion site redressed by specially trained nurses using meticulous aseptic precautions. In some institutions this may be a nursing responsibility. If so, the procedure is carried out according to hospital protocol.

The infusion is maintained at a constant rate by means of an infusion pump to ensure the proper concentrations of glucose and amino acids. Accurate calculation of the rate is required to deliver a measured amount in a given length of time. Because alterations in flow rate are relatively common, the drip should be checked frequently to ensure an even, continuous infusion. The TPN infusion rate should not be increased or decreased without the practitioner being informed, because alterations can cause hyperglycemia or hypoglycemia.

General assessments, such as vital signs, I&O measurements, and checking results of laboratory tests facilitate early detection of infection or fluid and electrolyte imbalance. Additional amounts of potassium and sodium chloride are often required in hyperalimentation; therefore, observation for signs of potassium or sodium deficit or excess is part of nursing care. This is rarely a problem except in children with reduced renal function or metabolic defects. Hyperglycemia may occur during the first day or two as the child adapts to the high-glucose load of the hyperalimentation solution. Although occurring infrequently, insulin may be required to assist the body's adjustment to the hyperglycemia. When this occurs, nursing responsibilities include blood glucose testing. To prevent hypoglycemia at the time the hyperalimentation is disconnected, the rate of the infusion and the amount of insulin are decreased gradually.

In addition to children's physical needs, their developmental needs must also be considered during the often long-term use of TPN. Regular assessment of development should be performed to assess the child's progress, and appropriate interventions should be instituted to encourage expected milestones. Delays in the areas of gross motor and language skills are found most often; therefore, special attention should be directed to these areas.

FAMILY TEACHING AND HOME CARE

When alternative feedings are needed for an extended period, the family may need to learn how to feed the child with a nasogastric, gastrostomy, or TPN feeding regimen. The same principles discussed earlier in this chapter for compliance, especially in terms of education (p. 725), and in Chapter 21 for discharge planning and home care are applied. Because of the numerous skills the family must learn for home TPN, ample time must be planned for the family to learn and perform the procedures under supervision before assuming full responsibility for the child's care.

The family may be referred to community agencies that provide support and practical assistance. The **Oley Foundation*** is a nonprofit research and education organization that assists persons receiving enteral nutrition and home TPN.

PROCEDURES RELATED TO ELIMINATION

ENEMA

The procedure for giving an enema to an infant or child does not differ essentially from that for an adult, except for the type and amount of fluid administered and the distance for inserting the tube into the rectum. Depending on the volume, the nurse uses a syringe with rubber tubing, an enema bottle, or an enema bag (see Guidelines box).

⚠ NURSING ALERT

Proper insertion of the catheter tip, especially in infants, is essential to prevent rectal damage and perforation (see Fig. 7-7, *B*). If insertion of the enema tip causes discomfort, remove the tip and notify the practitioner.

An isotonic solution is used in children. Plain water is not used because, being hypotonic, it can cause rapid fluid shift and fluid overload. The Fleet enema (pediatric or adult sized) is not advised for children because of the harsh action

*214 Hun Memorial, A23, Albany Medical Center, Albany, NY 12208; (800) 776-OLEY; website: web.wizvak.net/oleyfdn/index.html.

⸮ GUIDELINES

Administration of Enemas to Children

AGE	AMOUNT (mL)	INSERTION DISTANCE (cm [inches])
Infant	120-240	2.5 (1 inch)
2-4 years	240-360	5 (2 inches)
4-10 years	360-480	7.5 (3 inches)
11 years	480-720	10 (4 inches)

of its ingredients (sodium biphosphate and sodium phosphate). Commercial enemas can be dangerous to patients with megacolon and to dehydrated or azotemic children. The osmotic effect of the Fleet enema may produce diarrhea, which can lead to metabolic acidosis. Other potential complications are extreme hyperphosphatemia, hypernatremia, and hypocalcemia, which may lead to neuromuscular irritability and coma (Walton and others, 2000).

NURSING TIP

If prepared saline is not available, it can be made by adding 1 teaspoon of table salt to 500 mL (1 pint) of tap water.

Because infants and young children are unable to retain the solution after it is administered, the buttocks must be held together for a short time to retain the fluid. The enema is administered and expelled while the child is lying with the buttocks over the bedpan and with the head and back supported by pillows. Older children are usually able to hold the solution if they understand what to do and if they are not expected to hold it for too long. The nurse should have the bedpan handy or, for the ambulatory child, ensure that the bathroom is readily available before beginning the procedure. An enema is an intrusive procedure and thus threatening to the preschool child; therefore, a careful explanation is especially important to ease possible fear.

A preoperative bowel preparation solution given orally or through a nasogastric tube is increasingly being used instead of an enema. The polyethylene glycol–electrolyte lavage solution (Golytely) mechanically flushes the bowel without significant absorption, thereby avoiding potential fluid and electrolyte imbalances.

FYI

NuLytely, a modification of Golytely, has been found to have the same therapeutic advantage as Golytely and was developed to improve on the taste of Golytely (Diab and Marshall, 1996).

OSTOMIES

Children may require stomas for various health problems. The most frequent causes are necrotizing enterocolitis and imperforate anus in the infant (less often, Hirschsprung disease). In the older child the most frequent causes are inflammatory bowel disease, especially Crohn disease (regional enteritis), and ureterostomies for distal ureter or bladder defects.

Care and management of ostomies in the older child differ little from the care of ostomies in the adult patient. The major emphases in pediatric care are the preparation of the child for the procedure and teaching care of the ostomy to the child and family. The basic principles of preparation are the same as for any procedure (see p. 709). Simple, straightforward language is most effective, together with the use of illustrations and a replica model (e.g., drawing a picture of a child with a stoma on the abdomen and explaining it as "another opening where bowel movements [or any other term the child uses] will come out"). At another time the nurse can draw a pouch over the opening to demonstrate how the contents are collected. Using a doll to demonstrate the process is an excellent teaching strategy, and special books are available.*

Children with ileostomies are fitted immediately after surgery with an appliance to protect the skin from the proteolytic enzymes in the liquid stool. Parents are usually given a choice of caring for the colostomy with or without an appliance. Pediatric appliances are available in a variety of sizes to ensure an adequate fit.†

Ostomy equipment consists of a one- or two-piece system with a hypoallergenic skin barrier to maintain peristomal skin integrity. The pouch should be large enough to contain a moderate amount of stool and flatus but not so large as to overwhelm the infant or child. A backing helps minimize the risk of skin breakdown from moisture trapped between the skin and pouch. Small clips or rubber bands should be avoided to prevent choking in the young child. Granulation tissue may grow around an ostomy site (Fig. 22-39). This moist, beefy red tissue is not a sign of infection. However, if it continues to grow, the excess moisture can cause irritation of the surrounding skin.

Protection of the peristomal skin is a major aspect of stoma care. Well-fitting appliances are important to prevent leakage of contents. Before the appliance is applied, the skin is prepared with a skin sealant that is allowed to dry. Then stoma paste is applied around the base of the stoma or the back of the wafer. The sealant and paste work together to prevent peristomal breakdown.

In infants with a colostomy left unpouched, skin care is similar to that of any diapered child. However, the peristomal skin is protected with a wafer barrier, such as a hydrocolloid dressing (e.g., Duoderm) or a barrier substance (e.g., zinc oxide ointment [Desitin], karaya products, a mixture of the zinc oxide ointment and stoma [Stomahesive†] powder). A gauze dressing may be applied over the stoma and water to absorb stomal drainage. If the skin becomes inflamed, denuded, or infected, the care is similar to the interventions used for diaper dermatitis (see Chapter 30). A product that helps protect healthy skin, heal excoriated skin, and minimize pain associated with skin breakdown is Preshield Plus.‡ The skin protectant adheres to denuded weeping skin. It can be applied over topical antifungal and

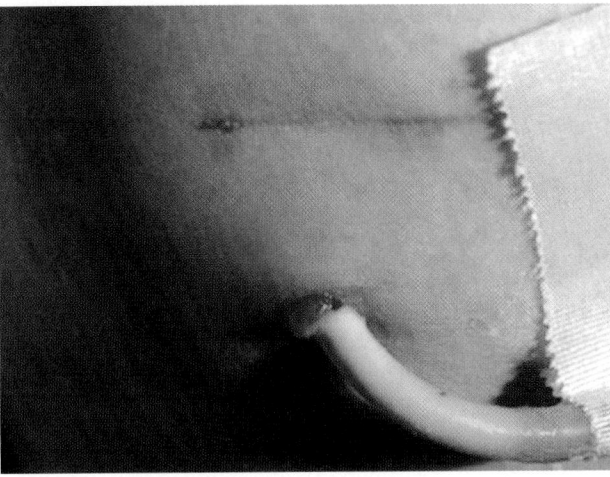

FIG. 22-39 ■ Appearance of healthy granulation tissue around stoma.

antibacterial agents if infection is present. "No-sting" barrier film* is a skin sealant that has no alcohol base and can be used on open skin without stinging.

With young children, protection of the pouch from being pulled off is also an important consideration. One-piece outfits keep exploring hands from reaching the pouch, and the loose waist prevents any pressure on the appliance. Keeping the child occupied with toys during the pouch change is also helpful. As children mature, their participation in ostomy care is encouraged. Even preschoolers can assist by holding supplies, pulling paper backings from the appliance, and helping clean the stoma area. Toilet training for bladder control needs to begin at the appropriate time as for any other child.

Older children and adolescents should eventually have total responsibility for ostomy care just as they would for usual bowel function. During adolescence, concerns for body image and the ostomy's impact on intimacy and sexuality emerge. The nurse should stress to teenagers that the presence of a stoma need not interfere with their activities. These youngsters can choose which ostomy equipment is best suited to their needs. Attractively designed and decorated pouch covers are well liked by teenagers.

An enterostomal therapy nurse specialist is an important member of the health care team and will have additional suggestions and skin care information and ostomy pouching options. Further information may be obtained by contacting the **Wound, Ostomy, and Continence Nurses Society (WOCN).**†

FAMILY TEACHING AND HOME CARE

Because these children are almost always discharged with a functioning colostomy, preparation of the family should begin as early as possible in the hospital. The family is instructed in the application of the device (if used), care of the skin, and appropriate action in case skin problems develop. Early evidence of skin breakdown or stomal complications, such as ribbonlike stools, excessive diarrhea, bleeding, prolapse, or failure to pass flatus or stool, is brought to the attention of the physician, the

---

Chris Has an Ostomy is available from **United Ostomy Association, Inc.,** 36 Executive Park, Suite 120, Irvine, CA 92714-6744; (800) 826-0826.

†**Little Ones Ostomy Products,** ConvaTec, CN 5254, Princeton, NJ 08543-5254; (800) 422-8811; website: www.convatec.com. Parents may find the following pamphlets helpful: *A Parent's Guide to Necrotizing Enterocolitis* or *Parent's Guide to Ostomy Care for Children,* available from ConvaTec.

‡**Healthpoint Medical,** 2600 Airport Freeway, Fort Worth, TX 76111; (800) 441-8227; website: www.healthpoint.com.

*3M, St. Paul, MN, (800) 228-3957.

†(888) 224-WOCN; website: www.wocn.org.

nurse, or the stoma specialist. The same principles are applied as discussed earlier in this chapter for compliance, especially in terms of education (p. 725), and in Chapter 21 for discharge planning and home care.

KEY POINTS

- Informed consent is valid when the person is capable of giving consent (is over the age of majority and is competent), is supplied with information needed to make an intelligent decision, and acts voluntarily when exercising freedom of choice.

- Informed consent is needed for major surgery, minor surgery, and diagnostic tests and medical treatments with an element of risk.

- The major tasks in psychologic preparation of the child for procedures are to establish trust, provide support, and give an explanation in easy-to-understand terms.

- Most parents and children want to be together during stressful procedures and should be offered this opportunity, along with guidance on how the parent can comfort the child.

- In the performance of a procedure the nurse should expect success, involve the child when possible in the procedure, provide distraction, and allow for expression of feelings.

- In giving postprocedural support, the nurse should encourage the child to express feelings and praise the youngster for completion of the procedure.

- Stressful times before and after surgery that produce anxiety in children include admission, blood tests, injection of preoperative medication (if used), transportation to the operating room, and return from the postanesthesia care unit.

- Assessment of compliance entails measuring factors that affect compliance through self-reporting, direct observation, monitoring of appointments and therapeutic response, pill counts, and chemical assay.

- Compliance strategies may be classified as organizational, educational, treatment, and behavioral.

- Knowledge of the sick child's eating habits and favorite foods can help in maintaining adequate nutrition.

- Control of fever may be accomplished by pharmacologic means (administration of antipyretics); hyperthermia is controlled by environmental means (minimum clothing, increased air circulation, cool compresses).

- Infection control is based on two systems. Standard precautions provide protection when the infected person is undiagnosed. Transmission-based precautions add extra interventions for patients diagnosed with or suspected to have an infection.

- Ensuring safety in the hospital setting is a major concern and can be achieved through environmental measures, limit setting, and safe transportation.

- Restraints are used cautiously and typically require a medical order. Therapeutic hugging can avoid the use of restraints.

- Factors that affect drug dosage determination include growth and maturation, difficulty in evaluating drug response, and body surface area.

- Family teaching regarding medication administration includes telling parents why the child is receiving the drug; its possible effects; and the amount, frequency, and length of time the drug is to be administered.

- The preferred sites for intramuscular injection in children are the vastus lateralis and ventrogluteal areas.

- Intermittent venous access is accomplished by a peripheral intermittent infusion device, a peripherally inserted central catheter, a central venous catheter, or an implanted port.

- Several safety catheters and needleless device systems are available to reduce the risk of needle-stick injuries in patients and caregivers.

- Nursing assessment of fluid and electrolyte disturbances entails observation of general appearance, vital signs, and measurement of intake and output.

- Oxygen can be administered by hood, mask, nasal cannula, incubator, or oxygen tent.

- Tracheostomy suctioning involves premeasured insertion of the catheter, application of suction for 5 seconds when withdrawing the catheter, and supplemental oxygen before and after suctioning.

- Alternative forms of feeding include gavage feeding, gastrostomy feeding, and total parenteral nutrition.

- In the care of children with ostomies, nurses play an important role in family support and instruction in care of the stoma site.

References

Algren C, Ireland D, Stewart E: Perioperative and perianesthesia care of the child. In Albers AC and others, editors: *Comprehensive care of the pediatric patient: prehospital through rehabilitation*, Park Ridge, Il, 1998, Emergency Nurses Association.

Algren C, Schwartz P: The application of nursing research to the child. In Albers AC and others, editors: *Comprehensive care of the pediatric patient: prehospital through rehabilitation*, Park Ridge, Il, 1998, Emergency Nurses Association.

American Academy of Pediatrics, Committee on Drugs: Guidelines for monitoring and management of pediatric patients during and after sedation for diagnostic and therapeutic procedures, *Pediatrics* 86(6):1110-1115, 1992.

American Academy of Pediatrics: Informed consent, parental permission, and assent in pediatric practice, *Pediatrics* 95(2):314-317, 1995.

American Academy of Pediatrics: Guidelines for monitoring and management of pediatric patients during and after sedation for diagnostic and therapeutic procedures: addendum, *Pediatrics* 110(4):836-838, 2002.

American Academy of Pediatrics: Consent for emergency medical services for children and adolescents, *Pediatrics* 111(3):703-705, 2003.

American Society of Anesthesiologists: Practice guidelines for sedation and analgesia by non-anesthesiologists, *Anesthesiology* 96:1004-1017, 2002.

Axelrod P: External cooling in the management of fever, *Clin Infect Dis* 31(suppl 5):S224-229, 2000.

Banerjee S and others: The intraosseous route is a suitable alternative to the intravenous route for fluid resuscitation in severely dehydrated children, *Indian Pediatr* 312:1511-1520, 1994.

Barker DP and others: Capillary blood sampling: should the heel be warmed? *Arch Dis Child Fetal Neonatal Ed* 74(2):F139-F140, 1996.

Barton S, Holmes S: A comparison of regeant strips and the refractometer for measurement of urine specific gravity in hospitalized children, *Pediatr Nurs* 23(5):480-482, 1998.

Beecroft PC and others: Intravenous lock patency in children: dilute heparin versus saline, *J Pediatr Pract* 2(4):211-233, 1997.

Berger JE, AAP Committee on Medical Liability: Consent by proxy for nonurgent pediatric care, *Pediatrics* 112(5):1186-1195, 2003.

Blackwood B: Normal saline instillation with endotracheal suctioning: primum non nocere (first do no harm), *J Adv Nurs* 29(4):928-934, 1999.

Blass EM, Watt L: Suckling-and sucrose-induced analgesia in human newborns, *Pain* 83(3):611-623, 1999.

Broome M: Consent (assent) for research with pediatric patients, *Semin Oncol Nurs* 15(2):96-103, 1999.

Broome M, Rehwaldt M, Fogg L: Relationship between cognitive behavioral techniques, temperament, observed distress, and pain reports in children and adolescents during lumbar puncture, *J Pediatr Nurs* 13(1):48-54, 1998.

Bryant RA, Doughty D, editors: *Acute and chronic wounds: nursing management*, ed 2, St Louis, 2000, Mosby.

Burke N: Alternative methods for newborn urine sample collection, *Pediatr Nurs* 21(6):546-549, 1995.

Calianno C: Patient hygiene. II. Skin care: keeping the outside healthy, *Nursing* 29(12 suppl):1-11, 1999.

Carlson D, Mowery BD: Standards to prevent complications of urinary catheterization in children: should and should-knots, *J Soc Pediatr Nurs* 2(1):37-41, 1997.

Carroll P: Closing in on safer suctioning, *RN* 61(5):22-27, 1998.

Carson SM: Chlorhexidine versus povidone-iodine for central venous catheter site care in children, *J Pediatr Nurs* (19)1:74-80, 2004.

Catudal R: Pediatric IV therapy: actual practice, *J Vasc Access Devices* 4(2):27-29, 1999.

Chung DH, Ziegler NM: Central venous catheter access, *Nutrition* 14(1):119-123, 1998.

Cohen HA and others: Urine samples from disposable diapers: an accurate method for urine cultures, *J Fam Pract* 44(3):290-292, 1997.

Connell F: The causes and treatment of fever: a literature review, *Nurs Stand* 12(11):40-43, 1997.

Coté CJ and others: Adverse sedation events in pediatrics: analysis of medications used for sedation, *Pediatrics* 106(4):633-644, 2000.

Cravero JP, Manzi DJA, Rice LJ: The management of procedure-related pain in the child. In Ashburn MA, Rice LJ, editors: *The management of pain*, Philadelphia, 1998, Churchill-Livingstone.

Diab FH, Marshall, JB: The palatability of five colonic lavage solutions, *Aliment Pharmacol Ther* 20(5):815-819, 1996.

Donaldson JS and others: Peripherally inserted central venous catheters: US-guided vascular access in pediatric patients, *Radiology* 197(2):542-544, 1995.

Dunn D: Malignant hypothermia, *AORN J* 65(4):728-754, 1997.

Eckler J: Combating infection, *Nursing* 27(10):20, 1997.

Ellett ML: Prevalence of feeding tube placement errors and associated risk factors in children, *MCN* 23(5):234-239, 1998.

El Radhi AS, Barry W: Do antipyretics prevent febrile convulsions? *Arch Dis Child* 88(7):641-642, 2003.

Engleman SG, Turnage-Carrier C: Tolerance of the Passy-Muir speaking valve in infants and children less than 2 years of age, *Pediatr Nurs* 23:571-573, 1997.

Essink-Tebbes CM and others: Safety of lidocaine-prilocaine cream application four times a day in premature neonates: a pilot study, *Eur J Pediatr* 158(5):421-423, 1999.

Fauroux B and others: Chest physiotherapy in cystic fibrosis: improved tolerance with nasal pressure support ventilation, *Pediatrics* 103(3): E32, 1999.

Fox MD: Measurement of urine output volume: accuracy of diaper weights in neonatal environments, *Neonat Netw* 11(3):11-18, 1992.

Frey AM: Pediatric peripherally inserted central catheter program report: a summary of 4,536 catheter days, *J Intraven Nurs* 18(6):280-291, 1995.

Frizzell J: Avoiding lab test pitfalls, *Am J Nurs* 98(2):34-37, 1998.

Gray M: Atraumatic urethral catheterization of children, *Pediatr Nurs* 22(4):306-310, 1996.

Gray L, Watt L, Blass EM: Skin-to-skin contact is analgesic in healthy newborns, *Pediatrics* 105(1):110-111, 2000; available at www.pediatrics.org/cgi/content/full/105/1/E14.

Groswasser J and others: Needle length and injection technique for efficient intramuscular vaccine delivery in infants and children evaluated through an ultrasonographic determination of subcutaneous and muscle layer thickness, *Pediatrics* 99(3 pt 1):400-402, 1997.

Guertler AT: Pearls, pitfalls, and updates: the clinical practice of emergency medicine, *Emerg Med Clin North Am* 15(2):303-313, 1997.

Hagelgans NA: Pediatric skin care issues for the home care nurse, *Pediatr Nurs* 19(5):499-507, 1993.

Hazinski MF: *Nursing care of the critically ill child*, ed 3, St Louis, 1996, Mosby.

Heilskov J and others: A randomized trial of heparin and saline for maintaining intravenous locks in neonates, *J Soc Pediatr Nurs* 3(3):111-116, 1998.

Heiney SP: Helping children through painful procedures, *Am J Nurs* 91(11):20-24, 1991.

Holden C and others: Enteral nutrition for children, *Nurs Stand* 11(32):49-54, 1997.

Huth M: Watch out: the bogeyman is in the hospital closet, *J Child Fam Nurs* 2(2):143-148, 1999.

Intravenous Nurses Society: Revised Intravenous Nursing Standards of Practice, *J Intraven Nurs* 21(1 suppl):S35, S46-S47, S59, 1998.

Jackson F: The ABC's of black hair and skin care, *ABNFJ* 9(5):100-104, 1998.

Janik JP, Wayne ER, Janik JS: Securing central lines in rambunctious toddlers, *Pediatrics* 96(3):523-524, 1995.

Joint Commission on Accreditation of Healthcare Organizations: Care of the patient: restraint and seclusion standards, *Comprehensive accreditation manual for hospitals*, TX.7.1-TX.7.5.5, 2001.

Kain Z, Caldwell-Andrews, A, Wang, S: Psychological preparation of the parent and pediatric surgical patient, *Anesthesia Clin North Am* 20(1):29-44, 2002.

Katsma D, Smith G: Analysis of needle path during intramuscular injection, *Nurs Res* 46(5):288-292, 1997.

Kearns GL, Leeder SJ, Wasserman GS: Acetaminophen overdose with therapeutic intent, *J Pediatr* 132(1):5-8, 1998.

Kennedy D: Medication "safety checks" in pediatric acute care, *J Intraven Nurs* 19(6):295-302, 1996.

Kinmonth AL, Fulton Y, Campbell MJ: Management of feverish children at home, *BMJ* 305(6862):1134-1136, 1992.

Kotter RW: Heparin vs saline for intermittent intravenous device maintenance in neonates, *Neonatal Netw* 15(6):43-47, 1996.

Krozek J, Scoggins SA: Restraints and seclusion policy . . . amended to comply with 2001 JCAHO standards, *Cinahl Information Sys* 9p, 2001.

Krueger H, Osborn L: Effects of hygiene among the uncircumcised, *J Fam Pract* 22(4):353-355, 1986.

Kubiak M and others: Comparison of stool containment in cloth and single-use diapers using simulated infant feces, *Pediatrics* 91(3): 632-636, 1993.

Larsson BA and others: Alleviation of the pain of venipuncture in neonates, *Acta Paediatr* 87(7):774-779, 1998.

Laurent C: And so to beds, *Nurs Times* 95(3):7-8, 1999.

Lee WE, Vallino LM: Intravenous insertion site protection: moisture accumulation in intravenous site protectors, *J Intraven Nurs* 29(4):194-197, 1996.

Lehmann M and others: Upright or lying down: is one better for doing a lumbar puncture (LP)? *Am J Dis Child* 144:427, 1990.

Liebman M, Barnsteiner J: Fever education: does it reduce parent fever anxiety? *Pediatr Emerg Care* 17(1):47-51, 2001.

Liptak GS: Enhancing compliance in pediatrics, *Pediatr Rev* 17(4): 128-134, 1996.

Long CA and others: Central line associated bacteremia in the pediatric patient, *Pediatr Nurs* 22(3):247-251, 1996.

Maki DG: Infections caused by intravascular devices used for infusion therapy: pathogenesis, prevention, and management. In Bisno AL, Waldvogel FA, editors: *Infections associated with indwelling medical devices*, ed 2, Washington, DC, 1994, American Society for Microbiology.

McIntosh N, van Veen L, Brameyer H: Alleviation of the pain of heel prick in preterm infants, *Arch Dis Child Fetal Neonatal Ed* 70(3):F177-F181, 1994.

McLane, KM and others: Comparison of interface pressures in the pediatric population among various support surfaces, *J Wound Ostomy Continence Nurs* 29(5):242-251, 2002.

Metheny N and others: pH, color, and feeding tubes, *RN* 61(1):25-27, 1998.

Montgomery LA and others: Guidelines for IV infiltrations in pediatric patients, *Pediatr Nurs* 25(2):167-180, 1999.

Moppett S, Parker M: Insertion of a suppository, *Nurs Times* 95 (23 suppl):1-2, 1999.

Moskop JC: Ethical issues in emergency medicine: informed consent in the emergency department, *Emerg Med Clin North Am* 17(2): 327-340, 1999.

Moureau N: Practical access, a back-to-basics review of intravenous therapy, *J Vasc Access Devices* 4(2 suppl):1-4, 1999.

O'Brien B and others: G-tube site care: a practical guide, *RN* 62(2):52-56, 1999.

Oncology Nursing Society, *Cancer chemotherapy guidelines and recommendations for practice*, ed 2, Pittsburgh, 1998, Oncology Nursing Press.

Orenstein R: The benefits and limitations of needle protectors and needleless intravenous systems, *J Intraven Nurs* 22(3):122-127, 1999.

Paisley MK and others: The use of heparin and normal saline flushes in neonatal intravenous catheters, *Pediatr Nurs* 23(5):521-527, 1997.

Pearson M: The Hospital Infection Control Practices Advisory Committee: Guidelines for prevention of intravascular-device-related infections, *Infect Control Hosp Epidemiol* 17:438-473, 1995.

Pearson M: Special communication: guidelines for prevention of intravascular device–related infections, parts I and II, *Am J Infect Control* 24(4):262-293, 1996.

Petitt J, Hughes K: Neonatal intravenous therapy practices, *J Vasc Access Devices* 4:7-16, 1999.

Polillio AM, Killy, J: Does a needleless injection system reduce anxiety in children receiving intramuscular injections? *Pediatr Nurs* 23(1):46-49, 1997.

Prandoni D and others: Assessment of urine collection techniques for microbial culture, *Am J Infect Control* 24(3):219-221, 1996.

Purssell E: The use of antipyretic medications in the prevention of febrile convulsions in children, *J Pediatr Nurs* 9(4):473-480, 2000.

Quigley, SM, Curley, MAQ: Skin integrity in the pediatric population: preventing and managing pressure ulcers, *J Soc Pediatr Nurses* 1(1):7, 1996.

Ratliff, CR, Rodheaver, GT: Pressure ulcer assessment and management, *Lippincott's Primary Care Pract* 3:242-258, 1999.

Reed T, Phillip S: Management of central venous catheter occlusion and repairs, *J Intraven Nurs* 19(6):289-294, 1996.

Rosenstock IM: Enhancing patient compliance with health recommendations, *J Pediatr Health Care* 2(2):67-72, 1988.

Rote N, Huether S. McCance K: Hypersensitivities, infection, and immunodeficiencies. In Huether S, McCance K, editors: *Understanding pathophysiology*, ed 2, St Louis, 2000, Mosby.

Russell B: Nosocomial infections, *Am J Nurs* 99(6):24J-24P, 1999.

Selekman J, Snyder B: Uses and alternatives to restraints in pediatric settings, *AACN Clin Issues* 7(4):603-610, 1996.

Selekman J, Snyder B: Institutional policies on the use of physical restraints on children, *Pediatr Nurs* 23(5):531-537, 1997.

Sharber J: The efficacy of tepid sponge bathing to reduce fever in young children, *Am J Emerg Med* 15(2):188-192, 1997.

Shinnar S and others: Short-term outcomes of children with febrile status epilepticus, *Epilepsia* 42(1):47-53, 2001.

Singer AJ, Konia N: Comparison of topical anesthetics and vasoconstrictors vs lubricants prior to nasogastric intubation: a randomized, controlled trial, *Acad Emerg Med* 6(3):184-190, 1999.

Vertanen H and others: An automatic incision device for obtaining blood samples from the heels of the preterm infants causes less damage than a conventional manual lancet, *Arch Dis Child Fetal Neonat Ed* 84:F53-F55, 2001.

Walton DM and others: Morbid hypocalcaemia associated with phosphate enema in a six week-old infant, *Pediatrics* 106:e37, 2000.

Wong DL, Baker CM: Pain in children: comparison of assessment scales, *Pediatr Nurs* 14(1):9-17, 1988.

Woolverton E: Practice pointers, *Sch Health Watch* 2(4):2, 1991.

23

The Child With Respiratory Dysfunction

MARILYN WINKELSTEIN

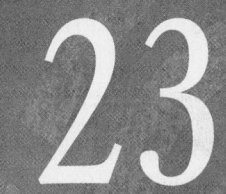

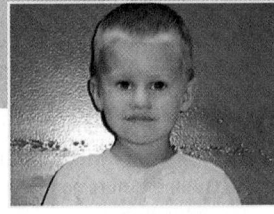

Remember to check out your companion CD-ROM

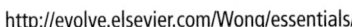

CHAPTER OUTLINE

RELATED TOPICS and ADDITIONAL RESOURCES

 IN TEXT

 CD COMPANION

 WEBSITE

WONG'S CLINICAL MANUAL OF PEDIATRIC NURSING, 6/E

RESPIRATORY INFECTION

GENERAL ASPECTS OF RESPIRATORY INFECTIONS

Infections of the respiratory tract are described according to the anatomic area of involvement. The **upper respiratory tract**, or **upper airway**, consists of the oronasopharynx, the pharynx, the larynx, and the upper part of the trachea. The **lower respiratory tract** consists of the lower trachea, mainstem bronchi, segmental bronchi, subsegmental bronchioles, terminal bronchioles, and the alveoli. In this discussion, the trachea is considered with lower tract disorders, and infections of the epiglottis and larynx are categorized as croup syndromes. However, respiratory infections seldom fall into discrete anatomic areas. Infections often spread from one structure to another because of the contiguous nature of the mucous membrane lining the entire tract. Consequently, respiratory tract infections involve several areas rather than a single structure, although the effect on one area may predominate in any given illness.

Etiology and Characteristics

Respiratory infections account for the majority of acute illnesses in children. The etiology and course of these infections are influenced by the age of the child, the season, living conditions, and preexisting medical problems.

Infectious Agents. The respiratory tract is subject to a wide variety of infective organisms. Viruses, such as the respiratory syncytial virus (RSV), cause most infections. Other agents involved in primary or secondary invasion include group A β-hemolytic streptococci, staphylococci, *Haemophilus influenzae*, *Chlamydia trachomatis*, *Mycoplasma*, and pneumococci.

Age. Infants younger than age 3 months have a lower infection rate, presumably because of the protective function of maternal antibodies. The infection rate increases from 3 to 6 months of age, the time between the disappearance of maternal antibodies and the infant's own antibody production. The viral infection rate remains high during the toddler and preschool years. By 5 years of age, viral respiratory infections are less frequent, but the incidence of *Mycoplasma pneumoniae* and group A β-streptococcal infections increases.

Some viral agents produce a mild illness in older children but severe lower respiratory tract illness or croup in infants.

For example, whooping cough is a relatively harmless tracheobronchitis in childhood but a serious disease in infancy.

Size. Anatomic differences influence the response to respiratory tract infections. The diameter of the airways is smaller in young children and subject to considerable narrowing from edematous mucous membranes and increased production of secretions. The distance between structures within the respiratory tract is also shorter in the young child, and organisms may move rapidly down the respiratory tract, causing more extensive involvement. The relatively short and open eustachian tube in infants and young children allows pathogens easy access to the middle ear.

Resistance. The ability to resist invading organisms depends on several factors. Deficiencies of the immune system place the child at risk for infection. Other conditions that decrease resistance are malnutrition, anemia, fatigue, and chilling of the body. Conditions that weaken defenses of the respiratory tract and predispose to infection also include allergies (e.g., allergic rhinitis), asthma, cardiac anomalies that cause pulmonary congestion, and cystic fibrosis. Day care attendance, especially if the caregivers smoke, increases the likelihood of infection (Blumer, 1998).

Seasonal Variations. The most common respiratory pathogens appear in epidemics during the winter and spring months. Mycoplasmal infections occur more often in autumn and early winter. Infection-related asthma (e.g., asthmatic bronchitis) occurs more frequently during cold weather, whereas winter and spring are typically the "RSV seasons."

Clinical Manifestations

Infants and young children, especially those between 6 months and 3 years of age, react more severely to acute respiratory tract infection than older children. Young children display a number of generalized signs and symptoms, as well as local manifestations (see Box 23-1).

Nursing Considerations

● *Assessment*

Assessment of the respiratory system follows the guidelines described in Chapter 7 (for assessment of the nose, mouth and throat, chest, and lungs). Special attention should also be given to the components and observations listed in Box 23-2.

BOX 23-1 ■ Signs and Symptoms Associated With Respiratory Infections in Infants and Small Children

FEVER
May be absent in newborn infants
Greatest at ages 6 months to 3 years
  Temperature may reach 39.5° to 40.5° C (103° to 105° F) even with mild infections
Often appears as first sign of infection
May be listless and irritable or somewhat euphoric and more active than normal, temporarily; some children talk with unaccustomed rapidity
Tendency to develop high temperatures with infection in certain families
  May precipitate febrile seizures (see Chapter 28)
  Febrile seizures uncommon after 3 or 4 years of age

MENINGISMUS
Meningeal signs without infection of the meninges
Occurs with abrupt onset of fever
Accompanied by:
  Headache
  Pain and stiffness in the back and neck
  Presence of Kernig and Brudzinski signs
Subsides as the temperature decreases

ANOREXIA
Common with most childhood illnesses
Frequently the initial evidence of illness
Persists to a greater or lesser degree throughout febrile stage of illness; often extends into convalescence

VOMITING
Small children vomit readily with illness
Clue to onset of infection
May precede other signs by several hours
Usually short-lived but may persist during the illness

DIARRHEA
Usually mild, transient diarrhea but may become severe
Often accompanies viral respiratory infections
Frequent cause of dehydration

ABDOMINAL PAIN
Common complaint
Sometimes indistinguishable from pain of appendicitis

Mesenteric lymphadenitis may be cause
Muscle spasms from vomiting may be a factor, especially in nervous, tense child

NASAL BLOCKAGE
Small nasal passages of infants easily blocked by mucosal swelling and exudation
Can interfere with respiration and feeding in infants
May contribute to the development of otitis media and sinusitis

NASAL DISCHARGE
Frequent occurrence
May be thin and watery (rhinorrhea) or thick and purulent
Depends on the type or stage of infection
Associated with itching
May irritate upper lip and skin surrounding the nose

COUGH
Common feature
May be evident only during acute phase
May persist several months after a disease

RESPIRATORY SOUNDS
Sounds associated with respiratory disease:
  Cough
  Hoarseness
  Grunting
  Stridor
  Wheezing
Auscultation:
  Wheezing
  Crackles
  Absence of sound

SORE THROAT
Frequent complaint of older children
Young children (unable to describe symptoms) may not complain even when highly inflamed
Child will often refuse to take oral fluids or solids

● Nursing Diagnoses

After a thorough assessment, several nursing diagnoses may be identified (see Nursing Care Plan, pp. 792-793). Others may be apparent in individual cases.

● Planning

The goals for the child with an acute respiratory infection and the family are as follows:

1 Child will exhibit normal respiratory efforts.
2 Child will receive adequate rest.
3 Child will remain comfortable.
4 Child will not spread primary infection to others.
5 Child's temperature will remain within normal limits.
6 Child will maintain normal hydration and adequate nutrition.

7 Child will experience no complications.
8 Child and family will receive information, especially for home care, and support.

● Implementation

Ease Respiratory Efforts.   Many acute respiratory infections are mild and cause few symptoms. Although children may feel uncomfortable and have a "stuffy" nose and some mucosal swelling, respiratory distress occurs infrequently. Interventions delivered at home are usually sufficient to relieve minor discomfort and ease respiratory efforts. However, children with croup or epiglottitis can develop sufficient swelling to obstruct the airway and may require hospitalization and more complex therapy.

Warm or cool mist is a common therapeutic measure for symptomatic relief of respiratory discomfort. The moisture

BOX 23-2 ■ Components for Assessing Respiratory Function

RESPIRATIONS

The pattern of respirations is observed for rate, depth, ease, and rhythm of breathing:

Rate—Rapid *(tachypnea),* normal, or slow for the particular child

Depth—Normal depth, too shallow *(hypopnea),* too deep *(hyperpnea);* usually estimated from the amplitude of thoracic and abdominal excursion

Ease—Effortless; labored *(dyspnea); orthopnea* (difficult breathing except in upright position); associated with intercostal or substernal retractions (inspiratory "sinking in" of soft tissues in relation to the cartilaginous and bony thorax); *pulsus paradoxus* (blood pressure falls with inspiration and rises with expiration); flaring nares; head bobbing (head of sleeping child with suboccipital area supported on caregiver's forearm bobs forward in synchrony with each inspiration); grunting; or wheezing

Labored breathing—Continuous, intermittent, becoming steadily worse, sudden onset, at rest or on exertion, associated with wheezing or grunting, associated with pain

Rhythm—Variation in rate and depth of respirations

OTHER OBSERVATIONS

In addition to respirations, particular attention is addressed to the following:

Evidence of infection—Check for elevated temperature, enlarged cervical lymph nodes, inflamed mucous membranes, and purulent discharges from the nose, ears, or lungs (sputum)

Cough—Observe the characteristics of the cough (if present); under what circumstances the cough is heard (e.g., night only, on arising), nature of the cough (paroxysmal with or without wheeze, "croupy" or "brassy"), frequency of cough, associated with swallowing or other activity, character of the cough (moist and dry), productivity

Wheeze—Expiratory or inspiratory, high-pitched or musical, prolonged, slowly progressive or sudden, associated with labored breathing

Cyanosis—Note distribution (peripheral, perioral, facial, trunk, and face), degree, duration, associated with activity

Chest pain—May be a complaint of older children. Note location and circumstances: localized or generalized, referred to base of neck or abdomen, dull or sharp, deep or superficial, associated with rapid, shallow respirations or grunting

Sputum—Older children may provide sputum sample by coughing, whereas young children may need use of bulb suction to provide a sample; note volume, color, viscosity, and odor

Bad breath—May be associated with some lung infections

soothes inflamed membranes and is beneficial when there is hoarseness or laryngeal involvement. However, the use of steam vaporizers in the home is discouraged because of the hazards related to their use and limited evidence to support their efficacy. Shallow pans with wide surface areas for evaporation increase humidity but should be placed where they do not pose a safety hazard.

A time-honored method of producing warm mist is the shower. Running a shower of hot water into the empty bathtub or open shower stall with the bathroom door closed produces a quick source of steam. Keeping a child in this environment for 10 to 15 minutes provides the same advantages as the mist tent without the fear and restraint associated with the confines of a tent. A small child can be held on the parent's lap. Older children can sit in the bathroom under the supervision of an adult.

Promote Rest. Children who have an acute febrile illness should be placed on bed rest. This is usually not difficult while the temperature is elevated but may become a problem when children begin to feel better. Often children will comply with bedrest if they are allowed to lie quietly on a couch where they can watch television or participate in a quiet activity. If children protest, allowing them to play quietly serves the purpose of rest better than allowing them to cry excessively in bed.

Promote Comfort. Older children are usually able to manage nasal secretions with little difficulty. Parents are instructed in the correct administration of nose drops and throat irrigations, if ordered. For very young infants, who normally breathe through their noses, an infant nasal aspirator or a rubber ear syringe is helpful in removing nasal secretions before feeding. This practice, followed by instillation of saline nose drops, may clear nasal passages and promote feeding. Saline nose drops can be prepared at home by dissolving 1 teaspoon of salt in 1 pint of warm water.

For older infants and children who can tolerate decongestants, vasoconstrictive nose drops may be administered 15 to 20 minutes before feeding and at bedtime. Two drops are instilled, and because this shrinks only the anterior mucous membranes, two more drops are instilled 5 to 10 minutes later. Phenylephrine (Neo-Synephrine) 0.25% and ephedrine 1% are frequently prescribed. Older cooperative children often prefer nasal sprays. They are taught to compress the plastic container at the moment of inspiration. Bottles of nose drops should be used for only for one child and one illness because they are easily contaminated with bacteria. To avoid rebound congestion, nose drops or sprays should not be administered for more than 3 days.

Hot or cold applications sometimes provide relief for children with painful cervical adenitis. An ice bag or heating pad applied to the neck may decrease the discomfort, but safety precautions must be observed to prevent burns. The ice bag or heating device must be covered, and the heating pad should not be set at high ranges.

Prevent Spread of Infection. Careful handwashing is carried out when caring for children with respiratory infections. Children and families are taught to use a tissue or their hand to cover their nose and mouth when they cough or sneeze and to dispose of tissues properly, as well as to wash their hands. Used tissues should be immediately thrown into the wastebasket, and tissues should not be allowed to accumulate in a pile. Children with respiratory infections should not share drinking cups, washcloths, or towels.

> **NURSING ALERT**
>
> To avoid contamination with respiratory viruses, wash hands and do not touch your eyes or nose.

Efforts should be made to separate affected children from contact with other children. Parents should keep affected children out of school and day care settings to prevent the spread of infection. Ideally, ill children should be isolated in a separate bedroom at the first sign of illness. However, this is a problem when living arrangements are crowded and there are several children in the family. Well children should be told to stay away from ill children.

Reduce Temperature.

If the child has a significantly elevated temperature, controlling the fever is important. Parents should know how to take a child's temperature and read the thermometer accurately. Nurses should not assume that all parents can read a thermometer. Parents who cannot perform this skill should receive instruction.

If the practitioner prescribes acetaminophen or ibuprofen, parents may need help giving the drug. Most parents can read the label and calculate the desired dose, but some may require careful instruction. It is important to emphasize accuracy in determining both the amount of drug to be given and the time intervals for administration. Cool liquids are given to reduce the temperature and minimize the chances of dehydration. (See Controlling Elevated Temperatures, Chapter 22.)

Promote Hydration.

Dehydration is always a hazard when children are febrile or anorexic, especially when vomiting or diarrhea is present. Offering small amounts of favorite fluids at frequent intervals encourages adequate fluid intake. High-calorie liquids, such as colas, fruit juices, water flavored and sweetened with corn syrup, or similar drinks prevent catabolism and dehydration but should be avoided if diarrhea is present. Oral rehydration solutions, such as Infalyte or Pedialyte, should be considered for infants, and sports drinks, such as Gatorade, are recommended for older children. Fluids should not be forced, and children should not be awakened to take fluids. Forcing fluids creates the same problem as urging unwanted food. Gentle persuasion with preferred beverages is usually more successful.

To assess a child's level of hydration (see Chapters 9 and 24), parents are advised to observe the frequency of voiding and to notify the nurse or practitioner if voiding is insufficient. Counting the number of wet diapers in a 24-hour period is a satisfactory method to assess output in infants and toddlers.

Provide Nutrition.

Loss of appetite is characteristic of children with acute infections. In most cases, children can be permitted to determine their own need for food. Many children show no decrease in appetite, and others respond well to foods such as gelatin, soup, and puddings (see Feeding the Sick Child, Chapter 22). Urging foods on anorexic children may precipitate nausea and vomiting and cause an aversion to feeding that may extend into the convalescent period and beyond.

Family Support and Home Care.

Young children with respiratory infections are irritable and difficult to comfort; therefore, the family needs support, encouragement, and practical suggestions concerning comfort measures and administration of medication. In addition to antipyretics and nose drops, the child may require antibiotic therapy. Parents of children receiving oral antibiotics must understand the importance of regular administration and of continuing the drug for the prescribed length of time, regardless of whether the child appears ill. Parents are cautioned against giving their child any medications that are not approved by the health practitioner. Adverse effects have been noted in children who have received preparations intended for adults such as long-acting nose drops (Neo-Synephrine II) and dextromethorphan cough squares that are often mistaken for candy. Parents should not give antibiotics left over from a previous illness. Self-medication with unprescribed antibiotics can produce serious side effects, and adverse reactions (see Chapter 22 for administration of medications and teaching parents).

● Evaluation

Continual reassessment and evaluation determine the effectiveness of nursing interventions. The nurse should use the following guidelines:

1 Observe child's respiratory effort and movement.
2 Observe signs and symptoms for progress toward health status before illness.
3 Observe child's behavior and activity.
4 Observe other family members and contacts for evidence of infection.
5 Take temperature.
6 Observe for signs of adequate hydration.
7 Observe eating behavior.
8 Assess for complications such as dehydration, weight loss, or spread of infection to other areas of the body.
9 Observe family's behavior and interview members regarding their feelings and concerns.

The *expected outcomes* are described in the Nursing Care Plan on pp. 792-793.

UPPER RESPIRATORY TRACT INFECTIONS

NASOPHARYNGITIS

Acute nasopharyngitis or the equivalent of the "common cold" is caused by the rhinovirus, RSV, adenovirus, influenza virus, and the parainfluenza virus. Symptoms are more severe in infants and children than in adults. Fever is common in young children, and older children have low-grade fevers, which appear early in the course of the illness. Other clinical manifestations are listed in Box 23-3.

Therapeutic Management

Children with nasopharyngitis are managed at home. There is no specific treatment, and effective vaccines are not available. Antipyretics are prescribed for mild fever and discomfort (see Chapter 22 for management of fever). Rest is recommended until the child is free of fever for at least 1 day. Decongestants may be prescribed for children and infants older than 6 months of age to shrink swollen nasal passages. The decongestants that exert their effect by vasoconstriction are usually less effective when taken orally than when applied topically as nose drops. Because these drugs affect all vascular beds, they should be given with caution to children with diabetes.

NURSING DIAGNOSIS ■ Ineffective breathing pattern related to inflammatory process

PATIENT GOAL 1: Will exhibit normal respiratory function

NURSING INTERVENTIONS/*RATIONALES*

Position for maximum ventilation (i.e., open airway and permit maximum lung expansion)

Allow position of comfort (e.g., tripod position of child with epiglottitis or maintain head elevation of at least 30 degrees)

Check child's position frequently to ensure child does not slide down *to avoid compressing the diaphragm*

Avoid constricting clothing or bedding

Use pillows and padding to maintain open airway (e.g., in infant or child with hypotonia)

*Provide increased humidity and supplemental oxygen by placing child in small tent or hood (infant) or administer via nasal cannula or mask (preferred methods for children older than infants because of safety issues)

Promote rest and sleep by scheduling appropriate activity and rest periods

Encourage relaxation techniques

Teach child and family measures to ease respiratory efforts (i.e., appropriate positioning)

For most respiratory illnesses, use cool-mist humidifier in child's room
 For spasmodic croup, create warm mist by running hot water in a closed bathroom (warm mist, often used for children with spasmodic croup, may be helpful because of its relaxing effect, but mostly because child is being held upright in the shower)

EXPECTED OUTCOMES

Respirations remain within normal limits (see inside back cover for normal variations)

Respirations are unlabored

Child rests and sleeps quietly

PATIENT GOAL 2: Will receive optimal oxygen supply

NURSING INTERVENTIONS/*RATIONALES*

Position for maximum ventilatory efficiency (see Goal 1, above)

Use pulse oximetry *to monitor oxygen saturations*

Place in a cool, humidified environment, using appropriate oxygen delivery system

*Provide oxygen as prescribed or needed

EXPECTED OUTCOMES

Child breathes easily

Respirations remain within normal limits (see inside back cover for normal variations)

Oxygen saturation is 95% or higher

NURSING DIAGNOSIS ■ Fear/anxiety related to difficulty breathing, unfamiliar procedures, and possibly environment (hospital)

PATIENT GOAL 1: Will experience reduction of fear/anxiety

NURSING INTERVENTIONS/*RATIONALES*

Explain unfamiliar procedures and equipment to child in developmentally appropriate terms

Establish rapport with child and parents

Remain with child and parents during procedures

Use calm, reassuring manner

Provide frequent attendance during acute phase of illness

Provide comfort measures child prefers (e.g., rocking, stroking, music)

Provide attachment objects (e.g., familiar toy, blanket)

Encourage family-centered care with increased parental attendance and, when possible, involvement

Do nothing to make child more anxious or fearful

Instill confidence in both parents and child

Try to avoid any intrusive or painful procedures

Be aware of child's rest/sleep cycle or pattern in planning nursing activities

Assess and implement appropriate pain management therapy (i.e., sedatives or analgesics) (see Pain Assessment; Pain Management, Chapter 21)

Provide diversional activities appropriate to child's cognitive ability and condition

*Administer medications that promote improved ventilation (e.g., bronchodilators, expectorants) as prescribed

EXPECTED OUTCOMES

Child exhibits no signs of respiratory distress or physical discomfort

Parents remain with child and provide comfort

Child engages in quiet activities appropriate for age, interest, condition, and cognitive level

NURSING DIAGNOSIS ■ Ineffective airway clearance related to mechanical obstruction, inflammation, increased secretions, and pain

PATIENT GOAL 1: Will maintain patent airway

NURSING INTERVENTIONS/*RATIONALES*

Position child in proper body alignment *to allow better lung expansion and improved gas exchange, as well as to prevent aspiration of secretions (prone, semiprone, side lying; for infants not at risk for aspiration, use supine or side-lying position for sleeping)*

Suction secretions from airway as needed
 Limit each suction attempt to 5 seconds with sufficient time between attempts to allow reoxygenation

Position supine with head in "sniffing" position with neck slightly extended and nose pointed to ceiling
 Avoid neck hyperextension

Assist child in expectorating sputum

*Administer expectorants if prescribed

Perform chest physiotherapy

Give nothing by mouth *to prevent aspiration of fluids* (e.g., child with severe tachypnea)

*Administer appropriate pain management

Have emergency equipment available *to avoid delay in treatment if needed*

Avoid throat examination and culture with suspected epiglottitis *because it could cause airway obstruction*

Assist child in splinting any incisional/injured area *to maximize effects of coughing and chest physiotherapy*

EXPECTED OUTCOMES

Airways remain clear

Child breathes easily; respirations are within normal limits (see inside back cover)

PATIENT GOAL 2: Will expectorate secretions adequately

NURSING INTERVENTIONS/*RATIONALES*

Ensure adequate fluid intake *to liquefy secretions*

Provide humidified atmosphere *to prevent crusting of nasal secretions and drying of mucous membranes*

Explain importance of expectoration to child and family

Assist child in coughing effectively; provide tissues

Remove accumulated mucus; suction if needed

*Administer pain medications as indicated before attempt to clear airway

Provide nebulization with appropriate solution and equipment as prescribed

*Dependent nursing action.

Continued

Assist with splinting *so child will experience minimal discomfort*
*Perform percussion, vibration, and postural drainage *to facilitate drainage of secretions*

EXPECTED OUTCOME
Older child expectorates secretions without undue stress and fatigue; younger child is able to have a productive cough

NURSING DIAGNOSIS ▨ **Risk for infection related to presence of infective organisms**

PATIENT GOAL 1: Will exhibit no signs of secondary infection

NURSING INTERVENTIONS/*RATIONALES*
Maintain aseptic environment, using sterile suction catheters and good handwashing
Isolate child as indicated *to prevent nosocomial spread of infection*
Administer antibiotics as prescribed *to prevent or treat infection*
Provide nutritious diet according to child's preferences and ability to consume nourishment *to support body's natural defenses*
Encourage good chest physiotherapy
Teach child or family manifestations of illness

EXPECTED OUTCOME
Child exhibits evidence of diminishing symptoms of infection

PATIENT GOAL 2: Will not spread infection to others

NURSING INTERVENTIONS/*RATIONALES*
Use standard precautions (see Infection Control, Chapter 22)
Instruct others (parents, members of staff) in appropriate precautions
Teach affected children protective methods to prevent spread of infection (e.g., handwashing, disposal of soiled tissues)
Limit the number of visitors/family members/siblings and screen for any recent illness in visitors
Try to keep infants and small children from placing hands and objects in contaminated areas
Assess home situation and implement protective measures as feasible in individual circumstances
*Administer antimicrobial medications if prescribed

EXPECTED OUTCOME
Others remain free from infection

NURSING DIAGNOSIS ▨ **Activity intolerance related to inflammatory process, imbalance between oxygen supply and demand**

PATIENT GOAL 1: Will maintain adequate energy levels

NURSING INTERVENTIONS/*RATIONALES*
Assess child's level of physical tolerance
Assist child in those activities of daily living that may be beyond tolerance
Provide diversional activities appropriate to child's age, condition, capabilities, and interest
Provide diversional play activities that promote rest and quiet but prevent boredom and withdrawal
Provide rest and sleep periods appropriate to age and condition
Instruct child to rest when feeling tired
Balance rest and activity when ambulatory

EXPECTED OUTCOMES
Child plays and rests quietly and engages in activities appropriate to age and capabilities (specify)

Child exhibits no evidence of increased respiratory distress
Child tolerates increasingly more activity

PATIENT GOAL 2: Will receive optimal rest

NURSING INTERVENTIONS/*RATIONALES*
Provide quiet environment
Organize activities for maximum sleep time
Do not perform nonessential treatments or procedures *to maximize rest*
Schedule visiting *to allow for sufficient rest*
Encourage parents to remain with child
Schedule treatments or other activities around child's needs *so that fatigue will be minimized.*
*Administer sedatives and analgesics as indicated if ordered for restlessness and pain
Encourage frequent rest periods and regular sleep times
Follow child's usual routine for bedtime and nap time
Implement measures to ensure sleep, such as a quiet, darkened room

EXPECTED OUTCOMES
Child remains calm, quiet, and relaxed
Child rests a sufficient amount (specify)

NURSING DIAGNOSIS ▨ **Pain related to inflammatory process, surgical incision**

PATIENT GOAL 1: Will experience no pain or reduction of pain/discomfort to level acceptable to child

NURSING INTERVENTIONS/*RATIONALES*
Use local measures (gargles, troches, heat, or cold) *to reduce throat pain*
Apply heat or cold as appropriate to affected area
*Administer analgesic as prescribed (see Pain Management, Chapter 21)
Assess response to pain control measures (see Pain Assessment, Chapter 21)
Encourage diversional activities appropriate to age, condition, capabilities

EXPECTED OUTCOME
Child has no pain or acceptable level of pain

NURSING DIAGNOSIS ▨ **Altered family processes related to illness or hospitalization of a child**

PATIENT (FAMILY) GOAL 1: Will experience reduction of anxiety and increased ability to cope

NURSING INTERVENTIONS/*RATIONALES*
Recognize parental concern and need for information and support
Explore family's feelings and "problems" surrounding hospitalization and child's illness
Explain therapy and child's behavior
Provide support as needed
Encourage family-centered care and encourage family to become involved in child's care

EXPECTED OUTCOME
Parents ask appropriate questions, discuss child's condition and care calmly, and become involved positively in child's care
See also:
　Nursing Care Plan: The Family of the Ill or Hospitalized Child, Chapter 21
　Nursing Care Plan: The Child in the Hospital, Chapter 21

*Dependent nursing action.

BOX 23-3 ■ Clinical Manifestations of Nasopharyngitis and Pharyngitis

NASOPHARYNGITIS
Younger Child
Fever
Irritability, restlessness
Sneezing
Vomiting or diarrhea

Older Child
Dryness and irritation of nose and throat
Sneezing, chilly sensation
Muscular aches
Cough, sometimes

Physical Signs
Edema and vasodilation of mucosa

PHARYNGITIS
Younger Child
Fever
General malaise
Anorexia
Moderate sore throat
Headache

Older Child
Fever (may reach 40° C [104° F])
Headache
Anorexia
Dysphagia
Abdominal pain
Vomiting

PHYSICAL SIGNS
Younger Child
Mild to moderate hyperemia

Older Child
Mild to fiery red, edematous pharynx
Hyperemia of tonsils and pharynx; may extend to soft palate and uvula
Often abundant follicular exudate that spreads and coalesces to form pseudomembrane on tonsils
Cervical glands enlarged and tender

BOX 23-4 ■ Early Evidence of Respiratory Complications

Parents are instructed to notify the health professional if any of the following are noted:
Evidence of earache (see p. 797)
Respirations faster than 50 to 60/min
Fever over 38.3° C (101° F)
Listlessness
Increasing irritability with or without fever
Persistent cough for 2 days or more
Wheezing
Crying
Refusal to eat
Restlessness and poor sleep patterns

Modified from National Association of Pediatric Nurse Associates and Practitioners (NAPNAP): *Baby's first cold*, New York, 1989, Winthrop Consumer Products. Copies available from NAPNAP, 1101 Kings Highway North, No. 206, Cherry Hill, NJ 08034; (609) 667-1773; website: www.napnap.org.

Cough suppressants may be prescribed for a dry, hacking cough. However, some cough preparations contain up to 22% alcohol, and should not be administered to young children continuously and must be stored securely away from the reach of children.

Antihistamines are largely ineffective. These drugs have a weak atropine-like effect that dries secretions, but they can cause drowsiness or, paradoxically, have a stimulatory effect on children. There is no support for the usefulness of expectorants. Antibiotics are usually not indicated.

Prevention. Nasopharyngitis is so widespread in the general population that it is impossible to prevent. Children are more susceptible because they have not yet developed resistance to many viruses. Very young infants are subject to serious complications such as pneumonia, and attempts should be made to protect them from exposure.

Nursing Considerations

A cold is often the parents' first introduction to an illness in their infant. Most discomfort of nasopharyngitis is related to the nasal obstruction, especially in small infants. Elevating the head of the bed or crib mattress assists with drainage of secretions. Suctioning and vaporization may also provide relief. Saline nose drops and gentle suction with a bulb syringe before feeding is useful.

Maintaining adequate fluid intake is essential. Although a child's appetite for solid foods is usually diminished for several days, it is important to offer favorite fluids to prevent dehydration. Fluids can be cool or warm, depending on individual preference.

Because nasopharyngitis is spread from secretions, the best means for prevention is avoiding contact with affected persons. This goal is difficult to accomplish in family settings, classrooms, and day care centers. Family members with a cold should try to "keep it to themselves" by carefully disposing of tissues; not sharing towels, glasses, or eating utensils; covering the mouth and nose with tissues when coughing or sneezing; and washing the hands thoroughly after nose blowing or sneezing. The most frequent carriers of infection are the human hands, which deposit viruses on doorknobs, faucets, and other everyday objects. Children should be taught to wash their hands thoroughly before putting them near their eyes, nose, or mouth.

Family Support. Support and reassurance are important elements of care for families of young children with recurrent upper respiratory infections (URIs). Because URIs are frequent in children less than 3 years of age, families may feel they are on an endless roller coaster of illness. They need reassurance that frequent colds are a normal part of childhood and that by 5 years of age, their children will have developed immunity to many viruses. Parents who work outside the home should expect to take time off to care for ill children during the fall and winter months. When children spend time routinely in day care centers, their infection rate is higher than if they are cared for in the home. Parents should know the signs of respiratory complications and should notify a health professional if complications occur or if the child does not improve within 2 or 3 days (Box 23-4).

PHARYNGITIS

Children who experience group A β-hemolytic streptococci (GABHS) infection of the upper airway *(strep throat)* are at risk for *acute rheumatic fever (ARF),* an inflammatory disease of the heart, joints, and central nervous system (see Chapter 25), and *acute glomerulonephritis,* an acute kidney infection (see Chapter 27). Permanent damage can result from these sequelae, especially ARF.

Clinical Manifestations

GABHS is generally a relatively brief illness that varies in severity from subclinical (no symptoms) to severe toxicity. The onset is often abrupt and characterized by pharyngitis,

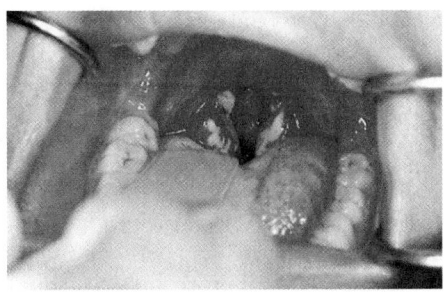

FIG. 23-1 ■ Tonsillitis and pharyngitis. (Courtesy Dr. Edward L. Applebaum, Head, Department of Otolaryngology, University of Illinois Medical Center, Chicago.)

headache, fever, and abdominal pain (especially in small children). The tonsils and pharynx may be inflamed and covered with exudate (Fig. 23-1), which usually appears by the second day of illness. However, streptococcal infections should be suspected in children older than 2 years of age who have pharyngitis without exudate (Thuma, 1997). Anterior cervical lymphadenopathy (in about 30% to 50% of cases) usually occurs early, and the nodes are often tender. Pain can be relatively mild to severe enough to make swallowing difficult. Clinical manifestations usually subside in 3 to 5 days unless complicated by sinusitis or parapharyngeal, peritonsillar, or retropharyngeal abscess. Nonsuppurative complications may appear after the onset of GABHS—acute nephritis in about 10 days and ARF in an average of 18 days.

Diagnostic Evaluation

Although 80% to 90% of all cases of acute pharyngitis are viral, a throat culture should be performed to rule out GABHS. Because some children normally harbor streptococci in their throats, a positive culture is not always conclusive evidence of active disease. Most streptococcal infections are short-term illnesses, and antibody responses appear later than symptoms and are useful only for retrospective diagnosis.

Rapid identification of GABHS with diagnostic test kits is possible in the office or clinic setting. Because of the very high specificity of these rapid tests, a positive test result generally does not require throat culture confirmation. However, the sensitivities of these kits vary considerably, and a confirmatory throat culture is recommended in patients who have a negative test result (American Academy of Pediatrics, 2003).

Therapeutic Management

If streptococcal sore throat infection is present, oral penicillin is prescribed in a dose sufficient to control the acute local manifestations and to maintain an adequate level for at least 10 days to eliminate any organisms that might remain to initiate ARF symptoms. Penicillin does not prevent the development of acute glomerulonephritis in susceptible children; however, it may prevent the spread of a nephrogenic strain of GABHS to others in the family. Penicillin usually produces a prompt response within 24 hours. Some patients require retreatment if the organism is not eradicated.

Intramuscular benzathine penicillin G is an appropriate therapy, but it is very painful and is not the first choice for children. Oral erythromycin is indicated for children allergic to penicillin. Other antibiotics used to treat GABHS are azithromycin, clarithromycin, oral cephalosporins, amoxicillin, and amoxicillin with clavulanic acid (McMillan and Feigin, 1999). A combination of penicillin and rifampin is more effective in eradicating GABHS than penicillin alone and is recommended for carriers.

Nursing Considerations

The nurse often obtains a throat swab for culture and instructs the parents about administering penicillin and analgesics as prescribed. Most children prefer to remain in bed during the acute phase of the illness. Cold or warm compresses to the neck may provide relief. In children who can cooperate, warm saline gargles offer relief of throat discomfort. Pain may interfere with oral intake, and children should not be forced to eat. Cool liquids or ice chips are usually more acceptable than solids.

Special emphasis is placed on correct administration of oral medication and completing the course of antibiotic therapy (see Administration of Medication; Compliance, Chapter 22). If injections are required, they must be administered deep into a large muscle mass (e.g., vastus lateralis or ventrogluteal muscle). To prevent pain, application of EMLA over the injection site for 2.5 hours before the injection is helpful (see Administration of Medication: Intramuscular Administration, Chapter 22). Parents also need to be aware of residual tenderness at the injection site, which may cause the child to limp for a day or two. Local applications of heat are helpful in relieving this discomfort.

Nurses play a key role in preventing the spread of disease. Children are considered noninfectious to others 24 hours after initiation of antibiotic therapy, but they should not return to school or day care until they have been taking antibiotics for a full 24-hour period.

> **⚠ NURSING ALERT**
>
> When nurses become aware that children have positive throat cultures for streptococcal infection, they should remind the children to discard their toothbrush and replace it with a new one after they have been taking antibiotics for 24 hours.

TONSILLITIS

The tonsils are masses of lymphoid tissue located in the pharyngeal cavity. They filter and protect the respiratory and alimentary tracts from invasion by pathogenic organisms and play a role in antibody formation. Although their size varies, children generally have much larger tonsils than adolescents or adults. This difference is thought to be a protective mechanism because young children are especially susceptible to URIs.

Pathophysiology

Several pairs of tonsils are part of a mass of lymphoid tissue encircling the nasal and oral pharynx, known as the *Waldeyer tonsillar ring* (Fig. 23-2). The *palatine,* or *faucial, tonsils* are located on either side of the oropharynx, behind and below the pillars of the fauces (opening from the mouth). A surface of the palatine tonsils is usually visible during oral examination. The palatine tonsils are those removed during

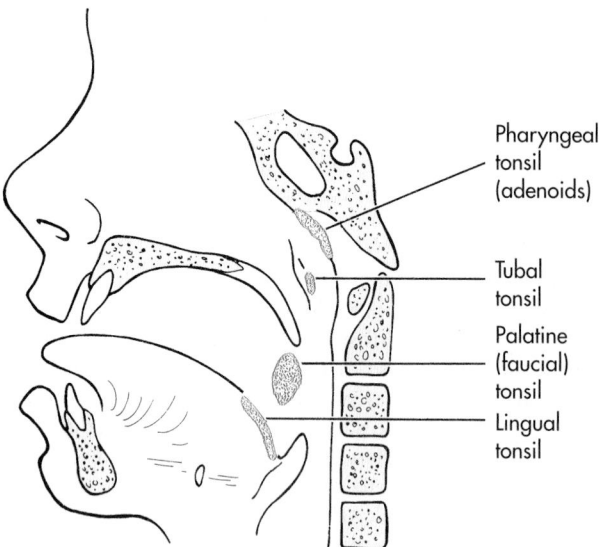

Pharyngeal tonsil (adenoids)

Tubal tonsil

Palatine (faucial) tonsil

Lingual tonsil

FIG. 23-2 ■ Location of various tonsillar masses.

tonsillectomy. The *pharyngeal tonsils,* also known as the *adenoids,* are located above the palatine tonsils on the posterior wall of the nasopharynx. Their proximity to the nares and eustachian tubes causes difficulties in instances of inflammation. The *lingual tonsils* are located at the base of the tongue. The *tubal tonsils,* found near the posterior nasopharyngeal opening of the eustachian tubes, are not part of the Waldeyer tonsillar ring.

Etiology

Tonsillitis often occurs with pharyngitis. The causative agent may be viral or bacterial. Because of the abundant lymphoid tissue and the frequency of URIs, tonsillitis is a common cause of morbidity in young children.

Clinical Manifestations

The manifestations of tonsillitis are caused by inflammation. As the palatine tonsils enlarge from edema, they may meet in the midline (kissing tonsils), obstructing the passage of air or food. The child has difficulty swallowing and breathing. When enlargement of the adenoids occurs, the space behind the posterior nares becomes blocked, making it difficult or impossible for air to pass from the nose to the throat. As a result, the child breathes through the mouth.

Therapeutic Management

Because tonsillitis is self-limiting, treatment of viral pharyngitis is symptomatic. Throat cultures positive for GABHS infection warrant antibiotic treatment. It is important to differentiate between viral and streptococcal infection in febrile exudative tonsillitis. Because most infections are of viral origin, early rapid tests can eliminate unnecessary antibiotic administration.

Tonsillectomy is the surgical removal of the palatine tonsils. Absolute indications for a tonsillectomy are malignancy and obstruction of the airway that result in cor pulmonale. *Adenoidectomy* (the surgical removal of the adenoids) is recommended for children who have hypertrophied adenoids that obstruct nasal breathing. The American Academy

of Otolaryngology-Head and Neck Surgery lists "3 or more infections of the tonsils or adenoids per year despite adequate medical therapy" as an indication for tonsillectomy or adenotonsillectomy (American Academy of Otolaryngology—Head and Neck Surgery, 2000). However, for some children the effectiveness of tonsillectomy or adenoidectomy is modest and may not justify the risk of surgery. In practice, most physicians rely on individualized decision making and do not subscribe to an absolute set of eligibility criteria for these surgical procedures (Paradise and others, 2002). Contraindications to either tonsillectomy or adenoidectomy are (1) cleft palate because tonsils help minimize escape of air during speech; (2) acute infections at the time of surgery because locally inflamed tissues increase the risk of bleeding; and (3) uncontrolled systemic diseases or blood dyscrasias.

Nursing Considerations

Nursing care involves providing comfort and minimizing activities or interventions that precipitate bleeding. A soft to liquid diet is preferred. A cool-mist vaporizer keeps the mucous membranes moist during periods of mouth breathing. Warm salt-water gargles, throat lozenges, and analgesic/antipyretic drugs such as acetaminophen are used to promote comfort. Combination nonopioid and opioid elixirs or tablets such as Tylenol with Codeine relieve pain and should be given routinely every 4 hours.

If surgery is needed, the child requires the same psychologic preparation and physical care as for any other surgical procedure (see Chapters 21 and 22). The following discussion focuses on postoperative nursing care for tonsillectomy and adenoidectomy (T&A), although both procedures may not be performed.

Until they are fully awake, children are placed on their abdomen or side to facilitate drainage of secretions. Suctioning is performed carefully to avoid trauma to the oropharynx. When alert, children may prefer sitting up, although they should remain in bed for the remainder of the day. They are discouraged from coughing frequently, clearing their throat, blowing their nose, or any other activity that may aggravate the operative site.

Some secretions are common, particularly dried blood from surgery. All secretions and vomitus are inspected for evidence of fresh bleeding (some blood-tinged mucus is expected). Dark brown (old) blood is usually present in the emesis, as well as in the nose and between the teeth. If parents do not expect this, they often become frightened at a time when they need to be calm and reassuring.

The throat is very sore after surgery. An ice collar provides relief, but many children find it bothersome and refuse to use it. Most children experience moderate pain after a T&A and need pain medication for at least the first 24 hours. Analgesics may be given rectally or intravenously to avoid the oral route. Because pain is continuous, analgesics should be administered at regular intervals. Local anesthetics, such as tetracaine lollipops or ice pops, and transdermal antiemetics such as promethazine (Phenergan) can be made by some pharmacists (see Pain Management, Chapter 21).

Food and fluids are restricted until children are fully alert and there are no signs of hemorrhage. Cool water, crushed ice, flavored ice pops, or diluted fruit juice is given, but fluids with a red or brown color are avoided to distinguish fresh or old blood in emesis from the ingested liquid. Citrus juice may cause discomfort and is usually poorly tolerated. Soft foods, particularly gelatin, cooked fruits, sherbet, soup, and mashed potatoes, are started on the first or second postoperative day or as the child tolerates feeding. The pain from surgery often inhibits intake, reinforcing the need for adequate pain control. Milk, ice cream, and pudding are usually not offered, because milk products coat the mouth and throat and may cause the child to clear the throat, which can initiate bleeding.

Postoperative hemorrhage is unusual but can occur. Therefore the nurse observes the throat directly for evidence of bleeding, using a good source of light and, if necessary, carefully inserting a tongue depressor. Signs of hemorrhage include increased pulse (greater than 120 beats/min), pallor, frequent clearing of the throat or swallowing by a younger child, and vomiting of bright red blood. Restlessness, an indication of hemorrhage, may be difficult to differentiate from general discomfort after surgery. Decreasing blood pressure is a late sign of shock.

NURSING ALERT

The most obvious early sign of bleeding is the child's continuous swallowing of the trickling blood. While the child is sleeping, note the frequency of swallowing. If continuous bleeding is suspected, notify the surgeon immediately.

Family Support and Home Care.   Discharge instructions include (1) avoiding irritating or highly seasoned foods, (2) avoiding gargles or vigorous toothbrushing, (3) discouraging coughing or clearing of the throat or putting objects in the mouth, (4) using analgesics or an ice collar for pain, and (5) limiting activity to decrease the potential for bleeding. Hemorrhage may occur up to 10 days after surgery as a result of tissue sloughing from the healing process. Any sign of bleeding warrants immediate medical attention.

INFLUENZA

Influenza, or "flu," is caused by three orthomyxoviruses, which are antigenically distinct: types A and B, which cause epidemic disease, and type C, which is unimportant from an epidemiologic standpoint. Influenza is spread from one individual to another by direct contact (large-droplet infection) or by articles recently contaminated by nasopharyngeal secretions. There is no predilection for a specific age-group, but attack rates are highest in young children who have had no previous contact with a strain. Influenza is frequently most severe in infants. During epidemics, infection among school-age children is believed to be a major source of transmission in a community. The disease is more common during the winter months and has a 1- to 3-day incubation period. Affected persons are most infectious for 24 hours before and after the onset of symptoms.

Clinical Manifestations

The manifestations of influenza may be subclinical, mild, moderate, or severe. Most patients have a dry throat and nasal mucosa, a dry cough, and a tendency toward hoarseness. A flushed face, photophobia, myalgia, hyperesthesia, and sometimes prostration accompany a sudden onset of fever and chills. Subglottal croup is common, especially in infants. The symptoms last for 4 to 5 days. Complications include severe viral pneumonia (often hemorrhagic), encephalitis, and secondary bacterial infections such as otitis media, sinusitis, or pneumonia.

Therapeutic Management

Uncomplicated influenza in children usually requires only symptomatic treatment: acetaminophen or ibuprofen for fever and sufficient fluids to maintain hydration. Children with influenza or other similar viruses should not receive aspirin because of its possible link with Reye syndrome. Amantadine hydrochloride is licensed for treatment of influenza in children. This medication has been effective in reducing symptoms associated with type A disease if administered within 24 to 48 hours after onset but is ineffective against type B or C influenza or other viral diseases. It should not be given to children younger than 1 year of age but is recommended for unvaccinated high-risk children. Zanamivir and rimantadine are two other drugs that have been approved for treatment of flu symptoms in children less than 18 years of age. Zanamivir is an inhaled medication that can cause bronchospasm and decreased lung function in children with asthma and chronic obstructive pulmonary disease. Zanamivir cannot be used for children less than 7 years of age, and rimantadine cannot be used for children less than 1 year of age (Palencia, 2000).

Prevention.   Inactivated influenza viral vaccines are safe and effective provided the antigens in the vaccine correlate with the circulating influenza viruses (see Immunizations, Chapter 10).

In 2003, the nasal spray flu vaccine was approved by the Food and Drug Administration. However, this preparation contains a live virus and should not be used in individuals who are immunocompromised or have cancer.

Nursing Considerations

Nursing care is the same as for any child with a URI, including implementing measures to relieve symptoms. The greatest danger to affected children is development of a secondary infection.

NURSING ALERT

Prolonged fever or appearance of fever during early convalescence is a sign of secondary bacterial infection and should be reported to the practitioner for antibiotic therapy.

OTITIS MEDIA

Otitis media (OM) is one of the most prevalent diseases of early childhood. Its incidence is highest in the winter months. Many cases of bacterial otitis media are preceded by a viral respiratory infection. The two viruses most likely to precipitate otitis media are the respiratory syncytial virus and influenza. Most episodes of acute otitis media (AOM) occur in the first 24 months of life, but the incidence decreases with age, except for a small increase at age 5 or 6 years when children enter school. OM occurs infrequently in children older than 7 years of age. Preschool-age boys are affected more frequently than preschool-age girls. Children who have siblings or parents with a history of chronic OM have a

BOX 23-5 ■ Standard Terminology for Otitis Media

Otitis media (OM)—An inflammation of the middle ear without reference to etiology or pathogenesis

Acute otitis media (AOM)—An inflammation of the middle ear space with a rapid onset of the signs and symptoms of acute infection—namely fever and otalgia (ear pain)

Otitis media with effusion (OME)—Fluid in the middle ear space without symptoms of acute infection

BOX 23-6 ■ Clinical Manifestations of Otitis Media

ACUTE OTITIS MEDIA
Follows an upper respiratory infection
Otalgia (earache)
Fever
Purulent discharge (otorrhea) may or may not be present

Infant or Very Young Child
Crying
Fussy, restless, irritable
Tendency to rub, hold, or pull affected ear
Rolls head from side to side
Difficulty comforting child
Loss of appetite

Older Child
Crying or verbalizes feelings of discomfort
Irritability
Lethargy
Loss of appetite

CHRONIC OTITIS MEDIA
Hearing loss
Difficulty communicating
Feeling of fullness, tinnitus, or vertigo may be present

higher incidence of OM. Children living in households with many members (especially smokers) are more likely to have OM than those living with fewer persons. Passive smoking increases the risk of persistent middle ear effusion by enhancing attachment of the pathogens that cause otitis to the respiratory epithelium in the middle ear space, by prolonging the inflammatory response and by impeding drainage through the eustachian tube (Berman and others, 2001; American Academy of Pediatrics, 2004). The standard terminology used to define OM is outlined in Box 23-5, and new AOM guidelines have been published (American Academy of Pediatrics, 2004a and 2004b).

Etiology

Streptococcus pneumoniae, Haemophilus influenzae, and *Moraxella catarrhalis* are the three most common bacteria causing AOM. The etiology of noninfectious OM is unknown, although OM may occur because of blocked eustachian tubes from the edema of URIs, allergic rhinitis, or hypertrophic adenoids. Chronic OM is frequently an extension of an acute episode.

A relationship between the incidence of OM and infant feeding methods has been noted. Breast-fed infants have a lower incidence than formula-fed infants. Breast-feeding may protect infants against respiratory viruses and allergy because breast milk contains secretory immunoglobulin (Ig) A, which limits the exposure of the eustachian tube and middle ear mucosa to microbial pathogens and foreign proteins. Reflux of milk up the eustachian tubes is also less likely to occur in breast-fed infants because of the semivertical positioning during breast-feeding.

Pathophysiology

OM is primarily the result of malfunctioning eustachian tubes. The eustachian tube, which connects the middle ear to the nasopharynx, is normally closed and flat, preventing organisms in the pharyngeal cavity from entering the middle ear. The eustachian tube opens to allow drainage of secretions produced by the middle ear mucosa and to equalize air pressure between the middle ear and the outside environment. Impaired drainage of the eustachian tube causes retention of secretions in the middle ear. Air is unable to escape through the obstructed tubes, is absorbed into the circulation, and causes negative pressure within the middle ear. If the tube opens, a difference in pressure causes bacteria to be swept into the middle ear chamber, where the organisms quickly proliferate and invade the mucosa.

Diagnostic Evaluation

Careful assessment of tympanic membrane mobility with a pneumatic otoscope is essential to differentiate AOM from otitis media with effusion (OME) (American Academy of Pediatrics, 2004b). If an accumulation of cerumen prevents adequate visualization of the tympanic membrane, the cerumen should be removed prior to inspection of the membrane. A diagnosis of AOM is made if visual inspection of the tympanic membrane reveals a purulent discolored effusion and a bulging or full, opacified, or very reddened immobile membrane (Pelton, 1998). An immobile tympanic membrane or an orange discolored membrane indicates OME. Clinical symptoms of otitis are also helpful in making the diagnosis (see Box 23-6). In AOM, symptoms such as acute ear pain, fever, and a bulging yellow or red tympanic membrane are usually present. In OME, these symptoms may be absent, and other nonspecific symptoms such as rhinitis, cough, or diarrhea are often present (American Academy of Pediatrics, 2004a and 2004b).

Therapeutic Management

Treatment for OM is one of the most common causes of antibiotic use in the ambulatory setting. Recently, however, concerns about drug-resistant *Streptococcus pneumoniae* and other drug resistances have caused infectious disease authorities to recommend careful and judicious use of antibiotics for treatment of this illness. Antibiotics are not required for initial treatment of OME but may be indicated for children with persistent effusion for more than 3 months (American Academy of Pediatrics, 2004b). It has been estimated that avoiding unnecessary treatment of OME with antibiotics would save millions of courses of antibiotics each year (American Academy of Pediatrics, 2004a). Recent reviews of the treatment of AOM reveal no clear evidence that antibiotics improve outcomes in children younger than 2 years of age with uncomplicated AOM (O'Neill, 2001). Current literature indicates waiting up to 72 hours for spontaneous resolution is safe and appropriate management of AOM in healthy infants and children (American Academy of Pediatrics, 2004a). However, the watchful waiting approach is not recommended for children younger than 2 years who have acute symptoms of fever and severe ear pain (Carlson and Scudder, 2004). In addition, all cases of AOM in infants younger than 6 months of age should be treated with antibiotics because of the infant's immature immune system and the potential for infection with bacteria other then the three most common organisms found in older infants and children with AOM.

When antibiotics are warranted, oral amoxicillin in high doses (80-90 mg/kg/day) is the treatment of choice for initial episodes of AOM in children who have not received antibiotics within the past month (Piglansky and others, 2003; Jackson, 2001; American Academy of Pediatrics, 2004a). The recommendation for the duration of antibiotic therapy is 10 to 14 days; in children 6 years and older, shorter courses may be sufficient (Iovino, 2003)

Second-line antibiotics used to treat otitis media include amoxicillin-clavulanate, azithromycin, and cephalosporins such as cefdinir, cefuroxime, and cefpodoxime. Intramuscular ceftriaxone is used when the causative organism is a highly resistant pneumococcus, and if the parents are noncompliant with the therapy. The use of steroids, decongestants, and antihistamines to treat acute AOM is not recommended.

Myringotomy, a surgical incision of the eardrum, may be necessary to alleviate the severe pain of AOM. A myringotomy is also performed to provide drainage of infected middle ear fluid in the presence of complications (mastoiditis, labyrinthitis, or facial paralysis) or to allow purulent middle ear fluid to drain into the ear canal for culture (DeRosa and Grundfast, 2002). Recently, a new minimally invasive laser-assisted myringotomy procedure has been performed in outpatient settings (Walker and Weber, 2001).

Tympanostomy tube placement and adenoidectomy are surgical procedures that may be done to treat recurrent otitis media. Tympanostomy tubes are pressure-equalizer (PE) tubes or grommets that facilitate continued drainage of fluid and allow ventilation of the middle ear. Myringotomy with or without insertion of PE tubes should *not* be performed for initial management of OME but may be recommended for children who have recurrent episodes of OME with a long cumulative duration (e.g., 6 months out of the previous 12) (American Academy of Pediatrics, 2004b). Adenoidectomy is never recommended for treatment of AOM and is only performed in children with recurrent AOM or chronic OME with nasal obstruction. Tonsillectomy either alone or with adenoidectomy is not considered an effective treatment of OME (Neill, 2002; American Academy of Pediatrics, 2004b).

In some children, residual middle ear effusions remain after episodes of AOM. Management options for OM with residual effusion include observation, antibiotics alone, or a combination of antibiotic and corticosteroid therapy. A hearing test should also be performed 3 months after the acute episode of AOM, and children with hearing loss should be referred to an otolaryngologist and should receive a speech and language evaluation as necessary.

Polyvalent pneumococcal polysaccharide vaccines have reduced the incidence of pneumococcal OM by 50% in children older than 2 years of age, but these vaccines are not effective in infants, who do not normally develop antibodies to polysaccharide vaccines (Andrews, 2001). For some high-risk infants, an immune globulin containing antibodies against bacterial polysaccharides (BPIG) has resulted in fewer cases of AOM caused by *Streptococcus pneumoniae.*

Nursing Considerations

Nursing objectives for the child with AOM include (1) relieving pain, (2) facilitating drainage when possible, (3) preventing complications or recurrence, (4) educating the family in care of the child, and (5) providing emotional support to the child and family.

Analgesic drugs such as acetaminophen and ibuprofen are used to treat mild pain. For more severe pain, the new Centers for Disease Control and Prevention and American Academy of Pediatrics guidelines recommend a stronger analgesic such as codeine (Iovino, 2003). An ice compress placed over the affected ear may also provide comfort and reduce edema and pressure.

If the ear is draining, the external canal may be cleaned with sterile cotton swabs or pledgets coupled with topical antibiotic treatment (Ramsey, 2002). If ear wicks or lightly rolled sterile gauze packs are placed in the ear after surgical treatment, they should be loose enough to allow accumulated drainage to flow out of the ear; otherwise, infection may be transferred to the mastoid process. The wicks need to stay dry during shampoos or baths. Occasionally, drainage is so profuse that the auricle and the skin surrounding the ear become excoriated from the exudate. This is usually prevented by frequent cleansing and application of various moisture barriers (e.g., Aloe Vesta, Proshield Plus) or petrolatum jelly (e.g., Vaseline).

Parents require anticipatory guidance regarding the temporary hearing loss that accompanies OM. The nurse should caution parents that their child is not ignoring them but may be unaware of being spoken to. Parents are instructed to speak louder, at closer proximity, and facing the child. Persistent difficulty in hearing beyond the acute stage should be evaluated.

Tympanostomy tubes may allow water to enter the middle ear, but recommendations for earplugs are inconsistent. Research indicates that swimming without earplugs poses no increased risk of infection. However, lake water is contaminated, and wearing earplugs while swimming in a lake prevents total flooding of the external canal. Bathwater and shampoo water should be kept out of the ear, if possible, because soap reduces the surface tension of water, and facilitates entry through the tube. Parents should be aware of the appearance of a grommet (usually a tiny, white, plastic spool-shaped tube) so that they can recognize it if it falls out. They are reassured that this is normal and requires no immediate intervention, although they should notify the practitioner.

Prevention of recurrence requires adequate education regarding antibiotic therapy. The symptoms of pain and fever usually subside within 24 to 48 hours, but nurses must emphasize that the infection is not completely eradicated until all of the prescribed medication is taken. Parents should be aware that potential complications of OM, such as hearing loss, can be prevented with adequate treatment and follow-up care.

Parents need to be taught ways to prevent OM, such as sitting or holding an infant upright during bottle-feeding and breast-feeding. Propping bottles is discouraged to avoid the supine position and to encourage human contact during feeding. Parents must recognize the initial signs of OM such as irritability and ear pulling. Eliminating tobacco smoke and known allergens from the environment is essential.

CROUP SYNDROMES

Croup is a general term applied to a symptom complex characterized by hoarseness, a resonant cough described as "barking" or "brassy" (croupy), varying degrees of inspiratory stridor, and varying degrees of respiratory distress resulting from swelling or obstruction in the region of the larynx. Acute infections of the larynx are important in infants and small children because of their increased incidence in these age-groups and because the small diameter of the airway in infants and children places them at risk for significant narrowing with inflammation.

Croup syndromes can affect the larynx, trachea, and bronchi. However, laryngeal involvement often dominates the clinical picture because of the severe effects on the voice and breathing. Croup syndromes are described according to the primary anatomic area affected (i.e., epiglottitis [or supraglottitis], laryngitis, laryngotracheobronchitis [LTB], and tracheitis). In general, LTB occurs in very young children, and epiglottitis is more common in older children. A comparison of croup syndromes is provided in Table 23-1.

ACUTE EPIGLOTTITIS

Acute epiglottitis, or *acute supraglottitis,* is a serious obstructive inflammatory process that occurs predominantly in children 2 to 5 years of age, but can occur from infancy to adulthood. The disorder requires immediate attention. The obstruction is supraglottic as opposed to the subglottic obstruction of laryngitis. The responsible organism is usually *Haemophilus influenzae.* LTB and epiglottitis do not occur together.

Clinical Manifestations

The onset of epiglottitis is abrupt and can rapidly progress to severe respiratory distress. The child usually goes to bed asymptomatic to awaken later, complaining of sore throat and pain on swallowing. The child has a fever; appears sicker than clinical findings suggest; and insists on sitting upright and leaning forward, with the chin thrust out, mouth open, and tongue protruding *(tripod position).* Drooling of saliva is common because of the difficulty or pain on swallowing and excessive secretions.

> ### ! NURSING ALERT
>
> Three clinical observations that have been found to be predictive of epiglottis are absence of spontaneous cough, presence of drooling, and agitation.

The child is irritable and extremely restless and has an anxious, apprehensive, and frightened expression. The voice is thick and muffled, with a froglike croaking sound on inspiration, but the child is not hoarse. Suprasternal and substernal retractions may be visible. The child seldom struggles to breathe, and slow, quiet breathing provides better air exchange. The sallow color of mild hypoxia may progress to frank cyanosis. The throat is red and inflamed, and a distinctive large, cherry red, edematous epiglottis is visible on careful throat inspection. *Throat inspection should be attempted only when immediate intubation can be performed if needed.*

Therapeutic Management

The course of epiglottitis may be fulminant, with respiratory obstruction appearing suddenly. Progressive obstruction leads to hypoxia, hypercapnia, and acidosis followed by decreased muscular tone, reduced level of consciousness, and, when obstruction becomes more or less complete, a rather sudden death. A presumptive diagnosis of epiglottitis constitutes an emergency.

The child who is suspected of having epiglottitis should be examined in a setting where emergency equipment is readily available. Examination of the throat with a tongue depressor is contraindicated until properly experienced personnel and equipment are at hand to proceed with immediate intubation or tracheostomy in the event that the examination precipitates further or complete obstruction.

TABLE 23-1 ■ Comparison of Croup Syndromes

	ACUTE EPIGLOTTITIS	ACUTE LARYNGOTRA-CHEOBRONCHITIS (LTB)	ACUTE SPASMODIC LARYNGITIS	ACUTE TRACHEITIS
Age-group affected	1-8 years	3 months-8 years	3 months-3 years	1 month-6 years
Etiologic agent	Bacterial, usually *Haemophilus influenzae*	Viral	Viral with allergic component	Bacterial, usually *Staphylococcus aureus*
Onset	Rapidly progressive	Slowly progressive	Sudden; at night	Moderately progressive
Major symptoms	Dysphagia	URI	URI	URI
	Stridor aggravated when supine	Stridor	Croupy cough	Croupy cough
	Drooling	Brassy cough	Stridor	Stridor
	High fever	Hoarseness	Hoarseness	Purulent secretions
	Toxic appearance	Dyspnea	Dyspnea	High fever
	Rapid pulse and respirations	Restlessness	Restlessness	No response to LTB therapy
		Irritability	Symptoms awaken child	
		Low-grade fever	Symptoms disappear during day	
		Nontoxic appearance	Tends to recur	
Treatment	Antibiotics	Humidity	Humidity	Antibiotics
	Airway protection	Racemic epinephrine		

URI, Upper respiratory infection.

If a lateral neck film is indicated, the same experienced personnel should accompany the child to the radiology department. Most practitioners prefer that the child not be transported but remain on the parent's lap in the examination area during portable radiology.

Endotracheal intubation or tracheostomy is usually considered for *H. influenzae* epiglottitis with severe respiratory distress. Intubation, tracheostomy, and any invasive procedure such as starting an intravenous (IV) infusion should be performed in the operating room. Whether or not there is an artificial airway, the child requires intensive observation by experienced personnel. The epiglottal swelling usually decreases after 24 hours of antibiotic therapy, and the epiglottis is near normal by the third day. Intubated children are generally extubated at this time.

Children with suspected bacterial epiglottitis are given antibiotics intravenously, followed by oral administration to complete a 7- to 10-day course. The use of corticosteroids for reducing edema may be beneficial during the early hours of treatment. Most intubated children receive a course of corticosteroids for 24 hours before extubation.

Prevention. The American Academy of Pediatrics (2003) recommends that all children beginning at 2 months of age receive the *H. influenzae* type B conjugate vaccine (see Immunizations, Chapter 10). Since administration of the vaccine has become a routine part of the regular immunization schedule, the incidence of epiglottitis has declined.

Nursing Considerations

Epiglottitis is a serious and frightening disease for the child and family. It is important to act quickly but calmly and to provide support without increasing anxiety. The child is allowed to remain in the position that provides the most comfort and security, and parents are reassured that everything possible is being done to obtain relief for their child.

> **!NURSING ALERT**
>
> Nurses who suspect epiglottitis should not attempt to visualize the epiglottis directly with a tongue depressor or take a throat culture but should refer the child for medical evaluation immediately (see Critical Thinking Exercise).

Acute care of the child is the same as that described for the child with LTB. Continuous monitoring of respiratory status, including pulse oximetry and blood gases, is an important part of nursing observations, and the IV infusion is maintained as described in Chapter 22.

ACUTE LARYNGITIS

Acute infectious laryngitis is a common illness in older children and adolescents. Infants and smaller children experience more generalized involvement (see the following section on LTB). Viruses are the usual causative agents, and the principal complaint is hoarseness, which may be accompanied by other upper respiratory symptoms (e.g., coryza, sore throat, nasal congestion) and systemic manifestations (e.g., fever, headache, myalgia, malaise). Associated complaints vary with the infecting virus. Adenoviruses and influenza viruses are responsible for more systemic involvement; parainfluenza viruses, rhinoviruses, and RSV cause more mild illness.

Therapeutic Management and Nursing Considerations

The disease is usually self-limited without long-term sequelae. Treatment is symptomatic with fluids and humidified air (see Nursing Care Plan, pp. 792-793).

ACUTE LARYNGOTRACHEOBRONCHITIS

LTB is the most common croup syndrome. It primarily affects children younger than 5 years of age, and the causative organisms are the parainfluenza virus, RSV, influenza A and B, and *Mycoplasma pneumoniae*. The disease is usually preceded by a URI, which gradually descends to adjacent structures. It is characterized by gradual onset of low-grade fever. Inflammation of the mucosa lining of the larynx and trachea causes a narrowing of the airway. When the airway is significantly

---

??? CRITICAL THINKING EXERCISE ???

Croup Syndrome

Kim, a 4 year old, is admitted to the emergency department with a sore throat, pain on swallowing, drooling, and a fever of 39° C (102.2° F). She looks ill, is agitated, and prefers to sit up and lean over. What nursing interventions should the nurse implement in this situation?

QUESTIONS

1. Evidence—Is there sufficient evidence to draw any conclusions about Kim's condition at this time?
2. Assumptions—Describe some underlying assumptions about each of the following:
   a. Epiglottitis in children
   b. Symptoms of epiglottitis
   c. Precautions to be taken when a child has suspected epiglottitis
   d. Immediate nursing interventions when caring for a child with epiglottitis
3. What priorities for nursing care can be drawn at this time?
4. Does the evidence objectively support your argument (conclusion)?
5. Are there alternative perspectives to your arguments? What are they?

ANSWERS

1. Yes, there are sufficient data to arrive at a possible conclusion in this situation.
2. a. Epiglottitis is a serious obstructive inflammatory process that occurs in children 2 to 5 years of age.
   b. Symptoms of epiglottitis include throat pain, restlessness, drooling, and a desire to sit upright and lean forward.
   c. Because epiglottitis can quickly progress to severe respiratory distress, the nurse should never examine the child's throat with a tongue depressor or take a throat culture.
   d. Nursing interventions for the child with epiglottitis include monitoring the child's respiratory status, allowing the child to remain in the position that is most comfortable, having a tracheostomy tray and emergency equipment available, and assisting with insertion of an IV line and administration of antibiotics.
3. The suspicion of epiglottitis constitutes an emergency. The priority for nursing care at this time is to maintain the child's airway.
4. Yes, the evidence supports the conclusion.
5. Alternative perspectives to this situation are not apparent at this time. However, after Kim's respiratory condition stabilizes and her treatment is begun, it would be worthwhile to determine whether her immunizations are up to date. Recently, the number of cases of epiglottitis has been reduced significantly by administration of the *Haemophilus influenzae* type B conjugate vaccine.

BOX 23-7 ■ Progression of Symptoms In Laryngotracheobronchitis

STAGE I
Fear
Hoarseness
Croupy cough
Inspiratory stridor when disturbed

STAGE II
Continuous respiratory stridor
Lower rib retraction
Retraction of soft tissue of neck
Use of accessory muscles of respiration
Labored respiration

STAGE III
Signs of anoxia and carbon dioxide retention
Restlessness
Anxiety
Pallor
Sweating
Rapid respiration

STAGE IV
Intermittent cyanosis
Permanent cyanosis
Cessation of breathing

From Walter EB, Shurin PA: Acute respiratory infections. In Krugman S and others: *Infectious diseases of children*, ed 9, St Louis, 1992, Mosby.

narrowed, the child struggles to inhale air past the obstruction and into the lungs, producing the characteristic inspiratory stridor and suprasternal retractions. The typical child with LTB is a toddler who develops the classic barking or seal-like cough and acute stridor after several days of coryza. When the child is unable to inhale a sufficient volume of air, symptoms of hypoxia become evident. Obstruction that is severe enough to prevent adequate exhalation of carbon dioxide can cause respiratory acidosis and eventual respiratory failure. The progression of symptoms is outlined in Box 23-7.

Therapeutic Management

The major objective in medical management is maintaining the airway and providing adequate respiratory exchange. Children with mild croup (no stridor at rest) are managed at home. Parents are taught the signs of respiratory distress and instructed to summon professional help early if needed. Children who progress to stage II respiratory symptoms should receive medical attention.

High humidity with cool mist provides relief for most children. A cool-air vaporizer can be used at home. In the hospital setting, hoods for infants or tents for toddlers may be used to provide increased humidity and supplemental oxygen.

⚠ NURSING ALERT

Children with severe respiratory distress (traditionally, a respiratory rate greater than 60 breaths/min for infants) should not be given anything by mouth to prevent aspiration and decrease the work of breathing.

Nebulized epinephrine (racemic epinephrine) is often used in children with severe disease, stridor at rest, retractions, or difficulty breathing. The α-adrenergic effects cause mucosal vasoconstriction and subsequently decrease subglottic edema. The onset of action is rapid, and the peak effect is observed in 2 hours. Additional doses may be administered every 20 to 30 minutes in the intensive care unit or 3 to 4 hours in the regular hospital unit (Wald, 1999). In a significant number of children, however, improvement persists and additional treatments are not necessary.

The use of corticosteroids is beneficial because the antiinflammatory effects decrease subglottic edema. The onset of action is clinically detectable as early as 6 hours after administration, with continued improvement over 12 to 24 hours.

It is essential to allow children with mild croup to drink beverages they like and to encourage their parents to try whatever comforting measures work best (e.g., holding their child, rocking, singing). If the child is unable to take oral fluids, IV fluid therapy may be indicated.

Nursing Considerations

The most important nursing function in the care of children with LTB is continuous, vigilant observation and accurate assessment of respiratory status. Cardiorespiratory monitoring and noninvasive pulse oximetry equipment supplement visual observations. Changes in therapy are frequently based on the nurses' observations and assessments, the child's response to therapy, and tolerance of procedures. The trend away from early intubation of children with LTB emphasizes the importance of nursing observations and the ability to recognize impending respiratory failure so that intubation can be implemented without delay. Intubation equipment must be readily accessible and taken with the child during transport to other areas (e.g., radiology, operating room).

⚠ NURSING ALERT

Early signs of impending airway obstruction include increased pulse and respiratory rate; substernal, suprasternal, and intercostal retractions; flaring nares; and increased restlessness.

To conserve energy, children are given every opportunity to rest. Infants or small children respond to being enclosed in a tent, coughing, having laryngeal spasms, and needing IV therapy as additional sources of distress. Most infants and small children prefer to be held and to sit upright. Children also need the security of their parent's presence. Crying increases respiratory distress and hypoxia, and an extremely fussy child may tolerate procedures better when held in the parent's lap with cool mist directed toward their face than in a mist tent.

The rapid progression of croup, the alarming sound of the cough and stridor, and the child's apprehensive behavior and ill appearance combine to create a frightening experience for the parents. Parents need reassurance regarding their child's progress and an explanation of treatments. They may feel guilty for not having suspected the seriousness of the condition sooner. The family should be allowed to remain with their child as much as possible, especially when this decreases the child's distress.

The nurse should provide the parents with an opportunity to express their feelings and should minimize any sense of blame or guilt. Parents need frequent reassurance pro-

TABLE 23-2 ■ Comparison of Conditions Affecting the Bronchi

	VIRAL-INDUCED ASTHMA*	BRONCHITIS	BRONCHIOLITIS
Description	Exaggerated response of bronchi to infection Bronchospasm, exudation, and edema of bronchi	Usually occurs in association with URI Seldom an isolated entity	More common infectious disease of lower airways Maximum obstructive impact at bronchiolar level
Age-group affected	Late infancy and early childhood	Affects children in first 4 years of life	Usually children 2-12 months of age; rare after age 2 Peak incidence approximately age 6 months
Etiologic agents	Most often viruses but may be any of a variety of URI pathogens	Usually viral Other agents (e.g., bacteria, fungi, allergic disorders, airborne irritants) can trigger symptoms	Viruses, predominantly respiratory syncytial viruses; also adenoviruses, parainfluenza viruses, and *Mycoplasma pneumoniae*
Predominant characteristics	Wheezing, productive cough	Persistent dry, hacking cough (worse at night) becoming productive in 2-3 days	Dyspnea, paroxysmal nonproductive cough, tachypnea with retractions and flaring nares, emphysema; may be wheezing
Treatment	Bronchodilators, corticosteroids	Cough suppressants if needed	Oxygen mist Ribavirin may be used for high-risk populations

*See Asthma, p. 813.
URI, Upper respiratory infection.

vided in a calm, quiet manner and education regarding what they can do to make their child more comfortable. Fortunately, as the crisis subsides and the child responds to therapy, breathing becomes easier and recovery is generally prompt. Home care includes continued humidity, adequate hydration, and nourishment.

ACUTE SPASMODIC LARYNGITIS

Acute spasmodic laryngitis (*spasmodic croup*, "midnight croup," or "twilight croup") is distinct from laryngitis and LTB and is characterized by paroxysmal attacks of laryngeal obstruction that occur chiefly at night. Signs of inflammation are absent or mild, and there is often a history of previous attacks lasting 2 to 5 days, followed by uneventful recovery. This condition usually affects children ages 1 to 3 years. Some children appear to be predisposed to the condition; allergies may be implicated in some cases.

The child goes to bed feeling well or with very mild respiratory symptoms but awakes suddenly with characteristic barking, metallic cough, hoarseness, noisy inspirations, and restlessness. The child appears anxious, frightened, and prostrated. Dyspnea is aggravated by excitement; but there is no fever, the attack subsides in a few hours, and the child appears well the next day.

Therapeutic Management and Nursing Considerations

Spasmodic croup is usually self-limited, and most children are managed at home. Cool mist is recommended for the child's room. Warm mist provided by steam from hot running water in a closed bathroom is also helpful. Sometimes the spasm is relieved by sudden exposure to cold air (as when the child is taken out into the night air to see the practitioner). Parents are usually advised to have the child sleep in humidified air until the cough has subsided to prevent subsequent episodes. Children with moderately severe symptoms may be hospitalized for observation and therapy

with cool mist and racemic epinephrine, as for LTB. Some patients respond to corticosteroid therapy.

BACTERIAL TRACHEITIS

Bacterial tracheitis, an infection of the mucosa of the upper trachea, is a distinct entity with features of both croup and epiglottitis. The disease occurs in children 1 month to 6 years of age and may be a serious cause of airway obstruction that is severe enough to cause respiratory arrest. It is believed to be a complication of LTB, and although *Staphylococcus aureus* is the most frequent organism responsible, group A β-hemolytic streptococci and *H. influenzae* have also been implicated.

The manifestations of bacterial tracheitis are similar to those of LTB but are unresponsive to LTB therapy. There is a history of previous URI with croupy cough, stridor unaffected by position, toxicity, and high fever. Another prominent symptom is the production of thick, purulent tracheal secretions. Respiratory difficulties are secondary to these copious secretions.

Therapeutic Management and Nursing Considerations

Bacterial tracheitis requires vigorous management with humidified oxygen, antipyretics, and antibiotics. Most children require endotracheal intubation and frequent tracheal suctioning to prevent airway obstruction. Early recognition to prevent catastrophic airway obstruction is essential.

INFECTIONS OF THE LOWER AIRWAYS

The *reactive portion* of the lower respiratory tract includes the bronchi and bronchioles in children. Cartilaginous support of the large airways is not fully developed until adolescence. Consequently, the smooth muscle in these structures represents a major factor in the constriction of the airway, particularly in the bronchioles, that portion that extends from the bronchi to the alveoli. Table 23-2 compares some of the major features of bronchial and bronchiolar infections.

BRONCHITIS

Bronchitis (sometimes referred to as *tracheobronchitis*) is inflammation of the large airways (trachea and bronchi), which is frequently associated with a URI. Viral agents are the primary cause of the disease, although *Mycoplasma pneumoniae* is a common cause in children older than 6 years of age. A dry, hacking, nonproductive cough that worsens at night and becomes productive in 2 to 3 days characterizes this condition.

Bronchitis is a mild, self-limiting disease that requires only symptomatic treatment, including analgesics, antipyretics, and humidity. Cough suppressants may be useful to allow rest but can interfere with clearance of secretions. Most patients recover uneventfully in 5 to 10 days.

RESPIRATORY SYNCYTIAL VIRUS AND BRONCHIOLITIS

Bronchiolitis is an acute viral infection with maximum effect at the bronchiolar level. The infection is rare in children older than 2 years of age. *RSV* is responsible for 80% or more of the cases during epidemic periods (Long, 1999). It is considered the single most important respiratory pathogen in infancy and early childhood. Infection begins in the late fall, reaches a peak during winter, and decreases in spring. It is easily spread from hand to eye, nose, or other mucous membranes.

Pathophysiology

In RSV, the bronchiole mucosa swell, and lumina are filled with mucus and exudate. The walls of the bronchi and bronchioles are infiltrated with inflammatory cells, and peribronchiolar interstitial pneumonitis is usually present. Varying degrees of obstruction produced in the small air passages lead to hyperinflation, obstructive emphysema resulting from partial obstruction, and patchy areas of atelectasis. Dilation of bronchial passages on inspiration allows sufficient space for intake of air, but narrowing of the passages on expiration prevents air from leaving the lungs. Thus air is trapped distal to the obstruction and causes progressive overinflation *(emphysema)*.

Clinical Manifestations

Bronchiolitis begins as a URI with symptoms of rhinorrhea and low-grade fever. Otitis media and conjunctivitis may also be present. In time a cough develops and, if the disease progresses, it becomes a respiratory tract infection with typical symptoms (see Box 23-8). Chest radiographs show hyperaeration and areas of consolidation that are difficult to differentiate from bacterial pneumonia. Apnea may be the first recognized indicator of RSV infection in very young infants. Severe disease is followed by a rise in arterial carbon dioxide tension ($PaCO_2$) (hypercapnia), leading to respiratory acidosis and hypoxemia.

Diagnostic Evaluation

Positive identification of RSV is accomplished by using either enzyme-linked immunosorbent assay (ELISA) or rapid immunofluorescent antibody (IFA) from direct aspiration of nasal secretions or nasopharyngeal washings (see Respiratory Secretion and Throat Specimens, Chapter 22).

Therapeutic Management

Bronchiolitis is treated symptomatically with high humidity, adequate fluid intake, and rest. Most children can be managed at home. Hospitalization is recommended for children

---

BOX 23-8 ■ Signs and Symptoms of Respiratory Syncytial Virus

INITIAL
Rhinorrhea
Pharyngitis
Coughing/sneezing
Wheezing
Possible ear or eye drainage
Intermittent fever

WITH PROGRESSION OF ILLNESS
Increased coughing and wheezing
Air hunger
Tachypnea and retractions
Cyanosis

SEVERE ILLNESS
Tachypnea, greater than 70 breaths/min
Listlessness
Apneic spells
Poor air exchange; poor breath sounds

---

with underlying lung or heart disease, associated debilitated states, or an inadequate caregiver. The child who is tachypneic, has marked retractions, seems listless, or has a history of poor fluid intake should also be admitted. Treatment involves mist therapy combined with oxygen administered by hood or tent in concentrations sufficient to alleviate dyspnea and hypoxia, after which mist alone is continued for mild dyspnea. Fluids by mouth may be contraindicated because of tachypnea, weakness, and fatigue; therefore, IV fluids are preferred until the acute crisis of the disease has passed.

Clinical assessments, noninvasive oxygen monitoring, and blood gas values guide therapy. Medical therapy for bronchiolitis is controversial. Bronchodilators, corticosteroids, cough suppressants, and antibiotics are not effective in uncomplicated disease and are not recommended for routine use.

Ribavirin has in vitro antiviral activity against RSV, but ribavirin aerosol treatment for RSV infection is highly controversial. Placebo-controlled clinical trials have failed to demonstrate efficacy of this drug, and there are concerns about the drug's cost and safety. The American Academy of Pediatrics (2003) recommends that decisions about ribavirin be made on the basis of the individual patient's clinical presentation and the physician's experience.

Prevention of RSV Infection

Two products, RSV immune globulin and palivizumab, are used to prevent RSV infection. *RSV immune globulin (RSV-IGIV)* is an IV preparation of immunoglobulin G that provides neutralizing antibodies against RSV. This drug is given in a monthly IV infusion beginning just before onset of the RSV season. The *monoclonal antibody, palivizumab,* is given monthly in an intramuscular (IM) injection. Both drugs have been licensed for prevention of RSV disease. The American Academy of Pediatrics (2003) recommends that RSV-IGIV be considered for infants and children younger than 24 months of age who have chronic lung disease (CLD) and who have required medical therapy for CLD within 6 months before the anticipated start of RSV season. Palivizumab is preferred for most high-risk children because of its ease of administration, safety, and effectiveness. Infants born at 32 weeks of gestation or earlier may benefit from RSV prophylaxis even if they do not have CLD. For these infants, the decision is based on their gestational age and their chronologic age at the start of RSV season. Infants born at 28 weeks' gestation or earlier may benefit by receiving the preventive drug during their first RSV season when it occurs in their first 12 months of life. Infants born at 29 to 32 weeks of gestation may benefit from prophylaxis until they are 6 months of age. Although these drugs have been shown to decrease the likelihood of hospitalization in infants born between 32 and 35 weeks' gestation, the cost of providing prophylaxis to this large group of infants should be considered carefully. The American Academy of Pediatrics (2003) recommends prophylaxis for infants born between 32 and 35 weeks' gestation if they are younger than 6 months of age at the start of the RSV season. Prophylaxis is also recommended if infants or children have two or more of the following additional risk factors: school-age siblings, crowding in the home, day care attendance, or exposure to tobacco smoke in the home. In addition, children who are 24 months of age or younger with hemodynamically significant cyanotic and acyanotic congenital heart disease are likely to benefit from palivizumab injections. RSV-IGIV is contraindicated in children with cyanotic congenital heart disease. Neither palivizumab nor RSV-IGIV has been evaluated for immunocompromised children.

Nursing Considerations

Children admitted to the hospital with suspected RSV infection should be assigned separate rooms or grouped with other RSV-infected children. The most important infection control measure in caring for these infants and children is consistent handwashing and the use of contact precautions (use of gloves, gowns, masks, and goggles). Another measure includes making patient assignments so that nurses assigned to children with RSV do not take care of other patients who are considered high risk.

If ribavirin is chosen for therapy, this drug is aerosolized and delivered via a small-particle aerosol generator (SPAG) through an oxygen hood, tent, mask, or ventilator. Care must be taken to decrease the escape of aerosolized ribavirin into the air.

> **❗NURSING ALERT**
>
> Because of concerns about potential toxic or teratogenic effects, pregnant health care providers should not care for a child receiving ribavirin.

Children receiving RSV-IVIG should be monitored for symptoms of fluid volume overload during IV administration. Antibodies in RSV-IVIG may interfere with the immune response to live virus vaccines (mumps, rubella, measles, and chickenpox); therefore, immunization with these vaccines should be deferred for 9 months after the last dose of RSV-IVIG infusion (American Academy of Pediatrics, 2003). Palivizumab does not interfere with response to vaccines. However, preparations of palivizumab do not contain a preservative, so the health care professional who administers this drug must arrange to administer it within 6 hours after opening a vial. To relieve the pain of IV infusions of RSV-IVIG and the IM injections of palivizumab, EMLA cream should be applied to the IV insertion site or the IM site before the procedure.

PNEUMONIAS

Pneumonia, inflammation of the pulmonary parenchyma, is common in childhood but occurs more frequently in infancy and early childhood. Clinically, pneumonia may occur either as a primary disease or as a complication of another illness. The various types of pneumonia include:

> **Lobar pneumonia**—All or a large segment of one or more pulmonary lobes is involved. When both lungs are affected, it is known as *bilateral* or *double pneumonia.*
> **Bronchopneumonia**—Begins in the terminal bronchioles, which become clogged with mucopurulent exudate to form consolidated patches in nearby lobules; also called *lobular pneumonia.*
> **Interstitial pneumonia**—The inflammatory process is more or less confined within the alveolar walls (interstitium) and the peribronchial and interlobular tissues.

Although the morphologic classification is typically used, the most useful classification of pneumonia is based on the etiologic agent (i.e., viral, bacterial, mycoplasmal, or aspiration of foreign substances) (see Aspiration Pneumonia, p. 811). Histomycosis, coccidioidomycosis, and other fungi also cause pneumonia. The causative agent is identified from the clinical history, the child's age, the general health history, the physical examination, radiography, and the laboratory examination.

Viral Pneumonia

Viral pneumonias, which occur more frequently than bacterial pneumonias, are seen in children of all ages and are often associated with viral URIs. Viruses that cause pneumonia include RSV in infants, and parainfluenza, influenza, and adenovirus in older children, There are few clinical symptoms that are unique to a specific virus, and differentiation among viruses is usually made by laboratory examination (Box 23-9).

The prognosis is generally good, although viral infections of the respiratory tract render the affected child more susceptible to secondary bacterial invasion, especially when there is denuded bronchial mucosa. Treatment is symptomatic and includes measures to promote oxygenation and comfort, such as oxygen administration with cool mist, chest physiotherapy and postural drainage, antipyretics for fever management, fluid intake, and family support. Some authorities recommend antimicrobial therapy in the hope of reducing or preventing secondary bacterial infection, but this therapy should be reserved for children in whom a bacterial infection is demonstrated by appropriate cultures.

Primary Atypical Pneumonia

Mycoplasma pneumoniae is the most common cause of pneumonia in children between ages 5 and 12 years. It occurs in the fall and winter months and is more prevalent in crowded living conditions. Most affected persons recover from acute illness in 7 to 10 days with symptomatic treatment followed by a week of convalescence. Hospitalization is rarely necessary.

Severe Acute Respiratory Syndrome

A severe form of atypical pneumonia identified as severe acute respiratory syndrome (SARS) was first reported in Asia in 2003. SARS is caused by a previously unrecognized

BOX 23-9 ■ General Signs of Pneumonia

Fever—Usually quite high
Respiratory
   Cough—Unproductive to productive with whitish sputum
   Tachypnea
   Breath sounds—Rhonchi or fine crackles
   Dullness with percussion
   Chest pain
   Retractions
   Nasal flaring
   Pallor to cyanosis (depends on severity)
Chest x-ray film—Diffuse or patchy infiltration with peribronchial distribution
Behavior—Irritable, restless, lethargic
Gastrointestinal—Anorexia, vomiting, diarrhea, abdominal pain

coronavirus called SARS Co-V. Clinical manifestations of this disorder include a fever greater than 100.4° F, headache, cough, shortness of breath, difficulty breathing, and after 2 to 7 days a dry, nonproductive cough and dyspnea. In some patients, the symptoms are severe enough to require intubation and mechanical ventilation. SARS is spread by close contact with a person with SARS. Most cases have involved people who have cared for or lived with someone with SARS or people who have traveled to areas with reported cases of SARS (O'Connor, 2003).

In children, two distinct forms of the illness have been observed. Teenagers have malaise, myalgia, chills, and rigor, whereas young children have mainly cough and runny nose. In younger children the clinical course seems to be milder and the disease resolves more quickly than in adolescents or adults (Hon and others, 2003)

Laboratory findings include lymphopenia, leukopenia, thrombocytopenia, elevated lactate dehydrogenase, aspartate aminotransferase, and creatinine kinase levels. The most reliable laboratory diagnostic test is positive antibodies for the SARS coronavirus 21 days after the illness. Chest radiographs in a substantial number of patients reveal focal interstitial infiltrates that progress to more generalized, patchy, interstitial infiltrates (Kuiken and others, 2003).

Treatment of SARS involves predominantly supportive care measures. Other therapies such as antibiotics, antiviral drugs, and steroids have been used with mixed results (O'Connor, 2003).

Nursing Considerations

The Centers for Disease Control and Prevention recommends that patients with SARS receive the same treatment as any patient with serious community-acquired atypical pneumonia. This includes the use of strict hand-washing, contact precautions, and airborne precautions (e.g., an isolation room with negative pressure relative to the surrounding area and the use of an N-95 filtering disposable respirator for persons entering the room). Recommendations for stopping the spread of SARS have also been developed. When triaging patients, nurses should place a surgical mask on any patient who has had close contact with SARS or who has a history of international travel to an area with cases of SARS. Health care workers who have had high-risk, unprotected exposure to SARS should be

excluded from duty and remain home from work to monitor their health for 10 days.

Bacterial Pneumonia

Streptococcus pneumoniae is the most common bacterial pathogen responsible for community-acquired pneumonia in both children and adults. During the last several decades, isolates of the *S. pneumoniae* organism that are resistant to penicillin and other antibiotics have become more prevalent (Tan and others, 2002). Other bacteria that cause pneumonia in children are group A streptococcus, *Staphylococcus aureus, M. catarrhalis,* and *Haemophilus influenzae.*

Beyond the neonatal period, bacterial pneumonias display distinct clinical patterns that facilitate their differentiation from other forms of pneumonia. The onset of illness is abrupt and generally follows a viral infection that disturbs the natural defense mechanisms of the upper respiratory tract.

Children with bacterial pneumonia appear ill. Symptoms include fever, malaise, rapid and shallow respirations, cough, and chest pain that is exaggerated by deep breathing. The pain of pneumonia may be referred to the abdomen and confused with appendicitis. Chills and meningeal symptoms *(meningism)* are common.

Older children with pneumococcal pneumonia can be treated at home if the condition is recognized and treatment is initiated early. Antibiotic therapy, bed rest, liberal oral intake of fluid, and administration of an antipyretic for fever are the principal therapeutic measures. Hospitalization is indicated when pleural effusion or empyema accompanies the disease. Pneumonia in the infant or young child is best treated in the hospital, because the course of illness is more variable and complications are more common in very young patients. IV fluids are frequently necessary, and oxygen is required if the child is in respiratory distress.

Complications.   Some children, especially infants, with staphylococcal pneumonia can develop empyema, pyopneumothorax, or tension pneumothorax. AOM and PE are also common in children with pneumococcal pneumonia. A recent report indicated that the frequency of children who are hospitalized with pneumococcal pneumonia complicated by necrosis, empyema, complicated pneumonic effusion, and lung abscess may be increasing (Tan and others, 2002). Reasons for this increase in complications are unknown.

When fluid is suspected in the pleural cavity, a diagnostic needle aspiration or thoracentesis is performed. Nonpurulent effusions do not require surgical drainage. Continuous closed-chest drainage may need to be instituted when purulent fluid is aspirated.

Prognosis.   The prognosis for pneumonia is generally good, with rapid recovery when symptoms are recognized and treated early. Streptococcal infections vary in duration but usually resolve spontaneously. The course of staphylococcal pneumonia is generally prolonged. The prognosis varies with the length of illness before treatment is begun, although early recognition and treatment are usually effective.

Prevention.   Use of pneumococcal polysaccharide vaccine is recommended for use in selected individuals, such as children older than age 2 years who are at risk of acquiring pneumococcal infection or are at risk of serious disease (see Immunizations, Chapter 10).

Nursing Considerations

Nursing care of the child with pneumonia is primarily supportive and symptomatic but necessitates thorough respiratory assessment and administration of oxygen and antibiotics. The child's respiratory rate and status, as well as general disposition and level of activity, are frequently assessed. Isolation procedures are instituted according to hospital policy. Relief of physical and psychologic stress encourages rest and conservation of energy. The child is disturbed as little as possible by clustering care to encourage the child's regular sleep cycle. If the cough is disturbing, judicious use of antitussives, especially before rest times and meals, is often helpful. To prevent dehydration, fluids are frequently administered intravenously during the acute phase. Oral fluids, if allowed, are given cautiously to avoid aspiration and to decrease the possibility of aggravating a fatiguing cough.

Children may be placed in a mist tent. Cool humidification moistens the airways and provides an atmosphere that aids in temperature reduction. Children in mist tents require frequent clothing and linen changes to prevent chilling in the damp atmosphere. They are usually comfortable in a semierect position but should be allowed to determine the position of comfort. Lying on the affected side (if pneumonia is unilateral) splints the chest on that side and reduces the pleural rubbing that often causes discomfort. Fever is usually controlled by administration of antipyretic drugs as prescribed, and temperature is monitored regularly to detect a rise that might trigger a febrile seizure.

Vital signs and breath sounds are monitored to assess the progress of the disease and to detect early signs of complications. Children with ineffectual cough or those who have difficulty handling secretions require suctioning to maintain a patent airway. A simple bulb syringe is usually sufficient for infants, but mechanical suction should be readily available if needed. Older children can usually handle secretions without assistance. Postural drainage and chest physiotherapy are generally prescribed every 4 hours or more often, depending on the child's condition.

The hospitalized child is apprehensive, and treatments and tests are frightening and stress-producing. Reducing anxiety and apprehension is essential. When the child is relaxed, respiratory efforts are lessened. Encouraging the presence of the caregiver provides the child with a customary source of comfort and support and often eases respiratory efforts in the child. The family needs support and reassurance. The child's dry, hacking cough can be tiring for the parents and often disturbs their sleep. Parents are kept informed of the child's progress and taught appropriate home care, such as use of a nasal aspirator and administration of antibiotics.

OTHER INFECTIONS OF THE RESPIRATORY TRACT

PERTUSSIS (WHOOPING COUGH)

Pertussis (whooping cough) is an acute respiratory infection caused by *Bordetella pertussis* that occurs chiefly in children younger than 4 years of age who have not been immunized.

It is highly contagious and is particularly threatening in young infants, who have a high morbidity and mortality rate. (See Table 14-1 for signs, symptoms, and management of pertussis and Chapter 10 for immunization.) The incidence is highest in the spring and summer months, and a single attack confers lifetime immunity. Pertussis vaccine is effective, but the immunity diminishes with time after the initial infection or immunization.

TUBERCULOSIS

Tuberculosis (TB) is the second leading cause of death from an infectious disease. Ten to 15 million persons in the United States are infected with TB. Case rates of TB for all ages are higher in urban, low-income areas and nonwhite racial and ethnic groups. In recent years, foreign-born children have accounted for more than one third of newly diagnosed cases of TB in children 14 years of age or younger in the United States (American Academy of Pediatrics, 2003).

TB is caused by the *Mycobacterium tuberculosis* organism. Children are susceptible to both the human *(M. tuberculosis)* and the bovine *(Mycobacterium bovis)* organisms. Human disease caused by *M. bovis* occurs in children who ingest unpasteurized milk or milk products. Although the causative agent for TB is the tubercle bacillus, other factors influence the degree to which the organism produces an altered state in the host. These factors include heredity (resistance to the infection may be genetically transmitted), gender (higher in adolescent girls), age (lower resistance in infants, higher incidence during adolescence), stress (emotional or physical), nutritional state, and intercurrent infection (especially human immunodeficiency virus [HIV], measles, and pertussis). Children with HIV infection have an increased incidence of tuberculosis disease, and all children with tuberculosis should be tested for HIV.

The source of tuberculosis infection in children is usually an infected member of the household or a frequent visitor to the home such as a baby-sitter or domestic worker. The lung is the usual portal of entry for the organism. In the lungs a proliferation of epithelial cells surround and encapsulate the multiplying bacilli in an attempt to wall it off, thus forming the typical tubercle. Extension of the primary lesion at the original site causes progressive tissue destruction as it spreads within the lung, discharges material from foci to other areas of the lungs (e.g., bronchi, pleura), or produces pneumonia. Erosion of blood vessels by the primary lesion can cause widespread dissemination of the tubercle bacillus to near and distant sites *(miliary tuberculosis)*. Areas that are frequently affected include the lymph nodes, meninges, and bone.

Diagnostic Evaluation

Diagnosis is based on information derived from physical examination, history, tuberculin skin testing, radiographic examinations, and cultures of the organism. The clinical manifestations of the disease are extremely variable (see Box 23-10).

The *tuberculin skin test* (TST) is the most important indicator of whether a child has been infected with the tubercle bacillus. The standard dose of purified protein derivative (PPD) is 5 tuberculin units, which is administered using a

27-gauge needle and a 1-mL syringe intradermally into the volar aspect of the forearm. Creation of a visible wheal is crucial to accurate testing. Recommendations for TST of children are listed in Box 23-11. Routine testing of children with no risk factors residing in communities with a low

prevalence of tuberculosis is not indicated (American Academy of Pediatrics, 2003).

A *positive reaction* indicates that the individual has been infected and has developed sensitivity to the tubercle bacillus. It does not, however, confirm the presence of active disease. Once individuals react positively, they will always react positively. A previously negative reaction that becomes positive indicates that the person has been infected since the last test. Guidelines for interpreting the tuberculin skin test are listed in Box 23-12. Prompt radiographic evaluation of all children with a positive TST reaction is recommended.

BOX 23-10 ■ Clinical Manifestations of Tuberculosis

May be asymptomatic or produce a broad range of symptoms:
  Fever
  Malaise
  Anorexia
  Weight loss
  Cough may or may not be present (progresses slowly over weeks
    to months)
  Aching pain and tightness in the chest
  Hemoptysis (rare)
With progression:
  Respiratory rate increases
  Poor expansion of lung on the affected side
  Diminished breath sounds and crackles
  Dullness to percussion
  Fever persists
  Generalized symptoms are manifested
  Pallor, anemia, weakness, and weight loss

> **⚠ NURSING ALERT**
>
> The American Academy of Pediatrics (2003) recommends that administration of the tuberculin skin test and interpretation of the results be performed and read by trained health care professionals.

The term *latent tuberculosis infection* (LTBI) is used to indicate infection in a person who has a positive TST, no physical findings of disease, and normal chest radiograph findings. The term *tuberculosis disease* is used when a child has clinical symptoms or radiographic manifestations caused by the *M. tuberculosis* organism. A diagnosis of LTBI or tuberculosis disease in a child is a sentinel event usually representing recent transmission of the *M. tuberculosis* organism.

BOX 23-11 ■ Tuberculin Skin Test (TST) Recommendations for Infants, Children, and Adolescents*

CHILDREN FOR WHOM IMMEDIATE TST IS INDICATED
Contacts of persons with confirmed or suspected contagious tuberculosis (contact investigation).
Children with radiographic or clinical findings suggesting tuberculosis disease.
Children immigrating from endemic countries (e.g., Asia, Middle East, Africa, Latin America).
Children with travel histories to endemic countries or significant contact with indigenous persons from such countries.

CHILDREN WHO SHOULD HAVE ANNUAL TST†
Children infected with human immunodeficiency virus (HIV).
Incarcerated adolescents.

CHILDREN WHO SOME EXPERTS RECOMMEND SHOULD BE TESTED EVERY 2 TO 3 YEARS†
Children with ongoing exposure to the following people: HIV-infected people, homeless people, residents of nursing homes, institutionalized adolescents or adults, users of illicit drugs, incarcerated adolescents or adults and migrant farm workers; foster children with exposure to adults in the preceding high-risk groups are included.

CHILDREN WHO SOME EXPERTS RECOMMEND SHOULD BE CONSIDERED FOR TST AT 4 TO 6 AND 11 TO 16 YEARS
Children whose parents immigrated (with unknown TST status) from regions of the world with high prevalence of tuberculosis;

continued potential exposure by travel to the endemic areas or household contact with persons from the endemic areas (with unknown TST status) should be an indication for repeat TST.

Children at Increased Risk for Progression of Infection to Disease
Children with other medical risk factors, including diabetes mellitus, chronic renal failure, malnutrition, and congenital or acquired immunodeficiencies deserve special consideration. Without recent exposure, these people are not at increased risk of acquiring tuberculosis infection. Underlying immune deficiencies associated with these conditions theoretically would enhance the possibility for progression to severe disease. Initial histories of potential exposure to tuberculosis should be included for all of these patients. If these histories or local epidemiologic factors suggest a possibility of exposure, immediate and periodic TST should be considered. **An initial TST should be performed before initiation of immunosuppressive therapy, including prolonged steroid administration, for any child with an underlying condition that necessitates immunosuppressive therapy.**

From American Academy of Pediatrics, Report of the Committee on Infectious Diseases: *2003 Red Book: report of the Committee on Infectious Diseases,* ed 26, Elk Grove Village, Il, 2003, The Academy.
*Bacille Calmette-Guérin (BCG) immunization is not a contraindication to tuberculin skin testing.
†Initial tuberculin skin testing is done at the time of diagnosis or circumstance, beginning at 3 months of age.

Therapeutic Management

Medical management of tuberculosis disease in children consists of adequate nutrition, chemotherapy, general supportive measures, prevention of unnecessary exposure to other infections that further compromise the body's defenses, prevention of reinfection, and sometimes surgical procedures.

Recommended drug therapy for treating tuberculosis disease includes combinations of isoniazid (INH), rifampin, and pyrazinamide (PZA). The American Academy of Pediatrics (2003) recommends a 6-month regimen consisting of INH, rifampin, and PZA given daily for the first 2 months, followed by INH and rifampin given 2 to 3 times a week by DOT (direct observation of therapy) for the remaining 4 months. DOT decreases the rates of relapse, treatment failures, and drug resistance and is recommended for treatment of children and adolescents with tuberculosis in the United States.

> **!NURSING ALERT**
>
> Direct observation of therapy means that a health care worker or other responsible, mutually agreed-on individual is present when medications are administered to the patient.

BOX 23-12 ■ Definition of Positive TST Results in Infants, Children, and Adolescents*

INDURATION ≥5 mm
Children in close contact with known or suspected contagious cases of tuberculosis disease
Children suspected to have tuberculosis disease:
   Findings on chest x-ray film consistent with active or previously active tuberculosis
   Clinical evidence of tuberculosis disease†
Children receiving immunosuppressive therapy‡ or immunosuppressive conditions, including HIV infection

INDURATION ≥10 mm
Children at increased risk of disseminated disease:
   Those younger than 4 years of age
   Those with other medical risk conditions, including Hodgkin disease, lymphoma, diabetes mellitus, chronic renal failure, or malnutrition
Children with increased exposure to tuberculosis disease:
   Those born, or whose parents were born, in high-prevalence regions of the world
   Those frequently exposed to adults who are HIV-infected, homeless, users of illicit drugs, residents of nursing homes, incarcerated or institutionalized, or migrant farm workers
   Those who travel to high-prevalence regions of the world

INDURATION ≥15 mm
Children 4 years of age or older without any risk factors

From American Academy of Pediatrics, Committee on Infectious Diseases: 2003 *Red Book: report of the Committee on Infectious Diseases*, ed 26, Elk Grove Village, Il, 2003, The Academy.
*These definitions apply regardless of previous Bacille Calmette-Guérin (BCG) immunization; erythema at TST site does not indicate a positive test result. TSTs should be read at 48 to 72 hours after placement.
†Evidence by physical examination or laboratory assessment that would include tuberculosis in the working differential diagnosis (e.g., meningitis).
‡Including immunosuppressive doses of corticosteroids.

When drug resistance is suspected, either ethambutol or an aminoglycoside is added to the therapeutic regimen until drug susceptibility results are available. Optimal therapy for tuberculosis in children with HIV infection has not been established, and consultation with a specialist is advised for HIV-infected children. Therapy should always include at least three drugs initially and be continued for at least 9 months. INH, rifampin, and PZA usually with ethambutol or an aminoglycoside should be given for at least the first 2 months. The three-drug regimen can be used after drug-resistant disease is excluded.

Preventive therapy is intended to keep latent infection from progressing and to prevent initial infection in persons in high-risk situations. INH given daily for 9 months is recommended for latent tuberculosis infection in children (American Academy of Pediatrics, 2003).

Surgical procedures may be required to remove the source of infection in tissues that are inaccessible to chemotherapy or that are destroyed by the disease. Orthopedic procedures may be performed for correction of bone deformities, and bronchoscopy may be done for removal of a tuberculous granulomatous polyp.

Prognosis.   Most children recover from primary TB infection and are often unaware of its presence. However, very young children have a higher incidence of disseminated disease. Tuberculosis is a serious disease during the first 2 years of life, during adolescence, and in children who are HIV-positive. Except in cases of tuberculous meningitis, death seldom occurs in treated children. Antibiotic therapy has decreased the death rate and the hematogenous spread from primary lesions.

Prevention.   The only definite means to prevent TB is to avoid contact with the tubercle bacillus. Maintaining an optimal state of health with adequate nutrition and avoiding fatigue and debilitating infections promote natural resistance but do not prevent infection. Pasteurization and routine testing of milk and elimination of diseased cattle have reduced the incidence of bovine tuberculosis.

Bacille Calmette-Guérin (BCG) vaccine is a live virus vaccine prepared from attenuated strains of bovine bacilli. In the United States, BCG vaccine is not routinely given and should be considered only in limited circumstances such as unavoidable risk of exposure to *M. tuberculosis* and failure or unfeasibility of other methods of control of tuberculosis.

Nursing Considerations

Children with TB receive their nursing care in ambulatory settings, outpatient departments, schools, and public health settings. Most children are not contagious and require only standard precautions. Children with no cough and negative sputum smears can be hospitalized on an open ward. However, airborne precautions and a negative-pressure room are required for children who are contagious and hospitalized with tuberculosis disease. Infection control for hospital personnel in contagious cases should include the use of a personally fitted air-purifying respirator (PAPR) for all patient contacts.

Children with tuberculosis can attend school or day care facilities if they are receiving chemotherapy. They can return to regular activities as soon as effective therapy has been instituted, adherence to therapy has been documented, and clinical symptoms have diminished. Children receiving chemotherapy for tuberculosis can receive measles and other age-appropriate live virus vaccines unless they are receiving high-dose corticosteroids, are severely ill, or have specific contraindications to immunization (American Academy of Pediatrics, 2003). Children with tuberculosis should also receive optimal nutrition and adequate rest.

Nurses assume several important roles in management of this disease, including assisting with radiographic examinations, performing skin tests, and obtaining specimens for laboratory examination. Skin tests must be performed correctly and the reaction determined in 48 to 72 hours. Sputum specimens are difficult or impossible to obtain from infants or young children, because they swallow mucus coughed from the lower respiratory tract. The best method for obtaining material for smears or culture is by *gastric washing* (i.e., aspiration of lavaged contents from the fasting stomach). The procedure is carried out and the specimen obtained early in the morning before the customary breakfast time.

Because the success of therapy depends on compliance with the drug regimen, parents are instructed about the importance and rationale for DOT. Case finding in the community and follow-up of known contacts—individuals from whom the affected child may have acquired the disease and persons who may have been exposed to the child with the disease—are essential control measures.

PULMONARY DYSFUNCTION CAUSED BY NONINFECTIOUS IRRITANTS

FOREIGN BODY ASPIRATION

Small children characteristically explore matter with their mouths and are prone to aspirate a foreign body (FB). FB aspiration can occur at any age but is most common in children 1 to 3 years of age. Severity is determined by the location, type of object aspirated, and extent of obstruction. For example, dry vegetable matter, such as a seed, nut, or piece of carrot or popcorn, that does not dissolve and that may swell when wet creates a particularly difficult problem. The high fat content of potato chips and peanuts may cause the added risk of lipoid pneumonia. "Fun foods" are the worst offenders in terms of potential for aspiration. Offending foods in the order of frequency of aspiration are hot dog, round candy, peanut or other nut, grape, cookie or biscuit, other meat, carrot, apple, and peanut butter.

A sharp or irritating object produces irritation and edema. A round, pliable object that does not break apart is more likely to occlude an airway than objects with different shapes. Latex balloons (uninflated, inflated, or in broken pieces) are especially hazardous, and a small piece of the pliable, impermeable latex can totally occlude the airway. A small object may cause little damage or pathologic changes, but objects of sufficient size to obstruct a passage can produce various changes, including atelectasis, emphysema, inflammation, and abscess.

Diagnostic Evaluation

The diagnosis of FB aspiration is suspected on the basis of the history and physical signs. Initially, an FB in the air passages produces choking, gagging, wheezing, or coughing. Laryngotracheal obstruction most commonly causes dyspnea, cough, stridor, and hoarseness because of decreased air entry. Cyanosis may occur if the obstruction becomes worse. Bronchial obstruction usually produces cough (frequently paroxysmal), wheezing, asymmetric breath sounds, decreased airway entry, and dyspnea. When an object is lodged in the larynx, the child is unable to speak or breathe. If the obstruction progresses, the child's face may become livid, and if the obstruction is total, the child can become unconscious and die of asphyxiation. If obstruction is partial, hours, days, or even weeks may pass without symptoms after the initial period. Secondary symptoms are related to the anatomic area in which the object is lodged and are usually caused by a persistent respiratory infection distal to the obstruction. FB should also be suspected in the presence of acute or chronic pulmonary lesions. Often, by the time secondary symptoms appear, the parents have forgotten the initial episode of coughing and gagging.

Radiographic examination reveals opaque FBs but is of limited use in localizing vegetable matter. Bronchoscopy is required for definitive diagnosis of objects in the larynx and trachea. Fluoroscopic examination is valuable in detecting and localizing FBs in the bronchi.

Therapeutic Management

FB aspiration may result in life-threatening airway obstruction, especially in infants because of the small diameters of their airways. Current recommendations for the emergency treatment of the choking child include the use of abdominal thrusts for children older than 1 year of age and back blows and chest thrusts for children younger than 1 year of age (see Airway Obstruction, p. 836).

A foreign body is rarely coughed up spontaneously. Most frequently, it must be removed instrumentally by endoscopy. This procedure should be carried out as quickly as possible, because the progressive local inflammatory process triggered by the foreign material hampers removal. A chemical pneumonia soon develops, and vegetable matter begins to macerate within a few days, causing it to be even more difficult to remove. After removal of the FB, the child is placed in a high-humidity atmosphere and any secondary infection is treated with appropriate antibiotics.

Nursing Considerations

A major role of nurses caring for a child who has aspirated an FB is to recognize the signs of FB aspiration and implement immediate measures to relieve the obstruction.

All persons working with children must be prepared to deal effectively with aspiration of an FB. Choking on food or other material should not be fatal. Back blows and the Heimlich maneuver are simple procedures that can be used by both health professionals and lay persons to save lives. It is the obligation of nurses to learn these techniques and to teach them to parents and other groups (see Fig. 23-8). To aid a child who is choking, nurses must recognize the signs of distress. Not every child who gags or coughs while eating is truly choking.

Prevention. Small children should not be allowed access to small objects that they might place in their mouth. Rubber balloons are high-risk items for children; Mylar balloons are the only safe variety for children. Aluminum tabs from soft drink cans, adhesive bandages, plastic tabs from protective coverings on containers, and price tags on clothing can all become FBs. Peanut butter, a staple in the diet of children, should never be given to a child unless it is spread thinly on bread or a cracker. A spoonful of peanut butter can obstruct the airway and stick to mucous membranes, becoming difficult or impossible for the child to dislodge.

Nurses are in a position to teach prevention in a variety of settings. They can educate parents about the hazards of FB aspiration in relation to the developmental level of their children and encourage them to teach their children safety. Parents should be cautioned about behaviors that their children might imitate (e.g., holding foreign objects, such as pins, nails, and toothpicks, in their lips or mouth). Prevention based on the child's age is discussed in Chapters 10 and 12.

ASPIRATION PNEUMONIA

Aspiration pneumonia occurs when food, secretions, inert materials, volatile compounds, or liquids enter the lung and cause inflammation and a chemical pneumonitis. Aspiration of fluid or foods is a particular hazard in the child who has difficulty with swallowing or is unable to swallow because of paralysis, weakness, debility, congenital anomalies, or absent cough reflex or the child who is force-fed, especially while crying or breathing rapidly.

Nursing Considerations

Care of the child with aspiration pneumonia is the same as that described for the child with pneumonia from other causes. However, the major thrust of nursing care is aimed at prevention of aspiration. Proper feeding techniques should be carried out for weak, debilitated, and uncooperative children, and preventive measures should be used to prevent aspiration of any material that might enter the nasopharynx.

Oily nose drops and oil-based vitamin preparations are not appropriate for infants and small children. Solvents, lighter fluid, and other hydrocarbon substances should be kept away from older infants and small children, who are apt to put anything in their mouths and who may be attracted by the slightly sweet smell. Use of talcum powder should be avoided. If used, careful application (placing it on the caregiver's hand and then the child's skin) and proper storage are essential.

Infants and debilitated children should be positioned on the right side after feedings to minimize the possibility of aspirating vomitus or regurgitated feeding.

ACUTE (ADULT) RESPIRATORY DISTRESS SYNDROME

Acute (adult) respiratory distress syndrome (ARDS) is recognized in children, as well as adults, and has been associated with clinical conditions and injuries such as sepsis, viral pneumonia, smoke inhalation, and near-drowning. It is a syndrome characterized by respiratory distress and hypoxemia that occur within 72 hours of a serious injury or surgery in a person with previously normal lungs.

The hallmark of ARDS is increased permeability of the alveolar-capillary membrane that results in pulmonary edema. The lungs become stiff, gas diffusion is impaired, and eventually there is bronchiolar mucosal swelling and congestive atelectasis. Surfactant secretion is reduced, and the atelectasis and fluid-filled alveoli provide an excellent medium for bacterial growth. The criteria for diagnosis of ARDS in children are an acute antecedent illness or injury, acute respiratory distress or failure, no evidence of prior cardiopulmonary disease, and diffuse bilateral infiltrates evidenced on chest radiography.

Treatment involves supportive measures, such as prevention of infection, maintenance of vascular volume and hydration, and cardiac output, adequate nutrition, comfort measures, and psychologic support. Definitive therapy is directed toward improvement of oxygenation. The use of endotracheal intubation and positive end-expiratory pressure (PEEP) may be required to ensure maximum oxygen delivery. Recent advances in the treatment of ARDS include (1) the use of lung-protective ventilator strategies, permissive hypercapnia, inhaled nitric oxide, high-frequency ventilation, and extracorporeal life support (Redding, 2001).

Prognosis. In spite of advances in treating ARDS, mortality in children varies greatly. The precipitating disorder influences the outcome; the worst prognosis is associated with uncontrolled sepsis, bone marrow transplantation, cancer, and multisystem involvement with hepatic failure.

Nursing care involves careful monitoring of cardiac output, heart rate, perfusion, capillary filling, and urine output, as well as assessment of respiratory status. Blood gas analysis and pulse oximetry are important evaluation tools. Respiratory distress is a frightening situation for both the child and the parents, and attention to their psychologic needs is a major element in the care of these children.

SMOKE INHALATION INJURY

A number of noxious substances that may be inhaled are toxic to humans. They are primarily products of incomplete combustion and cause more deaths from fires than flame injuries. The severity of the injury depends on the nature of the substances generated by the material burned, whether the victim is confined in a closed space, and the duration of contact with the smoke. Smoke inhalation results in three types of injury: heat, chemical, and systemic.

Heat injury involves thermal injury to the upper airway. Air has low specific heat; therefore, the injury goes no further than the upper airway. Reflex closure of the glottis prevents injury to the lower airway.

Chemical injury involves gases that may be generated during the combustion of materials such as clothing, furniture, and floor coverings. These synthetic materials are especially toxic. Irritant gases such as nitrous oxide or carbon dioxide combine with water in the lungs to form corrosive acids; aldehydes cause denaturation of proteins, cellular damage, and edema of pulmonary tissues.

Possible inhalation injury is suspected when there is a history of flames in a closed space whether burns are present or not. Sooty material around the nose or in the sputum, singed nasal hairs, or mucosal burns of the nose, lips, mouth, or throat are all signs that the affected person demands observation for possible pulmonary injury from inhalants. A hoarse voice and cough, inspiratory and expiratory stridor, and signs of respiratory distress are further evidence of airway involvement.

Systemic injury occurs from gases that are nontoxic to the airways (e.g., carbon monoxide [CO], hydrogen cyanide). However, these gases cause injury and death by interfering with or inhibiting cellular respiration. CO is responsible for more than half of all fatal inhalation poisonings in the United States. CO is a colorless, odorless gas with an affinity for hemoglobin 230 times greater than that of oxygen. When it enters the bloodstream, CO combines readily with hemoglobin to form carboxyhemoglobin (COHb). Because it is released less readily, tissue hypoxia reaches dangerous levels before oxygen is available to meet tissue needs.

> **⬤ NURSING ALERT**
>
> The oxygen saturation (Sao_2) obtained by pulse oximetry will be normal because the device measures only oxygenated and deoxygenated hemoglobin; it does not measure dysfunctional hemoglobin, such as COHb.

Accidental CO poisoning is most often a result of exposure to fumes of heaters or smoke from structural fires, although poorly ventilated recreational vehicles with improperly operated or maintained gas lamps or stoves and cooking in underventilated areas with charcoal grills or hibachis are also frequent causes. CO is produced by incomplete combustion of carbon or carbonaceous material such as wood or charcoal.

The signs and symptoms of CO poisoning are secondary to tissue hypoxia and vary with the level of COHb. Mild manifestations include headache, visual disturbances, irritability, and nausea, whereas more severe intoxication causes confusion, hallucinations, ataxia, and coma. The bright, cherry red lips and skin often described are less often observed; pallor and cyanosis are seen more frequently.

Therapeutic Management

Treatment of children with smoke inhalation injury is largely symptomatic. The most widely accepted treatment is placing the child on humidified 100% oxygen as quickly as possible and monitoring for signs of respiratory distress and impending failure. Baseline arterial blood gases and COHb levels are obtained. Surprisingly, arterial oxygen partial pressure (Pao_2) may be within normal limits unless there is marked respiratory depression. If CO poisoning is confirmed, 100% oxygen is continued until COHb levels fall to the nontoxic range of about 10%. The role of hyperbaric oxygen remains controversial.

Respiratory distress may occur early in the course of smoke inhalation as a result of hypoxia, or patients who are breathing well on admission may suddenly develop respiratory distress. Intubation or tracheostomy equipment should be available at the bedside. Transient edema of the airways can occur at any level in the tracheobronchial tree. Assessment and localization of the obstruction should be accomplished before severe swelling of the head, neck, or oropharynx occurs. Intubation is often necessary when (1) severe burns in the area of the nose, mouth, and face increase the likelihood of developing oropharyngeal edema and obstruction; (2) vocal cord edema causes obstruction; (3) the patient has difficulty handling secretions; and (4) progressive respiratory distress requires artificial ventilation. Controversy surrounds tracheostomy, but many prefer this procedure when the obstruction is proximal to the larynx and reserve nasotracheal intubation for lower tract involvement.

Corticosteroids have no established benefit and may increase the risk of infection. Prophylactic antibiotics offer no benefit and may lead to the development of resistant organisms (Sockrider, 1999).

Nursing Considerations

Nursing care of the child with inhalation injury is the same as that for any child with respiratory distress. Vital signs and other respiratory assessments are performed frequently, and the pulmonary status is carefully observed and maintained. Pulmonary physiotherapy is often part of the therapy, as well as mechanical ventilation if needed.

In addition to observation and management of the physical aspects of inhalation injury, the nurse also deals with the psychologic needs of a frightened child and distraught parents. As with any accidental injury, the parents feel overwhelming guilt, even when the injury occurred through no fault of their own. Parents need support, reassurance, and information regarding the child's condition, treatment, and progress.

PASSIVE SMOKING

Numerous investigations indicate that parental smoking is an important cause of morbidity in children. Children exposed to passive or environmental tobacco smoke have an increased number of respiratory illnesses, increased respiratory symptoms (i.e., cough, phlegm, and wheeze), and reduced performance on pulmonary function tests. Indoor exposure to environmental tobacco smoke has been linked to asthma in children (Morkjaroenpong and others, 2002). Among children with asthma, there is an association between parental cigarette smoking and asthma exacerbations, trips to the emergency department, medication use, and impaired recovery after hospitalization for acute asthma (Abulhosm and others, 1997). Maternal cigarette smoking is associated with increased respiratory symptoms and illnesses in children; decreased fetal growth; increased deliveries of low birth weight, preterm, and stillborn infants; and a greater incidence of sudden infant death syndrome (SIDS). Exposure to passive smoking during childhood may also contribute to the development of chronic lung disease in the adult.

Nursing Considerations

Nurses must provide information about the hazards of environmental smoke exposure in all their interactions with children and their family members. This information is especially important for children with respiratory and allergic illnesses.* In families where smokers refuse to quit, house rules should be established for reducing smoke in the child's environment (see Family Home Care box). Nurses should set an example for children and families and become advocates for "no smoking" ordinances in public places and prohibition of advertising tobacco products in the media.

LONG-TERM RESPIRATORY DYSFUNCTION

ASTHMA

Asthma is a chronic inflammatory disorder of the airways in which many cells (mast cells, eosinophils, and T lymphocytes) play a role. In susceptible children, inflammation causes recurrent episodes of wheezing, breathlessness, chest tightness, and cough, especially at night or in the early morning. These asthma episodes are associated with airflow limitation or obstruction that is reversible either spontaneously or with treatment. The inflammation also causes an increase in bronchial hyperresponsiveness to a variety of stimuli (National Asthma Education and Prevention Program, 1997).

Asthma is classified into four categories based on the symptom indicators of disease severity. These categories are mild intermittent, mild persistent, moderate persistent, and severe persistent. The mild intermittent category has the least number of symptoms; symptoms increase in frequency or intensity until the last category of severe persistent asthma (Box 23-13). These categories provide a stepwise approach to the pharmacologic management, environmental control, and educational interventions needed for each category (National Asthma Education and Prevention Program, 1997).

Asthma prevalence, morbidity, and mortality are increasing in the United States and other nations. These increases may result from increasing air pollution, poor access to medical care, or underdiagnosis and undertreatment. Asthma is the most common chronic disease of childhood, is the primary cause of school absences, and is responsible for a major proportion of pediatric admissions to emergency departments and hospitals.

Etiology

Studies of children with asthma indicate that allergy influences both the persistence and severity of the disease. Atopy, the genetic predisposition for the development of an

---

*For a copy of the EPA report *Respiratory health effects of passive smoking,* contact **CERI,** US EPA, 26 West Martin Luther King Drive, Cincinnati, OH 45268; (513) 569-7562.

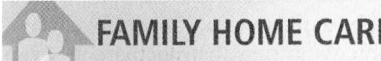

FAMILY HOME CARE

House Rules for Smoking Households

Maintain a smoke-free home.
Do not smoke around children.
Restrict smoking to an isolated, outdoor area.
Do not smoke in motor vehicles with children.
Do not smoke in rooms children use.
Do not allow visitors to smoke in the home.

IgE-mediated response to common aeroallergens, is the strongest predictor for developing asthma. Although allergens play an important role in asthma, 20% to 40% of children with asthma have no evidence of allergic disease (Eggleston, 1999). In addition to allergens, other substances and conditions can serve as triggers for asthma episodes (Box 23-14). Asthma is a complex disorder involving biochemical, immunologic, infectious, endocrine, and psychologic factors.

Pathophysiology

There is general agreement that inflammation contributes to increased airway reactivity in asthma. The mechanisms contributing to airway inflammation are multiple and involve a number of different pathways. However, recognition of the importance of inflammation has made the use of antiinflammatory agents a key component of asthma therapy.

Another important component of asthma is bronchospasm and obstruction. The mechanisms responsible for the obstructive symptoms in asthma include (Fig. 23-3): (1) inflammation and edema of the mucous membranes, (2) accumulation of tenacious secretions from mucous glands, and (3) spasm of the smooth muscle of the bronchi and bronchioles, which decreases the caliber of the bronchioles.

BOX 23-13 ■ Asthma Severity Classification in Children 5 Years of Age and Older: Clinical Features Before Treatment or Adequate Control*

STEP 4: SEVERE PERSISTENT ASTHMA
Continual symptoms
Frequent nighttime symptoms
Peak expiratory flow (PEF) or forced expiratory volume in 1 second (FEV_1) is ≤60% of predicted value
PEF variability >30%

STEP 3: MODERATE PERSISTENT ASTHMA
Daily symptoms
Nighttime symptoms >1 night / week
PEF or FEV_1 is >60% to <80% of predicted value
PEF variability >30%

STEP 2: MILD PERSISTENT ASTHMA
Symptoms >2 times a week, but <1 time a day
Nighttime symptoms >2 times a month
PEF or FEV_1 is ≥80% of predicted value
PEF variability 20% to 30%

STEP 1: MILD INTERMITTENT ASTHMA
Symptoms <2 times a week
Nighttime symptoms <2 times a month
PEF or FEV_1 is ≥80% of predicted value
PEF variability <20%

From National Asthma Education and Prevention Program: *Quick Reference NAEPP Expert Panel report: guidelines for the diagnosis and management of asthma: Update on Selected Topics 2002,* NIH pub no 02-5075, Bethesda, Md, 2003, National Heart, Lung, and Blood Institute.
*The presence of one clinical feature of severity is sufficient to place a patient in that category. An individual should be assigned to the most severe grade in which any feature occurs. The characteristics in this table are general and may overlap because asthma is highly variable. An individual's classification may change over time.

BOX 23-14 ■ Triggers Tending to Precipitate or Aggravate Asthmatic Exacerbations

Allergens
   Outdoor: trees, shrubs, weeds, grasses, molds, pollens, air pollution, spores
   Indoor: dust or dust mites, mold, cockroach antigen
Irritants: tobacco smoke, wood smoke, odors, sprays
Exposure to occupational chemicals
Exercise
Cold air
Changes in weather or temperature
Environmental change: moving to new home, starting new school, etc.
Colds and infections
Animals: cats, dogs, rodents, horses
Medications: aspirin, nonsteroidal antiinflammatory drugs (NSAIDs), antibiotics, β-blockers
Strong emotions: fear, anger, laughing, crying
Conditions: gastroesophageal reflux, tracheoesophageal fistula
Food additives: sulfite preservatives
Foods: nuts, milk/dairy products
Endocrine factors: menses, pregnancy, thyroid disease

BOX 23-15 ■ Clinical Manifestations of Asthma

COUGH
Hacking, paroxysmal, irritative, and nonproductive
Becomes rattling and productive of frothy, clear, gelatinous sputum

RESPIRATORY-RELATED SIGNS
Shortness of breath
Prolonged expiratory phase
Audible wheeze
May have a malar flush and red ears
Lips deep, dark red color
May progress to cyanosis of nail beds or circumoral cyanosis
Restlessness
Apprehension
Sweating may be prominent as the attack progresses
Older children may sit upright with shoulders in a hunched-over position, hands on the bed or chair, and arms braced
May speak with short, panting, broken phrases

CHEST
Hyperresonance on percussion
Coarse, loud breath sounds
Wheezes throughout the lung fields
Prolonged expiration
Crackles
Generalized inspiratory and expiratory wheezing; increasingly high pitched

WITH REPEATED EPISODES
Barrel chest
Elevated shoulders
Use of accessory muscles of respiration
Facial appearance: flattened malar bones, circles beneath the eyes, narrow nose, prominent upper teeth

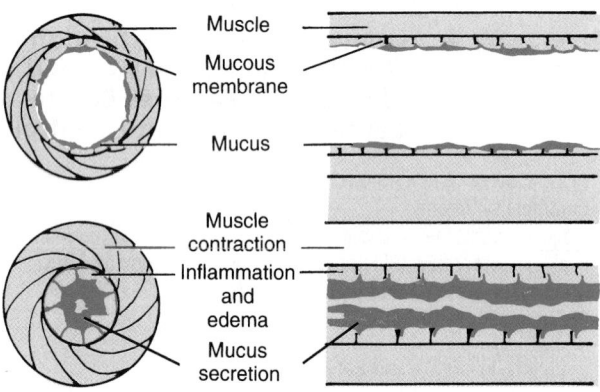

FIG. 23-3 ■ Mechanisms of obstruction in asthma.

> **! NURSING ALERT**
>
> Airflow is determined by the size of the airway lumen, degree of bronchial wall edema, mucus production, smooth muscle contraction, and muscle hypertrophy.

Bronchial constriction is a normal reaction to foreign stimuli, but in the child with asthma it is abnormally severe, producing impaired respiratory function. The smooth muscle arranged in spiral bundles around the airway causes narrowing and shortening of the airway, which significantly increases airway resistance to airflow. Because the bronchi normally dilate and elongate during inspiration and contract and shorten on expiration, the respiratory difficulty is more pronounced during the expiratory phase of respiration.

Increased resistance in the airway causes forced expiration through the narrowed lumen. The volume of air trapped in the lungs increases as airways are functionally closed at a point between the alveoli and the lobar bronchi.

This trapping of gas forces the individual to breathe at higher and higher lung volumes. Consequently, the person with asthma fights to inspire sufficient air. This expenditure of effort for breathing causes fatigue, decreased respiratory effectiveness, and increased oxygen consumption. The inspiration occurring at higher lung volumes hyperinflates the alveoli and reduces the effectiveness of the cough. As the severity of obstruction increases, there is a reduced alveolar ventilation with carbon dioxide retention, hypoxemia, respiratory acidosis, and, eventually, respiratory failure.

Diagnostic Evaluation

The classic manifestations of asthma are dyspnea, wheezing, and coughing. However, children may experience symptoms that range from acute episodes of shortness of breath, wheezing, and cough followed by a quiet period to a relatively continuous pattern of chronic symptoms that fluctuate in severity (Box 23-15). An attack may develop gradually or appear abruptly and may be preceded by a URI. The age of the child is often a significant factor, because the first attack frequently occurs between ages 3 and 8 years. In infancy an attack usually follows a respiratory infection. Some children may experience a prodromal itching at the front of the neck or over the upper part of the back just before an attack.

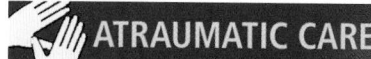

GUIDELINES

Interpreting Peak Expiratory Flow Rates*

- *Green (80% to 100% of personal best)* signals all clear. Asthma is under reasonably good control. No symptoms are present, and the routine treatment plan for maintaining control can be followed.
- *Yellow (50% to 79% of personal best)* signals caution. Asthma is not well controlled. An acute exacerbation may be present. Maintenance therapy may need to be increased. Call the practitioner if the child stays in this zone.
- *Red (below 50% of personal best)* signals a medical alert. Severe airway narrowing may be occurring. A short-acting bronchodilator should be administered. Notify the practitioner if the peak expiratory flow rate (PEFR) does not return immediately and stay in yellow or green zones.

*These zones are guidelines only. Specific zones and management should be individualized for each child.

! NURSING ALERT

Shortness of breath with air movement in the chest restricted to the point of absent breath sounds accompanied by a sudden rise in respiratory rate is an ominous sign indicating ventilatory failure and imminent asphyxia.

The diagnosis is determined primarily on the basis of clinical manifestations, history, physical examination, and, to a lesser extent, laboratory tests. Radiographic examinations are used primarily to rule out other diseases and to evaluate coexisting disease. Generally, chronic cough in the absence of infection or diffuse wheezing during the expiratory phase of respiration is sufficient to establish a diagnosis.

Pulmonary function tests (PFTs) provide an objective method of evaluating the presence and degree of lung disease, as well as the response to therapy. Spirometry can generally be performed reliably on children by the age of 5 or 6 years and includes either the traditional and simple mechanical spirometer often used in clinics, offices, and the home or new computerized versions. Another key measurement is the *peak expiratory flow rate (PEFR),* which measures the maximum flow of air that can be forcefully exhaled in 1 second. PEFR is measured in liters per minute using a *peak expiratory flow meter (PEFM).* Three zones of measurement are typically used to interpret PEFR. The zone system is patterned after a traffic light to make the categories easy to understand and remember (see Guidelines box). Each child needs to establish his or her *personal best value.* A personal best value should be established during a 2- to 3-week period when the child's asthma is stable. During this period, the child records their PEFR at least twice a day. After the personal best value has been established, the child's current PEFR on any occasion can be compared with the personal best value.

Skin testing is useful in identifying specific allergens. Information obtained by the puncture technique correlate better than intracutaneous tests with symptoms and measurements of specific IgE antibody (see Atraumatic Care box). *Provocative testing,* direct exposure of the mucous

ATRAUMATIC CARE

Skin Testing

To help allay children's fears of skin tests, give them a careful and thorough explanation of what is to be done and how many "pricks" are involved (usually series of 8 on each site, for a total of 30 tests). Very young, anxious patients may benefit from one prick on the arm to demonstrate how it feels. The skin is pierced with a stylet rather than a regular needle and syringe; then a drop of allergen is placed on the site. Another helpful strategy is to have the child count off the number of pricks with the nurse as a distraction. For intradermal skin injection, EMLA, a topical anesthetic, reduces or eliminates pain without altering test results.

membranes to a suspected antigen in increasing concentrations, helps to identify inhaled allergens. The radioallergosorbent test (RAST) helps identify antigens against various foods and is often useful in determining appropriate therapy.

Therapeutic Management

The overall goal of asthma management is to prevent disability, to minimize physical and psychologic morbidity, and to assist the child in living as normal and happy a life as possible. This includes facilitating the child's social adjustments in the family, school, and community and normal participation in recreational activities and sports. To accomplish these goals, the child and his or her family need to recognize symptoms, learn how to manage asthma exacerbations, visit a health care provider regularly, implement appropriate therapy, and identify and eliminate environmental irritants and allergens. Adherence to the prescribed regimen is essential to successful management.

Allergen Control.   Nonpharmacologic therapy is aimed at the prevention and reduction of exposure to airborne allergens and irritants. *House dust mites* and other components of house dust are one of the most frequent agents identified in children allergic to inhalants. The most important method to eliminate dust mites is to keep the humidity in the house lower than 50%, the level below which dust mites do not survive (Kaliner, Spector, and Wenzel, 1999). The *cockroach,* another common household inhabitant, is an important allergen in many locations. Exterminating live cockroaches, carefully cleaning kitchen floors and cabinets, putting food away after eating, and taking trash out in the evening are essential measures to control cockroaches. The mouse allergen is the most recent allergen to be identified in the homes of inner-city children with asthma. Researchers now recommend aggressive extermination of not only cockroaches, but also mice (Phipatanakul and others, 2000). Other recommendations for controlling allergens are found in the Family Home Care box on p. 816.

Skin testing identifies specific allergens and steps are taken to eliminate or avoid the offending allergens. Often, simply removing the offending environmental allergens or irritants (e.g., removal of a dog or cat from the home of a child sensitive to animal dander) will decrease the frequency

FAMILY HOME CARE

"Allergy-Proofing" the Home and Community

Keep humidity between 30% and 50%; use dehumidifier or air conditioner if available; keep air conditioners clean and free of mold; do not use vaporizers or humidifiers.

Encase pillows in zippered allergen-impermeable covers or wash pillows in hot water (at least 54.4° C [130° F]) every week.

Encase mattress and box springs in zippered allergen-impermeable cover.

Use foam rubber mattress and pillows or Dacron pillows and synthetic blankets.

Wash bed linens every 7 to 10 days in hot water (at least 54.4° C).

Encase polyester comforters in allergen-impermeable covers or wash in hot water (at least 54.4° C) every week; if possible, do not use comforters and use cotton blankets.

Do not use a canopy above the bed; children should not sleep on the bottom bunk of a bunk bed.

Store nothing under the bed; keep clothing in a closet with the door shut.

Use washable window shades; avoid heavy curtains; if curtains are used, launder them frequently.

Remove all carpeting if possible; if not possible, vacuum carpet once or twice a week while the child wears a mask; have child remain out of the room while vacuuming occurs and for 30 minutes after vacuuming.

If possible, use a central vacuum cleaner with a collecting bag outside of the home or use cleaner filters (e.g., high-efficiency particulate air [HEPA] filters).

Have air and heating ducts cleaned annually; change or clean filters monthly; cover heating vents with filter material (e.g., cheesecloth) to prevent circulation of dust, especially when heat is turned on after summer.

Remove unnecessary furniture, rugs, stuffed or real animals, toys, books, upholstered furniture, plants, aquariums, and wall hangings from child's room.

Use wipeable furniture (wood, plastic, vinyl, or leather) in place of upholstered furniture; avoid rattan or wicker furniture.

Cover walls with washable paint or wallpaper.

Limit child's exposure to animals (rabbits, gerbils, hamsters) at school; teach child to stay away from zoos, petting farms, and neighbor's pets.

Change child's clothes after playing outdoors; wash child's hair nightly if child is outside and pollen count is high.

Keep child indoors while lawn is being mowed, bushes/trees are being trimmed, or pollen count is high.

Keep windows and doors closed during pollen season; use air conditioner if possible or go to places that are air conditioned, such as libraries and shopping malls, when the weather is hot.

Wet-mop bare floors weekly; wet-dust and clean child's room weekly; child should not be present during cleaning activities.

Wash showers and shower curtains with bleach or Lysol at least once a month.

Limit or avoid child's exposure to tobacco and wood smoke; do not allow cigarette smoking in the house or car; select day care centers, play areas, and shopping malls that are smoke free.

Avoid odors or sprays (e.g., perfumes, talcum powder, room deodorizers, chalk dust at school, fresh paint, cleaning solutions).

Avoid cellar (basement) as a play area if it is damp, and use a dehumidifier in damp basement.

Cover all food, including pet food, and put food away in cabinets.

Store garbage in closed containers.

Use pesticide sprays, roach bait traps, and boric acid powder to kill cockroaches; if living in an apartment or adjacent housing, encourage neighbors to work together to get rid of cockroaches and mice.

Repair leaking or dripping faucets; seal cracks and crevices in cabinets and pantry areas.

---

of asthma episodes. Dehumidifiers or air conditioners control nonspecific factors that trigger an episode, such as extremes of temperature.

Drug Therapy.   Pharmacologic therapy is used to prevent and control asthma symptoms, reduce the frequency and severity of asthma exacerbations, and reverse airflow obstruction. A stepwise approach is recommended based on the severity of the child's asthma. Because inflammation is considered an early and persistent feature of asthma, therapy is directed toward long-term suppression of inflammation.

Asthma medications are categorized into two general classes: *long-term control medications (preventor medicines)* to achieve and maintain control of inflammation and *quick-relief medications (rescue medications)* to treat symptoms and exacerbations (National Asthma Education and Prevention Program, 2002).

Many asthma medications are given by inhalation with a nebulizer or a *metered-dose inhaler (MDI)*. The MDI should always be attached to a spacer when an inhaled corticosteroid is administered to prevent yeast infections in the mouth. Spacers are also important for children who have difficulty coordinating or learning proper inhalation technique (Togger and Brenner, 2001). Most pharmaceutical companies are currently striving to produce inhalers that do not contain chlorofluorocarbons (CFCs) as the propellant because CFCs have been linked to damage and depletion of the earth's ozone level. Several currently available CFC-free MDI devices, such as the Diskus inhaler and the Turbuhaler, use dry powder. These devices are breath-activated, and the child needs to inhale as quickly and deeply as possible to use them effectively. Infants and very young children who have difficulty using MDIs or other inhalers can receive their asthma medications via a *nebulizer.* When this device is used, the medication is mixed with saline and nebulized with compressed air. Children are instructed to breathe normally with the mouth open to provide a direct route to the trachea.

Corticosteroids are antiinflammatory drugs used to treat reversible airflow obstruction and to control symptoms and reduce bronchial hyperreactivity in chronic asthma. Corticosteroids may be administered parenterally, orally, or by inhalation. Oral medications are metabolized slowly, with an onset of action up to 3 hours after administration and peak effectiveness occurring within 6 to 12 hours. Oral systemic steroids may be given for short periods of time (i.e.,

3- or 10-day "bursts") to gain prompt control of inadequately controlled persistent asthma or to manage severe persistent asthma. These drugs should be given in the lowest effective dose. Long-term use poses the risk of adverse effects, such as osteoporosis, hypertension, Cushing syndrome, impaired immune mechanisms, and hypothalamic-pituitary-adrenal suppression (National Asthma Education and Prevention Program, 2002).

Inhaled steroids are used for long-term prevention of symptoms, as well as suppression, control, and reversal of inflammation. These medications have few side effects (cough, dysphonia, and oral thrush). There is strong evidence that these drugs improve the long-term outcomes for children of all ages with mild or moderate persistent asthma (National Asthma Education and Prevention Program, 2002). A recent study also indicated that regular use of low-dose inhaled corticosteroids is associated with a decreased risk of death from asthma (Suissa and others, 2000). Evidence from clinical trials that followed children for 6 years indicate that the use of inhaled corticosteroids at recommended doses does not have long-term significant effects on growth, bone mineral density, ocular toxicity, or suppression of the adrenal/pituitary axis (National Asthma Education and Prevention Program, 2002). However, primary care providers should monitor the growth of children and adolescents taking corticosteroids frequently (at least every 3 to 6 months) to assess the systemic effects of these drugs and make appropriate reductions in dosages or changes to other types of asthma therapy when necessary (Twarog, 1998).

Cromolyn sodium is a nonsteroidal antiinflammatory drug (NSAID) for asthma. It stabilizes mast cell membranes, inhibits activation and release of mediators from eosinophil and epithelial cells, and inhibits the acute airway narrowing after exposure to exercise, cold dry air, and sulfur dioxide. There is no way to reliably predict whether a child will respond to the drug. Cromolyn sodium has minimal side effects (occasional coughing on inhalation of the powder formulation) and may be given via nebulizer or MDI. *Nedocromil sodium* is another drug used for maintenance therapy in asthma. This drug has both antiallergic and antiinflammatory properties and few side effects.

β-Adrenergic agonists (primarily *albuterol, metaproterenol,* and *terbutaline*) are used for treatment of acute exacerbations and for the prevention of exercise-induced bronchospasm. They can be given via inhalation or as oral or parenteral preparations. The inhaled drug has a more rapid onset of action than the oral form. Inhalation also reduces troublesome systemic side effects: irritability, tremor, nervousness, and insomnia.

Inhaled β-adrenergic agents should not be taken more than three to four times daily for acute symptoms. *Salmeterol (Serevent)* is a long-acting bronchodilator that is used twice a day. This drug is added to antiinflammatory therapy and used for long-term prevention of symptoms, especially nighttime symptoms, and exercise-induced bronchospasm.

Methylxanthines, principally *theophylline,* have been used for decades to relieve symptoms and prevent asthma attacks. Theophylline, however, is now considered a third-line agent and unnecessary for treating asthma exacerbations. Theophylline may be taken IV, IM, orally, or rectally (seldom used). The drug is also available in sustained-release oral form. In addition to its bronchodilator effect, theophylline is a central respiratory stimulant and increases respiratory muscle contractility.

When theophylline is used, serum concentrations must be monitored. Therapeutic effects are maintained at plasma levels between 5 to 15 μg/mL. Maximum levels of 15 μg/mL are recommended for outpatient care (Eggleston, 1999).

> ### ❗ NURSING ALERT
> Theophylline toxicity can occur with serum levels 20 μg/mL or greater. Side effects from theophylline include nausea, vomiting, headache, irritability, and insomnia. Early signs of toxicity are nausea, tachycardia, and irritability; seizures and dysrhythmias occur at blood theophylline levels greater than 30 μg/mL.

Leukotriene Modifiers.   Leukotrienes are mediators of inflammation that cause increases in airway hyperresponsiveness. Leukotriene modifiers (such as zafirlukast, Zileuton, and montelukast sodium) block inflammatory and bronchospasm effects. These drugs are not used to treat acute episodes, but are given orally in combination with β-agonists and steroids to provide long-term control and prevention of symptoms in mild persistent asthma (Fost and Spahn, 1998).

Recently, the Food and Drug Administration approved the drug, omalizumab (Xolair), for treatment of asthma in patients older than 12 years of age. Omalizumab is a monoclonal antibody that blocks the binding of IgE to mast cells. Blocking this interaction eventually inhibits the inflammation that is associated with asthma. Because many patients with asthma are atopic and possess specific IgE antibodies to allergens responsible for airway inflammation, this drug is a promising adjunct to the treatment of asthma. The drug is administered once or twice a month via subcutaneous injection. Clinical trials of the drug indicate that it can be an effective therapy for patients with symptomatic moderate to severe allergic asthma that is poorly controlled with inhaled corticosteroids (Rosenwasser and Nash, 2003).

Exercise.   *Exercise-induced bronchospasm (EIB)* is an acute, reversible, usually self-terminating airway obstruction that develops during or after vigorous activity, reaches its peak 5 to 10 minutes after stopping the activity, and usually stops in another 20 to 30 minutes. Patients with EIB have cough, shortness of breath, chest pain or tightness, wheezing, and endurance problems during exercise, but an exercise challenge test in a laboratory is necessary to make the diagnosis.

The problem is rare in activities that require short bursts of energy (e.g., baseball, sprints, gymnastics, skiing) and more common in those that involve endurance exercise (e.g., soccer, basketball, distance running). Swimming is well tolerated by children with EIB, because they are breathing air fully saturated with moisture and because of the type of breathing required in swimming. Exhaling under water is beneficial because it prolongs expiration and increases the end-expiratory pressure within the respiratory tract (essentially pursed-lip breathing).

Children with asthma are often excluded from exercise by parents, teachers, and practitioners, as well as by the children themselves, because they are reluctant to provoke an attack. However, this practice can seriously hamper peer interaction and physical health. Exercise is advantageous for children with asthma, and most children can participate in activities at school and in sports with minimal difficulty, provided their asthma is under control. Participation should be evaluated on an individual basis. Appropriate prophylactic treatment with β-adrenergic agents or cromolyn sodium before exercise will usually permit full participation in strenuous exertion.

Chest Physiotherapy. Chest physiotherapy (CPT) includes breathing exercises and physical training. These therapies help produce physical and mental relaxation, improve posture, strengthen respiratory musculature, and develop more efficient patterns of breathing. For the motivated child, breathing exercises and controlled breathing are of value in preventing overinflation and improving efficiency of the cough. However, CPT is not recommended during acute, uncomplicated exacerbations of asthma.

Hyposensitization. The role of hyposensitization in childhood asthma has become controversial. In the past, immunotherapy was used for seasonal allergies and when single substances were identified as the offending allergen. It is not recommended for allergens that can be eliminated, such as foods, drugs, and animal dander.

Injection therapy is usually limited to clinically significant allergens. The initial dose of the offending allergen(s), based on the size of the skin reaction, is injected subcutaneously. The amount is increased at weekly intervals until a maximum tolerance is reached, after which a maintenance dose is given at 4-week intervals. This may be extended to 5- or 6-week intervals during the off-season for seasonal allergens. Successful treatment is continued for a minimum of 3 years and then stopped. If no symptoms appear, acquired immunity is assumed; if symptoms recur, treatment is reinstituted.

NURSING ALERT

Hyposensitization injections should be administered only with emergency equipment and medications readily available in the event of an anaphylactic reaction.

Prognosis. The outlook for children with asthma varies widely. Some children's asthma symptoms may improve at puberty, but up to two thirds of children with asthma continue to have symptoms through puberty and into adulthood. The prognosis for control or disappearance of symptoms varies in children from those who have rare and infrequent attacks to those who are constantly wheezing or are subject to status asthmaticus. In general, when symptoms are severe and numerous, when symptoms have been present for a long time, and when there is a family history of allergy, there is a greater likelihood of a poor prognosis. Many children who outgrow their exacerbations continue to have airway hyperresponsiveness and cough as adults. Furthermore, airway hyperresponsiveness in adults appears to be associated with decreased lung function.

Although death from asthma is rare, the death rate has increased in recent years. The adolescent age-group appears to be the most vulnerable, with the greatest increase occur-ring in ages 10 to 14 years. No reliable data exist to explain this increase. Factors that have been postulated include exposure of atopic persons to more allergens, change in severity of the disease, abuse of drug therapy (toxicity), failure of families and practitioners to recognize the severity of asthma, and psychologic factors such as denial and refusal to accept the disease. Risk factors for asthma deaths include early onset, frequent attacks, difficult-to-manage disease, adolescence, history of respiratory failure, psychologic problems (refusal to take medications), dependency on or misuse of drugs (high use), presence of physical stigmata (barrel chest, intercostal retractions), and abnormal pulmonary function tests (Capen and Sherman, 1998).

Status Asthmaticus. Children who continue to display respiratory distress despite vigorous therapeutic measures, especially use of sympathomimetics, are considered to be in *status asthmaticus.* The condition may develop gradually or rapidly, and often occurs with complicating conditions (e.g., pneumonia) that can influence the duration and treatment of the attack. A child with status asthmaticus is usually seen in the emergency department and frequently admitted to a pediatric intensive care unit for close observation and continuous cardiorespiratory monitoring.

NURSING ALERT

Status asthmaticus is a medical emergency that can result in respiratory failure and death if untreated. The child who sweats profusely, remains sitting upright, and refuses to lie down is in severe respiratory distress. Also, the child who suddenly becomes agitated, or the agitated child who suddenly becomes quiet, may be seriously hypoxic and requires immediate intervention.

Therapy for status asthmaticus is aimed at improvement of ventilation, correction of dehydration and acidosis, and treatment of any concurrent infection. Bronchospasm is relieved by giving inhaled aerosolized short-acting β2-agonists (either intermittently or continuously), along with corticosteroids (either orally or intravenously). For the child not responding to either of these therapies, subcutaneous epinephrine (1:1000) at a dose of 0.01 mL/kg, with a maximum dose of 0.3 mL, or subcutaneous terbutaline is administered. The child is given IV fluids and nothing by mouth except liquids if the condition permits. IV fluids are infused at maintenance rates, and the child is monitored for pulmonary edema.

NURSING ALERT

Dehydration should be corrected slowly; overhydration can increase the accumulation of interstitial pulmonary fluid to exacerbate small airway obstruction.

Correction of dehydration, acidosis, hypoxia, and electrolyte imbalance is guided by frequent monitoring of oxygenation (pulse oximetry), blood gases, and serum electrolytes. Nasal prongs, hood, or facemask are used to administer humidified oxygen. Because oxygen is a stimulus for respiration, high levels may significantly depress respirations.

The latest recommendations for the management of asthma state that antibiotics should not be used to treat acute asthma attacks except when a bacterial infection resulting from another condition such as pneumonia or sinusitis is present (National Asthma Education and Prevention Program, 2002). As the attack subsides, fluids and medications are given orally, adrenergic agonists are administered via an MDI, and plans for discharge and follow-up care are made.

Nursing Considerations

● Assessment

Physical assessment of asthma involves the same observations and techniques described in the general discussion of assessment of respiratory infection and physical assessment of the chest (see Chapter 7). In addition, some physical characteristics of chronic respiratory involvement are noted and evaluated, including chest configuration, posturing, and type of breathing.

Nurses assist with diagnostic tests, pulmonary function tests, and skin testing, as well as a general health assessment. Nurses also assess how asthma affects the child's everyday activities and self-concept, as well as the child and family's adherence to prescribed therapy. The nurse should determine any cultural or ethnic beliefs or practices that influence self-management and that may necessitate modifications in educational approaches to meet the needs of the family.

● Nursing Diagnoses

Based on a thorough assessment, several nursing diagnoses are identified. The more common diagnoses are included in the Nursing Care Plan below. Others may apply in specific situations.

● Planning

The goals for the child with asthma and the family include:

1 Child will not experience an asthmatic episode.
2 Child will exhibit improved ventilatory capacity.
3 Child will maintain optimal health.
4 Child will not develop complications.
5 Child will engage in normal activities for age.
6 Child and family will receive appropriate support and education regarding the disease and its management.

● Implementation

Avoid Allergens.   One goal of asthma management is avoidance of an exacerbation. Parents need to know how to avoid allergens and relieve asthma episodes. The nurse assists

---

NURSING CARE PLAN   The Child With Asthma

NURSING DIAGNOSIS ■ **Risk for suffocation related to interaction between individual and allergen(s)**

PATIENT GOAL 1: Will experience no asthmatic episode

NURSING INTERVENTIONS/RATIONALES
Teach child and family how to avoid conditions or circumstances that precipitate asthmatic episode
Assist parents in eliminating allergens or other stimuli that trigger exacerbation (see Family Home Care box, p. 816), such as:
  Meal planning to eliminate allergenic foods
  Removal of pets
  Modification of environment: "allergy-proof" home, especially no smoking in home
Avoid extremes of environmental temperature
  When child is exposed to cold air, recommend breathing through nose (not mouth) and wearing a mask or scarf, or cupping hand over nose and mouth *to create a reservoir of warm air to breathe*
Assist parents in obtaining or installing device to control environment (dehumidifier, air conditioner, electronic air filter)
Teach child and family to recognize early signs and symptoms *so that an impending episode can be controlled before it becomes distressful*
Teach child and family correct use of bronchodilators and antiinflammatory drugs (e.g., corticosteroids, cromolyn sodium), adverse effects, and dangers of overuse or underuse of drugs
Teach child to understand how equipment works
Teach child correct use of inhalers, nebulizers, and peak expiratory flow meters (PEFMs)
Teach child and family prophylactic treatment when appropriate (e.g., prevent exercise-induced bronchospasm by using medication before exercise)

Explain to child and family possible benefits of hyposensitization therapy when allergen(s) can be defined and cannot be avoided (e.g., pollen, mold) or controlled satisfactorily by drugs
*Administer hyposensitization therapy if prescribed

EXPECTED OUTCOMES
Family makes every effort to remove or avoid possible allergens or precipitating events
Child and family are able to detect signs of an impending episode early and implement appropriate actions
Child and family are able to administer medications and use inhalers and other equipment

PATIENT GOAL 2: Will experience optimal health

NURSING INTERVENTIONS/*RATIONALES*
Encourage sound health practices *to support body's natural defenses*
  Balanced, nutritious diet
  Adequate rest
  Good hygiene
  Appropriate exercise
  Follow-up care
Prevent respiratory infection, *because it can trigger an attack or aggravate the asthmatic state*
  Avoid exposure to infection
  Take meticulous care of equipment *to avoid bacterial or fungal growth*
  Use good handwashing technique

EXPECTED OUTCOMES
Child and parents practice sound health practices
Child exhibits no evidence of infection

*Dependent nursing action.

Continued

NURSING DIAGNOSIS ■ Ineffective airway clearance related to allergenic response and inflammation in the bronchial tree

PATIENT GOAL 1: Will exhibit evidence of improved ventilatory capacity

NURSING INTERVENTIONS/RATIONALES

Instruct or supervise breathing exercises and controlled breathing *to promote proper diaphragmatic breathing, side expansion, and improved chest wall mobility*

Use play techniques for breathing exercises with young children (e.g., blow a pinwheel or blow cotton balls on table) *to extend expiratory time and increase expiratory pressure*

Teach correct use of prescribed medications

Teach correct use of PEFM, nebulizer, and metered-dose inhaler (MDI) if indicated

Teach family to perform percussion and postural drainage and to encourage coughing if indicated

Encourage physical exercise

 Recommend activities requiring short bursts of energy (e.g., baseball, sprints, skiing), *because they may be better tolerated than those requiring endurance exercise* (e.g., soccer, distance running)

 Recommend swimming *because child breathes air saturated with moisture, and exhaling underwater prolongs expiration and increases end-expiratory pressure*

 Restrict physical activity only when child's condition makes it necessary

Encourage good posture *for maximum lung expansion*

Assist child and family in selecting activities appropriate to child's capabilities and preferences

EXPECTED OUTCOMES

Child breathes easily and without dyspnea

Child exhibits improved ventilatory capacity (specify)

Child engages in activities according to abilities and interest (specify)

NURSING DIAGNOSIS ■ Activity intolerance related to imbalance between oxygen supply and demand

PATIENT GOAL 1: Will receive optimal rest

NURSING INTERVENTIONS/RATIONALES

Encourage activities appropriate to child's condition and capabilities (specify)

Provide ample opportunities for sleep, rest, and quiet activities *to conserve oxygen supply*

EXPECTED OUTCOMES

Child engages in appropriate activities (specify)

Child appears rested

NURSING DIAGNOSIS ■ Interrupted family processes related to having a child with a chronic illness

PATIENT/FAMILY GOAL 1: Will exhibit positive adaptation to the condition

NURSING INTERVENTIONS/RATIONALES

Foster positive family relationships

Reinforce positive coping mechanisms of child and family

Use every opportunity to increase parents' and child's understanding of the disease and its therapies, *because adequate knowledge is related to family's timely use of preventive and emergency intervention*

Reinforce the need for responding to early signs of impending asthma episode, using prescribed medications as needed, *to decrease potential for a severe exacerbation*

Intervene appropriately if there is evidence of maladaptation

Be alert to signs of parental rejection or overprotection

Be alert to signs that child is depressed and make appropriate referral for psychologic support, *because depressed children, especially adolescents, may not comply with therapies as a means of passive suicide*

Teach child and family how to give respiratory treatments *to eliminate any confusion* regarding medication or inhalers/nebulizers

Encourage family to contact school personnel (e.g., nurse, teachers, coaches, principal) to develop a consistent plan of care for school setting

Refer family to appropriate support groups and community agencies

EXPECTED OUTCOME

Family copes with symptoms and effects of the disease and provides a normal environment for the child

STATUS ASTHMATICUS (SPECIAL NEEDS)

NURSING DIAGNOSIS ■ Risk for suffocation related to bronchospasm, mucus secretions, edema

PATIENT GOAL 1: Will experience cessation of bronchospasm

NURSING INTERVENTIONS/RATIONALES

Establish intravenous (IV) infusion *for administration of medication and hydration*

*Administer aerosolized bronchodilators and either oral or IV corticosteroids as prescribed *to relieve bronchospasm*

Closely monitor vital signs before, during, and after administration *for maximum efficacy and minimal side effects*

Interview parents to determine medications given before admission *to avoid possible overdose*

Have emergency equipment and medications readily available *to prevent delay in treatment*

EXPECTED OUTCOMES

Child breathes more easily

Child does not suffocate

PATIENT GOAL 2: Will exhibit normal respiratory function

NURSING INTERVENTIONS/RATIONALES

Administer humidified oxygen by tent, face mask, or cannula *to maintain satisfactory oxygenation*

Closely monitor oxygen saturations and blood gases via pulse oximetry *to detect early or impending hypoxia*

Closely monitor percentage of oxygen delivered, *since high levels may depress respirations*

Position *for optimal lung expansion*

 High-Fowler position

 Provide overbed table with pillows on which to lean if more comfortable for child

Implement measures to reduce fear/anxiety *to decrease respiratory efforts and oxygen consumption*

Encourage relaxation techniques *to decrease anxiety and promote lung expansion*

Organize activities to allow for rest, sleep, and minimal expenditure of energy

*Dependent nursing action.

NURSING CARE PLAN The Child With Asthma—*cont'd*

EXPECTED OUTCOMES

Child's respirations are unlabored and within normal limits (see inside back cover)

Child rests and sleeps comfortably

Child does not experience decreased oxygen saturations

PATIENT GOAL 3: Will successfully expel bronchial secretions

NURSING INTERVENTIONS/*RATIONALES*

Provide adequate hydration, orally or intravenously, *to liquefy secretions for easier removal*

Maintain NPO (nothing by mouth), if necessary, *to prevent aspiration of fluids and food*

Provide humidified atmosphere *to prevent drying of mucous membranes*

Encourage child to cough effectively

Provide tissues

Explain need to remove secretions

Suction, using correct technique, only when necessary

Do not use chest physiotherapy (CPT) during an acute episode, *because it will only agitate an already anxious, dyspneic child and aggravate the episode*

Position, if necessary, *to prevent aspiration of secretions*

Semiprone

Side lying

EXPECTED OUTCOMES

Secretions are adequately and easily expelled

Child coughs effectively

Child does not aspirate secretions, food, or fluids

NURSING DIAGNOSIS ■ **Risk for fluid volume deficit related to difficulty taking fluids, insensible fluid losses from hyperventilation, diaphoresis**

PATIENT GOAL 1: Will exhibit adequate hydration

NURSING INTERVENTIONS/*RATIONALES*

Maintain IV infusion at appropriate rate, *because fluid therapy will enhance liquefaction of secretions* (IV line usually run two-thirds to three-quarters maintenance unless dehydration present, *to minimize the risk of pulmonary edema because of high inspiratory pressures*)

Encourage oral fluids

Offer fluids when acute respiratory distress subsides *to decrease risk of aspiration*

Avoid cold liquids, *because they can trigger reflex bronchospasm*

Give fluids (and food) in small, frequent feedings *to avoid abdominal distention that might interfere with diaphragmatic excursion*

Use play techniques appropriate to child's age *to encourage fluid intake*

Measure intake and output

Correct dehydration slowly, *because overhydration can increase the accumulation of interstitial pulmonary fluid, leading to increased airway obstruction*

EXPECTED OUTCOME

Child exhibits adequate hydration

NURSING DIAGNOSIS ■ **Risk for injury (respiratory acidosis, electrolyte imbalance) related to hypoventilation, dehydration**

PATIENT GOAL 1: Will not experience acidosis

NURSING INTERVENTIONS/*RATIONALES*

Closely monitor blood pH, *because pH less than 7.25 impairs systemic, pulmonary, and coronary blood flow; normal pH enhances effect of bronchodilators*

*Administer sodium bicarbonate as ordered *to prevent or correct acidosis*

Maintain IV infusion *for administration of emergency medications and to prevent dehydration*

Prevent vomiting and subsequent dehydration; initially, child will experience alkalosis, but if vomiting becomes severe or uncontrolled, it can lead to acidosis

Implement measures to improve ventilation, *because hypoventilation may cause an accumulation of carbon dioxide, which will decrease pH*

EXPECTED OUTCOME

Child exhibits no evidence of respiratory acidosis

PATIENT GOAL 2: Will exhibit normal serum electrolytes

NURSING INTERVENTIONS/*RATIONALES*

Closely monitor serum electrolytes, *because dehydration, as well as medications, can alter normal serum electrolytes*

Maintain IV infusion at appropriate rate

Prevent dehydration and vomiting, *because they cause electrolyte imbalances*

EXPECTED OUTCOME

Child exhibits normal serum electrolytes

NURSING DIAGNOSIS ■ **Interrupted family processes related to emergency hospitalization of child**

PATIENT/FAMILY GOAL 1: Will experience reduction of anxiety

NURSING INTERVENTIONS/*RATIONALES*

Keep parents informed of child's condition

Encourage expression of feelings, especially regarding severity of condition and prognosis

Allow parents to be with child as much as possible by encouraging family-centered care concepts

Point out any evidence of improvement *to encourage positive coping behaviors*

If/when possible, schedule treatments and care to fit child's routines

Reduce sensory stimuli by maintaining quiet, relaxed environment

EXPECTED OUTCOMES

Family verbalizes concerns and spends time with child

Family exhibits no signs of distress

See also:

Nursing Care Plan: The Family of the Ill or Hospitalized Child, Chapter 21

Nursing Care Plan: The Child in the Hospital, Chapter 21

*Dependent nursing action.

FAMILY HOME CARE

Use of a Peak Expiratory Flow Meter

1. Before each use, make sure the sliding marker or arrow on the peak expiratory flow meter (PEFM) points to zero or is at the bottom of the numbered scale.
2. Stand up straight.
3. Remove gum or any food from the mouth.
4. Close your lips tightly around the mouthpiece. Be sure to keep your tongue away from the mouthpiece.
5. Blow out as hard and as quickly as you can, a "fast hard puff."
6. Note the number by the marker on the numbered scale.
7. Repeat entire routine three times; wait 30 seconds between each routine.
8. Record the highest of the three readings, not the average.
9. Measure the peak expiratory flow rate (PEFR) close to the same time and same way each day (e.g., morning and evening; before or 15 minutes after taking medication).
10. Keep a chart of your PEFRs.

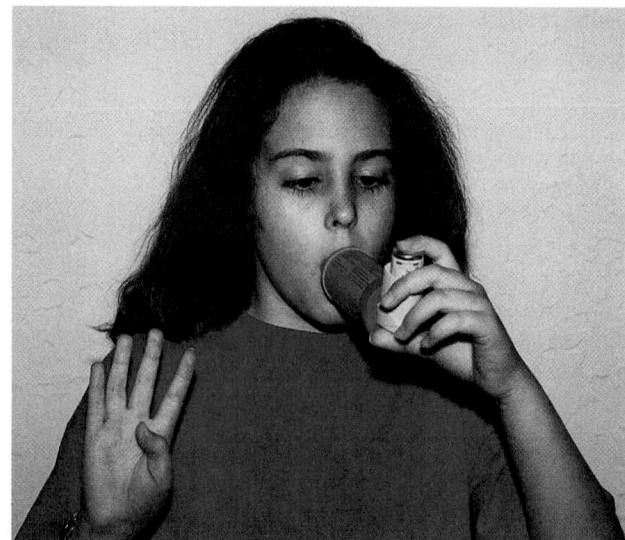

FIG. 23-4 ■ Child using metered-dose inhaler with spacer. Fingers are used for counting to 10 seconds.

the parent in modifying the environment to reduce contact with the offending allergen(s) (see Family Home Care box on p. 816). Parents are cautioned to avoid exposing a sensitive child to excessive cold, wind, or other extremes of weather, smoke, sprays, or other irritants. Foods known to provoke symptoms should be eliminated from the diet.

Approximately 2% to 6% of children with asthma are sensitive to aspirin; therefore, nurses should caution parents to use other analgesic/antipyretic drugs for discomfort or fever and to read package labeling. Although aspirin is rarely given to children in the United States, salicylate compounds are in other common medicines such as Pepto-Bismol. Children with aspirin-induced asthma may also be sensitive to NSAIDs and tartrazine (yellow dye number 5, a common food coloring).

Relieve Bronchospasm. Parents and older children are taught to recognize early signs and symptoms of an impending attack so that it can be controlled before symptoms become distressing. Most children can recognize prodromal symptoms well before an attack (about 6 hours), and implement preventive therapy. Objective signs that parents may observe include rhinorrhea, cough, low-grade fever, irritability, itching (especially in front of the neck and chest), apathy, anxiety, sleep disturbance, abdominal discomfort, and loss of appetite. A variety of easy-to-use, inexpensive PEFMs is available for use in the home and at school to assess changes in pulmonary function (see Family Home Care box above).

Children who use a nebulizer, MDI, Diskus, or Turbuhaler to deliver drugs need to learn how to use the device correctly. A study of school-age children with asthma indicated that only 7% of these children had effective MDI skills (Winkelstein and others, 2000). The MDI device (Fig. 23-4) delivers medication directly to the airways; therefore, the child needs to learn to breathe slowly and deeply for better distribution to narrowed airways (see Family Home Care box at right).

Young children and those who are unable to manipulate the MDI or coordinate breathing should use spacers. These devices allow the parent or child to deliver the medication

 **FAMILY HOME CARE**

Use of a Metered-Dose Inhaler*

STEPS FOR CHECKING HOW MUCH MEDICINE IS IN THE CANISTER
1. If the canister is new, it is full.
2. If the canister has been used repeatedly, it might be empty. (Check product label to see how many inhalations should be in each canister.)
3. The most accurate way to determine how many doses remain in an MDI is to count and record each actuation as it is used.
4. Many dry powder inhalers have a dose-counting device or dose indicator on the canister to let you know when the canister is empty.
5. Placing dry powder inhalers or MDIs with hydrofluoroalkanes in water will destroy these inhalers.

STEPS FOR USING THE INHALER
1. Remove the cap and hold inhaler upright.
2. Shake the inhaler.
3. Tilt the head back slightly and breathe out slowly.
4. With the inhaler in an upright position, position the mouthpiece:
   About 3 to 4 cm from the mouth *or*
   Insert into an AeroChamber *or* spacer (this method is recommended for young children and for people using corticosteroids)
5. At the end of a normal expiration, depress the top of the inhaler canister firmly to release the medication (into either the AeroChamber or the mouth), and breathe in slowly (about 3 to 5 seconds). Relax the pressure on the top of the canister.
6. Hold the breath for at least 5 to 10 seconds to allow the aerosol medication to reach deeply into the lungs.
7. Remove the inhaler and breathe out slowly through the nose.
8. Wait 1 minute between puffs (if additional one is needed).

Adapted from National Asthma Education and Prevention Program: *Expert Panel report II: guidelines for the diagnosis and management of asthma,* NIH pub no 97-4051, Bethesda, Md, 1997, National Heart, Lung, and Blood Institute.
*NOTE: Some inhaled dry-powder inhalers require a different inhalation technique. To use these dry-powder inhalers, it is important to close the mouth tightly around the mouthpiece of the inhaler and inhale rapidly and deeply.

from the MDI into the spacer, from which the child then inhales the medication. Spacers also prevent yeast infections in the mouth when inhaled corticosteroids are administered via an MDI.

The child and parents also need to be cautioned about the adverse effects of prescribed drugs and the dangers of overuse of β_2-agonists. They should know that it is important to use these drugs when needed but not indiscriminately or as a substitute for avoiding the symptom-provoking allergen. Parents are cautioned against purchasing over-the-counter preparations because these medications can place the children at risk for increased dosage of a drug and toxicity.

> **⚠ NURSING ALERT**
>
> Long-acting β-adrenergic inhalers (salmeterol [Serevent]) should be used only as directed (usually every 12 hours) and not more frequently. They are not intended to relieve acute asthmatic symptoms.

The family should obtain a PEFM and learn to use this device to monitor their child's asthma. A written asthma action plan that includes the three peak flow meter zones and the child's asthma medications should be obtained from the child's primary care provider. This action plan should be used to make decisions about asthma management at home and at school.

Parents are cautioned to avoid exposing the child with asthma to excessive cold, wind, or other extremes of weather and to smoke, sprays, or other irritants. Foods known to provoke symptoms should be eliminated from the diet, and parents are advised to read labels on prepared foods and snacks to determine the presence of allergens.

The child should be protected from a respiratory infection that can trigger an attack or aggravate the asthmatic state, especially in young children whose airways are mechanically smaller and more reactive. Annual influenza vaccinations are recommended for patients with persistent asthma (American Academy of Pediatrics, 2003). Equipment used for the child, such as nebulizers, must be kept absolutely clean to decrease the chances of contamination with bacteria and fungi.

Breathing exercises and controlled breathing are taught and encouraged for motivated youngsters, and the nurse should provide information concerning activities that promote diaphragmatic breathing, side expansion, and improved mobility of the chest wall. Play techniques that can be used for younger children to extend their expiratory time and increase expiratory pressure include blowing cotton balls or a Ping-Pong ball on a table, blowing a pinwheel, blowing bubbles, or preventing a tissue from falling by blowing it against the wall.

Self-care and asthma self-management programs are important in helping the child and family cope with asthma. Most asthma self-management programs for children convey several principles. First, asthma is a common disease that can be controlled with appropriate drug therapy, environmental control, education, and management skills. Second, it is much easier to prevent than to treat an asthma episode; adherence to a therapeutic program is necessary to prevent exacerbations. Third, children with asthma can live full and active lives.

Asthma camps provide an opportunity for children with asthma to engage in physical activity while learning about their disease in a controlled environment with their peers and health professionals. Children who attend asthma camps often demonstrate improved asthma self-management skills.

Several organizations provide education and services for health professionals and families of children with asthma.* Asthma education and awareness are important aspects of asthma management.

Provide Acute Asthma Care.   Children who are admitted to the hospital with acute asthma are ill, anxious, and uncomfortable. In many instances, they are admitted from the emergency department in status asthmaticus and in acute distress. Nebulized β-agonists with oxygen and a systematic corticosteroid are administered to relieve bronchospasm. The child is monitored closely and continuously during therapy for relief of respiratory distress and any side effects. Vital signs are checked frequently. An IV infusion may be started to provide a means for hydration and a route for medications.

Older children usually prefer the high-Fowler position, although they may be more comfortable sitting upright or leaning slightly forward. When possible, the nurse communicates in such a way that the child can reply in a few words to avoid fatigue, because shortness of breath makes talking difficult.

Children with acute asthma are apprehensive and anxious. The calm, efficient presence of a nurse helps to reassure them that they are safe and will be cared for during this stressful period. It is important to assure children that they will not be left alone and that their parents are allowed to remain with them.

Parents need reassurance and want to be informed of their child's condition and therapies. They may feel that they have in some way contributed to the child's condition or could have prevented the episode. Reassurance regarding their efforts expended on the child's behalf and their parenting capabilities can help alleviate their stress. Efforts to reduce parental apprehension will also reduce the child's distress. Anxiety is easily communicated to the child from parents and members of the staff.

Support Child and Family.   The nurse working with children with asthma can provide support in a number of ways. Many children voice frustration because their exacerbations interfere with their daily activities and social lives. They need education about what to do to prevent an asthma episode. These children also need reassurance from the health team that they can learn to control and cope with their asthma and live a normal life.

---

*Asthma and Allergy Foundation of America (AAFA),** 1125 15th Street, Washington, DC 20005; (202) 466-7643 or (800) 7-Asthma; website: www.aafa.org; **American Lung Association,** 1740 Broadway, New York, NY 10019; (212) 315-8700 or (800) Lung-USA; website: www.lungusa.org; **National Heart, Lung, and Blood Institute,** Information Center, Code AS-ASHA, PO Box 30105, Bethesda, MD 20824-0105; fax: (301) 251-1223; website: www.nhlbi.nih.gov/nhlbi.htm.

The short-term and long-term adaptation of children with asthma often depends on the family's acceptance of the disorder. The task of living day-to-day with affected children involves the family continually. There are periodic crises and the ever-present threat of a crisis, requiring parental vigilance; sleepless nights; frequent trips to the doctor, emergency department, or hospital; and often overwhelming medical expenses. Throughout these stresses, parents are encouraged to promote as normal a life as possible for their children.

Evaluation

Continual reassessment and evaluation determine the effectiveness of nursing interventions. The following observational guidelines and expected outcomes are important:

1 Interview family about removal or avoidance of known allergens.
2 Observe child for evidence of respiratory symptoms.
3 Assess child's general health.
4 Observe child and interview family about any infections or other complications.
5 Interview child about daily activities.
6 Determine the degree to which the family and child understand the child's condition and the extent to which the therapies are carried out.

The *expected outcomes* are described in the Nursing Care Plan on pp. 819-821.

CYSTIC FIBROSIS

Cystic fibrosis (CF) is inherited as an autosomal recessive trait; the affected child inherits the defective gene from both parents, with an overall incidence of 1:4 (see Appendix B). The mutated gene responsible for CF is located on the long arm of chromosome 7, along with its protein product, *cystic fibrosis transmembrane regulator (CFTR).*

Pathophysiology

CF is characterized by several clinical features: increased viscosity of mucous gland secretions, a striking elevation of sweat electrolytes, an increase in several organic and enzymatic constituents of saliva, and abnormalities in autonomic nervous system function. Although both sodium and chloride are affected, the defect appears to be primarily a result of abnormal chloride movement; the CFTR appears to function as a chloride channel. Children with CF demonstrate decreased pancreatic secretion of bicarbonate and chloride and an increase in sodium and chloride in both saliva and sweat. This characteristic is the basis for the sweat chloride diagnostic test.

The primary factor, and the one that is responsible for many of the clinical manifestations of the disease, is mechanical obstruction caused by the increased viscosity of mucous gland secretions (Fig. 23-5). Instead of forming a thin, freely flowing secretion, the mucous glands produce a thick, mucoprotein that accumulates and dilates them.

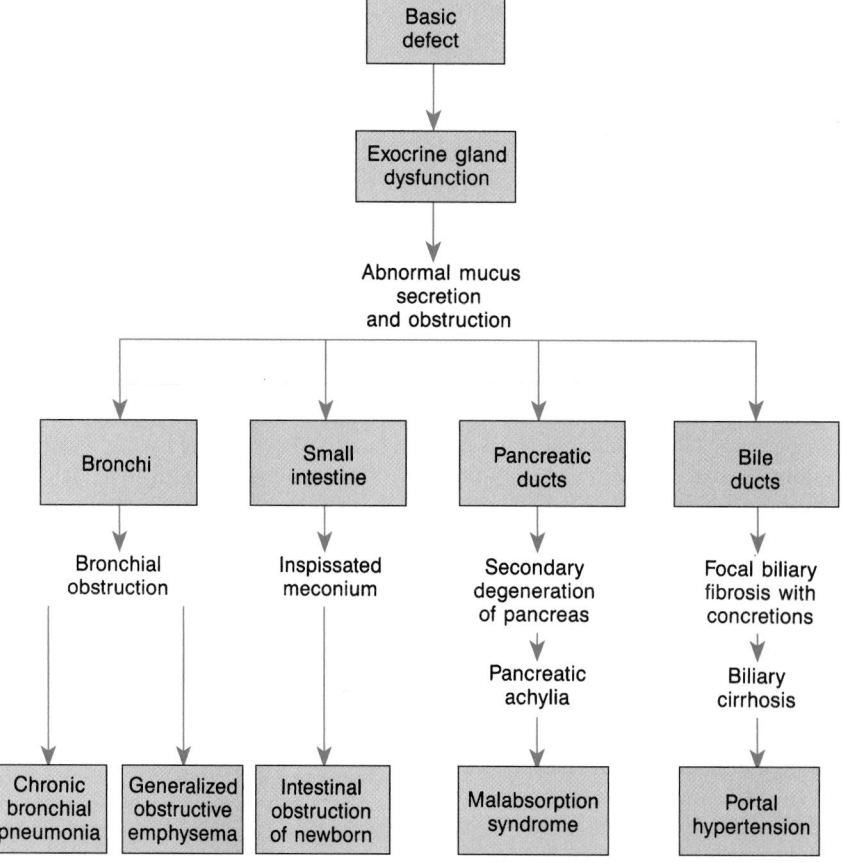

FIG. 23-5 ■ Various effects of exocrine gland dysfunction in cystic fibrosis.

Small passages in organs such as the pancreas and bronchioles become obstructed as secretions precipitate or coagulate to form concretions in glands and ducts. The earliest manifestation of CF is *meconium ileus* in the newborn, in which the small intestine is blocked with thick, puttylike, tenacious, mucilaginous meconium.

In the pancreas the thick secretions block the ducts, eventually causing *pancreatic fibrosis.* This blockage prevents essential pancreatic enzymes from reaching the duodenum, which causes marked impairment in the digestion and absorption of nutrients. The disturbed function is reflected in bulky stools that are frothy from undigested fat *(steatorrhea)* and foul smelling from putrefied protein *(azotorrhea).* The islands of Langerhans may decrease in number as pancreatic fibrosis progresses, and a type of diabetes called CF-related diabetes (CFRD) is a frequent finding in adolescents and adults with CF (Balinsky and Zhu, 2004). In the liver, localized biliary obstruction and fibrosis are common and become more extensive with time.

A common gastrointestinal (GI) complication associated with CF is *prolapse of the rectum,* which occurs in infancy and childhood, and is related to large, bulky stools, malnutrition, and increased intraabdominal pressure secondary to paroxysmal cough. Affected children of all ages are subject to intestinal obstruction from inspissated or impacted feces. Gumlike masses can obstruct the bowel and produce a partial or complete obstruction, a condition that is referred to as distal intestinal obstruction syndrome.

Pulmonary complications constitute the most serious threat to life in children with CF. Many children demonstrate respiratory symptoms before 1 year of age; others may not develop symptoms for weeks, months, or years. In the respiratory tract, bronchial and bronchiolar obstruction by the abnormally thick, tenacious mucus causes patchy atelectasis with hyperinflation. The child is unable to expectorate the mucus because of its increased viscosity. This retained mucus serves as an excellent medium for bacterial growth. Reduced oxygen–carbon dioxide exchange causes variable degrees of hypoxia, hypercapnia, and acidosis.

Diagnostic Evaluation

An initial evaluation is conducted with overall appraisal in the areas of general activity, physical findings, nutritional status, and findings on chest radiograms (see Box 23-16). The diagnosis of CF is established on the basis of (1) a history of the disease in the family, (2) absence of pancreatic enzymes, (3) increase in electrolyte concentration of sweat, and (4) chronic pulmonary involvement.

The consistent finding of abnormally high sodium and chloride concentrations in the sweat is a unique characteristic of CF. Parents frequently report that their infants taste "salty" when they kiss them. For diagnostic purposes the quantitative *sweat chloride test* is performed on sweat obtained by iontophoresis of pilocarpine. Normally the sweat chloride content is less than 40 mEq/L; a chloride concentration greater than 60 mEq/L is diagnostic of CF. In infants, a value greater than 40 mmol/L is highly suggestion of CF.

Chest radiography reveals characteristic patchy atelectasis and obstructive emphysema. PFTs are sensitive indexes of lung function, providing evidence of abnormal function of the small airways in CF. Other diagnostic tools that may aid in diagnosis include stool fat or enzyme analysis. Stool

analysis requires a 72-hour sample with accurate recording of food intake during that time. Radiographs, including barium enema, are used for diagnosis of meconium ileus.

Therapeutic Management

The improved survival rate of patients with CF is due to antibiotic therapy and improved nutritional management. Goals of therapy are to (1) prevent or minimize pulmonary complications, (2) ensure adequate nutrition for growth, (3) encourage appropriate physical activity, and (4) promote a reasonable quality of life for the child and the family. A multisystem approach to treatment is needed to accomplish these goals.

Management of Pulmonary Problems. Management of pulmonary problems is directed toward prevention and treatment of pulmonary infection by improving aeration, removing mucopurulent secretions, and administering antimicrobial agents. Most children develop respiratory symptoms by 3 years of age. The large amounts and viscosity of respiratory secretions in children with CF contribute to the likelihood of respiratory infections.

The most common pathogens responsible for pulmonary infections are *Pseudomonas aeruginosa, Burkholderia cepacia,*

BOX 23-16 ■ Clinical Manifestations of Cystic Fibrosis

MECONIUM ILEUS*
Abdominal distention
Vomiting
Failure to pass stools
Rapid development of dehydration

GASTROINTESTINAL MANIFESTATIONS
Large, bulky, loose, frothy, extremely foul-smelling stools
Voracious appetite (early in disease)
Loss of appetite (later in disease)
Weight loss
Marked tissue wasting
Failure to grow
Distended abdomen
Thin extremities
Sallow skin
Evidence of deficiency of fat-soluble vitamins A, D, E, and K
Anemia

PULMONARY MANIFESTATIONS
Initial signs:
    Wheezy respirations
    Dry, nonproductive cough
Eventually:
    Increased dyspnea
    Paroxysmal cough
    Evidence of obstructive emphysema and patchy areas of atelectasis
Progressive involvement:
    Overinflated, barrel-shaped chest
    Cyanosis
    Clubbing of fingers and toes
    Repeated episodes of bronchitis and bronchopneumonia

*In about 10% of cases.

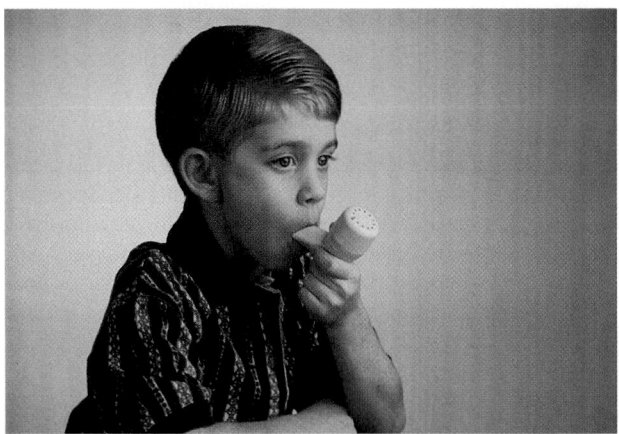

FIG. 23-6 ■ Child using Flutter mucus clearance device. (Courtesy Scandipharm, Inc.)

Staphylococcus aureus, Haemophilus influenzae, Escherichia coli, and *Klebsiella pneumoniae. P. aeruginosa* and *B. cepacia* are particularly pathogenic for children with CF, and infections with these organisms are difficult to clear. In addition, children with CF who are chronically colonized with these organisms have poorer survival rates than children who are not colonized (Rosenstein, 1999).

Prevention of infection involves a daily routine of CPT to maintain pulmonary hygiene. CPT is usually performed twice daily (on rising and in the evening) and more frequently if needed, especially during pulmonary infection. The *Flutter mucus clearance device** is a small, handheld plastic pipe with a stainless-steel ball on the inside that facilitates removal of mucus (Fig. 23-6). It has the advantage of increasing sputum expectoration and being used without an assistant.

Bronchodilator medication delivered in an aerosol opens bronchi for easier expectoration and is administered before CPT when the patient exhibits evidence of reactive airway disease or wheezing. Another aerosolized medication is *recombinant human deoxyribonuclease* (*D-Nase,* known generically as *dornase alfa (Pulmozyme),* which decreases the viscosity of mucus. It is well tolerated and has no major adverse effects; minor reactions are voice alterations and laryngitis. The drug causes improvement in PFTs and perceptions of well-being, as well as a reduction in the viscosity of sputum.

Physical exercise is an important adjunct to daily CPT. Exercise stimulates mucus secretion and provides a sense of well-being and increased self-esteem. Any aerobic exercise that is enjoyed by the patient should be encouraged. The ultimate aim of exercise is to establish an adequate breathing pattern.

Pulmonary infections are treated as soon as they are recognized. Some practitioners prefer to prescribe oral antibiotics prophylactically at the time of diagnosis; others begin therapy when pulmonary symptoms occur. Sputum culture and sensitivity guide the choice of antibiotic. Aerosolized antibiotics such as tobramycin, ticarcillin, and gentamicin are beneficial for patients with frequent pulmonary exacerbations.

---

*Manufactured by **Scandipharm, Inc.,** 22 Inverness Center Parkway, Birmingham, AL 35242; (205) 991-8085 or (800) 950-8085; website: www.scandipharm.com.

IV antibiotics are often administered at home as an alternative to hospitalization. Most children with CF have central venous access devices for home administration of IV medications. However, when pulmonary function does not improve with outpatient management, hospitalization may be recommended for continued antibiotic therapy and vigorous CPT. Oxygen administration is used for children with acute episodes but must be used cautiously because many children with CF have chronic carbon dioxide retention, and the unsupervised use of oxygen can be harmful (see Oxygen Therapy: Oxygen Toxicity, Chapter 22). Pneumothorax can occur in children and adolescents with more advanced disease if there is a rupture of subpleural blebs through the visceral pleura.

NURSING ALERT

Signs of a pneumothorax are usually nonspecific and include tachypnea, tachycardia, dyspnea, pallor, and cyanosis.

Management of Gastrointestinal Problems. The principal treatment for pancreatic insufficiency is replacement of pancreatic enzymes, which are administered with meals and snacks to ensure that digestive enzymes are mixed with food in the duodenum. Enteric-coated products prevent the neutralization of enzymes by gastric acids, thus allowing activation to occur in the alkaline environment of the small bowel. The amount of enzymes depends on the severity of the insufficiency, the response of the child to enzyme replacement, and the philosophy of the practitioner. Usually one to five capsules are administered with a meal, and a smaller amount is taken with snacks. Capsules can be swallowed whole or taken apart and the contents sprinkled on a small amount of food to be taken at the beginning of the meal. The amount of enzyme is adjusted to achieve normal growth and a decrease in the number of stools to one or two per day.

Children with CF require a well-balanced, high-protein, high-caloric diet (because of the impaired intestinal absorption). In fact, they often require up to 150% of the recommended daily allowances to meet their needs for growth. Breast-feeding with enzyme supplementation should be continued whenever possible for parents who prefer this method and, when necessary, supplemented with a higher-calorie-per-ounce formula. For formula-fed infants, commercial cow's milk formulas are usually adequate, although frequently a hydrolysate formula with medium-chain triglycerides (e.g., Pregestimil, Alimentum) may be recommended. Enzymes are mixed into cereal or fruit, such as applesauce. Because the uptake of fat-soluble vitamins is decreased, water-miscible forms of these vitamins (A, D, E, and K) are given, along with multivitamins and the enzymes. When high-fat foods are eaten, the child is encouraged to add extra enzymes. Sometimes patients will be placed on supplemental tube feedings or parenteral alimentation in an effort to build up nutritional reserves if there has been a history of inability to maintain weight.

Prognosis.   Despite considerable progress and a recent surge in new treatments, CF remains a progressive and incurable disease. The pulmonary involvement ultimately determines the patient's outcome, because pancreatic enzyme deficiency is less of a problem if adequate nutrition is ensured. With advances in technology, parents and adolescents are challenged to set future goals that include college, careers, social relationships, and marriage.

Screening.   In utero diagnosis of CF is possible based on detection of two CF mutations in the fetus. Newborn screening has been available since 1979. The standard method of diagnosis is detection of abnormal chloride secretions in sweat. Sometimes testing of DNA to detect the F508 gene may be substituted for the sweat test. Carrier screening is also available and reliable for siblings and family members of a child with CF (Balinsky and Zhu, 2004).

Nursing Considerations

Assessment of the child with CF involves both pulmonary and GI observations. Pulmonary assessment is the same as that described for asthma, with special attention to lung sounds, observation of cough, and evidence or degree of finger clubbing. GI assessment involves observing the frequency and nature of the stools and abdominal distention. The nurse should also be alert to evidence of failure to thrive (e.g., weight loss, wasting, pallor, fatigue). Family members are interviewed to determine the child's eating and eliminating habits, to determine salty perspiration, and to confirm a history of frequent respiratory infections or bowel obstruction in infancy.

On initial contact, which frequently occurs in the hospital setting, nurses are involved in performing or assisting with diagnostic tests, primarily sweat for laboratory analysis of chloride content and, less often, collection of stool specimens for trypsin and fat analyses.

Hospital Care.   When patients with CF are hospitalized, standard precautions with meticulous handwashing should be implemented to decrease the nosocomial spread of organisms among CF patients and to other patients in the hospital. Sputum and soiled tissues from all CF patients should be discarded in a covered no-touch receptacle whenever possible. In some hospitals, patients with CF who are colonized or infected with organisms with antimicrobial resistance are placed in a private room. In addition, CF patients who are colonized or infected with *Burkholderia cepacia* complex may be hospitalized in a private room on a separate nursing unit away from other CF patients and have limitations placed on their activities while in the hospital. Such limitations include not using the playroom or hospital cafeteria when other CF patients are present.

When the child with CF is hospitalized for diagnosis or treatment of pulmonary complications, aerosol therapy is instituted or continued. Respiratory therapists often initiate, supervise, and provide these treatments. If the hospital or institution does not have respiratory therapists assigned to this therapy, the nurse administers the aerosol therapy, performs CPT, and teaches breathing exercises. CPT should not be performed before or immediately after meals. Planning CPT so that it does not coincide with meals is difficult in the hospital situation, but essential to the effectiveness of this treatment.

Oxygen is cautiously administered to children in respiratory distress, and the child requires frequent assessment.

The hazard of *oxygen narcosis* is a constant threat in children with CF. The child requires close observation to assist with cough and expectoration.

The diet is implemented for the newly diagnosed child or continued for the child who is hospitalized for pulmonary disease. Children in the early stages of CF often have a good appetite, and some will eat excessively. With infection and increased lung involvement, their appetite diminishes, and eventually it becomes a challenge to tempt failing appetites. Some younger children may object to the extra fluids that are encouraged to prevent dehydration. Food is considered therapy for these patients. The caloric intake should be increased as necessary. Pancreatic enzymes are supplied for each meal or snack, and adequate salt is provided, especially for febrile children. (See Feeding the Sick Child, Chapter 22.)

Frequent skin care is performed to prevent irritation and skin breakdown over bony prominences. Particular attention is necessary after use of the bedpan or when the diaper is changed. Careful cleansing helps to reduce irritation and odor from offensive stools, and the use of moisture barriers protects the skin. (See Diaper Dermatitis, Chapter 30, and Maintaining Healthy Skin, Chapter 22.)

The child needs support during the many treatments and tests that are a part of the hospitalization. IV fluids and blood tests are almost always a part of the treatment, and the child soon associates hospitalization with these stress-provoking procedures. Because these children are usually quite thin with little muscle mass, careful selection of injection sites is required.

Providing support to both the child and the family is essential. The progressive nature of the disease makes each illness requiring hospitalization a potentially life-threatening event. Skilled nursing care and sympathetic attention to the emotional needs of the child and family help them cope with the stresses associated with repeated respiratory infections and hospitalization.

Home Care.   After the diagnosis is confirmed and after each hospitalization, home care is implemented. The plan of care should be flexible so that family activities are disrupted as little as possible. Parents need help finding and contacting the vendors who will provide home care equipment. They also need opportunities to learn how to use the equipment, as well as how to solve problems they may encounter while delivering therapy at home.

Patients and family members need education about the preferred diet of nutritious meals with tolerated fat, increased protein and carbohydrate, and the administration of pancreatic enzymes. For infants and young children, the enzymes can be mixed with pureed fruit, such as applesauce, and fed with a spoon. Capsules are usually suitable for older children. It is important to stress to parents that the enzymes, in the amount regulated to the child's needs, should be administered at the beginning of all meals and snacks. They are cautioned about not restricting salt, especially during hot weather, and ensuring an adequate fluid intake, because dehydration aggravates the thick mucus secretions. Oral hygiene is important because of interference with salivation and the increased susceptibility to oral infections.

One of the most important aspects of educating parents for home care is teaching CPT and breathing exercises. The success of a therapy program depends on conscientious performance of these treatments regularly as prescribed. The number of times these therapies are performed each day is determined on an individual basis, and often parents readily learn to adjust the number and intensity of the treatments to the child's needs. For the young child, postural drainage can be achieved with simple activities such as hanging by the knees from a bar or low-hanging trapeze, turning somersaults, or playing "wheelbarrow" with the child suspended head down and propelling with the hands while the adult holds on to the feet. Most children respond to a challenge, such as "How long can you stand on your head?" Small children can "stand on their heads" with their heads on the cushion of a large chair with or without an adult holding on to their feet. Parents soon learn to respond to cues from their children and incorporate spontaneous and "fun" activities into the treatment regimen.

Another important aspect of home care is the administration of IV antibiotics. As a result of the current use of venous access devices, such as peripherally inserted central catheter (PICC) lines, Infus-a-port, and central lines, parents and children can now assume responsibility for home administration of IV antibiotics.* When this occurs, families need detailed information about how to give the medications, their possible side effects, and how to troubleshoot any problems with the venous access device.

Children with CF should receive routine primary care with special attention to diet, growth and development, and immunizations. In addition to all recommended immunizations, patients with CF should receive the influenza vaccine starting at age 6 months and followed by a yearly booster (American Academy of Pediatrics, 2003).

The nurse can assist the family in contacting resources that provide help to families. Various child health services, many local clinics, private agencies, service clubs, and other community groups offer equipment and medications either free or at reduced rates. The **Cystic Fibrosis Foundation†** has chapters throughout the United States to provide education and services to families and professionals.

Family Support. The most challenging aspect of providing care for the family of a child with CF is meeting the emotional needs of the child and family. The diagnosis, treatment, and prognosis for CF are often associated with many problems and frustrations. The diagnosis can evoke feelings of guilt and self-recrimination in parents. These feelings may be particularly strong if the newly diagnosed child is the second affected child in the family and the par-

ents had been counseled about the 1:4 risk of such an event occurring.

The long-range problems for an infant, child, or adolescent with CF are those encountered in any chronic illness (see Chapter 18). Both the child and the family must make many adjustments, the success of which depends on their ability to cope and also on the quality and quantity of support they receive from outside sources. Combined efforts of a variety of health professionals are needed to provide the most comprehensive services to families. It is often the nurse who organizes and coordinates these services, assesses the home situation, and collects the data needed to evaluate the effectiveness of the services.

The persistent need for treatment several times a day places tremendous strain on the family. When the child is young, a family member must perform postural drainage and chest physiotherapy. Children often balk at these treatments, and the parents are placed in the position of insisting on adherence. The stress and anxiety related to this continual routine may produce feelings of resentment in both the child and the family members. When possible, occasional trusted respite care should be available to the parents to allow them the opportunity to leave the situation for short periods without undue anxiety about the child's welfare.

The affected child may become resentful about the disease, its relentless routine of therapy, and the necessary curtailment it places on activities and relationships. The child's activities are interrupted or built around treatments, medications, and diet. This imposes hardships and influences the child's quality of life. For example, the child may need to carry medication to school and other places if he or she eats away from home. Some aspects of the disease such as growth retardation and persistent coughing may be the cause of ridicule from other children. However, the child should be encouraged to attend school and to join age-appropriate peer groups to foster a life that is as normal and productive as possible.

As the disease progresses, family stress should be expected, and the patient may become angry and noncompliant. As the disease progresses, family members may become more aware of the possibility of death. It is important for the nurse to recognize the changing needs of the family and provide sources for counseling if necessary when stressful setbacks occur. Patients need to be guided into activities that enable them to express anger, sorrow, and fear without guilt. (See Ethical Case Study on facing page.)

Anticipatory grieving and other aspects related to care of a child with a terminal illness are another important part of nursing care. For example, it is important to prepare family members for end-of-life decisions and care. Families may need information about specific interventions such as hospice and treatments for pain and dyspnea (see Chapter 18 and the Ethical Case Study).

As life expectancy increases for children with CF, issues related to marriage, childbearing, and career choice become relevant. Men must be informed at some point that they will be unable to produce offspring. However, a distinction should be made between sterility and impotence. Normal sexual relationships can be expected. Female patients may be able to bear children but should be informed of the possible deleterious effects on the respiratory system created by

---

*Two excellent publications available from the **Cystic Fibrosis Foundation** are *What everyone should know about cystic fibrosis* and *Cystic fibrosis: a summary of symptoms, diagnosis, and treatment.* For information about specialized medications, such as Pulmozyme, equipment for CF or home infusions, contact **Home Infusion and Pharmacy Services,** a subsidiary of the **Cystic Fibrosis Pharmacy, Inc., HHCS Pharmacy Services,** 633 East Colonial Drive, Orlando, FL 32803; (800) 741-4427.

†6931 Arlington Road, Bethesda, MD 20814-3205; (800) FIGHT CF or (301) 951-4422; website: www.cff.org. In Canada: **Canadian Cystic Fibrosis Foundation,** 586 Eglinton Avenue East, Suite 204, Toronto, Ontario M4P 1P2.

✖ ETHICAL CASE STUDY

Ethical **Decision Making Model**	Michael, a 15-year-old boy, has cystic fibrosis. Since age 12 years, Michael's respiratory status has been getting progressively worse, and he has been hospitalized for multiple respiratory exacerbations. Last evening he was admitted to the adolescent unit in acute respiratory distress. Today, he told his favorite nurse: "I am so tired, I can't fight anymore. Can't they just let me go home now and be comfortable?" Michael lives with his father and his paternal grandmother. His mother died 6 years ago in a motor vehicle accident.
Evaluate the issue	Michael's pulmonary specialist, Dr A., believes Michael's illness is now terminal. Michael's paternal grandmother doesn't want Michael to suffer any more. She tells the nurse that she believes Michael is ready to die and she thinks a Do Not Resuscitate Order (DNR) and hospice care are best for Michael at this time. Michael's father does not believe Michael's condition has become progressively worse. He wants everything medically possible to be done for his son. He will not discuss a DNR order or hospice care.
Treat all involved with respect	Michael's wishes must be heard and acknowledged. He is 15 years old and sufficiently mature to deserve respectful honesty and consideration. By approximately age 14 years, adolescents demonstrate the same kind of reasoning abilities as adults concerning health care decisions. The father's concerns must also be addressed in an empathetic manner.
Hear all sides	The nurse has an obligation to be an advocate for her patient. However, the nurse should also consider the father's reasons for wanting everything possible to be done. Why is the father denying the seriousness of his son's condition? Does the father need more information, or is he overwhelmed and terrified at the prospect of losing his son and experiencing all the grief and emotions he felt when he lost his wife?
Initiate action	Which of the following actions is most appropriate for the nurse to take: ■ Talk to Michael's father about Michael's comments. ■ Tell the grandmother to try to get the father to agree to a DNR order and hospice. ■ Discuss Michael's comments with Dr. A.
Consider the outcome	The ethical dilemma is how to meet the needs of Michael and his father and grandmother. The nurse decided to share Michael's comments with Dr. A. and determine whether he is aware of both Michael's wishes and those of his father. After discussion with Dr. A., the nurse, and other health team members felt that Michael's father may need more information about his son's condition and feelings. The following plan was implemented: The family care coordinator will arrange a family conference in which all parties (including Michael) can exchange views and arrive at a decision about future care for Michael. If the family conference does not produce a consensus and Michael still maintains his position, the situation will need to be referred to the hospital ethics committee.

the burden of pregnancy. They also need to know that their children will be carriers of the CF gene.

Life as an independent adult, the goal that most families have for their children, should be encouraged for children with CF. From the time that children can take partial responsibility for their own care (e.g., CPT, taking enzymes), independence and accountability should be fostered. The prognosis for children with CF has improved, and many children with CF are well adjusted despite numerous hospitalizations and unpleasant complications.

RESPIRATORY EMERGENCY

RESPIRATORY FAILURE

In general, the term *respiratory insufficiency* is applied to two situations: (1) when there is increased work of breathing but gas exchange function is near normal and (2) when normal blood gas tensions cannot be maintained and hypoxemia and acidosis develop secondary to carbon dioxide retention.

Respiratory failure is defined as the inability of the respiratory apparatus to maintain adequate oxygenation of the blood, with or without carbon dioxide retention. *Respira-*

tory arrest is the cessation of respiration. *Apnea* is the cessation of breathing for more than 20 seconds or for a shorter period when associated with hypoxemia or bradycardia (Curley and Moloney-Harmon, 2001).

Effective pulmonary gas exchange requires clear airways, normal lungs and chest wall, and adequate pulmonary circulation. Anything that affects these functions or their relationships can compromise respiration.

Diagnostic Evaluation

Respiratory failure that occurs as a result of acute obstruction of a major airway or cardiac arrest is sudden and readily apparent. Gradual or progressive deterioration of respiratory function is less easily recognized. Nursing observation and judgment are vital to the recognition and early management of respiratory failure. Nurses must be able to assess a situation and initiate appropriate action within moments. Signs of respiratory failure are listed in Box 23-17.

Therapeutic Management

The interventions used in the management of respiratory failure are often dramatic, requiring special skills and emergency procedures. Some techniques used to assist ventilation

BOX 23-17 ■ Clinical Manifestations of Respiratory Failure

CARDINAL SIGNS
Restlessness
Tachypnea
Tachycardia
Diaphoresis

EARLY BUT LESS OBVIOUS SIGNS
Mood changes, such as euphoria or depression
Headache
Altered depth and pattern of respirations
Hypertension
Exertional dyspnea
Anorexia
Increased cardiac output and renal output
Central nervous system symptoms (decreased efficiency, impaired judgment, anxiety, confusion, restlessness, irritability, depressed level of consciousness)
Flaring nares
Chest wall retractions
Expiratory grunt
Wheezing or prolonged expiration

SIGNS OF MORE SEVERE HYPOXIA
Hypotension or hypertension
Dimness of vision
Somnolence
Stupor
Coma
Dyspnea
Depressed respirations
Bradycardia
Cyanosis, peripheral or central

include artificial ventilation, artificial airway, and cardiopulmonary resuscitation (CPR).

Artificial Ventilation.   A variety of methods for controlling or assisting ventilation are available. Temporary assistance involves the use of a manual self-inflating ventilation bag with a mask and valve to prevent rebreathing. With the mask placed over the child's nose and mouth, an open airway is established by correct positioning with the chin forward and the neck extended to the "sniffing" position. The bag is rhythmically compressed, forcing the gas from the bag into the child's lungs.

For prolonged assistance, mechanical ventilation is used to replace the bellows function of the diaphragm and thoracic wall muscles. The lungs are inflated by the application of either positive or negative pressure. The positive-pressure machine inflates the lung by increasing airway pressure above atmospheric pressure, and a negative-pressure ventilator creates a subatmospheric pressure around the chest wall while airway pressure remains atmospheric. Application of positive pressure by mechanical means usually improves the distribution of gas within the lung and often reinflates partially collapsed lung segments. The overall effect is the improvement of gas exchange.

Nursing Considerations

For families whose child has a respiratory arrest, support is aimed at keeping the family informed of the child's status and helping them to cope with a near-death experience or an actual death (see Chapter 18). Knowing that their child requires CPR is a frightening and often overwhelming experience for parents. Uncertainty regarding the outcome—both mortality and morbidity—is a primary concern. Traditionally, family members are not allowed to be present during resuscitation efforts. However, recent studies indicate that family presence during emergencies alleviates the family's anger about being separated from the patient during a crisis, reduces their anxiety, eliminates doubts about what was done to help the patient, and facilitates the grieving process when the patient dies (Tucker, 2003). Regardless of whether an institution permits parental presence during CPR, nurses must consider the needs, fears, and concerns of family members during an arrest situation. If family presence is not permitted, nurses should arrange for someone to remain with the family during the code. After the child's recovery or death, the family will continue to need support and thorough medical information regarding lifesaving measures, the prognosis if the child survives, and the cause of death if the child dies.

CARDIOPULMONARY RESUSCITATION

Cardiac arrest in children is less often of cardiac origin than from prolonged hypoxemia secondary to inadequate oxygenation, ventilation, and circulation (shock). Some causes of cardiac arrest include injuries, suffocation (e.g., FB aspiration), smoke inhalation, SIDS, or infection. Respiratory arrest has been associated with a better survival than cardiac arrest. After cardiac arrest occurs, the outcome of resuscitative efforts is poor.

Complete apnea signals the need for rapid, vigorous action to prevent cardiac arrest. In such situations, nurses must initiate action immediately. In the hospital, emergency equipment must be available and easily accessible in all patient care areas. The status of emergency equipment must be checked at least once daily. Regardless of the cause of the arrest, basic procedures are carried out and modified somewhat according to the child's size.

> **⚑ NURSING ALERT**
>
> Rescuers who have infections that may be transmitted by blood or saliva or who believe they have been exposed to such an infection should not perform mouth-to-mouth resuscitation if a barrier device or mask with a one-way valve is not available. If CPR efforts are anticipated in the workplace or other out-of-hospital settings, rescuers should have access to these devices (American Heart Association, 2000).

Outside the hospital situation the first action in an emergency is to quickly assess the extent of any injury and determine whether the child is unconscious. A child who is struggling to breathe but conscious should be transported immediately to an *advanced life support (ALS)* facility, with the child maintaining whatever position affords the most comfort. Attempting to transport a child by automobile wastes valuable time in obtaining help. Transport by an *emergency medical service (EMS)* is recommended. Services in most large communities can institute ALS immediately or en route to a medical facility.

An unconscious child is managed with care to prevent additional trauma if a head or spinal cord injury has been sustained. The circumstances in which the child is found offer clues to a possible injury. For example, a child who has been thrown from a bicycle or fallen from a tree is more likely to sustain trauma than a child who is discovered in bed. The child should be turned as a unit with firm support provided to the head and neck to prevent rolling, twisting, or tilting backward or forward.

Resuscitation Procedure

Current CPR guidelines incorporate the use of the automated external defibrillator (AED) in the treatment of cardiorespiratory arrest if the child has a weight greater than 25 kg or 55 pounds (approximately 8 years of age) (American Heart Association, 2000). In out-of-hospital situations, the use of AED defibrillation in children between 1 and 8 years is appropriate if the defibrillating machine is approved for use in children. In a hospital situation, where weight-based defibrillation dosing is possible, manual defibrillation is the mode of choice (American Heart Association, 2003). When using an AED, health care providers are advised to give adults and children older than 8 years a defibrillatory shock within 5 minutes of collapse outside the hospital and within 3 minutes in the hospital.

For effective CPR, the victim is placed on his or her back on a firm, flat surface, employing appropriate precautions (Fig. 23-7). *Unlike rescuers of adults, who initiate EMS first, pediatric rescuers provide 1 minute of basic life support (BLS) before activating EMS.* Because pediatric arrest is most commonly the result of a respiratory arrest, maintaining ventilation is a primary consideration. With loss of consciousness, the tongue, which is attached to the lower jaw, relaxes and falls back, obstructing the airway. To open the airway, the head is positioned with either the head tilt/chin lift or jaw thrust. Health professionals should be able to use both maneuvers. ***Head tilt*** is accomplished by placing one hand on the victim's forehead and applying firm, backward pressure with the palm to tilt the head back. The fingers of the free hand are placed under the bony portion of the lower jaw near the chin to lift and bring the chin forward *(chin lift).* This supports the jaw and helps tilt the head back (Fig. 23-8, *A*).

The *jaw thrust* is accomplished by grasping the angles of the victim's lower jaw and lifting with both hands, one on each side, displacing the mandible upward and outward (Fig. 23-8, *B*). In suspected neck injuries the jaw thrust method should be used while the cervical spine is completely immobilized. After restoration of a patent airway by removal of foreign material and secretions (if indicated), and if the child is not breathing, continuation of the airway is maintained and rescue breathing is initiated. To ventilate the lungs in the infant (birth to 1 year of age), the bag-valve-mask or operator's mouth is placed in such a way that both the mouth and the nostrils are covered (Fig. 23-8, *C*). Children (older than 1 year of age) are ventilated through the mouth while the nostrils are firmly pinched for airtight contact (Fig. 23-8, *D*).

> **! NURSING ALERT**
>
> The volume of air in an infant's lungs is small, and the air passages are considerably smaller, with resistance to flow potentially higher than in adults. Therefore small puffs of air are delivered.

If air enters freely and the chest rises, the airway is assumed to be clear. The correct volume for each breath must be provided without causing abdominal distention. Gastric distention, which interferes with diaphragmatic excursion, frequently occurs when more volume than necessary is delivered and the breaths are delivered too rapidly.

After the initial two breaths, the pulse is palpated to determine the presence of a heartbeat. The carotid is the most central and accessible artery in children older than 1 year of age (Fig. 23-8, *E*). However, the very short and often fat neck of the infant renders the carotid pulse difficult to palpate. Therefore, in the infant, it is preferable to use the brachial pulse, located on the inner side of the upper arm midway between the elbow and shoulder (Fig. 23-8, *F*). Absence of a carotid or brachial pulse is considered sufficient indication to begin external cardiac massage.

Chest Compression.   External chest compression consists of serial, rhythmic compressions of the chest to maintain circulation to vital organs until the child achieves spontaneous vital signs or ALS can be provided. *Chest compressions are always interspersed with ventilation of the lungs.* For optimal compressions, it is essential that the child's spine is supported on a firm surface during compressions of the sternum and that sternal pressure is forceful but not traumatic. For an infant the hard surface can be the rescuer's hand or forearm, with the palm supporting the infant's back. The child's head is positioned for optimal airway opening using the head tilt/chin lift maneuver. It is essential to prevent overextension of the head of small infants, because this tends to close the flexible trachea.

The placement of the fingers for compression in infants is at a point on the lower sternum one fingerbreadth below the intersection of the sternum and an imaginary line drawn between the nipples (Fig. 23-8, *G*). Compressions on the child 1 to 8 years of age are applied to the lower half of the sternum (Fig. 23-8, *H*). Sternal compression to infants is applied with two or three fingers on the sternum exerting a firm downward thrust; for children, pressure is applied with the heel of one hand. Current guidelines include the addition of the two-thumb technique for chest compressions for infants when two health care providers are present. In the two-thumb technique, one of the two rescuers places both thumbs side by side over the lower half of the infant's sternum; the remaining fingers encircle the infant's chest and support the back. The depth of compression is adapted to the child's size. The location, rate, and depth for children older than 8 years of age are the same as for adults.

CPR is continued at the appropriate ratio of breaths to compressions for age until signs of recovery appear. These signs include palpable peripheral pulses, return of pupils to normal size, the disappearance of mottling and cyanosis, and possibly return of spontaneous respiration.

	Objectives	ACTIONS		
		Adult (over 8 yr)	Child (1 to 8 yr)	Infant (under 1 yr)
A. AIRWAY	1. Assessment: Determine unresponsiveness.	Tap or gently shake shoulder.		
		Say, "Are you okay?"		Speak loudly.
	2. Get help.	Activate EMS.	Shout for help. If second rescuer available, have person activate EMS.	
	3. Position the victim.	Turn on back as a unit, supporting head and neck if necessary (4-10 sec).		
	4. Open the airway.	Head tilt/chin lift.		
B. BREATHING	5. Assessment: Determine breathlessness.	Maintain open airway. Place ear over mouth, observing chest. Look, listen, feel for normal breathing (no more than 10 sec).*		
	6. Give 2 rescue breaths.	Maintain open airway.		
		Pinch nose, seal mouth to mouth.		Mouth to nose and mouth.
		Give 2 slow effective breaths. Observe chest rise. Allow lung deflation between breaths.		
		2 sec each	1 to 1½ sec each	
	7. Option for obstructed airway.	a. Reposition victim's head. Try again to give rescue breaths.		
			b. Activate EMS.	
		c. Give 5 subdiaphragmatic abdominal thrusts (the Heimlich maneuver).		c. Give 5 back blows.
				c. Give 5 chest thrusts.
		d. Tongue-jaw lift and finger sweep.	d. Tongue-jaw lift, but finger sweep only if you see a foreign object.	
		If unsuccessful, repeat a, c, and d until successful.		
C. CIRCULATION	8. Assessment: Determine pulselessness.	Feel for carotid pulse with one hand; maintain head-tilt with other hand (no more than 10 sec).		Feel for brachial pulse: keep head tilt.
CPR	Pulse absent: Begin chest compressions: 9. Landmark check.	Use 2-3 fingers to locate lower margin of rib cage. Follow rib margin to base of sternum (xiphoid process).		Imagine a line drawn between the nipples.
	10. Hand position.	Place one hand above fingers of first hand on lower half of sternum.		Place 2 fingers on sternum 1 finger's width below line. Depress ½ -1 in.†
		Place other hand on top of hand on sternum. Depress 1½-2 in.	Use heel of one hand. Depress 1-1½ in.	
	11. Compression rate.	80-100 per min	100 per min	At least 100 per min
	12. Compressions to breaths.	2 breaths to every 15 compressions	1 breath to every 5 compressions	
	13. Number of cycles.	4	20 (approximately 1 min)	
	14. Reassessment.	Feel for carotid pulse.		Feel for brachial pulse.
		If no pulse, resume CPR, starting with compressions.	If alone, activate EMS. If no pulse, resume CPR, starting with compressions.	
	Pulse present; not breathing: Begin rescue breathing.	1 breath every 5 sec (12 per min)	1 breath every 3 sec (20 per min)	

* If victim is breathing or resumes breathing, place in recovery position: (1) move head, shoulders, and torso simultaneously; (2) turn onto side; (3) leg not in contact with ground may be bent and knee moved forward to stabilize victim; (4) victim should not be moved in any way if trauma is suspected and should not be placed in recovery position if rescue breathing or CPR is required.
† Use the 2 thumb–encircling hands technique if two rescuers are available for infant CPR.

FIG. 23-7 ■ One-rescuer CPR. (Modified from Stapleton ER and others: *BLS for healthcare providers*, Dallas, 2001, American Heart Association.)

Medications.   Medications are an important adjunct to CPR, especially cardiac arrest, and are used during and after resuscitation in children. Appropriate fluid therapy is initiated immediately in the hospital or by EMS personnel during transport (see Parenteral Fluid Therapy, Chapter 22, and Shock, Chapter 25). A complete supply of emergency medications is kept and maintained in all EMS vehicles and on all hospital units. The supply is checked on a regular basis (usually once on each 8-hour shift). Resuscitation medications are listed in Table 23-3.

NURSING ALERT

When administering drugs during CPR (or a "code"), use a saline flush between medications to prevent drug interactions. Document all drugs, dosages, and the time and route of administration.

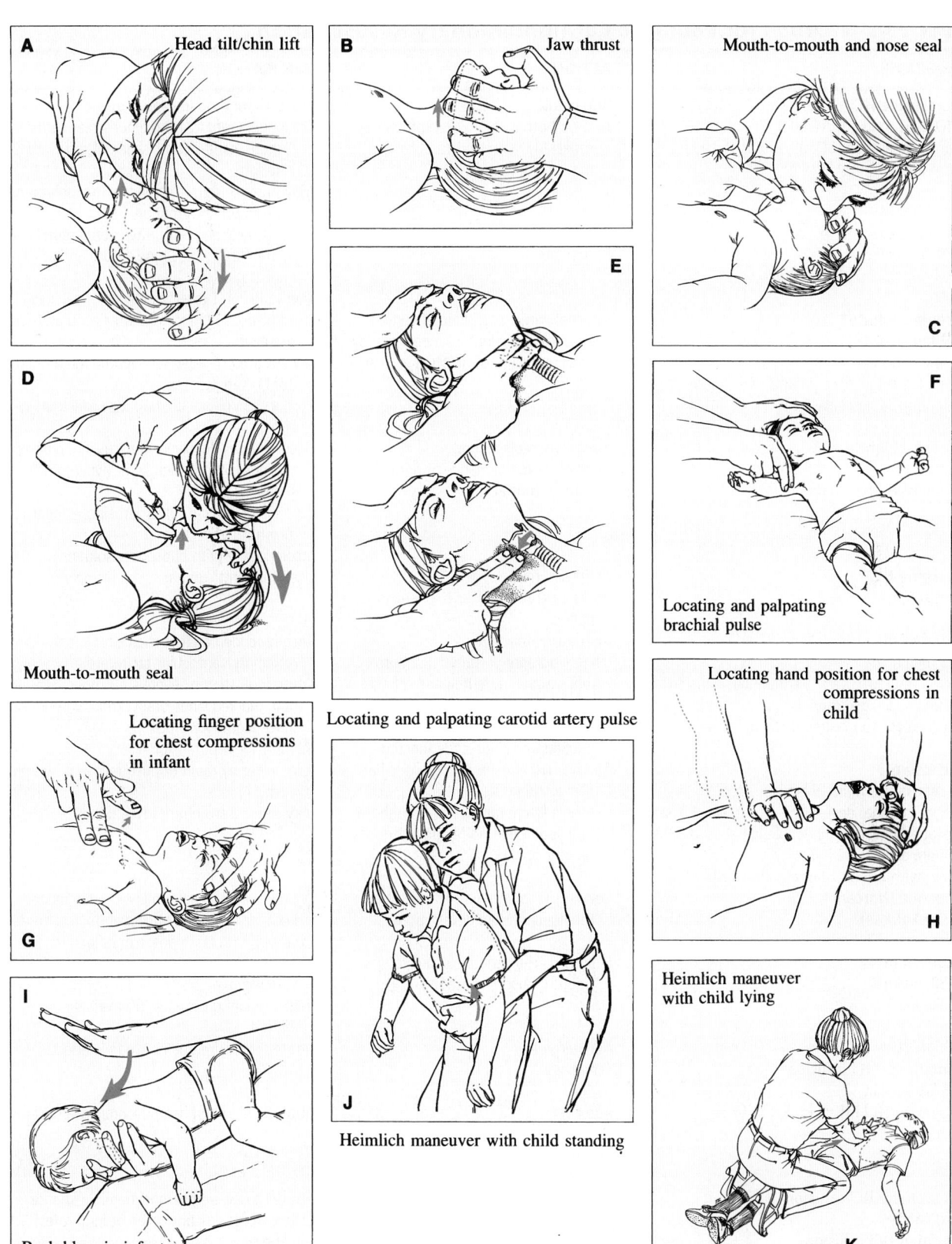

FIG. 23-8 ■ Procedures for cardiopulmonary resuscitation, **A** to **H**, and airway obstruction, **I** to **K**. (From Chandra NC, Hazinski MF, editors: *Textbook of basic life support for healthcare providers*, Dallas, 1997, American Heart Association.)

TABLE 23-3 ■ Drugs for Pediatric Cardiopulmonary Resuscitation

DRUG/DOSE	ACTION	IMPLICATION
Epinephrine HCl* IV/IO: 0.01 mg/kg (1:10,000) Endotracheal tube (ET): 0.1 mg/kg (1:1000) Repeat doses = 0.1 mL/kg (1:1000)	Adrenergic Acts on both α- and β-receptor sites, especially heart and vascular and other smooth muscle	Most useful drug in cardiac arrest Disappears rapidly from bloodstream after injection; instill 2-3 mL saline after ET administration May produce renal vessel constriction and decreased urine formation
Sodium bicarbonate IV/IO: 1 mEq/kg Newborn: 0.5 mEq/mL 2 mg/kg	Alkalinizer Buffers pH	Infuse slowly and only when ventilation is adequate; flush with saline before and after administration Don't mix with catecholamines or calcium
Atropine sulfate* 0.02 mg/kg/dose Minimum dose: 0.1 mg Maximum single dose: infants and children, 0.5 mg; adolescents, 1 mg	Anticholinergic-parasympatholytic Increases cardiac output, heart rate by blocking vagal stimulation in heart	Used to treat bradycardia after ventilatory assessment Always provide adequate ventilation and monitor O_2 saturation Produces pupillary dilation that constricts with light
Calcium chloride 10% 20 mg/kg IV 0.2 mg/kg/dose q 10 min	Electrolyte replacement Needed for maintenance of normal cardiac contractility	Used only for hypocalcemia, calcium blocker overdose, hyperkalemia, or hypermagnesemia Administer slowly; very sclerosing; administer in central vein Incompatible with phosphate solutions
Lidocaine HCl* 1 mg/kg/dose	Antidysrhythmic Inhibits nerve impulses from sensory nerves	Used for ventricular arrhythmias only
Amiodarone IV: 5 mg/kg Over 30 min followed by continuous infusion Starting at 5 μg/kg/min May increase to maximum 10 μg/kg/min	Antidysrhythmic agent Inhibits adrenergic stimulation; prolongs action potential and refractory period in myocardial tissues; decreased atrioventricular (AV) conduction and sinus node function	Recommended as first choice for shock-refractory ventricular tachycardia Contraindicated in severe sinus node dysfunction, marked sinus bradycardia, second- and third-degree AV block Monitor for hypotension
Adenosine 0.1 mg/kg as a rapid IV bolus Maximum initial dose: 6 mg (given over 1-2 sec) Repeat administration: double initial dose (Maximum dose = 12 mg) Follow with ≥5 mL normal saline flush	Antidysrhythmic, for supraventricular tachycardia (SVT) Causes a temporary block through the atrioventricular node and interrupts reentry circuits	Administer by rapid IV push followed by saline flush May cause transient bradycardia
Naloxone (Narcan)* 0.1 mg/kg/dose† May repeat q 2-3 min	Reverses respiratory arrest due to excessive opiate administration	Evaluate level of pain following administration because analgesic effects of opioids are reversed with large doses of naloxone
Magnesium 25-50 mg/kg Maximum: 2 g	Inhibits calcium channels and causes smooth muscle relaxation	Given by rapid IV infusion for suspected hypomagnesemia Have calcium gluconate (IV) available as antidote
INFUSIONS **Epinephrine HCl infusion** 0.05 μg/kg/min	Adrenergic See above	Titrated to desired hemodynamic effect
Dopamine HCl infusion 2 μg/kg/min	Agonist Acts on alpha receptors, causing vasoconstriction Increases cardiac output	Titrated to desired hemodynamic response
Dobutamine HCl infusion 2 μg/kg/min	Adrenergic direct-acting β_2 agonist Increases contractility and heart rate	Titrated to desired hemodynamic response Little vasoconstriction, even at high rates
Lidocaine HCl infusion 10 μg/kg/min	Antidysrhythmic Increases electrical stimulation threshold of ventricle	See above Lower infusion dose used in shock

*These drugs may be administered via the ET tube if an IV is not available.
†Dose of naloxone to reverse respiratory depression without reversing analgesia from opioids is 0.5 μg/kg in children <40 kg (American Pain Society, 1999).

		Actions		
Signs of life-threatening obstruction: truly choking child *cannot speak, becomes cyanotic,* and *collapses*				
	Objectives	**Adult (over 8 yr)**	**Child (1 to 8 yr)**	**Infant (under 1 yr)**
CONSCIOUS VICTIM	1. Assessment: Determine airway obstruction.	Ask, "Are you choking?" Determine if victim can cough or speak.		Observe breathing difficulty, ineffective cough, no strong cry.
	2. Act to relieve obstruction.	Perform up to 5 subdiaphragmatic abdominal thrusts (Heimlich maneuver).		Give 5 back blows.
				Give 5 chest thrusts.
	Be persistent.	Repeat Step 2 until obstruction is relieved or victim becomes unconscious.		
VICTIM WHO BECOMES UNCONSCIOUS	3. Position the victim: call for help.	Turn on back as a unit, supporting head and neck, face up, arms by sides. Call out, "Help!" Activate EMS. If second rescuer available, have person activate EMS.		
	4. Check for foreign body.	Perform tongue-jaw lift and finger sweep.	Perform tongue-jaw lift. Remove foreign object only if you actually see it.	
	5. Give rescue breaths.	Open the airway with head tilt/chin lift. Try to give rescue breaths. If airway is obstructed, reposition head and try to ventilate again.		
	6. Act to relieve obstruction.	Perform up to 5 subdiaphragmatic abdominal thrusts (Heimlich maneuver).		Give 5 back blows.
				Give 5 chest thrusts.
	7. Be persistent.	Repeat steps 4-6 until obstruction is relieved.		
UNCONSCIOUS VICTIM	1. Assessment: Determine unresponsiveness.	Tap or gently shake shoulder. Shout, "Are you okay?"	Tap or gently shake shoulder.	
		If unresponsive, activate EMS.		
	2. Call for help: position the victim.	Turn on back as a unit, supporting head and neck, face up, arms by sides.		
			Call out for help.	
	3. Open the airway.	Head-tilt/chin-lift.		Head tilt/chin lift, but do not tilt too far.
	4. Assessment: Determine breathlessness.	Maintain an open airway. Ear over mouth; observe chest. Look, listen, feel for breathing (no more than 10 sec).		
	5. Give rescue breaths.	Make mouth-to-mouth seal.		Make mouth-to-mouth-and-nose seal.
		Try to give rescue breaths.		
	6. If chest not rising, try again to give rescue breaths.	Reposition head. Try rescue breaths again.		
	7. Activate the EMS system.		If airway obstruction not relieved after about 1 min, activate EMS as rapidly as possible.	
	8. Act to relieve obstruction.	Perform up to 5 subdiaphragmatic abdominal thrusts (Heimlich maneuver).		Give 5 back blows.
				Give 5 chest thrusts.
	9. Check for foreign body.	Perform tongue-jaw lift and finger sweep.	Perform tongue-jaw lift. Remove foreign object only if you actually see it.	
	10. Rescue breaths.	Open the airway with head tilt/chin lift. Try again to give rescue breaths. If airway is obstructed, reposition head and try to ventilate again.		
	11. Be persistent.	Repeat steps 8-10 until obstruction is relieved.		

FIG. 23-9 ■ Foreign body airway obstruction management. (Modified from Stapleton ER and others: *BLS for healthcare providers,* Dallas, 2001, American Heart Association.)

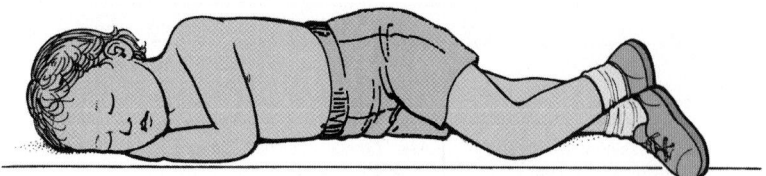

FIG. 23-10 ■ Recovery position for child after respiratory emergency.

AIRWAY OBSTRUCTION

Attempts at clearing the airway should be considered for (1) children in whom aspiration of a foreign body is witnessed or strongly suspected and (2) unconscious, nonbreathing children whose airways remain obstructed despite the usual maneuvers to open them. When aspiration is strongly suspected, the child is encouraged to continue coughing as long as the cough remains forceful. If the cough becomes ineffective, mechanical maneuvers should be used in an attempt to dislodge the object.

> **! NURSING ALERT**
>
> In a conscious choking child, attempt to relieve the obstruction only if:
> - The child is unable to make any sounds.
> - The cough becomes ineffective.
> - There is increasing respiratory difficulty with stridor.

Blind finger sweeps are avoided in both infants and children. A combination of *back blows* (over the spine between the shoulder blades) and *chest thrusts* (on the sternum, same location as for chest compressions) is recommended to relieve the foreign body obstruction in infants (Fig. 23-9). The Heimlich maneuver or abdominal thrusts are recommended for children older than 1 year of age.

Infants

A choking infant is placed face down over the rescuer's arm with the head lower than the trunk and the head supported (Fig. 23-8, *I*). For additional support the rescuer should support the arm firmly against the thigh. Up to five quick, sharp, back blows are delivered between the infant's shoulder blades with the heel of the rescuer's hand. Less force is required than would be applied to an adult. After delivery of the back blows, the rescuer's free hand is placed flat on the infant's back so that the infant is "sandwiched" between the two hands, making certain the neck and chin are well supported. While the rescuer maintains support with the infant's head lower than the trunk, the infant is turned and placed supine on the rescuer's thigh, where up to five quick downward chest thrusts are applied in rapid succession in the same location as external chest compressions described for CPR. Back blows and chest thrusts are continued until the object is removed or the infant becomes unconscious.

Children

The *Heimlich maneuver,* a series of *subdiaphragmatic abdominal thrusts,* is recommended for children older than 1 year of age. The maneuver creates an artificial cough that forces air, and with it the foreign body, out of the airway. The procedure is carried out with the child in a standing,

sitting, or lying position (Fig. 23-8, *J* and *K*). In the conscious choking child, upward thrusts are delivered to the upper abdomen with the fisted hand at a point just below the rib cage (Fig. 23-8, *J*). To prevent damage to the internal organs, the rescuer's hands should not touch the xiphoid process of the sternum or the lower margins of the ribs. Up to five thrusts are repeated in rapid succession until the foreign body is expelled.

It is neither necessary nor desirable to squeeze or compress the arms during the procedure. It is not a punch or a bear hug. The child may vomit after relief of the obstruction and should be positioned to prevent aspiration. After breathing is restored, the child should receive medical attention and be assessed for complications.

The success of the technique is primarily a result of the obstruction occurring at the end of a maximum respiration. The victim is most likely to choke on food during inspiration; therefore, the tidal volume plus expiratory reserve volume is present in the lungs. When pressure is exerted on the diaphragm by the maneuver, the food bolus is ejected with considerable force by this trapped air.

> **! NURSING ALERT**
>
> If the victim is breathing or resumes effective breathing after emergency interventions, place in the recovery position: move the head, shoulders, and torso simultaneously and turn onto the side. The leg not in contact with the ground may be bent and the knee moved forward to stabilize the victim (Fig. 23-10). The victim should not be moved in any way if trauma is suspected and should not be placed in the recovery position if rescue breathing or CPR is required.

KEY POINTS

- Acute infection of the respiratory tract is the most common cause of illness in infancy and childhood.

- The incidence and severity of respiratory tract infections are influenced by the infectious agents involved, the child's age, and the child's natural defenses.

- Common respiratory tract infections of childhood include nasopharyngitis, pharyngitis (including tonsillitis), influenza, and otitis media.

- Croup syndromes involve acute inflammation and variable degrees of obstruction of the epiglottis, larynx, or trachea.

- The primary goals in the care of children with croup are observation for signs of respiratory distress and relief of laryngeal obstruction.

- Common infections of the lower airways are bacterial tracheitis, bronchitis, and respiratory syncytial virus (RSV)/bronchiolitis.

- Pneumonias are classified according to site (lobar, bronchial, or interstitial) or by etiologic agent (viral, bacterial, mycoplasmal), or are associated with aspiration of foreign material).

- In tuberculosis, susceptibility to bacillus can be influenced by heredity, age, stress, poor nutrition, and intercurrent infection.

- Passive inhalation of or exposure to environmental tobacco smoke is a major environmental pollutant contributing to respiratory illness in children.

- Asthma is the leading cause of chronic illness in children.

- General therapeutic management of asthma includes allergen control, drug therapy, and sometimes hyposensitization.

- Support for the family of the child with asthma includes education about the disease and its therapy and facilitation of self-management.

- Cystic fibrosis is the most common inherited disease in children.

- The diagnosis of cystic fibrosis is based on the family history, increased sweat electrolyte content, absent pancreatic enzymes, and chronic pulmonary involvement.

- Choking and respiratory failure are respiratory emergencies that necessitate immediate intervention.

- The Heimlich maneuver is reserved for children in whom foreign body aspiration is witnessed or strongly suspected. A combination of back blows and chest thrusts is used for infants with foreign body aspiration.

- In a conscious choking child, attempts to relieve the obstruction are used only if the child is unable to make any sounds; the cough becomes ineffective; or the child has increasing respiratory difficulty with stridor.

References

Abulhosm RS and others: Passive smoke exposure impairs recovery after hospitalization for acute asthma, *Arch Pediatr Adolesc Med* 151:135-139, 1997.

American Academy of Otolaryngology—Head and Neck Surgery: *2000 Clinical indicators compendium*, Bulletin June 2000, 19:6, 2000.

American Academy of Pediatrics, and American Academy of Family Physicians: Clinical Practice Guidelines: Diagnosis and management of acute otitis media, *Pediatrics* 113(4):1451-1465, 2004.

American Academy of Pediatrics: Clinical Practice Guidelines: Otitis media with effusion, *Pediatrics* 113(5):1412-1429, 2004.

American Academy of Pediatrics, Committee on Infectious Diseases: *2003 Red Book: report of the Committee on Infectious Diseases*, ed 26, Elk Grove Village, Il, 2003, The Academy.

American Heart Association: Part 9: pediatric basic life support, *Resuscitation* 46:301-341, 2000.

American Heart Association, ILCOR Advisory Statement: *Use of automated external defibrillators for children: an update*, June 2003.

American Pain Society: *Principles of analgesic use in the treatment of acute pain and chronic cancer pain*, ed 3, Glenview, Il, 1992, The Society.

Andrews JS: Otitis media and otitis externa. In Hoekelman RA and others, editors: *Primary pediatric care*, ed 4, St Louis, 2001, Mosby.

Balinsky W, Zhu CW: Pediatric cystic fibrosis: evaluating costs and genetic testing, *J Pediatr Health Care* 18:30-34, 2004.

Berman S, Johnson C, Chan K, Kelley P: Ear, nose & throat. In Hay WW and other, editors: *Current pediatric diagnosis & treatment*, ed 15, New York, 2001, Lange Medical Books/McGraw-Hill.

Blumer JL: Traditional management of acute otitis media. In Klein JO, editor: *Otitis media management strategies for the 21st century*, Bala Cynwyd, Pa, 1998, Meniscus Educational Institute.

Capen CL, Sherman JM: Fatal asthma in children: a nurse managed model for prevention, *J Pediatr Nurs* 13(6):367-375, 1998.

Carlson L, Scudder L: Controversies in the management of pediatric otitis media: are more definitive answers on the horizon? *Adv Nurse Pract* 12(2):73-77, 2004

Curley MA, Moloney-Harmon PA: *Critical care nursing of infants and children*, Philadelphia, 2001, WB Saunders.

DeRosa J, Grundfast KM: Surgical management of otitis media, *Pediatr Ann* 31(12):814-820, 2002.

Eggleston PA: Asthma. In McMillan J and others, editors: *Oski's pediatrics, principles and practice*, ed 3, Philadelphia, 1999, Lippincott Williams & Wilkins.

Fost DA, Spahn JD: The leukotriene modifiers: a new class of asthma medication, *Contemp Pediatr* 15:95-107, 1998.

Hon KL and others: Clinical presentations and outcome of severe acute respiratory syndrome in children, *Lancet* 361(9370):1701-1703, 2003.

Iovino LA: New acute otitis media guidelines chart several new areas of care, *Infect Dis Child* 16(3):30-31, 2003.

Jackson PL: Healthy people 2010 objective: Reduce number and frequency of courses of antibiotics for ear infections in young children, *Pediatr Nurs* 27(6):591-593, 605, 2001.

Kaliner MA, Spector SL, Wenzel SE: Treating allergic rhinitis for better asthma control, *Patient Care N P*, pp 2-7, May 1999.

Kuiken T and others: Newly discovered coronavirus as the primary cause of severe acute respiratory syndrome, *Lancet* 362(9380): 263-270, 2003.

Long SS: Respiratory syncytial virus. In McMillan J and others, editors: *Oski's pediatrics: principles and practice*, ed 3, Philadelphia, 1999, Lippincott Williams & Wilkins.

McMillan JA, Feigin RD: Group A streptococcal infections. In McMillan J and others, editors: *Oski's pediatrics: principles and practice*, ed 3, Philadelphia, 1999, Lippincott Williams & Wilkins.

Morkjaroenpong V and others: Environmental tobacco smoke exposure and nocturnal symptoms among inner-city children with asthma, *J Allergy Clin Immunol* 110(1):147-153, 2002.

National Asthma Education and Prevention Program: *Expert Panel report II: guidelines for the diagnosis and management of asthma*, pub no 97-4051, Bethesda, Md, 1997, National Heart, Lung, and Blood Institute, National Institutes of Health.

National Asthma Education and Prevention Program: Guidelines for the diagnosis and management of asthma, update on selected topics 2002, *J Allergy Clin Immunol* 110(5):S145-S219, 2002.

Neill RA: What are the indications for tonsillectomy in children? *J Fam Pract* 51:314, 2002.

O'Connor BB: SARS—The latest menacing microbe, *Nurs Spectrum* 13(12DC), June 16, 2003.

O'Neill P: Acute otitis media: child health. In *Clinical evidence*, pp 181-188, London, 2001, BMJ Publishing Group.

Palencia S: Treating the flu: available medications, *Allergy Asthma Health*, pp 30-32, Fall 2000.

Paradise JL and others: Tonsillectomy and adenotonsillectomy for recurrent throat infection in moderately affected children, *Pediatrics* 110:7-15, 2002.

Pelton SI: Otoscopy for the diagnosis of otitis media, *Pediatr Infect Dis J* 17:540-543, 1998.

Phipatanakul W and others: Mouse allergen I: the prevalence of mouse allergen in inner-city homes, The National Cooperative Inner-City Asthma Study, *J Allergy Clin Immunol* 106(6):1070-1074, 2000.

Piglansky L and others: Bacteriologic and clinical efficacy of high dose amoxicillin for therapy of acute otitis media in children, *Pediatr Infect Dis J* 22(5):405-413, 2003.

Ramsey AM: Diagnosis and treatment of the child with a draining ear, *J Pediatr Health Care* 16(4):161-169, 2002.

Redding GJ: Current concepts in adult respiratory distress syndrome in children, *Curr Opin Pediatr* 13(3):261-266, 2001.

Rosenstein BJ: Cystic fibrosis. In McMillan J and others, editors: *Oski's pediatrics: principles and practice*, ed 3, Philadelphia, 1999, Lippincott Williams & Wilkins.

Rosenwasser LJ, Nash DB: Incorporating omalizumab into asthma treatment guidelines: Consensus Panel recommendations, *Pharmacy Therapeutics* 28(6):400-413, 2003.

Sockrider MM: Respiratory complications of burns and smoke inhalation (respiratory burns). In McMillan J and others, editors: *Oski's pediatrics: principles and practice,* ed 3, Philadelphia, 1999, Lippincott Williams & Wilkins.

Suissa S and others: Low-dose inhaled corticosteroids and the prevention of death from asthma, *N Engl J Med* 343(5):332-336, 2000.

Tan TQ and others: Clinical characteristics of children with complicated pneumonia caused by *Streptococcus pneumoniae, Pediatrics* 110(1):1-6, 2002.

Thuma PE: Pharyngitis and tonsillitis. In Hoekelman RA and others, editors: *Primary pediatric care,* ed 3, St Louis, 1997, Mosby.

Togger DA, Brenner PS: Metered dose inhalers, *Am J Nurs* 101(10):26-32, 2001.

Tucker TL: Open doors—family presence at codes, *Nurs Spectrum* 13(12DC):8-9, 2003.

Twarog FJ: Inhaled steroids for asthma—how safe? *Pediatr Alert* Dec 10, 1998.

Wald ER: Croup. In McMillan J and others, editors: *Oski's pediatrics: principles and practice,* ed 3, Philadelphia, 1999, Lippincott Williams & Wilkins.

Walker JA, Weber P: Laser assisted myringotomy, *Advance for Nurses,* Jan 29, 2001, DC/Baltimore.

Winkelstein ML and others: Factors associated with medication self—administration in children with asthma, *Clin Pediatr* 39(6):337-345, 2000.

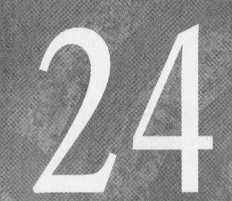

The Child With Gastrointestinal Dysfunction

CAROLYN V. DAIGNEAU

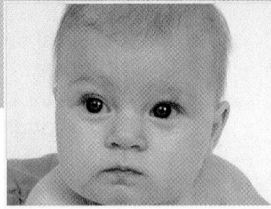

Remember to check out your companion CD-ROM

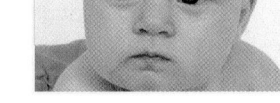

http://evolve.elsevier.com/Wong/essentials/

RELATED TOPICS and ADDITIONAL RESOURCES

 IN TEXT

Collection of Specimens, *Ch. 22*
Cystic Fibrosis, *Ch. 23*
Genitourinary Tract Disorders/Defects, *Ch. 27*
Diaper Dermatitis, *Ch. 30*
Encopresis, *Ch. 17*
Family-Centered Care of the Child During Illness and Hospitalization, *Ch. 21*
Infection Control, *Ch. 22*
Intestinal Parasitic Diseases, *Ch. 14*
Nursing Care of the High-Risk Newborn and Family, *Ch. 9*
Ostomies, *Ch. 22*
Pain Assessment; Pain Management, *Ch. 21*
Preparation for Procedures, *Ch. 22*
Procedures Related to Alternative Feeding Techniques, *Ch. 22*
Procedures Related to Elimination, *Ch. 22*

Recommendations for Routine Immunizations: Hepatitis, *Ch. 10*
Shock, *Ch. 25*
Surgical Procedures, *Ch. 22*
Total Parenteral Nutrition, *Ch. 22*

 CD COMPANION

Critical Thinking Exercises—Abdominal Pain; Constipation; Hematemesis; Home Care for the Adolescent; Ingestion of a Foreign Body
Case Studies—Appendicitis, Cleft Lip and Palate; Acute Diarrhea (Gastroenteritis); Dehydration and Diarrhea
Clinical Manifestations—Gastrointestinal Dysfunction in Children; Appendicitis; Hypertrophic Pyloric Stenosis
Nursing Care Plans
NCLEX-Style Review Questions

 WEBSITE

WebLinks
NCLEX-Style Review Questions

WONG'S CLINICAL MANUAL OF PEDIATRIC NURSING, 6/E

Nursing Care Plans—The Child With Hirschsprung Disease; The Child With Peptic Ulcer Disease; The Child With Acute Hepatitis; The Child With Hypertrophic Pyloric Stenosis; The Infant With an Anorectal Malformation; The Child With Celiac Disease
Community and Home Care Instructions—Caring for the Child With a Colostomy; Giving Gastrostomy Feedings; Caring for a Central Venous Catheter (for TPN)

LEARNING OBJECTIVES
On completion of this chapter the reader will be able to:

- Describe the characteristics of infants that affect their ability to adapt to fluid loss or gain.
- Formulate a plan of care for the infant with acute diarrhea.
- Compare and contrast the inflammatory diseases of the gastrointestinal tract.
- Describe the nursing care of the child with hepatitis.
- Formulate a plan for teaching parents preoperative and postoperative care of the child with a cleft lip or palate.
- Formulate a plan of care for the child with an obstructive disorder.
- Identify nutritional therapies for the child with a malabsorption syndrome.

GASTROINTESTINAL DYSFUNCTION

The extensive surface area of the gastrointestinal (GI) tract and its digestive function represent the major means of exchange between the human organism and the environment. Inflammatory and malabsorptive disorders impair the functional integrity of the GI tract. In addition, the intestine of the infant is extremely vulnerable to infection. Acute infectious diarrhea causes significant alterations in fluid and electrolyte balance in both infants and children.

Numerous observations provide clues to specific GI problems (Box 24-1). In any disorder that involves GI losses of large amounts of fluid, dehydration poses a serious threat to life and demands immediate attention.

DEHYDRATION

Dehydration is a common body fluid disturbance in infants and children and occurs whenever the total output of fluid exceeds the total intake, regardless of the cause. Dehydration may result from a number of diseases that cause insensible losses through the skin and respiratory tract, through increased renal excretion, and through the GI tract. Although dehydration can result from lack of oral intake (especially in elevated environmental temperatures), more often it is a result of abnormal losses, such as those that occur in vomiting or diarrhea, when oral intake only partially compensates for the abnormal losses. Other significant causes of dehydration are diabetic ketoacidosis and extensive burns.

Water Balance in Infants

Infants and young children have a greater need for water and are more vulnerable to alterations in fluid and electrolyte balance. Compared with older children and adults, infants have a greater fluid intake and output relative to size. Water and electrolyte disturbances occur more frequently and more rapidly, and infants and children adjust less promptly to these alterations.

The fluid compartments in the infant vary significantly from those in the adult, primarily because of an expanded extracellular compartment. The *extracellular fluid (ECF)* compartment constitutes more than half the total body water at birth and has a greater relative content of extracellular sodium and chloride. The infant loses a large amount of fluid at birth and maintains a larger amount of ECF than the adult until about 2 years of age. This contributes to greater and more rapid water loss during this age period.

Fluid losses create compartment deficits that are reflected throughout the duration of dehydration. In general, approximately 60% of fluid is lost from the ECF, and the remaining 40% comes from the *intracellular fluid (ICF)*. The amount of fluid lost from the ECF increases with acute illness and decreases with chronic loss.

Fluid losses vary with age and are divided into insensible, urinary, and fecal losses. Approximately two thirds of *insensible losses* occur through the skin; the remaining one third is lost through the respiratory tract. Heat and humidity, body temperature, and respiratory rate influence insensible fluid loss. Infants and children have a greater tendency to become highly febrile than do adults. Fever increases insensible water loss approximately 7 mL/kg/24 hr for each degree rise in temperature above 37.2° C (99° F). Fever and increased surface area relative to volume are factors that contribute to greater insensible fluid losses in young patients.

Body Surface Area. The infant's relatively greater body surface area (BSA) allows larger quantities of fluid to be lost in insensible perspiration through the skin. It is estimated that the BSA of the premature neonate is five times as great, and that of the newborn is two to three times as great, as that of the older child or adult. The proportionately longer GI tract in infancy is another source of fluid loss, especially from diarrhea.

Basal Metabolic Rate. The rate of metabolism in infancy is significantly higher than in adulthood because of the larger BSA in relation to the mass of active tissue. Consequently, there is a greater production of metabolic wastes that must be excreted by the kidneys. Any condition that increases metabolism causes greater heat production, insensible fluid loss, and an increased need for water for excretion. The basal metabolic rate (BMR) in infants and children is higher to support growth.

Kidney Function. The kidneys of the infant are functionally immature at birth and are inefficient in excreting waste products of metabolism. Of particular importance for fluid balance is the inability of the infant's kidneys to concentrate or dilute urine, to conserve or excrete sodium, and to acidify urine. The infant is less able to handle large quantities of solute-free water than is the older child, and infants are more likely to become dehydrated when given concentrated formulas or overhydrated when given excessive water or dilute formula.

BOX 24-1 ■ Clinical Manifestations of Gastrointestinal Dysfunction in Children

Failure to thrive—Weight consistently below the 3rd percentile or BMI (body mass index) below the 5th percentile or a decrease from established growth pattern.

Spitting up or **regurgitation**—Passive transfer of gastric contents into the esophagus or mouth

Vomiting—Forceful ejection of gastric contents; involves a complex process under central nervous system control that causes salivation, pallor, sweating, and tachycardia; usually accompanied by nausea

> *Projectile vomiting*—Vomiting accompanied by vigorous peristaltic waves and typically associated with pyloric stenosis or pylorospasm

Nausea—Unpleasant sensation vaguely referred to the throat or abdomen with an inclination to vomit

Constipation—Delay or difficulty with the passage of stools that is present for two or more weeks; associated with symptoms that may include blood-streaked stools and abdominal discomfort.

Encopresis—Involuntary overflow of incontinent stool causing soiling or incontinence secondary to fecal retention or impaction.

Diarrhea—Increase in the number of stools with an increased water content as a result of alterations of water and electrolyte transport by the gastrointestinal (GI) tract; may be acute or chronic

Hypoactive, hyperactive, or **absent bowel sounds**—Evidence of intestinal motility problems that may be caused by inflammation or obstruction

Abdominal distention—Protuberant contour of the abdomen that may be caused by delayed gastric emptying, accumulation of gas or stool, inflammation, or obstruction

Abdominal pain—Pain associated with the abdomen that may be localized or diffuse, acute or chronic; often caused by inflammation, obstruction, or hemorrhage

Gastrointestinal bleeding—May be from an upper or lower GI source and may be acute or chronic

> *Hematemesis*—Vomiting of bright red blood or denatured blood that results from bleeding in the upper GI tract or from swallowed blood from the nose or oropharynx

> *Hematochezia*—Passage of bright red blood per rectum, usually indicating lower GI tract bleeding

> *Melena*—Passage of dark-colored, "tarry" stools resulting from denatured blood, suggesting upper GI tract bleeding or bleeding from the right colon

Jaundice—Yellow coloration of the skin and sclerae associated with liver dysfunction

Dysphagia—Difficulty swallowing caused by abnormalities in the neuromuscular function of the pharynx or upper esophageal sphincter or by disorders of the esophagus

Dysfunctional swallowing—Impaired swallowing caused by central nervous system defects or structural defects of the oral cavity, pharynx, or esophagus; can cause feeding problems or aspiration

Fever—Common manifestation of illness in children with GI disorders; usually associated with dehydration, infection, or inflammation

BOX 24-2 ■ Daily Maintenance Fluid Requirements

1. Calculate weight of child in kilograms:

$$\frac{\text{Weight of child (in pounds)}}{\text{Divided by 2.2 pounds/kg}} = \text{Weight in kilograms}$$

2. Allow 100 mL/kg for first 10 kg.
3. Allow 50 mL/kg for second 10 kg.
4. Allow 20 mL/kg for remainder of weight in kilograms.
5. Divide total amount by 24 hours to obtain rate in milliliters per hour.

Fluid Requirements. Infants ingest and excrete a greater amount of fluid per kilogram of body weight than do older children. Because electrolytes are excreted with water and the infant has limited ability for conservation, maintenance requirements include both water and electrolytes. The daily exchange of ECF in the infant is greatly increased over that of older children, which leaves the infant little fluid volume reserve in dehydrated states. Fluid requirements depend on hydration status, size, environmental factors, and underlying disease (see Box 24-2 for Daily Maintenance Fluid Requirements).

Types of Dehydration

The pathophysiology of dehydration is understood by recognizing that the distribution of water between the ECF and ICF spaces depends on active transport of potassium into and sodium out of cells by energy-requiring processes. Sodium is the chief solute in ECF and is the primary determinant of ECF volume. Potassium is primarily intracellular. When ECF volume is reduced in acute dehydration, the total body sodium content is almost always reduced as well, regardless of serum sodium measurements. Replacement of fluid volume should therefore be accompanied by sodium repletion. Sodium depletion in diarrhea occurs in two ways: out of the body in stool and into the ICF compartment to replace potassium to maintain electrical equilibrium.

Dehydration is classified into three categories on the basis of osmolality and depends primarily on the serum sodium concentration: (1) isotonic, (2) hypotonic, and (3) hypertonic (Fann, 1998; Ledwith, 1997).

Isotonic (isosmotic or *isonatremic) dehydration,* the primary form of dehydration in children, occurs in conditions in which electrolyte and water deficits are present in approximately balanced proportions. Water and salt are lost in approximately equal amounts. The observable fluid losses are not necessarily isotonic, because losses from other avenues make adjustments so that the sum of all losses, or the net loss, is isotonic. There is no osmotic force between the ICF and the ECF, so the major loss is sustained from the ECF compartment. This significantly reduces the plasma volume and the circulating blood volume, which affects the skin, muscles, and kidneys. Shock is the greatest threat to life, and the child with isotonic dehydration displays symptoms characteristic of hypovolemic shock. Plasma sodium remains within normal limits, between 130 and 150 mEq/L.

Hypotonic (hyposmotic or *hyponatremic) dehydration* occurs when the electrolyte deficit exceeds the water deficit, leaving the serum hypotonic. Because ICF is more concentrated than ECF in hypotonic dehydration, water moves from the ECF to the ICF to establish osmotic equilibrium. This movement further increases the ECF volume loss, and shock is a frequent finding. Because there is a greater proportional loss of ECF in hypotonic dehydration, the physical signs tend to be more severe with smaller fluid losses than with isotonic or hypertonic dehydration. Serum sodium concentration is less than 130 mEq/L.

Hypertonic (*hyperosmotic* or *hypernatremic*) *dehydration* results from water loss in excess of electrolyte loss and is usually caused by a proportionally larger loss of water or a larger intake of electrolytes. This type of dehydration is the most dangerous and requires more specific fluid therapy. Hypertonic diarrhea may occur in infants who are given fluids by mouth that contain large amounts of solute, or in children who receive high-protein nasogastric tube feedings that place an excessive solute load on the kidneys. In hypertonic dehydration, fluid shifts from the lesser concentration of the ICF to the ECF. Plasma sodium concentration is greater than 150 mEq/L (Behrman, Kliegman, and Arvin, 2000).

Because the ECF volume is proportionally larger, hypertonic dehydration consists of a greater degree of water loss for the same intensity of physical signs. Shock is less apparent. However, neurologic disturbances, including alterations in consciousness, poor ability to focus attention, lethargy, increased muscle tone with hyperreflexia, and hyperirritability to stimuli are more likely to occur. Cerebral changes are serious and may result in permanent damage.

Diagnostic Evaluation

Diagnosis of the type and degree of dehydration is necessary to develop an effective plan of therapy. The degree of dehydration has been described as a percentage: 5% (mild), 10% (moderate), or 15% (severe). Water constitutes only 60% to 70% of the infant's weight. However, adipose tissue contains little water and is highly variable in individual infants and children. A more accurate means of describing dehydration is to reflect acute loss (over 48 hours or less) in milliliters per kilogram of body weight. For example, a loss of 50 mL/kg is considered to be a mild fluid loss, whereas a loss of 100 mL/kg produces severe dehydration. Weight is the most important determinant of the percent of total body fluid loss in infants and younger children. However, often the preillness weight is unknown. Other predictors of fluid loss include a changing level of consciousness (irritability to lethargy), response to stimuli, decreased skin elasticity and turgor, prolonged capillary refill, increased heart rate, and sunken eyes and fontanels. Clinical signs provide clues to the extent of dehydration (Table 24-1). Using multiple predictors increases the sensitivity of assessing the fluid deficit and early studies have shown a reasonably high degree of agreement between experienced observers in assessment of the level of dehydration. Objective signs of dehydration are present at a fluid deficit of less than 5%. Any two of the following signs—capillary refill of 2 seconds, absent tears, dry mucous membranes, and an ill general appearance—are predictors of a deficit of at least 5%. Generally, three or more clinical findings are present at a deficit of 5% to 9%, and six or more findings are found with a deficit of 10% or more (Gorelick, Shaw, and Murphy, 1997). Shock, tachycardia, and very low blood pressure are common features of severe depletion of ECF volume (see Shock, Chapter 25).

Therapeutic Management

See discussion on therapeutic management of diarrhea, p. 847.

Nursing Considerations

Nursing observation and intervention are essential to the detection and therapeutic management of dehydration. A variety of circumstances cause fluid losses in infants, and changes can take place quickly. An important nursing responsibility is observation for signs of dehydration. Nursing assessment should begin with observation of general appearance and proceed to more specific observations. Conditions in which dehydration may develop quickly include di-

TABLE 24-1 ■ **Evaluating Extent of Dehydration**

LEVEL OF DEHYDRATION	MILD	MODERATE	SEVERE
Weight loss—infants	5%	10%	15%
Weight loss—children	3%-4%	6%-8%	10%
Pulse	Normal	Slightly increased	Very increased
Blood pressure	Normal	Normal to orthostatic (>10 mm Hg change)	Orthostatic to shock
Behavior	Normal	Irritable, more thirsty	Hyperirritable to lethargic
Thirst	Slight	Moderate	Intense
Mucous membranes*	Normal	Dry	Parched
Tears	Present	Decreased	Absent, sunken eyes
Anterior fontanel	Normal	Normal to sunken	Sunken
External jugular vein	Visible when supine	Not visible except with supraclavicular pressure	Not visible even with supraclavicular pressure
Skin* (less useful in children >2 years)	Capillary refill >2 seconds	Slowed capillary refill (2-4 seconds [decreased turgor])	Very delayed capillary refill (>4 seconds) and tenting; skin cool, acrocyanotic or mottled
Urine specific gravity	>1.020	>1.020; oliguria	Oliguria or anuria

Adapted from Jospe N, Forbes G: Fluids and electrolytes—clinical aspects, *Pediatr Rev* 17(11):395-403, 1996.
*These signs are less prominent in patients who have hypernatremia.

arrhea; vomiting; sweating; fever; disorders such as diabetes, renal disease, and cardiac anomalies; administration of certain drugs (such as diuretics and steroids); and trauma (major surgery, burns, and other extensive injury).

Intake and Output.

Accurate measurements of fluid intake and output are vital to the assessment of dehydration. This includes oral and parenteral intake and losses from urine, stools, vomiting, fistulas, nasogastric suction, sweat, and wound drainage:

Urine—Frequency, color, consistency, and volume (when weighing diapers, approximately 1 g wet diaper weight equals 1 mL urine)

Stools—Frequency, volume, and consistency

Vomitus—Volume, frequency, and type

Sweating—Can be only estimated from frequency of clothing and linen changes

In addition to fluid intake and output, the following observations assist in assessment of dehydration:

Vital signs—Temperature (normal, elevated, or lowered depending on degree of dehydration), pulse (tachycardia), respirations (tachypnea), and blood pressure (hypotension)

Skin—Color, temperature, turgor, presence or absence of edema, and capillary refill

Mucous membranes—Moisture, color, and presence of and consistency of secretions

Body weight—Decreased in relation to degree of dehydration

Fontanel (infants)—Sunken, soft, or normal

Sensory alterations—Presence of thirst

For nursing interventions, see discussion under specific disorders.

DISORDERS OF MOTILITY

DIARRHEA

Diarrhea is a symptom that results from disorders involving digestive, absorptive, and secretory functions. Diarrhea is caused by abnormal intestinal water and electrolyte transport. Worldwide, there are an estimated 1.3 billion episodes of diarrhea. Approximately 24% of all deaths in children living in developing countries are related to diarrhea and dehydration. Most children living in developed countries have mild forms of gastroenteritis. However, in the United States, approximately 220,000 children younger than age 5 are hospitalized and approximately 300 children younger than 5 years die of diarrhea and dehydration each year (Endsley and Galbraith, 1998).

Diarrheal disturbances involve the stomach and intestines (gastroenteritis), the small intestine (enteritis), the colon (colitis), or the colon and intestines (enterocolitis). Diarrhea is classified as acute or chronic.

Acute diarrhea, a leading cause of illness in children younger than 5 years of age, is defined as a sudden increase in frequency and a change in consistency of stools, often caused by an infectious agent in the GI tract. It may be associated with upper respiratory or urinary tract infections, antibiotic therapy, or laxative use. Acute diarrhea is usually self-limited (less than 14 days duration) and subsides without specific treatment if dehydration does not occur. *Acute infectious di-*

arrhea (infectious gastroenteritis) is caused by a variety of viral, bacterial, and parasitic pathogens (Table 24-2).

Chronic diarrhea is defined as an increase in stool frequency and increased water content with a duration of more than 14 days. It is often caused by chronic conditions such as malabsorption syndromes, inflammatory bowel disease, immune deficiency, food allergy, lactose intolerance, or chronic nonspecific diarrhea, or as a result of inadequate management of acute diarrhea.

Intractable diarrhea of infancy is a syndrome that occurs in the first few months of life, persists for longer than 2 weeks with no recognized pathogens, and is refractory to treatment. The most common cause is acute infectious diarrhea that was not managed adequately.

Chronic nonspecific diarrhea (CNSD), also known as irritable colon of childhood and toddlers' diarrhea, is a common cause of chronic diarrhea in children 6 to 54 months of age. These children have loose stools, often with undigested food particles, and diarrhea greater than 2 weeks' duration. Children with CNSD grow normally and have no evidence of malnutrition, no blood in their stool, and no enteric infection (Huffman, 1999). Dietary indiscretions and food sensitivities have been linked to chronic diarrhea. The excessive intake of juices and artificial sweeteners such as sorbitol, a substance found in many commercially prepared beverages and foods, may be a factor.

Etiology

Most pathogens that cause diarrhea are spread by the fecal-oral route through contaminated food or water or are spread from person to person where there is close contact (e.g., day care centers). Lack of clean water, crowding, poor hygiene, nutritional deficiency, and poor sanitation are major risk factors, especially for bacterial or parasitic pathogens. The increased frequency and severity of diarrheal disease in infants is also related to age-specific alterations in susceptibility to pathogens. For example, the immune system of infants has not been exposed to many pathogens and has not acquired protective antibodies. Worldwide infectious agents, viruses, bacteria, and parasites are the most common causes of acute gastroenteritis. In developed nations, viruses, primarily rotavirus, cause 70% to 80% of infectious diarrhea.

Rotavirus is the most important cause of serious gastroenteritis among children and a significant nosocomial (hospital acquired) pathogen. Rotavirus disease is most severe in children 3 to 24 months of age. Children younger than 3 months of age have some protection from the disease because of maternally acquired antibodies. Approximately 25% of severe cases of rotavirus occur in older children (Coffin, 2001).

Salmonella, Shigella, and *Campylobacter* organisms are the most frequently isolated bacterial pathogens. *Salmonella* has the highest occurrence in infants; *Giardia* and *Shigella* have the highest incidence among toddlers. *Shigella* infection is uncommon in the United States, accounting for less than 5% of diarrheal illnesses in infants and toddlers. *Campylobacter* has a bimodal presentation (highest in children less than 12 months of age with a second rise in incidence at age 15 to 19 years). *Giardia* and *Cryptosporidium* organisms are parasites. *Giardia* represents 15% of nondysenteric illness in the United States; *Cryptosporidium* is often associated with outbreaks in

TABLE 24-2 ■ Infectious Causes of Acute Diarrhea

	PATHOLOGY	CHARACTERISTICS	COMMENTS
VIRAL AGENTS			
Rotavirus Incubation: 48 hours Diagnosis: enzyme immunoassay (EIA)	Fecal-oral transmission 7 groups (A-G): Most Group A Virus replicates in mature villus epithelial cells of small intestine; leads to (1) imbalance in ratio of intestinal fluid absorption to secretion and (2) malabsorption of complex carbohydrates	Mild to moderate fever Vomiting followed by the onset of watery stools: Fever and vomiting generally abate in approximately 2 days but diarrhea persists 5-7 days	Most common cause of diarrhea in children <5 years of age. Infants 6-12 months are most vulnerable. Peak occurrences in winter months. Important cause of nosocomial infections. Affects all ages; usually milder in children >3 years of age; immunocompromised children at greater risk for complications
Norwalk-Like Organisms Incubation: 12-48 hours Also called caliciviruses Diagnosis: EIA	Fecal-oral; contaminated water Pathology similar to rotavirus affects villus epithelial cells of small intestine leads to (1) imbalance in ratio of intestinal fluid absorption to secretion and (2) malabsorption of complex carbohydrates	Abdominal cramps; nausea vomiting, malaise, low-grade fever, watery diarrhea without blood; duration brief 2-3 days; tends to resemble so-called food poisoning symptoms with nausea predominating	Affects all ages Multiple strains often named for the location of outbreak (e.g., Norwalk, Sapporo, Snow Mountain, Montgomery)
BACTERIAL AGENTS			
Escherichia coli Incubation: 3-4 days Variable depending on strain Diagnosis: Sorbitol MacConkey Agar (SMAC agar) positive for blood but fecal leukocytes are absent or rare	*E. coli* strains produce diarrhea as result of enterotoxin production, adherence, or invasion (ETEC: enterotoxigenic-producing *E coli*) EHEC: Enterohemorrhagic *E. coli* Enteroaggregative *E. coli*)	Watery diarrhea 1-2 days then severe abdominal cramping and bloody diarrhea Can progress to hemolytic uremic syndrome (HUS)	Foodborne pathogen Traveler's diarrhea Highest incidence in summer Cause of nursery epidemics Symptomatic treatment Antibiotics may worsen course Antimotility agents and opioids should be avoided.
***Salmonella* groups** (nontyphoidal); Gram-negative rods, nonencapsulated nonsporulating Incubation 6-72 hours Diagnosis: gram-stained stool culture	Invasion of mucosa in the small and large intestine; edema of the lamina propria; focal acute inflammation with disruption of the mucosa and microabscesses	Nausea, vomiting, colicky abdominal pain, bloody diarrhea, fever; symptoms variable: mild to severe May have headache, and cerebral manifestations (e.g., drowsiness confusion, meningismus, seizures) Infants may be afebrile and nontoxic May result in life-threatening septicemia and meningitis Nausea/vomiting typically of short duration; diarrhea may persist as long as 2-3 weeks Typically shed virus for average of 5 weeks; cases reported up to a year	Incidence highest in warm months: July to November Foodborne outbreaks common Usually transmitted person to person but may transmit via undercooked meats, poultry Poultry and poultry products cause about half the cases. In children: pets (e.g., dogs, cats, hamsters, turtles) Communicable as long as organisms are excreted Antibiotics not recommended in uncomplicated cases Antimotility agents also not recommended—prolong transit time and carrier state Incidence decreasing over past 10 years
Salmonella typhi Produces enteric fever—systemic syndrome Incubation usually 7-14 days but could be 3-30 days depending on size of inoculum Diagnosis: positive blood cultures; also sometimes positive stool and urine Late stage: positive bone marrow culture	Bloodstream invasion; after ingestion, organism attaches to microvilli of ileal brush borders and bacteria invade the intestinal epithelium via Peyer's patches. Next is transported to intestinal lymph nodes and enters bloodstream via thoracic ducts, and circulating organisms reaches reticuloendothelial cells causing bacteremia	Manifestations depend on age Abdominal pain, diarrhea, nausea, vomiting, high fever, lethargy Must be treated with antibiotics	Incidence is much lower in developed countries; US has about 400 cases/year 65% of US cases acquired via international cases Ingestion of foods/water contaminated with human feces is most common mode of transmission Congenital and intrapartum transmission can occur Three vaccines are available

TABLE 24-2 ■ Infectious Causes of Acute Diarrhea—*cont'd*

	PATHOLOGY	CHARACTERISTICS	COMMENTS
***Shigella* groups** Gram-negative Nonmotile Anaerobic bacilli Incubation: 1-7 days Diagnosis: stool culture Loaded with polymorphonuclear leukocytes	Enterotoxins: invades the epithelium with superficial mucosal ulcerations	Patients appear sick Symptoms begin with fever, fatigue, anorexia Crampy abdominal pain precedes watery or bloody diarrhea Symptoms usually subside in 5-10 days	Most cases in children younger than 9 years with about one third of cases in children ages 1-4 weeks Antibiotics shorten illness and lower mortality All patients are at risk for dehydration Acute symptoms may persist for a week or more Antidiarrheal medications not recommended; may predispose to toxic mega colon
***Yersinia* enterocolitis** Incubation period: dose-dependent, 1-3 weeks Diagnosis: stool culture serology; (ELISA) Patients have leukocytosis; elevated sedimentation rate	Pathology is poorly understood; possibly production of enterotoxin	Mucoid diarrhea, sometimes bloody; abdominal pain suggestive of appendicitis; fever, vomiting	Seen more frequently in the winter months Transmitted by pets and food Antibiotics usually do not alter the clinical course in uncomplicated cases; antibiotics should be used in complicated infections and compromised hosts
Campylobacter jejuni Microaerophilic, motile, Gram-negative bacilli Incubation period: 1-7 days Ability to cause illness appears dose related. Diagnosis by stool culture, sometimes in the blood Commonly found in GI tract of wild or domestic animals	Not fully understood; possibly (1) adherence to intestinal mucosa by toxin; (2) invasion of the mucosa in the terminal ileum and colon; (3) translocation in which the organisms penetrate the mucosa and replicate in the lamina propria	Fever, abdominal pain, diarrhea, can be bloody; vomiting Watery, profuse, foul-smelling diarrhea Clinically like *Salmonella* or *Shigella* Fecal-oral transmission	Most infections in humans relate to consumption of contaminated foods or water; undercooked meats particularly chicken Also acquired from contaminated household pets (e.g., dogs, cats, hamsters) Bimodal peaks in infants <1 year and again at ages 15-29 Antibiotics do not prolong the carriage of bacteria and may eliminate organism more quickly Erythromycin is the drug of choice Antimotility agents not recommended and tend to prolong symptoms
Vibrio cholerae Gram-negative, motile, curved bacillus living in bodies of salt water Incubation 1-3 days Diagnosis by stool culture	Enters via oral route in contaminated food or water; if survives acid stomach environment, travels to the small intestine and adheres to the mucosa and produces toxin	Onset abrupt; vomiting, watery diarrhea without cramping or tenesmus Dehydration can occur quickly	More prevalent in developing countries Rehydration most important treatment Antibiotics can shorten diarrhea Despite continued efforts still no vaccine
Clostridium difficile Gram-positive anaerobic bacillus Diagnosis by detecting *C. difficile* toxin in stool culture.	Produces two important toxins (A and B) Toxin binds to the enterocyte surface receptor, resulting in alteration permeability, protein synthesis, and direct cytotoxicity	Mostly mild watery diarrhea lasting few days Some prolonged diarrhea and illness May cause pseudomembranous colitis Some individuals are extremely ill with high fever, leukocytosis, hypoalbuminemia	Associated with alteration of normal intestinal flora by antibiotics Adults tend to have more severe symptoms than children Treatment with antibiotics in symptomatic patients—metronidazole Resistant strains have developed Relapse is common

Continued

TABLE 24-2 ■ **Infectious Causes of Acute Diarrhea—*cont'd***

	PATHOLOGY	CHARACTERISTICS	COMMENTS
Clostridium perfringens Incubation period: 8-24 hours; anaerobic, gram-positive, spore-producing bacilli	Toxins produced in the intestine after ingestion of organism	Acute onset—watery diarrhea, crampy abdominal pain Fever, nausea, and vomiting rare Duration of illness usually 24 hours	Transmitted by contaminated food products, most often meats and poultry Usually self-limiting and medical intervention not needed Oral rehydration usually sufficient Antibiotics serve no purpose and should not be used
Clostridium botulinum Incubation period: 12-26 hours (range, 6 hours to 8 days) Gram-positive anaerobic spore-producing bacilli Blood and stool culture should be obtained and transmitted to special lab (usually state health department) to detect toxin	Botulism caused by binding of toxin to the neuromuscular junction	Clinical presentation related to age and the strain of the botulism GI abdominal pain, cramping, and diarrhea Other strains: respiratory, compromise CNS symptoms	Transmitted in contaminated food products Can be acquired via wound infection Treatment involves supportive care and neutralization of the toxin
Staphylococcus Incubation period is generally short, 1 to 8 hours Gram-positive nonmotile, aerobic, or facultative anaerobic bacteria Diagnosis by Identifying organism in food, blood, pus, aspirate	Direct tissue invasion and production of toxin	Clinical presentation depends on site of entry In food poisoning, profuse diarrhea, nausea, and vomiting	GI illness transmitted in inadequately cooked or refrigerated foods Self-limiting in GI illness Symptomatic treatment

young children in day care centers. *C. difficile, Plesiomonas,* and *Yersinia* are also parasites that are frequently responsible for causing diarrhea that lasts more than 10 days in a previously healthy adolescent. Traveler's diarrhea is also more common in adolescents than in other age-groups (Ramaswamy and Jacobson, 2001). (See also Intestinal Parasitic Diseases, Chapter 14).

Antibiotic administration is frequently associated with diarrhea because antibiotics alter the normal intestinal flora, resulting in an overgrowth of other bacteria such as *Clostridium difficile.* Antibiotic-associated diarrhea can also be caused by *Salmonella, Clostridium porringers* type A, and *Staphylococcus aureus* pathogens (Jabbar and Wright, 2003).

Pathophysiology

Invasion of the GI tract by pathogens results in increased intestinal secretion as a result of enterotoxins, cytotoxic mediators, or decreased intestinal absorption secondary to intestinal damage or inflammation. Enteric pathogens attach to the mucosal cells and form a cuplike pedestal on which the bacteria rest. The pathogenesis of the diarrhea depends on whether the organism remains attached to the cell surface resulting in a secretory toxin (noninvasive, toxin-producing, noninflammatory type diarrhea), or penetrates the mucosa (systemic diarrhea). Noninflammatory diarrhea is the most common diarrheal illness, resulting from the action of enterotoxin that is released after attachment to the

mucosa (Ramaswamy and Jacobson, 2001). The most serious and immediate physiologic disturbances associated with severe diarrheal disease are (1) dehydration, (2) acid-base imbalance with acidosis, and (3) shock that occurs when dehydration progresses to the point that circulatory status is seriously impaired.

Diagnostic Evaluation

Evaluation of the child with acute gastroenteritis begins with a careful history that seeks to discover the possible cause of diarrhea, to assess the severity of symptoms and the risk of complications, and to elicit information about current symptoms indicating other treatable illnesses that could be causing the diarrhea. The history should include questions about recent travel, exposure to untreated drinking or washing water sources, contact with animals or birds, day care center attendance, recent treatment with antibiotics, or recent diet changes. History questions should also explore the presence or absence of other symptoms such as the presence of fever, vomiting, frequency and character of stools (e.g., watery, bloody), urine output, dietary habits, and recent food intake (Burkhart, 1999).

Extensive laboratory evaluation is not indicated in children who have uncomplicated diarrhea and no evidence of dehydration because most diarrheal illnesses are self-limiting. Laboratory tests are indicated for children who are severely dehydrated and receiving intravenous therapy. Wa-

The Child With Gastrointestinal Dysfunction   CHAPTER 24   847

tery, explosive stools suggest glucose intolerance; foul-smelling, greasy, bulky stools suggest fat malabsorption. Diarrhea that develops after the introduction of cow's milk, fruits, or cereal may be related to enzyme deficiency or protein intolerance (Savilahti, 2000). Neutrophils or red blood cells in the stool indicate bacterial gastroenteritis or inflammatory bowel disease. The presence of eosinophils suggests protein intolerance or parasitic infection. There is debate about the benefit of obtaining stool cultures in children with domestically acquired gastroenteritis. Stool cultures should be performed when blood, mucus, or polymorphonuclear leukocytes are present in the stool; when symptoms are severe; when there is a history of travel to a developing country; and when there is suspicion of a specific pathogen. Gross blood or occult blood may indicate pathogens such as *Shigella, Campylobacter,* or hemorrhagic *Escherichia coli* strains. An enzyme-linked immunosorbent assay (ELISA) may be used to confirm the presence of rotavirus or *Giardia.* If there is a history of recent antibiotic use, the stool should be tested for *C. difficile* toxin. When bacterial and viral cultures are negative and when diarrhea persists for more than a few days, stools should be examined for ova and parasites. A stool specimen with a pH of less than 6 and the presence of reducing substances may indicate carbohydrate malabsorption or secondary lactase deficiency. Stool electrolyte measurements may help to identify children with secretory diarrhea.

Urine specific gravity should be determined if dehydration is suspected. A complete blood count (CBC), serum electrolytes, creatinine, and blood urea nitrogen (BUN) should be obtained in the child who requires hospitalization. The hemoglobin, hematocrit, creatinine, and BUN levels are usually elevated in acute diarrhea and should normalize with rehydration.

Therapeutic Management

The major goals in the management of acute diarrhea include (1) assessment of fluid and electrolyte imbalance, (2) rehydration, (3) maintenance fluid therapy, and (4) reintroduction of an adequate diet. Infants and children with acute diarrhea and dehydration should be treated first with *oral rehydration therapy (ORT).* ORT is one of the major worldwide health care advances of the past decade. It is more effective, safer, less painful, and less costly than intravenous (IV) rehydration. The American Academy of Pediatrics, World Health Organization, and Centers for Disease Control and Prevention all recommend ORT as the treatment of choice for most cases of dehydration caused by diarrhea (Nappert and others, 2000; American Academy of Pediatrics, 1996; Gastanaduy and Begue, 1999). Oral rehydration solutions (ORS) enhance and promote the reabsorption of sodium and water, and studies indicate that these solutions greatly reduce vomiting, volume loss from diarrhea, and the duration of the illness. Oral replacement solutions are available in the United States as commercially prepared solutions and are successful in treating the majority of infants with isotonic, hypotonic, or hypertonic dehydration. Guidelines for rehydration recommended by the American Academy of Pediatrics are included in Box 24-3.

BOX 24-3 ■ Model for Rehydration

Rehydration solution should consist of 75 to 90 mEq of sodium (Na+) per liter.

Give 40 to 50 mL/kg of rehydration solution over 4 hours.

Replacement and maintenance solution should consist of 40 to 60 mEq of Na+ per liter.

Reevaluate the need for further rehydration; initiate maintenance therapy using maintenance formulations, with daily volumes not to exceed 150 mL/kg/day.

In children with diarrhea without significant dehydration, the maintenance phase may be initiated without the need for rehydration solution (Acra and Ghishan, 1996).

If additional fluids are needed, use low-salt fluids such as breast milk or water.

Modified from American Academy of Pediatrics, Provisional Committee on Quality Improvement, Subcommittee on Acute Gastroenteritis: Practice parameter: the management of acute gastroenteritis in young children, *Pediatrics* 97(3):424-435, 1996.

After rehydration, ORS may be used during maintenance fluid therapy by alternating the solution with a low-sodium fluid such as water, breast milk, lactose-free formula, or half-strength lactose-containing formula. In older children ORS can be given and a regular diet continued. Ongoing stool losses should be replaced on a 1:1 basis with ORS. If the stool volume is not known, approximately 10 mL/kg (4 to 8 ounces) of ORS should be given for each diarrheal stool.

Solutions for oral hydration are useful in most cases of dehydration, and vomiting is not a contraindication. A child who is vomiting should be given an ORS at frequent intervals and in small amounts. In young children the fluid may be given with a spoon or small syringe in 5- to 10-mL increments every 1 to 5 minutes by the caregiver. An ORS may also be given via nasogastric or gastrostomy tube infusion. Infants without clinical signs of dehydration do not need ORT. They should, however, receive the same fluids recommended for infants with signs of dehydration in the maintenance phase and for ongoing stool losses.

! NURSING ALERT

Diarrhea is not managed by encouraging intake of clear fluids by mouth, such as fruit juices, carbonated soft drinks, and gelatin. These fluids usually have a high carbohydrate content, a very low electrolyte content, and a high osmolality (Lasche and Duggan, 1999). Caffeinated soda is avoided, because caffeine is a mild diuretic and may lead to increased loss of water and sodium. Chicken or beef broth is not given, because it contains excessive sodium and inadequate carbohydrate. A BRAT diet (bananas, rice, applesauce, and toast or tea) is contraindicated for the child and especially for the infant with acute diarrhea, because this diet has little nutritional value (low in energy and protein), is high in carbohydrates, and is low in electrolytes.

Early reintroduction of nutrients is desirable and is gaining more widespread acceptance. Continued feeding or early reintroduction of a normal diet has no adverse effects and actually lessens the severity and duration of the illness and improves weight gain when compared with the gradual reintroduction of foods (Lasche and Duggan, 1999). Infants who are breast-feeding should continue to do so, and ORS should be used to replace ongoing losses in these infants.

The use of nonhuman milk for infants and children with diarrhea remains controversial. Cow's milk and cow's milk formulas are of concern because poor digestion of lactose can occur in children with infectious diarrhea. However, some studies indicate that well-hydrated infants may resume full-strength nonhuman milk feeding immediately without adverse reactions (Hugger, Harkless, and Rentschler, 1998).

Many infants and children are safely managed with a diet containing cow's milk. Some practitioners advocate the use of a lactose-free formula only if milk or regular formula is not tolerated. In older children a regular diet can generally be offered after rehydration has been achieved. In toddlers there is no contraindication to continuing soft or pureed foods. A diet of easily digestible foods such as cereals, cooked vegetables, and meats is adequate for the older child.

In cases of severe dehydration and shock, IV fluids are initiated whenever the child is unable to ingest sufficient amounts of fluid and electrolytes to (1) meet ongoing daily physiologic losses, (2) replace previous deficits, and (3) replace ongoing abnormal losses. Patients who usually require IV fluids are those with severe dehydration, those with uncontrollable vomiting, those who are unable to drink for any reason (e.g., extreme fatigue, coma), and those with severe gastric distention.

The IV solution is selected on the basis of what is known regarding the probable type and cause of the dehydration—usually a saline solution containing 5% dextrose in water. Sodium bicarbonate may be added, because acidosis is usually associated with severe dehydration. Although the initial phase of fluid replacement is rapid in both isotonic and hypotonic dehydration, it is contraindicated in hypertonic dehydration because of the risk of water intoxication, especially in the brain cells.

After the severe effects of dehydration are under control, specific diagnostic and therapeutic measures are begun to detect and treat the cause of the diarrhea. Because of the self-limiting nature of vomiting and its tendency to improve when dehydration is corrected, the use of antiemetic agents is not recommended. The use of antibiotic therapy in children with acute gastroenteritis is controversial. Antibiotics may shorten the course of some diarrheal illnesses (e.g., those caused by *Shigella*). However, most bacterial diarrheas are self-limiting, and the diarrhea often resolves before the causative organism can be determined. Antibiotics may prolong the carrier period for bacteria such as *Salmonella*. Antibiotics may be considered, however, in patients with immunosuppression, severe symptoms or persistent disease, or patients who have had transplantation (Jabbar and Wright, 2003; Burkhart, 1999) (see Intestinal Parasitic Diseases, Chapter 14).

Nursing Considerations

Assessment

The nursing assessment of diarrhea begins with observation of the infant or child's general appearance and behavior. Physical assessment includes all the parameters described for assessment of dehydration, such as decreased urine output; decreased weight; dry mucous membranes; poor skin turgor,

sunken fontanel; and pale, cool, dry skin. With severe dehydration, increased pulse and respiration, decreased blood pressure, and a prolonged capillary refill time (>2 seconds) may indicate impending shock (see Table 24-1).

A history provides information about probable etiologic agents, such as introduction of a new food, exposure to infectious agents, travel to an area of high susceptibility, contact with foods that might be contaminated, and contact with pets known to be sources of enteric infections. An allergic, drug, and dietary history may indicate food allergies, use of laxatives or antibiotics, or sources of excess sorbitol and fructose (e.g., apple juice).

Nursing Diagnoses

Several nursing diagnoses are identified following a thorough physical assessment. The major diagnoses appropriate for the infant or child are described in the Nursing Care Plan on pp. 849-850. Other diagnoses may be evident depending on the age, condition, and etiology of the diarrhea.

Planning

The goals for the dehydrated infant or child and for the family are as follows:
1 Infant or child will maintain adequate hydration.
2 Infant or child will maintain appropriate nutrition for age.
3 Infant or child will not spread infection (if etiologic agent) to others.
4 Family will receive appropriate support and education, especially regarding home care.

Implementation

The management of most cases of acute diarrhea takes place in the home with education of the caregiver. Caregivers are taught to monitor for signs of dehydration (especially the number of wet diapers or voidings) and the amount of fluids taken by mouth, and to assess the frequency and amount of stool losses. Education relating to ORT, including the administration of maintenance fluids and replacement of ongoing losses, is important (see Critical Thinking Exercise). ORS should be administered in small quantities at frequent intervals. Vomiting is not a contraindication to ORT unless it is severe. Information concerning the introduction of a normal diet is essential. Parents need to know that a slightly higher stool output initially occurs with continuation of a normal diet and with ongoing replacement of stool losses. The benefits of a better nutritional outcome with fewer complications and a shorter duration of illness outweigh the potential increase in stool frequency. Parents' concerns should be addressed to ensure adherence to the treatment plan.

If the child with acute diarrhea and dehydration is hospitalized, an accurate weight must be obtained, as well as careful monitoring of intake and output. The child may be placed on parenteral fluid therapy with nothing by mouth (NPO) for 12 to 48 hours. Monitoring the IV infusion is an important nursing function. The nurse must ensure that the correct fluid and electrolyte concentration is infused, that the flow rate is adjusted to deliver the desired volume in a given time, and that the IV site is maintained.

Accurate measurement of output is essential to determine if renal blood flow is sufficient to permit the addition

NURSING CARE PLAN   The Child With Acute Diarrhea (Gastroenteritis)

NURSING DIAGNOSIS ■ **Fluid volume deficit related to excessive gastrointestinal (GI) losses in stool or emesis**

PATIENT GOAL 1: Will exhibit signs of rehydration and maintain adequate hydration

NURSING INTERVENTIONS/*RATIONALES*

*Administer an oral rehydration solution (ORS) *for both rehydration and replacement of stool losses*
  Give ORS frequently in small amounts, especially if child is vomiting, *because vomiting, unless severe, is not a contraindication to using ORS*
*Administer and monitor intravenous fluids as prescribed *for severe dehydration and vomiting*
*Administer antimicrobial agents as prescribed *to treat specific pathogens causing excessive GI losses*
Alternate ORS with a low-sodium fluid such as water, breast milk, or formula *for maintenance fluid therapy* (most authorities say formula should be lactose free only if infant is not tolerating formula)
After rehydration, offer child regular diet as tolerated *because studies show that early reintroduction of normal diet is beneficial in reducing number of stools and weight loss and shortening duration of illness*
Maintain a strict record of intake and output (urine, stool, and emesis) *to evaluate effectiveness of interventions*
Monitor urine specific gravity every 8 hours or as indicated *to assess hydration*
Weigh child daily *to assess for dehydration*
Assess vital signs, skin turgor, mucous membranes, and mental status every 4 hours or as indicated *to assess hydration*
Discourage intake of clear fluids such as fruit juices, carbonated soft drinks, and gelatin *because these fluids usually are high in carbohydrates and low in electrolytes, and have a high osmolality*
Instruct family in providing appropriate therapy, monitoring intake and output, and assessing for signs of dehydration *to ensure optimum results and improve compliance with the therapeutic regimen*

EXPECTED OUTCOME
Child exhibits signs of adequate hydration (specify)

NURSING DIAGNOSIS ■ **Altered nutrition: less than body requirements related to diarrheal losses, inadequate intake**

PATIENT GOAL 1: Will consume nourishment adequate to maintain appropriate weight for age

NURSING INTERVENTIONS/*RATIONALES*

After rehydration, instruct breast-feeding mother to continue feeding breast milk *because this tends to reduce severity and duration of illness*
Avoid giving BRAT diet (bananas, rice, applesauce, and toast or tea) *because this diet is low in energy and protein, too high in carbohydrates, and low in electrolytes*
Observe and record response to feedings *to assess feeding tolerance*
Instruct family in providing appropriate diet *to gain compliance with therapeutic regimen*

Explore concerns and priorities of family members *to improve compliance with therapeutic regimen*

EXPECTED OUTCOME
Child takes prescribed nourishment and exhibits a satisfactory weight gain

NURSING DIAGNOSIS ■ **Risk for transmitting infection related to microorganisms invading GI tract**

PATIENT (OTHERS) GOAL 1: Will not exhibit signs of GI infection

NURSING INTERVENTIONS/*RATIONALES*

Implement standard precautions or other hospital infection control practices, including appropriate disposal of stool and laundry and appropriate handling of specimens, *to reduce risk of spreading infection*
Maintain careful handwashing *to reduce risk of spreading infection*
Apply diaper snugly *to reduce likelihood of fecal spread*
Use superabsorbent disposable diapers *to contain feces and decrease chance of diaper dermatitis*
Attempt to keep infants and small children from placing hands and objects in contaminated areas
Teach children, when possible, protective measures *to prevent spread of infection,* such as handwashing after using toilet
Instruct family members and visitors in isolation practices, especially handwashing, *to reduce risk of spreading infection*

EXPECTED OUTCOME
Infection does not spread to others

NURSING DIAGNOSIS ■ **Impaired skin integrity related to irritation caused by frequent, loose stools**

PATIENT GOAL 1: Skin will remain intact

NURSING INTERVENTIONS/*RATIONALES*

Change diaper frequently *to keep skin clean and dry*
Cleanse buttocks gently with bland, nonalkaline soap and water or immerse child in a bath for gentle cleansing *because diarrheal stools are highly irritating to skin*
Apply ointment such as zinc oxide *to protect skin from irritation* (type of ointment may vary for each child and may require a trial period)
Expose slightly reddened intact skin to air whenever possible *to promote healing;* apply protective ointment to very irritated or excoriated skin *to facilitate healing*
Avoid using commercial baby wipes containing alcohol on excoriated skin *because they will cause stinging*
Observe buttocks and perineum for infection, such as *Candida,* so that appropriate therapy can be initiated
*Apply appropriate antifungal medication *to treat fungal infection of skin*

EXPECTED OUTCOME
Child has no evidence of skin breakdown

*Dependent nursing action.

Continued

NURSING DIAGNOSIS ▪ Anxiety/fear related to separation from parents, unfamiliar environment, distressing procedures

PATIENT GOAL 1: Will exhibit signs of comfort

NURSING INTERVENTIONS/*RATIONALES*

Provide mouth care and pacifier for infants *to provide comfort*

Encourage family visitation and participation in care as much as the family is able *to prevent stress associated with separation*

Touch, hold, and talk to child as much as possible *to provide comfort and relieve stress*

Provide sensory stimulation and diversion appropriate for child's developmental level and condition *to promote optimal growth and development*

EXPECTED OUTCOMES

Child exhibits minimal signs of physical or emotional distress

Family participates in child's care as much as possible

NURSING DIAGNOSIS ▪ Altered family processes related to situational crisis, knowledge deficit

PATIENT (FAMILY) GOAL 1: Family will understand about child's illness and its treatment and will be able to provide care

NURSING INTERVENTIONS/*RATIONALES*

Provide information to family about child's illness and therapeutic measures *to encourage compliance with therapeutic regimen, especially at home*

Assist family in providing comfort and support to child

Permit family members to participate in child's care as much as they desire *to meet needs of both child and family*

Instruct family regarding precautions *to prevent spread of infection*

Arrange for posthospitalization health care *for continued assessment and treatment*

Refer family to a community health care agency *for supervision of home care as needed*

EXPECTED OUTCOME

Family demonstrates ability to care for child, especially at home

---

?₂?₂ CRITICAL THINKING EXERCISE ???

Diarrhea

A mother brings her 8-month-old infant, Mary, to the primary care clinic. The mother reports that Mary has had a "cold" for about 2 days, and this morning she began to vomit and has had diarrhea for the past 8 hours. The mother states that Mary is still breast-feeding, but that she is not taking as much fluid as usual, and she is having three times as many stools as usual (the stools are watery in consistency). When the nurse practitioner examines Mary, she notes that her temperature is 100.4° F, her pulse and blood pressure are in the normal range, her mucous membranes are moist, and she has tears when she cries. The nurse practitioner also notes that Mary's weight has not changed from what it was when she was seen in the clinic 2 weeks ago for her well-child visit. What interventions should the nurse practitioner include in her initial management of Mary?

QUESTIONS

1. Evidence—Is there sufficient evidence for the nurse practitioner to draw any conclusions for her initial plan of management?
2. Assumptions—Describe some underlying assumptions about the following:
   a. Clinical manifestations of various levels of dehydration
   b. Management of acute diarrhea
   c. Breast-feeding and the management of acute diarrhea
   d. Use of antidiarrheal medications for acute diarrhea
3. What nursing interventions should the nurse practitioner implement at this time?
4. Does the evidence support the nurse practitioner's conclusion?
5. Are there any alternative perspectives that the nurse practitioner should consider?

ANSWERS

1. Yes, there are sufficient data for the nurse practitioner to arrive at some conclusions.
2. a. See Table 24-1, Evaluating Extent of Dehydration, and note the criteria for mild dehydration.
   b. Infants/children with mild dehydration are managed with oral rehydration therapy (ORS) and early reintroduction of an adequate diet. In cases of severe dehydration, or when infants and children have uncontrollable vomiting, intravenous fluids are used in the management of acute diarrhea.
   c. Breast-feeding generally can be continued in mild dehydration.
   d. Antidiarrheal medications are not recommended for the treatment of acute infectious diarrhea. These medications have adverse effects such as slowed motility and can prolong the illness.
3. At the present time, Mary meets all the criteria for mild dehydration. It is highly probable that she has acute infectious diarrhea because her mother noted that she has had a "cold" for several days, she is vomiting, having diarrhea, and has an elevated temperature. The priority for nursing care at this time is to provide rehydration via ORS. ORS is an effective, safe, and cost-effective way to treat mild dehydration. The nurse practitioner should provide the mother with instructions to give Mary ORS at frequent intervals and in small amounts. The mother should also be instructed to continue with breast-feeding and normal feedings. Early reintroduction of normal nutrients is desirable in cases of mild dehydration; delayed introduction of food may be harmful and can prolong the illness. Mary's mother should also be told to avoid the use of antidiarrheal medications.
4. Yes, the evidence supports this initial plan of management.
5. Mary's mother should be instructed to continue to monitor Mary for signs of improvement (an increase in the number of voidings or the number of wet diapers, and a decrease in vomiting). However, if Mary's condition does not improve, Mary's mother should be instructed to bring Mary back to the clinic or to the local emergency department. Mary's mother should be told to use frequent handwashing when caring for Mary to avoid transferring this infection to other members of the family.

of potassium to the IV fluids. The nurse is responsible for examination of stools and collection of specimens for laboratory examination (see Collection of Specimens, Chapter 22). Care should be taken when obtaining and transporting stools to prevent possible spread of infection. A clean tongue depressor can be used to obtain specimens for laboratory examination or as an applicator for transfer to a culture medium. Stool specimens should be transported to the laboratory in appropriate containers and media according to hospital policy.

Diarrheal stools are highly irritating to the skin, and extra care is needed to protect the skin of the diaper region from excoriation (see Diaper Dermatitis, Chapter 30). Rectal temperatures are avoided because they stimulate the bowel, increasing passage of stool.

Support for the child and family involves the same care and consideration given all hospitalized children (see Chapter 21). Parents are kept informed of the child's progress and instructed in the use of frequent and proper handwashing and the disposal of soiled diapers, clothes, and bed linen. Everyone caring for the child must be aware of "clean" areas and "dirty" areas, especially in the hospital, where the sink in the child's room is used for many purposes. Soiled diapers and linen should be discarded in receptacles close to the bedside. To remind caregivers to keep diapers and other soiled articles away from clean areas, place signs identifying "clean" (e.g., bed table) and "dirty" (e.g., sink, bathroom) areas. List the articles that may be stored in each area on these signs.

Prevention. The best intervention for diarrhea is prevention. The fecal-oral route spreads most infections, and parents need information about preventive measures such as personal hygiene, protecting the water supply from contamination, and careful food preparation.

> ### NURSING ALERT
>
> To reduce the risk of bacteria transmitted via food, encourage parents to:
>
> Quickly freeze or refrigerate all ground meat and other perishable foods.
>
> Never thaw food on the counter or let it sit out of the refrigerator for more than 2 hours.
>
> Wash hands, utensils, and work areas with hot, soapy water after contact with raw meat to keep bacteria from spreading.
>
> Check ground meat with a fork to make sure no pink is showing before taking a bite.
>
> Cook all dishes made with ground meat until brown or gray inside or to an internal temperature of 71° C (160° F).

Meticulous attention to perianal hygiene, disposal of soiled diapers, proper handwashing, and isolation of infected persons also minimizes the transmission of infection (see Infection Control, Chapter 22).

Parents need information about preventing diarrhea while traveling. They are cautioned against giving their children adult medications that are used to prevent traveler's diarrhea. Until vaccines or other prophylactic measures are proved to be safe for children, the best measure during travel to areas where water may be contaminated is to allow children to drink only bottled water and carbonated beverages (from the container through a straw supplied from home). Tap water, ice, unpasteurized dairy products, raw vegetables, unpeeled fruits, meats, and seafood should also be avoided.

● Evaluation

The effectiveness of nursing interventions is determined by continued reassessment according to the following observational guidelines:

1 Monitor fluid losses with careful intake and output measurements and daily weights.
2 Monitor food intake, especially calories.
3 Observe for evidence of complications from underlying disease (specify) or therapy.
4 Observe and interview family to determine extent and effectiveness of care.

The *expected outcomes* are described in the Nursing Care Plan on pp. 849-850.

CONSTIPATION

Constipation is an alteration in the frequency, consistency, or ease of passing stool. Parents often define constipation as 3 or more days without the passage of stool (Castiglia, 2001). It may also be defined as painful bowel movements, which are often blood streaked, or include the retention of stool, with or without soiling, even with a stool frequency of more than three stools per week (Loening-Baucke, 1995). The frequency of bowel movements, however, is not considered a diagnostic criterion because it varies widely among children. Having extremely long intervals between defecation is termed *obstipation.* Constipation with fecal soiling is referred to as *encopresis.*

Constipation may arise secondary to a variety of organic disorders or in association with a wide range of systemic disorders. Structural disorders of the intestine, such as strictures, ectopic anus, and Hirschsprung disease, may be associated with constipation. Systemic disorders associated with constipation include hypothyroidism, hypercalcemia resulting from hyperparathyroidism or vitamin D excess, and chronic lead poisoning. Constipation may be associated with drugs such as antacids, diuretics, antiepileptics, antihistamines, opioids, and iron supplementation. Spinal cord lesions may be associated with loss of rectal tone and sensation. Affected children are prone to chronic fecal retention and overflow incontinence.

The majority of children have *idiopathic* or *functional constipation,* because no underlying cause can be identified. Chronic constipation may occur as a result of environmental or psychosocial factors, or a combination of both. Transient illness, withholding and avoidance secondary to painful or negative experiences with stooling, and dietary intake with decreased fluid and fiber all play a role in the etiology of constipation.

Newborn Period

Normally the newborn infant passes a first meconium stool within 24 to 36 hours of birth. Any infant who does not do so should be assessed for evidence of intestinal atresia or stenosis, Hirschsprung disease (congenital aganglionic megacolon), hypothyroidism, meconium plugs, or meconium ileus.

??? CRITICAL THINKING EXERCISE

Constipation

Harry, an 8-month-old infant, is seen by the pediatric nurse practitioner for his well-child visit. Harry's mother states that he usually has one hard stool every 4 to 5 days, which causes discomfort when the stool is passed. He has also had one episode of diarrhea and two episodes of ribbonlike stools. Abdominal distention and vomiting have not accompanied the constipation, and Harry's growth has been normal. Currently, his diet consists of cow's milk formula only. Harry's mother reports that the infrequent passage of hard stools began approximately 6 weeks ago when she stopped breast-feeding. Which interventions should the nurse practitioner include in the initial management of Harry's problem?

QUESTIONS

1. Evidence—Is there sufficient evidence for the nurse practitioner to draw any conclusions about the management of Harry's problem?
2. Assumptions—Describe some underlying assumptions about the following:
   a. Causes of constipation in infants
   b. Factors associated with functional constipation in infants
   c. Management of functional constipation in infants
3. What interventions should the nurse practitioner implement at this time?
4. Does the evidence support these interventions?
5. Are there alternative perspectives that the nurse practitioner should consider? What are they?

ANSWERS

1. Yes, there are sufficient data to arrive at some conclusions for an initial plan of management.
2. a. Constipation in infancy can be caused by medical conditions such as Hirschsprung disease, hypothyroidism, or strictures, or it can be simple functional constipation.
   b. In infancy, changes in dietary practices such as a change from human milk to cow's milk may precipitate functional constipation.
   c. Functional constipation is usually treated by dietary modifications such as increasing the amount of carbohydrate, fruit, or vegetables in the infant's diet.
3. Initially, the nurse practitioner can tell Harry's mother that functional constipation may occur with changes in the diet (e.g., the change from breast-feeding 6 weeks ago to bottle-feeding of cow's milk). The nurse practitioner can recommend that Harry's mother slowly introduce cereal and prune juice into Harry's diet. Cereal and one or two offerings of fruit juice each day may help to prevent further constipation. Often, simple measures such as the introduction of solid foods or other dietary modifications help to remedy functional constipation.
4. The initial data seem to point to the conclusion that Harry has functional constipation. However, the one episode of diarrhea and the two episodes of passage of ribbonlike stools do not usually occur with functional constipation.
5. The nurse practitioner should remember that constipation can be caused by medical conditions such as Hirschsprung disease; therefore, a referral to a gastroenterologist for further evaluation is also warranted at this time.

Meconium plugs are caused by meconium that has reduced water content and are usually evacuated after digital examination but may require irrigations with a hypertonic solution or contrast medium.

Meconium ileus, the initial manifestation of cystic fibrosis, is the luminal obstruction of the distal small intestine by abnormal meconium. Treatment is the same as for a meconium plug; early surgical intervention may be needed to evacuate the small intestine.

Infancy

The onset of constipation frequently occurs during infancy, and may result from organic causes such as Hirschsprung disease, hypothyroidism, and strictures. It is important to differentiate these conditions from functional constipation. Constipation in infancy is often related to dietary practices. It is less common in breast-fed infants, who have softer stools than bottle-fed infants. Breast-fed infants may also have decreased stools because of more complete use of breast milk with little residue. When constipation occurs with a change from human milk or modified cow's milk to whole cow's milk, simple measures such as adding or increasing the amount of cereal, vegetables, and fruit in the diet of the infant usually corrects the problem. When a bottle-fed infant passes a hard stool that results in an anal fissure, stool-with-

holding behaviors may develop in response to pain on defecation (see Critical Thinking Exercise).

Childhood

Most constipation in early childhood is due to environmental changes or normal development when a child begins to attain control over bodily functions. A child who has experienced discomfort during bowel movements may deliberately try to withhold stool. Over time, the rectum accommodates to the accumulation of stool, and the urge to defecate passes. When the bowel contents are ultimately evacuated, the accumulated feces are passed with pain, thus reinforcing the desire to withhold stool.

Constipation in school-age children may represent an ongoing problem or a first-time event. The onset of constipation at this age is often the result of environmental changes, stresses, and changes in toileting patterns. A common cause of new-onset constipation at school entry is fear of using the school bathrooms, which are noted for their lack of privacy. Early and hurried departure for school immediately after breakfast may also impede bathroom use.

The management of simple constipation consists of a plan to promote regular bowel movements. Often this is as simple as changing the diet to provide more fiber and fluids, eliminating foods known to be constipating, and estab-

BOX 24-4 ■ High-Fiber Foods

BREAD, GRAINS
Whole-grain bread or rolls
Whole-grain cereals
Bran
Pancakes, waffles, and muffins with fruit or bran
Unrefined (brown) rice

VEGETABLES
Raw vegetables, especially broccoli, cabbage, carrots, cauliflower, celery, lettuce, and spinach
Cooked vegetables, such as those listed above, and asparagus, beans, Brussels sprouts, corn, potatoes, rhubarb, squash, string beans, and turnips

FRUITS
Raw fruits, especially those with skins or seeds, other than ripe banana or avocado
Raisins, prunes, or other dried fruits

MISCELLANEOUS
Nuts, seeds, legumes, popcorn
High-fiber snack bars

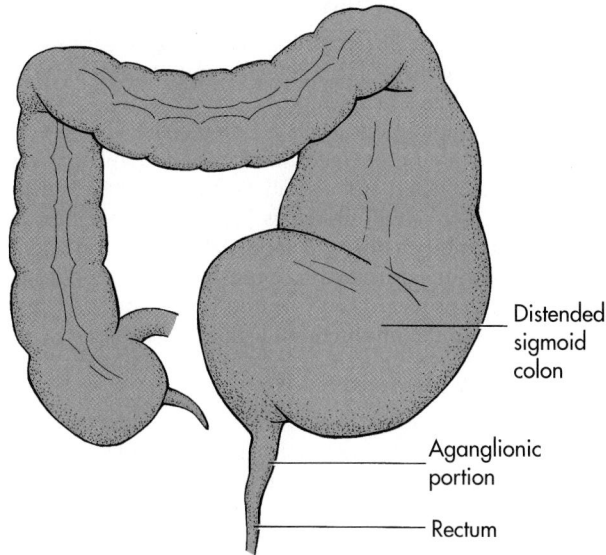

FIG. 24-1 ■ Hirschsprung disease.

lishing a bowel routine that allows for regular passage of stool. Stool-softening agents such as docusate or lactulose may also be helpful. If other symptoms such as vomiting, abdominal distention, or pain and evidence of growth failure are associated with the constipation, the condition should be investigated further.

Nursing Considerations

Constipation tends to be self-perpetuating. A child who has difficulty or discomfort when attempting to evacuate the bowels has a tendency to retain the bowel contents, and this may initiate a vicious circle. Nursing assessment begins with an accurate history of bowel habits, diet, events associated with the onset of constipation, drugs or other substances that the child may be taking, and the consistency, color, frequency, and other characteristics of the stool. If there is no evidence of a pathologic condition, the major task is to educate the parents regarding normal stool patterns and to participate in the education and treatment of the child.

Dietary modifications are essential in preventing constipation. During infancy, simply increasing the carbohydrate (sugar or corn syrup) in the infant's formula will often relieve the problem. During childhood the diet should contain increased amounts of fiber and fluid. Parents benefit from guidance in selecting foods that facilitate bowel movements (Box 24-4). They need reassurance concerning the benign nature of the condition. It is also important to discuss their attitudes and expectations regarding toilet habits.

When constipation persists despite dietary intervention, more aggressive management may be necessary. It is important to differentiate an acute episode of constipation from chronic functional constipation, which can result from chronic stool-withholding behavior. As the rectal vault becomes distended over time, further complications such as fecal impaction and encopresis may develop (see Chapter 17).

HIRSCHSPRUNG DISEASE

Hirschsprung disease *(congenital aganglionic megacolon)* is a mechanical obstruction caused by inadequate motility of part of the intestine. It accounts for about one fourth of all cases of neonatal obstruction, although it may not be diagnosed until later in infancy or childhood. The incidence is 1 in 5000 live births. It is four times more common in males than in females, and may follow a familial pattern in a small number of cases. Hirschsprung disease is usually an isolated birth defect but it has been associated with other syndromes including Down syndrome. Depending on its presentation, it may be an acute, life-threatening, or chronic condition (DiLorenzo, 2001).

Pathophysiology

The term *congenital aganglionic megacolon* describes the primary defect, which is the absence of ganglion cells in one or more segments of the colon. In Hirschsprung disease, there is an abnormal migration of the precursor ganglion cells that derive from the neural crest in the developing brain. The result is an impaired colonization of ganglion cells in the distal portion of the GI tract resulting in aganglionosis. In about 75% of cases the disease is limited to the rectosigmoid area with the aganglionic segment beginning at the internal anal sphincter and extending proximally, blending into the normal colon. Lack of enervation produces the functional defect that results in absence of propulsive movements (peristalsis). Stool accumulates with distention of the bowel proximal to the defect (megacolon). The internal sphincter fails to relax because the ganglion segment is missing the inhibitory neurotransmitter, nitric oxide. The result is an obstruction because the evacuation of stool, gas, and liquids is prevented (Fig. 24-1). Intestinal distention and ischemia may also occur as a result of distention of the bowel wall, which contributes to the development of *enterocolitis* (inflammation of the small bowel and colon). Enterocolitis is the leading cause of death in children with Hirschsprung disease (DiLorenzo, 2001).

Diagnostic Evaluation

Most children with Hirschsprung disease are diagnosed in the first few months of life. Clinical manifestations vary according to the age when symptoms are recognized and the presence of complications, such as enterocolitis (Box 24-5). In infants the findings include a distended abdomen, a contracted anal sphincter, and a small-caliber empty rectum. In older children, a careful history is helpful. Radiographs, an unprepped barium enema, and anorectal manometric examinations assist in the differential diagnosis, which is confirmed by a full-thickness rectal biopsy demonstrating the absence of ganglion cells in the myenteric and submucosal plexus.

Therapeutic Management

Treatment is primarily surgical to remove the aganglionic portion of the bowel to relieve obstruction and restore normal bowel motility and function of the internal anal sphincter. If the bowel is not significantly distended, this is accomplished in one surgery. However, in most cases two stages are required. First, a temporary ostomy is created proximal to the aganglionic segment to relieve obstruction and allow the normally enervated and dilated bowel to return to its normal size. Second, complete corrective surgery is performed usually when the child weighs approximately 9 kg (20 pounds). The various surgical procedures that can be performed are the Swenson, Duhamel, Boley, and Soave procedures. The Soave endorectal pull-through procedure, one of the most frequently used procedures, consists of pulling the end of the normal bowel through the muscular sleeve of the rectum, from which the aganglionic mucosa has been removed. The ostomy is usually closed at the time of the pull-through procedure.

Prognosis.   Most children with Hirschsprung disease require surgery rather than medical therapy. Once the patient is stabilized with fluid and electrolyte replacement, if needed,

BOX 24-5 ■ Clinical Manifestations of Hirschsprung Disease

NEWBORN PERIOD
Failure to pass meconium within 24 to 48 hours after birth
Refusal to feed
Bilious vomiting
Abdominal distention

INFANCY
Failure to thrive
Constipation
Abdominal distention
Episodes of diarrhea and vomiting
Signs of enterocolitis
    Explosive, watery diarrhea
    Fever
    Appears significantly ill

CHILDHOOD (SYMPTOMS APPEAR MORE CHRONIC)
Constipation
Ribbonlike, foul-smelling stools
Abdominal distention
Visible peristalsis
Easily palpable fecal mass
Undernourished anemic appearance

the temporary colostomy is performed and has a high rate of success. After the later pull-through procedure, anal stricture and incontinence are potential complications that may occur, requiring further therapy, including dilation or bowel-retraining therapy.

Nursing Considerations

The nursing concerns depend on the child's age and the type of treatment. If the disorder is diagnosed during the neonatal period, the main objectives are (1) to help the parents adjust to a congenital defect in their child, (2) to foster infant-parent bonding, (3) to prepare them for the medical/surgical intervention, and (4) to assist them in colostomy care after discharge.

Preoperative Care.   The child's preoperative care depends on the age and clinical condition. A child who is malnourished may not be able to withstand surgery until the physical status improves. Often this involves symptomatic treatment with enemas; a low-fiber, high-calorie, and high-protein diet; and in severe situations the use of total parenteral nutrition (TPN).

Physical preoperative preparation includes the same measures that are common to any surgery (see Surgical Procedures, Chapter 22). In the newborn, whose bowel is sterile, no additional preparation is necessary. However, in other children, preparation for the pull-through procedure involves emptying the bowel with repeated saline enemas and decreasing bacterial flora with systemic antibiotics and colonic irrigations using antibiotic solution. Oral antibiotics may also be prescribed.

Enterocolitis is the most serious complication of Hirschsprung disease. Emergency preoperative care includes frequent monitoring of vital signs and blood pressure for signs of shock; monitoring fluid and electrolyte replacements, as well as plasma or other blood derivatives; and observing for symptoms of bowel perforation, such as fever, increasing abdominal distention, vomiting, increased tenderness, irritability, dyspnea, and cyanosis.

Because progressive distention of the abdomen is a serious sign, the nurse measures abdominal circumference with a paper tape measure, usually at the level of the umbilicus or at the widest part of the abdomen. The point of measurement is marked with a pen to ensure reliability of subsequent measurements. Abdominal measurement can be obtained with the vital sign measurements and is recorded in serial order so that any change is obvious. To reduce stress to the acutely ill child when frequent measurements of abdominal circumference are needed, the tape measure can be left in place beneath the child rather than removed each time.

The child's age dictates the type and extent of psychologic preparation. Because a colostomy is usually performed, the child who is of at least preschool age is told about the procedure in concrete terms with the use of visual aids (see Chapter 22). It is important to time explanations appropriately to prevent the anxiety and confusion that could result from too much information. It is also important to stress to parents and older children that the colostomy for Hirschsprung disease is temporary, unless so much bowel is involved that a permanent ileostomy must be performed. In most instances the extent of bowel resection is known before surgery, although the nurse should be aware of those instances when doubt exists concerning repair. The nurse should remember that although a temporary colostomy is favorable in terms of future health and adjustment, it requires additional surgery, which may be very stressful to parents and children.

Postoperative Care.   Postoperative care is the same as that for any child or infant with abdominal surgery (see Surgical Procedures, Chapter 22). When a colostomy is part of the corrective procedure, stomal care is a major nursing task (see Ostomies, Chapter 22). To prevent contamination of the abdominal wound with urine in the infant, the diaper should be pinned below the dressing. Sometimes a Foley catheter is used in the immediate postoperative period to divert the flow of urine away from the abdomen.

Discharge Care.   After surgery, parents need instruction concerning colostomy care. Even a preschooler can be included in the care by handing articles to the parent, rolling up the colostomy pouch after it is emptied, or applying barrier preparations to the surrounding skin. Although the diagnosis of Hirschsprung disease is less frequent in school-age children or adolescents, children this age can often be involved in colostomy care to the point of total responsibility.

Some institutions and communities have enterostomal therapists who provide expert assistance in planning home care. If families require financial assistance and psychologic support, referral to a social worker, home health care agency, or community health nurse provides continuity of care.

VOMITING

Vomiting is the forceful ejection of gastric contents through the mouth. It is a well-defined, complex, coordinated process that is under central nervous system control and is often accompanied by nausea and retching. Vomiting may be divided into two categories, nonbilious and bilious. Some small intestinal reflux is common in all vomiting. In nonbilious vomiting, the majority of bile drains into the more distal portions of the intestine. If an obstruction is present, nonbilious vomiting suggests a more proximal obstruction. Bilious vomiting implies a disorder of motility or distal physical blockage. Causes of nonbilious vomiting include infectious, inflammatory, metabolic/endocrinologic, neurologic, and psychologic causes, and obstructive lesions. Causes of bilious vomiting include intestinal atresia and stenosis, malrotation with or without volvulus, ileus, intussusceptions, intestinal duplication, mass lesions, incarcerated inguinal hernia, and appendicitis. Vomiting may also be associated with other processes including acute infectious diseases, increased intracranial pressure (ICP), toxic ingestions, food intolerances and allergies, mechanical obstruction of the GI tract, metabolic disorders, and psychogenic problems. Vomiting is common in childhood, is usually self-limited, and requires no specific treatment. However, complications may occur, including dehydration and electrolyte disturbances, malnutrition, aspiration, and Mallory-Weiss syndrome (small tears in the distal esophageal mucosa).

Therapeutic Management

Management is directed toward detection and treatment of the cause of the vomiting and prevention of complications from the loss of fluid. Fluids are administered in the same manner and in a similar electrolyte composition to those ad-

ministered for diarrhea. Although most children respond to these measures, antiemetic drugs may be needed. Antiemetics such as ondansetron (Zofran) and trimethobenzamide (Tigan) block receptors in the chemoreceptor trigger zone; others such as metoclopramide (Reglan) enhance gastroduodenal peristalsis; still others such as promethazine (Phenergan) compete for H_1-receptor sites. For children who are prone to motion sickness, it is helpful to administer an appropriate dose of dimenhydrinate (Dramamine) before a trip.

Nursing Considerations

The major focus of nursing care is observation and reporting of vomiting behavior and associated symptoms and the implementation of measures to reduce the vomiting. Accurate assessment of the type of vomiting, the appearance of the vomitus, and the child's behavior in association with the vomiting helps to establish a diagnosis.

Nursing interventions are determined by the cause of the vomiting. When the vomiting is a manifestation of improper feeding methods, establishing proper techniques through teaching and example will usually correct the situation. If vomiting is believed to be an indication of obstruction, food is usually withheld or special feeding techniques are implemented. In situations in which vomiting is related to concurrent infection, dietary indiscretion, or emotional factors, efforts are directed toward maintaining hydration or preventing dehydration.

The thirst mechanism is the most sensitive guide to fluid needs, and ad libitum administration of a glucose-electrolyte solution to an alert child will restore water and electrolytes satisfactorily. It is important to include carbohydrate to spare body protein and avoid ketosis resulting from exhaustion of glycogen stores. Small, frequent feedings of fluids or foods are preferred. After vomiting has stopped, more liberal amounts of fluids are offered, followed by gradual resumption of the regular diet.

The vomiting infant or child is positioned on the side or semireclining to prevent aspiration and observed for evidence of dehydration. It is important to emphasize the need for the child to brush the teeth or rinse the mouth after vomiting to dilute hydrochloric acid that comes in contact with the teeth. A flavored mouthwash or tooth brushing will freshen the mouth. Careful monitoring of fluid and electrolyte status is necessary to prevent an electrolyte disturbance.

GASTROESOPHAGEAL REFLUX

Gastroesophageal reflux (GER) is defined as the transfer of gastric contents into the esophagus. Approximately 1 in 300 to 1 in 1000 children have gastroesophageal reflux. It is important to differentiate GER from *gastroesophageal reflux disease (GERD).* GERD represents symptoms or tissue damage that result from GER. However, GER may occur without reflux disease (GERD), and conversely GERD may occur without regurgitation (Orenstein, 1999). GER becomes a disease when complications such as failure to thrive, bleeding, or dysphagia develop. GERD is associated with respiratory symptoms, including apnea, bronchospasm, laryngospasm, and pneumonia (Zeiter and Hyams, 1999).

The causes of GER are related to dysfunction of the *lower esophageal sphincter (LES),* delay in gastric emptying, poor clearance of esophageal acid, and the susceptibility of esophageal mucosa to acid injury (Zeiter and Hyams,

1999). In the past, GER was thought to be the result of decreased LES tone. However, it now appears that *transient relaxation of the lower esophageal sphincter (TRLES)* is the mechanism the leads to GER. Factors that cause LES pressure to vary include gastric distention, increased abdominal pressure caused by coughing, central nervous system (CNS) disease, delayed gastric emptying, hiatal hernia, and gastrostomy placement.

Infants and children who are especially prone to GER include premature infants, infants with bronchopulmonary dysplasia, and children who have had tracheoesophageal or esophageal atresia repair, neurologic disorders, scoliosis, asthma, cystic fibrosis, or cerebral palsy.

Reflux of stomach contents into the esophagus predisposes the infant or child to aspiration and the development of respiratory symptoms, particularly pneumonia. Other concerns include the association of life-threatening apnea with GER; repeated irritation of the esophageal lining with gastric acid can lead to esophagitis and subsequent bleeding. Bleeding produces anemia, hematemesis, or melena (blood in stools). Heartburn is also a frequent symptom in children who are able to describe it (see also Box 24-6).

Diagnostic Evaluation

The history and physical examination is usually sufficiently reliable to establish the diagnosis of GER. However, the upper GI series is helpful to evaluate the presence of anatomic abnormalities (e.g., pyloric stenosis, malrotation, annular pancreas, hiatal hernia, esophageal stricture). Esophageal pH monitoring establishes the presence of acid reflux. Endoscopy may be helpful to assess the presence and severity of esophagitis and strictures and to exclude other disorders such as Crohn disease. *Scintigraphy* detects radioactive substances in the esophagus after a feeding of the compound and assesses gastric emptying.

Therapeutic Management

Therapeutic management of GER depends on its severity. No therapy is needed for the infant who is thriving and has no respiratory complications. Some children require small, frequent feedings of thickened formula and positioning therapy, which helps to minimize the symptoms until the child grows and a normal physiologic barrier to reflux develops.

Although more study continues on this topic, there is evidence to support a 1- to 2-week trial of a hypoallergenic formula in formula-fed infants. Controversies surround thickened feedings. Milk-thickening agents do not improve reflux index scores, but this therapy has been shown to decrease the number of episodes of vomiting and to increase the caloric density of the formula. Feedings thickened with 1 teaspoon to 1 tablespoon of rice cereal per ounce of formula may be recommended. This may benefit infants who are underweight as a result of GERD. Constant nasogastric feedings may be necessary for the infant with severe reflux and failure to thrive.

Several studies have examined the effectiveness of positioning therapy for infants. Esophageal pH monitoring has demonstrated that infants have significantly less GER in the prone position than in the supine position. Despite the potential benefit of the prone position in relationship to GERD, because of its association with sudden infant death syndrome (SIDS), the American Academy of Pediatrics recommends non-prone positioning for sleep (see Chapter 11). The prone position should only be considered in cases where the risk of death from the complications of GER outweighs the risk of SIDS. If the prone position is used, parents need to be cautioned to avoid soft bedding, which can increase the risk of SIDS. In children older than a year, there is a benefit to the left side position during sleep and the elevation of the head of the bed.

Pharmacologic therapy may be used as an adjunct therapy to treat infants and children with persistent symptoms of GER. H_2 antagonists, such as cimetidine (Tagamet), ranitidine (Zantac), or famotidine (Pepcid), have proved effective in reducing the amount of acid present in gastric contents and may prevent esophagitis. Proton pump inhibitors such as esomeprazole (Nexium), lansoprazole (Prevacid), omeprazole (Prilosec), pantoprazole (Protonix), and rabeprazole (Aciphex) are very effective in blocking acid production. Current investigations are ongoing to examine the effectiveness and potential side effects of these drugs in infants and children. Metoclopramide (Reglan) has been found to increase resting LES pressure mildly and to increase rates of gastric emptying. However, side effects, including restlessness, drowsiness, and extrapyramidal reaction, may occur, and in some patients, metoclopramide actually increases the number of reflux episodes. Bethanechol has been shown to increase LES pressure but has not been proved to decrease reflux by pH probe

---

BOX 24-6 ■ Clinical Manifestations and Complications of Gastroesophageal Reflux

SYMPTOMS IN INFANTS
Spitting up, regurgitation, vomiting (may be forceful)
Excessive crying, irritability, arching of the back, stiffening
Weight loss, failure to thrive
Respiratory problems (cough, wheeze, stridor, gagging, choking with feedings)
Hematemesis
Apnea or apparent life-threatening event (ALTE)

SYMPTOMS IN CHILDREN
Heartburn
Abdominal pain
Noncardiac chest pain
Chronic cough
Dysphagia
Nocturnal asthma
Recurrent pneumonia

COMPLICATIONS
Esophagitis
Esophageal stricture
Laryngitis
Recurrent pneumonia
Anemia
Barrett's esophagus

Adapted from Rudolph CD and others: Guidelines for evaluation and treatment of gastroesophageal reflux in infants and children: Recommendations of the North American Society for Pediatric Gastroenterology and Nutrition, *J Pediatr Gastroenterol Nutr* 32(suppl 2):S1-S31, 2001.

studies. Bethanechol has a side effect of respiratory symptoms such as wheezing. In practice, metoclopramide and bethanechol have not been shown to be effective in treating GERD in children (Rudolph and others, 2001).

Cisapride (Propulsid), a drug used to promote gastric emptying, was taken off the market in 2000 because of the risk of serious cardiac arrhythmias and death associated with its use. However, the drug is available through an investigational limited-access program.

Surgical management of GER is reserved for children with severe complications such as recurrent aspiration pneumonia, apnea, severe esophagitis, or failure to thrive, and for children who have failed to respond to medical therapy. The *Nissen fundoplication* (Fig. 24-2) is the most common surgical procedure. This surgery involves passage of the gastric fundus behind the esophagus to encircle the distal esophagus. The most recent surgical advance is the introduction of the laparoscopic Nissen fundoplication (Rothenberg, 1998; Trover and others, 1998). Complications following fundoplication include breakdown of the wrap, small bowel obstruction, gas-bloat syndrome, infection, retching, and dumping syndrome (Rudolph and others, 2001).

Prognosis. The majority of infants with GER have a mild problem that generally improves by 12 to 18 months of age and requires only conservative lifestyle changes or medical therapy. If GER is severe and remains unsuccessfully treated, multiple complications can occur. Esophageal strictures caused by persistent esophagitis with scarring is the most significant complication. Recurrent respiratory distress with aspiration pneumonia, another serious complication, is an indication for surgery. Failure to thrive caused by GER is generally managed with medical therapy and nutritional support.

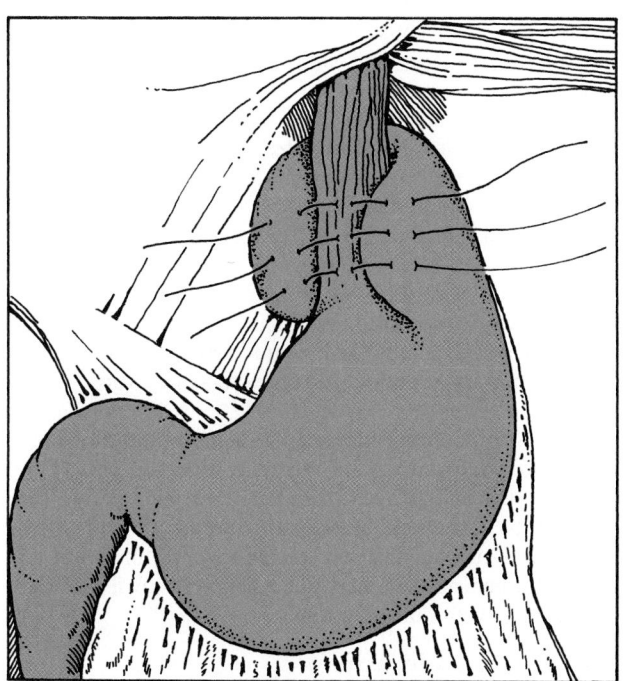

FIG. 24-2 ■ Nissen fundoplication sutures passing through esophageal musculature. (Redrawn from Campbell A, Ferrara B: *AORN J* 57:671-679, 1993.)

Nursing Considerations

Nursing care is directed at (1) identifying children with symptoms; (2) educating parents regarding home care, including feeding, positioning, and medications; and (3) if appropriate, providing care for the child undergoing surgical repair (see Surgical Procedures, Chapter 22). Early in the treatment program, parents should be reassured that most infants and children outgrow GER, and often conservative lifestyle changes are sufficient. Parents need support and reassurance to implement lifestyle changes. Although it is not known if lifestyle changes bring additional benefit to patients receiving pharmacologic interventions, some changes may be helpful. Older children and adolescents need to know that caffeine, chocolate, and spicy foods may weaken the LES and aggravate symptoms. Exposure to tobacco and alcohol are also associated with GER. Obesity increases abdominal pressure, and weight management may reduce GER symptoms. To help parents cope with the inconvenience of dealing with a child who spits up frequently, simple measures such as using bibs and protective cloths during and after feedings are beneficial. When medical management is necessary, parents need information about the medications and their potential side effects. Prokinetic medications must be given before feedings. Medications for acid control must be given regularly and timed to provide coverage two or three times a day as ordered.

INFLAMMATORY DISORDERS

ACUTE APPENDICITIS

Appendicitis, inflammation of the *vermiform appendix* (blind sac at the end of the cecum), is the most common cause of emergency abdominal surgery in childhood. In the Unites States, 60,000 to 80,000 cases are diagnosed each year. The average age of children with appendicitis is 10 years with boys and girls equally affected before puberty. Despite emphasis on early surgical intervention, the mortality of acute appendicitis in children is high. Death rates are 0.1% for nonperforated appendicitis and 5% for perforated appendicitis. Death is usually the result of complications associated with a delayed diagnosis. At the time of initial presentation, about one third of all cases involve an already perforated appendix. Abdominal pain is a common complaint in children, and perforation of the appendix can occur within approximately 48 hours of the initial complaint of pain. Early recognition is essential.

Etiology

The cause of appendicitis is obstruction of the lumen of the appendix usually by hardened fecal material (fecalith). Swollen lymphoid tissue, frequently occurring after a viral infection, can also obstruct the appendix. Another rare cause of obstruction is a parasite such as *Enterobius vermicularis* or pinworms, which can obstruct the appendiceal lumen.

Pathophysiology

With acute obstruction, the outflow of mucus secretions is blocked and pressure builds within the lumen, resulting in compression of blood vessels. The resulting ischemia is followed by ulceration of the epithelial lining and bacterial invasion. Subsequent necrosis causes perforation or rupture with fecal and bacterial contamination of the peritoneal cavity. The resulting inflammation spreads rapidly throughout the abdomen *(peritonitis),* especially in young children, who are unable to localize infection. Progressive peritoneal inflammation results in functional intestinal obstruction of the small bowel *(ileus)* because intense GI reflexes severely inhibit bowel motility. Because the peritoneum represents a major portion of total body surface, the loss of ECF to the peritoneal cavity leads to electrolyte imbalance and hypovolemic shock.

Diagnostic Evaluation

Diagnosis is not always straightforward. Numerous infections and inflammatory processes have similar features to that of appendicitis. Fever, vomiting, abdominal pain, and an elevated blood count are associated with appendicitis but are also seen in inflammatory bowel disease, pelvic inflammatory disease, gastroenteritis, urinary tract infection, right lower lobe pneumonia, constipation, mesenteric adenitis, Meckel diverticulum, and intussusception. Prolonged symptoms and delayed diagnosis often occur in preschoolage children, and the risk of perforation is greatest in this age-group because of their inability to verbalize their complaints.

The diagnosis is based primarily on the history and physical examination (Box 24-7). Pain, the cardinal feature, is initially generalized (usually periumbilical); however, it usually descends to the lower right quadrant. The most intense site of pain may be at **McBurney point,** located at a point midway between the anterior superior iliac crest and the umbilicus. Rebound tenderness is not a reliable sign and is extremely painful to the child. Referred pain, elicited by light percussion around the perimeter of the abdomen, indicates the presence of peritoneal irritation. Movement, such as riding over bumps in an automobile or gurney, aggravates the pain. In addition to pain, significant clinical manifestations include fever, a change in behavior, anorexia, and vomiting.

Laboratory studies usually include a complete blood count, urinalysis (to rule out a urinary tract infection), and in adolescent females, a serum human chorionic gonadotropin (to rule out an ectopic pregnancy). A white blood cell (WBC) count greater than 10,000/mm³ is common, but not necessarily specific for appendicitis. However,

a normal white blood count and a temperature less than 100.5° F may be helpful to exclude appendicitis. An elevated percentage of bands (often referred to as "a shift to the left") may indicate an inflammatory process. Recently, some primary care providers are adding the C-reactive protein (CRP) to the laboratory studies. CRP is an acute-phase reactant that rises within 12 hours of the onset of infection. However, the CRP test has low specificity, and any infectious process can cause an elevated CRP.

Ultrasonography (US) and a computed topography (CT) scan are helpful in differentiating pediatric abdominal pain from other causes. Findings such as visualization of the appendix and the presence of fluid around the appendix are important sonographic signs (Irish and others, 1998).

> **NURSING ALERT**
>
> Signs of peritonitis in addition to fever include sudden relief from pain after perforation, subsequent increase in pain (usually diffuse and accompanied by rigid guarding of the abdomen), progressive abdominal distention, tachycardia, rapid shallow breathing, pallor, chills, and irritability.

Therapeutic Management

Treatment of appendicitis before perforation includes rehydration, antibiotics, and surgical removal of the appendix *(appendectomy).* The operation is usually performed through a right lower quadrant incision (open appendectomy). Laparoscopic surgery is now commonly used to treat nonperforated acute appendicitis (Holcomb, 2001). Recovery is rapid, and, if no complications occur, the hospital stay is short.

Ruptured Appendix. Management of the child diagnosed with peritonitis caused by a ruptured appendix often begins preoperatively with IV administration of fluid and electrolytes, systemic antibiotics, and nasogastric suction. Postoperative management includes IV fluids, continued administration of antibiotics, and nasogastric suction for abdominal decompression until intestinal activity returns. The child with peritonitis is given antibiotics, including ampicillin, gentamicin, and clindamycin, for 7 to 10 days.

In some instances the wound is closed following irrigation of the peritoneal cavity. Many surgeons, however, leave the wound open (delayed closure) to prevent wound infection. A Penrose drain may be used to permit transperitoneal drainage. When delayed closure is used, wound irrigations and wet-to-dry dressings are a routine part of postoperative care.

Prognosis. Complications are uncommon following a simple appendectomy. The mortality rate for perforating appendicitis has improved from nearly certain death a century ago to 1% or less at present (Strahlman, 2001). The most common complications include wound infection and intraabdominal abscess. Early recognition of the illness is essential to prevent complications.

Nursing Considerations

Because abdominal pain is the most common childhood complaint with appendicitis, it is important to assess the severity of pain (see Pain Assessment, Chapter 21). One of

BOX 24-7 ■ Clinical Manifestations of Appendicitis

Right lower quadrant abdominal pain
Fever
Rigid abdomen
Decreased or absent bowel sounds
Vomiting (typically follows onset of pain)
Constipation or diarrhea may be present
Anorexia
Tachycardia, rapid shallow breathing
Pallor
Lethargy
Irritability
Stooped posture

NURSING CARE PLAN | **The Child With Appendicitis**

PREOPERATIVE CARE

NURSING DIAGNOSIS ▪ Pain related to inflamed appendix

PATIENT GOAL 1: Will experience no pain or reduction of pain to level acceptable to child

NURSING INTERVENTIONS/*RATIONALES*

See Pain Assessment; Pain Management, Chapter 21
Allow position of comfort (usually with legs flexed) *because it may vary among children*
Provide small pillow *for splinting of abdomen*
*Administer analgesia *to provide pain relief*

EXPECTED OUTCOME

Child rests quietly, reports or exhibits no evidence of discomfort

NURSING DIAGNOSIS ▪ Risk for fluid volume deficit related to decreased intake and losses secondary to loss of appetite, vomiting

PATIENT GOAL 1: Will receive fluids for adequate hydration

NURSING INTERVENTIONS/*RATIONALES*

Maintain NPO *to minimize losses through vomiting and minimize abdominal distention*
Maintain integrity of infusion site *for intravenous (IV) fluids and electrolytes*
*Administer IV fluids and electrolytes as prescribed
Monitor intake and output *to assess hydration*

EXPECTED OUTCOMES

Child receives sufficient fluids to replace losses
Child exhibits signs of adequate hydration (specify)

NURSING DIAGNOSIS ▪ Risk for infection related to possibility of rupture

PATIENT GOAL 1: Will experience minimized risk of infection

NURSING INTERVENTIONS/*RATIONALES*

Closely monitor vital signs, especially for increased heart rate and temperature and rapid, shallow breathing, *to detect ruptured appendix*
Observe for other signs of peritonitis (e.g., sudden relief of pain [sometimes] at time of perforation, followed by increased, diffuse pain and rigid guarding of the abdomen, abdominal distention, bloating, belching [from accumulation of air], pallor, chills, and irritability) *for appropriate treatment to be initiated*
Avoid administering laxatives or enemas, *because these measures stimulate bowel motility and increase risk of perforation*
Monitor white blood cell (WBC) count *as indicator of* infection

EXPECTED OUTCOMES

Child remains free of symptoms of peritonitis
Signs of peritonitis are recognized early (specify)

POSTOPERATIVE CARE

See Postoperative Care in Nursing Care Plan: The Child Undergoing Surgery, Chapter 22

*Dependent nursing action.

RUPTURED APPENDIX

NURSING DIAGNOSIS ▪ Risk for spread of infection related to presence of infective organisms in abdomen

PATIENT GOAL 1: Will experience minimized risk of spread of infection

NURSING INTERVENTIONS/*RATIONALES*

Provide wound care and dressing changes as prescribed *to prevent infection*
Monitor vital signs and WBC count *to assess presence of infection*
*Administer antibiotics as prescribed

EXPECTED OUTCOME

Child demonstrates resolution of peritonitis, as evidenced by lack of fever, clean wound, normal WBC count

NURSING DIAGNOSIS ▪ Risk for injury related to absence of bowel motility

PATIENT GOAL 1: Will not experience abdominal distention, vomiting

NURSING INTERVENTIONS/*RATIONALES*

Maintain NPO in early postoperative period *to prevent abdominal distention and vomiting*
Maintain nasogastric tube decompression *until bowel motility returns*
Assess abdomen for distention, tenderness, presence of bowel sounds *to assess presence of peristalsis*
Monitor passage of flatus and stool *as indicator of bowel motility*

EXPECTED OUTCOME

Child does not exhibit signs of discomfort; abdomen remains soft and nondistended; child does not vomit

NURSING DIAGNOSIS ▪ Altered family processes related to illness and hospitalization of child

PATIENT (FAMILY) GOAL 1: Will receive adequate support

NURSING INTERVENTIONS/*RATIONALES*

Encourage expression of feelings and concerns *to enhance coping*
Encourage child to discuss hospital admission and treatments *to clarify misconceptions*

EXPECTED OUTCOMES

Child and family express feelings and concerns
Child and family demonstrate understanding of hospitalization and treatments
See Nursing Care Plan: The Child in the Hospital, Chapter 21
See Nursing Care Plan: The Family of the Ill or Hospitalized Child, Chapter 21

the most reliable estimates is the degree of change in behavior. For example, a child who stays home from school and voluntarily lies down or refuses to play is much more likely to have considerable discomfort than the child who is absent from school but plays contentedly at home. The younger, nonverbal child will assume a rigid, motionless, side-lying posture with the knees flexed on the abdomen, and there is decreased range of motion of the right hip. Older children may exhibit all of these behaviors while complaining of abdominal pain. They can always indicate a point at which the pain is worse than at any other location.

> **⚠ NURSING ALERT**
>
> In any instance when severe abdominal pain is expected, be aware of the danger of administering laxatives or enemas or applying heat to the area. Such measures stimulate bowel motility and increase the risk of perforation.

Postoperative Care.   Postoperative care for the nonperforated appendix is the same as for most abdominal procedures. Care of the child with a ruptured appendix and peritonitis involves more complex care, and the course of recovery is considerably longer (usually 7 to 10 days of hospitalization). The child is maintained on IV fluids, allowed nothing by mouth, and kept on low continuous gastric decompression until there is evidence of intestinal activity. Listening for bowel sounds and observing for other signs of bowel activity (e.g., passage of stool) are part of the routine assessment. Management of IV therapy is the same as for any child receiving fluids and parenteral antibiotics. A drain is often placed in the wound during surgery, and frequent dressing changes with meticulous skin care are essential to prevent excoriation of the area surrounding the surgical site. Wound care includes irrigation with antibacterial solution.

Management of pain from the incision and repeated dressing changes and irrigations are an essential part of the child's care. Psychologic care of the child and parents is similar to that used in other emergency situations (see Emergency Admission, Chapter 21). Parents and older children need to express their feelings and concerns regarding the events surrounding the illness and hospitalization. The nurse can provide education and psychosocial support to promote adequate coping and alleviation of anxiety for both the child and the family. (See Nursing Care Plan on p. 859.)

MECKEL DIVERTICULUM

Meckel diverticulum is a remnant of the fetal omphalomesenteric duct that connects the yolk sac with the primitive midgut during fetal life. Normally this structure is obliterated by the seventh to eighth week of gestation, when the placenta replaces the yolk sac as the source of nutrition for the fetus. Failure of obliteration may result in an *omphalomesenteric fistula* (a fibrous band connecting the small intestine to the umbilicus, known as Meckel diverticulum).

Meckel diverticulum is a true diverticulum because it arises from the antimesenteric border of the small intestine, and all layers of the intestinal wall are present. The diverticulum is usually found within 100 cm (40 inches) of the ileocecal valve and averages 1 to 10 cm (2.625 to 4 inches) in length (Schwartz, 1999).

Meckel diverticulum is the most common congenital malformation of the GI tract and is present in 1% to 4% of the population (Schwartz, 1999). It is twice as common in males as in females, and complications are more frequent in males. Most symptomatic cases are seen in childhood. Patients requiring surgery are generally less than 10 years of age, and about 50% are less than 2 years of age (Schwartz, 1999).

Pathophysiology

The symptomatic complications of this condition are bleeding, obstruction, or inflammation; bleeding is the most common problem in children. Gastric mucosa is the most common ectopic tissue found in Meckel diverticulum. Bleeding is caused by peptic ulceration or perforation because of the unbuffered acidic secretion. Several other mechanisms can cause obstruction. Intussusception may be led by the diverticulum. Obstruction may also be caused by entanglement of the small intestine around a fibrous cord, trapping of a loop of intestine under the band, incarceration within a hernia sac, or volvulus of the intestinal segment containing the diverticulum. Diverticulitis occurs when peptic ulceration or obstruction leads to inflammation.

Diagnostic Evaluation

Diagnosis is usually based on the history, physical examination, and a specialized radiographic study. The most common clinical presentation in children includes painless rectal bleeding, abdominal pain, or signs of intestinal obstruction (Box 24-8). Bleeding, which may be mild or profuse, often appears as dark red or "currant jelly" stools; bleeding may be significant enough to cause hypotension. The more common obstructive symptoms in children are volvulus and intussusception. The Meckel scan, a radionucleotide *scintigraphy,* detects the presence of gastric mucosa with an overall diagnostic accuracy of 90%. Abdominal radiographs, barium enema, and arteriography are not successful diagnostic tools. Blood studies are performed to screen for bleeding disorders and anemia (Schwartz, 1999).

Therapeutic Management

The standard treatment is surgical removal of the diverticulum. When severe hemorrhage increases the surgical risk, interventions to correct hypovolemic shock, such as blood replacement, IV fluids, and oxygen, may be necessary. Antibiotics may be used preoperatively to control infection. If intestinal obstruction has occurred, appropriate preoperative measures are used to reverse electrolyte imbalances and prevent abdominal distention.

Prognosis.   If this condition is diagnosed and treated early, full recovery is likely. The mortality rate of untreated Meckel diverticulum ranges from 2.5% to 15%. Complications of untreated Meckel diverticulum include GI hemorrhage and bowel obstruction.

Nursing Considerations

Nursing objectives are similar to those for any child undergoing surgery (see Chapter 22). Because the onset of this condition is often rapid, parents require psychologic support. The massive intestinal bleeding that can accompany a

BOX 24-8 ■ Clinical Manifestations of Meckel Diverticulum

ABDOMINAL PAIN
Similar to appendicitis
May be vague and recurrent

BLOODY STOOLS*
Painless
Bright or dark red with mucus ("currant jelly" stool)
In infants, bleeding may be accompanied by pain

Sometimes
Severe anemia
Shock

*Often a presenting sign.

TABLE 24-3 ■ Clinical Manifestations of Inflammatory Bowel Diseases

CHARACTERISTICS	ULCERATIVE COLITIS	CROHN DISEASE
Rectal bleeding	Common	Uncommon
Diarrhea	Often severe	Moderate to severe
Pain	Less frequent	Common
Anorexia	Mild or moderate	May be severe
Weight loss	Moderate	May be severe
Growth retardation	Usually mild	May be severe
Anal and perianal lesions	Rare	Common
Fistulas and strictures	Rare	Common
Rashes	Mild	Mild
Joint pain	Mild to moderate	Mild to moderate

Meckel diverticulum is traumatic to both the child and the parents and may significantly affect their emotional reaction to hospitalization and surgery.

Specific preoperative considerations with intestinal bleeding include (1) frequent monitoring of vital signs and blood pressure for shock, (2) keeping the child on bed rest, and (3) recording the approximate amount of blood lost in stools. In the absence of frank hemorrhage, the nurse tests the stools for occult blood. Postoperatively, the child requires IV fluids, and a nasogastric tube for the decompression and evacuation of gastric contents.

INFLAMMATORY BOWEL DISEASE

Inflammatory bowel disease (IBD) is a term that is used for two forms of chronic intestinal inflammation—*ulcerative colitis (UC)* and *Crohn disease (CD).* Although UC and CD have similar epidemiologic, immunologic, and clinical features, they are two distinct conditions with very important differences (Table 24-3).

GI symptoms, extraintestinal and systemic inflammatory responses, and exacerbations and remissions without complete resolution characterize these diseases. Growth failure, particularly common in CD, is an important problem unique to the pediatric population. CD is more disabling, has more serious complications, and has less effective medical and surgical treatment than UC. Because UC is confined to the colon, theoretically it may be cured with a colectomy. Over the past 30 years, the incidence of CD has risen, whereas the incidence of UC in children has remained stable. The incidence of UC in children has been estimated as 3.5 new cases per 100,000 per year; the incidence of CD is 3.11 per 100,000 (Jackson and Grand, 1999)

Etiology

Despite decades of research, the etiology of IBD is not completely understood and there is no known cure. There is evidence to indicate a multifactorial etiology. It is proposed that IBD is the result of one or more environmental influences, such as infectious organisms, dietary habits, and environmental toxins that promote disease in genetically susceptible individuals. Research is focused on theories of defective immunoregulation of the inflammatory response to bacteria or viruses in the GI tract in individuals with a genetic predisposition. A familial tendency is apparent in approximately 20% to 25% of cases. Individuals from higher socioeconomic levels and more whites are affected, and the condition occurs more frequently among Jews living in Europe and North America, and among people living in urban settings. Males and females are affected equally (Leichtner, Jackson, and Grand, 1996). A primary role for psychologic factors has not been supported, although psychologic problems may occur as a result of IBD and psychologic problems may intensify symptoms and influence the course of the disease.

Pathophysiology: Ulcerative Colitis

The inflammation is limited to the colon and rectum, with the distal colon and rectum the most severely affected. Inflammation affects the mucosa and submucosa and involves continuous segments along the length of the bowel with varying degrees of ulceration, bleeding, and edema. The presentation may be mild, moderate, or severe, depending on the extent of mucosal inflammation and systemic symptoms. Most cases include bloody diarrhea or occult fecal blood, abdominal pain that is most intense during defecation, and varying degrees of systemic manifestations and growth abnormalities (Leichtner, Jackson, and Grand, 1996). Thickening of the bowel wall and fibrosis are unusual, but long-standing disease can result in shortening of the colon and strictures. Extraintestinal manifestations are less common in UC than in CD.

Pathophysiology: Crohn Disease

The chronic inflammatory process of CD involves any part of the GI tract from the mouth to the anus but most often affects the terminal ileum. The disease involves all layers of the bowel wall (transmural) in a discontinuous fashion, meaning that between areas of intact mucosa, there are areas of affected mucosa (skip lesions). The most common symptoms are abdominal pain with cramps, diarrhea, and weight loss. Other manifestations include fever; anorexia; rectal bleeding; and perineal discomfort, including anal fissures or fistulas. The presence of perianal disease is a strong indication for CD. Mild GI symptoms, poor growth, and extraintestinal manifestations may be present for several years before overt GI symptoms occur. The inflammation may result in ulcerations, fibrosis, and adhesions, stiffening of the bowel wall, stricture formation, and fistulas to other loops of bowel, bladder, vagina, or skin. Extraintestinal manifestations, including erythema nodosum, large joint arthritis, uveitis, mouth ulcers, liver disease, and renal calculi are common.

Diagnostic Evaluation

The diagnosis of UC and CD is derived from the history, physical examination, laboratory evaluation, and other diagnostic procedures. Because the diseases have similar symptoms, it is difficult to distinguish CD from UC. UC is confined to the large bowel and affects only the inner lining (the mucosa and submucosa). CD involves all layers of the bowel (transmural). Laboratory tests include a CBC to evaluate anemia and an erythrocyte sedimentation rate or CRP to assess the systemic reaction to the inflammatory process. Levels of total protein, albumin, iron, zinc, magnesium, vitamin B_{12}, and fat-soluble vitamins may be low in children with CD. Stools are examined for the presence of blood, leukocytes, and infectious organisms. A serologic panel is often used in combination with clinical findings to diagnose IBD and to differentiate between CD and UC. In IBD, autoantibodies called antineutrophil cytoplasm antibodies (ANCA) may be detected in the blood. The perinuclear antineutrophil cytoplasm antibody (pANCA) is associated with UC. Approximately 60% to 70% of patients with UC and 15% of those with CD are pANCA-positive. Anti–*Saccharomyces cerevisiae* antibodies (ASCA) have been found in 67% to 92% of individuals with CD (Baron, 2002).

In patients with CD, an upper GI series with small bowel follow-through reveals images that demonstrate narrowing or modularity of the small bowel. The terminal ileum may be narrowed or rigid with partial obstruction. In about one third of the patients, lesions pierce the walls of the small intestine and colon, creating tracts called fistulas between the intestine and adjacent structures such as the bladder, anus, vagina, or skin. Fistulas may become infected, causing discharge of pus and mucous. A CT scan is helpful in evaluating abscesses, fistulas, and bowel wall thickening. Endoscopy, direct visualization of the surface of the gastrointestinal tract with biopsies, is necessary to confirm the diagnosis and to assess the extent of inflammation and to evaluate for strictures. Endoscopy may be both upper and lower colonoscopy depending on the clinical presentation of the child.

Therapeutic Management

The goals of therapy are to (1) control the inflammatory process to reduce or eliminate the symptoms, (2) obtain long-term remission, (3) promote normal growth and development, and (4) allow as normal a lifestyle as possible. Treatment is individualized and managed according to the type and the severity of the disease, its location, and the response to therapy.

Medical Treatment

Drugs that mediate and control inflammation (corticosteroids, aminosalicylates, sulfasalazine, immunosuppressives, and biologic therapies) are used to treat IBD. *Corticosteroids,* such as prednisone and prednisolone, are used in short bursts to suppress the inflammatory response in moderate to severe IBD. These drugs inhibit the production of adhesion molecules, cytokines, and leukotrienes. Although these drugs reduce the acute symptoms of IBD, they have side effects that relate to long-term use, including growth suppression (adrenal suppression), weight gain, and decreased bone density (Baron, 2002). High doses of IV corticosteroids may be administered in acute episodes and tapered according to clinical response. *Aminosalicylates* are useful in decreasing the frequency of recurrences in mild cases of IBD. **Sulfasalazine** decreases inflammation by inhibiting prostaglandin synthesis. Because it is only active in the colon, it is not effective in the treatment of small bowel disease. Sulfasalazine may decrease the absorption of folic acid; therefore, daily supplements of folic acid are needed in long-term therapy. Side effects of this drug include headache, nausea, vomiting, neutropenia, and oligospermia. The side effects are caused primarily by the sulfapyridine component of the drug, so alternative nonabsorbable salicylate drugs such as olsalazine and mesalamine may be prescribed. Mesalamine comes in a variety of formulations that are active in different parts of the bowel. Asacol is active in the terminal ileum and the colon. Pentasa targets the jejunum, and Rowasa is a topical preparation administered rectally by enema to relieve inflammation of the distal colon and rectum.

Immunomodulatory medications are used when the symptoms of IBD persist despite the use of steroids or when the patient cannot be weaned from corticosteroids (e.g., when reducing the dose of steroids results in return of symptoms such as diarrhea, pain, and bleeding). *Azathioprine* and its metabolite *6-MP* block the synthesis of purine, thus inhibiting the ability of DNA and ribonucleic acid (RNA) to hinder lymphocyte function, especially that of T cells. Side effects include infection, pancreatitis, hepatitis, bone marrow toxicity, arthralgia, and malignancy. Other immunomodulatory medications include **methotrexate, cyclosporin,** and **mycophenolate mofetil.** Patients on these medications require regular monitoring of their CBC and differential to assess for changes that reflect suppression of the immune system.

Antibiotics, such as metronidazole and ciprofloxacin, may be used as an adjunctive therapy to treat complications such as perianal disease or small bowel bacterial overgrowth. Side effects of these drugs are peripheral neuropathy, nausea, and a metallic taste.

Biologic therapies act to regulate inflammatory and anti-inflammatory cytokines. Tumor necrosis factor-alpha (TNF-α) is believed to influence active inflammation. Infliximab (Remicade) is an antibody to TNF-α. This drug is given via IV infusions 6 to 12 weeks apart. Approximately 5% of patients have acute allergic reactions to infliximab and require premedication with prednisone and diphenhydramine before infusion to prevent reactions. Long intervals between infusions may predispose patients to serum sickness (an immune response causing fever, muscle pain, arthritis, and hives) (Baron, 2002). Severe complications of this drug include lupus-like syndrome or lymphoma. Other biologic medications include methotrexate, interleukin-10, and thalidomide.

Nutritional Support. Nutritional support is a primary component of the treatment of IBD. Growth failure is a common serious complication, especially in CD. Growth failure is characterized by weight loss, alteration in body composition, retarded height, and delayed sexual maturation. Malnutrition causes the growth failure, and its etiology is multifactorial. Malnutrition occurs as a result of inadequate dietary intake, excessive GI losses, malabsorption, drug-nutrient interaction, and increased nutritional requirements. Inadequate dietary intake occurs with anorexia and episodes of increased disease activity. Excessive loss of nutrients (protein, blood, electrolytes, and minerals) occurs secondary to intestinal inflammation and diarrhea. Carbohydrate, lactose, fat, vitamin, and mineral malabsorption, as well as vitamin B_{12} and folic acid deficiencies, occur with disease episodes and with drug administration and when the terminal ileum is resected. Finally, nutritional requirements are increased with inflammation, fever, fistulas, and during periods of rapid growth (e.g., adolescence).

The goals of nutritional support include (1) correction of nutrient deficits and replacement of ongoing losses, (2) provision of adequate energy and protein for healing, and (3) provision of adequate nutrients to promote normal growth. Nutritional support includes both enteral and parenteral nutrition. A well-balanced, high-protein, high-calorie diet is recommended for children whose symptoms do not prohibit an adequate oral intake. There is little evidence that avoiding specific foods influences the severity of the disease. Supplementation with multivitamins, iron, and folic acid is recommended.

Special enteral formulas, given either by mouth or continuous nasogastric infusion (often at night), may be required. Elemental formulas are completely absorbed in the small intestine with almost no residue. Several studies have demonstrated that a diet consisting only of elemental formula not only improved nutritional status but also induced disease remission, either without steroids or with a diminished dosage of steroids required. An elemental diet is a safe and potentially effective primary therapy for patients with CD.

TPN has also improved nutritional status in patients with IBD. Short-term remissions have been achieved after TPN, although complete bowel rest has not reduced inflammation or added to the benefits of improved nutrition by TPN (Leichtner, Jackson, and Grand, 1996). Nutritional support is less likely to induce a remission in UC than in CD. Improvement of nutritional status is important, however, in preventing deterioration of the patient's health status and in preparing the patient for surgery.

Surgical Treatment.   Surgery is indicated for UC when medical and nutritional therapies fail to prevent complications. Surgical options include a **subtotal colectomy** and **ileostomy** that leaves a rectal stump as a blind pouch. A reservoir pouch is created in the configuration of a J or S to help improve continence postoperatively. An ileoanal pull-through preserves the normal pathway for defecation. In many cases UC can be cured with a total colectomy.

Surgery may be required in children with CD when complications cannot be controlled by medical and nutritional therapy. Segmental intestinal resections are preformed for small bowel obstructions, strictures, or fistulas. Partial colonic resection is not curative, and the disease often recurs.

Prognosis.   IBD is a chronic disease. Relatively long periods of quiescent disease may follow exacerbations. The outcome of the disease is influenced by the regions and severity of involvement, as well as by appropriate therapeutic management. Malnutrition, growth failure, and bleeding are serious complications. The overall prognosis for UC is good.

The development of carcinoma of the colon is a long-term complication of IBD. In UC, removal of the diseased bowel prevents development of carcinoma. In CD, however, surgical removal of the affected bowel does not prevent bowel cancer, and routine screening of stool specimens is necessary for early detection.

Nursing Considerations

The nursing considerations in the management of IBD extend beyond the immediate period of hospitalization. These interventions involve (1) continued guidance of families in terms of dietary management, (2) coping with factors that increase stress and emotional lability, (3) adjusting to a disease of remissions and exacerbations, and (4) when indicated, preparing the child and parents for the possibility of diversionary bowel surgery.

Because nutritional support is an essential part of therapy, encouraging the anorectic child to consume sufficient quantities of food is often a challenge. Successful interventions include involving the child in meal planning; encouraging small, frequent meals or snacks rather than three large meals a day; serving meals around medication schedules when diarrhea, mouth pain, and intestinal spasm are controlled; and preparing high-protein, high-calorie foods such as eggnog, milkshakes, cream soups, puddings, or custard (if lactose is tolerated) (see Feeding the Sick Child, Chapter 22). Foods that are known to aggravate the condition are avoided. Using bran or a high-fiber diet for IBD is questionable. Bran, even in small amounts, has been shown to worsen the patient's condition. Occasionally the occurrence of aphthous stomatitis further complicates adherence to dietary management. Mouth care before eating and the selection of bland foods help relieve the discomfort of mouth sores.

When nasogastric feedings or TPN are indicated, nurses play an important role in explaining the purpose and the expected outcomes of this therapy. The nurse should acknowledge the anxieties of family members and give them adequate time to demonstrate the skills necessary to continue the therapy at home if needed (see Critical Thinking Exercise).

The importance of continued drug therapy despite remission of symptoms must be stressed to the child and family members. Failure to adhere to the pharmacologic regimen can result in exacerbation of the disease (see Compliance, Chapter 22).

Family Support.   The nurse should attend to the emotional components of the disease and assess any sources of stress. Frequently, the nurse can help children to adjust to problems of growth retardation, delayed sexual maturation, dietary restrictions, feelings of being "different" or "sickly," inability to compete with peers, and necessary absence from school during exacerbations of the illness (see Impact of Chronic Illness, Chapter 18).

If a permanent colectomy/ileostomy is required, the nurse can teach the child and family how to care for the ileostomy. The nurse can also emphasize the positive aspects of the surgery, particularly accelerated growth and sexual development, permanent recovery, and the eliminated risk of colonic cancer in UC, as well as the normality of life despite bowel diversion. Introducing the child and parents to other ostomy patients, especially those who are the same age, can

?? CRITICAL THINKING EXERCISE ??

Inflammatory Bowel Disease

Susan, a 13-year-old girl, was admitted to the hospital because of bloody diarrhea, abdominal pain, and weight loss. After a thorough evaluation, including laboratory tests, radiographic studies, and gastrointestinal endoscopy procedures, the diagnosis of Crohn disease (CD) was made. Medical treatment, including corticosteroid drugs and nutritional support, was implemented during this hospitalization.

Susan has improved considerably and is to be discharged home this week. Enteral formula administered by continuous nighttime nasogastric (NG) tube infusion will be continued at home, and both Susan and her family are eager to learn how to perform these feedings. You are the nurse who is responsible for Susan's discharge planning. Which interventions relating to these feedings should you include in Susan's preparations for discharge?

QUESTIONS
1. Evidence—Are there sufficient data to formulate any specific interventions for discharge?
2. Assumptions—Describe some underlying assumptions about the following:
    a. The goals of nutritional support for children with CD
    b. Teaching required by an adolescent or family member who is administering NG tube feedings at home
    c. Psychosocial issues related to CD
3. What are the priorities for discharge planning at this time?
4. Does the evidence support your conclusion?
5. Are there alternative perspectives to your conclusion? What are they?

ANSWERS
1. Yes, there is sufficient evidence to arrive at some conclusions about what to include in Susan's discharge planning.
2. a. The goals of nutritional support for a patient with CD include (1) correction of nutrient deficits and replacement of ongoing losses, (2) provision of adequate energy and protein for healing, and (3) provision of adequate nutrients to support normal growth.
    b. See Chapter 22, Gavage Feeding, p. 778.
    c. Adolescents who are diagnosed with CD must adjust to the fact that they have a chronic illness that is characterized by remissions and exacerbations. CD may affect their activities of daily living, their social interactions with peers, and their ability to attend school. An important goal of therapy for adolescents with CD is to allow them to have as normal a lifestyle as possible.
3. The most immediate priority for discharge is to teach Susan and her family how to insert the NG tube, how to administer the feedings, how to obtain the supplies needed for the tube feedings at home, and how to observe for any untoward effects of the NG feedings. As Susan's discharge nurse, you should have Susan and another family member insert the NG tube, demonstrate how to check the placement of the NG tube and how to start and stop the feedings while Susan is in the hospital. As Susan's nurse, you will also need to arrange for the appropriate vendors to deliver the feeding tube supplies and feeding pump to Susan's home prior to discharge so the supplies will be in place when Susan is discharged. While doing all this teaching, you should also be alert to any questions, worries, or anxieties that Susan or her family members may express.
4. Yes, Susan is to receive nighttime NG tube infusions at home, and her family has expressed a desire to perform this procedure at home. Therefore, this discharge teaching is needed and required.
5. Now that the acute disease exacerbation is under control, Susan will be able to resume school attendance and activities with her peers. However, some of her activities of daily living have been changed (e.g., the nighttime NG feedings), and she will need to adjust to remissions and exacerbations that characterize CD. To help Susan and her family cope with these changes, you should refer them to the services of the Crohn's and Colitis Foundation of America, Inc. Perhaps Susan can become involved in one of the adolescent peer-support groups that are sponsored by this group.

---

be effective in fostering eventual acceptance. Whenever possible, continent ostomies should be offered as options to the child, although they are not performed in all centers in the United States.

Because of the chronic and often lifelong nature of the disease, families benefit from the educational services provided by organizations such as the **Crohn's and Colitis Foundation of America, Inc. (CCFA).** * If diversionary bowel surgery is indicated, the **United Ostomy Association**† and the **Wound Ostomy and Continence Nurses Society**‡ are available to assist with ileostomy care and pro-

vide important psychologic support through their self-help groups. Adolescents often benefit by participating in peer-support groups, which are sponsored by the CCFA.

PEPTIC ULCER DISEASE

Peptic ulcers may be classified as acute or chronic, and peptic ulcer disease (PUD) is a chronic condition that affects the stomach or duodenum. Ulcers are described as gastric or duodenal and as primary or secondary. A *gastric ulcer* involves the mucosa of the stomach; a *duodenal ulcer* involves the pylorus or duodenum. Most *primary ulcers* occur in the absence of a predisposing factor and tend to be chronic, occurring more frequently in the duodenum. *Stress ulcers* result from the stress of a severe underlying disease or injury (e.g., severe burns, sepsis, intracranial disease, severe trauma, multisystem organ failure) and are more frequently acute and gastric.

About 1.7% of children in general pediatric practices have PUD, and the disease represents about 3.4% per 10,000 of pediatric hospital admissions. Primary ulcers are more common in children older than 6 years, and stress ulcers are more common in infants younger than 6 months.

---

*386 Park Avenue South, 17th Floor, New York, NY 10016; (800) 932-2423; website: www.ccfa.org.

†19772 MacArthur Boulevard, Suite 200, Irvine, CA 92612-2405; (714) 660-8624; website: www.uoa.org.

‡1550 South Coast Highway, Suite 201, Laguna Beach, CA 92651; (888) 224-9626; website: www.wocn.org. In Canada: **Crohn's and Colitis Foundation of Canada,** website: www.ccfc.ca; and **United Ostomy Association, Canada,** PO Box 825-50, Charles Street East, Toronto, Ontario M4Y 2N7; (416) 595-5452; fax: (416) 595-9924.

Except for very young children, the incidence is two to three times greater in boys than in girls (Motil, 1999).

Etiology

The exact cause is unknown, although infectious, genetic, and environmental factors are important. There is an increased familial incidence, and the disease is increased in persons with blood group O.

There is a significant relationship between the bacterium *Helicobacter pylori* (previously called *Campylobacter pylori*) and ulcers. *H. pylori* is known to colonize the gastric mucosa and has been identified in 90% to 100% of adult patients with PUD. It may cause ulcers by weakening the gastric mucosal barrier and allowing acid to damage the mucosa. It is believed that *H. pylori* is acquired via the fecal-oral route, and this hypothesis is supported by finding viable *H. pylori* in feces. The exact mechanism by which it causes gastric inflammation is unclear; however, the large amount of urease present in *H. pylori* may be a factor. Urease hydrolyses urea to ammonia and bicarbonate in the gastric mucosa, and ammonia can be toxic to gastric cells (Chelimsky and Czinn, 2001).

In addition to ulcerogenic drugs, both alcohol and smoking contribute to ulcer formation. There is no conclusive evidence to implicate particular foods, such as caffeine-containing beverages or spicy foods, but polyunsaturated fats and fiber may play a role in ulcer formation.

Psychologic factors may play a role in the development of PUD, and stressful life events, dependency, passiveness, and hostility have all been implicated as contributing factors.

Pathophysiology

Most likely, the pathology is due to an imbalance between the destructive (cytotoxic) factors and defensive (cytoprotective) factors in the GI tract. The toxic mechanisms include acid, pepsin, medications such as aspirin, nonsteroidal anti-inflammatory drugs (NSAIDs), bile acids, and infection with *H. pylori*. The defensive factors include the mucous layer, local bicarbonate secretion, epithelial cell renewal, and mucosal blood flow (Motil, 1999). Prostaglandins play a role in mucosal defense because they stimulate both mucus and alkali secretion. The primary mechanism that prevents the development of peptic ulcer is the secretion of mucus by the epithelial and mucus glands throughout the stomach. The thick mucus layer acts to diffuse acid from the lumen to the gastric mucosal surface, thus protecting the gastric epithelium. The stomach and the duodenum produce bicarbonate, and production of bicarbonate decreases acidity on the epithelial cells, thereby minimizing the effects of the low pH (Chelimsky and Czinn, 2001). When abnormalities in the protective barrier exist, the mucosa is vulnerable to damage by acid and pepsin. Exogenous factors, such as aspirin and NSAIDs, cause gastric ulcers by inhibition of prostaglandin synthesis. Zollinger-Ellison syndrome may occur in children who have multiple, large, or recurrent ulcers. This syndrome is characterized by hypersecretion of gastric acid, intractable ulcer disease, and intestinal malabsorption caused by a gastrin-secreting tumor of the pancreas (Motil, 1999).

Diagnostic Evaluation

Diagnosis is based on the history of symptoms, physical examination, and diagnostic testing. The focus is on symptoms such as epigastric abdominal pain, nocturnal pain, oral

---

BOX 24-9 ■ Characteristics of Peptic Ulcer

NEONATES
Usually gastric and secondary
Commonly has a history of prematurity, respiratory distress, sepsis, hypoglycemia, or an intraventricular hemorrhage
Perforation may be first sign that massive bleeding may occur

INFANTS TO 3-YEAR-OLD CHILDREN
Most likely to have a secondary ulcer located equally in the stomach or duodenum
Primary ulcers less common and usually located in stomach
Likely to present in relation to illness, surgery, or trauma
Hematemesis, melena, or perforation

2- TO 6-YEAR-OLD CHILDREN
Primary or secondary ulcers
Located equally in stomach and duodenum
Perforation more likely in secondary ulcers
Periumbilical pain, poor eating, vomiting, irritability, nighttime waking, hematemesis, melena

CHILDREN 6 YEARS AND OLDER
Usually primary and most often duodenal
More typical of adult type
Chance of recurrence greater
Often associated with *H. pylori*
Epigastric pain or vague abdominal pain
Nighttime waking, hematemesis, melena, and anemia may occur

---

regurgitation, heartburn, weight loss, hematemesis, and melena (Box 24-9). History should include questions relating to the use of potentially causative medications such as NSAIDS, corticosteroids, alcohol, and tobacco. Laboratory studies may include a CBC to detect anemia, stool analysis for occult blood, liver function tests, sedimentation rate, or CRP to evaluate inflammatory bowel disease, amylase and lipase to evaluate pancreatitis, and gastric acid measurements to identify hypersecretion. A lactose breath test may be performed to detect lactose intolerance.

Radiographic studies such as an upper GI series may be performed to evaluate obstruction or malrotation. An upper endoscopy is the most reliable procedure to diagnose PUD. A biopsy is taken to determine the presence of *H. pylori*. *H. pylori* can also be diagnosed by a blood test that identifies the presence of the antigen to this organism. The C urea breath test measures bacterial colonization in the gastric mucosa. This test is used to screen for *H. pylori* in adults and is now being evaluated for children.

Therapeutic Management

The major goals of therapy for children with PUD are to relieve discomfort, promote healing, prevent complications, and prevent recurrence. Management is primarily medical and consists of administration of medications to treat the infection and to reduce or neutralize gastric acid secretion.

Antacids are beneficial medications to neutralize gastric acid. However, in terms of healing the ulcer or eradication of *H. pylori*, antacids are not as effective as medications that inhibit acid secretion.

Histamine (H₂) receptor antagonists (antisecretory drugs) act to suppress gastric acid production. Cimetidine

(Tagamet), ranitidine (Zantac), and famotidine (Pepcid) are examples of these medications. These medications have few side effects.

Proton pump inhibitors (PPI), such as omeprazole and lansoprazole, act to inhibit the hydrogen ion pump in the parietal cells, thus blocking the production of acid. Controlled studies of these drugs have been done in adults, and these drugs are now commonly used to treat ulcers in children. They appear to be well tolerated and to have infrequent side effects (e.g., headache, diarrhea, nausea and vomiting).

Mucosal protective agents, such as sucralfate and bismuth-containing preparations, may be prescribed for PUD. Sucralfate is an aluminum-containing agent that forms a protective barrier over ulcerated mucosa to protect against acid and pepsin. Sucralfate is available in both pill and liquid forms. Because sucralfate blocks the absorption of other medications, it should be given separately from other medications.

Bismuth compounds are sometimes prescribed for the relief of ulcers, but they are used less frequently than PPIs. Although these compounds inhibit the growth of microorganisms, the mechanism of their activity is poorly understood. In combination with antibiotics, bismuth is effective against *H. pylori*. Although concern has been expressed about the use of bismuth salts in children because of potential side effects, none of these side effects have been reported when these compounds have been used in the treatment of *H. pylori* infection.

Triple drug therapy is the recommended treatment regimen for *H. pylori*. Combination therapy has demonstrated 90% effectiveness in eradication of *H. pylori* when compared with antibiotic monotherapy (Motil, 1999). Examples of drug combinations used in triple therapy are: (1) bismuth, clarithromycin, and metronidazole; (2) lansoprazole, amoxicillin, and clarithromycin; and (3) metronidazole, clarithromycin, and omeprazole.

In addition to medications, the child with PUD should be given a nutritious diet and advised to avoid caffeine. Adolescents are warned about gastric irritation associated with alcohol use and smoking.

Children with an acute ulcer who have developed complications, such as massive hemorrhage, require emergency care. The administration of IV fluids, blood, or plasma depends on the amount of blood loss. Replacement with whole blood or packed cells may be necessary for significant loss.

Surgical intervention may be required for complications such as hemorrhage, perforation, or gastric outlet obstruction. Ligation of the source of bleeding or closure of a perforation is performed. A vagotomy and pyloroplasty may be indicated in children with recurring ulcers despite aggressive medical treatment.

Prognosis. The long-term prognosis for PUD is variable. Many ulcers are successfully treated with medical therapy; however, primary duodenal peptic ulcers often recur. Complications such as GI bleeding can occur and extend into adult life. The effect of maintenance drug therapy on long-term morbidity remains to be established with further studies.

Nursing Considerations

The primary nursing goal is to promote healing of the ulcer through compliance with the medication regimen. If an analgesic/antipyretic is needed, acetaminophen, not aspirin or NSAIDs, is used. Critically ill neonates, infants, and children in intensive care units should receive antacids and H_2 blockers to prevent stress ulcers. Critically ill children receiving IV H_2 blockers should have their gastric pH values checked at frequent intervals and buffered with antacid if necessary.

The role of stress in ulcer formation should be considered for nonhospitalized children with chronic illnesses. In children, many ulcers occur secondarily to other conditions, and the nurse should be aware of family and environmental conditions that may aggravate or precipitate ulcers. Children may benefit from psychologic counseling and from learning how to cope constructively with stress.

HEPATIC DISORDERS

ACUTE HEPATITIS

Etiology

Hepatitis is an acute or chronic inflammation of the liver that can result from several different causes (e.g. a virus, chemical or drug reaction, or other diseases). Nonviral causes of hepatitis include autoimmune hepatitis, Wilson's disease, alpha-1 antitrypsin deficiency, and steatohepatitis. The following six viruses cause most cases (90%) of viral hepatitis (see Table 24-4):

- Hepatitis A virus (HAV)
- Hepatitis B virus (HBV)
- Hepatitis C virus (HCV)
- Hepatitis D virus (HDV)
- Hepatitis E virus (HEV)
- Hepatitis G virus (HGV)

Hepatitis A. HAV is the most common form of acute viral hepatitis in most parts of the world. It is a member of the picornavirus family. The virus produces a contagious disease transmitted primarily in contaminated stool spread via the fecal-oral route from person to person. HAV has been associated with miniepidemics in areas of poor hygiene and high population density. There is no chronic or carrier state. HAV infection affects individuals of all ages, but the highest incidence occurs among preschool- or school-age children younger than 15 years. Children may serve as the source of HAV infection in adults, such as in childcare center exposures. Usually HAV disease in children is mild. It is frequently anicteric and often subclinical. Infected children who show no symptoms may still spread the virus to others. HAV can be severe in children with immunodeficiency disorders. The incubation period is approximately 3 weeks. Although some cases may be prolonged, the prognosis is excellent. A highly effective vaccine for HAV was introduced in 1997 (Balistreri and others, 2002; Regev and Schiff, 2000).

Hepatitis B. HBV infection can occur as an acute or chronic infection and may range from being asymptomatic and limited to causing fatal fulminant (rapid and severe) hep-

TABLE 24-4 ■ Comparison of Types A, B, and C Hepatitis

CHARACTERISTICS	TYPE A	TYPE B	TYPE C
Incubation period	15-50 days, average 25-30 days	30-180 days, average 50 days	6-7 weeks, average 2 weeks-6 months
Period of communicability	Believed to be later half of incubation period to the first week after the onset of clinical illness	Variable Virus in blood or other body fluids during late incubation period and acute stage of disease; may persist in carrier state for years to lifetime	Begins before onset of symptoms May persist in carrier state for years
Mode of transmission	Principal route—fecal-oral Rarely—parenteral	Principal route—parenteral Less frequent route—oral, sexual, any body fluid Perinatal transfer—transplacental blood (last trimester), at delivery, or during breast-feeding, especially if mother has cracked nipples	Principal route—parenteral Nonparenteral spread possible
Clinical features			
Onset	Usually rapid, acute	More insidious	Usually insidious
Fever	Common and early	Less frequent	Less frequent
Anorexia	Common	Mild to moderate	Mild to moderate
Nausea and vomiting	Common	Sometimes present	Mild to moderate
Rash	Rare	Common	Sometimes present
Arthralgia	Rare	Common	Rare
Pruritus	Rare	Sometimes present	Sometimes present
Jaundice	Present (many cases anicteric)	Present	Present
Immunity	Present after one attack; no crossover to type B or C	Present after one attack; no crossover to type A or C	Present after one attack; no crossover to type A or B
Carrier state	No	Yes	Yes
Chronic infection	No	Yes	Yes
Prophylaxis			
Immune globulin (IG)	Passive immunity Successful, especially in early incubation period and preexposure prophylaxis	Passive immunity Inconsistent benefits; probably of no use	Not currently recommended by Centers for Disease Control and Prevention
HAV vaccine HBV immune globulin (HBIG)	Two inactivated vaccines are approved for children ages 2-18 years: Havrix and Vaqta; given in a 2-dose schedule (6-12 months between doses)		
HBV vaccine (see Box 7-2 and Table 10-4)	No benefit	Postexposure protection possible if given immediately after definite exposure Provides active immunity Universal vaccination recommended for all newborns	No benefit
Mortality	0.1%-0.2%	0.5%-2.0% in uncomplicated cases; may be higher in complicated cases	1%-2% in uncomplicated cases; may be higher in complicated cases

atitis. HBV varies greatly throughout the world. High-prevalence areas have been identified in Africa and Asia; the United States is considered a low-prevalence area. Transmission is usually via the parenteral route through the exchange of blood or any bodily secretion or fluid. Infections from blood transfusion have been reduced as a result of blood product–screening procedures. Transplantation of organs, intimate physical contact, transmission from mother to infant, and the splashing of contaminated fluids into the mouth or eyes are other sources of infection. Adults whose occupations are associated with exposure to blood or blood products (such as health care workers) are at increased risk for infection and should receive HBV vaccination.

Most HBV infection in children is acquired perinatally. Newborns are at risk for hepatitis if the mother is infected with HBV or was a carrier of HBV during pregnancy. Possible routes of maternal-fetal-infant transmission include (1) leakage of virus across the placenta late in pregnancy or during labor and (2) ingestion of amniotic fluid or maternal blood.

HBV infection occurs in children and adolescents in the following high-risk groups: (1) individuals with hemophilia and others who have received multiple transfusions, (2) children and adolescents involved in IV drug abuse, (3) institutionalized children and adolescents, (4) preschool-age children in endemic areas, and (5) individuals engaged in heterosexual or homosexual activity with infected partners. The incubation period of HBV infection varies from 45 to 160 days.

Hepatitis C. About 0.2% to 0.4% of children younger than 12 years of age are infected with HCV. It is estimated that 4 million people in the United States are anti–HCV-positive. Approximately 7% of HCV-infected mothers transmit the HCV virus to their newborns (Balistreri and others, 2002). The second most common route of infection is by percutaneous exposure, which occurs through transfusion of blood or blood products, transplantation of organs or tissues, or through sharing used needles. Transfusion-associated HCV infection is low, but a common cause of infection is injection drug use. The American Academy of Pediatrics (1998) suggests screening the following groups: (1) all infants born to HCV-infected women, (2) individuals who received blood products before 1992, (3) individuals involved in injection drug use, and (4) individuals who receive hemodialysis. The length of time that maternal antibody is present in infants born to HCV-infected women must be considered, and screening should be done after the infant is 12 months old. However, a routine screening program, such as that for HBV, is not recommended.

The clinical course of HCV infection is variable. Incubation averages 6 to 7 weeks, with a range of 2 weeks to 6 months. HCV causes acute hepatitis that progresses to chronic disease in more than 70% of affected individuals and can cause end-stage liver disease in 10% of these patients. However, both acute and chronic HCV infection often produce only mild nonspecific symptoms or no symptoms at all (Bonkovsky and Mehta, 2001)

Current recommendations are to evaluate HCV-infected children at regular intervals to monitor for chronic hepatitis. Most children will be asymptomatic with evidence of chronic hepatitis on liver biopsy. Liver enzyme levels may fluctuate between periods of normal and elevated values (Balistreri, 1999).

Hepatitis D. HDV is an important cause of acute and chronic liver disease. HDV is a defective RNA virus that requires the function of HBV. HDV infection occurs primarily in hemophiliac patients and IV drug abusers. The incubation period is 2 to 8 weeks. Both acute and chronic forms are more severe than HBV infection and can lead to cirrhosis. Testing for HDV infection is recommended in children with chronic HBV infection or severe liver disease and in children with acute exacerbation of a previously stable liver disease.

Hepatitis E. HEV infection is enterally transmitted. Transmission may occur through the fecal-oral route or from contaminated water. The incubation period is 2 to 9

weeks. This illness is uncommon in children, does not cause chronic liver disease, is not a chronic condition, and has no carrier state. The mortality rate resulting from submassive hepatic necrosis is low except in pregnant women in their third trimester, in whom mortality reaches 20%.

Hepatitis G. HGV is a blood-borne virus that may also be transmitted by organ transplantation. High-risk groups include transfusion recipients, IV drug users, and individuals infected with HCV. Individuals with the virus are often asymptomatic, and most infections are chronic. The incubation period is unknown.

Diagnostic Evaluation

Diagnosis is based on the history (especially regarding possible exposure to a hepatitis virus), physical examination, and serologic markers (antibodies or antigens) indicating the presence of active infection with hepatitis A, B, or C or previous infection. Because the liver has a large functional reserve, abnormal laboratory tests may be the only indication of hepatitis. However, liver function tests (LFTs) are not specific for the diagnosis of viral hepatitis. Although serum aspartate and alanine aminotransferase (AST and ALT) levels are markedly elevated in viral hepatitis, other diseases or conditions may cause their elevation. When hepatitis is severe, albumin levels are depressed and prothrombin times are increased. Serum bilirubin levels peak 5 to 10 days after clinical jaundice appears.

Diagnosis of viral hepatitis is based on the presence of specific viral markers. Diagnosis of acute HAV infection is based on the presence of anti-HAV immunoglobulin (Ig)M antibody in the serum. HBV diagnosis depends on the presence of hepatitis B surface antigen (HBsAG) or anti-HBV core (anti-HBc) IgM antibody. Chronic HBV infection is associated with the persistence of HBsAg and HBV DNA markers. The diagnosis of HCV is based on the detection of anti-HCV antibodies and confirmation by polymerase chain reaction for hepatitis C RNA.

Other diagnostic studies include a urinalysis to evaluate the bilirubinemia and to rule out other causes of hepatitis. An abdominal ultrasound provides measurement of liver size, detection of cystic lesions and stones, and imaging of the gallbladder. Cholescintigraphy radionuclide imaging detects abnormalities in liver uptake, concentration, and excretory function. Finally, a liver biopsy aids in assessing the severity of the disease.

Pathophysiology

Pathologic changes occur primarily in the parenchymal cells of the liver and result in varying degrees of swelling, infiltration of liver cells by mononuclear cells, subsequent degeneration, necrosis, and fibrosis.

Hepatitis can be self-limited, and complete regeneration of liver cells without scarring may occur. However, some forms of hepatitis do not result in complete return of liver function. These include *fulminant hepatitis,* which is characterized by a severe, acute course, and massive destruction of the liver, which results in liver failure and death in 1 to 2 weeks. *Subacute* or *chronic active hepatitis* is characterized by progressive liver destruction, uncertain regeneration, scarring, and potential cirrhosis.

The initial *anicteric* (absence of jaundice) *phase* usually lasts 5 to 7 days and is often mistaken for influenza. Symptoms include nausea, vomiting, extreme anorexia, malaise, easy fatigability, arthralgia, skin rashes, slight to moderate fever, and epigastric or upper right quadrant abdominal pain. Dark urine is a symptom of the *icteric* (jaundice) *phase.* Pruritus may accompany jaundice and can be bothersome, but many children with acute viral hepatitis do not develop jaundice.

Therapeutic Management

Treatment options for viral hepatitis are limited. The goals of management include early detection, recognition of chronic liver disease, support and monitoring, and prevention of spread of the disease.

HAV infection is an acute disease that resolves with support and management of symptoms. HBV and HCV treatment is directed at managing the viral load to prevent further destruction of the liver. Currently, interferons are used to treat HBV and HCV. Interferons are naturally occurring proteins that exert antiviral, antiproliferative, and immunomodulatory effects. A recent interferon formulation, pegylated interferon, can be administered once a week and has been found to sustain plasma levels and enhance viral suppression (Karnam and Reddy, 2003). Lamivudine and adefovir are two other interferon analogues that suppress the replication of HBV (Yuen and Lai, 2001). A combination of alpha interferon and ribavirin has resulted in a sustained response in some adult patients with HBV and HCV (Regev and Schiff, 2000).

Another important aspect of the therapeutic management of hepatitis involves hospitalization. Hospitalization is necessary if coagulopathy or fulminant hepatitis is present.

Prevention. Proper handwashing and standard isolation precautions can prevent the spread of hepatitis. Prophylactic use of standard immune globulin (IG) is effective in preventing HAV infection in situations of preexposure (e.g., anticipated travel to areas where HAV is prevalent) or in situations of postexposure during the early part of the incubation period. Hepatitis B immune globulin (HBIG) is effective in preventing HBV infection after exposure. IG must be administered less than 2 weeks after exposure.

Vaccines have been developed to prevent HAV and HBV infection. HBV vaccination is recommended for all newborns and for high-risk groups. HAV is also recommended for high-risk groups (see Immunizations, Chapter 10). Active immunizations are not available against HCV. It is possible to prevent HDV infection by preventing HBV infection.

Prognosis. The prognosis for children with hepatitis is variable and depends on the type of virus. HAV usually causes a mild and brief illness with no carrier state. HBV causes a wide spectrum of acute and chronic illness. Chronic HBV infection leads to cirrhosis in approximately one fourth to one third of the cases. Hepatocellular carcinoma is a potentially fatal complication of HBV infection. HCV infection frequently becomes chronic, and cirrhosis may develop in some patients. Chronic HCV infection is the leading indication for liver transplantation in adults in the United States (Regev and Schiff, 2000). Fulminant hepatic failure occurs in a small number of cases of viral hepatitis, regardless of the etiology, and is associated with a high mortality rate.

Nursing Considerations

Nursing objectives depend on the severity of the hepatitis, the medical management, and factors influencing the control and transmission of the disease. Children with benign viral hepatitis are frequently cared for at home, and the clinic or office nurse must explain the medical therapy and control measures. If further assistance is needed for parents to comply with therapy, a public health nursing referral may be necessary.

A well-balanced diet and a realistic schedule of rest and activity adjusted to the child's condition are encouraged. HAV is not infectious within a week after the onset of jaundice, and children may feel well enough to resume school. Parents are cautioned about administering any medication to the child, because normal doses of many drugs may become dangerous because of the liver's inability to detoxify and excrete them. Handwashing is the single most critical measure in reducing risk of transmission. The nurse should explain to parents and children the ways in which HAV (oral-fecal route) and HBV (parenteral route) are spread.

Children who are hospitalized are not usually isolated in a separate room unless they are fecally incontinent or their toys and other items become contaminated with feces. They are discouraged from sharing their toys. (For further discussion, see Infection Control, Chapter 22.)

Nurses who care for young people with HBV infection who have a known or suspected history of illicit drug use should help these teens to realize the dangers of drug abuse. Nurses should stress the parenteral mode of transmission of hepatitis and encourage them to seek counseling through a drug program. HBV and HCV are chronic diseases that require frequent monitoring and management. Many communities have multidisciplinary clinics dedicated to the management of these diseases.

CIRRHOSIS

Cirrhosis occurs at the end stage of many chronic liver diseases, including biliary atresia and chronic hepatitis. Cirrhosis can also result from infectious, autoimmune, or toxic factors and from chronic diseases such as hemophilia and cystic fibrosis. A cirrhotic liver is irreversibly damaged.

Clinical manifestations in children are similar to those seen with all chronic liver disorders. Children exhibit jaundice, poor growth, anorexia, muscle weakness, and lethargy. Ascites, edema, GI bleeding, anemia, and abdominal pain may be present with impaired intrahepatic blood flow. Pulmonary function may be impaired because of pressure against the diaphragm from hepatosplenomegaly and ascites. Dyspnea and cyanosis may occur, especially on exertion. Intrapulmonary arteriovenous shunts may develop and cause hypoxemia. Spider angiomas and prominent blood vessels are often present on the upper torso.

Therapeutic Management

Therapy is directed toward (1) frequent assessment of liver status with physical examination and liver function tests and (2) management of specific complications. The only successful treatment for end-stage liver disease and liver failure may be *liver transplantation,* which has improved the prognosis substantially for many children with cirrhosis. Currently, the 1-year survival rate for liver transplantation is 85%. Increasing numbers of recipients are reaching their

FAMILY FOCUS

End-Stage Liver Disease

In many cases the child and family must cope with an uncertain progression of the disease. The only hope for long-term survival may be liver transplantation. Transplantation can be very successful, but the waiting period may be long, and there are many more children in need of organs than there are donors. The procedure is very expensive and is performed only at designated medical centers that are often far from the family's home. The nurse should recognize the unique stresses of coping with end-stage liver disease and waiting for transplantation and assist the family in coping with these stressors. The assistance of social workers and support from other parents can be very beneficial.

BOX 24-10 ■ Clinical Manifestations of Extrahepatic Biliary Atresia

Jaundice
   Earliest manifestation and most striking feature of disorder
   First observed in sclera
   May be present at birth
   Usually not apparent until age 2 to 3 weeks
Urine dark and stains diaper
Stools lighter than expected or white or tan
Hepatomegaly and abdominal distention common
Splenomegaly occurs later
Poor fat metabolism results in:
   Poor weight gain
   General failure to thrive
Pruritus
Irritability
Difficult to comfort infant

---

second decade after transplant. The increasing lifespan after transplantation is due to advances in surgical techniques and improved preoperative, intraoperative, and postoperative care (Atkison and others, 2002).

Prognosis.   Liver transplantation has revolutionized the approach to liver cirrhosis. Liver failure and cirrhosis are indications for transplantation. Liver transplantation reflects the failure of other medical and surgical measures to prevent or treat cirrhosis. Careful monitoring of the child's condition and quality of life is necessary to evaluate the need for and timing of transplantation (see Family Focus box).

Nursing Considerations

Nursing care of the child with cirrhosis is determined by the cause of the cirrhosis, the severity of complications, and the prognosis. The prognosis for life is poor unless successful liver transplantation occurs. Nursing care of this child is similar to that for any child with a life-threatening illness (see Chapter 18). Hospitalization is usually required when complications occur.

BILIARY ATRESIA

Biliary atresia, or *extrahepatic biliary atresia (EHBA),* is a progressive inflammatory process that causes both intrahepatic and extrahepatic bile duct fibrosis, resulting in obstructed bile flow. EHBA has been detected in 1 in 10,000 to 1 in 15,000 live births. The disorder is more common in girls and premature infants. In the United States, the incidence is twice as high in African Americans as in white infants, and more common in Chinese than in either Japanese or white populations. If untreated, EHBA usually leads to cirrhosis, liver failure, and death in the first 2 years of life.

Etiology/Pathophysiology

The exact cause of biliary atresia is unknown. Because EHBA has two distinct forms, postnatal and fetal/embryonic, different pathogenic mechanisms are suggested. Postnatal EHBA represents 65% to 90% of cases and is probably the result of infection or an immune-mediated mechanism. Direct hyperbilirubinemia first appears after the resolution of physiologic jaundice. Histology demonstrates bile duct remnants and a progressive inflammatory process. In the fetal embryonic form, which represents 10% to 35% of cases, there is a con-

genital absence of biliary ductal patency and an absence of bile duct remnants. Many infants have associated congenital anomalies. The pathology of EHBA varies. Varying degrees of cholestasis occur, resulting in retention of irritants and toxins. Cholestasis is the accumulation of compounds that cannot be excreted because of occlusion or obstruction of the biliary tree. Injury to the liver occurs as the result of the inflammation caused by homeostasis.

Diagnostic Evaluation

Early diagnosis is the key to the survival of the child with EHBA. Infants who undergo surgery in the first 60 days of life have an 80% chance of establishing bile flow. Between 60 to 90 days of life, the chance of reestablishing flow drops to 50% and after 90 days to 10% (Sinatra, 2001). Growth parameters and nutritional status should be assessed, because many infants and children have nutritional deficiencies and poor growth. Several clinical signs may indicate the presence of EHBA (Box 24-10). Blood tests should include a CBC, electrolytes, bilirubin, and liver enzymes. Additional laboratory analyses include alpha$_1$-antitrypsin level, TORCH titers (see Maternal Infections, Chapter 9), hepatitis serology, alpha-fetoprotein, urine cytomegalovirus, and a sweat test, which is indicated to rule out other conditions that cause persistent cholestasis and jaundice. Abdominal ultrasonography allows inspection of the liver and biliary system. Hepatobiliary scintigraphy demonstrates biliary patency but does not provide diagnostic certainty. Endoscopic retrograde cholangiopancreatography (ERCP) is performed in very young infants. This procedure, which is done using general anesthesia, has an 80% reported diagnostic accuracy. Percutaneous liver biopsy is highly reliable when the biopsy contains specimens from a number of portal areas. Definitive diagnosis of EHBA is obtained during surgical laparotomy and an intraoperative cholangiogram.

Therapeutic Management

The primary treatment of biliary atresia is *hepatic portoenterostomy (Kasai procedure),* in which a segment of intestine is anastomosed to the resected porta hepatis to attempt bile drainage. Bile drainage is achieved in approximately 80% to 90% of infants who undergo surgery when younger than 10 weeks of age (Halamek and Stevenson, 1997). However, progressive cirrhosis still occurs in many children, and up to 80% to 90% eventually require liver transplantation (Andres, 1996). Prophylactic antibiotics are given following the Kasai procedure to minimize the risk of ascending cholangitis.

Medical management is primarily supportive. It includes nutritional support with infant formulas that contain medium-chain triglycerides and essential fatty acids. Supplementation with fat-soluble vitamins, a multivitamin, and minerals, including iron, zinc, and selenium, is usually required. Aggressive nutritional support with continuous tube feedings or TPN is indicated for moderate to severe failure to thrive. The enteral solution should be low in sodium. Ursodeoxycholic acid is used to treat pruritus and hypercholesterolemia.

Prognosis.   Untreated biliary atresia results in progressive cirrhosis and death in most children by 2 years of age. The Kasai procedure improves the prognosis but is not a cure. Biliary drainage can often be achieved if the surgery is done before the intrahepatic bile ducts are destroyed. Long-term survival has been reported in children who receive the Kasai procedure; however, even with successful bile drainage, many children ultimately develop liver failure.

Advances in surgical techniques and the use of immunosuppressive and antifungal drugs have improved the success of transplantation. The major obstacle continues to be a shortage of donor livers. Reduced-size, split-liver transplantation, retransplantation, and increased public awareness may improve donor organ availability in the future.

Nursing Considerations

Nursing interventions for the child with biliary atresia include support of the family before, during, and after surgical procedures as well as education regarding the treatment plan. In the postoperative period of a portoenterostomy, nursing care is similar to that after major abdominal surgery. Family members need education relating to the proper administration of medications and nutritional therapy, including special formulas, vitamin and mineral supplements, tube feedings, or parenteral nutrition. Pruritus can often be relieved by drug therapy or comfort measures such as baths and trimming of fingernails.

Children and their families also need psychosocial support. The uncertain prognosis, discomfort, and waiting for transplantation produces stress, and hospitalizations, pharmacologic therapy, and nutritional therapy impose financial burdens on the family. Families can receive help from the **Children's Liver Disease Foundation,** * an organization that provides educational materials, programs, and support systems.

STRUCTURAL DEFECTS

CLEFT LIP OR CLEFT PALATE

Clefts of the lip (CL) and palate (CP) are facial malformations that occur during embryonic development and are the most common congenital deformity of the head and neck. They may appear separately or, more often, together. CL re-

---

*36 Great Charles Street, Birmingham, B33 JY, United Kingdom; (0121) 212-3839; fax: (0121) 212-4300; website: www.childliverdisease.org.

sults from failure of the maxillary and median nasal processes to fuse; CP is a midline fissure of the palate that results from failure of the two sides to fuse. This discussion is concerned primarily with cleft lip and palate (CL/P).

CL may vary from a small notch to a complete cleft extending into the base of the nose (Fig. 24-3). Clefts can be unilateral or bilateral. Deformed dental structures are associated with CL. CP alone occurs in the midline and may involve the soft and hard palates. When associated with CL, the defect may involve the midline and extend into the soft palate on one or both sides.

CL/P is more common than CP and varies by ethnicity. The occurrence is 1:1000 births in whites; 1:500 births in Native Americans and Asians, and 1:2000 births in African Americans. CP occurs alone in only 1:2500 cases and does not display variation by ethnicity (Wilkins-Haug, 2003). Approximately 60% to 80% of children born with cleft lip and palate are male. Females have a higher frequency of isolated clefts of the secondary palate. Unilateral clefts are nine times more common than bilateral clefs and occur twice as frequently on the left side. Isolated bilateral CLs are uncommon; approximately 86% present with palatal clefts. Approximately 68% of unilateral CLs have an associated palatal cleft (Kirschner and LaRossa, 2000).

Etiology

Cleft deformities may be an isolated anomaly, or they may occur with a recognized syndrome. CL with or without CP is distinct from isolated CP. Clefts of the secondary palate alone are more likely to be associated with syndromes than isolated CL or CL and CP.

CL and CP may be caused by exposure to teratogens such as alcohol, anticonvulsants, and isotretinoin, but there is little evidence to link isolated clefts to any single teratogenic agent with the exception of phenytoin. Use of phenytoin during pregnancy is associated with a tenfold increase in the incidence of CL. The incidence of CL among mothers who smoke during pregnancy is twice as great as the incidence in mothers who do not smoke during pregnancy (Kirschner and LaRossa, 2000).

Pathophysiology

Cleft deformities represent a genetic defect in cell migration that results in a failure of the maxillary and premaxillary processes to come together between the third and twelfth week of embryonic development. Although often appearing together, CL and CP are distinct malformations embryologically, occurring at different times during the developmental process. Merging of the upper lip at the midline is completed between the seventh and eleventh weeks of gestation. Fusion of the secondary palate (hard and soft palate) takes place later, between the seventh and twelfth weeks of gestation. In the process of migrating to a horizontal position, they are separated by the tongue for a short time. If there is delay in this movement, or if the tongue fails to descend soon enough, the remainder of development proceeds but the palate never fuses.

Diagnostic Evaluation

CL with or without CP is apparent at birth. The defect elicits severe emotional reactions in parents. CP is less obvious than CL and may not be detected without a thorough

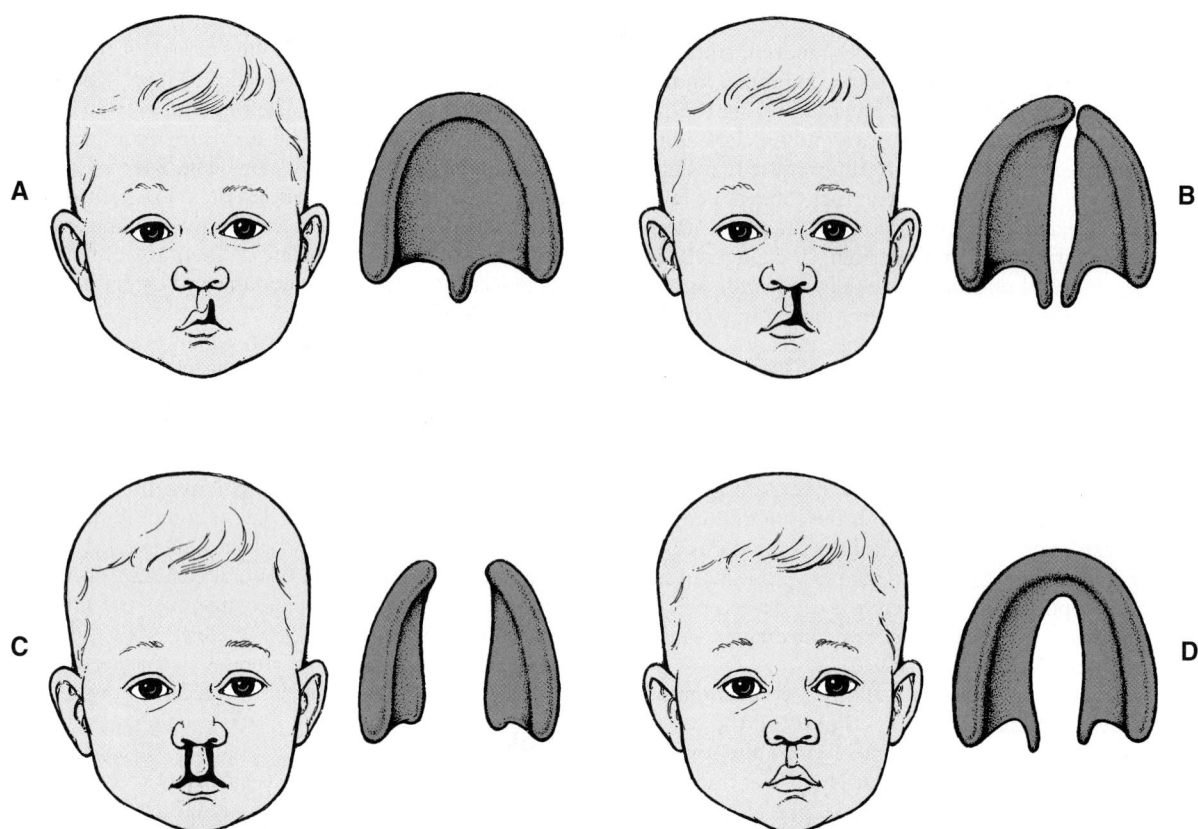

FIG. 24-3 ■ Variations in clefts of lip and palate at birth. **A,** Notch in vermilion border. **B,** Unilateral cleft lip and palate. **C,** Bilateral cleft lip and palate. **D,** Cleft palate.

assessment of the mouth. CP is identified when the examiner places a finger directly on the palate. Clefts of the hard palate form a continuous opening between the mouth and the nasal cavity. The severity of the CP has an impact on feeding; the infant is unable to generate negative pressure and create suction in the oral cavity. This impairs feeding, even though in most cases the infant's ability to swallow is normal.

Prenatal diagnosis with fetal ultrasound is not reliable until the soft tissues of the fetal face can be visualized at 13 to 14 weeks. The sensitivity of fetal ultrasound for facial clefting is almost 100% when CL/P is associated with other structural anomalies. In isolated CL/P, sensitivity may be 50% with CP; an intact lip is the most difficult to diagnose prenatally (Wilkins-Haug, 2003).

Therapeutic Management

Treatment of the child with CL is surgical and involves no long-term interventions other than possible scar revision. The management of CP involves the cooperative efforts of a multidisciplinary health care team, including pediatrics, plastic surgery, orthodontics, otolaryngology, speech/language pathology, audiology, nursing, and social work. Management is directed toward closure of the cleft(s), prevention of complications, and facilitation of normal growth and development in the child. Until recently, repair of cleft deformities in the neonate was not considered safe. Surgery is now possible in younger neonates because of advances in

pediatric anesthesiology and neonatology. However, the infant must be free of any oral, respiratory, or systemic infections. In deformities of both the lip and palate, the palate is repaired first to avoid disrupting the lip after it has been repaired.

Surgical correction: CL. The two most common procedures for repair of CL are the Tennison-Randall triangular flap (Z-plasty) and the Millard rotational advancement technique. The difference between these two is that the Tennison-Randall procedure crosses the philtral line and the Millard procedure advances a triangle of tissue in the upper third of the lip and does not cross the midline. Surgeons often use a combination of these two techniques to address individual differences. Improved surgical techniques have minimized scar retraction, and in the absence of infection or trauma, healing occurs with little scar formation. Optimal cosmetic results, however, are difficult to obtain in severe defects. Additional revisions may be necessary at a later age.

Surgical correction: CP. CP repair was previously postponed until a later age than the repair of the CL to take advantage of palatal changes that take place with normal growth. With advanced surgical and anesthesia techniques, many surgeons are currently performing palatal repairs in the neonatal period (Sandberg, Magee, and Denk, 2002). The timing of repair remains controversial. Most surgeons prefer to close the cleft before the child develops faulty speech habits.

Prognosis.   Even with good anatomic closure, most children with CL/P have some degree of speech impairment that requires speech therapy. Physical problems result from inefficient functioning of the muscles of the soft palate and nasopharynx, improper tooth alignment, and varying degrees of hearing loss. Improper drainage of the middle ear, as a result of inefficient function of the eustachian tube, contributes to recurrent otitis media with scarring of the tympanic membrane, which leads to hearing impairment in many children with CP. Upper respiratory infections require immediate and meticulous attention, and extensive orthodontics and prosthodontics may be needed to correct problems of malposition of teeth and maxillary arches.

Long-term problems are related to social adjustment of the child. The better the physical care, the better is the chance for emotional and social adjustment, although the presence of the defect and the degree of residual disability are not always directly related to a satisfactory adjustment. Physical defects are a threat to the self-image, and abnormal speech quality is an impediment to social expression.

Nursing Considerations

● Assessment

The lip defect is visible at birth, and assessment involves describing the location and extent of the defect; the CP is estimated by visualization during crying. CP without CL is detected by palpating the palate with the finger during the newborn assessment. The emotional impact of the birth of a child with a cosmetic and functional disability is especially traumatic to the family. Consequently, nursing assessment is also concerned with the emotional reaction of the family.

● Nursing Diagnoses

Based on a thorough physical assessment, a number of nursing diagnoses are evident and described in the Nursing Care Plan on pp. 875-876.

● Planning

The goals of care are related to preoperative care, short-term postoperative care, and long-term management. Goals for the infant and family include:

Preoperative care:

1 Family will cope with the impact of an infant with a defect.
2 Infant will receive optimum nutrition.
3 Infant will be prepared for surgery.

Postoperative care:

1 Infant will experience no trauma and minimal or no pain.
2 Infant will receive optimum nutrition.
3 Infant will experience no complications.
4 Infant and family will receive adequate support.
5 Family will be prepared for care at home and long-term needs of a child with CP.

● Implementation

The immediate nursing problems for an infant with CL/P deformities are related to feeding and dealing with the parental reaction to the defect. Facial deformities are particularly disturbing to parents. CL is a visible defect that may produce a strong negative response in parents, which could influence maternal-infant attachment. However, a study of infants with CL or CP indicated that maternal-infant attachment was not negatively affected when measured at 1 year of age (Speltz and others, 1997). During the initial phase following birth, it is important for the nurse to place emphasis not only on the infant's physical needs, but also on the parents' emotional needs (Speltz and others, 1997). The manner of handling the infant should convey to the parents that the infant is a precious human being. (See Chapter 18 for interventions in assisting parents in accepting a birth defect.) Throughout the course of therapy, parents need explanations of the immediate and long-range problems associated with CP. They may be unaware that more is involved than repairing the defect. Whenever possible, they should be referred to a comprehensive CP team.

Feeding.   Feeding the infant presents a challenge to nurses and parents. Growth failure in infants with CL or CP has been attributed to preoperative feeding difficulties. After surgical repair, most infants who have isolated CL or CP with no associated syndromes gain weight or achieve adequate weight and height for age (Lee, Nunn, and Wright, 1997).

CL or CP reduces the infant's ability to suck, making bottle-feeding and breast-feeding difficult. In breast-feeding the CL or CP interferes with compression of the areola. Liquid taken into the mouth escapes via the cleft through the nose. Feeding is best accomplished with the infant's head in an upright position, either held in the caregiver's hand or cradled in the arm. Normal nipples are unsuitable for these infants, who are unable to generate the suction required. A variety of special "cleft palate" nipples have been devised and used with some success. However, large, soft nipples with large holes; Nursettes; or the long, soft lamb's nipples appear to offer the best means for nipple feeding (Fig. 24-4). The newer "gravity flow" nipple* attached to a squeezable plastic bottle allows formula to be deposited directly into the mouth in the same manner as with a bulb syringe. Success has also been achieved by modification of a standard nipple. A single small slit or crosscut is made in the end of the nipple with a sharp surgical blade or pair of sharp, thin scissors. The enlarged opening, which can be adjusted to the infant's individual needs, allows the infant to swallow the formula easily, bypassing the suction problem.

The ESSR feeding technique also works well with these infants. The steps in ESSR are 1) *enlarge* the nipple, 2) *stimulate* the suck reflex, 3) *swallow* fluid appropriately, and 4) *rest* when the infant signals with facial expression. Infants fed with the ESSR method revealed a significantly greater increase in their mean weight before surgery than infants fed with traditional methods (Richard, 1994).

Using special or modified nipples or feeding techniques helps to meet the infant's sucking needs. Muscle development is important for later development of speech. During feeding, the nipple is positioned so that it is compressed by the infant's tongue and existing palate. If a single-slit nipple is used, the slit is placed vertically so that the infant will be able to produce and stop a flow of milk by alternately open-

---

*Ross Laboratories,** 625 Cleveland Avenue, Columbus, OH 43216.

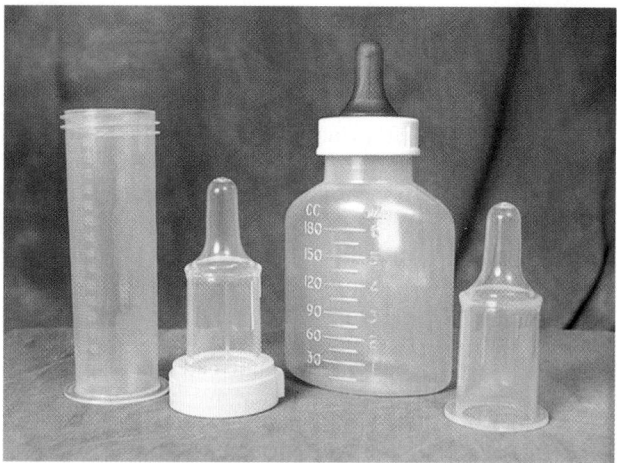

FIG. 24-4 ■ Some devices used to feed an infant with a cleft lip and palate. (Photo by Paul Vincent Kuntz, Texas Children's Hospital.)

ing and closing the opening. No matter which type of nipple is used, gentle, steady pressure on the base of the bottle reduces the chance of choking or coughing. The person feeding should resist the temptation to remove the nipple because of the noise the infant makes or for fear that the infant will choke. These infants swallow excessive amounts of air, and they require frequent burping.

When the infant has trouble with nipple feeding, a rubber-tipped medicine dropper, Asepto syringe, or Breck feeder (a large syringe with soft rubber tubing) provides an efficient, safe feeding device. The rubber extension should be long enough to extend back into the mouth to reduce the likelihood of regurgitation through the nose. The formula is deposited on the back of the tongue, and the flow is controlled by bulb or syringe compression that is adjusted to the infant's needs. With some infants, spoon feeding works best, especially if the formula is slightly thickened with cereal. After feeding, the infant is given water to rinse the mouth.

Breast-feeding is also an option. The nipple is positioned and stabilized well back in the oral cavity so that tongue action facilitates milk expression. The suction required to stimulate milk may be absent initially, and a breast pump may be useful before nursing to stimulate the let-down reflex.

Regardless of the feeding method used, the mother should begin feeding the infant as soon as possible, preferably after the initial nursery feeding. When maternal feeding is initiated early, the mother can help to determine the method best suited to her and the infant and can become adept in the technique before discharge from the hospital.

Preoperative Care. In preparation for surgical repair, parents are frequently taught to accustom the infant to the needs of the early postoperative period, especially if surgery is delayed for several months. It is mandatory for the infant to be positioned on the back or side postoperatively. Most infants tolerate these positions well because they are accustomed to being supine for sleeping. It is also helpful to place the infant or child in arm restraints periodically before admission and to feed the infant with a rubber-tipped Asepto syringe or other device that will be used postoperatively.

Postoperative Care: CL. The major efforts in the postoperative period are directed toward protecting the operative site. After CL repair *(cheiloplasty),* a metal appliance or adhesive strips are securely taped to the cheeks to relax the surgical site and prevent tension on the suture line caused by crying or other facial movement. Elbow restraints are used to prevent the infant from rubbing or disturbing the suture line and are applied immediately after surgery. It is advisable to pin the cuff of the restraints to the infant's clothing to keep the restraints in place. Older infants who roll over will require a jacket restraint in addition to restricting arm movement to prevent rolling on the abdomen and rubbing the face on the sheet, especially if the repair involves the lip. It is important to remove the elbow restraints periodically to exercise the arms, to provide relief from restrictions, to observe the skin for signs of irritation, and to provide an opportunity for cuddling and body contact. Restraints should be released one at a time. Sitting the infant in an infant seat provides a change of position and a different view of the environment. Adequate analgesia is required to relieve postoperative pain and to prevent restlessness.

Clear liquids are offered when the infant has fully recovered from the anesthesia, and feeding is resumed when tolerated. The suture site is carefully cleansed of formula or serosanguineous drainage as needed with a cotton-tipped swab dipped in saline. A thin layer of antibiotic ointment may be prescribed for application to the suture line after cleansing. Meticulous care of the suture line is essential because inflammation or infection will interfere with optimal healing and the ultimate cosmetic effect of the surgical repair. Gentle aspiration of mouth and nasopharyngeal secretions may be necessary to prevent aspiration and respiratory complications. An upright or infant seat position is helpful in the immediate postoperative period (especially for the infant who has difficulty in handling secretions).

Postoperative Care: CP. The child with CP repair *(palatoplasty)* is allowed to lie on the abdomen immediately postoperatively. The child may resume feeding by bottle, breast, or cup shortly after surgery.

> **⚠ NURSING ALERT**
>
> Avoid the use of suction or other objects in the mouth, such as tongue depressors, thermometers, spoons, or straws.

Oral packing may be secured to the palate after palatoplasty; this packing is usually removed after 2 to 3 days. Sometimes the infant will have difficulty breathing following surgery, because it is often necessary to alter an established pattern of breathing and adjust to breathing through the nose. This is frustrating but seldom requires more than positioning and support. The elbows may be restrained to keep the child's hands away from the mouth. Parents are instructed to maintain elbow restraints at home until the palate is healed, usually in 4 to 6 weeks. They are instructed to remove the restraints (one at a time) frequently to allow the child to exercise the arms.

The nurse must assess the infant or child's level of postoperative pain. Opioids may be prescribed initially, and acetaminophen may be given as needed thereafter.

The older infant or child may be discharged on a blenderized or soft diet, and parents are instructed to continue the diet until the surgeon directs them otherwise. Parents are cautioned against allowing the child to eat hard items (such as toast, hard cookies, and potato chips) that can damage the repaired palate.

Long-Term Care.   Children with CL/P often require a variety of services during recovery. Family members need support and encouragement by health professionals and guidance in activities that facilitate a normal outcome for their child. Financial stress is frequently cited as a difficult issue by parents. With the combined efforts of the family and the health team, most children achieve a satisfactory outcome. Many children with CL/P have surgical correction that creates a near-normal–appearing lip and permits good function. Parents need to understand the function of therapy and the purpose and care of all appliances, as well as the importance of establishing good mouth care and proper brushing habits.

Throughout the child's development, an important goal is the development of a healthy personality and self-esteem. Many communities have CP parents' groups that offer help and support to families. Agencies that provide services and information for children with CL/P and their families include the **American Cleft Palate Association, The Cleft Palate Foundation,** the **Association of Birth Defect Children,** the **March of Dimes–Birth Defects Foundation,** and the various state **Children's Medical Services.**

● *Evaluation*

To determine the effectiveness of nursing intervention, continual reassessment and evaluation of care are based on the following observational guidelines:

Preoperative care:

1 Observe and interview family members about their understanding, feelings, and concerns regarding the defect, any anticipated surgery, and their interactions with the infant.
2 Observe infant during feeding.
3 Complete preoperative checklist.

Postoperative care:

1 Inspect operative site, including the protective device.
2 Observe for behavioral and physiologic indicators of pain and response to analgesics.
3 Observe infant during feeding, measure intake and output, and weigh infant daily.
4 Observe operative site for evidence of infection, bleeding, sloughing, or irritation.
5 Observe and interview family regarding their understanding and concerns about the infant, including long-term needs.

The *expected outcomes* are described in the Nursing Care Plan below.

ESOPHAGEAL ATRESIA WITH TRACHEOESOPHAGEAL FISTULA

Congenital atresia of the esophagus and tracheoesophageal fistula (TEF) are rare malformations that are believed to result from failed separation of the esophagus and trachea by a septum that forms by the fourth week of gestation. These defects occur as separate entities or in combination (Fig. 24-5). They have a fatal outcome without early diagnosis and treatment.

Etiology

Esophageal atresia (EA) with or without an associated TEF is the most common esophageal malformation. It occurs in 1:2000 to 1:5000 live births. There appears to be an equal sex incidence, but the birth weight of most affected infants is significantly lower than average, and there is an unusually high incidence of prematurity in infants with EA. A history of maternal polyhydramnios is present in approximately 50% of infants with the defects. EA/TEF is often present with the VATER or VACTERL syndromes. VATER and VACTERL are acronyms that describe the associated anomalies. These syndromes involve a combination of vertebral, anorectal, cardiovascular, tracheoesophageal, renal, and limb abnormalities. The cardiac anomalies occur most frequently with EA/TEF.

NURSING CARE PLAN   The Child With Cleft Lip or Cleft Palate

PREOPERATIVE CARE

NURSING DIAGNOSIS ▪ **Altered nutrition: less than body requirements related to physical defect**

PATIENT GOAL 1: Will consume adequate nourishment

NURSING INTERVENTIONS/*RATIONALES*
Administer diet appropriate for age (specify)
Assist mother with breast-feeding if this is mother's preference, because the newborn with either defect can breast-feed
 Position and stabilize nipple well back in oral cavity *so that tongue action facilitates milk expression*
 Stimulate let-down reflex manually or with breast pump before nursing, *because suction required to stimulate milk may be absent initially*
Modify feeding techniques to adjust to defect, *because infant's ability to suck is reduced*
 Hold child in upright (sitting) position *to minimize risk of aspiration*

Use special feeding appliances *that compensate for infant's feeding difficulty*
 Try to feed infant using nipple *to meet infant's need for sucking and to promote muscle development for speech*
 Position nipple between infant's tongue and existing palate *to facilitate compression of nipple*
 When using devices without nipples (e.g., Breck feeder, Asepto syringe), deposit formula on back of tongue *to facilitate swallowing* and adjust flow according to infant's swallowing *to prevent aspiration*
Bubble (burp) frequently *because of tendency to swallow excessive amounts of air*
Encourage parents to begin feeding infant as soon as possible *so that they become adept in feeding technique before discharge*
Monitor weight *to assess adequacy of nutritional intake*

EXPECTED OUTCOMES
Infant consumes an adequate amount of nutrients (specify amount)
Infant exhibits appropriate weight gain

Continued

NURSING CARE PLAN The Child With Cleft Lip or Cleft Palate—*cont'd*

NURSING DIAGNOSIS ◾ **Risk for altered parenting related to infant with a highly visible physical defect**

PATIENT (FAMILY) GOAL 1: Will demonstrate acceptance of infant

NURSING INTERVENTIONS/RATIONALES
Allow expression of feelings *to encourage family's coping*
Convey attitude of acceptance of infant and family *because parents are sensitive to affective attitudes of others*
Indicate by behavior that child is a valuable human being *to encourage acceptance of infant*
Describe results of surgical correction of defect
    Use photographs of satisfactory results *to encourage feeling of hope*
Arrange meeting with other parents who have experienced a similar situation and coped successfully

EXPECTED OUTCOMES
Family discusses feelings and concerns regarding child's defect, its repair, and future prospects
Family exhibits an attitude of acceptance of infant
See also Nursing Care Plan: The Child Undergoing Surgery, Preoperative Care, Chapter 22

POSTOPERATIVE CARE

NURSING DIAGNOSIS ◾ **Risk for trauma of the surgical site related to surgical procedure, dysfunctional swallowing**

PATIENT GOAL 1: Will experience no trauma to operative site

NURSING INTERVENTIONS/RATIONALES
Position on back or side or in infant seat (cleft lip [CL]) *to prevent trauma to operative site*
Maintain lip-protective device (CL) *to protect the suture line*
Use nontraumatic feeding techniques *to minimize risk of trauma*
Restrain elbows *to prevent access to operative site*
    Use jacket restraints on older infant *to prevent rolling onto abdomen and rubbing face on sheet*
    Avoid placing objects in the mouth after cleft palate (CP) repair (suction catheter, tongue depressor, straw, pacifier, small spoon) *to prevent trauma to operative site*
    Prevent vigorous and sustained crying, *which can cause tension on sutures*
    Cleanse suture line gently after feeding and as necessary in manner ordered by surgeon (CL), *because inflammation or infection will interfere with healing and the cosmetic effect of surgical repair*
Teach cleansing and restraining procedures, especially when infant will be discharged before suture removal, *to minimize complications after discharge*

EXPECTED OUTCOME
Operative site remains undamaged

PATIENT GOAL 2: Will exhibit no evidence of aspiration

NURSING INTERVENTIONS/RATIONALES
Position *to allow for drainage of mucus* (partial side-lying position, semi-Fowler position) and to *prevent aspiration of formula*

EXPECTED OUTCOME
Child manages secretions and formula without aspiration

NURSING DIAGNOSIS ◾ **Altered nutrition: less than body requirements related to difficulty eating following surgical procedure**

PATIENT GOAL 1: Will consume adequate nourishment

NURSING INTERVENTIONS/RATIONALES
Monitor intravenous fluids (if prescribed)
Administer diet appropriate for age and as prescribed for postoperative period (specify)
Involve family in determining best feeding methods, *because family assumes feeding responsibility at home*
Modify feeding techniques *to adjust to defect and surgical repair*
    Feed in sitting position *to minimize risk of aspiration*
    Use special appliances *that compensate for feeding difficulties without causing trauma to operative site*
    Bubble frequently *because of tendency to swallow large amounts of air*
    Assist with breast-feeding if method of choice
Teach feeding and suctioning techniques to family *to ensure optimal home care*

EXPECTED OUTCOMES
Infant consumes an adequate amount of nutrients (specify amounts)
Family demonstrates ability to carry out postoperative care
Infant exhibits appropriate weight gain

NURSING DIAGNOSIS ◾ **Pain related to surgical procedure**

PATIENT GOAL 1: Will experience optimal comfort level

NURSING INTERVENTIONS/RATIONALES
Assess behavior and vital signs for evidence of pain
*Administer analgesics or sedatives as ordered
Remove restraints periodically while supervised *to exercise arms, provide relief from restrictions, and observe skin for signs of irritation*
Provide cuddling and tactile stimulation and other nonpharmacologic interventions *as needed for optimal comfort*
Involve parents in infant's care *to provide comfort and sense of security*

EXPECTED OUTCOME
Infant appears comfortable and rests quietly

NURSING DIAGNOSIS ◾ **Altered family processes related to child with a physical defect, hospitalization**

PATIENT (FAMILY) GOAL 1: Will receive adequate support

**NURSING INTERVENTIONS/RATIONALES
AND EXPECTED OUTCOMES**
Refer family to appropriate agencies and support groups
See Nursing Care Plan: The Family of the Ill or Hospitalized Child, Chapter 21

*Dependent nursing action.

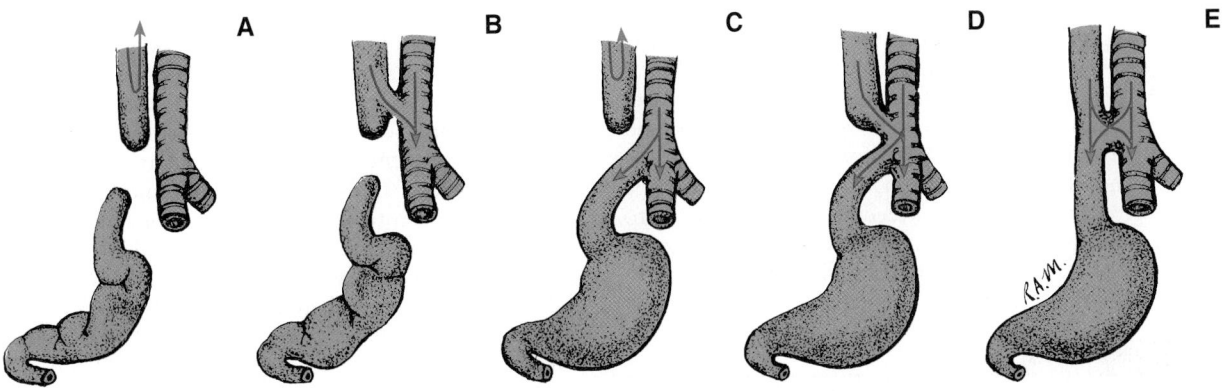

FIG. 24-5 ■ Five most common types of esophageal atresia and tracheoesophageal fistula.

Pathophysiology

The cause of EA/TEF is unknown. In the most frequently encountered form of esophageal atresia and TEF (80% to 95% of cases), the proximal esophageal segment terminates in a blind pouch, and the distal segment is connected to the trachea or primary bronchus by a short fistula at or near the bifurcation (Fig. 24-5, *C*). The second most common variety (5% to 8%) consists of a blind pouch at each end, widely separated and with no communication to the trachea (Fig. 24-5, *A*). Less frequently, an otherwise normal trachea and esophagus are connected by a common fistula (Fig. 24-5, *E*). Extremely rare anomalies involve a fistula from the trachea to the upper esophageal segment (Fig. 24-5, *B*) or to both the upper and the lower segments (Fig. 24-5, *D*).

Diagnostic Evaluation

The disorder is suspected on the basis of clinical manifestations (Box 24-11). EA should also be suspected in cases of maternal polyhydramnios. Although the diagnosis is established on the basis of clinical signs and symptoms, the exact type of anomaly is determined by radiographic studies. A radiopaque catheter is inserted into the hypopharynx and advanced until it encounters an obstruction. Chest films are taken to ascertain esophageal patency or the presence and level of a blind pouch. Sometimes fistulas are not patent, which makes their presence more difficult to diagnose. The presence of gas in the stomach or small bowel is indicative of a coexisting TEF.

Therapeutic Management

EA is a surgical emergency. The treatment includes maintenance of a patent airway, prevention of pneumonia, gastric or blind pouch decompression, and surgical repair of the anomaly. When EA/TEF is suspected, the infant is immediately taken off oral intake, started on IV fluids, and placed in the position least likely to cause aspiration of either mouth or stomach secretions. Removal of secretions from the mouth and upper pouch requires frequent or continuous suction. Because aspiration pneumonia is almost inevitable and appears early, broad-spectrum antibiotic therapy is often instituted.

Primary surgical correction consists of a thoracotomy with division and ligation of the TEF and an end-to-side anastomosis of the esophagus. This may consist of one operation or be staged with two or more procedures. For infants who are

---

BOX 24-11 ■ **Clinical Manifestations of Tracheoesophageal Fistula**

Excessive salivation and drooling
Three Cs of tracheoesophageal fistula (TEF)
 Coughing
 Choking
 Cyanosis
Apnea
Increased respiratory distress after feeding
Abdominal distention

---

premature, have multiple anomalies, or are in very poor condition, a staged procedure is preferred that involves palliative measures, including gastrostomy, ligation of the TEF, and provision of constant drainage of the esophageal pouch. A delayed esophageal anastomosis is usually attempted after several weeks to months when the upper pouch elongates. Further surgical techniques may be performed later to facilitate esophageal lengthening. If an esophageal anastomosis still cannot be accomplished, a *cervical esophagostomy* (to allow drainage of saliva) and gastrostomy are performed.

A primary anastomosis may be impossible because of insufficient length of the two segments of the esophagus. In these cases, an esophageal replacement procedure using a part of the colon or gastric tube interposition may be necessary to bridge the missing esophageal segment. Endotracheal intubation may be required, because many infants (10% to 20%) also have *tracheomalacia,* a weakness in the tracheal wall that occurs when a dilated proximal pouch compresses the trachea in early fetal life or when the trachea does not develop normally because of a loss of intratracheal pressure.

Complications of a primary repair include an anastomotic leak, strictures resulting from tension or ischemia, esophageal motility disorders causing dysphagia, and gastroesophageal reflux.

Prognosis. The prognosis is related to the birth weight, associated congenital anomalies, and time of diagnosis. The survival rate is nearly 100% in full-term infants without severe respiratory distress or other anomalies. In premature low-birth-weight infants with associated anomalies, the incidence of complications is high. The overall mortality is 50% (Ryckman, Flake, and Balistreri, 1997).

Nursing Considerations

Nursing responsibility for detection of this malformation begins *immediately* after birth. Ideally, the diagnosis should be made before the initial feeding, but often it is not. If fed, the infant swallows normally but suddenly coughs and struggles, and the fluid is aspirated or returns through the nose and mouth. For this reason, it is customary for the nurse to give the infant the first feeding of plain water or to be present when a parent feeds the child to observe the infant's response. Early breast-feeding should not be prevented unless there is a strong suspicion of EA.

> **NURSING ALERT**
>
> Any infant who has an excessive amount of frothy saliva in the mouth or difficulty with secretions and unexplained episodes of cyanosis should be suspected of having an EA/TEF and referred *immediately* for medical evaluation.

Cyanosis is usually the result of laryngospasm caused by overflow of saliva into the larynx from the proximal esophageal pouch. It normally clears after removal of the secretions from the oropharynx by suctioning. Any suspicion of TEF is reported immediately. The infant is placed in an incubator or a radiant warmer, and oxygen is administered to help relieve respiratory distress. Intubation and assisted mechanical ventilation may be necessary if the infant is in respiratory distress. When a newborn is suspected of having a TEF, the most desirable position is supine with the head elevated on an inclined plane of at least 30 degrees. This position minimizes the reflux of gastric secretions up the distal esophagus into the trachea and bronchi.

It is imperative that the source of aspiration be removed at once. Oral fluids are withheld, and the infant's fluid needs are met parenterally or via gastrostomy. Until surgery the blind pouch is kept empty by intermittent or continuous suction through an indwelling nasal catheter that extends to the end of the pouch. The catheter needs attention because it has a tendency to become clogged with mucus. It is usually replaced daily by the practitioner. In the event that a staged repair is performed, a gastrostomy tube is inserted and left open so that air entering the stomach through the fistula can escape, thus minimizing the danger that gastric contents will be regurgitated into the trachea. The tube empties by gravity drainage. Feedings through the gastrostomy tube and irrigations with fluid are contraindicated before surgery in the infant with a distal TEF. Nursing interventions include respiratory assessment, airway management, thermoregulation, fluid and electrolyte management, and potential nutritional support.

Postoperative Care.

Postoperative care is essentially the same as the care of any high-risk newborn (see Nursing Care of the High-Risk Newborn and Family, Chapter 9). The infant is returned to the radiant heater, and the gastrostomy tube is connected to gravity drainage until the infant can tolerate feedings. At this time, the tube is elevated and secured at a point above the level of the stomach. This allows gastric secretions to pass to the duodenum, and swallowed air can escape through the open tube. Tracheal suction should only be done using a premeasured catheter and with extreme caution to avoid injury to the suture line. If tolerated, gastrostomy feedings may be started and continued until the esophageal anastomosis is healed. Before oral feedings are initiated and the chest tube is removed, a contrast study or esophagram is performed to verify the integrity of the esophageal anastomosis.

The initial attempt at oral feeding must be carefully observed to make sure that the infant can swallow without choking. Oral feedings are begun with sterile water, followed by frequent small feedings of formula. Until the infant can take a sufficient amount by mouth, gastrostomy feedings or parenteral nutrition may supplement oral intake. Infants are usually not discharged until they are taking oral fluids well and the gastrostomy tube is removed. However, the infant who has palliative surgery will be discharged with the gastrostomy tube in place. The nurse is responsible for making certain that the caregiver is educated and has practiced the care of the gastrostomy (see Chapter 22).

Special Problems.

Upper respiratory complications are a threat to life in both the preoperative and the postoperative period. In addition to pneumonia, there is a constant danger of respiratory distress resulting from atelectasis, pneumothorax, and laryngeal edema. Any persistent respiratory difficulty after removal of secretions is reported to the surgeon immediately. The infant is monitored for anastomotic leaks, as evidenced by purulent chest tube drainage, increased WBC count, and temperature instability.

In the infant awaiting esophageal replacement surgery, the catheter is removed and the upper esophageal segment is drained through a cervical esophagostomy. An esophagostomy is difficult to care for because the skin becomes irritated by moisture from the continuous discharge of saliva. Frequent removal of drainage and application of a layer of protective ointment may remedy the problem. A dressing or ostomy appliance may be applied to collect the drainage, and an enterostomal therapist can provide additional guidance to prevent or treat skin breakdown.

For the infant who requires esophageal replacement, nonnutritive sucking is provided by a pacifier. Sometimes small amounts of water or formula are given orally, and although the liquid drains from the esophagostomy, this process allows the infant to develop mature sucking patterns. Other appropriate oral stimulation prevents feeding aversions. Infants who remain NPO for an extended period or who have not received oral stimulation have difficulty with eating by mouth after corrective surgery and may develop oral hypersensitivity and food aversion. They require patient, firm guidance to learn how to take food into the mouth and swallow after repair. A referral to a multidisciplinary feeding behavior program is often necessary.

As with any congenital anomaly, parents need support in adjusting to the child's condition (see Chapter 18). One difficulty is the immediate transfer of the sick newborn to the intensive care unit and the length of hospitalization. Encouraging parents to visit the infant, participate in care when appropriate, and express their feelings regarding the infant's condition facilitates the attachment process. The nurse in the intensive care unit should assume responsibility for ensuring that the parents are kept fully informed of the infant's progress.

Preparing parents for discharge involves teaching them skills that they will need at home. Parents are taught to observe for behaviors that indicate the need for suctioning, as well as signs of respiratory distress and constriction of the esophagus (e.g., poor feeding, dysphasia, drooling, regurgitation of undigested food). Discharge planning also includes obtaining the necessary equipment and home nursing services to provide home care.

HERNIAS

A *hernia* is a protrusion of a portion of an organ or organs through an abnormal opening. The danger from herniation arises when the organ protruding through the opening is constricted to the extent that circulation is impaired or when the protruding organs encroach on and impair the function of other structures. A hernia that cannot be reduced easily is called an *incarcerated hernia*. A *strangulated hernia* is one in which the blood supply to the herniated organ is impaired. The herniations of concern are those that protrude through the diaphragm, the abdominal wall, or the inguinal canal (see also Genitourinary Tract Disorders/Defects, Chapter 27). The other hernias of significance to the pediatric age-groups are outlined in Table 24-5.

TABLE 24-5 ■ Summary Outline of Hernias

TYPE	MANIFESTATIONS/ DIAGNOSTIC EVALUATION	MANAGEMENT
DIAPHRAGMATIC Protrusion of abdominal organs through opening in diaphragm	***Symptoms:*** Mild to severe respiratory distress within a few hours after birth; tachypnea, cyanosis, dyspnea, absent breath sounds in affected area; impaired cardiac output; possible symptoms of shock, severe acidosis ***Diagnosis*** suspected on basis of symptoms—confirmed by radiographic study; often diagnosed prenatally as early as twenty-fifth week of gestation	***Therapeutic:*** Supportive treatment of respiratory distress and correction of acidosis; possible use of endotracheal intubation, gastrointestinal (GI) decompression, and extracorporeal membrane oxygenation (ECMO) Prophylactic antibiotic administration Surgical reduction of hernia and repair of defect ***Nursing:*** *Preoperative:* Reduce stimulation—environmental/care activities Prompt recognition; resuscitation and stabilization Maintain suction, oxygen, and intravenous (IV) fluids Positioning—head up Administer medications *Postoperative:* Carry out routine postoperative care and observation Relieve pain and provide comfort Support family because this is a critical illness
HIATAL **Sliding:** Protrusion of an abdominal structure (usually stomach) through esophageal hiatus	***Symptoms:*** Dysphagia, failure to thrive, vomiting, neck contortions, frequent unexplained respiratory problems, bleeding; usually associated with gastroesophageal reflux (GER); may cause gastric volvulus and obstruction ***Diagnosis*** made by fluoroscopy	***Therapeutic:*** Management of GER symptoms; positioning; pharmacologic treatment; and dietary management Surgical treatment when complications are related to GER despite medical management ***Nursing:*** Be alert to significant signs and carry out routine postoperative care
ABDOMINAL **Umbilical:** Weakness in abdominal wall around umbilicus; incomplete closure of abdominal wall, allowing intestinal contents to protrude through opening	***Symptoms:*** Noted by inspection and palpation of the abdomen High incidence in premature and African-American infants Usually closes spontaneously by 1-2 years of age	***Therapeutic:*** No treatment of small defects Operative repair if persists to age 4-6 years or if defect is >1.5-2.0 cm by age 2 Strangulation requires immediate attention ***Nursing:*** Discourage use of home remedies (e.g., belly bands, coins) Reassure parents
Omphalocele: Protrusion of intraabdominal viscera into base of umbilical cord; sac is covered with peritoneum without skin **Gastroschisis:** Protrusion of intraabdominal contents through defect in abdominal wall lateral to umbilical ring; there is never a peritoneal sac	***Symptoms:*** Obvious on inspection Observe for other malformations	***Therapeutic:*** Surgical repair of defect Preoperative: Large lesions—gradual reduction of abdominal contents Prophylactic antibiotic administration ***Nursing*** (preoperative): Keep sac or viscera moist with saline-soaked pads Use overhead warming unit Carry out routine care of IV line Nasogastric suction NPO

OBSTRUCTIVE DISORDERS

Obstruction in the GI tract occurs when the passage of nutrients and secretions is impeded by a constricted or occluded lumen or when there is impaired motility *(paralytic ileus)*. Obstructions may be congenital or acquired. Many congenital obstructions such as atresia, imperforate anus, meconium plug, and meconium ileus usually appear in the neonatal period. Other obstructions of congenital etiology such as malrotation, Hirschsprung disease, volvulus, incarcerated hernia, and Meckel diverticulum appear after the first few weeks of life. Intestinal obstruction from acquired causes such as intussusception, pyloric stenosis, and tumors may occur in infancy or childhood. Intestinal obstructions from any cause are characterized by similar signs and symptoms (Box 24-12).

HYPERTROPHIC PYLORIC STENOSIS

Hypertrophic pyloric stenosis (HPS) occurs when the circumferential muscle of the pyloric sphincter becomes thickened, resulting in elongation and narrowing of the pyloric channel. This produces an outlet obstruction and compensatory dilation, hypertrophy, and hyperperistalsis of the stomach. This condition usually develops in the first few weeks of life, causing projectile vomiting, dehydration, metabolic alkalosis, and failure to thrive. The precise etiology is unknown. There is a genetic predisposition, and siblings and offspring of affected persons are at increased risk of developing HPS. Firstborn children and males are affected five times more frequently than females. HPS is more common in full-term than in premature infants, and it is seen less frequently in African-American and Asian infants than in Caucasian infants.

Pathophysiology

The circular muscle of the pylorus thickens as a result of hypertrophy (increased size) and hyperplasia (increased mass). This produces severe narrowing of the pyloric canal be-

---

BOX 24-12 ■ Clinical Manifestations of Mechanical/Paralytic Intestinal Obstruction

Colicky abdominal pain—From peristalsis attempting to overcome the obstruction

Abdominal distention—As a result of accumulation of gas and fluid above the level of the obstruction

Vomiting—Often the earliest sign of a high obstruction; a later sign of lower obstruction (may be bilious or feculent)

Constipation and obstipation—Early signs of low obstructions; later signs of higher obstructions

Dehydration—From losses of large quantities of fluid and electrolytes into the intestine

Rigid and boardlike abdomen—From increased distention

Bowel sounds—Gradually diminish and cease

Respiratory distress—Occurs as the diaphragm is pushed up into the pleural cavity

Shock—Plasma volume diminishes as fluids and electrolytes are lost from the bloodstream into the intestinal lumen

Sepsis—Caused by bacterial proliferation with invasion into the circulation

---

tween the stomach and the duodenum, causing partial obstruction of the lumen (Fig. 24-6, *A*). Over time, inflammation and edema further reduce the size of the opening, resulting in complete obstruction. The hypertrophied pylorus may be palpable as an olive-like mass in the upper abdomen. Pyloric stenosis is not a congenital disorder. Evidence suggests that local innervation is involved in the pathogenesis. In most cases this is an isolated lesion; however, it may be associated with intestinal malrotation, esophageal and duodenal atresia, and anorectal anomalies.

Diagnostic Evaluation

The diagnosis of HPS is often made after the history and physical examination. The olive-like mass is easily palpated when the stomach is empty, the infant is quiet, and the abdominal muscles are relaxed. Vomiting usually occurs 30 to 60 minutes after feeding and becomes projectile as the obstruction progresses. Emesis is nonbilious, usually consisting of stale milk. Often these infants become dehydrated and lethargic and appear significantly malnourished.

If the diagnosis is inconclusive from the history and physical signs (Box 24-13), ultrasonography will demonstrate an elongated, sausage-shaped mass with an elongated pyloric channel. If ultrasound fails to demonstrate a hyper-

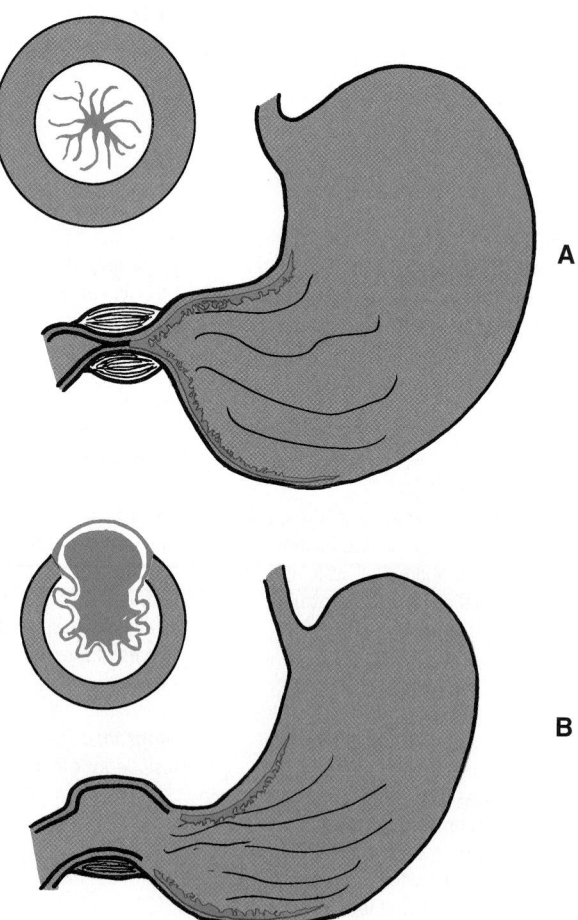

FIG. 24-6 ■ Hypertrophic pyloric stenosis. **A,** Enlarged muscular area nearly obliterates pyloric channel. **B,** Longitudinal surgical division of muscle down to submucosa establishes adequate passageway.

trophied pylorus, then upper GI radiography should be done to rule out other causes of vomiting. Laboratory findings reflect the metabolic alterations created by severe depletion of both fluid and electrolytes from extensive and prolonged vomiting. There are decreased serum levels of both sodium and potassium, although these may be masked by the hemoconcentration from ECF depletion. Of greater diagnostic value is a decrease in serum chloride levels and increases in pH and bicarbonate (carbon dioxide content) characteristic of metabolic alkalosis. The BUN level will be elevated as evidence of dehydration.

Therapeutic Management

Surgical relief of the pyloric obstruction by *pyloromyotomy* (sometimes called *Fredet-Ramstedt procedure*) is the standard treatment for this disorder. The procedure is performed through a right upper quadrant incision (laparotomy) and consists of a longitudinal incision through the circular muscle fibers of the pylorus down to, but not including, the submucosa (Fig. 24-6, *B*). The procedure has a high success rate when infants receive careful preoperative preparation to correct fluid and electrolyte imbalances.

Feedings are usually begun 4 to 6 hours postoperatively, beginning with small, frequent feedings of glucose water or electrolyte solutions. If clear fluids are retained, about 24 hours after surgery, formula is started in stepwise increments, with the amount and interval between feedings gradually increased until a full feeding schedule is reinstated (usually over a 48-hour period). The infant is discharged from the hospital by about the second or third postoperative day.

Another procedure, *laparoscopy,* may be performed for infants with HPS. The use of a small incision for the laparoscope results in shorter surgical time, more rapid postoperative feeding, and quicker discharge.

Prognosis.   Most infants recover completely and rapidly after pyloromyotomy. Postoperative complications include persistent pyloric obstruction and wound dehiscence. Some infants also have GER.

BOX 24-13 ■ Clinical Manifestations of Hypertrophic Pyloric Stenosis

Projectile vomiting
 May be ejected 3 to 4 feet from the child when in a side-lying position, 1 foot or more when in a back-lying position
 Occurs shortly after a feeding (may not occur for several hours)
 May follow each feeding or appear intermittently
 Nonbilious vomitus; may be blood-tinged
Infant hungry, avid nurser; eagerly accepts a second feeding after vomiting episode
No evidence of pain or discomfort except that of chronic hunger
Weight loss
Signs of dehydration
Distended upper abdomen
Readily palpable olive-shaped tumor in the epigastrium just to the right of the umbilicus
Visible gastric peristaltic waves that move from left to right across the epigastrium

Nursing Considerations

The diagnosis of HPS is considered in the very young infant who appears alert but fails to gain weight and has a history of vomiting after meals. Assessment is based on observation of eating behaviors and evidence of other characteristic clinical manifestations.

Preoperative Care.   Preoperatively the emphasis is placed on restoring hydration and electrolyte balance. Infants are usually given no oral feedings and receive IV fluids with glucose and electrolyte replacement based on laboratory serum electrolyte values. Careful monitoring of the IV infusion and diligent attention to intake, output, and urine specific gravity measurements are important. Vomiting and the number and character of stools are observed and recorded accurately.

Observations also include assessment of vital signs, particularly those that might indicate fluid or electrolyte imbalances. These infants are prone to metabolic alkalosis from loss of hydrogen ions and to potassium, sodium, and chloride depletion. The skin and mucous membranes, as well as daily weight, are assessed for alterations in hydration status and water gain or loss.

If stomach decompression and gastric lavage are used preoperatively, the nurse is responsible for ensuring that the tube is patent and functioning properly and for measuring and recording the type and amount of drainage. The infant is usually positioned flat or with the head slightly elevated. Infants who are receiving IV fluids and/or have a nasogastric tube for continuous drainage must be observed to prevent the needle or tube from becoming dislodged.

General hygienic care, with attention to the skin and mouth in dehydrated infants, is essential. Protection from infection is also important, because infants with impaired nutritional status are more susceptible than normal newborns. Parental involvement is encouraged and promoted.

Postoperative Care.   Postoperative vomiting may occur, and most infants, even with successful surgery, exhibit some vomiting during the first 24 to 48 hours. IV fluids are administered until the infant can retain adequate amounts by mouth. Observation of physical signs, monitoring of IV fluids, careful observation, and recording of intake and output are maintained. The infant is also observed for evidence of pain, and appropriate analgesics are given. The nasogastric tube may be maintained after surgery for a variable time.

Feedings are usually instituted soon after surgery, beginning with clear liquids containing glucose and electrolytes. They are offered slowly, in small amounts, and at frequent intervals as ordered by the practitioner. If the infant has been breast-fed, breast milk, expressed by the mother, is given by bottle when the infant is able to tolerate feedings. Breast-feeding is resumed as soon as feasible. Observation and recording of feedings and the infant's responses to feedings are a vital part of postoperative care. Positioning with the head elevated is usually continued postoperatively. Care of the operative site consists of observation for any drainage or signs of inflammation and care of the incision as directed by the surgeon.

Parents are encouraged to remain with their child and become involved in the child's care. Vomiting of a projec-

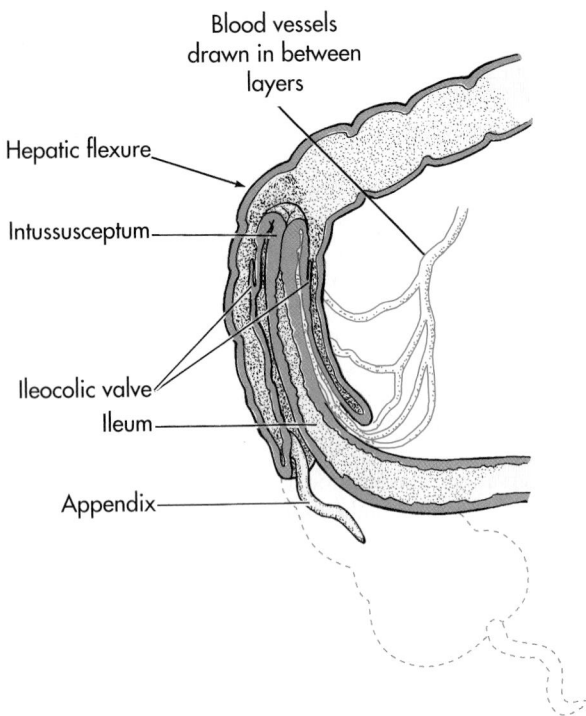

Blood vessels drawn in between layers

Hepatic flexure

Intussusceptum

Ileocolic valve

Ileum

Appendix

FIG. 24-7 ■ Ileocolic intussusception.

tile nature is frightening to parents, and they often believe that they may have done something wrong or that surgery was not successful. Most parents need support and reassurance that the condition is caused by a structural problem and is in no way a reflection on their parenting skills and capacities.

INTUSSUSCEPTION

Intussusception is one of the most frequent causes of intestinal obstruction in children between the ages of 3 months and 3 years. The peak occurrence is between the ages of 5 and 9 months (Brandt, 1999). Intussusception is more common in males than in females and in children with cystic fibrosis. Although specific intestinal lesions can be found in a small percentage of these children, the cause is usually not known. More than 90% of intussusceptions do not have a pathologic lead point, such as a polyp, lymphoma, or Meckel diverticulum. The idiopathic cases are most likely a result of hypertrophy of intestinal lymphoid tissue secondary to viral infection.

Pathophysiology

Intussusception occurs when a proximal segment of the bowel telescopes into a more distal segment, pulling the mesentery with it. The mesentery is compressed and angled, resulting in lymphatic and venous obstruction. As edema from the obstruction increases, pressure within the area of intussusception increases. When the pressure equals the arterial pressure, arterial blood flow stops, resulting in ischemia and the pouring of mucus into the intestine. Venous engorgement also leads to leaking of blood and mucus into the intestinal lumen, forming the classic currant jelly stools (Brandt, 1999). The most common site is the

BOX 24-14 ■ Clinical Manifestations of Intussusception

Sudden acute abdominal pain
Child screams and draws the knees onto the chest
Child appears normal and comfortable during intervals between episodes of pain
Vomiting
Lethargy
Passage of red, currant jelly–like stools (stool mixed with blood and mucus)
Tender, distended abdomen
Palpable sausage-shaped mass in upper right quadrant
Empty lower right quadrant (Dance sign)
Eventual fever, prostration, and other signs of peritonitis

ileocecal valve (ileocolic), where the ileum invaginates into the cecum and colon (Fig. 24-7). Other forms include ileoileal (one part of the ileum invaginates into another section of the ileum), and colocolic (one part of the colon invaginates into another area of the colon) usually in the area of the hepatic or splenic flexure or at some point along the transverse colon.

NURSING ALERT

The classic signs (e.g., severe colicky abdominal pain in a child with vomiting, currant jelly stools) may not be present. A more chronic picture, characterized by diarrhea, anorexia, weight loss, occasional vomiting, and periodic pain, may be present. Because intussusception is potentially life-threatening, the nurse should be aware of alternate presentations and observe these children closely and refer them for further evaluation.

Diagnostic Evaluation

Frequently the diagnosis can be made on subjective findings alone (Box 24-14). However, definitive diagnosis is based on a barium enema, which clearly demonstrates the obstruction to the flow of barium. Initially, however, an abdominal radiograph is obtained to detect intraperitoneal air from a bowel perforation, which would contraindicate a barium enema. A rectal examination reveals mucus, blood, and, occasionally, a low intussusception itself.

Therapeutic Management

In most cases the initial treatment of choice is nonsurgical hydrostatic reduction traditionally by barium enema. In this procedure, correction of the invagination is carried out at the same time as the diagnostic testing. The force exerted by the flowing barium is usually sufficient to push the invaginated portion of the bowel into its original position, similar to pushing an inverted "finger" out of a glove. This procedure is not recommended if there are clinical signs of shock or perforation.

The use of barium as the contrast agent is becoming less routine, and a high percentage of radiologists use water-soluble contrast and air pressure to reduce intussusceptions. The increased use of water-soluble contrast reflects concern regarding the risk of barium peritonitis. The administration of air pressure to reduce intussusception is as successful as, and more rapid than, barium without the risk of peritonitis, and with decreased exposure to radiation. Some use carbon dioxide instead of air. It has the advantage of being absorbed by the gut and is associated with less discomfort. It also eliminates the risk of an air embolism. IV fluids, nasogastric decompression, and antibiotic therapy may be used before hydrostatic reduction is attempted. If these procedures are not successful, the child may require surgical intervention. Surgery involves manually reducing the invagination and, when indicated, resecting any nonviable intestine.

Prognosis. Nonoperative reduction is successful in approximately 75% of cases. Surgery is required for patients in whom the contrast enema is unsuccessful. With early diagnosis and treatment, serious complications and death are uncommon.

Nursing Considerations

The nurse can help establish a diagnosis by listening to the parent's description of the child's physical and behavioral symptoms. It is not unusual for parents to express that they felt something was seriously wrong before others shared their concerns. The description of the child's severe colicky abdominal pain combined with vomiting is a significant sign of intussusception.

As soon as a possible diagnosis of intussusception is made, the nurse prepares the parents for the immediate need for hospitalization, the nonsurgical technique of hydrostatic reduction, and the possibility of surgery. It is important to explain the basic defect of intussusception. A model of the defect is easily demonstrated by pushing the end of a finger on a rubber glove back into itself or using the example of a telescoping rod. The principle of reduction by hydrostatic pressure can be simulated by filling the glove with water, which pushes the "finger" into a fully extended position.

Physical care of the child does not differ from that for any child undergoing abdominal surgery. Even though nonsurgical intervention may be successful, the usual preoperative procedures, such as withholding of fluids by mouth, routine laboratory testing (CBC and urinalysis), signed parental consent, and preanesthetic sedation, are performed. For the child with signs of electrolyte imbalance, hemorrhage, or peritonitis, additional preparation, such as replacement fluids, whole blood or plasma, and nasogastric suctioning may be needed. Before surgery the nurse monitors all stools.

> ### NURSING ALERT
> **Passage of a normal brown stool usually indicates that the intussusception has reduced itself. This is immediately reported to the practitioner, who may choose to alter the diagnostic/therapeutic plan of care.**

Postprocedural care includes observations of vital signs, blood pressure, intact sutures and dressing, and the return of bowel sounds. After hydrostatic reduction or autoreduction, the nurse observes for passage of barium or water-soluble contrast material and the stool patterns, because there may be recurrences of the intussusception. Children may be admitted to the hospital or monitored on an outpatient basis. A recurrence of intussusception is treated with hydrostatic reduction, but a laparotomy is considered for multiple recurrences.

Because hospitalization may be the child's first separation from the parents, it is important to preserve the parent-child relationship by encouraging rooming-in or extended visiting. It may be the parents' first experience with hospitalization, necessitating their preparation for procedures such as IV therapy, frequent vital sign and blood pressure monitoring, dressings, and special orders, such as NPO. Because of the rapidity of the onset, diagnosis, and treatment, parents may feel stunned or numb. They may ask few questions, or they may constantly make inquiries, sometimes the same ones several times. If the nurse realizes the circumstances surrounding this condition, the parents' reactions are more likely to be understood and accepted.

MALROTATION AND VOLVULUS

Malrotation of the intestine is due to the abnormal rotation of the intestine around the superior mesenteric artery during embryologic development. Malrotation may present in utero or may be asymptomatic throughout life. Infants with malrotation have intermittent vomiting, recurrent abdominal pain, distention, or lower GI bleeding. Malrotation is the most serious type of intestinal obstruction, because if the intestine undergoes complete volvulus (the intestine twisting around itself), compromise of the blood supply will result in intestinal necrosis, peritonitis, perforation, and death.

Diagnostic Evaluation

It is imperative that malrotation and volvulus be diagnosed promptly and surgical treatment instituted quickly. Any infant with bilious vomiting should be evaluated carefully for malrotation, volvulus, and obstruction. An upper GI series is the definitive procedure to diagnose this condition.

Therapeutic Management

Surgery is indicated to remove the affected area. Because of the extensive nature of some lesions, short-gut syndrome is a postoperative complication.

Nursing Considerations

Preoperatively the nursing care is the same as that provided to an infant or child with intestinal obstruction. Postoperatively the nursing care is similar to that provided to the infant or child who has undergone abdominal surgery.

ANORECTAL MALFORMATIONS

Anorectal malformations include a number of anomalies of the genitourinary and pelvic organs. These malformations are among the more common congenital malformations caused by abnormal development, with an incidence of 1 in 2000 to 5000 live births (Hendren, 1998). The anus and rectum originate from an embryologic structure called the *cloaca*. Lateral growth of the cloaca forms the urorectal septum that separates the rectum dorsally from the urinary tract ventrally. The rectum and urinary tract separate completely by the seventh week of gestation. Anomalies that occur reflect the stage of development of these processes.

Imperforate anus includes several forms of malformation without an obvious anal opening. Many have a fistula from the distal rectum to the perineum or genitourinary system. Anorectal malformations may occur in isolation or as part of the VACTERL or VATER syndromes.

A persistent cloaca is a complex anorectal malformation in which the rectum, vagina, and urethra drain into a common channel that opens onto the perineum via the usual urethral site. *Cloacal exstrophy* is a rare, severe defect in which there is externalization of the bladder and bowel through the abdominal wall. Often the genitalia are indefinite, and chromosome studies are necessary to determine the child's sex. Gender assignment is almost always female. The exstrophic bladder is separated into two halves by the cecum; other features may include an omphalocele, imperforate anus, and, at times, a neural tube defect. With improved surgical techniques, survival rates for this condition are 88% to 90% in some centers (Smith and others, 1997).

Anorectal anomalies are classified according to sex and abnormal anatomic features, including genitourinary and associated pelvic anomalies. The level of rectal descent is determined by the relationship of the termination of the bowel to the puborectalis sling of the levator ani musculature. Anorectal malformations are also classified according to the level of the malformation (high, intermediate, and low) (Table 24-6). About 50% of children with anorectal anomalies have a urologic problem.

Diagnostic Evaluation

Checking for patency of the anus and rectum is a routine part of the newborn assessment and should include observations regarding the passage of meconium. Inspection of the perineal area reveals absence of the normal anal opening; however, the appearance of the perineum alone does not accurately predict the level of the lesion. Genitourinary and pelvic anomalies associated with anorectal malformations should be considered.

In the newborn the presence of meconium on the perineum does not always indicate anal patency (particularly in girls), because a fistula may be present and allow evacuation of meconium through the vagina. Fistulas may not be apparent at birth but may become obvious as peristalsis gradually forces the meconium through the fistula. Rectourinary

fistulas should be suspected if there is meconium in the urine. Anal stenosis may not be identified until the child is older and presents with a history of difficult defecation, abdominal distention, and ribbonlike stools.

Abdominal ultrasound is performed to determine the existence of other malformations. An intravenous pyelogram (IVP) and voiding cystourethrogram are recommended for the infant with a high malformation to identify anomalies of the urinary tract. Further examination is also indicated when there is evidence of urinary tract infection or other symptoms. If a syndrome is suspected, cardiac evaluation and spinal films should be obtained.

Therapeutic Management

Successful treatment for anal stenosis is generally accomplished by manual dilations. The procedure is initiated by a physician and repeated on a regular basis by the nurses in the hospital. Parents are taught to continue the dilations at home. Perineal fistulas are treated by anoplasty during the newborn period. The opening is moved to the center of the external sphincter, and dilations are begun. More extensive defects are usually managed with a colostomy and corrective surgical repair performed later in the first year (Pena, 2000).

The type of defect, the sacral anatomy, and the quality of muscles influence the long-term prognosis. In general, if the newborn presents with a deep midline groove, two well-formed buttocks, and an anal dimple, the prognosis for bowel control is better than if the infant has a flat or "rocker" bottom and no midline groove because of associated neurologic problems (Flake and Ryckman, 1997). A functioning interior anal sphincter is important to achieve continence. In its absence, the child may need a bowel program to achieve socially acceptable bowel continence. Other potential complications after surgical treatment include strictures, recurrent rectourinary fistula, mucosal prolapse, and constipation.

Nursing Considerations

The first nursing responsibility is identification of undetected anorectal malformations. A poorly developed anal dimple, a genitourinary fistula, or vertebral abnormalities suggest a high lesion. A newborn who does not pass a stool

TABLE 24-6 ■ Classification of Anorectal Malformations

LEVEL	MALE	FEMALE
High	Anorectal agenesis	Anorectal agenesis
	With rectoprostatic-urethral fistula	With rectovaginal fistula
	Without fistula	Without fistula
	Rectal atresia	Rectal atresia
Intermediate	Recto-bulbar-urethral fistula	Rectovestibular fistula
		Rectovaginal fistula
Low	Agenesis without fistula	Agenesis without fistula
	Anocutaneous fistula	Anovestibular fistula
	Anal stenosis	Anocutaneous fistula
	Rare malformations	Anal stenosis
		Cloaca
		Rare malformations

From Stephens FD and others: *Pediatr Surg Int* 1:200, 1986.

within 24 hours of birth requires further assessment. In addition, meconium that appears at an inappropriate orifice is reported. Preoperative care includes diagnostic evaluation, GI decompression, and IV fluids.

Nursing care after an anorectoplasty is directed toward healing the surgical site without infection or complications. Care involves keeping the anal area as clean as possible with scrupulous perineal care. A temporary dressing and drain may be placed initially to manage the continuous passage of stool. Protective ointments such as zinc oxide and occlusive dressings such as hydrocolloids decrease skin irritation from frequent loose stools. The preferred position is a side-lying prone position with the hips elevated or a supine position with the legs suspended at a 90-degree angle to the trunk to prevent pressure on perineal sutures.

There may be a nasogastric tube for abdominal decompression and IV feedings. The infant is given formula when normal peristalsis is noted. Care of the infant with a colostomy involves frequent dressing changes, meticulous skin care, and correct application of a collection device (see Chapter 22).

Family Support, Discharge Planning, and Home Care.
Long-term follow-up is important for children with high malformations. After the definitive pull-through procedure, toilet training is delayed, and complete continence is seldom achieved at the usual age of 2 to 3 years of age. Prevention of constipation is important, and breast-feeding is encouraged postoperatively. If a cow's milk–based formula is used, a laxative may be prescribed. Bowel habit training, diet modification, and administration of stool softeners or fiber are important aspects of bowel management. Optimum bowel function may not be achieved until late childhood or adolescence. Support and reassurance are important during the slow progression to normal function.

Parents are instructed in perineal and wound care or care of the colostomy. Anal dilations may be necessary for some infants. Parents are advised to observe stooling patterns and notify the physician if there are any signs of anal stricture or complications.

MALABSORPTION SYNDROMES

Chronic diarrhea and malabsorption of nutrients characterize malabsorption syndromes. An important complication of malabsorption syndromes in children is failure to thrive. Most cases are classified according to the location of the supposed anatomic or biochemical defect. The term *celiac disease* is often used to describe a symptom complex with four characteristics: (1) steatorrhea (fatty, foul, frothy, bulky stools), (2) general malnutrition, (3) abdominal distention, and (4) secondary vitamin deficiencies.

Digestive defects are conditions in which the enzymes necessary for digestion are diminished or absent, such as (1) cystic fibrosis, in which pancreatic enzymes are absent; (2) biliary or liver disease, in which bile flow is affected; or (3) lactase deficiency, in which there is congenital or secondary lactose intolerance.

Absorptive defects are conditions in which the intestinal mucosal transport system is impaired. This may occur because of a primary defect (e.g., celiac disease) or secondary to inflammatory disease of the bowel that results in impaired absorption because bowel motility is accelerated (e.g., ulcerative colitis). Obstructive disorders (e.g., Hirschsprung disease) also cause secondary malabsorption from enterocolitis.

Anatomic defects, such as extensive resection of the bowel or "short-bowel syndrome," affect digestion by decreasing the transit time of substances and affect absorption by severely compromising the absorptive surface.

CELIAC DISEASE

Celiac disease (CD), also known as *gluten-induced enteropathy, gluten-sensitive enteropathy (GSE),* and *celiac sprue,* is a disease of the proximal small intestine characterized by abnormal mucosa and permanent intolerance to gluten. CD is second only to cystic fibrosis as a cause of malabsorption in children. The age that this condition first appears and its prevalence have changed over the past 30 to 40 years. Celiac sprue used to be considered a disease of childhood, but adult presentation is becoming more common. It is seen more frequently in Europe than in America and is rarely reported in Asians or blacks. Although previous figures suggested that CD affected 1 in 6000 individuals, recent studies suggest the prevalence is more likely to be 1 in 250 individuals (American Gastroenterological Association Medical Position Statement, 2001). The exact cause of CD is unknown, but there appears to be an inherited predisposition with an influence by environmental factors.

Pathophysiology

The disease is characterized by intolerance to the protein *gluten,* found in wheat, barley, rye, and oats. Although the pathologic process is still obscure, susceptible individuals are unable to digest the gliadin component of gluten, resulting in an accumulation of a toxic substance that is damaging to the mucosal cells.

Diagnostic Evaluation

Symptoms of CD are usually noted several months after the introduction of gluten-containing grains into the diet, typically between the ages of 1 and 5 years (Box 24-15). The clinical manifestations are usually insidious and chronic. The first evidence may be failure to thrive and diarrhea.

The diagnosis of celiac disease is based on a biopsy of the small intestine demonstrating the characteristic changes of mucosal inflammation, crypt hyperplasia, and villous atrophy (Dieterich, Esslinger, and Schuppan, 2003). Within a day or two of instituting the diet, most children with CD demonstrate a favorable response, including weight gain and improved appetite. Within a few weeks there is resolution of the diarrhea and steatorrhea.

Serologic testing to detect antibodies to connective tissue (endomysium and reticulin) and to gliadin are available. The presence of antigliadin, antireticulin, and antiendomysial IgG and IgA antibodies (and the disappearance of these antibodies when gluten is removed from the diet) aids in diagnosis (Walker-Smith, 1996). The autoantibodies of IgA antireticulin and antiendomysial IgA are more specific markers for active celiac disease than circulating IgA antigliadin antibodies, which may be present in other diseases and conditions. A more specific test is the enzyme tissue transglutaminase (tTG), which has been found to be the autoantigen recog-

BOX 24-15 ■ Clinical Manifestations of Celiac Disease

IMPAIRED FAT ABSORPTION
Steatorrhea (excessively large, pale, oily, frothy stools)
Exceedingly foul-smelling stools

IMPAIRED ABSORPTION OF NUTRIENTS
Malnutrition
Muscle wasting (especially prominent in legs and buttocks)
Anemia
Anorexia
Abdominal distention

BEHAVIORAL CHANGES
Irritability
Fretfulness
Uncooperativeness
Apathy

CELIAC CRISIS*
Acute, severe episodes of profuse watery diarrhea and vomiting
May be precipitated by:
    Infections (especially gastrointestinal)
    Prolonged fluid and electrolyte depletion
    Emotional disturbance

*In very young children.

nized by antiendomysial antibody (Walker-Smith and others, 2000). Although these markers are useful in the diagnosis and screening of CD, they vary in sensitivity and specificity and are usually followed by a biopsy to confirm the diagnosis (Murray, 1999).

Therapeutic Management

Treatment of chronic CD is primarily dietary. Although the diet is called "gluten free," it is actually *low* in gluten, because it is impossible to remove every source of this protein. Studies indicate that most patients can tolerate restricted amounts of gluten. Because gluten is found primarily in the grains of wheat and rye, but also in smaller quantities in barley and oats, these four foods are eliminated. Corn and rice become substitute grain foods.

Children with untreated celiac disease may have associated lactose intolerance related to intestinal mucosal lesions, which usually improve with gluten withdrawal and intestinal healing. Specific nutritional deficiencies are treated with appropriate supplements, including vitamins, iron, and calories.

Prognosis.   CD is regarded as a chronic disease. Its extent varies among children. The most severe symptoms usually occur in early childhood and again in adult life. Strict dietary avoidance of gluten prevents symptoms and may minimize the risk of developing lymphoma, the most serious complication of the disease.

Nursing Considerations

The main nursing consideration is helping the child adhere to dietary management. Considerable time is involved in explaining to the child and the parents the disease process, the specific role of gluten in aggravating the condition, and

those foods that must be restricted. It is especially difficult to maintain a diet indefinitely when the child has no symptoms and temporary transgressions result in no difficulties. However, evidence indicates that most individuals who relax their diet experience a relapse of their disease and possibly exhibit growth retardation, anemia, or osteomalacia. There is also the risk of developing malignant lymphoma of the small intestine or other GI malignancies.

Although the chief source of gluten is cereal and baked goods, grains are frequently added to processed foods as thickeners or fillers. Gluten is also added to many foods as "hydrolyzed vegetable protein." The nurse must advise parents to read carefully all ingredients on labels to avoid hidden sources of gluten. Many gluten-containing products are easily eliminated from the infant's or young child's diet, but monitoring the diet of a school-age child or adolescent is more difficult. Many "favorite" foods, such as hot dogs, pizza, and spaghetti, are chief offenders. Luncheon preparation away from home is particularly difficult, because bread, luncheon meats, and instant soups are not tolerated.

In addition to restricting gluten, other dietary alterations may be necessary initially. For example, in some children who have more severe mucosal damage, disaccharide digestion is impaired, especially lactose. Therefore, these children often need a temporary lactose-free diet, which necessitates eliminating all milk products.

Generally, management includes a diet high in calories and proteins, with simple carbohydrates, such as fruits and vegetables, but low in fats. Initially the bowel may be inflamed as a result of the pathologic process, so high-fiber foods, such as nuts, raisins, raw vegetables, and raw fruits with skin, are avoided until inflammation has subsided.

Several organizations and resources are available to help families cope with this condition. The **Celiac Sprue Association/United States of America*** is an organization that provides support, guidance, and educational materials to families concerning a gluten-free diet, food sources, recipes, and travel information. There are also several published cookbooks that contain gluten-free recipes.†

SHORT BOWEL SYNDROME

Short bowel syndrome (SBS) is a malabsorptive disorder that occurs when there is decreased mucosal surface area, usually as a result of extensive resection of the small intestine. The most common causes of SBS in children include congenital anomalies (jejunal and ileal atresia, gastroschisis), ischemia (necrotizing enterocolitis), and trauma or vascular injury (volvulus [twisting of bowel on itself]). Other causes include volvulus that results in massive resection, long-segment Hirschsprung disease, and omphalocele. The prognosis for infants and children with SBS has dramatically improved in the

---

*PO Box 31700, Omaha, NE 68131-0700; (402) 558-0600; website: www.csaceliacs.org. In Canada: **Canadian Celiac Association, Inc.,** 190 Britannia Road East, Unit 11, Mississauga, Ontario, L4Z 1W6; (905) 507-6208; website: www.celiac.ca.
†A booklet, *Pointers for parents: coping with celiac sprue,* provides information on shopping, cooking, and living with an affected child and is available from the Clinical Dietetics Department, Children's Memorial Hospital, 2300 Children's Plaza, Chicago, IL 60614; (773) 880-4793.

past 25 years as a result of advances in parenteral nutrition and enteral feeding. Both the amount and the location of bowel lost are important in determining the severity of the condition. The preservation of the terminal ileum and ileocecal valve influences fluid and nutrient absorption and may avoid problems of bacterial overgrowth by preventing the entrance of bacteria from the colon into the small intestine.

The small intestine has significant capacity for adaptation after resection. During the *adaptation process,* the villus height increases (villus hyperplasia), and the cell number and absorptive surface area are also increased. As villus length and the number of enterocytes available for absorption per centimeter of bowel increase, nutrient absorption increases. Intraluminal enteral feedings stimulate the adaptation process and maintain the structural and functional integrity of the small intestine.

Therapeutic Management

The goals of treatment are (1) to preserve as much length of bowel as possible during surgery; (2) to maintain the child's nutritional status, growth, and development while intestinal adaptation occurs; (3) to stimulate intestinal adaptation with enteral feeding; and (4) to minimize complications related to the disease process and therapy.

Nutritional support is the long-term focus of care. The *initial phase* of therapy includes TPN as the primary source of nutrition. Complications associated with SBS and long-term TPN include central venous catheter infection or occlusion, catheter migration, thrombosis or emboli, bacterial overgrowth, metabolic complications, cholestasis, and liver dysfunction (see Chapter 22).

The *second phase* is the introduction of enteral feeding, which usually begins as soon as possible after surgery. Elemental formulas containing glucose, sucrose and glucose polymers, hydrolyzed proteins, and medium-chain triglycerides facilitate absorption. Usually these formulas are given by continuous infusion through a nasogastric or gastrostomy tube. As the enteral feedings are advanced, the TPN solution is decreased in terms of calories, amount of fluid, and total hours of infusion per day.

The *final phase* of nutritional support occurs when growth and development are sustained exclusively by enteral feedings. When TPN is discontinued, there is a risk of nutritional deficiency secondary to malabsorption of fat-soluble vitamins (A, D, E, K) and trace minerals (iron, selenium, zinc). Serum vitamin and mineral levels should be obtained, and enteral supplementation of vitamins and minerals may be required. Pharmacologic agents have been used to reduce secretory losses. H_2 blockers, proton pump inhibitors, and octreotide inhibit gastric or pancreatic secretion. Cholestyramine is often prescribed to improve diarrhea that is associated with bile salt malabsorption. Growth factors have also been used to hasten adaptation and to enhance mucosal growth, but these uses are still experimental.

Numerous complications are associated with SBS and long-term TPN (see Chapter 22). Infectious, metabolic, and technical complications can occur. Catheter sepsis can occur after improper care of the catheter. The GI tract can also be a source of microbial seeding of the catheter. Bowel atrophy may foster increased intestinal permeability of bacteria. A lack of adequate sites for central lines may become a significant problem for the child in need of long-term TPN. Hepatic dysfunction, hepatomegaly with abnormal liver function tests, and cholestasis may also occur.

Bacterial overgrowth is likely to occur when the ileocecal valve is absent or when stasis exists as a result of a partial obstruction or a dilated segment of bowel with poor motility. Alternating cycles of broad-spectrum antibiotics are used to reduce bacterial overgrowth. This treatment may also decrease the risk of bacterial translocation and subsequent central venous catheter infections. Other complications of bacterial overgrowth and malabsorption include metabolic acidosis and gastric hypersecretion.

Many surgical interventions, including intestinal valves, tapering enteroplasty or stricturoplasty, intestinal lengthening, and interposed segments, have been used to slow intestinal transit, reduce bacterial overgrowth, or increase mucosal surface area. *Intestinal transplantation* has been performed successfully in children. However, the experience is limited, and the long-term results are unknown. Only children with a permanent dependence on TPN or severe complications of long-term parenteral nutrition are candidates for transplantation.

Prognosis.   The prognosis for infants with SBS has improved with advances in TPN and with the understanding of the importance of intraluminal nutrition. Improved surgical techniques for the management of therapy-related problems and the development of more specific immunosuppressive medications for transplantation have all contributed to improved management. The prognosis depends in part on the length of the residual small intestine. An intact ileocecal valve also improves the prognosis. Infants and children with SBS usually die of TPN-related problems, such as fulminant sepsis or severe TPN cholestasis.

Nursing Considerations

The most important components of nursing care are administration and monitoring of nutritional therapy. During TPN therapy, care must be taken to minimize the risk of complications related to the central venous access device (i.e., catheter infections, occlusions, dislodgment, or accidental removal). Care of the enteral feeding tubes and monitoring of enteral feeding tolerance are also important nursing responsibilities.

When long-term parenteral nutrition is required, preparing the family for home care is a major nursing responsibility that should be initiated early to prevent a lengthy hospitalization with subsequent problems such as family dysfunction and developmental delays. Many infants and children can be successfully cared for at home with enteral and parenteral nutrition when the family is prepared and provided with adequate support services. Follow-up by a multidisciplinary nutritional support service is essential. The nurse plays an active and important role in the success of a home nutrition program. Home infusion companies provide portable equipment, which enables the child and family to maintain a more normal lifestyle.

When hospitalization is prolonged, the child's developmental and emotional needs must be met. This often requires special planning to promote normal family adjustment and adaptation of the hospital routines. Care of the hospitalized child is discussed in Chapter 21.

KEY POINTS

- Infants are subject to fluid depletion because of their greater surface area relative to body mass, high rate of metabolism, and immature kidney function.

- Dehydration can be classified as isotonic, hypotonic, and hypertonic.

- Vomiting and diarrhea account for significant fluid depletion, especially in infants and small children.

- The amount, frequency, and characteristics of stool and vomitus are important nursing observations.

- Diarrhea can be caused by an inflammatory process of infectious origin, a toxic reaction to ingestion of poisonous substances, dietary indiscretions, or infections outside the alimentary tract. The primary treatment of diarrhea is the use of oral rehydrating solution.

- Hirschsprung disease requires surgical removal of aganglionic segments of bowel.

- Postoperative care of the child with abdominal surgery involves assessing the abdomen, providing hydration and nutrition, intravenous fluids, proper positioning, wound care, and psychologic support.

- Nursing care of gastrointestinal (GI) reflux is aimed at identifying children with suggestive symptoms, helping parents with home care feeding and positioning, and caring for the child undergoing surgical intervention.

- Although the cause of appendicitis is poorly understood, it is typically a result of obstruction of the lumen, usually by a fecalith. Common signs and symptoms are right lower quadrant abdominal pain, tenderness, and fever.

- Meckel diverticulum is a congenital malformation of the GI tract characterized by bloody stools.

- Inflammatory bowel disease refers to ulcerative colitis and Crohn disease. Chronic diarrhea is the most common feature. It is treated by dietary management and medication, although surgery is needed in some cases.

- Peptic ulcers are poorly understood, but contributing factors include interference with the normal protective mechanisms of the mucosal lining and the presence of *Helicobacter pylori.*

- Viral hepatitis is caused by six types of virus: hepatitis A virus, hepatitis B virus, hepatitis C virus, hepatitis D virus, hepatitis E virus, and hepatitis G virus.

- Hepatitis A virus is spread by the fecal-oral route, whereas hepatitis B and C viruses are transmitted primarily by the parenteral route. The most effective measure in prevention and control of hepatitis in any setting is handwashing.

- Structural disorders of the GI tract include cleft lip, cleft palate, esophageal atresia with tracheoesophageal fistula, anorectal malformations, and biliary atresia.

- Biliary atresia is a serious disorder, often causing progressive liver failure, which is an indication for liver transplantation.

- Cleft lip and palate, the most common facial malformation, may involve nutritional, dental, and speech problems.

- Hernias related to the GI tract can be minor (umbilical) or life-threatening (diaphragmatic, gastroschisis, omphalocele).

- General signs of obstruction include colicky abdominal pain, nausea and vomiting, abdominal distention, and decreased stool output.

- Hypertrophic pyloric stenosis is recognized by characteristic projectile vomiting, malnutrition, dehydration, and a palpable mass in the epigastrium and is relieved by pyloromyotomy.

- Intussusception is one of the most common causes of intestinal obstruction during infancy and is characterized by abdominal pain and blood in stools. Treatment is either nonsurgical hydrostatic reduction or surgical reduction.

- Malabsorption syndromes are disorders associated with some degree of impaired digestion or absorption. They include digestive defects, absorptive defects, and anatomic defects.

- Celiac disease is characterized by an intolerance to gluten. It is thought to be either an inborn error of metabolism or an immunologic response.

- Short-bowel syndrome is characterized by a loss of intestine resulting in a diminished ability to absorb a regular diet normally. Specialized enteral and parenteral nutrition is a major element of care for these children.

References

American Academy of Pediatrics, Committee on Infectious Diseases: Hepatitis C virus infection, *Pediatrics* 101(3):481-485, 1998.

American Academy of Pediatrics, Provisional Committee on Quality Improvement, Subcommittee on Acute Gastroenteritis: Practice parameter: the management of acute gastroenteritis in young children, *Pediatrics* 97(3):424-435, 1996.

American Gastroenterological Association Medical Position Statement: Celiac sprue, *Gastroenterology* 120(6):1522-1525, 2001.

Andres JM: Neonatal hepatobiliary disorders, *Clin Perinatol* 23(2): 321-352, 1996.

Atkison RP and others; Long-term results of pediatric liver transplantation in a combined pediatric and adult transplant program, *Can Med Assoc J* 166(13):1663-1671, 2002.

Balistreri AF: Hepatitis C—pediatric implications, presented at the Thirty-Fourth Annual Pediatric Postgraduate Course—Perspective in Pediatrics, Bal Harbour, Fla, Feb 5-11, 1999.

Balistreri WF and others: Acute and chronic hepatitis: Working group report of the First World Congress of Pediatric Gastroenterology, Hepatology, and Nutrition, *J Pediatr Gastroenterol Nutr* 35(suppl 2): S62-S73, 2002.

Baron ML: Crohn disease in children: this chronic illness can be painful and isolating, but new treatments may help, *Am J Nurs* 102(10): 26-34, 2002.

Behrman RE, Kliegman RM, Arvin AM: *Nelson textbook of pediatrics,* ed 16, Philadelphia, 2000, WB Saunders.

Bonkovsky HL, Mehata S: Hepatitis C: a review and update, *J Am Acad Dermatol* 44(2):159-182, 2001.

Brandt ML: Intussusception. In McMillan JA and others, editors: *Oski's pediatrics: principles and practice,* ed 3, Philadelphia, 1999, Lippincott Williams & Wilkins.

Burkhart DM: Management of acute gastroenteritis in children, *Am Fam Physician* 60(9):2555-2563, 2565-2566, 1999.

Castiglia PT: Constipation in children, *J Pediatr Health Care* 15(4):200-202, 2001.

Chelimsky G, Czinn S: Peptic ulcer disease in children, *Pediatr Rev* 22(10):349-355, 2001.

Coffin SE: Future vaccines: recent advances and future prospects, *Primary Care* 28(4):869-887, 2001.

Dieterich W, Esslinger B, Schuppan D: Pathomechanisms in celiac disease, *Int Arch Allergy Immunol* 132(2):98-108, 2003.

DiLorenzo C: Disorders of the anorectum: pediatric anorectal disorders, *Gastroenterol Clin* 30(1):269-287, 2001.

Endsley S, Galbraith A: Are you overlooking oral rehydration therapy in childhood diarrhea? It's not just for use in developing countries, *Postgrad Med* 104(4):159-162, 1998.

Fann B: Fluid and electrolyte balance in the pediatric patient, *J Intraven Nurs* 21(3):153-159, 1998.

Flake AW, Ryckman FC: Selected anomalies and intestinal obstruction. In Fanaroff AA, Martin RJ, editors: *Neonatal-perinatal medicine: diseases of the fetus and infant,* ed 6, St Louis, 1997, Mosby.

Gastanaduy AS, Begue RE: Acute gastroenteritis, *Clin Pediatr* 38(1):1-12, 1999.

Gorelick MH, Shaw KN, Murphy KO: Validity and reliability of clinical signs in the diagnosis of dehydration in children, *Pediatrics* 99(5):e6, 1997.

Halamek LP, Stevenson DK: Neonatal jaundice and liver disease. In Fanaroff AA, Martin RJ, editors: *Neonatal-perinatal medicine: diseases of the fetus and infant,* ed 6, St Louis, 1997, Mosby.

Hendren WH: Pediatric rectal and perineal problems, *Pediatr Clin North Am* 45(6):1353-1371, 1998.

Holcomb GW: Minimally invasive surgery. In Hoekelman RA and others, editors: *Primary pediatric care,* ed 4, St Louis, 2001, Mosby.

Huffman S: Toddler's diarrhea, *J Pediatr Health Care* 13:32-33, 1999.

Hugger J, Harkless G, Rentschler D: Oral rehydration therapy for children with acute diarrhea, *Nurse Pract* 23(12):52-62, 1998.

Irish MS and others: The approach to common abdominal diagnoses in infants and children, *Pediatr Clin North Am* 45(4):729-772, 1998.

Jabbar A, Wright RA: Gastroenteritis and antibiotic-associated diarrhea, *Primary Care* 30(1):63-80, 2003.

Jackson WD, Grand RJ: Crohn's disease. In McMillan JA and others, editors: *Oski's pediatrics: principles and practice,* ed 3, Philadelphia, 1999, Lippincott Williams & Wilkins.

Karnam US, Reddy KR: Pegylated interferons, *Clin Liver Dis* 7(1):139-148, 2003.

Kirschner RE, LaRossa D: Cleft lip and palate, *Otolaryngol Clin North Am* 33(6):1191-1215, 2000.

Lasche J, Duggan C: Managing acute diarrhea: what every pediatrician needs to know, *Contemp Pediatr* 16(2):74-83, 1999.

Ledwith C: Fluids and electrolytes In Merenstein G, Kaplan D, Rosenberg A, editors, *Handbook of pediatrics,* Stamford, Conn, 1997, Appleton & Lange.

Lee J, Nunn J, Wright C: Height and weight achievement in cleft lip and palate, *Arch Dis Child* 76(1):70-72, 1997.

Leichtner AM, Jackson WD, Grand RJ: Ulcerative colitis. In Walker WA and others, editors: *Pediatric gastrointestinal disease: pathophysiology, diagnosis, management,* ed 2, St Louis, 1996, Mosby.

Loening-Baucke V: Functional constipation, *Semin Pediatr Surg* 4(10):26-34, 1995.

Motil K: Peptic ulcer disease, In McMillan JA and others, editors: *Oski's pediatrics: principles and practice,* ed 3, Philadelphia, 1999, Lippincott, Williams & Wilkins.

Murray JA: The widening spectrum of celiac disease, *Am J Clin Nutr* 69:354-365, 1999.

Nappert G and others: Oral rehydration solutions therapy in the management of children with rotavirus diarrhea, *Nutr Rev* 58(3):80-87, 2000.

Orenstein SR: Gastroesophageal reflux, *Pediatr Rev* 20(1):24-28, 1999.

Pena A: Anorectal Malformations, In Behrman RE, Kliegman RM, Jenson HB, editors: *Nelson textbook of pediatrics,* ed 16, Philadelphia, 2000, WB Saunders.

Ramaswamy K, Jacobson K: Infectious diarrhea in children, *Gastroenterol Clin* 30(3):611-624, 2001.

Regev A, Schiff ER: Viral hepatitis A, B, and C, *Clin Liver Dis* 4(1): 47-71, 2000.

Richard ME: Weight comparisons of infants with complete cleft lip and palate, *Pediatr Nurs* 20(20):191-196, 1994.

Rothenberg SS: Experience with 220 consecutive laparoscopic Nissen fundoplication in infants and children, *J Pediatr Surg* 33(2):274-278, 1998.

Rudolph CD and others: Guidelines for evaluation and treatment of gastroesophageal reflux in infants and children: recommendations of the North American Society for Pediatric Gastroenterology and Nutrition, *J Pediatr Gastroenterol Nutr* 32 (suppl 2):S1-S31, 2001.

Ryckman F, Flake AW, Balistreri WF: Upper gastrointestinal disorders. In Fanaroff AA, Martin RJ, editors: *Neonatal-perinatal medicine: diseases of the fetus and infant,* ed 6, St Louis, 1997, Mosby.

Sandberg SJ, Magee WP, Denk MJ: Neonatal cleft lip and cleft palate repair, *AORN Online* 75(3):488, 490-499, 501, 503-504, 506-508, 2002.

Savilahti E: Food-induced malabsorption syndromes, *J Pediatr Gastroenterol Nutr* 30(S1):S61-S66, 2000.

Schwartz MZ: Meckel diverticulum. In Wyllie R, Hyams JS, editors: *Pediatric gastrointestinal disease: physiology, diagnosis, management,* ed 2, Philadelphia, 1999, WB Saunders.

Sinatra FR: Liver transplantation for biliary atresia, *Pediatr Rev* 22(5): 166-180, 2001.

Smith EA and others: Current urologic management of cloacal exstrophy: experience with 11 patients, *J Pediatr Surg* 32(2):256-262, 1997.

Speltz ML and others: Early predictors of attachment in infants with cleft lip and/or palate, *Child Dev* 68(1):12-25, 1997.

Strahlman RS: Appendicitis. In Hoekelman RA and others, editors: *Primary pediatric care,* ed 4, St Louis, 2001, Mosby.

Trover JA: Functional results of laparoscopic fundoplication in children, *J Pediatr Gastroenterol Nutr* 26(4):429-431, 1998.

Walker-Smith J: Celiac disease. In Walker WA and others, editors: *Pediatric gastrointestinal disease: pathophysiology, diagnosis, management,* ed 2, St Louis, 2000, Mosby.

Wilkins-Haug L: Prenatal diagnosis of orofacial clefts, *Up to Date,* Jan 7, 2003; www.uptodate.com.

Yuen MF, Lai CL: Treatment of chronic hepatitis B, *Lancet Infect Dis* 1(4):383-393, 2001.

Zeiter DK, Hyams JS: Gastroesophageal reflux: pathogenesis, diagnosis, and treatment, *Allergy Asthma Proc* 20(1):45-49, 1999.

25

The Child With Cardiovascular Dysfunction

PATRICIA O'BRIEN

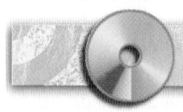

Remember to check out your companion CD-ROM

http://evolve.elsevier.com/Wong/essentials/

CHAPTER OUTLINE

RELATED TOPICS and ADDITIONAL RESOURCES

 IN TEXT

 CD COMPANION

 WEBSITE

- Design a plan for assisting a child during a cardiac diagnostic procedure.
- Demonstrate an understanding of the hemodynamics, distinctive manifestations, and therapeutic management of congenital heart disease.
- Outline a plan of care for an infant or child with congestive heart failure.
- Describe the care for a child who has hypoxia.

- Describe the care for an infant or a child with a congenital heart defect and its surgical repair.
- Discuss the role of the nurse in helping the child and family cope with congenital heart disease.
- Differentiate between rheumatic fever and rheumatic heart disease.
- List the criteria for selected cholesterol screening of children.

- Discuss the assessment and management of hypertension in children and adolescents.
- Outline a plan of care for a child with Kawasaki disease.
- Describe the emergency treatment for shock, including anaphylaxis.

CARDIOVASCULAR DYSFUNCTION

Cardiovascular disorders in children are divided into two major groups: congenital heart disease and acquired heart disorders. *Congenital heart disease* includes primarily anatomic abnormalities present at birth that result in abnormal cardiac function. The clinical consequences of congenital heart defects fall into two broad categories: congestive heart failure and hypoxemia. *Acquired cardiac disorders* refer to disease processes or abnormalities that occur after birth and can be seen in the normal heart or in the presence of congenital heart defects. They result from various factors, including infection, autoimmune responses, environmental factors, and familial tendencies.

ASSESSMENT OF CARDIAC FUNCTION
History and Physical Examination

Taking an accurate health history is an important first step in assessing an infant or child for possible heart disease. Parents may have specific concerns such as poor feeding or fast breathing in their infant or that their 7-year-old can no longer keep up with friends on the soccer field. Others may not always realize that their child has a medical problem; their child has always been pale and a fussy baby.

Asking details about the mother's health history, pregnancy, and birth history are important in assessing infants. Mothers with chronic health conditions, such as diabetes or lupus, are more likely to have infants with heart disease. Some medications, such as Dilantin, are teratogenic to the fetus. Maternal alcohol use or illicit drug use increases the risk of congenital heart defects. Exposures to infections, such as rubella, early in pregnancy may result in congenital anomalies. Infants with low birth weight resulting from intrauterine growth retardation are more likely to have congenital anomalies. High-birth-weight infants have an increased incidence of heart disease.

A detailed family history is also important. There is an increased incidence of congenital cardiac defects if either parent of a sibling has a heart defect. Some diseases, such as Marfan syndrome, and some cardiomyopathies are hereditary. A family history of frequent fetal loss, sudden infant death, and sudden death in adults may indicate heart disease. Congenital heart defects are seen in many syndromes such as Down syndrome and Turner syndrome.

The physical assessment of suspected cardiac disease begins with observation of general appearance, then proceeds with more specific observations. The following are supplementary to the general assessment techniques described for physical assessment of the chest and heart in Chapter 7.

Inspection

Nutritional state. Failure to thrive or poor weight gain is associated with heart disease.
Color. Cyanosis is a common feature of congenital heart disease, and pallor is associated with poor perfusion.
Chest deformities. An enlarged heart sometimes distorts the chest configuration.
Unusual pulsations. Visible pulsations of the neck veins are seen in some patients.
Respiratory excursion. This refers to the ease or difficulty of respiration (e.g., tachypnea, dyspnea, presence of expiratory grunt).
Clubbing of fingers. This is associated with cyanosis.

Palpation and Percussion

Chest. These maneuvers help discern heart size and other characteristics (e.g., thrills) associated with heart disease.
Abdomen. Hepatomegaly and/or splenomegaly may be evident.
Peripheral pulses. Rate, regularity, and amplitude (strength) may reveal discrepancies.

Auscultation

Heart rate and rhythm. Listen for fast heart rates (tachycardia), slow heart rates (bradycardia), or irregular rhythms.
Character of heart sounds. Listen for distinct or muffled sounds, murmurs, and additional heart sounds.

Diagnostic Evaluation

A variety of invasive and noninvasive tests may be used in the diagnosis of heart disease (Table 25-1). Some of the more common diagnostic tools that require nursing assessment and intervention are described here.

Bedside cardiac monitoring with the electrocardiogram (ECG) is commonly used in pediatrics, especially in the care of children with heart disease. The bedside monitor provides valuable information about heart rate and rhythm through a graphic display of the ECG tracing and a digital display. An alarm can be set with parameters for individual

TABLE 25-1 ■ **Procedures for Cardiac Diagnosis**

PROCEDURE	DESCRIPTIVE
Chest radiograph (x-ray)	Provides information on heart size and pulmonary blood flow patterns
Electrocardiography (ECG)	Graphic measure of electrical activity of heart
Holter monitor	24-hour continuous ECG recording used to assess dysrhythmias
Echocardiography	Use of high-frequency sound waves obtained by a transducer to produce an image of cardiac structures
Transthoracic	Done with transducer on chest
M-mode	One-dimensional graphic view used to estimate ventricular size and function
Two-dimensional (2-D)	Real-time, cross-sectional views of heart used to identify cardiac structures and cardiac anatomy
Doppler	Identifies blood flow patterns and pressure gradients across structures
Fetal	Imaging fetal heart in utero
Transesophageal (TEE)	Transducer placed in esophagus behind heart to obtain images of posterior heart structures or in patients with poor images from chest approach
Cardiac catheterization	Imaging study using radiopaque catheters placed in a peripheral blood vessel and advanced into heart to measure pressures and oxygen levels in heart chambers and visualize heart structures and blood flow patterns
Hemodynamics	Measures pressures and oxygen saturations in heart chambers
Angiography	Use of contrast material to illuminate heart structures and blood flow patterns
Biopsy	Use of special catheter to remove tiny samples of heart muscle for microscopic evaluation; used in assessing infection, inflammation, or muscle dysfunction disorders; also to evaluate for rejection after heart transplant
Electrophysiology(EPS)	Special catheters with electrodes employed to record electrical activity from within heart; used to diagnose rhythm disturbances
Exercise stress test	Monitoring of heart rate, blood pressure, electrocardiogram (ECG), and oxygen consumption at rest and during progressive exercise on a treadmill or bicycle
Cardiac magnetic resonance imaging (MRI)	Noninvasive imaging technique; used in evaluation of vascular anatomy outside of heart (i.e., coarctation of the aorta, vascular rings), estimates of ventricular mass and volume; uses for MRI are expanding

patient requirements and will sound if the heart rate is above or below the set parameters. Gelfoam electrodes are commonly used and placed on the right side of the chest (above the level of the heart) and on the left side of the chest, and a ground electrode is placed on the abdomen. Electrodes should be changed every 1 to 2 days because they are irritating to the skin. Bedside monitors are an adjunct to patient care and should never be substituted for direct assessment and auscultation of heart sounds. The nurse should assess the patient, not the monitor.

NURSING TIP

Electrodes for cardiac monitoring are often color coded: white for right, green (or red) for ground, and black for left. Always check to ensure that these colors are placed correctly.

Echocardiography. Echocardiography is one of the most frequently used tests for detecting cardiac dysfunction in children. Recent improvements in echocardiographic techniques have made it increasingly possible to confirm the diagnosis without resorting to cardiac catheterization. In increasing instances a prenatal diagnosis of congenital heart disease can be made by fetal echocardiography.

Echocardiography involves the use of ultra-high-frequency sound waves to produce an image of the heart's structure. A transducer placed directly on the chest wall delivers repetitive pulses of ultrasound and processes the returned signals (echoes).

Although the test is noninvasive, painless, and associated with no known side effects, it can be stressful for children. The child must lie quietly in the standard echocardiographic positions; crying, nursing, or sitting up often leads to diag-

nostic errors or omissions. Therefore infants and young children may need a mild sedative; older children benefit from psychologic preparation for the test. The distraction of a video or movie is often helpful.

Cardiac Catheterization. Cardiac catheterization is the most invasive diagnostic procedure in which a radiopaque catheter is inserted through a peripheral blood vessel into the heart (Uzark, 2001). The catheter is usually introduced through percutaneous technique, in which the catheter is threaded through a large-bore needle that is inserted into the vein. The catheter is guided through the heart with the aid of fluoroscopy. After the tip of the catheter is within a heart chamber, contrast material is injected, and films are taken of the dilution and circulation of the material *(angiography).* Types of cardiac catheterizations include:

Diagnostic catheterizations. These studies are used to diagnose congenital cardiac defects, particularly in symptomatic infants and before surgical repair. They are divided into right-sided catheterizations, in which the catheter is introduced through a vein (usually the femoral vein) and threaded to the right atrium (most common), and left-sided catheterizations, in which the catheter is threaded through an artery into the aorta and into the heart.

Interventional catheterizations (therapeutic catheterizations). A balloon catheter or other device is used to alter the cardiac anatomy. Examples include dilating stenotic valves or vessels or closing abnormal connections (Table 25-2).

Electrophysiology studies. Catheters with tiny electrodes that record the impulses of the heart directly from the conduction system are used to evaluate dysrhythmias and sometimes destroy accessory pathways that cause some tachydysrhythmias.

TABLE 25-2 ■ Current Interventional Cardiac Catheterization Procedures in Children

INTERVENTION	DIAGNOSIS
Balloon atrioseptostomy (BAS) Well established in newborns May also be done under echo guidance	Transposition of great arteries Some complex single-ventricle defects

Balloon dilation
Treatment of choice
	Valvular pulmonic stenosis
	Branch pulmonary artery stenosis
	Congenital valvular aortic stenosis
	Rheumatic mitral stenosis
	Recurrent coarctation of aorta
	Further follow-up required in:
	    Native coarctation of aorta in patients >7 months
	    Congenital mitral stenosis

Coil occlusion Accepted alternative to surgery	Patent ductus arteriosus (<4 mm)
Transcatheter device closure Several devices in clinical trials	Atrial septal defect
Stent placement	Pulmonary artery stenosis Other lesions investigational
Radio-frequency ablation	Some tachydysrhythmias

Data from Allen HD and others: Pediatric therapeutic cardiac catheterization: AHA Scientific Statement, *Circulation* 97:609-625, 1998.

Nursing Considerations

Cardiac catheterization has become a routine diagnostic procedure and may be done on an outpatient basis. However, it is not without risks, especially in neonates and seriously ill infants and children. Typical reactions include acute hemorrhage from the entry site (more likely with interventional procedures because larger catheters are used), low-grade fever, nausea, vomiting, loss of pulse in the catheterized extremity (usually transient, resulting from a clot, hematoma, or intimal tear), and transient dysrhythmias (generally catheter induced) (Uzark, 2001). Rare risks include stroke, seizures, tamponade, and death.

Preprocedural Care. A complete nursing assessment is necessary to ensure a safe procedure with minimum complications. This assessment should include accurate height (essential to correct catheter selection) and weight. Obtaining a history of allergic reactions is important, because some of the contrast agents are iodine-based. Specific attention to signs and symptoms of infection is crucial. Severe diaper rash may be a reason to cancel the procedure if femoral access is required. Because assessment of pedal pulses is important after catheterization, the nurse should assess and mark pulses (dorsalis pedis, posterior tibial) before the child goes to the catheterization room. The presence and quality of pulses in both feet are clearly documented. Baseline oxygen saturation using pulse oximetry in children with cyanosis is also recorded.

Preparing the child and family for the procedure is the joint responsibility of the physician, nurse, and parents. School-age children and adolescents benefit from a description of the catheterization laboratory and a chronologic explanation of the procedure, emphasizing what they will see, feel, and hear. Older children and adolescents may bring earphones and favorite music so they can listen during the catheterization procedure. Preparation materials such as picture books, videotapes, or tours of the catheterization laboratory may be helpful. Preparation should be geared to the child's developmental level. The child's caregivers often benefit from the same explanations. Additional information, such as the expected length of the catheterization, description of the child's appearance after catheterization, and usual postprocedure care, should be outlined.

Methods of sedation vary among institutions and may include oral or intravenous (IV) medications (see Chapter 22). The child's age, heart defect, clinical status, and type of catheterization procedure planned are considered when sedation is determined. General anesthesia may be needed for some interventional procedures. Children are allowed nothing by mouth (NPO) for 4 to 6 hours or more before the procedure according to institutional guidelines. Infants and patients with polycythemia may need IV fluids to prevent dehydration and hypoglycemia.

Postprocedural Care. Patients may recover from the procedure in a recovery unit, their hospital room, or, occasionally, intensive care may be required. Patients are usually placed on a cardiac monitor and a pulse oximeter for the first few hours of recovery. The most important nursing responsibility is observation of the following for signs of complications:

- Pulses, especially below the catheterization site, for equality and symmetry (pulse distal to the site may be weaker for the first few hours after catheterization but should gradually increase in strength)
- Temperature and color of the affected extremity, because coolness or blanching may indicate arterial obstruction
- Vital signs, which are taken as frequently as every 15 minutes, with special emphasis on heart rate, which is counted for 1 full minute for evidence of dysrhythmias or bradycardia
- Blood pressure, especially for hypotension, which may indicate hemorrhage from cardiac perforation or bleeding at the site of initial catheterization
- Dressing, for evidence of bleeding or hematoma formation in the femoral or antecubital area

■ Fluid intake, both IV and oral, to ensure adequate hydration (blood loss in the catheterization laboratory, the child's NPO status, and diuretic actions of dyes used during the procedure put children at risk for hypovolemia and dehydration)

■ Hypoglycemia, especially in infants, who should receive dextrose-containing IV fluids; blood glucose levels should be checked

> ### ▮ NURSING ALERT
>
> **If bleeding occurs, direct continuous pressure is applied 2.5 cm (1 inch) above the percutaneous skin site to localize pressure over the vessel puncture.**

Depending on hospital policy, the child may be kept in bed with the affected extremity maintained straight for 4 to 6 hours after venous catheterization and 6 to 8 hours after arterial catheterization to facilitate healing of the cannulated vessel. If younger children have difficulty complying, they can be held in the parent's lap with the leg maintained in the correct position. The child's usual diet can be resumed as soon as tolerated, beginning with sips of clear liquids and advancing as the condition allows. The child is encouraged to void to clear the contrast material from the blood. Generally, there is only slight discomfort at the percutaneous site. To prevent infection, the catheterization area is protected from possible contamination. If the child wears diapers, the dressing can be kept dry by covering it with a piece of plastic film and sealing the edges of the film to the skin with tape. However, the nurse must be careful to continue to observe the site for any evidence of bleeding (see Family Home Care box and Critical Thinking Exercise).

CONGENITAL HEART DISEASE

The incidence of congenital heart disease (CHD) in children is generally believed to be 5 to 8 per 1000 live births (Behrman, Kliegman, and Jenson, 2000). About 2 to 3 in 1000 infants will be symptomatic during the first year of life. CHD is the major cause of death (other than prematurity) in the first year of life. Although there are more than 35 well-recognized defects, the most common heart anomaly is ventricular septal defect (VSD).

The exact etiology of 90% of the congenital cardiac defects is unknown. Most are thought to be a result of multifactorial inheritance: a complex interaction of genetic and

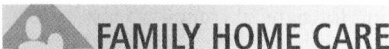

▮ FAMILY HOME CARE

After Cardiac Catheterization

Remove pressure dressing the day after catheterization. Cover site with an adhesive bandage strip for several days.

Keep site clean and dry. Avoid tub baths for several days; may shower.

Observe site for redness, swelling, drainage, and bleeding. Monitor for fever. Notify practitioner if these occur.

Avoid strenuous exercise for several days. May attend school.

Resume regular diet without restrictions.

Use acetaminophen or ibuprofen for pain.

Keep follow-up appointments per practitioner's instruction.

Modified from Children's Hospital (Boston) Cardiovascular Program, 1994.

environmental factors. The tremendous amount of information being discovered in molecular biology and the human genome project will likely increase our understanding of the genetic etiologies of congenital heart defects.

Some risk factors are known to increase the incidence of congenital heart defects. Maternal factors include chronic illnesses such as diabetics or poorly controlled phenylketonuria (PKU), alcohol consumption, and exposure to en-

??? CRITICAL THINKING EXERCISE ???

Cardiac Catheterization

Tommy, a 4-year-old with tetralogy of Fallot, has just returned to his hospital room from the cardiac catheterization recovery room. His mother calls you to the bedside to tell you that he is vomiting and bleeding. You arrive to find Tommy anxious, pale, crying, and sitting in a puddle of blood.

QUESTIONS

1. Evidence—Is there sufficient evidence to draw conclusions about Tommy's situation?
2. Assumptions—Describe an underlying assumption about each of the following:
   a. Risks of cardiac catheterization
   b. Association between vomiting and bleeding following heart catheterization
   c. Concerns related to acute blood loss
3. What priorities for nursing care should be established for Tommy?
4. Does the evidence support your nursing interventions?
5. What alternative perspectives might you have?

ANSWERS

1. Yes. This patient has just undergone an invasive surgical procedure. Bleeding is a potential risk after cardiac catheterization.
2. a. Complications after cardiac catheterization can include acute hemorrhage from the catheterization entry site, low-grade fever, nausea and vomiting, loss of pulses in the catheterized extremity, and transient dysrhythmias.
   b. Nausea and vomiting can occur after heart catheterization but are not directly related to acute blood loss. However, if the child had significant vomiting occurring immediately after the procedure and was not able to keep his leg straight, the vomiting might have increased the chance of bleeding at the catheterization entry site.
   c. Significant blood loss can occur in a short time after the use of an artery for cardiac catheterization.
3. The first priority is to prevent bleeding. Pressure is applied above the visible catheterization site where the vessel was accessed. Place the child flat in bed to decrease the effect of gravity on the rate of bleeding. Notify the practitioner immediately. Replacement fluids may need to be administered, and pharmacologic control of emesis is important.
4. This may be an arterial bleed, and Tommy is at risk for losing a large amount of blood in a short time. Your first priority should be to control the bleeding. Appropriate measures are to treat the patient like a shock patient by immediately lying the child flat to help with the control of bleeding.
5. In this case it is essential for the nurse to understand the complications associated with heart catheterization. Observation of acute blood loss at the site of catheter entry does not provide other alternative perspectives but supports an immediate need to control bleeding.

vironmental toxins and infections. Family history of a cardiac defect in a parent or sibling increases the likelihood of a cardiac anomaly. The risk of congenital heart disease increases if a first-degree relative (parent or sibling) is affected (Behrman, Kliegman, and Jenson, 2000). The familial risk is higher with left-sided obstructive lesions.

Congenital heart anomalies are often associated with chromosomal abnormalities, syndromes, or congenital defects in other body systems. Down syndrome (trisomy 21) and trisomy 13 and 18 are highly correlated with congenital heart defects.

Recent research in gene mapping has identified deletion of part of chromosome 22 (22q11), which is present in the majority of patients with DiGeorge syndrome, velocardiofacial syndrome (VCFS), and conotruncal anomaly face syndrome. The features of these syndromes include congenital cardiac defects, soft palate abnormalities, dysmorphic facial features, and speech and developmental delays. Mild immunologic abnormalities of T cells, absence or hypoplasia of the thymus, and parathyroid abnormalities resulting in hypocalcemia are seen with DiGeorge syndrome. Commonly associated cardiac defects are interrupted aortic arch, truncus arteriosus, tetralogy of Fallot, and posterior malaligned ventricular septal defects (Goldmuntz and others, 1998). There is a very variable clinical expression of this syndrome with some patients minimally affected and others having all characteristics.

Circulatory Changes at Birth

During fetal life, blood carrying oxygen and nutritive materials from the placenta enters the fetal system through the umbilicus via the large umbilical vein. Oxygenated blood enters the heart by way of the inferior vena cava. Because of the higher pressure of blood entering the right atrium, it is directed posteriorly in a straight pathway across the right atrium and through the *foramen ovale* to the left atrium. In this way the better-oxygenated blood enters the left atrium and ventricle to be pumped through the aorta to the head and upper extremities. Blood from the head and upper extremities entering the right atrium from the superior vena cava is directed downward through the tricuspid valve into the right ventricle. From here it is pumped through the pulmonary artery, where the major portion is shunted to the descending aorta via the *ductus arteriosus.* Only a small amount flows to and from the nonfunctioning fetal lungs (Fig. 25-1, *A*).

Before birth the high pulmonary vascular resistance created by the collapsed fetal lung causes greater pressures in the right side of the heart and the pulmonary arteries. At the same time, the free-flowing placental circulation and the ductus arteriosus produce a low vascular resistance in the remainder of the fetal vascular system. With the cessation of placental blood flow from clamping of the umbilical cord and the expansion of the lungs at birth, the hemodynamics of the fetal vascular system undergo pronounced and abrupt changes (Fig. 25-1, *B*).

With the first breath, the lungs are expanded, and increased oxygen causes pulmonary vasodilation. Pulmonary pressures start to fall as systemic pressures, given the removal of the placenta, start to rise. Normally the foramen ovale closes as the pressure in the left atrium exceeds the pressure in the right atrium. The ductus arteriosus starts to close in the presence of increased oxygen concentration in the blood and other factors.

Altered Hemodynamics

To appreciate the physiology of heart defects, it is necessary to understand the role of pressure gradients, flow, and resistance within the circulation. As with any fluid, blood flows from an area of high pressure to one of lower pressure

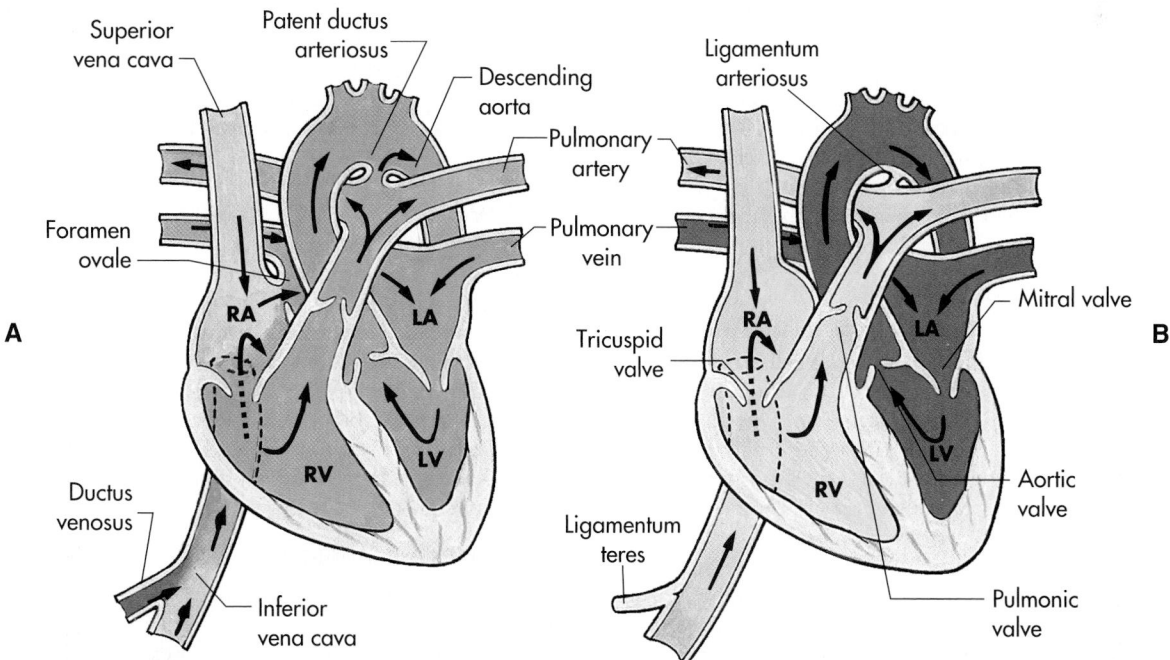

FIG. 25-1 ■ Changes in circulation at birth. **A,** Prenatal circulation. **B,** Postnatal circulation. Arrows indicate direction of blood flow. Although four pulmonary veins enter the *LA,* for simplicity this diagram shows only two. *RA,* Right atrium; *LA,* left atrium; *RV,* right ventricle; *LV,* left ventricle.

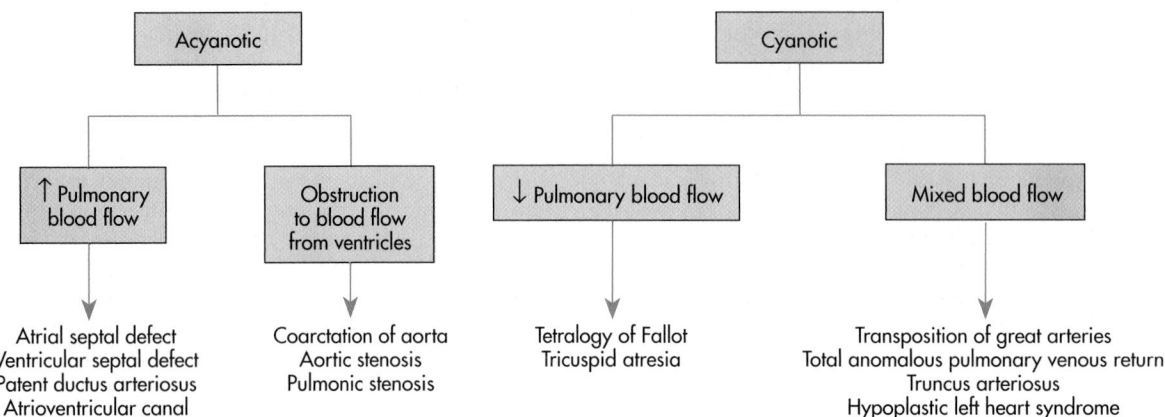

FIG. 25-2 ■ Comparison of acyanotic-cyanotic and hemodynamic classification systems of congenital heart disease.

and toward the path of least resistance in response to the pumping action of the heart. In general, the higher the pressure gradient, the greater the rate of flow; the higher the resistance, the lesser the rate of flow.

Normally the pressure on the right side of the heart is lower than that on the left side, and the resistance in the pulmonary circulation is less than that in the systemic circulation. Vessels entering or exiting these chambers have corresponding pressures. Therefore, if an abnormal connection exists between the heart chambers (such as a septal defect), blood will necessarily flow from an area of higher pressure (left side) to one of lower pressure (right side). Such a flow of blood is termed a *left-to-right shunt.* Anomalies resulting in cyanosis may result from a change in pressure so that the blood is shunted from the right to the left side of the heart *(right-to-left shunt)* because of either increased pulmonary vascular resistance or obstruction to blood flow through the pulmonic valve and artery. Cyanosis may also result from a defect that allows mixing of oxygenated and deoxygenated blood within the heart chambers or great arteries, such as occurs in truncus arteriosus.

CLASSIFICATION OF DEFECTS

Congenital heart defects have been divided into two categories. Traditionally, cyanosis, a physical characteristic, has been used as the distinguishing feature, dividing the anomalies into *acyanotic defects* and *cyanotic defects.* In clinical practice this system is problematic because children with acyanotic defects may develop cyanosis. Also, more often, those with cyanotic defects may appear pink and have more clinical signs of congestive heart failure (CHF).

A more useful classification system is based on hemodynamic characteristics (blood flow patterns within the heart). These blood flow patterns are (1) *increased pulmonary blood flow,* (2) *decreased pulmonary blood flow,* (3) *obstruction to blood flow* out of the heart, and (4) *mixed blood flow,* in which saturated and desaturated blood mix within the

heart or great arteries. As a comparison, both classification systems are outlined in Fig. 25-2.

With the hemodynamic classification system, the clinical manifestations of each group are more uniform and predictable. Defects that allow blood flow from the higher pressure left side of the heart to the lower pressure right side (left-to-right shunt) result in increased pulmonary blood flow and cause CHF. Obstructive defects impede blood flow out of the ventricles; obstruction on the left side of the heart results in CHF, whereas severe obstruction on the right side causes cyanosis. Defects that cause decreased pulmonary blood flow result in cyanosis. Mixed lesions present a variable clinical picture based on the degree of mixing and amount of pulmonary blood flow; hypoxemia (with or without cyanosis) and CHF usually occur together. This system is used in the following discussion.

DEFECTS WITH INCREASED PULMONARY BLOOD FLOW

In this group of cardiac defects, intracardiac communications along the septum or an abnormal connection between the great arteries allows blood to flow from the higher pressure left side of the heart to the lower pressure right side of the heart (Fig. 25-3). Increased blood volume on the right side of the heart increases pulmonary blood flow at the expense of systemic blood flow. Clinically, patients demonstrate signs and symptoms of CHF. Atrial and ventricular septal defects and patent ductus arteriosus are typical anomalies in this group (Box 25-1).

OBSTRUCTIVE DEFECTS

Obstructive defects are those in which blood exiting the heart meets an area of anatomic narrowing *(stenosis),* causing obstruction to blood flow. The pressure in the ventricle and in the great artery before the obstruction is increased, and the pressure in the area beyond the obstruction is de-

Text continued on p. 899.

BOX 25-1 ■ Defects With Increased Pulmonary Blood Flow

ATRIAL SEPTAL DEFECT (ASD)

Description: Abnormal opening between the atria, allowing blood from the higher pressure left atrium to flow into the lower pressure right atrium. There are three types:

Ostium primum (ASD 1)—Opening at lower end of septum; may be associated with mitral valve abnormalities

Ostium secundum (ASD 2)—Opening near center of septum

Sinus venosus defect—Opening near junction of superior vena cava and right atrium; may be associated with partial anomalous pulmonary venous connection

Pathophysiology: Because left atrial pressure slightly exceeds right atrial pressure, blood flows from the left to the right atrium, causing an increased flow of oxygenated blood into the right side of the heart. Despite the low pressure difference, a high rate of flow can still occur because of low pulmonary vascular resistance and the greater distensibility of the right atrium, which further reduces flow resistance. This volume is well tolerated by the right ventricle because it is delivered under much lower pressure than in a ventricular septal defect. Although there is right atrial and ventricular enlargement, cardiac failure is unusual in an uncomplicated ASD. Pulmonary vascular changes usually occur only after several decades if the defect is unrepaired.

Clinical manifestations: Patients may be asymptomatic. They may develop congestive heart failure (CHF). There is a characteristic murmur. Patients are at risk for atrial dysrhythmias (probably caused by atrial enlargement and stretching of conduction fibers) and pulmonary vascular obstructive disease and emboli formation later in life from chronic increased pulmonary blood flow.

Surgical treatment: Surgical Dacron patch closure of moderate to large defects similar to closure of ventricular septal defects.

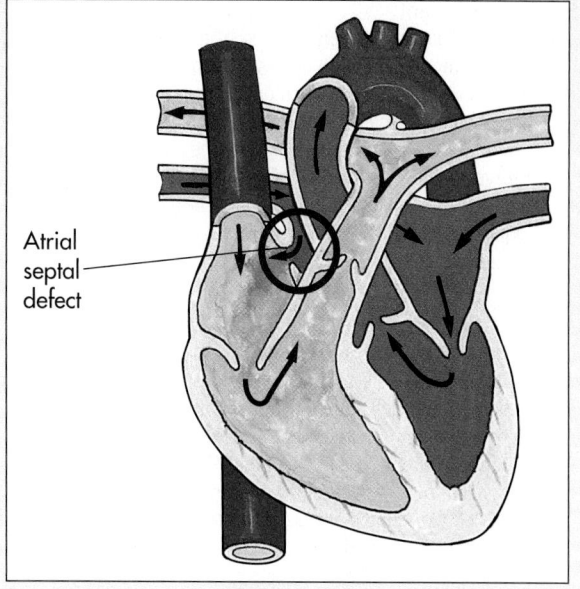

Atrial septal defect

Open repair with cardiopulmonary bypass is usually performed before school age. In addition, the sinus venosus defect requires patch placement, so the anomalous right pulmonary venous return is directed to the left atrium with a baffle. The ASD 1 may require repair or, rarely, replacement of the mitral valve.

Nonsurgical treatment: ASD 2 may also be closed using devices during cardiac catheterization. This technique is in clinical trials in some centers (Uzurk, 2001).

Prognosis: Very low operative mortality, less than 1%.

VENTRICULAR SEPTAL DEFECT (VSD)

Description: Abnormal opening between the right and left ventricles. May be classified according to location: membranous (accounting for 80%) or muscular. May vary in size from a small pinhole to absence of the septum, resulting in a common ventricle. Frequently associated with other defects, such as pulmonary stenosis, transposition of the great vessels, patent ductus arteriosus, atrial defects, and coarctation of the aorta. Many VSDs (20% to 60%) are thought to close spontaneously. Spontaneous closure is most likely to occur during the first year of life in children having small or moderate defects. A left-to-right shunt is caused by the flow of blood from the higher pressure left ventricle to the lower pressure right ventricle.

Pathophysiology: Because of the higher pressure within the left ventricle and because the systemic arterial circulation offers more resistance than the pulmonary circulation, blood flows through the defect into the pulmonary artery. The increased blood volume is pumped into the lungs, which may eventually result in increased pulmonary vascular resistance. Increased pressure in the right ventricle as a result of left-to-right shunting and pulmonary resistance causes the muscle to hypertrophy. If the right ventricle is unable to accommodate the increased workload, the right atrium may also enlarge as it attempts to overcome the resistance offered by incomplete right ventricular emptying. In severe defects Eisenmenger syndrome may develop (p. 914).

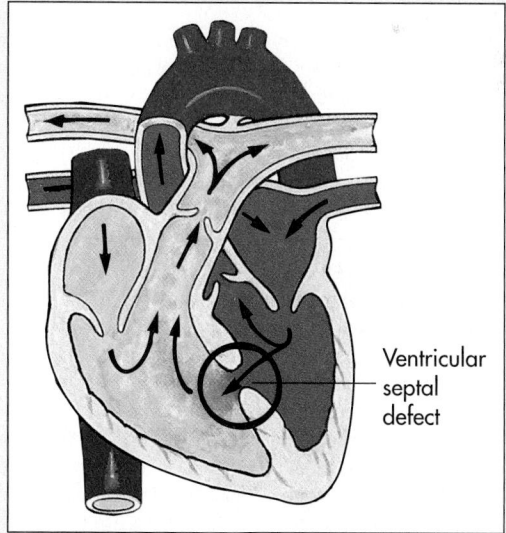

Ventricular septal defect

Clinical manifestations: CHF is common. There is a characteristic murmur. Patients are at risk for bacterial endocarditis and pulmonary vascular obstructive disease. In severe defects, Eisenmenger syndrome may develop.

Continued

BOX 25-1 ■ Defects With Increased Pulmonary Blood Flow—*cont'd*

Surgical treatment:
Palliative: Pulmonary artery banding (placing a band around the main pulmonary artery to decrease pulmonary blood flow) in infants in severe CHF was common in the past. It is unusual now because improvements in surgical techniques and postoperative care make complete repair in infancy the preferred approach.

Complete repair (procedure of choice): Small defects are repaired with a purse-string approach. Large defects usually require a knitted Dacron patch sewn over the opening. Both procedures are performed via cardiopulmonary bypass. The repair is generally approached through the right atrium and the tricuspid valve. Postoperative complications include residual VSD and conduction disturbances.

Nonsurgical treatment: Device closure during cardiac catheterization is under clinical trials in some centers for closure of muscular defects that carry a high operative risk.

Prognosis: Risks depend on the location of the defect, number of defects, and other associated cardiac defects. Single membranous defects have a low mortality (less than 5%); multiple muscular defects can have a risk of more than 20%.

ATRIOVENTRICULAR CANAL (AVC) DEFECT

Description: Incomplete fusion of endocardial cushions. Consists of a low atrial septal defect that is continuous with a high ventricular septal defect and clefts of the mitral and tricuspid valves, creating a large central atrioventricular (AV) valve that allows blood to flow between all four chambers of the heart. The directions and pathways of flow are determined by pulmonary and systemic resistance, left and right ventricular pressures, and the compliance of each chamber, although flow is generally from left to right. It is the most common cardiac defect in children with Down syndrome.

Pathophysiology: The alterations in the hemodynamics depend on the defect's severity and the child's pulmonary vascular resistance. Immediately after birth, while the newborn's pulmonary vascular resistance is high, there is minimum shunting of blood through the defect. After this resistance falls, left-to-right shunting occurs and pulmonary blood flow increases. The resultant pulmonary vascular engorgement predisposes to development of CHF.

Clinical manifestations: Patients usually have moderate to severe CHF. There is a characteristic murmur. There may be mild cyanosis that increases with crying. Patients are at high risk for developing pulmonary vascular obstructive disease.

Surgical treatment:
Palliative: Pulmonary artery banding for infants with severe symptoms that are caused by increased pulmonary blood flow in some centers. Most centers perform complete repair in infancy.

Complete repair: Surgical repair consists of patch closure of the septal defects and reconstruction of the AV valve tissue (either repair of the mitral valve cleft or fashioning two AV valves). If the mitral valve defect is severe, a valve replacement may be needed. Postoperative complications include heart block, CHF, mitral regurgitation, dysrhythmias, and pulmonary hypertension.

Prognosis: Operative mortality is less than 10%. A potential later problem is mitral regurgitation, which may require valve replacement.

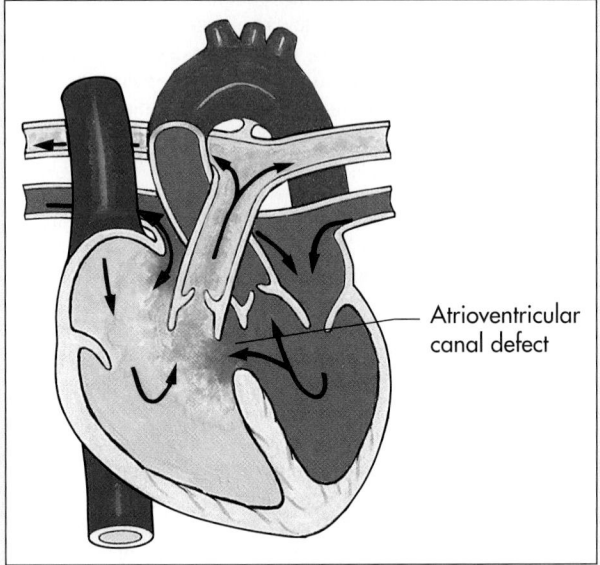

Atrioventricular canal defect

PATENT DUCTUS ARTERIOSUS (PDA)

Description: Failure of the fetal ductus arteriosus (artery connecting the aorta and pulmonary artery) to close within the first weeks of life. The continued patency of this vessel allows blood to flow from the higher pressure aorta to the lower pressure pulmonary artery, causing a left-to-right shunt.

Pathophysiology: The hemodynamic consequences of PDA depend on the size of the ductus and the pulmonary vascular resistance. At birth the resistance in the pulmonary and systemic circulations is almost identical, thus equalizing the resistance in the aorta and pulmonary artery. As the systemic pressure exceeds the pulmonary pressure, blood begins to shunt from the aorta, across the duct, to the pulmonary artery (left-to-right shunt). The additional blood is recirculated through the lungs and returned to the left atrium and left ventricle. The effect of this altered circulation is increased workload on the left side of the heart, increased pulmonary vascular congestion and possibly resistance, and potentially increased right ventricular pressure and hypertrophy.

Clinical manifestations: Patients may be asymptomatic or show signs of CHF. There is a characteristic machinery-like murmur. A widened pulse pressure and bounding pulses result from runoff of blood from the aorta to the pulmonary artery. Patients are at risk for bacterial endocarditis and pulmonary vascular obstructive disease in later life from chronic excessive pulmonary blood flow.

BOX 25-1 ■ Defects With Increased Pulmonary Blood Flow—*cont'd*

PATENT DUCTUS ARTERIOSUS (PDA)—*cont'd*

Medical management: Administration of indomethacin (prostaglandin inhibitor) has proved successful in closing a patent ductus in premature infants and some newborns (Pham and Carlos, 2002).

Surgical treatment: Surgical division or ligation of the patent vessel via a left thoracotomy. A newer technique, visual-assisted thoracoscopic surgery (VATS), uses a thoracoscope and instruments placed through three small incisions on the left side of the chest to place a clip on the ductus. It is used in some centers and eliminates the need for a thoracotomy, thereby speeding postoperative recovery.

Nonsurgical treatment: Use of coils to occlude the PDA in the catheterization laboratory is done in many centers. Small infants (with small-diameter femoral arteries) and those patients with large or unusual PDAs may require surgery.

Prognosis: Both procedures can be done at low risk with less than 1% mortality.

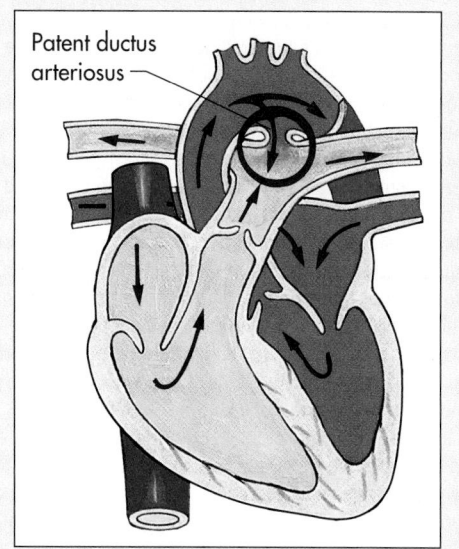

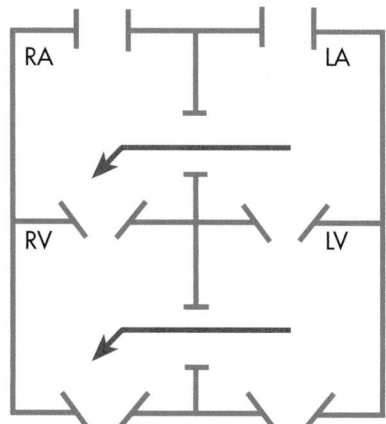

FIG. 25-3 ■ Hemodynamics in defects with increased pulmonary blood flow. See Fig. 25-1 for abbreviations.

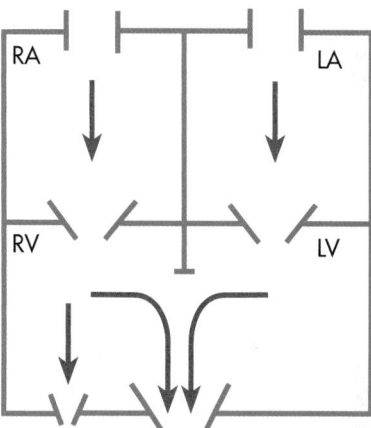

FIG. 25-5 ■ Hemodynamic defects with decreased pulmonary blood flow. See Fig. 25-1 for abbreviations.

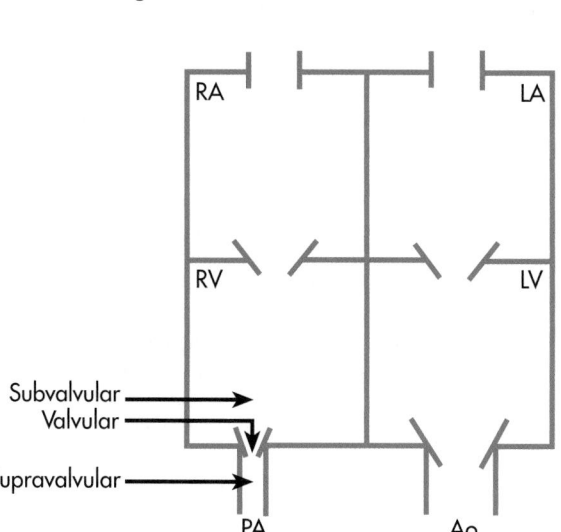

FIG. 25-4 ■ Obstruction to ventricular ejection can occur at the valvular level (shown), below the valve (subvalvular), or above the valve (supravalvular). Pulmonary stenosis is shown here. See Fig. 25-1 for abbreviations.

creased. The location of the narrowing is usually near the valve (Fig. 25-4), as follows:

> **Valvular**—At the site of the valve itself
> **Subvalvular**—Narrowing in the ventricle below the valve (also referred to as the *ventricular outflow tract*)
> **Supravalvular**—Narrowing in the great artery above the valve

Coarctation of the aorta (narrowing of the aortic arch), aortic stenosis, and pulmonic stenosis are typical defects in this group (Box 25-2). Hemodynamically, there is a pressure load on the ventricle and decreased cardiac output. Clinically, infants and children exhibit signs of CHF. Children with mild obstruction may be asymptomatic. Rarely, as in severe pulmonic stenosis, hypoxemia may be seen.

DEFECTS WITH DECREASED PULMONARY BLOOD FLOW

In this group of defects, there is obstruction of pulmonary blood flow and an anatomic defect (atrial septal defect [ASD] or VSD) between the right and left sides of the heart (Fig. 25-5). Because blood has difficulty exiting the right

BOX 25-2 ■ Obstructive Defects

COARCTATION OF THE AORTA (COA)

Description: Localized narrowing near the insertion of the ductus arteriosus, resulting in increased pressure proximal to the defect (head and upper extremities) and decreased pressure distal to the obstruction (body and lower extremities).

Pathophysiology: The effect of a narrowing within the aorta is increased pressure proximal to the defect and decreased pressure distal to it. In the preductal type of COA the lower half of the body is supplied with blood by the right ventricle through the ductus arteriosus. In the postductal type, right ventricular outflow cannot maintain blood flow to the descending aorta. Therefore collateral circulation develops during fetal life to maintain flow from the ascending to the descending aorta.

Clinical manifestations: There may be high blood pressure and bounding pulses in arms, weak or absent femoral pulses, and cool lower extremities with lower blood pressure. There are signs of congestive heart failure (CHF) in infants. Often these patients' hemodynamic condition deteriorates rapidly and they are admitted to the intensive care unit near death, usually severely acidotic and hypotensive. Mechanical ventilation and inotropic support are often necessary before surgery. Older children may experience dizziness, headaches, fainting, and epistaxis resulting from hypertension. Patients are at risk for hypertension, ruptured aorta, aortic aneurysm, or stroke.

Surgical treatment: Either resection of the coarcted portion with an end-to-end anastomosis of the aorta or enlargement of the constricted section using a graft of prosthetic material or a portion of the left subclavian artery. Because this defect is outside the heart and pericardium, cardiopulmonary bypass is not required and a thoracotomy incision is used. Postoperative hypertension (greater than 160 mm Hg) is treated with intravenous sodium nitroprusside or amrinone, followed by oral medications, such as captopril, hydralazine, and/or propranolol. Residual permanent hypertension after repair of COA seems to be related to age and time of repair. To prevent both hypertension at rest and exercise-provoked systemic hypertension after repair, elective surgery for COA is advised within the first 2 years of life. There is a 5% to 10% risk of recurrent narrowing in pa-

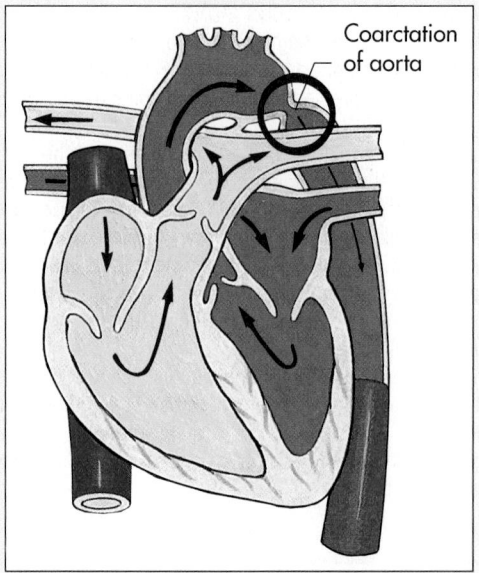

Coarctation of aorta

tients who underwent surgical repair as infants (Hougen and Sell, 1995). Percutaneous balloon angioplasty techniques have proved to be very effective in relieving residual postoperative coarctation gradients.

Nonsurgical treatment: Balloon angioplasty as a primary intervention for COA is being performed in some centers, but concerns about inadequate relief of gradients, risk of aneurysm formation, and restenosis have limited its widespread use. Recent studies have demonstrated that balloon angioplasty is effective in children and that aneurysm formation is rare. The high restenosis rate in infants younger than 7 months of age limits its application in this group, and further study is needed (Uzurk, 2001; Allen and others, 1998).

Prognosis: Less than 5% mortality in patients with isolated coarctation; increased risk in infants with other complex cardiac defects.

AORTIC STENOSIS (AS)

Description: Narrowing or stricture of the aortic valve, causing resistance to blood flow in the left ventricle, decreased cardiac output, left ventricular hypertrophy, and pulmonary vascular congestion. The prominent anatomic consequence of AS is the hypertrophy of the left ventricular wall, which eventually will lead to increased end-diastolic pressure, resulting in pulmonary venous and pulmonary arterial hypertension. Left ventricular hypertrophy also interferes with coronary artery perfusion and may result in myocardial infarction or scarring of the papillary muscles of the left ventricle, causing mitral insufficiency. *Valvular stenosis,* the most common type, is usually caused by malformed cusps resulting in a bicuspid rather than tricuspid valve or fusion of the cusps. *Subvalvular stenosis* is a stricture caused by a fibrous ring below a normal valve; *supravalvular stenosis* occurs infrequently. Valvular AS is a serious defect for the following reasons: (1) the obstruction tends to be progressive; (2) sudden episodes of myocardial ischemia, or low car-

diac output, can result in sudden death; and (3) surgical repair rarely results in a normal valve. This is one of the rare instances in which strenuous physical activity may be curtailed because of the cardiac condition.

Pathophysiology: A stricture in the aortic outflow tract causes resistance to ejection of blood from the left ventricle. The extra workload on the left ventricle causes hypertrophy. If left ventricular failure develops, left atrial pressure will increase; this causes increased pressure in the pulmonary veins, resulting in pulmonary vascular congestion (pulmonary edema).

Clinical manifestations: Infants with severe defects demonstrate signs of decreased cardiac output with faint pulses, hypotension, tachycardia, and poor feeding. Children show signs of exercise intolerance, chest pain, and dizziness when standing for a long period. There is a characteristic murmur. Patients are at risk for bacterial endocarditis, coronary insufficiency, and ventricular dysfunction.

BOX 25-2 ■ **Obstructive Defects**—*cont'd*

Valvular Aortic Stenosis

Surgical treatment: Aortic valvotomy under inflow occlusion (Uzurk, 2001).

Prognosis: Aortic valvotomy in critically ill neonates and infants still carries a mortality of 10% to 20% in major medical centers (Hawkins and others, 1998). Results of aortic valvotomy in older children are very good, with mortality close to 0%. However, aortic valvotomy remains a palliative procedure, and approximately 25% of patients require additional surgery within 10 years for recurrent stenosis. A valve replacement may be required at the second procedure. An aortic homograft with a valve may also be used *(extended aortic root replacement)*, or the pulmonary valve may be moved to the aortic position and replaced with a homograft valve *(Ross procedure)*.

Nonsurgical treatment: Dilating narrowed valve with balloon angioplasty in the catheterization laboratory.

Prognosis: Complications include aortic insufficiency or valvular regurgitation, tearing of the valve leaflets, and loss of pulse in the catheterized limb. Relief of obstruction is similar to that for surgical valvotomy (Allen and others, 1998).

Subvalvular Aortic Stenosis

Surgical treatment: May involve incising a membrane if one exists or cutting the fibromuscular ring. If the obstruction results from narrowing of the left ventricular outflow tract and a small aortic valve annulus, a patch may be required to enlarge the

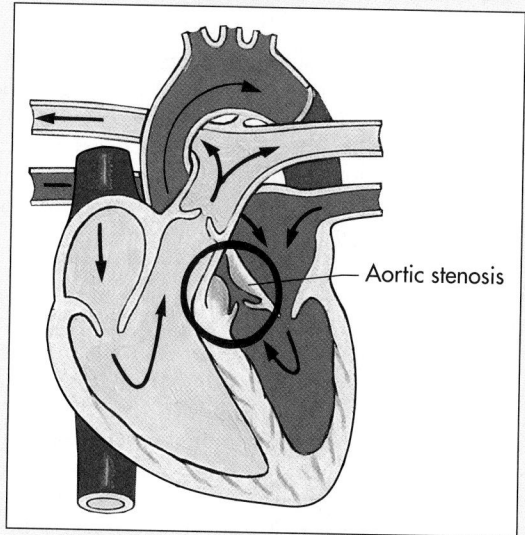

Aortic stenosis

entire left ventricular outflow tract and annulus and replace the aortic valve, an approach known as the *Konno* procedure.

Prognosis: Mortality from surgical repairs of subvalvular AS is less than 5% in major centers; however, about 20% of these patients develop recurrent subaortic stenosis and require additional surgery (Freed, 2001).

PULMONIC STENOSIS (PS)

Description: Narrowing at the entrance to the pulmonary artery. Resistance to blood flow causes right ventricular hypertrophy and decreased pulmonary blood flow. *Pulmonary atresia* is the extreme form of PS in that there is total fusion of the commissures and no blood flows to the lungs. The right ventricle may be hypoplastic.

Pathophysiology: When PS is present, resistance to blood flow causes right ventricular hypertrophy. If right ventricular failure develops, right atrial pressure will increase, and this may result in reopening of the foramen ovale, shunting of unoxygenated blood into the left atrium, and systemic cyanosis. If PS is severe, congestive heart failure (CHF) occurs, and systemic venous engorgement will be noted. An associated defect such as a patent ductus arteriosus (PDA) partially compensates for the obstruction by shunting blood from the aorta to the pulmonary artery and into the lungs.

Clinical manifestations: Patients may be asymptomatic; some have mild cyanosis or CHF. Newborns with severe narrowing will be cyanotic. There is a characteristic murmur. Cardiomegaly is evident on chest x-ray film. Patients are at risk for bacterial endocarditis, with progressive narrowing causing increased symptoms.

Surgical treatment: In infants, transventricular (closed) valvotomy **(Brock)** procedure. In children, pulmonary valvotomy with cardiopulmonary bypass. Need for surgical treatment is uncommon with widespread use of balloon angioplasty techniques (Uzurk, 2001).

Nonsurgical treatment: Balloon angioplasty in the cardiac catheterization laboratory to dilate the valve. A catheter is inserted across the stenotic pulmonic valve into the pulmonary artery, and a balloon at the end of the catheter is inflated and rapidly passed through the narrowed opening (see figure at right). The procedure is associated with few complications and has proved to be highly effective. It is the treatment of choice for discrete PS in most centers and can be done safely in neonates.

Prognosis: Low risk for both procedures; less than 2% mortality. Both balloon dilation and surgical valvotomy leave the pulmonic valve incompetent because they involve opening the fused valve leaflets; however, these patients are clinically asymptomatic. Long-term problems with restenosis or valve incompetence may occur.

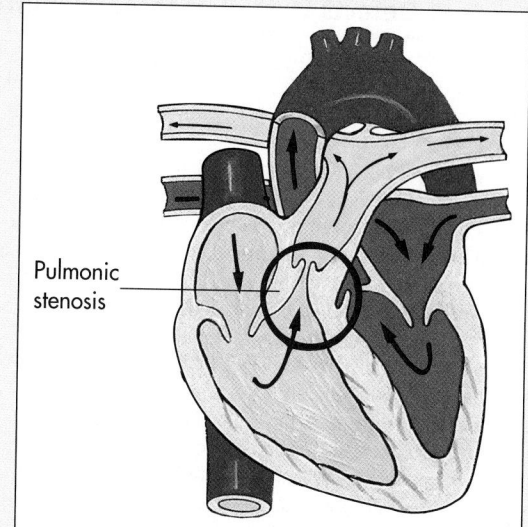

Pulmonic stenosis

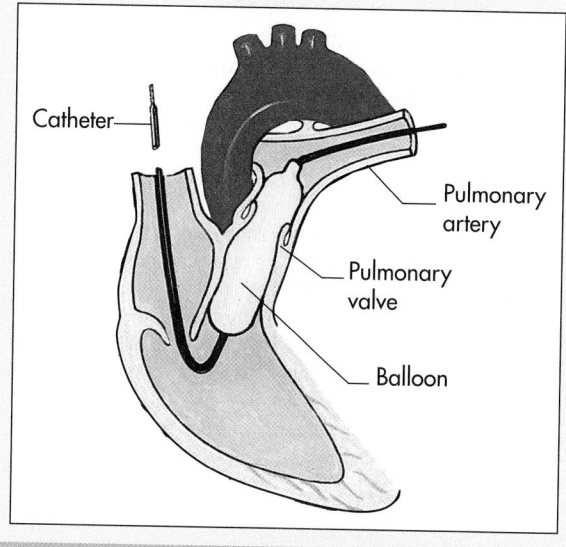

Catheter

Pulmonary artery

Pulmonary valve

Balloon

side of the heart via the pulmonary artery, pressure on the right side increases, exceeding left-sided pressure. This allows desaturated blood to shunt right to left, causing desaturation in the left side of the heart and in the systemic circulation. Clinically, these patients are hypoxemic and usually appear cyanotic. Tetralogy of Fallot and tricuspid atresia are the more common defects in this group (Box 25-3).

MIXED DEFECTS

Many complex cardiac anomalies are classified together in the *mixed* category (Box 25-4) because survival in the postnatal period depends on mixing of blood from the pulmonary and systemic circulations within the heart chambers. Hemodynamically, fully saturated systemic blood flow mixes with the desaturated pulmonary blood flow, causing a relative desaturation of the systemic blood flow. Pulmonary congestion occurs because the differences in pulmonary artery pressure and aortic pressure favor pulmonary blood flow. Cardiac output decreases because of a volume load on the ventricle. Clinically, these patients have a variable picture that combines some degree of desaturation (although cyanosis is not always visible) and signs of CHF.

Some defects, such as transposition of the great arteries, cause severe cyanosis in the first days of life and later cause CHF. Others, such as truncus arteriosus, cause severe CHF in the first weeks of life and mild desaturation.

CLINICAL CONSEQUENCES OF CONGENITAL HEART DISEASE

CONGESTIVE HEART FAILURE

CHF is the inability of the heart to pump an adequate amount of blood to the systemic circulation at normal filling pressures to meet the metabolic demands of the body. In children, CFH most frequently occurs secondary to structural abnormalities (e.g., septal defects) that result in increased blood volume and pressure within the heart. It can also result from myocardial failure in which the contractility of the ventricle is impaired. This can occur with cardiomyopathy, dysrhythmias, or severe electrolyte disturbances. CHF can also occur because of excessive demands on a normal heart muscle, such as in sepsis or severe anemia. *Text continued on p. 906.*

BOX 25-3 ■ Defects With Decreased Pulmonary Blood Flow

TETRALOGY OF FALLOT (TOF)

Description: The classic form includes four defects: (1) ventricular septal defect, (2) pulmonic stenosis, (3) overriding aorta, and (4) right ventricular hypertrophy.

Pathophysiology: The altered hemodynamics vary widely, depending primarily on the degree of pulmonary stenosis, but also on the size of the ventricular septal defect (VSD) and the pulmonary and systemic resistance to flow. Because the VSD is usually large, pressures may be equal in the right and left ventricles. Therefore the shunt direction depends on the difference between pulmonary and systemic vascular resistance. If pulmonary vascular resistance is higher than systemic resistance, the shunt is from right to left. If systemic resistance is higher than pulmonary resistance, the shunt is from left to right. Pulmonic stenosis decreases blood flow to the lungs and, consequently, the amount of oxygenated blood that returns to the left side of the heart. Depending on the position of the aorta, blood from both ventricles may be distributed systemically.

Clinical manifestations:

Infants: Some infants may be acutely cyanotic at birth; others have mild cyanosis that progresses over the first year of life as the pulmonic stenosis worsens. There is a characteristic murmur. There may be acute episodes of cyanosis and hypoxia, called blue spells or tet spells (p. 914). Anoxic spells occur when the infant's oxygen requirements exceed the blood supply, usually during crying or after feeding.

Surgical treatment:

Palliative shunt: In infants who cannot undergo primary repair, a palliative procedure to increase pulmonary blood flow and increase oxygen saturation may be performed. The preferred procedure is the *Blalock-Taussig* or *modified Blalock-Taussig shunt,* which provides blood flow to the pulmonary arteries from the left or right subclavian artery (see Table 25-4). In general, however, shunts are avoided because they may result in pulmonary artery distortion.

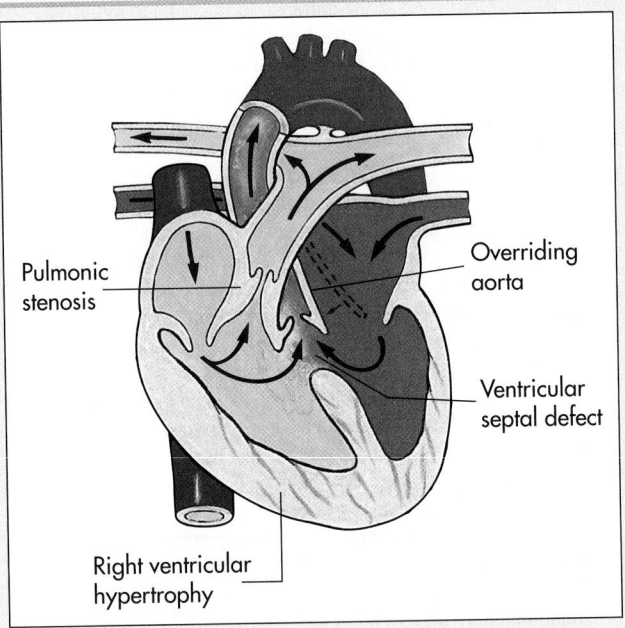

Pulmonic stenosis
Overriding aorta
Ventricular septal defect
Right ventricular hypertrophy

Complete repair: Elective repair is usually performed in the first year of life. Indications for repair include increasing cyanosis and the development of hypercyanotic spells. Complete repair involves closure of the VSD and resection of the infundibular stenosis, with a pericardial patch to enlarge the right ventricular outflow tract. The procedure requires a median sternotomy and the use of cardiopulmonary bypass.

Prognosis: The operative mortality for total correction of TOF is less than 5%. With improved surgical techniques there is a lower incidence of dysrhythmias and sudden death; surgical heart block is rare. Congestive heart failure may occur postoperatively.

BOX 25-3 ■ Defects With Decreased Pulmonary Blood Flow—*cont'd*

TRICUSPID ATRESIA

Description: Failure of the tricuspid valve to develop; consequently, there is no communication from the right atrium to the right ventricle. Blood flows through an atrial septal defect (ASD) or a patent foramen ovale to the left side of the heart and through a VSD to the right ventricle and out to the lungs. It is often associated with pulmonic stenosis and transposition of the great arteries. There is complete mixing of unoxygenated and oxygenated blood in the left side of the heart, resulting in systemic desaturation and varying amounts of pulmonary obstruction, causing decreased pulmonary blood flow.

Pathophysiology: At birth the presence of a patent foramen ovale (or other atrial septal opening) is required to permit blood flow across the septum into the left atrium; the patent ductus arteriosus allows blood flow to the pulmonary artery into the lungs for oxygenation. A VSD allows a modest amount of blood to enter the right ventricle and pulmonary artery for oxygenation. Pulmonary blood flow usually is diminished.

Clinical manifestations: Cyanosis is usually seen in the newborn period. There may be tachycardia and dyspnea. Older children have signs of chronic hypoxemia with clubbing. Patients are at risk for bacterial endocarditis, brain abscess, and stroke.

Therapeutic management: For the neonate whose pulmonary blood flow depends on the patency of the ductus arteriosus, a continuous infusion of prostaglandin E_1 is started until surgical intervention can be arranged.

Surgical treatment: *Palliative* treatment is the placement of a shunt *(pulmonary-to-systemic artery anastomosis)* to increase blood flow to the lungs. If the ASD is small, an atrial septostomy is done during cardiac catheterization. Some children have increased pulmonary blood flow and require *pulmonary artery banding* to lessen the volume of blood to the lungs. A *bidirectional Glenn shunt* (cavopulmonary anastomosis) may be performed at 6 to 9 months as a second stage.

Modified Fontan procedure: Systemic venous return is directed to the lungs without a ventricular pump through surgical connections between the right atrium and the pulmonary artery. A fenestration (opening) in the right atrial baffle is sometimes done to relieve pressure. The patient must have normal ventricular function and a low pulmonary vascular resistance for the procedure to be successful. The modified Fontan procedure separates oxygenated and unoxygenated blood inside the heart and eliminates the excess volume load on the ventricle but does not restore normal anatomy or hemodynamics (O'Brien and Boisvert, 2001).

Prognosis: Surgical mortality varies. It is less than 10% in many centers and increases with more complex anatomy and other risk factors. Postoperative complications include dysrhythmias, systemic venous hypertension, pleural and pericardial effusions, and ventricular dysfunction. Although initial results have been encouraging, long-term survival and morbidity must await future studies.

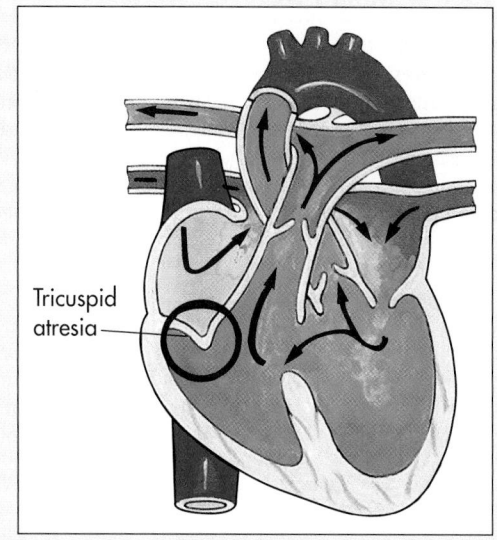

Tricuspid atresia

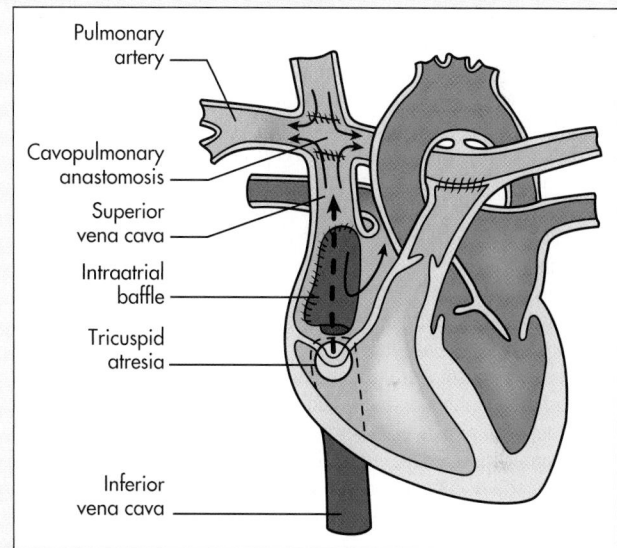

Pulmonary artery
Cavopulmonary anastomosis
Superior vena cava
Intraatrial baffle
Tricuspid atresia
Inferior vena cava

BOX 25-4 ■ Mixed Defects

TRANSPOSITION OF THE GREAT ARTERIES (TGA) OR TRANSPOSITION OF THE GREAT VESSELS (TGV)

Description: The pulmonary artery leaves the left ventricle, and the aorta exits from the right ventricle, with no communication between the systemic and pulmonary circulations.

Pathophysiology: Associated defects such as septal defects or patent ductus arteriosus (PDA) must be present to permit blood to enter the systemic circulation and/or the pulmonary circulation for mixing of saturated and desaturated blood. The most common defect associated with TGA is a patent foramen ovale. At birth there is also a PDA, although in most instances this closes after the neonatal period. Another associated anomaly may be a ventricular septal defect (VSD). The presence of these defects increases the risk of congestive heart failure (CHF), because they often produce high pulmonary blood flow under high pressure. For example, a large VSD permits blood to flow from the right to the left ventricle, into the pulmonary artery, and finally to the lungs. However, it also produces high pulmonary blood flow under high pressure, which can result in pulmonary vascular resistance. The same series of events occurs with a large PDA, because blood directly from the aorta flows under high pressure into the pulmonary artery and lungs.

Continued

BOX 25-4 ■ Mixed Defects—*cont'd*

TRANSPOSITION OF THE GREAT ARTERIES (TGA) OR TRANSPOSITION OF THE GREAT VESSELS (TGV)—*cont'd*

Clinical manifestations: Depend on the type and size of the associated defects. Children with minimum communication are severely cyanotic and depressed at birth. Those with large septal defects or a PDA may be less severely cyanotic but may have symptoms of CHF. Heart sounds vary according to the type of defect present. Cardiomegaly is usually evident a few weeks after birth.

Therapeutic management:

To provide intracardiac mixing: The administration of intravenous prostaglandin E_1 may be initiated to temporarily increase blood mixing if systemic and pulmonary mixing is inadequate to provide an oxygen saturation of 75% or to maintain cardiac output. During cardiac catheterization a balloon atrial septostomy *(Rashkind procedure)* may also be performed to increase mixing and maintain cardiac output over a longer period.

Surgical treatment:

Arterial switch procedure: Procedure of choice performed in first weeks of life. Involves transecting the great arteries and anastomosing the main pulmonary artery to the proximal aorta (just above the aortic valve) and anastomosing the ascending aorta to the proximal pulmonary artery. The coronary arteries are switched from the proximal aorta to the proximal pulmonary artery, creating a new aorta. Reimplantation of the coronary arteries is critical to the infant's survival, and they must be reattached without torsion or kinking to provide the heart with its supply of oxygen. The advantage of the arterial switch procedure is the reestablishment of normal circulation, with the left ventricle acting as the systemic pump. Potential complications of the arterial switch include narrowing at the great artery anastomoses or coronary artery insufficiency.

Intraatrial baffle repairs: Intraatrial baffle repairs are rarely performed, although many adolescents and adults survive today with repairs that were done 10 to 25 years ago. An intraatrial baffle is created to divert venous blood to the mitral valve and pulmonary venous blood to the tricuspid valve using the patient's atrial septum *(Senning procedure)* or a

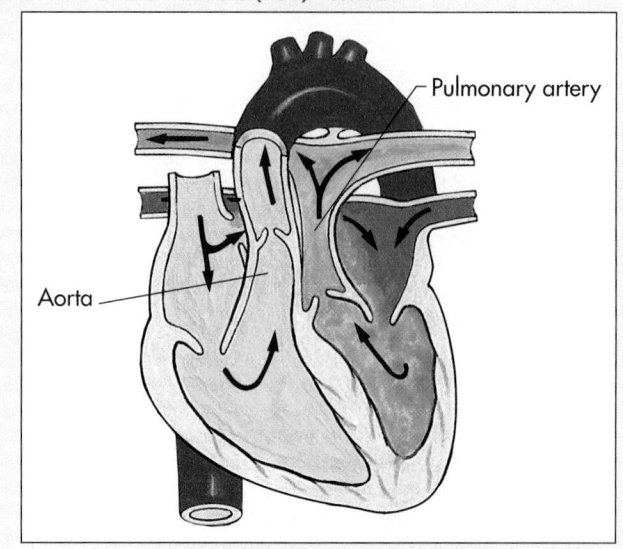

prosthetic material *(Mustard procedure).* They are performed in the first year of life. A disadvantage is the continuing role of the right ventricle as the systemic pump and the late development of right ventricular failure and rhythm disturbances. Other potential postoperative complications include loss of normal sinus rhythm, baffle leaks, and ventricular dysfunction.

Rastelli procedure: Operative choice in infants with TGA, VSD, and severe pulmonic stenosis (PS). It involves closure of the VSD with a baffle, directing left ventricular blood through the VSD into the aorta. The pulmonic valve is then closed, and a conduit is placed from the right ventricle to the pulmonary artery, creating a physiologically normal circulation. Unfortunately, this procedure requires multiple conduit replacements as the child grows.

Prognosis: Operative mortality is about 5% to 10% with all procedures; with atrial level repairs, there is a later risk of dysrhythmias and ventricular dysfunction.

TOTAL ANOMALOUS PULMONARY VENOUS CONNECTION (TAPVC)

Description: Rare defect characterized by failure of the pulmonary veins to join the left atrium. Instead, the pulmonary veins are abnormally connected to the systemic venous circuit via the right atrium or various veins draining toward the right atrium, such as the superior vena cava. The abnormal attachment results in mixed blood being returned to the right atrium and shunted from the right to the left through an atrial septal defect (ASD). The type of TAPVC is classified according to the pulmonary venous point of attachment as:

Supracardiac—Attachment above the diaphragm, such as to the superior vena cava (most common form)

Cardiac—Direct attachment to the heart, such as to the right atrium or coronary sinus

Infracardiac—Attachment below the diaphragm, such as to the inferior vena cava (most severe form)

TAPVC is also called total anomalous pulmonary venous return (TAPVR) or total anomalous pulmonary venous drainage (TAPVD).

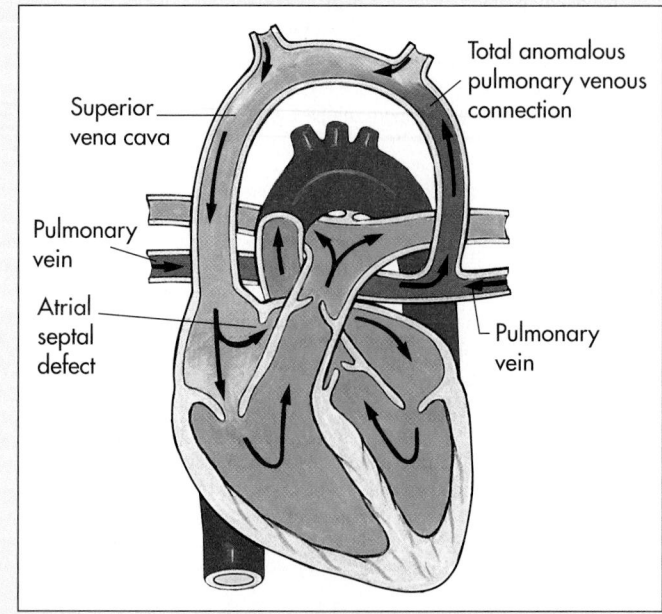

BOX 25-4 ■ Mixed Defects—*cont'd*

TOTAL ANOMALOUS PULMONARY VENOUS CONNECTION (TAPVC)

Pathophysiology: The right atrium receives all the blood that normally would flow into the left atrium. As a result, the right side of the heart hypertrophies, whereas the left side, especially the left atrium, may remain small. An associated ASD or patent foramen ovale allows systemic venous blood to shunt from the higher pressure right atrium to the left atrium and into the left side of the heart. As a result, the oxygen saturation of the blood in both sides of the heart (and ultimately, in the systemic arterial circulation) is the same. If the pulmonary blood flow is large, pulmonary venous return is also large and the amount of saturated blood is relatively high. However, if there is obstruction to pulmonary venous drainage, pulmonary venous return is impeded, pulmonary venous pressure rises, and pulmonary interstitial edema develops and eventually contributes to CHF. Infracardiac TAPVC is often associated with obstruction to pulmonary venous drainage and is a surgical emergency.

Clinical manifestations: Most infants develop cyanosis early in life. The degree of cyanosis is inversely related to the amount of pulmonary blood flow—the more pulmonary blood, the less cyanosis. Children with unobstructed TAPVC may be asymptomatic until pulmonary vascular resistance decreases during infancy, increasing pulmonary blood flow, with resulting signs of CHF. Cyanosis becomes worse with pulmonary vein obstruction; after obstruction occurs, the infant's condition usually deteriorates rapidly. Without intervention, cardiac failure will progress to death.

Surgical treatment: Corrective repair in early infancy. The surgical approach varies with the anatomic defect. In general, however, the common pulmonary vein is anastomosed to the left atrium, the ASD is closed, and the anomalous pulmonary venous connection is ligated. The cardiac type is most easily repaired; the infracardiac type has the highest morbidity and mortality because of the higher incidence of pulmonary vein obstruction. Potential postoperative complications include reobstruction; bleeding; dysrhythmias, particularly heart block; pulmonary artery hypertension; and persistent heart failure.

Prognosis: The cardiac type has a surgical mortality of less than 5%; morbidity and mortality are greater with the other types and increase with the presence of pulmonary vein obstruction.

TRUNCUS ARTERIOSUS (TA)

Description: Failure of normal septation and division of the embryonic bulbar trunk into the pulmonary artery and the aorta, resulting in a single vessel that overrides both ventricles. Blood from both ventricles mixes in the common great artery, causing desaturation and hypoxemia. Blood ejected from the heart flows preferentially to the lower pressure pulmonary arteries, causing increased pulmonary blood flow and reduced systemic blood flow. There are three types:

Type I—A single pulmonary trunk arises near the base of the truncus and divides into the left and right pulmonary arteries.

Type II—The left and right pulmonary arteries arise separately but in close proximity and at the same level from the back of the truncus.

Type III—The pulmonary arteries arise independently from the sides of the truncus.

Pathophysiology: Blood ejected from the left and right ventricles enters the common trunk, mixing pulmonary and systemic circulations. Blood flow is distributed to the pulmonary and systemic circulations according to the relative resistances of each system. The amount of pulmonary blood flow depends on the size of the pulmonary arteries and the pulmonary vascular resistance. Generally, resistance to pulmonary blood flow is less than systemic vascular resistance, resulting in preferential blood flow to the lungs. Pulmonary vascular disease develops at an early age in patients with truncus arteriosus.

Clinical manifestations: Most infants are symptomatic with moderate to severe CHF and variable cyanosis, poor growth, and activity intolerance. There is a characteristic murmur.

Surgical treatment: Early repair in the first few months of life. Corrective repair involves closing the VSD so that the truncus arteriosus receives the outflow from the left ventricle, excising the pulmonary arteries from the aorta, and attaching them to the right

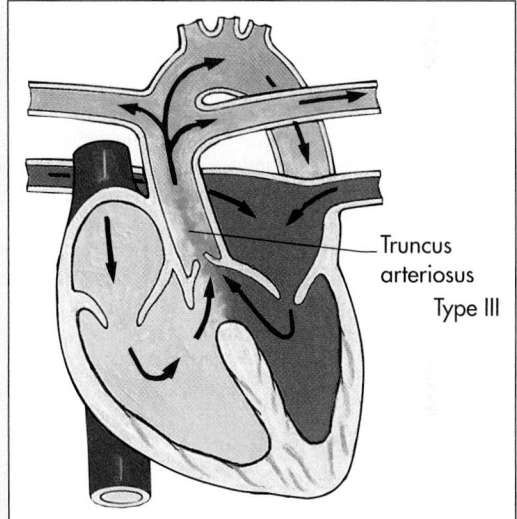

Truncus
arteriosus
Type III

ventricle by means of a homograft. Homografts (segments of cadaver aorta and pulmonary artery that are treated with antibiotics and cryopreserved) are preferred over synthetic conduits to establish continuity between the right ventricle and pulmonary artery. Homografts are more flexible and easier to use during the procedure and appear less prone to obstruction. Postoperative complications include persistent heart failure, bleeding, pulmonary artery hypertension, dysrhythmias, and residual VSD. These children require additional procedures to replace the conduit as its size becomes inadequate in relation to the children's growth.

Prognosis: Mortality is greater than 10%; future operations are required to replace the conduits.

Continued

BOX 25-4 ■ Mixed Defects—*cont'd*

HYPOPLASTIC LEFT HEART SYNDROME (HLHS)

Description: Underdevelopment of the left side of the heart, resulting in a hypoplastic left ventricle and aortic atresia. Most blood from the left atrium flows across the patent foramen ovale to the right atrium, to the right ventricle, and out the pulmonary artery. The descending aorta receives blood from the patent ductus arteriosus supplying systemic blood flow (O'Brien and Boisvert, 2001).

Pathophysiology: An ASD or patent foramen ovale allows saturated blood from the left atrium to mix with desaturated blood from the right atrium, and to flow through the right ventricle and out into the pulmonary artery. From the pulmonary artery the blood flows to the lungs, then through the ductus arteriosus into the aorta and out to the body. The amount of blood flow to the pulmonary and systemic circulations depends on the relationship between the pulmonary and systemic vascular resistances. The coronary and cerebral vessels receive blood by retrograde flow through the hypoplastic ascending aorta.

Clinical manifestations: Patients are usually symptomatic in the first week of life with cyanosis and CHF when the PDA starts to close with progressive deterioration and decreased cardiac output, leading to cardiovascular collapse. It is usually fatal in the first months of life without intervention.

Therapeutic management: Neonates require stabilization with mechanical ventilation and inotropic support preoperatively. A prostaglandin E₁ infusion is needed to maintain ductal patency, ensuring adequate systemic blood flow.

Surgical treatment: Several-staged approach. First stage is ***Norwood procedure:*** Anastomosis of the main pulmonary artery to the aorta to create a new aorta, placement of a shunt or inserting a conduit from the right ventricle to pulmonary artery to provide pulmonary blood flow, and creation of a large ASD. Postoperative complications include imbalance of systemic and pulmonary blood flow, bleeding, low cardiac output, and persistent heart failure. The second stage is often a ***bidirectional Glenn shunt*** done at 6 to 9 months of age to relieve cyanosis

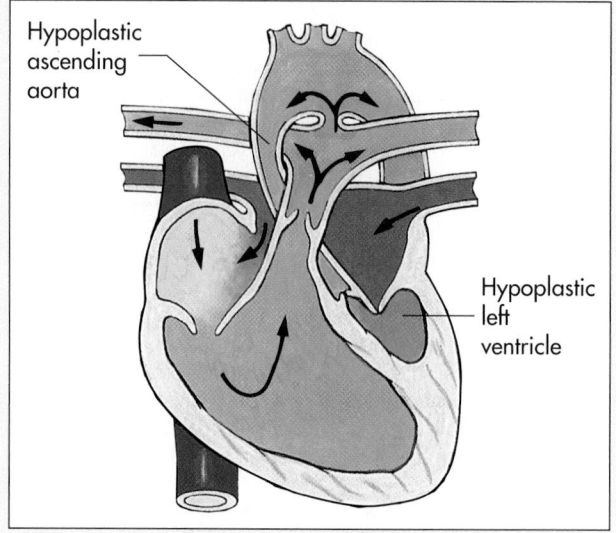

Hypoplastic ascending aorta

Hypoplastic left ventricle

and reduce the volume load on the right ventricle. The final repair is a ***modified Fontan procedure*** (see Tricuspid Atresia in Box 25-3).

Transplantation: Some programs believe that heart transplantation in the newborn period is the best option for these infants. Problems include the shortage of newborn organ donors, risk of rejection, long-term problems with chronic immunosuppression, and infection (see Heart Transplantation, p. 929).

Prognosis: Mortality risks of more than 25% with both surgery and transplantation. Results vary widely in different centers. This may improve in the future. Because of the high-risk nature of both surgical palliation and neonatal heart transplantation, some cardiologists continue to recommend no treatment for this defect.

Pathophysiology

Heart failure is often separated into two categories: right-sided and left-sided failure. In *right-sided failure* the right ventricle is unable to pump blood effectively into the pulmonary artery, resulting in increased pressure in the right atrium and systemic venous circulation. Systemic venous hypertension causes hepatosplenomegaly and occasionally edema. In *left-sided failure* the left ventricle is unable to pump blood into the systemic circulation, resulting in increased pressure in the left atrium and pulmonary veins. The lungs become congested with blood, causing elevated pulmonary pressures and pulmonary edema.

Although each type of heart failure produces different signs and symptoms, clinically it is unusual to observe solely right- or left-sided failure in children. Because each side of the heart depends on adequate function of the other side, failure of one chamber causes a reciprocal change in the opposite chamber.

If the abnormalities precipitating CHF are not corrected, the heart muscle becomes damaged. Despite compensatory mechanisms, the heart is unable to maintain an adequate cardiac output. Decreased blood flow to the kidneys continues to stimulate sodium and water reabsorption, leading to fluid overload, increased workload on the heart, and congestion in the pulmonary and systemic circulations (Fig. 25-6).

The signs and symptoms of CHF can be divided into three groups: (1) impaired myocardial function, (2) pulmonary congestion, and (3) systemic venous congestion (Box 25-5). Because these hemodynamic changes occur from different causes and at differing times, the clinical presentation may vary among children.

Diagnostic Evaluation

Diagnosis is made on the basis of clinical symptoms such as tachypnea and tachycardia at rest, dyspnea, retractions, activity intolerance (especially during feeding in infants), weight gain caused by fluid retention, and hepatomegaly. A chest x-ray film demonstrates cardiomegaly and increased pulmonary blood flow. Ventricular hypertrophy appears on the ECG. An echocardiogram is done to determine the cause of CHF such as a congenital heart defect or poor ventricular function.

Therapeutic Management

The goals of treatment are to (1) improve cardiac function (increase contractility and decrease afterload), (2) remove accumulated fluid and sodium (decrease preload), (3) de-

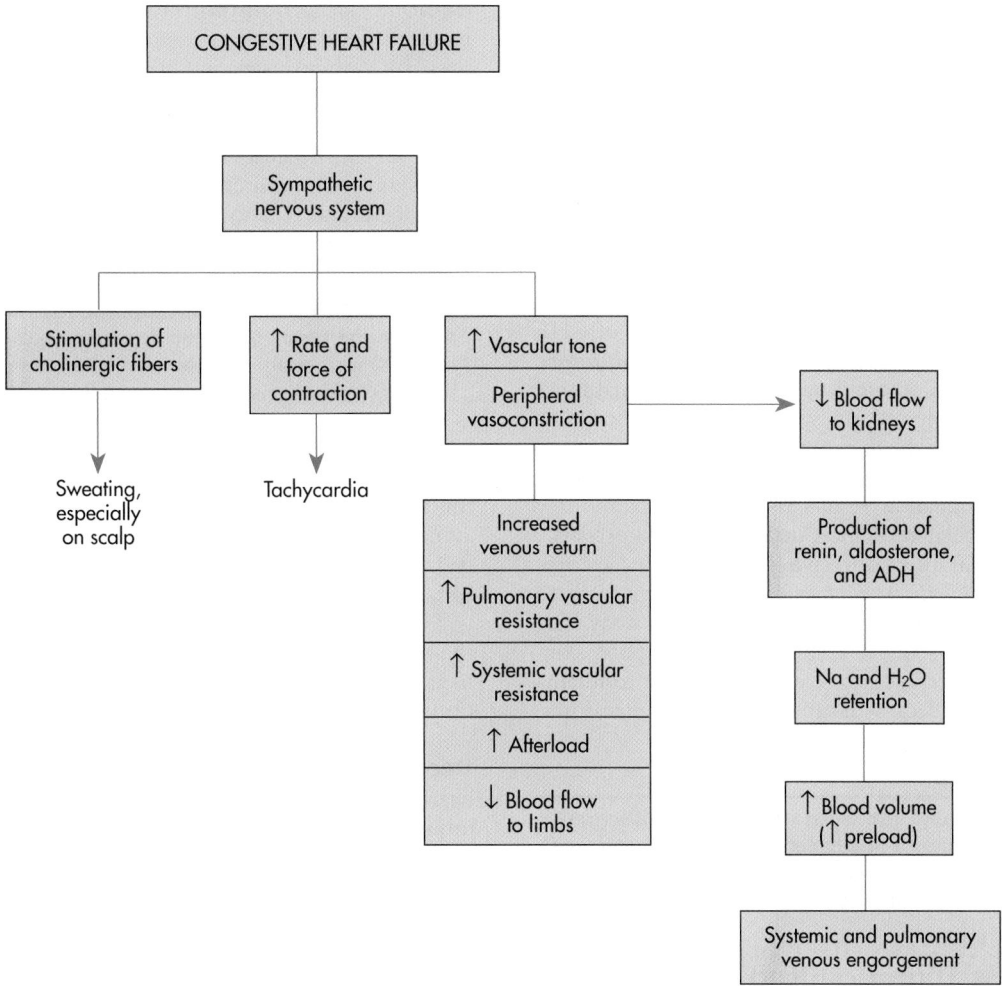

FIG. 25-6 ■ Pathophysiology of congestive heart failure.

BOX 25-5 ■ Clinical Manifestations of Congestive Heart Failure

IMPAIRED MYOCARDIAL FUNCTION	PULMONARY CONGESTION	SYSTEMIC VENOUS CONGESTION
Tachycardia	Tachypnea	Weight gain
Sweating (inappropriate)	Dyspnea	Hepatomegaly
Decreased urine output	Retractions (infants)	Peripheral edema, especially periorbital
Fatigue	Flaring nares	Ascites
Weakness	Exercise intolerance	Neck vein distention (children)
Restlessness	Orthopnea	
Anorexia	Cough, hoarseness	
Pale, cool extremities	Cyanosis	
Weak peripheral pulses	Wheezing	
Decreased blood pressure	Grunting	
Gallop rhythm		
Cardiomegaly		

crease cardiac demands, and (4) improve tissue oxygenation and decrease oxygen consumption. For most infants diagnosed with CHF, the cause is CHD. Infants are stabilized on medical therapy and then referred for surgical repair. For children newly diagnosed with CHF, the cause may be worsening ventricular function after a previous cardiac repair, cardiomyopathy, arrhythmia, or other causes. In addition to management of CHF, the underlying cause is treated if possible.

Improve Cardiac Function. Myocardial efficiency is improved through administration of digitalis glycosides. The beneficial effects are increased cardiac output, decreased heart size, decreased venous pressure, and relief of edema. In pediatrics, *digoxin (Lanoxin)* is used almost exclusively because of its more rapid onset. It is available as an elixir (0.05 mg/mL) for oral administration. For infants the dose is calculated in micrograms (1000 μg = 1 mg).

Treatment consists of a digitalizing dose, given orally or intravenously in divided doses over 24 hours to produce optimal cardiac effects, and a maintenance dose, given orally twice a day to maintain blood levels. During digitalization the child is monitored by means of an ECG to observe for the desired effects (prolonged P-R interval and reduced ventricular rate) and detect side effects, especially dysrhythmias.

A newer group of drugs used in the treatment of CHF are the *angiotensin-converting enzyme (ACE) inhibitors.* As their name implies, these drugs inhibit the normal function of the renin-angiotensin system in the kidney. The ACE inhibitors block the conversion of angiotensin I to angiotensin II so that, instead of vasoconstriction, vasodilation occurs. Vasodilation results in decreased pulmonary and systemic vascular resistance, decreased blood pressure, and a reduction in afterload. Two ACE inhibitors are frequently used in pediatrics: *captopril (Capoten),* given three times a day, and *enalapril (Vasotec),* given twice a day. The principal side effects of ACE inhibitors are hypotension, cough, and renal dysfunction. Captopril is given to infants and young children because it can be given in smaller doses.

> **NURSING ALERT**
>
> Because ACE inhibitors also block the action of aldosterone, the addition of potassium supplements or spironolactone (Aldactone) to the drug regimen of patients taking diuretics is usually not needed and may cause hyperkalemia.

Remove Accumulated Fluid and Sodium. Treatment consists of diuretics, possible fluid restriction, and possible sodium restriction. Diuretics are the mainstay of therapy to eliminate excess water and salt to prevent reaccumulation. The most frequently used agents are listed in Table 25-3. Because furosemide and the thiazides are potassium-losing diuretics, potassium supplements may be prescribed, and rich sources of the electrolyte are encouraged in the diet.

> **NURSING ALERT**
>
> A fall in the serum potassium level enhances the effects of digitalis, increasing the risk of digoxin toxicity. Therefore serum potassium levels must be carefully monitored.

Fluid restriction may be required in the acute states of CHF and must be carefully calculated to avoid dehydrating the child, especially if cyanotic CHD and significant polycythemia are present. Infants rarely need fluid restrictions because CHF makes feeding so difficult that they struggle to take maintenance fluids.

Sodium-restricted diets are used less often in children than in adults to control CHF because of their potential negative effects on appetite. If salt intake is restricted, additional table salt and highly salted foods are avoided.

Decrease Cardiac Demands. The workload on the heart is reduced when metabolic needs are kept to a minimum. This is accomplished by limiting physical activity (bed rest), preserving body temperature, treating any infections, reducing the effort of breathing (semi-Fowler position), and using medication to sedate an irritable child.

TABLE 25-3 ■ Diuretics Used in Congestive Heart Failure

ACTIONS	COMMENTS	NURSING CONSIDERATIONS
FUROSEMIDE (LASIX)		
Blocks reabsorption of sodium and water in proximal renal tubule and interferes with reabsorption of sodium	Drug of choice in severe congestive heart failure (CHF) Causes excretion of chloride and potassium (hypokalemia may precipitate digitalis toxicity)	Begin to record output as soon as drug is given Observe for dehydration caused by profound diuresis Observe for side effects (nausea and vomiting, diarrhea, ototoxicity, hypokalemia, dermatitis, postural hypotension) Encourage foods high in potassium and/or give potassium supplements Monitor chloride and acid-base balance with long-term therapy Observe for signs of digoxin toxicity
CHLOROTHIAZIDE (DIURIL)		
Acts directly on distal tubules to decrease sodium, water, potassium, chloride, and bicarbonate absorption	Less frequently used drug Causes hypokalemia, acidosis from large doses	Observe for side effects (nausea, weakness, dizziness, paresthesia, muscle cramps, skin eruptions, hypokalemia, acidosis) Encourage foods high in potassium and/or give potassium supplements
SPIRONOLACTONE (ALDACTONE)		
Blocks action of aldosterone, which promotes retention of sodium and excretion of potassium	Weak diuretic Has potassium-sparing effect; frequently used with thiazides, furosemide Poorly absorbed from gastrointestinal tract Takes several days to achieve maximum actions	Observe for side effects (skin rash, drowsiness, ataxia, hyperkalemia) Do not administer potassium supplements

Improve Tissue Oxygenation.   All of the preceding measures serve to increase tissue oxygenation, either by improving myocardial function or by lessening tissue oxygen demands. In addition, supplemental cool humidified oxygen may be administered to increase the amount of available oxygen during inspiration. Oxygen administration is especially helpful in patients with pulmonary edema, intercurrent respiratory infections, and increased pulmonary vascular resistance (oxygen is a vasodilator that decreases pulmonary vascular resistance).

> **⚠ NURSING ALERT**
>
> Oxygen is a drug and is administered only with an appropriate order. There are some uncommon circumstances in patients with complex hemodynamics in which oxygen can be detrimental.

An oxygen hood is preferred with young infants to provide increased concentration of the gas. A nasal cannula or face tent may be useful with older infants and children. Nasal cannulas are ideal for long-term oxygen administration because the child can be ambulatory and can easily eat and drink. Cool humidification is necessary to counteract the drying effect of oxygen. The amount of cool humidity is carefully regulated to prevent chilling.

Nursing Considerations

The infant or child with CHF is usually admitted to the hospital where intensive nursing care is available. The child is positioned for optimal ventilation and administered oxygen by the most effective means, IV access is established, and cardiac and respiratory function is monitored continuously using a cardiac monitor and pulse oximeter to monitor oxygen saturation. Urine output and serum electrolytes are evaluated frequently.

● Assessment

Nurses need to be alert to signs of CHF in infants and children with suspected or known congenital defects. Signs of CHF indicate a worsening clinical condition; the earlier they are detected, the sooner treatment can be begun.

● Nursing Diagnoses

Several nursing diagnoses are identified after a thorough assessment. Some of these are included in the Nursing Care Plan on pp. 913-914. Others may become apparent in special circumstances and with children in different age-groups.

● Planning

The goals for the infant or child with CHF and the family are as follows:

1 Child will exhibit improved cardiac output.
2 Child will experience decreased cardiac demands.
3 Child will exhibit improved respiratory function.
4 Child will maintain adequate nutritional status.
5 Child will exhibit no evidence of fluid excess.
6 Child and family will receive adequate support and education.

● Implementation

Although the objectives of nursing care are the same, interventions for infants differ from those for older children.

Assist in Measures to Improve Cardiac Function. The nurse's responsibility in administering digoxin includes observing for signs of toxicity, calculating and administering the correct dosage, and instituting parental teaching regarding drug administration at home. The child's apical pulse is always checked before administering digoxin. As a general rule, the drug is not given if the pulse is below 90 to 110 beats/min in infants and young children or below 70 beats/min in older children (the cutoff point for adults is 60). However, because the pulse rate varies in children in different age-groups, the written drug order should specify at what heart rate the drug is withheld. The nurse should also use judgment in evaluating the pulse rate. If it is significantly lower than the previous recording, the dose should be withheld until the practitioner is notified.

The apical rate is taken because a pulse deficit (radial pulse rate lower than apical) may be present with decreased cardiac output. It is auscultated for 1 full minute to evaluate alterations in rhythm. If the child is monitored by means of an ECG, a rhythm strip is obtained and attached to the chart for rate and rhythm analysis, such as abnormal lengthening of the P-R interval (more than a 50% increase over predigitalization interval) and dysrhythmias.

Digoxin is a potentially dangerous drug because the margin of safety of therapeutic, toxic, and lethal doses is very narrow. Many toxic responses are extensions of its therapeutic effects. Therefore the nurse must maintain a high index of suspicion for signs of toxicity when administering digoxin (Box 25-6).

Because digoxin toxicity can occur from accidental overdose, great care must be taken in properly calculating and measuring the dosage. When converting milligrams to micrograms to milliliters, the nurse carefully checks the placement of the decimal point, because an error causes a significant change in dosage. For example, 0.1 mg is 10 times the dosage of 0.01 mg.

> **⚠ NURSING ALERT**
>
> Infants rarely receive more than 1 mL (50 μg or 0.05 mg) in one dose; a higher dose is an immediate warning of a dosage error. To ensure safety, compare the calculation with another staff member's calculation before giving the drug.

These same principles are taught to parents in preparation for discharge, although the correct dose in milliliters is usually specified on the container, thus reducing potential errors in calculation. The nurse watches the parent measure the elixir in the dropper and stresses the level mark as the meniscus of the fluid that is observed at eye level. Other instructions for administering digoxin are listed in the Family Home Care box and the Critical Thinking Exercise.

Parents are also advised of the signs of toxicity. According to the practitioner's preference, they may be taught to

BOX 25-6 ■ Common Signs of Digoxin Toxicity in Children

GASTROINTESTINAL	CARDIAC
Nausea	Bradycardia
Vomiting	Dysrhythmias
Anorexia	

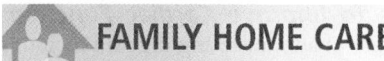

FAMILY HOME CARE

Administering Digoxin

Give digoxin at regular intervals, usually every 12 hours, such as 8 AM and 8 PM.

Plan the times so that the drug is given 1 hour before or 2 hours after feedings.

Use a calendar to mark off each dose that is given, or post a reminder, such as a sign on the refrigerator.

Have the prescription refilled before the medication is completely used.

Administer the drug carefully by slowly directing it on the side and back of the mouth.

Do not mix it with other foods or fluids, because refusal to consume these results in inaccurate intake of the drug.

If the child has teeth, give water after administering the drug; whenever possible, brush the teeth to prevent tooth decay from the sweetened liquid.

If a dose is missed and more than 4 hours has elapsed, withhold the dose and give the next dose at the regular time; if less than 4 hours has elapsed, give the missed dose.

If the child vomits, do not give a second dose.

If more than two consecutive doses have been missed, notify the practitioner.

Do not increase or double the dose for missed doses.

If the child becomes ill, notify the practitioner immediately.

Keep digoxin in a safe place, preferably a locked cabinet.

In case of accidental overdose of digoxin, call the nearest Poison Control Center immediately; the number is usually listed in the front of the telephone directory,

take the pulse before giving the drug. A return demonstration of the procedure from both parents or other principal caregiver is included as part of the teaching plan. Their level of anxiety in counting the pulse is assessed, because overconcern about the heart rate may result in excessive withholding of the drug.

Afterload reduction. For patients receiving ACE inhibitors for afterload reduction, the nurse should carefully monitor blood pressure before and after dose administration, observe for symptoms of hypotension, and notify the practitioner if blood pressure is low. Numerous medications affecting the kidney can potentiate renal dysfunction, so children taking multiple diuretics and an ACE inhibitor require careful assessment of serum electrolytes and renal function.

Decrease Cardiac Demands.
The infant requires rest and conservation of energy for feeding. Every effort is made to organize nursing activities to allow for uninterrupted periods of sleep. Whenever possible, parents are encouraged to stay with their infant to provide the holding, rocking, and cuddling that help children sleep more soundly. To minimize disturbing the infant, changing bed linen and complete bathing are done only when necessary. Feeding is planned to accommodate the infant's sleep and wake patterns. The child is fed when hungry, such as when sucking on fists rather than when crying for a bottle, because the stress of crying exhausts the limited energy supply. Because infants with CHF tire easily and may sleep through feed-

ings, smaller feedings every 3 hours may be helpful. Gavage feedings may be instituted to provide adequate nutrition and allow the infant to rest.

Every effort is made to minimize unnecessary stress. Older children need an explanation of what is happening to them to decrease anxiety about their illness and necessary treatments such as cardiac monitoring, oxygen administration, and medications. Outlining a plan for the day, preparing the child for tests and procedures, providing quiet activities, and providing adequate rest periods are all helpful interventions with older children. Some infants and children require sedation during the acute phase of illness to allow them to rest (Smith, 2001).

Temperature is carefully monitored because hyperthermia or hypothermia increases the need for oxygen. Febrile states are reported to the physician, because infection must be promptly treated. Maintaining body temperature is of special importance in children who are receiving cool, humidified oxygen and in infants who tend to be diaphoretic and lose heat by way of evaporation.

Skin breakdown from edema is prevented with a change of position every 2 hours (from side to side while in semi-Fowler position) and use of a pressure-relieving mattress or bed. The skin, especially over the sacrum, is checked for evidence of redness from pressure.

Reduce Respiratory Distress.
Careful assessment, positioning, and oxygen administration can reduce respiratory distress. Respirations are counted for 1 full minute during a resting state. Any evidence of increased respiratory distress is reported, because this may indicate worsening CHF.

Infants are positioned to encourage maximum chest expansion, with the head of the bed elevated; they should sit up in an infant seat or be held at a 45-degree angle. Children prefer to sleep on several pillows and remain in a semi-Fowler or high-Fowler position during waking hours. Shirts and diapers are pinned loosely to allow maximum chest expansion. Safety restraints, such as those used with infant seats, are applied low on the abdomen and loosely enough to provide both safety and maximum expansion.

The infant or child is often given humidified supplemental oxygen via oxygen hood or tent, nasal cannula, or mask. The child's response to oxygen therapy is carefully evaluated by noting respiratory rate, ease of respiration, color, and especially oxygen saturations, as measured by oximetry.

Respiratory infections can exacerbate CHF and should be appropriately treated and prevented if possible. The child should be protected from persons with respiratory infections and have a noninfectious roommate. With an older child, it is advantageous to choose a roommate who is also confined to bed and relatively quiet to promote a restful environment. Good handwashing is practiced before and after caring for any hospitalized child. Antibiotics may be given to combat respiratory infection. The nurse ensures that the drug is given at equally divided times over a 24-hour schedule to maintain high blood levels of the antibiotic.

Maintain Nutritional Status.
Meeting the nutritional needs of infants with CHF or serious cardiac defects is a nursing challenge. The metabolic rate of these infants is greater because of poor cardiac function and increased heart

??? CRITICAL THINKING EXERCISE ???

Digoxin Toxicity

You are visiting a 3-month-old infant at home who began receiving digoxin and Lasix (furosemide) 5 days ago for management of CHF. A brief assessment indicates that the infant the infant appears well but is not very active, has a weak suck reflex, and does not exhibit much spontaneous movement during interaction with the mother. The mother mentions that the infant is a good baby and does not cry much except when he is very hungry. She also mentions that he vomited several times yesterday and vomited twice this morning; this was not perceived as unusual because her 3-year-old did the same thing and was diagnosed with gastroesophageal reflux. Further assessment of the infant reveals an irregular heartbeat of 86 to 104 beats/min at rest, and the heart rhythm is also noted to be irregular. No murmur or other significant sounds are auscultated.

QUESTIONS

1. Evidence—Is there sufficient evidence to draw conclusions about this infant?
2. Assumptions—Describe an underlying assumption about each of the following:
   a. Side effects of Lasix (furosemide)
   b. Side effects of digoxin
   c. Infants with CHF
3. What priorities for nursing care should be established for this infant?
4. Does the evidence support your nursing interventions?
5. What alternative perspectives might you have?

ANSWERS

1. Yes. The infant has been vomiting since yesterday and has an irregular heartbeat.
2. a. Lasix is a diuretic that is a mainstay of therapy to eliminate excess water and salt to prevent reaccumulation of fluid. Side effects can include nausea and vomiting, diarrhea, ototoxicity, hypokalemia, and postural hypotension.
   b. Digoxin is a potentially dangerous drug because the margin of safety of therapeutic, toxic, and lethal doses is very narrow. Common signs of digoxin toxicity are bradycardia, anorexia, nausea, and vomiting. Dysrhythmias can occur with digoxin toxicity. The dose of digoxin must be calculated exactly.
   c. The goals of treatment for CHF are to improve cardiac output, remove excess fluid and stabilize the sodium level, decrease cardiac demands and improve tissue oxygenation, and decrease oxygen consumption. Digoxin is used because of its rapid onset and decreased risk of toxicity as a result of a relative short half-life compared with other digitalis preparations.
3. The home health nurse should notify the health care provider of the findings before giving digoxin. The assessment reveals a slow, irregular heartbeat and intermittent vomiting. These are common signs of digoxin toxicity in infants. Because the medication was started only 5 days ago, digoxin toxicity should be a major concern. Because Lasix (furosemide) is a non–potassium-sparing diuretic, a concomitant problem with the vomiting is hypokalemia, which is a common finding in children with CHF, Lasix administration, and vomiting. This should also be further evaluated at this visit.
4. Yes. The implications of the assessment are essential because the margin of safety for digoxin blood levels is narrow. Continuing to give the digoxin can cause a toxic reaction. Further evaluation is important.
5. Vomiting in a young child is a concern, but with a history of CHD and digoxin therapy, the first priority is to evaluate for digoxin toxicity. As noted above, hypokalemia is also a concern. The vomiting may cause fluid loss above that for which the infant is able to compensate, and the possibility of mild dehydration should be evaluated.

---

and respiratory rates. Their caloric needs are greater than those of the average infant because of their increased metabolic rate, yet their ability to take in adequate calories is hampered by their fatigue (Smith, 2001). Feeding for a fragile infant with serious CHD is similar to exercise in an adult, and these infants often do not have the energy or cardiac reserve to do extra work. The nurse seeks measures to enable the infant to feed easily without excess fatigue and to increase the caloric density of the formula.

The infant should be well rested before feeding and fed soon after awakening so as not to expend energy on crying. A 3-hour feeding schedule works well for many infants. (Feeding every 2 hours does not provide enough rest between feedings, and a 4-hour schedule requires an increased volume of feeding, which many infants are unable to take.) The feeding schedule should be individualized to the infant's needs. A soft preemie nipple or a slit in a regular nipple to enlarge the opening decreases the energy expenditure of the infant while sucking. Infants should be well supported and fed in a semiupright position. The infant may need to rest frequently and may need to have the jaw and cheeks stroked to encourage sucking. Generally, giving an infant about a half hour to complete a feeding is reasonable. Prolonging the feeding time can exhaust the infant and decrease the rest period between feedings.

Infants with feeding difficulties are often gavage fed using a nasogastric tube to supplement their oral intake and ensure adequate calories. If they are very stressed and fatigued, in respiratory distress, or tachypneic to 80 to 100 breaths/min, oral feedings may be withheld and all nutrition given by gavage feedings. Gavage feedings are usually a temporary measure until the infant's medical status improves and nutritional needs can be met through oral feedings. Some infants with severe CHF, neurologic deficits, or significant gastroesophageal reflux may need placement of a gastrostomy tube to allow adequate nutrition.

Increasing the caloric density of formulas by concentration and then adding corn oil, medium-chain triglycerides

(MCT oil), or Polycose is frequently done. Infant formulas provide 20 calories per ounce, and the use of additives can increase the calories to 30 calories or more per ounce. This allows the infant to obtain more calories despite a smaller volume intake of formula. The caloric density of the formula needs to be increased slowly (by two calories per ounce per day) to prevent diarrhea or formula intolerance. Breast-feeding mothers are encouraged to provide the infant with alternating feedings of breast milk and high-calorie formulas. Some lactating mothers will prefer to feed the child expressed breast milk that has been fortified with Similac or Enfamil powder, Polycose, or corn oil to increase caloric intake. A supplemental nurser may also be helpful. A diet plan specific to the individual infant's needs is calculated and prescribed by the nutritionist in collaboration with the other health personnel. The nurse needs to reinforce this information with the parents as necessary.

Assist in Measures to Promote Fluid Loss. When diuretics are given, the nurse records fluid intake and output and monitors body weight at the same time each day to evaluate benefit from the drug. Because profound diuresis may cause dehydration and electrolyte imbalance (loss of sodium, potassium, chloride, bicarbonate), the nurse observes for signs indicating either complication, as well as signs and symptoms suggesting reactions to the drugs. Diuretics should be given early in the day to children who are toilet trained to avoid the need to urinate at night. If potassium-losing diuretics are given, the nurse encourages foods high in potassium, such as bananas, oranges, whole grains, legumes, and leafy vegetables, and administers prescribed supplements. Serum potassium levels are checked frequently.

> **NURSING TIP**
>
> Mix the elixir with fruit juice (red punch or grape juice works well) to disguise the bitter taste and to prevent intestinal irritation from a concentrated solution.

Fluid restriction is rarely necessary in infants because of their difficulty in feeding. However, if fluids are restricted, the nurse plans fluid intake schedules for a 24-hour period, allowing for most fluids during waking hours. Toddlers and preschoolers should be given small amounts of liquid in small cups so that the containers appear full. It is also important to avoid leaving extra fluids at the bedside, because older children may help themselves to additional servings. Older children's cooperation is gained by placing them in charge of recording fluid intake.

If salt is limited, the nurse discusses food sources of sodium with the family and discourages their bringing salt-containing treats to the child. At mealtime the child's tray is checked to make sure the appropriate diet is given.

Support Child and Family. CHF is a serious complication of heart disease. Parents and older children are usually acutely aware of the critical nature of the condition. Because stress places additional demands on cardiac function, the nurse should focus on reducing anxiety through anticipatory preparation, frequent communication with the parent regarding the child's progress, and constant reassurance that everything possible is being done.

Home care involves many of the same interventions discussed under Plan for Discharge and Home Care (p. 921). The nurse teaches the family about the medications that need to be administered and alerts them to the signs of worsening CHF that require medical attention, such as increased sweating, decreased urine output (noted in fewer wet diapers or infrequent use of the toilet), or poor feeding. Compliance is a major issue, and every effort is extended to improve the family's adherence to the medication schedule (see Chapter 22). Written instructions regarding correct administration of digoxin are essential (see Family Home Care box, p. 910), including an explanation regarding signs of toxicity.

If CHF is the end stage of a severe heart defect, the nurse cares for this child as for any child who is terminally ill, using the principles discussed in Chapter 18.

● **Evaluation**

The effectiveness of nursing interventions for the family and the child with CHF is determined by continual reassessment and evaluation of care based on the following observational guidelines:

1. Monitor heart rate and quality, respiratory rate and efforts, and color, and observe behaviors that provide clues to expended effort.
2. Observe nutritional intake, feeding behaviors, and weight.
3. Monitor intake, output, and weight.
4. Interview and observe behaviors of family.

The **expected outcomes** are described in the Nursing Care Plan on pp. 913 and 914.

HYPOXEMIA

Hypoxemia refers to an arterial oxygen tension (or pressure, PaO_2) that is less than normal and can be identified by a decreased arterial saturation or a decreased PaO_2. *Hypoxia* is a reduction in tissue oxygenation that results from low oxygen saturations and PaO_2 and results in impaired cellular processes. *Cyanosis* is a blue discoloration in the mucous membranes, skin, and nail beds of the child with reduced oxygen saturation. It results from the presence of deoxygenated hemoglobin (hemoglobin not bound to oxygen) in a concentration of 5 g/dL of blood. Cyanosis is usually apparent when arterial oxygen saturations are 80% to 85%. Determination of cyanosis is subjective. It can vary depending on skin pigment, quality of light, color of the room, or clothing worn by the child. The presence of cyanosis may not accurately reflect arterial hypoxemia, because both oxygen saturation and the amount of circulating hemoglobin are involved. Children with severe anemia may not be cyanotic despite severe hypoxemia, because the hemoglobin level may be too low to produce the characteristic blue color. Conversely, patients with polycythemia may appear cyanotic despite a near-normal PaO_2. Heart defects that cause hypoxemia and cyanosis result from desaturated venous blood (blue blood) entering the systemic circulation without passing through the lungs.

Adolescents and young adults may become cyanotic because of unrepaired septal defects in which the increased pulmonary blood flow over many years results in pulmonary

NURSING CARE PLAN   The Child With Congestive Heart Failure

NURSING DIAGNOSIS ■ **Decreased cardiac output related to structural defect, myocardial dysfunction**

PATIENT GOAL 1: Will exhibit improved cardiac output

NURSING INTERVENTIONS/*RATIONALES*

*Administer digoxin (Lanoxin) as ordered, using established precautions *to prevent toxicity*
  Make certain dosage is within safe limits
  Infants rarely receive more than 1 mL (50 μg or 0.05 mg) in one dose; *a higher dose is an immediate warning of a dosage error*
  Ascertain correct preparation for route
  Check dosage with another nurse *to ensure safety*
  Count apical pulse for 1 full minute before giving drug
    Withhold medication and notify practitioner if pulse rate is less than 90 to 110 beats/min (infants) or 70 to 85 beats/min (older children), depending on previous pulse readings
  Recognize signs of digoxin toxicity (nausea, vomiting, anorexia, bradycardia, dysrhythmias)
  Often an ECG rhythm strip is taken *to assess cardiac status before administration*
  Ensure adequate intake of potassium
  Observe for signs of hypokalemia (muscle weakness, hypotension, dysrhythmias, tachycardia or bradycardia, irritability, drowsiness) or hyperkalemia (muscle weakness, twitching, bradycardia, ventricular fibrillation, oliguria, apnea)
  Monitor serum potassium levels *because decrease enhances digoxin toxicity*
*Administer medications to decrease afterload, as ordered
  Check blood pressure
    Observe for signs of hypotension
  Monitor electrolyte levels
  Attach cardiac monitor if ordered

EXPECTED OUTCOMES

Heartbeat is strong, regular, and within normal limits for age (see inside back cover)
Peripheral perfusion is adequate

NURSING DIAGNOSIS ■ **Ineffective breathing pattern related to pulmonary congestion**

PATIENT GOAL 1: Will exhibit improved respiratory function

NURSING INTERVENTIONS/*RATIONALES*

Place in inclined posture of 30 to 45 degrees *to encourage maximum chest expansion;* tilt mattress support of incubator; place older infant in infant seat
Avoid any constricting clothing or restraints around abdomen and chest
*Administer humidified oxygen as prescribed
Assess respiratory rate, ease of respiration, color, and oxygen saturations as measured by oximetry

EXPECTED OUTCOME

Respirations remain within normal limits, color is good, and child rests quietly (see inside back cover for normal variations in respirations)

PATIENT GOAL 2: Will experience reduction of anxiety

NURSING INTERVENTIONS/*RATIONALES*

Employ flexible feeding schedule *that reduces fretfulness associated with hunger*
Handle child gently
Hold and comfort infant
Employ comfort measures found effective for individual child
Encourage family to provide comfort and solace
Explain equipment and procedures to child *to decrease anxiety*

EXPECTED OUTCOME

Child rests quietly and breathes easily

NURSING DIAGNOSIS ■ **Fluid volume excess related to fluid accumulation (edema)**

PATIENT GOAL 1: Will exhibit no evidence of fluid excess

NURSING INTERVENTIONS/*RATIONALES*

*Administer diuretics as prescribed
Maintain accurate intake and output
Weigh daily at same time and on same scale *to assess fluid gain or loss*
Assess for evidence of increased or decreased edema
Maintain fluid restriction, if ordered
Provide skin care for children with edema
Change position frequently *to prevent skin breakdown associated with edema*
  Use alternating-pressure mattress

EXPECTED OUTCOME

Infant exhibits evidence of fluid loss (frequent urination, weight loss)

NURSING DIAGNOSIS ■ **Activity intolerance related to imbalance between oxygen supply and demand**

PATIENT GOAL 1: Will exhibit no additional respiratory or cardiac stress

NURSING INTERVENTIONS/*RATIONALES*

Maintain neutral thermal environment *because hypothermia or hyperthermia increases need for oxygen*
  Place newborn in incubator or under warmer
  Keep infant warm
  Treat fever promptly
Feed small volumes at frequent intervals (every 2 to 3 hours) using soft nipple with moderately large opening, *because infants with CHF tire easily*
Implement gavage feeding if infant becomes fatigued before taking an adequate amount
Time nursing activities to disturb child as little as possible
Implement measures to reduce anxiety
Respond promptly to crying or other expressions of distress

EXPECTED OUTCOME

Child rests quietly

*Dependent nursing action.

Continued

The Child With Congestive Heart Failure—*cont'd*

NURSING DIAGNOSIS ■ **Risk for infection related to reduced body defenses, pulmonary congestion**

See Infection Control, Chapter 22
See Nursing Care Plan: The Child With Congenital Heart Disease (*Wong's Clinical Manual of Pediatric Nursing,* ed 6)

NURSING DIAGNOSIS ■ **Altered family processes related to a child with a life-threatening illness**

PATIENT (FAMILY) GOAL 1: Will receive adequate support

NURSING INTERVENTIONS/*RATIONALES* AND EXPECTED OUTCOMES
See Nursing Care Plan: The Family of the Ill or Hospitalized Child, Chapter 21

PATIENT (FAMILY) GOAL 2: Will be prepared for home care

NURSING INTERVENTIONS/*RATIONALES*
Teach family:
  Medication administration and side/toxic effects
  Signs and symptoms of CHF and to report them to designated practitioner
  Feeding techniques and nutritional requirements
  Positioning
  Need for rest
  Growth and developmental considerations
    Growth is slowed
    Gross motor skills may be delayed more than fine motor skills
Refer to outpatient services and community resources as needed *for ongoing support*

EXPECTED OUTCOMES
Family demonstrates an understanding of the condition and required care at home
Family uses appropriate community resources

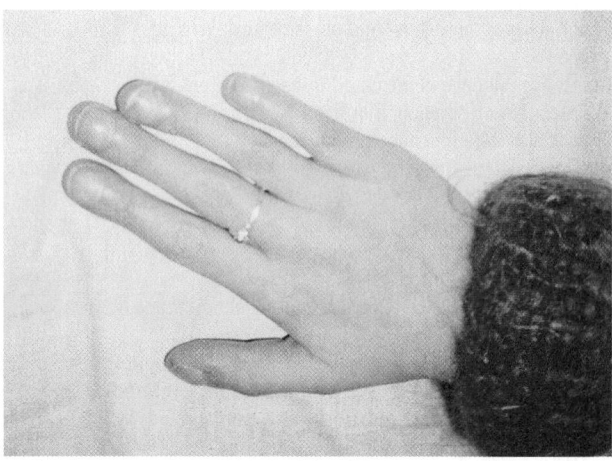
FIG. 25-7 ■ Clubbing of the fingers.

vascular changes. *Eisenmenger complex (syndrome)* refers to the clinical situation in which a left-to-right shunt becomes a right-to-left shunt because of a progressive increase in pulmonary vascular resistance. With increasing pulmonary vascular thickening, the resistance in the pulmonary circulation can exceed or equal that in the systemic circulation, causing a reversal of blood flow from the right to the left ventricle.

Clinical Manifestations

Over time, two physiologic changes occur in the body in response to chronic hypoxemia: polycythemia and clubbing. *Polycythemia,* an increased number of red blood cells, increases the oxygen-carrying capacity of the blood. However, anemia may result if iron is not readily available for the formation of hemoglobin. Polycythemia increases the viscosity of the blood and crowds out clotting factors. *Clubbing,* a thickening and flattening of the tips of the fingers and toes, is thought to occur because of chronic tissue hy-

poxemia and polycythemia (Fig. 25-7). Infants with mild hypoxemia may be asymptomatic except for cyanosis and exhibit near-normal growth and development. Those with more severe hypoxemia may exhibit fatigue with feeding, poor weight gain, tachypnea, and dyspnea. Severe hypoxemia resulting in tissue hypoxia is manifested by clinical deterioration and signs of poor perfusion.

Squatting, most characteristic of children with tetralogy of Fallot, is seen in toddlers and older children as an unconscious attempt to relieve chronic hypoxia, especially during exercise. Because of early surgical intervention during infancy, squatting is rarely seen.

Hypercyanotic spells, also referred to as *blue spells* or *tet spells* because they are often seen in infants with tetralogy of Fallot, may occur in any child whose heart defect includes obstruction to pulmonary blood flow and communication between the ventricles. The infant becomes acutely cyanotic and hyperpneic because sudden infundibular spasm decreases pulmonary blood flow and increases right-to-left shunting (the proposed mechanism in tetralogy of Fallot). Spells, rarely seen before 2 months of age, occur most frequently in the first year of life. They occur more often in the morning and may be preceded by feeding, crying, defecation, or stressful procedures (see Critical Thinking Exercise on the facing page). Because profound hypoxemia causes cerebral hypoxia, hypercyanotic spells require prompt assessment and treatment to prevent brain damage or possibly death.

Persistent cyanosis as a result of cyanotic cardiac defects places the child at risk for significant *neurologic complications.* Cerebrovascular accident (CVA, stroke), brain abscess, and developmental delays (especially in motor and cognitive development) may result from chronic hypoxia.

Therapeutic Management

Hypercyanotic spells occur suddenly, and prompt recognition and treatment are essential. In the hospital setting, spells are often seen during blood drawing or IV insertion,

❓❓❓ CRITICAL THINKING EXERCISE ❓❓❓

Hypercyanotic Spell

A 4-month-old infant known to have tetralogy of Fallot is seen in the emergency department because of a 2-day history of diarrhea, low-grade fever, and poor oral intake. When blood tests are obtained, he becomes acutely cyanotic with rapid shallow respirations.

QUESTIONS

1. Evidence—Is there sufficient evidence to draw conclusions about this infant's condition?
2. Assumptions—Describe an underlying assumption about each of the following:
   a. Symptoms associated with tetralogy of Fallot
   b. Diarrhea, low-grade fever, and poor oral intake in a 4-month-old infant
   c. Acute cyanotic episodes in a 4-month-old infant
3. What priorities for nursing care should be established for this infant?
4. Does the evidence support your nursing interventions?
5. What alternative perspectives might you have?

ANSWERS

1. Yes. The patient has a history of tetralogy of Fallot, which is associated with acute episodes of cyanosis and hypoxia. Hypercyanotic episodes occur suddenly and are common with crying.
2. a. Infants with tetralogy of Fallot may be acutely cyanotic at birth; others have mild cyanosis that progresses over the first year of life as pulmonic stenosis worsens.
   b. Symptoms of diarrhea, low-grade fever, and poor oral intake can be indicative of an acute infection in a young child. However, the hypercyanotic spell requires immediate attention.
   c. Acute cyanotic spells, called blue spells or "tet" spells, can occur suddenly when the infant's oxygen requirements exceed oxygen availability. This may occur during crying or after feeding.
3. The priorities are to immediately calm the infant, place in the knee-chest position, administer blow-by oxygen, and call for assistance.
4. Yes. The infant is having a hypercyanotic, or tet, spell, and the first actions should be to calm the infant, place in the knee-chest position, and give supplemental oxygen. A hypercyanotic spell will likely worsen without immediate intervention, so prompt action is needed. If the nurse fails to accept the conclusions, negative implications may result, because a severe hypercyanotic spell may require intravenous medications, hydration, and resuscitative measures to stabilize the infant. To decrease the pain at the phlebotomy site and possibly decrease the hypercyanotic spell, place EMLA or Elamax on the site 1 hour before procedure to decrease pain.
5. An alternative perspective is the concern for an infection because of a history of diarrhea and low-grade fever for the past 2 days. However, in the presence of a diagnosis of tetralogy of Fallot, the immediate presentation of a hypercyanotic episode needs immediate attention. There should be a record or notation on the plan of care of calming measures which have been effective in calming the child in the past—this information is crucial in the care of such children.

📋 GUIDELINES

Treating Hypercyanotic Spells

Place infant in knee-chest position (Fig. 25-8).
Employ calm, comforting approach.
Administer 100% oxygen by face mask.
Give morphine subcutaneously or through existing intravenous (IV) line.
Begin IV fluid replacement and volume expansion if needed.
Repeat morphine administration.

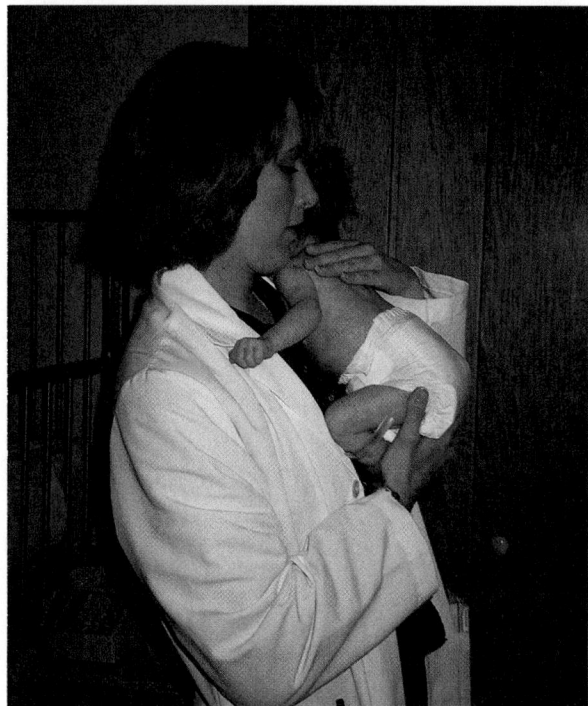

FIG. 25-8 ■ Infant held in knee-chest position.

surgical repair, a shunt may be created surgically to increase blood flow to the lungs. Several commonly used shunt procedures are described in Table 25-4 and Fig 25-9.

The cyanotic infant and child are well hydrated to keep the hematocrit and blood viscosity within acceptable limits to reduce the risk of CVAs. Fevers are carefully evaluated because bacteremia can result in bacterial endocarditis. The infant is monitored closely for anemia because of the risk of CVAs and the reduced arterial oxygen-carrying capacity that occurs. Iron supplementation and possibly blood transfusion are used as needed.

Respiratory infections or reduced pulmonary function from any cause can worsen hypoxemia in the cyanotic child. Aggressive pulmonary hygiene, chest physiotherapy, administration of antibiotics, and use of oxygen to improve arterial saturations are important interventions.

Nursing Considerations

The general appearance of infants and children with significant cyanosis poses unique concerns. Blue lips and fingernails are obvious signs of their hidden cardiac defect. Clubbing

when the child is highly agitated, or after cardiac catheterization. Treatment of a hypercyanotic spell is outlined in the Guidelines box. Morphine, administered subcutaneously or through an existing IV line, helps to reduce infundibular spasm. A spell indicates the need for prompt surgical treatment if possible. In infants with defects not amenable to

TABLE 25-4 ■ Selected Shunt Procedures for Children With Cardiac Defects

SHUNT LOCATION	COMMENTS
MODIFIED BLALOCK-TAUSSIG (BT) SHUNT	
Subclavian artery to pulmonary artery using Gore-Tex or Impra tube graft	Shunt flow sometimes excessive, requiring use of diuretics Possibility of thrombosis; antiplatelet therapy may be used postoperatively Easy to ligate at time of definitive correction Shunt size fixed and may become too small as child grows
CENTRAL SHUNT	
Ascending aorta to main pulmonary aorta using Gore-Tex graft	Length of shunt acts to restrict blood flow, limiting symptoms of congestive heart failure; may require diuretics Uncommon; used when modified BT shunt cannot be done Easy to perform and remove at time of repair
GLENN SHUNT	
Superior vena cava to side of right pulmonary artery, which is ligated from main pulmonary artery Blood flow to right lung only	Used as a second shunt procedure if complete repair is not possible High mortality in infants younger than age 6 months Superior vena cava syndrome may occur Pulmonary arteriovenous fistulas may occur many years later Difficult to take down at time of definitive repair
BIDIRECTIONAL GLENN (CAVOPULMONARY ANASTOMOSIS) SHUNT	
Superior vena cava to side of right pulmonary artery Blood flow to both lungs	Done as a second shunt; often as a staging step to a Fontan procedure Can be incorporated into eventual modified Fontan procedure Relieves cyanosis and decreases volume overload on ventricle

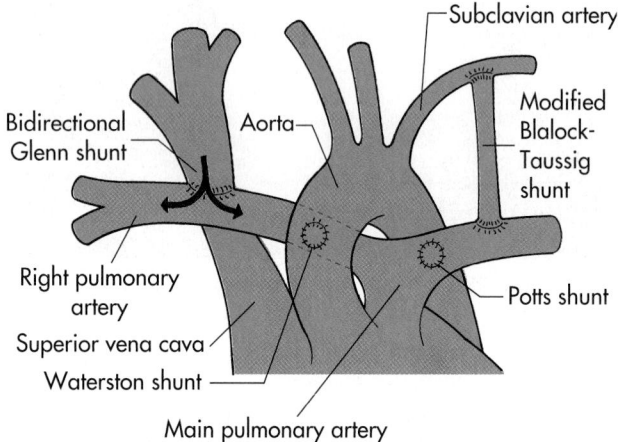

FIG. 25-9 ■ Schematic diagram of cardiac shunts. NOTE: Two early shunt procedures—Waterston shunt (ascending aorta to right pulmonary artery) and Potts shunt (descending aorta to left pulmonary artery)—are no longer performed because of problems with excessive pulmonary blood flow and distortion of the pulmonary arteries. Adult patients may have had these shunts done as their initial repair.

and small, thin stature in older children further indicate severe heart disease. Adolescents are especially concerned about their body image; children with cyanosis are often teased about their appearance and singled out as different. Many children, when asked what surgery will do, reply, "Make me pink." Their joy and excitement after surgery are evident when they see their pink fingers. Accentuating the normal and positive and being careful not to call attention to their cyanosis are helpful interventions. Meeting other children in the clinic or hospital who are cyanotic reassures them that they are not the only ones who are blue.

Parents are often fearful of their child's bluish color, because cyanosis is usually associated with lack of oxygen and severe illness. They also must deal with comments from relatives, friends, and strangers about their child's abnormal color. They need a simple explanation of hypoxemia and cyanosis and reassurance that cyanosis does not imply a lack of oxygen to the brain. Their questions and fears need to be addressed in a calm, supportive manner, and positive aspects of their child's growth and development are emphasized. They are taught the treatment for hypercyanotic spells (see Guidelines box, p. 915).

Dehydration must be prevented in hypoxemic children because it potentiates the risk of CVAs. Fluid status is carefully monitored, with accurate intake and output and daily weight measurements. Maintenance fluid therapy is the minimum requirement, supplemental fluids should be readily available, and gavage feeding or IV hydration is given to children unable to take adequate oral fluids. Fever, vomiting, and diarrhea can cause dehydration and require prompt treatment. Parents are instructed in the importance of adequate fluid intake and measures to prevent dehydration. An oral electrolyte solution should be available at home in the event that the infant is unable to tolerate the usual formula. The practitioner should be notified of fever, vomiting, diarrhea, or other problems.

Preventive measures and accurate assessment of respiratory infection are important nursing considerations. Any compromise in pulmonary function will increase the infant's hypoxemia. Good handwashing and protection from individuals with an obvious respiratory infection are important. Aggressive pulmonary hygiene, treatment with antibiotics or antiviral agents as indicated, and supplemental oxygen to decrease hypoxemia are necessary measures. Infants may need to be gavage fed or given parenteral hydration if respiratory distress prevents oral feeding.

> **! NURSING ALERT**
>
> Intracardiac shunting of blood from the right side (desaturated) to the left side of the heart allows air in the venous system to go directly to the brain, resulting in an air embolism. Therefore all IV lines should have filters in place to prevent air from entering the system, the entire tubing should be checked for air, all connections should be taped securely, and any air should be removed.

NURSING CARE OF THE FAMILY AND CHILD WITH CONGENITAL HEART DISEASE

When a child is born with a severe cardiac anomaly, the parents are faced with the immense psychologic and physical tasks of adjusting to the birth of a child with special needs. The reactions and nursing interventions required to support the family are similar to those of other parents whose children have serious chronic conditions and are discussed in Chapter 18.

The following discussion is primarily directed (1) toward the family of an infant who has a serious heart defect and requires home care before definitive repair and (2) toward preparation and care of the child and family when heart surgery is performed. For nursing care related to the child with hypoxemia and CHF, the reader should refer to earlier discussions of these topics.

Nursing care of the child with a congenital heart defect begins as soon as the diagnosis is suspected. Prenatal diagnosis of congenital heart defects is becoming increasingly frequent. Those with severe congenital cardiac defects are usually diagnosed in infancy.

Help Family Adjust to the Disorder

After parents learn of the heart defect, whether it is soon after the child's birth or at a later period, they are initially in a period of shock, followed by high anxiety and fear that the child will die. The family needs time to grieve before they can assimilate the meaning of the defect. Unfortunately, the demands for medical treatment may not allow this, instead necessitating that the parents immediately give informed consent for diagnostic/therapeutic procedures. The nurse can be instrumental in supporting parents in their loss, assessing their level of understanding, supplying information as needed, and helping other members of the health care team to understand the parents' reactions (see Family Focus box).

Severely distressed newborns usually remain in the hospital. This can seriously affect parent-infant attachment unless parents are encouraged to hold, touch, and look at their child. Every effort must be made by health personnel to foster attachment. (See Chapter 8 for suggestions on promoting attachment between parents and their hospitalized newborn.)

The effect of a child with a serious heart defect on the family is complex. No member, regardless of the degree of positive adjustment, is unaffected. Mothers frequently feel inade-

FAMILY FOCUS

The Diagnosis of Heart Disease

Remember, we don't have your experience. We don't see children everyday who have heart disease. We would have been upset finding out our child had to have his tonsils out. How could we ever be prepared for this? Please remember, we only know people who have trivial heart murmurs. How could we ever expect this to happen? And to us, this is the worst problem we've ever heard of.

We still fear most what we don't know and understand. Be honest with us. If you don't know either, tell us. But at least don't leave us wondering about what you know and we don't. Not knowing anything really can be worse than knowing something bad. Be honest, but don't strip us of hope. . . .

Please, remember we are trying to learn complex information in a moment of time. And trying to learn it in a context of great pain and emotional investment. This is our lives you're talking about. Please be thorough, but keep it simple. Tell us again, maybe even again and again, when we can hear better.

From Schrey C, Schrey M: A parent's perspective: our needs and our message, *Crit Care Nurs Clin North Am* 6(1):113-119, 1994.

quate in their mothering ability because they gave birth to a child with a defect and are unable to keep the child well. They often feel constantly exhausted from the pressures of caring for these children and the other family members. Fathers and siblings may feel neglected and resentful, a reaction similar to the feelings of family members toward other chronic conditions (see Chapter 18). Often, parents do not feel confident leaving the child in another's care. This often sets up a trap for parents, especially mothers, who become locked into the child's care with no relief. Although the fears are justified, they can be minimized by gradually teaching someone (a reliable relative or neighbor) how to care for the child.

The need to maintain discipline and set consistent limits cannot be overemphasized. Using behavior modification techniques, in the form of either concrete awards (e.g., a favorite activity) or social reinforcement (e.g., approval), can be effective. However, it is most beneficial if employed *before* the child learns to control the family. Therefore it is necessary to guide parents toward the need for discipline while the child is in infancy to prevent later problems.

Another issue that may develop within family relationships is the child's overdependency. This is often the result of parental fear that the child may die. The best approach to dealing with this dilemma is prevention. Parents need guidance to recognize the eventual hazards of continuing dependency and protectiveness as the child grows older, and the nurse can assist parents in learning ways to foster optimum development. Unless parents are shown what activities the child can do, they may focus on physical limitations and encourage dependency.

The child also needs opportunities for social development. These children do not need to be prevented from playing with other children because of concern regarding overexertion. Children usually limit their activities if allowed to set their own pace. Such practices foster increased dependency in the home environment. Parents need to be encouraged to seek appropriate social activity, especially before kindergarten.

A child with CHD may constitute a long-term family crisis. Frequently the continuing unremitting stresses of care—physical exhaustion, financial costs, emotional upset, fear of death, and concern for the child's future—are not fully appreciated by those caring for the family. Even when the child's condition is stabilized or corrected, the family may need to make new adjustments in their lifestyle. Introducing them to other families with similarly affected children can help them adjust to the daily stresses.*

Educate Family About the Disorder

When parents are ready to hear about the heart condition, they require a clear explanation based on their level of understanding. A review of the basic structure and function of the heart is helpful before describing the defect. A simple diagram, pictures, or a model of the heart can help parents visualize the heart and the congenital defect.† Parents appreciate receiving written information about the specific condition. A glossary of frequently used terms is also helpful. Parents also require information about prognosis and treatment options.

Increasingly, families are using the Internet as a source of information about heart disease in children.‡ They are also finding support through contacts with other parents and parent groups. Several Internet sites with pertinent information are listed in the footnote on this page. It is important for parents to realize that not all websites offer medically accurate information and that information from other parents might not be applicable to their own situation. Some children with rare, complex heart defects require individualized treatment plans, and general information on the Internet or in books may not apply to their child. Parents should use their health care team, in particular their cardiologist, to discuss information they have received from other sources.

Infants and children with CHD require good nutrition. Providing infants with adequate nutrition is especially difficult because of their high caloric requirements and inability to suck effectively because of fatigue and tachypnea. Instructing parents in feeding methods that decrease the work of the infant and giving high-calorie formula are important interventions. (See p. 910 for a discussion on feeding the infant with CHF.)

Children with severe cardiac defects are often anorexic. Encouraging them to eat can be a tremendous challenge. Because of the parents' concern over eating, children learn early to manipulate parents through eating, such as making unrealistic demands for foods that are not available. The nurse advises parents of the potential problem, because prevention yields greater success than intervention. For example, the child should be given a choice of available high-quality foods. Suggestions for feeding sick children are discussed in Chapter 22.

The family also needs to be knowledgeable regarding the therapeutic management of the disorder, especially in terms of the medications the child is receiving. Parents are taught the correct procedure for giving drugs and cautioned to keep them in a safe area to prevent accidental ingestion.

Children of various ages have different ideas about their heart. Children between ages 4 and 6 years have heard about the heart, know its approximate anatomic location in the chest or back, illustrate it as valentine-shaped, and characterize it by sounds such as *tick-tock* and *thump*. Children ages 7 to 10 have a clearer concept of the heart, realizing that it is not shaped like a valentine and that it has vital functions, such as "It makes you live." However, their knowledge of its integrated functions to pump blood through a system of vessels to all parts of the body is still hazy. By the age of 10 or 11, children have a much more involved concept of the heart, with knowledge of veins, valves, pumping action, and circulation. They are beginning to appreciate why death occurs when the heart stops.

Information given to the child must be tailored to the child's developmental age. As the child matures, the level of information is revised to meet the child's new cognitive level. Preschoolers need basic information about what they will experience more than what is actually occurring physiologically. School-age children benefit from a concrete explanation of the defect. Preadolescents and adolescents often appreciate a more detailed description of how the defect affects their heart. Children of all ages need to express their feelings concerning the diagnosis.

Help Family Cope With Effects of the Disorder

Parents should be aware of the symptoms of their child's cardiac condition (if the child is symptomatic). Parents of children who may develop CHF should be familiar with these symptoms and know when to contact the practitioner. Parents of children with cyanosis should be informed about fluid management and hypercyanotic spells. Parents should know how to contact their child's cardiologist at all times and know what to do in an emergency.

Another area of parental concern is the child's level of physical activity. Children do not need to restrict activity, and the best approach is to treat the child normally and allow self-limited activity. Exceptions to self-determined activity primarily involve strenuous recreational and competitive sports in children with specific cardiac problems. Activities and exercise restrictions should be discussed with the child's cardiologist. Deliberately attempting to prevent crying should be avoided because it can establish a maladaptive parental pattern of relating to the infant.

---

*Some local chapters of the American Heart Association have organized parent groups.

†The booklet *If your child has a congenital heart defect: a guide for parents,* as well as other information, is available from the **American Heart Association,** 7272 Greenville Avenue, Dallas, TX 75231; (214) 373-6300 or (800) AHA-USA1; website: www.americanheart.org.

‡**The Children's Health Information Network;** website: www.tchin.org; **PediHeart;** website: www.pediheart.org/parents/index.html; **NASPE** (information on arrhythmias); website: www.naspe.org; **Kids with Heart National Association for Children's Heart Disorders,** 1578 Careful Drive, Green Bay, WI 54304; website: www.kidswithheart.org.

NURSING ALERT

Although decisions regarding activity restrictions are made on an individual basis on the cardiologist's advice, children with moderate to severe aortic stenosis or insufficiency are usually not permitted to engage in strenuous activity (Koster, 1994).

Prepare Child and Family for Surgery

Few surgical procedures demand as much planning for preoperative preparation and postoperative care as heart surgery. The reader is urged to review the general principles for preparing children for procedures, such as surgery, discussed in Chapter 22. This discussion focuses on those measures specific to cardiovascular procedures. Preoperative preparation is often done in the outpatient setting, and children are admitted the day of surgery. Some infants and patients with other medical needs may be admitted the day before surgery.

No well-documented research exists on how extensive the preoperative preparation should be, and the nurse must use considerable judgment in planning the aspects of teaching. Preparation can be divided into three categories: environment, equipment, and procedures.

Introduce Child and Family to the Environment.

If a visit to the recovery room or intensive care unit (ICU) is planned, it should take place when there is least activity in the area, the parents can accompany the child, and the child is well-rested. Usually a day before surgery is ample time to allow the child to ask questions and to prevent undue fantasizing about the experience. If a visit is included in the teaching plan, the nurse can use a book, preferably with pictures or photographs of the actual rooms, to explain the environment to the child.

During the visit to the ICU, the child and parents should experience everything that directly affects the child's care, such as the sounds of ECG monitors, oxygen tents, and placement of the bed. All positive, nonfrightening aspects of the environment are emphasized, such as the play area, visitors' section, pictures or mobiles in the room, or television. If it is a pediatric ICU, the nurse can introduce the family to other children who may be recovering from surgery. The child should be protected from the frightening sights in the unit, and equipment not in view postoperatively, such as equipment located behind or below the bed, needs less attention. The child and parents are encouraged to ask questions or to explore further any equipment in the room, but they should not be pushed to assimilate more information than they appear to be tolerating.

Familiarize Child and Family With Equipment and Procedures.

Some of the equipment, such as the stethoscope, blood pressure apparatus, and thermometer, will already be familiar to the child and parents. However, the nurse emphasizes that procedures involving such equipment will be done more frequently. If monitoring devices, such as blood pressure or oximetry, are used, the child is told about the placement of the sensor on the skin.

Types of equipment new to many families are the oxygen mask, suction, chest tubes, endotracheal tubes, incentive spirometers, nasogastric tube, and IV tubing. Each of these is shown and demonstrated either on the child or on a doll, if he or she appears ready. With a younger child, miniaturized equipment suitable for use with a doll or puppet is often less anxiety-producing than the actual samples. If other children in the unit have an IV infusion or are in oxygen tents, the older child may benefit from seeing them, but this must be planned carefully to avoid frightening the child.

Several IV lines are inserted perioperatively: (1) an ordinary line for infusion of fluids, inserted in a peripheral vein; (2) a venous pressure line, inserted into the right subclavian or jugular vein; and (3) an arterial line for direct measurement of arterial pressure. Younger children need only know the location of each tubing. Older children may appreciate knowing the reason for each infusion. Because the lines are inserted during surgery, they are not painful; they only cause discomfort because movement is restricted.

The type and size of incision the child will have after surgery are discussed and can be shown on a doll. Usually one of two types of incisions is made: a *median sternotomy,* which splits the sternum, or a *lateral thoracotomy,* which extends from the midaxillary line to the scapula. Minimally invasive surgical techniques using a *mini-sternotomy* (opening the lower half of the sternum) are becoming more widely used to decrease postoperative pain and speed postoperative recovery. Frequently, no sutures are visible, because subcuticular, absorbable sutures may be used. If this is done, it should be pointed out to the child and parents, who may fear the incision will open.

An endotracheal (ET) tube is inserted during surgery and may be left in place for ventilatory assistance and tracheobronchial suctioning. However, it may be best to prepare older children for the ET tube only if *prolonged* ventilatory support is planned. The ET tube can be presented as a "breathing tube" that is placed in the nose or mouth. The nurse explains that while the tube is in, the child will feel it in the throat and will not be able to talk, but nothing is wrong. The child can express desires by pointing or using a picture communication board. At this point, communicating the amount of discomfort from the surgery can also be discussed, especially using measurement tools such as numbers or faces (see Pain Assessment, Chapter 21). The nurse stresses that the tube will be removed as soon as possible, often during the first postoperative day. The child may be told about chest tubes and their purpose in draining fluid from around the heart and lungs.

Preoperative physical care differs little, if any, from that for any other surgery and is discussed in Chapter 22. The child should be assured that the parents will be there when he or she wakes up; parents should be allowed to accompany their child as far as possible to the operating suite. After all the equipment and procedures have been explained, it is important to talk about "getting well" and going home. If a doll was used during the preparatory session, the tubes can be removed, and the doll can be dressed in regular clothes in anticipation of discharge.

Provide Postoperative Care

Immediate postoperative care is usually provided by specially trained nurses in ICUs. Many of the procedures, such as arterial pressure and central venous pressure (CVP) monitoring, and the observations related to vital functions require advanced educational training (the reader should refer to critical care texts for further information). However, nurses caring for the child before surgery and during the convalescent period need to be familiar with the major principles of care. Selected complications that may occur postoperatively are described in Box 25-7.

BOX 25-7 ■ Selected Complications After Cardiac Surgery and Treatment Approaches

CARDIAC
Congestive heart failure: Digoxin, diuretics (p. 902)
Low cardiac output: Intravenous inotropes (Shock, p. 932)
Dysrhythmias: Identification, drug treatment, possible pacing, cardioversion (p. 926)
Tamponade (blood or fluid in the pericardial space constricting the heart): Prompt removal of fluid by pericardiocentesis

RESPIRATORY
Atelectasis: Chest physiotherapy, coughing, deep breathing, ambulation
Pulmonary edema: Diuretics
Pleural effusions: Diuretics, possible chest tube drainage
Pneumothorax: Possible chest tube drainage

NEUROLOGIC
Seizures: Assessment, antiepileptic drugs
Cerebrovascular accident (stroke), cerebral edema, neurologic deficits: Assessment and treatment

INFECTIOUS DISEASE
Infections (especially wound, pneumonia, otitis media, and sepsis): Antibiotics

HEMATOLOGIC
Anemia: Iron supplementation, possible transfusion
Postoperative bleeding: Initially, clotting factors, blood products; may need repeat surgery to locate and ligate source of bleeding

OTHER
Postpericardiotomy syndrome (syndrome of fever, leukocytosis, friction rub, pericardial and pleural effusions, lethargy seen about 7 to 21 days after cardiac surgery; possible viral or autoimmune etiologies): Antipyretics, diuretics, antiinflammatory medications

Observe Vital Signs. Vital signs and blood pressure are recorded frequently until stable. Heart rate and respirations are counted for 1 full minute, compared with the ECG monitor, and recorded with activity. The heart rate is normally increased after surgery. The nurse observes cardiac rhythm and notifies the practitioner of any changes in regularity. Dysrhythmias may occur postoperatively secondary to anesthetics, acid-base and electrolyte imbalance, hypoxia, surgical intervention, or trauma to conduction pathways (p. 926).

At least hourly, the lungs are auscultated for breath sounds. Diminished or absent sounds most likely indicate an area of atelectasis, which necessitates further medical assessment. Temperature changes are typical during the early postoperative period. Hypothermia is expected immediately after surgery from hypothermia procedures, effects of anesthesia, and loss of body heat to the cool environment. During this period the child is kept warm to prevent additional heat loss. Infants may be placed under radiant heat warmers. During the next 24 to 48 hours the body temperature may rise to 37.7° C (100° F) or slightly higher as part of the in-

flammatory response to tissue trauma. After this period an elevated temperature is most likely a sign of infection and warrants immediate investigation for probable cause.

Maintain Respiratory Status. Infants usually require mechanical ventilation in the immediate postoperative period. Early extubation in the operating room or early postoperative period is becoming more common. Children may be extubated in the operating room or in the first few postoperative hours, especially children who did not require cardiopulmonary bypass. Suctioning is performed only as needed and performed carefully to avoid vagal stimulation (which can trigger cardiac dysrhythmias) and laryngospasm, especially in infants. Suctioning is intermittent and maintained for no more than 5 seconds at a time to prevent depleting the oxygen supply. Supplemental oxygen is administered with a manual resuscitation bag before and after the procedure to prevent hypoxia. The heart rate is monitored after suctioning to detect changes in rhythm or rate, especially bradycardia. The child should always be positioned facing the nurse to permit assessment of the child's color and tolerance of the procedure.

> **NURSING ALERT**
>
> During suctioning, observe for signs and symptoms of respiratory distress, such as tachypnea, use of accessory muscles for breathing, and restlessness.

When weaning and extubation are completed, humidified oxygen is delivered by mask, hood, or nasal cannula to prevent drying of mucosa. The child is encouraged to turn and deep breathe at least hourly. Every measure is employed to enhance ventilation and decrease pain, such as splinting of the operative site and use of analgesics. Chest tubes are inserted into the pleural or mediastinal space during surgery or in the immediate postoperative period to remove secretions and air to allow reexpansion of the lung. Drainage is checked hourly for color and quantity. Immediately after surgery the drainage may be bright red, but afterward it should be serous. The largest volume of drainage occurs in the first 12 to 24 hours and is greater in extensive heart surgery.

> **NURSING ALERT**
>
> Chest tube drainage greater than 3 mL/kg/hr for more than 3 consecutive hours or 5 to 10 mL/kg in any 1 hour is excessive and may indicate postoperative hemorrhage. The surgeon is notified immediately because cardiac tamponade can develop rapidly and is life-threatening.

Chest tubes are usually removed on the first to third postoperative day. Removal of chest tubes is a painful, frightening experience. Analgesics such as morphine sulfate, often combined with midazolam (Versed), should be given before the procedure. Older children are forewarned that they will feel a sharp, momentary pain. After the suture is cut, the tubes are quickly pulled out at the end of full inspiration to prevent intake of air into the pleural cavity. A purse-string suture (placed when the tubes were inserted) is pulled tight to close the opening. A petrolatum-covered gauze dressing is immediately applied over the wound and securely taped on all four sides to the skin so that an airtight seal is formed. The dressing is checked for signs of drainage and any evidence of infection.

Monitor Fluids.   Intake and output of all fluids must be accurately calculated. Intake is primarily IV fluids; however, a record of fluid used to flush the arterial and CVP lines or to dilute medications is also kept. Output includes hourly recordings of urine (usually a Foley catheter is inserted and attached to a closed collecting device), drainage from chest and nasogastric tubes, and blood drawn for analysis. Urine is analyzed for specific gravity to assess the concentrating ability of the kidneys and to assess approximately the body's degree of hydration. Renal failure is a potential risk from a transient period of low cardiac output.

NURSING ALERT

The signs of renal failure are decreased urine output (less than 1 mL/kg/hr) and elevated levels of blood urea nitrogen and serum creatinine.

Fluids are restricted during the immediate postoperative period to prevent hypervolemia, which places additional demands on the myocardium, predisposing to cardiac failure. To monitor fluid retention, the child is weighed daily, and the same scale is used at approximately the same time each day to avoid errors in measurement. The child is usually given nothing by mouth for the first 24 hours. If an ET tube is inserted, oral fluids are usually withheld until the child is extubated. Fluid restriction may be imposed even when oral fluids are given. The nurse calculates the distribution over a 24-hour period based on the child's preoperative weight and drinking habits. The distribution should allow for most fluid to be given during the child's most wakeful and active periods.

Provide Rest and Progressive Activity.   After heart surgery, rest should be provided to decrease the workload of the heart and promote healing. The simplest way to ensure individualized, efficient, high-quality care is to plan at the beginning of the shift the nursing procedures to be done, with periods of rest identified. The schedule should be shared with parents to allow them to visit at the most advantageous times, such as after a rest period when no special treatments are anticipated.

A progressive schedule of ambulation and activity is planned, based on the child's preoperative activity patterns and postoperative cardiovascular and pulmonary function. Ambulation is initiated early, usually by the second postoperative day, when chest tubes, arterial lines, and assisted ventilatory equipment may be removed. Activity progresses from sitting on the edge of the bed and dangling the legs to standing up and to sitting in a chair. Heart rate and respirations are carefully monitored to assess the degree of cardiac demand imposed by each activity. Tachycardia, dyspnea, cyanosis, desaturation, progressive fatigue, or dysrhythmias indicate the need to limit further energy expenditure.

Provide Comfort and Emotional Support.   Heart surgery is both painful and frightening for children, and comfort is a primary nursing concern. Continuous IV opi-

oid infusions, particularly morphine and fentanyl, are safe and effective analgesics. Patient-controlled analgesia may be used with children old enough to understand the concept. Nonsteroidal antiinflammatory drugs (NSAIDs) such as ketorolac (Toradol) may be used intravenously. Epidural morphine may be another option, because it affords very good pain control when a thoracotomy is performed. Paralyzing agents such as pancuronium (Pavulon) or metocurine (Metubine) may also be used with the analgesics for children who are very agitated or hemodynamically unstable.

Most patients need IV analgesics for pain control during the immediate postoperative period. After extubation and removal of lines and tubes, pain can be satisfactorily controlled with oral medications such as ibuprofen, codeine with acetaminophen (Tylenol), or oxycodone and acetaminophen (Tylox). Acetaminophen alone provides adequate pain relief for most children at discharge. Sternotomy incisions are usually well tolerated, with some discomfort when walking and coughing. Thoracotomy incisions are usually more painful because the incision is through muscle; a more aggressive pain management plan with around-the-clock medications for several days is often necessary to allow for adequate rest, ambulation, and pulmonary hygiene.

In addition to pharmacologic pain control, every effort is made to minimize the discomfort of procedures, such as using a firm pillow or favorite stuffed animal placed against the chest incision during movement and performing treatments *after* pain medication is given, preferably at a time that coincides with the drug's peak effect. Nonpharmacologic measures are used to lessen the perception of pain, and parents are encouraged to comfort their child as much as possible. (See also Pain Assessment; Pain Management, Chapter 21.)

Children may also be angry and uncooperative after surgery as a response to the physical pain and to the loss of control imposed by the surgery and treatments. They need an opportunity to express feelings, either verbally or through activity. Children also may express feelings of anger or rejection toward parents. The nurse must reassure parents that this is normal and that with continued support the anger will subside.

The nurse can support the parents by being available for information and explaining all the procedures to them. The first few postoperative days are particularly difficult because parents see their child in pain and realize the potential risks from surgery. They often are overwhelmed by the physical environment of the ICU and feel useless because they can do so little for their child. The importance of their presence in making the child feel more secure is stressed, even if they do not provide physical care.

Plan for Discharge and Home Care

Ideally, discharge planning begins on admission for cardiac surgery and includes an assessment of the parents' adjustment to the child's altered state of health. The family will need both verbal and written instructions on medication, nutrition, activity restrictions, subacute bacterial endocarditis, return to school, wound care, and signs and symptoms of infection or complications (see Family Home Care box). Referrals to community agencies may be warranted to assist parents in the transition from hospital to home and to reinforce the teaching.

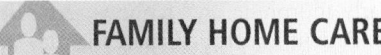

FAMILY HOME CARE

Topics to Include in Discharge Teaching After Cardiac Surgery

Medication teaching (for digoxin, see Family Home Care box, p. 910)
Activity restrictions
Diet and nutrition
Wound care (include dressings if any, suture removal, bathing)
Bacterial endocarditis prophylaxis (see Box 25-9)
Follow-up appointments (cardiologist, primary care provider)
   Community agencies as needed (visiting nurse service, early
     developmental intervention)
When to call practitioner; signs and symptoms of postoperative
   problems
Review of cardiac defect and surgical repair

The parents will also need clear instructions on when to seek medical care, such as for a change in the child's behavior or an unexplained fever. Follow-up with the cardiologist is also arranged before discharge. Appropriate identification, such as a MedicAlert device, is indicated for children with a pacemaker or a heart transplant and for those receiving anticoagulation therapy or antidysrhythmic medication.

The nurse also discusses common behavior disturbances that may occur after discharge, such as nightmares, sleep disturbances, separation anxiety, and overdependence. A supportive, consistent response is essential to allow the child to overcome the surgical experience. The child should be encouraged to work out feelings and fears through therapeutic play.

Although surgical correction of heart defects has improved dramatically, it is still not possible to completely repair many of the complex anomalies. For many children, repeat procedures are required to replace conduits or grafts or to manage complications such as restenosis. Consequently, the long-term prognosis is uncertain, and full recovery is not always possible. For these families, medical follow-up and continued emotional support are essential. The nurse can often serve as an important primary health professional and as a resource for referrals when needed.

ACQUIRED CARDIOVASCULAR DISORDERS

BACTERIAL (INFECTIVE) ENDOCARDITIS

Bacterial endocarditis (BE), or infective endocarditis (IE), also referred to as *subacute bacterial endocarditis (SBE),* is an infection of the valves and inner lining of the heart. Although it can occur without underlying heart disease, it is most often a sequela of bacteremia in the child with acquired or congenital anomalies of the heart or great vessels. It especially affects children with valvular abnormalities, prosthetic valves, recent cardiac surgery with invasive lines, and rheumatic heart disease with valve involvement. The most common causative agent is *Streptococcus viridans;* other causative agents are *Staphylococcus aureus,* gram-negative bacteria, and fungi such as *Candida albicans.*

BOX 25-8 ■ Clinical Manifestations of Infective Endocarditis

Onset usually insidious
Unexplained fever (low grade and intermittent)
Anorexia
Malaise
Weight loss
Characteristic findings caused by extracardiac emboli formation:
   Splinter hemorrhages (thin black lines) under the nails
   Osler nodes (red, painful intradermal nodes found on pads of
     phalanges)
   Janeway lesions (painless hemorrhagic areas on palms and soles)
   Petechiae on oral mucous membranes
May be present:
   Congestive heart failure
   Cardiac dysrhythmias
   New murmur or change in previously existing one

Pathophysiology

Organisms may enter the bloodstream from any site of localized infection. The most common portals of entry are oral from dental work *(S. viridans);* the urinary tract, such as from urinary tract infection after catheterization (gram-negative bacilli); the heart, from cardiac surgery, especially if synthetic material is used (valves, patches, conduits); and the bloodstream from long-term indwelling catheters. The microorganisms grow on the endocardium, forming vegetations (verrucae), deposits of fibrin, and platelet thrombi. The lesion may invade adjacent tissues, such as aortic and mitral valves, and may break off and embolize elsewhere, especially in the spleen, kidney, and central nervous system.

Diagnostic Evaluation

The diagnosis of IE is suspected on the basis of clinical manifestations (Box 25-8). Several laboratory findings may suggest IE (e.g., ECG changes [prolonged P-R interval], radiographic evidence of cardiomegaly, anemia, elevated erythrocyte sedimentation rate, leukocytosis, microscopic hematuria). Vegetations on the valve and abnormal valve function can often be visualized by echocardiography. Definitive diagnosis rests on growth and identification of the causative agent in the blood.

Therapeutic Management

Treatment should be instituted immediately and consists of administration of high doses of appropriate antibiotics intravenously for 2 to 8 weeks. Blood cultures are taken periodically to evaluate response to antibiotic therapy.

Prevention involves administration of prophylactic antibiotic therapy 1 hour before procedures known to increase the risk of entry of organisms. Drugs of choice include amoxicillin, ampicillin, clindamycin, cephalexin, cefadroxil, azithromycin, and clarithromycin (Box 25-9).

Nursing Considerations

Ideally, the objective of nursing care is to counsel parents of high-risk children concerning the need for prophylactic antibiotic therapy before procedures such as dental work. The

BOX 25-9 ■ Endocarditis Prophylaxis Recommendations

DENTAL PROCEDURES

Dental extractions

Periodontal procedures, including surgery, scaling and root planing, probing, and recall maintenance

Dental implant placement and reimplantation of avulsed teeth

Endodontic (root canal) instrumentation or surgery only beyond the apex

Subgingival placement of antibiotic fibers/strips

Initial placement of orthodontic bands but not brackets

Intraligamentary local anesthetic injections

Prophylactic cleaning of teeth or implants where bleeding is anticipated

OTHER PROCEDURES

Respiratory Tract

Surgeries that involve respiratory mucosa

Bronchoscopy with a rigid bronchoscope

Tonsillectomy and/or adenoidectomy

Gastrointestinal Tract

Sclerotherapy for esophageal varices

Esophageal stricture dilation

Endoscopic retrograde cholangiography with biliary obstruction

Biliary tract surgery

Surgical operations that involve intestinal mucosa

Genitourinary Tract

Prostatic surgery

Cystoscopy

Urethral dilation

From Dajani AS and others: Prevention of bacterial endocarditis: recommendations by the American Heart Association, *JAMA* 277:1794-1801, 1997.

family's regular dentist should be advised of existing cardiac problems in the child as an added precaution to ensure preventive treatment. These children should also maintain the highest level of oral health to reduce the chance of bacteremia from oral infections.

Parents should also have a high index of suspicion regarding potential infections. Without unduly alarming them, the nurse stresses that any unexplained fever, weight loss, or change in behavior (lethargy, malaise, anorexia) must be brought to the practitioner's attention. Such symptoms should not be self-diagnosed as a cold or flu. Early treatment is important in preventing further cardiac damage, embolic complications, and growth of resistant organisms.

Treatment of endocarditis requires long-term parenteral drug therapy. In many cases, IV antibiotics may be administered at home with nursing supervision for part of the treatment course. Nursing goals during this period are (1) preparation of the child for IV infusion, usually with an intermittent-infusion device, and several venipunctures for blood cultures; (2) observation for side effects of antibiotics, especially inflammation along venipuncture sites; (3) observation for complications, including embolism and CHF; and (4) education regarding the importance of follow-up visits for cardiac evaluation, echocardiographic monitoring, and blood cultures.

RHEUMATIC FEVER

Rheumatic fever (RF) is a poorly understood inflammatory disease that occurs after infection with group A β-hemolytic streptococcal pharyngitis. It is a self-limited illness that involves the joints, skin, brain, serous surfaces, and heart. Cardiac valve damage (referred to as *rheumatic heart disease*) is the most significant complication of RF. In developed countries RF and rheumatic heart disease have become uncommon. However, RF remains a devastating problem in developing (third world) countries and has reappeared in some parts of the United States (Gentles and others, 2001).

Etiology

Strong evidence supports a relationship between upper respiratory infection with group A streptococci and subsequent development of RF (usually within 2 to 6 weeks). In almost all cases of RF a previous infection with group A streptococci can be documented by laboratory evidence of rising antibody titers. Prevention or treatment of group A streptococcal infection prevents RF.

Diagnostic Evaluation

Diagnosis is based on a set of guidelines recommended by the American Heart Association. These guidelines, known as *modifications of the Jones criteria*, suggest that the presence of two major manifestations or one major and two minor manifestations, such as fever and arthralgia, with supportive evidence of recent streptococcal infection, indicates a high probability of RF (see Guidelines box).

Children suspected of having RF are tested for streptococcal antibodies. The most reliable and best standardized test is an elevated or rising *antistreptolysin-O (ASO or ASLO) titer*, which occurs in 80% of children with RF.

Therapeutic Management

The goals of medical management are (1) eradication of hemolytic streptococci, (2) prevention of permanent cardiac damage, (3) palliation of the other symptoms, and (4) prevention of recurrences of RF. Penicillin is the drug of choice, with erythromycin as a substitute in penicillin-sensitive children. Salicylates are used to control the inflammatory process, especially in the joints, and reduce the fever and discomfort. Bed rest is recommended during the acute febrile phase but need not be strict.

Prophylactic treatment against recurrence of RF is started after the acute therapy and involves monthly intramuscular injections of benzathine penicillin G (1.2 million U), two daily oral doses of penicillin (200,000 U), or one daily dose of sulfadiazine (1 g). The duration of long-term prophylaxis is uncertain.

Children who have had acute RF are susceptible to recurrent RF for the rest of their lives and should be followed medically for at least 5 years. Children and families must be aware of the need for continuing antibiotic prophylaxis for dental work, infection, and invasive procedures.

Nursing Considerations

The objectives of nursing care for the child with RF are to (1) encourage compliance with drug regimens, (2) facilitate recovery from the illness, (3) provide emotional support,

GUIDELINES

Diagnosis of Initial Attack of Rheumatic Fever (Jones Criteria, 1992 Update)*

MAJOR MANIFESTATIONS

Carditis
Tachycardia out of proportion to degree of fever
Cardiomegaly
New murmurs or change in preexisting murmurs
Muffled heart sounds
Pericardial friction rub
Chest pain
Changes in ECG (especially prolonged P-R interval)

Polyarthritis
Swollen, hot, red, painful joint(s)
After 1 to 2 days affects different joint(s)
Favors large joints—knees, elbows, hips, shoulders, wrists

Erythema Marginatum
Erythematous macules with clear center and wavy, well-demarcated border
Transitory
Nonpruritic
Primarily affects trunk and extremities (inner surfaces)

Chorea (St. Vitus Dance, Sydenham chorea)
Sudden aimless, irregular movements of extremities
Involuntary facial grimaces
Speech disturbances
Emotional lability
Muscle weakness (can be profound)
Muscle movements exaggerated by anxiety and attempts at fine motor activity; relieved by rest

Subcutaneous Nodes
Nontender swelling
Located over bony prominences
May persist for some time, then gradually resolve

Minor Manifestations
Clinical findings
  Arthralgia
  Fever

LABORATORY FINDINGS
Elevated acute-phase reactants
  Erythrocyte sedimentation rate
  C-reactive protein

SUPPORTING EVIDENCE OF ANTECEDENT GROUP A STREPTOCOCCAL INFECTION
Positive throat culture or rapid streptococcal antigen test
  Elevated or rising streptococcal antibody titer

From Special Writing Group of the Committee on Rheumatic Fever, Endocarditis, and Kawasaki Disease of the Council on Cardiovascular Disease in the Young of the American Heart Association: Guidelines for the diagnosis of rheumatic fever: Jones criteria, 1992 (update), *JAMA* 268:2069-2073, 1992.
*If supported by evidence of preceding group A streptococcal infection, the presence of two major manifestations or of one major and two minor manifestations indicates a high probability of acute rheumatic fever.

and (4) prevent the disease. Because compliance is a major concern in long-term drug therapy, every effort is made to encourage adherence to the therapeutic plan (see Compliance, Chapter 22). When compliance is poor, monthly injections may be substituted for daily oral administration of antibiotics, and children need preparation for this often-dreaded procedure.

Interventions during home care are primarily concerned with providing rest and adequate nutrition. Usually, after the febrile stage is over, children can resume moderate activity, and their appetite improves. If carditis is present, the family must be aware of any activity restrictions and may need help in choosing less strenuous activities for the child.

One of the most disturbing and frustrating manifestations of the disease is *chorea*. The onset is gradual and may occur weeks to months after the illness; it sometimes even occurs in children who have not been diagnosed with RF. It may be mistaken for nervousness, clumsiness, behavioral changes, inattentiveness, and learning disability. It is usually a source of great frustration to the child because the movements, incoordination, and weakness severely limit physical ability. The child needs an opportunity to verbalize feelings. Of utmost importance is stressing to parents and school-teachers the involuntary, sudden nature of the movements, that the chorea is transitory, and that all manifestations eventually disappear.

Nurses also have a role in prevention, primarily in screening school-age children for sore throats caused by group A streptococci. This may involve actively participating in throat culture screening programs or in referring children with a possible streptococcal infection for testing.

HYPERLIPIDEMIA (HYPERCHOLESTEROLEMIA)

Hyperlipidemia is a general term for excessive lipids (fat and fatlike substances); *hypercholesterolemia* refers to excessive cholesterol in the blood. High lipid or cholesterol levels are believed to play an important role in producing atherosclerosis (fatty plaques on the arteries), which eventually can lead to coronary artery disease, a primary cause of morbidity and mortality in the adult population. Research indicates that a presymptomatic phase of atherosclerosis begins in childhood. Preventive cardiology is focusing on the screening and management of lipid levels in childhood. The goal is to identify those children at high risk and intervene early.

Cholesterol is part of the lipoprotein complex in plasma that is essential for cellular metabolism. Triglycerides, natural fats synthesized from carbohydrates, are used for energy. Both are major lipids transported on *lipoproteins,* a combination of lipids and proteins, which include:

Low-density lipoproteins (LDLs)—Contain low concentrations of triglycerides, high levels of cholesterol, and moderate levels of protein. LDL is the major carrier of cholesterol to the cells. Cells use cholesterol for synthesis of membranes and steroid production. Elevated circulating LDL is a strong risk factor in cardiovascular disease.

High-density lipoproteins (HDLs)—Contain very low concentrations of triglycerides, relatively little cholesterol, and high levels of protein. They transport free cholesterol to the liver for excretion in the bile. High levels of HDL are thought to protect against cardiovascular disease.

**TABLE 25-5 ■ Classification of Choles-
terol Levels in Children
From Families With a
History of Heart Disease**

CATEGORY	TOTAL CHOLESTEROL (mg/dl)	LDL CHOLESTEROL (mg/dl)
Acceptable	<170	<110
Borderline	170-199	110-129
High	≥200	≥130

From National Cholesterol Education Program: Report of the Expert Panel on Blood Cholesterol Levels in Children and Adolescents, *Pediatrics* 89(3 pt 2):527, 1992.

Diagnostic Evaluation

Hyperlipidemia is diagnosed on the basis of analysis of blood for a full lipid profile. Two samples drawn in the fasting state (12 hours) should be analyzed, and the average of the values used for diagnosis. Blood samples should be collected after having the child sit for 5 minutes, and the tourniquet should be applied immediately before the needle puncture, because posture and vascular stasis may affect results. Diagnostic values for acceptable, borderline, and high total cholesterol and LDL cholesterol levels are listed in Table 25-5.

Screening children for hypercholesterolemia is a controversial issue, with some authorities advocating universal screening and others proposing selective screening. Guidelines recommended by the American Academy of Pediatrics' Committee on Nutrition (1998) recommend a strategy that combines two complementary approaches: (1) a *population approach* that aims to lower the average levels of blood cholesterol among all American children through population-wide changes in nutrient intake and eating patterns, and (2) an *individualized approach* based on selective screening. (See Evidence-Based Practice box.)

Therapeutic Management

Treatment of high cholesterol is primarily dietary. The American Academy of Pediatrics guidelines recommend a two-step dietary approach that restricts the intake of cholesterol and fat. Children with borderline LDL cholesterol are advised to follow the *step one diet.* It recommends the same nutrient intake as for the general population (i.e., less than 10% of total calories from saturated fatty acids, no more than 30% of calories from total fat, less than 300 mg/day of cholesterol, and adequate calories to support growth and development and to reach or maintain desirable body weight). Children with high LDL cholesterol levels initially are also placed on this diet. If these dietary modifications fail to achieve satisfactory levels of LDL after 3 months of therapy, the *step two diet* is initiated. These dietary restrictions include a further reduction of saturated fatty acid intake to 7% of calories and of cholesterol intake to less than 200 mg/day.

New research continues to support the benefit of diets low in saturated fats. Current thinking favors a "Mediterranean"-type diet. Whole grains, fruits, and vegetables form the foundation of this diet. In addition, this diet allows the use of monounsaturated fats, such as olive oil and canola oil,

EVIDENCE-BASED PRACTICE

Cholesterol Screening for Children

Practitioners' opinions differ regarding lipid screening in childhood. In 1992 the National Cholesterol Education Program (NCEP) issued a consensus statement that provides guidelines for cholesterol screening in the pediatric population. Currently, selective screening is recommended for children who have a family history of premature cardiovascular disease (<55 years old) or children who have at least one parent with a high blood cholesterol level (>240 mg/dL). In addition, if a child's complete family history is not available, practitioners may consider screening. Finally, cholesterol values should be obtained in children who have any individual risk factors, such as a history of diabetes, Kawasaki disease, hypertension, or obesity.

Selective screening is favored by many experts because high blood cholesterol levels aggregate in families as a result of shared genetic and environmental factors (American Academy of Pediatrics, 1998). In addition, the most severely affected children generally come from families in which there is a high incidence of early heart disease.

Advocates of selective screening oppose universal screening for various reasons. Screening is costly, and the laboratory data may vary significantly from center to center, resulting in inappropriate diagnosis.

Those favoring universal screening believe that selective screening is too limited and overlooks many children with hyperlipidemia. With varying family constellations a common situation today, family history may be incomplete. In addition, a negative history from a parent may be inaccurate, because approximately half of well-educated adults do not know their own cholesterol levels.

In your practice, how many adult family members know their "numbers"? Also, observe how often pediatric practitioners ask about parents' cholesterol levels and heart disease as part of the child's health assessment. From your observations do you believe that selective screening is being implemented?

which have beneficial effects on HDL-cholesterol values. The use of these fats also makes the diet more realistic.

> **! NURSING ALERT**
>
> The Report of the Expert Panel on Blood Cholesterol Levels in Children and Adolescents recommendations for fat intake are not intended for infants from birth to 2 years of age, whose fast growth requires a higher percentage of calories from fat. Toddlers 2 to 3 years of age may safely make the transition to the recommended eating pattern as they begin to eat with the family. No treatment recommendations are made for any child younger than 2 years of age.

For children with severe hypercholesterolemia who fail to respond to dietary modifications, drug therapy may be necessary. Two drugs recommended for treatment are the bile acid–binding resins or sequestrants *cholestyramine* and *colestipol.* These two drugs act by binding bile acids in the intestinal lumen. Because they are not absorbed by the intestine, they do not produce systemic toxicity and are safe for children. Cholestyramine (Questran) and colestipol (Colestid) are both powders that are mixed with water or juice just before ingestion. Some patients cannot tolerate the medication because of the taste and the side effects, the most significant being constipation, abdominal pain, gastrointestinal bloating, flatulence, and nausea.

Patients should be instructed to take one multivitamin supplement with iron daily, because cholestyramine may interfere with the absorption of fat-soluble vitamins. It may also interfere with the absorption of other medications, which should be given at least 1 hour before or 6 hours after the resin-binding agent is ingested.

Nursing Considerations

Nurses play an important role in the screening, education, and support of children with hyperlipidemia and their families. When a child is referred to a lipid clinic, it is essential that the family be adequately prepared for the first visit. Generally, the parents will be asked to keep a dietary history of the child before this visit. Sometimes they will need to complete a questionnaire regarding the child's normal dietary habits during the preceding year. Families should be instructed to keep their child fasting for at least 12 hours before screening. It is important to schedule the blood test early in the morning and to arrange for nourishment immediately thereafter. At the visit, a full family history should be taken, including the health of both parents and all first-degree relatives. Specific questions should be asked regarding early heart disease, hypertension, strokes (CVAs), sudden death, hyperlipidemia, diabetes, and endocrine abnormalities. Nurses may also uncover risk factors when obtaining a health history for other purposes. It is therefore important that nurses be familiar with current screening practices and the availability of resources for children with positive family histories.

Parents and extended families should be informed about cholesterol and hyperlipidemia. This education should include a brief introduction to the different lipoprotein categories, including cholesterol, HDL, LDL, and triglycerides. Also, behavioral risk factors for heart disease, such as smoking and exercise, should be reviewed. For management to be effective, parents need to understand the rationale for dietary and/or pharmacologic intervention. The key is prevention of future cardiovascular disease.

Stringent dietary guidelines may become an issue of control and a source of great stress for many families. Children should not be viewed as having a disease. Rather, the positive aspects of healthy eating, regular exercise, and avoiding smoking should be emphasized. Basic dietary changes should be encouraged for the whole family so that the affected child is not singled out. Cultural differences must be considered and recommendations individualized. Substitution rather than elimination needs to be emphasized. Visual aids are often helpful, especially for the children (e.g., test tubes depicting the amount of fat in a hot dog). Diets should be flexible and individually tailored by a nutritionist experienced in combining recommendations that meet both the nutritional demands of the growing child and the lipid modifications. Parents are encouraged to participate in dietary and educational sessions, ask questions, and share ideas and experiences.

Parents often feel guilty about the hereditary component of hyperlipidemia. Many also believe they have failed if the diet alone is not making a significant difference in their child's lipid profile. They need to be reassured that a dietary approach alone is often not sufficient, especially for children with values greater than the 95th percentile.

Parents of children who require pharmacologic therapy need to understand the purpose, dosage, and possible side effects of the various drugs. Medication schedules should remain flexible and should not interfere with the child's daily activities. For example, children of elementary school age may have better compliance if they take a resin-binding agent (e.g., cholestyramine, colestipol) twice a day (i.e., before school and at night) rather than the standard three times a day. Follow-up phone calls by the nurse between visits allow parents to discuss their concerns and ask any questions that have arisen.

CARDIAC DYSRHYTHMIAS

Dysrhythmias, or abnormal heart rhythms, can occur in children with structurally normal hearts, as features of some congenital heart defects, and in patients after surgical repair of congenital heart defects. They are also seen in patients with cardiomyopathy and with cardiac tumors. They can occur secondary to metabolic and electrolyte imbalances. They can be classified in several ways, including by heart rate characteristics (bradycardia and tachycardia) and by the origin of the dysrhythmia in the atria or ventricles (Hanisch, 2001). Some dysrhythmias are well-tolerated and self-limiting. Others may cause decreased cardiac output with associated symptoms. Some dysrhythmias can cause sudden death. Treatment depends on the cause of the dysrhythmia and its severity. Many advances have been made in the diagnosis and treatment of pediatric dysrhythmias in the past decade. Improvements in technology have allowed better diagnosis, the development of ablation techniques, and the expansion of pacemaker capabilities. New anti-arrhythmic medications have proven safe and effective in children. Radio-frequency ablation has offered a cure for some dysrhythmias. Pediatric electrophysiology has become a highly specialized field, and the student is referred to more detailed sources for an in-depth discussion. The following sections will address diagnostic studies and a general discussion of the most common tachycardia (supraventricular tachycardia, SVT) and the most common bradycardia (complete heart block) that require treatment in the pediatric population.

Diagnostic Evaluation

Nurses must be familiar with the standards of normal heart rate for the particular age-group (see inside back cover). An initial nursing responsibility is recognition of an abnormal heartbeat, either in rate or rhythm. When a dysrhythmia is suspected, the apical rate is counted for a full minute and compared with the radial rate, which may be lower because not all of the apical beats are felt. Consistently high or low heart rates should be regarded as suspicious. The patient should be placed on a cardiac monitor with recording capabilities. A 12-lead ECG yields more information than the monitor recording and should be done as soon as possible.

The basic diagnostic procedure is the ECG, including 24-hour Holter monitoring. *Electrophysiologic cardiac catheterization* allows for identification of the conduction disturbance and immediate investigation of drugs that may control the dysrhythmia. Another procedure that may be employed is *transesophageal recording*. An electrode catheter is passed to the lower esophagus and, when in position at a point proximal to the heart, is used to stimulate and record dysrhythmias.

Dysrhythmias can be classified according to various criteria, such as effect on heart rate and rhythm, as follows:

Bradydysrhythmias—abnormally slow rate
Tachydysrhythmias—abnormally rapid rate
Conduction disturbances—irregular heart rate

Bradydysrhythmias.   **Sinus bradycardia** (slower than normal rate) in children can be due to the influence of the autonomic nervous system, as with hypervagal tone, or in response to hypoxia and hypotension (Hanisch, 2001). Sinus bradycardias are also known to develop after some complex cardiac surgical repairs involving extensive atrial suture lines such as atrial baffle repairs (Mustrard and Senning repairs) and the Fontan procedure.

Complete atrioventricular block (AV block) is also referred to as **complete heart block.** This can be either congenital (occurring in children with structurally normal hearts) or acquired after surgery to repair cardiac defects. AV blocks are most often related to edema around the conduction system and resolve without treatment. Temporary epicardial wires are placed in most patients at surgery; if a rhythm disturbance occurs, temporary pacing can be employed. Several days after surgery, the health practitioner removes the wires by pulling slowly and deliberately down on them from the site of insertion.

A permanent pacemaker may be needed in some children. The pacemaker takes over or assists in the conduction function of the heart. The surgical implantation of a pacemaker is usually a low-risk procedure. After the wire has been introduced, a small incision is made and a pocket is formed under the muscle to house and protect the generator. Continuous ECG monitoring is necessary during the recovery phase to assess pacemaker function. The nurse should be aware of the programmed rate and expected individual generator variations. The pacemaker insertion site is monitored for signs of infection. Analgesics are given for pain.

Pacemaker functions have become more sophisticated, and some models can adjust heart rate to activity demands or be programmed for overdrive pacing or cardioversion.

When a pacemaker is implanted, the education of the parents and child includes an explanation of the device, a description of the component parts and the surgical procedure, and discharge teaching. For example, discharge teaching includes information about the signs and symptoms of infection, general wound care, and any specific limitations to activity. Instructions for telephone transmission of ECG readings are also given. Children with pacemakers should wear a MedicAlert device, and their parents should have a pacer identification card with specific pacer data in case of an emergency.

Discharge teaching includes information about the signs and symptoms of infection, general wound care, and activity restrictions. Parents and older children and adolescents should be taught to take a pulse and know the settings of the pacemaker. If the patient's low rate is set at 80 and the heart rate is only 68, there is a problem with the pacemaker that needs to be investigated. Instructions for telephone transmission of ECG readings are also given. Telephone trans-

mission can be used to transmit ECG strips and also to monitor battery life and pacemaker function. The pacemaker generator will have to be replaced periodically because of battery depletion. Children with pacemakers should wear a medical alert device, and their parents should have a pacemaker identification card with specific pacer data in case of emergency. CPR instruction is suggested for parents.

Tachydysrhythmias.   **Sinus tachycardia** (abnormally fast heart rate) secondary to fever, anxiety pain, anemia, dehydration, or any other etiologic factor requiring increased cardiac output should be ruled out first before diagnosing an increased heart rate as pathologic. SVT is the most common tachydysrhythmia found in children and refers to a rapid regular heart rate of 200 to 300 beats per minute (Hanisch, 2001). The onset of SVT is often sudden, the duration variable, and the rhythm may end abruptly and convert back to a normal sinus rhythm. Clinical signs in infants and young children are poor feeding, extreme irritability, and pallor. Children may experience palpitations, dizziness, chest pain, and diaphoresis. If SVT is sustained, signs of CHF may be seen.

The treatment of SVT depends on the degree of compromise imposed by the dysrhythmia. In some cases, vagal maneuvers, such as applying ice to the face, massaging the carotid artery (on one side of the neck only), or having an older child perform a Valsalva maneuver (e.g., exhaling against a closed glottis, blowing on a thumb as if it were a trumpet for 30 to 60 seconds), have terminated SVT. If vagal maneuvers fail or the child is hemodynamically unstable, adenosine (a drug that impairs AV conduction) may be used. Adenosine is given by rapid IV push with a saline bolus immediately after the drug because of its very short half-life. If this is unsuccessful or cardiac output is compromised, esophageal overdrive pacing or synchronized cardioversion (delivering an electrical shock to the heart) can be employed in the intensive care setting (Hanisch, 2001). Sedation is needed for both procedures. Cardioversion should never be done in a conscious patient. More long-term pharmacologic treatment includes digoxin or possibly Inderal or amiodarone for severe or recurrent SVT.

A primary focus of nursing care is education of the family regarding the symptoms of SVT and its treatment. SVT may occur again despite therapy. Parents should be taught to take a radial pulse for a full minute. If medication is prescribed, instructions regarding accurate dosage and the importance of administering the correct dose at specified intervals are stressed.

Radio-frequency ablation has become first-line therapy for some types of SVT. The procedure is done in the cardiac catheterization laboratory and begins with mapping of the conduction system to identify the arrhythmia focus. A catheter delivering radio-frequency current is directed at the site, and the area is heated to destroy the tissue in the area. These are lengthy procedures, often 6 to 8 hours, and sedation or general anesthesia is required. Preparation is similar to that for cardiac catheterization.

PULMONARY ARTERY HYPERTENSION

Pulmonary artery hypertension (PAH) describes a group of rare disorders that result in an elevation of pulmonary artery pressure above 25 mm Hg at rest after the neonatal period

(Barst, 1999). These disorders are poorly understood, and until recently there was no treatment beyond supportive care. PAH is a progressive, eventually fatal disease for which there is no known cure. It can be difficult to diagnose in the early stages. Often when patients become symptomatic and a diagnosis is made, their disease is rapidly progressing, treatment is unsuccessful, and death occurs within several years.

PAH can be caused by increased pulmonary blood flow or increased pulmonary vascular resistance. Why some children develop the disease and others do not is unclear. There are many possible causes of PAH. Cardiac causes occur primarily in patients with a large left-to-right shunt producing increased pulmonary blood flow. If these defects are not repaired early, the high pulmonary flow will cause changes in the pulmonary artery vessels and the vessels will lose their elasticity. Other causes of PAH include hypoxic lung diseases, thromboembolic diseases causing pulmonary vascular obstruction, collagen vascular diseases, and exposure to toxic substances. Many of the patients have no identifiable cause for PAH and have primary or idiopathic PAH.

Clinical Manifestations

The clinical manifestations include dyspnea with exercise, chest pain, and syncope. Dyspnea is the most common symptom and is caused by impaired oxygen delivery. Chest pain is the result of coronary ischemia in the right ventricle from severe hypertrophy. Syncope reflects a limited cardiac output leading to decreased cerebral blood flow. Right heart dysfunction is steadily progressive, and when symptoms of venous congestion and edema are present, prognosis is poor.

Therapeutic Management

Although no cure is known, several therapies have shown promise in slowing the progression of the disease and improving quality of life. In general, situations that may exacerbate the disease and cause hypoxia, such as exercise and high altitudes, are avoided. Supplemental oxygen, especially at night while sleeping, is commonly used to relieve hypoxia. Patients are at risk for thromboembolic events leading to pulmonary emboli so anticoagulation with Coumadin is often prescribed.

Vasodilator therapy (which relaxes vascular smooth muscle and reduces pulmonary artery pressure) has improved the survival of patients with PAH. Oral calcium-channel blockers have been successful in some children. Continuous IV prostacyclin or chronic inhaled nitric oxide have been used with some success in children who did not respond to oral therapy. Both these therapies, although promising, have only been used in small numbers of patients and are very expensive. Lung transplantation may be another treatment option.

CARDIOMYOPATHY

Cardiomyopathy refers to abnormalities of the myocardium in which the cardiac muscles' ability to contract is impaired. Cardiomyopathies are relatively rare in children. Possible etiologic factors include familial or genetic causes, infection, deficiency states, metabolic abnormalities, and collagen vascular diseases. Most cardiomyopathies in children are con-

sidered primary or idiopathic, in which the cause is unknown and the cardiac dysfunction is not associated with systemic disease. Some of the known causes of *secondary* cardiomyopathy are anthracycline toxicity (the antineoplastic agents doxorubicin [Adriamycin] and daunomycin), hemochromatosis (from excessive iron storage), Duchenne muscular dystrophy, Kawasaki disease, collagen diseases, and thyroid dysfunction.

Cardiomyopathies can be divided into three broad clinical categories according to the type of abnormal structure and dysfunction present: dilated cardiomyopathy, hypertrophic cardiomyopathy, and restrictive cardiomyopathy. *Dilated cardiomyopathy* is characterized by ventricular dilation and greatly decreased contractility resulting in symptoms of CHF. This is the most common type of cardiomyopathy in children. Its cause is often unknown. The clinical findings are of CHF with tachycardia, dyspnea, hepatosplenomegaly, fatigue, and poor growth. Dysrhythmias may be present and may be more difficult to control with worsening heart failure.

Hypertrophic cardiomyopathy is characterized by an increase in heart muscle mass without an increase in cavity size, usually occurring in the left ventricle and associated with abnormal diastolic filling. Half of these patients have a familial autosomal dominant genetic abnormality (Burch and Blair, 1999). Clinical symptoms usually present in the school-age period or adolescence and may include anginal chest pain, dysrhythmias, and syncope. Sudden death is possible. Presentation in infancy includes signs of CHF and has a poor prognosis. Chest radiography shows a mildly enlarged heart; the ECG demonstrates left ventricular (LV) hypertrophy, often with ST-T changes. The ECG is most helpful and demonstrates asymmetric septal hypertrophy and an increase in LV wall thickness, with a small LV cavity.

Restrictive cardiomyopathy, rare in children, describes a restriction to ventricular filling caused by endocardial or myocardial disease or both. It is characterized by diastolic dysfunction and absence of ventricular dilation or hypertrophy. Symptoms are of CHF (see p. 906).

Therapeutic Management

Treatment is directed toward correcting the underlying cause whenever feasible. However, in most affected children this is not possible, and treatment is aimed at managing CHF (p. 906) and dysrhythmias. Digoxin, diuretics, and aggressive use of afterload reduction agents have been found to be helpful in managing symptoms in those with dilated cardiomyopathy. Digoxin and inotropic agents are usually not helpful in the other forms of cardiomyopathy, because increasing the force of contraction may exacerbate the muscular obstruction and actually impair ventricular ejection. Beta blockers such as propranolol (Inderal) or calcium-channel blockers such as verapamil (Calan) have been used to reduce left ventricular outflow obstruction and improve diastolic filling in those with hypertrophic cardiomyopathy.

Careful monitoring and treatment of dysrhythmias is essential. Anticoagulants may be given to reduce the risk of thromboemboli, a complication of the sluggish circulation through the heart. For worsening heart failure and signs of poor perfusion, IV inotropic or vasodilating drugs may be needed. Severely ill children may require mechanical ventilation, oxygen administration, and IV medications. Heart transplantation may be a treatment option for patients who have worsening symptoms despite maximum medical therapy.

Nursing Considerations

Because of the poor prognosis in many children with cardiomyopathy, nursing care is consistent with that for any child with a life-threatening disorder (see Chapter 18). One of the most difficult adjustments for the child (especially the normally active youngster with hypertrophic cardiomyopathy) may be the realization of failing health and the need for restricted activity. The child should be included in decisions regarding activity and allowed to discuss feelings, particularly if the disease follows a progressively fatal course. After symptoms of CHF or dysrhythmias develop, the same nursing interventions are implemented as discussed on pp. 906 to 909. If cardiac transplantation is considered, the needs of the child and family are great in terms of psychologic preparation and postoperative care. The nurse plays an important role in assessing the family's understanding of the procedure and long-term consequences. Children of school age and older should be fully informed to give their assent to the procedure (see Informed Consent, Chapter 22).

HEART TRANSPLANTATION

Heart transplantation has become a treatment option for infants and children with worsening heart failure and a limited life expectancy despite maximum medical and surgical management. Indications for cardiac transplantation in children are cardiomyopathy and end-stage congenital heart disease. It is also an option for patients with some forms of complex congenital cardiac defects, such as hypoplastic left heart syndrome, for whom conventional surgical approaches have a high mortality (Luikart, 2001).

The heart transplant procedure may be orthotopic or heterotopic. *Orthotopic heart transplantation* refers to removing the recipient's own heart and implanting a new heart from a donor who has had brain death but a healthy heart. The donor and recipient are matched by weight and blood type. *Heterotopic heart transplantation* refers to leaving the recipient's own heart in place and implanting a new heart to act as an additional pump or "piggyback" heart; this type of transplant is rarely done in children.

Before transplantation, potential recipients undergo a careful cardiac evaluation to determine if there are any other medical or surgical options to improve the patient's cardiac status. Other organ systems are assessed to identify problems that might preclude or increase the risk of transplantation. A psychosocial evaluation of the patient and family is done to assess family function, support systems, and the family's ability to comply with the complex medical regimen after the transplant. Support services to help the family successfully care for their child are provided when possible. Parents and older adolescents need extensive education about the risks and benefits of transplantation so that they can make an informed decision (Higgins, 2001). Patients are listed on a national computer network organized by the **United Network for Organ Sharing (UNOS)** to match donors and recipients. (See also Organ or Tissue Donation/Autopsy, Chapter 18.)

The number of heart transplants in pediatric patients has been constant for the last decade, between 340 and 400 transplants per year (Boucek and others, 2001). This likely reflects a limit in the number of available donors. Infants are the largest group of pediatric transplant recipients. Recent data from the International Society for Heart and Lung Transplantation Registry for pediatric heart transplants between 1996 and 1999 showed a 1-year actuarial survival rate of 86% and a 4-year actuarial survival rate of 79% (Boucek and others, 2001). The largest minority is the early post-transplant period.

The post-transplant course is complex. Although heart function is greatly improved or normal after transplantation, the risk of rejection is serious. The leading cause of death after heart transplantation is rejection (Fortuna, Chinnock, and Bailey, 1999). Rejection of the heart is diagnosed primarily by endomyocardial biopsy in older children. Serial echocardiograms are often used in infants and young children to reduce the need for invasive biopsies. Immunosuppressants must be taken for life and have many systemic side effects (Luikart, 2001). Infection is always a risk. Potential long-term problems that may limit survival include chronic rejection, causing coronary artery disease; renal dysfunction and hypertension resulting from cyclosporine administration; lymphoma; and infection. In the short term, after successful transplantation, children are able to return to full participation in age-appropriate activities and appear to adapt well to their new lifestyle. Transplantation is not a cure, because patients must live with the lifetime consequences of chronic immunosuppression. The long-term prognosis is unknown because heart transplantation is a relatively new therapy in the pediatric population, begun in 1985.

Nursing Considerations

Nursing care after transplantation is demanding and complex, with careful attention to both the physical needs of the child and the emotional needs of the child and family. Successfully caring for a child after a heart transplant requires the expertise and dedication of many members of the health care team. Nurses play vital roles in assessment, coordination of care, psychosocial support, and patient and family education. The heart transplant recipient must be carefully monitored for signs of rejection, infection, and the side effects of the immunosuppressant medications. The patient and family's psychosocial well-being also needs to be assessed to identify issues such as increased family stress, depression, substance abuse, and school problems. Noncompliance with an intense medication regimen, especially during adolescence, can lead to serious medical problems and can be fatal. Immunosuppressants and nursing implications are discussed in Chapter 27 in relation to renal transplantation. Care of the immunosuppressed child is reviewed in Chapter 26. Psychosocial concerns and appropriate interventions for the child with a life-threatening disorder are presented in Chapter 18.

The first 6 months to 1 year after the transplant are most intense, because the risk of complications is greatest and the patient and family are adjusting to a new lifestyle. Patients are monitored closely by the health care team, with frequent visits and laboratory tests. Care is usually shared between local health care providers and the transplant center. Many patients are able to return to school and other age-appropriate activities within 2 to 3 months after the transplant.

VASCULAR DYSFUNCTION

SYSTEMIC HYPERTENSION

Hypertension is defined as the consistent elevation of blood pressure (BP) beyond values considered to be the upper limits of normal.

The two major categories are *essential hypertension* (no identifiable cause) and *secondary hypertension* (subsequent to an identifiable cause). Hypertension is the most common cause of CVAs and a major risk factor for myocardial infarction in adults. In recent years there has been increasing interest in this disorder in adolescents and children, particularly in terms of prevention of later morbidity and mortality. Routine BP measurements have detected hypertension with surprising frequency in asymptomatic children, especially teenagers. Although the prevalence of the condition in adolescents is difficult to evaluate, evidence is accumulating to indicate that the essential hypertension of adulthood may have its origin in childhood; thus, its early detection has significance for prevention and treatment.

Etiology

Most instances of hypertension observed in young children occur secondary to a structural abnormality or an underlying pathologic process, although this is being challenged by screening programs of relatively healthy children. The most common cause of secondary hypertension is renal disease, followed by cardiovascular, endocrine, and some neurologic disorders. As a rule, the younger the child and the more severe the hypertension, the more likely it is to be secondary.

The causes of essential hypertension are undetermined, but evidence indicates that both genetic and environmental factors play a role. The incidence of hypertension has been shown to be higher in children whose parents are hypertensive. American blacks have a higher incidence of hypertension than whites, and in these persons it develops earlier, is frequently more severe, and results in mortality at an earlier age. Environmental factors that contribute to the risk of developing hypertension include obesity, salt ingestion, smoking, and stress.

Diagnostic Evaluation

From the increasing numbers of hypertensive or potentially hypertensive children and adolescents being identified, a BP determination should be a routine part of annual assessment in children. Although clinical manifestations associated with hypertension depend largely on the underlying cause, some observations can provide clues to the examiner that an elevated BP may be a factor (Box 25-10). In infants and very young children who cannot communicate symptoms, observation of behavior provides clues, although gross behavioral changes may not be apparent until complications are present.

No definitive cutoff values are used in the diagnosis of hypertension in the pediatric patient. The National Institutes of Health (1996) has suggested the classification found on the inside back cover of this text. *Significant hypertension* is a BP persistently between the 95th and 99th percentiles for age, sex, and height. *Severe hypertension* is a

---

BOX 25-10 ■ Clinical Manifestations of Hypertension

ADOLESCENTS AND OLDER CHILDREN
Frequent headaches
Dizziness
Changes in vision

INFANTS OR YOUNG CHILDREN
Irritability
Head-banging or head-rubbing
May wake up screaming in the night

BP persistently at or above the 99th percentile for age, sex, and height. These newer guidelines take into account the differences in body size. It is important to note that a child who is large for his or her age may normally have a higher BP than a child of average size. Before a diagnosis is made, BP should be measured on at least three separate occasions.

A careful family history should be obtained to screen for other relatives with hypertension or other cardiovascular risk factors. In children with suspected primary hypertension, initial laboratory data are also obtained. This generally includes a urinalysis, renal function studies such as creatinine and blood urea nitrogen, a lipid profile, complete blood count, and electrolytes.

Therapeutic Management

Therapy for secondary hypertension involves diagnosis and treatment of the underlying cause. In cases amenable to surgical repair, the nature of the condition, the type of surgery, and the age of the child are all important considerations. Children or adolescents with consistently elevated BP readings from no known cause or those with secondary hypertension not amenable to surgical correction may be treated with a combination of nonpharmacologic and pharmacologic interventions. Dietary practices and lifestyle changes are important in the control of hypertension both for children and for adults. Nonpharmacologic measures, such as limitation of dietary salt, weight control, increased exercise, and avoidance of stress and smoking, carry no risk and should be instituted first, except in severe cases. Because the long-term effects of antihypertensive agents on children are not known, drug treatment of asymptomatic children with mild or borderline hypertension is not recommended.

Drug therapy is instituted with caution in children with significant elevations of BP resistant to nonpharmacologic intervention. The treatment should begin with one drug and should add other drugs only if control is not obtained. Compliance with antihypertensive drug regimens is extremely difficult. The oral antihypertensive drugs used most often in children include the beta blockers (propranolol), ACE inhibitors, diuretics, and occasionally a vasodilator (hydralazine). The goal is to achieve a normotensive state throughout the day without accompanying drug side effects.

Nursing Considerations

The nurse is active in detection, diagnosis, and therapy in many settings. Nurses are frequently the persons who operate well-child care and follow-up units and are usually the primary contact between health services and the child and family.

BP measurement should always be a part of the routine assessment of infants and children. To obtain an accurate reading, care is taken to quiet the child or relax the adolescent while the measurement is recorded to avoid false readings caused by excitement. The chief cause of falsely elevated BP readings is the use of improperly fitting, narrow cuffs. Therefore attention to correct measurement technique is essential (see Blood Pressure, Chapter 7).

Nursing counseling and guidance of affected children are challenges. Education aimed at understanding hypertension and its implication over the life span is essential in promoting patient and family compliance with both nonpharmacologic and pharmacologic therapies (see Compliance, Chapter 22).

Home BP measurements can facilitate surveillance in youngsters with chronic hypertension and can document effectiveness of therapy. A family member can be instructed in how to take and record accurate BP measurements, thus decreasing the number of trips to a health care facility. This individual needs to understand when to contact the practitioner regarding elevated values. The school nurse can often be a valuable resource in monitoring BP.

The nurse plays an important role in assessing individual families and providing targeted information regarding nonpharmacologic modes of intervention, such as diet, weight loss, smoking cessation, and exercise programs. If extensive dietary counseling is required, the child should be referred to a nutritionist with expertise in working with children and adolescents. Exercise regimens should be individualized. School children and young adolescents generally prefer team sports rather than individual training, which they may view as a burden rather than an enjoyable activity. If peers and family members can be encouraged to participate in any of the management strategies, the child's compliance is likely to be greater.

Young hypertensive women should avoid oral contraceptives because of their pressor effects. Other options need to be presented before this form of birth control is discontinued (see Contraception, Chapter 17).

If drug therapy is prescribed, the nurse needs to provide information to the family regarding the reasons for it, how the drug works, and possible side effects. General instructions for antihypertensive drugs include:

- Rise slowly from a horizontal position and avoid sudden position changes.
- Take drug as prescribed.
- Notify practitioner if unpleasant side effects occur, but do not discontinue drug.
- Avoid alcohol and stay on prescribed diet.

The need for follow-up is stressed, especially because antihypertensive therapy can sometimes be safely discontinued if BP remains under control over time.

KAWASAKI DISEASE (MUCOCUTANEOUS LYMPH NODE SYNDROME)

Kawasaki disease (KD) is an acute systemic vasculitis of unknown cause. It is seen in every racial group, and about 80% of the cases occur in children younger than the age of 5 years, with peak incidence in the toddler age-group. The

BOX 25-11 ■ Diagnostic Criteria for Kawasaki Disease

The child must exhibit five of the following six criteria, including fever:

1. Fever for 5 or more days (often diagnosed with shorter duration of fever if other symptoms are present)
2. Bilateral conjunctival injection (inflammation) without exudation
3. Changes in the oral mucous membranes, such as erythema, dryness, and fissuring of the lips; oropharyngeal reddening; or "strawberry tongue" (large papillae are exposed)
4. Changes in the extremities, such as peripheral edema, erythema of the palms and soles, and periungual desquamation (peeling) of the hands and feet
5. Polymorphous rash
6. Cervical lymphadenopathy (one lymph node >1.5 cm)

acute disease is self-limited. Without treatment, however, approximately 20% of children with KD develop cardiac sequelae. Infants younger than 1 year of age are most seriously affected by KD and are at the greatest risk for heart involvement.

The etiology of KD remains a mystery. Although it is not spread by person-to-person contact, several factors support infectious etiologic factors. It is often seen in geographic and seasonal outbreaks, with most cases reported in the late winter and early spring.

Pathophysiology

The principal area of involvement is the cardiovascular system. During the initial stage of the illness, extensive inflammation of the arterioles, venules, and capillaries occurs, which later progresses to the formation of coronary artery aneurysms in some children. When death occurs, it is usually the result of coronary thrombosis or severe scar formation and stenosis of the main coronary artery.

Clinical Manifestations

Because no specific diagnostic test exists for KD, the diagnosis is established on the basis of clinical findings and associated laboratory results (Box 25-11). These criteria should be used as guidelines. Many children with KD do not fulfill standard diagnosis criteria, and infants often have an atypical presentation. It is therefore important to consider KD as a possible diagnosis in any infant or child with prolonged elevated temperature that is unresponsive to antibiotics and is not attributable to another cause.

KD manifests in three phases: acute, subacute, and convalescent. The *acute phase* begins with the abrupt onset of high fever that is unresponsive to antibiotics and antipyretics. The child then develops the remaining diagnostic symptoms. During this stage the child is typically *very* irritable. The *subacute phase* begins with resolution of the fever and lasts until all clinical signs of KD have disappeared. During this phase the child is at greatest risk for the development of coronary artery aneurysms. Echocardiograms are used to monitor myocardial and coronary artery status. A baseline echocardiogram should be obtained at the time of diagnosis for comparison with future studies. Irritability persists during this phase. In the *convalescent phase,* all the clinical signs of KD have resolved, but the laboratory values have not returned to normal. This phase is complete when all blood values are normal (6 to 8 weeks after onset). At the end of this stage the child has regained his or her usual temperament, energy, and appetite.

Cardiac Involvement. The most serious complication of KD is the potential for myocardial infarction, which generally results from thrombotic occlusion of a coronary aneurysm. The main symptoms of acute myocardial infarction in children are abdominal pain, vomiting, restlessness, inconsolable crying, pallor, and shock.

Therapeutic Management

The current treatment of KD includes high-dose IV gamma globulin along with salicylate therapy. Gamma globulin has been demonstrated to be effective at reducing the incidence of coronary artery abnormalities when given within the first 10 days of the illness. A single, large infusion of 2 g/kg over 10 to 12 hours is recommended (American Academy of Pediatrics, 2000).

Aspirin is given initially in an antiinflammatory dose (80 to 100 mg/kg/day in divided doses every 6 hours) to control fever and symptoms of inflammation. After fever has subsided, aspirin is continued at an antiplatelet dose (3 to 5 mg/kg/day). Low-dose aspirin is continued in patients without echocardiographic evidence of coronary abnormalities until the platelet count has returned to normal (6 to 8 weeks). If the child develops coronary abnormalities, salicylate therapy is continued indefinitely. Additional anticoagulation with Coumadin may be indicated in children with giant aneurysms.

Prognosis. Most children with KD recover fully after treatment. However, when cardiovascular complications occur, serious morbidity may result. Death occurs rarely but almost always results from coronary thrombosis.

Nursing Considerations

In the initial phase the nurse must monitor the child's cardiac status carefully. Intake and output and daily weight measurements are recorded. Although the child may be reluctant to eat and therefore may be partially dehydrated, fluids need to be administered with care because of the usual finding of myocarditis. The child should be assessed frequently for signs of CHF, including decreased urine output, gallop rhythm (an additional heart sound), tachycardia, and respiratory distress.

Administration of gamma globulin should follow the same guidelines as for any blood product, with frequent monitoring of vital signs. Patients must be watched for allergic reactions (see Table 26-6). Cardiac status must be monitored because of the large volume being administered to patients with myocarditis and diminished left ventricular function.

Most nursing care focuses on symptomatic relief. To minimize skin discomfort, cool cloths, unscented lotions, and soft, loose clothing are helpful. During the acute phase, mouth care, including lubricating ointment to the lips, is important for the mucosal inflammation. Clear liquids and soft foods can be offered.

Patient irritability is perhaps the most challenging problem. These children need a quiet environment that promotes adequate rest. Their parents need to be supported in their efforts to comfort an often inconsolable child. They may need time away from their child, and nurses can often provide respite care for the family. Parents need to understand that irritability is a hallmark of KD and that they need not feel guilty or embarrassed about their child's behavior.

Discharge Teaching. Parents need accurate information about the progression of KD, including the importance of follow-up monitoring and when they should contact their practitioner. Irritability is likely to persist for up to 2 months after the onset of symptoms. Peeling of the hands and feet is painless and occurs primarily in the second and third weeks. Arthritis, especially of the larger weight-bearing joints, may persist for several weeks. Children are typically most stiff in the mornings, during cold weather, and after naps. Passive range of motion in the bathtub is often helpful in increasing flexibility. Any live immunizations (e.g., measles-mumps-rubella, varicella) should be deferred for 11 months after the administration of gamma globulin because the body might not produce the appropriate amount of antibodies (American Academy of Pediatrics, 2000). The decision to give the varicella (chickenpox) vaccine while the child is receiving aspirin therapy is made individually by the practitioner. Temperature should be recorded after discharge until the child has been afebrile for several days.

All parents should understand the unlikely but real possibility of myocardial infarction, as well as the signs and symptoms of cardiac ischemia, in a child. At discharge the ultimate cardiac sequela is generally not known, because changes occur up to a month after the onset of KD. In addition, the parents of children with known severe coronary artery sequelae may be taught cardiopulmonary resuscitation.

SHOCK

Shock, or *circulatory failure,* is a complex clinical syndrome characterized by inadequate tissue perfusion to meet the metabolic demands of the body, resulting in cellular dysfunction and eventual organ failure. Although the causes are different, the physiologic consequences are the same: hypotension, tissue hypoxia, and metabolic acidosis.

Circulatory failure in children is a result of hypovolemia, altered peripheral vascular resistance, or pump failure. Types of shock are listed in Box 25-12.

Pathophysiology

A healthy child's circulatory system is able to transport oxygen and metabolic substrates to body tissues, which require a constant source for these essential needs. The cardiac output and distribution to the various body tissues can change very rapidly in response to intrinsic (myocardial and intravascular) or extrinsic (neuronal) control mechanisms. In shock states these mechanisms are altered or challenged.

Reduced blood flow, as in hypovolemic shock, causes diminished venous return to the heart, low CVP, low cardiac output, and hypotension. Vasomotor centers in the medulla are signaled, causing a compensatory increase in the force and rate of cardiac contraction and constriction of arterioles and veins, thereby increasing peripheral vascular

BOX 25-12 ■ Types of Shock

HYPOVOLEMIC

Characteristics
Reduction in size of vascular compartment
Falling blood pressure
Poor capillary filling
Low central venous pressure

Most Frequent Causes
Blood loss (hemorrhagic shock)—trauma, gastrointestinal bleeding, intracranial hemorrhage
Plasma loss—increased capillary permeability associated with sepsis and acidosis, hypoproteinemia, burns, peritonitis
Extracellular fluid loss—vomiting, diarrhea, glycosuric diuresis, sunstroke

DISTRIBUTIVE

Characteristics
Reduction in peripheral vascular resistance
Profound inadequacies in tissue perfusion
Increased venous capacity and pooling
Acute reduction in return blood flow to the heart
Diminished cardiac output

Most Frequent Causes
Anaphylaxis (anaphylactic shock)—extreme allergy or hypersensitivity to a foreign substance
Sepsis (septic shock, bacteremic shock, endotoxic shock)—overwhelming sepsis and circulating bacterial toxins
Loss of neuronal control (neurogenic shock)—interruption of neuronal transmission (spinal cord injury)
Myocardial depression and peripheral dilation—exposure to anesthesia or ingestion of barbiturates, tranquilizers, opioids, antihypertensive agents, or ganglionic blocking agents

CARDIOGENIC

Characteristic
Decreased cardiac output

Most Frequent Causes
After surgery for congenital heart disease
Primary pump failure—myocarditis, myocardial trauma, biochemical derangements, congestive heart failure
Dysrhythmias—supraventricular tachycardia, atrioventricular block, and ventricular dysrhythmias; secondary to myocarditis or biochemical abnormalities (occasionally)

---

excess carbon dioxide. Prolonged vasoconstriction results in fatigue and atony of the peripheral arterioles, which leads to vessel dilation. Venules, less sensitive to vasodilator substances, remain constricted for a time, causing massive pooling in the capillary and venular beds, which further depletes blood volume.

Complications of shock create further hazards. Central nervous system hypoperfusion may eventually lead to cerebral edema, cortical infarction, or intraventricular hemorrhage. Renal hypoperfusion causes renal ischemia with possible tubular or glomerular necrosis and renal vein thrombosis. Reduced blood flow to the lungs can interfere with surfactant secretion and result in adult respiratory distress syndrome (ARDS), characterized by sudden pulmonary congestion and atelectasis with formation of a hyaline membrane. Gastrointestinal tract bleeding and perforation are always a possibility after splanchnic ischemia and necrosis of intestinal mucosa. Metabolic complications of shock may include hypoglycemia, hypocalcemia, and other electrolyte disturbances.

Diagnostic Evaluation

The etiology of shock can be discerned from the history and the physical examination. The severity of the shock is determined by measurements of vital signs, including CVP and capillary filling (Box 25-13). Shock can be regarded as a form of compensation for circulatory failure. Because of the progressive nature of shock, it can be divided into the following three stages or phases:

1 **Compensated shock.** Vital organ function is maintained by intrinsic compensatory mechanisms; blood flow is usually normal or increased but generally uneven or maldistributed in the microcirculation.
2 **Uncompensated shock.** Efficiency of the cardiovascular system gradually diminishes until perfusion in the microcirculation becomes marginal despite compensatory adjustments. The outcomes of circulatory failure that progress beyond the limits of compensation are tissue hypoxia, metabolic acidosis, and eventual dysfunction of all organ systems.
3 **Irreversible, or terminal, shock.** Damage to vital organs, such as the heart or brain, is of such magnitude that the entire organism will be disrupted regardless of therapeutic intervention. Death occurs even if cardiovascular measurements return to normal levels with therapy.

At all stages the principal differentiating signs are observed in the (1) degree of tachycardia and perfusion to extremities, (2) level of consciousness, and (3) BP. Additional signs or modifications of these more universal signs may be present depending on the type and cause of the shock. Initially the child's ability to compensate is effective; therefore, early signs are subtle. As the shock state advances, signs are more obvious and indicate early decompensation.

Additional signs may be present, depending on the type and etiology of the shock. In early septic shock there are chills, fever, and vasodilation, with increased cardiac output that results in warm, flushed skin (hyperdynamic or "hot" shock). A later and ominous development is disseminated intravascular coagulation (see Chapter 26), the major hematologic complication of septic shock. Anaphylactic shock is frequently accompanied by urticaria and angioneurotic edema, which is life-threatening when it involves the respiratory passages (see Anaphylaxis, p. 934.).

---

resistance. Simultaneously the lowered blood volume leads to the release of large amounts of catecholamines, antidiuretic hormone, adrenocorticosteroids, and aldosterone in an effort to conserve body fluids. This causes reduced blood flow to the skin, kidneys, muscles, and viscera to shunt the available blood to the brain and heart. Consequently, the skin feels cold and clammy, there is poor capillary filling, and glomerular filtration and urine output are significantly reduced.

As a result of impaired perfusion, oxygen is depleted in the tissue cells, causing them to revert to anaerobic metabolism, producing lactic acidosis. The acidosis places an extra burden on the lungs as they attempt to compensate for the metabolic acidosis by increased respiratory rate to remove

BOX 25-13 ■ Clinical Manifestations of Shock

COMPENSATED	UNCOMPENSATED
Apprehensiveness	Confusion and somnolence
Irritability	Tachypnea
Unexplained tachycardia	Moderate metabolic acidosis
Normal blood pressure	Oliguria
Narrowing pulse pressure	Cool, pale extremities
Thirst	Decreased skin turgor
Pallor	Poor capillary filling
Diminished urine output	
Reduced perfusion of extremities	**IRREVERSIBLE**
	Thready, weak pulse
	Hypotension
	Periodic breathing or apnea
	Anuria
	Stupor or coma

Laboratory tests that assist in assessment are blood gas measurements, pH, and sometimes liver function tests. Coagulation tests are evaluated when there is evidence of bleeding, such as oozing from a venipuncture site, bleeding from any orifice, or petechiae. Cultures of blood and other sites are indicated when there is a high suspicion of sepsis. Renal function tests are performed when impaired renal function is evident.

Therapeutic Management

Treatment of shock consists of three major thrusts: (1) ventilation, (2) fluid administration, and (3) improvement of the pumping action of the heart (vasopressor support). The first priority is to establish an airway and administer oxygen. After the airway is ensured, circulatory stabilization is the major concern.

Ventilatory Support. The lung is the organ most sensitive to shock. Decreased or redistribution of blood flow to respiratory muscles plus the increased work of breathing can rapidly lead to respiratory failure. Critically ill patients are unable to maintain an adequate airway. To place the lung at rest and improve ventilation, tracheal intubation is initiated early with positive-pressure ventilation. Supplemental oxygen is always given as soon as possible. Blood gases and pH are monitored frequently.

Increased extravascular lung water caused by edema contributes to the development of respiratory complications. Therapy is directed toward maintaining normal arterial blood gas measurements, normal acid-base balance, and circulation. Efforts are made to remove fluid and prevent its accumulation with the use of diuretics.

Cardiovascular Support. In most cases, rapid restoration of blood volume is all that is needed for resuscitation of the child in shock. An isotonic crystalloid solution (normal saline or Ringer's lactate) is the fluid of choice; colloids such as albumin are also used. Successful resuscitation is reflected by an increase in BP and a reduction in heart rate; increased cardiac output will result in improved capillary circulation and skin color. CVP measurements of right atrial pressure help guide fluid therapy, and urine output measurement is an important indicator of adequacy of circulation. Correction of acidosis, hypoxemia, hypoglycemia, hypothermia, and any metabolic derangements is mandatory.

Temporary pharmacologic support may be required to enhance myocardial contractility, to reverse metabolic or respiratory acidosis, and/or to maintain arterial pressure. The principal agents used to improve cardiac output and circulation are catecholamines, such as dopamine (Intropin) or epinephrine (Adrenalin). Vasodilators that are sometimes used include nitroprusside (Nipride) or milrinone.

Nursing Considerations

When shock is a likely complication, the child is observed carefully for any early signs, which are reported immediately for further medical evaluation.

> **NURSING ALERT**
>
> Early clinical signs include apprehension, irritability, normal BP, narrowing pulse pressure (difference between diastolic and systolic BP), thirst, pallor, diminished urine output, unexplained mild tachycardia, and a decrease in perfusion of the hands and feet.

The child who is in shock requires intensive observation and care. *The initial action is to ensure adequate tissue oxygenation.* The nurse should be prepared to administer oxygen by the appropriate route and to assist with any intubation and ventilatory procedures indicated. Other procedures and activities that require immediate attention are establishing an IV line, weighing the child, obtaining baseline vital signs, placing an indwelling catheter, obtaining blood gases and other measurements, and administering medications as indicated. The child is best positioned flat with the legs elevated.

The nurse's responsibilities are to monitor the IV infusion, intake and output, vital signs (including CVP), and general systems assessments on a routine basis. IV medications are titrated according to patient responses, and vital signs are taken every 15 minutes during the critical periods and thereafter as needed. Urine output is measured hourly; blood gases, hematocrit, pH, and electrolytes are monitored frequently to assess the status of the child and the efficacy of therapy. An apnea and cardiac monitor is attached and monitored continuously. In the initial stages of acute shock, the care of the child often requires the attendance of more than one nurse to manage all the necessary activities that must be carried out simultaneously (see Emergency Treatment box).

Throughout the intense activity the family must not be overlooked. Someone should contact family members at frequent intervals to inform them about what is being done and if there is any progress. Ideally, someone should remain with the parents to serve as liaison between them and the intensive care team. However, this is not always feasible in such a critical situation. As soon as possible, the family should be allowed to see the child. A member of the clergy may be called to help provide comfort and support.

ANAPHYLAXIS

Anaphylaxis is the acute clinical syndrome resulting from the interaction of an allergen and a patient who is hypersensitive to that allergen. When the antigen enters the circulatory sys-

EMERGENCY TREATMENT
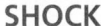

SHOCK

VENTILATION
Establish airway—be prepared for intubation
Administer oxygen, usually 100% by mask

FLUID ADMINISTRATION
Obtain vascular access (preferably IV, intraosseous in emergency)
Restore fluid volume as ordered
   (Initial volume resuscitation is 20 mL/kg of isotonic crystalloid [normal saline or Ringer's lactate] over 5 to 20 minutes)

CARDIOVASCULAR SUPPORT
Administer vasopressors, especially epinephrine IV (dose: 0.01 mg/kg = 0.1 mL/kg of 1:10,000 solution)
May repeat every 3 to 5 minutes in cardiac arrest

GENERAL SUPPORT
Continuous ECG monitoring
Monitor pulse oximetry
Keep child warm and calm

IN ADDITION:
Septic Shock: Administer broad-spectrum antibiotics IV
Anaphylaxis: Remove allergen if possible, intramuscular epinephrine, corticosteroids as ordered

Data from American Heart Association: *Pediatric advanced life support provider manual*, 2002.

---

tem, a generalized reaction rapidly takes place. Vasoactive amines (principally histamine or a histamine-like substance) are released and cause vasodilation, bronchoconstriction, and increased capillary permeability.

Severe reactions are immediate in onset, are often life-threatening, and frequently involve multiple systems, primarily the cardiovascular, respiratory, gastrointestinal, and integumentary systems. Exposure to the antigen can be by ingestion, inhalation, skin contact, or injection. Examples of common allergens associated with anaphylaxis include drugs (e.g., antibiotics, chemotherapeutic agents, radiologic contrast media), latex, foods, venoms from bees or snakes, and biologic agents (antisera, enzymes, hormones, blood products).

> ⚠ **NURSING ALERT**
>
> Penicillin allergy is associated with immediate onset (within an hour of administration) or accelerated onset (1 to 72 hours after administration) of skin eruption, especially a urticarial rash, or more serious symptoms such as laryngeal edema or anaphylactic shock.

Clinical Manifestations

The onset of clinical symptoms usually occurs within seconds or minutes of exposure to the antigen, and the rapidity of the reaction is directly related to its intensity: the sooner the onset, the more severe the reaction. The reaction may be preceded by symptoms of uneasiness, restlessness, irritability, severe anxiety, headache, dizziness, paresthesia, and disorientation. The patient may lose consciousness. Cutaneous signs of flushing and urticaria are common early signs, followed by

angioedema, most notable in the eyelids, lips, tongue, hands, feet, and genitalia.

Bronchiolar constriction may follow, causing narrowing of the airway; pulmonary edema and hemorrhage also may occur. Laryngeal edema with severe acute upper airway obstruction may be life-threatening and requires rapid intervention. Shock occurs as a result of mediator-induced vasodilation, which causes capillary permeability and loss of intravascular fluid into the interstitial space. Sudden hypotension and impaired cardiac output with poor perfusion are seen.

Therapeutic Management

Successful outcome of anaphylactic reactions depends on rapid recognition and institution of treatment. The goals of treatment are to provide ventilation, restore adequate circulation, and prevent further exposure by identifying and removing the cause when possible.

A mild reaction with no evidence of respiratory distress or cardiovascular compromise can be managed with subcutaneous administration of antihistamines, such as diphenhydramine (Benadryl) and epinephrine.

Moderate or severe distress presents a potentially life-threatening emergency. Establishing an airway is the first concern, as with all shock states. Epinephrine is given subcutaneously or intravenously as an antihistamine and to support the cardiovascular system and increase blood pressure. Other routes for giving epinephrine are intramuscular and via the airway, either nebulized or injected through an ET tube. In severe anaphylaxis, epinephrine by any route is better than none. Fluids are given to restore blood volume. Additional vasopressors may be given to improve cardiac output.

Prevention of a reaction is preferable. Preventing exposure is more easily accomplished in children known to be at risk, including those with (1) a history of previous allergic reaction to a specific antigen, (2) a history of atopy, (3) a history of severe reactions in immediate family members, and (4) a reaction to a skin test, although skin tests are not available for all allergens. Desensitization may be recommended in certain cases.

Nursing Considerations

The major nursing responsibility in anaphylaxis is anticipating which children are likely to develop a reaction, recognizing the early signs, and intervening appropriately. When an anaphylactic reaction is suspected, both immediate intervention and preparation for medical therapy are nursing responsibilities. Ventilation is ensured by placing the child in a head-elevated position, unless contraindicated by hypotension, to facilitate breathing and administer oxygen. If the child is not breathing, cardiopulmonary resuscitation (CPR) is initiated, and emergency medical services are summoned.

If the cause can be determined, measures are implemented to slow the spread of the offending substance. An IV infusion is established immediately. Emergency medications are given intravenously whenever possible; however, epinephrine may be given subcutaneously (see Emergency Treatment box). Vital signs and urine output are monitored frequently. Medications are administered as prescribed, with regular assessment to monitor effectiveness and to detect signs of side effects of medication and fluid overload.

To prevent an anaphylactic reaction, parents are always asked about possible allergic responses to foods, latex, medications, and environmental conditions. (See Guidelines box, Taking an Allergy History, p. 119). These are displayed prominently on the patient's chart. The specific allergen is noted, as is the type and severity of the reaction. Parents are excellent historians, especially when the child has displayed a pronounced reaction to a substance. Drugs, including related drugs (e.g., penicillin, nafcillin), and other items, such as latex, that have produced a reaction previously are *never* used. If the child is allergic to insect venom, the family is instructed to purchase an emergency kit to be kept with the child at all times. Both the family and the child, if the child is old enough, are taught how to use the equipment. Medical identification should be carried by the patient at all times.

TOXIC SHOCK SYNDROME

Toxic shock syndrome (TSS) is a relatively rare condition caused by the toxins produced by the *Staphylococcus* bacteria. First described in 1978, TSS can cause acute multisystem organ failure and a clinical picture that resembles septic shock. TSS became well known in 1980 because of the striking relationship between the disease and tampon use (Nakase, 2000). An aggressive health education campaign about the dangers of prolonged tampon use and a change in the chemical composition of tampons has markedly reduced the incidence of TSS in menstruating women. Cases of TSS have also been reported in men, older women, and children.

Diagnostic Evaluation

Diagnosis is established on the basis of the criteria established by the Centers for Disease Control and Prevention's toxic case definition (Box 25-14). A history of tampon use contributes to the diagnosis. Additional laboratory tests include cultures from blood, vagina, cervix, and any discharge. Other laboratory tests are those that facilitate the management of shock.

Therapeutic Management

The management of TSS is the same as management of shock of any etiology and may range from supportive care in mild cases to hospitalization and intensive care in severe cases. Appropriate parenteral antibiotics are usually administered after cultures are obtained.

Nursing Considerations

Nursing care and observation of the acutely ill patient are the same as those described for shock of any etiology. Because the disease is relatively rare, the major efforts of nursing are directed toward prevention. The association between the disease and the use of tampons provides some direction for education. Avoiding the use of tampons offers the most certain preventive measure, although this approach is probably unacceptable to most adolescent girls, who prefer the freedom, comfort, and inconspicuousness that tampons afford.

Adolescent girls who use tampons can be taught general hygiene measures, such as handwashing before insertion of the tampon and not to use a tampon that has been dropped or otherwise soiled. Tampons should be inserted carefully to avoid vaginal abrasion. Also, it is wise to modify their use. For example, tampons may be used intermittently during the menstrual cycle, alternating with sanitary napkins—perhaps using the napkins during the night, when at home during the day, and when flow is slight. Young girls are advised not to use superabsorbent tampons and not to leave any tampon in the body for more than 4 to 6 hours.

Patients who use tampons need to understand that they should remove the tampon and consult their health professional if they develop a sudden high fever, vomiting, diarrhea, muscle pain, dizziness, fainting or near fainting when standing up, or rash that resembles a sunburn.

BOX 25-14 ■ Criteria for Definition of Toxic Shock Syndrome

1. Fever of 38.9° C (102° F) or higher
2. Presence of diffuse macular erythroderma
3. Desquamation, particularly of palms and soles, 1 to 2 weeks after onset of illness
4. Hypotension, defined as a systolic blood pressure of 90 mm Hg or less for adults and below the 5th percentile for children younger than 16 years of age; or an orthostatic drop in diastolic blood pressure of 15 mm Hg or more with a change from lying to sitting; or orthostatic syncope; or orthostatic dizziness
5. Involvement of three or more of the following organ systems: gastrointestinal, muscular, mucous membrane, renal, hepatic, hematologic, or central nervous system

Toxic shock syndrome is probable when four of the five major criteria are fulfilled. In addition, if blood and cerebrospinal fluid cultures are obtained, they must be negative for any organisms other than *Staphylococcus aureus*. Serologic tests for Rocky Mountain spotted fever, leptospirosis, and measles also must be negative.

Modified from American Academy of Pediatrics, Committee on Infectious Diseases, Pickering L, editor: *2003 Red Book: report of the Committee on Infectious Diseases*, ed 26, Elk Grove Village, Il, 2003, The Academy.

KEY POINTS

■ Congenital heart disease (CHD) is the most common form of cardiac disease in children.

■ Major categories to investigate in the cardiac history are poor weight gain, poor feeding habits, and fatigue during feeding; frequent respiratory infections and difficulties; and evidence of exercise intolerance.

■ The most common tests used in assessing cardiac function are radiography, electrocardiography, echocardiography, and cardiac catheterization.

■ Cardiac catheterization procedures can be divided into three groups: (1) diagnostic procedures, including angiography, that measure pressures and saturations to establish cardiac diagnosis; (2) interventional procedures, in which catheters or balloon devices are used to correct cardiac defects; and (3) electrophysiology studies, in which catheters with electrodes are used to evaluate dysrhythmias.

■ Diagnostic cardiac catheterization provides important information about oxygen saturation of blood within the chambers and great vessels, pressure changes, changes in cardiac output or stroke volume, and anatomic abnormalities.

■ Several prenatal factors may predispose children to CHD: maternal rubella during pregnancy, maternal alcoholism, maternal age older than 40 years, and maternal type 1 diabetes.

■ Congenital heart defects can be divided into four main groups, as determined by hemodynamic patterns: (1) defects that result in increased pulmonary blood flow, (2) obstructive defects, (3) defects that result in decreased pulmonary blood flow, and (4) mixed defects.

- Clinical consequences of congenital heart defects include congestive heart failure (CHF) and hypoxemia. A child can have both hypoxemia and CHF, although usually they occur independently.

- Clinical manifestations of CHF are impaired myocardial function (tachycardia, cardiomegaly), pulmonary congestion (dyspnea, tachypnea, orthopnea, cyanosis), and systemic congestion (hepatosplenomegaly, edema, distended veins).

- Nursing measures in the care of a child with CHF are to assist in improving cardiac function, decrease cardiac demands, reduce respiratory distress, maintain nutritional status, promote fluid loss, and provide family support.

- Clinical manifestations of hypoxemia are cyanosis, polycythemia, clubbing, and delayed growth and development. The child is at increased risk for hypercyanotic spells, cerebrovascular accidents, brain abscess, and bacterial endocarditis.

- Caring for the child with CHD and the family requires helping them to adjust to the disorder and to cope with the effects of the defect, and fostering growth-promoting family relationships.

- Preoperative care of the child with a congenital heart defect involves introducing the child and family to the hospital and preparing them for preoperative and postoperative procedures.

- Providing postoperative care includes observing vital signs and arterial/venous pressures, maintaining respiratory status, allowing maximum rest, providing comfort, monitoring fluids, planning for progressive activities, giving emotional support, observing for complications of surgery, and planning for discharge and home care.

- Acquired cardiovascular disorders include bacterial endocarditis, rheumatic fever, hyperlipidemia (hypercholesterolemia), and cardiac dysrhythmias.

- Prevention of bacterial endocarditis in certain children with CHD involves administration of prophylactic antibiotics when specific procedures are performed.

- Acute rheumatic fever is a systemic inflammatory disease that can damage the cardiac valves and is associated with previous group A streptococcal infection. Its incidence has increased in some areas of the United States.

- Cholesterol screening in children is controversial; currently, children with known risk factors for hyperlipidemia are screened and treated as needed. The influence of childhood cholesterol levels on later development of coronary artery disease is under investigation.

- Common dysrhythmias in children include slow rhythms (bradycardias, heart block) and fast rhythms (sinus tachycardia, supraventricular tachycardia).

- Heart transplantation has been extended to infants and children with cardiomyopathy and complex congenital heart defects involving ventricular dysfunction, such as hypoplastic left heart syndrome.

- Education of the child with hypertension and the family focuses on drug therapy, diet control, and appropriate exercise.

- Kawasaki disease is an extensive inflammation of small vessels and capillaries that may progress to involve the coronary arteries, causing aneurysm formation. The administration of gamma globulin is an important aspect of treatment.

- Emergency treatment for shock includes ensuring ventilation; administering vasopressors, fluids/blood, and antibiotics as needed; and providing supportive measures such as correct positioning, warmth, and psychologic reassurance to the child and family.

- Persons at risk for anaphylaxis may be identified by a history of previous allergic reaction, history of atopy, history of severe reactions in family, and positive skin test to the allergen.

- Nursing management of the patient with toxic shock syndrome focuses on prevention primarily through education concerning safe tampon use.

References

Allen HD and others: Pediatric therapeutic cardiac catheterization, AHA Scientific Statement, *Circulation* 97:609-625, 1998.

American Academy of Pediatrics: Cholesterol in childhood, *Pediatrics* 101(1 part 1):141-147, 1998.

American Academy of Pediatrics, Committee on Infectious Diseases, Pickering L, editor: *2000 Red Book: report of the Committee on Infectious Diseases*, ed 25, Elk Grove Village, Il, 2000, The Academy.

Barst RJ: Recent advances in the treatment of pediatric pulmonary artery hypertension, *Pediatr Clin North Am* 46(2):333-345, 1999.

Beekman RH: Coarctation of the aorta. In Allen HD and others, editors: *Moss and Adams' heart disease in infants, children and adolescents*, ed 6, Philadelphia, 2001, Lippincott Williams & Wilkins.

Behrman RE, Kliegman RM, Jenson HA: *Nelson textbook of pediatrics*, ed 16, Philadelphia, 2000, WB Saunders.

Boucek MM and others: The registry of the International Society of Heart and Lung Transplantation: fourth official pediatric report 2000, *J Heart Lung Transplant* 20:39-52, 2001.

Burch M, Blair E: The inheritance of hypertrophic cardiomyopathy, *Pediatr Cardiol* 20(5):313-316, 1999.

Fortuna RS, Chinnock RE, Bailey LL: Heart transplantation among 233 infants during the first six months of life: the Loma Linda experience, *Clin Transpl* 1999:263-272, 1999.

Freed MD: Aortic stenosis. In Allen HD and others: *Moss and Adams' heart disease in infants, children, and adolescents*, ed 6, Philadelphia, 2001, Lippincott Williams & Wilkins.

Gentles T and others: Left ventricular mechanics during and after acute rheumatic fever: contractile dysfunction is closely related to valve regurgitation, *J Am Coll Cardiol* 37(1):201-207, 2001.

Goldmuntz E and others: Frequency of 22q11 deletion in patients with conotruncal defects, *J Am Coll Cardiol* 32:492-498, 1998.

Hanisch D: Pediatric arrhythmias, *J Pediatr Nurs* 16(5):351-362, 2001.

Hawkins JA and others: Late results and reintervention after aortic valvotomy for critical aortic stenosis, *Ann Thorac Surg* 65:1758-1762, 1998.

Higgins SS: Parental role in decision making about pediatric cardiac transplantation: Familial and ethical considerations, *J Pediatr Nurs* 16(5):332-337, 2001.

Hougen TJ, Sell J: Recent advances in the diagnosis and treatment of coarctation of the aorta, *Curr Opin Cardiol* 10(5):524-529, 1995.

Koster NK: Physical activity and congenital heart disease, *Nurs Clin North Am* 29(2):345-356, 1994.

Luikart, H: Pediatric cardiac transplantation management issues, *J Pediatr Nurs* 16(5):320-3331, 2001.

Nakase J: Update on emerging infections from the Centers for Disease Control and Prevention, *Ann Emerg Med* 36(3):268-270, 2000.

National Institutes of Health, National Heart, Lung, and Blood Institute: *Update on the Task Force Report (1987) on High Blood Pressure in Children and Adolescents*, Bethesda, Md, 1996, The Institutes.

O'Brien P, Boisvert JT: Current management of infants and children with single ventricle anatomy, *J Pediatr Nurs* 16(5):338-350, 2001.

Pham JT, Carlos MA: Current treatment strategies of symptomatic patent ductus arteriosus, *J Pediatr Health Care* 16(6):306-310, 2002.

Smith P: Primary care in children with congenital hearth disease, *J Pediatr Nurs* 16(5):308-319, 2001.

Uzurk K: Therapeutic cardiac catheterization for congenital heart disease: a new era in pediatric care, *J Pediatr Nurs* 16(5):300-307, 2001.

26

The Child With Hematologic or Immunologic Dysfunction

ROSALIND BRYANT

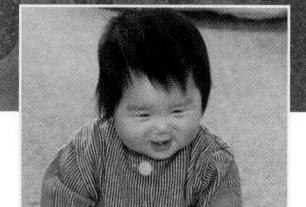

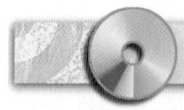 Remember to check out your companion CD-ROM

http://evolve.elsevier.com/Wong/essentials/

CHAPTER OUTLINE

RELATED TOPICS and ADDITIONAL RESOURCES

 IN TEXT

 CD COMPANION

 evolve **WEBSITE**

HEMATOLOGIC/IMMUNOLOGIC DYSFUNCTION

ASSESSMENT OF HEMATOLOGIC FUNCTION

Several tests can be performed to assess hematologic function, including additional procedures to identify the cause of the dysfunction. The following discussion is limited to a description of the most common and one of the most valuable tests, the *complete blood cell count (CBC)*. Other procedures, such as those related to iron, coagulation, and immune status, are discussed throughout the chapter as appropriate. The nurse should be familiar with the significance of the findings from the CBC (Table 26-1) and aware of normal values for age, which are listed in Appendix E.

As with any disorder, the history and physical examination are essential to identification of hematologic dysfunction, and the nurse is often the first person to suspect a problem based on information from these sources. Comments by the parent regarding the child's lack of energy, food diary of poor sources of iron, frequent infections, and bleeding that is difficult to control offer clues to the more common disorders affecting the blood. A careful physical appraisal, especially of the skin, can reveal findings (e.g., pallor, petechiae, bruising) that may indicate minor or serious hematologic conditions. Nurses need to be aware of the clinical manifestations of blood diseases to assist in recognizing symptoms and establishing a diagnosis.

FYI

A common term used in describing an abnormal CBC is *shift to the left*, which refers to the presence of immature neutrophils in the peripheral blood from hyperfunction of the bone marrow, as seen during a bacterial infection.

RED BLOOD CELL DISORDERS

ANEMIA

The term *anemia* describes a condition in which the number of red blood cells (RBCs) or the hemoglobin (Hgb or Hb) concentration is reduced below normal values for age. As a result of this decrease, the oxygen-carrying capacity of the blood is diminished, causing a reduction in the oxygen available to the tissues. Anemia is the most common hematologic disorder of infancy and childhood and is not a disease itself but an indication or manifestation of an underlying pathologic process.

Classification

Anemias are classified in relation to (1) *etiology* or *physiology,* manifested by erythrocyte or Hgb depletion, and (2) *morphology,* the characteristic changes in RBC size, shape, or color (Box 26-1). Although the morphologic classification is more useful in terms of laboratory evaluation of anemia, the etiologic approach provides direction for planning nursing care. For example, anemia with reduced Hgb concentration may be caused by a dietary depletion of iron, and the principal intervention is replenishing iron stores. The classification of anemias is found in Fig. 26-1.

Consequences of Anemia

The basic physiologic defect caused by anemia is a decrease in the oxygen-carrying capacity of blood and consequently a reduction in the amount of oxygen available to the cells. When the anemia has developed slowly, the child usually adapts to the declining Hgb level.

The effects of anemia on the circulatory system can be profound. Because the viscosity of blood depends almost entirely on the concentration of RBCs, the resulting hemodilution of severe anemia decreases peripheral resistance, causing greater quantities of blood to return to the heart. The increased circulation and turbulence within the heart may produce a murmur. Because the cardiac workload is greatly increased, especially during exercise, infection, or emotional stress, cardiac failure may ensue.

Children seem to have a remarkable ability to function quite well despite low levels of Hgb. *Cyanosis* (the result of the quantity of deoxygenated Hgb in arterial blood) is typically not evident. Growth retardation, resulting from decreased cellular metabolism and coexisting anorexia, is a common finding in chronic severe anemia and is frequently accompanied by delayed sexual maturation in the older child.

Diagnostic Evaluation

In general, anemia may be suspected from findings on the history and physical examination, such as lack of energy, easy fatigability, and pallor, but unless the anemia is severe, the first clue to the disorder may be alterations in the CBC, such

TABLE 26-1 ■ Tests Performed as Part of the Complete Blood Cell Count

TEST (AVERAGE VALUE)*	DESCRIPTION/COMMENTS
Red blood cell (RBC) count (4.5-5.5 million/mm³)	Number of RBCs/mm³ of blood
	Indirectly estimates Hgb content of blood
	Reflects function of bone marrow
Hemoglobin (Hgb) determination (11.5-15.5 g/dL)	Amount of Hgb/g/dL of whole blood
	Total blood Hgb primarily depends on number of circulating RBCs, but also on amount of Hgb in each cell
Hematocrit (Hct) (35%-45%)	Percentage or volume of packed RBCs to whole blood
	Indirectly measures Hgb content
	Is approximately three times Hgb content
RBC indexes	
Mean corpuscular volume (MCV) (77-95 μm³)	Average of mean volume (size) of a single RBC
	MCV values expressed as cubic microns (μm³) or femtoliters (fL)
Mean corpuscular hemoglobin (MCH) (25-33 pg/cell)	Average or mean quantity (weight) of Hgb in a single RBC
	MCH values expressed as picograms (pg) or micromicrograms (μμg)
	MCV and MCH depend on accurate counts of RBCs, whereas MCHC does not; therefore, MCHC is often more reliable
	All indexes depend on average cell measurements and do not show individual RBC variations (anisocytosis)
Mean corpuscular hemoglobin concentration (MCHC) (31%-37% Hgb [g]/dL RBC)	Average concentration of Hgb in a single RBC
	MCHC values expressed as % Hgb (g)/cell or Hgb (g)/dL RBC
RBC volume distribution width (RDW) (13.4% ± 1.2%)	Average size of RBCs
	Differentiates some types of anemia
Reticulocyte count (0.5%-1.5% erythrocytes)	% Reticulocytes to RBCs
	Index of production of mature RBCs by bone marrow
	Decreased count indicates depressed bone marrow function
	Increased count indicates erythrogenesis in response to some stimulus
	When reticulocyte count is extremely high, other forms of immature RBCs (normoblasts, even erythroblasts) may be present
	Indirectly estimates hypochromic anemia
	Usually elevated in patients with chronic hemolytic anemia
White blood cell (WBC) count (4.5-13.5 × 10³ cells/mm³)	Number of WBCs/mm³ of blood
	Total number of WBCs less important than differential count
Differential WBC count	Inspection and quantification of WBC types present in peripheral blood
	Values are expressed as percentages; to obtain absolute number of any type of WBC, multiply its respective percentage by total number of WBCs
Neutrophils (polys) (54%-62%) (3-5.8 × 10³ cells/mm³)	Primary defense in bacterial infection; capable of phagocytizing and killing bacteria
Bands (3%-5%) (0.15-0.4 × 10³ cells/mm³)	Immature neutrophil
	Increased numbers in bacterial infection
	Also capable of phagocytosis and killing
Eosinophils (1%-3%) (0.05-0.25 × 10³ cells/mm³)	Named for their staining characteristics with eosin dye
	Increased in allergic disorders, parasitic diseases, certain neoplasms, and other diseases
Basophils (0.075%) (0.015-0.030 cells/mm³)	Named for their characteristic basophilic stippling
	Contain histamine, heparin, and serotonin; believed to cause increased blood flow to injured tissues while preventing excessive clotting
Lymphocytes (25%-33%) (1.5-3.0 × 10³ cells/mm³)	Involved in development of antibody and delayed hypersensitivity
Monocytes (3%-7%)	Large phagocytic cells that are involved in early stage of inflammatory reaction
Absolute neutrophil count (ANC) (>1000)	% Neutrophils × WBC count
	Indicates body's capability to handle bacterial infections
Platelet count (150-400 10³/mm³)	Number of platelets/mm³ of blood
	Cellular fragments that are necessary for clotting to occur
Stained peripheral blood smear	Visual estimation of amount of Hgb in RBCs and overall size, shape, and structure of RBCs
	Various staining properties of RBC structures may be evidence of immature forms of erythrocytes
	Shows variation in size and shape of RBCs: microcytic, macrocytic, poikilocytic (variable shapes)

*See Appendix E for normal values according to ages.

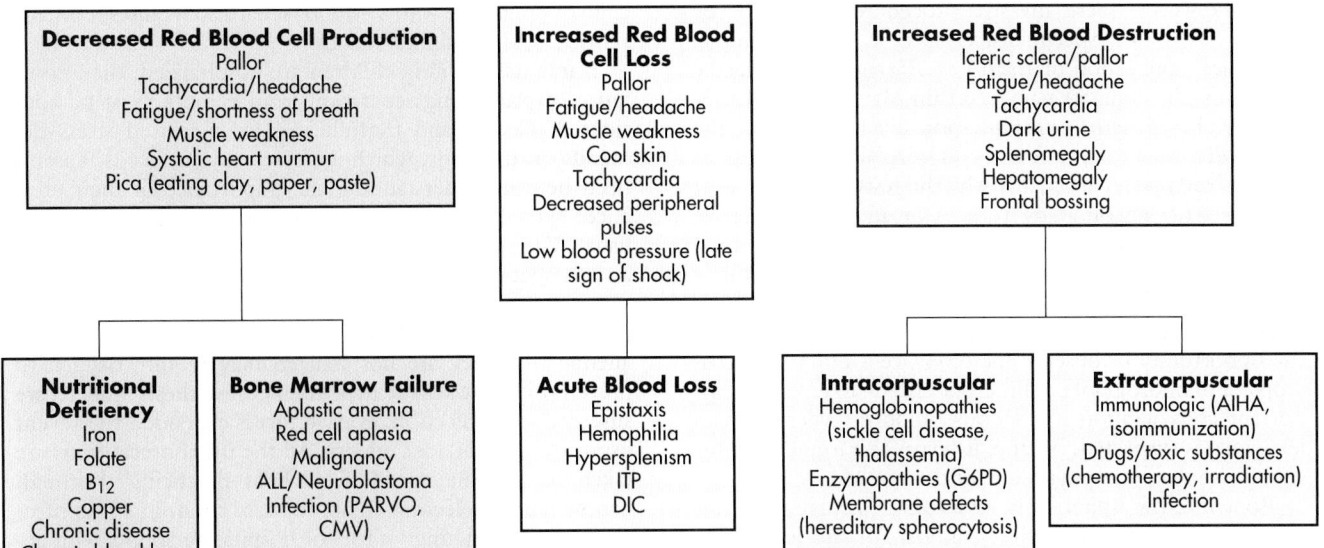

FIG. 26-1 ■ Classifications of anemias.

BOX 26-1 ■ Red Blood Cell (RBC) Morphology
Characteristics of RBCs

SIZE (CELL SIZE)
Variation in RBC sizes (anisocytosis)
   Normocytes (normal cell size)
   Microcytes (smaller than normal cell size)
   Macrocytes (larger than normal cell size)

SHAPE (IRREGULAR SHAPE)
Variation in RBC shapes (poikilocytes)
   Spherocytes (globular cells)
   Drepanocytes (sickle-shaped cells)
   Numerous other irregular-shaped cells

COLOR (STAINING CHARACTERISTICS)
Variation in hemoglobin concentration in the RBC
   Normochromic (sufficient or normal amount of hemoglobin per RBC)
   Hypochromic (reduced amount of hemoglobin per RBC)
   Hyperchromic (increased amount of hemoglobin per RBC)

as decreased RBCs, and decreased Hgb and hematocrit (Hct) levels (see Fig. 26-1). Although anemia is sometimes defined as an Hgb level below 10 or 11 g/dL, this arbitrary cutoff is inappropriate for all children, because Hgb levels normally vary with age (see Table 26-1 and Appendix E).

Other tests specific to a particular type of anemia are employed to determine the underlying cause of anemia. These are discussed in relation to the particular disorder.

Therapeutic Management

The objective of medical management is to reverse the anemia by treating the underlying cause and to make up for any deficiency of blood, blood component, or substance the blood needs for normal functioning. For example, blood or blood cells are replaced after hemorrhage; in nutritional anemias the specific deficiency is replaced.

In patients with severe anemia, supportive medical care may include oxygen therapy, bed rest, and replacement of intravascular volume with intravenous (IV) fluids. The prognosis for anemia depends on the correction of the cause.

Nursing Considerations

The assessment of anemia includes the basic techniques that are applicable to any condition. The age of the infant or child provides some clues regarding the possible etiology of the anemia. For example, iron deficiency anemia occurs more frequently in the toddler between 12 and 36 months of age and during the growth spurt of adolescence.

Racial or ethnic background is significant. For example, the anemias related to abnormal Hgb levels are found in Southeast Asians and persons of African or Mediterranean ancestry. These same groups may be genetically deficient in the enzyme lactase after the period of infancy. Affected individuals are unable to tolerate lactose in the diet, with consequent intestinal irritation and chronic blood loss.

Special emphasis is placed on a careful history to elicit any information that might help identify the cause of the anemia. For example, a statement such as "My child drinks lots of milk" is a frequent finding in toddlers with iron deficiency anemia. An episode of diarrhea may have precipitated a temporary lactose intolerance in a young child.

Stool examination for occult (microscopic) blood (Hemoccult test) can identify chronic intestinal bleeding that results from a primary or secondary lactase deficiency. It is also important to understand the significance of various blood tests (see Table 26-1).

Prepare Child and Family for Laboratory Tests.
Usually, several blood tests are ordered, but because they are generally done sequentially rather than at one time, the child is subjected to multiple finger or heel punctures or venipunctures. Laboratory technicians frequently are not aware of the trauma that repeated punctures represent to a

child. However, these invasive procedures need not be painful (see Blood Specimens, Chapter 22). For example, the topical application of **EMLA** or **Elamax** before needle punctures can eliminate pain (see Pain Management, Chapter 21). Therefore the nurse is responsible for preparing the child and family for the tests by (1) explaining the significance of each test, particularly why the tests are not done at one time; (2) encouraging parents or another supportive person to be with the child during the procedure; and (3) allowing the child to play with the equipment on a doll or participate in the actual procedure (e.g., by cleansing the finger with an alcohol swab). Older children may appreciate the opportunity to observe the blood cells under a microscope or in photographs. This experience is an especially important consideration if a serious blood disorder, such as leukemia, is suspected, because it serves as a foundation for explaining the pathophysiology of the disorder.

Bone marrow aspiration is not a routine hematologic test but is essential for definitive diagnosis of the leukemias, lymphomas, and certain anemias.

NURSING TIP

The following are suggested explanations for teaching children about blood components:
- Red blood cells—Carry the oxygen you breathe from your lungs to all parts of your body
- White blood cells—Help keep germs from causing infection
- Platelets—Small parts of cells that help make bleeding stop; platelets help your body stop bleeding by forming a clot (scab) over the hurt area
- Plasma—The liquid portion of blood; has clotting factors that help make bleeding stop

---

Decrease Tissue Oxygen Needs.   Because the basic pathology in anemia is a decrease in oxygen-carrying capacity, an important nursing responsibility is to assess the child's energy level and minimize excess demands. The child's level of tolerance for activities of daily living and play is assessed, and adjustments are made to allow as much self-care as possible without undue exertion. During periods of rest the nurse takes vital signs and observes behavior to establish a baseline of nonexertion energy expenditure. During periods of activity the nurse repeats these measurements and observations to compare them with resting values.

NURSING ALERT

Signs of exertion include tachycardia, palpitations, tachypnea, dyspnea, shortness of breath, hyperpnea, breathlessness, dizziness, light-headedness, diaphoresis, and change in skin color. The child looks fatigued (sagging, limp posture; slow, strained movements; inability to tolerate additional activity; difficulty sucking in infants).

Diversional activities are planned that promote rest but prevent boredom and withdrawal. Because short attention span, irritability, and restlessness are common in anemia and increase stress demands on the body, appropriate activities are planned, such as listening to music; using a tape recorder; watching television; reading or listening to stories or comics; continuing a favorite hobby, such as stamp collecting, coloring, or drawing; playing board and card games; or being wheeled in a carriage or chair. Choosing the appropriate roommate, such as a

child of similar age with a diagnosis that also requires restricted activity, is a helpful intervention.

If infants or young children are hospitalized, the importance of preventing separation from parents must be considered. Crying and fretfulness place increased stress demands on the body, which increases oxygen needs. Parents need help in understanding the importance of their presence, even though the child may be less responsive than usual. The nurse also explains the reason for mood changes and the necessity of allowing the child's dependency.

Prevent Complications.   Children who are so severely anemic that they are hospitalized may require oxygen to prevent or reduce tissue hypoxia. Because these children are susceptible to infection, every effort is expended to prevent exposure to infectious agents. All the usual precautions are taken to prevent infection, such as practicing thorough handwashing, selecting an appropriate room in a noninfectious area, restricting visitors or hospital personnel with active infection, and maintaining adequate nutrition. The nurse also observes for signs of infection, particularly temperature elevation and leukocytosis.

IRON-DEFICIENCY ANEMIA

Anemia caused by an inadequate supply of dietary iron is the most prevalent nutritional disorder in the United States and the most common mineral disturbance. Children 12 to 36 months of age are at risk for anemia as a result of cow's milk being a major staple of the child's diet (Segel, Hirsh, and Feig, 2002). The prevalence of iron deficiency anemia has decreased, probably in part because of families' participation in the Women, Infants, and Children (WIC) program, which provides iron-fortified formula for the first year of life and routine screening of Hgb levels during early childhood (Bogen, Krause, and Serwint, 2001). Premature infants are especially at risk because of their reduced fetal iron supply. Adolescents are also at risk because of their rapid growth rate combined with poor eating habits.

Pathophysiology

Iron-deficiency anemia can be caused by any number of factors that decrease the supply of iron, impair its absorption, increase the body's need for iron, or affect the synthesis of Hgb. Although the clinical manifestations and diagnostic evaluation are quite similar regardless of the cause, the therapeutic and nursing considerations depend on the specific reason for the iron deficiency. The following discussion is limited to iron-deficiency anemia resulting from inadequate iron in the diet.

During the last trimester of pregnancy, iron is transferred from mother to fetus. Most of the iron is stored in the circulating erythrocytes of the fetus, with the remainder stored in the fetal liver, spleen, and bone marrow. These iron stores are usually adequate for the first 5 to 6 months in a full-term infant but for only 2 to 3 months in premature infants or multiple births. If dietary iron is not supplied to meet the infant's growth demands after the fetal iron stores are depleted, iron-deficiency anemia results. Physiologic anemia should not be confused with iron-deficiency anemia resulting from nutritional causes.

Although most toddlers with iron-deficiency anemia are underweight, many infants are overweight because of excessive milk ingestion (known as *milk babies*). These children become anemic for two reasons: milk, a poor source of iron, is given almost to the exclusion of solid foods, and 50% of iron-deficient infants fed cow's milk have an increased fecal loss of blood.

Therapeutic Management

After the diagnosis of iron-deficiency anemia is made, therapeutic management focuses on increasing the amount of supplemental iron the child receives. This is usually done through dietary counseling and the administration of oral iron supplements.

In formula-fed infants the most convenient and best sources of supplemental iron are iron-fortified commercial formula and iron-fortified infant cereal. Iron-fortified formula provides a relatively constant and predictable amount of iron and is not associated with an increased incidence of gastrointestinal (GI) symptoms, such as colic, diarrhea, or constipation. Infants younger than 12 months of age should *not* be given fresh cow's milk because it may increase the risk of GI blood loss occurring from allergy to the milk protein or from GI mucosal damage resulting from a lack of cytochrome iron (heme protein) (Segel, Hirsh, and Feig, 2002). If GI bleeding is suspected, the child's stool should be guaiac tested on at least four or five occasions to identify any intermittent blood loss.

Dietary addition of iron-rich foods is usually inadequate as the sole treatment of iron-deficiency anemia, because the iron is poorly absorbed and thus provides insufficient supplemental quantities of iron. If dietary sources of iron cannot replace body stores, oral iron supplements are prescribed for approximately 3 months. Ferrous iron, more readily absorbed than ferric iron, results in higher Hgb levels. Ascorbic acid (vitamin C) appears to facilitate absorption of iron and may be given as vitamin C–enriched foods and juices with the iron preparation.

If the Hgb level fails to rise after 1 month of oral therapy, it is important to assess for persistent bleeding, iron malabsorption, noncompliance, improper iron administration, or other causes for the anemia. Parenteral (IV or intramuscular [IM]) iron administration is safe and effective, but painful, expensive, and occasionally associated with regional lymphadenopathy or allergic reaction (Andrews, 2003). Therefore parenteral iron is reserved for children who have iron malabsorption or chronic hemoglobinuria. Transfusions are indicated for the most severe anemia and in cases of serious infection, cardiac dysfunction, or surgical emergency when anesthesia is required. Packed RBCs (2 to 3 cc/kg), not whole blood, are used to minimize the chance of circulatory overload. Supplemental oxygen is administered when tissue hypoxia is severe.

Prognosis.   The prognosis for a child with this condition is very good. However, there is some evidence that if the iron-deficiency anemia is severe and long-standing, cognitive, behavioral, and motor impairment may result (Halterman and others, 2001; Andrews, 2003).

Nursing Considerations

An essential nursing responsibility is instructing parents in the administration of iron. Oral iron should be given as prescribed in two divided doses between meals, when the presence of free hydrochloric acid is greatest, because more iron is absorbed in the acidic environment of the upper GI tract. A citrus fruit or juice taken with the medication aids in absorption.

NURSING TIP

Cow's milk contains substances that bind the iron and interfere with absorption. Iron supplements should not be administered with milk or milk products (Carley, 2003).

An adequate dosage of oral iron turns the stools a tarry green color. The nurse advises parents of this normally expected change and inquires about its occurrence on follow-up visits. Absence of the greenish black stool may be a clue to poor administration of iron, either in schedule or in dosage. Vomiting or diarrhea can occur with iron therapy. If the parents report these symptoms, the iron can be given with meals and the dosage reduced and then gradually increased until tolerated.

Liquid preparations of iron may temporarily stain the teeth. If possible, the medication should be taken through a straw or given through a syringe or medicine dropper placed toward the back of the mouth. Brushing the teeth after administration of the drug lessens the discoloration.

If parenteral iron preparations are prescribed, iron dextran must be injected deeply into a large muscle mass using the Z-track method. The injection site is *not* massaged after injection to minimize skin staining and irritation. Because no more than 1 mL should be given in one site, the IV route should be considered to avoid multiple injections. Careful observation is required because of the risk of adverse reactions, such as anaphylaxis, with IV administration. A test dose is recommended before routine use.

Diet.   A primary nursing objective is to prevent nutritional anemia through family education. Because breast milk is a poor iron source after 5 months of lactation, the nurse must reinforce the importance of administering iron supplementation in the exclusively breast-fed infant by 4 to 6 months of age (Andrews, 2003; Griffins and Abrams, 2001).

In the formula-fed infant, the nurse discusses with parents the importance of using iron-fortified formula and the introduction of solid foods at the appropriate age during the first year of life. Traditionally, cereals are one of the first semisolid foods to be introduced into the infant's diet at approximately 4 months of age (Davidsson, 2003). The best solid-food source of iron is commercial iron-fortified cereals. It may be difficult at first to teach the infant to accept foods other than milk. The same principles are applied as those for introducing new foods (see Nutrition, Chapter 10), especially feeding the solid food before the milk. Predominantly milk-fed infants rebel against solid foods, and parents are cautioned about this and the need to be firm in not relinquishing control to the child. It may require intense problem solving on the part of both the family and the nurse to overcome the child's resistance.

A difficulty encountered in discouraging the parents from feeding milk to the exclusion of other foods is dispelling the popular myth that milk is a "perfect food." Many parents believe that milk is best for the infant and equate the weight gain with a "healthy child" and "good mothering." The nurse can also stress that overweight is not synonymous with good health.

Diet education of teenagers is especially difficult, especially because teenage girls are particularly prone to following weight-reduction diets. Emphasizing the effect of anemia on appearance (pallor) and energy level (difficulty maintaining popular activities) may be useful. (See Chapter 11—Mineral Disturbances and Table 11-2—for sources of iron-rich foods.)

SICKLE CELL ANEMIA

Sickle cell anemia (SCA) is one of a group of diseases collectively termed *hemoglobinopathies,* in which normal adult hemoglobin (hemoglobin A [HbA]) is partly or completely replaced by abnormal sickle hemoglobin (HbS). *Sickle cell disease (SCD)* includes all those hereditary disorders whose clinical, hematologic, and pathologic features are related to the presence of HbS. Even though SCD is sometimes used to refer to SCA, this use is incorrect. Other correct terms for SCA are *SS* and *homozygous sickle cell disease.*

The following are the most common forms of SCD in the United States:

Sickle cell anemia, the homozygous form of the disease (HbSS or SS).
Sickle cell–C disease, a heterozygous variant of SCD, including both HbS and HbC (SC).
Sickle cell–hemoglobin E disease, a variant of SCD in which glutamic acid has been substituted for lysine in the number-26 position of the β-chain (SE).
Sickle thalassemia disease, a combination of sickle cell trait and β-thalassemia trait (Sβthal). $β^+$ refers to the ability to still produce some normal HbA. $β^0$ indicates that there is no ability to produce HbA.

Of the SCDs, SCA is the most common form in African Americans, followed by sickle cell–C disease and sickle β-thalassemia.

SCA is found primarily in African Americans, Hispanics, and other ethnic groups. SCA occurs infrequently in Caucasians (especially those of Mediterranean descent). The incidence of the disease varies in different geographic locations. Among African Americans the incidence of sickle cell trait is about 8%. In West Africa the incidence is reported to be as high as 40% among native Africans. The high incidence of sickle cell trait in West Africans is believed by some to be the result of selective protection afforded trait carriers against one type of malaria.

The gene that determines the production of HbS is situated on an autosome and, when present, is always detectable and therefore dominant. Heterozygous persons who have both normal HbA and abnormal HbS are said to have *sickle cell trait.* Persons who are homozygous have predominantly HbS and have *sickle cell anemia.* The inheritance pattern is essentially that of an autosomal recessive disorder (see Appendix B). Therefore, when both parents have sickle cell trait, there is a 25% chance with each pregnancy of producing an offspring with SCA.

Although the defect is inherited, the sickling phenomenon is usually not apparent until later in infancy because of the presence of fetal hemoglobin (HbF). As long as the child has predominantly HbF, sickling does not occur because there is less HbS. The newborn with SCA is generally asymptomatic because of the protective effect of Hgb F (60% to 80% HbF), but this rapidly decreases during the first year, so the child is at risk for sickle cell–related complications (Dover and Platt, 2003).

Pathophysiology

The clinical features of SCA are primarily the result of (1) *obstruction* caused by the sickled RBCs and (2) increased RBC *destruction* (Fig. 26-2). The entanglement and enmeshing of rigid sickle-shaped cells with one another intermittently block the microcirculation, causing vaso-occlusion. The resultant absence of blood flow to adjacent tissues causes local hypoxia, leading to tissue ischemia and infarction (cellular death). Most of the complications seen in SCA can be traced to this process and its impact on various organs of the body. The effect of sickling and infarction on organ structures occurs in the following sequence (see also consequences in Box 26-2):

1 Stasis with enlargement
2 Infarction with ischemia and destruction
3 Replacement with fibrous tissue (scarring)

Clinical Manifestations

The clinical manifestations of SCA vary greatly in severity and frequency. The most acute symptoms of the disease occur during periods of exacerbation called *crises.* There are several types of episodic crises: vaso-occlusive, acute splenic sequestration, aplastic, hyperhemolytic, cerebrovascular accident (stroke), chest syndrome, and infection. The crises may occur individually or concomitantly with one or more other crises. The episode may be a *vaso-occlusive crisis,* preferably called a "painful episode," characterized by distal ischemia and pain; *sequestration crisis,* a pooling of blood in the liver and spleen with decreased blood volume and shock; *aplastic crisis,* diminished RBC production resulting in profound anemia; or *hyperhemolytic crisis,* an accelerated rate of RBC destruction characterized by anemia, jaundice, and reticulocytosis. This complication frequently suggests other coexisting conditions, such as viral illness or glucose-6-phosphate dehydrogenase (G6PD) deficiency.

Another serious complication is *acute chest syndrome,* which is clinically similar to pneumonia. It is the presence of a new pulmonary infiltrate and is associated with chest pain, fever, cough, tachypnea, wheezing, and hypoxia. A *cerebrovascular accident (CVA, stroke)* is a sudden and severe complication, often with no related illnesses. Sickled cells block the major blood vessels in the brain, resulting in cerebral infarction, which causes variable degrees of neurologic impairment. Repeat CVAs causing progressively greater brain damage occur in approximately 70% of untreated children who have already experienced one stroke (Dover and Platt, 2003).

Diagnostic Evaluation

Newborn screening for SCA is mandatory in most of the United States so that infants can be identified before symptoms occur. At birth the infant has up to 80% of HbF, which does not carry the defect. Because levels of HbS are low at birth, Hgb electrophoresis or other tests that measure Hgb concentrations are indicated. Early diagnosis (before 3 months of age) enables initiation of appropriate interventions to minimize complications. The family is taught to administer prophylactic antibiotics and identify early signs of infection to seek medical therapy as soon as possible.

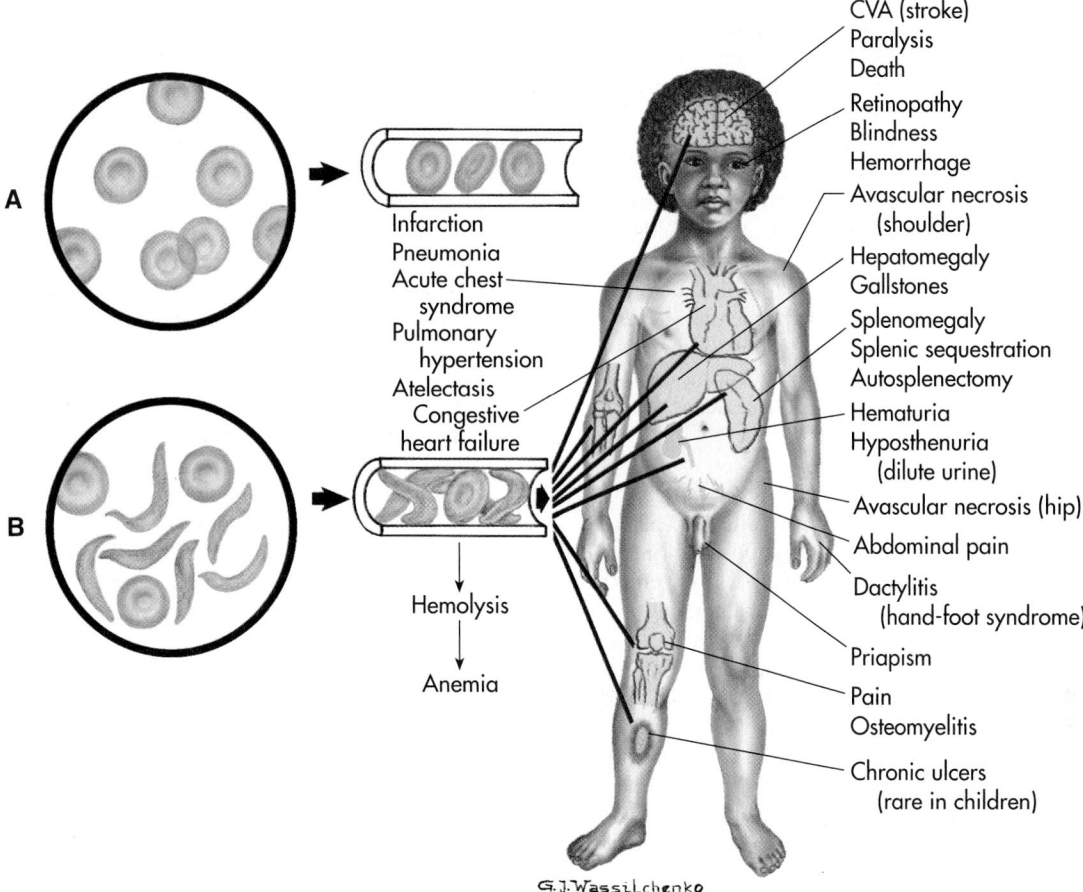

FIG. 26-2 ■ Differences between effects of **A,** normal and **B,** sickled red blood cells on circulation with related complications.

BOX 26-2 ■ Clinical Manifestations of Sickle Cell Anemia

GENERAL

Possible growth retardation

Chronic anemia (Hgb 6 to 9 g/dL)

Possible delayed sexual maturation

Marked susceptibility to sepsis

VASO-OCCLUSIVE CRISIS

Pain in area(s) of involvement

Manifestations related to ischemia of involved areas:

Extremities—painful swelling of hands and feet (sickle cell dactylitis, or "hand-foot syndrome"), painful joints

Abdomen—severe pain resembling acute surgical condition

Cerebrum—stroke, visual disturbances

Chest—symptoms resembling pneumonia, protracted episodes of pulmonary disease

Liver—obstructive jaundice, hepatic coma

Kidney—hematuria

Genital—priapism (painful penile erection)

SEQUESTRATION CRISIS

Pooling of large amounts of blood:

Hepatomegaly

Splenomegaly

Circulatory collapse

EFFECTS OF CHRONIC VASO-OCCLUSIVE PHENOMENA

Heart—cardiomegaly, systolic murmurs

Lungs—altered pulmonary function, susceptibility to infections, pulmonary insufficiency

Kidneys—inability to concentrate urine, progressive renal failure, enuresis

Liver—hepatomegaly, cirrhosis, intrahepatic cholestasis

Spleen—splenomegaly, susceptibility to infection, functional reduction in splenic activity progressing to autosplenectomy

Eyes—intraocular abnormalities with visual disturbances, sometimes progressive retinal detachment and blindness

Extremities—skeletal deformities such as lordosis and kyphosis, avascular necrosis of hip/shoulder, chronic leg ulcers, susceptibility to osteomyelitis

Central nervous system—hemiparesis, seizures

If SCA is not diagnosed in early infancy, it is likely to manifest symptoms during the toddler and preschool years. SCA is occasionally first diagnosed during a crisis that follows an acute respiratory or GI infection. Routine hematologic tests are done to evaluate the anemia. Several specific tests detect the presence of the abnormal Hgb in the heterozygote or the homozygote. For *screening* purposes the *sickle-turbidity test (Sickledex)* is frequently used because it can be performed on blood from a finger stick and yields accurate results in 3 minutes. However, if the test is positive, Hgb electrophoresis is necessary to distinguish between those children with the trait and those with the disease. *Hemoglobin electrophoresis* ("finger printing" of the protein) is an accurate, rapid, and specific test for detecting the homozygous and heterozygous forms of the disease, as well as the percentages of the various types of Hgb.

Therapeutic Management

The aims of therapy are (1) to prevent conditions that enhance sickling phenomena, which are responsible for the pathologic sequelae; and (2) to treat the medical emergencies of sickle cell crisis. Prevention consists of maintaining hemodilution. The successful implementation of this goal depends more often on nursing interventions than on medical therapies. Research is investigating hydroxyurea with and without erythropoietin, which may increase the concentration of fetal hemoglobin and ultimately reduce complications (Ferster and others, 2001; Charache and others, 1996). Hematopoietic stem cell transplantation with stabilization of prior organ damage is a possible cure for SCD (Karayalcin, 2000). Limiting factors include proper patient selection as well as the availability of suitable donors (Karayalcin, 2000). This technology raises many ethical issues regarding patient access and availability of therapy (Simon, Lobe, and Jackson, 1999; Platt and Guinan, 1996).

Medical management of a crisis is usually directed at supportive and symptomatic treatment. The main objectives are to provide (1) rest to minimize energy expenditure and oxygen use; (2) hydration through oral and IV therapy; (3) electrolyte replacement, because hypoxia results in metabolic acidosis, which also promotes sickling; (4) analgesics for the severe pain from vaso-occlusion; (5) blood replacement to treat anemia and hydration to reduce the viscosity of the sickled blood; and (6) antibiotics to treat any existing infection. (See Ethical Case Study.)

Administration of pneumococcal and meningococcal vaccines is recommended for these children because of their susceptibility to infection as a result of a functional asplenia. In addition to routine immunizations, the child with SCD should receive a yearly influenza vaccination. (See Immunizations, Chapter 10.) Oral penicillin prophylaxis is also recommended by 2 months of age (American Academy of Pediatrics, 2002; National Institutes of Health, National Heart, Lung, and Blood Institute [NIH/NHLBI], 2002; Segal and others, 2002).

Short-term oxygen therapy may be helpful if a child has symptoms of respiratory difficulty. Severe hypoxia must be prevented because this causes massive systemic sickling that can be fatal. Although oxygen may prevent more sickling, it usually is not effective in reversing sickling, because the oxygen is unable to reach the enmeshed sickled erythrocytes (Perkins, 2001; Chiocca, 1996) in clogged vessels. In addi-

tion, prolonged administration can depress bone marrow, further aggravating the anemia (Khoury and Grimsley, 1995).

Exchange transfusion, which reduces the number of circulating sickle cells and slows down the vicious circle of hypoxia, thrombosis, tissue ischemia, and injury, has been successful. The procedure is sometimes advocated as a possible preventive technique. A transcranial Doppler (TCD) test identifies the child with SCD who is high-risk for developing a CVA by monitoring the intracranial vascular flow (American Academy of Pediatrics, 2002; Segal and others, 2002). The TCD is performed yearly on children from 2 to 16 years of age. If the TCD is abnormal, then magnetic resonance imaging of the brain is done to detect cerebral arterial stenosis or ischemia. The recommended treatment for a confirmed abnormal TCD is chronic transfusion therapy (Segal and others, 2002). However, multiple transfusions carry the risk of transmission of viral infection, hyperviscosity, transfusion reactions, alloimmunization, and hemosiderosis (Orkin and Nathan, 2003; Karayalcin, 2000). After a CVA has occurred, blood transfusions are usually given every 3 to 4 weeks to help prevent a repeat stroke. To reduce iron overload, home subcutaneous chelation therapy may be started (see p. 950).

In children with recurrent life-threatening splenic sequestration, splenectomy may be a lifesaving measure. However, because the spleen usually atrophies on its own through progressive fibrotic changes *(functional asplenia)*, routine splenectomy is not recommended because of the risk of overwhelming infection. Any procedure that requires anesthesia has increased risk for these children. *Painful priapism (continual or intermittent erection)* may be treated by aspiration of the corpora cavernosum. This complication is particularly frequent in vaso-occlusive crises.

The most frequent problem for patients with SCA is *vaso-occlusive pain* (Fig. 26-3). The chronic nature of this pain can greatly affect the child's development. A multidisciplinary approach is best for its management. When mild to moderate pain is reported, ibuprofen or acetaminophen is used initially. If these drugs are not effective alone, codeine can be added. The dosages of both drugs are titrated (adjusted) to a therapeutic level. Opioids such as immediate- and sustained-release morphine, oxycodone, hydromorphone (Dilaudid), and methadone are administered intravenously or orally for severe pain and are given around the clock. Patient-controlled analgesia (PCA) has been used successfully for sickle cell–related pain. PCA reinforces the patient's role and responsibility in managing the pain and provides flexibility in dealing with pain, which may vary in severity over time. The use of high-dose IV methylprednisolone has decreased the duration of severe pain in children (Dover and Platt, 2003; Griffin, McIntire, and Buchanan, 1994). (See Pain Management, Chapter 21.)

!NURSING ALERT

Meperidine (pethidine [Demerol]) is not recommended. Normeperidine, a metabolite of meperidine, is a central nervous system stimulant that produces anxiety, tremors, myoclonus, and generalized seizures when it accumulates with repetitive dosing. Patients with SCD are particularly at risk for normeperidine-induced seizures (NIH/NHLBI, 2002; American Pain Society, 1999).

⚡ ETHICAL CASE STUDY

Ethical Decision Making Model	*Joey is a 7-year-old with sickle cell disease. His family belongs to a Jehovah's Witness church and indicates they are quite strong in their faith and beliefs. Joey has had several sickle cell pain crises this past year requiring hospitalization. He has never had a blood transfusion, yet the parents have been informed that a blood transfusion is often required to treat the physical problems associated with sickle cell disease. He arrives in the clinic today looking pale, and his hemoglobin is 4.9 (baseline Hgb is 8 g/dL), with a reticulocyte count of 1. He has had a cough, fever as high as 100° F, and runny nose for the past week. Physical examination reveals a grade II/VI systolic ejection murmur (SEM) with gallop at the left lower sternal border. His pulse is 120, respirations 20, blood pressure 102/60. Joey states he feels tired, has no appetite, and he appears quite listless.*
Evaluate the issue	The first priority is to evaluate Joey's condition. Children with sickle cell disease are anemic, but when their hemoglobin drops extremely low, the reticulocyte count should increase as the bone marrow tries to produce new red blood cells. When children with sickle cell disease experience aplastic crisis, the bone marrow does not respond to the decreasing hemoglobin, which is exemplified by Joey's low reticulocyte count. This often occurs after a viral illness, which is reflected in the symptoms experienced by Joey this past week. The treatment for aplastic crises in a child with sickle cell disease is blood transfusion because it can be several weeks before the bone marrow recovers and begins making new red blood cells again. On examination, Joey has clinical symptoms created by the decreasing hemoglobin.

Treat all involved with respect	The physician sits with Joey's parents to discuss the need for blood transfusion. The physician explains that without a blood transfusion, Joey's condition could become severe and he could die. Joey's mother becomes distraught and states she cannot give permission to transfuse her son with blood or blood products. The physician listens while the parents discuss their religious beliefs.
	
	    The controversy in this case is that Joey's family is Jehovah's Witness. Individuals of this faith believe that ingesting the blood of any flesh is forbidden and that blood transfusions are equivalent to oral ingestion of blood. Transfusion of whole blood, packed red blood cells, white blood cells, platelets, and plasma (fresh or frozen) is forbidden.
	
	    Consequences of parents giving consent for a blood transfusion require the family to leave the church, family, friends, and the Jehovah's Witness community. Refusal of blood transfusion and blood products is a basic component of the Jehovah's Witness faith, and if this covenant is broken, the individual loses eternal salvation. Families are often shunned by their church community, and the child is perceived as an outcast because his future beyond death is affected by the ingestion of the blood regardless of the eventual outcome of the child's health status.

Hear all sides	Joey's hematology nurse and social worker are asked to spend time with the parents, further exploring their concerns regarding the blood transfusion. It becomes evident that they cannot give permission for the transfusion. The physician is adamant that the child's best hope for recovery is to receive a blood transfusion.
Initiate action	For the parents' sake, it is better to obtain a court order for life-saving transfusion than to ask their permission. This removes the decision from the parents and prevents the parents and child from being ostracized, because the matter was removed from their control. The nurse's role is to be an advocate for the family and a resource to other members of the health care team regarding the family's beliefs.
Consider the outcome	The eventual outcome if Joey does not receive a blood transfusion is that his hemoglobin will likely continue to fall as red blood cells are lysed. He will become more ill with ensuing respiratory difficulty, propensity for systemic infections, and eventual cardiac failure and death. If his parents fail to give consent for a blood transfusion a court order may be obtained and Joey may be given the necessary blood transfusion, which will improve his health status. However, it is possible that Joey will become ill again at some point in the future and will require a blood transfusion, at which point a court order will again be necessary because the parents will not give consent for such therapy. It is unknown how Joey's parents and church family will react to him receiving a blood transfusion.

Prognosis.   The prognosis varies. Most of the time, children are without symptoms and participate in normal activities without restrictions. The greatest risk is usually in children younger than 5 years of age, and the majority of deaths in these children are caused by overwhelming infection. Consequently, SCA is a chronic illness with a potentially terminal outcome.

Individuals with higher levels of HbF are more likely to have fewer complications than those with lower levels (Steinberg and others, 2003; Segal and others, 2002). Long-term follow up of patients taking hydroxyurea alone revealed a 40% reduction in mortality (Steinberg and others, 2003).

Physical and sexual maturation are delayed in adolescents with SCA. Although adults achieve normal height, weight,

and sexual function, the delay may present problems to the adolescent (Dover and Platt, 2003; Gribbons, Zahr, and Opas, 1995). Hematopoietic stem cell transplantation offers the hope of a cure for some children, although the mortality rate is approximately 8% and the graft failures after transplantation range from 9% to 14% (Dover and Platt, 2003) (see p. 959).

Nursing Considerations

Educate family and child. Family education begins with an explanation of the disease and its consequences. After this explanation, the most important issues to teach the family are to (1) seek early intervention for problems, such as fever of 38.5° C (101.5° F) or greater; (2) give penicillin as ordered;

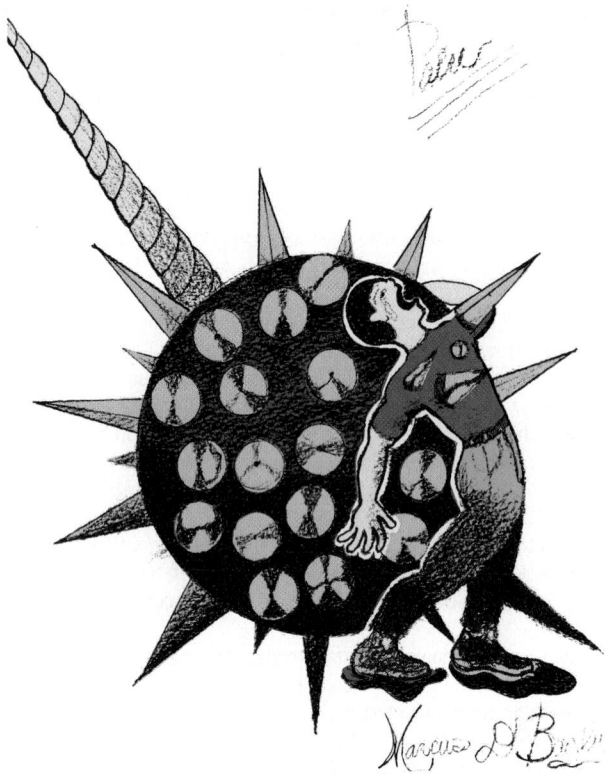

FIG. 26-3 ■ Drawing of sickle cell pain by a 17-year-old boy. When asked what message he would like to give health professionals about treating pain, he stated, "Tell them to listen to the patient and family. They know about the pain."

(3) recognize signs and symptoms of splenic sequestration, as well as respiratory problems that can lead to hypoxia; and (4) treat the child normally. The nurse tells the family that the child is normal but can get sick in ways that other children cannot.

NURSING TIP

One simple yet graphic way to demonstrate the effect of sickling is to roll rounded objects, such as marbles or beads, through a tube to simulate normal circulation and then roll pointed objects, such as screws or jacks, through the tube. The effect of sickling and clumping of the pointed objects is especially noticeable at a bend or slight narrowing of the tube.

The nurse emphasizes the importance of adequate hydration to prevent sickling and to delay the stasis-thrombosis-ischemia cycle in a crisis. It is not sufficient to advise parents to "force fluids" or "encourage drinking." They need specific instructions on how many daily glasses or bottles of fluid are required. Many foods are also a source of fluid, particularly soups, flavored ice pops, ice cream, sherbet, gelatin, and puddings.

Increased fluids combined with impaired kidney function result in the problem of *enuresis*. Parents who are unaware of this fact frequently employ the usual measures to discourage bed-wetting, such as limiting fluids at night, and may resort to punishment and shame to force bladder control. Enuresis is treated as a complication of the disease,

such as joint pain or some other symptom, to alleviate parental pressure on the child.

Promote Supportive Therapies During Crises. The success of many of the medical therapies relies heavily on nursing implementation. Management of pain is an especially difficult problem and often involves experimenting with various analgesics, including opioids, and schedules before relief is achieved. Unfortunately, these children tend to be undermedicated, resulting in their "clock watching" and demands for additional doses sooner than might be expected. Often this incorrectly raises suspicions of drug addiction, when in fact the problem is one of improper dosage (see Family Focus box). In choosing and scheduling analgesics, the goal should be *prevention* of pain.

NURSING ALERT

Advise parents to be particularly alert to situations in which dehydration may be a possibility, such as hot weather, and to recognize early signs of reduced intake, such as decreased urine output (e.g., fewer wet diapers) and increased thirst.

Any pain program should be combined with psychologic support to help the child deal with the depression, anxiety, and fear that may accompany the disease. This includes regular visits with the child to discuss any concerns during the hospitalization and positive reinforcement of coping skills, such as successful methods of dealing with the pain and compliance with treatment prescriptions. To reduce the negative connotation associated with the term "crisis," it is best to say "pain episode."

Frequently, heat to the affected area is soothing. Cold compresses are not applied to the area because this enhances sickling and vasoconstriction. Bed rest is usually well tolerated during a crisis, although actual rest depends greatly on pain alleviation and organized schedules of nursing care. Some activity, particularly passive range-of-motion exercises, is beneficial to promote circulation. Usually the best course of action is to let children dictate their activity tolerance.

If blood transfusions or exchange transfusions are given, the nurse has the responsibility of observing for signs of transfusion reaction (see Table 26-5). Because hypervolemia from too-rapid transfusion can increase the workload of the heart, the nurse also is alert to signs of cardiac failure.

In splenic sequestration the size of the spleen is gently measured by abdominal palpation (see Abdomen, Chapter

7). The nurse should be aware of spleen size because an increasing splenomegaly is an ominous sign. A decreasing spleen size denotes response to therapy. Vital signs and blood pressure are also closely monitored for impending shock. Anemia is typically not a presenting complication in vaso-occlusive crises but is a critical problem in other types of crises. The nurse monitors for evidence of increasing anemia and institutes appropriate nursing intervention (see p. 946). Oxygen is not beneficial in vaso-occlusive episodes unless hypoxemia is present (Karayalcin, 2000; Chiocca, 1996). It does not reverse sickled RBCs, and if used in the nonhypoxic patient, it will decrease erythropoiesis (Khoury and Grimsley, 1995). Because prolonged use of oxygen can aggravate the anemia, signs of lack of therapeutic benefit, such as restlessness, increased pallor, and continued pain, are reported.

Intake, especially of IV fluids, and output are recorded. The child's weight should be taken on admission, because it serves as a baseline for evaluating hydration. Because diuresis can result in electrolyte loss, the nurse also observes for signs of hypokalemia and should be familiar with normal serum electrolyte values to report changes.

Recognize Other Complications. Nurses also need to be aware of the signs of acute chest syndrome and CVA, both potentially fatal complications.

> **⚠ NURSING ALERT**
>
> Report signs of the following immediately:
> Acute chest syndrome:
>   Severe chest, back, or abdominal pain
>   Fever of 38.5° C (101.5° F) or higher
>   Very congested cough
>   Dyspnea, tachypnea
>   Retractions
>   Declining oxygen saturation (oximetry)
> Cerebrovascular accident (CVA, stroke):
>   Severe, unrelieved headaches
>   Severe vomiting
>   Jerking or twitching of the face, legs, or arms
>   Seizures
>   Strange, abnormal behavior
>   Inability to move an arm or leg
>   Stagger or an unsteady walk
>   Stutter or slurred speech
>   Weakness in the hands, feet, or legs
>   Changes in vision

Support Family. Families need the opportunity to discuss their feelings regarding transmitting a potentially fatal, chronic illness to their child. Because of the widely publicized prognosis for children with SCA, many parents express their prevalent fear of the child's death. Three manifestations of SCD that may appear in the first 2 years of life (dactylitis, severe anemia, leukocytosis) can be predictors of disease severity (Miller and others, 2000). However, nursing care for the family should be the same as for any family with a child with a life-threatening illness. Particular emphasis is placed on the siblings' reactions, the stress on the marital relationship, and the childrearing attitudes displayed toward the child (see Chapter 18). Sev-

eral resources are available to the family with a sickling disorder.*

The nurse advises parents to inform all treating personnel of the child's condition. The use of medical identification, such as a bracelet, is another way of ensuring awareness of the disease.

If family members have the SCD trait or SCA, genetic counseling is necessary. A primary goal is informing parents who carry the trait, in language they can understand, of the 25% chance with each pregnancy of having a child with the disease.

β-THALASSEMIA (COOLEY ANEMIA)

The term *thalassemia,* which is derived from the Greek word *thalassa,* meaning "sea," is applied to a variety of inherited blood disorders characterized by deficiencies in the rate of production of specific globin chains in Hgb. The name appropriately refers to descendants of or those people living near the Mediterranean sea, who have the highest incidence of the disease, namely Italians, Greeks, and Syrians. Evidence suggests that the high incidence of the disorders among these groups is a result of selective advantage of the trait to malaria, as is postulated in sickle cell disease. However, the disorder has a wide geographic distribution, probably as a result of genetic migration through intermarriage or possibly as a result of spontaneous mutation.

β-Thalassemia is the most common of the thalassemias and occurs in four forms: two heterozygous forms: *thalassemia minor,* an asymptomatic silent carrier, and *thalassemia trait,* which produces a mild microcytic anemia; *thalassemia intermedia,* which is manifested as splenomegaly and moderate to

---

*****National Association for Sickle Cell Disease, Inc.,** 3345 Wilshire Boulevard, Suite 1106, Los Angeles, CA 90010-1880; (800) 421-8453; website: www.sicklecelldisease.org; **Center for Sickle Cell Disease,** Howard University, 2121 Georgia Avenue NW, Washington, DC 20059; (202) 806-7930; **National Heart, Lung, and Blood Institute,** 9000 Rockville Pike, Building 31, Room 4A-21, Bethesda, MD 20892; (301) 496-4236; website: www.nhlbi.nih.gov. The **Agency for Healthcare Research Quality (AHRQ)** (formerly AHCPR) has published three booklets on sickle cell disease: *Sickle Cell Disease: Comprehensive Screening, Diagnosis, Management, and Counseling in Newborns and Infants,* Clinical Practice Guideline no 6, pub no AHCPR-0562; *Sickle Cell Disease: Comprehensive Screening and Management in Newborns and Infants,* Quick Reference Guide for Clinicians no 6, pub no AHCPR-0563; and *Sickle Cell Disease in Newborns and Infants: A Guide for Parents,* pub no AHCPR 93-0564. They are available from the AHCPR Publications Clearinghouse, PO Box 8547, Silver Spring, MD 20907; (800) 358-9295; website: www.ahcpr.gov. *Guideline for the Management of Acute and Chronic Pain in Sickle-Cell Disease* is available from the **American Pain Society,** 4700 West Lake Avenue, Glenview, IL 60025-1485; (847) 375-4715; fax: (847) 375-6315; email: info@ampainsoc.org; website: www.ampainsoc.org. *Clinical Reference Guide for Health Care Providers: Sickle Cell Related Pain: Assessment and Management—A Guide for Patients and Parents* is available from the **New England Regional Genetics Groups (NERGG),** No. 28 Clarendon Street, Newton, MA 02460; (617) 243-3033; email: maryaten@mediaone.net; website: www.nergg.org. A video, *Sickle Cell Disease Is More Than Pain Management,* is available from Maxishare, PO Box 2041, Milwaukee, WI 53201; (800) 444-7747. Information is also available from the **Sickle Cell Disease Association of America, Inc.,** 200 Cooperate Pointe, Suite 495, Culver City, CA 90230-8727; (310) 216-6363; website: www.sicklecelldisease.org.

severe anemia; and a homozygous form, *thalassemia major* (also known as *Cooley anemia*), which results in a severe anemia that would lead to cardiac failure and death in early childhood without transfusion support.

Pathophysiology

Normal postnatal Hgb is composed of 2 α- and 2 β-polypeptide chains. In β-thalassemia there is a partial or complete deficiency in the synthesis of the β-chain of the Hgb molecule. Consequently, there is a compensatory increase in the synthesis of α-chains, and γ-chain production remains activated, resulting in defective Hgb formation. This unbalanced polypeptide unit is very unstable; when it disintegrates, it damages RBCs, causing severe anemia.

To compensate for the hemolytic process, an overabundance of erythrocytes is formed unless the bone marrow is suppressed by transfusion therapy. Excess iron from hemolysis of supplemental RBCs in transfusions and from the rapid destruction of defective cells is stored in various organs *(hemosiderosis).*

Diagnostic Evaluation

The onset of thalassemia major may be insidious and not recognized until the latter half of infancy. The clinical effects of thalassemia major are primarily attributable to (1) defective synthesis of HbA, (2) structurally impaired RBCs, and (3) shortened life span of erythrocytes (Box 26-3).

Hematologic studies reveal the characteristic changes in RBCs (i.e., microcytosis, hypochromia, anisocytosis, poikilocytosis, target cells, and basophilic stippling of various stages). Low Hgb and Hct levels are seen in severe anemia, although they are typically lower than the reduction in RBC count because of the proliferation of immature erythrocytes. Hgb electrophoresis confirms the diagnosis, and radiographs of involved bones reveal characteristic findings.

Therapeutic Management

The objective of supportive therapy is to maintain sufficient Hgb levels to prevent bone marrow expansion and the resulting bony deformities, and to provide sufficient RBCs to support normal growth and normal physical activity. Transfusions are the foundation of medical management. Recent studies have evaluated the benefits of maintaining the child's Hgb level above 9.5 g/dL, a goal that may require transfusions as often as every 3 to 5 weeks. The advantages of this therapy include (1) improved physical and psychologic well-being because of the ability to participate in normal activities, (2) decreased cardiomegaly and hepatosplenomegaly, (3) fewer bone changes, (4) normal or near-normal growth and development until puberty, and (5) fewer infections.

One of the potential complications of frequent blood transfusions is iron overload. Because the body has no effective means of eliminating the excess iron, the mineral is deposited in body tissues. To minimize the development of hemosiderosis, *deferoxamine (Desferal),* an iron-chelating agent, is given with oral supplements of vitamin C. Vitamin C should be used only in patients who are ascorbate depleted and only while deferoxamine is being administered. As ferritin levels decrease toward normal, the role of vitamin C in increasing iron excretion disappears (Orkin and Nathan, 2003). Deferoxamine is given

BOX 26-3 ■ Clinical Manifestations of β-Thalassemia

ANEMIA (BEFORE DIAGNOSIS)
Pallor
Unexplained fever
Poor feeding
Enlarged spleen/liver

WITH PROGRESSIVE ANEMIA
Signs of chronic hypoxia
 Headache
 Precordial and bone pain
 Decreased exercise tolerance
 Listlessness
 Anorexia

OTHER FEATURES
Small stature
Delayed sexual maturation
Bronzed, freckled complexion (if not chelated)

BONE CHANGES (OLDER CHILDREN IF UNTREATED)
Enlarged head
Prominent frontal and parietal bosses
Prominent malar eminences
Flat or depressed bridge of the nose
Enlarged maxilla
Protrusion of the lip and upper central incisors and eventual malocclusion
Generalized skeletal osteoporosis

intravenously or subcutaneously, often at home using a portable infusion pump, over 8 to 24 hours (usually during sleep) for 5 to 7 days a week. It is also given intravenously over 4 hours at the time of blood transfusion in many centers. Creative strategies such as behavioral contracting have been used to assist the child in complying with the deferoxamine regimen.

In some children with severe splenomegaly who demonstrate increased transfusion requirements, a splenectomy may be necessary to decrease the disabling effects of abdominal pressure and to increase the lifespan of supplemental RBCs. Over time, the spleen may accelerate the rate of RBC destruction and thus increase transfusion requirements. After a splenectomy, children generally require fewer transfusions, although the basic defect in Hgb synthesis remains unaffected. A major postsplenectomy complication is severe and overwhelming infection. Therefore these children continue to receive prophylactic antibiotics with close medical supervision for many years and should receive the pneumococcal and meningococcal vaccines in addition to the regularly scheduled immunizations (see Immunizations, Chapter 10).

⚠ NURSING ALERT

Ensure that the family/patient understands the need to notify the health professional of all fevers of 38.5° C (101.5° F) or greater because of the risk of sepsis in a child with asplenia.

Prognosis.   Most children treated with blood transfusion and early chelation therapy survive well into adulthood. The most common cause of death is iron-induced heart disease, multiple organ failure, postsplenectomy sepsis, liver disease, and malignancy (Paley, 2000). Hematopoietic stem cell transplantation has the best results in the least symptomatic patients with a 75% rate of complication-free survival (Orkin and Nathan, 2003; Paley, 2000).

Nursing Considerations

The objectives of nursing care are to (1) promote compliance with transfusion and chelation therapy, (2) assist the child in coping with the anxiety-provoking treatments and the effects of the illness, (3) foster the child's and family's adjustment to a chronic illness, and (4) observe for complications of multiple blood transfusions. Basic to each of these goals is explaining to parents and older children the defect responsible for the disorder, its effect on RBCs, and the potential effects of untreated iron overload (such as diabetes and heart disease). Because the prevalence of this condition is high among families of Mediterranean descent, the nurse also inquires about the family's previous knowledge about thalassemia. All families with a child with thalassemia should be tested for the trait and referred for genetic counseling.

As with any chronic illness, the needs of the family must be met for optimal adjustment to the stresses imposed by the disorder (see Chapter 18). Sources of information for the family include the **Cooley's Anemia Foundation*** and the **Thalassemia Action Group.†** Genetic counseling for the parents and fertile offspring is mandatory, and both prenatal diagnosis using amniocentesis at 20 weeks of gestation or fetal blood sampling at 10 weeks and screening for thalassemia trait are available.

APLASTIC ANEMIA

Aplastic anemia (AA) refers to a bone marrow failure condition in which the formed elements of the blood are simultaneously depressed. The peripheral blood smear demonstrates pancytopenia or the triad of profound anemia, leukopenia, and thrombocytopenia. *Hypoplastic anemia* is characterized by a profound depression of RBCs, but normal or slightly decreased white blood cells (WBCs) and platelets.

Etiology

Aplastic anemia can be *primary* (*congenital,* or present at birth) or *secondary (acquired).* The best-known congenital disorder of which aplastic anemia is an outstanding feature is *Fanconi syndrome,* a rare hereditary disorder characterized by pancytopenia, hypoplasia of the bone marrow, and patchy brown discoloration of the skin resulting from the deposit of melanin and associated with multiple congenital anomalies of the musculoskeletal and genitourinary systems. The syndrome appears to be inherited as an autoso-

*129-09 26th Avenue, Suite 203, Flushing, NY 11354; (718) 321-2873 or (800) 522-7222; fax: (718) 321-3340; website: www.thalassemia.org.

†129-09 26th Avenue, Suite 203, Flushing, NY 11354; (718) 321-2873 or (800) 522-7222; fax: (718) 321-3340; website: http://www.cooleysanemia.org/sections.php?sec=2&tab=83.

BOX 26-4 ■ Common Causes of Acquired Aplastic Anemia

Infection with the human parvovirus (HPV), hepatitis, or overwhelming infection

Irradiation

Drugs such as the chemotherapeutic agents and several antibiotics, one of the most notable being chloramphenicol

Industrial and household chemicals, including benzene and its derivatives, which are found in petroleum products, dyes, paint remover, shellac, and lacquers

Infiltration and replacement of myeloid elements, such as in leukemia or the lymphomas

Idiopathic, in which no identifiable precipitating cause can be found

mal recessive trait with varying penetrance; therefore, affected siblings may demonstrate several different combinations of defects.

Several etiologic factors contribute to the development of acquired hypoplastic anemia; however, about 70% of all cases are considered idiopathic (Box 26-4). Acquired aplastic anemia is classified as either severe acquired aplastic anemia or moderate acquired aplastic anemia. The following discussion focuses on severe acquired aplastic anemia, which carries a poorer prognosis and follows a more rapidly fatal course than the primary types.

Diagnostic Evaluation

The onset of clinical manifestations, which include anemia, leukopenia, and decreased platelet count, is usually insidious. Definitive diagnosis is determined from bone marrow aspiration, which demonstrates the conversion of red bone marrow to yellow, fatty bone marrow. Severe AA is defined as less than 25% bone marrow cellularity with at least two of the following findings: absolute granulocyte count <500 mm^3, platelet count $<20,000$/mm^3, and absolute reticulocyte count $<40,000$/mm^3 (Shimamura and Guinan, 2003; Shende, 2000). Moderate AA is defined as more than 25% bone marrow cellularity with the presence of mild or moderate cytopenias (Shimamura and Guinan, 2003; Shende, 2000).

Therapeutic Management

The objectives of treatment are based on the recognition that the underlying disease process is failure of the bone marrow to carry out its hematopoietic functions. Therefore therapy is directed at restoring function to the marrow and involves two main approaches: (1) immunosuppressive therapy to remove the presumed immunologic functions that prolong aplasia or (2) replacement of the bone marrow through transplantation. Bone marrow transplantation is the treatment of choice for severe aplastic anemia when a suitable donor exists (see p. 959).

Antilymphocyte globulin (ALG) or *antithymocyte globulin (ATG)* is the principal drug treatment used for aplastic anemia. The rationale for using ATG is based on the theory that aplastic anemia may be a result of autoimmunity. ATG and cyclosporine suppress T cell–dependent autoimmune responses but does not cause bone marrow suppression.

Cyclosporine is administered orally for several weeks to months. The optimal schedule for ATG administration is still under investigation. It is usually given intravenously over 12 to 16 hours for 4 days, after a test dose to check for hypersensitivity. A course may be repeated, depending on the reduction in circulating lymphocytes and the patient's response. Because of the hypersensitivity response associated with ATG (i.e., fever, chills, myalgias), methylprednisolone is given intravenously to prevent these side effects. Colony-stimulating factor (CSF), and granulocyte-macrophage colony-stimulating factor (GM-CSF) given parenterally, may be used to enhance bone marrow production. Androgens may be used with ATG to stimulate erythropoiesis if the AA is nonresponsive to initial therapies. Cyclosporine may be administered in children who fail to respond to ATG, and success has also been achieved using high-dose methylprednisolone.

Hematopoietic stem cell transplantation should be considered early in the course of the disease if a compatible donor can be found. Transplantation is more successful when performed before multiple transfusions have sensitized the child to leukocyte and *human leukocyte antigens (HLA)*. Hematopoietic stem cell transplantation is associated with an 85% survival rate in untransfused patients compared with a 70% survival rate in transfused patients (Shende, 2000).

Nursing Considerations

The care of the child with aplastic anemia is similar to that of the child with leukemia (see p. 958)—specifically, preparing the child and family for the diagnostic and therapeutic procedures, preventing complications from the severe pancytopenia, and emotionally supporting them in terms of a potentially fatal outcome. Information and support are available from the **Aplastic Anemia and MDS International Foundation, Inc.***

Because each of these nursing considerations is discussed in the section on leukemia, only the exceptions are presented here. The drug ATG is usually administered by way of a central vein. If not, vigilant care must be directed to the IV infusion to prevent extravasation. Meticulous care of the venous access is essential because of the child's susceptibility to infection. CSFs are usually given by subcutaneous injection over several days. Chemotherapeutic agents have been reported in the treatment of the relapsed patient with AA after ATG/CSF therapy. Many of the side effects associated with chemotherapy such as nausea and vomiting, alopecia, and mucositis are experienced by children receiving treatment for AA. Specialized care is required for children who have *hematopoietic stem cell transplantation (HSCT)* (see p. 959).

DEFECTS IN HEMOSTASIS

Hemostasis is the process that stops bleeding when a blood vessel is injured. Vascular and plasma clotting factors, as well as platelets, are required. A complex system of clotting, anticlotting, and clot breakdown *(fibrinolysis)* mechanisms

---

*PO Box 613, Annapolis, MD 21404-0613; (800) 747-2828; fax: (410) 867-0240; website: www.aamds.org.

exists in equilibrium to ensure clot formation only in the presence of blood vessel injury and to limit the clotting process to the site of vessel wall injury. Dysfunction in these systems will lead to bleeding or abnormal clotting. Although the coagulation process is complex, clotting depends on three factors: (1) vascular influence, (2) platelet role, and (3) clotting factors.

HEMOPHILIA

The term *hemophilia* refers to a group of bleeding disorders in which there is a deficiency of one of the factors necessary for coagulation of the blood. Although the symptomatology is similar regardless of which clotting factor is deficient, the identification of specific factor deficiencies allows definitive treatment with replacement agents.

In about 80% of all cases of hemophilia, the inheritance pattern is demonstrated as X-linked recessive (see Appendix B). The two most common forms of the disorder are *factor VIII deficiency (hemophilia A,* or *classic hemophilia)* and *factor IX deficiency (hemophilia B,* or *Christmas disease). von Willebrand disease (vWD)* is another hereditary bleeding disorder characterized by a deficiency, abnormality, or absence of the protein called von Willebrand factor (vWF) and a deficiency of factor VIII. Unlike hemophilia, vWD affects both males and females. The following discussion is primarily concerned with factor VIII deficiency, which accounts for 80% to 85% of all hemophilia cases.

Pathophysiology

The basic defect of hemophilia A is a deficiency of *factor VIII (antihemophilic factor [AHF])*. AHF is produced by the liver and is necessary for the formation of thromboplastin in phase I of blood coagulation. The less AHF found in the blood, the more severe the disease. Individuals with hemophilia have two of the three factors required for coagulation: vascular influence and platelets. Therefore they may bleed for longer periods, but not at a faster rate.

Bleeding into subcutaneous and intramuscular tissue is common. Hemarthrosis, which is bleeding into a joint space, is the most frequent type of internal bleeding. Bony changes and crippling deformities occur after repeated bleeding episodes over several years. Signs of hemarthrosis are swelling, warmth, redness, pain, and loss of movement. Bleeding in the neck, mouth, or thorax is serious, because the airway can become obstructed. Intracranial hemorrhage can have fatal consequences and is one of the major causes of death. Hemorrhage anywhere along the GI tract can lead to anemia, and bleeding into the retroperitoneal cavity is especially hazardous because of the large space for blood to accumulate. Hematomas in the spinal cord can cause paralysis.

Diagnostic Evaluation

Overt, prolonged hemorrhage is readily apparent; bleeding into tissues is less apparent (Box 26-5). The diagnosis is usually made from a history of bleeding episodes, evidence of X-linked inheritance (only one third of the cases are new mutations), and laboratory findings. The tests specific for hemophilia plasma depend on specific factors for a reaction to occur, such as the partial thromboplastin time (PTT). Specific determination of factor deficiencies requires assay procedures normally performed in specialized laboratories.

BOX 26-5 ■ Clinical Manifestations of Hemophilia

Prolonged bleeding anywhere from or in the body
Hemorrhage from any trauma—loss of deciduous teeth, circumcision, cuts, epistaxis, injections
Excessive bruising—even from a slight injury, such as a fall
Subcutaneous and intramuscular hemorrhages
Hemarthrosis (bleeding into the joint cavities), especially the knees, ankles, and elbows
Hematomas—pain, swelling, and limited motion
Spontaneous hematuria

Carrier detection is possible in classic hemophilia using DNA testing and is an important consideration in families in which female offspring may have inherited the trait.

Therapeutic Management

The primary therapy for hemophilia is replacement of the missing clotting factor. The products available are *factor VIII concentrate* from pooled plasma or a genetically engineered recombinant, to be reconstituted with sterile water immediately before use, and *DDAVP (1-deamino-8-d-arginine vasopressin)*, a synthetic form of vasopressin that increases plasma factor VIII and vWF levels and is the treatment of choice in mild hemophilia and vWD if the child shows an appropriate response. DDAVP is not effective in the treatment of severe hemophilia A, severe vWD, or any form of hemophilia B. Vigorous therapy is instituted to prevent chronic crippling effects from joint bleeding.

Other drugs may be included in the therapy plan, depending on the source of the hemorrhage. Corticosteroids are given for hematuria, acute hemarthrosis, and chronic synovitis. Nonsteroidal antiinflammatory drugs (NSAIDs), such as ibuprofen, are effective in relieving pain caused by synovitis; however, they must be used with caution because they inhibit platelet function (National Hemophilia Foundation, 2003; Dragone and Karp, 1996). Oral administration or local application of epsilon-aminocaproic acid (Amicar) prevents clot destruction; however, its use is limited to mouth or trauma surgery, and a dose of factor concentrate must be given first.

A regular program of exercise and physical therapy is an important aspect of management. Physical activity within reasonable limits strengthens muscles around joints and may decrease the number of spontaneous bleeding episodes.

Treatment without delay results in more rapid recovery and a decreased likelihood of complications; therefore, most children are treated at home. The family is taught the technique of venipuncture and to administer the AHF to children older than 2 to 3 years of age. The child learns the procedure for self-administration at 8 to 12 years of age. Home treatment is highly successful, and the rewards, in addition to the immediacy, are less disruption of family life, fewer school or work days missed, and enhancement of the child's self-esteem and independence.

Primary prophylaxis in hemophilia patients has been practiced for many years in European countries (Fischer and others, 2001) and has proved to be effective in preventing arthropathy. Primary prophylaxis involves the infusion of factor VIII concentrate on a regular basis before the onset of joint damage. Secondary prophylaxis involves the infusion of factor VIII concentrate on a regular basis after the child experiences his first joint bleed. The infusions are given three times a week. Aggressive factor replacement may be a cost-effective alternative to primary prophylaxis. This involves the infusion of a high dose of factor VIII concentrate when a joint bleed occurs, followed by 2 days of more standard doses of factor VIII concentrate with consideration of additional treatment every other day for one week (Montgomery, Gill, and Scott, 2003; Nolan and others, 2003).

Prognosis. Although there is no cure for hemophilia, its symptoms can be controlled and its potentially crippling deformities greatly reduced or even avoided. Today many children with hemophilia function with minimal or no joint damage. They are normal children with an average life expectancy in every respect but one: they have a tendency to bleed, which is a significant inconvenience but not necessarily a life-threatening event.

Unfortunately, those individuals with hemophilia who were treated before current purification techniques for factor VIII concentrate (between 1979 and 1985) may have been exposed to the human immunodeficiency virus (HIV). It is estimated that more than 50% of these patients have seroconverted to HIV-positive status (Butler and others, 2003). As these individuals become sexually active, the issue of sexual transmission of HIV becomes increasingly important. The adolescent must be knowledgeable regarding safe sexual behavior. Individuals with hemophilia diagnosed and treated with factor concentrates since 1985 are at virtually no risk for developing HIV infection from treatment. Current manufacturing techniques have also greatly reduced the risk of hepatitis transmission.

Gene therapy may prove to be a treatment option in the future. This therapy involves introducing a working copy of the factor VIII gene into a patient who has a flawed copy of the gene. Problems exist with appropriate selection of the vector, identification of the cell for gene expression, and control of side effects (Montgomery, Gill, and Scott, 2003).

Nursing Considerations

The earlier a bleeding episode is recognized, the more effectively it can be treated. Signs that indicate internal bleeding are especially important to recognize. Children are aware of internal bleeding and are very reliable in telling the examiner where an internal bleed is. In addition to the manifestations described (see Box 26-5), the nurse maintains a high level of suspicion when a child with hemophilia demonstrates signs such as headache, slurred speech, loss of consciousness (from cerebral bleeding), and black tarry stools (from GI bleeding).

Prevent Bleeding. The goal of prevention of bleeding episodes is directed toward decreasing the risk of injury. Prevention of bleeding episodes is geared mostly toward appropriate exercises to strengthen muscles and joints and to allow age-appropriate activity. During infancy and toddlerhood the normal acquisition of motor skills creates innumerable opportunities for falls, bruises, and minor wounds. Restraining the child from mastering motor development can herald more serious long-term problems than allowing the behavior. However, the environment should be made as safe as possible, with close supervision maintained during playtime, to minimize incidental injuries.

For older children the family usually needs assistance in preparing for school. A nurse who knows the family can be instrumental in discussing the situation with the school nurse and in jointly planning an appropriate schedule of activity. Because almost all persons with hemophilia are boys, the physical limitations in regard to active sports may be a difficult adjustment, and activity restrictions must be tempered with sensitivity to the child's emotional, as well as physical, needs. Use of protective equipment, such as padding and helmets, is particularly important, and noncontact sports, especially swimming, walking, jogging, tennis, golf, fishing, and bowling are encouraged (National Hemophilia Foundation, 2003).

To prevent oral bleeding, some readjustment in terms of dental hygiene may be needed to minimize trauma to the gums, such as use of a water irrigating device, softening the toothbrush in warm water before brushing, or using a sponge-tipped disposable toothbrush. A regular toothbrush should be soft bristled and small in size.

Because any trauma can lead to a bleeding episode, all persons caring for these children must be aware of their disorder. These children should wear medical identification, and older children should be encouraged to recognize situations in which disclosing their condition is important, such as during dental extraction or injections. Health personnel need to take special precautions to prevent the use of procedures that may cause bleeding, such as IM injections. The subcutaneous route is substituted for IM injections whenever possible. Venipunctures for blood samples are usually preferred for these children. There is usually less bleeding after the venipuncture than after finger or heel punctures. Neither aspirin nor any aspirin-containing compound should be used. Acetaminophen (Tylenol) is a suitable aspirin substitute, especially for use during control of pain at home.

Recognize and Control Bleeding.

As noted, the earlier a bleeding episode is recognized, the more effectively it can be treated. Factor replacement therapy should be instituted according to established medical protocol, and supportive measures may be implemented, such as *RICE,* which is (1) *rest,* (2) *ice,* (3) *compression,* and (4) *elevation.* When parents and older children are taught such measures beforehand, they can be prepared to initiate immediate treatment. Plastic bags of ice or cold packs should be kept in the freezer for such emergencies. However, such measures do not take the place of factor replacement.

Prevent Crippling Effects of Bleeding.

As a result of repeated episodes of hemarthrosis, incompletely absorbed blood in the joints, and limitation of motion, bone and muscle changes occur that result in flexion contractures and joint fixation. During bleeding episodes the joint is elevated and immobilized. Active range-of-motion exercises are usually instituted after the acute episode. This allows the child to control the degree of exercise and discomfort. If an exercise program is instituted in the home, a physical therapist or public health nurse may need to supervise compliance with the regimen. Rarely, orthopaedic intervention, such as casting, application of traction, or aspiration of blood, may be necessary to preserve joint function. Diet is also an important consideration, because excessive body weight can increase the strain on affected joints, especially the knees, and predispose to hemarthrosis. Consequently, calories need to be supplied in accordance with energy requirements.

Support Family and Prepare for Home Care.

Genetic counseling is essential as soon as possible after diagnosis. Unlike many other disorders in which both parents carry the trait, the feeling of responsibility for this condition usually rests with the mother. Without an opportunity to discuss her feelings, the marital relationship can suffer. Technology is now available to identify carriers in approximately 80% of cases and may reduce the anxiety regarding childbearing in females who may be at risk of carrying the defective gene, such as sisters or maternal aunts of an affected male. The discovery of factor concentrates has greatly changed the outlook for these children. Bleeding can be minimized, and the child can live a much more normal, unrestricted life. Children are taught to take responsibility for their disease at an early age. They learn their limitations and other preventive measures, as well as self-administration of the prophylactic AHF.

The needs of families who have children with hemophilia are best met through a comprehensive team approach of physicians (pediatrician, hematologist, orthopedist), nurse practitioner, nurse, social worker, and physical therapist. Parent-group discussions are beneficial in meeting those needs often best met by similarly affected families. For example, with the improved prognosis for these children, parents and adolescents with hemophilia are faced with vocational and financial problems, in addition to concern over future childbearing. After children reach 21 years of age, many insurance companies will no longer carry them. This can be disastrous in terms of the cost of treatment. The **National Hemophilia Foundation*** and the **Canadian Hemophilia Society†** provide numerous services and publications for both health providers and families. Financial support is particularly important. A person with severe hemophilia may require factor replacement therapy and other medical treatments that cost in excess of $70,000 to $90,000 a year.

Children who have become infected with HIV through transfusions and factor replacement products are faced with the consequences of this dreaded disease. Consequently, they need the support of health professionals, especially in the areas of safe sexual practices to avoid disease transmission and public education regarding acquired immunodeficiency syndrome (AIDS) and ways to deal with public reactions to persons who have AIDS (see p. 978).

---

*116 West 43rd Street, 11th Floor, New York, NY 10001; (800) 42HANDI or (212) 328-3700; fax (212) 328-3777; email: info@hemophilia.org; website: www.hemophilia.org.
†625 President Kennedy, Suite 1210, Montreal, Quebec H3A 1K2; (514) 848-0503; e-mail: chs@odysee.net.

BOX 26-6 ■ Clinical Manifestations of Idiopathic Thrombocytopenic Purpura

Easy bruising
    Petechiae
    Ecchymoses
    Most often over bony prominences
Bleeding from mucous membranes
    Epistaxis
    Bleeding gums
    Internal hemorrhage evidenced by:
        Hematuria
        Hematemesis
        Melena
        Hemarthrosis
        Menorrhagia
Hematomas over lower extremities

BOX 26-7 ■ Criteria for Anti-D Antibody Therapy

Children between age 1 year and 19 years
Rh(D)-positive blood type
Normal white blood cell count and hemoglobin for age: platelets <30,000/μL
No active mucosal bleeding
No prior history of reaction to plasma products
No patient known to be immunoglobulin A deficient
No concurrent infection
No patient with Evans syndrome (characterized by the combination of idiopathic thrombocytopenia purpura and autoimmune hemolytic anemia)
No patient with suspected lupus or other collagen/vascular disorder

IDIOPATHIC THROMBOCYTOPENIC PURPURA

Idiopathic thrombocytopenic purpura (ITP) is an acquired hemorrhagic disorder characterized by (1) *thrombocytopenia,* excessive destruction of platelets, (2) *purpura,* a discoloration caused by petechiae beneath the skin, and (3) a *normal bone marrow with normal or increased number of immature platelets (megakaryocytes) and eosinophils.* Although the cause is unknown, it is believed to be an autoimmune response to disease-related antigens. It is the most frequently occurring thrombocytopenia of childhood. The greatest frequency of occurrence is between 2 and 10 years of age.

The disease occurs in one of two forms: an acute, self-limiting course or a chronic condition (greater than 6 months' duration). The acute form is most often seen after upper respiratory infections; after the childhood diseases measles, rubella, mumps, and chickenpox; or after infection with parvovirus B19.

Diagnostic Evaluation

The diagnosis is suspected on the basis of clinical manifestations (Box 26-6). In ITP the platelet count is reduced to below 20,000 mm³; therefore, tests that depend on platelet function, such as the tourniquet test, bleeding time, and clot retraction, are abnormal. Although there is no definitive test on which to establish a diagnosis of ITP, several are usually performed to rule out other disorders in which thrombocytopenia is a manifestation, such as systemic lupus erythematosus, lymphoma, or leukemia.

Therapeutic Management

Management of ITP is primarily supportive, because the course of the disease is self-limited in the majority of cases. Activity is restricted at the onset while the platelet count is low and while active bleeding or progression of lesions is occurring. Treatment for acute presentation is symptomatic and has included prednisone, IV immune globulin (IVIG), and anti-D antibody. These are not curative therapies. Some experts suggest that no therapy is necessary for the asymptomatic patient, with no difference in the recovery of platelet counts over time. *Anti-D antibody* is a relatively new ther-

apy for ITP. Infusion of anti-D antibody causes a transient hemolytic anemia in the patient. Along with the clearance of antibody-coated RBCs, there is prolonged survival of platelets resulting from the blockade of the Fc receptors of the reticuloendothelial cells. The platelet count does not increase until 48 hours after an infusion of anti-D antibody; therefore, it is not appropriate therapy for patients who are actively bleeding. The benefits of choosing anti-D antibody therapy over prednisone or IVIG is that anti-D antibody can be given in one dose over 5 to 10 minutes and is significantly less expensive than IVIG. Historically, patients who are treated with prednisone must first undergo a bone marrow examination to rule out leukemia. Therefore the use of anti-D antibody alleviates the need for a bone marrow examination. Patients must meet certain criteria before the administration of anti-D antibody (Box 26-7). Premedication with acetaminophen (such as Tylenol) 5 to 10 minutes before infusion is recommended.

⬤ NURSING ALERT

After administration of anti-D antibody, observe the child for a minimum of 1 hour and maintain a patent IV line. Obtain baseline vital signs before the infusion and again 5, 20, and 60 minutes after beginning the infusion. Fever, chills, and headache may occur during or shortly after the infusion. If fever, chills, or headache occurs, diphenhydramine (Benadryl) and Solu-Cortef should be given and the patient should be observed for an additional hour.

Splenectomy is reserved for those patients in whom ITP has persisted for 1 year or longer. It is the only treatment associated with long-term remission for 60% to 90% of children. Splenectomy removes the risk of hemorrhage but increases the risk of septicemia (Wilson, 2003; Bell, 2002; Chu and others, 2000). Before considering splenectomy, it is generally recommended to wait until the child is older than 5 years of age because of the increased risk of bacterial infection. Pneumococcal and meningococcal vaccines are recommended before splenectomy (see Immunizations, Chapter 10). The child also receives penicillin prophylaxis after splenectomy. The length of prophylactic therapy is controversial, but in general, a minimum of 3 years is recommended.

Prognosis. The majority of children have a self-limited course without major complications. Some children will develop chronic ITP and require ongoing therapy. A splenectomy may modify the disease process, and the child will be asymptomatic.

Nursing Considerations

Nursing care is largely supportive and should include teaching regarding possible side effects of therapy and limitation in activities while the child's platelet count is 50,000 to 100,000/mm³. Children with ITP should not participate in *any* contact sports, bike riding, skateboarding, in-line skating, gymnastics, climbing, or running. Parents are encouraged to engage their children in quiet activities and to prevent any injuries to the child's head. The harmful effects of using aspirin and NSAIDs to control pain are critical for these children; therefore, salicylate substitutes (such as acetaminophen) are always used. As in any condition with an uncertain outcome, the family needs emotional support.

DISSEMINATED INTRAVASCULAR COAGULATION

Disseminated intravascular coagulation (DIC), also known as ***consumption coagulopathy,*** is characterized by diffuse fibrin deposition in the microvasculature, consumption of coagulation factors, and endogenous generation of thrombin and plasmin. DIC is a secondary disorder of coagulation that occurs as a complication of a number of pathologic processes, such as hypoxia, acidosis, shock, and endothelial damage. It can result from many severe systemic diseases, such as congenital heart disease, necrotizing enterocolitis, gram-negative bacterial sepsis, rickettsial infections, and some severe viral infections.

Pathophysiology

DIC occurs when the first stage of the coagulation process is abnormally stimulated. Although no well-defined sequence of events occurs, two distinct phases can be identified. First, when the clotting mechanism is triggered in the circulation, thrombin is generated in greater amounts than can be neutralized by the body. Consequently, there is rapid conversion of fibrinogen to fibrin, with aggregation and destruction of platelets. If local and widespread fibrin deposition in blood vessels takes place, obstruction and eventual necrosis of tissues occur. Second, the fibrinolytic mechanism is activated, causing extensive destruction of clotting factors. With a deficiency of clotting factors the child is vulnerable to uncontrollable hemorrhage into vital organs. An additional complication is damage and hemolysis of RBCs (Fig. 26-4).

Diagnostic Evaluation

DIC is suspected when the patient has an increased tendency to bleed (Box 26-8). Hematologic findings include prolonged prothrombin time (PT), PTT, and thrombin time (TT). There is a profoundly depressed platelet count, fragmented RBCs, and depleted fibrinogen.

Therapeutic Management

Treatment of DIC is directed toward control of the underlying or initiating cause, which in most instances stops the coagulation problem spontaneously. Platelets and fresh-

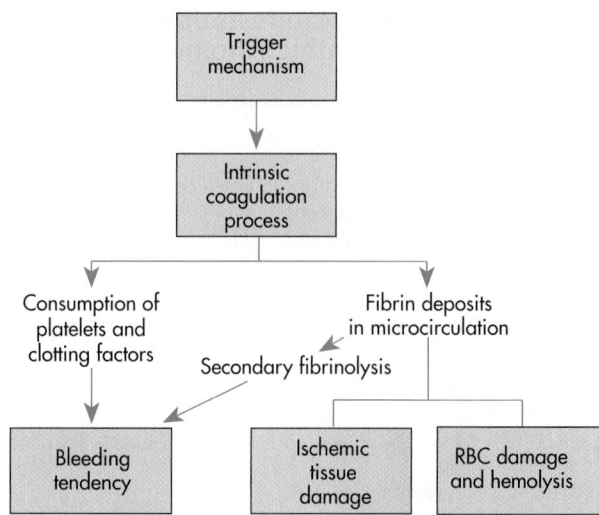

FIG. 26-4 ■ Effects of disseminated intravascular coagulation.

BOX 26-8 ■ Clinical Manifestations of Disseminated Intravascular Coagulation

Petechiae
Purpura
Bleeding from openings in the skin
    Venipuncture site
    Surgical incision
Bleeding from umbilicus, trachea (newborn)
Evidence of gastrointestinal bleeding
Hypotension
Organ dysfunction from infarction and ischemia

frozen plasma may be needed to replace lost plasma components, especially in the child whose underlying disease remains uncontrolled. The extremely ill newborn infant may require exchange transfusion with fresh blood. The IV administration of heparin to inhibit thrombin formation is most often restricted to patients who have not responded to treatment of the underlying disease or replacement of coagulation factors and platelets.

Nursing Considerations

The goals of nursing care are to be aware of the possibility of DIC in the severely ill child and to recognize signs that might indicate its presence. The skills needed to monitor IV infusion and blood transfusions and to administer heparin are the same as for any child receiving these therapies (see p. 978). (See Chapter 18 for care of the child with a life-threatening illness.)

EPISTAXIS (NOSEBLEEDING)

Isolated and transient episodes of epistaxis, or nosebleeding, are common in childhood. The nose, especially the septum, is a highly vascular structure, and bleeding usually results from direct trauma, including blows to the nose, foreign bodies, and nose picking, or from mucosal inflammation associated with allergic rhinitis and upper respiratory infections. The bleeding ordinarily stops spontaneously or with minimal pressure and requires no medical evaluation or therapy.

Recurrent epistaxis and severe bleeding may indicate an underlying disease, particularly vascular abnormalities, leukemia, thrombocytopenia, and clotting factor deficiency diseases (e.g., hemophilia, von Willebrand disease). Nosebleeds are sometimes associated with administration of aspirin, even in normal amounts. Persistent episodes of epistaxis require medical evaluation.

Nursing Considerations

In the event of a nosebleed, an essential intervention is to remain calm. Otherwise, the child will become more agitated, the blood pressure will increase, and the child will not cooperate. Although in most instances a nosebleed is not serious, it can be very upsetting to family members as well. They need reassurance that the loss of blood is not serious and that the bleeding usually stops within 10 to 15 minutes.

To control the bleeding, the child is instructed to sit up and lean forward (not to lie down) to avoid aspiration of blood. Most of the nosebleeding originates in the anterior part of the nasal septum and can be controlled by applying pressure to the soft lower portion of the nose with the thumb and forefinger (see Emergency Treatment box). During this time the child breathes through the mouth.

In the event that hemorrhage continues, the child should be evaluated by a practitioner, who may pack the nose with epinephrine-soaked gauze. After a nosebleed, petroleum or water-soluble jelly can be inserted into each nostril to prevent crusting of old blood and to lessen the likelihood of the child's picking at the nose and restarting the hemorrhage. If a child has numerous nosebleeds, factors believed to increase the likelihood of bleeds are eliminated, such as discouraging nose picking or altering the household humidity by placing a cool-mist humidifier in the child's room. Repeated bleeding episodes lasting longer than 30 minutes may be an indication to refer the child for evaluation for the possibility of a bleeding disorder.

NEOPLASTIC DISORDERS

Neoplastic disorders are the leading cause of death from disease in children past infancy, and almost half of all childhood cancers involve the blood or blood-forming organs. Leukemias and lymphomas are discussed here. Malignant solid tumors of childhood are discussed elsewhere in relation to the tissues or organs involved.

LEUKEMIAS

Leukemia, cancer of the blood-forming tissues, is the most common form of childhood cancer. The annual incidence is 3 to 4 cases per 100,000 white children younger than 15 years of age (Margolin, Steuber, and Poplack, 2002). It occurs more frequently in males than in females after age 1 year, and the peak onset is between 2 and 6 years of age. It is one of the forms of cancer that has demonstrated dramatic improvements in survival rates. Current long-term disease-free survival for children with acute lymphoid leukemia approaches 80% (Redner, 2000), whereas acute nonlymphoid leukemia has a 45% to 50% survival rate (Redner, 2000). (See also Prognosis, see p. 959.)

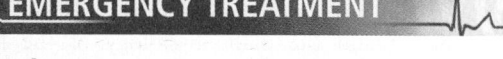

EMERGENCY TREATMENT

Epistaxis

Have child sit up and lean forward (not lying down).

Apply continuous pressure to nose with thumb and forefinger for at least 10 minutes.

Insert cotton or wadded tissue into each nostril, and apply ice or cold cloth to bridge of nose if bleeding persists.

Keep child calm and quiet.

Classification

Leukemia is a broad term given to a group of malignant diseases of the bone marrow and lymphatic system. Research has revealed that it is a complex disease of varying heterogeneity. Consequently, classification has become increasingly complex, sophisticated, and essential, because identification of the subtype of leukemia has therapeutic and prognostic implications. The following is a brief overview of the major classification systems currently being used.

Morphology. Two forms are generally recognized in children: *acute lymphoid leukemia (ALL)* and *acute nonlymphoid (myelogenous) leukemia (ANLL or AML).* Synonyms for ALL include lymphatic, lymphocytic, lymphoblastic, and lymphoblastoid leukemia. Usually the terms *stem cell* or *blast cell leukemia* also refer to the lymphoid type of leukemia. Synonyms for the AML type include granulocytic, myelocytic, monocytic, myelogenous, monoblastic, and monomyeloblastic.

> **Cytochemical markers.** Several chemical stains aid in differentiation between ALL and ANLL. For instance, terminal deoxynucleotidyl transferase (TdT) is able to differentiate between ALL and non-ALL (Margolin, Steuber, and Poplack, 2002).
>
> **Chromosome studies.** Chromosome analysis has become an important tool in the diagnosis of acute lymphoblastic leukemia. For example, children with trisomy 21 have 20 times the risk of other children for developing ALL. Children with more than 50 chromosomes on the leukemic cells (hyperdiploid) have the best prognosis (Margolin, Steuber, and Poplack, 2002). Translocations of chromosomes also found on the leukemic cells can denote good prognosis, as in the trisomies 4 and 10, or a poor prognosis, as in the t(9:22) or Philadelphia chromosome.
>
> **Cell-surface immunologic markers.** Cell-surface antigens have permitted differentiation of ALL into three broad classes: non-T, non-B ALL; B-cell ALL; and T-cell ALL. Children with non-T, non-B ALL have the best prognosis, especially if they have the common acute lymphocytic leukemia antigen, known as CALLA positive, on their cell surfaces (Margolin, Steuber, and Poplack, 2002).

Pathophysiology

Leukemia is an unrestricted proliferation of immature WBCs in the blood-forming tissues of the body. Although not a "tumor" as such, the leukemic cells demonstrate the same neoplastic properties as solid cancers. Therefore the resulting pathologic condition and clinical manifestations are caused by infiltration and replacement of any tissue of the body with nonfunctional leukemic cells. Highly vascular organs, such as the spleen and liver, are the most severely affected.

To understand the pathophysiology of the leukemic process, it is important to clarify two common misconceptions. First, although leukemia is an overproduction of WBCs, most often in the acute form the leukocyte count is low (thus the term *leukemia*). Second, these immature cells do not deliberately attack and destroy the normal blood cells or vascular tissues. Cellular destruction takes place by infiltration and subsequent competition for metabolic elements (Table 26-2).

In all types of leukemia the proliferating cells depress the production of formed elements of the blood in bone marrow by competing for and depriving the normal cells of the essential nutrients for metabolism. The most frequent presenting signs and symptoms of leukemia are a result of infiltration of the bone marrow. The three main consequences are (1) *anemia* from decreased RBCs, (2) *infection* from neutropenia, and (3) *bleeding* from decreased platelet production. The invasion of the bone marrow with leukemic cells gradually causes a weakening of the bone and a tendency toward fractures. As leukemic cells invade the periosteum, increasing pressure causes severe pain.

The spleen, liver, and lymph glands demonstrate marked infiltration, enlargement, and eventually fibrosis. Hepatosplenomegaly is typically more common than lymphadenopathy. The next most important site of involvement is the central nervous system (CNS) secondary to leukemic infiltration, which may cause increased intracranial pressure (see Box 28-1).

Leukemic cells may also invade the testes, kidneys, prostate, ovaries, GI tract, and lungs. With long-term survivors becoming more common, such sites of leukemia invasion, especially the testes, are becoming more important clinically.

Diagnostic Evaluation

Leukemia is usually suspected by the history, physical manifestations (see Table 26-2), and a peripheral blood smear that contains immature forms of leukocytes, frequently combined with low blood counts. Definitive diagnosis is based on flow cytometry of the cells obtained in the bone marrow aspiration or biopsy. Flow cytometry identifies the specific type of blast cell. Typically, the bone marrow is hypercellular, with primarily blast cells. After the diagnosis is confirmed, a lumbar puncture is performed to determine if there is any CNS involvement. A few of the children will have CNS involvement at diagnosis, although most are asymptomatic.

Therapeutic Management

Treatment of leukemia involves the use of chemotherapeutic agents, with or without cranial irradiation, in four phases: (1) *induction therapy,* which achieves a complete remission or less than 5% leukemic cells in the bone marrow; (2) *CNS prophylactic therapy,* which prevents leukemic cells from invading the CNS; (3) *intensification therapy* (consolidation), which eradicates residual leukemia cells, followed by delayed intensification, which prevents emergence of resistant leukemic clones; and (4) *maintenance therapy,* which serves to maintain the remission phase. Although the combination of drugs and radiation may vary according to institutions, the prognostic or risk characteristics of the patient, and the type of leukemia being treated, the following general principles for each phase are quite consistently employed.

> **Remission induction.** Almost immediately after confirmation of the diagnosis, induction therapy is begun and lasts for 4 to 6 weeks. The principal drugs used for induction in ALL are corticosteroids, vincristine, and L-asparaginase, with or without doxorubicin. Recent clinical trials have substituted dexamethasone for prednisone because of its effectiveness in crossing the blood-brain barrier and reducing CSF relapse (Colby-Graham, and Chordas, 2003). However, the toxicities of dexamethasone continue to be evaluated. Drug therapy for AML includes doxorubicin or daunorubicin (daunomycin) and cytosine arabinoside; various other drugs such as etoposide or thioguanine may be used.
>
> Because many of the drugs also cause myelosuppression of normal blood elements, the period immediately after a

TABLE 26-2 ■ Pathology and Related Clinical Manifestations of Leukemia

ORGAN OR TISSUE	CONSEQUENCES	MANIFESTATIONS
Bone marrow dysfunction	Decreased RBCs—anemia	Pallor, fatigue
	Neutropenia—infection	Fever
	Decreased platelets—bleeding tendencies	Hemorrhage (petechiae)
	Invasion of bone marrow—bone weakness; invasion of periosteum	Tendency toward fractures
		Pain
Liver	Infiltration, enlargement, eventual fibrosis	Hepatomegaly
Spleen		Splenomegaly
Lymph glands		Lymphadenopathy
Central nervous system: meninges	Increased intracranial pressure, ventricular enlargement	Severe headache
		Vomiting
		Irritability, lethargy
		Papilledema
	Meningeal irritation	Eventual coma
		Pain
		Stiff neck and back
Hypermetabolism	Cell deprivation of nutrients by invading cells	Muscle wasting
		Weight loss
		Anorexia
		Fatigue

remission can be critical. The body is defenseless against and highly susceptible to infection and spontaneous hemorrhage. Consequently, supportive therapy during this time is essential.

CNS prophylactic therapy. Treatment of the CNS consists of prophylactic therapy using intrathecal chemotherapy with methotrexate, cytarabine, and hydrocortisone. Sometimes methotrexate, as well as cytarabine, may be given as single agents intrathecally. Because of the concern regarding late effects of cranial irradiation, this treatment is reserved for high-risk patients and those with CNS disease.

Intensification or consolidation therapy. After complete remission is obtained, a period of intensified treatment is administered to eradicate residual leukemic cells; this is followed by delayed intensification to prevent emergence of resistant leukemic clones. Intrathecal along with systemic chemotherapy, including L-asparaginase, high-dose or intermediate-dose methotrexate, cytarabine, vincristine, and mercaptopurine, is administered over a period of several months.

Maintenance therapy. Maintenance therapy is begun after completion of successful induction and consolidation therapy to preserve the remission and further lessen the number of leukemic cells. Combined drug regimens, including daily mercaptopurine, weekly methotrexate, and periodic intrathecal therapy, are administered over the remaining 2-year period. Also, during maintenance therapy, periodic CBCs are taken to evaluate the marrow's response to the drugs.

Reinduction after relapse. The presence of leukemic cells in the bone marrow, CNS, or testes constitutes a relapse. Therapy for the child who has relapsed includes reinduction with prednisone and vincristine, along with a combination of other drugs not previously used. CNS preventive therapy and maintenance therapy follow as outlined previously, after remission occurs.

Hematopoietic stem cell transplantation (HSCT). HSCT has been used successfully for treating children who have ALL and AML. HSCT is *not* recommended for children with ALL during the first remission because of the excellent results possible with chemotherapy. Because of the poorer prognosis in children with AML, recent studies support HSCT during first remission. From 60% to 70% of children with AML who undergo HSCT experience long-term remission (Colby-Graham, and Chordas, 2003).

Bone marrow used for HSCT may not only be from antigen-matched related donors, but also from matched unrelated donors or mismatched donors. Peripheral blood stem cell transplants are capable of differentiating into specialized cells of the hematologic system and can be obtained from related or unrelated donors or from umbilical cord blood. Regardless of the type of transplant, it is accompanied by significant morbidity and mortality, including graft-versus-host disease (GVHD), overwhelming infection, or severe organ damage.

Prognosis

The most important prognostic factors for determining long-term survival for children with ALL (in addition to treatment) are (1) the initial WBC count, (2) the child's age at the time of diagnosis, (3) the type of cell involved, (4) the sex of the child, and (5) karyotype analysis. Children with a normal or low WBC count and who have non-T, non-B ALL and are CALLA positive have a much better prognosis than those with a high count or other cell types. Children diagnosed between 2 and 9 years of age have consistently demonstrated a better outlook than those diagnosed before 2 or after 10 years of age, and girls appear to have a more favorable prognosis than boys. Children with a deoxyribonucleic acid (DNA) index greater than 1.16 (hyperdiploid) and translocation of chromosomes 4 and 10 have a better prognosis (Margolin, Steuber, and Poplack, 2002).

Late Effects of Treatment

Although vigorous treatment of childhood cancers has resulted in dramatically improved survival rates, increasing concern surrounds late effects—adverse changes related to treatment modalities—and recurrence of the disease process. Almost no organ is exempt, and almost every antineoplastic agent, including and especially irradiation, is responsible for some adverse effect.

The most devastating late effect is development of a second malignancy. Children who received cranial irradiation at age 5 years or younger are most susceptible to developing brain tumors (Silverman and Sallan, 2003). Treatment with anthracycline is associated with cardiomyopathy; cranial irradiation and intrathecal chemotherapy are associated with cognitive and neuropsychologic deficits, which are just a few of the long-term sequelae. Consequently, close monitoring for late effects is essential, especially with the advent of additional clinical trials.

Nursing Considerations

Nursing care of the child with leukemia is directly related to the regimen of therapy. General psychologic interventions during each phase of therapy are discussed in Chapter 18.

● Assessment

The history and physical examination often yield the first clues to the presence of neoplastic disease. Vague complaints such as fatigue, pain in a limb, night sweating, lack of appetite, headache, and general malaise may be the earliest clues of leukemia.

● Nursing Diagnoses

Many nursing diagnoses become apparent after an assessment of the child with leukemia and the family. Some are considered in the Nursing Care Plan on pp. 966 to 970. Others will be identified in specific situations.

● Planning

The goals of nursing care of the child with leukemia and the family include:

1 Child will receive appropriate primary health care.
2 Child and family will be prepared for diagnostic and therapeutic procedures.
3 Child will experience minimal complications of myelosuppression.
4 Problems of irradiation and drug toxicity will be managed.
5 Child and family will receive adequate support and education.

● Implementation

Nursing care of the child with leukemia is directly related to the regimen of therapy. Nurses working with families of children with cancer have a significant supportive role in helping them understand the various therapies, preventing or managing expected side effects or toxicities, observing for late effects of treatment, and helping the child and family live as normal a life as possible and cope with the emotional aspects of the disease. Education is a constant feature of the nursing role, especially in terms of clinical trials and home care. Diagnosis of leukemia tends to generate anxiety in families and patients. The nurse is instrumental in providing support and reassurance, as well as accurate explanation regarding diagnostic tests, procedures, and treatment plans.

Prepare Child and Family for Diagnostic and Therapeutic Procedures.
From the time before diagnosis to cessation of therapy, children must undergo several tests; the most traumatic are bone marrow aspiration or biopsy and lumbar punctures. Multiple finger sticks and venipunctures for blood analysis and drug infusion are common occurrences. Therefore the child needs an explanation of each procedure and what can be expected. In addition, effective pharmacologic measures, including conscious and unconscious sedation, and nonpharmacologic strategies are used to reduce discomfort associated with these painful procedures.

Relieve Pain.
The effective use of analgesia is especially important when the malignant process is uncontrolled and causes acute pain. Dosages of opioids (narcotics) are adjusted or *titrated to the child's needs* and administered *around the clock* for optimal pain control. Nonpharmacologic strategies should be implemented as needed but are not substitutes for pharmacologic management. The reader is encouraged to review the principles of pain assessment and management presented in Chapter 21 and Preparation for Procedures in Chapter 22 when caring for a child with leukemia.

Prevent Complications of Myelosuppression.
The leukemic process and most of the chemotherapeutic agents cause myelosuppression. The reduced numbers of blood cells result in secondary problems of infection, bleeding tendencies, and anemia. Supportive care involves both medical and nursing management. Because these are so closely linked, they are discussed together rather than separately.

Infection. A frequent complication of treatment for childhood cancer is overwhelming infection secondary to neutropenia. The child is most susceptible to overwhelming infection during three phases of the disease: (1) at the time of diagnosis and relapse when the leukemic process has replaced normal leukocytes, (2) during immunosuppressive therapy, and (3) after prolonged antibiotic therapy that predisposes to the growth of resistant organisms. However, the use of granulocyte colony–stimulating factor (GCSF) has reduced the incidence and duration of infection in children receiving treatment for cancer.

The first defense against infection is prevention. When the child is hospitalized, the nurse employs all measures to control transfer of infection. These typically include the use of a private room, restriction of all visitors and health personnel with active infection, and strict handwashing technique with an antiseptic solution. In some research centers, special germ-free environments are available during complete myelosuppression from intensive chemotherapy or for bone marrow transplant.

NURSING ALERT

Because the usual viral infections of childhood are particularly dangerous, the child is not immunized against these diseases (measles, rubella, mumps, and polio) until the immune system is capable of responding appropriately to the vaccine. If given when the immune system is depressed, the attenuated virus can result in an overwhelming infection. The child can receive the Salk (inactivated) vaccine for poliomyelitis. Children with cancer should not routinely receive the varicella vaccine. Siblings and other family members can receive the varicella vaccine without risk to the child with cancer (American Academy of Pediatrics, 2003) (Chapter 10).

The child is evaluated for potential sites of infection (e.g., mucosal ulceration; skin abrasion; skin tear, such as a hangnail) and observed for any elevation in temperature. To identify the source of infection, chest radiographs and blood, stool, urine, and nasopharyngeal cultures are taken. IV antibiotics are administered, and if this therapy is prolonged, a venous access device, such as a peripherally inserted central catheter (PICC), intermittent infusion device (saline lock or PRN adaptor), catheter, or implanted infusion port, is used to maintain IV access.

Prevention of infection continues to be a priority after discharge from the hospital. Ordinarily, the child is allowed to return to school when the WBC count is at a satisfactory level, usually an absolute neutrophil count (ANC) greater than 500/mm³ (see Guidelines box). At all times, family members are encouraged to practice good handwashing to prevent introducing pathogens into the home. The child may need to be isolated from school contacts in the event of an outbreak of a childhood disease, especially chickenpox.

Nutrition is another important component of infection prevention. An adequate protein-caloric intake provides the child with better host defenses against infection and increased tolerance to chemotherapy and irradiation. However, providing optimal nutrition during periods of anorexia and vomiting from chemotherapy is a tremendous challenge (see Feeding the Sick Child, Chapter 22).

Hemorrhage. Before the use of transfused platelets, hemorrhage was a leading cause of death in patients with leukemia. Now most bleeding episodes can be prevented or controlled with the administration of platelet concentrates or platelet-rich plasma.

⸬ GUIDELINES

Calculating the Absolute Neutrophil Count

Determine the total percent of neutrophils ("polys" or "segs" and "bands").
Multiply white blood cell (WBC) count by percent of neutrophils.

Example:
 WBC = 1000, neutrophils = 7%, nonsegmented neutrophils (bands) = 7%
 Step 1: 7% + 7% = 14%
 Step 2: 0.14 × 1000 = 140 absolute neutrophil count (ANC)

Because infection increases the tendency toward hemorrhage, and because bleeding sites become more easily infected, skin punctures are avoided whenever possible. When finger sticks, venipunctures, IM injections, and bone marrow aspirations are performed, aseptic technique must be employed, as well as continued observation for bleeding. Meticulous mouth care is essential, because gingival bleeding with resultant mucositis is a frequent problem. Because the rectal area is prone to ulceration from various drugs, feces and urine are removed immediately, and the perianal area is washed. Using rectal temperatures is avoided to prevent trauma. Children are advised to avoid activities that might cause injury or bleeding, such as riding bicycles or skateboards, climbing trees or playground equipment, and playing contact sports.

Platelet transfusions are generally reserved for active bleeding episodes that do not respond to local treatment and that may occur during induction or relapse therapy. Epistaxis and gingival bleeding are the most common. The nurse teaches parents and older children measures to control nosebleeding (see p. 957). Pressure at the site without disturbing clot formation is the general rule.

During bleeding episodes the parents and child need much emotional support. Often parents will request a platelet transfusion, unaware of the need for trying local measures first. The nurse can be instrumental in allaying anxiety by acknowledging the feelings of the child and family and explaining the reason for delaying a platelet transfusion until absolutely necessary.

Anemia. Initially, anemia may be profound from complete replacement of the bone marrow by leukemic cells. During induction therapy, blood transfusions may be necessary. The usual precautions in caring for the child with anemia are instituted (see p. 941).

Use Precautions in Administering and Handling Chemotherapeutic Agents.

Many chemotherapeutic agents are vesicants (sclerosing agents) that can cause severe cellular damage if even minute amounts of the drug infiltrate surrounding tissue. Only nurses experienced with chemotherapeutic agents should administer vesicants. Guidelines are available* and must be followed exactly to prevent tissue damage to patients. Interventions for extravasation vary, but each nurse should be aware of the institution's policies and implement them at once.

In addition to extravasation, a potentially fatal complication is anaphylaxis, especially from L-asparaginase, teniposide (VM-26), etoposide (VP-16), bleomycin, and cisplatin. Nursing responsibilities include prevention of, recognition of, and preparation for serious reactions. Prevention begins with a careful history for known allergy.

In addition to the many responsibilities nurses must have in regard to the child and family, they must also use safeguards to protect themselves. Handling chemotherapeutic agents may present risks to handlers and to their offspring, although the exact degree of risk is not known.

Some children have a venous access device, which facilitates administration of IV drugs. During treatment and re-

mission, many drugs are taken orally at home. Compliance with the medication schedule is essential, and nurses play an important role in educating the family about the drugs and encouraging adherence to the plan.

> **NURSING ALERT**
>
> Chemotherapeutic drugs must be given through a free-flowing IV line. The infusion is stopped *immediately* if any sign of infiltration (pain, stinging, swelling, or redness at the cannulation site) occurs.

> **NURSING ALERT**
>
> When chemotherapeutic and immunologic agents are given, the child must be observed for 20 minutes after the infusion for signs of anaphylaxis (cyanosis, hypotension, wheezing, severe urticaria). Emergency equipment (especially blood pressure monitor and bag-valve-mask) and emergency drugs (especially oxygen, epinephrine, antihistamine, aminophylline, corticosteroids, and vasopressors) must be available. If a reaction is suspected, the drug is discontinued, the IV line is flushed with saline, and the child's vital signs and subsequent responses are monitored.

Manage Problems of Drug Toxicity. Chemotherapy presents several nursing challenges. The complexity of the treatment protocols is often overwhelming to families. In addition, each therapy is associated with a number of predictable side effects. Nurses must be aware of these side effects and use judgment in recognizing reactions, as well as toxicities (Box 26-9).

Nausea and vomiting. The nausea and vomiting that occur shortly after administration of several of the drugs and from cranial or abdominal radiation can be profound. The serotonin-receptor antagonists (e.g., ondansetron [Zofran]) are effective in the control of nausea and vomiting occurring after emetogenic chemotherapy and radiation therapy. When combined with dexamethasone, these agents are the treatment of choice in the prevention of cisplatin-induced delayed emesis (Bryant, 2003).

The most beneficial regimen for antiemetic control has been the administration of the antiemetic *before* the chemotherapy begins. The goal is to prevent the child from ever experiencing nausea or vomiting, thus preventing development of anticipatory symptoms (the conditioned response of developing nausea and vomiting before receiving the drug).

Anorexia. Loss of appetite is a direct consequence of the chemotherapy or irradiation. It is a major problem for parents because it is the one area they feel responsible for, particularly when so many other facets of care are outside their control. There are no universally successful techniques for encouraging a sick child to eat. However, the guidelines in Chapter 22 can be helpful during the anorexic period and can prevent additional problems during the remission.

Some children still do not eat despite these approaches. When loss of appetite and weight persist, the nurse should investigate the family situation to determine if any factors (e.g., conditioned aversion to food, environmental stress related to eating, controlling behavior, anger) might be contributing to the problem. Nasogastric tube feedings or total parenteral nutrition may be implemented for children with significant nutritional problems.

***Cancer Chemotherapy Guidelines* can be obtained from the **Oncology Nursing Society,** 501 Holiday Drive, Pittsburgh, PA 15220-2749; (412) 921-7373; website: www.ons.org.

BOX 26-9 ■ Summary of Selected Chemotherapeutic Agents Used in the Treatment of Childhood Leukemias and Lymphomas*

BLEOMYCIN (BLENOXANE)
Administration
IV, IM, SC

Side Effects and Toxicity
Allergic reaction—fever, chills, hypotension, anaphylaxis
Fever (nonallergic)
N/V (mild)†
Stomatitis
Cumulative dose effects include:
  Skin—rash, hyperpigmentation, thickening, ulceration, peeling, nail changes, alopecia
  Lungs—pneumonitis with infiltrate that can progress to fatal fibrosis

Comments and Specific Nursing Considerations
Should give test dose (SC) before therapeutic dose is administered
Have emergency drugs at bedside
Hypersensitivity occurs with first one to two doses
May give acetaminophen before drug to reduce likelihood of fever
Concentration of drug in skin and lungs accounts for toxic effects
Perform pulmonary function tests at baseline, during and following therapy

CYCLOPHOSPHAMIDE (CYTOXAN, CTX, NEOSAR)
Administration
PO, IV, IM

Side Effects and Toxicity
N/V (3 to 4 hours later) (severe at high doses)
BMD (10 to 14 days later)
Alopecia
Hemorrhagic cystitis
Severe immunosuppression
Stomatitis (rare)
Hyperpigmentation
Transverse ridging of nails
Infertility
Cardiac toxicity
SIADH

Comments and Specific Nursing Considerations
BMD has platelet-sparing effect
Give dose early in day to allow adequate fluids afterward
Force fluids before administering drug and for 2 days after to prevent chemical cystitis; encourage frequent voiding even during night
Warn parents to report signs of burning on urination or hematuria to practitioner
Mesna is given to prevent hemorrhagic cystitis

CYTOSINE ARABINOSIDE (ARA-C, CYTOSAR, CYTARABINE, ARABINOSYL CYTOSINE)
Administration
IV, IM, SC, IT

Side Effects and Toxicity
Alopecia
N/V (mild)
BMD (7 to 14 days later)
Mucosal ulceration

Immunosuppression
Hepatitis (usually subclinical)
Fever, conjunctivitis, and maculopapular rash with high doses

Comments and Specific Nursing Considerations
Crosses blood-brain barrier
Use with caution in patients with hepatic dysfunction
Administer steroid eye drops to prevent conjunctivitis with high doses

CORTICOSTEROIDS (HORMONES)
Administration
PO, IT; IM or IV rarely used

Side Effects and Toxicity, Short-Term
For short-term use, no acute toxicity
Usual side effects are mild: moon face, fluid retention, weight gain, mood changes, increased appetite, gastric irritation, insomnia, susceptibility to infection

Comments and Specific Nursing Considerations
Explain expected effects, especially in terms of body image, increased appetite, and personality changes
Monitor weight gain
Recommend moderate salt restriction
Administer with antacid and early in morning (sometimes given every other day to minimize side effects)
May need to disguise bitter taste (crush tablet and mix with syrup, jam, ice cream, or other highly flavored substance; use ice to numb tongue before administration; place tablet in gelatin capsule if child can swallow it)
Observe for potential infection sites; usual inflammatory response and fever are absent

Side Effects and Toxicity, Long-Term
Long-term effects of chronic steroid administration are mood changes, hirsutism, trunk obesity (buffalo hump), thin extremities, muscle wasting and weakness, osteoporosis, poor wound healing, bruising, potassium loss, gastric bleeding, hypertension, diabetes mellitus, growth retardation

Comments and Specific Nursing Considerations
Same as for short-term use; in addition, encourage foods high in potassium (bananas, raisins, prunes, coffee, chocolate)
Test stools for occult blood
Monitor blood pressure
Test blood for sugar and urine for acetone
Observe for signs of abrupt steroid withdrawal: flulike symptoms, hypotension, hypoglycemia, shock

DACARBAZINE (DTIC-DOME)
Administration
IV

Side Effects and Toxicity
N/V (especially after first dose) (severe)
BMD (7 to 14 days later)
Alopecia
Flulike syndrome
Burning sensation in vein during infusion (not extravasation)

*Includes principal drugs used in the treatment of childhood leukemias and lymphomas. Several other conventional and investigational chemotherapeutic agents may be employed in the treatment regimen.
†*N/V*, Nausea and vomiting. Mild, 20% incidence; moderate, 20% to 70% incidence; severe, >0.75% incidence.
IV, Intravenous; *IT*, intrathecal; *PO*, by mouth; *IM*, intramuscular; *SC*, subcutaneous; *BMD*, bone marrow depression.

BOX 26-9 ■ Summary of Selected Chemotherapeutic Agents Used in the Treatment of Childhood Leukemias and Lymphomas—*cont'd*

Comments and Specific Nursing Considerations
Vesicant‡ (less sclerosive)

Must be given cautiously in patients with renal dysfunction

Decrease IV rate or use warm, moist towels on IV site to decrease burning

DAUNORUBICIN (DAUNOMYCIN, RUBIDOMYCIN) AND DOXORUBICIN (ADRIAMYCIN, DOXORUBICIN)
Administration

IV

Side Effects and Toxicity

N/V (moderate)

Stomatitis

BMD (7 to 14 days later)

Fever, chills

Local phlebitis

Alopecia

Cumulative-dose toxicity includes:

    Cardiac abnormalities

    Electrocardiographic changes

    Heart failure

Comments and Specific Nursing Considerations
Vesicant (extravasation may not cause pain)

Use only sterile distilled water as a diluent

Observe for any changes in heart rate or rhythm and signs of failure

Cumulative dose must not exceed 375 mg/m² (less with radiation)

Warn parents that drug causes urine to turn red (for up to 12 days after administration); this is normal, not hematuria

L-ASPARAGINASE (ELSPAR)
Administration

SQ, IV

Side Effects and Toxicity

Allergic reactions (including anaphylactic shock)

Fever

N/V (mild)

Anorexia

Weight loss

Arthralgia

Toxicity:

    Liver dysfunction

    Hyperglycemia

    Renal failure

    Pancreatitis

    Coagulation abnormalities

Comments and Specific Nursing Considerations
Have emergency drugs at bedside

Record signs of allergic reaction, such as urticaria, facial edema, hypotension, or abdominal cramps

Check weight daily

Normally, blood urea nitrogen (BUN) and ammonia levels rise as a result of drug; not evidence of liver damage

Check urine for sugar and blood amylase

Observe for thrombotic events

MECHLORETHAMINE (NITROGEN MUSTARD, MUSTARGEN)
Administration

IV

Side Effects and Toxicity

N/V (30 minutes to 8 hours later) (severe)

BMD (2 to 3 weeks later)

Alopecia

Local phlebitis

Comments and Specific Nursing Considerations
Vesicant

MERCAPTOPURINE (6-MP, PURINETHOL)
Administration

PO, IV

Side Effects and Toxicity

N/V (mild)

Diarrhea

Anorexia

Stomatitis

BMD (4 to 6 weeks later)

Immunosuppression

Dermatitis

Less often may be hepatic dysfunction

Comments and Specific Nursing Considerations
6-MP is an analog of xanthine; therefore, allopurinol (Zyloprim) delays its metabolism and increases its potency, necessitating a lower dose (one-third to one-quarter) of 6-MP

METHOTREXATE (MTX, AMETHOPTERIN)
Administration

PO, IV, IM, IT

May be given in conventional doses (mg/m²) or high doses (g/m²)

Side Effects and Toxicity

N/V (severe at high doses)

Diarrhea

Mucosal ulceration (2 to 5 days later)

BMD (10 days later)

Immunosuppression

Dermatitis

Photosensitivity

Alopecia (uncommon)

Toxic effects include:

    Hepatitis (fibrosis)

    Osteoporosis

    Nephropathy

    Pneumonitis (fibrosis)

Neurologic toxicity with IT use—pain at injection site, meningismus (signs of meningitis without actual inflammation), especially fever and headache; potential sequelae—transient or permanent hemiparesis, seizures, dementia, death

---

‡Vesicants (sclerosing agents) can cause severe cellular damage if even minute amounts of the drug infiltrate surrounding tissue.

Continued

BOX 26-9 ■ Summary of Selected Chemotherapeutic Agents Used in the Treatment of Childhood Leukemias and Lymphomas—*cont'd*

Comments and Specific Nursing Considerations

Side effects and toxicity are dose-related

Potency and toxicity are increased by reduced renal function, salicylates, sulfonamides, and aminobenzoic acid; avoid use of these substances, such as aspirin

Avoid exposure to sun and use sun block

High-dose therapy:

Citrovorum factor (folinic acid or leucovorin) decreases cytotoxic action of MTX; used as an antidote for overdose and to enhance normal cell recovery after high-dose therapy; avoid use of vitamins containing folic acid during MTX therapy unless prescribed by physician

IT therapy:

Drug must be mixed with preservative-free diluent

Report signs of neurotoxicity immediately

PROCARBAZINE (MATULANE)
Administration
PO

Side Effects and Toxicity
N/V (moderate)

BMD (3 to 4 weeks later)

Lethargy

Dermatitis

Myalgia

Arthralgia

Less often:

Stomatitis

Neuropathy

Alopecia

Diarrhea

Amenorrhea

Comments and Specific Nursing Considerations

Central nervous system (CNS) depressants (phenothiazines, barbiturates) enhance CNS symptoms

Monoamine oxidase (MAO) inhibition sometimes occurs; therefore all other drugs are avoided unless medically approved; red wine, fava beans, and broad bean pods are avoided

VINCRISTINE (ONCOVIN) AND VINBLASTINE (VELBAN)
Administration
IV

Side Effects and Toxicity
Neurotoxicity (less severe with vinblastine)—paresthesia (numbness); ataxia; weakness; footdrop; hyporeflexia; constipation (dynamic ileus); hoarseness (vocal cord paralysis); abdominal, chest, and jaw pain; mental depression

Fever

N/V (mild)

BMD (minimal; 7 to 14 days later)

Alopecia

Syndrome of inappropriate antidiuretic hormone excretion (SIADH)

Comments and Specific Nursing Considerations
Vesicant

Report signs of neurotoxicity because they may necessitate cessation of drug

Individuals with underlying neurologic problems may be more prone to neurotoxicity

Monitor stool patterns closely; administer stool softener

Excreted primarily by liver into biliary system; administer cautiously to anyone with biliary disease

Maximum vincristine dose is 2 mg

Mucosal ulceration. One of the most distressing side effects of several drugs is GI mucosal cell damage, which can produce ulcers anywhere along the alimentary tract. Oral ulcers greatly compound anorexia because eating is extremely uncomfortable, but the following interventions may be helpful: (1) provide a bland, moist, soft diet appropriate for the child's age and preferences; (2) use a soft sponge toothbrush (Toothettes)* or cotton-tipped applicator; (3) provide frequent mouthwashes with normal saline (using a solution of 1 teaspoon of table salt and 1 pint of water) or sodium bicarbonate mouth rinses (using a solution of 1 teaspoon of baking soda in 1 quart of water); and(4) use local anesthetics (e.g., Chloraseptic lozenges) or nonprescription preparations without alcohol (e.g., Orabase, Ulcerease, Benadryl/Maalox solution). Although local anesthetics are effective in temporarily relieving the pain, many children dislike the taste and numb feeling they produce.

⚠ NURSING ALERT

Viscous lidocaine is not recommended for young children; if applied to the pharynx, it may depress the gag reflex, increasing the risk of aspiration. Seizures have been rarely associated with the use of oral viscous lidocaine (Cho, Cheng, and Cheng, 2000).

---

*Manufactured by **Halbrand, Inc.,** Willoughby, Ohio.

Other preparations that may be used to prevent or treat mucositis include chlorhexidine gluconate (Peridex) because of its dual effectiveness against candidal and bacterial infections, antifungal troches (lozenges) or mouthwash, and lip balm (e.g., Aquaphor) to keep the lips moist. Agents that should not be used include lemon glycerin swabs (irritate eroded tissue and can decay teeth), hydrogen peroxide (delays healing by breaking down protein), and milk of magnesia (dries mucosa).

Stomatitis may cause such difficulty with eating that the child may require hospitalization for hydration, parenteral nutrition, and pain control (often with IV morphine). The child will usually choose the foods that are best tolerated, and the nurse should encourage parents to relax any eating pressures. Because the stomatitis is a temporary condition, the child can resume good food habits after the ulcers heal. Dental hygiene can become a serious problem for children with orthodontic appliances. Sometimes it may be necessary to remove the braces to allow chemotherapy to continue.

Rectal ulcers are managed by meticulous toilet hygiene, warm sitz baths after each bowel movement, and use of an occlusive ointment or dressing applied to the ulcerated area to promote epithelialization. Stool softeners are necessary to prevent further discomfort. Parents are advised to record bowel movements, because the child may voluntarily avoid defecation to prevent discomfort. Rectal thermometers and suppositories are contraindicated because insertion may further traumatize the area.

Neuropathy.   Vincristine and, to a lesser extent, vinblastine can cause various neurotoxic effects. Nursing interventions for management of these effects include (1) administering stool softeners or laxatives for severe constipation caused by decreased bowel innervation; (2) maintaining good body alignment and, if on bed rest, using a footboard or high-top shoes to minimize or prevent footdrop; (3) carrying out safety measures during ambulation because of weakness and numbing of the extremities, which may cause difficulty in walking or fine hand movement; and (4) providing a soft or liquid diet for severe jaw pain.

Hemorrhagic cystitis.   Sterile hemorrhagic cystitis, a side effect of chemical irritation to the bladder from cyclophosphamide, can be decreased and often prevented by (1) a liberal fluid intake (at least one and a half times the recommended daily fluid requirement); (2) frequent voiding immediately after feeling the urge, before bed, and after arising; (3) administering the drug early in the day to allow for sufficient oral intake and voiding; and (4) administering mesna (an agent that provides protection to the bladder) as ordered. If oral home administration is prescribed, the family needs *specific* instructions regarding exactly how much fluid the child must have.

> **NURSING ALERT**
>
> If signs of cystitis occur, such as burning or bleeding on urination, prompt medical evaluation is needed.

Alopecia.   Hair loss is a common side effect of several chemotherapeutic drugs and cranial irradiation, although not all children lose their hair during drug therapy. It is better to warn children and parents of this side effect than to allow them to think that it is only a remote possibility. A soft cotton cap is the most comfortable head wear for children. Polyester increases perspiration and causes itching. Other options include scarves, hats, or a wig.

> **NURSING TIP**
>
> If the child chooses to wear a wig, encouraging a child to select one similar to the child's own hairstyle and color before the hair falls out is helpful in fostering later adjustment to hair loss.

The nurse should also inform the family that hair regrows in 3 to 6 months and may be of a different color and texture. Frequently the hair is darker, thicker, and curlier than before. If the child chooses not to wear a wig, attention to some type of head covering, especially in cold climates and during exposure to sun, and scalp hygiene are important. The scalp should be washed like any other body part.

Moon face.   Short-term steroid therapy produces no acute toxicities and produces two beneficial reactions: increased appetite and a sense of well-being. However, it does produce alterations in body image, which, although not clinically significant, can be extremely distressing to older children. One of these is moon face, in which the child's face becomes rounded and puffy. It is not unusual for other children to make fun of the child with such remarks as "Miss Piggy," "Porky Pig," or "fat face." It is helpful to reassure children who experience such name-calling that after cessation of the drug the facial changes will return to normal. Unlike hair loss, little can be done to camouflage this obvious change. If the child resumes activity early in the course of treatment, the change may be less noticeable to peers than after a long absence.

Mood changes.   Shortly after beginning steroid therapy, children experience a number of mood changes that range from feelings of well-being and euphoria to depression and irritability. If parents are unaware of these drug-induced changes, they may become unduly concerned. Therefore the nurse should warn them of the reactions and encourage them to discuss the behavioral changes with each other and the child.

Provide continued physical care and emotional support. Because of the improved survival of these children, continued monitoring of physical and intellectual growth and development is essential. Nurses should stress the importance of regular follow-up care.

An important aspect of continued emotional support involves the prognosis. Although leukemia is no longer invariably fatal, it must be remembered that survival statistics are only average estimates and apply to those children treated with the latest protocols since diagnosis. For the low-risk child the chances may be better, but for the high-risk child they may be significantly poorer. Of those who do survive after discontinuing therapy, some will relapse. Therefore, at present, only the passage of time is positive confirmation of the child's being ultimately "cured" of the disease. Remission, even in excess of 5 years, cannot be equated with a cure. With increasing concern regarding late effects of treatment, continued surveillance of the child's health status is needed. The nurse who is working with family members must individualize information regarding the "numbers" and the potential risks. An understanding of each member's emotional needs, as well as competent care of physical ones, is essential to the positive, growth-promoting support of the family. Comprehensive emotional support for the family of the child with a potentially fatal illness is discussed in Chapter 18.

● *Evaluation*

The effectiveness of nursing interventions is determined by continual reassessment and evaluation of care based on the following observational guidelines:

1 Compare number of visits for primary health with recommended schedule of health supervision.
2 Monitor growth, development, and other aspects of regular health assessment; check mouth for adequacy of dental hygiene; review immunization record for age-appropriate vaccines and use of non-live virus preparations.
3 Interview child and family regarding their understanding of treatments and diagnostic tests.
4 Employ pain assessment techniques for procedural pain.
5 Make careful observations of physical status.
   a Take vital signs regularly.
   b Observe for evidence of bleeding, infection, neuropathy, cystitis, and mucosal ulceration.
   c Observe and record intake and output.
6 Interview child and family and observe behaviors as a result of complications of therapies.
7 Interview child and family and observe behaviors that provide clues to their response to the disease, its therapy, and nursing interventions.

The *expected outcomes* are described in the Nursing Care Plan on pp. 966 to 970.

NURSING CARE PLAN **The Child With Cancer**

NURSING DIAGNOSIS ■ Risk for injury related to malignant process, treatment

PATIENT GOAL 1: Will experience partial or complete remission from disease

NURSING INTERVENTIONS/*RATIONALES*
*Administer chemotherapeutic agents as prescribed
Assist with radiotherapy as ordered
Assist with procedures for administration of chemotherapeutic agents (e.g., lumbar puncture for intrathecal administration)
†Prepare child and family for surgical procedure if appropriate

EXPECTED OUTCOME
Child achieves a partial or complete remission from disease

PATIENT GOAL 2: Will not experience complications of chemotherapy

NURSING INTERVENTIONS/*RATIONALES*
Follow guidelines for administration of chemotherapeutic agents
Observe for signs of infiltration at intravenous (IV) site: pain, stinging, swelling, redness
Immediately stop infusion if any sign of infiltration occurs *to prevent severe tissue damage*
Implement policies of institution *to treat infiltration*
Obtain careful history for known allergies *to prevent anaphylaxis*
Observe child for 20 minutes after infusion *for signs of anaphylaxis* (cyanosis, hypotension, wheezing, severe urticaria)
Stop infusion of drug and flush IV line with normal saline if reaction is suspected
Have emergency equipment (especially blood pressure monitor and manual resuscitation bag and mask) and emergency drugs (especially oxygen, epinephrine, antihistamine, aminophylline, corticosteroids, and vasopressors) readily available *to prevent delay in treatment*

EXPECTED OUTCOMES
Child will not experience complications of chemotherapy
Child will receive prompt, appropriate treatment of complications

NURSING DIAGNOSIS ■ Risk for infection related to depressed body defenses

PATIENT GOAL 1: Will experience minimized risk of infection

NURSING INTERVENTIONS/*RATIONALES*
Place child in private room *to minimize exposure to infective organisms*
Advise all visitors and staff to use good handwashing technique *to minimize exposure to infective organisms*
Screen all visitors and staff for signs of infection *to minimize exposure to infective organisms*
Use scrupulous aseptic technique for all invasive procedures
Monitor temperature *to detect possible infection*
Evaluate child for any potential sites of infection (e.g., needle punctures, mucosal ulceration, minor abrasions, dental problems)
Provide nutritionally complete diet for age *to support body's natural defenses*

Avoid giving live attenuated virus vaccines (e.g., measles, mumps, rubella, oral poliovirus) to child with depressed immune system *because these vaccines can result in overwhelming infection*
*Give inactivated virus vaccines (e.g., varicella [chickenpox], Salk polio, influenza) as prescribed and indicated *to prevent specific infections*
Administer antibiotics as prescribed
*Administer granulocyte colony-stimulating factor (GCSF) as prescribed

EXPECTED OUTCOMES
Child does not come in contact with infected persons or contaminated articles
Child consumes diet appropriate for age (specify)
Child does not exhibit signs of infection

NURSING DIAGNOSIS ■ Risk for injury (hemorrhage, hemorrhagic cystitis) related to interference with cell proliferation

PATIENT GOAL 1: Will exhibit no evidence of bleeding

NURSING INTERVENTIONS/*RATIONALES*
Use all measures to prevent infection, especially in ecchymotic areas, *because infection increases tendency toward bleeding*
Use local measures (e.g., apply pressure, ice) *to stop bleeding*
Restrict strenuous activity *that could result in accidental injury*
Involve child in responsibility for limiting activity when platelet count drops *to encourage compliance*
Avoid skin punctures when possible *to prevent bleeding*
Observe for bleeding after procedures such as venipuncture, bone marrow aspiration
Turn frequently and use pressure-reducing or pressure-relieving mattress *to prevent decubitus ulcers*
Teach parents and older child measures to control nosebleeding
Prevent oral and rectal ulceration *because ulcerated skin is prone to bleeding*
Avoid aspirin-containing medications *because aspirin interferes with platelet function*
*Administer platelets as prescribed *to raise platelet count*

EXPECTED OUTCOME
Child exhibits no evidence of bleeding

PATIENT GOAL 2: Will exhibit no evidence of hemorrhagic cystitis

NURSING INTERVENTIONS/*RATIONALES*
Observe for signs of cystitis (e.g., burning and pain on urination)
Report signs of cystitis to practitioner, *because prompt medical evaluation is needed*
Give liberal (3000 mL/m²/day) fluid intake (meters squared is calculated from West nomogram; see Administration of Medication, Chapter 22)
Encourage frequent voiding, including during nighttime, *to minimize metabolites' contact with bladder mucosa*
Administer drugs irritating to bladder early in the day *to allow for sufficient fluid intake and voiding*

EXPECTED OUTCOMES
Child voids without discomfort
No hematuria is present

*Dependent nursing action.
†Indicates content that is specific to a particular malignancy.

PATIENT GOAL 3: Will experience minimal effects of anemia

**NURSING INTERVENTIONS/*RATIONALES*
AND EXPECTED OUTCOMES**

See Nursing Care Plan: The Child With Anemia (*Wong's Clinical Manual of Pediatric Nursing*, ed. 6)

NURSING DIAGNOSIS ■ **Risk for fluid volume deficit related to nausea and vomiting**

PATIENT GOAL 1: Will experience no nausea or vomiting

NURSING INTERVENTIONS/*RATIONALES*

*Administer initial dose of antiemetic before chemotherapy begins *to prevent child from ever experiencing nausea and vomiting, thus preventing an anticipatory response*
*Administer antiemetic around the clock for as long as nausea and vomiting typically last *to prevent any episodes from occurring*
Assess child's response to antiemetic, *because no antiemetic drug is uniformly successful*
Avoid foods with strong odors *that may induce nausea and vomiting*
Uncover hospital food tray outside of child's room *to reduce food odors that may induce nausea*
Encourage frequent intake of fluids in small amounts, *because small portions are usually better tolerated*
*Administer IV fluid, as prescribed, *to maintain hydration*

EXPECTED OUTCOMES

Child retains food and fluid
Child does not experience nausea or vomiting

NURSING DIAGNOSIS ■ **Altered mucous membranes related to administration of chemotherapeutic agents**

PATIENT GOAL 1: Will not develop oral mucositis

NURSING INTERVENTIONS/*RATIONALES*

Inspect mouth daily for oral ulcers; report evidence of ulcers to practitioner *for early treatment*
Avoid oral temperatures *to prevent trauma*
Institute meticulous oral hygiene as soon as a drug is used that causes oral ulcers
    Use soft sponge toothbrush, cotton-tipped applicator, or gauze-wrapped finger *to avoid trauma*
    Administer frequent (at least every 4 hours and after meals) mouthwashes (normal saline with or without sodium bicarbonate solution) *to promote healing*
Apply local anesthetics to ulcerated areas before meals and as needed *to relieve pain*
    Avoid using viscous lidocaine for young children, *because if applied to pharynx, it may depress gag reflex, increasing risk of aspiration, and may cause seizures*
Apply lip balm *to keep lips moist and prevent cracking or fissuring*
Serve bland, moist, soft diet; offer food best tolerated by child
Encourage fluids; use a straw *to help bypass painful areas*
Encourage parents to relax any eating pressures, *because stomatitis is a temporary condition*
Avoid juices containing ascorbic acid and hot or cold or spicy foods if they cause further discomfort
Avoid using lemon glycerin swabs *(irritate eroded tissue and can decay teeth)*, hydrogen peroxide *(delays healing by breaking down protein)*, and milk of magnesia *(dries mucosa)*

Explain to parents that child may require hospitalization *for hydration, parenteral nutrition, and pain control (often with IV morphine)* if stomatitis interferes with food and fluid intake
*Administer antiinfective medication as ordered *to prevent or treat mucositis*
*Administer analgesics, including opioids, *to control pain*

EXPECTED OUTCOMES

Mucous membranes remain intact
Ulcers show evidence of healing
Child reports or exhibits no evidence of discomfort

PATIENT GOAL 2: Will not develop rectal ulceration

NURSING INTERVENTIONS/*RATIONALES*

Wash perianal area after each bowel movement *to lessen irritation*
Use warm sitz baths or tub baths *to promote healing*
Expose reddened but not ulcerated areas to air *to keep skin dry*
Apply protective skin barriers (transparent film dressings, occlusive ointment) to perineal area *to protect skin from direct contact with urine or feces and to promote healing*
Observe for constipation *resulting from child's voluntary refusal to defecate or from chemotherapy*
Record bowel movements; use stool softener *to prevent constipation;* may need stimulants *for evacuation*
Avoid rectal temperatures and suppositories *to prevent rectal trauma*

EXPECTED OUTCOMES

Rectal mucosa remains clean and intact
Ulcerated areas heal without complications
Child has regular bowel movements

NURSING DIAGNOSIS ■ **Altered nutrition: less than body requirements related to loss of appetite**

PATIENT GOAL 1: Will receive adequate nutrition

NURSING INTERVENTIONS/*RATIONALES*

Encourage parents to relax pressures placed on eating; explain that loss of appetite *is a direct consequence of nausea and vomiting and chemotherapy*
Allow child *any* food tolerated; plan to improve quality of food selections when appetite increases
Explain expected increase in appetite from steroids *to prepare child and parents for this change*
Take advantage of any hungry period: serve small "snacks," *because small portions are usually better tolerated*
Fortify foods with nutritious supplements, such as powdered milk or commercial supplements, *to maximize quality of intake*
Allow child to be involved in food preparation and selection *to encourage eating*
Make food appealing
Remember usual food practices of children in each age-group, such as food jags in toddlers or normal occurrence of physiologic anorexia, *to distinguish these expected changes from actual refusal to eat*
Assess family for additional problems (e.g., use of food by child as a control mechanism if appetite does not improve despite improved physical status) *to identify areas that require intervention*

EXPECTED OUTCOME

Nutritional intake is adequate

---

*Dependent nursing action.

Continued

NURSING DIAGNOSIS ■ **Impaired skin integrity related to administration of chemotherapeutic agents, radiotherapy, immobility**

PATIENT GOAL 1: Will maintain skin integrity

NURSING INTERVENTIONS/*RATIONALES*

Provide meticulous skin care, especially in mouth and perianal regions, *because they are prone to ulceration*

Change position frequently *to stimulate circulation and relieve pressure*

Encourage adequate caloric-protein intake *to prevent negative nitrogen balance*

EXPECTED OUTCOME

Skin remains clean and intact

PATIENT GOAL 2: Will experience minimal negative effects of therapy

NURSING INTERVENTIONS/*RATIONALES*

Select loose-fitting clothing over irradiated area *to minimize additional irritation*

Protect area from sunlight and sudden changes in temperature (avoid ice packs, heating pads) during radiotherapy or administration of methotrexate

EXPECTED OUTCOME

Child and family comply with suggestions (specify)

NURSING DIAGNOSIS ■ **Impaired physical mobility related to neuromuscular impairment (neuropathy)**

PATIENT GOAL 1: Will experience minimal negative effects of peripheral neuropathy

NURSING INTERVENTIONS/*RATIONALES*

Encourage ambulation when child is able

Alter activity, including school attendance, *to prevent injuries if weakness occurs*

Use footboard or high-top shoes *to prevent footdrop*

Provide fluids and soft foods *to lessen chewing movements with jaw pain*

EXPECTED OUTCOME

Child ambulates without incident or difficulty

NURSING DIAGNOSIS ■ **Body-image disturbance related to loss of hair, moon face, debilitation**

PATIENT/FAMILY GOAL 1: Will exhibit positive coping behaviors

NURSING INTERVENTIONS/*RATIONALES*

Introduce idea of wig before hair loss

Encourage child to select a wig similar to child's own hairstyle and color before hair falls out *to foster later adjustment to hair loss*

Provide adequate covering during exposure to sunlight, wind, or cold, *because natural protection is lost*

Suggest keeping thin hair clean, short, and fluffy *to camouflage partial baldness*

Explain that hair begins to regrow in 3 to 6 months and may be a slightly different color or texture *to prepare child and family for changes in appearance of new hair*

Explain that alopecia during a second treatment with same drug may be less severe

Encourage good hygiene, grooming, and sex-appropriate items (e.g., wig, scarves, hats, makeup, attractive sex-appropriate clothing) *to enhance appearance*

EXPECTED OUTCOMES

Child verbalizes concern regarding hair loss

Child helps determine methods to reduce effects of hair loss and applies these methods

Child appears clean, well-groomed, and attractively dressed

PATIENT GOAL 2: Will exhibit adjustment to altered facial appearance

NURSING INTERVENTIONS/*RATIONALES*

Encourage rapid reintegration with peers *to lessen contrast of changed facial appearance*

Stress that this reaction is temporary *to provide reassurance that usual appearance will return*

Evaluate weight gain carefully (*with weight gain resulting from administration of steroids, extremities remain thin*)

Encourage visits from friends before discharge *to prepare child for reactions and questions*

EXPECTED OUTCOMES

Family demonstrates understanding of consequences of therapies

Child resumes former activities and relationships within capabilities

PATIENT GOAL 3: Will express feelings

NURSING INTERVENTIONS/*RATIONALES*

Provide opportunities for child to discuss feelings and concerns

Provide materials for nonverbal expression (e.g., play, art)

EXPECTED OUTCOME

Child expresses feelings regarding altered body in words, play, art (specify)

NURSING DIAGNOSIS ■ **Pain related to diagnosis, treatment, physiologic effects of neoplasia**

PATIENT GOAL 1: Will experience no pain or reduction of pain to level acceptable to child

NURSING INTERVENTIONS/*RATIONALES*

Whenever possible, make use of procedures (e.g., noninvasive temperature monitoring, venous access device) *to minimize discomfort*

Assess need for pain management (see Chapter 21)

Evaluate effectiveness of pain relief with degree of alertness vs sedation *to determine need for change in dosage, time of administration, or drug*

Implement appropriate nonpharmacologic pain reduction techniques *as adjunct to analgesics*

*Administer analgesics as prescribed

Avoid aspirin or any of its compounds (e.g., other nonsteroidal antiinflammatory agents) *because aspirin increases bleeding tendency*

*Administer drugs on preventive schedule (around the clock) *to prevent pain from recurring*

Monitor effectiveness of therapy on pain assessment record

EXPECTED OUTCOME

Child rests quietly, reports or exhibits no evidence of discomfort, and verbalizes no complaints of discomfort

*Dependent nursing action.

NURSING CARE PLAN **The Child With Cancer**—*cont'd*

NURSING DIAGNOSIS ■ Fear related to diagnostic test, procedures, treatments

PATIENT GOAL 1: Will exhibit reduced fear related to diagnostic procedures and tests

NURSING INTERVENTIONS/*RATIONALES*

Explain procedure carefully at child's level of understanding *to reduce fear of the unknown*

Explain what will take place and what child will feel, see, and hear *to increase sense of control*

Use recall of each step *as method of distraction*

Explain special requests of child (e.g., need to remain motionless during test or radiotherapy) *to encourage cooperation*

Provide child with some means for involvement with procedure (e.g., holding a piece of equipment, such as bandage or tape, counting with the operator, answering questions) *to promote sense of control, encourage cooperation, and support child's coping skills*

Implement distracting techniques and pain reduction techniques as indicated

See also Preparation for Procedures, Chapter 22

EXPECTED OUTCOMES

Child readily responds to verbal directives

Child repeats information accurately

NURSING DIAGNOSIS ■ Fear related to diagnosis, prognosis

See Nursing Care Plan: The Child Who Is Terminally Ill or Dying, Chapter 18

NURSING DIAGNOSIS ■ Diversional activity deficit related to restricted environment (private room)

PATIENT GOAL 1: Will have opportunity to participate in diversional activities

NURSING INTERVENTIONS/*RATIONALES*

Provide age-appropriate toys that can be properly cleaned *to provide diversion without risk of infection*

Involve child-life specialist or other supportive services in planning diversional activities

EXPECTED OUTCOMES

Child engages in activities appropriate for age and interests

Suitable toys are provided

NURSING DIAGNOSIS ■ Altered family processes related to having a child with a life-threatening disease

PATIENT/FAMILY GOAL 1: Will demonstrate knowledge about diagnostic/therapeutic procedures

NURSING INTERVENTIONS/*RATIONALES*

Explain reason for each test and procedure

Explain reason for radiotherapy, chemotherapy

Explain operative procedure honestly (if appropriate)

Avoid overemphasis on benefits, which may not be immediately evident (applies primarily to brain tumors), *to avoid unrealistic expectations*

See also Preparation for Procedures, Chapter 22

EXPECTED OUTCOME

Child and family demonstrate understanding of procedures (specify learning and manner of demonstration)

PATIENT (FAMILY) GOAL 1: Will receive adequate support

NURSING INTERVENTIONS/*RATIONALES*

Teach parents about disease process

Explain all procedures that will be done to child

Schedule time for family to be together, without interruptions from staff, *to encourage communication and expression of feelings*

Help family plan for future, especially for helping child live a normal life, *to promote child's optimal development*

Encourage family to discuss feelings regarding child's course before diagnosis and child's prognosis

Discuss with family how they will tell child about outcome of treatment and need for additional treatment (if appropriate) *to maintain open and honest communication*

Refer to local chapter of American Cancer Society or other organizations

EXPECTED OUTCOMES

Family demonstrates knowledge of child's disease and treatments (specify methods of learning and evaluation)

Family expresses feelings and concerns and spends time with child

See also:

Nursing Care Plan: The Child in the Hospital, Chapter 21

Nursing Care Plan: The Family of the Ill or Hospitalized Child, Chapter 21

NURSING DIAGNOSIS ■ Altered family processes related to a child undergoing therapy

PATIENT (FAMILY) GOAL 1: Will demonstrate understanding of side effects or complications of treatment

NURSING INTERVENTIONS/RATIONALES

Advise family of expected side effects versus toxicities; clarify which demand medical evaluation (mucosal ulceration, hemorrhagic cystitis, peripheral neuropathy, evidence of infection or dehydration) *to prevent delay in treatment*

Reassure family that such reactions are not caused by return of cancer cells *to minimize undue concern*

Interpret prognostic statistics carefully, realizing family's temporary need to interpret them as they see necessary, *to present a realistic, but hopeful, future*

Prepare family for expected mood changes from steroids

Interpret mood changes based on drugs or reactions to disease/treatment *to prevent any unwarranted negative reaction to child (e.g., punishment)*

EXPECTED OUTCOMES

Family demonstrates knowledge of instructions (specify methods of learning and evaluation)

Family demonstrates understanding of behavior changes

Continued

NURSING CARE PLAN   The Child With Cancer—*cont'd*

PATIENT GOAL 2: Will receive adequate support during treatment

NURSING INTERVENTIONS/*RATIONALES*
Explain reason for antibiotics or transfusions, particularly why platelets are reserved for acute, uncontrolled bleeding episodes
Observe for signs of transfusion reaction (see Table 26-5)
Record appropriate time for hemostasis to occur after administration of platelets *to determine if transfusions are becoming less effective*

EXPECTED OUTCOME
Child demonstrates understanding of procedures and tests (specify methods of learning and evaluation)

PATIENT (FAMILY) GOAL 3: Will be prepared for home care

NURSING INTERVENTIONS/*RATIONALES*
Teach preventive measures at discharge (e.g., handwashing, isolation from crowds) *to prevent infection*
Stress importance of isolating child from any known cases of chickenpox or other childhood diseases; work with school nurse and physician to determine optimal time for school reattendance *to prevent unnecessary absences or risk of infection*
Teach home care instructions specific to child's needs

EXPECTED OUTCOME
Family demonstrates ability to provide home care for child (specify)

NURSING DIAGNOSIS ■ **Anticipatory grief related to perceived potential loss of a child**

PATIENT (FAMILY) GOAL 1: Will acknowledge and cope with possibility of child's death

NURSING INTERVENTIONS/*RATIONALES*
Provide consistent contact with family *to establish a trusting relationship that encourages communication*
Clarify, refocus, and supply information as needed
Help family plan care of child, especially at terminal stage (e.g., extent of extraordinary lifesaving measures) *to ensure that their wishes are implemented*
Provide or arrange for hospice care if family desires it
Arrange for spiritual support in accordance with family's beliefs or affiliations

EXPECTED OUTCOMES
Family remains open to counseling and nursing contact
Family and child discuss their fears, concerns, needs, and desires at terminal stage
Family investigates hospice care
Appropriate religious representative is contacted (specify)

PATIENT (FAMILY) GOAL 2: Will receive adequate support

NURSING INTERVENTIONS/*RATIONALES*
AND EXPECTED OUTCOMES
See Nursing Care Plan: The Child Who Is Terminally Ill or Dying (Chapter 18)

LYMPHOMAS

Pediatric lymphomas are the third most common group of malignancies in children and adolescents. The lymphomas, a group of neoplastic diseases that arise from the lymphoid and hemopoietic systems, are divided into Hodgkin disease and non-Hodgkin lymphoma (NHL). These diseases are further subdivided according to tissue type and extent of disease. NHL is more prevalent in children younger than 14 years of age, whereas Hodgkin disease is prevalent in adolescence and the young adult period, with a striking increase between ages 15 and 19 years.

HODGKIN DISEASE

Hodgkin disease is a neoplastic disease that originates in the lymphoid system and primarily involves the lymph nodes. It predictably metastasizes to nonnodal or extralymphatic sites, especially the spleen, liver, bone marrow, and lungs, although no tissue is exempt from involvement (Fig. 26-5). It is classified according to four histologic types: (1) lymphocytic predominance, (2) nodular sclerosis, (3) mixed cellularity, and (4) lymphocytic depletion. Accurate staging of the extent of disease is the basis for treatment protocols and expected prognoses.

The Ann Arbor staging system (Box 26-10) assigns stage based on the number of sites of lymph node involvement, presence of extranodal disease, and history of any symptoms. Patients are classified as A if asymptomatic and as B if they have the following symptoms: temperature of 38° C (100.4° F) or higher for 3 consecutive days, drenching night sweats, or unexplained loss of body weight (10% or more) over the preceding 6 months (Hudson and Donaldson, 2002).

Asymptomatic enlarged cervical or supraclavicular lymphadenopathy is the most common presentation of Hodgkin disease (Box 26-11). Other systemic symptoms, including fever, weight loss, and night sweats, as well as cough, abdominal discomfort, anorexia, nausea, and pruritus, may be manifested. Because multiple organs may be involved, diagnosis is based on several tests and the extent of metastatic disease. Tests include a CBC, erythrocyte sedimentation rate, serum copper, ferritin level, fibrinogen, immunoglobulins, uric acid level, liver function tests, T-cell function studies, and urinalysis. Radiographic tests include computed tomography (CT) scans of the neck, chest, abdomen, and pelvis; a gallium scan (identifies metastatic/recurrent disease); a chest x-ray film; and, if clinically indicated, a bone scan to identify metastatic disease. With the advent of CT and gallium scans, a lymphangiogram may not be needed, although elimination is controversial.

Although used rarely, *lymphangiography* may be performed. This is visualization of the lymphatic circulation of the lower extremities, groin, ileopelvic and abdominal-aortic regions, and thoracic duct by way of a radiopaque medium injected in the feet or hands.

A lymph node biopsy is essential to establish histologic diagnosis and staging. The presence of Reed-Sternberg cells is

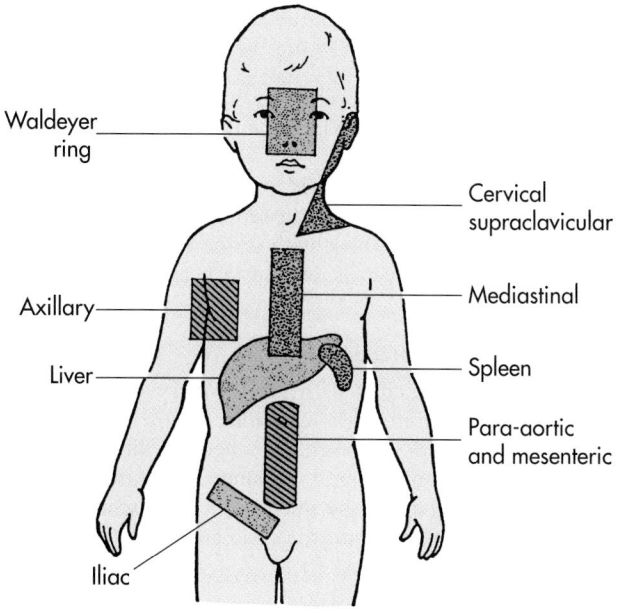

Waldeyer ring

Cervical supraclavicular

Axillary

Mediastinal

Liver

Spleen

Para-aortic and mesenteric

Iliac

FIG. 26-5 ■ Main areas of lymphadenopathy and organ involvement in Hodgkin disease.

characteristic of Hodgkin disease. These large cells, which are multilobed and nucleated with abundant cytoplasm and a typically halolike clear zone around the nucleolus, are often described as having an "owl's eyes" appearance (Hudson and Donaldson, 2002). A bone marrow aspiration or biopsy is usually performed. With the advent of CT and gallium scans to identify metastatic disease and multiagent chemotherapy to eradicate metastatic disease, a laparotomy without splenectomy is avoided except in a few selected cases.

Therapeutic Management

The primary modalities of therapy are radiation and chemotherapy. Each may be used alone or in combination based on the clinical staging. Radiation may involve only the involved field (IF), an extended field (EF) (involved areas plus adjacent nodes), or total nodal irradiation (TNI), depending on the extent of involvement.

An effective combination of chemotherapy widely used is MOPP (mechlorethamine, vincristine [Oncovin], procarbazine, prednisone) or ABVD (adriamycin, bleomycin, vinblastine, dacarbazine). However, this therapy combination has caused severe late effects, especially secondary malignancies. At present, use of ABVD with COPP (cyclophosphamide, vincristine, prednisone, procarbazine) as a substitute for MOPP has minimized late effects.

Follow-up care of children no longer receiving therapy is essential to identify relapse and secondary cancers. In children with splenectomy resulting from laparotomy or splenic irradiation, prophylactic antibiotics are administered for an indefinite period. Also, immunizations against pneumococci and meningococci are recommended before the splenectomy.

Prognosis.   Long-term survival for all stages of Hodgkin disease is excellent. Early-stage disease can have survival rates greater than 90%, with advanced stages having rates between 65% and 75%.

Nursing Considerations

Nursing care involves the same objectives as for patients with other types of cancer—specifically, (1) preparation for diagnostic and operative procedures, (2) explanation of treatment side effects (see Box 26-9), and (3) child and family support (see Chapter 18). Because this is most often a disease of adolescents and young adults, the nurse must have an appreciation of their psychologic needs and reactions during the diagnostic and treatment phases (see Nursing Care Plan, pp. 966 to 970).

Once the child is hospitalized for suspected Hodgkin disease, a battery of diagnostic tests is ordered. The family needs an explanation of why each test is performed, because many of them, such as bone marrow aspiration and lymph node biopsy are invasive procedures.

The most common side effect of irradiation is fatigue. This is particularly difficult for active, outgoing school-age children and adolescents, because it prevents them from keeping up with their peers. Sometimes adolescents will push themselves to the point of physical exhaustion rather than admit and succumb to the decreased activity tolerance. The nurse cautions parents to observe for behavior such as extreme fatigue at the end of the day, falling asleep at the dinner table, inability to concentrate on homework, or an increased susceptibility to infection. A regular bedtime and scheduled rest periods are important for these children, especially during chemotherapy, when myelosuppression increases the risk of infection and debilitation. Before discharge the nurse should discuss a feasible school schedule with the parents and child.

An area of concern for adolescents is the high risk of sterility from irradiation and chemotherapy. Both drugs, particularly procarbazine and alkylating agents, and irradiation to the gonads can lead to infertility. Adolescents should be informed of these side effects early in the course of the diagnosis and treatment. Sperm banking is now offered at many cancer centers before the initiation of treatment in adolescent boys. Sexual function is not altered, although the appearance of secondary sexual characteristics and menstruation may be delayed in the pubescent child. Delayed sexual maturation may be an extremely sensitive and stressful issue for children (see Chapter 17).

NON-HODGKIN LYMPHOMA

Non-Hodgkin lymphoma (NHL) occurs more frequently in children than Hodgkin disease. NHL is diagnosed in approximately 750 to 800 children each year in the United States (Link and Donaldson, 2003). Histologic classification of childhood NHL is strikingly different from that of Hodgkin disease, as demonstrated in the following statements:

- The disease is usually diffuse rather than nodular.
- The cell type is either undifferentiated or poorly differentiated.
- Dissemination occurs early, more often, and rapidly.
- Mediastinal involvement and invasion of meninges are common.

NHL exhibits a variety of morphologic, cytochemical, and immunologic features, not unlike the diversity seen in leukemia. Classification is based on the histologic pattern: (1) lymphoblastic, (2) Burkitt or non-Burkitt, or (3) large cell. Immunologically these cells are also classified as T cells; B cells; or non-T, non-B cells (lacking immunologic properties).

The clinical staging system used in Hodgkin disease is of little value in NHL, although it has been modified and other systems have been developed.

Diagnostic Evaluation

Because the clinical presentation of most children with NHL is widespread disseminated disease, thorough pathologic staging is unnecessary. Clinical manifestations depend on the anatomic site and extent of involvement. These manifestations include many of those seen in Hodgkin disease and leukemia, as well as organ symptoms related to pressure from enlargement of adjacent lymph nodes, such as intestinal or airway obstruction, cranial nerve palsies, and spinal paralysis.

Recommendations for staging include a surgical biopsy of an enlarged node, histopathologic confirmation of disease with cytochemical and immunologic evaluation, bone marrow examination, radiographic studies (especially tomograms of the lungs and GI organs), and lumbar puncture.

Therapeutic Management

The treatment protocols for NHL include aggressive use of irradiation and chemotherapy. Similar to leukemic therapy, the protocols include induction, consolidation, and mainte-

nance phases, some with intrathecal chemotherapy. Several antineoplastic agents used in the treatment of NHL include vincristine, prednisone, L-asparaginase, methotrexate, 6-mercaptopurine, cytarabine, cyclophosphamide, anthracyclines, and teniposide or etoposide (Link and Donaldson, 2003).

Prognosis. The prognosis is excellent for children with localized disease, and long-term remissions are possible in many patients, even in those with disseminated disease. Because relapse after 2 years is rare, survival after 24 months is considered a cure.

Nursing Considerations

Nursing care of the child with NHL is very similar to that required for children with leukemia. Many of the same drugs are employed, although the schedules differ. Because of the intense chemotherapy, nursing care is primarily directed toward managing the side effects of these agents and providing supportive care to the child and family (see Nursing Care Plan, pp. 966 to 970).

IMMUNOLOGIC DEFICIENCY DISORDERS

A number of disorders can cause profound, often life-threatening alterations within the body's immune system. The most serious are those conditions that completely depress immunity, such as severe combined immunodeficiency disease. However, the one disorder that generates the most anxiety, within both the family and the community at large, is HIV infection/AIDS.

Several classifications of immune dysfunction exist. *AIDS,* severe combined immunodeficiency syndrome (SCID), and *Wiskott-Aldrich syndrome* are syndromes wherein the body is unable to mount an immune response. The immune response can also be misdirected. In *autoimmune disorders,* antibodies, macrophages, and lymphocytes attack healthy cells.

HUMAN IMMUNODEFICIENCY VIRUS INFECTION AND ACQUIRED IMMUNODEFICIENCY SYNDROME

Since the first cases of AIDS were identified in the early 1980s, HIV infection has generated intense medical investigation. Research has led to early diagnosis of and improved medical treatments for HIV infection, changing this disease from a rapidly fatal one to a chronic, but terminal, disease of childhood.

Epidemiology

The first AIDS cases in the pediatric population in the United States were identified in children born to HIV-infected mothers and in children who received blood products. More than 90% of these children acquired the disease perinatally from their mothers. Smaller numbers of children were infected through the transfusion of contaminated blood/blood products before 1985 or were infected through sexual abuse. In contrast, sexual activity and IV drug use are major sources of HIV infection in adolescents.

The estimated number of children with perinatally acquired AIDS peaked during 1992; subsequent years have seen significant declines. This trend is a result of implementation of recommended HIV counseling and voluntary testing practices and the use of zidovudine therapy to prevent perinatal transmission. Zidovudine therapy in HIV-infected pregnant women, and subsequently in their infants, has significantly reduced the transmission of HIV (Lyall, 2002; Ioannidis and others, 2001). The effectiveness of other HIV drugs such as Nevirapine to prevent perinatal transmission is being studied (Meldrum, 2003; Merchant and Keshavarz, 2001). Routine HIV counseling and voluntary testing for pregnant women are recommended (American Academy of Pediatrics, 2000), and guidelines for the use of antiretroviral drugs in HIV-infected pregnant women to reduce perinatal transmission are available (Lyall, 2002).

Etiology

HIV is a retrovirus that is transmitted by lymphocytes and monocytes. It is found in the blood, semen, vaginal secretions, and breast milk. It has an incubation period of months to years (Ezekowitz and Stockman, 2003). There are different strains of HIV. HIV-2 is prevalent in Africa, whereas HIV-1 is the dominant strain in the United States and elsewhere. *Horizontal transmission* of HIV occurs through intimate sexual contact or parenteral exposure to blood or body fluids containing visible blood. *Perinatal (vertical) transmission* occurs when an HIV-infected pregnant woman passes the infection to her infant. There is no evidence that *casual* contact between infected and uninfected individuals can spread the virus.

Pathophysiology

The HIV virus primarily infects a specific subset of T lymphocytes, the CD_4^+ T cells. The virus takes over the machinery of the CD_4^+ lymphocyte, using it to replicate itself, rendering the CD_4^+ cell dysfunctional. The CD_4^+ lymphocyte count gradually decreases over time, leading to progressive immune deficiency. The count eventually reaches a critical level below which there is substantial risk of opportunistic illnesses followed by death.

Clinical Manifestations

Common clinical manifestations of HIV infection in children are varied (Box 26-12). The diagnosis of AIDS is associated with certain illnesses or conditions. The most common AIDS-defining conditions observed among American children are listed in Box 26-13. Other problems in these children may include short stature, malnutrition, and cardiomyopathy. CNS abnormalities resulting from HIV infection may include neuropsychologic deficits; developmental disabilities; and deficits in motor skills, communication, and behavioral functioning.

Diagnostic Evaluation

For children 18 months of age and older, the HIV enzyme-linked immunosorbent assay (ELISA) and Western blot immunoassay are performed to determine HIV infection. In infants born to HIV-infected mothers, these assays will be positive because of the presence of maternal antibodies derived transplacentally. Maternal antibodies may persist in the infant up to 18 months of age. Therefore other diagnostic tests are employed, most commonly the HIV polymerase

---

BOX 26-12 ■ Common Clinical Manifestations of HIV Infection in Children

Lymphadenopathy
Hepatosplenomegaly
Oral candidiasis
Chronic or recurrent diarrhea
Failure to thrive
Developmental delay
Parotitis

BOX 26-13 ■ Common AIDS-Defining Conditions in Children

Pneumocystis carinii pneumonia (PCP)
Lymphoid interstitial pneumonitis (LIP)
Recurrent bacterial infections
Wasting syndrome
HIV encephalopathy
Candidal esophagitis
 Cytomegalovirus disease
 Mycobacterium avium-intracellulare complex infection
 Severe herpes simplex infection
 Pulmonary candidiasis
Cryptosporidiosis

---

chain reaction (PCR) for detection of proviral DNA. With this technique, more than 95% of infected infants can be diagnosed by 1 month of age (Ezekowitz and Stockman, 2003).

The Centers for Disease Control and Prevention (CDC) (1994) has developed a classification system to describe the spectrum of HIV disease in children (Table 26-3). The system indicates the severity of clinical signs and symptoms and the degree of immunosuppression. Mild signs and symptoms include lymphadenopathy, parotitis, hepatosplenomegaly, and recurrent or persistent sinusitis or otitis media. Moderate signs and symptoms include lymphoid interstitial pneumonitis (LIP) and a variety of organ-specific dysfunctions or infections. Severe signs and symptoms include AIDS-defining illnesses with the exception of LIP. Children with LIP have a better prognosis than those with other AIDS-defining illnesses. In children whose HIV infection is not yet confirmed, the letter *E* (vertically exposed) is placed in front of the classification. The immune categories are based on CD_4^+ lymphocyte counts and percentages. Age adjustment of these numbers is necessary because normal counts, which are relatively high in infants, decline steadily until 6 years of age, when they reach adult norms (Table 26-4).

Therapeutic Management

The goals of therapy for HIV infection include slowing the growth of the virus, preventing and treating opportunistic infections, and providing nutritional support and symptomatic treatment. *Antiretroviral drugs* work at various stages of the HIV life cycle to prevent reproduction of functional new virus particles. Although not a cure, these drugs can suppress viral replication, preventing further deterioration of the immune system, and thus delay disease progression. Classes of

TABLE 26-3 ■ Pediatric HIV Classification*

IMMUNOLOGIC CATEGORIES	N: NO SIGNS/ SYMPTOMS	A: MILD SIGNS/ SYMPTOMS	B: MODERATE SIGNS/ SYMPTOMS†	C: SEVERE SIGNS/ SYMPTOMS†
No evidence of suppression	N1	A1	B1	C1
Evidence of moderate suppression	N2	A2	B2	C2
Severe suppression	N3	A3	B3	C3

From Centers for Disease Control and Prevention: 1994 Revised classification system for human immunodeficiency virus infection in children less than 13 years of age, *MMWR* 43(RR-12):1-10, 1994.
*Children whose HIV infection status is not confirmed are classified by using the above table with the letter *E* (for perinatally exposed) placed before the appropriate classification code (e.g., EN2).
†Both category C and lymphoid interstitial pneumonitis in category B are reportable to state and local health departments as AIDS.

TABLE 26-4 ■ Immunologic Categories Based on Age-Specific CD_4^+ T-Lymphocyte Counts and Percent of Total Lymphocytes

	AGE OF CHILD					
	<12 MONTHS		1-5 YEARS		6-12 YEARS	
	μL	(%)	μL	(%)	μL	(%)
IMMUNOLOGIC CATEGORY						
No evidence of suppression	≥1500	(≥25)	≥1000	(≥25)	≥500	(≥25)
Evidence of moderate suppression	750-1499	(15-24)	500-999	(15-24)	200-499	(15-24)
Severe suppression	<750	(<15)	<500	(<15)	<200	(<15)

From Centers for Disease Control and Prevention: 1994 Revised classification system for human immunodeficiency virus infection in children less than 13 years of age, *MMWR* 43(RR-12):1-10, 1994.

antiretroviral agents include nucleoside reverse transcriptase inhibitors (e.g., zidovudine, didanosine, stavudine, lamivudine, abacavir), nonnucleoside reverse transcriptase inhibitors (e.g., nevirapine, delavirdine, efavirenz), nucleotide reverse transcriptase inhibitors (e.g., adefovir), protease inhibitors (e.g., indinavir, saquinavir, ritonavir, nelfinavir, amprenavir), and adjunctive antiretrovirals (e.g., hydroxyurea). Combinations of these drugs are used to forestall the emergence of drug resistance. Antiretroviral therapy regimens and guidelines are continually evolving. Therapy is lifelong, making adherence difficult. Laboratory markers (CD_4^+ lymphocyte count, viral load) assist in monitoring both disease progression and response to therapy.

Pneumocystis carinii pneumonia (PCP) is the most common opportunistic infection of children infected with HIV. It occurs most frequently between 3 and 6 months of age. All infants born to HIV-infected women should receive prophylaxis during the first year of life according to guidelines set by the CDC (1995) and the American Academy of Pediatrics (2000). After 1 year of age, the need for prophylaxis is determined by the presence of severe immunosuppression or a history of PCP (National Institute of Allergy and Infectious Diseases/NIH, 2003; CDC, 1995). Trimethoprim-sulfamethoxazole (TMP-SMZ) is the agent of choice. If adverse effects are experienced with TMP-SMZ, dapsone or pentamidine can be used.

Prophylaxis is often employed for other opportunistic infections, such as disseminated *Mycobacterium avium-intracellulare* complex (MAC), candidiasis, or herpes simplex. IV immunoglobulin has been helpful in preventing recurrent or serious bacterial infections in some HIV-infected children.

Immunization against common childhood illnesses is recommended for all children exposed to and infected with HIV (American Academy of Pediatrics, 2000). Varicella (chickenpox) vaccine and measles-mumps-rubella (MMR) vaccine can be administered if there is no evidence of severely immunocompromised close contacts. The pneumococcal and influenza vaccines are recommended. Because antibody production to vaccines may be poor or decrease over time, immediate prophylaxis after exposure to several vaccine-preventable diseases (e.g., measles, varicella) is warranted. It should be recognized that children receiving IV gamma globulin prophylaxis may not respond to the MMR vaccine (Morbidity and Mortality Weekly Report [MMWR], 2003).

HIV infection often leads to marked failure to thrive and multiple nutritional deficiencies. Nutritional management may be difficult because of recurrent illness, diarrhea, and other physical problems. Intensive nutritional interventions should be instituted when the child's growth begins to slow or weight begins to decrease.

Prognosis. Early recognition and improved medical care have changed HIV disease from a rapidly fatal illness to a chronic disease. After the introduction of combination antiretroviral therapy, the numbers of new AIDS cases and deaths declined substantially. Between 1995 and 1998, the annual number of AIDS cases declined by 38% and deaths declined by 63% (MMWR, 2003). The annual number of AIDS cases and deaths has remained stable since 1998 (CDC, 2001). The number of children with AIDS attributed to perinatal HIV transmission peaked in 1992 at 954 cases and declined by 89% to 101 cases in 2001 (CDC, 2001).

Nursing Considerations

Education concerning transmission and control of infectious diseases, including HIV infection, is essential for children with HIV infection and anyone involved in their care. The basic tenets of standard precautions should be presented in an age-appropriate manner, with careful consideration of the educational levels of the individuals (see Infection Control, Chapter 22). Safety issues, including appropriate storage of special medications and equipment (e.g., needles and syringes), are emphasized. Unfortunately, relatives, friends, and others in the general public may be fearful of contracting HIV infection, and criticism and ostracism of the child and family may occur. In an effort to protect the child, the family may limit the child's activities outside the home. Although certain precautions are justified in limiting exposure to sources of infections, they must be tempered with concern for the child's normal developmental needs. Both the family and the community need ongoing education about HIV to dispel many of the myths that have been perpetuated by uninformed persons.*

Prevention is a key component of HIV education. Educating adolescents about HIV is essential in preventing HIV infection in this age-group. Education should include the routes of transmission, the hazards of IV and other recreational drug use, and the value of sexual abstinence and safe sex practices. Such education should be a part of anticipatory guidance provided to all adolescent patients. Nurses can also encourage adolescents at risk to undergo HIV counseling and testing. In addition to identifying infected teenagers and getting them into care, such counseling affords adolescents an opportunity to learn about, and possibly change, their risk behaviors.

The nurse's role in the care of the child with HIV is multifaceted (see Nursing Care Plan, pp. 976 to 977). The nurse serves as educator, direct care provider, case manager, and advocate. As with all chronic illnesses, these children will have much involvement with the health care system. The need for HIV medications is lifelong. Nurses are instrumental in encouraging and empowering these children (and their caretakers) to adhere to their medication regimens. Clinic visits and hospitalizations may become frequent as the disease progresses. The physiologic care of the child is directed at minimum exposure to infections; nutritional support; comfort measures, including pain management; and assessment and recognition of changes in status that may indicate new complications. The scope of nursing care will change with new symptoms, changes in treatment, and disease progression. The unpredictability of the course of pediatric HIV infection is a continual source of stress to these children and their caretakers. Psychologic interventions will vary with the unique circumstances of each child and family.

The multiple complications associated with HIV disease are potentially painful (Ezekowitz and Stockman, 2003; Sullivan and Woda, 2003). Aggressive pain management is essential for these children to have an acceptable quality of

---

*Additional information is available from the **AIDS Hotline:** (800) 342-2437 (AIDS); and from the **National Pediatric and Family HIV Resource Center,** 30 Bergen Street, ADMC 4, Newark, NJ 07103; (973) 972-0410 or (800) 362-0071; website: www.pedhivaids.org.

 FAMILY FOCUS

Caregivers and the Infant With HIV Infection

Unlike other fatal pediatric diseases, HIV infection is associated with special family alterations. The infant infected in utero faces multiple physical and parental problems. Because the mother is infected, she may be ill or dying and therefore unable to care for the child. If possible, grandparents or other relatives may assume care. Foster care is often difficult to arrange because of the nature of the disease, especially in relation to the social stigma and the child's multiple medical needs. These children may require frequent hospitalizations with progression of their HIV disease. When children remain in the hospital, the importance of consistent caregivers, especially primary nurses, who attend to the youngsters' physical, developmental, and emotional needs cannot be overemphasized. However, primary nurses may face the risk of overinvolvement and must be aware of the boundaries of a therapeutic relationship.

life. Their pain may be due to infections (e.g., otitis media, dental abscess), encephalopathy (e.g., spasticity), adverse effects of medications (e.g., peripheral neuropathy), or an unknown source (e.g., deep musculoskeletal pain). Sources of pain are related not only to disease processes, but also to various treatments these children often undergo, including venipunctures, lumbar punctures, biopsies, and endoscopies. Ongoing assessment of pain is crucial and is most easily accomplished in older children who are able to communicate. Nonverbal and developmentally delayed children are more difficult to assess. Be alert for other signs of pain: emotional detachment, lack of interactive play, irritability, and depression. Effective pain management depends on the appropriate use of pharmacologic agents, including EMLA cream, acetaminophen, NSAIDs, muscle relaxants, and opioids. Tolerance to opioids may indicate increased dosing; monitored use ensures safety. Nonpharmacologic interventions (guided imagery, hypnosis, relaxation and distraction techniques) are useful adjuncts.

Common psychosocial concerns include disclosure of the diagnosis to the child, making custody plans when the parent is infected, and anticipating the loss of a family member. Other stressors may include financial difficulties, HIV-associated stigma, striving to keep the diagnosis secret, other infected family members, and the multiple losses associated with HIV. Most mothers of these children are single mothers who are also HIV-infected. As primary caretakers, they often attend to the needs of their child first, neglecting their own health in the process (see Family Focus box). The nurse can encourage the mother to receive regular health care. Family members are often involved in the care of the child, particularly if the mother has symptomatic illness. After the death of the mother, a grandparent or other relative typically assumes responsibility for the care of the child. Nursing can provide support and encouragement for the new surrogate parent, particularly during the transition phase. If no family member is available, the child may be placed in a foster or group home. Nursing is an integral part of the multidisciplinary team necessary for the successful management of the complex medical and social problems of these families.

NURSING DIAGNOSIS ■ **Risk for infection related to impaired body defenses, presence of infective organisms**

PATIENT GOAL 1: Will experience minimized risk of infection

NURSING INTERVENTIONS/RATIONALES

Use thorough handwashing technique *to minimize exposure to infective organisms*

Advise visitors to use good handwashing technique *to minimize exposure to infective organisms*

Place child in room with noninfectious children or in private room

Restrict contact with persons who have infections, including family, other children, friends, and members of staff; explain that child is highly susceptible to infection *to encourage cooperation and understanding*

Observe medical asepsis as appropriate *to decrease risk of infection*

Encourage good nutrition and adequate rest *to promote body's remaining natural defenses*

Explain to family and older child importance of contacting health professional if exposed to childhood illnesses (e.g., chickenpox, measles) *so that appropriate immunizations can be given*

*Administer appropriate immunizations as prescribed *to prevent specific infections*

*Administer antibiotics as prescribed

EXPECTED OUTCOMES

Child does not come in contact with infected persons or contaminated articles

Child and family apply good health practices

Child exhibits no evidence of infection

PATIENT GOAL 2: Will not spread disease to others

NURSING INTERVENTIONS/RATIONALES

Implement and carry out standard precautions *to prevent spread of virus* (see Infection Control, Chapter 22)

Instruct others (e.g., family, staff members) in appropriate precautions; clarify any misconceptions about communicability of virus, *because this is a frequent problem and may interfere with use of appropriate precautions*

Teach affected children protective methods *to prevent spread of infection* (e.g., handwashing, handling genital area, care after using bedpan or toilet)

Endeavor to keep infants and small children from placing hands and objects in contaminated areas

Place restrictions on behaviors and contacts for affected children who bite or who do not have control of their bodily secretions

Assess home situation and implement protective measures as feasible in individual circumstances

EXPECTED OUTCOME

Others do not acquire the disease

NURSING DIAGNOSIS ■ **Altered nutrition: less than body requirements related to recurrent illness, diarrheal losses, loss of appetite, oral candidiasis**

PATIENT GOAL 1: Will receive optimum nourishment

NURSING INTERVENTIONS/RATIONALES

Provide high-calorie, high-protein meals and snacks *to meet body requirements for metabolism and growth*

Provide foods child prefers *to encourage eating*

Fortify foods with nutritional supplements (e.g., powdered milk, commercial supplements) *to maximize quality of intake*

Provide meals when child is most likely to eat well

Use creativity to encourage child to eat (see Feeding the Sick Child, Chapter 22)

Monitor child's weight and growth *so that additional nutritional interventions can be implemented if growth begins to slow or weight drops*

*Administer antifungal medication as ordered *to treat oral candidiasis*

EXPECTED OUTCOME

Child consumes a sufficient amount of nutrients (specify)

NURSING DIAGNOSIS ■ **Impaired social interaction related to physical limitations, hospitalizations, social stigma toward HIV infection**

PATIENT GOAL 1: Will participate in peer-group and family activities

NURSING INTERVENTIONS/RATIONALES

Assist child in identifying personal strengths *to facilitate coping*

Educate school personnel and classmates about HIV infection *so that child is not unnecessarily isolated*

Encourage child to participate in activities with other children and family

Encourage child to maintain phone contact with friends during hospitalization *to lessen isolation*

EXPECTED OUTCOME

Child participates in activities with peer group and family

NURSING DIAGNOSIS ■ **Impaired social interaction related to physical limitations, hospitalizations, social stigma toward HIV infection**

PATIENT GOAL 1: Will participate in peer-group and family activities

NURSING INTERVENTIONS/RATIONALES

Assist child in identifying personal strengths *to facilitate coping*

Educate school personnel and classmates about HIV infection *so that child is not unnecessarily isolated*

Encourage child to participate in activities with other children and family

Encourage child to maintain phone contact with friends during hospitalization *to lessen isolation*

EXPECTED OUTCOME

Child participates in activities with peer group and family

NURSING DIAGNOSIS ■ **Altered sexuality patterns related to risk of disease transmission**

PATIENT GOAL 1: Will exhibit healthy sexual behavior

NURSING INTERVENTIONS/RATIONALES

Educate adolescent about the following *so that adolescent has adequate information to identify safe, healthy expressions of sexuality:*

Sexual transmission

Risks of perinatal infection

Dangers of promiscuity

Abstinence, use of condoms

Avoidance of high-risk behaviors

Encourage adolescent to talk about feelings and concerns related to sexuality *to facilitate coping*

EXPECTED OUTCOMES

Adolescent exhibits a positive sexual identity

Adolescent does not infect other individuals

*Dependent nursing action.

NURSING CARE PLAN   The Child and Adolescent With HIV Infection—*cont'd*

NURSING DIAGNOSIS ■ **Chronic pain related to disease process (i.e., encephalopathy, treatments)**

PATIENT GOAL 1: Will exhibit minimal or no evidence of pain or irritability

NURSING INTERVENTIONS/*RATIONALES*

Assess pain (see Pain Assessment, Chapter 21)

Use nonpharmacologic strategies *to help child manage pain*
  For infants, may try general comfort measures (i.e., rocking, holding, swaddling, reducing environmental stimuli [may or may not be effective because of encephalopathy])

Use pharmacologic strategies (see Pain Management, Chapter 21)
  Plan preventive schedule if analgesics are effective in relieving continuous pain
  Encourage use of premedication for painful procedures *to minimize discomfort* (i.e., use of EMLA)
  Child may benefit from use of adjunctive analgesics (e.g., antiepileptics) that are effective against neuropathic pain

Use pain assessment record *to evaluate effectiveness of pharmacologic and nonpharmacologic interventions*

EXPECTED OUTCOME

Child exhibits absence of or minimal evidence of pain or irritability

NURSING DIAGNOSIS ■ **Interrupted family processes related to having a child with a dreaded and life-threatening disease**

PATIENT (FAMILY) GOAL 1: Will receive adequate support and will be able to meet needs of child

**NURSING INTERVENTIONS/*RATIONALES*
AND EXPECTED OUTCOMES**

See Nursing Care Plan: The Family of the Child Who Is Ill or Hospitalized, Chapter 21

NURSING DIAGNOSIS ■ **Anticipatory grief related to having a child with a potentially fatal illness**

See Nursing Care Plan: The Child Who Is Terminally Ill or Dying, Chapter 18

Children with HIV infection attend day care centers and schools. It is well established that the risk of HIV transmission in these settings is minimal. These institutions are required to follow CDC and Occupational Safety Health Administration (OSHA) guidelines for infection control measures. Standard precautions describing proper management of blood and body fluids should also be followed. It is recommended that school personnel receive current HIV information and include it in the health education curriculum for kindergarten through twelfth grade (American Academy of Pediatrics, 2000; American Academy of Pediatrics, 1999). School nurses play a vital role in educating the school staff, students, and parents. They are also invaluable in monitoring the needs of known affected children.

Confidentiality is a major issue in day care or school attendance. Parents and legal guardians have the right to decide whether they inform these agencies of their child's HIV diagnosis. Unfortunately, myths about HIV infection continue to exist, and the family often wishes to avoid any potential criticism or ostracism of the child.

Nursing care of the child with HIV infection is summarized in the Nursing Care Plan on p. 976 and above.

SEVERE COMBINED IMMUNODEFICIENCY DISEASE

SCID is a defect characterized by absence of both humoral and cell-mediated immunity. The terms *Swiss-type lymphopenic agammaglobulinemia* (an autosomal recessive form of the disease) and *X-linked lymphopenic agammaglobulinemia* have been used to describe this disorder, which, as the names imply, can follow either mode of inheritance.

Susceptibility to infection occurs early in life, most often in the first month of life. The child suffers from chronic infection, fails to completely recover from an infection, is frequently reinfected, and is infected with unusual agents. Failure to thrive is a consequence of the persistent illnesses.

Diagnosis is usually based on a history of recurrent, severe infections from early infancy; a familial history of the disorder; and specific laboratory findings, which include lymphopenia, lack of lymphocyte response to antigens, and absence of plasma cells in the bone marrow. Documentation of immunoglobulin (Ig) deficiency is difficult during infancy because of the normally delayed response of infants in producing their own immunoglobulins and material transfer of IgG.

Therapeutic Management

The only definitive treatment for SCID is HSCT from a histocompatible donor (usually a sibling), a haplo-identical donor (usually a parent), or a matched unrelated donor. IVIG infusions and PCP prophylaxis are used to augment the humoral immunity until the transplant is performed. Several investigators are attempting gene therapy with some success, but there is a potential complication of insertional mutagenesis (Buckley, 2002).

Nursing Considerations

Nursing care focuses on the prevention of infection and supporting the child and family. The care is consistent with that needed for HSCT for any condition (see p. 959). Because the prognosis for SCID is very poor if a compatible bone marrow donor is not available, nursing care is directed at supporting the family in caring for a child with a life-threatening illness (see Chapter 18). Genetic counseling is essential because of the modes of transmission in either form of the disorder.

WISKOTT-ALDRICH SYNDROME

The Wiskott-Aldrich syndrome (WAS) is an X-linked recessive disorder characterized by a triad of abnormalities: (1) thrombocytopenia, (2) eczema, and (3) immunodeficiency of selective functions of B lymphocytes and T lymphocytes. A defective gene has been identified and designated the

WAS protein (Bonilla and Geha, 2003). At birth the presenting symptoms may be bloody diarrhea as a result of thrombocytopenia. As the child grows older, recurrent infection and eczema become more severe, and the bleeding becomes less frequent.

Eczema is typical of the allergic type and easily becomes superinfected. Chronic infection with herpes simplex is a frequent problem and may lead to chronic keratitis of the eye with loss of vision. Chronic pulmonary disease, sinusitis, and otitis media result from repeated infections. In those children who survive the bleeding episodes and overwhelming infections, malignancy presents an additional risk to survival.

Medical treatment involves the following:

1. Counteracting the bleeding tendencies with platelet transfusions
2. Using IV gamma globulin to provide passive immunity
3. Administering prophylactic antibiotics to prevent and control infection.

Splenectomy alone or HSCT may extend the survival to adulthood (Bonilla and Geha, 2003; Champi, 2002).

Nursing Considerations

Because of the poor prognosis for these children, the main nursing consideration is supporting the family in the care of a fatally ill child (see Chapter 18). Physical care is directed at controlling the problems imposed by the disorder. The measures used to control bleeding are similar to those for hemophilia and vWD (see previous discussions). Another major goal is prevention or control of infection. Because eczema is a troublesome problem, nursing measures specific to this condition are especially important (see Chapter 30). The genetic implications of this X-linked recessive disorder differ little from those of any other X-linked disorder.

TECHNOLOGIC MANAGEMENT OF HEMATOLOGIC/IMMUNOLOGIC DISORDERS

BLOOD TRANSFUSION THERAPY

Technologic advances in blood banking and transfusion medicine enable the administration of only the blood component needed by the child, such as packed RBCs in anemia or platelets for bleeding disorders. However, regardless of the blood component infused, all transfusions have some risks. Therefore nurses need to be aware of the possible complications and the appropriate interventions. Table 26-5 summarizes the major hazards of transfusions, the signs and symptoms typically associated with each, and nursing responsibilities. General guidelines that apply to all transfusions include:

- Take vital signs, including blood pressure, *before* administering blood to establish baseline data for intratransfusion and posttransfusion comparison, then every 15 minutes for 1 hour while blood is infusing.
- Check the identification of the recipient with the donor's blood group and type, regardless of the blood product being used.
- Administer the first 50 mL of blood or 20% of the volume (whichever is smaller) *slowly* and stay with the child.

- Administer with normal saline on a piggyback setup or have normal saline available.
- Administer blood through an appropriate filter to eliminate particles in the blood and prevent the precipitation of formed elements; gently shake the container frequently.
- Use blood within 30 minutes of its arrival from the blood bank; if it is not used, return to the blood bank—do not store in the regular unit refrigerator.
- Infuse a unit of blood (or the specified amount) within 4 hours. If the infusion will exceed this time, the blood should be divided into appropriately sized quantities by the blood bank, and the unused portion refrigerated under controlled conditions.
- If a reaction of any type is suspected, take vital signs, stop the transfusion, maintain a patent IV line with normal saline and new tubing, notify the practitioner, and do not restart the transfusion until the child's condition has been medically evaluated.

Although hemolytic reactions are rare, ABO incompatibility remains the most common cause of death from blood transfusion, and human error is usually responsible (administration of the wrong type to the patient or mislabeling of the blood product) (Norville and Bryant, 2002). Hemolysis can also cause the release of large quantities of phospholipids, which are capable of stimulating disseminated intravascular coagulation (see p. 956). Acute kidney shutdown and eventual renal failure are a result of renal vasoconstriction from antigen-antibody complexes derived from the RBC surface.

Blood is usually administered to children by infusion pump; therefore, the usual precautions and management related to pumps apply. When the blood is started with a standard transfusion set, the filter chamber is filled to allow the total filter to be used. The drip chamber is partially filled with blood to permit counting of the drops. In adjusting the flow rate, it is important to remember that blood administration sets do not use microdrops (60 drops/mL) but regular drops (usually 10 or 15 drops/mL). Therefore this must be considered when calculating the flow rate.

HEMATOPOIETIC STEM CELL TRANSPLANTATION

HSCT is used to establish healthy hematopoiesis in both malignant and nonmalignant disease. Candidates for transplantation are children who have disorders that are unlikely to be cured by other means. Most HSCT patients undergo ablative therapy that is intensive using high-dose combination chemotherapy with or without total body irradiation (Ryan and others, 2002). After the body is free of cells and the immune system is suppressed to prevent rejection of the transplanted marrow, the stem cells harvested from the bone marrow, peripheral blood, or the umbilical vein of the placenta are given to the patient by IV transfusion. The newly transfused stem cells will begin to repopulate the ablative bone marrow. In essence, a new blood-forming organ will be accepted by the recipient.

The selection process of a suitable donor and the potential complications in transplantation are related to the *HLA system complex*. Some of the major HLA antigens are A, B, C, D, and DR. There is a wide diversity for each of these HLA loci. There are more than 20 different HLA-A antigens that can be inherited and more than 40 different HLA-B antigens.

TABLE 26-5 ■ **Nursing Care of the Child Receiving Blood Transfusions**

COMPLICATION	SIGNS/SYMPTOMS	PRECAUTIONS/NURSING RESPONSIBILITIES
IMMEDIATE REACTIONS		
Hemolytic reactions		
Most severe type, but rare	Chills	Identify donor and recipient blood types and groups before transfusion is begun; verify with another nurse or practitioner
Incompatible blood	Shaking	
Incompatibility in multiple transfusions	Fever	Transfuse blood slowly for first 15-20 minutes or initial 20% of blood volume; remain with patient
	Pain at needle site and along venous tract	Stop transfusion immediately in event of signs or symptoms, maintain patent intravenous line, and notify practitioner
	Nausea/vomiting	
	Sensation of tightness in chest	Save donor blood to re-crossmatch with patient's blood
	Red or black urine	Monitor for evidence of shock
	Headache	Insert urinary catheter and monitor hourly outputs
	Flank pain	Send sample of patient's blood and urine to laboratory for presence of hemoglobin (indicates intravascular hemolysis)
	Progressive signs of shock or renal failure	
	Sudden severe headache	Observe for signs of hemorrhage resulting from disseminated intravascular coagulation (DIC)
		Support medical therapies to reverse shock
Febrile reactions		
Leukocyte or platelet antibodies	Fever	May give acetaminophen for prophylaxis
Plasma protein antibodies	Chills	Leukocyte poor red blood cells (RBCs) are less likely to cause reaction
		Stop transfusion immediately; report to practitioner for evaluation
Allergic reactions		
Recipient reacts to allergens in donor's blood	Urticaria	Give antihistamines for prophylaxis to children with tendency toward allergic reactions
	Pruritus	
	Flushing	Stop transfusions immediately
	Asthmatic wheezing	Administer epinephrine for wheezing or anaphylactic reaction
	Laryngeal edema	
Circulatory overload		
Too rapid transfusion (even a small quantity)	Precordial pain	Transfuse blood slowly
	Dyspnea	Prevent overload by using packed RBCs or administering divided amounts of blood
Excessive quantity of blood transfused (even slowly)	Rales	
	Cyanosis	Use infusion pump to regulate and maintain flow rate
	Dry cough	Stop transfusion immediately if signs of overload
	Distended neck veins	Place child upright with feet in dependent position to increase venous resistance
	Hypertension	
Air emboli		
May occur when blood is transfused under pressure	Sudden difficulty in breathing	Normalize pressure before container is empty when infusing blood under pressure
	Sharp pain in chest	
	Apprehension	Clear tubing of air by aspirating air with syringe at nearest Y connector if air is observed in tubing; disconnect tubing and allow blood to flow until air has escaped only if a Y connector is not available
Hypothermia		
	Chills	Allow blood to warm at room temperature (less than 1 hour)
	Low temperature	Use approved mechanical blood warmer or electric warming coil to warm blood rapidly; never use microwave oven
	Irregular heart rate	
	Possible cardiac arrest	Take temperature if patient complains of chills; if subnormal, stop transfusion
Electrolyte disturbances		
Hyperkalemia (in massive transfusions or in patients with renal problems)	Nausea, diarrhea	Use washed RBCs or fresh blood if patient is at risk
	Muscular weakness	
	Flaccid paralysis	
	Paresthesia of extremities	
	Bradycardia	
	Apprehension	
	Cardiac arrest	

Continued

TABLE 26-5 ■ **Nursing Care of the Child Receiving Blood Transfusions—*cont'd***

COMPLICATION	SIGNS/SYMPTOMS	PRECAUTIONS/NURSING RESPONSIBILITIES
DELAYED REACTIONS		
Transmission of infection		
Hepatitis	Signs of infection (e.g., jaundice)	Blood is tested for antibiotics to HIV, hepatitis C virus (HCV), and
Human immunodeficiency virus (HIV)	Toxic reaction: high fever, severe	hepatitis B core antigen (HBcAg); in addition, blood is tested
Malaria	headache or substernal pain,	for hepatitis B surface antigen (HBsAg) and alanine amino-
Syphilis	hypotension, intense flushing,	transferase (ALT), and a serology test is performed for syphilis;
Bacteria or viruses	vomiting/diarrhea	positive units are destroyed; individuals at risk for carrying cer-
Other alloimmunization	Increased risk of hemolytic,	tain viruses are deferred from donation
Antibody formation	febrile, and allergic reactions	Report any sign of infection and, if occurring during transfusion,
Occurs in patients receiving multiple		stop transfusion immediately, send sample for culture and sen-
transfusions		sitivity tests, and notify practitioner
		Use limited number of donors
		Observe carefully for signs of reactions
Delayed hemolytic reaction	Destruction of RBCs and fever	Observe for posttransfusion anemia and decreasing benefit from
	5-10 days after transfusion	successive transfusion

The genes are inherited as a single unit or *haplotype.* A child inherits one unit from each parent; thus, a child and each parent have one identical and one nonidentical haplotype. Because the possible haplotype combinations among siblings follow the laws of mendelian genetics, there is a 1-in-4 chance that two siblings have two identical haplotypes and are perfectly matched at the HLA loci.

The importance of HLA matching is to prevent the serious complication known as *GVHD.* Because the child's immune system is essentially rendered nonfunctional, there is little difficulty with bone marrow rejection by the recipient. However, the donor's marrow may contain antigens not matched to the recipient's antigens, which begin attacking body cells. The more closely the HLA systems match, the less likely GVHD is to develop. However, it can occur even with a perfect HLA match, because there are as yet unidentified and thus unmatched histocompatibility antigens (Guinan, Krance, and Lehmann, 2002).

Different types of HSCT are now performed in children with cancer. *Allogeneic HSCT* involves the matching of a histocompatible donor with the recipient. However, allogeneic HSCT is limited by the presence of a suitable marrow donor.

Because of the limited numbers of patients having HLA-identical siblings, other types of allogeneic transplants have evolved. *Umbilical cord blood stem cell transplantation* is an established, rich source of hematopoietic stem cells for use in children with cancer (Ryan and others, 2002). Because stem cells can be found with high frequency in the circulation of newborns, cord blood transplantation has become an alternative for some children (Ryan and others, 2002). The benefit of using umbilical cord blood is the blood's relative immunodeficiency at birth, allowing for partially matched unrelated cord blood transplants to be successful, with a lower risk of GVHD-related problems (Ryan and others, 2002).

Autologous HSCTs use the patient's own marrow that was collected from disease-free tissue, frozen, and sometimes treated to remove malignant cells. Children with solid tumors such as neuroblastoma, Hodgkin disease, NHL, rhabdomyosarcoma, Ewing sarcoma, and Wilms tumor have been treated with autologous HSCTs.

Peripheral stem cell transplants (PSCTs) are also used in children with cancer. PSCT, a type of autologous transplant, differs in the way stem cells are collected from the patient. CSF is first given to stimulate the production of many stem cells (Ryan and others, 2002). After the WBC count is high enough, the stem cells are collected by an "apheresis" machine. This machine filters out peripheral stem cells from whole blood, returning the remainder of the blood cells and plasma to the child. Stem cells have been collected in very small children without problems (Guinan, Krance, and Lehmann, 2002). The peripheral stem cells are then frozen until the patient is ready for the PSCT.

Nursing Considerations

The care of children undergoing HSCT is similar to that of any child receiving chemotherapy and radiotherapy. The hospitalization is typically 3 to 6 weeks in an isolated environment, during which time the child is subjected to numerous procedures and side effects of therapy. Throughout this long ordeal there is the family's concern for successful engraftment and fear of fatal complications (see Family Focus box). Consequently, nurses involved with the child and family need to provide sensitive care and maintain a supportive attitude during the many crises that may arise. If the procedure is not successful, the care needed by these families is consistent with that required by the family of any child with a life-threatening disorder (see Chapter 18).

APHERESIS

Apheresis is the removal of blood from an individual, separation of the blood into its components, retention of one or more of these components, and reinfusion of the remainder of the blood into the individual. Apheresis is most often used to remove large quantities of platelets from healthy adult donors. These transfusion products have greatly prolonged the survival of patients with hematologic and oncologic diseases.

This technique is used to remove peripheral blood stem cells (PBSCs) from children before they receive HSCT or high-dose chemotherapy or radiation therapy, which is severely toxic to the bone marrow. These PBSCs can then be used to restore the child's bone marrow. Apheresis is also

The Decision for a Hematopoietic Stem Cell Transplant

A family's decision for a child to undergo hematopoietic stem cell transplantation (HSCT) may be fraught with challenges. Often the child is facing certain death from the malignancy. The preparation of the child for the transplant also places the patient at great medical risk.

Once the preparatory regimen is begun and the child's immune system is destroyed, there is no turning back. Unlike kidney transplantation, HSCT does not have a "rescue" procedure, such as dialysis, for supportive therapy. If the donor is a sibling, the issue of his or her marrow "saving" the brother or sister can be a concern, especially if the transplant fails. Parents often must leave the home to stay at the transplant center and encounter additional stressors such as arranging childcare, taking a leave from work, and managing finances. The patient faces the greatest stress—fear of HSCT failure or life-threatening complications.

used as a therapeutic modality. The blood component that is diseased or toxic is separated from the blood, and the remainder is returned to the individual. Therapeutic apheresis is considered part of standard therapy for many diseases. Plasma is selectively removed from individuals with hyperviscosity, life-threatening complications of myasthenia gravis, Guillain-Barré syndrome, thrombotic thrombocytopenic purpura, and certain drug overdoses. WBCs are removed from individuals with high-WBC-count leukemia.

Nursing Considerations

Difficult venous access and small blood volume can limit the ability to use this therapy in the infant and young child. Education of the family and child focuses on the purposes of the therapy, as well as the technology.

Specially trained individuals perform the apheresis procedure. Attention focuses on rate of removal, blood component separation, and reinfusion of blood into the child. Vital signs are monitored, and the child is continuously observed for any adverse reactions secondary to the circulatory volume changes and the anticoagulant used.

When apheresis components are infused, nursing measures will differ depending on whether the product is autologous (blood component from the child) or allogeneic (blood component from another individual). Autologous components are the child's own blood; therefore, a major precaution is proper identification to ensure the correct component. The rate of infusion should be adjusted to the child's tolerance. If the product is allogeneic, all precautions for blood transfusions apply.

KEY POINTS

■ Anemia is defined as reduction of red blood cells or hemoglobin concentration to levels below normal for age; disorders are classified either by etiology/physiology or by morphology.

■ The role of the nurse in treatment of anemia is to assist in establishing a diagnosis, prepare the child for laboratory tests, ad-

minister prescribed medications, decrease tissue oxygen needs, implement safety precautions, and observe for complications.

■ The main nursing goal in prevention of nutritional anemia is parent education regarding correct feeding practices.

■ Sickle cell anemia is a hereditary hemoglobinopathy caused by normal adult hemoglobin (Hgb A) being partly or completely replaced by sickle hemoglobin (Hgb S).

■ Nursing care of the child with sickle cell anemia is focused on teaching the family how to prevent and recognize sickle cell problems, manage pain during crises, and help the child and parents adjust to a lifelong, chronic disease.

■ Nursing care of the child with thalassemia includes observing for complications of multiple blood transfusions, assisting the child in coping with the effects of illness, and fostering parent-child adjustment to long-term illness.

■ Causes of acquired aplastic anemia include irradiation, drugs, industrial and household chemicals, infections, and infiltration and replacement of myeloid elements; however, the majority of the causes are idiopathic.

■ Clotting depends on three processes: vascular spasm, platelet aggregation, and coagulation and clot formation.

■ Nursing care of the child with hemophilia involves preventing bleeding by decreasing the risk of injury, recognizing and managing bleeding with factor replacement, preventing the crippling effects of joint degeneration, and preparing and supporting the child and family for home care.

■ Goals in the care of the child with leukemia are to prepare the family for diagnostic and therapeutic procedures, prevent complications of myelosuppression, manage problems of irradiation and drug toxicity, and provide continued emotional support.

■ The lymphomas include Hodgkin and non-Hodgkin lymphoma and are disorders involving the lymphoid system.

■ Immunodeficiency disorders render the affected individual unable to fight infectious organisms.

■ HIV infection is primarily acquired in infants from a parent with HIV infection and in adolescents from engaging in high-risk behaviors.

■ Blood transfusions supply needed blood components.

■ Hematopoietic stem cell transplantation replaces the diseased or malfunctioning bone marrow with viable blood stem cells.

■ Apheresis is the selective removal of a blood component. It can be used to supply cellular elements needed for therapy (i.e., platelets or stem cells) or to remove diseased components.

References

American Academy of Pediatrics, Section of Hematology/Oncology, Committee on Genetics: Health supervision for children with sickle cell disease, *Pediatrics* 109(3):526-536, 2002.

American Academy of Pediatrics, Committee on Pediatric AIDS: Identification and care of HIV-exposed and HIV-infected infants, children, and adolescents in foster care, *Pediatrics* 106(1):149-153, 2000.

American Academy of Pediatrics and the Committee on Pediatric AIDS: Technical report: perinatal human immunodeficiency virus testing and prevention of transmission, *Pediatrics* 106(6):1-12, 2000.

American Academy of Pediatrics, Committee on Pediatric AIDS and Committee on Infectious Diseases: Issues related to human immunodeficiency virus transmission in schools, child care, medical settings, the home, and community, *Pediatrics* 104(2):318-324, 1999.

American Academy of Pediatrics, Committee on Infectious Diseases, Pickering L, editor: *2003 Red Book: report of the Committee on Infectious Diseases*, ed 26, Elk Grove Village, Il, 2003, The Academy.

American Pain Society: *Guidelines for the management of acute and chronic pain in sickle-cell disease*, Glenview, Il, 1999, American Pain Society.

Andrews NC: Disorders of iron metabolism and sideroblastic anemia. In Nathan D, Orkin SH, Ginsburg D, Look AT, editors: *Nathan and Oski's hematology of infancy and childhood*, ed 6, Philadelphia, 2003, WB Saunders.

Bell WR: Role of splenectomy in immune (idiopathic) thrombocytopenic purpura, *Blood Rev* 16:39-41, 2002.

Bogen DL, Krause JP, Serwint JR: Outcome of children identified as anemic by routine screening in an inner-city clinic, *Arch Pediatr Adolesc Med* 155:366-371, 2001.

Bonilla FA, Geha RS: Primary immunodeficiency diseases. In Nathan D, Orkin SH, Ginsburg D, Look AT, editors: *Nathan and Oski's hematology of infancy and childhood*, ed 6, Philadelphia, 2003, WB Saunders.

Bryant, R: Managing side effects of childhood cancer treatment, *J Pediatr Nurs* 18(2):113-125, 2003.

Buckley RH: Gene therapy for SCID—a complication after remarkable progress, *Lancet* 360:1185-86, 2002.

Butler RB and others: Promoting safer sex among HIV-positive youth with haemophilia: theory, intervention, and outcome, *Haemophilia* 9(2):214-222, 2003.

Carley A: Anemia: when is it iron deficiency? *Pediatr Nurs* 29(2): 127-133, 2003.

Centers for Disease Control and Prevention: 1994 revised classified system for human immunodeficiency virus infection in children less than 13 years of age, *MMWR* 43(RR-12):1-10, 1994.

Centers for Disease Control and Prevention: 1995 revised guidelines for prophylaxis against *Pneumocystis carinii* pneumonia for children infected with or perinatally exposed to human immunodeficiency virus, *MMWR* 44(RR-4):1-11, 1995.

Centers for Disease Control and Prevention: *HIV/AIDS surveillance report*, 2001, 13:2, 2001.

Champi C: Primary immunodeficiency disorders in children: prompt diagnosis can lead to lifesaving treatment, *J Pediatr Health Care* 16:16-21, 2002.

Charache S and others: Hydroxyurea and sickle cell anemia: clinical utility of a myelosuppressive switching agent, *Medicine* 75(6):300-326, 1996.

Chiocca EM: Sickle cell crisis: severe pain and potential tissue necrosis are the major concerns, *Am J Nurs* 96(9):49, 1996.

Cho S, Cheng AC, Cheng MCK: Oral care for children with leukemia, *Hong Kong Med J* 6(2):203-208, 2000.

Chu YW, Korb J, Sakamoto KM: Idiopathic thrombocytopenia purpura, *Pediatr Rev* 21(3):95-104, 2000.

Colby-Graham MF, Chordas C: The childhood leukemias, *J Pediatr Nurs* 18(2):87-95, 2003.

Davidsson L: Approaches to improve iron bioavailability from complementary foods, *J Nutr* 133(5 suppl 1):1560S-2S, 2003.

Dover GJ, Platt OS: Sickle cell disease. In Nathan D, Orkin SH, Ginsburg D, Look AT, editors: *Nathan and Oski's hematology of infancy and childhood*, ed 6, Philadelphia, 2003, WB Saunders.

Dragone MA, Karp S: Bleeding disorders. In Jackson PL, Vessey JA, editors: *Primary care of the child with a chronic condition*, ed 2, St Louis, 1996, Mosby.

Ezekowitz RAB, Stockman III JA: Hematologic manifestations of systemic diseases. In Nathan D, Orkin SH, Ginsburg D, Look AT, editors: *Nathan and Oski's hematology of infancy and childhood*, ed 6, Philadelphia, 2003, WB Saunders.

Ferster A and others: Five years of experience with hydroxyurea in children and young adults with sickle cell disease, *Blood* 97(11): 3628-3632, 2001.

Fischer K and others: Changes in treatment strategies for severe haemophilia over the last 3 decades: effects of clotting factor consumption and arthropathy, *Haemophilia* 7:446-452, 2001.

Gribbons D, Zahr LK, Opas SR: Nursing management of children with sickle cell disease: an update, *J Pediatr Nurs* 10(4):232-242, 1995.

Griffin TC, McIntire D, Buchanan GR: High-dose intravenous methylprednisolone therapy for pain in children and adolescents with sickle cell disease, *N Engl J Med* 330(11):733-737, 1994.

Griffins IJ, Abrams SA: Iron and breastfeeding, *Pediatr Clin North Am* 48:401, 2001.

Guinan ED, Krance RA, Lehmann LE: Stem cell transplantation in pediatric oncology. In Pizzo PA, Poplack DG, editors: *Principles and practice of pediatric oncology*, ed 4, Philadelphia, 2002, JB Lippincott.

Halterman JS and others: Iron deficiency and cognitive achievement among school-aged children and adolescents in the United States, *Pediatrics* 107(6):1381-1386, 2001.

Hudson MM, Donaldson SS: Hodgkins disease. In Pizzo PA, Poplack DG, editors: *Principles and practice of pediatric oncology*, ed 4, Philadelphia, 2002, JB Lippincott.

Ioannidis JP and others: Perinatal transmission of human immunodeficiency virus type I by pregnant women with RNA virus loads <1000 copies 1 ml, *J Infect Dis* 183:539-545, 2001.

Karayalcin G: Hemolytic anemia (sickle cell anemia). In Lanzkowsky P, editor: *Manual of pediatric hematology and oncology*, ed 3, San Diego, 2000, Academic Press.

Khoury H, Grimsley E: Oxygen inhalation in nonhypoxic sickle cell patients during vaso-occlusive crisis, *Blood* 86(10):3998, 1995.

Link MP, Donaldson SS: The lymphomas and lymphadenopathy. In Nathan D, Orkin SH, Ginsburg D, Look AT, editors: *Nathan and Oski's hematology of infancy and childhood*, ed 6, Philadelphia, 2003, WB Saunders.

Lyall EGH: Paediatric HIV in 2002—a treatable and preventable infection, *J Clin Virol* 25:107-119, 2002.

Margolin JF, Steuber CP, Poplack DG: Acute lymphoblastic leukemia. In Pizzo PA, Poplack DG, editors: *Principles and practice of pediatric oncology*, ed 4, Philadelphia, 2002, JB Lippincott.

Meldrum J: Nevirapine efficacy underestimated for protecting babies from HIV? *AIDSmap* retrieved August 18, 2003, from www.aidsmap.com.

Merchant RC, Keshavarz R: Human immunodeficiency virus postexposure prophylaxis for adolescents and children *Pediatrics* 108(2): 1-13, 2001.

Miller ST and others: Prediction of adverse outcomes in children with sickle cell disease, *N Engl J Med* 342(2):83-89, 2000.

Montgomery RR, Gill JC, Scott JP: Hemophilia and von Willebrand disease. In Nathan D, Orkin SH, Ginsburg D, Look AT, editors: *Nathan and Oski's hematology of infancy and childhood*, ed 6, Philadelphia, 2003, WB Saunders.

Morbidity and Mortality Weekly Report: Advancing HIV prevention: new strategies for a changing epidemic—United States, *MMWR* 52(15):329-332, 2003.

National Hemophilia Foundation, Bleeding Disorders Information Center: Newly diagnosed: parents FAQ 2003. Retrieved August 23, 2003, from www.hemophilia.org/bdi/bdi_newly7c.htm.

National Institute of Allergy and Infectious Diseases, National Institutes of Health (NIAID/NIH): HIV infection and AIDS: an overview, *Anthrax, NIAID fact sheet*, 2003. Retrieved August 18, 2003, from www.niaid.nih.gov/factsheets/hivinf.htm.

National Institutes of Health; National Heart, Lung, and Blood Institute (NIH/NHLBI), Division of Blood Disease and Resources: *The management of sickle cell disease*, NIH pub no 02-2117, Bethesda, Md, 2002, NHLBI Health Information Network.

Nolan B and others: Unsuspected haemophilia in children with a single swollen joint, *Br Med J* 326:151-152, 2003.

Norville R, Bryant R: Blood component deficiencies. In Baggott C and others, editors: *APON nursing care of children and adolescents with cancer*, ed 3, Philadelphia, 2002, WB Saunders.

Orkin SH, Nathan DG: The thalassemias. In Nathan D, Orkin SH, Ginsburg D, Look AT, editors: *Nathan and Oski's hematology of infancy and childhood*, ed 6, Philadelphia, 2003, WB Saunders.

Paley C: Hemolytic anemia (thalassemias). In Lanzkowsky P, editor: *Manual of pediatric hematology and oncology*, ed 3, San Diego, 2000, Academic Press.

Perkins S: Disorders of hematopoiesis. In Collins RD, Swerdlow SH, editors: *Pediatric hematopathology,* ed 1, Philadelphia, 2001, Churchill Livingstone.

Platt OS, Guinan EC: Bone marrow transplantations in sickle cell anemia: the dilemma of choice, *N Engl J Med* 335(6):426-427, 1996.

Redner A: Leukemias. In Lanzkowsky P, editor: *Manual of pediatric hematology and oncology,* ed 3, San Diego, 2000, Academic Press.

Ryan LG and others: Hematopoietic stem cell transplantation. In Baggott CR, Kelly KP, Fochtman D, Foley CV, editors: *Nursing care of children and adolescents with cancer,* ed 3, Philadelphia, 2002, WB Saunders.

Segel GB, Hirsch MG, Feig SA: Managing anemia in a pediatric office practice: part 1, *Pediatr Rev* 23(3):75-83, 2002.

Segel GB, Hirsch MG, Feig SA: Managing anemia in a pediatric office practice: part 2, *Pediatr Rev* 23(4):111-121, 2002.

Shende A: Bone marrow failure. In Lanzkowsky P, editor: *Manual of pediatric hematology and oncology,* ed 3, San Diego, 2000, Academic Press.

Shimamura A, Guinan EC: Acquired aplastic anemia. In Nathan D, Orkin SH, Ginsburg D, Look AT, editors: *Nathan and Oski's hematology of infancy and childhood,* ed 6, Philadelphia, 2003, WB Saunders.

Silverman LB, Sallan SE: Acute lymphoblastic leukemia. In Nathan D, Orkin SH, Ginsburg D, Look AT, editors: *Nathan and Oski's hematology of infancy and childhood,* ed 6, Philadelphia, 2003, WB Saunders.

Simon K, Lobo ML, Jackson S: Current knowledge in the management of children and adolescents with sickle cell disease: part 1, physiological issues, *J Pediatr Nurs* 14(5):281-295, 1999.

Steinberg MH and others: Effect of hydroxyurea on mortality and morbidity in adult sickle cell anemia: risks and benefits up to 9 years of treatment, *JAMA* 289(13):1645-1651, 2003.

Sullivan JL, Woda BA: Lymphohistiocytic disorders. In Nathan D, Orkin SH, Ginsburg D, Look AT, editors: *Nathan and Oski's hematology of infancy and childhood,* ed 6, Philadelphia, 2003, WB Saunders.

Wilson DB: Acquired platelet defects. In Nathan D, Orkin SH, Ginsburg D, Look AT, editors: *Nathan and Oski's hematology of infancy and childhood,* ed 6, Philadelphia, 2003, WB Saunders.

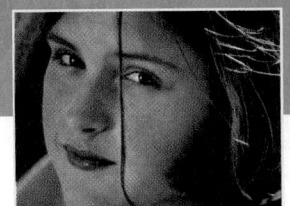

27

The Child With Genitourinary Dysfunction

BARBARA MONTAGNINO and HELEN CURRIER

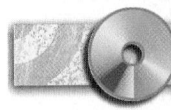
Remember to check out your companion CD-ROM

http://evolve.elsevier.com/Wong/essentials/

CHAPTER OUTLINE

RELATED TOPICS and ADDITIONAL RESOURCES

 IN TEXT

Administration of Medication, *Ch. 22*
Anemia, *Ch. 26*
Collection of Specimens, *Ch. 22*
Impact of Chronic Illness, Disability, or
   Death on the Child and Family, *Ch. 18*
Infection Control, *Ch. 22*
Physical Examination: Genitalia, *Ch. 7*
Preparation for Procedures, *Ch. 22*
Surgical Procedures, *Ch. 22*
Systemic Hypertension, *Ch. 25*

 CD COMPANION

Guidelines—Prevention of Urinary Tract
   Infections
Clinical Manifestations—Urinary Tract
   Disorders or Disease; Acute Renal
   Failure; Chronic Renal Failure
Nursing Care Plan
NCLEX-Style Review Questions

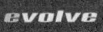 WEBSITE

WebLinks
NCLEX-Style Review Questions
   **WONG'S CLINCAL MANUAL
   OF PEDIATRIC NURSING, ED 6**

Community and Home Care
   Instructions—Giving Medications to
   Children; Collecting a Urine Sample
Nursing Care Plan—The Child With Uri-
   nary Tract Infection

GENITOURINARY DYSFUNCTION

ASSESSMENT OF RENAL FUNCTION

Assessment of kidney and urinary tract integrity and diagnosis of renal or urinary tract disease are based on several evaluative tools. Physical examination, history taking, and observation of symptoms are the initial procedures. In suspected urinary tract diseases or disorders, further assessment by laboratory, radiologic, and other evaluative methods is carried out.

Clinical Manifestations

As in most disorders of childhood, the incidence and type of kidney or urinary tract dysfunction change with the age and maturation of the child. In addition, the presenting complaints and the significance of these complaints vary with maturation. For example, a complaint of enuresis has greater significance at age 8 years than at age 4. In the newborn, urinary tract disorders are associated with a number of obvious malformations of other body systems, including the curious and unexplained but frequent association between malformed or low-set ears and urinary tract anomalies.

Many of the clinical manifestations of renal disease are common to a variety of childhood disorders, but their presence is an indication to obtain further information from the child's history, family history, and laboratory studies as part of a complete physical examination. Suspected renal disease can be further evaluated by means of radiographic studies and renal biopsy (Table 27-1).

Laboratory Tests

Both urine and blood studies contribute vital information for detection of renal problems. The single most important test is probably routine urinalysis. Specific urine and blood tests provide additional information. Because nurses are usually the persons who collect the specimens for examination and who often perform many of the screening tests, they should be familiar with the test, its function, and factors that can alter or distort the results of the test. The major urine and blood tests are outlined in Tables 27-2 and 27-3.

Nursing Considerations

Nursing responsibilities in assessment of genitourinary disorders or diseases begin with observation of the child for any manifestations that might indicate dysfunction. Many conditions have specific characteristics that distinguish them from other disorders. These are discussed as appropriate throughout the chapter.

The nurse is generally the one who is responsible for preparing infants, children, and parents for tests and for collection of urine and (sometimes) blood specimens (see Preparation for Procedures, Chapter 22, and Collection of Specimens, Chapter 22) for observation and laboratory analysis. An important nursing responsibility is to maintain careful *intake and output* measurements and *blood pressure* on most children with genitourinary dysfunction and those who might be at risk for developing renal complications (e.g., children in shock, postoperative patients). For example, any significant degree of renal disease can diminish the glomerular filtration rate, a measure of the amount of plasma from which a given substance is totally cleared in 1 minute. A number of substances can be used, but the most useful clinical estimation of glomerular filtration is the clearance of *creatinine,* an end product of protein metabolism in muscle and a substance that is freely filtered by the glomerulus and secreted by renal tubular cells. The nurse's responsibility in this test is collection of urine, usually a 12- or 24-hour specimen.

GENITOURINARY TRACT DISORDERS/DEFECTS

URINARY TRACT INFECTION

Infection of the genitourinary tract is one of the most common conditions of childhood. Up to 10% of children will have a febrile urinary tract infection (UTI) during the first 2 years of life (Rosenthal, 2004). UTI may involve the urethra and bladder (lower urinary tract), or the ureters, renal pelvis, calyces, and renal parenchyma (upper urinary tract). Because it is often impossible to localize the infection, the broad designation UTI is applied to the presence of significant numbers of microorganisms anywhere within the urinary tract, except the distal third of the urethra, which is usually colonized with bacteria. The peak incidence of UTI not caused by structural anomalies occurs between 2 and 6 years of age, and except for the neonatal period, females have a higher risk for developing UTI (Table 27-4). This coincides with toilet training and establishing voiding habits.

TABLE 27-1 ■ Radiologic and Other Tests of Urinary System Function

TEST	PROCEDURE	PURPOSE	COMMENTS AND NURSING RESPONSIBILITIES
Urine culture and sensitivity	Collection of sterile specimen	Determines presence of pathogens and the drugs to which they are sensitive	Does not require specific parental permission Send specimen to laboratory immediately after collection Catheterization, clean-catch, or suprapubic specimen
Renal/bladder ultrasound	Transmission of ultrasonic waves through renal parenchyma, along ureteral course, and over bladder	Allows visualization of renal parenchyma, renal pelvis without exposure to external beam radiation or radioactive isotopes Visualization of dilated ureters and bladder wall also possible	Noninvasive procedure
Testicular (scrotal) ultrasound	Transmission of ultrasonic waves through scrotal contents and testis	Allows visualization of scrotal contents, including testis Testicular ultrasound is used to identify masses, and Doppler-enhanced ultrasound is used to differentiate hyperemia of epididymo-orchitis from ischemia or torsion	Noninvasive procedure
Scout film	Flat plate roentgenogram of abdomen and pelvis for kidney, ureters, bladder (KUB)	Detects and establishes renal outlines, presence of calculi, or opaque foreign bodies in bladder	Prepare as for routine x-ray film
Voiding cysto-urethrography	Contrast medium injected into bladder through urethral catheter until bladder is full; films taken before, during, and after voiding	Visualizes bladder outline and urethra, reveals reflux of urine into ureters, and shows complications of bladder emptying	Prepare child for catheterization
Radionuclide (nuclear) cystogram	Radionuclide-containing fluid injected through urethral catheter until bladder is full; images generated before, during, and after voiding	Alternative to voiding cystourethrography in children with allergy to intravesical contrast material Allows evaluation of reflux, although visualization of anatomic details is relatively poor	Prepare child for catheterization Reassure patient and parents that allergic response to contrast materials is avoided by use of radionuclide
Radioisotope imaging studies	Contrast medium injected intravenously; computer analysis to measure uptake or washout (excretion) for analysis of organ function	DTPA radioisotope used to measure glomerular filtration rate; estimate of differential renal function and renal washout to determine presence and location of upper urinary tract obstruction DMSA radioisotope allows visualization of renal scars and differential renal function; ureters and bladder are not visualized MAG 3 radioisotope combines features of DTPA (evaluation of upper urinary tract obstruction) with features of DMSA radioisotope (differential renal function)	Insert or assist with insertion of intravenous infusion Monitor intravenous infusion Urethral catheterization may accompany DTPA radioisotope scan; prepare child for catheterization when indicated
Intravenous pyelography (IVP) (intravenous urogram; excretory urogram)	Intravenous injection of a contrast medium Medium secreted and concentrated by tubules X-ray films made 5, 10, and 15 minutes after injection; delayed films (30, 60 minutes, etc.), are obtained if obstruction suspected	Defines urinary tract Provides information about integrity of kidneys, ureters, and bladder Retroperitoneal masses visualized when they shift position of ureters	Preparation for test: Infants less than 2 years of age—no solid food, omit one bottle on morning of examination; studies should be performed early to avoid withholding of fluids Children age 2-14 years of age—give cathartic evening before examination, nothing orally after midnight, enema (soapsuds) morning of examination

TABLE 27-1 ■ Radiologic and Other Tests of Urinary System Function—*cont'd*

TEST	PROCEDURE	PURPOSE	COMMENTS AND NURSING RESPONSIBILITIES
Computed tomography (CT)	Narrow-beam x-rays and computer analysis provide precise reconstruction of area	Visualizes vertical or horizontal cross section of kidney. Especially valuable to distinguish tumors and cysts	Noncontrast scan is noninvasive. Contrast-enhanced CT scan preparation is similar to IVP
Cystoscopy	Direct visualization of bladder and lower urinary tract through small scope inserted via urethra	Investigation of bladder and lower tract lesions; visualizes ureteral openings, bladder wall, trigone, and urethra	Give nothing orally after midnight. Carry out preoperative preparations. Prepare the child for cystoscopy
Retrograde pyelography	Contrast medium injected through ureteral catheter	Visualizes pelvic calyces, ureters, and bladder	
Renal angiography	Contrast medium injected directly into renal artery via catheter placed in femoral artery (or umbilical artery in newborn) and advanced to renal artery	Visualizes renal vascular system, especially for renal arterial stenosis	Give cathartic if ordered. Give preoperative medication if ordered. Observe for reaction to contrast medium. Monitor vital signs after procedure
Whitaker perfusion test	Injection of contrast material through renal pelvis and ureters. Pressures are measured in renal pelvis and urinary bladder	Determine presence of obstruction causing upper urinary tract dilation	Prepare child for insertion of a spinal needle or perfusion catheter in renal pelvis (anesthetic often required)
Renal biopsy	Removal of kidney tissue by open or percutaneous technique for study by light, electron, or immunofluorescent microscopy	Yields histologic and microscopic information about glomeruli and tubules; helps to distinguish between types of nephritic syndromes. Distinguishes other renal disorders	Give nothing orally 4-6 hours before test. Premedicate as ordered. Prepare setup for procedure. Assist with procedure. Take vital signs. Apply pressure to area with pressure dressing and, if feasible, a sandbag. Bed rest for 24 hours. Observe for abdominal pain, tenderness. Monitor input and output; surgical incision may be required in infants
Urodynamics	Set of tests designed to measure bladder filling, storage, and evacuation functions. Uroflowmetry is a test to determine efficiency of urination. Cystometrogram is a graphic comparison of bladder pressure as a function of volume. Voiding pressure study is a comparison of detrusor contraction pressure, sphincter electromyelogram, and urinary flow	Determine characteristic of voiding dysfunction. Used to identify type (cause) of incontinence or urinary retention. Especially valuable for voiding dysfunction complicated by urinary infection, urinary retention, or neurogenic bladder dysfunction	Prepare child for catheterization. Insertion of a rectal tube will produce feelings of rectal fullness or pressure. Insertion of needles may be required for sphincter electromyography

TABLE 27-2 ■ Urine Tests of Renal Function

TEST	NORMAL RANGE	DEVIATIONS	SIGNIFICANCE OF DEVIATIONS
PHYSICAL TESTS			
Volume	Age-related. Newborn: 30-60 mL. Children: Bladder capacity (oz) = Age (years) + 2	Polyuria	Osmotic factors (urinary glucose level in diabetes mellitus)
		Oliguria	Retention caused by obstructive disease. Inadequate bladder emptying caused by neurogenic bladder or obstructive disorder
		Anuria	Obstruction of urinary tract; acute renal failure

Continued

TABLE 27-2 ■ **Urine Tests of Renal Function—*cont'd***

TEST	NORMAL RANGE	DEVIATIONS	SIGNIFICANCE OF DEVIATIONS
Specific gravity	With normal fluid intake: 1.016-1.022 Newborn: 1.001-1.020	High	Dehydration Presence of protein or glucose Presence of radiopaque contrast medium after radiologic examinations
	Others: 1.001-1.030	Low	Excessive fluid intake Distal tubular dysfunction Insufficient antidiuretic hormone Diuresis
Osmolality	Newborn: 50-600 mOsm/L Thereafter: 50-1400 mOsm/L	Fixed at 1.010 High or low	Chronic glomerular disease Same as for specific gravity More sensitive index than specific gravity
Appearance	Clear pale yellow to deep gold	Cloudy Cloudy reddish pink to reddish brown Light Dark Red	Contains sediment Blood from trauma or disease Myoglobin after severe muscle destruction Dilute Concentrated Trauma

CHEMICAL TESTS

TEST	NORMAL RANGE	DEVIATIONS	SIGNIFICANCE OF DEVIATIONS
pH	Newborn: 5-7 Thereafter: 4.8-7.8 Average: 6	Weak acid or neutral	If associated with metabolic acidosis, suggests tubular acidosis If associated with metabolic alkalosis, suggests potassium deficiency Urinary infection
		Alkaline	Metabolic alkalosis
Protein level	Absent	Present	Abnormal glomerular permeability (e.g., glomerular disease, changes in blood pressure) Most kidney disease Orthostatic in some individuals
Glucose level	Absent	Present	Diabetes mellitus Infusion of concentrated glucose-containing fluids Glomerulonephritis Impaired tubular reabsorption
Ketone levels	Absent	Present	Conditions of acute metabolic demand (stress) Diabetic ketoacidosis
Leukocyte esterase	Absent	Present	Can identify both lysed and intact white blood cells via enzyme detection
Nitrites	Absent	Present	Most species of bacteria convert nitrates to nitrites in the urine

MICROSCOPIC TESTS

TEST	NORMAL RANGE	DEVIATIONS	SIGNIFICANCE OF DEVIATIONS
White blood cell count	Less than 1 or 2	More than 5 polymorphonuclear leukocytes/field	Urinary tract inflammatory process
		Lymphocytes	Allograft rejection Malignancy
Red blood cell count	Less than 1 or 2	4-6/field in centrifuged specimen	Trauma Stones Glomerular injury Infection Neoplasms
Presence of bacteria	Absent to a few	More than 100,000 organisms/mL in centrifuged specimen	Urinary tract infection
Presence of casts	Occasional	Granular casts	Tubular or glomerular disorders Degenerative process in advanced renal disease

		Cellular casts
		   White blood cell
		   Red blood cell
		Hyaline casts
			Pyelonephritis
			Glomerulonephritis
			Proteinuria; usually transient

TABLE 27-3 ■ Blood Tests of Renal Function

TEST	NORMAL RANGE (mg/dl)	DEVIATIONS	SIGNIFICANCE OF DEVIATIONS
Blood urea nitrogen (BUN)	Newborn: 4-18 Infant, child: 5-18	Elevated	Renal disease—acute or chronic (the higher the BUN, the more severe the disease) Increased protein catabolism Dehydration Hemorrhage High protein intake Corticosteroid therapy
Uric acid Creatinine	Child: 2.0-5.5 Infant: 0.2-0.4 Child: 0.3-0.7 Adolescent: 0.5-1.0	Increased Increased	Severe renal disease Severe renal impairment

TABLE 27-4 ■ Sex Ratio of Urinary Tract Infections

	FEMALES	MALES
Neonate	0.4	1
1-6 months	1.5	1
6-12 months	4.0	1
1-3 years	10.0	1
3-11 years	9.0	1
11-16 years	2.0	1

From Belman AB, Kaplan GW: *Genitourinary problems in pediatrics*, Philadelphia, 1981, WB Saunders; modified from Winberg J and others: Epidemiology of symptomatic urinary tract infection in childhood, *Acta Paediatr Scand Suppl* 252:1, 1974.

Classification

Infection of the urinary tract may be present with or without clinical symptoms. As a result, the site of infection is often difficult to pinpoint with any degree of accuracy. Various terms used to describe urinary tract disorders include:

Bacteriuria—Presence of bacteria in the urine
Asymptomatic bacteriuria—Significant bacteriuria with no evidence of clinical infection (usually defined as greater than 100,000 colony-forming units [CFUs])
Symptomatic bacteriuria—Bacteriuria accompanied by physical signs of urinary infection (dysuria, suprapubic discomfort, hematuria, fever)
Recurrent UTI—Repeated episode of bacteriuria or symptomatic UTI
Persistent UTI—Persistence of bacteriuria despite antibiotic treatment
Febrile UTI—Bacteriuria accompanied by fever and other physical signs of urinary infection; presence of a fever typically implies a pyelonephritis
Cystitis—Inflammation of the bladder
Urethritis—Inflammation of the urethra
Pyelonephritis—Inflammation of the upper urinary tract and kidneys
Urosepsis—Febrile urinary tract infection coexisting with systemic signs of bacterial illness; blood culture reveals presence of urinary pathogen

Etiology

A variety of organisms can be responsible for UTI. *Escherichia coli* (80% of cases) and other gram-negative enteric organisms are most frequently implicated; these organisms are usually found in the anal and perineal region. Other organisms associated with UTI include *Proteus, Pseudomonas, Klebsiella, Staphylococcus aureus, Haemophilus,* and coagulase-negative *Staphylococcus.* Several factors contribute to the development of UTI in childhood.

Anatomic and Physical Factors. The structure of the lower urinary tract is believed to account for the increased incidence of bacteriuria in females (Rosenthal, 2004). The short urethra, which measures about 2 cm (0.75 inch) in young girls and 4 cm (1.5 inches) in mature women, provides a ready pathway for invasion of organisms. In addition, the closure of the urethra at the end of micturition may return contaminated bacteria to the bladder. The longer male urethra (as long as 20 cm [8 inches] in an adult) and the antibacterial properties of prostatic secretions inhibit the entry and growth of pathogens.

> **FYI**
>
> Considerable evidence suggests there are fewer UTIs among circumcised male infants than among uncircumcised male infants, but the difference is not significant enough to recommend routine circumcision in newborns (American Academy of Pediatrics, 1999).

The single most important host factor influencing the occurrence of UTI is ***urinary stasis.*** Ordinarily, urine is sterile, but at 37° C (98.6° F) it provides an excellent culture medium. Under normal conditions the act of completely and repeatedly emptying the bladder flushes away any organisms before they have an opportunity to multiply and invade surrounding tissue. However, urine that remains in the bladder allows bacteria from the urethra to rapidly become established in the rich medium. Incomplete bladder emptying (stasis) may result from *reflux* (see Vesicoureteral Reflux), anatomic abnormalities (especially those involving the ureters), dysfunction of the voiding mechanism, or extrinsic ureteral or bladder compression that may be caused by constipation. The key to preventing UTI is to maintain adequate blood supply to the bladder wall by avoidance of overdistention and high bladder pressure.

Altered Urine and Bladder Chemistry. Several mechanical and chemical characteristics of the urine and bladder mucosa help maintain urinary sterility. An increased fluid intake promotes flushing of the normal bladder and lowers the concentration of organisms in the infected bladder. Diuresis also seems to enhance the antibacterial properties of the renal medulla.

Most pathogens favor an alkaline medium. Normally, urine is slightly acidic. A urine pH of about 5 hampers bacterial multiplication, although the acidification rarely eliminates the bacteriuria. Much has been reported about the use of cranberry juice for the prevention of UTI. This mechanism was initially thought to result from increased urine acidity. However, a study of children with neurogenic bladder shows ingestion of cranberry juice results in a median pH of only 6.0. Urine is bacteriostatic to *E. coli* at a pH of 5.0 (attainable only by injection of pure hippuric acid). Further findings from this study suggest the antiadherence properties of cranberries are most often observed in UTI caused by fimbriated *E. coli* strains, which are more common in healthy patients with UTI and less common in patients with chronic medical illnesses or urinary tract anomalies (Schlager and others, 1999). Further research is needed to determine the efficacy of cranberry products in children with UTI.

Diagnostic Evaluation

The clinical manifestations of UTI depend on the age of the child (Box 27-1). Diagnosis of UTI is confirmed by detection of bacteriuria in urine culture, but urine collection is often difficult, especially in infants and very small children. Several factors may alter a urine specimen, and contamination of a specimen by organisms from sources other than the urine, such as perineal and perianal flora in bag specimens, is the most frequent cause of false-positive results. Unless the specimen is a first morning sample, a recent high fluid intake may indicate a falsely low organism count. Therefore children should not be encouraged to drink large volumes of water in an attempt to obtain a specimen quickly.

> **NURSING ALERT**
>
> A child who exhibits the following should be evaluated for UTI:
> Incontinence in a toilet-trained child
> Strong-smelling urine
> Frequency or urgency

More accurate estimates of bacterial content are obtained from *suprapubic aspiration* (in children younger than 2 years of age) and properly performed bladder catheterization (as long as the first few milliliters are excluded from collection). The specimen should be taken directly to the laboratory for culture immediately.

Tests to detect bacteriuria are being used with increased frequency in screening for UTI. The dipstick tests that test for leukocyte esterase or nitrite are quick and inexpensive methods for detecting infection before obtaining final culture results.

Localization of the infection site may involve more specific tests, including percutaneous kidney taps and bladder washout procedures. Other tests such as ultrasonography, voiding cystourethrogram (VCUG), intravenous pyelogram (IVP), and DSMA (dimercaptosuccinic acid) scan may be performed after the infection subsides to identify anatomic

BOX 27-1 ■ Signs and Symptoms of Urinary Tract Disorders or Disease at Different Ages

NEONATAL PERIOD (BIRTH TO 1 MONTH)
Poor feeding
Vomiting
Failure to gain weight
Rapid respiration (acidosis)
Respiratory distress
Spontaneous pneumothorax or pneumomediastinum
Frequent urination
Screaming on urination
Poor urine stream
Jaundice
Seizures
Dehydration
Other anomalies or stigmata
Enlarged kidneys or bladder

INFANCY (1 TO 24 MONTHS)
Poor feeding
Vomiting
Failure to gain weight
Excessive thirst
Frequent urination
Straining or screaming on urination
Foul-smelling urine
Pallor
Fever
Persistent diaper rash
Seizures (with or without fever)
Dehydration
Enlarged kidneys or bladder

CHILDHOOD (2 TO 14 YEARS)
Poor appetite
Vomiting
Growth failure
Excessive thirst
Enuresis, incontinence, frequent urination
Painful urination
Swelling of face
Seizures
Pallor
Fatigue
Blood in urine
Abdominal or back pain
Edema
Hypertension
Tetany

abnormalities contributing to the development of infection and existing kidney changes from recurrent infection.

Therapeutic Management

The objectives of treatment of children with UTI are (1) to eliminate current infection, (2) to identify contributing factors to reduce the risk of recurrence, (3) to prevent systemic spread of the infection, and (4) to preserve renal function. Antibiotic therapy should be initiated on the basis of identification of the pathogen, the child's history of antibiotic use, and the location of the infection. Several antimicrobial drugs are available for treating UTI, but all of them can occasionally be ineffective because of resistance of organisms. Common antiinfective agents used for UTI include the penicillins, sulfonamide (including trimethoprim and sulfisoxazole in combination), the cephalosporins, and nitrofurantoin.

If anatomic defects such as primary reflux or bladder neck obstruction are present, surgical correction of these abnormalities may be necessary to prevent recurrent infection. Follow-up study is an important component of medical management, because the relapse rate is high and recurrent infection tends to occur 1 to 2 months after termination of treatment. The aim of therapy and careful follow-up is to reduce the chance of renal scarring. However, recurrent infection of the urinary bladder predisposes the individual to transient episodes of vesicoureteral reflux (VUR).

Vesicoureteral Reflux.   VUR refers to the abnormal retrograde flow of bladder urine into the ureters. During voiding, urine is swept up the ureters and then flows back into the empty bladder, where it acts as a reservoir for bacterial growth until the next void. *Primary reflux* results from congenitally abnormal insertion of ureters into the bladder; *secondary reflux* occurs as a result of an acquired condition.

It is not clear that reflux necessarily causes infections. What is clear is that reflux is more likely to be associated with recurring kidney infections rather than simple bladder infections (cystitis). In the presence of reflux, infected urine (bacteria) from the bladder has access to the kidney, resulting in kidney infections (pyelonephritis). These children are usually very symptomatic with high fevers, vomiting, and chills. Reflux when associated with UTI is the most common cause of renal scarring in children. Renal scarring may occur with the first episode of febrile UTI. Reflux in the presence of sterile urine does not cause renal damage. Therefore the most important concept in managing VUR is preventing bacteria from reaching the kidneys. VUR is managed conservatively with daily low-dose antibiotic therapy. A urine culture should be done every 2 to 3 months and any time the child has a fever. This method of management requires a motivated, reliable, and cooperative family. Many children will outgrow the reflux over a period of years. An annual voiding cystourethrogram is done to assess the status of the reflux.

Indications for surgical intervention include significant anatomic abnormality at the ureterovesical junction, recurrent UTIs, severe forms of VUR, noncompliance with medical therapy, intolerance to antibiotics, and VUR after puberty in females.

Prognosis.   With prompt and adequate treatment at the time of diagnosis, the long-term prognosis for UTI is usually excellent. However, the hazard of progressive renal injury is greatest when infection occurs in young children (especially those younger than 2 years of age) and is associated with congenital renal malformations and reflux. Therefore early diagnosis of children at risk is particularly important during infancy and toddlerhood.

Nursing Considerations

Nurses should instruct parents to observe regularly for clues suggesting UTI. Unfortunately, the signs of UTI are not as evident as those of upper respiratory tract infection. Therefore many cases go undetected because no one thought to investigate this very common problem.

Because infants and young children often are unable to express their feelings and sensations verbally, it is difficult to detect discomfort they may be experiencing from dysuria. A careful history regarding voiding habits, stooling pattern, and episodes of unexplained irritability may assist in detecting less obvious cases of UTI. Consequently, parents should be cautioned to observe for specific clues of UTI in suspected cases.

> **NURSING TIP**
>
> Check the diaper every half hour. This increases the opportunity for observing the stream for such findings as straining or fretting before voiding begins, signs of discomfort before and during urinating, starting and stopping the stream intermittently, and frequent dripping of small amounts of urine.

When infection is suspected, collecting an appropriate specimen is essential. It is the nurse's responsibility to take every precaution to obtain acceptable clean-voided specimens to avoid the use of other collecting procedures except when absolutely indicated. Because of the unreliability of a specimen obtained via a urine collection bag, suprapubic aspiration of urine or sterile catheterization should be done in the infant or young child who presents with fever.

Frequently, additional tests are performed to detect anatomic defects. Children are prepared for these tests as appropriate for their age. This includes an explanation of the procedure, its purpose, and what the children will experience (see Preparation for Procedures, Chapter 22). Sometimes a simple description of the urinary system is helpful. Especially for preschool children, the nurse must clarify that the urinary tract is separate from any sexual function and that the test is for a problem that they did not cause. Children may associate blame for perceived wrongdoing (e.g., masturbation) or unacceptable thoughts with the reason for the illness or the tests. For children younger than 3 to 4 years of age, the procedure can be explained on a doll. For those who are older, a simple drawing of the bladder, urethra, ureters, and kidneys makes the procedure more understandable.

Handling actual equipment when feasible can be helpful in allaying anxiety in children of all ages. Anticipatory instruction on distraction techniques such as deep breathing, storytelling, and imagery may help the child relax and be more cooperative during the actual procedures. If surgery is indicated, the child will be able to encounter the impending procedure with facts and understanding of the procedure that will help to decrease his or her fear and anxiety concerning more extensive medical-surgical intervention.

Because antibacterial drugs are indicated in UTI, the nurse advises parents of proper dosage and administration. When antiseptics such as nitrofurantoin are used for prolonged therapy to maintain urine sterility, parents need an explanation of the drug's continued necessity when no signs of infection are present. For all children an adequate or increased fluid intake is encouraged.

GUIDELINES

Prevention of Urinary Tract Infection

FACTORS PREDISPOSING TO DEVELOPMENT
Short female urethra close to vagina and anus
Incomplete emptying (reflux) and overdistention of bladder
Concentrated urine

MEASURES OF PREVENTION
Perineal hygiene: wipe from front to back.
Avoid tight clothing or diapers; wear cotton panties rather than nylon.
Check for vaginitis or pinworms, especially if child scratches between legs.
Avoid "holding" urine; encourage child to void frequently, especially before long trip or other circumstances in which toilet facilities are not available.
Empty bladder completely with each void. Have the child "double void" (void, wait a few minutes and void again). Severe cases may require clean, intermittent catheterization or biofeedback instruction.
Avoid straining during defecation and avoid constipation.
Encourage generous fluid intake.

Prevention. Prevention is the most important goal in both primary and recurrent infection, and most preventive measures are simple hygienic habits that should be a routine part of daily care (see Guidelines box). For example, parents are taught to cleanse their infant's genital areas from front to back to avoid contaminating the urethral area with fecal organisms. Female children are taught to wipe from front to back after voiding or defecating. Children should void as soon as they feel the urge (see Critical Thinking Exercise).

Sexually active adolescent females are advised to urinate as soon as possible after they have intercourse to flush out bacteria introduced during the activity. Children who have recurrent UTIs or neurogenic bladder are frequently maintained on daily low-dose antibiotics. Giving the dose at bedtime allows the drug to remain in the bladder overnight. The nurse should reinforce the importance of compliance to parents and older children.

OBSTRUCTIVE UROPATHY

Structural or functional abnormalities of the urinary system that obstruct the normal flow of urine can produce renal disorders. When there is interference with urine flow, the backup of urine above the obstruction causes *hydronephrosis* (dilation of the renal pelvis from distention) with eventual pressure destruction of renal parenchyma, although the dilating ureters form a reservoir that reduces the effect on the kidneys for a long time.

Obstruction may be congenital or acquired, unilateral or bilateral, complete or incomplete, and the manifestations may be acute or chronic. The obstruction can occur at any level of the upper or lower urinary tract (Fig. 27-1). Partial obstruction may not be symptomatic unless there is a water or solute diuresis. Boys are affected more frequently than girls, and malformations should be suspected when patients have some other congenital defects (e.g., prune belly syn-

??? CRITICAL THINKING EXERCISE ???

Urinary Tract Infection and Constipation

During your assessment of Ginger, a 4-year-old admitted to the hospital for a severe urinary tract infection (UTI), her mother tells you that Ginger has bowel movements every third to fourth day. They are usually large, hard-formed stools, and Ginger sometimes has trouble evacuating the stool.

QUESTIONS
1. Evidence—Is there sufficient evidence to draw a conclusion about Ginger's UTI and constipation?
2. Assumptions—Describe an underlying assumption about each of the following:
   a. Urinary tract infections and females
   b. Normal bowel patterns for 4-year-old children
   c. Association between UTIs and constipation
3. What priorities for nursing care should be established for Ginger?
4. Does the evidence support your nursing intervention?
5. What alternative perspectives might you have?

ANSWERS
1. Yes. Ginger's mother reports a history of constipation with large, hard, formed stools occurring only every 3 to 4 days. She was diagnosed with a UTI severe enough to be admitted to the hospital.
2. a. The structure of the lower urinary tract is believed to account for the increased incidence of bacteriuria in females.
   b. A history of hard, large stools occurring every 3 to 4 days is not a normal elimination pattern for 4-year-old children.
   c. The presence of a large stool mass within the colon is likely to cause pressure on the bladder and urethra and not allow the bladder to empty completely. Stasis of the urine can lead to infection.
3. The first priority at this time is to begin treatment for the UTI. Ginger's diet and fluid intake should be evaluated, and a plan to prevent constipation in the future should be developed.
4. Yes. Ginger's history reflects chronic problems with constipation that must be addressed.
5. Ginger might have other risk factors associated with UTIs in children, and this should be explored further. The single most important host factor influencing the occurrence of UTI is urinary stasis. Other possible causes of urinary stasis may need to be considered.

drome, chromosomal anomalies, anorectal malformations, defects of the pinna of the ear).

Damage to distal nephrons in chronic uropathy alters the ability to concentrate urine, contributing to increased urine flow and metabolic acidosis occurring from decreased excretion of acid secondary to impaired ability of the distal nephron to secrete hydrogen ions. Partial obstruction results in progressive loss of renal function as a result of irreversible damage to the nephrons. Pooled urine serves as a medium for bacterial growth; therefore, UTIs further increase the extent of renal damage.

Early diagnosis and surgical correction or procedures that divert the flow of urine to bypass the obstruction, such as placement of a temporary percutaneous nephrostomy tube or cutaneous ureterostomy, are essential to prevent progressive renal damage. Medical complications of acute or chronic renal failure or infection are managed as described for those disorders.

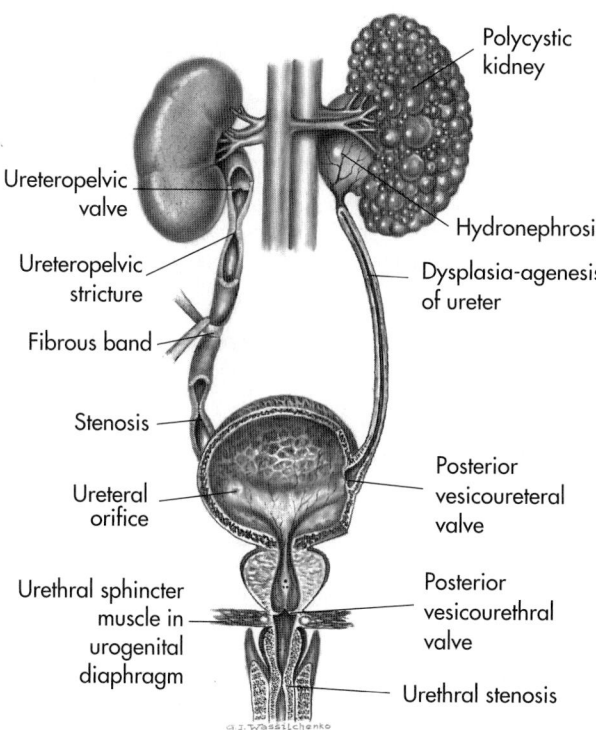

Polycystic
kidney

Ureteropelvic
valve

Ureteropelvic
stricture

Hydronephrosis

Fibrous band

Dysplasia-agenesis
of ureter

Stenosis

Ureteral
orifice

Posterior
vesicoureteral
valve

Urethral sphincter
muscle in
urogenital
diaphragm

Posterior
vesicourethral
valve

Urethral stenosis

FIG. 27-1 ■ Major sites of urinary tract obstruction.

Nursing Considerations

Nursing goals in urinary tract obstruction include helping to identify cases, assisting with diagnostic procedures, and caring for children with complications (described elsewhere). Preparing parents and children for procedures is a major nursing responsibility. Preparation for urinary diversion procedures is of special importance (see Preparation for Procedures, Chapter 22).

Parents and children need emotional support and counseling during the lengthy management of these disorders. Many children are discharged with ureteral drainage systems in place that must be protected from damage, and the danger of infection is a constant concern. Parents are taught to care for the equipment and recognize the signs of possible obstruction or infection within the system. Maintaining adequate urine flow is imperative. Fluids should be encouraged. The tube should be observed frequently for indications of obstruction resulting from sediment, small blood clots, or kinking. The physician should inspect any drainage from around the tube.

Children with external diversional systems will need psychologic support and guidance, especially as they reach adolescence and body image concerns assume more prominence. Those with progressive renal deterioration may face the prospect of dialysis and/or transplantation and the emotional aspects that accompany these procedures.

EXTERNAL DEFECTS

Defects of the external genitourinary tract are serious conditions primarily because of the psychologic impact on the child. Satisfactory surgical repair is successful for the more common disorders and is carried out or initiated as early as possible. The major anomalies of the lower genitourinary tract, their description, and their management are outlined in Table 27-5.

Psychologic Problems Related to Genital Surgery

Surgery involving sexual organs can be particularly disruptive to children, especially preschoolers fearing punishment, retaliation, body mutilation, or castration. Some of the problems of hospitalization, separation, and anxiety can be eased by hospital practices that are sensitive to the needs of the child (see Chapter 21).

The body image of a child is largely derived as a result of feedback from the primary caregivers, and parental anxiety regarding an acceptable physical appearance and adequate future sexual competency is readily communicated to an affected child. Therefore children with birth defects are at risk for developing a distorted body image that reflects the caregiver's subtly communicated evaluation of their bodies. The trend toward repair of visible genital defects is based in large part on these psychologic variables. The earlier a repair can be achieved, the more likely the possibility that the child will develop a normal body image.

During the years from 3 to 6, the phallic-oedipal period, children show a strong interest and concern about the genital area, sex differences, and genital normality or its lack. It is also a time when children are frightened of what they perceive to be threats to their body and bodily function. They also view any untoward happening as a punishment for real or imagined wrongdoing or unacceptable sexual feelings, such as masturbation, sex play, or erotic feelings. Surgical repair is recommended before these fears and anxieties develop.

After extensive review of the emotional, cognitive, and body-image problems that may occur in children undergoing surgical reconstruction of a genital deformity, it was recommended that surgery be accomplished between the ages of 6 and 15 months to minimize the psychologic effects of surgery and anesthesia (Kass, 1996).

Nursing Considerations

Preparing children and their families for diagnostic and surgical procedures (see Preparation for Procedures, Chapter 22) and for home care is a major nursing function. Most postoperative care involves care of the surgical site. Tub baths are discouraged for 1 week after simple surgeries. The surgical site is kept clean and otherwise protected from infection and is inspected for signs of infection. Dressings, if any, are inspected regularly. More complex surgeries require additional care and observation (e.g., catheter care for urethral reconstruction and care of urinary diversion stomas and collection devices).

Some older children's activities, such as pushing, lifting, playing with straddle toys or in sandboxes, swimming, and rough activities, may be restricted for some types of surgical repairs. Precise restrictions depend on the specific type of surgery. Activities of infants and toddlers are not limited.

In most cases the results of surgery are quite satisfactory. However, in some of the more severe defects, such as exstrophy and those that require stomas, additional emotional interventions may be needed. A major concern of parents and children is related to surgery affecting the genitalia directly. Concerns about penile size, appearance of the genitalia, po-

TABLE 27-5 ■ Defects of the Genitourinary Tract

DEFECT	THERAPEUTIC MANAGEMENT	DEFECT	THERAPEUTIC MANAGEMENT
INGUINAL HERNIA Protrusion of abdominal contents through inguinal canal into scrotum	Detected as painless inguinal swelling of variable size Surgical closure of inguinal defect	**EXSTROPHY OF BLADDER** Eversion of posterior bladder through anterior bladder wall and lower abdominal wall; associated with open pubic arch (a severe defect)	Potential objectives of surgical correction: Preserve renal function Attain urinary control Adequate reconstructive repair Improve sexual function (especially in males)
HYDROCELE Fluid in scrotum	Surgical repair indicated if spontaneous resolution not accomplished in 1 year		
PHIMOSIS Narrowing or stenosis of preputial opening of foreskin	Mild cases: manual retraction of foreskin and proper cleansing of area Severe cases: circumcision or vertical division and transverse suturing of foreskin	**AMBIGUOUS GENITALIA** Types: Masculinized female (female pseudohermaphrodite)	Therapeutic management: Gender assignment—female; assign gender while avoiding irreversible surgery, realizing some children may change gender later in life; family participation essential
HYPOSPADIAS Urethral opening located behind glans penis or anywhere along ventral surface of penile shaft	Objectives of surgical correction: Enable child to void in standing position and direct stream voluntarily in usual manner Improve physical appearance of genitalia Produce a sexually adequate organ	Incompletely masculinized male (male pseudohermaphrodite)	Assign gender while avoiding irreversible surgery, realizing some children may change gender later in life; family participation essential
		True hermaphrodite (both ovaries and testes)	Assign gender while avoiding irreversible surgery, realizing some children may change gender later in life; gender assignment depends on predominant characteristics; family participation essential
CHORDEE Ventral curvature of penis, often associated with hypospadias	Surgical release of fibrous band causing the deformity	Mixed gonadal dysgenesis	Assign gender while avoiding irreversible surgery, realizing some children may change gender later in life; gender assignment depends on predominant characteristics; family participation essential
EPISPADIAS Meatal opening located on dorsal surface of penis	Surgical correction, usually including penile and urethral lengthening and bladder neck reconstruction (if necessary)		
CRYPTORCHIDISM Failure of one or both testes to descend normally through inguinal canal	Detected by inability to palpate testes within scrotum Medical: administration of human chorionic gonadotropin (older child) Surgical: orchiopexy Objectives of therapy: Prevent damage to undescended testicle Decrease incidence of malignant tumor formation Avoid trauma and torsion Close inguinal canal Prevent cosmetic and psychologic disability from empty scrotum		

tential ability to procreate, and rejection by peers (especially the opposite sex) are potential fears that require psychologic adjustment, particularly during adolescence.

GLOMERULAR DISEASE

NEPHROTIC SYNDROME

Nephrotic syndrome is a clinical state that includes massive proteinuria, hypoalbuminemia, hyperlipemia, and edema. The disorder can occur as (1) a primary disease known as *idiopathic nephrosis, childhood nephrosis,* or *minimal-change nephrotic syndrome (MCNS);* (2) a secondary disorder that occurs as a clinical manifestation after or in association with glomerular damage of known or presumed etiology; or (3) a congenital form inherited as an autosomal recessive disorder. The disorder is characterized by increased glomerular permeability to plasma protein, which results in massive urinary protein loss. The glomerulus is responsible for the initial step in the formation of urine, and the filtration rate depends on an intact glomerular membrane. This discussion is devoted to MCNS because it constitutes 80% of nephrotic syndrome cases.

Pathophysiology

The onset of MCNS can occur at any age but predominantly occurs in children between 2 and 7 years of age. It is rare in children younger than 6 months of age, uncom-

mon in infants younger than 1 year of age, and unusual after the age of 8. Patients with MCNS are twice as likely to be male.

The pathogenesis of MCNS is not understood. There may be a metabolic, biochemical, physiochemical, or immune-mediated disturbance that causes the basement membrane of the glomeruli to become increasingly permeable to protein, but the cause and mechanisms are only speculative.

The glomerular membrane, normally impermeable to albumin and other proteins, becomes permeable to proteins, especially albumin, which leak through the membrane and are lost in urine *(hyperalbuminuria).* This reduces the serum albumin level *(hypoalbuminemia),* decreasing the colloidal osmotic pressure in the capillaries. As a result, the vascular hydrostatic pressure exceeds the pull of the colloidal osmotic pressure, causing fluid to accumulate in the interstitial spaces *(edema)* and body cavities, particularly in the abdominal cavity *(ascites).* The shift of fluid from the plasma to the interstitial spaces reduces the vascular fluid volume *(hypovolemia),* which in turn stimulates the renin-angiotensin system and the secretion of antidiuretic hormone and aldosterone. Tubular reabsorption of sodium and water is increased in an attempt to increase intravascular volume. The elevation of serum lipids is unexplained. The sequence of events in nephrotic syndrome is diagrammed in Fig. 27-2.

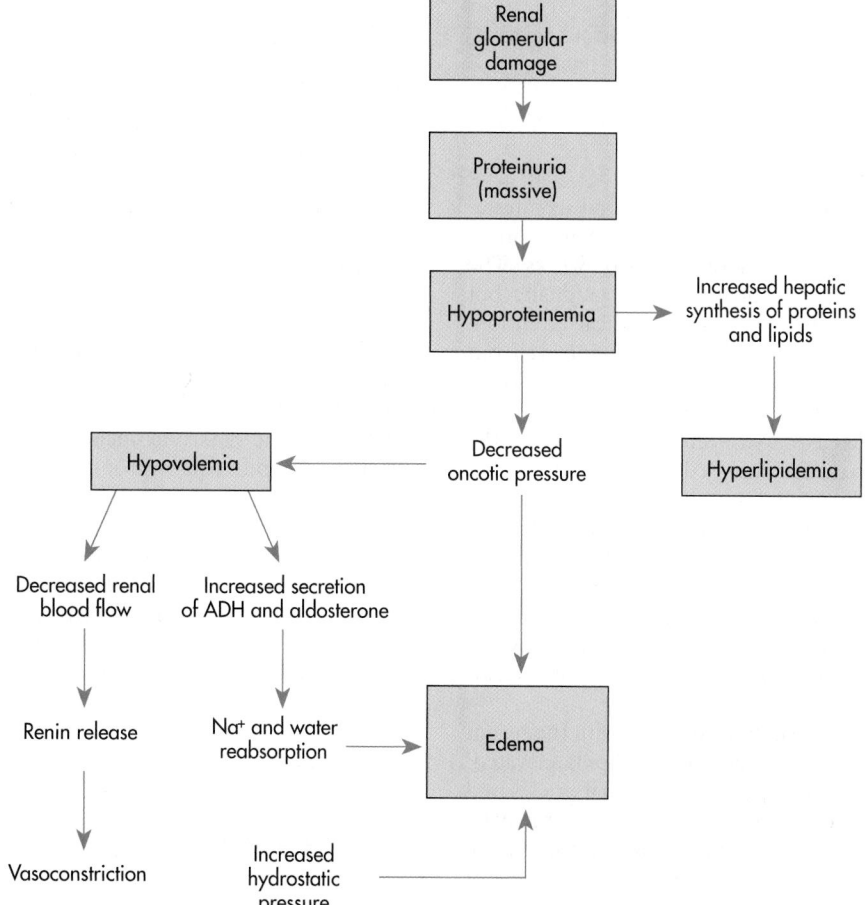

FIG. 27-2 ■ Sequence of events in nephrotic syndrome.

BOX 27-2 ■ Clinical Manifestations of Nephrotic Syndrome

Weight gain
Puffiness of face (facial edema):
    Especially around the eyes
    Apparent on arising in the morning
    Subsides during the day
Abdominal swelling (ascites)
Pleural effusion
Labial or scrotal swelling
Edema of intestinal mucosal may cause:
    Diarrhea
    Anorexia
    Poor intestinal absorption
Ankle/leg swelling
Irritability
Easily fatigued
Lethargic
Blood pressure normal or slightly decreased
Susceptibility to infection
Urine alterations:
    Decreased volume
    Frothy

❗NURSING ALERT

A child who exhibits the following should be evaluated for the possibility of nephrotic syndrome:
    Weight gain over that expected based on previous pattern
    Parent observation that the child's clothes fit tightly
    Decreased urine output
    Pallor, fatigue

Diagnostic Evaluation

The disease is suspected on the basis of clinical manifestations (Box 27-2), especially when weight gain in a previously well child increases slowly over days or weeks. The generalized edema may develop rapidly or gradually but eventually prompts the family to seek medical attention. Parents usually give a history of the child being well but steadily gaining weight and then becoming anorexic, irritable, and less active.

The diagnosis of MCNS is suspected on the basis of the history and clinical manifestations (edema, proteinuria, hypoalbuminemia, and hypercholesterolemia in the absence of hematuria and hypertension) in children between the ages of 2 and 8 years. The hallmark of MCNS is massive proteinuria (higher than 3+ on urine dipstick). Hyaline casts, oval fat bodies, and a few red blood cells can be found in the urine of some affected children, although there is seldom gross hematuria. The glomerular filtration rate is usually normal or high.

Total serum protein concentration is low, with the serum albumin significantly reduced and plasma lipids elevated. Hemoglobin and hematocrit are usually normal or elevated as a result of hemoconcentration. The platelet count may be elevated. Serum sodium concentration may be low. If the patient does not respond to a 4- to 8-week course of steroids, a renal biopsy may be needed to distinguish between other types of nephrotic syndrome. The biopsy re-

sults of children with MCNS are remarkable for effacement of the foot processes of the epithelial cells lining the basement membrane, but otherwise the kidney tissue is normal.

Therapeutic Management

Objectives of therapeutic management include (1) reducing excretion of urinary protein, (2) reducing fluid retention in the tissues, (3) preventing infection, and (4) minimizing complications related to therapies. Dietary restrictions include a low-salt diet and fluid restriction. If complications of edema develop, diuretic therapy may be initiated to provide temporary relief from edema. Sometimes infusions of 25% albumin are used. Acute infections are treated with appropriate antibiotics.

Corticosteroids are the first line of therapy for MCNS. The starting dose for prednisone is usually 2 mg/kg body weight per day, in one or more divided doses. In most children this response occurs within 7 to 21 days. The medication is then tapered over a period of several weeks and eventually stopped if the child remains asymptomatic. About two thirds of children with MCNS have a relapse, heralded first by increased urine protein. Relapses can be diagnosed early if parents are taught routine home monitoring of urine protein by dipstick. Relapses are treated with a repeated course of high-dose steroid therapy. Side effects of the steroids include weight gain, rounding of the face, and increased appetite. Long-term therapy may result in hirsutism, growth retardation, cataracts, hypertension, gastrointestinal bleeding, bone demineralization, infection, and hyperglycemia. Children who do not respond to steroid therapy, those who have frequent relapses, and those in whom the side effects threaten their growth and general health may be considered for a course of therapy using other immunosuppressant medications (cyclophosphamide, chlorambucil, or cyclosporine).

MCNS episodes, both the first episode and relapse, often happen in conjunction with a viral or bacterial infection. Relapses can also be triggered by allergies and immunizations. Relapses in children with MCNS may continue over many years.

Complications of nephrotic syndrome include infection, circulatory insufficiency secondary to hypovolemia, and thromboembolism. Infections that may be seen in children with nephrotic syndrome include peritonitis, cellulitis, and pneumonia and require prompt recognition and vigorous treatment with appropriate antibiotic therapy.

Prognosis. The prognosis for ultimate recovery in most cases is good. It is a self-limiting disease, and in children who respond to steroid therapy the tendency to relapse decreases with time. With early detection and prompt implementation of therapy to eradicate proteinuria, progressive basement membrane damage is minimized, so that when the tendency to exacerbations is past, renal function is usually normal or near normal. It is estimated that approximately 80% of affected children have this favorable prognosis.

Nursing Considerations

Continuous monitoring of fluid retention or excretion is an important nursing function. Strict intake and output records are essential but may be difficult to obtain from very young children. Application of collection bags is highly irritating to edematous skin that is readily subject to breakdown. Application of diapers or weighing wet pads may be necessary.

Another strategy for obtaining a daily urine protein is to place cotton balls in the diaper at night before bedtime and then squeeze them out in the morning.

Other methods of monitoring progress include urine examination for albumin, daily weight, and measurement of abdominal girth. Assessment of edema (e.g., increased or decreased swelling around the eyes and dependent areas), the degree of pitting, and the color and texture of skin are part of nursing care. Vital signs are monitored to detect any early signs of complications such as shock or an infective process.

Infection is a constant source of danger to edematous children and those receiving corticosteroid therapy. These children are particularly vulnerable to upper respiratory infection; therefore, they must be kept warm and dry, active, and protected from contact with infected individuals (i.e., roommates, visitors, and personnel). Vital signs are monitored to detect any early signs of an infective process.

Loss of appetite accompanying active nephrosis creates a perplexing problem for nurses. During this time the combined efforts of nurse, dietitian, parents, and the child are needed to formulate a nutritionally adequate and attractive diet. Salt is usually restricted (but not eliminated) during the edema phase, and fluid restriction (if prescribed) is limited to short-term use during massive edema. Every effort should be made to serve attractive meals with preferred foods and a minimum of fuss, but it usually requires a considerable amount of ingenuity and enticement to get the child to eat (see Feeding the Sick Child, Chapter 22).

Children usually adjust activities according to their tolerance level. However, they may require guidance in selecting play activities. Suitable recreational and diversional activities are an important part of their care. Irritability and mood swings that accompany steroid therapy are not unusual in these children and may create an additional challenge to the nurse and the family.

Family Support and Home Care.   Continuous support of the child and family is one of the major nursing considerations. Many children are treated at home during exacerbations. Parents are taught to detect signs of relapse and to call for changes in treatment at the earliest indications. Unless the edema and proteinuria are severe or the parents, for some reason, are unable to care for the ill child, *home care is preferred*. Parents are instructed in testing urine for albumin, administration of medications, and general care. Parents are also instructed regarding avoiding contact with infected playmates, but the child should attend school.

The prolonged course of the relapsing form of nephrotic syndrome is taxing to both the child and the family. The up-and-down course of remissions and exacerbations with periodic disruption of family life by hospitalization places a severe strain on the child and the family, both psychologically and financially. Reassurance regarding this characteristic of the course of the disease, with emphasis on the importance of long-term care, needs to be provided to parents and children to gain their cooperation. A satisfactory response is more likely when relapses are detected and therapy is instituted early, and remissions are prolonged when instructions are carried out faithfully. Continuous support of the child and family is one of the major nursing considerations (see Chapter 18).

ACUTE GLOMERULONEPHRITIS

Acute glomerulonephritis (AGN) may be a primary event or a manifestation of a systemic disorder that can range from minimal to severe. Common features include oliguria, edema, hypertension and circulatory congestion, hematuria, and proteinuria. Most cases are postinfectious and have been associated with pneumococcal, streptococcal, and viral infections. *Acute poststreptococcal glomerulonephritis (APSGN)* is the most common of the postinfectious renal diseases in childhood and the one for which a cause can be established in the majority of cases. APSGN can occur at any age but affects primarily early school-age children, with a peak age of onset of 6 to 7 years. It is uncommon in children younger than 2 years of age, and males outnumber females 2:1.

Etiology

APSGN is an immune-complex disease that occurs after an antecedent streptococcal infection with certain strains of the group A β-hemolytic streptococcus. Most streptococcal infections *do not* cause APSGN. A latent period of 10 to 21 days occurs between the streptococcal infection and the onset of clinical manifestations. Disease secondary to streptococcal pharyngitis is more common in the winter or spring, but when APSGN is associated with pyoderma (principally *impetigo*), it may be more prevalent in later summer or early fall, especially in warmer climates. Second episodes of AGN are rare.

Pathophysiology

The pathophysiology of APSGN is still uncertain. Immune complexes are deposited in the glomerular basement membrane. The glomeruli become edematous and infiltrated with polymorphonuclear leukocytes, which occlude the capillary lumen. The resulting decrease in plasma filtration results in an excessive accumulation of water and retention of sodium that expands plasma and interstitial fluid volumes, leading to circulatory congestion and edema. The cause of the hypertension associated with AGN cannot be completely explained by fluid retention. Excess renin may also be produced.

Diagnostic Evaluation

Typically, affected children are in good health until they experience the streptococcal infection. In some instances there is a history of only a mild cold or no previous infection at all. The onset of nephritis appears after an average latent period of about 10 days (Box 27-3). Because the child appears to be well during the latent period, the association is not recognized by the parents. The edema is relatively moderate and may not be appreciated by someone unfamiliar with the child's normal appearance.

Urinalysis during the acute phase characteristically shows hematuria and proteinuria. Proteinuria generally parallels

BOX 27-3 ■ Clinical Manifestations of Acute Poststreptococcal Glomerulonephritis

Edema:
  Especially periorbital
  Facial edema more prominent in the morning
  Spreads during the day to involve extremities and abdomen
Anorexia
Urine:
  Cloudy, smoky brown (resembles tea or cola)
  Severely reduced volume
Pallor
Irritability
Lethargy
Child appears ill
Child seldom expresses specific complaints
Older children may complain of:
  Headaches
  Abdominal discomfort
  Dysuria
Vomiting possible
Mild to moderately elevated blood pressure

the hematuria and may be 3+ or 4+ in the presence of gross hematuria. Gross discoloration of the urine reflects red blood cell and hemoglobin content. Microscopic examination of the sediment shows many red blood cells, leukocytes, epithelial cells, and granular and red blood cell casts. Bacteria are not seen.

Azotemia that results from impaired glomerular filtration is reflected in elevated blood urea nitrogen and creatinine levels in at least 50% of cases. Occasionally proteinuria is excessive and the patient may have nephrotic syndrome (i.e., hypoproteinemia and hyperlipidemia).

Cultures of the pharynx are rarely positive for streptococci, because the renal disease occurs weeks after the infection.

NURSING ALERT

A child who exhibits the following should be evaluated for possible AGN:
  Orbital edema, which parents report is worse in the morning
  Loss of appetite
  Decreased output
  Dark-colored urine
  Antecedent streptococcal infection

Some serologic tests are necessary to make the diagnosis of AGN. Circulating serum antibodies to streptococcus indicate the presence of a previous infection. The antistreptolysin O (ASO) titer is the most familiar and readily available test for streptococcal infection. Other antibodies that may aid in diagnosis are elevated antihyaluronidase (AHase), antideoxyribonuclease B (ADNase-B), and streptozyme.

All patients with APSGN have reduced serum complement (C3) activity in the early stages of the disease. Rising C3 levels are used as a guide to indicate improvement of the disease and should be normal in almost all patients 8 weeks after the disease onset.

Studies that may be useful include chest x-ray examination, which generally shows cardiac enlargement, pulmonary congestion, or pleural effusion during the edematous phase of acute disease. Renal biopsy for diagnostic purposes is seldom required but may be useful in the diagnosis of atypical cases.

Therapeutic Management

Management consists of general supportive measures and early recognition and treatment of complications. Children who have normal blood pressure and a satisfactory urine output can generally be treated at home. Those with substantial edema, hypertension, gross hematuria, or significant oliguria should be hospitalized because of the unpredictability of complications.

Dietary restrictions depend on the stage and severity of the disease, especially the extent of edema. Moderate sodium restriction and even fluid restriction may be instituted for children with hypertension and edema. Foods with substantial amounts of potassium are generally restricted during the period of oliguria.

Regular measurement of vital signs, body weight, and intake and output is essential to monitor the progress of the disease and to detect complications that may appear at any time during the course of the disease. *A record of daily weight is the most useful means for assessing fluid balance.* Rarely, children with AGN will develop acute renal failure with oliguria that significantly alters the fluid and electrolyte balance (resulting in hyperkalemia, acidosis, hypocalcemia, and/or hyperphosphatemia). These children require careful management. Peritoneal dialysis or hemodialysis is seldom needed.

Acute hypertension must be anticipated and identified early. Blood pressure measurements are taken every 4 to 6 hours. A variety of antihypertensive medications, as well as diuretics, are used to control hypertension. Antibiotic therapy is indicated only for those children with evidence of persistent streptococcal infections. It is used to prevent transmission of nephritogenic streptococci to other family members.

Prognosis. Almost all children correctly diagnosed as having APSGN recover completely, and specific immunity is conferred, so that subsequent recurrences are uncommon. Some of these children have been reported to develop chronic disease, but most of these cases are now believed to be different glomerular diseases misdiagnosed as poststreptococcal disease.

Nursing Considerations

Nursing care of the child with glomerulonephritis involves careful assessment of the disease status, with regular monitoring of vital signs (including frequent measurement of blood pressure), fluid balance, and behavior.

Vital signs provide clues to the severity of the disease and early signs of complications. They are carefully measured, and any deviations are reported and recorded. The volume and character of urine are noted, and the child is weighed daily. Children with restricted fluid intake, especially those who are not severely edematous or those who have lost weight, are observed for signs of dehydration.

Assessment of the child's appearance for signs of cerebral complications is an important nursing function, because the severity of the acute phase is variable and unpredictable.

The child with edema, hypertension, and gross hematuria may be subject to complications, and anticipatory preparations such as seizure precautions and intravenous equipment are included in the nursing care plan.

For most children a regular diet is allowed, but it should contain no added salt. Foods high in sodium and salted treats are eliminated, and parents and friends are advised not to bring snacks such as potato chips or pretzels. However, the total amount of salt ingested is usually less than prescribed because of the child's poor appetite. Fluid restriction, if prescribed, is more difficult, and the amount permitted should be evenly divided throughout the waking hours. Meal preparation and service require special attention, since the child is indifferent to meals during the acute phase. Again, collaboration with parents and the dietitian and special consideration for food preferences facilitate meal planning.

During the acute phase children are generally quite content to lie in bed. As they begin to feel better and their symptoms subside, they will want to be up and about. Activities should be planned to allow for frequent rest periods and avoidance of fatigue. Children who have mild edema and no hypertension, as well as convalescent children who are being treated at home, need follow-up care. Parents are instructed regarding general measures, including diet, and prevention of infection.

Health supervision is continued with weekly, followed by monthly, visits for evaluation and urinalysis. Parent education and support in preparation for discharge and home care include education in home management and the need for follow-up care and health supervision.

MISCELLANEOUS RENAL DISORDERS

HEMOLYTIC-UREMIC SYNDROME

Hemolytic-uremic syndrome (HUS) is an uncommon, acute renal disease that occurs primarily in infants and small children between the ages of 6 months and 5 years. HUS is the most frequent cause of acquired acute renal failure in children (Brandt and others, 1994). The clinical features of the disease include acquired hemolytic anemia, thrombocytopenia, renal injury, and central nervous system symptoms. The etiology of HUS is thought to be associated with bacterial toxins, chemicals, and viruses. The appearance of the disease has been associated with *Rickettsia*, viruses (especially coxsackie virus, echovirus, and adenovirus), *Escherichia coli*, pneumococci, *Shigella*, and *Salmonella* and may represent an unusual response to these infections. Multiple cases of HUS caused by enteric infection of the *E. coli* 0157:H7 serotype have been traced to undercooked meat, especially ground beef. Often sources are unpasteurized milk or fruit juice, especially apple; alfalfa sprouts; lettuce; and salami; and drinking or swimming in sewage-contaminated water. The clinical presentation is usually a history of a prodromal illness (most often gastroenteritis or an upper respiratory infection) followed by the sudden onset of hemolysis and renal failure.

Pathophysiology

The primary site of injury appears to be the endothelial lining of the small glomerular arterioles, which become swollen and occluded with deposits of platelets and fibrin clots (intravascular coagulation). Red blood cells are damaged as they at-

BOX 27-4 ■ Clinical Manifestations of Hemolytic Uremic Syndrome
Vomiting
Irritability
Lethargy
Marked pallor
Hemorrhagic manifestations:
Bruising
Petechiae
Jaundice
Bloody diarrhea
Oliguria or anuria
Central nervous system involvement:
Seizures
Stupor/coma
Signs of acute heart failure (sometimes)

tempt to move through the partially occluded blood vessels. These damaged cells are removed by the spleen, causing acute hemolytic anemia. The platelet aggregation within the damaged blood vessels or the damage and removal of platelets produce the characteristic thrombocytopenia.

Diagnostic Evaluation

The triad of anemia, thrombocytopenia, and renal failure is sufficient for diagnosis (Box 27-4). Renal involvement is evidenced by proteinuria, hematuria, and the presence of urinary casts; blood urea nitrogen and serum creatinine levels are elevated. A low hemoglobin and hematocrit and a high reticulocyte count confirm the hemolytic nature of the anemia.

Therapeutic Management

The goals of therapy are early diagnosis and aggressive, supportive care of the acute renal failure and hemolytic anemia. The most consistently effective treatment of HUS is hemodialysis or peritoneal dialysis, which is instituted in any child who has been anuric for 24 hours or who demonstrates oliguria with uremia or hypertension and seizures. Other treatments include use of pharmacologic agents, fresh-frozen plasma, and plasma pheresis. Blood transfusions with fresh, washed packed cells are administered for severe anemia but are used with caution to prevent circulatory overload from added volume.

Prognosis.   With prompt treatment the recovery rate is about 95%, but residual renal impairment ranges from 10% to 50% in various areas. Long-term complications include chronic renal failure, hypertension, and central nervous system disorders. Death is usually caused by residual renal impairment or central nervous system injury.

Nursing Considerations

Nursing care is the same as that provided in acute renal failure and, for children with continued impairment, includes management of chronic disease. Because of the sudden and life-threatening nature of the disorder in a previously well child, parents are often ill-prepared for the impact of hospitalization and treatment. Therefore support and understanding are especially important aspects of care.

WILMS TUMOR*

Wilms tumor, or nephroblastoma, is the most common malignant renal and intraabdominal tumor of childhood. Its frequency is estimated to be 7.6 cases per million white children less than 15 years of age (Grundy and others, 2002). Wilms tumor occurs about three times more often in blacks than in East Asians in the United States. The peak age at diagnosis is approximately 3 years, and occurrence is slightly more frequent in boys than in girls. The majority of patients with Wilms tumor are diagnosed at younger than 5 years of age, with 1% to 2.5% having a familial origin. Unfortunately, there is no method of identifying gene carriers at this time.

Etiology

Wilms tumor probably arises from a malignant, undifferentiated cluster of primordial cells capable of initiating the regeneration of an abnormal structure. Its occurrence slightly favors the left kidney, which is advantageous because surgically this kidney is easier to manipulate and remove. In about 10% of cases both kidneys are involved. Studies have shown that development of Wilms tumor is frequently associated with aniridia, hemihypertrophy, Beckwith-Wiedemann syndrome, or genitourinary anomalies (Kline and Sevier, 2003; Grundy and others, 2002).

Diagnostic Evaluation

In a child suspected of having Wilms tumor, special emphasis is placed on the history and physical examination for the presence of congenital anomalies, a family history of cancer, and signs of malignancy (e.g., weight loss, size of liver and spleen, indications of anemia, lymphadenopathy). Most children with Wilms tumor are brought to the practitioner because of abdominal swelling or an abdominal mass (Box 27-5). Specific tests include radiographic studies, including abdominal ultrasound, abdominal and chest computed tomography scan, hematologic studies, biochemical studies, and urinalysis. Studies to demonstrate the relationship of the tumor to the ipsilateral kidney and the presence of a normal functioning kidney on the contralateral side are essential. If a large tumor is present, an inferior venacavagram is necessary to demonstrate possible tumor involvement adjacent to the vena cava. A bone marrow aspiration may be performed to rule out metastasis, which is rare in children with Wilms tumor.

> **⚠ NURSING ALERT**
>
> To reinforce the need for caution, it may be necessary to post a sign on the bed that reads "DO NOT PALPATE ABDOMEN." Careful bathing and handling are also important in preventing trauma to the tumor site.

Therapeutic Management

Combined treatment of surgery and chemotherapy with or without radiation is based on the histologic pattern and clinical stage (Box 27-6).

Surgery is scheduled as soon as possible after confirmation of a renal mass, usually within 24 to 48 hours of admission. A

---

*Rosalind Bryant, MN, RN, CS, PNP, revised this section.

BOX 27-5 ■ Clinical Manifestations of Wilms Tumor

Abdominal swelling or mass:
  Firm
  Nontender
  Confined to one side
Hematuria (less than one fourth of cases)
Fatigue/malaise
Hypertension (occasionally)
Weight loss
Fever
Manifestations resulting from compression of tumor mass
Secondary metabolic alterations from tumor or metastasis
If metastasis, symptoms of lung involvement:
  Dyspnea
  Cough
  Shortness of breath
  Chest pain (sometimes)

BOX 27-6 ■ Staging of Wilms Tumor

Stage I: Tumor is limited to kidney and completely resected.
Stage II: Tumor extends beyond kidney but is completely resected.
Stage III: Residual nonhematogenous tumor is confined to abdomen.
Stage IV: Hematogenous metastases; deposits are beyond stage III, namely, to lung, liver, bone, and brain.
Stage V: Bilateral renal involvement is present at diagnosis.

---

large transabdominal incision is performed for optimal visualization of the abdominal cavity. The tumor, affected kidney, and adjacent adrenal gland are removed. Great care is taken to keep the encapsulated tumor intact, because rupture can seed cancer cells throughout the abdomen, lymph channel, and bloodstream. The contralateral kidney is carefully inspected for evidence of disease or dysfunction. Regional lymph nodes are inspected, and a biopsy is performed when indicated. Any involved structures, such as part of the colon, diaphragm, or vena cava, are removed. Metal clips are placed around the tumor site for exact marking during radiotherapy.

If both kidneys are involved, the child may be treated with radiotherapy or chemotherapy before surgery to decrease the size of the tumor, allowing more conservative surgery. It may be possible to perform a partial nephrectomy on the less affected kidney, with a total nephrectomy on the opposite side. When a transplant is feasible, such as from a twin, sibling, or parent, bilateral nephrectomy is considered as a last resort.

Postoperative radiation therapy is indicated for children with large tumors, metastasis, residual postoperative disease, unfavorable histology, or recurrence. Chemotherapy is indicated for all stages. The most effective agents for treating Wilms tumor are actinomycin D (dactinomycin), vincristine, and Adriamycin with the addition of cyclophosphamide for unfavorable histology or advanced disease (Grundy and others, 2002). The duration of therapy varies, ranging from 6 to 15 months.

Prognosis.   Survival rates for Wilms tumor are the highest among all childhood cancers. Children with localized tumor (stages I and II) have a 90% chance of cure with multimodal therapy. Factors that favorably affect the success of further therapy include initial treatment with only vincristine and dactinomycin, relapse to the lungs only, relapse in the abdomen of a patient who received no prior abdominal irradiation, and relapse more than 12 months after diagnosis. Wilms tumor may recur, especially in the lungs. Both chemotherapy and radiation therapy can induce second tumors, usually in areas that have been irradiated (Gundy and others, 2002).

Nursing Considerations

Nursing care of the child with Wilms tumor is similar to that of children with other cancers treated with surgery, irradiation, and chemotherapy. However, there are some significant differences; these are discussed for each phase of nursing intervention.

Preoperative Care.   The preoperative period is one of swift diagnosis. The nurse is faced with the challenge of preparing the child and parents for all laboratory and operative procedures within 24 to 48 hours of admission. Because of the minimal amount of available preparatory time, explanations should be simple, repetitive, and focused on the child's actual experiences. In addition to the usual preoperative observations, blood pressure is monitored, because hypertension from excess renin production is a possibility.

There are several special preoperative concerns, the most important of which is that the *tumor is not palpated unless absolutely necessary,* because manipulation of the mass may cause dissemination of cancer cells to adjacent and distant sites.

Because radiotherapy and chemotherapy are usually begun immediately after surgery, parents need an explanation of what to expect, such as major benefits and side effects. The timing of the information should be considered to avoid overwhelming the family. Ideally, the nurse should be present during physician-parent conferences to answer questions as they arise. It is usually better to postpone telling the child about these side effects until after surgery. Alopecia, usually of most concern to older children, does not occur until approximately 2 weeks after the initial treatment regimen. Therefore the child can be prepared for the hair loss postoperatively.

Postoperative Care.   Despite the extensive surgical intervention necessary in many children with Wilms tumor, the recovery is usually rapid. The major nursing responsibilities are the same as those after any abdominal surgery (see Surgical Procedures, Chapter 22). Because these children are at risk for intestinal obstruction from vincristine-induced ileus, radiation-induced edema, and postsurgical adhesion formation, gastrointestinal activity, such as bowel movements, bowel sounds, distention, vomiting, and pain, are carefully monitored.

The nurse also monitors blood pressure, urine output, and signs of infection, as well as instituting pulmonary hygiene to prevent postoperative pulmonary complications.

Family Support.   The postoperative period is frequently difficult for parents. The shock of seeing their child immediately after surgery may be the first realization of the seriousness of the diagnosis. It also marks the confirmation of the stage of the tumor. During this period, the nurse should be with the parents to assure them of the child's recovery after surgery and to assess the parent's understanding of the total experience. They need an opportunity to express their feelings and need to be provided the same emotional care discussed in Chapter 18 for families who have a child with a life-threatening disorder.

Older children need an opportunity to deal with their feelings concerning the many procedures to which they have been subjected in rapid succession. Play therapy with dolls or puppets or through drawing can be extremely beneficial in helping them adjust. It is not unusual for children to feel angry because of the extent of surgery, the need for additional therapy, or the seriousness of the disorder.

> **!NURSING ALERT**
>
> Because the child is left with one kidney, certain precautions, such as avoiding contact sports, are recommended to prevent injury to the remaining organ. Prompt detection and treatment of any genitourinary signs or symptoms are mandatory.

RENAL FAILURE

Renal failure is the inability of the kidneys to excrete waste material, concentrate urine, and conserve electrolytes. It can occur suddenly *(acute renal failure [ARF])* in response to inadequate perfusion, kidney disease, or urinary tract obstruction, or it can develop slowly *(chronic renal failure)* as a result of long-standing kidney disease or an anomaly.

Azotemia and uremia are terms often used in relation to renal failure. *Azotemia* is the accumulation of nitrogenous waste within the blood. *Uremia* is a more advanced condition in which retention of nitrogenous products produces toxic symptoms. Azotemia is not life-threatening, whereas uremia is a serious condition that often involves other body systems.

ACUTE RENAL FAILURE

ARF is said to exist when the kidneys suddenly are unable to regulate the volume and composition of urine appropriately in response to food and fluid intake and the needs of the organism. The principal feature of ARF is oliguria* associated with azotemia, metabolic acidosis, and diverse electrolyte disturbances. ARF is not common in childhood, but the outcome depends on the cause, associated findings, and prompt recognition and treatment.

The pathologic conditions that produce ARF caused by glomerulonephritis and hemolytic-uremic syndrome have been discussed in relation to those disorders. ARF can also develop as a result of a large number of related or unrelated clinical conditions: poor renal perfusion, urinary tract

---

*The definition of oliguria varies extensively in the literature, from 1.8 to 4 dL/m²/24 hr.

obstruction, acute renal injury, or the final expression of chronic, irreversible renal disease. The most common cause in children is transient renal failure resulting from severe dehydration or other causes of poor perfusion that may respond to restoration of fluid volume.

Pathophysiology

ARF is usually reversible, but the deviations of physiologic function can be extreme, and mortality in the pediatric age-group remains high. There is severe reduction in the glomerular filtration rate, an elevated blood urea nitrogen level, and a significant reduction in renal blood flow.

The clinical course is variable and depends on the cause. In reversible ARF there is a period of severe oliguria, or a low-output phase, followed by an abrupt onset of diuresis, or a high-output phase, and then a gradual return to, or toward, normal urine volumes.

Diagnostic Evaluation

In many instances of ARF the infant or child is already critically ill with the precipitating disorder, and the explanation for development of oliguria may or may not be readily apparent (Box 27-7). When a previously well child develops ARF without obvious cause, a careful history is taken to reveal symptoms that may be related to glomerulonephritis, obstructive uropathy, or exposure to nephrotoxic chemicals (e.g., ingestion of heavy metals, inhalation of carbon tetrachloride or other organic solvents or drugs known to be toxic to the kidneys). Significant laboratory measurements during renal shutdown that serve as a guide for therapy are blood urea nitrogen, serum creatinine, pH, sodium, potassium, and calcium.

> **! NURSING ALERT**
>
> Diminished urine output and lethargy in a child who is dehydrated, in shock, or recently postoperative should be evaluated for possible acute kidney failure.

> **! NURSING ALERT**
>
> Any of the following signs of hyperkalemia constitute an emergency and are reported immediately:
>   Serum potassium concentrations in excess of 7 mEq/L
>   Presence of electrocardiographic abnormalities, such as prolonged QRS complex, depressed ST segment, high peaked T waves, bradycardia, or heart block

Therapeutic Management

Treatment of ARF is directed toward (1) treatment of the underlying cause, (2) management of the complications of renal failure, and (3) provision of supportive therapy within the constraints imposed by the renal failure.

Treatment of poor perfusion resulting from dehydration consists of volume restoration, as described in Chapter 24 in treatment of dehydration. If oliguria persists after restoration of fluid volume or if the renal failure is caused by intrinsic renal damage, the physiologic and biochemical abnormalities that have resulted from kidney dysfunction must be corrected or controlled. Initially a Foley catheter is inserted to rule out urine retention, to collect available urine for analysis, and to monitor results of diuretic admin-

---

BOX 27-7 ■ Clinical Manifestations of Acute Renal Failure

Specific:
    Oliguria
    Anuria uncommon (except in obstructive disorders)
Nonspecific (may develop):
    Nausea
    Vomiting
    Drowsiness
    Edema
    Hypertension
Manifestations of underlying disorder or pathologic condition

---

istration. The catheter may or may not be removed during the oliguric phase.

The amount of exogenous water provided should not exceed the amount needed to maintain zero water balance. It is calculated on the basis of estimated endogenous water formation and losses from sensible (primarily gastrointestinal) and insensible sources. No allotment is calculated for urine as long as oliguria persists.

When the output begins to increase, either spontaneously or in response to diuretic therapy, the intake of fluid, potassium, and sodium must be monitored and adequate replacement provided to prevent depletion and its consequences. Some patients pass enormous amounts of electrolyte-rich urine.

Complications. The child with ARF has a tendency to develop water intoxication and hyponatremia, which makes it difficult to provide calories in sufficient amounts to meet the needs of the child and reduce the tissue catabolism, metabolic acidosis, hyperkalemia, and uremia. If the child is able to tolerate oral foods, food sources high in concentrated carbohydrate and fat but low in protein, potassium, and sodium may be provided. However, many children have functional disturbances of the gastrointestinal tract, such as nausea and vomiting; therefore, the intravenous (IV) route is generally preferred and usually consists of essential amino acids or a combination of essential and nonessential amino acids administered by the central venous route.

Control of water balance in these patients requires careful monitoring of feedback information, such as accurate intake and output, body weight, and electrolyte measurements. In general, during the oliguric phase, no sodium, chloride, or potassium is given unless there are other large, ongoing losses. Regular measurement of plasma electrolyte, pH, blood urea nitrogen, and creatinine levels is required to assess the adequacy of fluid therapy and to anticipate complications that require specific treatment.

Hyperkalemia is the most immediate threat to the life of the child with ARF. Hyperkalemia can be minimized and sometimes avoided by eliminating potassium from all food and fluid, by reducing tissue catabolism, and by correcting acidosis. Measures employed for the reduction of serum potassium levels are oral or rectal administration of an ion-exchange resin such as sodium polystyrene sulfonate (Kayexalate) and peritoneal dialysis or hemodialysis (p. 1008). The resin produces its effect by exchange of its sodium for the potassium, thus binding potassium for removal from the body. This increased sodium concentration may contribute to fluid overload, hypertension, and cardiac failure. Dialysis removes potassium and other waste products from the serum by diffusion through a semipermeable membrane.

Hypertension is a frequent and serious complication of ARF, and to detect it early, blood pressure measurements are made every 4 to 6 hours. The most common cause of hypertension in ARF is overexpansion of extracellular fluid and plasma volume together with activation of the renin-angiotensin system. Hypertension is controlled with antihypertensive drugs. Other measures that may be used include limiting fluids and salt.

Anemia is frequently associated with ARF, but transfusion is not recommended unless the hemoglobin drops below 6 g/dL. Transfusions, if used, consist of fresh, packed red blood cells given slowly to reduce the likelihood of increasing blood volume, hypertension, and hyperkalemia.

Seizures occur rather often when renal failure progresses to uremia and are also related to hypertension, hyponatremia, and hypocalcemia. Treatment is directed to the specific cause when known. More obscure causes are managed with antiepileptic drugs.

Cardiac failure with pulmonary edema is almost always associated with hypervolemia. Treatment is directed toward reduction of fluid volume, with water and sodium restriction and administration of diuretics.

Prognosis.

The prognosis of ARF depends largely on the nature and severity of the causative factor or precipitating event and the promptness and competence of management. The outcome is least favorable in children with rapidly progressive nephritis and cortical necrosis. Children in whom ARF is a result of hemolytic-uremic syndrome or acute glomerulitis may recover completely, but residual renal impairment or hypertension is more often the rule. Complete recovery is usually expected in children whose renal failure is a result of dehydration, nephrotoxins, or ischemia. ARF following cardiac surgery is less favorable. It is often impossible to assess the extent of recovery for several months.

Nursing Considerations

Meticulous attention to fluid intake and output is mandatory and includes all of the physical measurements discussed previously in relation to problems of fluid balance. Monitoring fluid balance and vital signs is a continuous process, and observers are constantly on the alert for signs of complications so that appropriate interventions can be implemented. Because these children require intensive observation and, often, specialized treatment, such as dialysis, they are usually admitted to an intensive care unit in which needed equipment and trained personnel are available.

Limiting fluid intake requires ingenuity on the part of caregivers to cope with the child who is thirsty. Rationing the daily intake in small amounts of fluid served in containers that give the impression of larger volumes is one strategy. Older children who understand the rationale of fluid limits can help determine how their daily ration should be distributed.

Meeting nutritional needs is sometimes a problem; the child may be nauseated, and encouraging concentrated foods without fluids may be difficult. When nourishment is provided by the IV route, careful monitoring is essential to prevent fluid overload. In addition, nursing measures such as maintaining an optimal thermal environment, reducing any elevation of body temperature, and reducing restlessness and anxiety are employed to decrease the rate of tissue catabolism.

The nurse must be continually alert for changes in behavior that indicate the onset of complications. Infection from reduced resistance, anemia, and general morbidity is a constant threat. Fluid overload and electrolyte disturbances can precipitate cardiovascular complications such as hypertension and cardiac failure. Fluid and electrolyte imbalances, acidosis, and accumulation of nitrogenous waste products can produce neurologic involvement manifested by coma, seizures, or alterations in sensorium.

Although children with ARF are usually quite ill and voluntarily diminish their activity, infants may become restless and irritable, and children are often anxious and frightened. There are frequent, painful, and stress-producing treatments and tests that must be performed. The presence of a supportive, empathetic nurse can provide comfort and stability in a threatening and unnatural environment.

Family Support.

Providing support and reassurance to parents is among the major nursing responsibilities. The seriousness of ARF and its emergency nature are stressful to parents, and most feel some degree of guilt regarding the child's condition, especially when the illness is a result of ingestion of a toxic substance, dehydration, or a genetic disease. They need reassurance and a sympathetic listener. They also need to be kept informed of the child's progress and provided explanations regarding the therapeutic regimen. The equipment and the child's behavior are sometimes frightening and anxiety provoking. Nurses can do much to help parents comprehend and deal with the stresses of the situation.

CHRONIC RENAL FAILURE

The kidneys are able to maintain the chemical composition of fluids within normal limits until more than 50% of functional renal capacity is destroyed by disease or injury. Chronic renal insufficiency or failure (CRF) begins when the diseased kidneys can no longer maintain the normal chemical structure of body fluids under normal conditions. Progressive deterioration over months or years produces a variety of clinical and biochemical disturbances that eventually culminate in the clinical syndrome known as *uremia.*

A variety of diseases and disorders can result in CRF. The most frequent causes are congenital renal and urinary tract malformations, vesicoureteral reflux associated with recurrent urinary tract infection, chronic pyelonephritis, hereditary disorders, chronic glomerulonephritis, and glomerulonephropathy associated with systemic diseases such as anaphylactoid purpura and lupus erythematosus.

Pathophysiology

Early in the course of progressive nephrotic destruction, the child remains asymptomatic with only minimal biochemical abnormalities. Unless the presence of CRF is detected in the process of routine assessment, signs and symptoms that indicate advanced renal damage frequently emerge only late in the course of the disease. Midway in the disease process, as increasing numbers of nephrons are totally destroyed and most others are damaged to varying degrees, the few that remain intact are hypertrophied but functional. These few normal nephrons are able to make sufficient adjustments to stresses to maintain reasonable degrees of fluid and electrolyte balance. Definitive biochemical examination at this time will reveal restricted tolerance to excesses or restrictions. As the disease progresses to the end stage, because of a severe reduction in the number of functioning nephrons, the kidneys are no longer able to maintain fluid and electrolyte balance, and the features of uremic syndrome appear.

The accumulation of various biochemical substances in the blood, those that result from diminished renal function, produces complications such as the following:

Retention of waste products, especially the blood urea nitrogen and creatinine
Water and sodium retention, which contributes to edema and vascular congestion
Hyperkalemia of dangerous levels
Metabolic acidosis of a sustained nature because of continual hydrogen ion retention and bicarbonate loss
Calcium and phosphorus disturbances, resulting in altered bone metabolism, which in turn causes growth arrest or retardation, bone pain, and deformities known as *renal osteodystrophy*
Anemia caused by hematologic dysfunction, including shortened life span of red blood cells, impaired red blood cell production related to decreased production of erythropoietin, prolonged bleeding time, and nutritional anemia
Growth disturbance, probably caused by such factors as renal osteodystrophy, poor nutrition associated with dietary restrictions and loss of appetite, and biochemical abnormalities

Children with CRF seem to be more susceptible to infection, especially pneumonia, urinary tract infection, and septicemia, although the reason for this is unclear. These children become extraordinarily sensitive to changes in vascular volume that may cause pulmonary overload, central nervous system symptoms, hypertension, and cardiac failure.

Diagnostic Evaluation

The diagnosis of CRF is usually suspected on the basis of any number of clinical manifestations, a history of prior renal disease, and/or biochemical findings. The onset is usually gradual, and the initial signs and symptoms are vague and nonspecific (Box 27-8).

Laboratory and other diagnostic tools and tests are of value in assessing the extent of renal damage, biochemical disturbances, and related physical dysfunction (see Tables 27-1 to 27-3). Often they can help establish the nature of the underlying disease and differentiate between other disease processes and the pathologic consequences of renal dysfunction.

Therapeutic Management

In irreversible renal failure the goals of medical management are to (1) promote maximum renal function, (2) maintain body fluid and electrolyte balance within safe biochemical limits, (3) treat systemic complications, and (4) promote as active

---

BOX 27-8 ■ Clinical Manifestations of Chronic Renal Failure

Early signs:
  Loss of normal energy
  Increased fatigue on exertion
  Pallor, subtle (may not be noticed)
  Elevated blood pressure (sometimes)
As the disease progresses:
  Decreased appetite (especially at breakfast)
  Less interest in normal activities
  Increased or decreased urine output with compensatory intake of fluid
  Pallor more evident
  Sallow, muddy appearance of skin
Child may complain of:
  Headache
  Muscle cramps
  Nausea
Other signs and symptoms:
  Weight loss
  Facial edema
  Malaise
  Bone or joint pain
  Growth retardation
  Dryness or itching of the skin
  Bruised skin
  Sensory or motor loss (sometimes)
  Amenorrhea (common in adolescent girls)
Uremic syndrome (untreated):
  Gastrointestinal symptoms
    Anorexia
    Nausea and vomiting
  Bleeding tendencies
    Bruises
    Bloody diarrheal stools
    Stomatitis
    Bleeding from lips and mouth
  Intractable itching
  Uremic frost (deposits of urea crystals on skin)
  Unpleasant "uremic" breath odor
  Deep respirations
  Hypertension
  Congestive heart failure
  Pulmonary edema
  Neurologic involvement
    Progressive confusion
    Dulled sensorium
    Coma (ultimately)
    Tremors
    Muscular twitching
    Seizures

---

and normal a life as possible for the child for as long as possible. The child is allowed unrestricted activity and is allowed to set his or her own limits regarding rest and extent of exertion. School attendance is encouraged as long as the child is able. When the effort is too great, home tutoring is arranged.

Diet regulation is the most effective means, short of dialysis, for reducing the quantity of materials that require renal excretion. The goal of the diet in renal failure is to provide sufficient calories and protein for growth while limiting the excretory demands made on the kidney, to minimize metabolic bone disease *(osteodystrophy),* and to minimize fluid and electrolyte disturbances. Dietary protein intake is limited only to the recommended daily allowance (RDA) for the child's age. Restriction of protein intake below the RDA is believed to negatively affect growth and neurodevelopment. Malnutrition may develop in patients with CRF even before they need dialysis (Steiber, 1999).

Sodium and water are not usually limited unless there is evidence of edema or hypertension, and potassium is not usually restricted. However, restrictions of any or all three may be imposed in later stages or at any time that abnormal serum concentrations are evident.

Dietary phosphorus is controlled to prevent or correct the calcium/phosphorus imbalance by the reduction of protein and milk intake. Phosphorus levels can be further reduced by oral administration of calcium carbonate preparations that combine with the phosphorus to decrease gastrointestinal absorption and thus the serum levels of phosphate. At the same time that serum calcium levels are increased from the calcium carbonate, vitamin D therapy is begun to increase calcium absorption.

Metabolic acidosis is alleviated through administration of alkalizing agents such as sodium bicarbonate or a combination of sodium and potassium citrate.

Growth failure is one major consequence of CRF, especially in the preadolescent. These children grow poorly both before and after the initiation of hemodialysis. The use of recombinant human growth hormone to accelerate growth in children with growth retardation secondary to CRF has been successful (Mehls and others, 2002; Schaefer and others, 1999). *Osseous deformities* that result from renal osteodystrophy, especially those related to ambulation, are troublesome and require correction if they occur. *Dental defects* are common in children with CRF, and the earlier the onset of the disease, the more severe are the dental manifestations (including hypoplasia, hypomineralization, tooth discolorization, alteration in size and shape of teeth, malocclusion, and ulcerative stomatitis). Therefore regular dental care is especially important in these children.

Anemia in children with CRF is related to decreased production of erythropoietin. Recombinant human erythropoietin (rHuEPO) is being offered to these children as thrice-weekly or weekly subcutaneous injections and is replacing the need for frequent blood transfusions. The drug corrects the anemia and in turn increases appetite, activity, and general well-being in the children who receive it.

Hypertension of advanced renal disease may be managed initially by cautious use of a low-sodium diet, fluid restriction, and perhaps diuretics such as hydrochlorothiazide or furosemide. Severe hypertension requires the use of antihypertensive agents, singly or in combinations.

Intercurrent infections are treated with appropriate antimicrobials at the first sign of infection; however, any drug eliminated through the kidneys is administered with caution. Other complications are treated symptomatically (e.g., central-acting antiemetics for *nausea,* antiepileptics for *seizures,* and diphenhydramine [Benadryl] for *pruritus*).

Once evidence of *end-stage renal disease (ESRD)* appears in a child, the disease runs its relentless course and results in death in a few weeks, unless waste products and tox-ins are removed from body fluids by dialysis or kidney transplantation. Because these techniques have been adapted for infants and small children, these alternatives have been implemented in most cases of renal failure after conservative management is no longer effective (see Technologic Management of Renal Failure, p. 1008).

Prognosis. Dialysis and transplantation are the only treatments currently available for children with ESRD. Although children may survive on dialysis, it is not an ideal long-term modality. Complications include infection of access sites, growth failure, and disruption of normal socialization. Many pediatric centers encourage families of children with ESRD to consider renal transplantation. The North American Renal Transplantation in Children Report of the Pediatric Renal Transplant Cooperative Study reports a graft survival of 90% at 1 year and 74% at 6 years for living donor kidneys, and 80% at 1 year and 58% at 6 years for cadaver kidneys (Benfield and others, 2003).

Posttransplant complications include infection, hypertension, steroid toxicity, hyperlipidemia, aseptic necrosis, malignancy, and growth retardation (Suthanthiran and Strom, 1994). Long-term graft survival is not guaranteed, and many children require a second or third transplant. Successful renal transplantation does improve rehabilitation of children with CRF, both educationally and psychologically. Increasing use of primary or preemptive renal transplants is becoming the optimal form of renal replacement therapy, leading to substantial improvement in quality of life (Laine and others, 1998).

Nursing Considerations

Assessment

Assessment of the child with CRF is primarily one of observation for signs of complications and evidence of improvement through therapy. Some of the first changes observed are growth failure, developmental delay, bone disease, and hypertension.

Nursing Diagnoses

A number of nursing diagnoses become evident on assessment of the child. The most relevant in the majority of cases are outlined in the Nursing Care Plan on p. 1007. Others will be appropriate for individual children and their families.

Planning

The goals of care for the child with CRF, especially one in ESRD, and the family are as follows:

1 Child will receive encouragement in his or her normal growth and development, minimizing the impact of the disease process.
2 Child will remain free of complications.
3 Child and family will receive appropriate support, guidance, and education.

Implementation

The multiple complications of ESRD are managed according to medical protocols prescribed for the care of those specific problems. However, progressive disease places a number of stresses on the child and family, including those of a potentially fatal illness (see Chapter 18). There is a continuing need for repeated examinations that often entail painful procedures, side effects, and frequent hospitalizations. Diet therapy becomes progressively more restricted and intense, and the child is required to take a variety of medications. Ever present in all aspects of the treatment regimen is the agonizing realization that without treatment, death is inevitable.

Some specific stresses related to ESRD and its treatment are predictable. When it first becomes apparent that ESRD is inevitable, both parents and child experience depression and anxiety. Acceptance is particularly difficult if renal failure progresses rapidly after diagnosis. Denial and disbelief are usually pronounced, especially among the parents. After kidney failure is established and symptoms become progressively more distressing, the initiation of dialysis is usually perceived as a positive experience, and after experiencing initial concerns regarding the treatment, the child begins to feel better and parental anxiety is relieved for a time.

Initiating a dialysis regimen is a traumatic and anxiety-provoking experience for most children, because it involves surgery for implantation of a graft, fistula, or peritoneal catheter. The initial experience with the dialysis procedure is frightening to most children. They need reassurance about the nature of the preparations for dialysis and the conduct of the treatment.

Both the graft and the fistula require needle insertions at each dialysis. The goal is to perform pain-free venipuncture. Using buffered lidocaine with a small-gauge needle (30 gauge) to anesthetize the area before venipuncture of the graft/fistula is one method. Using an anesthetizing topical preparation such as EMLA (eutectic mixture of local anesthetics [lidocaine and prilocaine]) 1 hour before venipuncture is another approach (see Pain Management, Chapter 21).

External dual-lumen venous access devices eliminate the need for needles but are more prone to infection and other central line complications.

Adolescents, with their increased need for independence and their urge for rebellion, usually adapt less well. They resent the control and enforced dependence imposed by the rigorous and unrelenting therapy program. They resent being dependent on hemodialysis technology, their parents, and the professional staff. Depression or hostility is common in adolescents undergoing hemodialysis.

The availability of home peritoneal dialysis has offered a greater degree of freedom for persons undergoing long-term dialysis. The nurse is responsible for teaching the family about (1) the disease, its implications, and the therapeutic plan; (2) the possible psychologic effects of the disease and the treatment; and (3) the technical aspects of the procedure. The family learns to manage the various aspects of the dialysis procedure, how to maintain accurate records, and how to observe for signs of complications that need to be reported to the proper persons.

Body changes related to the disease process, such as skin color, growth retardation, and lack of sexual maturation, are stress provoking. Dietary restrictions are particularly burdensome for both children and parents. Children feel deprived when they are unable to eat foods previously enjoyed and that are unrestricted for other family members. Consequently, failure to cooperate may occur. Diet restrictions may be interpreted as punishment. Some children, unable

FAMILY FOCUS

Family Priorities

Families who have children with long-term chronic illnesses, such as end-stage renal disease, spend much time in hospitals, outpatient clinics, and primary health care facilities. When they miss appointments or respond less quickly than anticipated, sometimes they are quickly labeled "noncompliant." It is important to remember that families have to develop priorities for the unit as a whole. Sometimes the family may decide that it is more important for the parent to go to work or to attend a sibling's school performance than to attend an appointment scheduled for them by health care personnel. The chronically ill child cannot and should not always be the number one priority for the family. The professional staff who works with the family can help the parents prioritize the needs of the ill child within the needs of the family constellation.

Teresa Hall, MS, RN
Hathaway Children's Services
Sylmar, Calif

to understand fully the purpose of restrictions, will sneak forbidden food items at every opportunity. Allowing children, especially adolescents, maximum participation in and responsibility for their own treatment program is helpful.

After months or years of dialysis, the parents and child feel anxiety associated with the prognosis and continued pressures of the treatment. The relentless need for treatment interferes with family plans. The time spent in transportation to and from the dialysis unit and the time spent undergoing dialysis treatments cut into time for outside activities, including school. Graft and fistula problems, as well as peritoneal catheter exit site infections, may develop and present a common source of aggravation (see Family Focus box).

The possibility of renal transplantation often provides hope for relief from the rigors of hemodialysis and peritoneal dialysis. Most children and families respond well to a kidney transplant, and most children can be successfully rehabilitated.

The **National Kidney Foundation*** and other agencies provide a number of services and information for families of children with renal disease.

● Evaluation

The effectiveness of nursing interventions is determined by continual reassessment and evaluation of care based on the following observational guidelines:

1. Observe and interview family regarding their compliance with the medical and dietary regimen.
2. Monitor vital signs, growth measurements, laboratory reports, behavior, and appearance.
3. Observe and interview child and family regarding their feelings, concerns, and fears; observe reactions to therapies and prognosis.

The *expected outcomes* are described in the Nursing Care Plan on p. 1007.

---

*30 East 33rd Street, New York, NY 10016; (212) 889-2210 or (800) 622-9010; website: www.kidney.org. In Canada: **Kidney Foundation of Canada,** 300-5165, Sherbrooke Street West, Montreal, QC H4A 1T6; (514) 369-4806 or (800) 361-7494; website: www.kidney.ca.

NURSING DIAGNOSIS ▪ **Risk for injury related to accumulated electrolytes and waste products**

PATIENT GOAL 1: Will maintain near-normal electrolyte levels

NURSING INTERVENTIONS/RATIONALES

*Assist with dialysis *to maintain excretory function*

*Administer Kayexalate as prescribed *to reduce serum potassium levels*

Provide diet low in potassium, sodium, and phosphorus, if prescribed, *to reduce excretory demand on kidneys*

Observe for evidence of accumulated waste products (hyperkalemia, hyperphosphatemia, uremia) *to ensure prompt treatment*

EXPECTED OUTCOME

Child exhibits no evidence of waste product accumulation

NURSING DIAGNOSIS ▪ **Fluid volume excess related to failure of renal regulatory mechanisms**

PATIENT GOAL 1: Will maintain appropriate fluid volume

NURSING INTERVENTIONS/RATIONALES

*Assist with dialysis *to maintain excretory function*

Monitor progress *to assess adequacy of therapy and detect possible complications*

EXPECTED OUTCOME

Child exhibits no evidence or complications of accumulated fluid between dialysis sessions

PATIENT GOAL 2: Will maintain appropriate fluid volume through regulation of fluid intake

NURSING INTERVENTIONS/RATIONALES

*Administer oral fluids as prescribed

Use strategies to prevent undesirable intake

Review daily fluid restrictions with parents and child *to encourage cooperation*

Suggest ways to divide total volume of fluid into small quantities to be spread over entire day

Keep mouth moist by other means, such as hard candy, ice chips, fine mist spray of cool water, *to prevent feeling of dryness*

EXPECTED OUTCOME

Child exhibits minimal evidence of fluid gain

NURSING DIAGNOSIS ▪ **Altered nutrition: less than body requirements related to restricted diet**

PATIENT GOAL 1: Will consume appropriate diet

NURSING INTERVENTIONS/RATIONALES

Provide dietary instructions for foods *that reduce excretory demands on kidney and provide sufficient calories and protein for growth*

*Limit phosphorus, salt, and potassium as prescribed

Encourage intake of carbohydrates *to provide calories for growth* and foods high in calcium *to prevent bone demineralization*

Arrange for renal dietitian to meet with family to review allowable foods and assist in dietary planning *so that family understands dietary needs of child*

Help hemodialysis patients to fill out menu requests for meals

EXPECTED OUTCOME

Child consumes an adequate amount of appropriate foods

Child shows no evidence of deficiencies or weight loss

NURSING DIAGNOSIS ▪ **Body-image disturbance related to chronic illness, impaired growth, and perception of being "different"**

PATIENT GOAL 1: Will develop positive self-esteem and understanding of disease

NURSING INTERVENTIONS/*RATIONALES*

Provide education about CRF, including management, treatment, and long-term outcome

Encourage child's independence with care and management of CRF *because independence helps child develop positive self-esteem*

Allow child to participate in dialysis procedures

Allow child to participate in making decisions when appropriate

Promote self-esteem in child with CRF

Organize patient support group or suggest counseling as needed

Provide positive reinforcement during dialysis procedures and follow-up visits

EXPECTED OUTCOME

Child demonstrates an understanding of CRF and complies with therapies

Child exhibits signs of positive self-esteem

NURSING DIAGNOSIS ▪ **Altered family processes related to a child with a chronic disease**

PATIENT (FAMILY) GOAL 1: Will exhibit positive coping behaviors

NURSING INTERVENTIONS/*RATIONALES*

Assist parents in diet planning and support their efforts to adjust diet to meet needs of all family members

Provide anticipatory guidance regarding probable and expected events, such as symptoms, diet, and effects of medications

Assist parents in decision making regarding dialysis and transplantation *because these are the alternatives after other measure are no longer effective*

Prepare child and family for hemodialysis or kidney transplantation *because preparation is essential for positive coping*

Prepare child and family for home hemodialysis or continuous home peritoneal dialysis

Maintain periodic contact with family *for ongoing support*

Refer family to special agencies and support groups *for long-term support*

EXPECTED OUTCOME

Child and family demonstrate ability to cope with stresses of illness (specify)

See also:

Nursing Care Plan: The Child in the Hospital, Chapter 21

Nursing Care Plan: The Family of the Ill or Hospitalized Child, Chapter 21

Nursing Care Plan: The Child Who Is Terminally Ill or Dying, Chapter 18

*Dependent nursing action.

TECHNOLOGIC MANAGEMENT OF RENAL FAILURE

DIALYSIS

Dialysis is the process of separating colloids and crystalline substances in solution by the difference in their rate of diffusion through a semipermeable membrane. Methods of dialysis currently available for clinical management of renal failure are *peritoneal dialysis,* wherein the abdominal cavity acts as a semipermeable membrane through which water and solutes of small molecular size move by osmosis and diffusion according to their respective concentrations on either side of the membrane, and *hemodialysis,* in which blood is circulated outside the body through artificial membranes that permit a similar passage of water and solutes. A third type of dialysis is *hemofiltration,* in which blood filtrate is circulated outside the body by hydrostatic pressure exerted across a semipermeable membrane with simultaneous infusion of a replacement solution. Types of hemofiltration include *continuous venovenous hemofiltration (CVVH), continuous venovenous hemodialysis (CVVHD),* and *continuous venovenous hemodiafiltration (CVVHDF).* These continuous renal replacement therapies are used in ARF, severe fluid overload, inborn errors of metabolism, or after bone marrow transplant (Goldstein, 2003).

Peritoneal dialysis is the preferred form of dialysis for infants, children and parents who wish to remain independent, families who live a long distance from the medical center, and children who prefer fewer dietary restrictions and a gentler form of dialysis. Chronic peritoneal dialysis is most often performed at home. The two types of peritoneal dialysis are *continuous ambulatory peritoneal dialysis (CAPD)* and *continuous cycling peritoneal dialysis (CCPD).* In both methods, commercially available sterile dialysis solution is instilled into the peritoneal cavity through a surgically implanted indwelling catheter tunneled subcutaneously and sutured into place. The warmed solution is allowed to enter the peritoneal cavity by gravity and remains a variable length of time according to the rate of solute removal and glucose absorption in individual patients. The care and management of the procedure are the responsibility of the parents of young children. Use of home health nurses to give parents respite from care has been initiated in some centers (Cascio and others, 1994). Older children and adolescents can carry out the procedure themselves, which provides them with some control and less dependency. This is especially important for adolescents.

> ## ⚠ NURSING ALERT
>
> Observe for changes in the color of the dialysate draining from the child. The spent solution should be clear. If the color is cloudy, notify the practitioner immediately (Schaefer, 2003).

Hemodialysis requires the creation of a vascular access and the use of special dialysis equipment—the hemodialyzer, or so-called artificial kidney. Vascular access may be one of three types: fistulas, grafts, or external vascular access devices. An *atriovenous fistula* is an access in which a vein and artery are connected surgically. The preferred site is the radial artery and a forearm vein that produces dilation and thickening of the superficial vessels of the forearm to pro-

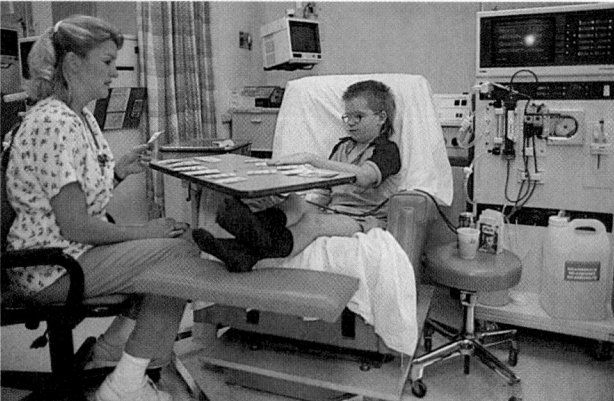

FIG. 27-3 ■ Diversional activities help lessen the boredom children can experience during hemodialysis.

vide easy access for repeated venipuncture. An alternative is the creation of a subcutaneous (internal) *arteriovenous graft* by anastomosing artery and vein, with a synthetic prosthetic graft for circulatory access. The most commonly used material is expanded polytetrafluoroethylene (ePTFE). Both the graft and the fistula require needle insertions with each dialysis treatment.

For external vascular access devices, percutaneous catheters are inserted in the femoral, subclavian, or internal jugular veins, even in very small children. A more permanent form of external access is available via a central catheter inserted surgically into the internal jugular vein. This catheter has a dual lumen, which allows a larger volume of blood flow with minimum recirculation. Catheters eliminate the need for skin punctures but may require some home care.

Hemodialysis is best suited to children who do not have someone in the family who is able to perform home peritoneal dialysis and to those who live close to a dialysis center. The procedure is usually performed three times per week for 4 to 6 hours, depending on the size of the child. Hemodialysis achieves rapid correction of fluid and electrolyte abnormalities but can cause problems in association with this rapid change, such as muscle cramping and hypotension. Disadvantages include school absence during dialysis and strict fluid and dietary restrictions between dialysis sessions. Boredom for the child and family is often a problem during dialysis, and planned activities should be introduced (Fig. 27-3) (Currier and Brewer, 1999).

Most children show rapid clinical improvement with the implementation of dialysis, although it is directly related to the duration of uremia before dialysis and good nutrition. Growth rate and skeletal maturation improve, but recovery of normal growth occurs infrequently. In many cases, sexual development, although delayed, progresses to completion.

TRANSPLANTATION

Renal transplantation is now an acceptable and effective means of therapy in the pediatric age-group. Although peritoneal dialysis and hemodialysis are life preserving, both require major alterations in lifestyle. Transplantation offers the opportunity for a relatively normal life and is the preferred form of treatment for children with ESRD. Primary or preemptive transplants maintain the greatest amount of normalcy in the family's life.

Kidneys for transplant are available from two sources: a *living related donor (LRD),* usually a parent or a sibling, or a *cadaver donor (CAD),* wherein the family of a dead or brain-dead patient consents to donation of a healthy kidney. Retransplantation occurs frequently.

The primary goal in transplantation is the long-term survival of grafted tissue by securing tissue that is antigenically similar to that of the recipient and by suppressing the recipient's immune mechanism. The immunosuppressant therapy of choice has been corticosteroids (Prednisone) in conjunction with cyclosporine and azathioprine. Other therapies include antilymphoblast globulin or monoclonal antibodies. New immunosuppressant medications are rapidly coming into clinical trials and into use in large transplant centers. It is important for the nurse to learn about the medications used in the antirejection protocol(s) and their side effects. Because the immunosuppressant medications are taken indefinitely, transplant patients experience many side effects of the drugs, including hypertension, growth retardation, cataracts, risk of infection, obesity, characteristics of Cushing syndrome, and hirsutism (Currier, McCarley, and Brewer, 2001).

> **! NURSING ALERT**
>
> The child with a recent kidney transplant (a few days) or one who was grafted approximately 6 months previously who exhibits any of the following should be evaluated immediately for possible rejection:
>   Fever
>   Swelling and tenderness over graft area
>   Diminished urine output
>   Elevated blood pressure

Rejection of the transplanted kidney is the most common cause of transplant failure. Rejection is treated aggressively with immunosuppressant medications and can often be reversed. Some patients do not respond to treatment of acute rejection or develop chronic rejection and must eventually return to dialysis or undergo another kidney transplant.

KEY POINTS

- Common inflammatory disorders of the genitourinary tract include urinary tract infection, nephrotic syndrome, and acute glomerulonephritis.
- Management of urinary tract infections is directed at eliminating infection, detecting and correcting functional or anatomic abnormalities, preventing recurrences, and preserving renal function.
- Vesicoureteral reflux is the retrograde flow of bladder urine into the ureters.
- Obstructive uropathy is a result of structural or functional abnormalities of the urinary system that obstruct the normal flow of urine.
- The more common defects of the genitourinary tract include phimosis, cryptorchidism, inguinal hernia, hydrocele, and hypospadias.
- Body-image concerns and castration anxiety are particularly intense in children with defects in the genital area.

- Nephrotic syndrome is characterized by increased glomerular permeability to protein, with massive urinary loss of protein resulting in hypoproteinemia and edema.
- Management of nephrotic syndrome is aimed at reducing excretion of protein, reducing or preventing fluid retention by tissues, and preventing infection and other complications.
- Common features of acute glomerulonephritis are oliguria, edema, hypertension, circulatory congestion, hematuria, and proteinuria.
- Therapeutic management of acute glomerulonephritis is maintenance of fluid balance, treatment of hypertension, and antibiotic therapy.
- Management of hemolytic-uremic syndrome is aimed at control of complications and hematologic manifestations of renal failure.
- Wilms tumor is the most common malignant neoplasm of the kidney in infants and children.
- In acute renal failure, management is directed at determining treatment of the underlying cause, management of complications of renal failure, and supportive therapy.
- Abnormalities in chronic renal failure are waste product retention, water and sodium retention, hyperkalemia, acidosis, calcium and phosphorus disturbance, anemia, and growth disturbances.
- The types of dialysis used in end-stage renal disease are peritoneal dialysis and hemodialysis.
- When the child will need home dialysis, the nurse educates the family about the disease, its implications, the therapeutic plan, possible psychologic effects of the disease, and the treatment and technical aspects of the procedure.
- The major concerns in renal transplantation are tissue matching and prevention of rejection; psychologic concerns involve self-image as related to possible body changes as a result of the effects of corticosteroid therapy.

References

American Academy of Pediatrics: Task Force on Circumcision, *Pediatrics* 103(3):686-693, 1999.

Benfield MR, McDonald RA, Bartosh S and others: Changing trends in pediatric transplantation: 2001 annual report of the North American Pediatric Renal Transplant Cooperative Study, *Pediatr Transplant* 7(4):321-335, 2003.

Brandt JR and others: More on *E. coli*–induced hemolytic-uremic syndrome, *J Pediatr* 125(4):519-526, 1994.

Cascio C and others: Use of private duty nurses for daily CCPD and family relief in pediatric PD patients, *Adv Perit Dial* 10:304-306, 1994.

Currier H, Brewer ED: Pediatric hemodialysis. In Gutch CF, Stoner MH, Corea AL, editors: *Review of hemodialysis for nurses and dialysis personnel,* ed 6, St Louis, 1999, Mosby.

Currier H, McCarley PB, Brewer ED: The pediatric renal failure-dialysis-transplant patient. In Lancaster L, editor: *ANNA core curriculum,* ed 4, Pitman, NJ, 2001, American Nephrology Nurses' Association.

Goldstein SL: Overview of pediatric renal replacement therapy in AFT, *Artificial Organs* 27(9):770-783, 2003.

Grundy PE and others: Wilms tumor. In Pizzo PA, Poplack DP, editors: *Principles and practices of pediatric oncology,* ed 4, Philadelphia, 2002, JB Lippincott.

Kass E: Timing of elective surgery on the genitalia of male children with particular reference to the risks, benefits, and psychological effects of surgery and anesthesia, *Pediatrics* 97(4):590-594, 1996.

Kline NE, Sevier N: Solid tumors in children, *J Pediatr Nurs* 18(2):96-102, 2003.

Laine J and others: Pediatric kidney transplantation, *Ann Med* 30(1):45-57, 1998.

Mehls O and others: Effectiveness of growth hormone treatment in short children with chronic renal failure, *J Pediatr* 141(1):147-148, 2002.

Rosenthal M: Current concept in managing UTIs in children, *Infect Dis Child* 17(3):30-31, 2004.

Schaefer F: Management of peritonitis in children receiving chronic peritoneal dialysis, *Paediatr Drugs* 5(5):315-325, 2003.

Schaefer F and others: Long-term experience with growth hormone treatment in children with chronic renal failure, *Perit Dial Int* 19(suppl 2):S467-S472, 1999.

Schlager TA and others: Effect of cranberry juice on bacteriuria in children with neurogenic bladder receiving intermittent catheterization, *J Pediatr* 135(6):698-702, 1999.

Steiber AL: Clinical indicators associated with poor oral intake of patients with chronic renal failure, *J Ren Nutr* 9(2):84-88, 1999.

Suthanthiran M, Strom TB: Renal transplantation, *N Engl J Med* 331(6):365-375, 1994.

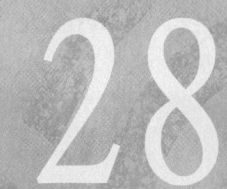

The Child With Cerebral Dysfunction

ROSALIND BRYANT

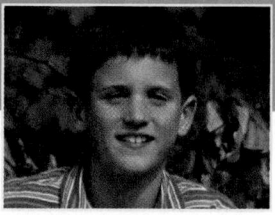

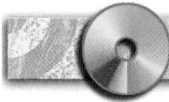

Remember to check out your companion CD-ROM

http://evolve.elsevier.com/Wong/essentials/

CHAPTER OUTLINE

RELATED TOPICS and ADDITIONAL RESOURCES

 IN TEXT

 CD COMPANION

Critical Thinking Exercise—Seizures
Case Studies—Meningitis; Hydrocephalus
   With Myelomeningocele
Clinical Manifestations—Increased
   Intracranial Pressure in Infants and
   Children; Acute Head Injury;
   Posttraumatic Syndromes; Bacterial
   Meningitis; Rabies
Nursing Care Plans
NCLEX-Style Review Questions

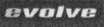 WEBSITE

WebLinks
NCLEX-Style Review Questions

 WONG'S CLINICAL MANUAL
   OF PEDIATRIC NURSING, 6/E

Community and Home Care
   Instructions—Caring for an
   Intermittent Infusion Device;
   Administering Oral and Rectal
   Medications
Nursing Care Plan—The Child With
   Acute Bacterial Meningitis

CEREBRAL DYSFUNCTION

ASSESSMENT OF CEREBRAL FUNCTION

Most of the information about the status of the brain is obtained by indirect measurements. Some of these measurements are discussed elsewhere in relation to numerous aspects of childcare (e.g., as part of assessments of health [Chapter 7], newborn status [Chapter 8], mental retardation [Chapter 19], hypoxic injury [cerebral palsy, Chapter 32], and attainment of developmental milestones at each stage of development). Since increased intracranial pressure and altered states of consciousness have such prominent places in neurologic dysfunction, they are described here, followed by techniques for neurologic assessment and diagnostic tests.

General Aspects

Children younger than 2 years of age require special evaluation, since they are unable to respond to directions designed to elicit specific neurologic responses in infants. Early neurologic responses in infants are primarily reflexive; these responses are gradually replaced by meaningful movement in the characteristic cephalocaudal direction of development. This evidence of progressive maturation reflects more extensive myelinization and changes in neurochemical and electrophysiologic properties.

Most information about infants and small children is gained by observing their spontaneous and elicited reflex responses as they develop increasingly complex locomotor and fine motor skills and by eliciting progressively sophisticated communicative and adaptive behaviors. Delay or deviation from expected milestones helps identify high-risk children. Persistence or reappearance of reflexes that normally disappear indicates a pathologic condition. In evaluating the infant or young child, it is also important to obtain the pregnancy and delivery history to determine the possible effect of intrauterine environmental influences known to affect the orderly maturation of the central nervous system (CNS). These influences include maternal infections, chemicals, trauma, and metabolic insults.

General aspects of assessment that provide clues to the etiology of dysfunction include the following:

Family history—Sometimes offers clues regarding possible genetic disorders with neurologic manifestations
Health history—May provide valuable clues regarding the cause of dysfunction (e.g., an injury, short febrile illness, encounter with an animal or insect, ingestion of neurotoxic substances, inhalation of chemicals, a past illness, or known diabetes mellitus)

Physical evaluation of infants—Includes observation of the following:
  Size and shape of the head
  Spontaneous activity and postural reflex activity
  Sensory responses
  Attitude—normal flexed posture, extreme extension, opisthotonos, hypotonia
  Symmetry in movement of extremities
  Excessive tremulousness or frequent twitching movements
  Altered expiratory cycle:
    Prolonged apnea
    Ataxic breathing
    Paradoxic chest movement
    Hyperventilation
  Skin and hair texture
  Distinctive facial features
  Presence of a high-pitched, piercing cry
  Abnormal eye movements
  Inability to suck or swallow
  Lip smacking
  Asymmetric contraction of facial muscles
  Yawning (may indicate cranial nerve involvement)
  Muscular activity and coordination
  Level of development

Increased Intracranial Pressure

The brain, tightly enclosed in the solid bony cranium, is well protected but highly vulnerable to pressure that may accumulate within the enclosure. The cranium's total volume—brain (80%), cerebrospinal fluid (CSF) (10%), and blood (10%)—must remain approximately the same at all times. A change in the proportional volume of one of these components (e.g., increase or decrease in intracranial blood) must be accompanied by a compensatory change in another. In this way the volume and pressure normally remain constant. Examples of compensatory changes are reduction in blood volume, decrease in CSF production, increase in CSF absorption, or shrinkage of brain mass by displacement of intracellular and extracellular fluid. Children with open fontanels compensate by skull expansion and widened sutures. However, at any age the capacity for spatial compensation is limited. An increase in intracranial pressure (ICP) may be caused by tumors or other space-occupying lesions, accumulation of fluid within the ventricular system, bleeding, or edema of cerebral tissues. Once compensation is exhausted, any further increase in volume will result in a rapid rise in ICP.

Early signs and symptoms of increased ICP are often subtle and assume many patterns (Box 28-1). As pressure

BOX 28-1 ■ Clinical Manifestations of Increased Intracranial Pressure in Infants and Children

INFANTS
Tense, and/or bulging fontanel
Separated cranial sutures
Macewen sign (cracked-pot sound on percussion)
Irritability
High-pitched cry
Increased occipitofrontal circumference
Distended scalp veins
Changes in feeding
Crying when disturbed
Setting-sun sign

CHILDREN
Headache
Nausea
Vomiting
Diplopia, blurred vision
Seizures

PERSONALITY AND BEHAVIOR SIGNS
Irritability, restlessness
Indifference, drowsiness
Decline in school performance
Diminished physical activity and motor performance
Increased sleeping
Memory loss
Inability to follow simple commands
Lethargy and drowsiness

LATE SIGNS
Bradycardia
Lowered level of consciousness
Decreased motor response to command
Decreased sensory response to painful stimuli
Alterations in pupil size and reactivity
Decerebrate or decorticate posturing
Cheyne-Stokes respirations
Papilledema
Coma

BOX 28-2 ■ Levels of Consciousness

Full consciousness—Awake and alert; oriented to time, place, and person; behavior appropriate for age
Confusion—Impaired decision making
Disorientation—Disorientation to time and place, decreased level of consciousness
Lethargy—Limited spontaneous movement, sluggish speech, drowsy
Obtundation—Arousable with stimulation
Stupor—Remains in a deep sleep, responsive only to vigorous and repeated stimulation
Coma—No motor or verbal response to noxious (painful) stimuli
Persistent vegetative state (PVS)—The permanently lost function of the cerebral cortex—eyes follow objects only by reflex or when attracted to the direction of loud sounds, all four limbs are spastic but can withdraw from painful stimuli, hands show reflexive grasping and groping, the face can grimace, some food may be swallowed, and the child may groan or cry but utters no words.

Modified from Seidel HM and others, editors: *Mosby's guide to physical examination*, ed 5, St Louis, 2003, Mosby.

Levels of Consciousness. Assessment of level of consciousness (LOC) remains the earliest indicator of improvement or deterioration in neurologic status. LOC is determined by observations of the child's responses to the environment. Other diagnostic tests, such as motor activity, reflexes, and vital signs, are more variable and do not necessarily directly parallel the depth of the comatose state. The most consistently used terms are described in Box 28-2.

Coma Assessment. Several scales have been devised in an attempt to standardize the description and interpretation of the degree of depressed consciousness. The most popular of these is the *Glasgow Coma Scale (GCS),* which consists of a three-part assessment: eye opening, verbal response, and motor response (Fig. 28-1). When LOC is being assessed in young children, it is often useful to have a parent present to help elicit a desired response. An infant or child may not respond in an unfamiliar environment or to unfamiliar voices. Children older than 3 years of age should be able to give their name, although they may not be cognizant of place or time.

Numeric values of 1 through 5 are assigned to the levels of response in each category. The sum of these numeric values provides an objective measure of the patient's LOC. The lower the score, the deeper the coma. A person with an unaltered LOC would score the highest, 15; a score of 8 or below is generally accepted as a definition of coma; the lowest score, 3, indicates deep coma. The Task Force for the Determination of Brain Death in Children has established physical examination criteria for cases of irreversible coma.

NURSING ALERT

Lack of response to painful stimuli is abnormal and should be reported immediately.

Neurologic Examination

The purpose of the neurologic examination is to establish an accurate, objective baseline of neurologic information. It is essential that the neurologic examination be documented in

increases, signs and symptoms become more pronounced and the level of consciousness deteriorates.

Altered States of Consciousness

Consciousness implies awareness—the ability to respond to sensory stimuli and have subjective experiences. There are two components of consciousness: *alertness,* an arousal-waking state, including the ability to respond to stimuli; and *cognitive power,* including the ability to process stimuli and produce verbal and motor responses.

An altered state of consciousness usually refers to varying states of unconsciousness that may be momentary or may extend for hours, days, or indefinitely. *Unconsciousness* is depressed cerebral function—the inability to respond to sensory stimuli and have subjective experiences. *Coma* is defined as a state of unconsciousness from which the patient cannot be aroused even with powerful stimuli.

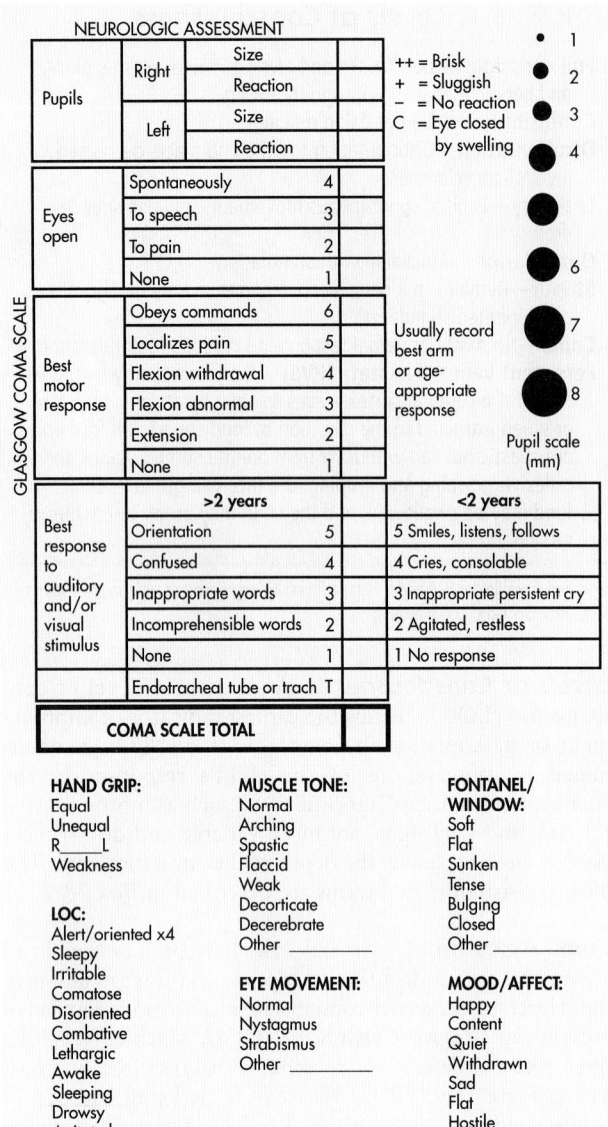

FIG. 28-1 ■ Pediatric coma scale.

a fashion that is able to be reproduced by others. This allows for a comparison of the findings that allows the observer to detect subtle changes in the neurologic status that might not otherwise be evident. Descriptions of behaviors should be simple, objective, and easily interpreted: "Drowsy but awake and conversationally rational/oriented"; "Sleepy but arousable with vigorous physical stimuli. Pressure to nail base of right hand results in upper extremity flexion/lower extremity extension."

Vital Signs. Pulse, respiration, and blood pressure provide information regarding the adequacy of circulation and the possible underlying cause of altered consciousness. Autonomic activity is most intensively disturbed in cases of deep coma or brainstem lesions.

Body temperature is often elevated, and sometimes the elevation may be extreme. Coma of a toxic origin may produce hypothermia. High temperature is most frequently a sign of an acute infectious process or heat stroke but may be caused by ingestion of some drugs (especially salicylates, al-

cohol, and barbiturates) or by intracranial bleeding, especially subarachnoid hemorrhage. Hypothalamic involvement may cause elevated or decreased temperature.

The *pulse* is variable and may be rapid, slow and bounding, or feeble. *Blood pressure* may be normal, elevated, or at shock levels. The Cushing reflex, or pressor response, which causes a slowing of the pulse and an increase in blood pressure, is uncommon in children; when it occurs, it is a very late sign. Vital signs are also affected by medications. For assessment purposes, actual *changes* in pulse and blood pressure are more important than the direction of the change.

Respirations are often slow, deep, and irregular. Slow, deep breathing is often seen in the heavy sleep caused by sedatives, after seizures, or in cerebral infections. Slow, shallow breathing may result from sedatives or opioids (narcotics). Hyperventilation (deep and rapid respirations) is usually a result of metabolic acidosis or abnormal stimulation of the respiratory center in the medulla caused by salicylate poisoning, hepatic coma, or Reye syndrome.

Breathing patterns have been described with a number of terms (e.g., apneustic, cluster, ataxic, Cheyne-Stokes). However, it is better to describe what is being observed rather than placing a label on it because the traditional terms are often used and interpreted incorrectly. Periodic or irregular breathing is an ominous sign of brainstem (especially medullary) dysfunction that often precedes complete apnea. The *odor* of the breath may provide additional clues (e.g., the fruity, acetone odor of ketosis; the foul odor of uremia; the fetid odor of hepatic failure; or the odor of alcohol).

Skin. The skin may offer clues to the cause of unconsciousness. The body surface should be examined for the presence of injury, needle marks, petechiae, bites, and ticks. Evidence of toxic substances may be found on the hands, face, mouth, and clothing—especially in small children.

Eyes. Pupil size and reactivity are assessed (Fig. 28-2; see also Fig. 28-1). Pinpoint pupils are commonly observed in poisoning, such as opiate or barbiturate poisoning, or in brainstem dysfunction. Widely dilated and reactive pupils are often seen after seizures and may involve only one side. Dilated pupils may also be caused by eye trauma. Widely dilated and fixed pupils suggest paralysis of cranial nerve III secondary to pressure from herniation of the brain through the tentorium. A unilateral fixed pupil usually suggests a lesion on the same side. If pupils are fixed bilaterally for more than 5 minutes, brainstem damage is usually implied. Dilated and nonreactive pupils are also seen in hypothermia, anoxia, ischemia, poisoning with atropine-like substances, or prior instillation of mydriatic drugs.

> **! NURSING ALERT**
>
> **The sudden appearance of a fixed and dilated pupil(s) is a neurosurgical emergency.**

The description of eye movements should indicate whether one or both eyes are involved and how the reaction was elicited. The parents should be asked about preexisting strabismus, which will cause the eyes to appear normal under compromise. A posttraumatic strabismus indicates cranial nerve VI damage.

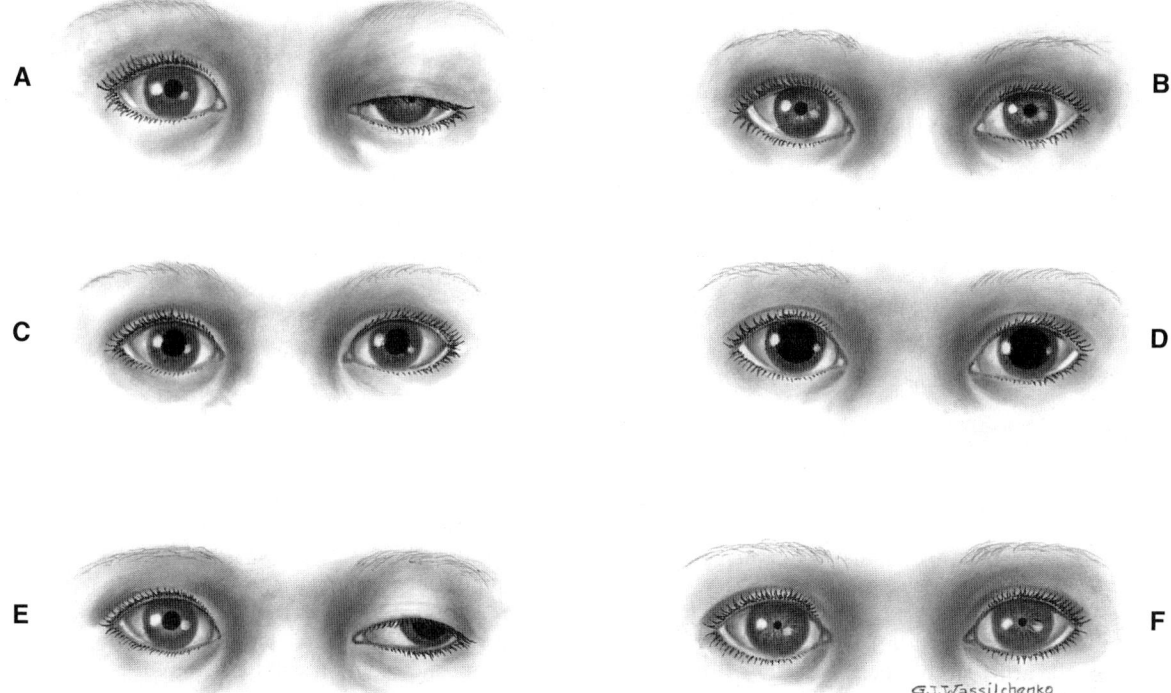

FIG. 28-2 ■ Variations in pupil size with altered states of consciousness. **A,** Ipsilateral pupillary constriction with slight ptosis. **B,** Bilateral small pupils. **C,** Midposition, light fixed to all stimuli. **D,** Bilateral dilated and fixed pupils. **E,** Dilated pupils, left eye abducted with ptosis. **F,** Pinpoint pupils.

Special tests, usually performed by qualified persons, include the following:

Doll's head maneuver—Elicited by rotating the child's head quickly to one side and then to the other. Conjugate (paired or working together) movement of the eyes in the direction opposite to the head rotation is normal. Absence of this response suggests dysfunction of the brainstem or oculomotor nerve (cranial nerve III).

> **! NURSING ALERT**
>
> Any tests that require head movement are not attempted until after cervical spine injury has been ruled out.

Caloric test, or oculovestibular response—Elicited with the child's head up (head of bed is elevated 30 degrees) by irrigating the external auditory canal with 10 mL of ice water for 20 seconds, which normally causes conjugate movement of the eyes toward the side of stimulation. This movement is lost when the pontine centers are impaired, thus providing important information in assessment of the comatose patient.

> **! NURSING ALERT**
>
> The caloric test is painful and is never performed on a child who is awake or on an individual with a ruptured tympanic membrane.

Funduscopic examination—Reveals additional clues. Papilledema will not be evident early in the course of unconsciousness because it takes 24 to 48 hours to develop, if it develops at all. Papilledema is characterized by optic disc swelling, indistinct optic disc margins, hemorrhage, tortuosity of vessels, and absence of venous pulsations. The presence of preretinal (subhyaloid) hemorrhages in children is almost invariably a result of acute trauma with intracranial bleeding, usually subarachnoid or subdural hemorrhage.

Motor Function. Observing spontaneous activity, posture, and response to painful stimuli provides clues to the location and extent of cerebral dysfunction. Even subtle movements (e.g., the outward rotation of a hip) should be noted and the child observed for other signs. Asymmetric movements of the limbs or absence of movement suggests paralysis. In hemiplegia the affected limb lies in external rotation and will fall uncontrollably when lifted and allowed to drop. These observations should be described rather than labeled.

In the deeper comatose states there is little or no spontaneous movement, and the musculature tends to be flaccid. There is considerable variability in the motor behavior in lesser degrees of coma. For example, the child may be relatively immobile or restless and hyperkinetic; muscle tone may be increased or decreased. Tremors, twitching, and spasms of muscles are common observations. The patient may display purposeless plucking or tossing movements. Combative or negativistic behavior is not uncommon. Hyperactivity is more common in acute febrile and toxic states than in cases of increased ICP. Seizures are common in children and may be present in coma from any cause. Any repetitive or seizure movements should be described.

Posturing. Since cortical control over motor function is lost in brain dysfunction, primitive postural reflexes emerge. These reflexes are evident in posturing and motor movements directly related to the area of the brain involved. *Decorticate posturing* (Fig. 28-3, *A*) is seen when there is severe dysfunction of the cerebral cortex. Typical decorti-

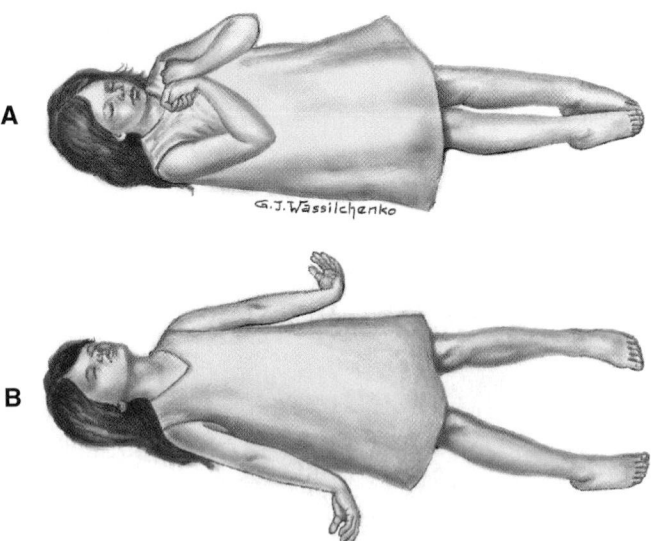

G.J.Wassilchenko

FIG. 28-3 ■ **A,** Decorticate posturing. **B,** Decerebrate posturing.

cate posturing includes adduction of the arms at the shoulders, flexion of the arms on the chest with the wrists flexed and the hands fisted, and extension and adduction of the lower extremities. *Decerebrate posturing* (Fig. 28-3, *B*), a sign of dysfunction at the level of the midbrain, is characterized by rigid extension and pronation of the arms and legs. The posturing may not be evident when the child is quiet but can usually be elicited by applying painful stimuli, such as a blunt object pressed on the base of the nail.

Reflexes. Testing of some reflexes may be of limited value. In general, the corneal, pupillary, muscle-stretch, superficial, and plantar reflexes tend to be absent in deep coma. The state of reflexes is variable in lighter grades of unconsciousness and depends on the underlying pathologic process and the location of the lesion. Absence of corneal reflexes and presence of a tonic neck reflex are associated with severe brain damage. The Babinski reflex (see Extremities, Chapter 7) may be of value if it is found to be present consistently in children older than 18 months. A positive Babinski reflex is significant in assessment of pyramidal tract lesions when it is unilateral and associated with other pyramidal signs.

⚠ NURSING ALERT

Three key reflexes that demonstrate neurologic health in young infants are the Moro, tonic neck, and withdrawal reflexes.

Special Diagnostic Procedures

Numerous diagnostic procedures are used for assessment of cerebral function. Laboratory tests that may help to determine the cause of unconsciousness include blood glucose, urea nitrogen, and electrolyte (pH, sodium, potassium, chloride, calcium, and bicarbonate) tests; clotting studies, hematocrit, and a complete blood cell count; liver function tests; blood cultures (if fever is present); and sometimes studies to detect lead or other toxic substances, such as drugs.

Highly sophisticated tests are carried out with specialized equipment by skilled personnel. Most of these tests are out-

lined in Box 28-3. Because such tests can be threatening to children, a child will need preparation for, and support and reassurance during, the tests (see Preparation for Procedures, Chapter 22).

Children who are old enough to understand will require careful explanation of the procedure, why it is being done, what they will experience, and how they can help. School-age children usually appreciate a more detailed description of why contrast material is injected. The importance of lying still for tests must be stressed. Children unfamiliar with the machines can be shown a picture beforehand. Although radiographic examinations are not painful, the machinery is often so frightening in appearance that the child protests because of anxiety.

Tests such as computed tomography (CT) and magnetic resonance imaging (MRI) require that children be immobilized. Chin and cheek pads are sometimes used to prevent the slightest head movement, and straps are applied to the body to prevent any change in body position. The nurse can explain these events to a frightened child by comparing them to an astronaut's preparation for a space flight. It is very important to emphasize to the child that at no time is the procedure painful.

Usually young children are developmentally unable to cooperate, and sedation will be required. Numerous agents are used for sedation during diagnostic procedures; chloral hydrate remains a safe and frequently used medication before diagnostic imaging tests. The suggested oral chloral hydrate dose is as follows (Lee, Nechyba, and Gunn, 2002):

- 75 to 100 mg/kg (to a maximum dose of 1 g for infants and 2 g for children).
- If child is still awake after 20 minutes, supplementary doses of 100 mg/kg may be given up to a total dose of 1g for infants and 2 g for children.
- The drug should be given 35 to 45 minutes before the anticipated imaging time.

It is helpful for nurses to become acquainted with the equipment and the general environment in which the test will take place so that they can better explain the procedure to children at their level of understanding. Equipment is often strange and ominous to children and may be perceived as a frightening monster. They need constant reassurance from a trusted companion. Since children are particularly frightened of needles, they need to be informed of any medication or contrast media to be administered intravenously.

Physical preparation may involve administering a sedative or providing IV access for infusion of contrast material. If so, children should be given a local topical anesthetic such as EMLA before the IV is placed and helped through the preparation and administration and assured that someone will remain with them (if possible). Children will need continual support and reinforcement during procedures for which they remain conscious. Vital signs and physiologic response to the procedure are monitored throughout. Conscious sedation records become part of the child's chart. Many diagnostic procedures performed on an outpatient basis require sedation, and children need recovery time and observation. Written instructions should be reviewed with parents if the child is discharged to home following a procedure.

Children who have undergone a procedure while under general anesthesia require postanesthesia care, including posi-

BOX 28-3 ■ Procedures Used in Cerebral Assessment

LUMBAR PUNCTURE (LP)
Diagnostic: measures spinal fluid pressure, obtains cerebrospinal fluid (CSF) for visualization and laboratory analysis

SUBDURAL TAP
Helps rule out subdural effusions
Relieves intracranial pressure

ELECTROENCEPHALOGRAPHY (EEG)
Measures electric activity of cerebral cortex
Detects electric abnormalities
Used to determine brain death

VIDEO EEG
Split-screen simultaneous visualization of whole-body, facial, and EEG recording

COMPUTED TOMOGRAPHY (CT) SCAN
Visualizes horizontal and vertical cross section of brain at any axis
Distinguishes density of various intracranial tissues and structures—congenital abnormalities, hemorrhage, tumors, and demyelinating and inflammatory processes

NUCLEAR BRAIN SCAN
Test material accumulates in areas where blood-brain barrier is defective
Identifies focal brain lesions (e.g., tumors, abscesses)
Positive uptake of material with encephalitis and subdural hematoma
Visualizes CSF pathways

TRANSILLUMINATION
Varying degrees of localized glowing may be seen in abnormal fluid accumulation in various areas of head

ECHOENCEPHALOGRAPHY
Identifies shifts in midline structures from their normal positions as a result of intracranial lesions
May show ventricular dilation

RADIOGRAPHY
Shows fractures, dislocations, spreading suture lines, and craniostenosis
Shows degenerative changes, bone erosion, and calcifications

MAGNETIC RESONANCE IMAGING (MRI)
Permits visualization of morphologic features of target structures
Permits tissue discrimination unavailable with many other techniques

POSITRON EMISSION TRANSAXIAL TOMOGRAPHY (PETT)
OR POSITRON EMISSION TOMOGRAPHY (PET)
Detects and measures such functions as blood volume and flow in brain, metabolic activity, and biochemical changes within tissues

REAL-TIME ULTRASONOGRAPHY (RTUS)
Allows high-resolution anatomic visualization in a variety of imaging planes

DIGITAL SUBTRACTION ANGIOGRAPHY (DSA)
Visualizes vasculature of target tissue
Visualizes finite vascular abnormalities

---

tioning to prevent aspiration of secretions and frequent assessment of vital signs and LOC. In addition, other neurologic functions, such as pupillary responses, motor strength, and movement, are tested at regular intervals. Any surgical wound resulting from the test is checked for bleeding, CSF leakage, and other complications. Children who undergo repeated subdural taps should have their hematocrit measured daily to detect any blood loss from the procedure.

Children's emotional reactions to procedures are also considered. They should be allowed to express their feelings about their experiences verbally and through the use of therapeutic play. Parents also seek—and are entitled to—an explanation of results of tests and procedures performed on their children. Nurses are in a unique position to provide support and education to parents regarding procedures.

NURSING CARE OF THE UNCONSCIOUS CHILD

The unconscious child requires continuous nursing attendance, with observation, recording, and evaluation of changes in objective signs. These observations provide valuable information regarding the patient's progress. Often they serve as a guide to diagnosis and treatment. Therefore careful and detailed observations are essential for the patient's welfare. In addition, vital functions must be maintained and complications prevented through conscientious and meticulous nursing care. The outcome of unconsciousness may be early with complete recovery, death within a few hours or days, persistent and permanent unconsciousness, or recovery with varying degrees of residual mental and/or physical disability. The outcome and recovery of the unconscious child may depend on the level of nursing care and observational skills.

Emergency measures are directed toward ensuring a patent airway, treatment of shock, and reduction of ICP (if present). Delayed treatment often leads to increased damage. As soon as emergency measures have been implemented—and in many cases concurrently—therapies for specific causes are begun. Because nursing care is closely related to medical management, both are considered here.

● Assessment

Continual observation of LOC, pupillary reaction, and vital signs is essential to management of CNS disorders. Regular assessment of neurologic signs is a vital part of nursing comatose children. Vital signs are measured and recorded regularly. The frequency depends on the cause of coma, the status, and the progression of cerebral involvement. Intervals may be as short as every 15 minutes or as long as every 2 hours. Significant alterations are reported immediately. Temperature is taken every 2 to 4 hours, depending on the patient's condition.

An elevated temperature may occur in children with CNS dysfunction; therefore a light covering is sufficient. Vigorous efforts, such as tepid sponge baths or application of a hypothermia blanket, are needed to prevent brain damage if temperature exceeds 40° C (104° F) rectally.

The LOC is assessed periodically, including size, equality, and reaction of pupils to light; as well as signs of meningeal irritation such as nuchal rigidity. Other aspects of LOC assessment include response to vocal commands, spontaneous behavior, resistance to care, and response to painful stimuli. Motions of any type, changes in muscle tone or strength, and body position are noted. Seizure activity is described according to the type and length of seizure and body areas involved (see Box 28-13). An antiepileptic drug such as phenytoin (Dilantin) or phenobarbital is ordered for control of seizure activity.

Pain management for the comatose child requires astute nursing observation and management. Signs of pain include changes in behavior (e.g., increased agitation and rigidity, alterations in physiologic parameters); increased heart rate, respiratory rate, and blood pressure; and decreased oxygen saturation. Since these findings are not specific for pain, the nurse should observe for their appearance during times of induced or suspected pain and their disappearance after the inciting procedure or the administration of analgesia. A pain assessment record should be used to document indications of pain and the effectiveness of interventions (see Pain Assessment, Chapter 21).

The use of opioids, such as morphine, to relieve pain is controversial because they may mask signs of altered consciousness or depress respirations. However, unrelieved pain activates the stress response, which can elevate ICP. In order to block the stress response, some authorities advocate the use of analgesics, sedatives, and, in some cases such as head injury, paralyzing agents via continuous IV infusion. A frequently used combination is fentanyl (Sublimaze), midazolam (Versed), and vecuronium (Norcuron). If there are concerns about assessing the LOC or respiratory depression, naloxone can be used to reverse the opioid effects. Acetaminophen and codeine may also be effective analgesics for mild to moderate pain. Regardless of which drugs are used, adequate dosage and regular administration are essential in order to provide optimal pain relief (see Pain Management, Chapter 21).

Other measures to relieve discomfort include providing a quiet, dimly lit environment; limiting visitors to a minimum; preventing any sudden, jarring movement, such as banging into the bed; and preventing an increase in ICP. The last is most effectively achieved by proper positioning and prevention of straining, such as during coughing, vomiting, or defecating.

> **NURSING ALERT**
>
> When opioids are used, bowel elimination must be closely monitored because of the potential constipating effect. Stool softeners should be given with laxatives as needed to prevent constipation.

Nursing Diagnoses

Based on a thorough assessment, several nursing diagnoses are identified. The more common diagnoses for the unconscious child are included in the Nursing Care Plan on pp. 1022 to 1024. Others may apply in specific situations.

Planning

The goals for the unconscious child and the family include:

1. Child will maintain respiratory integrity.
2. Child will not experience increasing ICP.
3. Child will have basic needs (hygiene, nutrition, hydration, elimination) met.
4. Child will not experience complications of immobility.
5. Family will receive adequate support and education.

Implementation

Respiratory Management

Respiratory effectiveness is the primary concern in the care of the unconscious child, and establishment of an adequate airway is *always* the first priority. Carbon dioxide has a potent vasodilating effect and will increase cerebral blood flow (CBF) and ICP. Cerebral hypoxia that lasts longer than 4 minutes nearly always causes irreversible brain damage.

> **NURSING ALERT**
>
> Respiratory obstruction and subsequent compromise leads to cardiac arrest. Maintaining an adequate, patent airway is of the utmost importance.

Children in lighter states of coma may be able to cough and swallow, but those in deeper states are unable to handle secretions, which tend to pool in the throat and pharynx. Dysfunction of cranial nerves IX and X places the child at risk for aspiration and cardiac arrest; therefore the child is positioned to prevent aspiration of secretions, and the stomach is emptied to reduce the likelihood of vomiting. In infants, blockage of air passages from secretions can happen in seconds. In addition, upper airway obstruction from laryngospasm is a frequent complication in comatose children.

An oral airway can be used for the child who is suffering a temporary loss of consciousness, such as after a contusion, seizure, or anesthesia. For children who remain unconscious for a longer time, a nasotracheal or orotracheal tube is inserted to maintain the open airway and facilitate removal of secretions. A tracheostomy is performed in cases in which laryngoscopy for introduction of an endotracheal tube would be difficult or dangerous. Suctioning is used only as needed to clear the airway, exerting care to prevent increasing ICP. Respiratory status is observed and evaluated regularly. Signs of respiratory embarrassment may be an indication for ventilatory assistance.

When the respiratory center is involved, mechanical ventilation is usually indicated (see Chapter 22). Blood gas analysis is performed regularly, and oxygen is administered when indicated. Moderately severe hypoxia and respiratory acidosis are often present but are not always evident from clinical manifestations. Hyperventilation frequently accompanies unconsciousness and may lead to respiratory alkalosis, or it may represent the body's attempt to compensate for metabolic acidosis. Therefore blood gas and pH determinations are essential guides for electrolyte therapy. Chest physiotherapy is carried out on a regular basis, and the child's position is changed at least every 2 hours to prevent pulmonary complications.

Intracranial Pressure Monitoring

Management of the child with increased ICP is possibly the most formidable task and the most controversial subject in pediatric critical care. It appears that the outcome in pediatric neurologic injury may reflect the initial cerebral damage more than the subsequent intracranial hypertension. Of note, ICP gives little indication of the severity of the initial insult (Bayir, Kochanek, and Clark 2003).

When increased ICP is a result of accumulation of CSF from obstruction of CSF flow, a ventricular tap will provide relief quickly and effectively. Evacuation of a hematoma reduces pressure from this source. Indications for inserting an ICP monitor are as follows:

1 Glasgow Coma Scale evaluation of 8
2 Glasgow Coma Scale evaluation of less than 8 with respiratory assistance
3 Deterioration of condition
4 Subjective judgment regarding clinical appearance and response.

Four major types of ICP monitors are

1 Intraventricular catheter with fibroscopic sensors attached to a monitoring system
2 Subarachnoid bolt (Richmond screw)
3 Epidural sensor
4 Anterior fontanel pressure monitor.

Transducers for both ventricular and subarachnoid monitoring should be set up without the use of a flush device. Direct ventricular pressure measurement remains the gold standard of ICP monitoring.

The catheter method involves introduction of a catheter into the lateral ventricle on the nondominant side, if known, or placement in the subdural space. The catheter has the advantage of providing a means of extraventricular (or continuous) drainage to reduce pressure. A drainage bag attached to the system is kept at the level of the ventricles and can be lowered to decrease ICP (see Critical Thinking Exercise).

> **NURSING ALERT**
>
> If the external ventricular drain (EVD) is unclamped for CSF drainage, carefully monitor the level of the collection container. If the container is too low, improper CSF decompression could lower ICP too rapidly, causing bleeding and pain.

?? CRITICAL THINKING EXERCISE

Hydrocephalus

Three-year-old Emma is 5 days postoperative for removal of a posterior fossa tumor. Although an external ventricular drain (EVD) was placed to treat her hydrocephalus, she continues to demonstrate signs of increased ICP, including holding the back of her head, anorexia, crying when moved or when strangers enter the room, and intermittent lethargy. On examination, fluid drainage is noted on the mother's clothes, and Emma is experiencing repetitive, rapid eyelid blinking.

QUESTIONS

1. Evidence—Is there sufficient evidence to draw conclusions about Emma's behavior, physical assessment findings, and ICP?
2. Assumptions—Describe any underlying assumption about each of the following:
   a. A preschool-age child who had a posterior fossa tumor removed 5 days ago
   b. A preschool-age child who has an EVD placed to treat the hydrocephalus
   c. A preschool-age child with an EVD who continues to demonstrate physical signs associated with increased ICP after recent surgery
3. What priorities for nursing care should be established?
4. Does the evidence support your nursing intervention?
5. What alternative perspectives might you have?

ANSWERS

1. Yes. Emma's fussiness, holding the back of her head, intermittent periods of lethargy, and repetitive, rapid eye blinking are signs of increased ICP.
2. a. Emma's posterior fossa tumor removal places her at risk for cerebral edema with associated increased ICP.
   b. Emma's EVD may be occluded and should be assessed. Positioning of the EVD is important to evaluate since the CSF drains by gravity; repositioning may be necessary to promote adequate drainage and decrease ICP.
   c. The physical signs and behavior are indicative of increased ICP, which may occur if Emma's EVD is obstructed or is draining improperly. There is evidence that CSF is draining on the mother's clothing, which is an abnormal finding with an EVD; the EVD is a closed system, and breakage or malfunction may cause the child further harm if bacteria colonize the reservoir.
3. The nurse should inspect the EVD site, assess Emma's neurologic status, and notify the medical provider of the findings. A transparent dressing should be placed over the EVD site to observe for CSF drainage, an abnormal finding. The EVD should remain positioned so that gravity drainage of CSF is enhanced (at the level of the external auditory meatus with the head at a 20- to 30-degree elevation); rapid CSF drainage is undesirable since it may result in subdural complications. A CT scan may be useful in determining the status of the drainage device.
4. Yes. Emma's signs of increased ICP and CSF drainage on her mother's clothes support the nurse's actions.
5. Another consideration for some of Emma's fussiness in the postoperative period is discomfort and pain. However, pain management should be monitored closely to avoid masking the signs of increased ICP. Once it is evident that the ICP is elevated, pain management measures should be performed, including an assessment of what Emma has taken previously to relieve pain. In addition, the nurse should explain the signs of elevated ICP to the mother and convey that obstruction of CSF flow from the EVD can cause these clinical signs and behaviors. Reassurance that the increased ICP will subside with removal of the EVD obstruction is important.

With the bolt method the end of the bolt is placed into the subarachnoid space. The bolt cannot be adequately secured in a small child's pliant skull, although special modifications have been developed for children younger than 6 years of age.

NURSING ALERT

The bolt is stabilized with dressings, but these are not changed or disturbed, even to check the site.

The placement of the bolt is not adjusted by anyone except the neurosurgeon who placed the device. The neurosurgeon is notified if a satisfactory waveform is not observed.

An epidural sensor can be placed between the dura and the skull through a burr hole and connected to a stopcock assembly and a transducer, which provides a readout of the pressure. Correlation of pressure readings is less invasive but may be inconsistent. In infants a fontanel transducer can be used to detect impulses from a pressure sensor and convert them to electrical energy. The electrical energy is then converted to visible waves or numeric readings on an oscilloscope. ICP measurement from the anterior fontanel is noninvasive but may prove to be inaccurate if the equipment is poorly placed or inconsistently recalibrated. The intraparenchymal pressure monitoring device (e.g., Camino) is a result of fiberoptic technology and performs reliably.

ICP can be increased by instillation of solutions; therefore antibiotics are administered systemically if a positive CSF culture is obtained. However, IV ICP monitoring rarely causes infection. Since CSF is a body fluid, standard precautions are implemented according to hospital policy (see Infection Control, Chapter 22).

Nurses caring for patients with intracranial monitoring devices must be acquainted with the system, assist with insertion, interpret the monitor readings, and be able to distinguish between danger signals and mechanical dysfunction.

For increased ICP resulting from cerebral edema, several medical measures are available. Osmotic diuretics may provide rapid relief in emergency situations. Although their effect is transient, lasting only about 6 hours, they can be lifesaving in emergencies. These substances are rapidly excreted by the kidneys and carry with them large quantities of sodium and water. Mannitol (or sometimes urea) administered intravenously is the drug most frequently used for rapid reduction. The infusion is generally given slowly but may be pushed rapidly in cases of herniation or impending herniation. Because of the profound diuretic effect of the drug, an indwelling catheter is inserted to ensure bladder emptying. Adrenocorticosteroids are not recommended for cerebral edema secondary to head trauma. $PaCO_2$ should be maintained at 25 to 30 mm Hg to produce vasoconstriction, which reduces CSF, thereby decreasing ICP.

Nursing Activities. In cases of high levels of increased ICP, nursing procedures tend to trigger reactive pressure waves in many patients. For example, increased intrathoracic or abdominal pressure will be transmitted to the cranium. Particular care should be taken in positioning these patients to avoid neck vein compression, which may further increase ICP by interfering with venous return.

The child can be propped to one side or the other, and the use of an alternating-pressure mattress reduces the chance of prolonged pressure to vulnerable areas. Frequent clinical assessment of the child cannot be replaced by an ICP monitoring device.

NURSING ALERT

The head of the bed is elevated 15 to 30 degrees, and the child is positioned so that the head is maintained in midline to facilitate venous drainage and avoid jugular compression. Turning side to side is contraindicated because of the risk of jugular compression.

It is important to avoid activities that may increase ICP by causing pain or emotional stress. Gentle range-of-motion exercises can be carried out but should not be performed vigorously. Nontherapeutic touch can cause an increase in ICP. Any disturbing procedures to be performed should be scheduled to take advantage of therapies that reduce ICP, such as osmotherapy and sedation. Efforts are taken to minimize or eliminate environmental noise. Assessment and intervention to relieve pain are important nursing functions to decrease ICP. Individualizing nursing activities and minimizing environmental stimuli by decreasing noxious procedures help to control ICP (El Bashir and others, 2003; Vernon-Levett, 1998).

Suctioning. Suctioning and percussion are poorly tolerated and are therefore contraindicated unless concurrent respiratory problems exist. Hypoxia and the Valsalva maneuver associated with cough both acutely elevate ICP. Vibration, which does not increase ICP, accomplishes excellent results and should be tried first if treatment is needed. If suctioning is necessary, it should be brief and preceded by hyperventilation with 100% oxygen, which can be monitored during suctioning with a pulse oxygen sensor reading to determine oxygen saturation.

Nutrition and Hydration

Fluids and calories are supplied initially by the IV route (see Chapter 22). An IV infusion is started early, and the type of fluid administered is determined by the general condition of the patient. Fluid therapy requires careful monitoring and adjustment based on neurologic signs and electrolyte determinations. Often, comatose children are unable to cope with the same amounts of fluid they could tolerate at other times, and overhydration must be avoided to prevent fatal cerebral edema.

Later, nutrition is provided in a balanced formula given by nasogastric or gastrostomy tube. The nasogastric tube is usually taped in place with care to prevent pressure on the nares. Most children have continuous feedings, but if bolus feedings are used, the tube is rinsed with water after each feeding. Tubes are replaced according to unit policy. Nostrils are alternated with each replacement to prevent nasal irritation and pressure. Overfeeding should be avoided to prevent vomiting with its potential danger of aspiration. Stomach contents are aspirated and measured before feeding to ascertain the amount remaining in the stomach. If the residual volume is excessive (depending on the size of the child), the dietitian and physician should be consulted regarding alteration of the formula composition to provide the needed calories and nutrients in a smaller volume. The aspirated contents should always be refed.

Hydration is maintained in the same manner (initially by IV and later by feeding tube). When cerebral edema is a threat, fluids may be restricted to reduce the chance of fluid overload. Skin and mucous membranes are examined for signs of dehydration. Observation for signs of altered fluid balance related to abnormal pituitary secretions is a part of nursing care.

Altered Pituitary Secretion. An altered ability to handle fluid loads is attributed in part to the syndrome of inappropriate antidiuretic hormone secretion (SIADH) and diabetes insipidus (DI) resulting from hypothalamic dysfunction (see Chapter 29). SIADH frequently accompanies CNS diseases such as head injury, meningitis, encephalitis, brain abscess, brain tumor, and subarachnoid hemorrhage. In the patient with SIADH, scant quantities of urine are excreted, electrolyte analysis reveals hyponatremia and hyposmolality, and manifestations of overhydration are evident. It is important to evaluate all parameters, since the reduced urine output might be erroneously interpreted as a sign of dehydration.

The treatment of SIADH consists of restriction of fluids until serum electrolytes and osmolality return to normal levels. Since SIADH frequently occurs with meningitis in children, fluid restriction is often prescribed. Likewise, DI may occur following intracranial trauma. There is increased urine volume and the accompanying danger of dehydration (see Table 28-1 for comparison of fluid changes in SIADH and DI). Adequate replacement of fluids is essential, and observation of electrolyte balance is necessary to detect signs of hypernatremia and hyperosmolality. Exogenous vasopressin may be administered.

Medications

The cause of unconsciousness determines specific drug therapies. Children with infectious processes are given antibiotics appropriate to the disease and the infecting organism, and corticosteroids are prescribed for inflammatory conditions and edema. Cerebral edema is an indication for osmotherapy with osmotic diuretics. Sedatives or antiepileptics are prescribed for seizure activity (see p. 1050). Sedation in the combative child provides amnesic and anxiolytic properties in conjunction with a paralytic agent. The combination decreases ICP and allows treatment of cerebral edema. Usual drugs include morphine, midazolam (Versed), and pancuronium (Pavulon). Midazolam is attractive because of its short half-life.

Deep coma, induced by administration of barbiturates, is controversial in the management of ICP. Barbiturates are currently reserved for the reduction of increased ICP when all else has failed. Barbiturates decrease the cerebral metabolic rate for oxygen and protect the brain during times of reduced cerebral perfusion pressure (CPP). Barbiturate coma requires extensive monitoring, cardiovascular and respiratory support, and ICP monitoring to assess response to therapy. Paralyzing agents such as pancuronium also may be needed to aid in performing diagnostic tests, improving effectiveness of therapy, and reducing risks of secondary complications. Elevation of ICP and/or heart rate of patients who are being given paralyzing agents or are under sedation may indicate the need for another dose of either or both medications.

Thermoregulation

Hyperthermia often accompanies cerebral dysfunction; if it is present, measures are implemented to reduce the temperature to prevent brain damage and to reduce metabolic demands generated by the increased body temperature. Antipyretics are the method of choice for fever reduction; cooling devices are used for hyperthermia. Laboratory tests and other methods are used in an attempt to determine the cause, if any, of the hyperthermia.

Elimination

A retention catheter is usually inserted in the acute phase, although diapers may be used and weighed to record urine output. The child who formerly had bowel and bladder control is generally incontinent. If the child remains comatose for a long period, the indwelling catheter may be removed and periodic bladder emptying accomplished by intermittent catheterization. Stool softeners are usually sufficient to maintain bowel function, but suppositories or enemas may be needed occasionally for adequate elimination and to prevent an impaction. The passage of liquid stool after a period of no bowel activity is usually a sign of an impaction. To avoid this preventable problem, daily recording of bowel activity is essential.

Hygienic Care

Routine measures for cleansing and maintaining skin integrity are an integral part of nursing care of the unconscious child. Skinfolds require special attention to prevent excoriation. The child who is unable to move is prone to develop tissue breakdown and pressure necrosis; therefore the child may be placed on a pressure-reducing or pressure-relieving device to prevent pressure on prominent areas of the body. The goal is prevention by regular change of position and inspection of vulnerable areas, such as the ankle, trochanter, and shoulder. Since unconscious children undergo numerous invasive procedures, these skin sites require special assessment and intervention to promote healing and to prevent infection. Bed linen and any clothing are kept dry and free of wrinkles. If the child requires surgery or radiography, the nurse checks all dressings, bony sites, catheters, and IV access lines. (See also Maintaining Healthy Skin, Chapter 22.)

Mouth care is performed at least twice daily, since the mouth tends to become dry or coated with mucus. The

TABLE 28-1 ■ Effects of Altered Pituitary Secretion

MEASUREMENT	DIABETES INSIPIDUS	SYNDROME OF INAPPROPRIATE ANTIDIURETIC HORMONE SECRETION
Urine output	Increased	Decreased
Specific gravity	Decreased	Increased
Serum sodium	Increased (hypernatremia)	Decreased (hyponatremia)

NURSING DIAGNOSIS ■ **Risk for suffocation (aspiration): ineffective airway clearance related to depressed sensorium, impaired motor function**

PATIENT GOAL 1: Will maintain patent airway

NURSING INTERVENTIONS/*RATIONALES*

Position for optimal ventilation
   Insert oral airway if indicated
   Position with neck slightly extended and nose in "sniffing" position *to open trachea fully*
   Avoid neck hyperextension, *which can block airway*
   Place in semiprone or side-lying position *to prevent aspiration*
Remove accumulated secretions promptly *to prevent aspiration*
Provide routine care of endotracheal tube or tracheostomy if appropriate; have equipment available for emergency insertion if indicated for respiratory distress *to prevent delay in treatment*
Monitor artificial ventilation

EXPECTED OUTCOME

Airway remains patent

NURSING DIAGNOSIS ■ **Risk for injury related to physical immobility, depressed sensorium, intracranial problem**

PATIENT GOAL 1: Will maintain stable intracranial pressure (ICP)

NURSING INTERVENTIONS/*RATIONALES*

Elevate head of bed 15 to 30 degrees with child's head in midline position *to facilitate venous drainage and avoid jugular compression*
Avoid positions or activities that increase ICP
   Pressure on neck veins
      Turning side-to-side is contraindicated *because of risk of jugular compression*
   Flexion or hyperextension of neck
   Head rotation
   Valsalva maneuver
   Painful stimuli
   Respiratory procedures (especially suctioning, percussion)
Prevent constipation (*Valsalva maneuver increases ICP*)
   *Administer stool softener as prescribed
   Closely monitor bowel elimination when child is receiving codeine *because of its constipating effect*
Minimize emotional stress and crying *because they cause increased ICP*
   Provide quiet, subdued environment
   Reduce environmental noise (e.g., placing earphones over child's ears *has been shown to lower ICP, heart rate, and blood pressure*)
   Provide pleasant auditory experiences
   Use therapeutic touch
   Avoid emotionally stressful conversation (e.g., about pain, condition, prognosis)
   *Administer sedation, if ordered, for extreme agitation or restlessness
Prevent or relieve pain, *since pain causes increased ICP*
   Closely observe child for signs of pain, especially changes in behavior (e.g., agitation); increased heart rate, respiratory rate, and blood pressure (*usually increase with pain*); decreased oxygen saturation
   Observe child's response during times of induced or suspected pain
   Observe child's response following a painful procedure or the administration of analgesia
   Use pain assessment record (see Chapter 21)
   *Administer paralyzing and analgesic agents if prescribed

Schedule disturbing procedures to take advantage of therapies that reduce ICP (e.g., bathe child after sedation or osmotherapy)
Monitor ICP monitoring device

EXPECTED OUTCOMES
ICP remains within safe limits
Child shows no evidence of sustained increased ICP

PATIENT GOAL 2: Will exhibit no signs of cerebral hypoxia

NURSING INTERVENTIONS/*RATIONALES*

Maintain patent airway *because respiratory obstruction leads to cardiac arrest, and cerebral hypoxia lasting longer than 4 minutes nearly always causes irreversible brain damage*
Provide oxygen as indicated by objective signs or as ordered
*Hyperventilate at prescribed intervals if ordered
Monitor blood gases and pH
If child is on mechanical ventilation:
   Monitor for correct settings, proper functioning
   Prepare to provide artificial ventilation in case of ventilatory failure; have manual resuscitation bag at bedside
*Administer medications as ordered *to prevent cerebral edema and improve cerebral circulation*

EXPECTED OUTCOME

Child breathes easily; respirations are within normal limits (see inside back cover)

PATIENT GOAL 3: Will exhibit no evidence of cerebral edema

NURSING INTERVENTIONS/*RATIONALES*

Elevate head of bed to 15 to 30 degrees *to facilitate venous drainage*
Maintain intravenous (IV) fluids as prescribed
   Avoid overhydration *to prevent cerebral edema*
Monitor intake and output
Monitor electrolyte balance and specific gravity *to detect signs of hypernatremia and hyperosmolality because diabetes insipidus (DI) and the syndrome of inappropriate antidiuretic hormone secretion (SIADH) frequently occur with central nervous system (CNS) diseases and trauma*
*Administer hyperosmolar fluids as prescribed
*Administer corticosteroids as ordered

EXPECTED OUTCOME

Child exhibits no signs of sustained increased ICP

PATIENT GOAL 4: Will experience no seizures

NURSING INTERVENTIONS/*RATIONALES*

Avoid stimulation that precipitates undesirable responses
Schedule nursing activities for minimal disturbance
*Administer antiepileptic drugs as prescribed
   IV fosphenytoin (Cerebyx) is often used to treat seizures instead of IV phenytoin because of the potential for complications with IV phenytoin
   If IV phenytoin is ordered, administer carefully and observe the following precautions:
      Infuse completely in 1 hour *because drug tends to precipitate*
      Never mix phenytoin with 5% dextrose; *drug will precipitate*
      Do not exceed 0.5mg/kg/min in the neonate or 1mg/kg/min in infants and children
      Dilute phenytoin with normal saline *to decrease vein irritation and pain*

EXPECTED OUTCOME

Child exhibits no seizure activity or undue restlessness and agitation

*Dependent nursing action.

NURSING CARE PLAN   The Unconscious Child—*cont'd*

PATIENT GOAL 5: Will exhibit stable body temperature

NURSING INTERVENTIONS/*RATIONALES*

Closely monitor child's temperature *because elevations often occur with CNS dysfunction*
Remove excess coverings
*Administer antipyretics if prescribed for fever
Give tepid sponge bath, if indicated, only for hyperthermia, not for fever, *because it may induce shivering*
Apply and monitor hypothermia blanket if indicated and ordered; administer antishivering agents, if ordered, *because shivering increases ICP and metabolic rate*

EXPECTED OUTCOME

Body temperature remains within safe limits (see inside back cover)

PATIENT GOAL 6: Will exhibit no evidence of respiratory tract infection

NURSING INTERVENTIONS/*RATIONALES*

Turn frequently—at least every 2 hours, as tolerated, unless contraindicated by increased ICP
Keep persons with upper respiratory tract infection away from child
Use good handwashing technique
Keep all equipment in contact with child clean or sterile
Provide good oral hygiene *to decrease presence of infective organisms*
Perform chest physiotherapy if prescribed and as tolerated; avoid percussion *because it can increase ICP*

EXPECTED OUTCOME

Child exhibits no evidence of pulmonary dysfunction

PATIENT GOAL 7: Will experience no corneal irritation

NURSING INTERVENTIONS/*RATIONALES*

Patch eye, if indicated, *for protection*
Keep lids completely closed *to protect corneas when corneal reflexes are absent*
Instill "artificial tears" *to lubricate eyes*
Assess eyes carefully for early signs of irritation or inflammation

EXPECTED OUTCOME

Corneas remain clear and moist

PATIENT GOAL 8: Will exhibit no breakdown in mucous membrane integrity

NURSING INTERVENTIONS/*RATIONALES*

Provide meticulous mouth care, *since mouth tends to become dry or coated with mucus*
Avoid drying products (e.g., lemon and glycerin swabs)

EXPECTED OUTCOME

Mucous membranes remain clear, moist, and free of irritation

PATIENT GOAL 9: Will experience no physical injury

NURSING INTERVENTIONS/*RATIONALES*

Keep side rails up *to prevent falls*
Pad hard surfaces *that may injure extremities during spontaneous or involuntary movements*

EXPECTED OUTCOME

Child remains free of physical injury

PATIENT GOAL 10: Will maintain limb flexibility and full range of motion

NURSING INTERVENTIONS/*RATIONALES*

Perform passive range-of-motion exercises *to prevent contractures*
Position *to reduce contractures*
    Place small, rolled pad in palms *to maintain proper position of fingers*
    Use footboard or ankle-high shoes *to prevent footdrop*
    Splint joints, if needed, *to prevent severe contractures of wrists, knees, and ankles*

EXPECTED OUTCOME

Joints remain flexible and retain full range of motion

NURSING DIAGNOSIS ▪ **Risk for impaired skin integrity related to immobility, body secretions, invasive procedures**

PATIENT GOAL 1: Will maintain skin integrity

NURSING INTERVENTIONS/*RATIONALES*

Place child on pressure-reducing surface *to prevent tissue breakdown and pressure necrosis*
Change position frequently unless contraindicated by increased ICP
Protect pressure points (e.g., trochanter, sacrum, ankle, heels, shoulder, occiput)
Inspect skin surfaces regularly for signs of irritation, redness, evidence of pressure
Cleanse skin regularly, at least once daily
Protect skinfolds and surfaces that rub together *to prevent excoriation;* keep these areas dry and free of moisture
Keep clothing and linen clean, dry, and free of wrinkles
Carry out good perineal care
Gently massage skin with lotion or other lubricating substance, unless on existing reddened pressure areas, *to stimulate circulation and prevent drying*
Protect lips with cream or ointment *to prevent drying and cracking*

EXPECTED OUTCOME

Skin remains clean, intact, and free of irritation

NURSING DIAGNOSIS ▪ **Feeding, bathing/hygiene, toileting self-care deficits (level 4) related to physical immobility, perceptual and cognitive impairment**

PATIENT GOAL 1: Will receive optimal nutrition

NURSING INTERVENTIONS/*RATIONALES*

Provide nourishment in manner suitable to child's condition
Monitor IV feedings when ordered
Record intake and output
*Feed prescribed formula by means of nasogastric or gastrostomy tube
Weigh daily or as ordered

EXPECTED OUTCOME

Child obtains sufficient nourishment

*Dependent nursing action.

Continued

NURSING CARE PLAN The Unconscious Child—*cont'd*

PATIENT GOAL 2: Will receive proper hygienic care

NURSING INTERVENTIONS/*RATIONALES*
Bathe daily or more often if indicated
Dress appropriately
Keep hair clean

EXPECTED OUTCOME
Child appears clean and as well groomed as possible within limitations of condition

PATIENT GOAL 3: Will void and defecate adequately

NURSING INTERVENTIONS/*RATIONALES*
Provide sufficient liquid intake, unless contraindicated by cerebral edema or if overhydration is a threat
*Apply urine-collecting device or insert indwelling catheter (if ordered)
Provide proper catheter care
Clean skin well after each elimination *to prevent skin irritation*
Diaper as needed *to contain stool and urine*
Check abdomen for evidence of distention
    Measure abdominal girth *to detect enlargement*
*Administer stool softener *to prevent constipation*
*Administer laxatives, suppositories, or enemas as indicated *to promote evacuation*

EXPECTED OUTCOMES
Child eliminates sufficient urine (specify)
Bowel is evacuated daily
Child's diaper area remains clean and free of irritation

NURSING DIAGNOSIS ▪ Disturbed sensory/perceptual alterations (visual, auditory, kinesthetic, gustatory, tactile, olfactory) related to CNS impairment, bed rest

PATIENT GOAL 1: Will receive appropriate sensory stimulation

NURSING INTERVENTIONS/*RATIONALES*
Provide tactile stimulation as tolerated
Provide auditory stimulation (e.g., by voice, radio, music box)
Provide visual stimuli appropriate for age

*Dependent nursing action.

Provide proprioceptive stimulation (e.g., by rocking, cuddling)
Encourage family to participate in stimulation program
Demonstrate for family how and where to touch child

EXPECTED OUTCOMES
Child receives sensory stimulation appropriate to age and condition
Child appears relaxed and rests quietly
Stimulation does not induce seizures or increase ICP

PATIENT GOAL 2: Will exhibit no evidence of pain

NURSING INTERVENTIONS/*RATIONALES*
Assess for evidence of pain
Use pain assessment record *to document effectiveness of interventions*
Administer pain medication as needed

EXPECTED OUTCOME
Child exhibits no evidence of pain

NURSING DIAGNOSIS ▪ Interrupted family processes related to a child hospitalized with a potentially fatal condition or permanent disability

PATIENT (FAMILY) GOAL 1: Will receive adequate support

NURSING INTERVENTIONS/*RATIONALES*
AND EXPECTED OUTCOMES
See Nursing Care Plan: The Family of the Ill or Hospitalized Child, Chapter 21

PATIENT (FAMILY) GOAL 2: Will express feelings and concerns

NURSING INTERVENTIONS/*RATIONALES*
Provide needed information
Answer family's questions; encourage expression of feelings
Refer to persons or agencies for further information and clarification
Support parents' decisions

EXPECTED OUTCOME
Family verbalizes feelings and concerns

teeth are carefully brushed with a soft toothbrush or cleaned with gauze saturated with saline. Commercially prepared cleansing devices, such as Toothettes, are convenient for cleansing the mouth and teeth. Lips are coated with ointment or other preparations to protect them from drying, cracking, or blistering.

The deeply comatose child is also prone to eye irritation. The corneal reflexes are absent; therefore the eyes are easily irritated or damaged by linen, dust, or other substances that may come in contact with them. There is excessive dryness as a result of incomplete closure of the eyes and/or decreased secretions, especially if the child is undergoing osmotherapy to reduce or prevent brain edema.

⚑ **NURSING ALERT**

The eyes should be examined regularly and carefully for early signs of irritation or inflammation. Artificial tears (methylcellulose) are placed in the eyes every 1 to 2 hours. Eye dressings may sometimes be needed to protect the eyes from possible damage.

The hair is combed and styled neatly. Long hair is usually braided and secured with ponytail bands. The scalp should be kept clean with dry or wet shampoos as needed. The child's head may be shaved for tests or surgical procedures. If so, the hair is saved, if possible, and given to the family.

Positioning and Exercise

The unconscious child is positioned to prevent aspiration of saliva, nasogastric secretions, and vomitus, and to minimize ICP. The head of the bed is elevated, and the child is placed in a side-lying or semiprone position. A small, firm pillow is placed under the head, and the uppermost limbs are flexed and supported with pillows. The weight of the body should not rest on the dependent arm. In the semiprone position the child lies with the dependent arm at the side behind the body, the opposite side supported on pillows, and the uppermost arm and leg flexed and resting on the pillows. This position prevents undue pressure on the dependent extremities. The dependent position of the face encourages drainage of secretions and prevents the flaccid tongue from obstructing the airway.

Normal range-of-motion exercises help to maintain function and prevent contractures of joints. Exercises should be done gently and with full range of motion. A small rolled pad can be placed in the palms to help maintain proper position of fingers; footboards or boots can be used to help prevent footdrop; splinting may be needed to prevent severe contractures of the wrist, knee, or ankle in decerebrate children.

Stimulation

Sensory stimulation is important in the care of the unconscious child, just as it is in the care of the alert child. For the temporarily unconscious or semiconscious child, sensory stimulation helps to arouse the child to the conscious state and orient the child in terms of time and place. Auditory and tactile stimulation are especially valuable. Tactile stimulation is not appropriate for the child in whom it may elicit an undesirable response. However, for other children tactile contact often has a relaxing and calming effect. When the child's condition permits, holding or rocking has a soothing effect and provides the body contact needed by young children.

The auditory sense is often present in a state of coma. Hearing is the last sense to be lost and the first one to be regained; therefore the child should be spoken to as any other child. Conversation around the child should not include thoughtless or derogatory remarks. A radio playing soft music or a music box or CD player is frequently used to provide auditory stimulation. Singing the child's favorite songs or reading a favorite story is a tactic used to maintain the child's contact with a familiar world. Playing songs or stories recorded in the parents' voices can provide a continuous source of familiar stimulation.

Regaining Consciousness.

Awakening from a coma is a gradual process; however, sometimes children regain consciousness within a short time. Regaining orientation involves knowing person, place, and time, in that order.

Certain behaviors have been observed when children awaken from the unconscious state. The stress and anxiety they appear to feel in a strange and unfamiliar environment are consistently expressed in silent and withdrawn behavior. Children respond to basic questioning but usually do not display their prehospitalization personality and social behavior until they are transferred from the critical care area.

Family Support

Helping parents of an unconscious child cope with the situation is especially difficult. They may demonstrate all the guilt, fear, hostility, and anxiety of any parent of a seriously ill child (see Chapter 18). In addition, these parents are faced with the uncertain outcome of the cerebral dysfunction. The fear of death, mental retardation, or other permanent disability is present. Nursing intervention with parents depends on the nature of the pathologic condition, the personality of the parents, and the parent-child relationship before the injury or illness.

If there is little or no residual effect, the child will be dismissed to home care fairly soon. The parents need the most intensive nursing intervention during the period of crisis and uncertainty. During the recovery phase they are given information, information is clarified, and they are encouraged to become involved in the child's care. Often the child's hospitalization is brief; however, some children require extended hospitalization for intensive therapy and rehabilitation.

The parents of children who die within hours or days require the support and guidance that the parents of any dying child would need in coping with the reality of the death and resolving their grief (see Chapter 18).

Probably the most difficult situations are those that involve children who are unconscious permanently or for an indefinite period. Unlike parents who lose a child through death, the finality is lacking for these parents, often leaving them in a state of suspended grief. The presence of the child renders the parents unable to resolve the loss. Like parents of dying children, parents of the comatose child search for any signs of hope. Well-meaning friends and relatives relate instances of miraculous recoveries. The parents seek confirmation and support for such possibilities and assign erroneous meanings to any sign in the child, such as reflexive muscle contractions, that might be interpreted as evidence of recovery.

At these times nurses need to respond with compassion and gentle honesty. They can acknowledge that miraculous recoveries do occur, but they are rare. The important message is to maintain open communication with the family.

Like parents who lose a child through death, the parents of the child lost to their world attempt to reconstitute a representation of the child. They bring items that belong to the child, such as favorite toys, music, and other objects cherished by the child. This is interpreted as an attempt to provide stimulation for the child in the hope of eliciting a response, to let the hospital staff know the child as the unique individual he or she was so that the parents' distress can be better appreciated, and to reconstitute an image of the child "lost" to them and for whom they mourn. An awareness of these behaviors and coping mechanisms provides nurses with the understanding that helps them support the parents in their grief process.

Superimposed on the process of grieving for the "lost" child, parents may be faced with difficult decisions. When the child's brain is so severely damaged that vital functions must be maintained by artificial means, the parents must make the final decision to remove life-support systems. Since the decision is so difficult for parents, the practitioner is frequently placed in a position of making the decision indirectly. After providing the parents with all of the information, the practitioner will suggest that the child be removed from the life support to "see if the child can make it without help." The approach relieves the parents of the decision and can be effective, but it is based on an evaluation of the parents' intellectual level and emotional state. Sometimes parents may even choose to refuse treatment if they believe it to be best for the child and the family (informed dissent). At other times parents request that "everything possible" be done for the child.

The nurses can be instrumental in providing guidance and clarifying information—a valued but demanding undertaking. It is not unusual for the family to ask the same questions and to compare responses elicited from different staff members. A child's death is an intensely personal issue that deserves direct involvement by the nurse and auxiliary support systems.

When the child has survived the illness or injury that produced the brain damage but is left unconscious permanently, the parents must decide whether to place the child in a chronic care facility or arrange to care for the child at home. The nurse can listen to the parents' discussions regarding alternatives, provide information when appropriate, and support the family in their decision. The nurse can help the family prepare for the transfer of the child and make referrals to persons or agencies that can provide additional assistance.

When the child has survived the cerebral insult and is not comatose, but physical and/or mental capacity is limited, either minimally or severely, families must cope with the long and tedious rehabilitation process and the uncertain outcome. The drain on financial, emotional, and social resources can be enormous.

For parents who choose to care for their child at home, planning for home care begins early in the process of recovery. The family should become involved with the care of the child as soon as they indicate an interest and ability to do so. They need education and support in learning to care for the child, regular follow-up observation and assessment of the home management, and planning for some respite care of the child. Parents need to understand that it is important to plan for periodic relief from the continual care of the child (see Preparing for Discharge and Home Care, Chapter 21; and Family-Centered Home Care, Chapter 20).

● Evaluation

The effectiveness of nursing interventions for the unconscious child is determined by continual reassessment and evaluation of care based on the following observational guidelines:

1. Monitor child's neurologic signs, vital signs, and behavior.
2. Observe child's response to nursing activities, therapies, and diagnostic procedures; monitor ICP.
3. Observe child's color, position, and motor activity; measure fluid and nutritional intake and output.
4. Monitor status of child's respiratory, renal, and gastrointestinal systems and skin.
5. Observe family behaviors and interview members regarding their understandings and their feelings and concerns.

The *expected outcomes* are described in the Nursing Care Plan on pp. 1022 to 1024.

CEREBRAL TRAUMA

HEAD INJURY

Head injury is a pathologic process involving the scalp, skull, meninges, or brain as a result of mechanical force. According to national statistics and the **Safe Kids Campaign,*** injuries are the number-one health risk for children and the leading cause of death in children older than 1 year of age. Yearly, 1 in 4 children in the United States will suffer an injury serious enough to require medical attention. Tragically, 8000 children are killed every year by injuries. It has been estimated that 300 per 100,000 children per year have a traumatic brain injury and that 10 per 100,000 children per year die as a result of the brain injury. Studies indicate that as many as three fourths of the childhood deaths caused by mechanical trauma are the direct result of a brain injury.

Etiology

The three major causes of brain damage in childhood in order of importance are falls, motor vehicle injuries, and bicycle injuries. Neurologic injury accounts for the highest mortality, with boys affected twice as often as girls. In motor vehicle accidents children younger than 2 years of age are almost exclusively injured as passengers, whereas older children may also be injured as pedestrians or cyclists. The majority of deaths from brain trauma caused by bicycle injuries occur between the ages of 5 and 19 years. Bicycle helmet laws have been effective in reducing the risk of head injury by 85% and brain injury by 88% (Rivara and Grossman, 2004).

The exposed nature of the head renders it particularly vulnerable to external violence, and many of the physical characteristics of children predispose them to craniocerebral trauma. For example, infants are frequently left unattended on beds, in high chairs, and in other places from which they can fall. Because the head of an infant or toddler is proportionately larger and heavier in relation to other body parts, it is the most likely to be injured. Incomplete motor development contributes to falls at young ages, and the natural curiosity and exuberance of children also increase their risk of injury.

Pathophysiology

The pathology of brain injury is directly related to the force of impact. Intracranial contents (brain, blood, CSF) are damaged because the force is too great to be absorbed by the skull and musculoligamentous support of the head. The elastic, pliable skull of the infant and young child absorbs much of the direct energy of physical impact to the head and affords some protection to intracranial structures. Although nervous tissue is delicate, it usually requires a severe blow to cause significant damage.

A child's response to head injury is different from that of an adult. The larger head size and insufficient musculoskeletal support render the very young child particularly vulnerable to acceleration-deceleration injuries.

Primary head injuries are those that occur at the time of trauma and include skull fracture, contusions, intracranial hematoma, and diffuse injury. Subsequent complications include hypoxic brain damage, increased ICP, infection, and cerebral edema. The predominant feature of a child's brain

---

1301 Pennsylvania Avenue NW, Suite 1000, Washington, DC 20004-1707; (202) 662-0600; website: www.safekids.org.

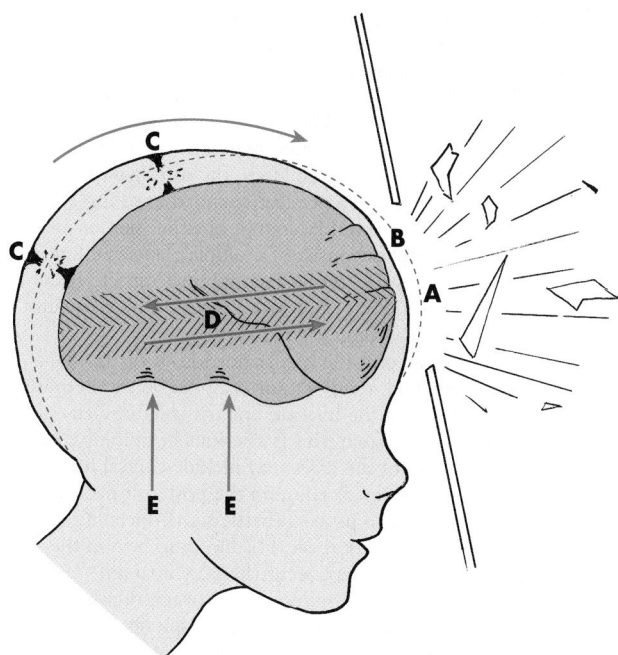

FIG. 28-4 ■ Mechanical distortion of cranium during closed head injury. **A,** Preinjury contour of skull. **B,** Immediate postinjury contour of skull. **C,** Torn subdural vessels. **D,** Shearing forces. **E,** Trauma from contact with floor of cranium. (Redrawn from Grubb RL, Coxe WS: Central nervous system trauma: cranial. In Eliasson SG, Presky AL, Hardin WB Jr, editors: *Neurological pathophysiology,* New York, 1974, Oxford University Press.)

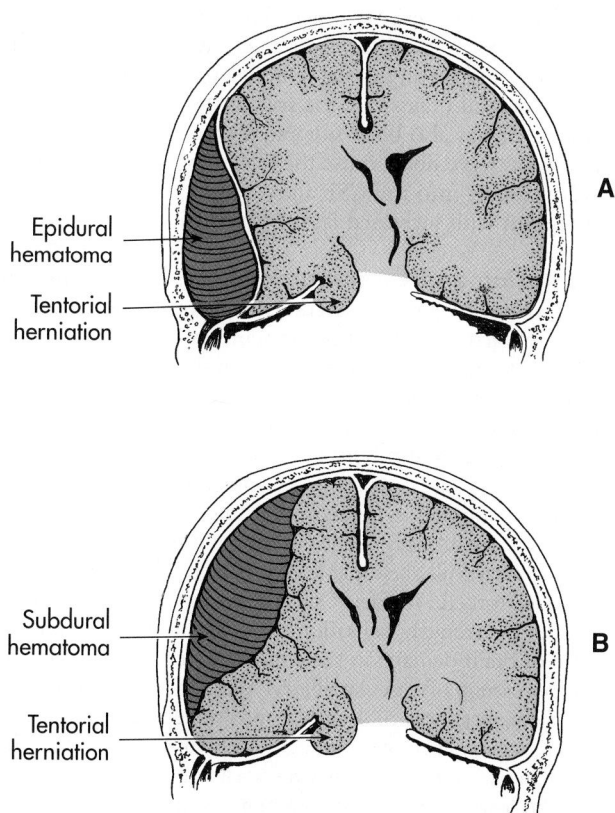

FIG. 28-5 ■ **A,** Epidural (extradural) hematoma and compression of temporal lobe through tentorial hiatus. **B,** Subdural hematoma.

injury is the amount of diffuse swelling that occurs. Hypoxia and hypercapnia threaten the energy requirements of the brain and increase cerebral blood flow. The added volume across the blood-brain barrier, along with the loss of autoregulation, exacerbates cerebral edema. Pressure inside the skull that is greater than arterial pressure results in inadequate perfusion.

Cerebral hyperemia occurs more often in children, and this volume expansion may account for their tendency to develop intracranial hypertension. However, because the cranium of very young children has the ability to expand and the thin skull is more compliant, they may tolerate increases in ICP better than older children and adults do. Children have a significantly higher percentage of good outcomes and a lower mortality rate, as well as a lower incidence of surgical mass lesions after severe head trauma. However, their thinner, softer skull may sustain greater long-term damage than previously suggested.

Physical forces act on the head through *acceleration, deceleration,* or *deformation.* Acceleration or deceleration is more descriptive of the circumstances responsible for most head injuries. When the stationary head receives a blow, the sudden acceleration causes deformation of the skull and mass movement of the brain. Continued movement of the intracranial contents allows the brain to strike parts of the skull (e.g., the sharp edges of the sphenoid or the irregular surface of the anterior fossa) or the edges of the tentorium.

Although the brain volume remains unchanged, significant distortion takes place as the brain changes shape in response to the force of impact to the skull. This movement can cause

bruising at the point of impact *(coup)* and/or at a distance as the brain collides with the unyielding surfaces far removed from the point of impact *(contrecoup)* (Fig. 28-4). Thus a blow to the occipital region can cause severe injury to the frontal and temporal areas of the brain. Sudden deceleration, such as takes place during a fall, causes the greatest cerebral injury at the point of impact. Children with an acceleration/deceleration injury demonstrate diffuse generalized cerebral swelling produced by increased blood volume or a redistribution of cerebral blood volume (cerebral hyperemia) rather than by increased water content (edema), as seen in adults.

Another effect of brain movement is shearing stresses, which may tear small arteries and cause subdural hemorrhages. Damage can also occur when severe compression of the skull causes the brain to be forced through the tentorial opening. This can produce irreparable damage to the brainstem (Fig. 28-5).

Concussion. The most common head injury is *concussion,* a transient and reversible neuronal dysfunction, with instantaneous loss of awareness and responsiveness, that results from trauma to the head and persists for a relatively short time, usually minutes or hours. It is generally followed by amnesia for the moment of the injury and a variable period after the injury. The common misconception that loss of consciousness is the hallmark of concussion is not true, especially for children. Concussion is correctly defined as "a traumatically induced alteration in mental status." Confusion and amnesia following head injury are the hallmarks of concussion.

The pathogenesis of concussion is still unclear but may be a result of shearing forces that cause stretching, compression, and tearing of nerve fibers, particularly in the area of the central brainstem, the seat of the reticular activating system. It has also been suggested that the anatomic alterations of nerve fibers cause the release of large quantities of acetylcholine into the CSF and a reduction in oxygen consumption with increased lactate production.

Contusion and Laceration. The terms *contusion* and *laceration* are used to describe visible bruising and tearing of cerebral tissue. Contusions represent petechial hemorrhages along the superficial aspects of the brain at the site of impact (coup injury) and/or a lesion remote from the site of direct trauma (contrecoup injury). In serious accidents there may be multiple sites of injury.

The major areas of the brain susceptible to contusion or laceration are the occipital, frontal, and temporal lobes. Also, the irregular surfaces of the anterior and middle fossae at the base of the skull are capable of producing bruises or lacerations on forceful impact. Contusions may cause focal disturbances in strength, sensation, or visual awareness. The degree of brain damage in the contused areas varies according to the extent of vascular injury. Signs will vary from mild, transient weakness of a limb to prolonged unconsciousness and paralysis. However, the signs and symptoms may be clinically indistinguishable from those of concussion.

The lower incidence of cerebral contusion in infancy has been attributed to the infant's pliable skull with less convolutional markings of the inner space between brain tissue and bone. In addition, the infant's brain tissue has a softer consistency, which also reduces surface injury. However, infants who are roughly shaken (shaken baby syndrome) can sustain profound neurologic impairment, seizures, retinal hemorrhages, and intracranial subarachnoid or subdural hemorrhages. In addition to these classic injuries, high cervical spinal cord hemorrhages and contusions can occur.

Cerebral lacerations are generally associated with penetrating or depressed skull fractures. However, they may occur without fracture in small children. When brain tissue is actually torn, with bleeding into and around the tear, usually more severe and prolonged unconsciousness and paralysis occur, leaving permanent scarring and some degree of disability.

Fractures. Because of its flexibility, the immature skull is able to sustain a greater degree of deformation than the adult skull before it incurs a fracture. A great deal of force is required to produce a fracture in the skull of an infant. However, the undersurface of the skull contains grooves in which the meningeal arteries lie. A fracture that runs through one of these grooves may tear the artery and produce severe and damaging hemorrhage. Hypovolemic hypotension can occur in infants with skull fractures.

The types of fractures that occur are as follows:

> **Linear fractures** are those in which the lines of the fracture are predetermined by the site and velocity of the impact, as well as by the strength of the bone. These are uncommon before 2 to 3 years of age but constitute the majority of childhood skull fractures. Most linear skull fractures are associated with an overlying hematoma or soft-tissue swelling (Schutzman and Greenes, 2001).

> **Depressed fractures** are those in which the bone is locally broken, usually into several irregular fragments that are pushed inward, causing pressure on the brain. The inner portion of the bone is more extensively fragmented than the outer portion, which almost invariably produces tears in the dura. These are uncommon before 2 to 3 years of age. In infants and very young children, the soft, malleable bone may become dented in a peculiar rounded or "Ping-Pong ball" depression, without laceration of either skin or dura.

> **Comminuted fractures** consist of multiple associated linear fractures. They usually result from intense impact. These types of fractures often result from repeated blows against an object and may suggest child abuse.

> **Basilar fractures** involve the basilar portion of the frontal, ethmoid, sphenoid, temporal, or occipital bones. Because of the proximity of the fracture line to structures surrounding the brainstem, this is a serious head injury. Approximately 80% of the cases may include clinical features such as subcutaneous bleeding in the posterior neck area and over the mastoid process (battle sign). Bleeding around the eyes (raccoon eyes) or bleeding behind the tympanic membrane may occur (hemotympanum).

> **Open fractures** cause communication between the skull and the scalp or the surfaces of the upper respiratory tract. Open fractures increase the risk of central nervous system infection. They may have an overlying laceration called a *compound fracture.* Open fractures can also create an opening in the paranasal sinuses or middle ear that can lead to CSF rhinorrhea or otorrhea. Facial paralysis, vertigo, tinnitus, or hearing loss may develop.

> **Diastatic fractures** are traumatic separations of the cranial sutures. These most frequently affect the lambdoid suture and are rarely seen beyond the first 3 years of life. They require no specific treatment but should be observed for "growing fractures." Growing fractures are skull fractures associated with an underlying dural tear that may be caused by a leptomeningeal cyst, dilated ventricles, or a herniated brain. Neurologic symptoms include headache, seizures, and asymmetric cranial growth (Schutzman and Greenes, 2001). Infants and young children who have isolated skull fractures should be evaluated for growing skull fractures from 1 to 2 months after the injury (Schutzman and Greenes, 2001).

Complications

The major complications of trauma to the head are hemorrhage, infection, edema, and herniation through the tentorium. Infection is always a hazard in open injuries, and edema is related to tissue trauma. Vascular rupture may occur even in minor head injuries, causing hemorrhage between the skull and cerebral surfaces. Compression of the underlying brain produces effects that can be rapidly fatal or insidiously progressive.

❗NURSING ALERT

Posttraumatic meningitis should be suspected in children with increasing drowsiness and fever who also have basilar skull fractures.

Epidural Hemorrhage. The blood accumulates between the dura and the skull to form a hematoma, which, because of the difficulty with which dura is stripped from bone, forces the underlying brain contents downward and inward as the brain expands (see Fig. 28-5, *A*). Since bleeding is generally arterial, brain compression occurs rapidly. Most often the expanding hematoma is located in the parietotemporal region, forcing the medial portion of the temporal lobe under the edge of the tentorium, where it causes pressure on nerves and blood vessels. The lower incidence of epidural hematoma in childhood has been attributed to the fact that the middle meningeal artery is not embedded in the bone surface of the skull until approximately 2 years of age. Therefore a fracture of the temporal bone is less likely to lacerate the artery. Second, the dura closely adheres to the inner table of the skull, especially at the level of the sutures, making separation from bleeding less likely. However, a child's skull can be indented with sufficient force to tear the middle meningeal artery and rebound intact without causing a fracture. Hemorrhage can also derive from dural veins or the dural sinuses, especially in infants and small children, in whom fracture is less likely to occur. In 20% to 40% of children a skull fracture is not detectable. The classic clinical picture of epidural hemorrhage (momentary unconsciousness followed by a normal period, then lethargy or coma) is seldom evident in children (see Box 28-4 for clinical manifestations). The period of impaired consciousness is frequently lacking, and the symptom-free period is atypical because of nonspecific complaints such as irritability, headache, and vomiting. When it does occur, the symptom-free period frequently lasts longer than 48 hours. Clinically significant epidural hematomas are uncommon in children younger than 4 years of age. These differences may be caused by the decreased tendency of the resilient skull to fracture; the ability of blood to escape through widened sutures, an open fontanel, or a fracture; bleeding from smaller vessels with less rapid and massive bleeding; lower systolic blood pressure in children; and possibly the decreased susceptibility of the child's brain to pressure changes.

Subdural Hemorrhage.   A subdural hemorrhage is bleeding between the dura and the cerebrum, usually as a result of rupture of cortical veins that bridge the subdural space (see Fig. 28-5, *B*). Subdural hematomas are 10 times more frequent than epidural hematomas, occurring most often in infancy, with a peak incidence at 6 months.

Unlike epidural hemorrhage, which develops inwardly against the less resistant brain tissue, subdural hemorrhage tends to develop more slowly and spreads thinly and widely until it is limited by the dural barriers—the falx and tentorium. Subdural hematoma is fairly common in infants, frequently as a result of birth trauma, falls, assaults, or violent shaking. The small subdural space and dura firmly attached to the skull in this area are highly vulnerable to increased ICP.

❗NURSING ALERT

Children with a subdural hematoma and retinal hemorrhages should be evaluated for the possibility of child abuse, especially shaken baby syndrome (SBS).

Repeated subdural taps often provide relief in the infant, as revealed by follow-up CT scans, improved neurologic status, and a flat anterior fontanel. Surgical evacuation of the hematoma is the treatment of choice in the older child and is frequently required in infants.

Cerebral Edema.   Some degree of brain edema is expected, especially 24 to 72 hours after craniocerebral trauma. Cerebral edema caused by direct cellular injury or

BOX 28-4 ■ Clinical Manifestations of Acute Head Injury

MINOR INJURY
May or may not lose consciousness
Transient period of confusion
Somnolence
Listlessness
Irritability
Pallor
Vomiting

SIGNS OF PROGRESSION
Altered mental status (e.g., difficulty rousing child)
Mounting agitation
Development of focal lateral neurologic signs (p. 1013)
Marked changes in vital signs

SEVERE INJURY
Signs of increased intracranial pressure (see Box 28-1)
Increased head size (infant)
Bulging or full fontanel (infant)
Retinal hemorrhage
Extraocular palsies (especially cranial nerve VI)
Hemiparesis
Quadriplegia
Elevated temperature
Unsteady gait (older child)
Papilledema (older child)
Retinal hemorrhages

ASSOCIATED SIGNS
Scalp trauma
Other injuries (e.g., to extremities)

vascular injury induces vascular stasis, anoxia, and further vasodilation. If the progression continues unchecked, ICP exceeds arterial pressure and fatal anoxia ensues, and/or the pressure causes herniation of a portion of the brain over the edge of the tentorium, compressing the brainstem and occluding the posterior cerebral arteries. Diffuse cerebral swelling and changes in CBF are common patterns following head injury in children.

❗NURSING ALERT

If a child loses consciousness or vomits more than three times, medical attention should be sought.

Diagnostic Evaluation

A detailed history, especially a health history, both past and present, is essential in evaluating the child with a craniocerebral trauma. Certain disorders, such as drug allergies, hemophilia, diabetes mellitus, or epilepsy, may produce similar symptoms. Furthermore, even minor traumatic injury can aggravate a preexisting disease process. Events surrounding the injury often supply significant data. It must be determined whether the infant or child exhibited alterations in consciousness, and any other signs and behaviors exhibited by the child must be noted. Since head injuries are frequently accompanied by injuries in other areas, the examination is performed with care to avoid further damage.

Initial Assessment. Priorities in the initial stabilization phase of a child with a head injury include assessment of the ABCs (airway, breathing, circulation); evaluation for shock; a neurologic examination, especially LOC; pupillary symmetry and response to light; and seizures (Bayir Kochanek, and Clark, 2003). The assessment is carried out quickly in relation to vital signs (see Emergency Treatment box). Excited and irritable children may have a rapid pulse, hyperventilate, appear pale, and feel clammy shortly after an injury.

Ocular signs such as fixed and dilated pupils, fixed and constricted pupils, and pupils that are poorly reactive or nonreactive to light and accommodation indicate increased ICP or brainstem involvement. It is important to remain with the child who demonstrates fixed and dilated pupils, since these are ominous signs, with the probability of respiratory arrest. Dilated, nonpulsating blood vessels indicate increased ICP before the appearance of papilledema. Retinal hemorrhages are seen in acute head injuries.

Less urgent but important additional assessments include examination of the scalp for lacerations and palpation for other abnormalities. A significant amount of blood loss can occur from scalp lacerations.

An accurate assessment of clinical signs provides baseline information. Serial evaluations, preferably by a single observer, help to detect changes in the neurologic status. Alterations in mental status, evidenced by increased difficulty in rousing the child, mounting agitation, development of focal lateral neurologic signs, or marked changes in vital signs, usually indicate extension or progression of the basic pathologic process.

Special Tests. After a thorough clinical examination, a variety of diagnostic tests are helpful in providing a more definitive diagnosis of the type and extent of the trauma. The severity of a head injury may not be apparent on clinical examination of a child, but it will be detectable on a CT

EMERGENCY TREATMENT

Head Injury

Assess child:
  A—Airway (with cervical-spine immobilization)
        Use jaw thrust to open airway
  B—Bleeding
  C—Circulation
Clean any abrasions with soap and water.
  Apply clean dressing.
  If bleeding, apply ice to relieve pain and swelling.
Keep NPO until instructed otherwise.
Assess pain, but do not give analgesics or sedatives.
Check pupil reaction every 4 hours (including twice during night) for 48 hours.
Awaken twice during the night to check level of consciousness.
Seek medical attention if any of the following apply:
  Injury sustained:
    At high speed (e.g., automobile)
    Fall from a significant distance (e.g., roof, tree, or height greater than that of the child)
    From great force (e.g., baseball bat)
    Under suspicious circumstances
  Loss of consciousness
  Amnesia
  Discomfort (crying) more than 10 minutes after injury
  Headache that is severe, worsening, interferes with sleep
  Fluid leak from ears or nose
  Vomiting three or more times
  Swelling in front of or above earlobe or increased swelling
  Confused or not behaving normally
  Difficult to rouse from sleep
  Difficulty speaking
  Blurred vision or seeing double
  Unsteady gait
  Difficulty using extremities
  Neck pain
  Pupils dilated, unequal, or fixed
  Infant with full or bulging fontanel
  Bruising below the eyes

scan. Whenever the child has a history consistent with a serious head injury (unrestrained occupant in a severe motor vehicle accident or a fall from a significant height), it is important that a scan be performed even if the child initially appears alert and oriented. All children with head injuries who have any alteration of consciousness, headache, vomiting, skull fracture, seizure, or a predisposing medical condition should also undergo CT scanning.

MRI and neurobehavioral assessment following early head injury may be useful in documenting cognitive impairment in relation to structural alterations in the young brain. MRI provides details of soft tissues better than any other noninvasive device. Electroencephalography is not particularly helpful for early diagnosis but is useful for defining seizure activity or focal destructive lesions after the acute phase of illness. Lumbar puncture is rarely used in craniocerebral trauma and is contraindicated in the presence of increased ICP because of the possibility of herniation. In some centers monitoring ICP is part of the assessment.

Posttraumatic Syndromes. Posttraumatic syndromes can be clinically manifested because of structural complications resulting from a head injury and through the signs and symptoms demonstrated by the child. Structural complications can include hydrocephalus and focal deficits such as optic atrophy, cranial nerve palsies, motor deficits, diabetes insipidus, aphasia, and seizures. Behavioral disturbances include sleep disturbances, phobias, emotional lability, altered school performance, and changes related to aggressiveness or withdrawal. ***Postconcussion syndrome*** is a common sequela to brain injury and can occur within minutes to an hour after a head injury. The manifestations vary with the age of the child. The syndrome occurs very frequently in children younger than 1 year of age. The syndrome in adolescents is similar to that in adults. The duration of manifestations can vary from several days to several months. Death from concussion is preventable unless overwhelming secondary brain injury has occurred (Durkin and others, 1998; Gennarelli, 1999).

Posttraumatic seizures occur in a number of children who survive a head injury and are more common in children than in adults. Seizures are more likely to occur within the first few days of the head injury (Chiaretti and others, 2000). ***Structural complications*** (e.g., hydrocephalus) may occur following a head injury. The type of residual effect depends on the location and nature of the disorder. True mental retardation occurs only after severe injuries.

Therapeutic Management

The majority of children with mild to moderate concussion who have not lost consciousness can be cared for and observed at home after careful examination reveals no serious intracranial injury. Nurses should provide parents with clear explanations and instructions and should encourage them to ask questions both before and after leaving the medical facility if clarification is needed (see Family Focus box).

The parents are instructed to check the child every 2 hours to determine any changes in responsiveness. The sleeping child should be wakened to see if he or she can be roused normally. Parents are advised to maintain contact with the health professional, who usually wishes to examine the child again in 1 or 2 days. The manifestations of epidural hematoma in children do not generally appear until 24 hours or more after injury.

Children with severe injuries, those who have lost consciousness for more than a few minutes, and those with prolonged and continued seizures or other focal or diffuse neurologic signs must be hospitalized until their condition is stable and their neurologic signs have diminished.

The child is maintained on nothing by mouth or restricted to clear liquids, if able to take fluids by mouth, until it is determined that vomiting will not occur. IV fluids are indicated in the child who is comatose or displays dulled sensorium and/or in the child with persistent vomiting. Fluid balance is closely monitored by daily weights; accurate intake and output measurements; and serum osmolality to detect early signs of water retention, excessive dehydration, and states of hypertonicity or hypotonicity.

The volume of IV fluid is carefully monitored to avoid aggravating any cerebral edema and to minimize the possibility of overhydration in case of SIADH. However, damage

FAMILY FOCUS

Maintaining Contact

Maintaining contact with parents for continued observation and reevaluation of the child, when indicated, facilitates early diagnosis and treatment of possible complications from head injury, such as hematoma, hydrocephalus, cysts, and posttraumatic seizures. Children are generally hospitalized for 24 to 48 hours' observation if their family lives far from medical facilities or lacks transportation or a telephone that would provide access to immediate help. Other circumstances such as language or other communication barriers, or even emotional trauma, may hinder learning and make it difficult for families to feel confident in caring for their child at home.

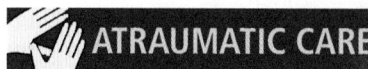

ATRAUMATIC CARE

Noninvasive Local Anesthesia

The use of topical lidocaine, epinephrine, and tetracaine (LET) solution (Pasero and McCaffery, 1999) or lidocaine, adrenaline, and tetracaine (LAT) gel provides noninvasive anesthesia for suturing (Ernst and others, 1997). Both of these preparations provide an acceptable alternative to tetracaine, adrenaline, and cocaine (TAC), which is more expensive, is a restricted narcotic, and carries a higher potential for toxicity (Pasero and McCaffery, 1999).

to the hypothalamus or pituitary gland may produce diabetes insipidus with its accompanying hypertonicity and dehydration.

Restlessness can be satisfactorily managed, if necessary, with mild sedation, and headache is usually controlled with acetaminophen (Tylenol). Antiepileptics are used for seizure control and frequently in cases of suspected contusion or laceration. Antibiotics may be administered if lacerations, CSF leakage, or excessive cerebral tissue damage is present. Prophylactic tetanus toxoid is given as appropriate. Cerebral edema is managed as described for the unconscious child. Hyperthermia is controlled with tepid sponges or a hypothermia blanket.

Surgical Therapy. Scalp lacerations are sutured after the underlying bone is carefully examined (see Atraumatic Care box). Depressed fractures require surgical reduction and removal of bone fragments. Torn dura is sutured. "Ping-Pong ball" skull fractures in very young infants ordinarily correct themselves within a few weeks and do not require specific treatment, although they can be reduced by pressure against the bone.

Prognosis. The outcome of craniocerebral trauma depends on the extent of injury and complications. However, the outlook is generally more favorable for children than for adults (Faillace, 2002; Masson and others, 2003). More than 90% of children with concussions or simple linear fractures recover without symptoms after the initial period. The incidence of fatalities and neurologic sequelae is lower in children than in adults, even in those with severe head injuries. The prognosis for recovery is primarily related to the duration of coma and the degree of injury. The combination of impaired consciousness and skull fracture carries the highest risk of complication.

The concern regarding outcome is increasingly focused on cognitive, emotional, and/or mental problems. Recent studies indicate that children experience a higher frequency of psychologic disturbances following head injury, whereas adults are more prone to complaints of a physical nature.

Children may be more vulnerable than adults to long-term cognitive and behavioral dysfunction after diffuse brain injury. Even with recovery, the effects of brain injury on a child's potential can never be known.

True coma (not obeying commands, eyes closed, and not speaking) usually does not last more than 2 weeks. A child's eventual outcome can range from brain death to a persistent vegetative state to complete recovery. However, even the best recovery may be associated with personality changes, including mood lability and loss of confidence, impaired short-term memory, headaches, and subtle cognitive impairments. Many children are left with significant disabilities after head injury that appear months later as learning difficulties, behavioral changes, or emotional disturbances (Faillace, 2002). Generally, within 6 months to 1 year after the injury, 90% of the long-term neurologic outcome has been achieved.

Nursing Considerations

The hospitalized child requires careful neurologic assessment and evaluation (including vital signs) repeated at frequent intervals to provide information needed to establish a correct diagnosis, reveal signs and symptoms of increased ICP, determine clinical management, prevent many complications, and provide support to the child and family during the recovery phases.

The child is placed on bed rest, usually with the head of the bed elevated slightly, and appropriate safety measures, such as side rails kept up for older children and seizure precautions for children of all ages, are implemented. For the extremely restless child, hard surfaces may have to be padded and restraint used to prevent the possibility of further injury. Care is individualized according to the specific needs of the child. The unconscious child is managed as described in the previous section, but most childhood head injuries are those causing momentary stunning or temporary unconsciousness. Children may be restless and irritable, but more often their reaction is to fall asleep when left undisturbed. A quiet environment helps reduce the restlessness and irritability. Shining bright lights directly into the child's face is irritating and often aggravates the child, making assessment of ocular responses difficult.

Frequent examinations of vital signs, neurologic signs, and LOC are extremely important nursing observations. When possible, they should be performed by a single observer to better detect subtle changes that may indicate worsening of neurologic status. Pupils are checked for size, equality, reaction to light, and accommodation. After the initial elevations usually seen following injury, the vital signs generally return to normal unless there is brainstem involvement. An axillary measurement of temperature is the safest method, since seizures are not uncommon and vomiting is a frequent response in children, especially when the child is disturbed.

The most important nursing observation is assessment of the child's LOC. Alterations in consciousness appear earlier in the progression of an injury than alterations of vital signs or focal neurologic signs. Some expected responses may be misinterpreted as deviations from the normal. Frequent examinations of alertness are fatiguing to the child; therefore the child often desires to fall asleep, which may be confused with depressed consciousness. When left alone, the child promptly dozes. It is not uncommon to observe ocular divergence through the partially closed eyelids.

A key nursing role is to provide sedation and analgesia for the child. The conflict between the need to promote comfort and relieve anxiety in the child versus the need to be able to assess for neurologic changes presents a dilemma. However, both goals can be achieved with close observation of the child's LOC and response to analgesics, use of a pain assessment record, and effective communication with the practitioner. To differentiate between sedation from an opioid and sedation from the injury, naloxone (Narcan) can be given *slowly* to reverse the opioid's sedative effect. Decreasing restlessness after administration of an analgesic most likely reflects pain control rather than a decreasing LOC.

Observations of position and movement provide additional information. Any abnormal posturing is noted, as well as whether it occurs continuously or intermittently. Are the child's handgrips strong and equal in strength? Are there any signs of decerebrate or decorticate posturing? What is the child's response to stimulation? Is movement purposeful, random, or absent? Are movement and/or sensation equal on both sides or restricted to one side only?

The child may complain of headache or other discomfort. The child who is too young to describe a headache will be fussy and resist being handled. The child who suffers from vertigo will often assume a position of comfort and vigorously resist efforts to be moved. Forcible movement causes the child to vomit and display spontaneous nystagmus. Seizures, relatively common in children with craniocerebral trauma, may be of any type but are more often generalized, regardless of the type of injury. Any seizure activity should be carefully observed and described in detail. Children in postictal (post-seizure) states are lethargic, with sluggish pupils.

Drainage from any orifice is noted. Bleeding from the ear suggests the possibility of a basal skull fracture. The amount and characteristics of the drainage are observed, and since the auditory canal may be a source of infection, dry, sterile cotton can be placed loosely at the orifice and changed when soiled.

> ### ◗ NURSING ALERT
>
> Suctioning through the nares is contraindicated because there is a risk of the catheter entering the brain parenchyma through a fracture in the skull.

Head trauma is frequently accompanied by other undetected injuries; therefore any bruises, lacerations, or evidence of internal injuries or fractures of the extremities are noted and reported. Associated injuries are evaluated and treated appropriately.

The child with normal LOC is usually allowed clear liquids unless fluid is restricted. If the child has an IV infusion, it is maintained as prescribed. The diet is advanced to that appropriate for the child's age as soon as the condition permits. Intake and output are measured and recorded, and any incontinence of bowel or bladder is noted in the child who has been toilet trained.

The child should be observed for any unusual behavior, but behavior should be interpreted in relation to the child's normal behavior. For example, urinary incontinence during sleep would be of no consequence in a child who routinely wets the bed but would be highly significant for one who is always dry. In addition, a child who is subject to nightmares might cry out and demonstrate agitated behavior at night. Parents are valuable resources. Information obtained from parents at or shortly after admission is helpful in evaluating the child's behavior (e.g., the case with which the child is roused normally, the usual sleeping position, how much the child sleeps during the day, motor activity the child is capable of [rolling over, sitting up, climbing], hearing and visual acuity, appetite, and manner of eating [spoon, bottle, cup]). There would be less concern about a child who falls asleep several times during the day if this were consistent with the child's usual behavior.

Family Support.   The emotional and educational support of the family of children who have suffered head injury presents a formidable, challenging aspect to nursing care. Witnessing the parents' ordeal of grief and helplessness on seeing their child in an intensive care unit connected to monitoring equipment in an altered state evokes empathy. The nurse can encourage the family to be involved in the child's care, to bring in familiar belongings, or to make a tape recording of familiar voices and sounds. Parents may need a demonstration on how to touch or cuddle their child and may want to talk about their grief. The nurse can listen attentively, reinforce what is being done to assist the child, and direct parents toward signs and symptoms of recovery to instill hope without promises. A common phenomenon is for families to seek information from all health care providers, asking, "What will she be like? What do you know?" as they search for some clue that the child is recovering. Honesty and kindness, along with competent care, distinguish excellent nursing abilities.

When the child is discharged, the parents are advised of probable posttraumatic symptoms that may be expected, such as behavioral changes, sleep disturbances, phobias, and seizures. They should understand observations that should be made and how to contact the physician, nurse, or health facility in case the child develops any unusual signs or symptoms. The importance of follow-up evaluation should be emphasized. It is often advisable to refer the family to a public health agency for home follow-through to be certain that the child receives posthospital evaluation.

Rehabilitation.   The rehabilitation and management of the child with permanent brain injury are essential aspects of care. Rehabilitation of brain-injured children is begun as soon as feasible and usually involves the family and a rehabilitation team. Careful assessment of the child's capabilities, limitations, and probable potential is made as early as possible, and appropriate interventions are implemented to maximize the residual capacities. The **Brain Injury Associ-**ation of America* "arose from the mutual frustration and sense of hopelessness experienced by families in their search for appropriate facilities and support to return head-injured loved ones to their maximum functioning potential." It provides information and listings of rehabilitation services and support groups throughout the country.

Pediatric trauma rehabilitation is a national concern. Coordinating care and services for early rehabilitation involves identifying the child and family's response to the traumatic injury and disability, securing available resources, and recognizing the parental role in the process.

The child with a disability resulting from head trauma requires assessment on a physical, cognitive, emotional, and social level. The child has experienced separation, pain, sensory deprivation and overload, changes in circadian cycle, and fear of the unknown. Recovery and transition require new coping strategies at the same time that regressive and acting-out behavior may start. Parents and children need honest communication for decision making. A rehabilitation facility or home rehabilitation is advocated when the child has progressed beyond what can be provided in a hospital setting. The Rancho Los Amigos Scale provides a systematic assessment of the possible progress a child may achieve following a severe head injury.

Prevention.   Tremendous strides have been taken in the prevention of cerebral damage after head injury in children. New developments requiring research point to the prevention of cellular injury or the primary insult. However, the greatest benefit lies in prevention of head injuries. Nurses can exert a valuable influence on behalf of children through education. The reason injuries remain preventable is that unnecessary risks go unchecked. Inadequate supervision combined with a child's natural sense of indestructibility and exploration can lead to lethal results. Nurses are in the unique position of influencing caregivers in terms of growth and development. Banning the use of infant walkers is an example. This equipment does not help develop motor skills but places infants at risk for head and neck injuries from falls, especially down steps. Public education, coupled with legislative support, can prevent childhood injuries. (For extensive discussions of childhood injuries, see the discussions on injury prevention in Chapters 10, 12, 13, 15, and 16. See also Childhood Mortality, Chapter 1.)

NEAR-DROWNING

Drowning ranks second as a cause of accidental death in children. Most cases of drowning are accidental, usually involving the following individuals:

1 Children who are helpless in water, such as inadequately attended children in or near swimming pools or infants in bathtubs
2 Small children who fall into ponds, streams, and flooded excavations, usually near home
3 Occupants of pleasure boats who fail to wear life preservers
4 Children who have diving accidents
5 Children who are able to swim but overestimate their endurance.

---

*105 North Alfred Street, Alexandria, VA 22314; (703) 236-6000; fax: (703) 236-6001; website: www.biausa.org.

Accidental drowning occurs five times more often in boys than in girls; almost 40% of children are younger than age 5, and 90% of cases occur in private swimming pools (Kallas, 2004).

Drowning can take place in any body of water, including such unlikely ones as a pail of water. Top-heavy toddlers fall head first into a pail of water, their arms become trapped, and they are unable to free themselves. Hot tubs and whirlpool spas have been implicated in childhood drowning injury. The suction created at the outlet is strong enough to trap even larger children underwater. Drowning as a form of fatal child abuse has also been recognized as a problem. Homicidal drownings are unwitnessed, they usually occur in the home, and the victims are either infants or toddlers. With expeditious treatment many children are being saved. For purposes of this discussion, two terms need clarification:

Drowning—Death from asphyxia while submerged, regardless of whether fluid has entered the lungs

Near-drowning—Survival at least 24 hours after submersion in a fluid medium

Pathophysiology

The major pulmonary changes that occur in drowning are directly related to the length of submersion (regardless of the type and amount of fluid aspirated), the physiologic response of the victim, and the development and degree of immersion hypothermia. In addition, cerebral recovery depends on the effectiveness of initial resuscitation and subsequent critical care measures to support cerebral salvage.

Physiologic factors that influence the extent of damage from immersion include resistance to asphyxia and anoxia, which shows some individual variation. There is greater resistance with diminishing age; young children can withstand longer periods of submersion. More important is the drowning, or diving, reflex. This neurologic response is triggered by immersion of the face in cold water. Blood is shunted away from the periphery, and the flow is concentrated to the brain and heart predominantly.

The problems created by near-drowning are (1) hypoxia and asphyxiation, (2) aspiration, and (3) hypothermia (except near-drowning in hot tubs). Cardiopulmonary arrest is secondary to asphyxiation.

Hypoxia is the primary problem because it results in global cell damage, and different cells tolerate variable lengths of anoxia. Neurons, especially cerebral cells, sustain irreversible damage after 4 to 6 minutes of submersion. The heart and lungs can survive up to 30 minutes. Regardless of the amount of water aspirated, there is arterial hypoxemia (resulting from atelectasis with shunting of blood through the nonventilated alveoli) and a combined respiratory acidosis (resulting from retained carbon dioxide) and metabolic acidosis (caused by buildup of acid metabolites from anaerobic metabolism). The pathologic events are directly related to the duration of submersion. The major difficulty is acute ventilatory insufficiency. Approximately 10% of drowning victims die without aspirating fluid but succumb from acute asphyxia as a result of prolonged reflex laryngospasm.

Aspiration of fluid occurs in the majority of drownings. The aspirated fluid results in pulmonary edema, atelectasis, airway spasm, and pneumonitis, which aggravates the hypoxia. It was previously thought that submersion in salt water versus fresh water altered the physiologic response to near-drowning. However, there is no clinically significant difference in the response of human survivors, and the type of water does not alter the therapy or outcome.

Hypothermia occurs rapidly in infants and children, partly because of their large surface area relative to body mass and partly as a result of the cold water itself. Water is an excellent heat conductor, and the contact with the skin is increased by struggling. Hypothermia may make resumption or maintenance of cardiac function possible if body temperature is less than 30° C (86° F). Profound hypothermia is usually evidence of lengthy submersion.

Therapeutic Management

Resuscitative measures should begin at the scene of a drowning, and the victim should be transported to the hospital with maximal ventilatory and circulatory support. Many victims need care for some time after aspiration of fluid. In the hospital, intensive pulmonary care is implemented and continued according to the needs of the patient.

In general, the management of the near-drowning victim is based on the degree of cerebral insult (Box 28-5). The first priority is to restore oxygen delivery to the cells and prevent further hypoxic damage. A spontaneously breathing child will do well in an oxygen-enriched atmosphere; the more severely affected child will require endotracheal intubation and mechanical ventilation. Blood gases and pH are monitored frequently as a guide to oxygen, fluid, and electrolyte therapies.

> **! NURSING ALERT**
>
> All children who have a near-drowning experience should be admitted to the hospital for observation. Although many patients do not appear to have suffered adverse effects from the event, complications (e.g., respiratory compromise, cerebral edema) may occur 24 hours after the incident.

BOX 28-5 ■ Clinical Manifestations of Near-Drowning

CATEGORY	CHARACTERISTICS
A	Awake, minimal injury
	Fully conscious; may have mild hypothermia, mild chest radiograph changes, mild arterial blood gas abnormalities
B	Blunted sensorium, moderate injury
	Obtund, stuporous, purposeful response to painful stimuli, mild to moderate hypothermia, frequent respiratory distress, abnormal chest radiographs, arterial blood gas abnormalities
C	Comatose, severe anoxia
	Unarousable, abnormal response to pain, abnormal respiratory pattern, seizures, shock, marked arterial blood gas abnormalities, abnormal chest radiographs, arrhythmias, metabolic acidosis, hyperkalemia, hyperglycemia, disseminated intravascular coagulation
C1	Decorticate, Cheyne-Stokes respirations
C2	Decerebrate, central hyperventilation
C3	Flaccid, apneic, or cluster breathing
C4	Flaccid, apneic, no detectable circulation

Aspiration pneumonia is a frequent complication that occurs about 48 to 72 hours after the episode. Bronchospasm, alveolocapillary membrane damage, atelectasis, abscess formation, and acute respiratory distress syndrome are other complications that occur after aspiration of fluid.

Prognosis. Studies report that the best predictors of a good outcome were length of submersion in non-icy water (>5° C [41° F]) for less than 5 minutes and the presence of sinus rhythm, reactive pupils, and neurologic responsiveness at the scene. The worst prognoses—for death or severe neurologic impairment—were in children submerged for more than 10 minutes and not responding to advanced life support within 25 minutes. All children without spontaneous, purposeful movement and normal brainstem function 24 hours after near-drowning suffered severe neurologic deficits or death (Zuckerman, Gregory, and Santos-Damiani, 1998; Kallas, 2004).

Nursing Considerations

Nursing care depends on the condition of the child. A child who survives may need intensive respiratory nursing care with attention to vital signs, mechanical ventilation and/or tracheostomy, blood gas determination, chest therapy, and IV infusion. Frequently the child is comatose for an indefinite period and requires the same care as an unconscious child. A difficult aspect in the care of the child victim of near-drowning is helping the parents cope with severe guilt reactions. The magnitude of the event is so great that efforts to provide comfort and support are of only limited success. Parents need to hear that everything possible is being done to treat the child, and this message needs to be repeated often.

The parents of the child who is saved from death are also faced with the anxiety of not knowing what the outcome will be, and sometimes they wish for the death of the child. Because their situation generates such intense feelings of loneliness, it is important for families to know that they are not alone. They need to be reminded frequently that there are caring people to assist them both during the crisis and later. Additional sources of support that can be recommended are psychiatric and social work consultants, community services, and religious support. Self-help groups are excellent if these are available in the community.

Nurses often have difficulty relating to the parents if obvious neglect has precipitated the accident and subsequent problems; therefore it is important for those who care for these children and their families to assess their own feelings about the situation, as well as the coping abilities and resources of the family. Caring for near-drowning victims and their families requires nurses to be sensitive to the needs of the child and the family and to recognize their own reactions and emotions.

Prevention. Most drownings, particularly of infants or small children, can be prevented with adequate supervision. Water safety and survival training should be required for all school-age children, and nurses can be active advocates in their communities. Nurses are also in a position to emphasize the importance of adequate adult supervision when children are in the water. Aquatic programs for infants and toddlers do not decrease the risk of drowning; young children should never be left unattended when in or near the water (American Academy of Pediatrics, 2000; Kallas, 2004). Parents with pools should know cardiopulmonary resuscitation (CPR) techniques. See also Injury Prevention, Chapters 10, 12, 13, 15, and 16.

NERVOUS SYSTEM TUMORS

Brain tumor and neuroblastoma are two major forms of childhood cancer derived from neural tissue. CNS tumors account for approximately 20% of all childhood cancers, and approximately 65 cases per million occur in children under 15 years of age (Redner, 2000). Both of these tumors are difficult to treat and have not demonstrated the dramatic improvements in survival seen in other forms of childhood cancer.

BRAIN TUMORS

Brain tumors are the most common solid tumors in children and are the second most common childhood cancer. The majority of tumors (about 60%) are *infratentorial* (below the tentorium cerebelli), which means that they occur in the posterior third of the brain, primarily in the cerebellum or brainstem. This anatomic distribution accounts for the frequency of symptoms resulting from increased ICP. The other tumors are *supratentorial,* or within the anterior two thirds of the brain, mainly the cerebrum.

Brain tumors, whether benign or malignant, can arise from any cell within the cranium. Consequently, the cranial cells' origin provides a histologic classification for major tumors. For instance, astrocytes (cells that form the supportive tissue for neurons) may form a common glial tumor called an astrocytoma. The major infratentorial tumors are medulloblastomas, cerebellar astrocytomas, brainstem gliomas, and ependymomas, and the major supratentorial tumors are astrocytomas, hypothalamic tumors, optic pathway tumors, and craniopharyngiomas.

Diagnostic Evaluation

The signs and symptoms of brain tumors are directly related to their anatomic location and size and, to some extent, the age of the child. In infants, whose cranial sutures are still open, virtually no early detectable symptoms develop. It is not until spinal fluid obstruction causes markedly increased head size that a lesion may be suspected. Even in older children, clinical manifestations are nonspecific. However, the most common symptoms are headache, especially on awakening, and vomiting that is not related to feeding. The common clinical manifestations and assessment of brain tumors are presented in Table 28-2.

Diagnosis of a brain tumor is based subjectively on presenting clinical signs and objectively on neurologic tests and histologic diagnosis via surgery. Because the signs and symptoms are vague and easily overlooked, early diagnosis necessitates a high index of suspicion during history taking. A number of tests may be used in the neurologic evaluation, but the most common diagnostic procedure is MRI, which determines the location and extent of the tumor. Other tests that may be used include CT, angiography, electroencephalography, and cerebral lumbar puncture. Lumbar puncture is

TABLE 28-2 ■ Clinical Manifestations and Assessment of Brain Tumors

SIGNS AND SYMPTOMS	ASSESSMENT
HEADACHE	
Recurrent and progressive	Record description of pain, location, severity, and duration
In frontal or occipital areas	Use pain rating scale to assess severity of pain (see Chapter 21)
Usually dull and throbbing	Note changes in relation to time of day and activity
Worse on arising, less during day	Observe changes in behavior in infants (persistent irritability, crying, head rolling)
Intensified by lowering head and straining, such as during bowel movement, coughing, sneezing	
VOMITING	
With or without nausea or feeding	Record time, amount, and relationship to feeding, nausea, and activity
Progressively more projectile	
More severe in morning	
Relieved by moving about and changing position	
NEUROMUSCULAR CHANGES	
Incoordination or clumsiness	Test muscle strength, gait, coordination, and reflexes (see Chapter 7)
Loss of balance (use of wide-based stance, falling, tripping, banging into objects)	
Poor fine motor control	
Weakness	
Hyporeflexia or hyperreflexia	
Positive Babinski sign	
Spasticity	
Paralysis	
BEHAVIORAL CHANGES	
Irritability	Observe behavior regularly
Decreased appetite	Compare observations with parental reports of normal behavioral patterns
Failure to thrive	Monitor growth and food intake
Fatigue (frequent naps)	Monitor activity and sleep
Lethargy	
Coma	
Bizarre behavior (staring, automatic movements)	
CRANIAL NERVE NEUROPATHY	
Cranial nerve involvement varies according to tumor location	Assess cranial nerves, especially VII (facial), IX (glossopharyngeal), X (vagus), V (trigeminal, sensory roots), and VI (abducens) (see Chapter 7)
Most common signs:	Assess visual acuity, binocularity, and peripheral vision (see Chapter 7)
Head tilt	
Visual defects (nystagmus, diplopia, strabismus, episodic "graying out" of vision, visual field defects)	
VITAL SIGN DISTURBANCES	
Decreased pulse and respiration	Measure vital signs frequently
Increased blood pressure	Monitor pulse and respirations for 1 full minute
Decreased pulse pressure	Record pulse pressure (difference between systolic and diastolic blood pressure)
Hypothermia or hyperthermia	
OTHER SIGNS	
Seizures	Record seizure activity
Cranial enlargement*	Measure head circumference daily (infant and young child)
Tense, bulging fontanel at rest*	Perform funduscopic examination if skilled in procedure
Nuchal rigidity	
Papilledema (edema of optic nerve)	

*Present only in infants and young children.

dangerous in the presence of increased ICP because of the possibility of brainstem herniation following a sudden release of pressure. The definitive diagnosis is based on brain tissue specimens obtained during surgery.

Therapeutic Management

Treatment may involve the use of surgery, radiation therapy, and chemotherapy. All three may or may not be used, depending on the type of tumor. The treatment of choice is total removal of the tumor without residual neurologic damage. Patients with the most complete tumor removal have the greatest chance of survival. Radiation therapy is used to treat most tumors and to shrink the size of the tumor before attempting surgical removal. Chemotherapy has emerged in the past decade to delay radiation in children younger than 3 years of age because of the rapid brain development occurring in the first 3 years of life (Murray-Ryan and Petriccione, 2002; Strother and others, 2002). Chemotherapy is also used as adjunct therapy for residual tumor, nonresectable tumor, or recurrent tumor. Water-soluble agents are able to penetrate the disrupted blood-brain barrier and attack brain tumor cells (Murray-Ryan and Petriccione, 2002; Strother and others, 2002). Typically, the most commonly used chemotherapy is cisplatin, carboplatin, vincristine, cyclophosphamide, lomustine, carmustine, etoposide, ifosfamide, and topotecan. Surgery (biopsy, resection, laser, or stereotactic), radiation therapy (hyperfractionated, fractionated, or stereotactic), and/or multi-agent chemotherapy are all instrumental in the treatment of brain tumors.

Prognosis.   The prognosis for the child with a brain tumor depends on the type of brain tumor, the size of the tumor, the extent of the disease, and the age of the child. Problems associated with treatment and a relatively poor prognosis, primarily in infants and young children, are compounded by serious late effects of therapy. A decline in incidence of children with medulloblastoma has been significantly linked with a protective effect of maternal folate, iron, and multivitamin supplementation. Along with the recent advances of surgical instrumentation allowing aggressive surgical intervention (e.g., stereotactic surgery, radiosurgery), modifications in radiation (e.g., hyperfractionation, brain mapping) and use of chemotherapy (e.g., intrathecal, intratumoral) have increased the long-term survival rates for many children with brain tumors (Alston and others, 2003; Gupta and Berger, 2003; Murray-Ryan and Petriccione, 2002; Strother and others, 2002).

Nursing Considerations

A brain tumor is often suspected in a child admitted to the hospital with neurologic dysfunction, although the actual diagnosis may not as yet be confirmed. Establishing a baseline of data with which to compare preoperative and postoperative changes is an essential step toward planning physical care and preventing complications. It also allows the nurse to assess the degree of physical incapacity and the family's emotional reaction to the diagnosis.

Vital signs, including blood pressure and pulse pressure (the difference between systolic and diastolic pressures), are taken routinely and more often when any change is noted.

Any sudden variations are reported immediately. It is especially important to note a change in vital signs during or after diagnostic procedures. A routine neurologic assessment is also performed at the same time as vital signs, and head circumference is measured on infants and very young children.

The child is observed for evidence of headache, vomiting, and any seizure activity. The location, severity, and duration of the headache are noted, as well as its relationship to activity and time of day. Behaviors such as lying flat and facing away from light or refusing to engage in play are clues to discomfort in the nonverbal child. The child's gait is observed at least once daily. Head tilt and other changes in posturing are always noted.

Prepare Child and Family for Diagnostic/Operative Procedures.   The child's preparation for the diagnostic tests depends on his or her age and previous experience. Since most of the tests involve x-ray equipment, the child may be familiar with the procedure. By the time most children are late preschoolers, they know that the head and brain are important parts of their bodies. It may be helpful to have them draw their concept of the brain in order to clarify misconceptions and base the explanation on their level of understanding.

Although the temptation is to justify the need for surgery by stating that removing the tumor will take away various symptoms, the nurse should refrain from emphasizing this point too strenuously. Postsurgery headaches and cerebellar symptoms, such as ataxia, may be aggravated rather than improved. Surgery may not improve vision. With optic gliomas the child will be blind in one eye. Finally, surgical removal of the mass may be impossible, and after surgery there may be temporary deterioration of functioning. Being honest before surgery most often makes honesty after the operation easier because no false hopes were created.

However, honesty does not negate instilling hope. A truthful explanation regarding the operation is: "The surgeon will see exactly where the tumor is. If it is small and in one place, it will be removed. If it is large, as much of it as possible will be removed so that some of your symptoms will go away." It is best to deliver information in small amounts and let the child pursue additional answers. For example, some children will ask about what happens when part of the tumor is left in. An honest reply is that after surgery the practitioner will attempt to destroy the remaining tumor with radiation and/or chemotherapy. A further explanation of radiation or chemotherapy should be delayed until a decision regarding these treatments is made.

The hair may be shaved in the operating room just before surgery or in the child's room, usually the night before surgery. When shaving is done with the child awake, the procedure is approached in a sensitive, positive way. If the child's hair is long, it should be braided so that the long swatch can be saved. Showing children how they look at different stages of the process helps them prepare for the final appearance.

Once the hair is clipped very short or shaved, the child can be given a cap or scarf to wear to camouflage the baldness. Every precaution is taken to provide privacy during the procedure and to protect the child from teasing or ridicule by other children before surgery. It is also emphasized that the hair will regrow shortly after surgery. Depending on the child's immediate adjustment to the hair loss, the nurse may introduce the idea of wearing a wig until the hair is grown in, particularly if additional irradiation or chemotherapy is anticipated.

The child is also told about the size of the dressing. Usually the entire scalp is covered to maintain a tight wound closure, even if only a small incision is made. Infratentorial head dressings may be attached to the upper back and extend forward on the neck to maintain slight extension and alignment as a precaution against wound rupture. Applying a similar dressing or "special hat" to a doll is often a less traumatic way of demonstrating the physical appearance.

The child also needs a brief explanation of how he or she will feel after surgery and where he or she will be. Ordinarily children will return to a special intensive care unit, which they should visit beforehand. The child should be aware that he or she may be sleepy for some time after surgery and that a headache is likely, although it should last only a few days.

Parents need similar explanations before surgery, especially in terms of special equipment used in the intensive care unit, dressings, and their child's behavior. For example, they should know that it is not unusual for the child to be comatose or lethargic for a few days after surgery. The nurse may wish to encourage less frequent visiting during this period so that parents can rest and be able to provide support when the child awakens.

The nurse should participate in preoperative conferences with the physician and parents. The nurse needs to know what information the parents have been given in order to be able to give further explanations or emotional support when necessary.

Prevent Postoperative Complications. Usually the surgeon will prescribe specific orders for vital signs, neurologic checks, positioning, fluid regulation, and medication. These vary somewhat, depending on the location of the craniotomy. The following are general principles of care for infratentorial or supratentorial surgery. Additional aspects of care that are discussed elsewhere may include care of the child with seizures and care of the unconscious child in terms of neurologic assessment.

Vital signs are taken as frequently as every 15 to 30 minutes until stable. Temperature measurement is particularly important because of hyperthermia resulting from surgical intervention in the hypothalamus or brainstem and from some types of general anesthesia. To prepare for this reaction, a cooling blanket should be placed on the bed *before* the child returns to the unit so that it is ready for use when needed. The temperature is monitored carefully when any cooling measures are taken because hypothermia can occur suddenly. Recognizing signs of other complications such as increased ICP, meningitis, and respiratory tract infection is imperative.

> **NURSING ALERT**
>
> When temperature is elevated, an infectious process must always be suspected, particularly if the febrile state occurs 1 to 2 days after surgery.

Neurologic checks are an essential aspect of care and include pupillary reaction to light, LOC, sleep patterns, and response to stimuli. Although children may be comatose for a few days, once they regain consciousness, there should be a steady increase in alertness. Regression to a lethargic, irritable state indicates increasing pressure, possibly caused by meningitis or cerebral edema.

> **NURSING ALERT**
>
> Sluggish, dilated, or unequal pupils are reported immediately because they may indicate increased ICP and potential brainstem herniation, a medical emergency.

Observations for function are not instituted until the child regains consciousness. However, as soon as possible the nurse should begin testing reflexes, handgrip, and functioning of the cranial nerves. Muscle strength is usually diminished as a result of general weakness after surgery but should improve daily. Ataxia may be significantly worse with cerebellar intervention, but it will slowly improve. Edema near the cranial nerves may depress important functions such as the gag, blink, or swallowing reflex.

Dressings are observed for evidence of drainage. If soiled, the dressing is not removed but is reinforced with dry sterile gauze. The approximate amount of drainage is estimated and recorded. A drain may be placed in the operative site.

> **NURSING ALERT**
>
> To keep an accurate account of drainage, the soiled area is circled with a pen every hour or so. In this way, continuous bleeding is easily recognized. The presence of colorless drainage is reported immediately, since it most likely is CSF from the incisional area. A foul odor from the dressing may indicate an infection. Such a finding is reported, and a culture is taken.

Once the younger child is alert, the arms may need to be restrained to preserve the dressing. Even a child who has been cooperative before surgery must be closely supervised during the initial stages of regaining consciousness, when disorientation and restlessness are common. Correct positioning after surgery is critical to prevent pressure against the operative site, reduce ICP, and avoid the danger of aspiration. If a large tumor was removed, the child is not placed on the operated side, since the brain may suddenly shift to that cavity, causing trauma to the blood vessels, linings, and the brain itself. The nurse confers with the surgeon to be certain of the correct position, including degree of neck flexion. The first 24 to 48 hours after brain surgery are critical. If the child's position is restricted, notice of this is posted above the head of the bed. When the child is turned, every precaution is used to prevent jarring or malalignment in order to prevent undue strain on the sutures. Two nurses are needed—one supporting the head and the other supporting the body. The use of a turning sheet may facilitate turning a heavy child.

The child with an infratentorial procedure is usually positioned flat and on either side. Pillows should be placed against the child's back, not head, to maintain the desired position. Ordinarily the head and neck are kept in midline with the body and slightly extended. In a supratentorial craniotomy the head is usually elevated above the heart to facilitate CSF drainage and decrease excessive blood flow to the brain to prevent hemorrhage.

> **! NURSING ALERT**
>
> The Trendelenburg position is contraindicated in both infratentorial and supratentorial surgeries because it increases ICP and the risk of hemorrhage. If shock is impending, the practitioner is notified immediately, before the head is lowered.

With an infratentorial craniotomy the child is allowed nothing by mouth for at least 24 hours, or longer if the gag and swallowing reflexes are depressed or the child is comatose. With a supratentorial operation, clear fluids may be resumed soon after the child is alert, sometimes within 24 hours. If the child vomits, oral liquids are stopped. Vomiting not only predisposes to aspiration, but also increases ICP and the potential for incisional rupture.

The child should be fed to conserve energy and minimize movement. If there is any sign of facial paralysis, the child is fed slowly to prevent choking or aspiration. Sometimes gavage feeding is necessary when body functions are too depressed to permit safe oral feedings or when the child refuses to eat or drink. IV fluids are continued until oral fluids are well tolerated. Because of the postoperative cerebral edema and danger of increased ICP, fluids are carefully monitored.

Headache may be severe and is largely a result of cerebral edema. Measures to relieve some of the discomfort include providing a quiet, dimly lit environment; restricting visitors to a minimum; preventing any sudden jarring movement, such as banging into the bed; and preventing an increase in ICP. Avoiding increased ICP is most effectively achieved by proper positioning and prevention of straining, such as during coughing, vomiting, or defecating. The use of opioids, such as morphine, to relieve pain is controversial because it is thought that they may mask signs of altered consciousness or depress respirations. However, they can be given safely, since naloxone can be used to reverse opioid effects, such as sedation or respiratory depression. Acetaminophen and codeine are also effective analgesics for mild to moderate pain. Regardless of the drugs used, adequate dosage and regular administration are essential to providing optimal pain relief. (See also Pain Assessment; Pain Management, Chapter 21.) Placing an ice bag on the forehead may also provide some headache relief, especially if facial edema is severe.

Bowel movements are monitored to prevent constipation. Stool softeners may be given as soon as liquids are tolerated to facilitate easy passage of stool. Saline drops, or artificial tears, may be needed to prevent corneal ulceration if the eyelids do not close completely.

Support Child and Family.
The emotional needs of the family are immense when the diagnosis is a brain tumor, and feelings are influenced by the extent of surgery, any neurologic deficits, the expected prognosis, and additional therapy. Since few definitive answers can be given before surgery, the surgeon's report is a significant finding that can vary from a completely benign, resected neoplasm to a highly malignant, invasive, and only partially removed tumor. Although parents try to prepare themselves for a potentially fatal diagnosis, it is a shock for them.

Ideally, a nurse should be with the parents when the physician visits with them to discuss the expected prognosis and plan of therapy. Although parents may hear only a fraction of what they are told, they can begin to put the future into perspective. While some children will be cured, those with residual tumor may live for several years or die within a relatively short period of time. Regardless of the future prospects, the parents' thinking must be directed toward helping the child recover and resume a normal life to his or her maximal potential.

It is also a time to encourage parents to verbalize their feelings about the diagnosis. Often they express tremendous guilt for attributing the insidious onset of symptoms, such as ataxia, visual difficulty, or headache, to "minor complaints" by the child. Any comments that insinuate that the parents should have sought medical advice sooner are avoided, since such remarks only add to the parents' guilt feelings.

During this period the nurse should also discuss with parents what they plan to tell the child. If the child was prepared honestly, as described previously, the diagnosis can be expressed in a similar manner. During recovery the child will need additional explanation about the treatment, as well as the reason for any residual neurologic effects, such as ataxia or blindness.

Promote Return to Optimal Functioning.
The ultimate goal is a cured child who has maximal functioning. As soon as possible, the child should resume usual activities within tolerable limits, especially returning to school.* Until the skull is completely healed, the child may need to wear a helmet when engaging in any active sport. The school nurse and teacher should confer with the parents to discuss activity restrictions, such as physical education, and the reactions of schoolmates to the child's appearance. Since children often equate brain surgery with "going crazy," it is important to prepare the child for possible remarks to this effect. As one child told a classmate, "It's *your* head they should have fixed, because you're crazy. Can't you see that I'm all better?"

After discharge, the family needs continuing medical and emotional support from health care personnel. Children who are long-term survivors after treatment for a brain tumor may have residual disabilities, such as growth retardation, cranial nerve palsies, sensory defects, motor abnormalities (especially ataxia), intellectual deficits, memory loss, dysphagia, dysgraphia, and behavioral problems. The high frequency of late effects attests to the tremendous need for follow-up care despite successful treatment of the tumor. See Nursing Care Plan: The Child With Cancer, Chapter 26.

---

*Excellent publications are available from the **National Brain Tumor Foundation,** 414 13th Street, Suite 700, Oakland, CA 94712; (800) 934-CURE; fax: (510) 839-9779; website: www.braintumor.org. The pamphlet *When Your Child Is Ready to Return to School* is available from the **American Brain Tumor Association,** 2720 River Road, Des Plaines, IL 60018; (847) 827-9910; fax: (847) 827-9918; website: www.abta.org.

NEUROBLASTOMA

Neuroblastomas are the most common malignant extracranial solid tumors in children, accounting for 8% to 10% of all childhood cancers (Brodeur and Maris, 2002). They occur in about 1 per 10,000 live births, with a slightly higher incidence in males. The majority of children with neuroblastoma present before 10 years of age, with the median age of occurrence at 22 months (Brodeur and Maris, 2002). These tumors originate from embryonic neural crest cells that normally give rise to the adrenal medulla and the sympathetic ganglia. Consequently, the majority of tumors develop in the adrenal gland or the retroperitoneal sympathetic chain. Other sites may be in the head, neck, chest, or pelvis.

Neuroblastoma is a "silent" tumor. In more than 70% of cases, diagnosis is made after metastasis occurs, with the first signs caused by involvement in the nonprimary site, usually the lymph nodes, bone marrow, skeletal system, skin, or liver.

Diagnostic Evaluation

The objective of diagnosis is to locate the primary site and areas of metastasis. The signs and symptoms of neuroblastoma depend on the location and stage of the disease. Most presenting signs are caused by compression of adjacent structures (Box 28-6). Skeletal survey; skull, neck, chest, abdominal, and bone CT scans; and bilateral bone marrow aspirations and biopsies are used to locate a tumor mass and/or metastasis. A metaiodobenzylguanidine (MIBG)

scan is used to determine involvement of bone and/or tissue; however, it is only available at certain centers.

Urinary excretion of catecholamines is detected in approximately 95% of children with adrenal or sympathetic tumors. Analyzing the breakdown products excreted in the urine, namely vanillylmandelic acid (VMA), homovanillic acid (HVA), dopamine, and norepinephrine permits detection of suspected tumor before and after medical/surgical intervention (Kline and Sevier, 2003; Broder and Maris, 2002). Amplification of proto-oncogene, known as the *N-myc* gene, and chromosomal abnormalities correlates strongly with advanced-stage disease, rapid tumor progression, and a poor prognosis (Brodeur and Maris, 2002).

Therapeutic Management

Accurate clinical staging is important for establishing initial treatment. Therefore surgery is used both to remove as much of the tumor as possible and to obtain biopsies. In early stages, complete surgical removal of the tumor is the treatment of choice (Box 28-7). If the tumor is large, partial resection is attempted, with a course of irradiation postoperatively to shrink the tumor in the hope of complete removal at a later date. Surgery is usually limited to biopsy in stages III and IV because of the extensive metastasis, although the use of additional surgery to assess tumor regression or remove a regressed tumor is not unlikely (Box 28-7).

The precise role of radiation therapy is unclear. It does not appear to be of any benefit in children with stage I and II disease. It is commonly used with stage III disease; although it may not improve survival expectancy, it may make a large tumor operable. Radiation therapy provides emergency management of a massive neuroblastoma that is causing spinal cord compression (Kline and Sevier, 2003; Nguyen and others, 2000). Radiation therapy also offers palliation for metastatic lesions in the bones, lung, liver, or brain.

Chemotherapy is the mainstay of therapy for extensive local or disseminated disease. Agents used in various combinations include cyclophosphamide, doxorubicin, cisplatin, etoposide, vincristine, ifosfamide, carboplatin, topotecan, and teniposide. In children with high-risk disease or recurrent disease, retinoic acid, radiation therapy, and myeloablative chemotherapy with peripheral stem cell rescue may be used to

---

BOX 28-6 ■ Clinical Manifestations of Neuroblastoma

ABDOMINAL TUMORS
Firm, nontender, irregular mass
Crosses the midline
Compression of kidney, ureter, or bladder may cause urinary frequency or retention

DISTANT METASTASIS
Ocular:
 Supraorbital ecchymosis
 Periorbital edema
 Proptosis (exophthalmos) from invasion of retrobulbar soft tissue
Lymphadenopathy, especially cervical and supraclavicular
Skeletal: bone pain may or may not be present
Intracranial: neurologic impairment
Thoracic: respiratory obstruction
Spinal cord: varying degrees of paralysis
Adrenal:
 Increased catecholamine excretion
 Flushing
 Hypertension
 Tachycardia
 Diaphoresis

WIDESPREAD METASTASIS
Pallor
Weakness
Irritability
Anorexia
Weight loss

BOX 28-7 ■ Staging System for Neuroblastoma

Stage I: Localized tumor confined to the area of origin; local excision with or without microscopic disease; negative lymph nodes
Stage II: Unilateral tumor with incomplete gross excision; lymph nodes negative
Stage III: Tumor infiltrating across the midline with or without regional lymph node involvement; unilateral tumor with regional involvement; midline tumor with bilateral regional lymph node involvement
Stave IV: Dissemination of tumor to distant lymph nodes, bone, bone marrow, liver, or other organs
Stage IV-S: Localized primary tumor as defined for stage I or II with dissemination limited to liver, skin, or bone marrow but not to bone

obtain a longer remission, even though a poor overall survival rate is seen (Kline and Sevier, 2003; Brodeur and Maris, 2002).

Prognosis.   If all stages are grouped together, the 5-year disease-free survival rates range from 88% to 90% for children in the low-risk stage, and from 22% to 30% in children in the high-risk stage (Brodeur and Maris, 2002). Generally, the younger the child at diagnosis (especially younger than 1 year of age), the better the survival rate. Neuroblastoma is one of the few tumors that demonstrate spontaneous regression (especially stage IV-S), possibly as a result of maturity of the embryonic cell or the development of an active immune system.

Nursing Considerations

Nursing considerations are similar to those discussed for leukemia and brain tumors, including psychologic and physical preparation for diagnostic and operative procedures; prevention of postoperative complications for abdominal, thoracic, or cranial surgery; and explanation of chemotherapy and radiation therapy and their side effects.

Since this tumor carries a poor prognosis for many children, every consideration must be given the family in terms of coping with a life-threatening illness (see Chapter 18). Because of the high degree of metastasis at the time of diagnosis, many parents suffer substantial guilt for not having recognized signs earlier. Parents need much support in dealing with these feelings and expressing them to the appropriate people.

INTRACRANIAL INFECTIONS

The nervous system and its coverings are subject to infection by the same organisms that affect other organs of the body. However, the nervous system is limited in the ways in which it responds to injury. Infectious processes share virtually the same clinical and pathologic features. They differ primarily in the growth and virulence of the specific organism. It is generally difficult to distinguish between the various etiologic agents by looking at clinical manifestations. Laboratory studies are needed to identify the causative agent. The inflammatory process can affect the meninges *(meningitis),* the brain *(encephalitis),* or the spinal cord *(myelitis).*

Meningitis is the most common infection of the CNS. It can be caused by a variety of organisms, but the three main types are the following:

1 **Bacterial,** or pyogenic, caused by pus-forming bacteria, especially the meningococcus, pneumococcus, and *Haemophilus* organisms
2 **Tuberculous,** caused by the tubercle bacillus
3 **Viral,** or aseptic, caused by a wide variety of viral agents

BACTERIAL MENINGITIS

Bacterial meningitis is an acute inflammation of the meninges and the CNS. The advent of antimicrobial therapy has had a marked effect on the course and prognosis of the illness, although the use of conjugate vaccines against *Haemophilus influenzae* type B (Hib vaccine) beginning in 1990 has led to the most dramatic change in the epidemiology of bacterial meningitis (Bonthius and Karacay, 2002; CDC, 2002). In the early 1990s, the incidence of *H. influenzae* decreased from 41 cases per 100,000 children to 3 cases per 100,000 children younger than 5 years of age (CDC, 2002). Today *H. influenzae* type B infection has virtually been eradicated in areas of the world where the vaccine is administered routinely (Bonthius and Karacay, 2002; CDC, 2002). However, bacterial meningitis caused by other organisms remains a serious illness in children. It is significant because of the residual damage caused by undiagnosed and untreated or inadequately treated cases. The majority of reported cases occur in children between 1 month and 5 years of age (Bonthius and Karacay, 2002; Saez-Llorens and McCracken, 2003).

Bacterial meningitis can be caused by any of a variety of bacterial agents. *Streptococcus pneumoniae* (pneumococcal) and *Neisseria meningitidis* (meningococcal) organisms are responsible for bacterial meningitis in 95% of children older than 2 months of age. The leading causes of neonatal meningitis are the group B streptococci and *Escherichia coli* organisms. *E. coli* infection is seldom seen beyond infancy. Meningococcal (epidemic cerebrospinal) meningitis occurs in epidemic form and is the only form readily transmitted to others. It is transmitted by droplet infection from nasopharyngeal secretions. Although it may develop at any age, the risk of meningococcal infection increases with the number of contacts; therefore it occurs predominantly in school-age children and adolescents.

Pathophysiology

Meningitis appears to occur as an extension of a variety of bacterial infections, probably as a result of the lack of acquired resistance to the various causative organisms. The most common route of infection is by vascular dissemination from a focus of infection elsewhere. Organisms also gain entry by direct implantation after penetrating wounds, skull fractures that provide an opening into the skin or sinuses, lumbar puncture or surgical procedures, anatomic abnormalities such as spina bifida, or foreign bodies such as a ventricular shunt. Once implanted, the organisms spread into the CSF, which serves as a conduit for spread of infection throughout the subarachnoid space.

The infective process is that seen in any bacterial infection—inflammation, exudation, white blood cell accumulation, and varying degrees of tissue damage. The brain becomes hyperemic and edematous, and the entire surface of the brain is covered with a layer of purulent exudate. As infection extends to the ventricles, thick pus, fibrin, or adhesions may occlude the narrow passages, obstructing the flow of CSF.

> **! NURSING ALERT**
>
> Any child who is ill and develops a purpuric or petechial rash may have overwhelming meningococcemia and must receive medical attention immediately (Box 28-8).

Diagnostic Evaluation

A lumbar puncture (LP) is the definitive diagnostic test. The fluid pressure is measured, and samples are obtained for culture, Gram stain, blood cell count, and determination of glucose and protein content. The findings are usually diag-

BOX 28-8 ■ Clinical Manifestations of Bacterial Meningitis

CHILDREN AND ADOLESCENTS
Usually abrupt onset
Fever
Chills
Headache
Vomiting
Alterations in sensorium
Seizures (often the initial sign)
Irritability
Agitation
May develop:
   Photophobia
   Delirium
   Hallucinations
   Aggressive behavior
   Drowsiness
   Stupor
   Coma
Nuchal rigidity
   May progress to opisthotonos
Positive Kernig and Brudzinski signs
Hyperactive but variable reflex responses
Signs and symptoms peculiar to individual organisms:
   Petechial or purpuric rashes (meningococcal infection), espe-
     cially when associated with a shocklike state
   Joint involvement (meningococcal and *H. influenzae* infection)
   Chronically draining ear (pneumococcal meningitis)

INFANTS AND YOUNG CHILDREN
Classic picture (above) rarely seen in children between 3 months
   and 2 years of age
Fever
Poor feeding

Vomiting
Marked irritability
Frequent seizures (often accompanied by a high-pitched cry)
Bulging fontanel
Nuchal rigidity may or may not be present
Brudzinski and Kernig signs are not helpful in diagnosis
   Difficult to elicit and evaluate in this age-group
Subdural empyema (*H. influenzae* infection)

NEONATES: SPECIFIC SIGNS
Extremely difficult to diagnose
Manifestations vague and nonspecific
Well at birth but within a few days begins to look and behave
   poorly
Refuses feedings
Poor sucking ability
Vomiting or diarrhea
Poor tone
Lack of movement
Weak cry
Full, tense, and bulging fontanel may appear late in course of ill-
   ness
Neck usually supple

NEONATES: NONSPECIFIC SIGNS THAT MAY BE PRESENT
Hypothermia or fever (depending on the maturity of the infant)
Jaundice
Irritability
Drowsiness
Seizures
Respiratory irregularities or apnea
Cyanosis
Weight loss

nostic. Culture and stain are needed to identify the causative organism. Spinal fluid pressure is usually elevated, but interpretation is often difficult when the child is crying. Sedation with meperidine (Demerol) or fentanyl (Sublimaze) and midazolam (Versed) can alleviate the child's pain and fear associated with this procedure. EMLA, a topical anesthetic cream applied to the skin overlying L3 to L5 an hour before LP, reduces pain for children undergoing this procedure.

There is generally an elevated white blood cell count, predominantly polymorphonuclear leukocytes, but it may be extremely variable. The glucose level is reduced, generally in proportion to the duration and severity of the infection. The protein concentration is usually increased. A blood culture is advisable for all children with suspected meningitis and occasionally proves positive when results of CSF culture are negative. Nose and throat cultures may provide helpful information in some cases.

Therapeutic Management

Acute bacterial meningitis is a medical emergency that requires early recognition and immediate institution of therapy to prevent death and avoid residual disabilities. The initial therapeutic management includes the following:

   ■ Isolation precautions
   ■ Initiation of antimicrobial therapy

   ■ Maintenance of optimal hydration
   ■ Maintenance of ventilation
   ■ Reduction of increased ICP
   ■ Management of bacterial shock
   ■ Control of seizures
   ■ Control of extremes of temperature
   ■ Correction of anemia
   ■ Treatment of complications

The child is isolated from other children, usually in an intensive care unit for close observation. An IV infusion is started to facilitate the administration of antimicrobial agents, fluids, antiepileptic drugs, and blood if needed. The child is placed on a cardiac monitor.

The choice of antibiotic is based on the known sensitivity of the organism. Except under special circumstances, the drugs are administered intravenously throughout the course of treatment. They are given in large doses, and the period of therapy is determined by CSF findings (normal glucose level and negative culture) and the child's clinical condition. Dexamethasone is currently recommended for the treatment of *H. influenzae* type b meningitis to decrease the risk of neurologic sequelae, and it should be considered for use in other types of bacterial meningitis (American Academy of Pediatrics, 2003; Bonthius and Karacay, 2002; El Bashir and others, 2003). It should not be used if aseptic or nonbacterial meningitis is suspected (Bonthius and Karacay, 2002).

Maintaining hydration is a prime concern, and the decision to administer IV fluids and the type and amount of fluid are determined by the patient's condition. Optimal hydration involves correction of any fluid deficits followed by maintenance hydration at minimal levels to prevent cerebral edema. Electrolyte disturbances and cerebral edema are complications associated with poor neurologic outcomes (Bonthius and Karacay, 2002). If indicated, measures are taken to reduce ICP as described previously (p. 1020).

Complications are treated appropriately, such as aspiration of subdural effusion in infants and heparin therapy for children who develop disseminated intravascular coagulation syndrome. If shock occurs, it is managed by restoration of blood volume and maintenance of electrolyte balance. Seizures, which occur in a large number of children, are controlled with anticonvulsants.

Lumbar puncture is carried out as needed to determine the effectiveness of therapy. The patient is evaluated neurologically during the convalescent period and at regular intervals during the succeeding year.

Prognosis.   The age of the child, the type of organism, the severity of the infection, the duration of the illness before the onset of therapy, and the sensitivity of the organism to antimicrobial drugs are important factors in determining the prognosis. Sequelae are most commonly seen when the disease occurs in the first 2 months of life and least often in children with meningococcal meningitis. The residual deficits in infants are primarily a result of communicating hydrocephalus and the greater effects of cerebritis on the immature brain. In older children the residual effects are related to the inflammatory process itself or result from vasculitis associated with the disease. The mortality rate and incidence of poor neurologic outcome are highest in patients with pneumococcal meningitis (Prober, 2004; Saez-Llorens and McCracken, 2003). Evaluation of cranial nerve VIII is needed for at least a 6-month follow-up period to assess for possible hearing loss.

Prevention.   Vaccines are available for types A, C, Y, and W-135 meningococci and *H. influenzae* type b. Routine meningococcal vaccination of children is not recommended. However, routine vaccinations for *H. influenzae* type b are recommended for all children beginning at 2 months of age (see Immunizations, Chapter 10). Pneumococcal conjugate vaccine is also recommended for all children beginning at 2 months of age (American Academy of Pediatrics, 2003; Kaplan, 2002).

Nursing Considerations

Nurses should take necessary precautions to protect themselves and others from possible infection. Parents are taught the proper procedures and supervised in their application.

! NURSING ALERT

A major priority of nursing care of a child with suspected meningitis is to administer the antibiotic as soon as it is ordered. The child is also placed on respiratory isolation for at least 24 hours after implementation of antimicrobial therapy.

The room should be kept as quiet as possible, and environmental stimuli kept at a minimum, because most affected children are sensitive to noise, bright lights, and other external stimuli. Most children are more comfortable without a pillow and with the head of the bed slightly elevated. A side-lying position is more often assumed because of nuchal rigidity. The nurse should avoid actions, such as lifting the child's head, that cause pain or increase discomfort. Measures are taken to ensure safety because children with meningitis are often restless and subject to seizures.

The nursing care of the child with meningitis is determined by the child's symptoms and treatment. Observation of vital signs, neurologic signs, LOC, urine output, and other pertinent data is carried out at frequent intervals. The child who is unconscious is managed as described previously (see p. 1018), and all children are observed carefully for signs of complications just described, especially signs of increased ICP, shock, or respiratory distress. Head circumference is measured on the infant because subdural effusions and obstructive hydrocephalus can develop as a complication of meningitis.

Fluids and nourishment are determined by the child's status. The child with dulled sensorium is usually given nothing by mouth. Other children are allowed clear liquids initially and progressed to a diet suitable for their age. Careful monitoring and recording of intake and output are needed to determine deviations that might indicate impending shock or increasing fluid accumulation, such as cerebral edema or subdural effusion.

One of the problems in nursing care of children with meningitis is maintaining the IV infusion for the length of time needed to provide adequate antimicrobial therapy (usually 10 days). Since continuous IV fluids are usually not necessary, an intermittent infusion device is used. In some cases children who are recovering uneventfully are sent home with the device, and parents are taught IV drug administration.

Family Support.   The sudden onset of the illness makes emotional support of the child and parents extremely important. Parents are very upset and concerned about their child's condition and frequently feel guilty for not having suspected the seriousness of the illness sooner. They need much reassurance that the natural onset of meningitis is sudden and that they acted responsibly in seeking medical assistance when they did. The nurse encourages them to openly discuss their feelings to minimize blame and guilt. They also are kept informed of the child's progress and of all procedures and treatments. In the event that the child's condition worsens, they need the same psychologic care as parents facing the possible death of their child (see Chapter 18; see also Family Focus box).

NONBACTERIAL (ASEPTIC) MENINGITIS

Aseptic meningitis is caused by a number of agents, principally viruses, and is frequently associated with other diseases, such as measles, mumps, herpes, and leukemia. Enteroviruses and mumps viruses account for a large number of cases.

The onset may be abrupt or gradual. The initial manifestations are headache, fever, malaise, gastrointestinal symptoms, and signs of meningeal irritation that develop a day or

FAMILY FOCUS

Preventing Bacterial Meningitis

With immunization schedules calling for administration of Hib vaccine and pneumococcal conjugate vaccine to infants at 2 months of age, parents should be encouraged to bring their child to a health facility so that the full series of inoculations is completed. With the 10% to 15% mortality rate associated with bacterial meningitis, early immunization can prevent families from experiencing the tragic death of a child. Nurses play a significant role in educating families regarding preventive measures, such as early vaccination.

BOX 28-9 ■ Clinical Manifestations of Encephalitis

ONSET: SUDDEN OR GRADUAL	SEVERE CASES
Malaise	High fever
Fever	Stupor
Headache	Seizures
Dizziness	Disorientation
Apathy	Spasticity
Lethargy	Coma (may proceed to death)
Neck stiffness	Ocular palsies
Nausea and vomiting	Paralysis
Ataxia	
Tremors	
Hyperactivity	
Speech difficulties: mutism	
Altered mental status	

two after the onset of illness. Abdominal pain and nausea and vomiting are common; back and leg pain, sore throat, chest pain, photophobia, and generalized muscular aches or pains are found occasionally. A maculopapular rash may be present. These symptoms usually subside spontaneously and rapidly, and the child is well in 3 to 10 days, with no residual effects.

Diagnosis is based on clinical features and CSF findings, which include increased lymphocytes, predominantly mononuclear cells. It is important to differentiate this self-limited disorder from the more serious form of meningitis and to diagnose and treat any disease of which it is a manifestation.

Treatment is primarily symptomatic, such as acetaminophen for headache and muscle pain and positioning for comfort. Antimicrobial agents may be administered and isolation enforced until a definitive diagnosis is made as a precaution against the possibility that the disease might be of bacterial origin.

Nursing care is similar to nursing care of the child with bacterial meningitis.

ENCEPHALITIS

Encephalitis is an inflammatory process of the CNS that produces altered function of various portions of the brain and spinal cord. Encephalitis can be caused by a variety of organisms, including bacteria, spirochetes, fungi, protozoa, helminths, and viruses. Most infections are associated with viruses, and this discussion is limited to these etiologic agents.

Etiology

Encephalitis can occur as a result of either direct invasion of the CNS by a virus or postinfectious involvement of the CNS after a viral disease. Often the specific type of encephalitis in a particular child may not be identified for some time or at all. The majority of cases of known etiology are associated with childhood viral diseases. Most other viral infections are those involved with arthropod vectors and those associated with hemorrhagic fevers. The vector reservoirs for most agents pathogenic for humans and detected in the United States are mosquitos and ticks; therefore most cases of encephalitis appear during the hot summer months.

Herpes simplex encephalitis is an uncommon disease, but 30% of cases involve children. The initial clinical findings are nonspecific (fever, altered mental status), but most cases evolve to demonstrate focal neurologic signs and symptoms. Children may experience focal seizures. The CSF is abnor-mal in most cases. Because of a rise in the number of children with herpes simplex virus encephalitis, suspected cases require prompt attention, especially since the diagnosis can be difficult. The clinical diagnosis can be confirmed by the rapid appearance of IgM antibody to herpes simplex virus type 1 in CSF and serum. The early use of IV acyclovir reduces mortality and morbidity.

Diagnostic Evaluation

The clinical features are similar, regardless of the agent involved. Manifestations can range from a mild, benign form that resembles aseptic meningitis, lasts a few days, and is followed by rapid and complete recovery, to a fulminating encephalitis with severe CNS involvement (Box 28-9).

The diagnosis is made on the basis of clinical findings, circumstances associated with the disease, and (when possible) identification of the specific virus. Arboviruses are rarely detected in the blood or spinal fluid, but viruses of herpes, mumps, measles, and enteroviruses may be found in CSF. Serologic diagnosis may be reached by means of a variety of antibody tests. The first blood for testing should be drawn as soon after onset as possible, with the second 2 or 3 weeks later. Laboratory detection of herpes simplex virus DNA in CSF may be used to expedite diagnosis of herpes simplex encephalitis.

Therapeutic Management

Patients with suspected encephalitis are hospitalized promptly for skilled nursing care and observation. Treatment is primarily supportive, including conscientious nursing care, control of cerebral manifestations, and adequate nutrition and hydration, with observations and management as for other disorders involving cerebral injury. Follow-up care with periodic reevaluation and rehabilitation are important requisites to survivors with residual effects of the disease.

Prognosis. The prognosis for the child afflicted with encephalitis depends on the child's age, the type of organism, and residual neurologic damage. Very young children (younger than 2 years of age) may exhibit increased neurologic disability, including learning difficulties and seizure disorders.

Nursing Considerations

Nursing care of the child with encephalitis is the same as for any unconscious child and the child with meningitis. Neurologic monitoring, administration of medications, and support of the child and parents are the major aspects of care.

REYE SYNDROME

Reye syndrome (RS) is a disorder defined as toxic encephalopathy associated with other characteristic organ involvement. It is characterized by fever, profoundly impaired consciousness, and disordered hepatic function.

The etiology of the disorder is obscure, but most cases of RS follow a common viral illness, most frequently influenza or varicella. The potential association between aspirin therapy for the treatment of fever in children with varicella or influenza and the development of RS precludes its use in these patients (Bhutta and others, 2003; McGovern and others, 2001).

Pathophysiology

RS has been defined by the Centers for Disease Control and Prevention (CDC) as an acute noninflammatory encephalopathy and hepatopathy, with no reasonable explanation for the cerebral and hepatic abnormalities. The pathology of RS is a mitochondrial insult induced by different viruses, drugs, exogenous toxins, and genetic factors.

Diagnostic Evaluation

Elevated ammonia levels tend to correlate with the clinical manifestations and prognosis. Definitive diagnosis is established by liver biopsy (Box 28-10). Children who in the past would have been diagnosed with RS are now given other diagnoses, such as metabolic disorders, as a result of improved diagnostic techniques.

Therapeutic Management

The most important aspect of successful management of the child with RS is early diagnosis and aggressive therapy. Rapid progression through coma stages and high peak ammonia concentrations are associated with a more serious prognosis. Cerebral edema with increased ICP represents the most immediate threat to life. Recovery from RS is rapid and usually without sequelae if diagnosis is determined early and implementation of therapy is prompt.

Prognosis. Although the incidence of Reye syndrome has markedly decreased, health professionals must remind parents and caregivers to avoid using both aspirin and non-aspirin–containing salicylates during febrile illnesses in children (Bhutta and others, 2003; Kamienski, 2003). Survivors may have subtle neuropsychologic deficits. Generally, recovery is good given the gravity of the disease (Bhutta and others, 2003; Kamienski, 2003).

Nursing Considerations

The child who is acutely ill with RS requires continuous and intensive nursing care. In addition to appraising vital functions and neurologic status, the nurse assists with a lumbar puncture, obtains blood for laboratory examination, and inserts various IV lines such as peripheral, arterial, and central venous pressure. A retention catheter and a nasogastric tube are inserted, and when respirations are compromised, an

---

BOX 28-10 ■ Staging Criteria for Reye Syndrome

Stage I: Vomiting, lethargy, and drowsiness; liver dysfunction; type I electroencephalogram (EEG); follows commands; pupillary reaction brisk

Stage II: Disorientation, combativeness, delirium, hyperventilation, hyperactive reflexes, appropriate responses to painful stimuli; evidence of liver dysfunction; type I EEG; pupillary reaction sluggish

Stage III: Obtunded, coma, hyperventilation, decorticate rigidity, preservation of pupillary light reaction and oculovestibular reflexes (although sluggish); type II EEG

Stage IV: Deepening coma, decerebrate rigidity, loss of oculocephalic reflexes, large and fixed pupils, loss of doll's eye reflex, loss of corneal reflexes; minimal liver dysfunction; type III or IV EEG; evidence of brainstem dysfunction

Stage V: Seizures, loss of deep tendon reflexes, respiratory arrest, flaccidity; type IV EEG; usually no evidence of liver dysfunction

---

endotracheal tube is inserted and attached to a ventilator for controlled respirations.

Care and observations are implemented as for any child with an altered state of consciousness (p. 1013) and increasing ICP. Accurate and frequent monitoring of intake and output is essential for adjusting fluid volumes to prevent both dehydration and cerebral edema. The child who is paralyzed and in a drug-induced coma is totally dependent on the caregivers, and meticulous vigilance and attention to all biologic needs are mandatory. Since hypovolemic shock is a constant danger in children with controlled fluid intake and osmotic diuresis, vital signs, including central venous pressure and/or cardiac output (Swan-Ganz catheter), are monitored frequently. Because of related liver dysfunction, the nurse must observe for signs of impaired coagulation such as prolonged bleeding time.

Family Support. Parents of children with RS need a great deal of emotional support. They are usually frightened by the child's appearance, the treatment, and the life-threatening severity and suddenness of the illness. Their distress is increased if they believe that their actions may have contributed to a delay in diagnosis. They need to be kept informed regarding the child's progress, to have diagnostic procedures and therapeutic management explained, and to be given concerned and sympathetic support.

The **National Reye's Syndrome Foundation*** was established by the parents of a child who died of this disease in hope of encouraging research on the disease and of educating parents and health professionals.

HUMAN IMMUNODEFICIENCY VIRUS ENCEPHALOPATHY

Children with human immunodeficiency virus (HIV) encephalopathy, a complication of acquired immunodeficiency syndrome (AIDS), present a nursing challenge. Progressive encephalopathy has been greatly reduced in infants and children as a result of a dramatic decrease in perinatal HIV transmission and the availability of combination antiretroviral therapy (American Academy of Pediatrics, 2003).

---

*PO Box 829; Bryan, OH 43506-0829; (800) 233-7397; fax: (419) 636-9897; website: www.reyessyndrome.org.

Neurologic manifestations in children suggest that the progressive encephalopathy is a result of primary and persistent infection of the brain with the virus. Unexplained neurodevelopmental regression and focal seizures are the dominant clinical features of the disorder. Others include progressive motor dysfunction and atypical CNS infections. These manifestations indicate a poor prognosis and, almost invariably, a fatal outcome. However, earlier implementation of therapies for AIDS may allow for slower progression of these neurologic complications.

Appropriate precautions are practiced by nurses when caring for these children. Careful handling of the child is a hallmark of excellent nursing, since these children may experience pain, isolation, social stigma, susceptibility to infection, and abandonment resulting in less than minimum sensorimotor stimulation. Nursing assessment and intervention warrant planning time to meet developmental needs, especially if it means holding, rocking, and comforting the child. Pain management is essential and may require use of several drugs to effectively treat the neuropathic pain (see Pain Assessment and Pain Management, Chapter 21). (See Chapter 26 for a more extensive discussion of AIDS.)

RABIES

Rabies is an acute infection of the nervous system caused by a virus that is almost invariably fatal if left untreated. It is transmitted to humans by the saliva of an infected mammal introduced through a bite or skin abrasion. After entry into a new host, the virus multiplies in muscle cells and is spread through neural pathways without stimulating a protective host immune response.

Approximately 88% of rabies cases come from wild animals, and 12% from domestic animals. Emergency departments across the country have observed that the majority of dog bites occurring in children were found to be provoked (Brady, 2000). The risk of infection from a dog bite is 5%, compared to a 20% to 50% risk of infection from a cat bite (Avner, 1999). Cats are now the most common domestic animals and should be the target of rabies vaccination programs. Carnivorous wild animals (especially raccoons, skunks, and foxes) and bats are the animals most often infected with rabies and the cause of most indigenous cases of human rabies in the United States (CDC, 2001). The likelihood of human exposure to a rabid domestic animal has decreased greatly. The circumstances of a biting incident are important. An unprovoked attack is more likely to indicate a rabid animal than a provoked attack. Bites inflicted on a child attempting to feed or handle an apparently healthy animal can generally be regarded as provoked. Any child bitten by a wild animal is assumed to be exposed to rabies.

NURSING ALERT

Unusual behavior in an animal is cause for suspicion; children should be warned to beware of wild animals that appear friendly.

The disease is uncommon in humans, but the highest incidence occurs in children younger than 15 years of age. The incubation period usually ranges from 1 to 3 months but may be as short as 10 days or as long as 8 months. Only 10% to 15% of persons bitten develop the disease, but once

symptoms are present, rabies progresses inexorably to a fatal outcome. Diagnosis is made on the basis of the history and clinical features (Box 28-11). Although treatment is of little avail once symptoms appear, the long incubation period allows time for induction of active and passive immunity before the onset of illness.

Therapeutic Management

Two types of immunizing products are available for use in humans: the *inactivated rabies vaccines,* which induce an active immune response; and the *globulins,* which contain preformed antibodies. The two types of products should be used concurrently for postexposure rabies treatment when prophylaxis is indicated.

The current therapy for a rabid animal bite consists of thorough cleansing of the wound and passive immunization with *human rabies immune globulin (HRIG)* as soon as possible after exposure. A tetanus shot should be administered and antibiotics given if indicated (CDC, 1999; Molf, 2002).

Postexposure active immunity is conferred by administration of the *human diploid cell rabies vaccine (HDCV).* The first dose of the vaccine is given at the same time as the immune globulin and followed by intramuscular injections on days 3, 7, 14, and 28 after the first dose (Molf, 2002). An additional dose in 90 days is recommended by the World Health Organization. Before antirabies prophylaxis is initiated, the local or state health department is consulted.

Nursing Considerations

Both parents and children are frightened by the urgency and seriousness of the situation. They need anticipatory guidance for the therapy and support and reassurance regarding the efficacy of the preventive measures for this dreaded disease. Animal bites require treatment in an emergency department to allow for wound care and rabies prophylaxis. Prevention strategies for young children include close supervision of interactions between children and animals (Bernardo and others, 2002). Certain circumstances may warrant vaccination, such as when a child is being taken

BOX 28-11 ■ Clinical Manifestations of Rabies

INITIAL SIGNS
General malaise
Fever
Sore throat

EXCITEMENT PHASE
Hypersensitivity
Increased reaction to external stimuli
Seizures
Maniacal behavior
Choking

SEVERE SPASM OF RESPIRATORY MUSCLES*
Apnea
Cyanosis
Anoxia

---

*From attempts at swallowing (characteristics from which the term *hydrophobia* was derived).

to an area of the world where rabies in stray dogs is still a problem.

SEIZURE DISORDERS

Seizures are caused by malfunctions of the brain's electrical system that result from cortical neuronal discharge. The manifestations of seizures are determined by the site of origin and may include unconsciousness or altered consciousness; involuntary movements; and changes in perception, behaviors, sensations, and posture. Seizures are the most commonly observed neurologic dysfunction in children and can occur with a wide variety of conditions involving the CNS.

EPILEPSY

Seizures result from paroxysmal discharges in cortical neurons and are symptoms of abnormal brain function. They are considered to be a symptom of an underlying disease process. Once it is determined that the child has had a seizure, it is important to distinguish whether the episode was an epileptic or a non-epileptic seizure. Seizures are the indispensable characteristic of epilepsy; however, not every seizure is epileptic. Epilepsy is a chronic seizure disorder with recurrent and unprovoked seizures.

Etiology

Seizure disorders have numerous and varied causes (e.g., tumors, infections, neoplasms). Most seizures are *idiopathic*. Although the cause of idiopathic epilepsy is unknown, genetic factors may in some way alter the seizure threshold to influence neuronal discharge. A seizure disorder also can be *acquired* as a result of brain injury during prenatal, perinatal, or postnatal periods. This injury may be caused by trauma, hypoxia, infections, exogenous or endogenous toxins, and a variety of other factors. Biochemical events (e.g., hypoglycemia, hypocalcemia, and certain nutritional deficiencies) produce seizure activity.

The incidence of causative factors associated with childhood seizures is frequently related to the age of the child. Seizures are more common during the first 2 years of life than during any other period of childhood. In very young infants the most frequent causes are birth injuries—such as intracranial trauma, hemorrhage, or anoxia—and congenital defects of the brain. Acute infections are a frequent cause of seizures in late infancy and early childhood but become an infrequent cause in middle childhood. In children older than 3 years of age the most common factor is idiopathic epilepsy.

Seizure activity is believed to be caused by spontaneous electric discharge initiated by a group of hyperexcitable cells referred to as the *epileptogenic focus.* These cells display increased electric excitability in response to any of a variety of physiologic stimuli, such as cellular dehydration, abnormal blood glucose levels, electrolyte imbalance, fatigue, emotional stress, and endocrine changes. When neuronal excitation from the epileptogenic focus spreads to the brainstem, a generalized seizure develops. Seizures are designated as *focal (localized), focal with rapid generalization,* and *generalized,* on the basis of the characteristic neuronal discharges. In a large proportion of children focal seizures

spread to other areas, ultimately becoming generalized with loss of consciousness.

Classification

There are many different types of epileptic seizures, and each has unique characteristics. The onset of a seizure is abrupt, paroxysmal, and transitory, and signs are highly variable. The current classification system divides seizures into two major categories: partial and generalized (Box 28-12). Some of these are described in the following section.

Partial seizures are caused by abnormal electric discharges from epileptogenic foci limited to a more-or-less circumscribed region of the cerebral cortex. Focal seizures may arise from any area of the cerebral cortex, but the frontal, temporal, and parietal lobes are the ones that are most often affected. The area of cerebral involvement is reflected by clinical manifestations. Partial seizures are subdivided into three types. *Simple partial seizures* have elementary or simple symptoms and are accompanied by no alteration of consciousness (also called an *aura*). *Complex partial seizures* involve complex symptoms and impairment of consciousness. These seizures may begin with an *aura,* a simple partial seizure that is usually a sensation or sensory phenomenon that reflects the complicated connections and integrative functions of that area of the brain. The aura is part of the seizure event and is associated with electroencephalogram (EEG) changes (Johnston, 2004; Shafer, 1999). *Simple* or *complex seizures secondarily generalized* develop into generalized seizures, usually a tonic-clonic event.

Generalized seizures without a focal onset appear to arise in the reticular formation, and the clinical observations indicate that the initial involvement is from both hemispheres. Frequently loss of consciousness occurs and is the initial clinical manifestation. Unlike partial seizures that become generalized, there is no aura. Episodes occur at any time, day or night, and the interval between episodes may be minutes, hours, weeks, or even years. Most affected persons first experience seizures in childhood, and children whose seizures begin before age 4 years have mental retardation and behavioral and learning problems more frequently than those whose seizures begin after age 4.

Diagnostic Evaluation

Establishing a diagnosis is critical. The process of diagnosis in a child with a seizure disorder has two major foci: (1) to ascertain the type of seizure the child has experienced and (2) to attempt to understand the cause of the events. The assessment and diagnosis rely heavily on a thorough history, skilled observation, and use of several diagnostic tests.

During the assessment process it is unusual to observe the child having a seizure; therefore, a complete, accurate, and detailed history should be obtained from a reliable and knowledgeable informant. This history involves prenatal, perinatal, and neonatal periods, including any instances of infection, apnea, colic, or poor feeding, and information regarding any previous accidents or serious illnesses.

Another treatment for refractory seizures is the use of the *ketogenic diet,* which severely restricts carbohydrate and protein intake and uses fat as the primary fuel to produce ketosis. A recent review of the effects of the diet supports

BOX 28-12 ■ Classification and Clinical Manifestations of Seizures

PARTIAL SEIZURES

Simple Partial Seizures With Motor Signs

Characterized by:

Localized motor symptoms

Somatosensory, psychic, autonomic symptoms

Combination of these

Abnormal discharges remain unilateral

Manifestations:

Aversive seizure (most common motor seizure in children)

Eye or eyes and head turn away from the side of the focus

Awareness of movement or loss of consciousness

Rolandic (Sylvan) seizure

Tonic-clonic movements involving the face

Salivation

Arrested speech

Most common during sleep

Jacksonian march (rare in children)

Orderly, sequential progression of clonic movements beginning in a foot, hand, or face and moving or "marching" to adjacent body parts

Simple Partial Seizures With Sensory Signs

Characterized by various sensations, including:

Numbness, tingling, prickling, paresthesia, or pain originating in one area (e.g., face or extremities) and spreading to other parts of the body

Visual sensations or formed images

Motor phenomena such as posturing or hypertonia

Uncommon in children younger than 8 years of age

Complex Partial Seizures (Psychomotor Seizures)

Observed more often in children from 3 years through adolescence

Characterized by:

Period of altered behavior

Amnesia for event (no recollection of behavior)

Inability to respond to environment

Impaired consciousness during event

Drowsiness or sleep usually follows seizure

Confusion and amnesia may be prolonged

Complex sensory phenomena (aura)

Most frequent sensation—strange feeling in the pit of the stomach that rises toward the throat

Often accompanied by:

Odd or unpleasant odors or tastes

Complex auditory or visual hallucinations

Ill-defined feelings of elation or strangeness (e.g., déjà vu, a feeling of familiarity in a strange environment)

May be strong feelings of fear and anxiety, distorted sense of time and self

Small children may emit a cry or attempt to run for help

Patterns of motor behavior:

Stereotypic

Similar with each subsequent seizure

May suddenly cease activity, appear dazed, stare into space, become confused and apathetic, and become limp or stiff or display some form of posturing

May be confused

May perform purposeless, complicated activities in a repetitive manner (automatisms), such as walking, running, kicking, laughing, or speaking incoherently, most often followed by postictal confusion or sleep; may be oropharyngeal activities, such as smacking, chewing, drooling, swallowing, and nausea or abdominal pain followed by stiffness, a fall, and postictal sleep; rarely manifests as rage or temper tantrums; aggressive acts uncommon during seizure

GENERALIZED SEIZURES

Tonic-Clonic Seizures (Formerly Known as *Grand Mal*)

Most common and most dramatic of all seizure manifestations

Occur without warning

Tonic phase: lasts approximately 10 to 20 seconds

Manifestations:

Eyes roll upward

Immediate loss of consciousness

If standing, falls to floor or ground

Stiffens in generalized, symmetric tonic contraction of entire body musculature

Arms usually flexed

Legs, head, and neck extended

May utter a peculiar piercing cry

Apneic, may become cyanotic

Increased salivation and loss of swallowing reflex

Clonic phase: lasts about 30 seconds but can vary from only a few seconds to a half hour or longer

Manifestations:

Violent jerking movements as the trunk and extremities undergo rhythmic contraction and relaxation

May foam at the mouth

May be incontinent of urine and feces

As event ends, movements become less intense, occur at longer intervals, then cease entirely

Status epilepticus: series of seizures at intervals too brief to allow the child to regain consciousness between the time one event ends and the next begins

Requires emergency intervention

Can lead to exhaustion, respiratory failure, and death

Postictal state:

Appears to relax

May remain semiconscious and difficult to arouse

May awaken in a few minutes

Remains confused for several hours

Poor coordination

Mild impairment of fine motor movements

May have visual and speech difficulties

May vomit or complain of severe headache

When left alone, usually sleeps for several hours

On awakening is fully conscious

Usually feels tired and complains of sore muscles and headache

No recollection of entire event

Absence Seizures (Formerly Called *Petit Mal* or *Lapses*)

Characterized by:

Onset usually between 4 and 12 years of age

More common in girls than in boys

Usually cease at puberty

Brief loss of consciousness

Minimal or no alteration in muscle tone

May go unrecognized because of little change in child's behavior

Abrupt onset; suddenly develops 20 or more attacks daily

BOX 28-12 ■ Classification and Clinical Manifestations of Seizures—cont'd

Event often mistaken for inattentiveness or daydreaming

Events can be precipitated by hyperventilation, hypoglycemia, stresses (emotional and physiologic), fatigue, or sleeplessness

Manifestations:

Brief loss of consciousness

Appear without warning or aura

Usually last about 5 to 10 seconds

Slight loss of muscle tone may cause child to drop objects

Able to maintain postural control; seldom falls

Minor movements such as lip smacking, twitching of eyelids or face, or slight hand movements

Not accompanied by incontinence

Amnesia for episode

May need to reorient self to previous activity

Atonic and Akinetic Seizures (Also Known As *Drop Attacks*)

Characterized by:

Onset usually between 2 and 5 years of age

Sudden, momentary loss of muscle tone and postural control

Events recur frequently during the day, particularly in the morning hours and shortly after awakening

Manifestations:

Loss of tone causes child to fall to the floor violently

Unable to break fall by putting out hand

May incur a serious injury to the face, head, or shoulder

Loss of consciousness only momentary

Myoclonic Seizures

A variety of seizure episodes

May be isolated as benign essential myoclonus

May occur in association with other seizure forms

Characterized by:

Sudden, brief contractures of a muscle or group of muscles

Occur singly or repetitively

No postictal state

May or may not be symmetric

May or may not include loss of consciousness

Infantile Spasms

Also called *infantile myoclonus, massive spasms, hypsarrhythmia, salaam episodes,* or *infantile myoclonic spasms*

Most commonly occur during the first 6 to 8 months of life

Twice as common in males as in females

Child may have numerous seizures during the day without postictal drowsiness or sleep

Outlook for normal intelligence is poor

Manifestations:

Possible series of sudden, brief, symmetric, muscular contractions

Head flexed, arms extended, and legs drawn up

Eyes may roll upward or inward

May be preceded or followed by a cry or giggling

May or may not include loss of consciousness

Sometimes flushing, pallor, or cyanosis

Infants who are able to sit but not stand:

Sudden dropping forward of the head and neck with trunk flexed forward and knees drawn up—the "salaam" or "jack-knife" seizure

Less often: alternate clinical forms observed

Extensor spasms rather than flexion of arms, legs, and trunk, and head nodding

Lightning events involving a single, momentary, shocklike contraction of the entire body

---

that some children have reduced seizures during treatment, but the long-term effects, such as increased blood lipid levels, are not known (Lefevre and Aronson, 2000).

History of the seizure(s) should be equally detailed, including the type of seizure or description of the child's behavior during the event(s), the age at onset, and the time at which the seizure occurs (e.g., early morning, before meals, while awake, or during sleep). Any factors that may have precipitated the seizure are important, including fever, infection, falls that may have caused trauma to the head, anxiety, fatigue, activity (e.g., hyperventilation), and environmental events (exposure to strong stimuli such as bright, flashing lights or loud noises). If the child can describe any sensory phenomena, these are recorded. The duration and progression of the seizure (if any) and the *postictal* (period after the seizure) feelings and behavior, such as confusion, inability to speak, amnesia, headache, and sleep, are recorded. The ability to identify seizure types accurately has resulted from the technologic advances in video recording and long-term EEG monitoring.

A complete physical and neurologic examination, including developmental assessment of language, learning, behavior, and motor abilities, often provides clues to neurologic disturbances. A family history can offer clues to paroxysmal disorders such as migraine, breath-holding spells, febrile seizures, or neurologic diseases that may be related to the seizure disorder.

Laboratory studies that may prove to be of value include a complete blood cell count and white blood cell count (for signs of infection). Blood and CSF glucose may give evidence of hypoglycemic episodes or infection, and serum electrolytes, blood urea nitrogen, calcium, and other blood studies might indicate metabolic disturbances. Lumbar puncture can confirm a suspected diagnosis of cerebrospinal infection.

Skull radiographs, CT scans, and other studies help to identify skull abnormalities, separation of sutures, and intracranial calcifications. Focal seizures in children younger than 1 year of age are indications for MRI to rule out a supratentorial tumor. An EEG is obtained for all children with seizure activity and is the most useful tool for evaluating seizure disorders. The EEG is carried out under varying conditions—with the child asleep, awake, awake with provocative stimulation (flashing lights, noise), and hyperventilating. Stimulation elicits abnormal electrical activity, which is recorded on the EEG.

Variations of the EEG are video recordings and simultaneous polygraphs of the patient during waking and/or sleeping. These techniques can be used concurrently and are especially valuable in differentiating epileptic activity from paroxysmal behavior or non-epileptic motor events.

Therapeutic Management

The objectives of treatment of seizure disorders are to (1) control the seizures or reduce their frequency, (2) discover and correct the cause when possible, and (3) help the child who has recurrent seizures to live as normal a life as possible. Seizures of a recurrent nature are treated as soon as the diagnosis is established. If the seizure activity is a manifestation of an infectious, traumatic, or metabolic process, the seizure therapy is instituted as a part of the general therapeutic regimen. Seizure control is considered to prevent secondary brain cell injury from the neuronal discharge and hypoxia.

It is known that persons predisposed to epilepsy have seizures when their basal level of neuronal excitability exceeds a critical point or threshold; no event occurs if the excitability is maintained below this threshold. The administration of antiepileptic drugs serves to raise this threshold and prevent seizures. Consequently, the primary therapy for seizure disorders is the administration of the appropriate antiepileptic drug or combination of drugs in a dosage that provides the desired effect without causing undesirable side effects or toxic reactions.

Numerous drugs are available for control of seizures. The primary drugs prescribed for partial seizures and/or generalized tonic-clonic seizures are carbamazepine (Tegretol), phenytoin (Dilantin), fosphenytoin (Cerebyx), and valproic acid (Depakote or Depakene). The drug of choice for absence seizures is ethosuximide (Zarontin) and valproic acid. The dosage is determined by monitoring serum drug levels. Complete control can be achieved in only 50% to 75% of affected children, however, even with careful attention to details of therapy.

There is increasing evidence that diminishing polypharmacy can bring about a better quality of life; therefore single-drug therapy is recommended. Several new drugs have also increased seizure control for many children. These include gabapentin (Neurontin), lamotrigine (Lamictal), and Felbamate (Felbatol). The use of Felbamate is controversial because of the side effects of aplastic anemia or hepatic failure.

Once seizures are controlled, the drug or drugs are continued for a prolonged time. However, periodic reevaluation of the drug is important to assess the continued effectiveness and to alter the dosage if indicated. The dosage will need to be increased as the child grows.

Withdrawal of antiepileptic therapy follows a predesigned protocol, usually begun when the child has been seizure free for at least 2 years with a normal EEG. Recurrence is most likely within the first year after discontinuance of the medication. When a medication is discontinued, the dosage should be reduced gradually over 1 to 2 weeks. Sudden withdrawal of a drug can cause an increase in the number and severity of seizures, often precipitating status epilepticus. If the time for reducing the medication coincides with puberty or, in younger children, occurs during periods when the child is subject to frequent infections, the drug is continued for a longer period. Repeat EEGs are generally obtained every 6 months to 2 years.

When seizure activity is determined to be caused by a hematoma, tumor, or other progressive cerebral lesion, surgical removal is the treatment. Surgery also may be indicated for those who suffer from repetitive, incapacitating seizures that are caused by a focal brain abnormality, if removal of the lesion does not result in significant loss of vital functions, such as speech and movement. The risks of brain surgery cannot be underestimated. Also, the costs of surgical interventions must be taken into consideration, as well as the numerous tests necessary to assess the child before surgery.

Status Epilepticus. Status epilepticus is a continuous seizure that lasts more than 30 minutes or a series of seizures from which the child does not regain a premorbid level of consciousness. The initial treatment is directed toward support and maintenance of vital functions, including maintaining an adequate airway, administration of oxygen, and hydration, followed by IV administration of either diazepam (Valium) or phenobarbital. Rectal diazepam is a simple, effective, and safe treatment for prehospital management (Lee and others, 2002; Mitchell and others, 1999). Lorazepam (Ativan) may be replacing IV diazepam as the drug of choice. It has a longer duration of action and causes less respiratory distress in children older than 2 years of age.

> **NURSING ALERT**
>
> Fosphenytoin (Cerebyx) is often used to treat seizures instead of IV phenytoin because of possible complications and drug interactions associated with IV phenytoin. If IV phenytoin is used, it should be administered via slow IV push and at a rate that does not exceed 50 mg/min. Because phenytoin precipitates when mixed with glucose, only normal saline is used to flush the tubing or catheter. Fosphenytoin may be given in saline or glucose solutions at a rate of up to 150 mg PE (phenytoin equivalent)/min, and it may be given intramuscularly if necessary.

The child must be closely monitored during administration to detect early alterations in vital signs that may indicate impending cardiac arrest or respiratory depression. When diazepam is ineffective, phenobarbital, often in extremely high levels that may require respiratory support, is given intravenously as the initial medication. Patients who do not respond to drug therapy may require the use of IV lidocaine, general anesthesia, or a potent skeletal muscle relaxant such as curare. This should be administered by an anesthesiologist.

> **NURSING ALERT**
>
> Status epilepticus is a medical emergency requiring immediate intervention to prevent permanent injury to the brain, respiratory failure, and death.

Prognosis. The course and prognosis for children with seizures depend on the etiology, type of seizure, age at onset, and family and medical histories. At diagnosis the best predictors of long-term remission were children with idiopathic syndromes, younger than 9 years of age at onset, and no prior neonatal seizures before treatment (Berg and others, 2001).

Risk factors associated with recurrence of epilepsy include the following:

1 Adolescent age and older
2 Family history of epilepsy

3 Frequent seizures on antiepileptic medication

4 Multiple antiepileptic therapy (polytherapy)

5 Abnormal EEG

6 Seizures that result from past injury or insult (Berg and others, 2001).

The prognosis following treatment for status epilepticus is more favorable than previously reported. The majority of children will probably have no intellectual impairment. The highest morbidity is found in patients with a non-idiopathic, non-febrile cause, compared to children with idiopathic or febrile status epilepticus who have a more favorable outcome (Johnston, 2004; Barnard and Wirrell, 1999).

Nursing Considerations

An important nursing function during a seizure is observing the seizure and describing its pertinent features. Any alterations in behavior and characteristics of the seizure, such as sensory-hallucinatory phenomena (e.g., an aura), motor effects (e.g., eye movements, muscular contractions, laterality, and complex activities), alterations in consciousness, and postictal state, are noted and recorded (Box 28-13).

Generalized seizures and others with dramatic manifestations are easily detected, but absence seizures may be more difficult to detect. They are easily misinterpreted as inattention. Any unusual behavior, even seemingly inconsequential behavior such as a momentary interruption of activity, staring, or mental blankness, should be described. The more detailed these descriptions, the more valuable they are for assessment. The nurse notes the time that the seizure began and the duration of the seizure.

History taking is a vital tool for helping to identify factors that are significant in establishing a cause of the seizures. Interviewing the child and family helps to elicit problems related to the psychologic impact of the disorder on their lives.

The child must be protected from injury during the seizure (see Emergency Treatment box). It is impossible to halt a seizure once it has begun, and no attempt should be made to do so. The nurse must remain calm, stay with the child, and prevent the child from sustaining any harm during the seizure. If possible, the child should be isolated from the view of others by closing a door or pulling screens. A seizure can be very upsetting to the child, other visitors, and their families. If other persons are present, they should be assured that everything is being done for the child. After the seizure, they can be given a simple explanation about the event as needed.

BOX 28-13 ■ General Observations of the Child During a Seizure

OBSERVE SEIZURE

Describe

Order of events (before, during, and after)

Duration of seizure

Tonic-clonic—from first signs of event until jerking stops

Absence—from loss of consciousness until consciousness regained

Complex partial—from first sign of unresponsiveness, motor activity, automatisms until signs of responsiveness to environment return

Onset

Time of onset

Significant preseizure precipitating events—bright lights, noise, excitement, stress

Behavior

Change in facial expression

Cry or other sound

Stereotyped or automatous movements

Random activity (wandering)

Position of eyes, head, body, extremities

Unilateral or bilateral posturing of one or more extremities

Movement

Change of position, if any

Site of commencement—hand, thumb, mouth, generalized

Tonic phase—length, parts of body involved

Clonic phase—twitching or jerking movements, parts of body involved, sequence of parts involved, generalized, change in character of movements

Lack of movement or muscle tone of body part or entire body

Face

Color change—pallor, cyanosis, flushing

Perspiration

Mouth—position, deviating to one side, teeth clenched, tongue bitten, frothing at mouth, flecks of blood or bleeding

Lack of expression

Asymmetric expression

Eyes

Position—straight ahead, deviation upward or outward, conjugate or divergent gaze

Pupils—change in size, equality, reaction to light and accommodation

Respiratory Effort

Presence and length of apnea

Other

Incontinence of urine or stool

OBSERVE POSTICTALLY

Duration of postictal period

State of consciousness

Orientation

Arousable

Motor ability

Any change in motor function

Ability to move all extremities

Paresis or weakness

Speech

Sensations

Complaint of discomfort or pain

Any sensory impairment

Recollection of preseizure sensations, aura

∿ EMERGENCY TREATMENT

Seizures

TONIC-CLONIC SEIZURE
During the Seizure
Remain calm.
Time the seizure episode.
If child is standing or seated, ease child down to the floor.
Place pillow or folded blanket under child's head.
Loosen restrictive clothing.
Remove eyeglasses.
Clear area of any hazards or hard objects.
Allow seizure to end without interference.
If vomiting occurs, turn child to one side.
Do not:
    Attempt to restrain child or use force
    Put anything in child's mouth
    Give any food or liquids

After the Seizure
Time the postictal period.
Check for breathing. Check position of head and tongue. Reposition if head is hyperextended. If child is not breathing, give rescue breathing and call emergency medical service (EMS).
Keep child on side.
Remain with child.
Do not give food or liquids until fully alert and swallowing reflex has returned.
Call EMS when necessary.
Look for medical identification and determine what factors occurred before onset of seizure that may have been triggering factors.
Check head and body for possible injuries.
Check inside of mouth to see if tongue or lips have been bitten.

COMPLEX PARTIAL SEIZURE
During the Seizure
Do not restrain.
Remove harmful objects from area.
Redirect to safe area.
Do not agitate; instead, talk in calm, reassuring manner.
Do not expect child to follow instructions.
Watch to see if seizure generalizes.

After the Seizure
Stay with child and reassure until fully conscious.

CALL EMERGENCY MEDICAL SERVICES IF:
Child stops breathing
There is evidence of injury or child is diabetic or pregnant
Seizure lasts for more than 5 minutes (unless duration of that child's seizures is typically longer than 5 minutes) and written medical order is present.
Status epilepticus occurs
Pupils are not equal in size after seizure
Child vomits continuously 30 minutes after seizure has ended (sign of possible acute problem)
Child cannot be awakened and is unresponsive to painful stimuli after seizure has ended
Seizure occurs in water
This is child's first seizure

Modified from *Seizure recognition and first aid*, 2001, Epilepsy Foundation; website: www.efa.org.

❗NURSING ALERT

Do not move or forcefully restrain the child during a tonic-clonic seizure and do not place a solid object between the teeth.

If the nurse is able to reach the child in time, a child who is standing or is seated in a chair (including a wheelchair) is eased to the floor immediately. During and sometimes after the tonic-clonic seizure, the swallowing reflex is lost, salivation increases, and the tongue is hypotonic. Therefore the child is at risk for aspiration and airway obstruction. Placing the child on the side facilitates drainage and helps to maintain a patent airway. If the child becomes cyanotic, oxygen is administered. After the seizure the child is kept on the side in bed to allow the youngster to sleep. When feasible, the child is reintegrated into the environment as soon as possible. Sending a child with a chronic seizure disorder home from school is not necessary, unless the parents request this.

Children who are known to have seizures or who are under observation for seizures will require some precautions. The extent of these measures depends on the type and frequency of the seizure (Box 28-14).

Long-Term Care. Care of the child with a recurrent seizure disorder involves physical care and instruction regarding the importance of the drug therapy and, probably more significant, the problems related to the emotional aspects of the disorder. There are few diseases that generate as much anxiety among relatives as epilepsy. Fears and misconceptions about the disease and its treatment abound in the layperson's mind. For many it represents the archetype of severe hereditary affliction. Therefore the foci of nursing care are directed toward helping the child and the family to deal with the psychologic and sociologic problems related to the disorder and educating the child, the family, peers, and the public toward a more realistic and liberal view of the disease.

Children subject to seizures are placed on some type of drug therapy. The nurse can help the parents plan the administration of the medication at convenient times to minimize disruption to the family routine. The most convenient times for administration seem to be with meals or at bedtime. Although antiepileptic drugs are available in liquid ex-

BOX 28-14 ■ Seizure Precautions

Extent of precautions depends on type, severity, and frequency of seizures
May include the following:
    Side rails raised when child is sleeping or resting
    Side rails and other hard objects padded
    Waterproof mattress/pad on bed/crib
    Appropriate precautions during potentially hazardous activities:
        Swimming with a companion
        Use of protective helmet and padding during bicycle riding, skateboarding, in-line skating
        Supervision during use of hazardous machinery/equipment
Have child carry or wear medical identification
Alert other caregivers to need for any special precautions
Identify and avoid triggering factors whenever possible

tracts or emulsions, the tablet form is preferred by neurologists. The unequal distribution of the drug in the solute and the increased likelihood of inaccurate measurements make liquid medication less desirable. For small children the tablet of the proper dosage can be crushed and administered in syrup, jelly, or other palatable substances.

> **NURSING ALERT**
>
> Children taking phenobarbital and/or phenytoin should receive adequate vitamin D and folic acid, since deficiencies of both have been associated with these antiepileptics. Phenytoin should not be taken with milk.

It is important to impress on the family the need to continue the medication regularly without interruption for as long as required. The parents and the child will need to know the common side effects of the drug prescribed and observe for signs that might indicate unfavorable reactions.

Parents need to be warned of possible behavioral changes as the seizures are controlled in children taking primidone, phenobarbital, or phenytoin. Changes in personality, indifference to school activities and family, hyperactivity, or even psychotic behavior may sometimes be observed. The potential effects of antiepileptics on learning and behavior should be considered. Progressive intellectual deterioration in a child with epilepsy requires investigation of present medication plus the role of the underlying cerebral pathology. Parents should notify the health professional if the child has an illness, including vomiting or fever. Vomiting can interfere with drug absorption; fever may increase metabolic requirements; both can precipitate seizure activity.

Rectal preparations of some medications are highly useful and effective when a child is unable to take oral medications because of repeated vomiting, gastrointestinal surgery, or status epilepticus. Administration of rectal drugs can be learned by parents for home treatment during a seizure. Rectal Ativan is useful as an adjunctive home treatment for children at risk for prolonged seizures.

The degree to which activities are restricted is individualized for each child and depends on the following factors:

1 Type, frequency, and severity of the seizures
2 The child's response to therapy
3 The length of time the seizures have been controlled.

Normal healthy activities are encouraged for children, and participation in competitive sports is determined on an individual basis. With encouragement, most older children can accept the restrictions placed on activities. Only essential restrictions should be placed on children regarding sports and peer activity to reduce the likelihood of needlessly accentuating differences.

Because the child is encouraged to attend school, camp, and other normal activities, the school nurse and the teacher should be made aware of the child's condition and therapy. They can help to ensure regularity of medication and any special care the child might need. Teachers, childcare providers, camp counselors, youth organization leaders, coaches, and other adults who assume responsibility for children should be instructed regarding care of the child during a seizure so that they can act in a calm manner to promote the welfare of the child and to positively influence the attitude of the child's peers.*

Triggering Factors.   Careful and detailed documentation of seizures over a period of time may reveal a pattern. When this occurs, the nurse or responsible adult may intervene to identify the triggering factors and make changes in the environment that may prevent the seizures or decrease their frequency. The necessary changes are often very simple and cost free but can make an enormous difference in the child's and family's lives (see Critical Thinking Exercise).

Factors that may trigger seizures in children include the following:

- Changes in dark-light patterns, such as those that occur with a flash on a camera, automobile headlights, passing a picket fence, reflections of light on snow or water, or rotating blades on a fan
- Sudden loud noises, specific voices, songs, or nursery rhymes
- Startling or sudden movements
- Extreme or drastic changes in temperature
- Dehydration
- Fatigue
- Hyperventilation
- Hypoglycemia
- Ingestion of caffeine
- Insufficient protein in the diet (protein is needed to metabolize some antiepileptic drugs)

Although there have been reports of seizures triggered by flashing video games, this relationship has not been confirmed by controlled studies. Seizures may be caused by the length of playing time, which may cause sleep deprivation, fatigue, excitement, or photosensitivity (Johnston, 2004). On the basis of current knowledge, the overwhelming majority of children with seizures can play video games without the risk of seizures.†

If a child is photosensitive, avoiding such things as wallpaper with stripes, ceiling fans, and blinking lights may be necessary; viewing the TV screen from a distance of at least 2 yards and covering one eye may be beneficial.

Family Support.   Parental attitudes and management of a child with a seizure disorder are as varied as those of other parents of children with a chronic disorder, and they are subject to the same long-term problems (see Chapter 18). Whether the seizures result from illness, injury, or unknown etiology, the parents may feel guilt, anxiety, and often humiliation. They want to know if the condition will affect the child's mental capacities. To many persons, epilepsy is erroneously associated with mental deficiency. Seizures do frequently accompany other manifestations of severe brain damage from disease or injury, but the majority of children with seizures, like any population of healthy children, display a wide range of intelligence.

---

*An excellent resource is Santilli N, Dodson WE, Walton AV: *Students With Seizures: A Manual for School Nurses,* ed 2, 2001, Landover, Md, Epilepsy Foundation of America.
†For more information on video games and epilepsy, contact the **Epilepsy Foundation** National Office, 4351 Garden City Drive, Landover, MD 20785; (301) 459-3700 or (800) EFA-1000; website: www.efa.org.

??? CRITICAL THINKING EXERCISE ???

Seizures

Since age 2 years, Jane Little has had epilepsy that is well controlled with medication. However, now that she has begun elementary school, her seizures have returned. On the way home Jane usually has a seizure on the bus; however, on weekends and holidays she is seizure free. Jane's parents are concerned that a triggering factor at school may bring on the seizures and are considering taking her out of school. As the school nurse, what should you advise Jane's parents to do?

QUESTIONS
1. Evidence—Is there sufficient evidence to draw conclusions about the recurrence of Jane's seizures when riding on the school bus?
2. Assumptions—Describe an underlying assumption about each of the following:
   a. A 6-year-old school-age girl diagnosed with epilepsy and seizures at 2 years of age
   b. A school-age child whose seizures are no longer totally controlled, despite adequate pharmacologic management
   c. A school-age child with epilepsy who is exposed to a seizure trigger when she rides the school bus and attends school
3. What priorities for nursing care should be established?
4. Does the evidence support your nursing intervention?
5. What alternative perspectives might you have?

ANSWERS
1. Yes. Jane is a school-age child with previously controlled seizures who is now having seizures while riding on the school bus. There appears to be a pattern to the seizure activity; however, until further assessment is performed, the exact reason for the seizure activity may not be found.
2. a. Jane's seizures have been controlled in the past with anticonvulsant medication.
   b. This abrupt onset of seizures after having control for years needs further evaluation. With the consistent pattern and abrupt onset of the seizures, seeking medical reevaluation should be advised if no triggering event is identified.
   c. There are many environmental factors that may trigger seizures in children who have had adequate pharmacologic management of seizures. These include but are not necessarily limited to the following: changes in dark-light patterns such as a camera flash, automobile lights, reflections on light surfaces such as snow or water, or rotating fan blades; sudden noises or startling movements; drastic changes in temperature; dehydration; fatigue; hypoglycemia; caffeine; and inadequate amounts of protein in the diet. Since the seizures appear to have a pattern, that is, when Jane rides the bus home from school, further investigation and assessment are required.
3. Your first priority is to help the family identify triggering events that would yield pertinent and necessary information. Because the bus ride appears to be a focal event surrounding the recurrence of seizures, this must be assessed for potential triggers. At your suggestion, Mrs. Little rode the school bus home with Jane. As on previous rides Jane began to seize as a long white picket fence was passed; her mother noted that the child stared intently at the fence and that is when the seizure activity started. Because the fence was perceived as a potential triggering factor, actions were taken to minimize exposure to the repetitive motion of observing the white picket fence as the bus passed. Once Jane was seated on the other side of the bus, the seizure episodes stopped. As the school nurse, it would be appropriate for you to continue discussing Jane's progress with her parents and explore their feelings about taking her out of school. With a thorough assessment of their feelings about the matter and reassurance that the trigger for the recurrence of seizure activity is removed, the parents may be more amenable to leaving Jane in school. Parents of children with chronic illness such as epilepsy are encouraged to make the child's life as normal as possible, and taking her out of school would not promote that goal.
4. An accurate interpretation of the information is that it is not within the scope of nursing practice for the school nurse to change the dosage of the antiepileptic medication. As Jane grows, adjustments in medication will be necessary when she visits her primary care practitioner. An option that was explored was having the parents take Jane to school in their car; however, the seizures may still occur if Jane sits in the same position as on the school bus and is exposed to the fence that was the triggering mechanism in this case.
5. One alternate perspective that may need to be explored is whether the antiepileptic medication is within the therapeutic range for the size of the child. If recent antiepileptic drug levels have not been obtained, this may be something to consider. A visit to the primary care practitioner is encouraged.

Parents also wonder how the illness will affect the child's future and need reassurance that it will not shorten the life of the child and that the child can attend school, marry, and elect to have children. The child will need vocational guidance, and the parents should become familiar with the laws in their state regarding any limitations that might be imposed on the child because of the disorder. It should be emphasized that seizures can be controlled or greatly reduced in the majority of children and that new studies hold the promise of progress in future treatment. Parents also need reassurance that there is less stigma attached to the disease than there has been in the past.

It is important to encourage a healthy attitude toward the child and the disease and to help the parents feel competent in their ability to meet their responsibilities. The child should be reared as any normal child, with natural concern tempered by the understanding of the need of the child not to be overprotected. Many parents refrain from correcting or punishing the child, especially if they have had the experience of such an emotional stress precipitating a seizure. The child must not be made to feel different in any way. Parents should be encouraged to be honest and open about the disorder with the child and with others. Some parents are tempted to try to conceal the nature of the child's illness because of their belief that the disorder is shameful or a disgrace to the family.

Restrictions on the child's activities will be necessary for safety, but this area can be approached in a positive way in terms of what the child *can* do rather than what the child cannot do. Sometimes parents curtail the child's activities more than necessary. The child needs to experience the maturing influences of play and work. The **Epilepsy Foundation*** is a national organization that works toward and for the welfare of persons with epilepsy and their families, helps with employment and legal problems, and provides education to patients, families, and communities.

The Child With Epilepsy.   The child who is provided the security of a loving family, rewards and punishments no different from those of other children, and support in acquiring self-esteem is more apt to have a positive attitude toward the disease. Children derive their self-concept and self-esteem from observations of others' reactions to them and their own perception of their capabilities. The suddenness and unpredictability of seizures and the reactions of others further influence their feelings. When others consider children to be different, inferior, or objects of ridicule, they come to view themselves as different, inferior, and incapable.

Children with epilepsy need to learn about their disease and the role that the medication plays in contributing to their prolonged well-being. As soon as they are old enough, children should assume responsibility for taking their own medication and be advised to carry medical identification with pertinent information about their condition. Planning activities with children and emphasizing the activities in which they can engage rather than those in which they cannot will help them succeed and gain satisfaction in their achievements. They should be offered opportunities and encouraged to exercise judgment in their daily lives.

The adolescent period may be a trying time for the child with epilepsy. Limits imposed on the young person's activities at a time when freedom and independence are desired may bring the disability into sharp focus. For example, some states do not allow persons with epilepsy to obtain a driver's license, even when the disease is controlled; in others there are restrictions on employment insurance.

Epilepsy should not be a severe impairment to most youngsters, and the nurse, by assuming the role of patient advocate, helping to educate the public regarding the disease, working toward making opportunities available to persons with the disorder, and lobbying for legislation that recognizes the needs of the individual with a seizure disorder, can help to erase the stigma that still remains regarding the disease. See Nursing Care Plan: The Child With Epilepsy.

FEBRILE SEIZURES

Febrile seizures are transient disorders of children that occur in association with a fever. They are one of the most common neurologic disorders of childhood, affecting about 4% of children. Most febrile seizures occur after 6 months of age and usually before age 3 years, with increased frequency in children younger than 18 months. They are unusual after 5 years of age. Boys are affected about twice as often as girls, and there appears to be an increased susceptibility in families. Most febrile seizures are generalized and last less than 5 minutes (Johnston, 2004; Fishman, 1999).

***Epilepsy Foundation** National Office, 4351 Garden City Drive, Landover, MD 20785; (301) 459-3700 or (800) EFA-1000; website: www.efa.org.

The cause of febrile seizures is still uncertain. In most children the severity but not the rapidity of the temperature elevation seems to be a factor. The fever usually exceeds 38.8° C (101.8° F) and occurs during the temperature rise rather than after a prolonged elevation. Sometimes it constitutes the dramatic beginning of an illness. Febrile seizures usually accompany an upper respiratory or gastrointestinal infection. Although pertussis and the MMR vaccine do not cause febrile seizures, these immunizations can be precipitating factors in initial episodes of febrile seizures in children prone to having seizures (Barlow and others, 2001).

Most febrile seizures have stopped by the time the child is taken to a medical facility. However, if the seizure continues, treatment consists of controlling the seizure with diazepam (Valium) and reducing the temperature by administration of acetaminophen. In children with simple febrile seizures, prophylactic antiepileptic therapy is not recommended. The most important interventions are parental education and emotional support (American Academy of Pediatrics, 1999; Johnston, 2004). Little risk of neurologic deficit, epilepsy, mental retardation, or altered behavior has been observed as sequelae of febrile seizures.

Parents need reassurance of the *benign* nature of febrile seizures (almost 95% of children with febrile seizures will not develop epilepsy or any neurologic damage). They should be told that their child is in no danger of dying during a febrile seizure. They also need education regarding protecting the child from harm and observing exactly what happens to the child during the event. Attempts to lower the temperature with acetaminophen or to use diazepam to prevent a seizure are of no benefit in most children (Uhari and others, 1995). Tepid sponge baths are ineffective in significantly lowering the temperature; the shivering effect further increases metabolic output, and cooling causes discomfort in the child.

! **NURSING ALERT**

If a febrile seizure lasts more than 5 minutes, parents should seek medical attention immediately. Parents should call for emergency assistance (911) and not try to take a child in a car if he or she is actively seizing.

CEREBRAL MALFORMATIONS

CRANIAL DEFORMITIES

In the normal newborn the cranial sutures are separated by membranous seams several millimeters wide. For the first few hours to 1 to 2 days after birth, the cranial bones are highly mobile, which allows them to mold and slide over one another, adjusting the circumference of the head to accommodate to the changing shape and character of the birth canal. The principal sutures in the infant's skull are the sagittal, coronal, and lambdoidal sutures, and the major soft areas at the juncture of these sutures are the anterior and posterior fontanels (see Fig. 8-5).

Following birth, growth of the skull bones occurs in a direction *perpendicular* to the line of the suture, and normal closure occurs in a regular and predictable order. Although there are wide variations in the age at which closure takes place in individual children, normally all sutures and fontanels are ossified by the following ages:

8 weeks: Posterior fontanel closed
6 months: Fibrous union of suture lines and interlocking of serrated edges
18 months: Anterior fontanel closed
12 years: Sutures unable to be separated by increased ICP

Solid union of all sutures is not completed until very late childhood. Closure of a suture before the expected time inhibits the perpendicular growth. Since normal increase in brain volume requires expansion, the skull is forced to grow in a direction *parallel* to the fused suture. This alteration in skull growth always produces a distortion of the head shape when the underlying brain growth is normal. The small head with closed and normal shape is a result of deficient brain growth; the suture closure is secondary to this brain growth failure. Failure of brain growth is not secondary to suture closure.

Various types of cranial deformities are encountered in early infancy. These include the enlarged head with frontal protrusion (bossing; characteristic of hydrocephalus), the parietal bossing that is seen in chronic subdural hematoma, the small head, and a variety of skull deformities (Box 28-15). Some occur during prenatal development; in others, head circumference is usually within normal limits at birth, and the deviation from normal development becomes apparent with advancing age.

Prognosis. The majority of infants presenting with craniosynostosis have normal brain development. The exceptions are those genetic disorders that involve brain pathology.

BOX 28-15 ■ Cranial Deformities

Microcephaly—Head circumference more than 2 standard deviations below average for age, sex, and gestation; caused by failure of brain development
  Management—No treatment available
Craniosynostosis—Premature closure of single or multiple sutures of cranial vault, face, and base of skull
  Scaphocephaly—Premature closure of sagittal suture causes skull to become elongated in an anteroposterior direction, with a high cranial vault and a subnormal transverse diameter
  Brachycephaly—Premature closure of coronal sutures causes skull to become shortened in an anteroposterior direction, with flattening of occiput and forehead
  Oxycephaly—Premature closure of both coronal and sagittal sutures causes an excessively high and narrow skull that tapers upward on all sides
  Plagiocephaly—Unilateral closure of one coronal or lambdoidal suture causes skull to become asymmetric
  Craniofacial dysostosis (Crouzon disease)—Premature closure of any or all cranial sutures, most frequently the coronal, and a typical facial deformity (widely spaced eyes, hypoplastic maxilla, and beaklike nose; tongue appears large and protruding; frequently with exophthalmos)
    Management—Surgical release of closed sutures; Crouzon disease—surgical correction of major facial deformities

Nursing Considerations

Nursing care of families in which there is a child with a cranial defect involves identifying children with deformities and referring them for evaluation. Since there is no therapy available for children with microcephaly, nursing care is directed toward helping parents adjust to rearing a child with brain damage (see Chapter 19).

Caring for infants who benefit from surgery requires special emphasis on observation for signs of decreased hematocrit and hemoglobin because of the large blood loss during surgery (see Family Focus box). A cardiac monitor may demonstrate a resting heart rate of 200. Nursing care includes observation for signs of hemorrhage, infection, pain, and swelling, as well as parental education for suture care and safety. Surgical sutures should remain dry and intact. Parents need to observe for any signs of redness, drainage, or swelling and report any temperature greater than 38.4° C (101° F).

Early surgical management of craniosynostosis allows proper expansion of the brain and the creation of an acceptable appearance. Parents require special support and education during this time, especially from the health care team (Stal, Chebret, and McElroy, 1998).

HYDROCEPHALUS

Hydrocephalus is a condition caused by an imbalance in the production and absorption of CSF in the ventricular system. When production is greater than absorption, CSF accumulates within the ventricular system, usually under increased pressure, producing passive dilation of the ventricles.

Pathophysiology

The two mechanisms by which CSF is formed include secretion by the choroid plexuses and lymphatic-like drainage by the extracellular fluid of the brain. CSF circulates throughout the ventricular system and then is absorbed within the subarachnoid spaces by a mechanism that is not entirely clear. Prenatal diagnosis is undoubtedly having an impact on the current prevalence at birth of hydrocephalus. The advent of MRI and CT scanning has provided valuable information about the pathophysiology of various diseases. The causes are diverse; they are either congenital (maldevelopment or intrauterine infection) or acquired (neoplasm, hemorrhage, or infection).

Hydrocephalus is a symptom of an underlying brain disorder resulting in either (1) impaired absorption of CSF within the subarachnoid space (ventricles communicate; *communicating hydrocephalus*) or (2) obstruction to the flow of CSF within the ventricles (ventricles do not communicate; *noncommunicating hydrocephalus*). Any imbal-

FAMILY FOCUS

Blood Donation

Parents may wish to provide a compatible blood donor for their infant undergoing a planned surgical correction for craniosynostosis. Nurses need to inform and guide parents through this blood bank procedure.

ance of secretion and absorption causes an increased accumulation of CSF in the ventricles, which become dilated and compress the brain substance against the surrounding rigid bony cranium. When this occurs before fusion of the cranial sutures, it produces enlargement of the skull, as well as dilation of the ventricles (Fig. 28-6). In children younger than 10 to 12 years of age, previously closed suture lines, especially the sagittal suture, may become diastatic or opened.

Most cases of noncommunicating hydrocephalus are a result of developmental malformations. Although the defect usually is apparent in early infancy, it may become evident at any time from the prenatal period to late childhood or early adulthood. Other causes include neoplasms, infections, and trauma. An obstruction to the normal flow can occur at any point in the CSF pathway to produce increased pressure and dilation of the pathways proximal to the site of obstruction.

Developmental defects (e.g., Arnold-Chiari malformations [ACMs], aqueduct stenosis, aqueduct gliosis, and atresia of the foramina of Luschka and Magendie [Dandy-Walker syndrome]) account for most cases of hydrocephalus from birth to 2 years of age. Hydrocephalus is so often associated with myelomeningocele that all such infants should be observed for its development. In the remainder of cases there is a history of intrauterine infection, perinatal hemorrhage, and neonatal meningoencephalitis. In older children hydrocephalus is most often a result of space-occupying lesions, intracranial infections, hemorrhage, or preexisting developmental defects, such as aqueduct stenosis or the *Arnold-Chiari malformation* (a congenital anomaly in which the cerebellum and medulla oblongata extend down through the foramen magnum).

Diagnostic Evaluation

The two factors that influence the clinical picture in hydrocephalus are the time of onset and the presence of preexisting structural lesions. In infancy, before closure of the cra-

nial sutures, head enlargement is the predominant sign, whereas in older infants and children the lesions responsible for hydrocephalus produce other neurologic signs through pressure on adjacent structures before causing CSF obstruction (Box 28-16).

In infancy the diagnosis of hydrocephalus is based on head circumference that crosses one or more grid lines on the measurement chart within a period of 2 to 4 weeks and on associated neurologic signs that are present and progressive. However, other diagnostic studies are needed to localize the site of CSF obstruction. Routine daily head circumference measurements are carried out in infants with myelomeningocele and intracranial infections. In evaluation of a premature infant, specially adapted head circumference charts are consulted to distinguish abnormal head growth from rapid head growth that takes place normally.

The signs and symptoms in early to late childhood are caused by increased ICP, and specific manifestations are related to the focal lesion. Most commonly resulting from posterior fossa neoplasms and aqueduct stenosis, the clinical manifestations are primarily those associated with space-occupying lesions.

The primary diagnostic tools for detecting hydrocephalus are CT and MRI. Sedation is required, since the child must remain absolutely still for an accurate picture to be produced. Diagnostic evaluation of children who have symptoms of hydrocephalus after infancy is similar to that used in those with suspected intracranial tumor. In the neonate, echoencephalography is useful in comparing the ratio of lateral ventricle to cortex.

Therapeutic Management

The treatment of hydrocephalus is directed toward relief of the hydrocephalus, treatment of complications, and management of problems related to the effect of the disorder on psychomotor development. The treatment is, with few ex-

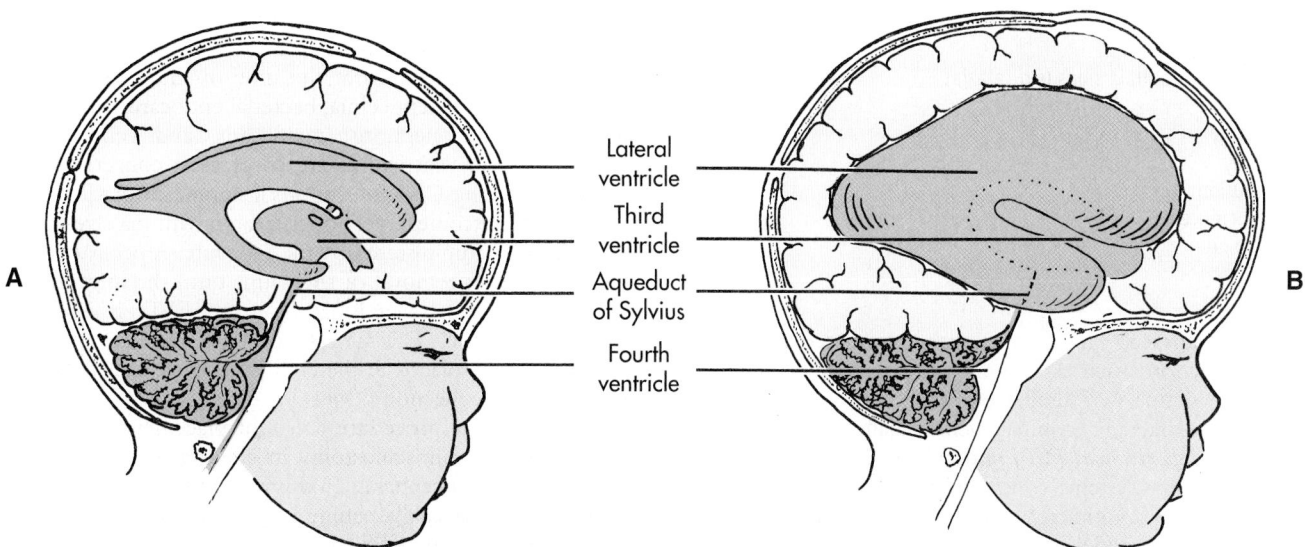

A

Lateral ventricle
Third ventricle
Aqueduct of Sylvius
Fourth ventricle

B

FIG. 28-6 ■ Hydrocephalus: a block in flow of cerebrospinal fluid. **A,** Patent cerebrospinal fluid circulation. **B,** Enlarged lateral and third ventricles caused by obstruction of circulation—stenosis of aqueduct of Sylvius.

BOX 28-16 ■ Clinical Manifestations of Hydrocephalus

INFANCY (EARLY)
Abnormally rapid head growth
Bulging fontanels (especially anterior) sometimes without head enlargement:
  Tense
  Nonpulsatile
Dilated scalp veins
Separated sutures
Macewen sign (cracked-pot sound on percussion)
Thinning of skull bones

INFANCY (LATER)
Frontal enlargement, or bossing
Depressed eyes
Setting sun sign (sclera visible above the iris)
Pupils sluggish, with unequal response to light

INFANCY (GENERAL)
Irritability
Lethargy
Infant cries when picked up or rocked and quiets when allowed to lie still
Early infantile reflex acts may persist
Normally expected responses fail to appear
May display:
  Change in level of consciousness
  Opisthotonos (often extreme)
  Lower extremity spasticity
  Vomiting
Advanced cases:
  Difficulty in sucking and feeding
  Shrill, brief, high-pitched cry
  Cardiopulmonary embarrassment

CHILDHOOD
Headache on awakening; improvement following emesis or upright posture
Papilledema
Strabismus
Extrapyramidal tract signs (e.g., ataxia)
Irritability
Lethargy
Apathy
Confusion
Incoherence
Vomiting

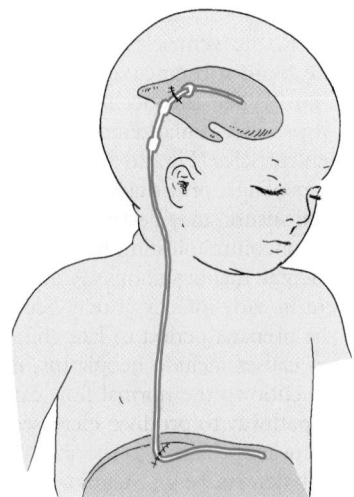

FIG. 28-7 ■ Ventriculoperitoneal shunt. Catheter is threaded beneath the skin.

The initial shunt is placed when necessary to relieve CSF obstruction, and revisions are needed when signs of malfunction appear. In all mechanisms the initial success rate is relatively high; however, shunts are associated with complications that interfere with continued shunt function or threaten the life of the child.

The major complications of VP shunts are infection and malfunction. All shunts are subject to mechanical difficulties, such as kinking, plugging, or separation or migration of the tubing. Malfunction is most often caused by mechanical obstruction either within the ventricles from particulate matter (tissue or exudate) or at the distal end from thrombosis or displacement as a result of growth. The child with a shunt obstruction is often first seen in an emergency department with clinical manifestations of increased ICP, frequently accompanied by worsening neurologic status.

The most serious complication, shunt infection, can occur at any time, but the period of greatest risk is 1 to 2 months after placement. The infection is generally a result of intercurrent infections at the time of shunt placement. Infections include septicemia, bacterial endocarditis, wound infection, shunt nephritis, meningitis, and ventriculitis. Meningitis and ventriculitis are of greatest concern, since any complicating CNS infection is a significant predictor of intellectual outcome. Infection is treated with massive doses of antibiotics administered by the IV route. A persistent infection requires removal of the shunt until the infection is controlled. External ventricular drainage (EVD) is used until CSF is sterile. The EVD allows for removal of CSF through a tube placed in the child's ventricle that flows by gravity into a collection device.

An alternative procedure to shunt placement is the endoscopic third ventriculostomy in children with noncommunicating hydrocephalus. In this procedure, an endoscope is used to make a small opening in the floor of the third ventricle that allows the CSF to flow freely through the previously blocked ventricle. Aldana and others (2003) have shown that endoscopic septal fenestration has an overall patency rate of 81%, which may eliminate the need for a CSF

ceptions, surgical. This is accomplished by direct removal of an obstruction (such as a tumor) or placement of a shunt that provides primary drainage of the CSF from the ventricles to an extracranial compartment, usually the peritoneum *(ventriculoperitoneal [VP] shunt)* (Fig. 28-7).

Most shunt systems consist of a ventricular catheter, a flush pump, a unidirectional flow valve, and a distal catheter. In all models the valves are designed to open at a predetermined intraventricular pressure and close when the pressure falls below that level, thus preventing backflow of secretions.

shunt. The complication rate of the endoscopic septal fenestration procedure was 9.3% and included intraventricular hemorrhage, sterile meningitis, and septostomy failure (Aldana and others, 2003).

Prognosis.   The prognosis of children with treated hydrocephalus depends largely on the rate at which hydrocephalus develops, the duration of increased ICP, the frequency of complications, and the cause of the hydrocephalus. For example, malignant tumors may have a high mortality regardless of other complicating factors.

Surgically treated hydrocephalus with continued neurosurgical and medical management has a survival rate of about 80%, with the highest incidence of mortality occurring within the first year of treatment. Of the surviving children, approximately one third are both intellectually and neurologically normal, and one half have neurologic disabilities.

Nursing Considerations

Preoperatively the infant with diagnosed or suspected hydrocephalus is observed carefully for signs of increasing ICP. In infants the head is measured daily at the point of largest measurement—the occipitofrontal circumference (OFC) (see Head Circumference, Chapter 7, for technique). Fontanels and suture lines are gently palpated for size, signs of bulging, tenseness, and separation. An infant with normal ICP will display bulging under certain circumstances such as straining or crying; therefore such accompanying behavior should be noted. Irritability, lethargy, or seizure activity, as well as altered vital signs and feeding behavior, may indicate an advancing pathologic condition.

In older children, who are usually admitted to the hospital for elective or emergency shunt revision, the most valuable indicator of increasing ICP is an alteration in the child's LOC and the way in which the child interacts with the environment. Changes are identified by observation and by comparison of present behavior with customary behavior, sleep patterns, developmental capabilities, and habits, all obtained through a detailed history and a baseline assessment. This baseline information serves as a guide for postoperative assessment and evaluation of shunt function.

General nursing care of the infant with hydrocephalus may present special problems. Maintaining adequate nutrition often requires flexible feeding schedules to accommodate diagnostic procedures, since feeding before or after handling can precipitate an episode of vomiting. Small feedings at more frequent intervals are often better tolerated than larger ones spaced farther apart. These infants are often difficult to feed and require extra time and innovation.

The nurse is responsible for preparing the child for diagnostic tests such as tomography and for assisting the practitioner with procedures such as a ventricular tap, which is often performed to relieve excessive pressure during the preoperative period and for CSF examination. Sedation is required, since the child must remain absolutely still during diagnostic testing. IV pentobarbital or oral chloral hydrate is commonly used for these procedures. (See Chapter 22 for information about preparing children for procedures.)

> **! NURSING ALERT**
>
> If surgery is anticipated, IV lines should not be placed in a scalp vein on a child with hydrocephalus.

Fortunately, almost all affected children are recognized, and treatment is begun early. For those children with significant head enlargement, care must be exercised to see that the head is well supported when the infant is fed or moved to prevent extra strain on the infant's neck, and measures must be taken to prevent development of pressure areas. As the hydrocephalus progresses, untreated children become increasingly helpless and prone to the multiple problems of immobility (e.g., pressure sores and contracture deformities). Not infrequently, infants with irreversible brain damage or with severe developmental defects such as hydranencephaly, in which both cerebral hemispheres fail to develop and are replaced with a membranous sac filled with CSF, are placed in long-term care facilities.

Postoperative Care.   Routine postoperative care and observation are instituted. In addition, the infant or child is positioned carefully on the unoperated side to prevent pressure on the shunt valve and pressure areas. The child is kept flat to help avert complications resulting from too-rapid reduction of intracranial fluid. When the ventricular size is reduced too rapidly, the cerebral cortex may pull away from the dura and tear the small interlacing veins, producing a subdural hematoma. This is not a problem in children with elective shunt revision, since their intraventricular size and pressure have been normal. The surgeon indicates the position to be maintained and the extent of activity allowed. If there is increased ICP, the surgeon will prescribe elevation of the head of the bed and/or that the child be allowed to sit up to enhance gravity flow through the shunt. Pain management can usually be achieved with acetaminophen with or without codeine for mild-to-moderate pain and opioids for severe pain (see Pain Management, Chapter 21).

Observation is continued for signs of increased ICP, which indicates obstruction of the shunt. Neurologic assessment includes evaluation of pupillary dilation (pressure causes compression or stretching of the oculomotor nerve, producing dilation on the same side as the pressure) and blood pressure (hypoxia to the brainstem causes variability in these vital signs).

> **! NURSING ALERT**
>
> Arbitrary pumping of the shunt may cause obstruction or other problems and should not be performed unless indicated by the neurosurgeon.

The child is also observed for abdominal distention, because CSF may cause peritonitis or a postoperative ileus as a complication of distal catheter placement. In addition, intake and output are carefully monitored. Children may be placed on fluid restriction with nothing by mouth for 24 hours. The IV infusion is closely monitored to prevent fluid overload. Routine feeding is resumed after the prescribed NPO period, but the presence of bowel sounds is determined before feeding a child with a VP shunt.

Since infection is the greatest hazard of the postoperative period, nurses are continually on the alert for the usual manifestations of CSF infection, which may include elevated vital signs, poor feeding, vomiting, decreased responsiveness, and seizure activity. There may be signs of local inflammation at the operative sites and along the shunt tract. The child's diaper should be kept off the peritoneal dressing site or suture line. Antibiotics are administered by the IV route as ordered, and the nurse may also need to assist the practitioner with intraventricular instillation. The incision site is inspected for leakage, and any suspected drainage is tested for glucose, an indication of CSF.

Meticulous skin care is continued postoperatively, with extra care taken to prevent tissue damage from pressure. A pressure-reducing mattress or overlay pad underneath the child helps prevent pressure on prominent areas. Skin is inspected regularly for any signs of pressure, irritation, or infection.

Family Support. Specific needs and concerns of parents during periods of hospitalization are related to the reason for the child's hospitalization (shunt revision, infection, diagnosis) and the diagnostic and/or surgical procedures to which the child must be subjected. Often parents have very little understanding of anatomy; therefore they need further exploration and reinforcement of information that was given to them by the physician and neurosurgeon, as well as information about what they can expect. They are especially frightened of any procedure that involves the brain, and the fear of retardation or brain damage is very real and pervasive. Nurses can do much to allay their anxiety by explaining the rationale underlying the various nursing and medical activities, such as positioning or testing, and by simply being available and willing to listen to their concerns.

To prepare for the child's discharge and home care, the parents are instructed on how to recognize signs that indicate shunt malfunction or infection and how to pump the shunt, if necessary. Active children may have accidents, such as a fall, that can damage the shunt, and the tubing may pull out of the distal insertion site or become disconnected during normal growth.

Safe transportation is an essential issue to discuss with parents. The tendency for the enlarged head to fall forward and to turn to the side, combined with poor head control, influences the type of child restraint system needed. Small infants can be restrained reclining in an approved car-restraint bed.

The management of hydrocephalus in a child is a demanding task for both family and health professionals, and helping a family cope with the child is an important nursing responsibility. It is important to emphasize that hydrocephalus is a lifelong problem and that the child will require evaluation on a regular basis. The overall aim is to establish realistic goals and an appropriate educational program that will help the child to achieve his or her optimal potential.

Anticipatory guidance will prepare parents for possible problems and help them to avoid being overprotective of the child. Few restrictions (mainly contact sports) need be placed on the child's activities, and the child should be encouraged to live as would any other child of the same age and abilities. Parents need support and encouragement in coping with the child and with problems the child may encounter in relationships with peers and others. Reactions of other children when the child has a noticeably enlarged head or requires shaving at the times of revision are stressful situations for both child and parents. (See Chapter 18 for a discussion on problems and coping with the child with a disability.)

Families can be referred to community agencies for support and guidance. The **National Hydrocephalus Foundation (NHF)*** and the **Hydrocephalus Association†** provide information on the condition for families and assist interested groups in establishing local organizations. Helpful booklets are available from these and other sources.

KEY POINTS

- Level of consciousness (LOC) is the most important indicator of neurologic health; altered levels include full consciousness, confusion, disorientation, lethargy, obtundation, stupor, coma, and persistent vegetative state.

- Complete neurologic examination includes LOC; posture; motor, sensory, cranial nerve, and reflex testing; and vital signs.

- Nursing care of the unconscious child focuses on ensuring respiratory management; performing neurologic assessment; monitoring intracranial pressure (ICP); supplying adequate nutrition and hydration; providing drug therapy; promoting elimination, hygienic care, proper positioning, exercise, and stimulation; and providing family support.

- Fractures resulting from head injuries may be classified as depressed, compound, basilar, and diastatic.

- Primary head injury involves features that occur at the time of trauma, including fractured skull, contusions, intracranial hematoma, and diffuse injury. Secondary complications include hypoxic brain damage, increased ICP, infection, cerebral edema, and posttraumatic syndromes.

- The young child's response to head injury is different because of the following features: larger head size, expandable skull, larger blood volume to the brain, small subdural spaces, and thinner, softer brain tissue.

- Problems resulting from near-drowning include hypoxia and asphyxiation, aspiration, and hypothermia.

- Nursing care of the child with a brain tumor includes observing for signs and symptoms related to the tumor, preparing the child and family for diagnostic tests and operative procedures, preventing postoperative complications, planning for discharge, and promoting a return to optimal health.

- Nursing care of the child with meningitis includes administering antibiotics, taking isolation precautions, removing environmental stimuli, ensuring correct positioning, monitoring vital signs, administering intravenous therapy, promoting adequate fluid and nutritional status, and providing supportive care to the family.

- Routine immunization of infants with *Haemophilus influenzae* type B and pneumococcal conjugate vaccines has reduced the incidence of bacterial meningitis.

---

*12413 Centralia Road, Lakewood, CA 90715-1623; (562) 402-3523 or (888) 857-3434; fax: (562) 924-6666; website: www.nhfonline.org.
†870 Market Street, Suite 955, San Francisco, CA 94102; (415) 732-7040; website: www.hydroassoc.org. A booklet entitled *About Hydrocephalus: A Book for Parents* is available in English or Spanish.

- Encephalitis may result from direct invasion of the central nervous system by a virus or from involvement of the central nervous system after viral disease.
- A seizure is a symptom of an underlying pathologic condition and may be manifested by sensory-hallucinatory phenomena, motor effects, sensorimotor effects, or loss of consciousness.
- Partial seizures are categorized as simple (without associated impairment of consciousness) or complex (with impaired consciousness); both types may become generalized.
- Generalized seizures are categorized as tonic-clonic convulsive absence, atonic and akinetic, myoclonic, and infantile spasms.
- Long-term care of the child with recurrent seizure disorders includes physical care as well as education regarding the importance of drug therapy and problems related to emotional aspects of the disorder.
- Febrile seizures are the most common type of childhood seizure.
- Many cranial deformities are amenable to surgical correction.
- Hydrocephalus is a symptom of underlying brain pathology demonstrated by impaired absorption of cerebrospinal fluid (CSF) or obstruction to the flow of CSF within the ventricles.
- Therapy for hydrocephalus involves relief of the hydrocephalus, treatment of the underlying brain disorder if possible, prevention and/or treatment of complications, and management of problems related to psychomotor development.

References

Aldana PR, Kestle JRW, Brockmeyer DL, Walker ML: Results of endoscopic septal fenestration in the treatment of isolated ventricular hydrocephalus, *Pediatr Neurosurg* 38(6):286-294, 2003.

Alston RD, Newton R, Kelsey A and others: Childhood medulloblastoma in northwest England, 1954 to 1977: incidence and survival, *Dev Med Child Neurol* 45(5):308-314, 2003.

American Academy of Pediatrics, Committee on Infectious Diseases (Pickering L, editor): *2003 red book: report of the Committee on Infectious Diseases,* ed 26, Elk Grove Village, Il, 2003, The Academy.

American Academy of Pediatrics: Committee on Quality Improvement, Subcommittee on Febrile Seizures: Practice parameter: long-term treatment of the child with simple febrile seizures, *Pediatrics* 103(6):1307-1309, 1999.

American Academy of Pediatrics: Committee on Sports Medicine and Fitness and Committee on Injury and Poison Prevention: Swimming programs for infants and toddlers, *Pediatrics* 105(4):868-870, 2000.

Avner JR: Animal and human bites and bite-related infections. In Burg FD, Ingelfinger JR, Wald WR, editors: *Gellis and Kagan's current pediatric therapy,* ed 16, Philadelphia, 1999, WB Saunders.

Barlow WE, Davis RL, Glassen JM and others: The risks of seizures after receipt of whole-cell pertussis or measles, mumps and rubella vaccine, *N Engl J Med* 345(9):656-661, 2001.

Barnard C, Wirrell E: Does status epilepticus cause developmental deterioration and development of epilepsy? *J Child Neurol* 14(12):787-794, 1999.

Bayir H, Kochanek PM, Clark RS: Traumatic brain injury in infants and children: mechanisms of secondary damage and treatment in the intensive care unit, *Crit Care Clin* 19(3):529-549, 2003.

Berg AT, Shinnar S, Levy SR, Testa FM: Two-year remission and subsequent relapse in children with newly diagnosed epilepsy, *Epilepsia* 42(12):1553-1562, 2001.

Bernardo LM, Gardner MJ, Rosenfield RL and others: A comparison of dog bite injuries in younger and older children treated in a pediatric emergency department, *Pediatr Emerg Care* 18(3):247-249, 2002.

Bhutta AT, Van Savell H, Schexnayder SM: Reye's syndrome: down but not out, *South Med J* 96(1):43-45, 2003.

Bonthius DJ, Karacay B: Meningitis and encephalitis in children: an update, *Neurol Clin* 20(4):1013-1038, 2002.

Brady M: Common injuries. In Burns CE, Brady M, Dunn AM, Starr NB, editors: *Pediatric primary care, a handbook for nurse practitioners,* ed 2, Philadelphia, 2000, WB Saunders.

Brodeur GM, Maris JM: *Neuroblastoma.* In Pizzo PA, Polack DG, editors: *Principles and practice of pediatric oncology,* ed 4, Philadelphia, 2002, Lippincott-Raven.

Centers for Disease Control and Prevention: Progress toward elimination of *Haemophilus influenza* type b invasive disease among infants and children—United States, 1998-2000, *MMWR* 51:234-239, 2002.

Centers for Disease Control and Prevention: Compendium of animal rabies prevention and control, 2001, National Association of State Public Health Veterinarians, Inc, *MMWR* 50(RR-8):1-9, 2001.

Centers for Disease Control and Prevention: Human rabies prevention—United States, 1999, *MMWR* 48(RR-1):1-21, 1999.

Chiaretti A and others: Early post-traumatic seizures in children with head injury, *Childs Nerv Syst* 16(12):862-866, 2000.

Durkin MS and others: The epidemiology of urban pediatric neurological trauma: evaluation of, and implications for, injury prevention programs, *Neurosurgery* 42(2):300-310, 1998.

El Bashir H, Laundy M, Booy R: Diagnosis and treatment of bacterial meningitis, *Arch Dis Child* 88(7):814-819, 2003.

Faillace WJ: Management of childhood neurotrauma, *Surg Clin North Am* 82(2):349-363, 2002.

Fishman MA: Febrile seizures. In McMillan JA and others, editors: *Principles and practice of pediatrics,* ed 3, Philadelphia, 1999, JB Lippincott.

Gennarelli TA: Trauma to the head: general considerations. In Schwartz GR, editor: *Principles and practices of emergency medicine,* ed 4, Philadelphia, 1999, Lippincott Williams & Wilkins.

Gupta N, Berger MS: Brain mapping for hemispheric tumors in children, *Pediatr Neurosurg* 38(6):302-306, 2003.

Johnston MV: Seizures in childhood. In Behrman RE, Kliegman RM, Jenson HTS, editors: *Nelson textbook of pediatrics,* ed 17, Philadelphia, 2004, WB Saunders.

Kallas HJ: Drowning and near-drowning. In Behrman RE, Kliegman RM, Jenson HTS, editors: *Nelson textbook of pediatrics,* ed 17, Philadelphia, 2004, WB Saunders.

Kamienski MC: Reye syndrome, *Am J Nurs* 103(7):54-57, 2003.

Kaplan SL: Management of pneumococcal meningitis, *Pediatr Infect Dis J* 21(6):589-591, 2002.

Kline NE, Sevier N: Solid tumors in children, *J Pediatr Nurs* 18(2):96-102, 2003.

Lee C, Nechyba C, Gunn V: *Drug doses.* In The John Hopkins Hospital (Gunn V, Nechyba C, editors): *The Harriet Lane handbook,* ed 16, Philadelphia, 2002, Mosby.

Lefevre F, Aronson N: Ketogenic diet for the treatment of refractory epilepsy in children: a systematic review of efficacy, *Pediatrics* 105(4):e46, 2000; available at www.pediatrics.org/cgi/content/full/105/4/e46.

Masson F, Thicoipe M, Mokni T and others: Epidemiology of traumatic comas: a prospective population-based study, *Brain Inj* 17(4):279-293, 2003.

McGovern MC, Glasgow JFT, Stewart MC: Lesson of the week: Reye's syndrome and aspirin: lest we forget, *Br Med J* 322(7302):1591-1592, 2001.

Mitchell WG and others: An open-label study of repeated use of diazepam rectal gel (Diastat) for episodes of acute breakthrough seizures and clusters: safety, efficacy, and tolerance, *North Am Diastat Group, Epilepsia* 40(11):1610-1617, 1999.

Molf I: *Immunoprophylaxis.* In The John Hopkins Hospital (Gunn V, Nechyba C, editors): *The Harriet Lane handbook,* ed 16, Philadelphia, 2002, Mosby.

Murray-Ryan J, Petriccione MM: Central nervous system tumors. In Baggott CR, Kelly KP, Fochtman D, Foley GV, editors: *Nursing care of children and adolescents with cancer,* ed 3, Philadelphia, 2002, WB Saunders.

Nguyen NP and others: Neuroblastoma producing spinal cord compression: rapid relief with low dose of radiation, *Anticancer Res* 20(6c):4687-4690, 2000.

Pasero C, McCaffery M: Procedural pain management. In McCaffery M, Pasero C, editors: *Pain clinical manual,* ed 2, St Louis, 1999, Mosby.

Prober CG: Central nervous system infections. In Behrman RE, Kliegman RM, Jenson HTS, editors: *Nelson textbook of pediatrics,* ed 17, Philadelphia, 2004, WB Saunders.

Redner A: Central nervous system malignancies. In Lanzkowsky P, editor: *Manual of pediatric hematology and oncology,* ed 3, San Diego, 2000, Academic Press.

Rivara FP, Grossman D: Injury control. In Behrman RE, Kliegman RM, Jenson HTS, editors: *Nelson textbook of pediatrics,* ed 17, Philadelphia, 2004, WB Saunders.

Saez-Llorens X, McCracken GH Jr: Bacterial meningitis in children, *Lancet* 361(9375):2139-2148, 2003.

Schutzman SA, Greenes DS: Pediatric minor head trauma, *Ann Emerg Med* 37(1):65-74, 2001.

Shafer PO: Epilepsy and seizures: advances in seizure assessment, treatment, and self-management, *Nurs Clin North Am* 34(3):743-759, 1999.

Stal S, Chebret L, McElroy C: The team approach in the management of congenital and acquired deformities, *Clin Plast Surg* 25(4):485-491, 1998.

Strother DR, Pollack IF, Fisher PG and others: Tumors of the central nervous system. In Pizzo PA, Pollack DG, editors: *Principles and practice of pediatric oncology,* ed 4, Philadelphia, 2002, Lippincott-Raven.

Uhari M and others: Effect of acetaminophen and of low intermittent doses of diazepam on prevention of recurrences of febrile seizures, *J Pediatr* 126(6):991-995, 1995.

Vernon-Levett P: Neurologic system. In Slota MC, editor: *Core curriculum for pediatric critical care nursing,* Philadelphia, 1998, WB Saunders.

Zuckerman GB, Gregory PM, Santos-Damiani SM: Predictors of death and neurologic impairment in pediatric submersion injuries: the pediatric risk of mortality score, *Arch Pediatr Adolesc Med* 152:134-140, 1998.

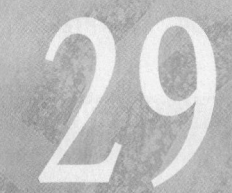

The Child With Endocrine Dysfunction

29

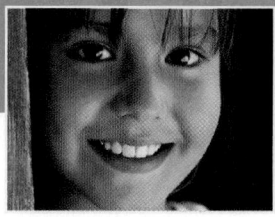

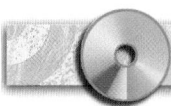 Remember to check out your companion CD-ROM

http://evolve.elsevier.com/Wong/essentials/

CHAPTER OUTLINE

RELATED TOPICS and ADDITIONAL RESOURCES

 IN TEXT

 CD COMPANION

Critical Thinking Exercise—Hypothyroidism
Case Study—Diabetes Mellitus
Clinical manifestations—Panhypopituitarism; Hyperparathyroidism; Hypoparathyroidism; Type 1 Diabetes Mellitus
Nursing Care Plan
NCLEX-Style Review Questions

evolve WEBSITE

WebLinks
NCLEX-Style Review Questions

WONG'S CLINICAL MANUAL OF PEDIATRIC NURSING, 6/E

Community and Home Care Instructions—Giving Intramuscular or Subcutaneous Injections

- Differentiate between the disorders caused by hypopituitary and hyperpituitary dysfunction.
- Describe the manifestations of thyroid hypofunction and hyperfunction and the management of children with the disorders.

- Distinguish between the manifestations of adrenal hypofunction and hyperfunction.
- Differentiate among the various categories of diabetes mellitus.
- Discuss the management and nursing care of the child with diabetes mellitus in the acute care setting.

- Distinguish between a hypoglycemic and a hyperglycemic reaction.
- Design a teaching plan for a child with diabetes mellitus.
- Formulate a teaching plan for instructing the parents of a child with diabetes mellitus.

DISORDERS OF PITUITARY FUNCTION

The *pituitary gland,* or *hypophysis,* is often referred to as the *master gland* because of its role in regulating other endocrine glands. Under the influence of secretions from the hypothalamus, the anterior lobe of the pituitary (adenohypophysis) releases or withholds seven hormones (Table 29-1). These hormones control the secretion of hormones from other endocrine glands and influence somatic and sexual development. Because of this relationship, a dysfunction observed in target tissues can be a result of malfunction of the hypothalamus, the pituitary gland, or the target gland. If the tropic hormones are involved, the resulting disorder reflects the altered stimulus to the target gland. For example, if thyroid-stimulating hormone is deficient, thyroid hormone is also deficient, and the child displays the manifestations of hypothyroidism. Overproduction of pituitary hormone is thought to be caused by hyperplasia of the pituitary cells or by a primary hypothalamic defect that results in excess production of the hormone's releasing factor.

Deficiencies of the anterior pituitary hormones may be a result of organic defects or of idiopathic etiology and may occur as a single hormonal problem or in combination with other hormonal deficiencies. The clinical manifestations depend on the hormones involved and the age of onset. This

TABLE 29-1 ■ Endocrine Glands and Their Function

HORMONE	PRIMARY EFFECT	HORMONE	PRIMARY EFFECT
ADENOHYPOPHYSIS (ANTERIOR PITUITARY GLAND)		**ADRENAL CORTEX**	
Growth hormone (GH)	Promotes growth of bone and soft tissues	Aldosterone	Regulates sodium retention and excretion
Thyroid-stimulating hormone (TSH)	Stimulates thyroid hormone secretion	Sex hormones	Influence development of bones, reproductive organs, and secondary sex characteristics
Adrenocorticotropic hormone (ACTH)	Stimulates adrenal cortex to secrete glucocorticoids and androgens	Glucocorticoids	Promote metabolism
			Mobilize body defenses during stress
Gonadotropins	Stimulate gonads to mature and pro-		Suppress inflammatory reaction
Follicle-stimulating hormone (FSH)	duce sex hormones and germ cells	**ADRENAL MEDULLA**	
Luteinizing hormone (LH)		Catecholamines	Produce a sympathetic response
Prolactin	Stimulates milk secretion		Increase blood pressure and blood glucose levels
Melanocyte-stimulating hormone (MSH)	Promotes pigmentation of skin	**ISLETS OF LANGERHANS OF PANCREAS**	
		Insulin	Promotes utilization of glucose by cells; decreases blood glucose levels
NEUROHYPOPHYSIS (POSTERIOR PITUITARY GLAND)		Glucagon	Increases blood glucose levels
Antidiuretic hormone (ADH)	Acts on kidney tubules to reabsorb water		Accelerates glyconeogenesis
Oxytocin	Stimulates uterine contractions	Somatostatin	Inhibits secretion of insulin and glucagon
	Causes milk ejection reflex	**OVARIES**	
		Estrogen	Stimulates ripening of ova
THYROID GLAND			Produces female secondary sex characteristics
Thyroid hormones	Regulate metabolic rate		Promotes epiphyseal closure of bones
	Control rate of body cell growth	Progesterone	Prepares uterus for fertilization
Thyrocalcitonin	Influences ossification and development of bone	**TESTES**	
		Testosterone	Stimulates spermatogenesis
PARATHYROID GLANDS			Produces male secondary sex characteristics
Parathyroid hormone (PTH)	Regulates calcium metabolism		Promotes epiphyseal closure of bones

discussion is limited to dysfunction related primarily to the secretion of growth hormone.

HYPOPITUITARISM: GROWTH HORMONE DEFICIENCY

Hypopituitarism is primarily a disorder associated with deficient secretion of *GH (somatotropin)*. It may be caused by a variety of conditions: development defects; destructive lesions such as tumors, trauma, vascular abnormalities, or surgery; certain hereditary disorders; or functional disorders such as anorexia nervosa or psychosocial dwarfism. In more than half of children with hypopituitarism, no lesion is evident and the cause is unknown and is called *idiopathic hypopituitarism* or *idiopathic pituitary growth failure.*

GH deficiency inhibits somatic growth in all body cells (Fig. 29-1). The primary site of dysfunction in the syndrome appears to be in the hypothalamus. The extent of idiopathic GH deficiency may be complete or partial, but the cause is unknown. It is frequently associated with other pituitary hormone deficiencies and is treated more frequently in boys than in girls.

Diagnostic Evaluation

Only a small number of children with delayed growth or short stature have hypopituitary dwarfism. In the majority of instances the cause is constitutional delay (see Chapter 17). Although children with hypopituitarism are normal at birth, they show growth patterns that progressively deviate

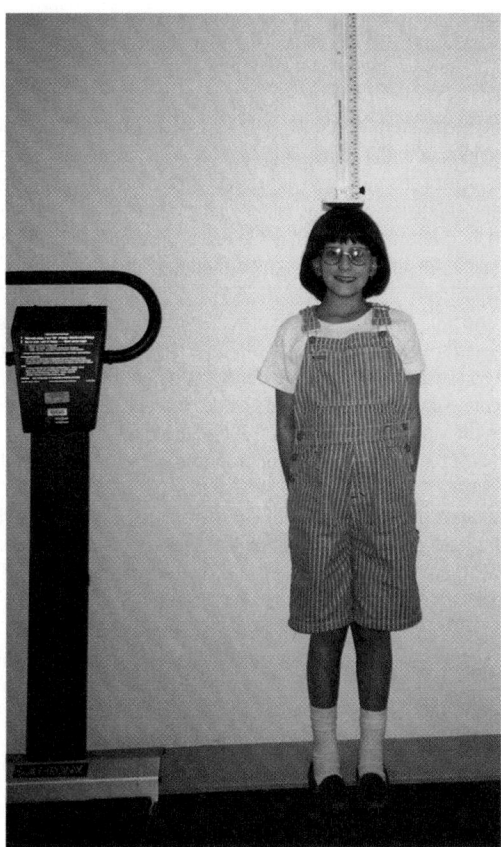

FIG. 29-1 ■ Thirteen-year-old girl with short stature. Height is 133 cm. Normal height for age is 145 to 168 cm.

from the normal growth rate, often beginning in infancy. The chief complaint in most instances is short stature (Box 29-1). Growth deceleration over time is an important measure for which to assess because it may be an indicator of a pathologic process (Halac and Zimmerman, 2004).

A complete diagnostic evaluation should include a family history, a history of the child's growth patterns and previous health status, physical examination, psychosocial evaluation, drug intake, parental heights, birth size, nutritional state, review of systems, radiographic surveys, and endocrine studies. Many endocrinologists recommend a magnetic resonance image of the brain before starting growth hormone therapy to rule out a pituitary abnormality or lesion (Arends and others, 2002). The diagnosis is based on radioimmunoassay of plasma GH levels stimulated pharmacologically with two different stimulation tests. GH levels below 10 ng/mL after two provocative tests help to establish the diagnosis (Miller and Zimmerman, 2004; Guyda, 2000; Shulman and Bercu, 1998). Serum levels of the hormones directly responsible for skeletal growth (insulin-like growth factor 1, insulin-like growth factor-binding protein 3) are now used to evaluate GH deficiency error (Durham, 2003). (See Ethical Case Study.)

Radiographic examination of the hand and wrist for centers of ossification is an important procedure in evaluating growth. Endocrine studies to detect tropic hormone deficiencies are also performed if there is evidence of hypothyroidism, hypersecretion of cortisol, or gonadal aplasia.

Therapeutic Management

Treatment of GH deficiency caused by organic lesions is directed toward correction of the underlying disease process (e.g., surgical removal or irradiation of a tumor). The definitive treatment of GH deficiency is replacement of GH. *Biosynthetic GH* prepared by recombinant DNA technology is the therapy of choice (Miller and Zimmerman, 2004). The Food and Drug Administration (FDA) has approved recombinant GH therapy for the following conditions: GH-deficient (GHD), chronic renal insufficiency before transplantation, Turner syndrome, short stature from Prader-Willi syndrome, children with a history of intrauter-

BOX 29-1 ■ Clinical Manifestations of Hypopituitarism

Presenting complaint—short stature
  Usually normal growth first year
  Growth during second year drops below established percentile
  Growth measurements below 5th percentile
Premature aging common in later life
Height may be retarded more than weight
Appear well nourished
Skeletal proportions normal
Tend to be relatively inactive
Less apt to participate in aggressive, sporting-type activities
Bone age nearly always retarded but closely related to height age
Usually primary teeth appear at expected age; eruption of permanent teeth delayed
Teeth are overcrowded and malpositioned (because of underdeveloped jaw)
Sexual development usually delayed but normal

✖ ETHICAL CASE STUDY

Ethical Decision Making Model	*Johnny is an 11-year-old white male who is in the 3rd percentile for height for his age. He has been evaluated by a pediatric endocrinologist for short stature, and the work-up was negative for growth hormone deficiency or an underlying etiology causing growth failure. Johnny's father is 6'2" tall and was a college basketball star and has been discussing growth hormone (GH) treatment with the pediatric endocrinologist for several months. His mother, who is small and petite at 5'1", is defensive and voices concerns that she does not want Johnny to receive hormone shots. Johnny is a quiet boy who does well in school and is an excellent chess player, placing first on the school's chess team last year. When discussing the benefits and risks associated with GH therapy, Johnny is quiet except for expressing his desire to be tall enough to play basketball like his father. The family returns to the clinic to discuss GH therapy further.*
Evaluate the issue	The first step in evaluating this case is to determine how the diagnosis of idiopathic short stature was established. The work-up for GH deficiency should include assessment of Johnny's height, bone age, adjusted growth velocity, and responses to GH provocative testing. When possible, the child's growth patterns since birth should be evaluated, especially growth velocity. Evaluation of Johnny's parents' adult height is important because heredity plays a major factor in height predisposition. A careful prenatal history should be performed to rule out maternal disorders that may have influenced intrauterine growth. Prematurity is also a cause for concern. If no underlying etiology is found, the diagnosis becomes one of idiopathic short stature.
	The next important step is to become knowledgeable of the GH literature. A recent meta-analysis of studies evaluating GH therapy in children with idiopathic short stature revealed that 1 year of therapy causes an increase in growth velocity and suggests that long-term GH therapy may increase adult height (Finkelstein and others, 2002). However, controversy continues as to whether GH has an effect on short-term growth only and not on final adult height (Saenger, 2000; Bercu, 1996). The issues surrounding GH therapy include the benefits obtained from therapy, cost associated with treatment, and, most importantly, disagreement among professionals as to whether idiopathic short stature should even be classified as a treatable problem. Side effects reported in the literature include allergy, impaired glucose tolerance, pseudotumor cerebri, hyperlipidemia, slipped capital femoral epiphysis, transient peripheral edema, exaggeration of scoliosis, and even leukemia (Bercu, 1996; Finkelstein and others, 2002).
	Studies have documented that GH therapy costs more than $35,000 per 2.54 cm of height gained (Finkelstein and others, 1998; Bercu, 1996). Controversy exists as to the appropriateness of GH therapy in preventing psychosocial problems caused by an individual's short stature. Several researchers found no relationship between short stature and the amount of psychosocial risk factors experienced by these individuals (Kranzler and others, 2000; Gilmore and Skuse, 1996; Sandberg, Brook, and Campos, 1994). Some researchers feel that short stature as an isolated physical characteristic is of limited value as a predictor of a child's psychologic adaptation or quality of life (Sandberg and Voss, 2002; Voss, 2000; Bercu, 1996). What is apparent is that careful evaluation of the need for GH treatment in children is essential (Sandberg and Voss, 2002; Voss, 2000).
Treat all involved with respect	It is evident that the issue of GH therapy is highly controversial among medical professionals, and this conflict can easily be transferred to anxious parents and the child. What is most important in working with this family is to listen to all concerns and to address specific questions the parents and child might have. The parents do not seem to be in agreement with a decision to administer GH therapy, and there is no evidence as to the position the pediatric endocrinologist has taken on the matter. When therapies are available that are questionable as to their clinical importance and long-term value, a family's interests must be heard and the treatment information available must be given in a manner that will allow the best decision for the child to be made.
Hear all sides	Children will not understand the risks and benefits of GH therapy and will not be able to express their thoughts and concerns. One should therefore ask whether it is appropriate to make such decisions for children, based on the experiences and expectations of adults. Health care professionals must be aware that there is a danger that some parents, including those with children within the normal range for height, may seek GH therapy because they perceive tallness as desirable. Treatment may be motivated less by concern for the child than by the parents' wishes for a perfect child (Voss, 2000). Careful assessment by listening to the desires of the parents and by discussing GH therapy with the child in an age-appropriate manner is essential.
Initiate action	In this case study, action evolves around appropriate assessment of the risks and benefits of GH therapy for a child with idiopathic short stature. Because it is evident that a great deal of controversy continues in the medical specialty regarding this intervention, parents must be informed of the risks and benefits of GH therapy and the reasons why medical professionals differ in their opinions. Careful evaluation of the cost of treatment and the family's resources must be considered.
Consider the outcome	The outcome for GH therapy in children with idiopathic short stature remains unanswered. Those who believe strongly that GH therapy should not be administered in otherwise healthy children believe that GH intervention requires better evidence than a deviation from the mean in stature (Voss, 2000). Those in strong support of GH therapy for idiopathic short stature are equally strong in their belief that short stature below the 3rd percentile on the growth curve is simply not normal (Saenger, 2000). The evidence supports that careful consideration must take place before GH therapy is administered to children with idiopathic short stature.

ine growth restriction who have not reached a normal height range by age 2 years, and children with idiopathic short stature who are >2.25 standard deviations below the mean in height and who are unlikely to catch up in height (Wilson and others, 2003). Children with other hormone deficiencies require replacement therapy to correct the specific disorders. This may involve administration of thyroid extract, cortisone, testosterone, or estrogens and progesterone. The sex hormones are usually begun during adolescence to promote normal sexual maturation. Much controversy exists over the use of GH in children who are short but not GHD.

Prognosis.   GH replacement is successful in 80% to 90% of affected children. Children who respond to therapy typically increase their growth rate from 3.5 to 4 cm/year before treatment to 8.7 ± 1.5 cm/year. Young children, obese children, and severely GHD children respond best. Growth responses to GH will vary depending on age, length of treatment, frequency of administration, dosage, weight, and GH receptor amount (Blethen and others, 1996). Overall studies have noted improved actual or near-final adult height. Early diagnosis and initiation of therapy is important to successful therapy (August, Julius, and Blethen, 1998). Recent investigation revealed that patients diagnosed with GHD in childhood are no longer GHD at the end of therapy after attainment of final height (Thomas and others, 2003).

Nursing Considerations

Nursing care is primarily directed toward assisting in establishing the diagnosis and providing emotional support to the child and family (see Chapter 17). Because these children appear younger than their chronologic age, others frequently relate to them in childish ways. Parents and teachers benefit from guidance directed toward realistic expectations of the child based on age and abilities (Zimet and others, 1997).

Children undergoing hormone replacement require additional support, such as preparation for daily subcutaneous injections and education for self-management during the school-age years (see the Critical Thinking Exercise on p. 1090).

> **NURSING ALERT**
>
> **Injections are given at bedtime to most closely approximate physiologic release of GH.**

Even when hormone replacement is successful, these children attain their eventual adult height at a slower rate than their peers; thus they need assistance in setting realistic expectations regarding the expected outcome. Professionals and families may find education and support from the **Human Growth Foundation.*** The treatment is expensive—up to $20,000 to $30,000 per year depending on dosage.

PITUITARY HYPERFUNCTION

Excess GH before closure of the epiphyseal shafts results in proportional overgrowth of long bones until the individual reaches a height of 8 feet or more. Vertical growth is ac-

companied by rapid and increased development of muscles and viscera. Weight is increased but is usually in proportion to height. Proportional enlargement of head circumference also occurs and may result in delayed closure of the fontanels. Children with a pituitary-secreting tumor may also demonstrate signs of increasing intracranial pressure, especially headache.

If hypersecretion of GH occurs after epiphyseal closure, growth is in the transverse direction, producing a condition known as *acromegaly.* Typical facial features include overgrowth of the head, lips, nose, tongue, jaw, and paranasal and mastoid sinuses; separation and malocclusion of the teeth in the enlarged jaw; disproportion of the face to the cerebral division of the skull; increased facial hair; and thickened, deeply creased skin.

Diagnostic Evaluation

Diagnosis is based on a history of excessive growth during childhood and evidence of increased levels of GH. Radiologic studies may reveal a tumor in an enlarged sella turcica; normal bone age; enlargement of bones, such as the paranasal sinuses; and evidence of joint changes. Endocrine studies to confirm excess of other hormones, such as cortisol and sex hormones, are also included in the differential diagnosis.

Therapeutic Management

If a lesion is present, surgical treatment, including cryosurgery or hypophysectomy, may be warranted to remove the tumor whenever feasible. Other therapies that destroy pituitary tissue include external irradiation and radioactive implants. Depending on the extent of surgical extirpation and the degree of pituitary insufficiency, hormone replacement with thyroid extract, cortisone, and sex hormones may be necessary.

Nursing Considerations

The primary nursing consideration is early identification of children with excessive growth rates. Although medical management does not diminish the height already attained, it can retard further growth. The earlier the treatment is begun, the better the chance to attain a normal adult height.

Children with excessive growth rates require as much emotional support as those with short stature. However, girls may suffer from the effects of excessive height much more than boys, who may find their height an asset when pursuing sports such as basketball. A compassionate nurse can be very supportive to these children, especially before adolescence, when they are larger than their peers. The nurse can emphasize to a tall girl that as boys grow older, they become taller, and she will not always be looking down at them. Because early adolescence is a time of idol worship, the nurse can point out marriages of celebrities in which the woman is taller than the man to help the girl gain a perspective that not all heterosexual relationships must follow stereotypic models.

PRECOCIOUS PUBERTY

Manifestations of sexual development before age 9 years in boys or age 8 years in girls are considered precocious and should be investigated (Midyett and others, 2003; Kempers

---

*997 Glen Cove Avenue, Glen Head, NY 11545; (800) 451-6434; website: hgf1 www.hgfound.org.

and Otten, 2002). Girls with a higher percent of body fat at 5 years of age are more likely to exhibit earlier pubertal development (Davison, Susman, and Birch, 2003). African-American girls usually enter puberty first, followed by Mexican-American and then white girls (Anderson, Dallal, and Must 2003; Chumlea and others, 2003; Wu, Mendola, and Buck, 2002). Early sexual development can have a number of causes and may result from a disorder of the gonad, the adrenal gland, or the hypothalamic-pituitary gonadal axis. The disorder occurs far more frequently in girls than in boys. No causative factor can be found in 80% to 90% of girls. A central nervous system insult or structural injury in boys is more common (Root, 2000).

True, or *complete, precocious puberty* is always isosexual and results from premature activation of the hypothalamic pituitary-gonadal axis, which produces early maturation and development of the gonads with secretion of sex hormones, development of secondary sex characteristics, and sometimes production of mature sperm or ova. Precocious puberty is explained only as an unusually early activation of the maturation process that is regarded as a normal course of events at a later age. There is early acceleration of linear growth with early epiphyseal fusion and ultimate height less than what would have been anticipated with later pubertal onset. *Precocious pseudopuberty,* or *incomplete puberty,* differs from true sexual precocity in that there is no early secretion of gonadotropin. Most cases result from early overproduction of sex hormone, usually caused by a tumor of the ovary or testis, a tumor or hyperplasia of the adrenal gland, or exogenous sources of androgens or estrogens.

Therapeutic Management

Treatment of precocious pseudopuberty is directed toward the specific cause when known. Precocious puberty of central origin is managed with monthly subcutaneous injections of a synthetic analog of *luteinizing hormone–releasing hormone* (LHRH; Lupron), which regulates pituitary secretions. This therapy slows the prepubertal growth to normal rates in affected children. Treatment is discontinued at a chronologically appropriate time, allowing pubertal changes to resume.

Nursing Considerations

Psychologic support and guidance of the child and family are the most important aspects of management. Parents need a detailed explanation and reassurance of the benign nature of the condition. Dress and activities for the physically precocious child should be appropriate to the chronologic age.

Despite the early sexual development, maturation of the gonads and the appearance of secondary sexual characteristics proceed in the usual order. After puberty, physical differences from peers are no longer present. Heterosexual interest is not usually advanced beyond the child's chronologic age; however, the nurse should emphasize to parents that the child is fertile. No form of contraception is necessary, however, unless the child is sexually active.

DIABETES INSIPIDUS

The principal disorder of posterior pituitary hypofunction is diabetes insipidus (DI), also known as *neurogenic DI.* The disease is a result of hyposecretion of *antidiuretic hormone*

(ADH), or *vasopressin,* which produces a state of uncontrolled diuresis. Primary causes are familial or idiopathic; secondary causes include trauma (accidental or surgical), tumors, granulomatous disease, infections (meningitis or encephalitis), or vascular anomalies (aneurysm). The disorder is not to be confused with nephrogenic DI, a rare hereditary disorder caused by unresponsiveness of the renal tubules to the hormone.

Clinical Manifestations

The cardinal signs of DI are polyuria and polydipsia. In the older child excessive urination accompanied by a compensatory insatiable thirst may be so intense that the child does little other than drink fluids and void (Cheetham and Baylis, 2002). Not infrequently, the first sign is enuresis. In the infant the initial symptom is irritability that is relieved with feedings of water but not milk. The infant is also prone to dehydration, electrolyte imbalance, hyperthermia, azotemia, and potential circulatory collapse.

> **! NURSING ALERT**
>
> The child with DI complicated by congenital absence of the thirst center must be encouraged to drink sufficient quantities of liquid to prevent electrolyte imbalance.

Diagnostic Evaluation

The simplest test used to diagnose this condition is restriction of oral fluids and observation of consequent changes in urine volume and concentration. In DI, fluid restriction has little or no effect on urine formation but causes weight loss from dehydration. If this test is positive, the child should be given a test dose of injected *aqueous vasopressin (Pitressin),* which should alleviate the polyuria and polydipsia. Unresponsiveness to exogenous vasopressin usually indicates nephrogenic DI.

> **! NURSING ALERT**
>
> Small children require close supervision during fluid restriction to prevent them from drinking, even from toilet bowls, plants, or other unlikely sources of fluid.

Therapeutic Management

The usual treatment requires daily hormone replacement of vasopressin. The drug of choice is *desmopressin acetate (DDAVP),* a synthetic analog of vasopressin. DDAVP may also be given orally. Recent studies have found this to be an effective alternative (Boulgourdjian and others, 1997). Nasal DDAVP has widely replaced the use of vasopressin tannate in peanut oil. The injectable form has the advantage of lasting 48 to 72 hours, which affords the child a full night's sleep. However, it has the disadvantages of requiring frequent injections and proper preparation of the drug.

> **! NURSING ALERT**
>
> To be effective, vasopressin must be thoroughly resuspended in the oil by being held under warm running water for 10 to 15 minutes and shaken vigorously before being drawn into the syringe. If this is not done, the oil may be injected without ADH. Small brown particles, which indicate drug dispersion, must be seen in the suspension.

DDAVP is available and administered intranasally by way of a flexible tube to achieve adequate control. It is usually administered twice daily. The response pattern of the child is variable, with duration ranging from 8 to 20 hours. Children receiving DDAVP need to be observed for a possible overdose of the drug. The signs of overdosage are those of water intoxication and are similar to manifestations of inappropriate antidiuretic hormone secretion.

Nursing Considerations

The initial objective of care is identification of the disorder. After confirmation of the diagnosis, parents need a thorough explanation of the condition, with special emphasis on distinguishing between diabetes insipidus and diabetes mellitus. The parents must realize that treatment is lifelong. If the child is to receive the injectable vasopressin, ideally both parents, and children who are older than 7 years of age, should be taught the correct procedure for preparation and administration of the drug. After children are old enough, they should be encouraged to assume full responsibility for care.

For emergency purposes these children should wear medical alert identification. Older children are advised to carry the nasal vasopressin spray with them for temporary relief of symptoms. School personnel should be made aware of the problem so that the child is granted unrestricted use of the lavatory and drinking water. Failure to permit this may result in embarrassing accidents that often result in the child's unwillingness to attend school.

SYNDROME OF INAPPROPRIATE ANTIDIURETIC HORMONE SECRETION

Hypersecretion of the posterior pituitary ADH (vasopressin) produces the disorder known as *syndrome of inappropriate antidiuretic hormone secretion (SIADH).* SIADH is observed with increased frequency in a variety of conditions, especially those involving infections, tumors, and trauma of the central nervous system.

The manifestations observed are directly related to fluid retention and hypotonicity. Increased secretion of ADH causes the kidneys to reabsorb water, which increases the fluid volume and decreases serum osmolality. When serum sodium levels are lowered to 120 mEq/L, the child displays anorexia, nausea (sometimes vomiting), stomach cramps, irritability, and personality changes. With progressive reduction in sodium, other neurologic signs, stupor, and seizures may be evident. The symptoms disappear when the underlying disorder is corrected. Immediate management consists of restricting fluids.

> **! NURSING ALERT**
>
> Children with SIADH develop an expanded circulatory volume but do not form edema, which is an excess of both water and sodium.

Nursing Considerations

The first goal of nursing management is recognizing the presence of SIADH from symptoms described in patients at risk. Accurately measuring intake, output, and daily weight, and observing for signs of fluid overload are primary nursing functions, especially in the child receiving intravenous (IV) fluids.

Seizure precautions are implemented, and the child and family need education regarding the rationale for fluid restriction. The rare child with chronic SIADH will be placed on a long-term regimen of ADH-antagonizing medication and will require instructions for its administration.

DISORDERS OF THYROID FUNCTION

The thyroid gland secretes two types of hormones: *thyroid hormone,* which consists of the hormones *thyroxine (T4)* and *triiodothyronine (T3),* and *thyrocalcitonin.* The secretion of thyroid hormones is controlled by *thyroid-stimulating hormone (TSH)* from the anterior pituitary. Hypothyroidism or hyperthyroidism may result from a defect in the target gland or from a disturbance in secretion of TSH or its releasing factor in the hypothalamus.

Because the functions of T_3 and T_4 are qualitatively the same, the term *thyroid hormone (TH)* is used throughout this discussion.

The synthesis of TH depends on available sources of dietary iodine and tyrosine. The thyroid is the only endocrine gland capable of storing excess amounts of hormones for release as needed. The main physiologic action of TH is to regulate the basal metabolic rate and thereby control the processes of growth and tissue differentiation.

Thyrocalcitonin helps maintain blood calcium levels by decreasing the calcium concentration. Its effect is the opposite of parathormone; it inhibits skeletal demineralization and promotes calcium deposition in the bone.

JUVENILE HYPOTHYROIDISM

Hypothyroidism is one of the most common endocrine problems of childhood. It may be either congenital (see Chapter 9) or acquired and represents a deficiency in secretion of TH. Hypothyroidism from dietary insufficiency of iodine is rare in the United States because iodized salt is a readily available source of the nutrient. This discussion is limited to the juvenile form of hypothyroidism.

Beyond infancy, primary hypothyroidism may be caused by a number of defects. For example, a congenital hypoplastic thyroid gland may provide sufficient amounts of TH during the first year or two but be inadequate when rapid body growth increases demands on the gland. A partial or complete thyroidectomy for cancer or thyrotoxicosis can leave insufficient thyroid tissue to furnish hormones for body requirements. Irradiation for Hodgkin disease or other malignancies or infectious processes may be a cause of hypothyroidism (Pizzo and Poplack, 2001).

Clinical manifestations depend on the extent of dysfunction and the age of the child at the onset (Box 29-2). Because brain growth is nearly complete by 2 to 3 years of age, mental retardation or neurologic sequelae are not associated with juvenile hypothyroidism.

Therapy is oral TH replacement, the same as for hypothyroidism in the infant, although the prompt treatment needed for brain growth in the infant is not required in the child. In children with severe symptoms, the restoration of euthyroidism is achieved more gradually, with administration of increasing amounts of L-thyroxine over 4 to 8 weeks to avoid symptoms of hyperthyroidism that can occur with treatment of chronic hypothyroidism.

BOX 29-2 ■ Clinical Manifestations of Juvenile Hypothyroidism

Decelerated growth	Constipation
Less when acquired at later age	Sleepiness
Myxedematous skin changes	Mental decline
Dry skin	
Puffiness around eyes	
Sparse hair	

BOX 29-3 ■ Clinical Manifestations of Lymphocytic Thyroiditis

ENLARGED THYROID GLAND	**HYPERTHYROIDISM (POSSIBLE)**
Usually symmetric	Nervousness
Firm	Irritability
Freely movable	Increased sweating
Nontender	Hyperactivity
TRACHEAL COMPRESSION	
Sense of fullness	
Hoarseness	
Dysphagia	

Nursing Considerations

The importance of early recognition in the infant is discussed in Chapter 9. Cessation or retardation of growth in a child whose growth has previously been normal should alert the observer to the possibility of hypothyroidism. After diagnosis and implementation of thyroxine therapy, the importance of compliance and periodic monitoring of the response to therapy should be stressed to the parents. Children should learn to take responsibility for their health as soon as they are old enough, at about 9 to 10 years of age.

GOITER

A goiter is an enlargement or hypertrophy of the thyroid gland. It can be congenital or acquired. Congenital disease usually occurs as a result of antithyroid drugs or iodides administered to the mother during pregnancy. The acquired disease can result from increased secretion of pituitary thyrotropic hormone in response to decreased circulating levels of TH, neoplastic or inflammatory processes, or dietary iodine deficiency.

Enlargement of the thyroid gland may be mild and noticeable only when there is an increased demand for TH (e.g., during periods of rapid growth). Enlargement of the thyroid at birth can be sufficient to cause severe respiratory distress. TH replacement is necessary to treat the hypothyroidism and reverse the TSH effect on the gland.

Nursing Considerations

Large goiters are identified by their obvious appearance. Smaller nodules may be evident only on palpation. Nurses in ambulatory settings need to be aware of the possibility of neck enlargement from goiters and report such findings.

> **! NURSING ALERT**
>
> If an infant is born with a goiter, immediate precautions are instituted for emergency ventilation, such as supplemental oxygen and a tracheostomy set. Positioning the child with the neck hyperextended often facilitates breathing.

Immediate surgery to remove part of the gland may be lifesaving. When thyroid replacement is necessary, parents have the same needs regarding its administration as discussed for the parents of children who have hypothyroidism.

LYMPHOCYTIC THYROIDITIS

Lymphocytic thyroiditis (*Hashimoto disease, juvenile autoimmune thyroiditis*) is the most common cause of thyroid disease in children and adolescents, and it accounts for the largest percentage of juvenile hypothyroidism. It also accounts for many of the enlarged thyroid glands formerly designated as thyroid hyperplasia of adolescence, or "adolescent goiter." The disease is more common in girls than in boys and in whites than in African Americans. It occurs more frequently after age 6, reaching a peak incidence in adolescence; there is evidence that the disease is self-limited.

Pathophysiology

There is a strong genetic predisposition to the development of autoimmune thyroiditis, although no mode of inheritance has been delineated and the basic stimulus or autoimmune defect is unknown. The disease is characterized by lymphocytic infiltration of the gland, inflammation, and, in many patients, replacement with fibrous tissue. In the early stages there may be only hyperplasia.

Diagnostic Evaluation

The enlarged thyroid gland may be detected by the practitioner during a routine examination, although it may be noted by parents when the youngster swallows. Most children are euthyroid, but some display symptoms of hypothyroidism. Others have signs that suggest hyperthyroidism (Box 29-3).

Thyroid function tests are usually normal, although TSH levels may be slightly or moderately elevated. With progressive disease the T_4 decreases, followed by a decrease in T_3 levels and an increase in TSH. A variety of abnormalities in radioactive iodine uptake may be noted. The majority of children have serum antibody titers to thyroid antigens, but fewer children have a positive red blood cell hemagglutination test. When both tests are used, almost all children with thyroid autoimmunity are detected.

Therapeutic Management

In many cases the goiter is transient and asymptomatic and regresses spontaneously within a year or two. Therapy of a nontoxic diffuse goiter is usually simple, uncomplicated, and effective. Oral administration of TH depresses TSH, thus decreasing the size of the gland significantly. Surgery is contraindicated in this disorder.

Nursing Considerations

Nursing care consists of identifying the youngster with thyroid enlargement, reassuring the child that the condition is probably only temporary, and reinforcing instructions for thyroid therapy.

HYPERTHYROIDISM (GRAVES DISEASE)

The largest percentage of hyperthyroidism in childhood is caused by Graves disease, which is usually associated with an enlarged thyroid gland and exophthalmos (Streetman and Khanderia, 2004; Thompson, 2002). The peak incidence of the disease occurs between 12 and 14 years of age, but it may be present at birth in children of thyrotoxic mothers. The incidence is five times higher in girls than in boys. The disease is apparently caused by a serum thyroid-stimulating immunoglobulin, but no specific etiology has been identified. There is definitive evidence for familial association; a large number of persons with the disease possess the histocompatibility antigen HLA-B8.

Diagnostic Evaluation

The development of manifestations is highly variable (Box 29-4). Manifestations develop gradually, with an interval between onset and diagnosis of approximately 6 to 12 months. Diagnosis is established on the basis of increased levels of T_4 and T_3. Thyrotropin (TSH) is suppressed to unmeasurable levels. Other tests are rarely indicated.

Therapeutic Management

Therapy for hyperthyroidism is controversial, but all methods are directed toward retarding the rate of hormone secretion. The three acceptable modes available are (1) the antithyroid drugs, which interfere with the biosynthesis of TH, including propylthiouracil (PTU) and methimazole (MTZ, Tapazole); (2) subtotal thyroidectomy; and (3) ablation with radioiodine (^{131}I-iodide) (Streetman and Khanderia, 2004; Rivkees and Cornelius, 2003). When affected children exhibit signs and symptoms of hyperthyroidism, their activity should be limited. Vigorous exercise is restricted until thyroid levels are decreased to normal or near-normal values.

Thyrotoxicosis (thyroid "crisis" or thyroid "storm") may occur from sudden release of the hormone. Although it is unusual in children, a crisis can be life-threatening. A crisis may be precipitated by acute infection, surgical emergencies, or discontinuation of antithyroid therapy. Treatment, in addition to antithyroid drugs, is administration of β-adrenergic blocking agents (propranolol), which provide relief from the disturbing side effects of the reaction.

Nursing Considerations

The initial nursing objective is identification of children with hyperthyroidism. Because the clinical manifestations often appear gradually, the goiter and ophthalmic changes may not be noticed, and the excessive activity may be attributed to behavioral problems. Nurses in ambulatory settings, particularly those caring for children in school, need to be alert to signs that suggest this disorder, especially weight loss despite an excellent appetite, academic difficulties resulting from a short attention span and inability to sit still, unexplained fatigue and sleeplessness, and difficulty with fine motor skills (such as writing). Exophthalmos may develop long before the onset of signs and symptoms of hyperthyroidism and may be the only presenting sign (Thompson, 2002).

Much of the care during diagnosis and initial medical therapy is related to the physical symptoms. The child needs a quiet, unstimulating environment that is conducive to rest, and sometimes hospitalization is necessary during the imme-

BOX 29-4 ■ Clinical Manifestations of Hyperthyroidism (Graves Disease)

CARDINAL SIGNS
Emotional lability
Physical restlessness, characteristically at rest
Decelerated school performance
Voracious appetite with weight loss in 50% of cases
Fatigue

PHYSICAL SIGNS
Tachycardia
Widened pulse pressure
Dyspnea on exertion
Exophthalmos (protruding eyeballs)
Wide-eyed, staring expression with lid lag
Tremor
Goiter (hypertrophy and hyperplasia)
Warm, moist skin
Accelerated linear growth
Heat intolerance (may be severe)
Hair fine and unable to hold a curl
Systolic murmurs

THYROID STORM
Acute onset:
  Severe irritability and restlessness
  Vomiting
  Diarrhea
  Hyperthermia
  Hypertension
  Severe tachycardia
  Prostration
May progress rapidly to:
  Delirium
  Coma
  Death

diate treatment phase. A regular routine is beneficial, with frequent rest periods, minimizing the stress of coping with unexpected demands and meeting the child's needs promptly. Physical activity is restricted. For example, school physical education classes are discontinued. Despite the excessive activity of these children, they tire easily, experience muscle weakness, and are unable to relax to recoup their strength.

After therapy is instituted, the nurse explains the drug regimen, emphasizing the importance of observing for side effects of antithyroid drugs. Untoward effects of propylthiouracil and related compounds include skin rash, drug fever, enlargement of the salivary and cervical lymph glands, diminished sense of taste, hepatitis, and edema of the lower extremities.

NURSING ALERT

Children being treated with propyl-thiouracil must be carefully monitored for side effects of the drug. Because sore throat and fever accompany the grave complication of leukopenia, these children should be seen by a practitioner if such symptoms occur. Parents and children should be taught to recognize and report symptoms immediately.

Parents should also be aware of the signs of hypothyroidism, which can occur from overdose of the drugs. The most common indications are lethargy and somnolence.

Surgical Care.
If surgery is anticipated, iodine is usually administered for a few weeks before the procedure. Because oral iodine preparations are unpalatable, they should be mixed with a strong-tasting fruit juice, such as grape or punch flavors, and be given through a straw. Compliance with iodine therapy is essential to avoid the danger of thyroid crisis after sudden discontinuation.

Psychologic preparation of children for thyroidectomy is similar to that for any other surgical procedure (see Chapter 22). However, of special consideration is the site of the incision. The fear of having the throat cut is very real and in older children is associated with death. The nurse should explain that the throat is not cut, only the skin, to allow for removal of the gland. Showing children a picture of the anatomic location of the thyroid around the trachea is often helpful. Children should be prepared for the dressing around the neck and the possibility of an endotracheal or "breathing" tube after surgery.

Postoperative care involves positioning with the neck slightly flexed to avoid strain on the sutures and observation for bleeding and complications. The children are taught to support the neck in this position when they sit up. Damage to the recurrent laryngeal nerve is evidenced by severe stridor or hoarseness, although some hoarseness is expected. Observation for signs of hypoparathyroidism, which causes hypocalcemia, should be implemented in the immediate postoperative period.

✦ NURSING ALERT

The earliest indication of hypoparathyroidism may be anxiety and mental depression, followed by paresthesia and evidence of heightened neuromuscular excitability, such as:

Chvostek sign—Facial muscle spasm elicited by tapping the facial nerve in the region of the parotid gland

Trousseau sign—Carpal spasm elicited by pressure applied to nerves of the upper arm

Tetany—Carpopedal spasm (sharp flexion of wrist and ankle joints), muscle twitching, cramps, seizures, and sometimes stridor

---

DISORDERS OF PARATHYROID FUNCTION

The parathyroid glands secrete *parathormone (PTH),* whose main function, along with vitamin D, is to maintain homeostasis of blood calcium concentration. PTH exerts its effect by (1) increasing the release of calcium and phosphate from the bone (bone demineralization), (2) increasing the absorption of calcium and the excretion of phosphate by the kidneys, and (3) promoting calcium absorption in the gastrointestinal tract. The net result of these actions is to increase the plasma calcium concentration while lowering the plasma phosphate concentration.

HYPOPARATHYROIDISM

Two classic forms of hypoparathyroidism are observed during childhood. *Autoimmune hypoparathyroidism,* in which there is deficient production of PTH, may occur as a component of multiglandular failure, usually in relation to autoimmune phenomena. Familial hypoparathyroidism is inherited as an autosomal recessive trait, with early onset, usually in the first month of life. In *pseudohypoparathyroidism,* production of PTH is increased but end-organ responsiveness to the hormone is deficient. Pseudohypoparathyroidism is also thought to be inherited as an X-linked dominant trait with variable expressivity. Transient hypoparathyroidism may also be observed in infants born to mothers with the disease or in infants fed a milk formula with a high phosphate-to-calcium ratio (see Chapter 9).

Diagnostic Evaluation

The diagnosis of hypoparathyroidism is made on the basis of clinical manifestations associated with *decreased serum calcium* and *increased serum phosphorus levels* (Box 29-5). Levels of plasma PTH are low in idiopathic hypoparathyroidism but high in pseudohypoparathyroidism. End-organ responsiveness is tested by the administration of PTH with

---

BOX 29-5 ■ Clinical Manifestations of Hypoparathyroidism

PSEUDOHYPOPARATHYROIDISM
Short stature
Round face
Short, thick neck
Short, stubby fingers and toes
Dimpling of skin over knuckles
Subcutaneous soft tissue calcifications
Mental retardation a prominent feature

IDIOPATHIC HYPOPARATHYROIDISM
None of the above physical characteristics observed
Papilledema may be seen
May be mental retardation

BOTH TYPES
Dry, scaly, coarse skin with eruptions
Hair often brittle
Nails thin and brittle with characteristic transverse grooves
Dental and enamel hypoplasia
Muscle contractions:
　Tetany
　Carpopedal spasm
　Laryngospasm (laryngeal stridor)
　Muscle cramps and twitching
　Positive Chvostek sign or Trousseau sign (see Nursing Alert at left)
　Paresthesias, tingling
Neurologic:
　Headache
　Seizures (generalized, absence, or focal)
　Swings of emotion
　Loss of memory
　Depression
　Confusion can occur
Gastrointestinal:
　Muscle cramps
　Diarrhea
　Vomiting
Retarded skeletal growth

measurement of urinary cyclic adenosine monophosphate (cAMP). Kidney function tests are included in the differential diagnosis to rule out renal insufficiency. Although bone radiographs are usually normal, they may demonstrate increased bone density and suppressed growth.

Therapeutic Management

The objective of treatment is to maintain normal serum calcium and phosphate levels with a minimum of complications. Acute or severe tetany is corrected immediately by IV and oral administration of calcium gluconate and follow-up daily doses to achieve normal levels. When the diagnosis is confirmed, *vitamin D therapy* is begun. Long-term management consists of administration of massive doses of vitamin D; oral calcium supplementation may be useful, although it is not essential.

Nursing Considerations

The initial objective is recognition of hypocalcemia. Unexplained seizures, irritability (especially to external stimuli), gastrointestinal symptoms (e.g., diarrhea, vomiting, abdominal cramps), and positive signs of tetany should lead the nurse to suspect this disorder. Much of the initial nursing care is related to the physical manifestations and includes institution of seizure and safety precautions, reduction of environmental stimuli (e.g., sudden noises or movements, bright lights), and observation for signs of laryngospasm.

NURSING ALERT

Signs of *laryngospasm* are stridor, hoarseness, and a feeling of tightness in the throat. A tracheostomy set and injectable calcium gluconate should be placed near the bedside for emergency use. The IV administration of calcium gluconate requires precautions against extravasation of the drug and tissue destruction.

After initiation of treatment, the nurse discusses with the parents the need for continuous daily administration of calcium salts and vitamin D. Because vitamin D toxicity can be a serious consequence of therapy, parents are advised to watch for signs, which include weakness, fatigue, lassitude, headache, nausea, vomiting, and diarrhea. Early renal impairment is manifested by polyuria, polydipsia, and nocturia.

HYPERPARATHYROIDISM

Hyperparathyroidism is rare in childhood but can be primary or secondary. The most common cause of primary hyperparathyroidism is adenoma of the gland. The most common causes of secondary hyperparathyroidism are chronic renal disease, renal osteodystrophy, and congenital anomalies of the urinary tract. The common factor is hypercalcemia. The manifestations of hyperparathyroidism are listed in Box 29-6.

Diagnostic Evaluation

Blood studies to confirm *elevated calcium* and *lowered phosphorus levels* are routinely performed. Measurement of PTH, as well as several tests to isolate the cause of the hypercalcemia, such as renal function studies, should be included. Other procedures employed to substantiate the physiologic consequences of the disorder include electrocardiography and radiographic bone surveys.

BOX 29-6 ■ Clinical Manifestations of Hyperparathyroidism

GASTROINTESTINAL
Nausea
Vomiting
Abdominal discomfort
Constipation

CENTRAL NERVOUS SYSTEM
Delusions
Confusion
Hallucinations
Impaired memory
Lack of interest and initiative
Depression
Varying levels of consciousness

NEUROMUSCULAR
Weakness
Easy fatigability
Muscle atrophy (especially proximal muscles of lower limbs)
Tongue twitching
Paresthesias in extremities

SKELETAL
Vague bone pain
Subperiosteal resorption of phalanges
Spontaneous fractures
Absence of lamina dura around teeth

RENAL
Polyuria
Polydipsia
Renal colic
Hypertension

Therapeutic Management

Treatment depends on the cause. The treatment of primary hyperparathyroidism is surgical removal of the tumor or hyperplastic tissue. Treatment of secondary hyperparathyroidism is directed at the underlying contributing cause, thus subsequently restoring the serum calcium balance. However, in some instances, the underlying disorder is irreversible, such as in chronic renal failure (see Chapter 27). In this instance treatment is the same as the treatment for renal osteodystrophy.

Nursing Considerations

Because surgical removal is the major treatment modality, nursing care is similar to that discussed for the child with hyperthyroidism (p. 1072). Because hypocalcemia is a potential complication, observation for signs of tetany, institution of seizure precautions, and having calcium gluconate available for emergency use are part of the nursing care.

DISORDERS OF ADRENAL FUNCTION

The *adrenal cortex* secretes three main groups of hormones collectively called *steroids* and classified according to their biologic activity: (1) *glucocorticoids* (cortisol, corticosterone), (2) *mineralocorticoids* (aldosterone), and (3) *sex steroids* (androgens, estrogens, and progestins). Alterations in the levels of these hormones produce significant dysfunction in a variety of body tissues and organs. Because the adrenocortical cells are capable of producing any of the steroids, pathologic conditions may result in a deficiency or an excess of more than one type of hormone. However, most are rare in children.

The *adrenal medulla* secretes the *catecholamines epinephrine* and *norepinephrine.* Both hormones have essentially the same effects on various organs as those caused by direct sympathetic stimulation, except that the hormonal effects last several times longer. Catecholamine-secreting tumors are the primary cause of adrenal medullary hyperfunction.

ACUTE ADRENOCORTICAL INSUFFICIENCY

The acute form of adrenocortical insufficiency *(adrenal crisis)* may result from a number of causes during childhood. Although it is a rare disorder, some of the more common etiologic factors include hemorrhage into the gland from trauma, which may be caused by a prolonged, difficult labor; fulminating infections, such as meningococcemia, which result in hemorrhage and necrosis (Waterhouse-Friderichsen syndrome); abrupt withdrawal of exogenous sources of cortisone or failure to increase exogenous supplies during stress; or congenital adrenogenital hyperplasia of the salt-losing type.

Diagnostic Evaluation

There is no rapid, definitive test for confirmation of acute adrenocortical insufficiency. Routine procedures such as measurement of plasma cortisol levels are too time consuming to be practical. Therefore diagnosis is usually based on clinical symptoms (Box 29-7). Improvement with cortisol therapy confirms the diagnosis.

Therapeutic Management

Treatment involves replacement of cortisol, replacement of body fluids to correct dehydration and hypovolemia, administration of glucose solutions to correct hypoglycemia, and specific antibiotic therapy in the presence of infection. If hemorrhage has been severe, whole blood may be replaced. In the event that these measures do not reverse the circulatory collapse, vasopressors are used for immediate vasoconstriction and elevation of blood pressure. After the child's condition is stabilized, oral doses of cortisone, fluids, and salt are given, similar to the regimen used for chronic adrenal insufficiency.

Nursing Considerations

Because of the abrupt onset and potentially fatal outcome of this condition, prompt recognition is essential. Vital signs and blood pressure are measured often to monitor the hyperpyrexia and shocklike state. Seizure precautions are instituted, because seizures from the elevated temperature are not uncommon. As soon as therapy is instituted, the nurse monitors the child's response to fluid and cortisol replacement, being alert to too-rapid administration of fluids and drugs. Overtreatment with cortisol and sodium chloride can precipitate complications such as an ascending flaccid paralysis. The nurse should observe for signs of hypokalemia and should evaluate serum electrolyte levels. The condition is rapidly corrected with IV and oral potassium replacement. Intake and urine output are measured and recorded.

BOX 29-7 ■ Clinical Manifestations of Acute Adrenocortical Insufficiency

EARLY SYMPTOMS
Increased irritability
Headache
Diffuse abdominal pain
Weakness
Nausea and vomiting
Diarrhea

GENERALIZED HEMORRHAGIC MANIFESTATIONS (WATERHOUSE-FRIDERICHSEN SYNDROME)
Fever—increases as condition worsens
Central nervous system signs
   Nuchal rigidity
   Seizures
   Stupor
   Coma

SHOCKLIKE STATE
Weak, rapid pulse
Decreased blood pressure
Shallow respirations
Cold, clammy skin
Cyanosis
Circulatory collapse (terminal event)

NEWBORN
Hyperpyrexia
Tachypnea
Cyanosis
Seizures
Gland may be evident as palpable retroperitoneal mass (hemorrhagic)

⚠ NURSING ALERT

Monitor serum electrolyte levels and observe for signs of hypokalemia or hyperkalemia, (e.g., weakness, poor muscle control, paralysis, cardiac dysrhythmias, apnea).

NURSING TIP

When the oral preparation is given, potassium supplement should be mixed with a small amount of strongly flavored fruit juice to disguise its bitter taste.

The sudden, severe nature of this disorder requires considerable emotional support for the child and family. The child is usually in an intensive care unit, where the surroundings are strange and frightening. Because recovery within 24 hours is often dramatic, the nurse should keep the parents apprised of the child's condition, emphasizing signs of improvement, such as a lowered temperature and elevated blood pressure. If paralysis occurs, the nurse should assure them that this condition is temporary and quickly reversed.

CHRONIC ADRENOCORTICAL INSUFFICIENCY (ADDISON DISEASE)

Chronic adrenocortical insufficiency is rare in children. When it does occur, it is usually caused by a destructive lesion of the adrenal glands or a neoplasm or it has an idiopathic cause.

BOX 29-8 ■ Clinical Manifestations of Chronic Adrenocortical Insufficiency

NEUROLOGIC SYMPTOMS
Muscular weakness
Mental fatigue
Irritability, apathy, and negativism
Increased sleeping, listlessness

PIGMENTARY CHANGES
Previous scars
Palmar creases
Mucous membranes
Hair
Hyperpigmentation over pressure points (elbows, knees, or waist)
Less frequently, vitiligo (loss of pigmentation)

GASTROINTESTINAL SYMPTOMS
Dehydration
Anorexia
Weight loss

CIRCULATORY SYMPTOMS
Hypotension
Small heart size
Dizziness
Syncopal (fainting) attacks

HYPOGLYCEMIA
Headache
Hunger
Weakness
Trembling
Sweating

OTHER SIGNS (SEEN IN SOME CHILDREN)
Recurrent, unexplained seizures
Intense craving for salt
Acute abdominal pain
Electrolyte imbalances

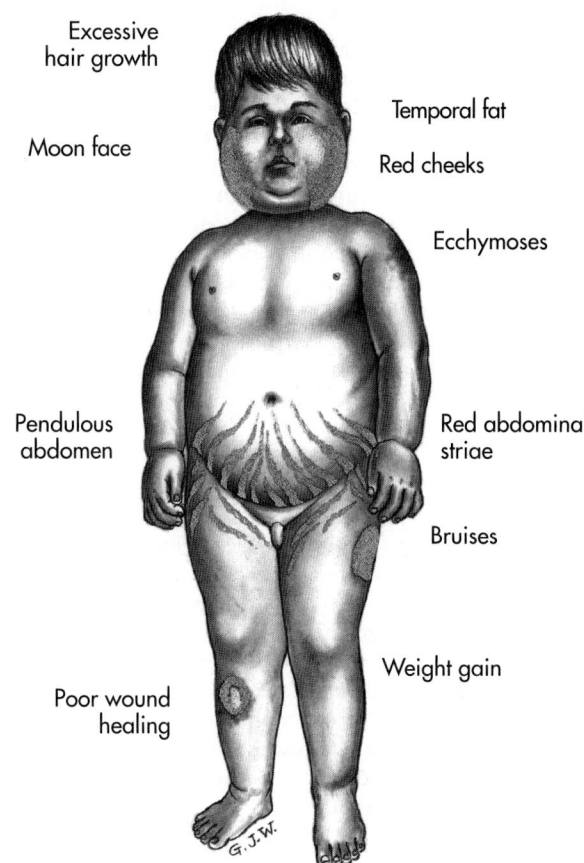

FIG. 29-2 ■ Characteristics of Cushing syndrome.

Evidence of this disorder is usually gradual in onset, because 90% of adrenal tissue must be nonfunctional before signs of insufficiency are manifested (Box 29-8). However, during periods of stress, when demands for additional cortisol are increased, symptoms of acute insufficiency may appear in a previously well child.

Definitive diagnosis is based on measurements of functional cortisol reserve. The cortisol and urinary 17-hydroxycorticosteroid levels are low and fail to rise, whereas plasma *adrenocorticotropic hormone (ACTH)* levels are elevated with corticotropin stimulation, the definitive test for the disease.

Therapeutic Management

Treatment involves replacement of *glucocorticoids (cortisol)* and *mineralocorticoids (aldosterone)*. Some children are able to be maintained solely on oral supplements of cortisol (cortisone or hydrocortisone preparations) with a liberal intake of salt. Other forms of therapy include monthly injections of desoxycorticosterone acetate or implantation of desoxycortico-

sterone acetate pellets subcutaneously every 9 to 12 months. During stressful situations, such as infection, emotional upset, or surgery, the dosage must be tripled to accommodate the body's increased need for glucocorticoids. Failure to meet this requirement will precipitate an acute crisis. Overdosage produces cushingoid signs (Fig. 29-2).

Nursing Considerations

After the disorder is diagnosed, parents need guidance concerning drug therapy. They must be aware of the continuous need for cortisol replacement. Sudden termination of the drug because of inadequate supplies or inability to ingest the oral form because of vomiting places the child in danger of an acute adrenal crisis. Ideally, the parents should have a prefilled syringe of hydrocortisone in the home and should be taught the proper technique for intramuscular administration of the drug in case of a crisis. Unnecessary administration of cortisone will not harm the child but, if needed, may be lifesaving. Any evidence of acute insufficiency is reported to the practitioner immediately.

Because the body cannot supply endogenous sources of cortical hormones during times of stress, the home environment should be stable and relatively unstressful. Parents need to be aware that during periods of emotional or physical crisis the child requires additional hormone replacement. The child should wear medical identification to permit medical personnel to adjust the requirements during emergency care.

CUSHING SYNDROME

Cushing syndrome is a characteristic group of manifestations caused by excessive circulating free cortisol. It can result from a variety of etiologies, which generally fall into one of five categories (Box 29-9). Cushing syndrome in young children may be due to an adrenal tumor (Moshang, 2003).

Cushing syndrome is uncommon in children. When seen, it is often caused by excessive or prolonged steroid therapy, which produces a cushingoid appearance (Box 29-10; see also Fig. 29-2). This condition is reversible after steroids are discontinued. Abrupt withdrawal may precipitate acute adrenal insufficiency; gradual withdrawal of exogenous supplies is necessary to allow the anterior pituitary an opportunity to secrete increasing amounts of ACTH to stimulate the adrenals to produce cortisol.

Diagnostic Evaluation

Several tests are helpful in confirming excess cortisol levels. These include fasting blood glucose levels for hyperglycemia, serum electrolyte levels for hypokalemia and alkalosis, 24-hour urinary levels of elevated 17-hydroxycorticoids and 17-ketosteroids, and radiographic studies of bone for evidence of osteoporosis and of the skull for enlargement of the sella turcica. Administration of an exogenous supply of cortisone normally suppresses ACTH production. However, in individuals with Cushing syndrome, cortisol levels remain elevated. This test is helpful in differentiating between children who are obese and those who appear to have cushingoid features.

Therapeutic Management

Treatment of Cushing syndrome depends on the cause. In most cases surgical intervention involves bilateral adrenalectomy and postoperative replacement of the cortical hormones (the therapy for this is the same as that outlined for chronic adrenal insufficiency). If a pituitary tumor is found, surgical extirpation or irradiation may be chosen. In either of these instances treatment of panhypopituitarism with replacement of growth hormone, thyroid extract, antidiuretic hormone, gonadotropins, and steroids may be necessary for an indefinite period.

Nursing Considerations

Nursing care also depends on the cause. When cushingoid features are caused by steroid therapy, the effects may be lessened with administration of the drug early in the morning and on an alternate-day basis. Giving the drug early in the day maintains the normal diurnal pattern of cortisol secretion. If given during the evening, the drug is more likely to produce symptoms, because endogenous cortisol levels are already low and the additional supply exerts more pronounced effects. An alternate-day schedule allows the anterior pituitary an opportunity to maintain more normal hypothalamic-pituitary-adrenal control mechanisms.

If an organic cause is found, nursing care is related to the treatment regimen. Although a bilateral adrenalectomy permanently solves one condition, it also produces another syndrome. Before surgery, parents need to be adequately informed of the operative benefits and disadvantages. Postoperative teaching regarding drug replacement is a nursing function.

BOX 29-9 ■ Etiology of Cushing Syndrome

Pituitary—Cushing syndrome with adrenal hyperplasia, usually attributed to an excess of adrenocorticotropin hormone (ACTH)

Adrenal—Cushing syndrome with hypersecretion of glucocorticoids, generally a result of adrenocortical neoplasms

Ectopic—Cushing syndrome with autonomous secretion of ACTH, most often caused by extrapituitary neoplasms

Iatrogenic—Cushing syndrome, frequently a result of administration of large amounts of exogenous corticosteroids

Food dependent—Inappropriate sensitivity of adrenal glands to normal postprandial increases in secretion of gastric inhibitory polypeptide (Magiakou and others, 1994)

BOX 29-10 ■ Clinical Manifestations of Cushing Syndrome

Centripetal fat distribution
   Truncal obesity
   Supraclavicular fat pads
   Fat pads on neck and back ("buffalo hump")
Rounded or "moon" face
Muscular wasting
   Thin extremities
   Pendulous abdomen
   Muscle weakness
Thin skin and subcutaneous tissue
Poor wound healing
Increased susceptibility to infection
Decreased inflammatory response
Excessive bruising
Petechial hemorrhages
Facial plethora ("red cheeks")
Reddish purple abdominal striae
Hypertension
Hypokalemia
Alkalosis
Osteoporosis
   Compression fractures of vertebrae
   Kyphosis
   Backache
   Retarded linear growth
Hypercalciuria—renal calculi
Psychoses
   Irritability
   Insomnia
   Euphoria
   Depression
   Frank psychoses
Peptic ulcer
Hyperglycemia
   Glycosuria
   Latent or overt diabetes
Virilization
   Hirsutism (excessive body hair)
   Acne
   Deepening of voice
   Clitoral enlargement
   Tendency toward male physique in female
Amenorrhea
Impotence

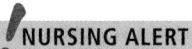

NURSING ALERT

Postoperative complications of adrenalectomy are related to the sudden withdrawal of cortisol. Observe for signs of a shocklike state, especially hypotension and hyperpyrexia.

CONGENITAL ADRENOGENITAL HYPERPLASIA

Congenital adrenogenital hyperplasia (CAH) is a family of disorders caused by decreased enzyme activity required for cortisol production in the adrenal cortex. The most common defect is 21-hydroxylase deficiency, which constitutes more than 90% of all cases of CAH (Levine, 2000). This deficiency occurs in approximately 1 per 12,000 to 1 per 15,000 births and causes overproduction of the adrenal androgens, resulting in virilization of the female fetus.

Pathophysiology

Interference in the biosynthesis of cortisol during fetal life results in an increased production of ACTH, which stimulates hyperplasia of the adrenal gland. Depending on the enzymatic defect, increased quantities of cortisol precursors and androgens are secreted. There are six major types of biochemical defects. In each there is excess production of androgens, which causes ambiguous genitalia in females and precocious genital development in males. In both sexes, linear growth is accelerated and epiphyseal closure is premature, ultimately resulting in short stature. Other forms of CAH do not result in excess production of androgens but cause various degrees of hypoaldosteronism or hyperaldosteronism.

The most common biochemical defect is partial or complete *21-hydroxylase deficiency.* With partial deficiency, enough aldosterone is produced to preserve sodium and adequate cortisol is produced to prevent signs of adrenocortical insufficiency. In the complete or salt-losing form, insufficient amounts of aldosterone and cortisol are produced, so that circulatory collapse occurs without immediate replacement of the mineralocorticoids and glucocorticoids.

Diagnostic Evaluation

Clinical diagnosis is initially based on congenital abnormalities that lead to difficulty in assigning sex to the newborn (Box 29-11) and on signs and symptoms of adrenal insufficiency or hypertension. Definitive diagnosis is confirmed by evidence of increased 17-ketosteroid levels in most types of CAH (Levine, 2000). Blood electrolytes demonstrate loss of sodium and chloride and elevation of potassium. A karyotype for positive sex determination should always be done in any case of ambiguous genitalia.

Ultrasonography can also be used to visualize the presence of pelvic structures. It is especially useful in CAH to identify the absence or presence of female reproductive organs in a newborn or child with ambiguous genitalia. Because it yields immediate results, it has the advantage of determining the child's gender long before the more complex laboratory results for chromosome analysis or steroid levels are available.

Therapeutic Management

The initial medical objective is to confirm the diagnosis and assign a sex to the child, usually according to the genotype. In both sexes cortisone is administered to sup-

---

BOX 29-11 ■ Clinical Manifestations of Adrenogenital Hyperplasia

Female: Masculinization
   Enlarged clitoris (appears as small phallus)
   Fusion of labia (saclike structure resembling a scrotum)
   Vaginal orifice usually closed by fused labia
Male: Precocious genital development
   Genital enlargement (macrogenitosomia precox)
   Frequent erections
Untreated: Early sexual maturation
   Enlargement of external sexual organs
   Development of axillary, pubic, and facial hair
   Deepening of voice
   Acne
   Marked increase in musculature (changes toward an adult male physique)
   Accelerated linear growth
   Premature epiphyseal closure (short stature by end of puberty)
Female:
   No breast development
   Females remain amenorrheic and infertile
Male:
   Testes remain small

---

press the abnormally high secretions of ACTH. Cortisone depresses the secretion of ACTH by the adenohypophysis, which in turn inhibits the secretion of adrenocorticosteroids, which stems the progressive virilization. If cortisol is given early enough, the signs and symptoms of masculinization in the female gradually disappear, and excessive early linear growth is slowed. Puberty occurs normally at the appropriate age.

Because these children are unable to produce cortisol in response to stress, the dosage is increased during episodes of infection, fever, or other stresses. Acute emergencies require immediate IV or intramuscular administration. Children with the salt-losing type of CAH require aldosterone replacement and supplementary dietary salt.

Depending on the degree of masculinization in the female, reconstructive surgery may be required to reduce the size of the clitoris, separate the labia, and create a vaginal orifice. This should be done after the infant is physically able to tolerate the procedure and before she is old enough to be aware of the abnormal genitalia. Plastic surgery is generally done in stages and yields excellent cosmetic results. The capacity for orgasm is not necessarily impaired and fertility is preserved.

Unfortunately, not all children with CAH are diagnosed at birth and raised in accordance with their genetic sex. Particularly in the case of affected females, masculinization of the external genitalia may have led to sex assignment as a male. In these situations it is advisable to continue rearing the child as a male in accordance with the assigned sex and phenotype. Hormone replacement may be required to permit linear growth and to initiate male pubertal changes. Surgery is usually indicated to remove the female organs and reconstruct the phallus for satisfactory sexual relations. These individuals are not fertile. Males with the non–salt-losing variant of CAH may go undiagnosed until early childhood when premature virilism occurs.

Nursing Considerations

The nursing care of the child with CAH and the family is concerned primarily with identifying the condition and providing support and assistance. Of major importance is recognition of ambiguous genitalia in newborns. If there is any question regarding assignment of sex, the parents need to be told immediately to prevent the embarrassing situation of informing family members of the child's sex and then having to change the announcement. As with any congenital defect, the parents require an adequate explanation of the condition and a period of time to grieve for the loss of perfection. Parents need an explanation regarding this disorder that facilitates their explaining it to others. The external genitalia are referred to as sex organs, and the similarity between the penis/clitoris and scrotum/labia during fetal development is emphasized to help parents understand that too much male hormone secretion caused some organs to overdevelop. Using a correct vocabulary allows parents to explain the abnormalities to others in a straightforward manner, just as if the defect involved the heart or an extremity. As soon as the sex is determined, parents are informed of the findings and encouraged to choose an appropriate name, and the child is identified as a male or female, with no reference to ambiguous sex. If the appearance of the enlarged genitalia in a female child concerns the parents, they are encouraged to discuss their feelings.

Nursing considerations regarding cortisol and aldosterone replacement are the same as those for chronic adrenocortical insufficiency. A follow-up visit by a home health nurse may be desirable to ensure that parents understand and comply with the treatment regimen. Likewise, nurses in well-child facilities should assume responsibility for guidance and supervision regarding this aspect of care during each visit.

Because these infants are especially prone to dehydration and salt-losing crises, parents need to be aware of signs of dehydration and the urgency of immediate medical intervention to stabilize the child's condition. Parents, and later the child, need to understand that the medical regimen must be a lifelong commitment; therefore, they should be provided with the education and counseling that is most likely to ensure informed and willing compliance. They also need to know that growth retardation that may have occurred before therapy cannot be overcome and that normal stature is not a realistic expectation, even though growth velocity may improve with medication. The parents are also taught to give necessary injections (see Chapter 22).

In the unfortunate situation in which the sex is erroneously assigned and the correct sex determined later, parents need a great deal of help in understanding the reason for the incorrect sex identification and the options for sex reassignment or medical/surgical intervention.

> **⚠ NURSING ALERT**
>
> The parents should be advised that there is no physical harm in treating for suspected adrenal insufficiency that is not present, whereas the consequence of not treating acute adrenal insufficiency can be fatal (Ruble, 1996).

Because the hereditary form of adrenogenital hyperplasia is an autosomal-recessive disorder, parents should be referred to genetic counseling before conceiving another child. Prenatal treatment with glucocorticoid (dexamethasone) can be offered to the mother during subsequent pregnancies to prevent the occurrence of sex ambiguity. Likewise, affected offspring also require genetic counseling, since both sexes are generally able to reproduce. (See genetic counseling in Chapter 9 and Appendix B.)

HYPERALDOSTERONISM

Excessive secretion of aldosterone may be caused by an adrenal tumor; also, in some types of adrenogenital syndromes, symptoms are caused by increased sodium levels, water retention, and potassium loss. The clinical diagnosis is suspected when there are findings of hypertension, hypokalemia, and polyuria that fail to respond to antidiuretic hormone administration.

Therapeutic Management

Temporary treatment of the disorder involves replacement of potassium and administration of *spironolactone (Aldactone),* a diuretic that blocks the effects of aldosterone. Definitive treatment is similar to that for chronic adrenocortical insufficiency.

Nursing Considerations

An important nursing consideration is recognition of the syndrome, particularly in children who demonstrate high blood pressure. After the diagnosis, nursing care is related to the treatment regimen, such as education about the diuretic and potassium supplements (see Nursing Tip, p. 1074). Parents need to be aware of the signs of hypokalemia and hyperkalemia (see Nursing Alert, p. 1074).

PHEOCHROMOCYTOMA

Pheochromocytoma is an adrenal tumor characterized by secretion of catecholamines. The tumor most commonly arises from the chromaffin cells of the adrenal medulla but may occur wherever these cells are found, such as along the paraganglia of the aorta or thoracolumbar sympathetic chain. In children this type of tumor is most frequently bilateral or multiple and is generally benign. Often there is a familial transmission of the condition as an autosomal-dominant trait that tends to favor males. The clinical manifestations of pheochromocytoma are caused by an increased production of catecholamines, and they mimic those of other disorders, such as hyperthyroidism, diabetes mellitus, or functional hyperventilation (Box 29-12).

Therapeutic Management

Definitive treatment consists of surgical removal of the tumor. In children the tumors may be bilateral, requiring a bilateral adrenalectomy and lifelong glucocorticoid and mineralocorticoid therapy.

Nursing Considerations

An initial nursing objective is identification of children with this disorder. Outstanding clues are hypertension and hypertensive attacks. Preoperative nursing care involves frequent monitoring of vital signs and observing for evidence of hypertensive attacks and congestive heart failure. Urine should be tested at least daily for glucose and ketones. Any signs of hyperglycemia are noted and reported immediately.

BOX 29-12 ■ Clinical Manifestations of Pheochromocytoma

Hypertension	Polyuria
Tachycardia	Polydipsia
Headache	Hyperventilation
Decreased gastrointestinal activity; resultant constipation	Nervousness
	Heat intolerance
Anorexia	Diaphoresis
Weight loss	Signs of congestive heart
Hyperglycemia	failure in severe cases

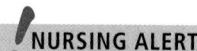

NURSING ALERT

DO NOT PALPATE MASS. Preoperative palpation may facilitate release of catecholamines, which can stimulate severe hypertension and tachyarrhythmias.

The environment should be conducive to rest and free of emotional stress. This requires adequate preparation during hospital admission and before surgery. Parents are encouraged to room-in with their child and to participate in the care. Play activities need to be tailored to the child's energy level but should not be overly strenuous or challenging, because these can increase the metabolic rate and promote frustration and anxiety.

After surgery the child is observed for signs of shock from removal of excess catecholamines. If a bilateral adrenalectomy was performed, the nursing interventions are those discussed for chronic adrenocortical insufficiency.

DISORDERS OF PANCREATIC HORMONE FUNCTION

The islets of Langerhans of the pancreas have three major functioning cells:

1 The *alpha cells* produce *glucagon,* which increases the blood glucose levels by stimulating the liver and other cells to release stored glucose (glycogenolysis).
2 The *beta cells* produce *insulin,* which lowers blood glucose levels by facilitating the entrance of glucose into the cells for metabolism.
3 The *delta cells* produce *somatostatin,* which is believed to regulate the release of insulin and glucagon.

The discussion of disorders of pancreatic hormone secretion is limited to diabetes mellitus.

DIABETES MELLITUS

Diabetes mellitus (DM) is a disease of metabolism characterized by a total or partial deficiency of the hormone *insulin,* resulting in a metabolic adjustment or physiologic change in almost all areas of the body. It is the most common endocrine disorder of childhood, with the peak incidence reached during early adolescence (Ross, 2003).

Classification

Traditionally DM had been classified according to the type of treatment needed. The old categories were insulin-dependent diabetes mellitus (IDDM), or type I, and non–insulin-dependent diabetes mellitus (NIDDM), or type II. In 1997 these terms were eliminated because treatment can vary (some people with NIDDM require insulin) and because the terms do not indicate the underlying problem. The new terms are type 1 and type 2, using Arabic symbols to avoid confusion (e.g., type II could be read as type eleven) (American Diabetes Association, 2001).

Type 1 diabetes is characterized by destruction of the pancreatic beta cells, which produce insulin: this usually leads to absolute insulin deficiency. Type 1 diabetes has two forms. *Immune-mediated diabetes mellitus* results from an autoimmune destruction of the beta cells. It typically starts in children or young adults who are slim, but it can arise in adults of any age. *Idiopathic type 1* refers to rare forms of the disease that have no known cause.

Type 2 diabetes usually arises because of insulin resistance, in which the body fails to use insulin properly, combined with relative (rather then absolute) insulin deficiency. People with type 2 can range from predominantly insulin resistant with relative insulin deficiency to predominantly deficient in insulin secretion with some insulin resistance. In the past, type 2 diabetes occurred in those who were older than age 45, were overweight and sedentary, and had a family history of diabetes.

Changes in food consumption and exercise patterns have increased the rate of type 2 diabetes mellitus in children and adolescents in the United States (Ramchandani, 2004; Kiess and others, 2003; Steinberger and Daniels, 2003; Stephenson, 2003).

Etiology

The clinical syndrome of DM results from a large variety of etiologic and pathogenic mechanisms. Type 1 DM is now believed to be an autoimmune disease that arises when a person with a genetic predisposition is exposed to a precipitating event, such as a viral infection.

Genetic Factors.   Type 1 DM is not inherited, but heredity is a prominent factor in the etiology. A variety of genetic mechanisms have been proposed, but most authorities favor a multifactorial inheritance or a recessive gene somehow linked to the human lymphocyte antigen (HLA). However, the genetic influence in type 1 DM and type 2 DM appears to differ in several ways. Studies of type 2 DM in identical twins demonstrate a 90% to 100% concordance throughout the lifespan, whereas studies of type 1 DM in identical twins demonstrate a 30% to 50% concordance rate (Stephenson, 2003; Redondo, Fain, and Elisenbath, 2001). Children diagnosed with type 1 diabetes before 5 years of age may have different autoimmune and genetic characteristics related to their diabetes than older children (Hathout and others, 2003).

Autoimmune Mechanisms.   An autoimmune process is involved in persons who develop type 1 DM. The current theory is that the presence of the HLA genes causes a defect in the immune system that renders the possessor susceptible to a trigger event, which can be a dietary source (Kimpimaki and others, 2001), virus, bacterium, or chemical irritant. The predisposing event initiates an autoimmune process that gradually destroys beta cells. Without beta cells, no insulin can be produced. There is also a strong association between type 1 DM and other autoimmune endocrine disorders, such as thyroiditis and Addison disease.

Pathophysiology

Insulin is needed to support the metabolism of carbohydrates, fats, and proteins, primarily by facilitating the entry of these substances into the cell, with the exception of nerve cells and vascular tissue. With a deficiency of insulin, glucose is unable to enter the cell, and its concentration in the bloodstream *(hyperglycemia)* increases. The increased concentration of glucose produces an osmotic gradient that causes the movement of body fluid from the intracellular space to the extracellular space; from there the body fluid is excreted by the kidneys. When the serum glucose level exceeds the renal threshold (±180 mg/dL), glucose "spills" into the urine *(glycosuria),* along with an osmotic diversion of water *(polyuria),* a cardinal sign of diabetes. The urinary fluid losses cause the excessive thirst *(polydipsia)* observed in diabetes. As might be expected, this water washout results in a depletion of other essential chemicals.

Protein is also wasted during insulin deficiency. Because glucose is unable to enter the cells, protein is broken down and converted to glucose by the liver *(glucogenesis);* this glucose then contributes to the hyperglycemia. Without the use of carbohydrates for energy, fat and protein stores are depleted as the body attempts to meet its energy needs. The hunger mechanism is triggered, but the increased food intake *(polyphagia)* enhances the problem by further elevating the blood glucose.

Ketoacidosis.

When insulin is absent, glucose is unavailable for cellular metabolism and the body chooses alternate sources of energy, principally fat. Consequently, fats break down into fatty acids, and glycerol in the fat cells and liver is converted to ketone bodies (β-hydroxybutyric acid, acetoacetic acid, acetone). The ketone bodies can be used as an alternative source of fuel for glucose, but they are used in the cells at a limited rate. Any excess is eliminated in the urine *(ketonuria)* or the lungs (acetone breath). The ketone bodies in the blood *(ketonemia)* are strong acids that lower serum pH, producing *ketoacidosis.* The respiratory system attempts to eliminate the excess carbon dioxide by increased depth and rate—*Kussmaul respirations,* the hyperventilation characteristic of metabolic acidosis.

With cellular death, potassium is released from the cell into the interstitial spaces and then into the bloodstream. It is then excreted by the kidney, where the loss is accelerated by osmotic diuresis. The total-body potassium level is then decreased, even though the serum potassium level may be elevated as a result of the decreased fluid volume in which it circulates. Alteration in serum and tissue potassium can make cardiac arrest a potential problem.

If these conditions are not reversed by insulin therapy in combination with correction of the fluid deficiency and electrolyte imbalance, progressive deterioration occurs, with dehydration, electrolyte imbalance, acidosis, coma, and death. *Diabetic ketoacidosis (DKA)* is a pediatric emergency and should be diagnosed promptly, with therapy instituted.

Long-Term Complications.

Long-term complications of diabetes involve the small, and the larger, blood vessels. The principal microvascular complications are *nephropathy* and *retinopathy.* The process appears to be one of *glycosylation,* wherein proteins from the blood become deposited in the basement membrane of small vessels (e.g., glomeruli, retina), where they become trapped by "sticky" glucose compounds (glycosyl radicals). The buildup of these substances over time causes narrowing of the vessels with subsequent interference with microcirculation to the affected areas. With poor control, vascular changes appear as early as 2.5 to 3 years after diagnosis; with good control, changes have been postponed for 20 or more years.

Neuropathy appears to be an identical process, but glycosylation occurs on the sheath of nerves, interrupting neurotransmission of stimuli. Macrovascular disease may develop after 25 years of diabetes and creates the predominant complications in patients with type 2 DM. Intensive insulin therapy appears to delay the onset and slow the progression of clinically important retinopathy (including vision loss), nephropathy, and neuropathy by 35% to more than 70% (Wunderlich and others, 1998).

> **!NURSING ALERT**
>
> Recurrent urinary tract and vaginal infections, especially with *Candida albicans,* are often an early sign of type 1 DM, especially in adolescents.

Diagnostic Evaluation

Three groups of children who should be considered at risk for diabetes are (1) those who have glycosuria, polyuria, and a history of weight loss or failure to gain despite a hearty appetite; (2) those with transient or persistent glycosuria; and (3) those who display manifestations of metabolic acidosis, with or without stupor or coma. Clinical manifestations of type 1 DM are outlined in Box 29-13. Diabetes is a great imitator; influenza, gastroenteritis, and appendicitis are the conditions most often diagnosed.

An 8-hour fasting blood glucose level ≥126 mg/dL, a random blood glucose value of ≥200 accompanied by classic signs of diabetes, or an oral glucose tolerance test (OGTT) finding ≥200 mg/dL in the 2-hour sample is almost certain to indicate diabetes (Hoffman, 2003; American Diabetes Association, 2001). Postprandial blood glucose determinations and the traditional OGTTs have yielded low detection rates in children and are not usually necessary for establishing a diagnosis. Serum insulin levels may be normal or moderately elevated at the onset of diabetes; delayed insulin response to glucose indicates the presence of impaired glucose tolerance.

Ketoacidosis must be differentiated from other causes of acidosis or coma, including hypoglycemia, uremia, gastroenteritis with metabolic acidosis, salicylate intoxication encephalitis, and other intracranial lesions. DKA is a state of relative insulin insufficiency and may include the presence of hyperglycemia (blood glucose level ≥330 mg/dL), ketonemia (strongly positive), acidosis (pH <7.30 and bicarbonate <15 mmol/L), glycosuria, and ketonuria (Magee and Bhatt, 2001). Tests used to determine glycosuria and ketonuria include glucose oxidase tapes (Keto-Diastix).

BOX 29-13 ■ Clinical Manifestations of Type 1 Diabetes Mellitus

Polyphagia
Polyuria
Polydipsia
Weight loss
Enuresis or nocturia
Irritability and "not himself" or "herself"
Shortened attention span
Lowered frustration tolerance
Fatigue
Dry skin
Blurred vision
Poor wound healing
Flushed skin
Headache

Frequent infections
Hyperglycemia:
  Elevated blood glucose levels
  Glucosuria
  Diabetic ketosis:
    Ketones, as well as glucose, in urine
  Dehydration may or may not be present
  Diabetic ketoacidosis:
    Dehydration
    Electrolyte imbalance
    Acidosis
    Deep, rapid breathing (Kussmaul)

Therapeutic Management

The definitive treatment is replacement of insulin. However, insulin needs are affected by nutritional intake, activity, emotions, and other life events, such as illnesses and puberty. Medical and nutritional guidance are primary, but management also includes continuing diabetes education, family guidance, and emotional support.

Insulin Therapy. Insulin is available in highly purified pork preparations and in human insulin manufactured by biosynthesis. Most clinicians suggest human insulin as the treatment of choice. It is available in rapid-, short-, intermediate-, and long-acting preparations, and all are packaged in the strength of 100 units/mL (see Box 29-14). (Other dosages are available for situations in which extraordinarily large or small dosages are required.)

NURSING TIP

Insulin comes dissolved in liquids at different strengths. Most people use U-100 insulin. This means it has 100 units of insulin per milliliter (mL) of fluid. Be sure that the syringe you use matches the insulin strength. U-100 insulin needs a U-100 syringe.

Daily insulin is administered subcutaneously by twice-daily injections, by multiple-dose injections, or by means of a portable pump. Diabetes can be controlled satisfactorily in most children with a ***twice-daily insulin*** regimen consisting of a combination of ***rapid-acting (lispro)*** or ***short-acting (regular)*** and ***intermediate-acting (NPH or Lente)*** insulin given in the same syringe before breakfast and before the evening meal. The amount of insulin is determined by measurements of the blood glucose level after the peak effect of the insulin has occurred. For example, the amount of regular insulin at breakfast is determined by a pattern of the previous lunchtime blood glucose values. Regular insulin is best given at least 30 minutes before meals to allow sufficient time for absorption. On the other hand, lispro insulin is best given no more than 10 to 15 minutes before the meal. Some children require more frequent administration of insulin. This includes children with difficult-to-control diabetes and children during

BOX 29-14 ■ Types of Insulin

There are four types of insulin, based on the following criteria:
■ How soon the insulin starts working (onset)
■ When the insulin works the hardest (peak time)
■ How long the insulin lasts in your body (duration).
However, each person responds to insulin in his or her own way. That is why onset, peak time, and duration are given as ranges.

Rapid-acting insulin (Lispro) reaches the blood within 15 minutes after injection. The insulin peaks 30 to 90 minutes later and may last as long as 5 hours.

Short-acting (regular) insulin usually reaches the blood within 30 minutes after injection. The insulin peaks 2 to 4 hours later and stays in the blood for about 4 to 8 hours.

Intermediate-acting (NPH and lente) insulins reach the blood 2 to 6 hours after injection. The insulins peak 4 to 14 hours later and stay in the blood for about 14 to 20 hours.

Long-acting (ultralente) insulin takes 6 to 14 hours to start working. It has no peak or a very small peak 10 to 16 hours after injection. The insulin stays in the blood between 20 to 24 hours.

Some insulins come mixed together. For example, you can buy regular insulin and NPH insulins already mixed in one bottle, which makes it easier to inject two kinds of insulin at the same time. However, you can't adjust the amount of one insulin without also changing how much you get of the other insulin.

the adolescent growth spurt. An intensive insulin management program has been shown to reduce microvascular complications in young, healthy patients who have type 1 DM.

NURSING TIP

Never store insulin at very cold (less than 36° F) or very hot (more than 86° F) temperatures. Extreme temperatures destroy insulin.

Insulin may lose some potency if the bottle has been opened for more than 30 days. Look at the bottle of insulin closely to make sure the insulin looks normal. Regular insulin should be perfectly clear—no floating pieces or color. NPH or lente insulin should be cloudy, with no floating pieces or crystals on the bottle.

The ***insulin pump*** is designed to deliver fixed amounts of regular or lispro insulin continuously, thereby more closely imitating the release of the hormone by the islet cells (Olohan and Zappitelli, 2003). The system consists of a syringe to hold the insulin, a plunger, and a computerized mechanism to drive the plunger. The insulin flows from the syringe through a catheter to a needle inserted into subcutaneous tissue (the abdomen or thigh), and the lightweight device is worn on a belt or a shoulder holster. The tubing and catheter are changed every 48 hours by the child or parent, using aseptic technique, and taped in place.

Although the pump provides more even insulin release, it has disadvantages. It should not be removed for more than 1 to 2 hours, which may limit some activities, such as bathing and swimming, although some water-safe models are now available; skin infections are common; and, as with any other mechanical device, it is subject to malfunction. However, the pumps are equipped with alarms that signal problems that may arise, such as depleted batteries, an occluded needle or tubing, or a microprocessor malfunction.

Researchers are experimenting with *intranasal* and *inhaled insulin administration* (Skyler and others, 2001). Given nasally or deep into the lungs, the insulin is able to cross the mucosa to increase serum levels. The duration of action is not long enough to be a total replacement for injections but may be of value as insulin supplementation at mealtime.

Islet cell or *whole pancreas transplantation* may offer hope to patients in the future. Viable insulin-producing cells have been injected into the portal vein, where they take root in the liver and eventually produce up to two thirds of the needed insulin. The major use of transplants has been in persons who have serious complications, particularly those whose deteriorating kidneys require renal transplants and who are receiving immunosuppression therapy. However, islet cell and pancreatic transplants tend not to be sustainable over time despite continuation of therapy. The use of nonhuman islets encapsulated in immunoprotective, semipermeable membranes may have a future in the treatment of type 1 DM (Robertson and others, 2000; Lanza and others, 1999).

Monitoring.   *Self-blood glucose monitoring (SBGM)* has improved diabetes management and is used successfully by children from the onset of their diabetes. By testing their own blood, children and parents are able to change their insulin regimen to maintain their glucose level in the euglycemic (normal) range of 80 to 120 mg/dL. Diabetes management depends to a great extent on SBGM. Table 29-2 provides an overview of the features of several glucose monitoring units. Two new devices that measure and record blood glucose levels automatically have been approved by the FDA for use in children (Chase and others, 2003; Olohan and Zappitelli, 2003; Cox, 2002). The GlucoWatch Biographer uses reverse iontophoresis to draw interstitial fluid through the skin to measure the glucose level with an electrochemical sensor (Chase and others, 2003; Olohan and Zappitelli, 2003; Plotnick, 2003).

Laboratory measurement of *glycosylated hemoglobin (hemoglobin A_{1c})* levels reflects the average blood glucose levels during the previous 2 to 3 months and is of value in assessing glucose control in any person with diabetes. As red blood cells circulate in the bloodstream, glucose molecules gradually attach to the hemoglobin A molecules and remain there for the lifetime of the red blood cell, approximately 120 days. Nondiabetic hemoglobin A_{1c} values are generally between 4% and 6% but can vary by laboratory. Acceptable diabetes control for children is typically a hemoglobin A_{1c} value of 7.5%.

Urine testing for glucose is no longer used for diabetes management; there is poor correlation between simultaneous glycosuria and blood glucose concentrations. However, urine testing can be carried out to detect evidence of ketonuria.

Nutrition.   Essentially the nutritional needs of children with diabetes are no different from those of unaffected children. Children with diabetes require no special foods or supplements. They need sufficient calories to balance daily expenditure for energy and to satisfy the requirement for growth and development. They also need consistent intake and timing of food, especially carbohydrates.

Normally insulin is secreted in response to food intake. However, insulin injected subcutaneously has a relatively predictable time of onset, peak effect, duration of action, and absorption rate, depending on the type of insulin used. Consequently, the timing of food consumption is regulated to correspond to the time and action of the insulin prescribed. Meals and snacks must be eaten at the same times each day, and the total number of calories and proportions of basic nutrients must be consistent from day to day. The

TABLE 29-2 ■ Features of Eight Popular Glucose Monitoring Meters

METER	ACCUCHECK ADVANTAGE	ACCUCHECK COMPLETE	FREESTYLE	GLUCOMETER DEX2	GLUCOMETER ELITE XL	ONE TOUCH ULTRA	PRECISION
Manufacturer	Roche Diagnostics	Roche Diagnostics	TheraSense	Bayer	Bayer	Lifescan	Abbott Laboratories
Sample size (microliters)	4	4	0.3	4	2	1	2.5
Weight (ounces)	2	1.6	2.2	3.5	2.1	1.5	2.79
Memory: number of test results stored with date and time obtained	100	1000	250	100	120	1.50	450
Recommended (°F) temperature range	57°-104°	57°-104°	50°-95°	50°-104°	50°-104°	43°-111°	0°-131°
Test time (seconds)	26	26	5-15	30	30	5	20
Approved for alternate site testing	No	No	Yes	Yes	Yes	Yes	No
Blood ketone analysis	No	No	No	No	No	No	Yes
Altitude limit recommendations (feet)	10,150	10,150	10,400	8,800	8,800	10,000	7,200
Website	www.accucheck.com	www.accucheck.com	www.therasense.com	www.glucometer.com	www.glucometer.com	www.LifeScan.com	www.MediSense.com

From Trecroci D, 2002. Adapted with permission from King Publishing, Inc. (For complimentary issue or subscription information, contact 800-488-8468.)

distribution of calories, especially carbohydrates, is determined to fit the activity pattern of each child. Alterations in food intake are made so that food, insulin, and exercise are balanced. Extra food is needed for extra activity.

There's no one diet for diabetes. General guidelines exist, such as "eat less fat and saturated fat" and "eat more whole grains, fruits, and vegetables." Sugars and sweets, or "simple sugars," don't raise blood glucose any quicker than starches, or "complex carbohydrates." Provide healthy nutrition advice—eat sugars and sweets in moderation. Diabetes meal plans must be based on individual needs and developed with expert assistance from a registered dietitian.

Exercise.   Exercise is encouraged and never restricted unless indicated by other health conditions, because it lowers blood glucose levels. It is included as part of diabetes management and is planned around the child's interests and capabilities. However, in most instances, children's activities are unplanned, and the resulting decrease in the blood glucose level can be compensated for by providing extra snacks before (and, if prolonged, during) the activity. Besides providing a feeling of well-being, regular exercise aids in the body's use of food and often decreases insulin requirements.

Hypoglycemia.   Even a child with well-controlled diabetes may often experience mild symptoms of hypoglycemia, but if the signs and symptoms are recognized early (see Table 29-3) and relieved promptly by appropriate therapy, the child's activity should not be interrupted for more than a few minutes.

! NURSING ALERT

Hypoglycemic episodes most commonly occur before meals, or when the insulin effect is peaking.

The most common causes of hypoglycemia, *insulin reaction,* are bursts of physical activity without additional food, or delayed, omitted, or incompletely consumed meals or snacks. Reglycosalation of muscles and replenishment of liver glycogen may occur over the ensuing 24 hours; therefore, particular vigilance related to hypoglycemia may be necessary during the night after a day's vigorous exertion.

In the majority of cases, simple concentrated sugar, such as honey, that can be held in the mouth for a short time will elevate the blood glucose level and alleviate hypoglycemic symptoms. The simpler the carbohydrate, the more rapidly it will be absorbed. For a mild reaction, low-fat milk is a good food to use in children. It supplies them with lactose or milk sugar, as well as providing a more prolonged action from the protein and fat (aids in decreased absorption). All children with diabetes should carry with them a source of glucose, such as glucose tablets, Insta-glucose, hard candy, or sugar cubes. The rapid-releasing sugar is followed by a complex carbohydrate and protein, such as a slice of bread or a cracker spread with peanut butter.

Glucagon is sometimes prescribed for home treatment of severe hypoglycemia. It is available by prescription as a prefilled syringe and is administered intramuscularly or subcutaneously. Glucagon functions by releasing stored glycogen from the liver and requires about 10 minutes to elevate the blood glucose level. After the child is responsive, the lost glycogen stores are replaced by small amounts of sugar-containing fluid administered frequently until the child feels comfortable about trying solid foods.

! NURSING ALERT

Vomiting may occur after administration of glucagon; therefore, precautions against aspiration must be taken (e.g., placing the child on his or her side), because the child will be unconscious.

The *Somogyi effect* should be recognized as a separate response from hypoglycemia. This phenomenon occurs when the blood glucose level decreases to the point where stress hormones (epinephrine, growth hormone, and corticosteroids) are released, causing a rebound hyperglycemia. Prevention consists of increasing the amount of food eaten or decreasing the insulin.

Illness Management.   Illness alters diabetes management. Maintaining blood glucose control is usually related to the seriousness of the illness. As the illness runs its course, the goal of diabetes management is to maintain some euglycemia while recognizing and treating urinary ketones and preventing dehydration. Some hyperglycemia and ketonuria are expected in most illnesses, even with diminished food intake, and indicate the need for increased insulin. Insulin should never be omitted during an illness, although dosage requirements may increase, decrease, or remain unchanged, depending on the severity of the illness and the child's appetite. In addition, supplemental doses of lispro or regular insulin are often used to manage the hyperglycemia associated with illness. Illness management must always include careful attention to fluid balance. Hyperglycemia contributes to dehydration, and the child will require extra oral fluids while ill.

Management of Diabetic Ketoacidosis.   DKA, the most complete state of insulin deficiency, is a life-threatening situation. The child is admitted to an intensive care facility for management, which consists of rapid assessment, adequate insulin to reduce the elevated blood glucose level, fluids to overcome dehydration, and electrolyte replacement (especially potassium). The preferred method for administering insulin to the child with ketoacidosis is a continuous IV infusion of low-dose regular insulin.

Current trends suggest cautious fluid resuscitation and blood glucose management to reduce risk of cerebral edema. The fluid deficit is replaced evenly over 24 to 48 hours. Serum potassium levels may be normal on admission, but rapid return of potassium to cells after initiation of fluid and insulin can seriously deplete serum levels, with the attendant risk of cardiac arrhythmias. A cardiac monitor is employed as a guide to therapy and to determine changes that might indicate alterations in potassium concentration.

! NURSING ALERT

Potassium must never be given until the serum potassium level is known to be normal or low and voiding of urine is observed. All maintenance IV fluids should include 20 to 40 mEq/L of potassium. Never give potassium as a rapid IV bolus, or cardiac arrest may result.

When the critical period is over, the task of regulating insulin dosage to diet and activity is begun. Children should be actively involved in their own care and are given responsibility according to their ability and guidance of the nurse.

⚠ NURSING ALERT

Because insulin can chemically bind to plastic tubing and in-line filters, thereby reducing the amount of the medication reaching the bloodstream, an insulin mixture is run through the tubing to saturate the insulin binding sites before the infusion is begun.

● Assessment

Daily monitoring of blood glucose levels; periodic urine analysis for ketones; and observation for signs of hypoglycemia, hyperglycemia, or other complications is part of the daily life of the child with diabetes and the family. Diabetes should be suspected in any child who exhibits the manifestations outlined in Box 29-13, and the child should be referred for further assessment and appropriate testing.

The signs and symptoms of hypoglycemia are caused by both increased adrenergic activity and impaired brain function, and it is often difficult to distinguish between hyperglycemia and a hypoglycemic reaction (Table 29-3). Because the symptoms are similar and usually begin with changes in behavior, the simplest way to differentiate between the two is to test the blood glucose level (low in hypoglycemia; elevated in hyperglycemia).

Education is the cornerstone of diabetes management and the major responsibility in diabetes nursing care. Whether teaching is conducted on an outpatient basis or in a preparatory, in-depth manner on an inpatient basis, the ability and readiness of the individual learner must be accurately assessed. This includes assessment of the educational background and emotional stability of the individual(s) involved and the use of appropriate measurement tools, such as a pretest or an objective assessment of the learner's educational level and literacy.

● Nursing Diagnoses

A number of nursing diagnoses are prominent in the nursing management of type 1 DM, and others specific to individual cases become evident. The most common are outlined in the Nursing Care Plan on pp. 1091 to 1093.

● Planning

The goals of care for the child with DM and the family are as follows:

1 Child and family will be educated about the disease, assessment techniques, and therapy.
2 Child will experience a minimum of complications of diabetes.
3 Child will develop a positive self-image.
4 Child and family will receive adequate support.

● Implementation

After the child with diabetes is diagnosed and insulin therapy initiated, the major nursing responsibility is the education of the family and reinforcement of information. The parents must supervise and manage the child's therapeutic program, but the child should assume responsibility for self-management as soon as he or she is capable. Children can assist with blood glucose testing at a relatively young age (4 to 5 years),

TABLE 29-3 ■ Comparison of Manifestations of Hypoglycemia and Hyperglycemia

VARIABLE	HYPOGLYCEMIA	HYPERGLYCEMIA
Onset	Rapid (minutes)	Gradual (days)
Mood	Labile, irritable, nervous, weepy	Lethargic
Mental status	Difficulty concentrating, speaking, focusing, coordinating	Dulled sensorium Confused
Inward feeling	Nightmares	Thirst
	Shaky feeling, hunger	Weakness
	Headache	Nausea/vomiting
	Dizziness	Abdominal pain
Skin	Pallor	Flushed
	Sweating	Signs of dehydration
Mucous Membranes	Normal	Dry, crusty
Respirations	Shallow, normal	Deep, rapid (Kussmaul)
Pulse	Tachycardia, palpitations	Less rapid, weak
Breath odor	Normal	Fruity, acetone
Neurologic	Tremors	Diminished reflexes
	Late: hyperreflexia, dilated pupils, seizure	Paresthesia
Ominous signs	Shock, coma	Acidosis, coma
Blood:		
Glucose	Low: below 60 mg/dL	High: 250 mg/dL or more
Ketones	Negative	High/large
Osmolarity	Normal	High
pH	Normal	Low (7.25 or less)
Hematocrit	Normal	High
HCO3	Normal	Less than 20 mEq/L
Urine:		
Output	Normal	Polyuria (early) to oliguria (late) Enuresis, nocturia
Glucose	Negative	High
Ketones	Negative/trace	High
Visual	Diplopia	Blurred vision

and most should be able to administer their own insulin with supervision at about 9 years of age. In situations in which the parents are inconsistent or unreliable, the child is taught self-care at an earlier age and additional adult support is sought.

Several organizations are prepared to assist with education and dissemination of knowledge about diabetes. The **American Diabetes Association, Inc.,*** **Canadian Diabetes Association,†** **Juvenile Diabetes Foundation International,‡**

---

*1701 North Beauregard Street, Alexandria, VA 22311; (800) 232-3472; website: www.diabetes.org.
†15 Toronto Street, Suite 800, Toronto, Ontario M5C 2E3; (416) 363-3373 or (800) BANTING; website: www.diabetes.ca.
‡120 Wall Street, New York, NY 10005; (800) 223-1138; website: www.jdf.org.

Juvenile Diabetes Research Foundation—Canada,* and American Association of Diabetes Educators† are valuable resources for a variety of educational materials. The **National Diabetes Information Clearinghouse‡** publishes a number of comprehensive annotated bibliographies, including *Educational Materials for and About Young People With Diabetes* (a compilation of resource materials for children, siblings, parents, teachers, and health professionals) and *Sports and Exercise for People With Diabetes.*

Self-management, the ultimate goal for the child with diabetes, is more likely to occur when the child understands the disorder and the care it requires. Properly educated and with adequate resources, any family should be able to follow a program of regulated control satisfactorily. The following information will allow the family to manage the daily aspects of care.

Identification.   One of the first issues to raise with parents is the need for the child to wear medical identification. This essential and immediate information could save the child's life. Identification tags come in a variety of forms, including neck chains, bracelets, and tags for shoes.

Nature of Diabetes.   The better the parents understand the pathophysiology of diabetes and the function and action of insulin and glucagon in relation to caloric intake and exercise, the better their understanding of the disease and its effect on the child. Parents need answers to a number of questions (voiced or unvoiced), because those answers will provide them with an increased feeling of security in coping with the disease. Parents initially may worry about what diabetes is, how their child developed diabetes, and if their other children are at risk of developing diabetes. In addition, they will worry about what to tell family, friends, and school personnel. They may have fears about complications and about how they will afford the cost of diabetes care.

Meal Planning.   Normal nutrition is a major aspect of the family education program. Diet instruction is usually conducted by the nutritionist, with reinforcement and guidance from the nurse. Learning about foods within specific food groups helps in making choices. Weights and measures of foods, used as eye-training devices in defining portion sizes, should be practiced repeatedly, with gradual conversion to estimating foods. Members of the family are also guided in reading labels for the nutritional value of foods and food contents. Meals and snacks are modified to suit the child and the present food menu, preserving cultural patterns and preferences as much as possible.

Lists of popular fast-food items and items served at the major fast-food chains can be obtained from the American Diabetes Association to help guide food selections. Children are advised to use sugar substitutes with moderation in

items such as soft drinks. "Sugar-free" chewing gum and candy made with sorbitol may be used in moderation. However, sorbitol is metabolized to fructose and then to glucose, and large amounts of sorbitol can cause an osmotic diarrhea. Dietetic foods that contain sorbitol are more expensive than regular foods, and often the total carbohydrate content of the food is the same or even greater.

Insulin.   Families need to understand the treatment method and the insulin prescribed, including the effective duration, onset, and peak action. They also need to know the characteristics of the various types of insulins, and the proper mixing and dilution of insulins. Insulin, after it has been opened, should be discarded in 1 month (even if refrigerated). Unopened insulin is good until the expiration date on the bottle.

Injection Procedure.   Learning to give the insulin injections is a source of anxiety for the family and the child. It is helpful for the learner to know that this important aspect of care will become as routine as brushing the teeth. First, the basic injection technique is taught, using an orange or similar item and normal saline for practice. To gain the confidence of the child, the nurse demonstrates the technique by giving a skillful injection to the parent, who then returns the demonstration by giving the nurse an injection. With practice, family members soon are able to give the insulin injection to the child. Both parents should participate, and as little time as possible should elapse between instruction and the actual injection, especially with parents and the teenage learner.

Insulin is injected at a 90-degree angle into subcutaneous tissue, where it is slowly absorbed (Fig. 29-3). Newly diagnosed children may have lost adipose tissue, and care should be exercised not to inject into the muscle. The pinch technique is the most effective method for obtaining skin tightness to allow easy entrance of the needle into subcutaneous tissues in children. The site selected will sometimes depend on whether the child or parent administers the insulin. The upper arms, thighs, hips, and abdomen are usual injection sites for insulin. The child can reach the thighs, abdomen, and part of the hip and arm easily but may require help to inject other sites. For example, a parent can pinch a loose fold of skin on the arm while the child injects the insulin.

Injections are rotated to various areas of the body to enhance absorption, because insulin absorption is slowed by the fat pads that develop in overused areas of injection. The parents and child are helped to work out a rotation pattern, which involves giving about four to six injections in one area (each injection about 1 inch, or the diameter of the insulin vial, from the previous injection) and then moving to another area. In this way injection sites for an entire month can be planned in advance on a simple chart or illustration, such as an outline of a body or a teddy bear. It is a good idea for the parents each to give one or two injections a week in the areas that are difficult to reach to keep in practice.

It is important to remember that the absorption rate varies in different parts of the body (Table 29-4). Methodically using one anatomic area and then moving to another minimizes variation in absorption rates. Recommendations sug-

*89 Granton Drive, Richmond Hill, Ontario L4B 2N5; (800) 668-0274; website: www.jdfc.ca.
†100 West Monroe, Suite 400, Chicago, IL 60603; (800) 338-3633; website: www.aadenet.org.
‡1 Information Way, Bethesda, MD 20892-3560; (301) 654-3327; fax: (301) 907-8906; e-mail: ndic www.niddk.nih.gov/health/diabetes/ndic.htm.

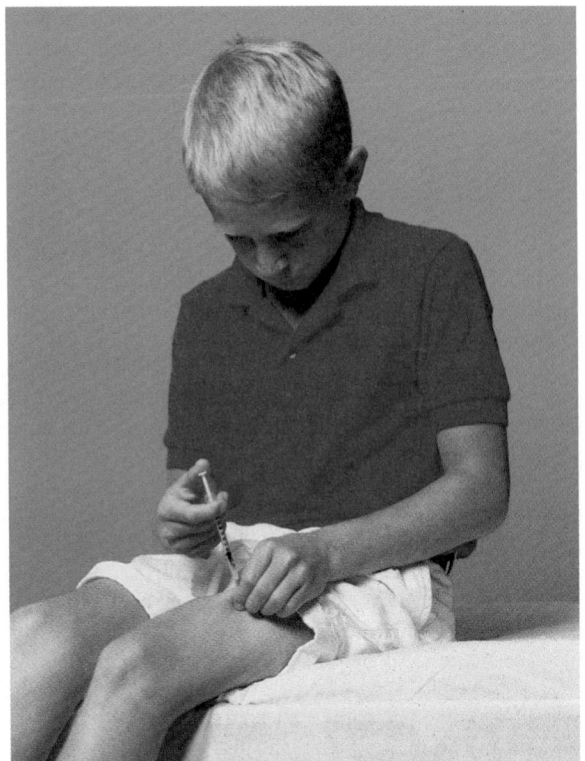

FIG. 29-3 ■ School-age children are able to administer their own insulin.

TABLE 29-4 ■ Onset and Duration of Action Related to Injection Site

	SITE OF INJECTION			
	ABDOMEN	ARM	LEG	BUTTOCK
Rate	Very fast	Fast	Slow	Very slow
Duration	Very short	Short	Long	Very long

From Albisser AM, Sperlich M: Adjusting insulins, *Diabetes Educ* 18(3):211-218, 1992.

gest rotating injections within an anatomic area (Fleming, 1999). An example of this would be using the abdomen for morning injections and the thighs for evening injections. This may assist with obtaining more consistent blood glucose levels. Injecting *small* doses of insulin also minimizes changes in plasma glucose levels. Absorption is also altered by vigorous exercise, which enhances absorption from exercised muscles. Therefore it is recommended that excess exercise be avoided during the time the insulin is expected to peak or that other sites be used.

Teaching includes the proper way to equalize pressure in the bottle by injecting an amount of air equal to the amount of solution withdrawn and how to remove air bubbles from the syringe. When insulin dosages are small, an air bubble in the syringe can displace a significant amount of medication. Since the introduction of $\frac{5}{10}$-mL and $\frac{3}{10}$-mL syringes, the risk of incorrect dosage has diminished. However, insulin injections of less than 2 units of U100 have an unacceptably large error. Diluted insulin should be used if the prescribed dose is less than 2 units (Gnanalingham, Newland, and Smith, 1998). Aspiration for blood before injecting the insulin is not routinely done.

Insulin syringes should be compared for accuracy, comfort, and strength. The family or child should be able to choose both "their" insulin and "their" syringe from a variety of samples. Use of the same type of syringe (even during hospitalization) is recommended to prevent errors in dosage caused by varying markings and amounts of dead space among syringes.

When the child's dosage requires the injection of both rapid- or short-acting and intermediate-acting insulin at the same time, most families prefer to mix the two and use a single injection. However, there are some problems associated with this accepted practice, and the family should understand what happens when insulins are mixed. Longer-acting insulins contain ingredients that bind to insulin, allowing for gradual release after injection. Some brands contain extra binding compounds that can bind with rapid- or short-acting insulin, blunting the action of the quicker insulin and altering the effect on blood glucose. The degree of alteration depends on the type of longer-acting insulin, the ratio of rapid- or short-acting insulin to long-acting insulin, and how long the mixture is allowed to stand before injection. The mixture should be injected less than 5 minutes after mixing (before the zinc content of the long-acting insulin affects the action time of the rapid- or short-acting insulin) or longer than 15 minutes after mixing (to allow the insulins to resume long-acting and short-acting properties).

To obtain the maximum benefit from mixing insulins, the recommended practice is to:

1. Inject the measured amount of air (equivalent to the dosage) into the longer-acting insulin (cloudy).
2. Inject the measured amount of air into the rapid- or short-acting (clear) insulin and, without removing the needle, withdraw the clear insulin.
3. Insert the needle (already containing the clear insulin) into the longer-acting insulin and withdraw the desired amount.

⚠ NURSING ALERT

When mixing types of insulin, always withdraw the clear insulin first, then the longer-acting insulin next to avoid contaminating the clear insulin with the longer-acting insulin.

It has become acceptable practice (though not recommended by all professionals) to reuse disposable needles and syringes. Bacteria counts are unaffected, and there is a considerable cost saving. It is important to stress the importance of vigorous handwashing before handling any equipment, as well as capping the syringe immediately after use. Syringes may be stored at room temperature. Nurses should also teach proper disposal of equipment after use in the home. Although it is not standard practice in the hospital, the use of a needle clipper is recommended to safely remove and house the used needle. In addition, the syringe plunger can be broken before disposal. An excellent means for syringe disposal is use of an opaque, puncture-resistant container, such as an empty coffee can, bleach bottle, or milk carton that is labeled "biohazardous waste" and is discarded with similar material only, not with household refuse. Many pharmacies now carry commercially produced sharps containers.

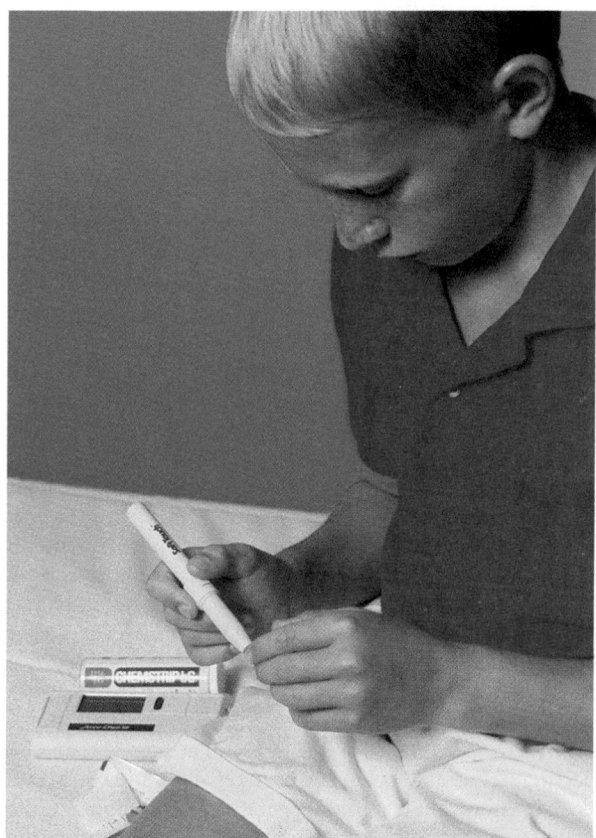

FIG. 29-4 ■ Child using finger-stick device to obtain blood sample. Blood glucose monitor and reagent strips are nearby.

ATRAUMATIC CARE

Minimizing Pain of Blood Glucose Monitoring

To enhance blood flow to the finger, hold it under warm water for a few seconds before the puncture.

When obtaining blood samples, use the ring finger or thumb (blood flows more easily to these areas), and puncture the finger just to the side of the finger pad (more blood vessels and fewer nerve endings).

To prevent a deep puncture, press the platform of the lancet device lightly against the skin and avoid steadying the finger against a hard surface.

Use glucose monitors that require very small blood samples to avoid repunctures, (e.g., Glucometer Elite).

Apply EMLA or LMX to the puncture site, especially when the child is newly diagnosed and the skin is still very sensitive (see Pain Management, Chapter 21).

Other devices are available for insulin injection and may offer advantages to some children. Children who do not wish to give themselves injections can be taught to use a syringe-loaded injector *(Inject-Ease)*. With the device, puncture is always automatic. Adolescents respond well to a self-contained and compact device resembling a fountain pen (e.g., *NovoPen*), which eliminates conventional vials and syringes. Preloaded pens may also cause less pain, because the needle is not blunted by piercing the rubber top of the insulin vial (Lteif and Schwenk, 1999).

Some children are considered candidates for continuous subcutaneous insulin infusion with a portable insulin pump. The child and the parents are taught to operate the device, including the mechanics of the pump, battery changes, and alarm systems. They learn how to load the syringe, insert the catheter, adjust the insulin flow for routine needs and for illnesses, and connect and disconnect the catheter. Nurses who work where insulin pumps are part of the therapeutic regimen should become familiar with the operation of the specific device being used and the protocol of the regimen.

Glucose Monitoring. Nurses should also be prepared to teach and supervise blood glucose monitoring. Blood for testing can be obtained by two different methods: manually or with a spring-loaded puncturing device. The automatic lancet device is recommended because its precise puncture depth produces better blood flow and less pain. However,

the child and family should learn to use both methods in the event of mechanical failure. Several lancet devices are available from which to choose, and each provides a means for obtaining enough blood for testing (Fig. 29-4). Many lancet devices may be adjusted for depth of puncture.

NURSING ALERT

Caution children not to allow anyone else to use their lancet or lancet device because of the risk of contracting hepatitis B virus or human immunodeficiency virus (HIV) infection.

Repeated finger punctures can be painful, but most children become accustomed to the procedure (see Atraumatic Care box). However, persistent signs of redness and soreness at the puncture site should be investigated. It may be evidence of poor technique or poor skin healing relative to poor control. Alternative site testing (AST) meters were approved by the FDA in 1999; however, results of AST on comparison with fingertip measures haven't been consistent (Seley, 2003; Lock and others, 2002). Further studies need to be conducted.

The least expensive testing method uses a visually read reagent strip to which blood is applied. After blotting, the color change is compared with a color scale for an estimation of the blood glucose level. The strips can be cut in half (although this is not recommended by all professionals) to obtain two readings per strip. This method might be ideal for use at school, where expensive equipment can be lost or broken.

Many types of glucose monitors are available for home use. The family should be shown features of several meters, including advantages and disadvantages, and allowed to choose equipment that best meets their needs. One important consideration is the amount of blood needed. Choosing devices that require small amounts may prevent repunctures.

Urine Testing. Urine ketone testing is easily taught but requires careful attention to technique. The test strip must be used accurately and the test timed precisely. Because the test strip is visually read, there must be adequate lighting available. Testing for ketones is recommended during times of illness or when glucose readings are high. Because moisture will cause changes to take place in both glucose and ketone strips, families are instructed to discard strips that are discolored, that have been open for a specified time, or after an expiration date. Test strips are available for testing both glucose and ketones.

Hyperglycemia and Hypoglycemia. Severe hyperglycemia is most often caused by illness, growth, emotional upset, or inaccurate or missed insulin doses. With careful glucose monitoring, most elevations can be managed by adjustment of insulin or food intake. Parents should understand how to adjust food, activity, and insulin at the time of illness or when the child is treated for an illness with a medication known to raise the blood glucose level, such as cough syrup or steroids. The hyperglycemia is managed by increasing insulin soon after the increased glucose is noted.

Hypoglycemia is caused by imbalances of food intake, insulin, and activity. Ideally, hypoglycemia should be prevented, and parents need to be prepared to prevent, recognize, and treat the problem. They should be familiar with the signs of hypoglycemia and instructed in treatment, including care of the child with seizures (see Chapter 28). Hypoglycemia can be managed effectively as outlined in the Emergency Treatment box.

Exercise. Exercise should be planned (as may be necessary for the sedentary teenager) or observed (as in most active children). If the child is more active at one time of the day than at another, food or insulin can be altered to meet the activity pattern of the individual. Food should be increased in the summer, when children tend to be more active. Decreased activity on return to school may require a decrease in food intake. The child who is active in team sports will need additional food intake on the days of activity in the form of a carbohydrate snack about a half-hour before the anticipated activity. Races or other competition may call for a slightly higher food intake than practice times.

Food will usually need to be repeated for prolonged activity periods, often as frequently as every 45 minutes to 1 hour. Families should be informed that if increased food is not tolerated, decreased insulin is the next course of action. If the blood glucose level is elevated ($\geq$240 mg/dL) and ketone values are positive before planned exercise, the activity should be postponed until the blood glucose is controlled. Moderate to large ketone values should be reported to the practitioner.

Record Keeping. Recording information about food, insulin, blood glucose measurements, and ketonuria is useful to the practitioner, as well as to the family. Insulin reactions are noted, including the time, severity, treatment, and response to treatment. Dietary variations are noted so that an increased blood glucose level can be analyzed in relation to the insulin dose, food intake, and activity level. Record keeping should also include identified stresses, such as school exams, birthday parties, and injuries.

Self-Management. Self-management is the key to close control. Being able to make changes at the time they are needed rather than waiting until the next contact with health professionals is important for self-management and gives the child and parents the feeling that they have control over the disease. As children grow and assume more and more responsibility for self-management, they develop confidence in their ability to manage their disease and in themselves as persons. Self-management techniques to be mastered are the testing of blood and urine, administration of insulin, and adjustment of insulin and diet with alterations in day-to-day activities and unusual occurrences.

Hygiene. All aspects of personal hygiene are emphasized for the child with diabetes. The child should be cautioned against wearing shoes without socks, wearing sandals, or walking barefoot. The correct method of nail and extremity care instituted for each particular child (with the guidance of a podiatrist) can begin health practices that last a lifetime. Eyes should be checked once per year, unless the child wears glasses, and then as directed by the ophthalmologist. Regular dental care is emphasized, and cuts and scratches should be treated with plain soap and water unless otherwise indicated.

Acute Care. Children with diabetes may be admitted to the hospital at the time of their initial diagnosis, during illness or surgery, or during episodes of DKA—especially in the small number who exhibit a degree of metabolic lability or who have repeated episodes of DKA. Most children with diabetes are able to keep the disease under control with periodic assessment and adjustment of insulin, diet, and activity as needed under health supervision.

The child with DKA requires intensive nursing care. On admission to the hospital, usually to an intensive care unit,

EMERGENCY TREATMENT

Hypoglycemia

MILD REACTION: ADRENERGIC SYMPTOMS
Give child 10 to 15 g of simple carbohydrate (preferably liquid; e.g., 3 to 6 ounces of orange juice).
Follow with starch-protein snack.

MODERATE REACTION: NEUROGLYCOPENIC SYMPTOMS
Give child 10 to 15 g of simple carbohydrate as discussed previously.
Repeat in 10 to 15 minutes if symptoms persist.
Follow with larger snack.
Watch child closely.

SEVERE REACTION: UNRESPONSIVE, UNCONSCIOUS, OR SEIZURES
Administer glucagon as prescribed.
Follow with planned meal or snack when child is able to eat, or add a snack.

NOCTURNAL REACTION
Give child 10 to 15 g of simple carbohydrate.
Follow with a snack.

an IV infusion is started immediately to hydrate the child and to administer insulin, usually as a continuous infusion (see Management of Diabetic Ketoacidosis, p. 1083). The blood glucose level is monitored at regular intervals, and the insulin administered as ordered.

Sodium, potassium, and bicarbonate levels are monitored and replaced as indicated. Because potassium and sodium reenter the cells rapidly after administration of insulin, depletion of these electrolytes can be a serious consequence. The child is attached to a cardiac monitor for continual assessment of cardiac status, especially when potassium levels are markedly altered.

Careful and accurate records are maintained, including vital signs, blood pressure, IV fluids, electrolytes, insulin, blood glucose level, intake and output, and weight. A urine collection device is used to obtain the urine measurements, which include volume, specific gravity, and glucose and ketone values. The volume relative to the glucose content is important, because 5% glucose in a 300-mL sample is a significantly greater amount than a similar reading from a 75-mL sample. A diabetic flow sheet maintained at the bedside provides an ongoing record of the vital signs, urine and blood tests, amount of insulin given, and intake and output of the patient. The level of consciousness is assessed and recorded at frequent intervals. Any change or deterioration in the level of consciousness must be reported to the health care provider. Such changes may indicate an increase in intracranial pressure and must be managed aggressively. The comatose child generally regains consciousness fairly soon after initiation of therapy but is managed as is any unconscious child during that time.

Family Support.   In any educational program the psychologic needs of the child are just as important as the physical needs. Adjustment to a chronic illness is difficult and follows the grief process (see Chapter 18). A noticeable adjustment cycle occurs during the week-long education course. First, there is interest and perhaps some anger and doubt, followed by denial and accompanied by the overwhelming feeling of "Why me?" There are doubts regarding the ability to absorb so much essential information. Then there are the acceptance and synthesis of material, as the learners realize that they are able to state and demonstrate their understanding of the material.

Young children usually adjust well to problems related to the disease. However, challenges exist, such as providing regular feedings to the sick infant or to the negative toddler. With toddlers and preschoolers, insulin injections and glucose testing may be difficult at first. However, they usually accept the procedures when the parents use a matter-of-fact approach without calling attention to a "hurt" and treat the procedure like any other routine part of the child's life. After the injection, time with some special and positive attention, such as reading, talking, or some other pleasant activity, is one way to convert children who initially refuse injections to those who accept them.

School-age children tend to accept their condition more easily than adolescents. School-age children can understand the basic concepts related to their disease and its treatment. They are able to test blood glucose and urine; recognize food groups; give injections; keep records; and distinguish

between feelings of fear, excitement, and hypoglycemia. They understand how to recognize, prevent, and treat hypoglycemia. However, they still need considerable parental involvement.

Adolescents appear to have the most difficulty in adjusting. Adolescence is a time when there is much stress toward being "perfect" and being like peers and, no matter what others say, having diabetes is being different. Some youngsters are more upset about not being able to have a candy bar than about injections, diet, and other aspects of management. If children can accept the difference as a part of life, in other words, that each person is different in some way, then with adequate family support they should be able to adjust well (see Family Focus box and Critical Thinking Exercise).

For all families, daily compliance with numerous procedures and structured living schedules is difficult. Maintaining good blood glucose control requires ongoing motivation. Nurses can encourage families to adhere to treatment regimens and lifestyle adjustments by emphasizing the benefits of preventing complications such as hypoglycemia. In some families complications can have a favorable impact. After parents experience the child's having a severe insulin reaction with a seizure or the adolescent has one in a public place, the desire to maintain better control is reinforced. They must understand how to prevent problems and how to handle problems calmly if they occur. (See Compliance, Chapter 22.)

> **NURSING TIP**
>
> Ongoing motivation to adhere to a regimen is difficult. An older child and parent (or another caregiver) may enjoy negotiating a day off when the responsibility for testing and recording blood glucose is delegated from the child to the caregiver (or vice versa).

Camps for children with diabetes and other special groups are very useful. In the special camp these children learn that they are not alone. As a result, most children become more independent and resourceful outside the camp setting. Camp time also provides parents a respite from the child's daily regimen. Information about such camps and organizations can be obtained from the American Diabetes Association. A free list of accredited camps specifically for children and teenagers with diabetes is also available.*

● *Evaluation*

The effectiveness of nursing interventions is determined by continual reassessment and evaluation of care based on the following observational guidelines:

1 Interview family to determine their understanding of the disease; have child and family demonstrate and discuss the needed assessment and therapeutic techniques.
2 Interview family regarding their understanding of tight control; analyze and evaluate management records.
3 Discuss child's disease with him or her.
4 Interview family and child regarding their feelings and concerns about the disease.

The *expected outcomes* are described in the Nursing Care Plan on pp. 1091 to 1093.

---

*Camp Directory, 1701 North Beauregard Street, Alexandria, VA 22311; (800) 232-3472.

The Adolescent With Type 1 Diabetes Mellitus

As a nurse caring for adolescents with type 1 diabetes mellitus (DM), I am constantly aware of the wide range of adolescent behaviors that affect the course of this disease. Education of the child and the parents can often make the difference between a disease in control of the teenager and a teenager in control of the disease.

I have cared for many adolescent girls who have episodes of hyperglycemia at the time of menstruation that can result in diabetic ketoacidosis (DKA). I have found that education regarding sick-day protocol with sliding-scale, rapid-acting insulin instituted at the first sign of hyperglycemia, which may occur 1 to 2 days before onset of menses, can keep the adolescent girl out of the intensive care unit and in control of her diabetes.

Eating disorders, such as bulimia or anorexia nervosa, in the teenager with type 1 DM pose a serious health hazard. Also, insulin manipulation or omission has been identified as a weight loss method used by some adolescents (Barber and Lowes, 1998). Poor disease control may also be used by depressed teens as a method of suicide. Nurses working with these adolescents must be aware of the hazards and openly discuss the risks with the young person. A referral for specialized intervention may be needed.

Another group of adolescents with diabetes who are at risk are those who drink alcohol. I have found that confusion about the effects of alcohol on blood glucose is common. Teenagers may believe that alcohol will increase blood glucose levels, when in fact the opposite occurs. Ingestion of alcohol inhibits the release of glycogen from the liver, thereby resulting in hypoglycemia. Teenagers with diabetes who drink alcohol may become hypoglycemic but may be treated as if they were inebriated (drunk). Behaviors may be similar, such as shakiness, combativeness, slurred speech, and loss of consciousness.

Education regarding the effects of alcohol is important and must be included in a teaching plan. If teenagers insist on drinking alcohol, they can be cautioned to use sweetened mixers or eat snacks when consuming alcoholic beverages.

Episodes of hyperglycemia or hypoglycemia may become a serious issue for adolescents who are leaving home for the first time. One teenager confided that her mother always recognized her combative, antisocial behavior as impending hypoglycemia and treated her with the appropriate intervention. The teenager feared that a college roommate might be offended by the behavior and might leave her alone with impending hypoglycemia.

One young man realized he could not live alone when he "took a nap because of feeling tired" and woke up 4 days later in the hospital. Fortunately, his family realized he was in a coma and summoned emergency medical service. The fatigue signaled the beginning of a viral infection, which led to a blood glucose level of 410 mg/dL. Nurses need to address these fears openly and facilitate ways in which the teenager can enlist the aid of significant peers who may be available during hyperglycemic or hypoglycemic episodes.

Susan Zekauskas, MSN, RN, PNP

Type 1 Diabetes Mellitus

Rebecca is a 15-year-old with a 3-year history of type 1 diabetes mellitus and has been admitted to the pediatric intensive care unit for treatment of diabetic ketoacidosis (DKA). This is her fifth hospital admission for DKA in the past year. Rebecca's parents are divorced, and she has four younger siblings, none of whom has diabetes. Rebecca's mother has maintained two jobs for the past 5 years and frequently leaves Rebecca in charge of the household. In anticipation of her discharge you are to plan a patient education program for Rebecca and her mother. What important issues regarding Rebecca's unstable diabetic management must you consider to plan the education program?

QUESTIONS
1. Evidence—Is there sufficient evidence to draw conclusions about Rebecca's recurrent episodes of DKA?
2. Assumptions—Describe an underlying assumption about each of the following:
    a. Type 1 diabetes mellitus in adolescence
    b. Type 1 diabetes mellitus and menses
    c. Emotional stress and elevated blood glucose levels
    d. Blood glucose monitoring for insulin management
3. What priorities for nursing care should be established for Rebecca?
4. Does the evidence support your nursing intervention?
5. What alternative perspectives might you have?

ANSWERS
1. Yes. Rebecca has had five hospital admissions for DKA in the past year. Numerous factors must be involved with her unstable disease.
2. a. The normal tasks of adolescence can play a significant role in blood glucose instability.
    b. Adolescent girls with diabetes have frequent fluctuations of blood glucose levels immediately before, during, or after their menses.
    c. Rebecca's personal loss from the divorce, her mother's absence because of a heavy work schedule, and the added responsibilities of the household may cause significant stress, resulting in elevated blood glucose levels.
    d. Careful, frequent, consistent monitoring of blood glucose levels is essential for effective insulin management during adolescence.
3. The first priority would be to focus directly on the issues of hyperglycemia. Determination of Rebecca's practice of monitoring and management of her diabetes at home is essential. Areas of diabetic management that should be emphasized include careful dietary management, an appropriate exercise program, conscientious self-testing of blood glucose, appropriate administration of daily insulin, and adherence to sliding-scale insulin therapy. Discussion of the emotional stressors she identifies at this time is appropriate.
4. Yes, Rebecca's history of DKA over the past year supports her inability to monitor and manage her diabetes.
5. It would be appropriate to make a referral for special support services for counseling and possible home care follow-up to assess her diabetic management skills at home.

NURSING CARE PLAN   The Child With Diabetes Mellitus

HOSPITAL CARE

NURSING DIAGNOSIS ■ **Risk for injury related to insulin deficiency**

PATIENT GOAL 1: Will exhibit normal blood glucose levels

NURSING INTERVENTIONS/*RATIONALES***

Obtain blood glucose level *to determine most appropriate dose of insulin*

*Administer insulin as prescribed *to maintain normal blood glucose level*

Understand the action of insulin

    Understand the differences in composition, time of onset, and duration of action for the various insulin preparations *to ensure accurate insulin administration*

Employ aseptic techniques when preparing and administering insulin

    Subcutaneous injection; depth according to thickness of subcutaneous tissue

    Rotation of sites *to enhance absorption of insulin*

EXPECTED OUTCOME

Child demonstrates normal blood glucose levels

NURSING DIAGNOSIS ■ **Risk for injury related to hypoglycemia**

PATIENT GOAL 1: Will exhibit no evidence of hypoglycemia

NURSING INTERVENTIONS/*RATIONALES***

Recognize signs of hypoglycemia early

    Be particularly alert at times when blood glucose levels are lowest (before meals and snacks; 2 to 4 AM; after bursts of physical activity without additional food; or with delayed, omitted, or incompletely consumed meal or snack)

    Test blood glucose

Offer 10 to 15 g of readily absorbed carbohydrates, such as orange juice, hard candy, or milk, *to elevate blood glucose level and alleviate symptoms of hypoglycemia*

Follow with complex carbohydrate and protein, such as bread or cracker spread with peanut butter or cheese, *to maintain blood glucose level*

*Administer glucagon to unconscious or combative child *to elevate blood glucose level;* position child *to minimize risk of aspiration, because vomiting may occur*

EXPECTED OUTCOMES

Child ingests an appropriate carbohydrate

Child displays no evidence of hypoglycemia

PREPARATION FOR HOME CARE

NURSING DIAGNOSIS ■ **Knowledge deficit (diabetes management) related to care of a child with newly diagnosed diabetes mellitus**

PATIENT/FAMILY GOAL 1: Will accept teaching provided

NURSING INTERVENTIONS/*RATIONALES***

Select methods, vocabulary, and content appropriate to learner's level *to maximize learning*

Allow time for family and child to begin to adjust to initial impact of the diagnosis

Select an environment conducive to learning

Allow ample time for the education process *to prevent overwhelming the learner*

Restrict length of teaching sessions *because this is how people learn best*

    Child—15 to 20 minutes

    Parents—45 to 60 minutes

Involve all senses and employ a variety of teaching strategies, especially participation, *because it is usually the most effective method for learning*

Provide pamphlets or other supplementary materials *for future referral*

EXPECTED OUTCOME

Child or family display attitude conducive to learning

PATIENT/FAMILY GOAL 2: Will demonstrate understanding of disease and its therapy

NURSING INTERVENTIONS/*RATIONALES***

Provide information regarding the pathophysiology of diabetes and the function and actions of insulin and glucagon in relation to caloric intake and exercise

Answer questions and clarify misconceptions *to ensure optimal learning*

Explain the function and expected effects of procedures and tests, *because these are a necessary part of diabetes management*

EXPECTED OUTCOME

Child or family demonstrate an understanding of the disease and its therapy (specify indicators)

PATIENT/FAMILY GOAL 3: Will demonstrate understanding of meal planning

NURSING INTERVENTIONS/*RATIONALES***

Enlist the services of a dietitian *to teach meal planning*

Emphasize relationship between normal nutritional needs and the disease *to encourage a sense of normalcy*

Become familiar with family's culture and food preferences *so that these are included in meal planning*

Teach or reinforce learners' understanding of the basic food groups and the meal plan prescribed

Help child and family estimate portion sizes by volume, *because this is more practical than weighing food*

Suggest low-carbohydrate snack items

Guide family in assessing labels of food products for carbohydrate content, *because consistency in carbohydrate portions is essential*

Teach or reinforce an understanding of the concept of exchanges, *because exchanges ensure day-to-day consistency in total intake while allowing a choice of foods*

Relate constant carbohydrate equivalents to familiar foods

Retain cultural patterns and family preferences as much as possible, *so that child and family are more likely to adhere to diet requirements*

EXPECTED OUTCOME

Child or family demonstrate an understanding of meal planning and food selection (specify indicators)

*Dependent nursing action.

Continued

NURSING CARE PLAN The Child With Diabetes Mellitus—*cont'd*

PATIENT/FAMILY GOAL 4: Will demonstrate knowledge of and ability to administer insulin

NURSING INTERVENTIONS/*RATIONALES*

Teach child and family the characteristics of the insulins prescribed for child, *because there are several insulin preparations*

Teach proper mixing of insulins *to prevent contaminating the vials*

Teach injection procedure

Impress on learners that the procedure will be a routine part of child's life *to decrease anxiety and increase cooperation*

Involve caregivers and child, if old enough, *so that more than one person learns the procedure*

Teach basic techniques using an orange or similar item *so that learner can gain confidence before injecting a person*

Use demonstration and return demonstration techniques on another before injecting child, *because this is usually less stressful*

Help families and child work out a set rotational pattern, *because this is important for maximum absorption of insulin and prevention of hypertrophy at injection site*

Teach proper care of insulin and equipment

Teach management of continuous infusion pump (if used)

EXPECTED OUTCOMES

Child or family demonstrate an understanding of insulin, its various forms, and action (specify indicators)

Child or family demonstrate injection technique correctly

Child or family develop a rotation plan

Child or family demonstrate correct use of pump and care of injection site

PATIENT/FAMILY GOAL 5: Will demonstrate ability to test blood glucose level

NURSING INTERVENTIONS/*RATIONALES*

Teach family and child, if old enough:

Blood glucose monitoring or use of equipment selected for use

Interpretation of results *so that they learn how to adjust insulin based on blood glucose level*

Care and maintenance of equipment

EXPECTED OUTCOME

Child and/or family demonstrate correct use of glucose monitoring equipment

PATIENT/FAMILY GOAL 6: Will demonstrate ability to test urine

NURSING INTERVENTIONS/*RATIONALES*

Teach family and child, if old enough:

Urine ketone testing and interpretation of results

Proper care of test strips

EXPECTED OUTCOME

Child or family demonstrate urine testing and interpretation

PATIENT/FAMILY GOAL 7: Will demonstrate understanding of proper hygiene

NURSING INTERVENTIONS/*RATIONALES*

Emphasize importance of personal hygiene *so that child establishes health practices that last a lifetime*

Encourage regular dental care and yearly ophthalmologic examinations, *because these are important for child's general health*

Teach proper care of cuts and scratches *to minimize risk of infection*

Teach proper foot care, *because this will become a high priority during adulthood*

EXPECTED OUTCOME

Child and family demonstrate an understanding of importance of proper hygiene

PATIENT/FAMILY GOAL 8: Will demonstrate understanding of importance of exercise regimen

NURSING INTERVENTIONS/*RATIONALES*

Arrange for occupational therapy program that includes physical activity, *because this is an important part of diabetic management*

Work with child, family, and others (e.g., coaches) to help plan a home exercise program

Reiterate practitioner's instructions regarding adjustment of food or insulin to meet child's activity pattern; reinforce with examples *so that child and family are adequately prepared*

EXPECTED OUTCOME

Child and family outline and carry out a regular exercise program

PATIENT/FAMILY GOAL 9: Will demonstrate understanding and management of hyperglycemia and hypoglycemia

NURSING INTERVENTIONS/*RATIONALES*

Instruct learners in how to recognize signs of hyperglycemia and hypoglycemia (especially hypoglycemia) *to prevent delay in treatment*

Explain relationship of insulin needs to illness, activity, and intense emotion (either positive or negative)

Teach how to adjust food, activity, and insulin at times of illness and during other situations that alter blood glucose levels

Suggest carrying source of carbohydrate, such as sugar cubes or hard candy, in pocket or handbag *so that it is readily available to treat hypoglycemia*

Instruct parents and child in how to treat hypoglycemia with food, simple sugars, or glucagon

EXPECTED OUTCOME

Child and family demonstrate an understanding of signs and management of a hypoglycemic reaction (specify)

PATIENT/FAMILY GOAL 10: Will wear medical identification

NURSING INTERVENTIONS/*RATIONALES*

Encourage acquisition of a means of identification, such as an identification bracelet, that explains child's condition *in case of emergency*

Explain to child why identification is important *so that child is more likely to comply*

EXPECTED OUTCOME

Family acquires and child wears medical identification

NURSING CARE PLAN   The Child With Diabetes Mellitus—*cont'd*

PATIENT/FAMILY GOAL 11: Will keep proper records of insulin administration and testing procedures

NURSING INTERVENTIONS/*RATIONALES*

Help child and family to design a form for keeping records of the following, *because this information is useful to both practitioner and family in managing diabetes:*
Insulin administered
Blood and urine tests
Food intake
Marked variation in exercise
Illness

EXPECTED OUTCOME

Family and child keep an accurate record of insulin administration, glucose testing, etc.

PATIENT/FAMILY GOAL 12: Will engage in self-management

NURSING INTERVENTIONS/*RATIONALES*

Encourage honesty in recording, such as eating a forbidden candy bar, *so that recording is accurate and useful*
Encourage independence in applying concepts learned in teaching sessions, *because diabetes management is a lifelong endeavor*
Instruct when to seek assistance from medical personnel *to prevent delay in treatment*

EXPECTED OUTCOME

Child takes responsibility for management of disease commensurate with age and capabilities

KEY POINTS

- The endocrine system has three components: the cell, which sends a chemical message via a hormone; target cells, which receive the message; and the environment through which the chemical is transported from the site of synthesis to the sites of cellular action.

- Pituitary dysfunction is manifested primarily by growth disturbance.

- The main physiologic action of thyroid hormone is to regulate the basal metabolic rate and control the processes of growth and tissue differentiation.

- Disorders of thyroid function include hypothyroidism, autoimmune thyroiditis, goiter, and hyperthyroidism.

- Therapy for hyperthyroidism is directed at retarding the rate of hormone secretion and may include drug therapy, thyroidectomy, or radioiodine therapy.

- Classic forms of hypoparathyroidism in childhood are idiopathic—deficient production of parathyroid hormone (PTH)—and pseudohypoparathyroidism—increased PTH production with end-organ unresponsiveness to PTH.

- The adrenal cortex secretes three important groups of hormones: glucocorticoids, mineralocorticoids, and sex steroids.

- Disorders of adrenal function include acute adrenocortical insufficiency, chronic adrenocortical insufficiency, Cushing syndrome, congenital adrenogenital hyperplasia, and hyperaldosteronism.

- Four categories of Cushing syndrome are pituitary, adrenal, ectopic, and iatrogenic.

- Management of congenital adrenogenital hyperplasia includes assignment of a sex according to genotype, administration of cortisone, and, possibly, reconstructive surgery.

- Diabetes mellitus is categorized as type 1 diabetes and type 2 diabetes.

- Education of families includes explanation of diabetes, meal planning, administering insulin injection, monitoring, general hygienic practices, promoting exercise, record keeping, and observing for complications.

References

American Diabetes Association: Report of the Expert Committee on the Diagnosis and Classification of Diabetes Mellitus, *Diabetes Care* 24(suppl 1):S5-S20, 2001.

Anderson SE, Dallal GE, Must A: Relative weight and race influence average age at menarche: results from two nationally representative surveys of US girls studied 25 years apart, *Pediatrics* 111(4):844-850, 2003.

Arends NJT and others: MRI findings of the pituitary gland in short children born small for gestational age (SGA) in comparison with growth hormone-deficient (GHD) children and children with normal stature, *Clin Endocrinol* 57:719-724, 2002.

August GP, Julius JR, Blethen SL: Adult height in children with growth hormone deficiency who are treated with biosynthetic growth hormone: The National Cooperative Growth Study Experience, *Pediatrics* 102(2):512-516, 1998.

Barber CJ, Lowes L: Eating disorders and adolescent diabetes: is there a link? *Br J Nurs* 7(7):398-402 1998.

Bercu B: The growing conundrum: growth hormone treatment of the non–growth hormone deficient child, *JAMA* 276(7):567-568, 1996.

Blethen SL and others: Safety of recombinant deoxyribonucleic acid-derived growth hormone, *J Clin Endocrinol Metab* 81(5):1704-1710, 1996.

Boulgourdjian EM and others: Oral desmopressin treatment of central diabetes insipidus in children, *Acta Pediatr* 86:1261-1262, 1997.

Chase HP and others: Use of the GlucoWatch Biographer in children with type 1 diabetes, *Pediatrics* 111(4):790-794, 2003.

Cheetham T, Baylis PH: Diabetes insipidus in children: pathophysiology, diagnosis and management, *Paediatr Drugs* 4(12):785-796, 2002.

Chumlea WC and others: Age at menarche and racial comparisons in US girls, *Pediatrics* 111(1):110-113, 2003.

Cox M: A better mousetrap: what's new in blood glucose monitoring? *J Pediatr Health Care* 16(3):314-316, 2002.

Davison KK, Susman EJ, Birch LL: Percent body fat at age 5 predicts earlier pubertal development among girls at age 9, *Pediatrics* 111(4):815-821, 2003.

Durham E: Growth hormone deficiency in children, a change in diagnostic approach, *Adv Nurse Practitioners* 11(1):41-67, 2003.

Finkelstein BS, Imperiale TF, Speroff T and others: Effect of growth hormone therapy on height in children with idiopathic short stature, *Arch Pediatr Adolesc Med* 156(3): 230-240, 2002.

Fleming DF: Challenging traditional insulin injection practices, *Am J Nurs* 99(2):72-74, 1999.

Gilmore J, Skuse D: Short stature—the role of intelligence in psychosocial adjustment, *Arch Dis Child* 75(6):25-31, 1996.

Gnanalingham MG, Newland P, Smith CP: Accuracy and reproducibility of low dose insulin administration using pen-injectors and syringes, *Arch Dis Child* 79(1):59-62, 1998.

Guyda HJ: Growth hormone testing and the short child, *Pediatr Res* 48(5):579-580, 2000.

Halac I, Zimmerman D: Evaluation of short stature in children, *Pediatr Ann* 33(3):171-176, 2004.

Hathout EH and others: Clinical, autoimmune, and HLA characteristics of children diagnosed with type 1 diabetes before 5 years of age, *Pediatrics* 111(4):860-863, 2003.

Hoffman RP: Juvenile diabetes: avoiding problems during therapy, *Clinical Advisor* May, pp 70-75, 2003.

Kempers MJE, Otten BJ: Idiopathic precocious puberty versus puberty in adopted children: auxological response to gonadotrophin-releasing hormone agonist treatment and final height, *Eur J Endocrinol* 147: 609-616, 2002.

Kiess W and others: Type 2 diabetes mellitus in children and adolescents: a review from a European perspective, *Horm Res* 59(suppl 1):77-84, 2003.

Kimpimaki T and others: Short term exclusive breastfeeding predisposes young children to increased genetic risk of type 1 diabetes to progressive beta-cell autoimmunity, *Diabetologia* 44(1):63-69, 2001.

Kranzler JH and others: Is short stature a handicap? A comparison of the psychosocial functioning of referred and nonreferred children with normal short stature and children with normal stature, *J Pediatr* 136(4):96-102, 2000.

Lanza RP and others: Xenotransplantation of cells using biodegradable microcapsules, *Transplant* 67(8):1105-1111, 1999.

Levine LS: Congenital adrenal hyperplasia, *Pediatr Rev* 21(5):159-170, 2000.

Lock JP and others: Whole-blood glucose testing at alternative sites: glucose values and hematocrit of capillary blood drawn from fingertip and forearm, *Diabetes Care* 25(6):961-964, 2002.

Lteif AN, Schwenk WF: Accuracy of pen injectors versus insulin syringes in children with type 1 diabetes, *Diabetes Care* 22(10):137-140, 1999.

Magee MF, Bhatt BA: Management of decompensated diabetes: diabetic ketoacidosis and hyperglycemic hyperosmolar syndrome, *Crit Care Clin* 17(1):75-106, 2001.

Magiakou MA and others: Cushing's syndrome in children and adolescents: presentation, diagnosis, and therapy, *N Engl J Med* 331(10):629-636, 1994.

Midyett LK and others: Are pubertal changes in girls before age 8 benign? *Pediatrics* 111(1):47-51, 2003.

Miller BS, Zimmerman D: Idiopathic short stature in children, *Pediatr Ann* 33(3):177-181, 2004.

Moshang T: Editorial: Cushing's disease, 70 years later . . . and the beat goes on, *J Clin Endocrinol Metab* 88(1):31-33, 2003.

Olohan K, Zappitelli D: The insulin pump: making life with diabetes easier, *Am J Nurs* 103(4):48-56, 2003.

Pizzo PA, Poplack DG: *Principles and theories of pediatric oncology*, Philadelphia, 2001, Lippincott Williams & Wilkins.

Plotnick LP: The next step in blood glucose monitoring? *Pediatrics* 111(4):885, 2003.

Ramchandani N: Type 2 diabetes in children, *Am J Nurs* 104(3):65-68, 2004.

Redondo M, Fain P, Eisenbarth G: Genetics of type 1A diabetes, *Recent Prog Horm Res* 58:69-89, 2001.

Rivkees SA, Cornelius EA: Influence of iodine-131 dose on the outcome of hyperthyroidism in children, *Pediatrics* 111(4):745-748, 2003.

Robertson RP and others: Pancreas and islet transplantation for patients with diabetes (technical review), *Diabetes Care* 23:112-116, 2000.

Root AW: Precocious puberty, *Pediatr Rev* 21(1):10-19, 2000.

Ross LF: Minimizing risks: the ethics of predictive diabetes mellitus screening research in newborns, *Arch Pediatr Adolesc Med* 157:89-95, 2003.

Ruble JA: Congenital adrenal hyperplasia. In Jackson PL, Vessey JA, editors: *Primary care of the child with a chronic condition*, ed 2, St Louis, 1996, Mosby.

Saenger P: The case in support of GH therapy, *J Pediatr* 36(1):106-109, 2000.

Sandberg DE, Brook AE, Campos SP: Short stature: a psychosocial burden requiring growth hormone therapy? *Pediatr* 94(6 pt 1):832-840, 1994.

Sandberg DE, Voss LD: The psychosocial consequences of short stature: a review of the evidence, *Best Pract Res Clin Endocrinol Metab* 16(3):449-463, 2002.

Seley J: Giving the fingers a rest, alternative site testing eases blood glucose monitoring, *Am J Nurs* 103(3):73-77, 2003.

Shulman DI, Bercu BB: Growth hormone therapy: an update, *Contemp Pediatr* 15(8):95-108, 1998.

Skyler J and others: Efficacy of inhaled human insulin in type 1 diabetes mellitus: a randomized proof-of-concept study, *Lancet* 357(9253): 324-325, 2001.

Steinberger J and Daniels SR: Obesity, insulin resistance, diabetes, and cardiovascular risk in children, *Circulation* 107:1448-1453, 2003.

Stephenson M: Type 2 diabetes: a growing epidemic in children, *Infect Dis Child* 16(4):34, 36-37, 2003.

Streetman DD, Khanderia U: Diagnosis and treatment of Graves disease, *Am J Nurse Practit* 8(1):27-36, 2004.

Thomas M and others: Growth hormone (GH) secretion in patients with childhood-onset GH deficiency: retesting after one year of therapy and at final height, *Horm Res* 59:7-15, 2003.

Thompson GB: Surgical management in Graves' disease, *Panminerva Med* 44(4):287-293, 2002.

Voss LD: Growth hormone therapy for the short normal child: who needs it and who wants it? *J Pediatr* 36(1):103-106, 2000.

Wilson TA and others: Update of guidelines for the use of growth hormone in children: the Lawson Wilkins pediatric endocrinology society drug and therapeutics committee, *J Pediatr* 143:415-421, 2003.

Wu T, Mendola P, Buck GM: Ethnic differences in the presence of secondary sex characteristics and menarche among US girls: the third national health and nutrition examination survey, 1988-1994, *Pediatrics* 110(4):752-756, 2002.

Wunderlich RP and others: Pathophysiology and treatment of painful diabetic neuropathy of the lower extremity, *South Med J* 91(10): 894-898, 1998.

Zimet GD and others: Psychosocial outcome of children evaluated for short stature, *Arch Pediatr Adolesc Med* 151(10):1017-1023, 1997.

The Child With Integumentary Dysfunction

MARILYN L. WINKELSTEIN

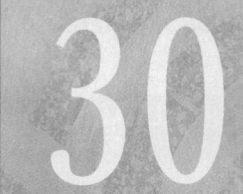

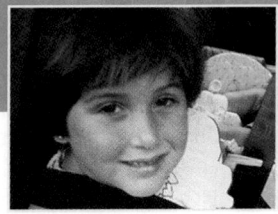

30

Remember to check out your companion CD-ROM

http://evolve.elsevier.com/Wong/essentials/

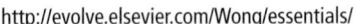

CHAPTER OUTLINE

RELATED TOPICS and ADDITIONAL RESOURCES

- Describe the distribution and configuration of the various skin lesions.
- List the benefits of a moist environment for wound healing.
- Discuss the nursing care related to therapies for skin disorders.
- Contrast the manifestations of and therapies for bacterial, viral, and fungal infections of the skin.
- Compare the skin manifestations related to age in children.
- Outline a plan of care to prevent and treat diaper dermatitis.
- Outline a plan of care for a child with atopic dermatitis.
- Formulate a teaching plan for an adolescent with acne.
- Describe the methods for assessing a burn wound.
- Discuss the physical and emotional care of a child with a severe burn wound.

INTEGUMENTARY DYSFUNCTION

SKIN LESIONS

Lesions of the skin result from a variety of etiologic factors. Skin lesions originate from (1) contact with injurious agents (infective organisms, toxic chemicals, and physical trauma); (2) hereditary factors; (3) external factors (e.g., allergens); or (4) systemic diseases (e.g., measles, lupus erythematosus, nutritional deficiency diseases). Responses to these agents or factors are highly individualized. An agent that may be harmless to one individual may be damaging to another, and a single agent may produce different responses in different individuals.

An important factor in the etiology of skin manifestations is the age of the child. Infants are subject to "birthmark" malformations and atopic dermatitis that appear early in life; the school-age child is susceptible to ringworm of the scalp; and acne is a characteristic skin disorder of puberty. Contact dermatitis, such as poison ivy, is seen only when the noxious agent is found in the environment. Tension and anxiety may produce, modify, or prolong skin conditions.

Skin of Younger Children

The major skin layers arise from different embryologic origins. Early in the embryonic period, a single layer of epithelium forms from the ectoderm, while simultaneously the corium develops from the mesenchyme. In the infant and small child the epidermis is loosely bound to the dermis.

This poor adherence causes the layers to separate easily during an inflammatory process to form blisters. This is especially true in preterm infants, who have a propensity to blister formation and separation of the skin during careless handling (such as removal of adhesive tape). In contrast, the skin of the older child is thinner, and the cells of all the strata are more compressed.

Pathophysiology of Dermatitis

More than half of the dermatologic problems in children are forms of dermatitis. This implies a sequence of inflammatory changes in the skin that is grossly and microscopically similar but diverse in course and causation. Acute responses produce intercellular and intracellular edema, the formation of intradermal vesicles, and an initial infiltration of inflammatory cells into the epidermis. In the dermis there is edema, vascular dilation, and early perivascular cellular infiltration. The location and manner of these reactions produce the lesions characteristic of each disorder. The changes are usually reversible, and the skin ordinarily recovers without blemish unless complicating factors such as ulceration from the primary irritant, scratching, and infection are introduced or underlying vascular disease develops. In chronic conditions permanent effects are seen that vary according to the disorder, the general condition of the affected individual, and the available therapy.

Diagnostic Evaluation

Although the history and subjective symptoms of skin lesions are explored first, the obvious objective characteristics of the lesions are often noted simultaneously. Many skin lesions are easily diagnosed after careful inspection.

History and Subjective Symptoms. Many cutaneous lesions are associated with local symptoms. The most common local symptom is itching *(pruritus)*, which varies in intensity. Pain or tenderness often accompanies some skin lesions. Other skin sensations such as burning, prickling, stinging, or crawling are also described. Alterations in local feeling include absence of sensation *(anesthesia)*, excessive sensitivity *(hyperesthesia)*, diminished sensation *(hypesthesia* or *hypoesthesia)*, or abnormal sensation, such as burning or prickling *(paresthesia)*. These symptoms may remain localized or migrate, may be constant or intermittent, and may be aggravated by a specific activity, such as exposure to sunlight.

It is important to determine whether the child has an allergic condition such as asthma or hay fever or history of a previous skin disease. Atopic dermatitis, often associated with allergies, frequently begins in infancy. Important questions for the parent include when the lesion or symptom first appeared, whether it occurred with ingestion of a food or other substance, including any medication, and whether the condition was related to activity such as contact with plants, insects, or chemicals.

Objective Findings. The distribution, size, morphology, and arrangement of skin lesions provide significant information. Extrinsic causes usually result from physical, chemical, or allergic irritants or from an infectious agent such as bacteria, fungi, viruses, or animal parasites. Skin manifestations are also produced by intrinsic causes such as an infection (measles or chickenpox), drug sensitization, or other allergic phenomena.

Lesion. Skin lesions assume distinct characteristics that are related to the pathologic process. Nurses should become familiar with the common terms that are applied to skin lesions because these terms are used in the processes of record keeping and communication. These terms include:

1 **Erythema**—A reddened area caused by increased amounts of oxygenated blood in the dermal vasculature
2 **Ecchymoses (bruises)**—Localized red or purple discolorations caused by extravasation of blood into dermis and subcutaneous tissues
3 **Petechiae**—Pinpoint, tiny, and sharp circumscribed spots in the superficial layers of the epidermis
4 **Primary lesions**—Skin changes produced by a causative factor; common primary lesions in pediatric skin disorders are macules, papules, and vesicles (Fig. 30-1)
5 **Secondary lesions**—Changes that result from alteration in the primary lesions, such as those caused by rubbing, scratching, medication, or involution and healing (Fig. 30-2)
6 **Distribution pattern**—The pattern in which lesions are distributed over the body, whether local or generalized, and the specific areas associated with the lesions
7 **Configuration and arrangement**—The size, shape, and arrangement of a lesion or groups of lesions (e.g., ***discrete, clustered, diffuse,*** or ***confluent***)

Laboratory Studies. If a skin problem is related to a systemic disease (e.g., collagen or immunodeficiency disease) laboratory studies are performed to identify these conditions. Diagnostic techniques include microscopic examination, cultures, skin scrapings or biopsy, cytodiagnosis, patch testing, Wood light examination, allergic skin testing, and other laboratory tests such as blood count and sedimentation rate.

WOUNDS

Wounds are structural or physiologic disruptions of the skin that activate normal or abnormal tissue repair responses. Wounds are classified as acute or chronic. ***Acute wounds*** are those that heal uneventfully within 2 to 3 weeks. ***Chronic wounds*** are those that do not heal in the expected time frame or are associated with complications. Cofactors that disrupt or delay wound healing include compromised perfusion, malnutrition, and infection. In children, most wounds are acute and can be prevented from becoming chronic wounds through appropriate nursing care. Wounds are also classified as surgical and nonsurgical and then further classified in the same manner as burns: superficial, partial-thickness, full-thickness (complex wounds that include muscle or bone).

Epidermal Injuries

Abrasions are the most common epidermal wounds in children, usually in the form of a skinned knee or elbow. In most injuries the margins of the abraded area are superficial, involving only the outer layers of epidermis, although the central portion may extend into the dermis. Epithelial

Macule—flat; nonpalpable; circumscribed; less than 1 cm in diameter; brown, red, purple, white, or tan in color
Examples: Freckles; flat moles; rubella; rubeola

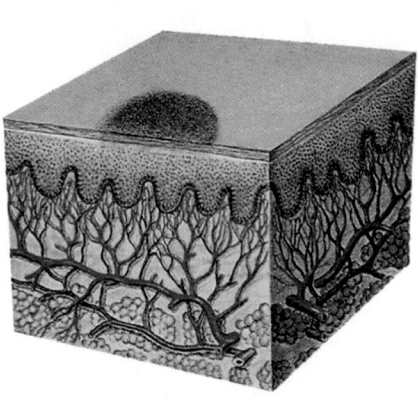

Plaque—elevated; flat topped; firm; rough; superficial papule greater than 1 cm in diameter; may be coalesced papules
Examples: Psoriasis; seborrheic and actinic keratoses

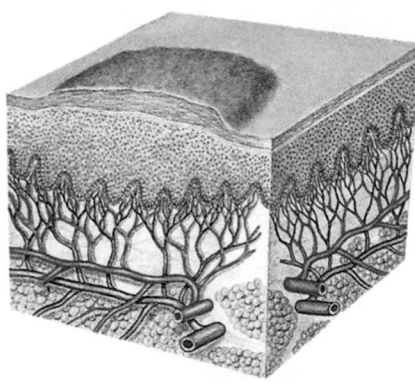

Patch—flat; nonpalpable; irregular in shape; macule that is greater than 1 cm in diameter
Examples: Vitiligo; port-wine marks

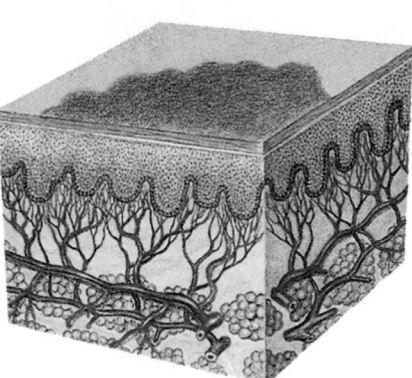

Wheal—elevated, irregularly shaped area of cutaneous edema; solid, transient, changing, variable diameter; pale pink with lighter center
Examples: Urticaria; insect bites

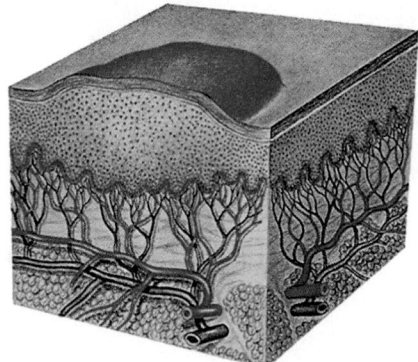

FIG. 30-1 ■ Primary skin lesions. (From Seidel HM and others: *Mosby's guide to physical examination,* ed 5, St Louis, 2003, Mosby.)

continued

Papule—elevated; palpable; firm; circumscribed; less than 1 cm in diameter; brown, red, pink, tan, or bluish red in color
Examples: Warts; drug-related eruptions; pigmented nevi

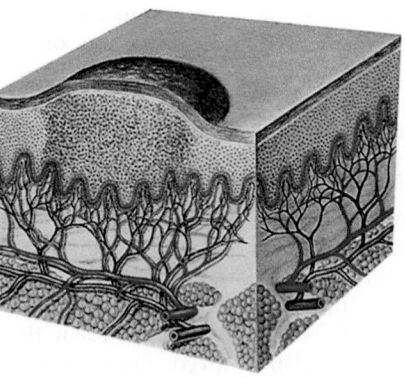

Nodule—elevated; firm; circumscribed; palpable; deeper in dermis than papule; 1 to 2 cm in diameter
Examples: Erythema nodosum; lipomas

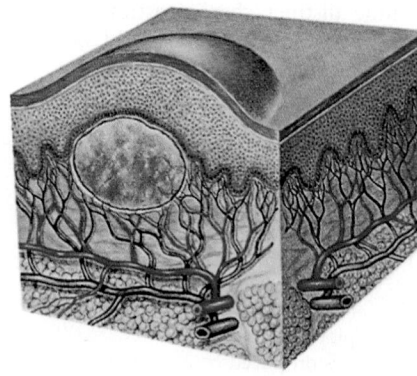

Vesicle—elevated; circumscribed; superficial; filled with serous fluid; less than 1 cm in diameter
Examples: Blister; varicella

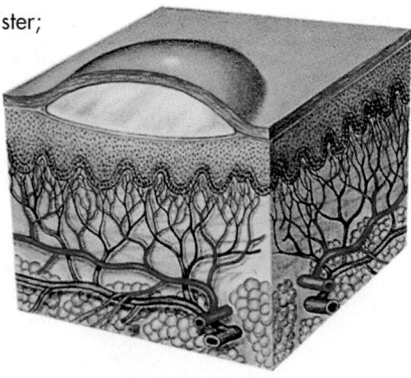

Pustule—elevated; superficial; similar to vesicle but filled with purulent fluid
Examples: Impetigo; acne; variola

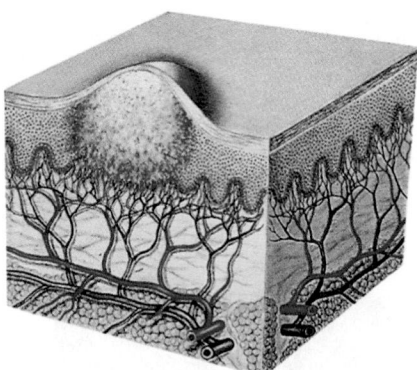

Bulla—vesicle greater than 1 cm in diameter
Examples: Blister; pemphigus vulgaris

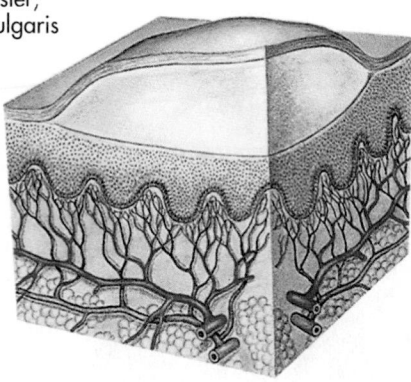

Cyst—elevated; circumscribed; palpable; encapsulated; filled with liquid or semisolid material
Example: Sebaceous cyst

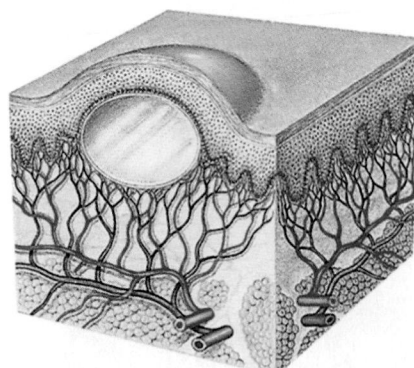

FIG. 30-1, cont'd ■ Primary skin lesions.

tissue is composed of labile cells, which are constantly destroyed and replaced throughout the lifespan. Therefore, epidermal injuries usually result in rapid uneventful healing and recovery.

Injury to Deeper Tissues

Tissues composed of *permanent cells* such as muscle and nerve cells are unable to regenerate. These tissues repair themselves by substituting fibrous connective tissue for the injured tissue. This fibrous tissue, or *scar,* serves as a patch to preserve or restore the continuity of the tissue. Wounds involving permanent cells include surgical incisions, lacerations, ulcers, evulsions, and full-thickness burns.

Process of Wound Healing

When the skin is injured, its normal protective barrier function is broken. In the healthy immunocompetent individual, acute traumatic abrasions, lacerations, and superficial skin and soft-tissue injuries heal spontaneously without complications. The process of tissue healing involves complex cellular interactions and biochemical reactions. The healing process is segregated into four phases that are characterized by the particular cells involved and the chemicals produced. The four stages of wound healing include hemostasis, inflammation, proliferation, and remodeling (Krasner, Rodeheaver, and Sibbald, 2001). Some authorities combine the first two phases. In the *hemostasis* phase, platelets act to seal off the damaged blood vessels and to form a stable clot. Hemostasis occurs within minutes of the initial injury to the skin unless there is an underlying clotting disorder.

Inflammation, the second stage of wound healing, presents a clinical picture that involves erythema, swelling, and warmth often associated with pain at the wound site. This stage usually lasts up to 4 days after injury. The inflammation phase involves white blood cells such as the neutrophils, monocytes, and macrophages. These cells mount an initial defense against microbial invasion and secrete proteolytic enzymes that destroy nonviable tissue and microorganisms in the wound area.

The *proliferative* phase, which includes *granulation* and *contracture,* is the third stage of healing. This phase lasts from 4 to 21 days in acute wounds depending on the size of the wound. The phase involves the replacement of dermal tissues and subdermal tissues in deep wounds as well as the contraction of the wound. The phase is characterized clinically by the presence of granulation tissue, the "beefy," pebbled red tissue in the wound base. Fibroblasts or immature connective tissue cells secrete collagen, which provides the foundation for dermal regeneration. Angiocytes regenerate the outer layers of capillaries and endothelial cells produce the lining in a process called angiogenesis. The formation of granulation tissue, which provides the foundation for the wound, is dependent on angiogenesis. The keratinocytes are responsible for epithelialization. In the final

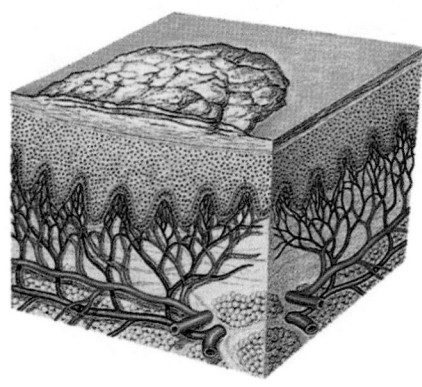

Scale—heaped-up keratinized cells; flaky exfoliation; irregular; thick or thin; dry or oily; varied size; silver, white, or tan in color
Examples: Psoriasis; exfoliative dermatitis

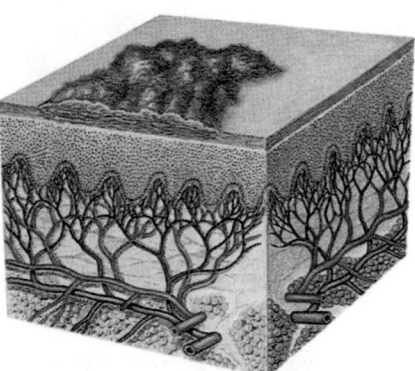

Crust—dried serum, blood, or purulent exudate; slightly elevated; size varies; brown, red, black, tan, or straw in color
Examples: Scab on abrasion; eczema

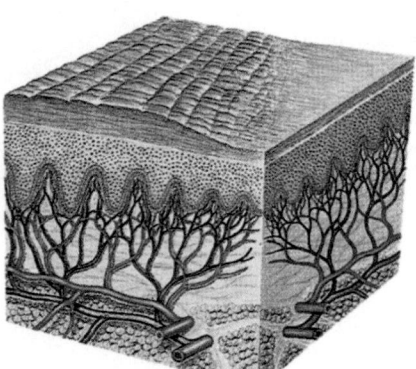

Lichenification—rough, thickened epidermis; accentuated skin markings caused by rubbing or irritation; often involves flexor aspect of extremity
Example: Chronic dermatitis

FIG. 30-2 ■ Secondary skin lesions. (From Seidel HM and others: *Mosby's guide to physical examination,* ed 5, St Louis, 2003, Mosby.)

continued

Scar—thin to thick fibrous tissue replacing injured dermis; irregular; pink, red, or white in color; may be atrophic or hypertrophic
Example: Healed wound or surgical incision

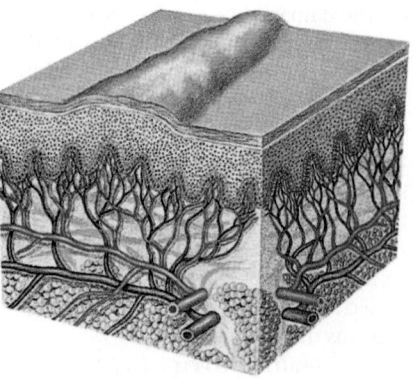

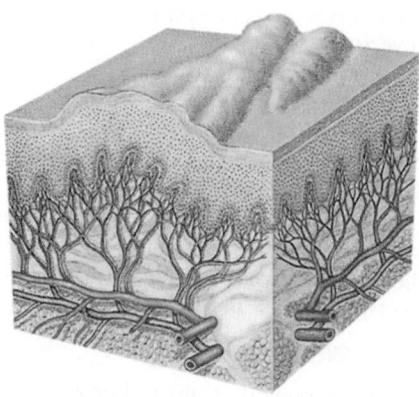

Keloid— irregularly shaped, elevated, progressively enlarging scar; grows beyond boundaries of wound; caused by excessive collagen formation during healing
Example: Keloid from ear piercing or burn scar

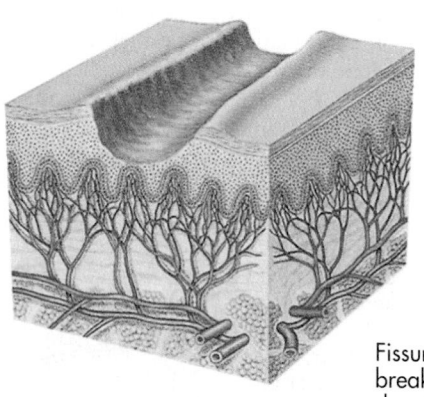

Excoriation—loss of epidermis; linear or hollowed-out crusted area; dermis exposed
Examples: Abrasion; scratch

Fissure—linear crack or break from epidermis to dermis; small; deep; red
Examples: Athlete's foot; cheilosis

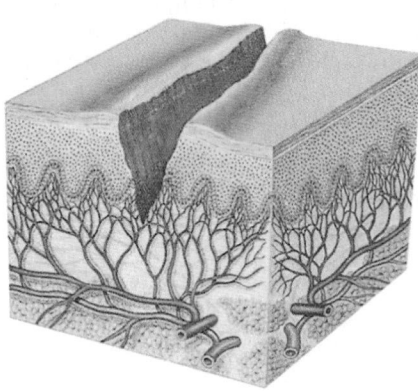

Erosion—loss of all or part of epidermis; depressed; moist; glistening; follows rupture of vesicle or bulla; larger than fissure
Examples: Varicella; variola following rupture

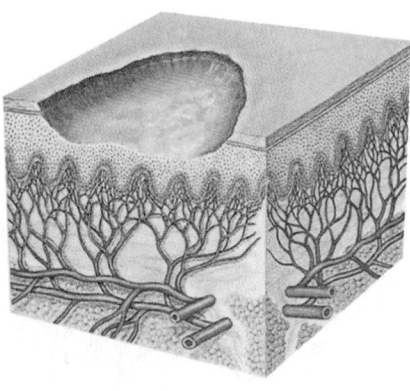

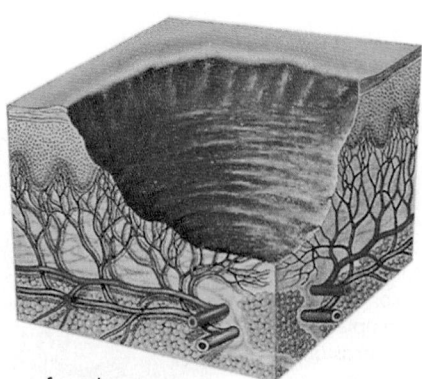

Ulcer—loss of epidermis and dermis; concave; varies in size; exudative; red or reddish blue
Examples: Decubiti; stasis ulcers

FIG. 30-2, cont'd ■ Secondary skin lesions.

stage of epithelialization, contracture occurs as the keratinocytes differentiate and form the protective outer layer or stratum corneum of the skin.

Remodeling or *maturation* is the final phase of the healing process. This phase occurs in the dermis as fibroblasts increase the tissue tensile strength and gradually replace Type 3 collagen in the scar tissue with Type 1 collagen, thicken the collagen fibers, and reorient the collagen fibers along the lines of tissue tension. Fibroblasts disappear as the wound becomes stronger. The wound edges are brought closer together, and a mature scar is formed. Children heal aggressively with abundant scar tissue, especially during growth spurts. The highly elastic quality of children's skin pulls on the wound, and the wound defends against this pull by forming scar tissue. Remodeling and maturation occurs over several months and can take up to 2 years. Thus some wounds that appear to be completely healed can break down suddenly if attention is not paid to the initial causative factors.

The phases of wound healing are complex and may be interrupted by disease conditions, medications, and other systemic and local factors that influence the healing process. When a wound does not follow the *"normal wound healing trajectory,"* it may become stuck in one of the stages and become a chronic wound. It is important that health care providers understand and address the factors that influence wound healing and prevent the development of chronic wounds.

Factors That Influence Healing

A revolution in wound healing has occurred in the last two decades. Emphasis has shifted from interventions aimed at maintaining a dry environment to those that promote a moist, crust-free environment that enhances the migration of epithelial cells across the wound and facilitates remodeling. An acute full-thickness wound kept in a moist environment usually reepithelializes in 12 to 15 days, whereas the same wound when kept open to the air heals in about 25 to 30 days.

Numerous factors can delay healing (Table 30-1). For example, traditional practices, such as the use of antiseptics (hydrogen peroxide and povidone-iodine [Betadine] solu-

TABLE 30-1 ■ Factors That Delay Wound Healing

FACTOR	EFFECT ON HEALING
Dry wound environment	Allows epithelial cells to dry out and die; impairs migration of epithelial cells across wound surface
Nutritional deficiencies	
Vitamin A	Results in inadequate inflammatory response
Vitamin B₁	Results in decreased collagen formation
Vitamin C	Inhibits formation of collagen fibers and capillary development
Protein	Reduces supply of amino acids for tissue repair
Zinc	Impairs epithelialization
Immunocompromise	Results in inadequate or delayed inflammatory response
Impaired circulation	Inhibits inflammatory response and removal of debris from wound area
	Reduces supply of nutrients to wound area
Stress (pain, poor sleep)	Releases catecholamines that cause vasoconstriction
Antiseptics	
Hydrogen peroxide	Toxic to fibroblasts; can cause subcutaneous gas formation (mimics gas-forming infection)
Povidone-iodine	Toxic to white and red blood cells and fibroblasts
Chlorhexidine	Toxic to white blood cells
Medications	
Corticosteroids	Impair phagocytosis
	Inhibit fibroblast proliferation
	Depress formation of granulation tissue
	Inhibit wound contraction
Chemotherapy	Interrupts the cell cycle, damages DNA or prevents DNA repair
Antiinflammatory drugs	Decrease the inflammatory phase
Foreign bodies	Increase inflammatory response
	Inhibit wound closure
Infection	Increases inflammatory response
	Increases tissue destruction
Mechanical friction	Damages or destroys granulation tissue
Fluid accumulation	Accumulation in area inhibits tissues from approximating
Radiation	Inhibits fibroblastic activity and capillary formation
	May cause tissue necrosis
Diseases	
Diabetes mellitus	Inhibits collagen synthesis
	Impairs circulation and capillary growth
	Hyperglycemia impairs phagocytosis
Anemia	Reduces oxygen supply to tissues
Peripheral vascular disease	Reduces oxygen supply to wounds
Uremia	Decreases collagen and granulation tissue

tions), which were once thought to prevent infection, are now known to have a cytotoxic effect on healthy cells and minimal effect on controlling infections. Povidone-iodine may also be absorbed through the skin in neonates and young children.

GENERAL THERAPEUTIC MANAGEMENT

Some skin disorders demand aggressive therapy, but by and large the major aim of treatment is to prevent further damage, eliminate the cause, prevent complications, and provide relief from discomfort while tissues undergo healing. Factors that contribute to the development of dermatitis and that prolong the course of the disease should be eliminated when possible. The most common causative agents of dermatitis in infants, children, and adolescents are environmental factors (soaps, bubble baths, shampoos, rough or tight clothing, wet diapers, blankets, and toys) and the natural elements (such as dirt, sand, heat, cold, moisture, and wind). Dermatitis may also result from home remedies and medications.

Dressings

No one dressing meets the needs of all wounds. The traditional *dry* gauze dressing should not be used on open wounds, because it allows the wound surface to dry, does little to prevent bacterial invasion, and adheres to the dried scab so that removal disturbs the newly regenerating epithelial cells. In most instances, traditional gauze dressings have been replaced with moist wound healing dressings (see Table 30-2). Moist wound healing increases the rate of collagen synthesis and reepithelialization and decreases pain and inflammation. It also creates an environment for autolytic débridement of necrotic tissue, which creates a clean wound bed and enhances granulation. However, a balance must be achieved between creating a moist wound bed and maintaining a dry periwound area that protects the skin and wound from maceration. The dressing type and frequency of dressing changes help to achieve this balance. The frequency of dressing changes is based on the presence of infection, the type of dressing, the location of the wound, and the amount of drainage. Dressings should always be changed when they are loose or soiled. They should be changed more frequently in areas where contamination is likely (e.g., the sacral area, the buttocks, the tracheal area) or when wound infection is suspected or present.

Topical Therapy

Several agents and methods are available for treatment. In selecting a therapeutic regimen, the practitioner considers (1) the choice of active ingredient, (2) the proper vehicle or base, (3) the cosmetic effect, (4) the cost, and (5) instructions for use. Several basic concepts must also be considered. Overtreatment is avoided. For example, when the dermatitis is acute, topical applications should be mild and bland to avoid further irritation. Broken or inflamed skin, especially in children, is more absorbent than intact skin, and chemicals that are nonirritating to intact skin may be quite irritating to inflamed skin.

Topical applications may be applied to treat the disorder, reduce itching, decrease external stimuli, or apply external heat or cold. The emollient action of soaks, baths, and lo-

tions provides a soothing film over the skin surface that reduces external stimuli. Ordinarily, lukewarm, tepid, or cool applications offer the greatest relief.

> **⏐ NURSING ALERT**
>
> Application of heat tends to aggravate most conditions, and its use is usually reserved for reducing specific inflammatory processes, such as folliculitis and cellulitis.
>
> Ointments in a petrolatum base provide protection from moisture. Therefore, this type of ointment is indicated around gastrostomy tubes, in skinfolds, and in the diaper area. Creams are absorbed by the skin and are used for areas where a nongreasy "feel" is desired (e.g., face, hands).

Topical Corticosteroid Therapy. Glucocorticoids are the therapeutic agents used most frequently for skin disorders. Their local antiinflammatory effects are merely palliative, so the medication must be applied until the condition undergoes a remission or the causative agent is eliminated. Corticosteroids are applied directly to the affected area, are essentially nonsensitizing, and have only minor side effects. As with the use of any steroids, their use in large amounts may mask signs of infection, and symptoms may be exacerbated after termination of the drug. Families are cautioned that the medication cannot be used for all skin disorders. The concentrations available without prescription are not adequate for stubborn skin conditions (e.g., psoriasis) and may cause worsening of inflammation caused by fungus or bacteria. Most parents and children apply too much topical hydrocortisone; therefore, they should be counseled that it is both effective and economical to apply only a thin film and to massage it into the skin. Parents and children should also be advised to use the application for no more than 5 to 7 days because these agents may cause depigmentation and other changes in the skin.

Other Topical Therapies. Other topical treatments include chemical cautery (especially useful for warts), cryosurgery, electrodesiccation (chiefly used for warts, granulomas, and nevi), ultraviolet therapy (primarily used in psoriasis and acne), laser therapy (especially for birthmarks), and acne therapies such as dermabrasion and chemical peels. New drugs called topical immunomodulators are very effective in reducing the itching of atopic dermatitis (eczema) and preventing the recurrence of "flares."

Systemic Therapy

Systemic drugs may be used as an adjunct to topical therapy in some dermatologic disorders. The drugs most frequently used are corticosteroids, antibiotics, and antifungal agents. Corticosteroids are valuable because of their capacity to inhibit inflammatory and allergic reactions. Dosage is carefully adjusted and gradually tapered to the minimum dose that is effective and tolerated. In infants and children, dosage is larger than is usually calculated from body weight ratios. However, prolonged use may temporarily suppress growth.

Antibiotics are used in severe or widespread skin infections. However, because these drugs tend to produce hypersensitivity in some patients, they are used with caution. Antifungal agents are the only means for treating systemic fungal infections.

TABLE 30-2 ■ **Properties of Commonly Used Dressings and Other Products**

EXAMPLES	INDICATIONS	ADVANTAGES	DISADVANTAGES	CONSIDERATIONS
POLYURETHANE FILMS Op-Site, Tegaderm, Bioclusive, BlisterFilm, Acu-derm, Polyskin II, Transorb, Epi View	Protection of partial-thickness red wounds Cover dressing for hydrophilic preparations and hydrogels Autolytic débridement of wounds with dry eschar	Transparent; good adhesion; reduces pain, minimizes friction forces to wound; time saving; easy to store; cost-effective Moisture, vapor, and oxygen transmission Impermeable to water and bacteria	Adhesive injury to intact and new skin; nonabsorbent; some products difficult to apply; variable barrier function; can promote wound infection Unsuitable for electrical stimulation wound healing	Protect wound margins; avoid in wounds with infection, copious drainage, tracts or fragile skin surrounding lesion Change only if dressing leaks or at least every 7 days Contraindicated in third-degree burns
POLYMERIC FOAMS Allevyn, Allevyn Adhesive, Allevyn Cavity, Nu-Derm, Lyofoam, PolyMem	Used when a nonadherent dressing is needed (good for absorption around G tubes and tracheostomies) Used for wounds with moderate to heavy exudates	Moisture is absorbed into foam; maceration is decreased Removal does not cause reinjury to wound Comfortable, easy to apply; cushions and protects wound	Requires an additional dressing to secure if the foam does not have an adhesive surface	Do not use on infected wounds Contraindicated for third-degree burns
HYDROCOLLOIDS Duoderm CGF, Duoderm Extra Thin, Comfeel, Restore, Tegasorb, SignaDress, Cutinova Hydro, Ultec, Actiderm, RepliCare	Protection of superficial and small, deep red wounds Autolytic débridement of small, noninfected yellow wounds* Partial thickness, stages 2 and 3; shallow full thickness, granulating with minimal to moderate exudates, stage 4	Absorbent; nonadhesive to healing tissue; waterproof; reduces pain; easy to apply; time-saving; easy to store Moldable to area; occlusive; provides insulation; maintains moist wound surface; wet-to-dry adherence	Nontransparent; may soften and lose shape with heat or friction; odor and brown drainage on removal (melted dressing material)	Frequency of changes depends on amount of exudates (change as needed for leakage) or at least every 7 days DO NOT USE for heavily exudative wounds, sinus tracts, or infected wounds; shape dressing to wound area Contraindicated in third-degree burns
HYDROGELS/SHEETS Vigilon, Elastogel, Aquasorb, Nu-Gel, Duoderm Gel, Second Skin, Hypergel, Intra-Site Gel, Carrasyn	Protection of superficial and moderately deep red wounds Autolytic débridement of small, noninfected yellow or black wounds* Delivery system for topical antimicrobial creams (increases penetration) Partial and full thickness	Absorbent; nonadhesive; reduces pain; compatible with topicals; good conformity; easy to store Maintains a moist wound surface, has a "cooling" effect	Poor barrier; semitransparent; requires cover dressing to secure; can promote growth of *Pseudomonas* and other gram-negative bacteria and yeast Unused portion will desiccate Not for weight-bearing ulcers Expensive; nonadhesive High water content can macerate surrounding skin	Avoid in infected wounds; change dressing as needed for leakage Cut and shape to wound DO NOT REMOVE poly backing Monitor wound for over-hydration and skin maceration around wound edges

Modified from Bryant RA: *Acute and chronic wounds, nursing management,* St Louis, 2000, Mosby; McCulloch JM, Kloth LC, Feedar JA: *Wound healing alternatives in management,* Philadelphia, 1995, FA Davis.
*NOTE: Users should read package inserts for any contraindications to use of these products. Some dressings, such as Duoderm CGF, have been approved for application to infected wounds if wound is cultured and treated for infection. Many products should not be used on third-degree burns.   *Continued*

TABLE 30-2 ■ Properties of Commonly Used Dressings and Other Products—*cont'd*

EXAMPLES	INDICATIONS	ADVANTAGES	DISADVANTAGES	CONSIDERATIONS
HYDROCOLLOID ABSORPTION POWDERS, PASTES, BEADS, AND GRANULES				
Bard absorption dressing, Comfeel Ulcus paste, Comfeel Ulcus powder, Multidex powder and gel, Debrisan	Used on uneven and exudating ulcers	Controls bacteria Cleanses wound Reduces odor Cost-effective		Cleanse with lukewarm water or saline to remove Contraindicated in third-degree burns
ALGINATES				
Sorbsan, Kaltostat, Curasorb, Restore, CalciCare, Fibrocal, Aquacel	Used for leg ulcers, donor sites, infected traumatic or exudating wounds	Nonallergenic; biodegradable; little to no local tissue reaction Decreases pain at wound site	Expensive; easily displaced by mechanical forces Permeable to bacteria, urine	Change daily after proper cleansing if used on infected wounds Requires a secondary cover dressing Contraindicated in third-degree burns

NURSING CARE OF THE CHILD WITH A SKIN DISORDER

The child's subjective symptoms and the parent's history provide valuable information to help establish a diagnosis. Older children often describe the condition as painful, itching, or tingling or in other descriptive terms. However, much can be determined by also observing the younger child's behavior. Does the child scratch? Is the child restless or irritable? Does the child favor or avoid using a body part? A careful history provides important clues. Has the child had access to chemicals or been in the woods or around a woodpile? Has the child eaten a new food? Is the child taking medication? Has the child any known allergy? Do siblings or playmates have similar lesions? What soap or bubble bath is used for bathing?

It is important for nurses to not only describe, but also to assess skin lesions and wounds. The color, shape, and distribution of lesions and wounds are important. Individual lesions are described according to standard terminology. Sometimes two descriptors are used to describe a particular characteristic (e.g., maculopapular rash). To confirm or amplify the findings made by inspection, the skin may be gently palpated to detect characteristics such as temperature, moisture, texture, elasticity, and the presence of edema. Wounds are assessed for depth of tissue damage, evidence of healing, and signs of infection.

❗ NURSING ALERT

Signs of wound infection are:
- Increased erythema, especially beyond the wound margin
- Edema
- Purulent exudate
- Pain
- Increased temperature

The frequency of wound assessment depends on the severity and complexity of the wound. For example, simple or chronic wounds are assessed weekly; infected or complex wounds are assessed daily. Wounds are measured at least weekly (height, width, and depth). The wound bed is assessed for color, drainage, odor, necrosis, granulation tissue, fibrin slough, undermining and condition of the wound edges, and the color and condition of the surrounding skin.

Therapeutic programs are designed to include general measures such as rest, protection, and relief of discomfort and specific treatments such as medication and physical techniques. Only a few skin diseases are contagious; therefore, it is usually not necessary to isolate the affected child unless there is a danger of acquiring a secondary infection (e.g., the child receiving large doses of corticosteroids or other immunosuppressant drugs or the child with an immunologic deficiency disorder). However, if the skin manifestation is caused by a viral exanthema, such as measles or chickenpox, the child is prevented from exposing other susceptible children.

Wound Care

Parents can generally manage small skin lesions or wounds at home. The parents are instructed to wash their hands and then wash the wound gently with mild soap and water or normal saline. They are cautioned to avoid Betadine, alcohol, and hydrogen peroxide because these products are toxic to wounds.

❗ NURSING ALERT

Do not put anything in a wound that you would not put in the eye. The safest solution is normal saline.

Open wounds are covered with a dressing, such as a commercial adhesive bandage, although larger wounds may benefit from the use of occlusive dressings (see Table 30-2). If occlusive dressings are applied, parents should learn how to apply and remove the dressings correctly. For example, hydrocolloid dressings adhere best if a wide margin is left around the wound and the dressing is pressed against intact skin until it adheres.* If a dressing needs to be secured, a non-alcohol skin barrier can be applied to protect the skin,

---

*Information on the use of the hydrocolloid dressing Duoderm is available from **ConvaTec Professional Services,** PO Box 5254, Princeton, NJ 08543; (800) 422-8811; fax: (908) 281-2405; website: www.convatec.com.

ATRAUMATIC CARE

Painless Suturing and Wound Cleansing

A variety of topical anesthetic solutions, such as lidocaine, adrenaline, and tetracaine (LAT) combined and tetracaine-phenylephrine (tetraphen), applied to wounds, especially on the head, scalp, and face, provide anesthesia in 10 to15 minutes (Smith and others, 1996). Tetracaine, adrenaline, and cocaine (TAC) combined or AC (without tetracaine) should not be used because of the potential for lethal cocaine intoxication. LAT is as effective, is safer, and is much less expensive than TAC. If further anesthesia is required or if the topical preparations are not available, using buffered lidocaine administered with a 30-gauge needle reduces the stinging and burning of the injection (see Pain Management, Chapter 21). The use of a noninvasive tissue adhesive (e.g., Dermabond*) provides a faster and less painful method of facial laceration repair with cosmetic results comparable to those obtained with suturing (Osmond, Klassen, and Quinn, 1995).

*Manufactured by **Closure Medical Corporation,** 5250 Greens Dairy Road, Raleigh, NC 27616; (919) 876-7800.

or the wound can be "picture framed" with a hydrocolloid and dressing tape can be secured to the hydrocolloid. This method of securing the dressing protects the skin when the tape is removed. Montgomery straps or stretch netting can also be used to secure dressings and to avoid the use of tape.

NURSING ALERT

Advise parents that the yellow gel forming under hydrocolloid dressings may look like pus and has a distinct odor (somewhat fruity) but is normal leakage.

Dressings are removed carefully to protect intact skin and the epithelial surface of the wound. When removing transparent or hydrocolloid dressings, the nurse or parent should raise one edge of the dressing and pull *parallel* to the skin to loosen the adhesive. The longer the dressings are left on, the easier they are to remove. Less frequent dressing changes decrease wound contamination.

Lacerations present a special challenge. The injured child and family are usually very distressed by the bleeding. In particular, scalp lacerations tend to bleed profusely. Parental guilt and shock usually accompany the injury. The initial nursing intervention is to apply pressure to the area and to attempt to calm the child before further examination. Unless there is bleeding from a severed artery, the wound is cleansed with a forced jet of sterile tepid water or saline (via syringe) and examined for extent, depth, and presence of foreign material such as dirt, glass, or fabric fragments.

The location of the wound facilitates assessment. Wounds over bony areas may contain bone chips, and clear fluid seeping from severe head wounds may indicate cerebrospinal fluid. A pressure dressing is applied for transfer to medical care. After the child is in a medical facility, he or she is prepared for suturing (see Atraumatic Care box).

Puncture wounds that do not require a tetanus booster are soaked in warm water and soap for several minutes. Causing the wound to rebleed may be helpful. An adhesive bandage can be applied if desired. Puncture wounds of the head, chest, or abdomen or those that could still contain a portion of the puncturing object must be evaluated carefully.

Parents are cautioned against opening blisters or kissing a wound "to make it better." The wound can easily become contaminated from germs in the human mouth. If scabs form, they are allowed to slough off without assistance; picking or early removal may cause scarring and secondary infection. Parents are advised to seek medical help if there is evidence of infection.

Relief of Symptoms

Most therapeutic regimens for skin lesions are directed toward relief of pruritus, the most common subjective complaint. Cooling the affected area and increasing the skin pH with cool baths or compresses and alkaline applications (e.g., baking soda baths) are helpful in cooling the affected area and reducing the itching. Clothing and bed linen should be soft and lightweight to decrease the irritation from friction and stimulation.

During treatment, both the affected and unaffected skin is protected from damage and secondary infection. Preventing scratching is very importance. Older children can cooperate, although they may need to be reminded to stop scratching or rubbing. However, small or uncooperative children may require the use of devices such as mittens (especially during sleep) or special coverings. Keeping fingernails clean, short, and trimmed reduces the risk of secondary infection.

Antipruritic medications, such as diphenhydramine (Benadryl) or hydroxyzine (Atarax), may be prescribed for severe itching, especially if it disturbs the child's rest. Pain and discomfort are usually managed with nonpharmacologic measures and mild analgesia. Severe pain requires more potent medication. Occlusive dressings over wounds reduce pain. For suturing wounds a topical anesthetic or intradermal buffered lidocaine should be used (see Pain Management, Chapter 21).

Topical Therapy

The specific type of topical therapy and the mode of application depend on the nature and location of the lesion. It is especially important to wash the hands before and after application of any topical therapy. The skin is assessed before the application and reassessed after treatment. Any observed changes are noted and described.

Wet compresses or *dressings* cool the skin by evaporation, relieve itching and inflammation, and cleanse the area by loosening and removing crusts and debris. A variety of ingredients, such as plain water or Burow solution (available without a prescription), can be applied on Kerlix gauze, plain gauze, or (preferably) soft cotton cloths such as freshly laundered handkerchiefs or strips from diaper, sheeting, or pillowcase material.

Dressings immersed in the desired solution are wrung out slightly and applied to the affected area wet but not dripping. They are applied flat and smooth in such a way that motion is not totally restricted—fingers are wrapped separately, and arms and legs are wrapped so that elbows and knees can bend. Dressings are held in place by Kerlix or other cotton wrap, tubular stockinette, mittens, and socks (two pairs—one to hold the dressings in place, the other to take up movement). When evaporation begins to dry them, the dressings are removed, rewet in the solution, and reapplied using aseptic technique. The solution is *not* poured or applied with a syringe directly over the dressings. As fluid evaporates, the solution becomes more concentrated, and this occurrence could damage sensitive lesions.

Fresh solution at room temperature is applied at 2-, 3-, or 4-hour intervals and allowed to remain on the lesion from 30 to 90 minutes. Wet dressings are seldom continued after about 48 hours. The child is protected against chilling during treatment, and no more than 20% of the body is covered at one time to avoid the risk of hypothermia. After treatment, the skin is dried thoroughly by patting with a towel. Lotion or other medication (if prescribed) is applied at this time.

When children are uncooperative in the use of wet dressings, *soaks* are often used for removal of crusts and for their mild astringent action. The same solutions are used as for wet compresses. Gaining young children's cooperation for hand or foot soaks is difficult unless the procedure is accompanied by play. Older infants and toddlers delight in playing with brightly colored objects or poker chips scattered over the bottom of the receptacle, and preschoolers can be challenged to hold a floating item beneath the water's surface. However, these activities require supervision; infants and small children place items in their mouths, and children easily lose control with water play. Washing dishes, cars, dolls, or doll clothes will also occupy time during soaks.

Although older children can cooperate, they, too, need something to do during the procedure, such as listening to music or a story, or watching television. Placing the solution and the extremity in a plastic sealable bag is an effective method to soak a hand or foot.

Baths are useful in the treatment of widespread dermatitis by evenly distributing the soothing antipruritic and antiinflammatory effects of the solution, usually oatmeal or mineral oil preparations. The solution is added to a tub of lukewarm water. The temperature of the bath is tepid, and the treatment usually lasts 15 to 30 minutes. Therapeutic baths are more interesting when toy boats or other items for water play accompany the procedure.

Topical applications are applied to skin lesions to ease discomfort, prevent further injury, and facilitate healing. A thin application of the ointment or cream may be covered with a plastic film and anchored with adhesive, covered with a commercial transparent dressing or wrapped in Kerlix gauze and held in place by a stretchy net dressing. Topical preparations are applied systematically with the contour of the body surface (not simply up and down). Children love to be "painted," and lotion applications can be fun when an ordinary paintbrush is used. Regardless of the type of preparation used, parents need detailed information on how to apply it and how long the preparation should remain on the skin.

! NURSING ALERT

Provide written instructions and demonstrate to parents the correct amount of topical medication to apply (e.g., size of a pea; thin film to cover). If more than one preparation is applied, mark the containers with numbers so the parents remember the correct order of application. Stress that more is not necessarily better with some medications, such as steroids.

HOME CARE AND FAMILY SUPPORT

Dermatologic conditions always involve the family, but few situations require hospitalization and most care is delivered at home. Because the family members must carry out the treatment plan, their cooperation is essential. Regimens that are simple to accomplish in the clinic, hospital, or primary care provider's office may be frustrating and baffling at home. The family may also need assistance in adapting equipment available for home therapy.

It is important that the child and family be given as detailed explanations as possible about both the expected and unexpected results of treatment, including any ill effects that might occur. If unexplained reactions develop, the family is directed to discontinue treatment and report the reactions to the appropriate person. The use of over-the-counter medicines is discouraged unless the preparations have been discussed with the health care provider and have received approval.

Because the skin is the most visible portion of the body, defects in its surface alter its appearance and cause distress for the child. Skin problems may also result in rejection by others. Parents of other children may fear that their children will "catch" the disorder. Occasionally the affected child's own family members reduce their interaction or physical contact with the child. This is seldom a problem with dermatitis of short duration, but chronic conditions can frequently create problems and affect the child's self-esteem (see Family Focus box).

INFECTIONS OF THE SKIN

BACTERIAL INFECTIONS

Normally, the skin harbors a variety of bacterial flora, including the major pathogenic varieties of staphylococci and streptococci. The degree of pathogenicity of the organism depends on its invasiveness and toxicity, the integrity of the

👥 FAMILY FOCUS

Skin Lesions and Self-Esteem in the School-Age Child

When I was 8 years old, a lot of small, oval, tannish brown spots developed, especially around my neck and waist. The dermatologist said it was a rare condition and it should disappear by the time I was 11 or 12. They actually disappeared when I was 10. Because the spots were kind of unusual, the dermatologist invited me to attend a dermatology meeting where people with strange skin problems were placed in private clinic rooms and doctors came in and looked at each person's skin. They were all nice, but I felt a little like an animal in the zoo. The thing I mostly remember about the spots was that I always tried to keep them covered. People stared, and kids made fun of me. The spots didn't hurt or itch, but I always knew they were there. I would not wear a two-piece swimsuit, even though my friends wore them. My mom and I tried to think of anything that might have caused the spots, but I never knew why they developed on me. I remember thinking it wasn't fair that it happened to me. I learned that many times, people cannot prevent the bad things that happen to them.

Marissa White, age 16
Tulsa, Oklahoma

skin, and the immune and cellular defenses of the host. Children with congenital or acquired immunodeficiency disorders (such as AIDS), those in a debilitated condition, those receiving immunosuppressant therapy, and those with a generalized malignancy such as leukemia or lymphoma are at risk for developing bacterial infections.

Because of the characteristic "walling-off" process of the inflammatory reaction (abscess formation), staphylococci are more difficult to treat, and the local infected area is associated with an increase in bacteria all over the skin surface that serves as a source of continuing infection. Staphylococcal infections occur most often in younger children, and the incidence decreases with advancing age. Common bacterial skin disorders are outlined in Table 30-3.

Nursing Considerations

The major nursing interventions related to bacterial skin infections are to prevent the spread of infection and to prevent complications. Handwashing is mandatory before and after contact with an affected child, and this practice is emphasized to all those who care for the child. The child should be provided with towels separate from those of other family members. Impetigo contagiosa is easily spread by self-inoculation; therefore, children with this condition must be cautioned against touching the involved area. This is difficult to accomplish. Although distraction or reminders are useful, these measures do not work when children are unsupervised or sleeping.

Children and parents are often tempted to squeeze follicular lesions. They must be warned that squeezing will not

TABLE 30-3 ■ Bacterial Infections

DISORDER/ORGANISM	MANIFESTATIONS	MANAGEMENT	COMMENTS
Impetigo contagiosa (Fig. 30-3)—*Staphylococcus*	Begins as a reddish macule Becomes vesicular Ruptures easily, leaving superficial, moist erosion Tends to spread peripherally in sharply marginated irregular outlines Exudate dries to form heavy, honey-colored crusts Pruritus common Systemic effects: minimal or asymptomatic	Careful removal of undermined skin, crusts, and debris by softening with 1:20 Burow solution compresses Topical application of bactericidal ointment Systemic administration of oral or parenteral antibiotics (penicillin) in severe or extensive lesions	Tends to heal without scarring unless secondary infection Autoinoculable and contagious Very common in toddler, preschooler May be superimposed on eczema
Pyoderma—*Staphylococcus, Streptococcus*	Deeper extension of infection into dermis Tissue reaction more severe Systemic effects: fever, lymphangitis	Soap and water cleansing Wet compresses Bathing with antibacterial soap as prescribed	Autoinoculable and contagious May heal with or without scarring
Folliculitis (pimple), **furuncle** (boil), **carbuncle** (multiple boils)—*Staphylococcus aureus*	Folliculitis: infection of hair follicle Furuncle: larger lesion with more redness and swelling at a single follicle Carbuncle: more extensive lesion with widespread inflammation and "pointing" at several follicular orifices Systemic effects: malaise, if severe	Skin cleanliness Local warm, moist compresses Topical application of antibiotic agents Systemic antibiotics in severe cases Incision and drainage of severe lesions, followed by wound irrigations with antibiotics or suitable drain implantation	Autoinoculable and contagious Furuncle and carbuncle tend to heal with scar formation A lesion should never be squeezed
Cellulitis—*Streptococcus, Staphylococcus, Haemophilus influenzae* (Fig. 30-4)	Inflammation of skin and subcutaneous tissues with intense redness, swelling, and firm infiltration Lymphangitis "streaking" frequently seen Involvement of regional lymph nodes common May progress to abscess formation Systemic effects: fever, malaise	Oral or parenteral antibiotics Rest and immobilization of both affected area and child Hot moist compresses to area	Hospitalization may be necessary for child with systemic symptoms Otitis media may be associated with facial cellulitis
Staphylococcal scalded skin syndrome—*S. aureus*	Macular erythema with "sandpaper" texture of involved skin Epidermis becomes wrinkled (in 2 days or less), and large bullae appear	Systemic administration of antibiotics Gentle cleansing with saline, Burow solution, or 0.25% silver nitrate compresses	Infant subject to fluid loss, impaired body temperature regulation, and secondary infection, such as pneumonia, cellulitis, and septicemia Heals without scarring

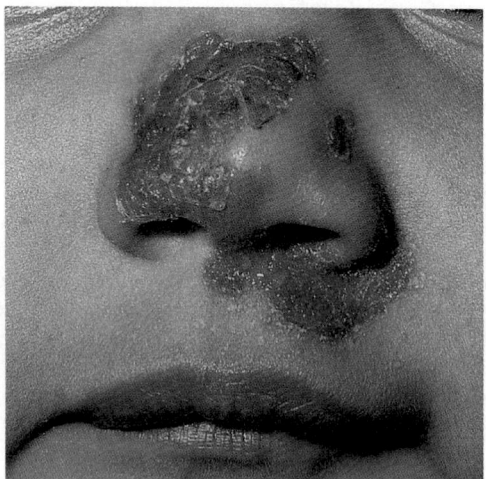

FIG. 30-3 ■ Impetigo contagiosa. (From Weston WL, Lane AT, Morelli JG: *Color textbook of pediatric dermatology,* ed 3, St Louis, 2002, Mosby.)

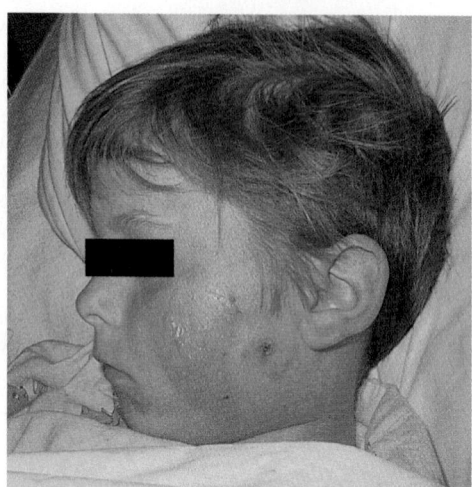

FIG. 30-4 ■ Cellulitis of cheek from puncture wound. (From Weston WL, Lane AT, Morelli JG: *Color textbook of pediatric dermatology,* ed 3, St Louis, 2002, Mosby.)

hasten the resolution of the infection and that there is a risk of making the lesion worse or spreading the infection. No attempt should be made to puncture the surface of the pustule with a needle or sharp instrument. A child with a sty may waken with the eyelids of the affected eye sealed shut with exudate. The child or the parents are instructed to gently wipe the lid from the inner to the outer edge with warm water and a clean washcloth until the exudate is removed.

The child with limited cellulitis of an extremity is usually managed at home on a regimen of oral antibiotics and warm compresses. The parents are taught the procedures and instructed in administration of the medication. Children with more extensive cellulitis, especially around a joint with lymphadenitis or on the face, are usually admitted to the hospital for parenteral antibiotics with continued treatment at home. Nurses are responsible for teaching the family to administer the medication and apply compresses.

VIRAL INFECTIONS

Viruses are intracellular parasites that produce their effect by using the intracellular substances of the host cells. Composed of only a DNA or RNA core enclosed in an antigenic protein shell, viruses are unable to provide for their own metabolic needs or to reproduce themselves. After a virus penetrates a cell of the host organism, it sheds the outer shell and disappears within the cell, where the nucleic acid core stimulates the host cell to form more virus material from its intracellular substance. In a viral infection the epidermal cells react with inflammation and vesiculation (as in herpes simplex) or by proliferating to form growths (warts).

Many of the communicable viral diseases of childhood are associated with rashes, and each rash is characteristic. The type of lesion and the configuration of rubeola, rubella, and chickenpox are described in Table 14-1. Other common viral disorders of the skin are outlined in Table 30-4.

DERMATOPHYTOSES (FUNGAL INFECTIONS)

The dermatophytoses (ringworm) are infections caused by a group of closely related filamentous fungi that invade primarily the stratum corneum, hair, and nails. These are su-

perficial infections that live on, not in, the skin. They are confined to the dead keratin layers and are unable to survive in the deeper layers. Because the keratin is desquamated constantly, the fungus must multiply at a rate that equals the rate of keratin production to maintain itself; otherwise, the infection would be shed with the discarded skin cells. Common dermatophytoses are outlined in Table 30-5.

Dermatophytoses are designated by the Latin word *tinea,* with further designation related to the area of the body where they are found (e.g., tinea capitis [ringworm of the scalp]). Dermatophyte infections are most often transmitted from one person to another or from infected animals to humans. Diagnosis is made from microscopic examination of scrapings taken from the advancing periphery of the lesion, which almost always produces a scale.

Nursing Considerations

When teaching families how to care for ringworm, the nurse should emphasize good health and hygiene. Because of the infectious nature of the disease, affected children should not exchange grooming items, headgear, scarves, or other articles of apparel that have been in proximity to the infected area with other children. Affected children are provided with their own towels and directed to wear a protective cap at night to avoid transmitting the fungus to bedding, especially if they sleep with another person. Because the infection can be acquired by animal-to-human transmission, all household pets should be examined for the presence of the disorder. Other sources of infection are seats with headrests (theater seats), seats in public transportation vehicles, helmets, and gymnasium mats.

Treatment with the drug griseofulvin frequently continues for weeks or months, and because subjective symptoms subside, children or parents may be tempted to decrease or discontinue the drug. The nurse should emphasize to family members the importance of maintaining the prescribed dosage schedule and of taking the medication with high-fat foods for best absorption. They are also instructed regarding possible drug side effects, such as headache, gastrointestinal upset, fatigue, insomnia, and photosensitivity. For children who take the drug over many months, periodic

TABLE 30-4 ■ **Viral Infections**

INFECTION	MANIFESTATIONS	MANAGEMENT	COMMENTS
Verruca (warts) Cause: human papillomavirus (various types)	Usually well-circumscribed, gray or brown, elevated, firm papules with a roughened, finely papillomatous texture Occur anywhere, but usually appear on exposed areas such as fingers, hands, face, and soles May be single or multiple Asymptomatic	Not uniformly successful Local destructive therapy, individualized according to location, type, and number—surgical removal, electrocautery, curettage, cryotherapy (liquid nitrogen), caustic solutions (lactic acid and salicylic acid in flexible collodion, retinoic acid, salicylic acid plasters), x-ray treatment, laser	Common in children Tend to disappear spontaneously Course unpredictable Most destructive techniques tend to leave scars Autoinoculable Repeated irritation will cause to enlarge Apply topical anesthetic EMLA
Verruca plantaris (plantar wart)	Located on plantar surface of feet and, because of pressure, are practically flat; may be surrounded by a collar of hyperkeratosis	Apply caustic solution to wart, wear foam insole with hole cut to relieve pressure on wart; soak 20 minutes after 2-3 days; repeat until wart comes out	Destructive techniques tend to leave scars, which may cause problems with walking Apply topical anesthetic EMLA
Herpes simplex virus Type I (cold sore, fever blister) Type II (genital)	Grouped, burning, and itching vesicles on inflammatory base, usually on or near mucocutaneous junctions (lips, nose, genitals, buttocks) Vesicles dry, forming a crust, followed by exfoliation and spontaneous healing in 8-10 days May be accompanied by regional lymphadenopathy	Avoidance of secondary infection Burow solution compresses during weeping stages Topical therapy (penciclovir) can shorten duration of cold sores Oral antiviral (acyclovir) for initial infection or to reduce severity in recurrence Valacyclovir (Valtrex), an oral antiviral used for episodic treatment of recurrent genital herpes, reduces pain, stops viral shedding, and has a more convenient administration schedule than acyclovir	Heal without scarring unless secondary infection Type I cold sores can be prevented by using sunscreens protecting against ultraviolet A (UVA) and ultraviolet B (UVB) light to prevent lip blisters Aggravated by corticosteroids Positive psychologic effect from treatment May be fatal in children with depressed immunity
Varicella-zoster virus (herpes zoster; shingles)	Caused by same virus that causes varicella (chickenpox) Virus has affinity for posterior root ganglia, posterior horn of spinal cord, and skin; crops of vesicles usually confined to dermatome following along course of affected nerve Usually preceded by neuralgic pain, hyperesthesias, or itching May be accompanied by constitutional symptoms	Symptomatic Analgesics for pain Mild sedation sometimes helpful Local moist compresses Drying lotions may be helpful Ophthalmic variety: systemic corticotropin (adrenocorticotropic hormone [ACTH]) or corticosteroids Acyclovir Lidoderm topical anesthetic	Pain in children usually minimal Postherpetic pain does not occur in children Chickenpox may follow exposure; isolate affected child from other children in a hospital or school May occur in children with depressed immunity; can be fatal
Molluscum contagiosum Cause: pox virus Small, benign tumors	Flesh-colored papules with a central caseous plug (umbilicated) Usually asymptomatic	Cases in well children resolve spontaneously in about 18 months Treatment reserved for troublesome cases Apply topical anesthetic EMLA and remove with curette Use tretinoin gel 0.01% or cantharidin (Cantharone) liquid Curettage or cryotherapy	Common in school-age children Spread by skin-to-skin contact, including autoinoculation and fomite-to-skin contact

testing is required to monitor leukopenia and assess liver and renal function.

SYSTEMIC MYCOTIC (FUNGAL) INFECTIONS

Mycotic (systemic or deep fungal) infections have the capacity to invade the viscera, as well as the skin. The most common infections are the lung diseases, which are usually acquired by inhalation of fungal spores. These fungi produce a variable spectrum of disease, and some are quite common in certain geographic areas. They are not transmitted from person to person but appear to reside in the soil, from which their spores are airborne. The cutaneous lesions caused by deep fungal infections are granulomatous and appear as ulcers, plaques, nodules, fungating masses, and abscesses. The course of deep fungal diseases is chronic with slow progression that favors sensitization (Table 30-6).

TABLE 30-5 ■ Dermatophytoses (Fungal Infections)

DISEASE/ORGANISM	MANIFESTATIONS	MANAGEMENT	COMMENTS
Tinea capitis— *Trichophyton tonsurans, Microsporum audouinii, Microsporum canis* (Fig. 30-5, *A*)	Lesions in scalp but may extend to hairline or neck Characteristic configuration of scaly, circumscribed patches or patchy, scaling areas of alopecia Generally asymptomatic, but severe, deep inflammatory reaction may occur that manifests as boggy, encrusted lesions (kerions) Pruritic Microscopic examination of scales is diagnostic	Oral griseofulvin Oral ketoconazole for difficult cases Selenium sulfide shampoos Topical antifungal agents (e.g., clotrimazole, haloprogin, miconazole)	Person-to-person transmission Animal-to-person transmission Rarely, permanent loss of hair *M. audouinii* transmitted from one human being to another directly or from personal items; *M. canis* usually contracted from household pets, especially cats Atopic individuals more susceptible
Tinea corporis— *Trichophyton rubrum, Trichophyton mentagrophytes, M. canis, Epidermophyton* (see Fig. 30-5, *B*)	Generally round or oval, erythematous scaling patch that spreads peripherally and clears centrally; may involve nails (tinea unguium) Diagnosis: direct microscopic examination of scales Usually unilateral	Oral griseofulvin Local application of antifungal preparation such as tolnaftate, haloprogin, miconazole, clotrimazole; apply 1 inch beyond periphery of lesion; continual application 1 to 2 weeks after no sign of lesion	Usually of animal origin from infected pets Majority of infections in children caused by *M. canis* and *M. audouinii*
Tinea cruris ("jock itch")— *Epidermophyton floccosum, T. rubrum, T. mentagrophytes*	Skin response similar to tinea corporis Localized to medial proximal aspect of thigh and crural fold; may involve scrotum in males Pruritic Diagnosis: same as for tinea corporis	Local application of tolnaftate liquid Wet compresses or sitz baths may be soothing	Rare in preadolescent children Health education regarding personal hygiene

Tinea pedis ("athlete's foot")— *T. rubrum, Trichophyton interdigitale, E. floccosum*	On intertriginous areas between toes or on plantar surface of feet
	Lesions vary:
	  Maceration and fissuring between toes
	  Patches with pinhead-sized vesicles on plantar surface
	  Pruritic
	  Diagnosis: direct microscopic examination of scrapings
		Oral griseofulvin
		Local applications of tolnaftate liquid and antifungal powder containing tolnaftate
		Acute infections: compresses or soaks followed by application of glucocorticoid cream
		Elimination of conditions of heat and perspiration by clean, light socks and well-ventilated shoes; avoidance of occlusive shoes
			Most frequent in adolescents and adults; rare in children, but occurrence increases with wearing of plastic shoes
			Transmission to other individuals rare despite general opinion to contrary
			Ointments not successful

Candidiasis (moniliasis)— *Candida albicans*	Grows in chronically moist areas Inflamed areas with white exudate, peeling, and easy bleeding Pruritic Diagnosis: characteristic appearance	Amphotericin B, nystatin ointment, or other antifungal preparations to affected areas	Common form of diaper dermatitis (see Fig. 30-11) Oral form common in infants (see Chapter 9) Vaginal form in older females May be disseminated in immunosuppressed children

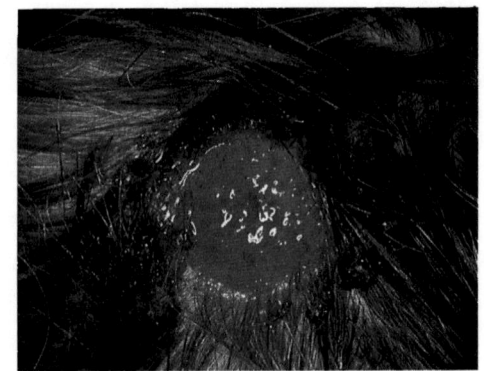 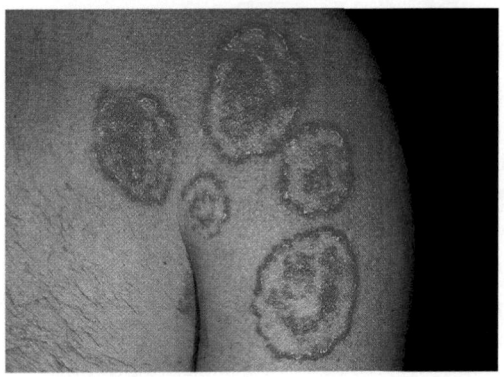

FIG. 30-5 ■ **A,** Tinea capitis. **B,** Tinea corporis. Both infections are caused by *Microsporum canis,* the "kitten" or "puppy" fungus. (From Habif TP: *Clinical dermatology: a color guide to diagnosis and therapy,* ed 4, St Louis, 2004, Mosby.)

TABLE 30-6 ■ Systemic Mycoses

DISORDER/ ORGANISM	SKIN MANIFESTATIONS	SYSTEMIC MANIFESTATIONS	TREATMENT	COMMENTS
North American blastomycosis— *Blastomyces dermatitidis*	Chronic granulomatous lesions and microabscesses in any part of body Initial lesion is a papule; undergoes ulceration and peripheral spread	Pulmonary symptoms, such as cough, chest pain, weakness, and weight loss May have skeletal involvement, with bone destruction and formation of cutaneous abscesses	Intravenous (IV) administration of amphotericin B	Usual portal of entry is lungs Source of infection unknown Noninfectious Pulmonary infections may be mild and self-limiting and require no treatment Progressive disease often fatal
Cryptococcosis— *Cryptococcus neoformans (Torula histolytica)*	Usually on face; acneiform, firm, nodular, painless eruption	Central nervous system (CNS) manifestations: headache, dizziness, stiff neck, and signs of increased intracranial pressure Low-grade fever, mild cough, lung infiltration	IV amphotericin B; may be administered intrathecally for CNS involvement 5-Flurocytosine for meningitis Excision and drainage of local lesions	Acquired by inhalation of dust but may enter through skin Prognosis serious Noninfectious Increased incidence in persons receiving corticosteroids with lymphoreticular malignancies, or type 2 diabetes
Histoplasmosis— *Histoplasma capsulatum*	Not distinctive or uniform but most appear as punched-out or granulomatous ulcers	General systemic symptoms may include pallor, diarrhea, vomiting, irregular spiking temperature, hepatosplenomegaly, and pulmonary symptoms Any tissue of body may be involved with related symptoms	IV amphotericin B for severe cases Oral ketoconazole	Organism cultured from soil, especially where contaminated with fowl droppings Fungus enters through skin or mucous membranes of mouth and respiratory tract Endemic in Mississippi and Ohio River valleys Disseminated diseases most common in infants and children
Coccidioidomycosis (valley fever)— *Coccidioides immitis*	Erythema nodosum Erythema multiforme Erythematous maculopapular rash	Primary lung disease usually asymptomatic May be sign of acute febrile illness Disseminated disease is very serious	IV amphotericin B IV miconazole (synthetic imidazole) Intraventricular miconazole plus oral ketoconazole for CNS involvement Surgical resection of persistent pulmonary cavities	Inhalation of aerospores from soil Endemic in southwestern United States Usually resolves spontaneously Increased incidence in dark-skinned races (Filipino, black, Mexican, Asian)

SKIN DISORDERS RELATED TO CHEMICAL OR PHYSICAL CONTACTS

CONTACT DERMATITIS

Contact dermatitis is an inflammatory reaction of the skin to chemical substances, natural or synthetic, that evokes a hypersensitivity response or direct irritation. The initial reaction occurs in an exposed region, most commonly the face and neck, backs of the hands, forearms, male genitalia, and lower legs. Early in the reaction, there is usually a sharp delineation between inflamed and normal skin that ranges from a faint, transient erythema to massive bullae on an erythematous swollen base. Itching is a constant symptom.

The cause may be a primary irritant or a sensitizing agent. A *primary irritant* is one that irritates any skin. A *sensitizing agent* produces an irritation on those individuals who have met the irritant or something chemically related to it, have undergone an immunologic change, and have become sensitized. Prior exposure is not necessarily a factor in the reaction. A sensitizer irritates in relatively low concentrations only persons who are allergic to it.

In infants, contact dermatitis occurs on the convex surfaces of the diaper area (see Diaper Dermatitis, p. 1121). Other agents that produce contact dermatitis include plants (poison ivy, oak, or sumac), animal irritants (wool, feathers, and furs), metal (nickel found in jewelry and the snaps on sleepers and denim), vegetable irritants (oleoresins, oils, and turpentine), synthetic fabrics (e.g., shoe components), dyes, cosmetics, perfumes, and soaps (including bubble baths). The list is endless.

The major goal in treatment is to prevent further exposure of the skin to the offending substance. Provided there is no further irritation, the normal recuperative powers of the skin will often produce healing without treatment. Otherwise, treatment of contact dermatitis is based on severity. Mild cases are treated with topical steroids. Mild to moderately severe cases may require a 2-week course of strong topical corticosteroids. Very severe cases require systemic corticosteroids (Kronemyer, 2003).

Nursing Considerations

Nurses frequently detect evidence of contact dermatitis during routine physical assessments. Skin manifestations in specific areas suggest limited contact, such as around the eyes (mascara), areas of the body covered by clothing but not protected by undergarments (wool), or areas of the body not covered by clothing (ultraviolet injury). Generalized involvement is more likely to be caused by bubble bath or soap. Often nurses can determine the offending agent and counsel families regarding management. However, if the lesions persist, are extensive, or show evidence of infection, medical evaluation is indicated.

POISON IVY, OAK, AND SUMAC

Contact with the dry or succulent portions of any of three poisonous plants (ivy, oak, and sumac) produces localized, streaked or spotty, oozing, and painful impetiginous lesions. The offending substance in these plants is an oil, *urushiol,* that is extremely potent. Sensitivity to urushiol is not inborn but is developed after one or two exposures and may change over a lifetime. All parts of the plants contain the oil,

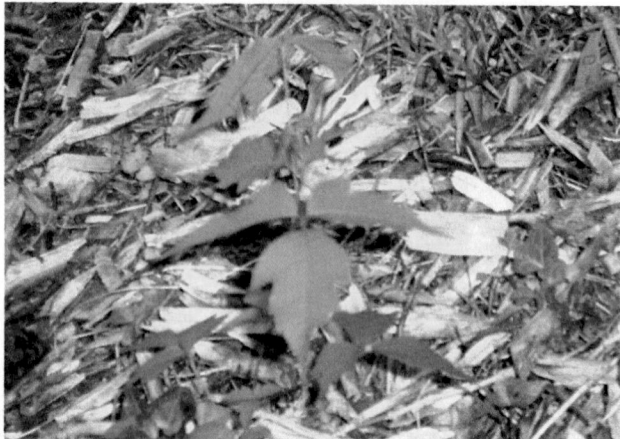

FIG. 30-6 ■ Poison ivy.

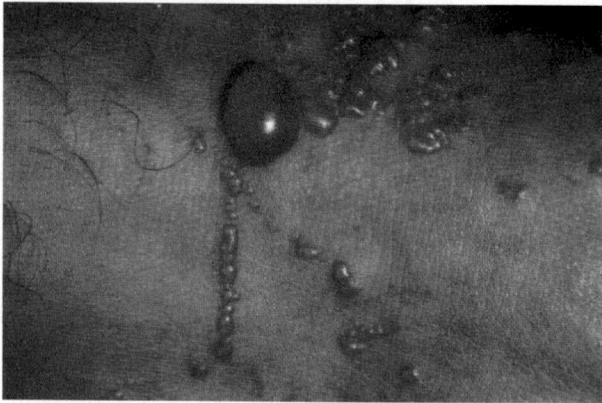

FIG. 30-7 ■ Poison ivy; note "streaked" blisters surrounding one large blister. (From Habif TP: *Clinical dermatology: a color guide to diagnosis and therapy,* ed 4, St Louis, 2004, Mosby.)

including dried leaves and stems (Fig. 30-6). Even smoke from burning brush piles can produce a reaction.

Animals do not seem to be affected by the oil; however, dogs or other animals that have run or played in the plants may carry the sap on their fur, and animals that eat the plants can transfer the oil in their saliva. Shoes, tools, and toys can transfer the oil. Golf balls that have been in the rough are another source of contact.

Urushiol takes effect as soon as it touches the skin. It penetrates through the epidermis and bonds with the dermal layer, where it initiates an immune response. The full-blown reaction is evident after about 2 days, with redness, swelling, and itching at the site of contact. Several days later, streaked or spotty blisters oozing serum from damaged cells produce the characteristic impetiginous lesions (Fig. 30-7). The lesions dry and heal spontaneously, and itching stops by 10 to 14 days.

Therapeutic Management

Treatment of the lesions includes calamine lotion, soothing Burow solution compresses, or Aveeno baths to relieve discomfort. Topical corticosteroid gel is very effective for prevention or relief of inflammation, especially when applied

⁇⁇ CRITICAL THINKING EXERCISE ⁇⁇

Poison Ivy

While at an overnight camp near a stream, Billy, age 9, runs up to the campfire and shows the nurse some leaves he has picked in the woods. The nurse recognizes the leaves as poison ivy. One of the adolescent assistants wants to throw the leaves on the campfire, and scrub Billy's hands vigorously with soap. Billy's cabin mates ask the nurse: "Is poison ivy catching? Are we going to get it too?" What nursing actions should the camp nurse implement?

QUESTIONS
1. Evidence—Is there sufficient evidence to draw any conclusions at this time?
2. Assumptions—Describe some underlying assumptions about the following:
    a. The agent that causes poison ivy
    b. Effects of poison ivy on the skin
    c. Immediate treatment for poison ivy
    d. Contraindicated treatments for poison ivy
3. What implications and priorities for nursing care can be drawn at this time?
4. Does the evidence support this conclusion?
5. Are there alternative perspectives to your arguments?

ANSWERS:
1. Yes, there are sufficient data to determine an effective intervention.
2. **a.** The leaves and stems of the poison ivy plant contain urushiol, an oil, that produces an immune reaction in the skin.
    b. When urushiol comes in contact with the skin, it penetrates the epidermis and bonds with the dermal layer. After about 2 days, localized, oozing, and painful impetiginous lesions are produced in the skin.
    c. When a child has contact with any part of the poison ivy plant, the skin areas should be immediately flushed with cold running water to neutralize the urushiol, and calamine lotion should be applied. Clothing that has come in contact with the plant should be removed and thoroughly laundered in hot water and detergent.
    d. Harsh soap is contraindicated because it removes the protective skin oils and dilutes the urushiol, allowing it to spread; hard scrubbing irritates the skin.
3. The most important immediate intervention is to rinse Billy's hands in cool water and apply calamine lotion. Because Billy's camp is near a stream, he can enter the water where it is shallow, and allow the water to rinse the oil of the poison ivy from his hands as well as his clothes. The leaves should not be burned because contact with the smoke can cause a skin reaction and is also dangerous to the lungs if it is inhaled. Billy's clothes should be washed in hot water with detergent. Poison ivy lesions are not contagious so the camp nurse should tell Billy's cabin mates that they will not "catch" his poison ivy.
4. Yes, the evidence supports these interventions.
5. The camp nurse should use this experience as an opportunity to provide the young campers and the adolescent assistants with education about common hazardous plants, insects, and ticks found in the outdoor environment, strategies to prevent contact with these agents and first aid measures to implement if contact does occur.

---

before blisters form. Oral corticosteroids may be needed for severe reactions, and a sedative such as diphenhydramine (Benadryl) may be ordered.

Nursing Considerations

When it is known that the child has made contact with the plant, the area is immediately flushed (preferably within 15 minutes) with *cold* running water to neutralize the urushiol not yet bonded to the skin. If there is a stream nearby, an effective method is to have the child enter the water (clothes and all) and allow the water to rinse the oil from both skin and clothing. Harsh soap is contraindicated because it removes protective skin oils and dilutes the urushiol, allowing it to spread; hard scrubbing irritates the skin. All clothing that has come in contact with the plant is removed with care and thoroughly laundered in hot water and detergent. Every effort is made to prevent the child from scratching the lesions. Although the lesions do not spread by contact with the blister serum or from scratching, they can become secondarily infected (see Critical Thinking Exercise).

Prevention.   Prevention is best accomplished by avoiding contact and removing the plant from the environment. All children, especially those known to be sensitive, should be taught to recognize the plant. Information regarding means for destroying plants can be obtained from the US Department of Agriculture or Forestry Service. A cream that protects exposed skin from poison oak and ivy is Stokogard.*

DRUG REACTIONS

Adverse reactions to drugs are seen more often in the skin than in any other organ, although any organ of the body can be affected. The reaction may be a result of toxicity related to drug concentration, individual intolerance to the average dosage of the drug, or an allergic or idiosyncratic response. The manifestations may be associated with side effects or secondary effects of a drug, either of which are unrelated to its primary pharmacologic actions.

---

*Distributed in the United States by **Stockhausen, Inc.,** 2401 Doyle Street, Greensboro, NC 27406; (800) 334-0242.

Although any drug is capable of producing a reaction in the susceptible individual, some drugs have a tendency to produce a particular reaction consistently, and others are more likely to produce an untoward effect. Many are allergenic responses that occur after a previous administration of the drug, even a topical application. Other factors influence a drug response in a particular individual. For example, the incidence increases with the amount and number of drugs given.

> **NURSING ALERT**
>
> Intravenous (IV) drugs are more likely to cause a reaction than oral drugs. Stop the drug, but maintain the infusion with normal saline.

Manifestations of drug reactions may be delayed or immediate. A period of 7 days is usually required for a child to develop sensitivity to a drug that has never been administered previously. With prior sensitivity the manifestations appear almost immediately. Rashes are the most common manifestation of adverse drug reactions in children. However, individual drug reactions may vary from a single lesion to extensive, generalized epidermal necrosis such as that seen in Stevens-Johnson syndrome (see Table 30-9). Cutaneous manifestations can resemble almost any skin disease and can be seen in almost any degree of severity. With few exceptions, the distribution of a drug eruption is widespread, because it results from a circulating agent, appears as an inflammatory response with itching, is sudden in onset, and may be associated with constitutional symptoms such as fever, malaise, gastrointestinal upsets, anemia, or liver and kidney damage.

In most cases treatment for simple cutaneous reactions consists of discontinuing the drug. Sometimes a decision is made to continue the drug (such as an antibiotic in an infant or small child) until the cause of the rash is clearly indicated. In urticarial-type eruptions antihistamines may be ordered, and for widespread and severe lesions corticosteroids are beneficial. Severe anaphylactic reactions are a medical emergency (see Anaphylaxis, Chapter 25).

Nursing Considerations

The most effective means of management is prevention. Parents always remember a severe reaction. A careful history will elicit evidence of a previous drug reaction. The history should include the name of the drug, nature of the reaction, drug dose, and how soon after administration the reaction occurred (see Chapter 6).

Nurses who suspect that a rash is caused by a medication should withhold any further dose and report the eruption to the practitioner. Frequent offenders in drug reactions are penicillin and sulfonamides, and nurses must be alert to this possibility. However, even commonplace drugs, including aspirin, barbiturates, chemical agents in some foods, flavoring agents, and preservatives, are capable of producing an undesired response. Persons who have severe reactions should wear an identification bracelet or chain in case of emergency or inadvertent administration of the offending drug.

FOREIGN BODIES

Parents can remove small wooden splinters with a needle and tweezers that have been sterilized with alcohol or a flame. The area around the sliver is washed with soap and water before removal is attempted. The sliver is exposed with the needle, then grasped firmly by the tweezers and pulled out. Some foreign bodies, such as a fishhook, pieces of glass, a difficult-to-see object, or a deeply embedded object (such as a needle in a foot or near a joint), require medical evaluation.

Small cactus prickles or spines are troublesome to remove, but the following methods may prove helpful:

- Apply a thin layer of water-soluble household glue and cover with gauze; when the glue dries, peel off the gauze.
- Apply hair removal wax or body sugar (Aplon*), let dry, and remove.
- Place cellophane tape, sticky side down, over the spines and lift off.

SKIN DISORDERS RELATED TO INSECT AND ANIMAL CONTACTS

SCABIES

Scabies is an endemic infestation caused by the scabies mite, *Sarcoptes scabiei*. Lesions are created as the impregnated female burrows into the stratum corneum of the epidermis (never into living tissue) to deposit her eggs and feces. The inflammatory response and intense itching occur after the host becomes sensitized to the mite, approximately 30 to 60 days after initial contact. If the person has been previously sensitized to the mite, the response occurs within 48 hours after exposure. After this time, the areas over which the mite has traveled will begin to itch and develop the characteristic eruption (Box 30-1). Consequently, mites will not necessarily be located at all sites of eruption.

There is great variability in the type of lesions. Infants often develop an eczematous eruption; therefore, the observer must look for discrete papules, burrows, or vesicles.

Nursing Considerations

The treatment of scabies is the application of a scabicide. Currently, permethrin 5% cream (Elimite) is the drug. Alternative drugs are 1% lindane cream or lotion and 10% crotamiton. Permethrin is preferred because it is safer, it avoids the risk of neurotoxicity, and it is more effective than lindane. Nurses instructing families in the use of scabicides should emphasize the importance of following directions carefully.

---

*Zoulla, Inc., PO Box 160, Greenville, MI 48838; (616) 754-3333; fax: (616) 754-3337; website: www.zoulla.com.

BOX 30-1 ■ Clinical Manifestations of Scabies

LESION
Children—minute grayish-brown, threadlike (mite burrows), pruritic
Black dot at end of burrow (mite)
Infants—eczematous eruption, pruritic

DISTRIBUTION
Generally in intertriginous areas—interdigital, axillary-cubital, popliteal, inguinal
Children older than 2 years of age—primarily hands and wrists
Children younger than 2 years—primarily feet and ankles

Permethrin is applied to all skin surfaces (not just areas with rash, but also areas between the fingers and toes, the umbilicus, and the cleft of the buttocks). The cream should remain on the skin for 8 to 14 hours and then be removed by bathing. Lindane is removed by bathing after 8 to 12 hours. One application of permethrin and lindane is sufficient. Lindane should not be used for premature infants, young infants, people with known seizure disorders, people with hypersensitivity to the product, patients with crusted scabies, or patients with extensive dermatitis. Lindane should not be used immediately after a bath or shower. Crotamiton is applied once a day for 2 days, followed by a cleansing bath 48 hours after the last application. Families need to know that although the mite that causes scabies will be killed with these treatments, the rash and the itch will not be eliminated until the stratum corneum is replaced in approximately 2 to 3 weeks. Soothing ointments or lotions can be applied for itching. Antibiotics may be given for secondary infection.

Another prescription drug used to treat scabies is ivermectin (Frankowski and Weiner, 2002). Ivermectin is administered orally in a single dose for treatment of severe or crusted scabies. It should be considered for patients whose infestation is refractory or those who can not tolerate topical scabicides (Offidani and others, 1999). However, the safety and efficacy of ivermectin for pediatric patients younger than 5 years of age or children weighing less than 15 kg (33 lb) is not established. This drug is not currently licensed for treatment of scabies by the US Food and Drug Administration (American Academy of Pediatrics, 2003).

PEDICULOSIS CAPITIS

Pediculosis capitis (head lice) is an infestation of the scalp by *Pediculus humanus capitis,* a common parasite in school-age children. The adult louse lives only about 48 hours when away from a human host, and the lifespan of the average female is 1 month. The female lays her eggs at night at the junction of a hair shaft and close to the skin because the eggs need a warm environment. The *nits,* or eggs, hatch in approximately 7 to 10 days. Itching is usually the only symptom. Common areas involved are the occipital area, behind the ears, and the nape of the neck (Box 30-2).

Diagnostic Evaluation

Diagnosis is made by observation of the white eggs (nits) firmly attached to the hair shafts (Fig. 30-8). Because of their brief lifespan and mobility, adult lice are more difficult to locate. Nits must be differentiated from dandruff, lint, hair spray, and other items of similar size and shape. Scratch

BOX 30-2 ■ Clinical Manifestations of Pediculosis

Pruritus (caused by crawling insects and insect saliva on skin)
Nits observable on hair shaft (see Fig. 30-8)

DISTRIBUTION
Occipital area
Behind ears
Nape of neck
Eyebrows and eyelashes (occasionally) (caused by pubic lice)

marks or inflammatory papules, caused by secondary infection, may also be found on the scalp in the vulnerable areas.

Therapeutic Management

Treatment consists of the application of pediculicides and manual removal of nit cases. The drug of choice for infants and children is permethrin 1% creme rinse (Nix), which kills adult lice and nits. This product and preparations of pyrethrin with piperonyl butoxide (RID or A-200 Pyrinate) can be obtained without a prescription and are more effective and safer than lindane. The **United States Food and Drug Administration (FDA)** has issued a warning regarding the use of Lindane because of the potential for neurotoxicity (FDA, 2003). Although the FDA believes that the benefits of Lindane outweigh the risks when used as directed, patients should be treated with these medications when other treatments are not tolerable or have failed. Another product, Malathion 0.5% (Ovide) approved for treatment of head lice is available only by prescription. However, Malathion contains flammable alcohol, must remain on the hair for 8 to 12 hours, and is not recommended for children younger than 2 years of age.

Nursing Considerations

An important nursing role is providing the parents with education about pediculosis. Nurses should emphasize that *anyone* can get pediculosis; it has no respect for age, socio-

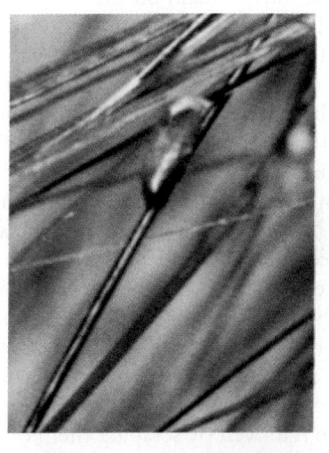
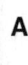
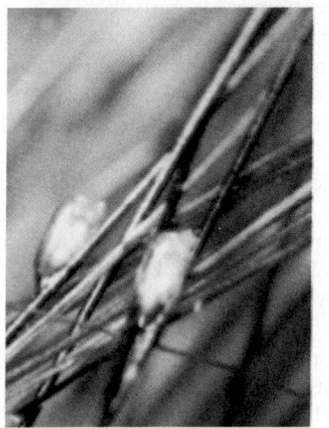

FIG. 30-8 ■ A, Empty nit case. **B,** Viable nits. (From *The contemporary approach to the control of head lice in schools and communities,* Pittsburgh, 1991, SmithKline Beecham.)

economic level, or cleanliness. The louse does not jump or fly, but it can be transmitted from one person to another on personal items. Lice are more apt to infest white children, those with straight hair, and girls. Children are cautioned against sharing combs, hair ornaments, hats, caps, scarves, coats, and other items used on or near the hair. Children who share lockers are more likely to become infested, and slumber parties place children at risk. Lice are not carried or transmitted by pets.

Nurses or parents should carefully inspect children who scratch their head more than usual for bite marks, redness, and nits. The hair is systematically spread with two flat-sided sticks or tongue depressors, and the scalp is observed for any movement that indicates a louse. Nurses should wear gloves when examining the hair. Lice are small and grayish tan, have no wings, and are visible to the naked eye. The nits, or eggs, appear as tiny whitish oval specks adhering to the hair shaft about ¼ inch from the scalp. The adherent nature of the nits distinguishes them from dandruff, which falls off readily. *Empty nit cases,* indicating hatched lice, are translucent rather than white and are located more than ¼ inch from the scalp (see Fig. 30-8).

If evidence of infestation is found, it is important to treat the child according to the directions on the label of the pediculicide. Parents are advised to read the directions carefully before beginning treatment. The child is made as comfortable as possible during the application process, because the pediculicide must remain on the scalp and hair for several minutes. Playing "beauty parlor" during the shampoo is a useful strategy. The child lies supine, with the head over a sink or basin, and covers the eyes with a dry towel or washcloth. This prevents medication, which can cause chemical conjunctivitis, from splashing into the eyes. If eye irritation occurs, the eyes must be flushed well with tepid water. It is not necessary to remove the nits after treatment because only live lice cause infestation. However, because none of the pediculicides are 100% effective in killing all the eggs, the makers of some pediculicides recommend manual removal of the nits after treatment. An extra-fine-tooth comb that is included in many commercial pediculicides or is available at community pharmacies facilitates manual removal. If the comb is ineffective in removing the nit cases, they should be removed by scraping them off the strands of hair with the examiner's fingernails.

Live lice survive for up to 48 hours away from the host, but nits are shed into the environment and are capable of hatching in 7 to 10 days. Therefore measures must be taken to prevent further infestation (see Community Focus box). Spraying with insecticide is not recommended because of the danger to children and animals. Families should also be advised that the pediculicide is relatively expensive, especially when several members of the household require treatment.

The psychologic effects of lice infestations are stressful to children. They are influenced by the reactions of others, including their parents, school nurses, and officials. Some children feel ashamed or guilty. Parents are strongly cautioned against cutting a child's hair or, worse, shaving a child's head. Lice infest short hair as readily as long hair, and these actions only compound the child's distress and serve as a continual reminder to peers, who are prone to taunt children who have a different appearance.

COMMUNITY FOCUS

Preventing the Spread and Recurrence of Pediculosis

Machine wash all washable clothing, towels, and bed linens in hot water, and dry in a hot dryer for at least 20 minutes. Dry clean nonwashable items.

Thoroughly vacuum carpets, car seats, pillows, stuffed animals, rugs, mattresses, and upholstered furniture.

Seal nonwashable items in plastic bags for 14 days if unable to dry clean or vacuum.

Soak combs, brushes, and hair accessories in lice-killing products for 1 hour or in boiling water for 10 minutes.

In day care centers, store children's clothing items such as hats and scarves and other headgear in separate cubicles.

Discourage the sharing of items such as hats, scarves, hair accessories, combs, and brushes among children in group settings such as day care centers.

Avoid physical contact with infested individuals and their belongings, especially clothing and bedding.

Inspect children in a group setting regularly for head lice.

Provide educational programs on the transmission of pediculosis, its detection, and treatment.

Modified from Chin J, editor: *Control of communicable diseases manual,* Washington, DC, 2000, American Public Health Association.

Prevention. The increasing incidence of pediculosis in schoolchildren is a serious concern for school nurses, parents, and community health agencies. However, school head lice screening programs have not proven to have a significant effect on the incidence of head lice in the school setting; parent education programs may be more helpful in the management of head lice. Children with head lice should be allowed to return to school after proper treatment. Both the American Academy of Pediatrics and the National Association of School Nurses discourage a "no nit" policy for schools (Frankowski and Weiner, 2002).

ARTHROPOD BITES AND STINGS

Bites and stings account for a significant amount of mild to moderate discomfort in children. Most bites and stings are managed by simple symptomatic measures, such as compresses, calamine lotion, and prevention of secondary infection. *Arthropods* include insects and arachnids, such as mites, ticks, spiders, and scorpions. Most arthropods in the United States are relatively harmless, including tarantulas. Although all spiders produce venom that is injected via fangs, some are unable to pierce the skin and others produce venom that is insufficiently toxic to be harmful. Only scorpions and two spiders—the brown recluse and the black widow—inject venom deadly enough to require immediate attention. Children bitten by these arachnids must receive medical attention as soon as possible. Major offending creatures, their manifestations, and management are outlined in Table 30-7.

When a hymenopteran (bees in particular) stings, its barbed stinger penetrates into the skin. As long as the stinger remains in the skin, the muscles push the stinger deeper and the venom is pumped into the wound. The best approach is to remove the stinger as quickly as possible and

TABLE 30-7 ■ Skin Lesions Caused by Arthropods

MECHANISM/CHARACTERISTIC	MANIFESTATIONS	MANAGEMENT
INSECT BITES—FLIES, GNATS, MOSQUITOES, FLEAS		
Mechanism: Foreign protein in insects' saliva introduced when skin is penetrated for a blood-sucking meal *Distribution:* Almost everywhere—fleas, mosquitoes, ants Suburbs and rural areas—bees Urban areas—hornets, wasps, yellow jackets	Hypersensitivity reaction Papular urticaria Firm papules; may be capped by vesicles or excoriated Little or no reaction in nonsensitized person	*Treatment:* Use antipruritic agents and baths Administer antihistamines Prevent secondary infection *Prevention:* Avoid contact Remove focus, such as treating furniture, mattresses, carpets, and pets, where insects may live Apply insect repellent when exposure is anticipated
CHIGGERS—HARVEST MITES		
Mechanism: Attach with claws and secrete a digestive substance that liquefies the host's epidermis *Manifestations:* Erythematous papules Intense itching	Same as insect bites Favor warm areas of body, especially intertriginous areas and areas covered with clothing	Avoid contact, especially in areas of tall grass and underbrush Apply insect repellant when exposure is anticipated; insecticides such as diazinon can also be sprayed in yards May require systemic steroids for extensive bites
HYMENOPTERANS—BEES, WASPS, HORNETS, YELLOW JACKETS, FIRE ANTS		
Mechanism: Injection of venom through stinging apparatus Venom contains histamine, allergenic proteins, and often a spreading factor, hyaluronidase Severe reactions caused by hypersensitivity or multiple stings	Local reaction: small red area, wheal, itching, and heat Systemic reactions: may be mild to severe, including generalized edema, pain, nausea and vomiting, confusion, respiratory embarrassment, and shock	*Treatment:* Carefully scrape off stinger or pull out stinger as quickly as possible Cleanse with soap and water Apply cool compresses Apply common household product (e.g., lemon juice, paste made with aspirin or baking soda) Administer antihistamines Severe reactions: administer epinephrine, corticosteroids; treat for shock *Prevention:* Teach child to wear shoes; to avoid wearing bright clothing, flowery prints, shiny jewelry, or perfumed grooming products (cologne, scented hairspray), which might attract the insect; and to avoid places where the insect may be contacted Hypersensitive children should wear medical identification to indicate allergy and therapy needed; family should keep emergency medication and be taught its administration
BLACK WIDOW SPIDER		
Mechanism: Venom injected through a clawlike appendage; has neurotoxic action *Characteristics:* Spider is shiny black, with a body about 1.25 cm (0.5 inch) long and a red or orange hourglass-shaped marking on underside Avoids light and bites in self-defense	Mild sting at time of bite Area becomes swollen, painful, and erythematous Dizziness, weakness, and abdominal pain May produce delirium, paralysis, seizures, and (if large amount of venom absorbed) death	*Treatment:* Cleanse wound with antiseptic Apply cool compresses Administer antivenin Administer muscle relaxant, such as calcium gluconate; analgesics or sedatives; hydrocortisone or diazepam intravenously *Prevention:* Teach children to avoid places that harbor the spider (e.g., woodpiles)

Continued

TABLE 30-7 ■ Skin Lesions Caused by Arthropods—cont'd

MECHANISM/CHARACTERISTIC	MANIFESTATIONS	MANAGEMENT
BROWN RECLUSE SPIDER		
Mechanism:	Mild sting at time of bite	*Treatment:*
Venom injected via fangs	Transient erythema followed by bleb or	Apply cool compresses locally
Venom contains powerful necrotoxin	blister; mild to severe pain in 2-8	Administer antibiotics, corticosteroids
Characteristics:	hours; purple, star-shaped area in 3-4	Relieve pain
Spider is slender, with long legs and	days; necrotic ulceration in 7-14 days	Wound may require skin graft
body length of 1 to 2 cm; color is	(Fig. 30-9)	*Prevention:*
fawn to dark brown; recognized by	Systemic reactions may include fever,	Teach children to avoid possible nesting sites
fiddle-shaped mark on head	malaise, restlessness, nausea, vomit-	
Shy; bites only when annoyed or	ing, and joint pain	
surprised	Generalized petechial eruption	
Prefers dark areas where seldom	Wounds heal with scar formation	
disturbed		
SCORPIONS		
Mechanism:	Intense local pain, erythema, numbness,	*Treatment:*
Sting by means of a hooked caudal	burning, restlessness, vomiting	Delay absorption of venom by keeping child
stinger that discharges venom	Ascending motor paralysis with	quiet; place involved area in dependent
Venom of more venomous species	seizures, weakness, rapid pulse, ex-	position
contains hemolysins,	cessive salivation, thirst, dysuria, pul-	Administer antivenin
endotheliolysins, and neurotoxins	monary edema, coma, and death	Relieve pain
Characteristics:	Some species produce only local tissue	Admit to pediatric intensive care unit for
Usual habitat is southwestern	reaction with swelling at puncture	surveillance
United States	site (distinctive)	*Prevention:*
	Symptoms subside in a few hours	Teach children to avoid possible nesting sites
	Deaths occur among children younger	
	than 4 years of age, usually in first	
	24 hours	
TICKS		
Mechanism:	Tick usually attached to skin, head em-	*Treatment:*
In process of sucking blood, head and	bedded	Grasp tick with tweezers (forceps) as close as
mouth parts are buried in skin	Produce firm, discrete, intensely pruritic	possible to point of attachment
Characteristics:	nodules at site of attachment	Pull straight up with steady, even pressure; if
Feed on blood of mammals	May cause urticaria or persistent local-	bare hands, use a tissue to touch tick during
Significant in humans because of	ized edema	removal; wash hands thoroughly with soap
pathologic organism carried		and water
May be vectors of various infectious		Remove any remaining part (e.g., head) with
diseases, such as Rocky Mountain		sterile needle
spotted fever, Q fever, tularemia,		Cleanse wounds with soap and disinfectant
relapsing fever, Lyme disease, tick		*Prevention:*
paralysis		Teach children to avoid areas where prevalent
Must attach and feed for 1-2 hours to		Inspect skin (especially scalp) after being in
transmit disease		wooded areas
Usual habitat is very wooded area		

to get away from the vicinity of other insects to prevent further injury. Children who have become sensitized to hymenopteran bites may demonstrate a severe systemic response that can be life threatening. One sting can produce generalized urticaria, respiratory difficulty (from laryngeal edema), hypotension, and death. Intramuscular administration of epinephrine provides immediate relief and must be available for emergency use.

Hypersensitive children should wear a medical identification bracelet. They should also have a kit that contains epinephrine and a hypodermic syringe. Families are reminded to check the expiration date on the kit and to replace an outdated one. They should determine if a nurse is available at the school and the school policy regarding administration of drugs. If a school nurse is not present, someone at the school should be designated to inject the epinephrine in case of an emergency.

INFECTIONS TRANSMITTED BY ARTHROPODS

The organisms responsible for a number of disorders are transmitted to human beings via arthropods (Table 30-8). Mammals become infected only through the bites of infected

TABLE 30-8 ■ Eruptions Caused by Rickettsiae

DISORDER/ORGANISM/HOST	MANIFESTATIONS	MANAGEMENT	COMMENTS
Rocky Mountain spotted fever—*R. rickettsii* Arthropod: tick Transmission: tick Mammal source: wild rodents; dogs	Gradual onset: fever, malaise, anorexia, myalgia Abrupt onset: rapid temperature elevation, chills, vomiting, myalgia, severe headache Maculopapular or petechial rash primarily on extremities (ankles and wrists) but may spread to other areas, characteristically on palms and soles	Control: protection from tick bite by wearing proper apparel, tick repellent Tetracycline or chloramphenicol Vigorous supportive therapy	Usually self-limited in children Onset in children may resemble any infectious disease Severe disease rare in children Children and dogs should be inspected regularly if they play in wooded areas See Table 30-7 for management of ticks
Epidemic typhus—*R. prowazekii* Arthropod: body louse Transmission: infected feces into broken skin Mammal source: humans	Abrupt onset of chills, fever, diffuse myalgia, headache, malaise Maculopapular rash becomes petechial 4 to 7 days later, spreading from trunk outward	Control: immediate destruction of vectors Tetracycline or chloramphenicol Supportive treatment	Patient should be isolated until deloused See discussion on p. 1115 for management of pediculosis Excreta from infected lice also in dust—disinfect patient's clothing, bedding, and possessions and wash in hot water
Endemic typhus—*R. typhi* Arthropod: rat fleas or lice Transmission: flea bite; inhaling or ingesting flea excreta Mammal source: rats	Headache, arthralgia, backache followed by fever; may last 9-14 days Maculopapular rash after 1-8 days of fever; begins in trunk and spreads to periphery; rarely involves face, palms, soles	Control: eliminate rat reservoir, insect vectors, or both Tetracycline or chloramphenicol Supportive treatment	Fairly common in United States Shorter duration than epidemic typhus Mild, seldom fatal illness Difficult to distinguish from epidemic typhus
Rickettsialpox—*R. akari* Arthropod: mouse mite Transmission: mite Mammal source: house mouse	Maculopapular rash following primary lesion; eschar at site of bite; fever, chills, headache	Control: eradication of rodent reservoir and mite vector Tetracycline or chloramphenicol Supportive treatment	Self-limited nonfatal disease Endemic in New York City Found in many cities in United States

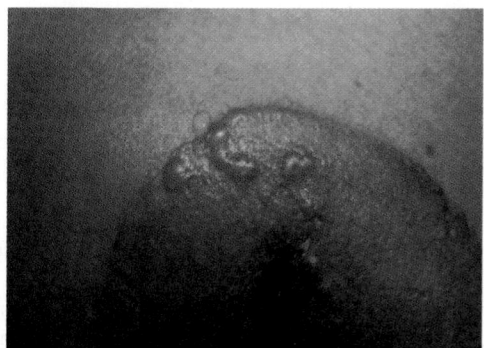

FIG. 30-9 ■ Brown recluse spider bite; note central necrosis surrounded by purplish area and blisters. (From Weston WL, Lane AT: *Color textbook of pediatric dermatology,* St Louis, 1991, Mosby.)

lice, fleas, ticks, and mites, all of which serve as both infectors and reservoirs. Rickettsiae are intracellular parasites, similar in size to bacteria that inhabit the alimentary tract of a wide range of natural hosts. Rickettsial diseases are more common in temperate and tropical climates where humans live in association with arthropods. Infection in humans is incidental (except epidemic typhus) and not necessary for the survival of the rickettsial species. However, after the organism invades a human, it causes a disease that varies in intensity from a benign, self-limiting illness to a disease that is fulminating and fatal.

LYME DISEASE

Lyme disease (LD) is the most common tick-borne disorder in the United States. It is caused by the spirochete *Borrelia burgdorferi,* which enters the skin and bloodstream through the saliva and feces of ticks, especially the deer tick. Most cases of Lyme disease are reported in the Northeast from southern Maine to northern Virginia. The disease may present in any of three stages. *Stage 1* consists of the tick bite at the time of inoculation, followed in 3 to 31 days by the development of *erythema migrans* at the site of the bite (Fig. 30-10). *Stage 2,* the most serious stage of the disease, is characterized by systemic involvement of neurologic, cardiac, and musculoskeletal systems that appears several weeks after the cutaneous phase is completed. *Stage 3,* or the late stage, includes musculoskeletal pain that involves the tendons, bursae, muscles, and synovia. Arthritis may occur, and late neurologic problems include deafness and chronic encephalopathy.

Diagnostic Evaluation

Diagnosis is best made clinically during the early stages by recognizing the characteristic rash, erythema migrans. Serologic testing may be used to establish the diagnosis in later stages of the disease.

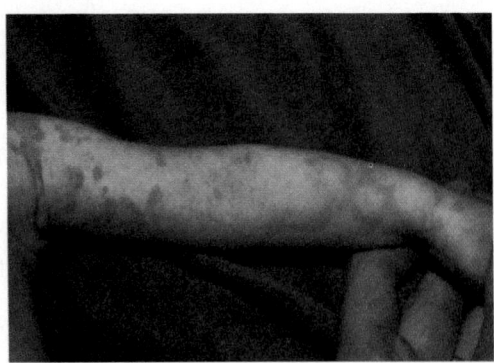

FIG. 30-10 ■ Lyme disease. Note annular red rings in erythema chronicum migrans. (From Weston WL, Lane AT: Color textbook of pediatric dermatology, St Louis, 1991, Mosby.)

Therapeutic Management

Early and appropriate treatment is essential to prevent complications. Children older than 8 years of age are treated with oral doxycycline; amoxicillin is recommended for children younger than 8 years of age (American Academy of Pediatrics, 2003). For patients allergic to penicillin, alternative drugs include cefuroxime or erythromycin (Wade, 2000). Most experts treat individuals with early Lyme disease for 14 to 21 days. Treatment of erythema migrans almost always prevents development of later stages of Lyme disease.

In 1998, the FDA licensed a Lyme disease vaccine for people 15 to 70 years of age. However, the vaccine was withdrawn in 2002 because of low market demand and is no longer available.

Nursing Considerations

The major thrust of nursing care should be educating parents to protect their children from exposure to ticks. Children should avoid tick-infested areas or wear light-colored clothing so that ticks can be spotted easily, tuck pant legs into socks, and wear a long-sleeved shirt tucked into pants when in wooded areas. Grass and shrubbery where ticks may be lurking should be avoided, and children and adults should walk in the center of trails. Parents and children need to perform regular tick checks when they are in infested areas. After a hike, a bare skin check (with special attention to the scalp, neck, armpits, and groin areas) is important to spot any ticks and remove them. Parents should also be alert for signs of the skin lesion, especially if their children have been in tick-infested areas. Insect repellents containing diethyltoluamide (DEET) and permethrin can protect against ticks, but parents should use these chemicals cautiously. Although there have been reports of serious neurologic complications in children resulting from frequent and excessive application of DEET repellants, the risk is low when they are used properly. Products with DEET should be applied sparingly according to label instructions and not applied to a child's face, hands, or any areas of irritated skin. After the child returns indoors, treated skin should be washed with soap and water. Information about Lyme disease can be obtained from the **American Lyme Disease Foundation, Inc.***

---

*Mill Pond Offices 293, Route 100, Suite 204, Somers, NY 10589; (914) 277-6970 or (800) 876-LYME; fax: (914) 277-6974; website: www.aldf.com.

ANIMAL BITES

Animal bites are common in childhood. However, children are bitten more often by animals belonging to the family or to neighbors than by stray animals. More than half the victims of dog bites are younger than 5 years of age; boys are bitten more frequently than girls (Bernardo and others, 2000). Most dog or cat injuries are to the upper extremities. Small children are likely to be bitten or scratched on the head, face, and neck because they tend to put their heads near the animal's head and flail their arms rather than protecting their heads. Animal bites are potentially serious because of the likelihood of significant infection. Injuries vary in intensity from small puncture wounds to complete evulsion of tissue that is associated with significant crush injury.

Therapeutic Management

General wound care consists of rinsing the wound with copious amounts of saline or Ringer's lactate under pressure via a large syringe and of washing the surrounding skin with mild soap. A clean pressure dressing is applied, and the extremity is elevated if the wound is bleeding. Medical evaluation is advised, because there is danger of tetanus and rabies, although dogs in most urban areas must be immunized against rabies. Bites from wild animals, such as squirrels, bats, raccoons, foxes, and skunks, are also dangerous.

Prophylactic antibiotics are indicated for puncture wounds and wounds in areas that may prove to be cosmetically or functionally impaired if infected. Extensive lacerations are débrided and loosely sutured to allow for drainage in the event of infection. Tetanus toxoid is administered according to standard guidelines (see Immunizations, Chapter 10), and rabies protocol is followed (see Rabies, Chapter 28). Injuries to poorly vascularized areas, such as the hands, are more likely to become infected than those in more vascularized areas, such as the face; puncture wounds are more apt to become infected than lacerations.

Nursing Considerations

The most important aspect related to animal bites is prevention. Children should understand animal behavior and develop respect for animals (see Community Focus box). Parents should monitor their children's behavior with a dog and instruct them not to tease or surprise a dog, invade its territory, interfere with its feeding or sleeping, take its toy, or interact with a sick or injured dog or a dog with pups. Parents who are considering getting a pet, especially a dog, for themselves or their children should select a dog that has a high level of sociability with, and is unlikely to be a danger to, children.

HUMAN BITES

Children often acquire lacerations from the teeth of other humans in rough play, during fights, or as victims of child abuse. Many preschool children bite others out of frustration or anger. Because human dental plaque and gingiva harbor pathogenic organisms, all human bites should receive attention. Delayed treatment increases the risk of infection.

If the laceration is less than 0.25 inch in length, the wound can be treated at home. The wound is washed vigorously with soap and water, and a pressure dressing is applied to stop bleeding. Ice applications minimize discomfort

COMMUNITY FOCUS

Animal Safety

Teach children to avoid all strange animals, especially wild, sick, or injured ones, who may be carriers of rabies (use the same techniques employed in teaching children not to talk to strangers).

Teach children to avoid dangerous and nervous animals in the neighborhood.

Vaccinate your own dog against rabies.

Never permit children to break up an animal fight, even when their own pet is involved. Use a rake, broom, or garden hose to separate animals.

Teach children the danger of mistreating or teasing pets (animals will bite if mauled, annoyed, or frightened).

Spay or neuter your pets (spaying or neutering reduces aggression, not protectiveness).

Avoid direct eye contact with a threatening dog, and remain motionless until a threatening dog leaves the area.

Never hold your face close to an animal.

Teach children not to disturb an animal that is eating, sleeping, or caring for young puppies, kittens, etc.

Never tease, pull the tail, or take away food, a bone, or a toy with which an animal is playing.

Never approach a strange dog that is confined or restrained; do not keep animals confined with short ropes or chains (this can make them aggressive or vicious, especially when teased).

Do not run, ride a bicycle, or skate in front of a dog (it will startle the dog); teach children the importance of avoiding bike routes where dogs are known to chase vehicles.

Do not allow an inexperienced child or adult to feed a dog (if the person pulls back when the animal moves to take the food, this can frighten and startle the animal).

If a dog is asleep or unaware of your presence, or has not seen you approach, speak to the animal to make it aware of your presence and to avoid startling the animal.

Allow a dog to see and sniff a child before attempting to pet the animal.

Do not permit a child to lead a large dog.

Train or socialize a dog for appropriate behavior; avoid aggressive play with pets.

Do not adopt pets for children until children demonstrate their maturity and ability to handle and care for pets.

From The Humane Society of the United States: *Preventing and avoiding dog bites,* Washington, DC, 1998, The Society.

and swelling. Increased pain or redness at the wound site is an indication that the child should receive medical attention for antibiotic therapy. Tetanus toxoid is needed if the child is insufficiently immunized. Wounds larger than 0.25 inch should receive medical attention.

CAT SCRATCH DISEASE

Cat scratch disease (CSD) is the most common cause of regional lymphadenitis in children and adolescents. It usually follows the scratch or bite of an animal (a cat or kitten in 99% of cases). The disease is usually a benign, self-limiting illness that resolves spontaneously in about 2 to 4 months. Diagnosis is made on the basis of (1) history of contact with a cat or kitten; (2) the presence of regional lymphadenopathy for several days; and (3) serologic identification of the causative organism by indirect fluorescent antibody assay or polymerase chain reaction test. The disease may persist for

several months before gradual resolution. In some children, especially those who are immunocompromised, the adenitis may progress to suppuration and serious complications. Treatment is primarily supportive, but antibiotic therapy may hasten the resolution of adenopathy in the disease (Centers for Disease Control and Prevention, 2002).

MISCELLANEOUS SKIN DISORDERS

A number of miscellaneous skin lesions occur in children. Some occur as a result of congenital disorders and are inherited as an autosomal-dominant trait (Table 30-9). *Ichthyoses* are a heterogeneous group of disorders characterized by scaling that create challenging problems in treatment. These disorders are not discussed in detail here because of their wide variability.

SKIN DISORDERS ASSOCIATED WITH SPECIFIC AGE-GROUPS

Several common dermatologic conditions are confined to children in specific age-groups. These conditions include diaper, atopic, and seborrheic dermatitis that occurs predominantly in infants and acne, which is most common in adolescence.

DIAPER DERMATITIS

Diaper dermatitis is very common in infants and one of several acute inflammatory skin disorders caused either directly or indirectly by the wearing of diapers. The peak age of occurrence is 9 to 12 months of age, and the incidence is greater in bottle-fed infants than in breast-fed infants.

Pathophysiology and Clinical Manifestations

Diaper dermatitis is caused by prolonged and repetitive contact with an irritant (e.g., urine, feces, soaps, detergents, ointments, friction). Although the irritant in the majority of cases is urine and feces, the specific components that contribute to irritation include a combination of factors.

Prolonged contact of the skin with diaper wetness produces higher friction, greater abrasion damage, increased transepidermal permeability, and increased microbial counts. Healthy skin is less resistant to potential irritants.

Although ammonia was once thought to cause diaper rash because of the association between the strong odor on diapers and dermatitis, ammonia alone is not sufficient. The irritant quality of urine is related to an increase in pH from the breakdown of urea in the presence of fecal urease. The increased pH promotes the activity of fecal enzymes, principally the proteases and lipases, which act as irritants. Fecal enzymes also increase the permeability of skin to bile salts, another potential irritant in feces.

The eruption of diaper dermatitis is manifested primarily on convex surfaces or in folds. The lesions represent a variety of types and configurations. Eruptions involving the skin in most intimate contact with the diaper (e.g., the convex surfaces of buttocks, inner thighs, mons pubis, scrotum) but sparing the folds are likely to be caused by chemical irritants, especially from urine and feces (Fig. 30-11). Other causes are detergents or soaps from inadequately rinsed cloth diapers or the chemicals in disposable wipes. Perianal

TABLE 30-9 ■ Miscellaneous Skin Disorders

DISEASE/CAUSATIVE AGENT	LOCAL MANIFESTATIONS	MANAGEMENT	COMMENTS
Urticaria— Usually allergic response to drugs or infection	Development of wheals Vary in size and configuration and tend to appear quickly, spread irregularly, and fade within a few hours May be constant or intermittent, sparse or profuse, small or large, discrete or confluent May be acute, chronic, or recurrent in acute attacks	Local soothing and antipruritic applications Antihistamines Epinephrine or ephedrine Cortisone in severe cases Severe upper respiratory involvement may require tracheostomy	Known etiologic agents should be avoided May be accompanied by malaise, fever, lymphadenopathy Severe cases may involve mucous membranes, internal organs, and joints Obstruction to air passages constitutes medical emergency (see Chapter 25)
Intertrigo— Mechanical trauma and aggravating factors of excessive heat, moisture, and sweat retention	Red, inflamed, moist, partially denuded, marginated areas, the shape of which is determined by location Appears where opposing skin surfaces rub together, such as intergluteal folds, groin, neck, and axilla Excessive moisture and obesity are often factors	Affected areas kept clean and dry Skinfolds kept separated with a generous supply of nonmedicated powder Expose to air and light Remove excess clothing	A form of diaper irritation Prevent recurrence by keeping susceptible areas clean and dry Frequently associated with overheating from too much clothing; common in tracheostomy patients with short necks and copious secretions
Psoriasis— Unknown; hereditary predisposition; may be triggered by stress	Round, thick, dry, reddish patches covered with coarse, silvery scales over trunk and extremities; first lesions commonly appear in scalp; facial lesions more common in children than in adults Affected cells proliferate at a much more rapid rate than normal cells	Tar preparations in combination with ultraviolet (UV) B light or natural sunlight Topical corticosteroids Topical vitamin D analog calcipotriene Phenol and saline solutions followed by a tar shampoo to remove scales Keratolytic agents (salicylic acid) Acitretin Emollients may provide relief	Uncommon in children younger than age 6 years Persons are otherwise healthy individuals Coal tar acts synergistically with UV light Keratolytic agents enhance absorption of corticosteroids Humidifiers may help in winter

involvement is usually the result of chemical irritation from feces, especially diarrheal stools. *Candida albicans* infection produces perianal inflammation and a maculopapular rash with satellite lesions that may cross the inguinal fold (Fig. 30-12). It is seen in up to 90% of infants with chronic diaper dermatitis and should be considered in diaper rashes that are recalcitrant to treatment.

Nursing Considerations

Nursing interventions are aimed at altering the three factors that produce dermatitis—wetness, pH, and fecal irritants. The most significant factor amenable to intervention is the moist environment created in the diaper area. Changing the diaper as soon as it becomes wet eliminates a large part of the problem, and removing the diaper to expose healthy skin to air facilitates drying. The use of a hair dryer or heat lamp is not recommended because these devices can cause burns.

Diaper construction has a significant impact on the incidence and severity of diaper dermatitis. Superabsorbent disposable paper diapers reduce diaper dermatitis. They contain an absorbent gelling material that binds water tightly to decrease skin wetness, maintains pH control by providing a buffering capacity, and decreases skin irritation by preventing mixing of urine and feces in the diaper. Another advance in diapers is the addition of an inner layer or top sheet that is impregnated with petrolatum (as in Ultra Pampers with Tender Touch Liner*).

Guidelines for controlling diaper rash are presented in the Family Home Care box. A common misconception about using cornstarch on skin is that it promotes the growth of *Candida albicans*. Neither cornstarch nor talc promotes the growth of fungi under conditions normally found in the diaper area. Cornstarch is more effective in reducing friction and tends to cake less than talc when the skin is wet. On the basis of these properties and its safety in terms of inhalation injury, cornstarch is the preferred product. Talc should not be used.

ATOPIC DERMATITIS (ECZEMA)

Eczema or eczematous inflammation of the skin refers to a descriptive category of dermatologic diseases and not to a specific etiology. Atopic dermatitis (AD) is a type of pruritic

---

*Manufactured by **Procter & Gamble Company**, 1 Procter & Gamble Plaza, Cincinnati, OH 45224; (800) 285-6064; website: www.pampers.com.

TABLE 30-9 ■ **Miscellaneous Skin Disorders**—*cont'd*

DISEASE/CAUSATIVE AGENT	LOCAL MANIFESTATIONS	MANAGEMENT	COMMENTS
Alopecia*—			
Alopecia areata	Sudden onset of asymptomatic, noninflammatory, round, bald patches in hairy parts of body	Psychologic support Inducement of allergic contact dermatitis to stimulate growth of hair Minoxidil (peripheral vasodilator)	Family history in 10% to 26% of cases Some concern regarding drug therapy safety Refer to support groups*
Traumatic alopecia	Traction alopecia around scalp margins from tight hair styles (e.g., braids, pony tails, corn rows)	Counseling regarding hair styling, use of hair cosmetics, hot combs, rollers	More prevalent in black children and adolescents Prolonged traction can produce fibrosis of hair root and permanent loss
Trichotillomania	Compulsive hair pulling	Determine and treat cause	Chronic hair pulling may require psychologic therapy
Tinea capitis	See Table 30-5	See Table 30-5	See Table 30-5
Erythema multiforme (Stevens-Johnson syndrome)— Unknown; associated with ingestion of some drugs; often follows upper respiratory infection	Erythematous papular rash Lesions enlarge by peripheral expansion; develop central vesicle Involves most skin surfaces except scalp May extend to mucous membranes, especially oral, ocular, and urethral	Symptomatic and supportive Maintain adequate intake of fluids (oral or intravenous), calories, and protein Moist wound care, hydrogels such as CarraGauze, Vaseline, or Aquaphor Appropriate treatment of complications Diligent monitoring of urine volume and specific gravity, hemoglobin and hematocrit, serum electrolyte levels, total body weight	Rash often preceded by fever and malaise Complications include renal failure and severe eye disease Respiratory involvement in a number of cases Self-limiting, but recovery may extend for weeks; skin lesions may subside without scarring; mucous membrane lesions may persist for months Recurrence rate 20%; mortality as high as 10%
Neurofibromatosis— Inherited disorder; autosomal-dominant inheritance pattern	Café-au-lait spots, pigmented nevi, axillary freckling Slow-growing cutaneous and subcutaneous neurofibromas	Symptomatic treatment of associated manifestations (e.g., speech defects, seizures, skeletal defects [scoliosis, kyphosis], learning disabilities) Surgical removal of troublesome tumors	High mutation rate Refer to support groups† Family needs to know about genetic implications

*National Alopecia Areata Foundation, 710 C Street, Suite 11, San Rafael, CA 94901; (415) 456-4644; fax: (415) 456-4274; e-mail: 74301.1642@compuserve.com.
†National Neurofibromatosis Foundation, Inc., 95 Pine Street, 16th Floor, New York, NY 10005; (800) 323-7938 or (212) 344-6633; fax: (212) 747-0004; e-mail: nnff@nf.org; website: www.nf.org.

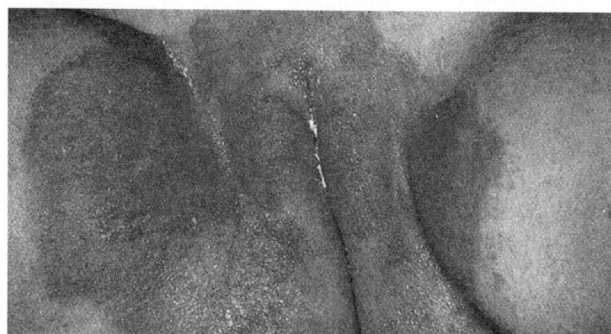

FIG. 30-11 ■ Irritant diaper dermatitis. Note sharply demarcated edges. (From Habif TP: *Clinical dermatology: a color guide to diagnosis and therapy,* ed 3, St Louis, 1996, Mosby.)

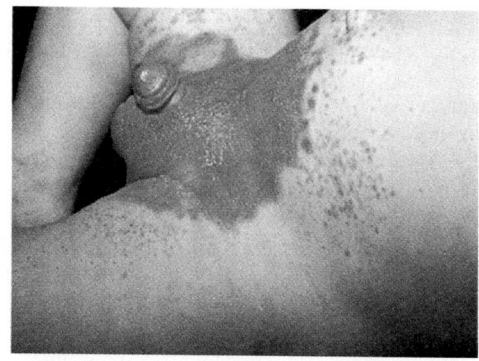

FIG. 30-12 ■ Candidiasis of diaper area. Note beefy red central erythema with satellite pustules. (From Weston WL, Lane AT, Morelli JG: *Color textbook of pediatric dermatology,* ed 2, St Louis, 1996, Mosby.)

 **FAMILY HOME CARE**

Controlling Diaper Rash

Keep skin dry.*
 Use superabsorbent disposable diapers to reduce skin wetness.
 If using cloth diapers, use only overwraps that allow air to circulate; avoid rubber pants.
 Change diapers as soon as soiled—especially with stool—whenever possible, preferably once during the night.
 Expose healthy or only slightly irritated skin to air, not heat, to dry completely.
Apply ointment, such as zinc oxide or petrolatum, to protect skin, especially if skin is very red or has moist, open areas.
 Avoid removing skin barrier cream with each diaper change; remove waste material and reapply skin barrier cream.
 To completely remove ointment, especially zinc oxide, use mineral oil; do not wash vigorously.
Avoid overwashing the skin, especially with perfumed soaps or commercial wipes, which may be irritating.
 May use a moisturizer or nonsoap cleanser, such as cold cream or Cetaphil, to wipe urine from skin.
 Gently wipe stool from skin using water and mild soap, such as Dove.
 When traveling fill an old baby wipe container with soft paper towels and warm water.

*Powder helps keep the skin dry, but talc is very dangerous if breathed into the lungs. Plain cornstarch or cornstarch-based powder is safer. When using any powder product, shake it first into your hand, then apply it to the diaper area. Store the container away from the infant's reach; keep the container closed when not in use.

eczema that usually begins during infancy and is associated with allergy with a hereditary tendency *(atopy)*. AD presents in three forms based on the age of the child and the distribution of lesions:

1 **Infantile (infantile eczema)**—Usually begins at 2 to 6 months of age; generally undergoes spontaneous remission by 3 years of age.
2 **Childhood**—May follow the infantile form; occurs at 2 to 3 years of age; 90% of children have manifestations by age 5 years.
3 **Preadolescent and adolescent**—Begins at about 12 years of age; may continue into the early adult years or indefinitely.

The diagnosis of AD is based on a combination of history and morphologic findings (Box 30-3). Children with AD have a lower threshold for cutaneous itching, and many authorities believe the dermatologic manifestations appear subsequent to scratching from the intense pruritus. For example, infants rub their faces against bed linen, and their crawling (a form of scratching) results in irritation of knees and elbows. Lesions disappear if the scratching is stopped.

The majority of children with infantile AD have a family history of eczema, asthma, food allergies, or allergic rhinitis, which strongly supports a genetic predisposition. The cause is unknown but appears to be related to abnormal function of the skin, including alterations in perspiration, peripheral vascular function, and heat tolerance. Manifestations of the chronic disease improve in humid climates and get worse in the fall and winter, when homes are heated and environmental humidity is lower. The disorder can be controlled but not cured.

BOX 30-3 ■ Clinical Manifestations of Atopic Dermatitis

DISTRIBUTION OF LESIONS
Infantile form—generalized, especially cheeks, scalp, trunk, and extensor surfaces of extremities (Fig. 30-13)
Childhood form—flexural areas (antecubital and popliteal fossae, neck), wrists, ankles, and feet
Preadolescent and adolescent form—face, sides of neck, hands, feet, face, and antecubital and popliteal fossae (to a lesser extent)

APPEARANCE OF LESIONS
Infantile form:
 Erythema
 Vesicles
 Papules
 Weeping
 Oozing
 Crusting
 Scaling
 Often symmetric
Childhood form:
 Symmetric involvement
 Clusters of small erythematous or flesh-colored papules or minimally scaling patches
 Dry and may be hyperpigmented
 Lichenification (thickened skin with accentuation of creases)
 Keratosis pilaris (follicular hyperkeratosis) common
Adolescent/adult form:
 Same as childhood manifestations
 Dry, thick lesions (lichenified plaques) common
 Confluent papules

OTHER PHYSICAL MANIFESTATIONS
Intense itching
Unaffected skin dry and rough
African-American children likely to exhibit more papular or follicular lesions than are Caucasian children
May exhibit one or more of the following:
 Lymphadenopathy, especially near affected sites
 Increased palmar creases (many cases)
 Atopic pleats (extra line or groove of lower eyelid)
 Prone to cold hands
 Pityriasis alba (small, poorly defined areas of hypopigmentation)
 Facial pallor (especially around nose, mouth, and ears)
 Bluish discoloration beneath eyes ("allergic shiners")
 Increased susceptibility to unusual cutaneous infections (especially viral)

Therapeutic Management

The major goals of management are to (1) hydrate the skin, (2) relieve pruritus, (3) reduce flare-ups or inflammation, and (4) prevent and control secondary infection. The general measures for managing AD focus on reducing pruritus, as well as other aspects of the disease. Management strategies include avoiding exposure to skin irritants or allergens, avoiding overheating, avoiding skin hydration, and administrating medications such as antihistamines, topical steroids, and (sometimes) mild sedatives as indicated.

Enhancing skin hydration and preventing dry, flaky skin is accomplished in a number of ways, depending on the child's

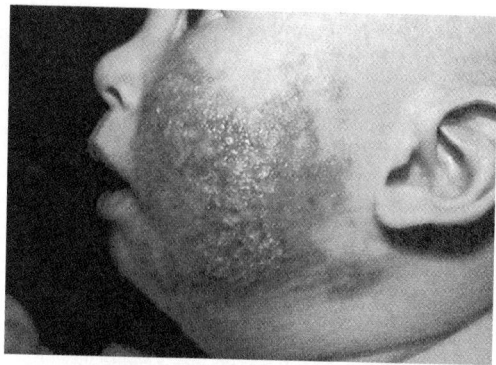

FIG. 30-13 ■ Infantile atopic dermatitis with oozing and crusting of lesions. (From Weston WL, Lane AT, Morelli JG: *Color textbook of pediatric dermatology*, ed 3, St Louis, 2002, Mosby.)

skin characteristics and individual needs. A tepid bath with a mild soap (Dove or Neutrogena), no soap, or an emulsifying oil, followed immediately by application of an emollient (within 3 minutes) assists in trapping moisture and preventing moisture loss. Bubble baths and harsh soaps should be avoided. The bath may need to be repeated once or twice daily, depending on the child's status; excessive bathing without emollient application only dries out the skin. Some lotions are not effective, and emollients should be chosen carefully to prevent excessive skin drying. Aquaphor, Cetaphil, and Eucerin are acceptable lotions for skin hydration. A nighttime bath, followed by emollient application and dressing in soft cotton pajamas, may help alleviate most nighttime pruritus.

Sometimes colloid baths, such as the addition of 2 cups of cornstarch to a tub of warm water, provide temporary relief of itching and may help the child sleep if given before bedtime. Cool wet compresses are soothing to the skin and provide antiseptic protection.

Oral antihistamine drugs such as hydroxyzine (Atarax) or diphenhydramine (Benadryl) usually relieve moderate or severe pruritus. Nonsedating antihistamines such as loratadine (Claritin) or fexofenadine (Allegra) may be preferred for daytime pruritus relief. Because pruritus increases at night, a mildly sedating antihistamine may be needed.

Occasional flare-ups require the use of topical steroids to diminish inflammation. Low-, moderate-, or high-potency topical corticosteroids are prescribed, depending on the degree of involvement, the area of the body to be treated, the age of the child, the potential for local side effects (striae, skin atrophy, and pigment changes), and the type of vehicle to be used (e.g., cream, lotion, ointment). Topical immunomodulators, a new nonsteroidal treatment for atopic dermatitis are best used at the beginning of a "flare up" just as the skin becomes red and itches. Two new immunomodulator medications used in children with AD are tacrolimus and pimecrolimus (Kronemyer, 2003). Tacrolimus is available in two ointment strengths (0.03% and 0.1%); the 0.03% concentration has been approved for use in children 2 years of age and older. Tacrolimus is recommended for intermittent therapy in patients who are not adequately responsive to, or are intolerant of, conventional therapy (Yetman and Parks, 2002). Pimecrolimus is available in a 1% cream that has no systemic accumulation or effects. This drug is approved for use in children with mild to moderate AD. Both drugs can be used freely on the face without worrying about steroid side effects

If secondary skin infections occur in children with AD, these infections are managed with appropriate systemic antibiotics.

Nursing Considerations

● Assessment

Assessment of the child with AD includes a family history for evidence of atopy, a history of previous involvement, and any environmental or dietary factors associated with the present and previous exacerbations. The skin lesions are examined for type, distribution, and evidence of secondary infection. Parents are interviewed regarding the child's behavior, especially in relation to scratching, irritability, and sleeping patterns. Exploration of the family's feelings and methods of coping is also important.

● Nursing Diagnoses

Nursing diagnoses identified for the child with AD include Impaired skin integrity related to eczematous lesions, Risk for infection related to risk of secondary infection of primary lesions, and Interrupted family processes related to the child's discomfort and lengthy therapy. Other diagnoses will be apparent in individual cases.

● Planning

The objectives for nursing care of the child with AD and the family are:

1 Child will experience no or minimal pruritus.
2 Child will receive appropriate treatment for skin hydration.
3 Child will experience no complications.
4 Child and family will receive adequate support.

● Implementation

The nursing care of the child with AD is challenging. Controlling the intense pruritus is imperative if the disorder is to be successfully managed, because scratching leads to new lesions and may cause secondary infection. In addition to the medical regimen, other measures can be taken to prevent or minimize the scratching. Fingernails and toenails are cut short, kept clean, and filed frequently to prevent sharp edges. Gloves or cotton stockings can be placed over the hands and pinned to shirtsleeves. One-piece outfits with long sleeves and long pants also decrease direct contact with the skin. If gloves or socks are used, the child needs time to be free from such restrictions. An excellent time to remove gloves, socks, or other protective devices is during the bath or after receiving sedative or antipruritic medication.

Conditions that increase itching are eliminated when possible. Woolen clothes or blankets, rough fabrics, and furry stuffed animals are removed from the child's environment. Because heat and humidity cause perspiration (which intensifies itching), proper dress for climatic conditions is essential. Pruritus is often precipitated by exposure to the irritant effects of certain components of common products such as soaps, detergents, fabric softeners, perfumes, and powders. Most children experience less itching when soft cotton fabrics are worn next to the skin. During cold months, synthetic fabrics (not wool) should be used for overcoats, hats, gloves, and snowsuits. Exposure to latex products, such as gloves and balloons, should also be avoided.

Clothes and sheets are laundered in a mild detergent and rinsed thoroughly in clear water (without fabric softeners or antistatic chemicals). Putting the clothes through a second complete wash cycle without using detergent reduces the amount of residue remaining in the fabric.

Preventing infection is usually accomplished by preventing scratching. Baths are given as prescribed, the water is kept tepid, and soaps (except as indicated) and bubble baths are avoided, as are oils or powders. Skinfolds and diaper areas need frequent cleansing with plain water. A room humidifier or vaporizer may benefit children with extremely dry skin. The skin lesions are examined for signs of infection—usually the presence of honey-colored crusts with surrounding erythema. Any signs of infection are reported to the practitioner.

NURSING ALERT

If the child is being treated with baths for hydration, it is imperative that the emollient preparation be applied immediately after bathing (while the skin is still slightly moist) to prevent drying.

Wet soaks and compresses are applied and medications for pruritus or infection are administered as directed. The family is given explicit instructions on the preparation and use of soaks, special baths, and topical medications, including the order of application if more than one is prescribed. It is important to emphasize that one thick application of topical medication is *not* equivalent to several thin applications, and that excessive use of an agent (particularly steroids) can be hazardous. If children have difficulty remaining still for a 10- or 15-minute soak, bath, or dressing application, these can be carried out at naptime or when the child is engrossed in watching television, listening to a story, or playing with tub toys.

Because adequate rest is important for these children, who are usually fretful and irritable, planning meals, baths, medications, and treatments during periods when they are awake is essential. Sleepy, tired children are normally cranky, and such behavior only intensifies the urge to scratch. During periods of irritability, these children tend to have a poor appetite, which is worsened by restriction of their usual foods.

Diet modification is another source of frustration to parents. When a hypoallergenic diet is prescribed, parents need help to understand the reason for the diet and the guidelines for avoiding hyperallergic foods (see Guidelines box). Because hypoallergenic diets take time before visible effects are apparent, parents need reassurance that results may not be seen immediately. If airborne allergens make eczema worse, the family is counseled about "allergy proofing" the home (see Asthma, Chapter 23).

Family Support.   Parents are assured that the lesions will not produce scarring (unless secondarily infected) and that the disease is not contagious. However, the child may have repeated exacerbations and remissions. Spontaneous and permanent remission takes place at approximately 2 to 3 years of age in most children with the infantile disorder.

During acute phases, emotional stress can become intense for the family. They need time to discuss negative feel-

GUIDELINES

Preventing Atopy in Children

IDENTIFY CHILDREN AT RISK
Family history of allergy
Increased immunoglobulin E in cord blood and postnatal serum
Dry, flaky skin

PRENATAL PRECAUTIONS (LAST TRIMESTER)
Avoid any known food allergens
Avoid milk and other dairy products, peanuts, and eggs
Minimize ingestion of other hyperallergenic foods

POSTNATAL PRECAUTIONS
Breast milk or casein/whey hydrolysate formula (e.g., Nutramigen, Pregestimil, Alimentum) exclusively for at least 6 months
No solid food for first 6 months
No cow's milk or soy formula for 12 months
No eggs, fish, corn, citrus, peanuts, nuts, or chocolate for 12 to 18 months
One new food added at 5- to 7-day intervals to identify possible reaction

ENVIRONMENTAL CONTROL
Limited exposure to dust, molds, furry animals, and cigarette smoke

Data from Johnstone D: Strategy for intervention of food allergy in infants, *Int Pediatr* 4(4):319-325, 1989; Zeiger R and others: Effectiveness of dietary manipulation in the prevention of food allergy in infants, part II, *J Allergy Clin Immunol* 78(1 pt 2):224-238, 1986; Wood RA: Prospects for the prevention of allergy in children, *Curr Opin Pediatr* 8(6):601-605, 1995.

ings and to be reassured that these feelings are normal. Stress tends to aggravate the severity of the condition. Therefore, efforts to relieve as much anxiety as possible in both the parents and the child have a beneficial emotional and physical effect.

Evaluation

The effectiveness of nursing interventions is determined by continual reassessment and evaluation of care based on the following observational guidelines:

1 Observe child's behavior, clothing, and activities.
2 Examine skin for evidence of dryness.
3 Examine skin lesions for evidence of secondary infection.
4 Interview aspects of family and encourage dialogue regarding the child and aspects of care.

Expected Outcomes

1 Child does not scratch and rests or plays quietly.
2 Skin appears well hydrated.
3 There is no evidence of secondary infection.
4 Family members comply with the therapeutic regimen, freely discuss their feelings and concerns, and appear to be coping with the inconveniences imposed by the disorder (specify).

SEBORRHEIC DERMATITIS

Seborrheic dermatitis is a chronic, recurrent, inflammatory reaction of the skin. It occurs most commonly on the scalp (cradle cap) but may involve the eyelids (blepharitis), external ear canal (otitis externa), nasolabial folds, and inguinal region. The cause is unknown, although it is more common in early infancy, when sebum production is increased. The lesions are characteristically thick, adherent, yellowish, scaly, oily patches that may or may not be mildly pruritic. Unlike atopic dermatitis, seborrheic dermatitis is not associated with a positive family history for allergy and is very common in infants shortly after birth and in adolescents after puberty. Diagnosis is made primarily on the basis of the appearance and the location of the crusts or scales.

Nursing Considerations

Cradle cap may be prevented with adequate scalp hygiene. Not infrequently, parents omit shampooing the infant's hair for fear of damaging the "soft spots," or fontanels. The nurse should discuss how to shampoo the infant's hair and emphasize that the fontanel is like skin anywhere else on the body—it does not puncture or tear with mild pressure.

When seborrheic lesions are present, the treatment is directed at removing the crusts. Parents are taught the appropriate procedure to clean the scalp. Education may need to include a demonstration. Shampooing should be done daily with a mild soap or commercial baby shampoo; medicated shampoos are not necessary, but an antiseborrheic shampoo containing sulfur and salicylic acid may be used. Shampoo is applied to the scalp and allowed to remain on the scalp until the crusts are softened. Then the scalp is thoroughly rinsed. A fine-tooth comb or a soft facial brush after shampooing helps to remove the loosened crusts from the strands of hair after shampooing.

ACNE

Acne vulgaris is the most common skin problem treated by physicians during patients' adolescence. Acne involves anatomic, physiologic, biochemical, genetic, immunologic, and psychologic factors.

One half of the adolescent population experiences acne by the end of the teenage years. Although the disorder can appear before the age of 10 years, the peak incidence occurs in middle to late adolescence (at age 16 to 17 years in females and 17 to 18 years in males). It is more common in males than in females. The degree to which an individual is affected may range from nothing more than a few isolated comedones to a severe inflammatory reaction. Although the disease is self-limited and not life-threatening, it has great significance to the adolescent. Health professionals should not underestimate the impact that acne has on teens.

Numerous factors affect the development and course of acne. Its distribution in families and a high degree of concordance in identical twins suggest hereditary factors. Premenstrual flares of acne occur in nearly 70% of adolescent girls, suggesting a hormonal cause. Studies do not indicate a clear association between stress and acne, but adolescents commonly cite stress as a cause for acne outbreaks. Cosmetics containing lanolin, petrolatum, vegetable oils, lauryl alcohol, butyl stearate, and oleic acid can increase comedone production. Exposure to oils in cooking grease can be a precursor in adolescents who work over fast-food restaurant hot oils. There is no known link between dietary intake and the development or worsening of acne.

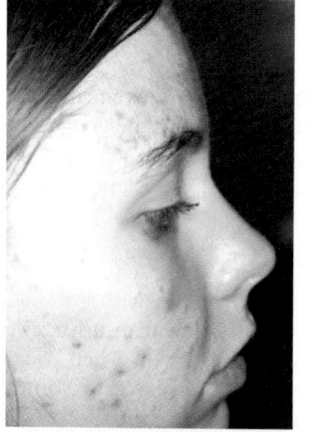

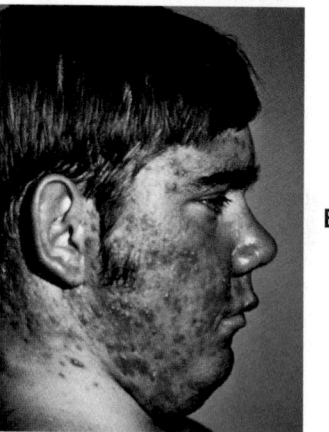

FIG. 30-14 ■ Acne vulgaris. **A,** Comedones with a few inflammatory pustules. **B,** Papulopustular acne. (From Weston WL, Lane AT: *Color textbook of pediatric dermatology,* St Louis, 1991, Mosby.)

Pathophysiology

Acne is a disease that involves the ***pilosebaceous follicles*** (the hair follicle and sebaceous gland complex) of the face, neck, chest, and upper back. Three pathophysiologic factors are involved in the development of acne: excessive sebum production, comedogenesis, and the overgrowth of *Propionibacterium acnes* (Mancini, 2000).

Comedogenesis (formation of comedones) results in a noninflammatory lesion that may be either an ***open comedone*** ("blackhead") or a ***closed comedone*** ("whitehead"). Inflammation occurs with the proliferation of *Propionibacterium acnes,* which draws in neutrophils, causing inflammatory papules, pustules, nodules, and cysts (Fig. 30-14).

Therapeutic Management

Successful management of acne depends on a cooperative effort between the health care provider, the adolescent, and the parents. Unlike many other dermatologic conditions, acne lesions resolve slowly, and improvement may not be apparent for at least 6 weeks. Individual comedones can take several weeks to months to resolve, and papules and pustules usually resolve in about 1 week. The multifactorial causes of acne necessitate a combined approach for successful treatment. Treatment consists of general measures of care and specific treatments determined by the type of lesions involved.

General Measures. Improvement of the adolescent's overall health status is part of the general management. Adequate rest, moderate exercise, a well-balanced diet, reduction of emotional stress, and elimination of any foci of infection are all part of general health promotion.

Cleansing. Dirt or oil on the surface of the skin does not cause acne. Gentle cleansing with a mild cleanser once or twice daily is usually sufficient. Antibacterial soaps are ineffective and may be too drying when used in combination with topical acne medications. For some adolescents hygiene of the hair and scalp appears to be related to the clinical activity of the acne. Acne on the forehead may improve with brushing the hair away from the forehead and more frequent shampooing.

Medications. Treatment success depends on commitment from the adolescent. Before prescribing treatment, the adolescent's level of comfort and readiness to begin treatment should be determined.

Tretinoin (Retin-A) is the only drug that effectively interrupts the abnormal follicular keratinization that produces microcomedones, the invisible precursors of the visible comedones. Tretinoin alone is usually sufficient for management of comedonal acne (Russell, 2000). Tretinoin is available as a cream, gel, or liquid. This drug can be extremely irritating to the skin and requires careful patient education for optimal usage. The patient should be instructed to begin with a pea-sized dot of medication, which is divided into the three main areas of the face and then gently rubbed into each area. The medication should not be applied for at least 20 to 30 minutes after washing to decrease the burning sensation. The avoidance of sun and the daily use of sunscreen must be emphasized, because sun exposure can result in severe sunburn. Adolescents should be advised to apply the medication at night and to use a sunscreen with a sun protection factor (SPF) of at least 15 in the daytime.

Topical *benzoyl peroxide* is an antibacterial agent that inhibits the growth of *P. acnes* organisms. It is effective against both inflammatory and noninflammatory acne and is an effective first-line agent. This medication is available as a cream, lotion, gel, or wash. The patient should be informed that the medication may have a bleaching effect on sheets, bedclothes, and towels. The adolescent can be reassured that skin bleaching will not occur. Accommodation to the medication can be gained with a gradual increase in the strength and frequency of application.

When inflammatory lesions accompany the comedones, a *topical antibacterial agent* may be prescribed. These agents are used to prevent new lesions as well as to treat preexisting acne. Clindamycin, erythromycin, metronidazole, azelaic acid, and the combination of either benzoyl peroxide and erythromycin (Benzamycin) or benzoyl peroxide and glycolic acid are all choices for topical antibacterial therapy (Leyden, 1997). The combination of 5% benzoyl peroxide and 3% erythromycin is especially beneficial, although the exact mechanism of action is not understood

(Burkhart, Specht, and Neckers, 2000). Tretinoin improves the penetration of other topical agents, and combination therapy with tretinoin and an antibacterial treatment is the only way to address three of the pathogenic causes of acne: keratinization, *P. acnes,* and inflammation (Laude, 2000).

Systemic antibiotic therapy is used when moderate to severe acne does not respond to topical treatments. Oral antibiotics are considered safe to use to treat acne. These antibiotics include tetracycline, erythromycin, minocycline, doxycycline, clindamycin, and trimethoprim-sulfamethoxazole (Leyden, 1997).

Females with mild to moderate acne may respond well to topical treatment and the addition of an *oral contraceptive pill (OCP).* OCPs reduce the endogenous androgen production and decrease the bioavailability of the woman's circulating androgens. Both of these actions result in decreased acne.

Isotretinoin, 13-cis retinoic acid (Accutane), is a very potent and effective oral agent that is reserved for severe cystic acne that has not responded to other treatments. Isotretinoin is the only agent available that affects factors involved in the development of acne. However, treatment with isotretinoin should be managed *only* by a dermatologist. Adolescents with multiple, active, deep dermal or subcutaneous cystic and nodular acne lesions are treated for 20 weeks. Multiple side effects can occur, including dry skin and mucous membranes, nasal irritation, dry eyes, decreased night vision, photosensitivity, arthralgia, headaches, mood changes, aggressive or violent behaviors, depression, and suicidal ideation. Adolescents on this drug should be monitored for depression, depressive symptoms, and suicidal ideation (Jacobs, Deutsch, and Brewer, 2001). The drug should be given only at the recommended doses for no longer than the recommended duration. The most significant side effects of this drug are the teratogenic effects. Isotretinoin is absolutely contraindicated in pregnant women. Sexually active young women must be using an effective contraceptive method during treatment and for 1 month after treatment. Patients receiving isotretinoin should also be monitored for elevated cholesterol and triglyceride levels. Significant elevation may require discontinuation of the medication.

Nursing Considerations

Because acne is so common and its appearance may seem so mild, the health care provider may underestimate the relative importance of the disease to the adolescent. The nurse should assess the individual adolescent's level of distress, current management, and perceived success of any regimen before initiating a referral. If adolescents do not perceive the acne to be a problem, motivation to follow the treatment plan may be absent.

The nurse can provide ongoing support for the adolescent when a treatment plan is initiated. The family is also encouraged to support the adolescent in his or her efforts. Use of medications and basic skin care information should be discussed in detail with the adolescent. Written instructions should accompany the verbal discussion. Information to dispel myths regarding the use of abrasive cleansing products can prevent unnecessary costs and trauma to the skin.

Teenagers need education about the factors that aggravate and damage the skin, such as too vigorous scrubbing.

In addition, picking, squeezing, and manual expression with fingernails breaks down the ductal walls of lesions and causes the acne to worsen. Mechanical irritation, such as vinyl helmet straps that rub areas predisposed to acne, can also cause the development of lesions.

THERMAL INJURY*

BURNS

Burn injuries are usually attributed to extreme heat sources but may also result from exposure to cold, chemicals, electricity, or radiation. Most burns are relatively minor and do not require definitive medical treatment. However, burns involving a large body surface area, critical body parts, or the geriatric or pediatric population often benefit from treatment in specialized burn centers. The American Burn Association has established criteria to guide decisions regarding the severity of injury and the need for transfer for specialized care. Burn prevention is also discussed in Chapters 10, 12, 15, and 16.

When burns are characterized by patients' age and type of injury, the following patterns become apparent: (1) hot-water scalds are most frequent in toddlers; (2) flame-related burns are more common in older children; (3) 10% to 20% of documented cases of child abuse include burn injuries (Herndon and others, 2002); and (4) children playing with matches or lighters account for 1 in 10 house fires.

The extent of tissue destruction is determined by the intensity of the heat source, the duration of contact or exposure, the conductivity of the tissue involved, and the rate at which the heat energy is dissipated by the skin. A brief exposure to high-intensity heat from a flame can produce burn injuries similar to those induced by long exposure to less intense heat in hot water.

Characteristics of Burn Injury

The physiologic responses, therapy, prognosis, and disposition of the injured child are all directly related to the *amount of tissue destroyed*. Therefore the severity of the burn injury is assessed on the basis of the percentage of surface burned and the depth of the burn. Among children in the school age–group or younger age-groups, a burn that is 10% of the **total body surface area (TBSA)** can be life-threatening if not treated correctly. Other important factors in determining the seriousness of the injury are the location of the wounds, the age of the child, the causative agent, the presence of respiratory involvement, the general health of the child, and the presence of any associated injury or condition.

Type of Injury. The majority of burns result from contact with thermal agents such as a flame, hot surfaces, or hot liquids. Electrical injuries caused by household current have the greatest incidence in young children, who insert conductive objects into electrical outlets and bite or suck on connected electrical cords (Herndon and others, 2002). These burns occur most commonly during the spring and summer months and are also associated with risk-taking be-

haviors in boys. Direct contact with high- or low-voltage current, as well as lightning strikes, is the most frequent mechanism of injury. The resistance of the tissue and the path of the electric current are responsible for the damage incurred. Electric current travels through the body following the path of least resistance, which involves the tissues, fluid, blood vessels, and nerves. A more localized burn is produced if skin resistance is high at the area of contact, and a more systemic pattern of injury is produced if skin resistance is low. Often compared with a crush injury, serious electrical trauma results from current passing through vital organs, muscle compartments, and nerve or vascular pathways. Loss of limbs, cardiac fibrillation, respiratory collapse, and burns are common occurrences after exposure to electrical energy.

Chemical burns are seen in the pediatric population and can cause extensive injury. The severity of injury is related to the chemical agent (acid, alkali, or organic compound) and the duration of contact. The mechanism of injury differs from other burns in that there is a chemical disruption and alteration of the physical properties of the exposed body area. Noxious agents exist in many cleaning products commonly found in the home. In addition to concern for localized damage, the potential for systemic toxicity must be addressed. Of particular concern is the exposure of the eyes to chemical agents, the ingestion of caustic substances, and inhalation of toxic gases produced from chemicals.

Extent of Injury. The extent of a burn is expressed as a percentage of the TBSA. This is most accurately estimated by using specially designed age-related charts (Fig. 30-15). It is more efficient to use a chart designed to assign body proportions to children of different ages.

Depth of Injury. A thermal injury is a three-dimensional wound that is also assessed in relation to depth of injury. Traditionally the terms *first-, second-,* and *third-degree* have been used to describe the depth of tissue injury. However, with the current emphasis on wound healing, these have been replaced by more descriptive terms based on the extent of destruction to the epithelializing elements of the skin (Fig. 30-16).

Superficial (first-degree) burns are usually of minor significance. With these burns, there is often a latent period followed by erythema. Tissue damage is minimal, the protective functions of the skin remain intact, and systemic effects are rare. Pain is the predominant symptom, and the burn heals in 5 to 10 days without scarring. Mild sunburn is an example of a superficial first-degree burn.

Partial-thickness (second-degree) injuries involve the epidermis and varying degrees of the dermis. These wounds are painful, moist, red, and blistered. Superficial partial-thickness burns involve the epidermis and part of the dermis. Dermal elements are intact, and the wound should heal in approximately 14 days with variable amounts of scarring (Fig. 30-17). The wound is extremely sensitive to temperature changes, exposure to air, and light touch. Although classified as second-degree or partial-thickness burns, deep dermal burns resemble full-thickness injuries in many respects. Sweat glands and hair follicles remain intact. The burn may appear mottled, with pink, red, or waxy white areas exhibiting blisters and edema formation. Systemic ef-

---

*Rose U. Baker, MSN, RN-CS, and Mary Mondozzi, MSN, RN, CS, revised this section.

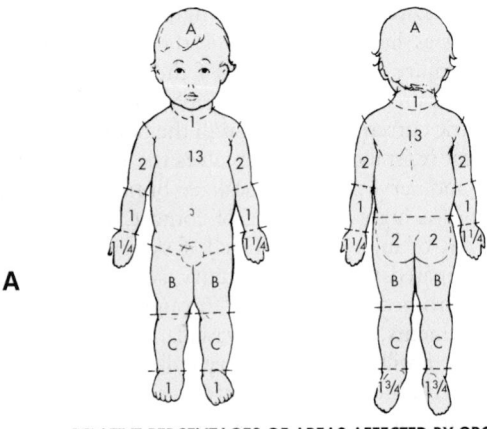

A

RELATIVE PERCENTAGES OF AREAS AFFECTED BY GROWTH

AREA	BIRTH	AGE 1 YR	AGE 5 YR
A = 1/2 of head	9 1/2	8 1/2	6 1/2
B = 1/2 of one thigh	2 3/4	3 1/4	4
C = 1/2 of one leg	2 1/2	2 1/2	2 3/4

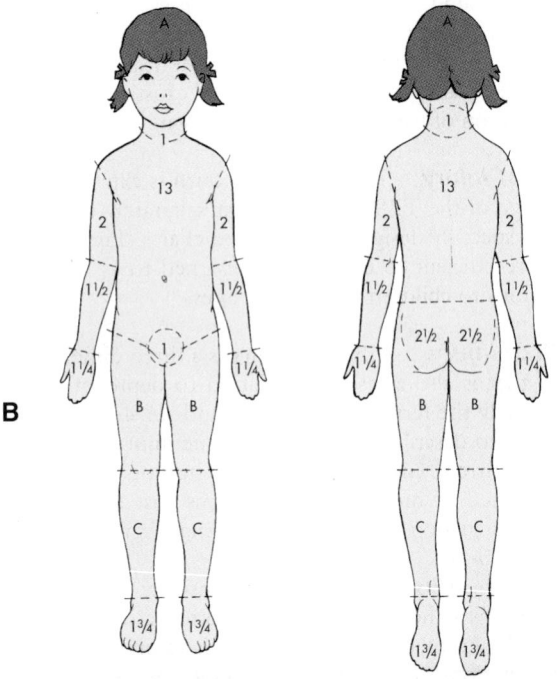

B

RELATIVE PERCENTAGES OF AREAS AFFECTED BY GROWTH

AREA	AGE 10 YR	AGE 15 YR	ADULT
A = 1/2 of head	5 1/2	4 1/2	3 1/2
B = 1/2 of one thigh	4 1/2	4 1/2	4 3/4
C = 1/2 of one leg	3	3 1/4	3 1/2

FIG. 30-15 ■ Estimation of distribution of burns in children. **A,** Children from birth to age 5 years. **B,** Older children.

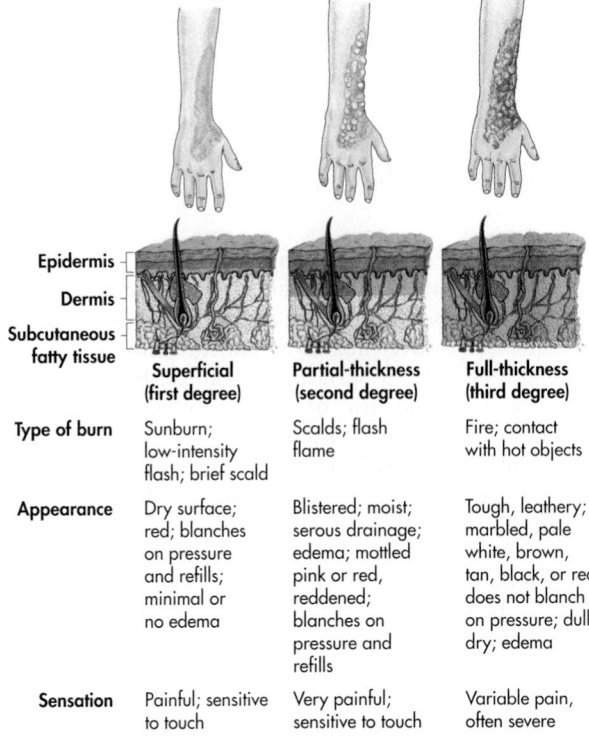

	Superficial (first degree)	Partial-thickness (second degree)	Full-thickness (third degree)
Type of burn	Sunburn; low-intensity flash; brief scald	Scalds; flash flame	Fire; contact with hot objects
Appearance	Dry surface; red; blanches on pressure and refills; minimal or no edema	Blistered; moist; serous drainage; edema; mottled pink or red, reddened; blanches on pressure and refills	Tough, leathery; marbled, pale white, brown, tan, black, or red; does not blanch on pressure; dull, dry; edema
Sensation	Painful; sensitive to touch	Very painful; sensitive to touch	Variable pain, often severe

FIG. 30-16 ■ Classification of burn depth. (Redrawn from Grant HD, Murray RH: *Emergency care*, ed 7, Upper Saddle River, NJ, 1995, Prentice-Hall.)

and is distinguished by a dry, leathery appearance (Fig. 30-18). Normally, full-thickness burns lack sensation in the area of injury because of the destruction of nerve endings. However, most full-thickness burns have superficial and partial-thickness burned areas at the periphery of the burn, where nerve endings are intact and exposed. Excised eschar and donor sites also cause exposed nerve fibers. As the peripheral fibers regenerate, painful sensations return. Consequently, children often experience severe pain related to the size and depth of the burn. Full-thickness wounds are not capable of reepithelialization and require surgical excision and grafting to close the wound.

Fourth-degree burns are full-thickness injuries that involve underlying structures such as muscle, fascia, and bone. The wound appears dull and dry, and ligaments, tendons, and bone may be exposed (Fig. 30-19).

Severity of Injury. Burns are classified as minor, moderate, or major, which is useful in determining the disposition of the patient for treatment. Burn patients are categorized as (1) those with a *major burn injury,* who require the services and facilities of a specialized burn center; (2) those with a *moderate burn,* who may be treated in a hospital with expertise in burn care; and (3) those with *minor injuries,* who may be treated on an outpatient basis. The extent and depth of the burn (Table 30-10), the causative agent, and the body area involved, the patient's age, and concomitant injuries and illnesses determine the severity of the injury.

Because the skin of infants is so thin, it is likely to sustain deeper injuries. Children younger than 2 years of age, especially 6 months or younger, have a significantly higher mor-

fects are similar to those encountered with full-thickness burns. Although many of these wounds heal spontaneously, they often heal with extensive scarring.

Full-thickness (third-degree) burns are serious injuries that involve the entire epidermis and dermis and extend into subcutaneous tissue (see Fig. 30-16). Nerve endings, sweat glands, and hair follicles are destroyed. The burn varies in color from red to tan, waxy white, brown, or black

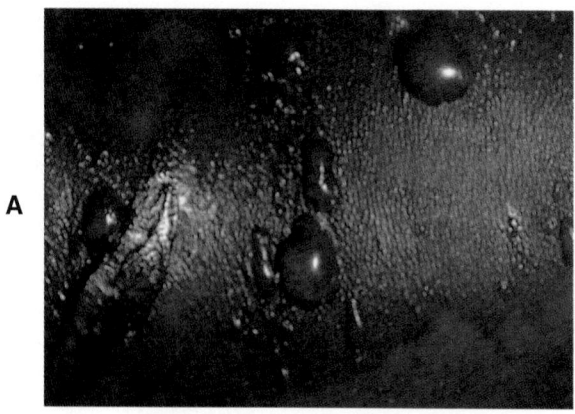
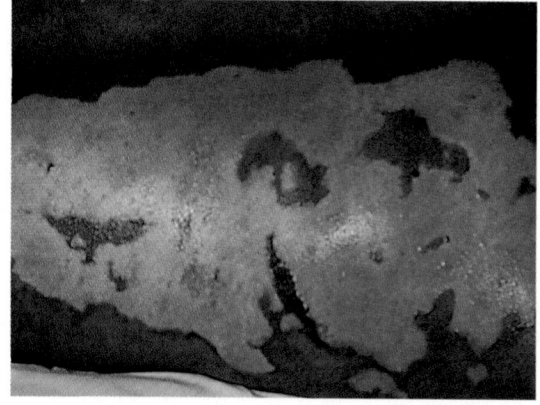

FIG. 30-17 ■ Superficial partial-thickness burns on black child. **A,** Blisters intact. **B,** Blisters removed. (Courtesy Hillcrest Medical Center, Tulsa, Okla.)

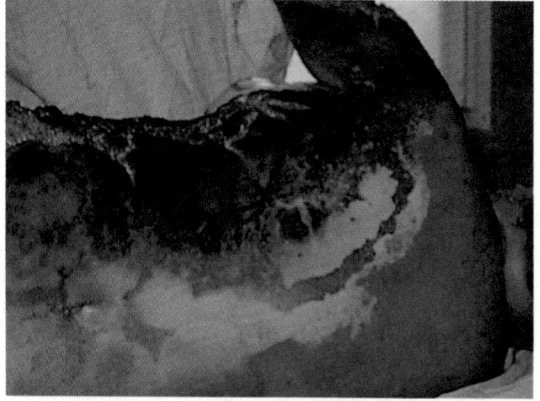
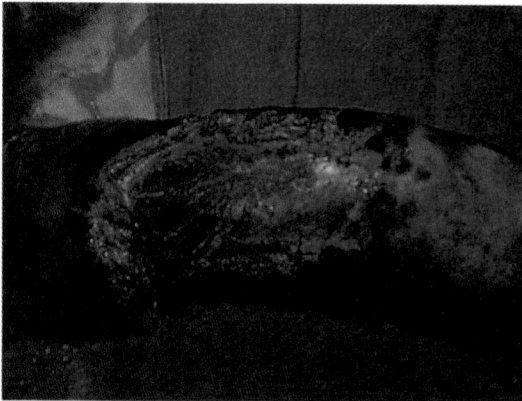

FIG. 30-18 ■ *Bottom to top:* Deep partial-thickness burn (red area); full-thickness burn (white area); full-thickness burn with eschar (brown area). (Courtesy Hillcrest Medical Center, Tulsa, Okla.)

FIG. 30-19 ■ Full-thickness burn with muscle and fascia involved. (Courtesy Hillcrest Medical Center, Tulsa, Okla.)

TABLE 30-10 ■ Severity Grading System Adopted by the American Burn Association

	MINOR*	MODERATE*	MAJOR*
Partial-thickness burns	<10% of total body surface area (TBSA)	>10% to 20% of TBSA	>20% of TBSA
Full-thickness burns			All
Treatment	Usually outpatient; may require 1- to 2-day admission	Admission to hospital, preferably one with expertise in burn care	Admission to a burn center

From Vaccaro P, Trofino RB: Care of the patient with minor to moderate burns. In Trofino RB, editor: *Nursing care of the burn-injured patient,* Philadelphia, 1991, FA Davis.
*Minor burns exclude any burn involving the face, hands, feet, perineum, or crossing joints; electrical burns; any injury complicated by the presence of inhalation injury or concomitant trauma; children with psychosocial factors affecting the injury.

tality rate than older children with burns of similar magnitude. Acute or chronic illnesses or superimposed injuries also complicate burn care and response to treatment.

Inhalation Injury.   Trauma to the tracheobronchial tree often follows inhalation of the heated gases and toxic chemicals produced during combustion. Although direct thermal injury to the upper airway may occur, heat damage below the vocal cords is rare. Inspired heated air is cooled in the upper airway before reaching the trachea. Reflex closure of the cords and laryngeal spasm also prevent full inhalation.

However, evidence of direct thermal injury to the upper airway includes burns of the face and lips, singed nasal hairs, and laryngeal edema. Clinical manifestations may be delayed as long as 24 to 48 hours. Wheezing, increasing secretions, hoarseness, wet rales, and carbonaceous secretions are signs of respiratory tract involvement. Upper airway obstruction is often associated with burn shock and fluid resuscitation. In such situations, endotracheal intubation may also be necessary to preserve a patent airway.

Inhalation of carbon monoxide is suspected when the injury has occurred in an enclosed space. Mucosal erythema and edema followed by sloughing of the mucosa are manifestations of respiratory injury. A mucopurulent membrane replaces the mucosal lining and seriously compromises respiration and ventilation.

Early in the postburn period most pulmonary infections result from nosocomial exposure, immobility, and abdominal distention. The hematogenous variety occurs later and is related to the septic burn wound or other foci, such as phlebitis at the site of an invasive IV line. A significant increase in mortality has been observed when inhalation injury and pneumonia are both present.

Deep burns, especially those circling the thorax, may cause restriction of chest excursion as a result of edema and inelastic eschar formation. Young children are particularly at risk because of the pliability of the skeletal structure. Hypoxia is relieved by an escharotomy incision, which allows expansion of the chest wall to facilitate ventilation.

Pathophysiology

Thermal injuries produce both local and systemic effects that are related to the extent of tissue destruction. In superficial burns the tissue damage is minimal. In partial-thickness burns there is considerable edema and more severe capillary damage. With a major burn greater than 30% of the TBSA, there is a systemic response involving an increase in capillary permeability, allowing plasma proteins, fluids, and electrolytes to be lost. Maximum edema formation in a small wound occurs about 8 to 12 hours after injury. After a larger injury, hypovolemia, associated with this phenomenon, will slow the rate of edema formation, with maximum effect at 18 to 24 hours.

Another systemic response is anemia, caused by direct heat destruction of red blood cells, hemolysis of injured red blood cells, and trapping of red blood cells in the microvascular thrombi of damaged cells. A long-term decrease in the number of red blood cells may occur as a result of increased red blood cell fragility. Initially there is an increased blood flow to the heart, brain, and kidneys, with decreased blood flow to the gastrointestinal tract. There is an increase in metabolism to maintain body heat, providing for the increased energy needs of the body.

Complications. Thermally injured children are subject to a number of serious complications, both from the wound and from systemic alterations resulting from the injury. The immediate threat to life is related to airway compromise and profound shock. During healing, infection—both local and systemic sepsis—is the primary complication. Mortality associated with thermal trauma in children increases with the severity of injury and decreases as age advances. In children older than 3 years, the mortality rate is similar to that of adults. Below this age, the survival rate with burns and their associated complications lessens considerably.

A less apparent respiratory injury is inhalation of carbon monoxide. Carbon monoxide has a greater affinity for hemoglobin than does oxygen, thereby depriving peripheral tissues and oxygen-dependent organs (such as the heart and brain) of the oxygen needed for survival. Treatment for either of these two problems is 100% oxygen, which reverses the situation rapidly.

Pulmonary problems are a major cause of fatality in children with either thermal burns or complications in the respiratory tract. Respiratory problems include inhalation injuries, aspiration in unconscious patients, bacterial pneumonia, pulmonary edema, pulmonary embolus, posttraumatic pulmonary insufficiency, and atelectasis. The most common cause of respiratory failure in the pediatric age-group is bacterial pneumonia, which requires prolonged intubation and sometimes necessitates a tracheostomy. Tracheostomies increase the incidence of serious complications and are performed only in extreme cases.

A less common complication is pulmonary edema resulting from fluid overload or acute respiratory distress syndrome (ARDS) in association with gram-negative sepsis. This syndrome results from pulmonary capillary damage and leakage of fluid into the interstitial spaces of the lung. A loss of compliance and interference with oxygenation are the consequences of pulmonary insufficiency in conjunction with systemic sepsis.

Wound Sepsis. Sepsis is a critical problem in the treatment of burns and an ever-present threat following the shock phase. Initially, burn wounds are relatively pathogen free unless they are contaminated with potentially infectious material, such as dirt or polluted water. However, dead tissue and exudate provide a fertile field for bacterial growth. On approximately the third postburn day, early colonization of the wound surface by a preponderance of gram-positive organisms (primarily staphylococci) changes to predominantly gram-negative opportunistic organisms, particularly *Pseudomonas aeruginosa.* By the fifth postburn day, bacterial invasion is well under way beneath the surface of the burn wound. Early surgical excision of eschar together with placement of autograft reduces the incidence of sepsis.

Therapeutic Management

Emergency Care. The initial management of the burn patient begins at the scene of injury. The first priority is to stop the burning process (see Emergency Treatment box). The child should then be transported immediately to the nearest medical facility for treatment and evaluation. The child and the family are usually extremely frightened and anxious; sensitivity to their emotional state and reassurance should be provided during the transport process.

Stop the burning process. The chief aim of rescue in flame burns is to smother the fire, not fan it. Children tend to panic and run, which spreads the flames and makes assistance more difficult. The injured child should be placed in a horizontal position and rolled in a blanket, rug, or similar article, with care taken not to cover the head and face because of the danger of inhalation of toxic fumes. If nothing is available, the victim should lie down and roll over slowly to extinguish the flames. Remaining in the vertical position may cause the hair to ignite or the inhalation of flames, heat, or smoke.

Major burns with large amounts of denuded skin should not be cooled. Heat is rapidly lost from burned areas, and additional cooling leads to a drop in core body temperature and potential circulatory collapse. Wet dressings also promote vasoconstriction because of cooling, resulting in impaired circulation to the burned area and increased tissue damage. Chemical burns require continuous flushing with large amounts of water before transport to a medical facility. The use of neutralizing agents on the skin is contraindi-

EMERGENCY TREATMENT

Burns

MINOR BURNS

Stop the burning process:

Apply cool water to the burn or hold the burned area under cool running water. Do not use ice.

Do not disturb any blisters that form, unless the injury is from a chemical substance.

Do not apply anything to the wound.

Cover with a clean cloth if risk of damage or contamination.

Remove burned clothing and jewelry.

MAJOR BURNS

Stop the burning process:

Flame burns—smother the fire.

Place victim in the horizontal position.

Roll victim in a blanket or similar object; avoid covering the head.

Assess for an adequate airway and breathing.

If not breathing, begin mouth-to-mouth resuscitation.

Remove burned clothing and jewelry.

Cover wound with a clean cloth.

Keep victim warm.

Transport to medical aid.

Begin intravenous and oxygen therapy as prescribed.

---

cated, because a chemical reaction is initiated and further injury may result. If the chemical is in powder form, the addition of water may spread the caustic agent. The powder should be brushed off if possible.

Burned clothing is removed to prevent further damage from smoldering fabric and hot beads of melted synthetic materials. Jewelry is removed to eliminate the transfer of heat from the metal and constriction resulting from edema formation. This also provides access to the wound and prevents painful removal later.

Assess the victim's condition.   As soon as the flames are extinguished, the child is assessed. Airway, breathing, and circulation are the primary concerns. Cardiopulmonary complications may result from exposure to electric current, inhalation of toxic fumes and smoke, hypovolemia, and shock. Emergency measures are instituted as appropriate.

Cover the burn.   The burn wound should be covered with a clean cloth to prevent contamination, decrease pain by eliminating air contact, and prevent hypothermia. No attempt should be made to treat the burn. Application of topical ointments, oils, or other home remedies is contraindicated.

Transport the child to medical aid.   The child with an extensive burn is not given anything by mouth to avoid aspiration in the presence of paralytic ileus and upper airway edema and to prevent water intoxication. The child is transported to the nearest medical facility. If this cannot be accomplished within a relatively short period, IV access should be established, if possible, with a large-bore catheter. Oxygen is administered, if available, at 100%. A report of the initial assessment and any interventions implemented is given to the medical facility assuming care of the child.

Provide reassurance.   Providing reassurance and psychologic support to both the family and the child helps immeasurably during the period of postinjury crisis. Reducing anxiety conserves energy the family and child will need to cope with the physiologic and emotional stress of injury.

Minor Burns.   Treatment of burns classified as minor can usually be managed adequately on an outpatient basis when it is determined that the parent can be relied on to carry out instructions for care and observation. Patients with less than optimum circumstances may require close follow-up to ensure adherence with treatment.

The wound is cleansed with a mild soap and tepid water. Débridement of the wound includes removal of any embedded debris, chemicals, and devitalized tissue. Removal of intact blisters remains controversial. Some authorities argue that blisters provide a barrier against infection; others maintain that blister fluid is an effective medium for the growth of microorganisms. However, blisters should be broken if the injury is due to a chemical agent to control absorption. Most practitioners favor covering the wound with an antimicrobial ointment to reduce the risk of infection and to provide some form of pain relief. The dressing consists of nonadherent fine-mesh gauze placed over the ointment and a light wrap of gauze dressing that avoids interference with movement. This helps to keep the wound clean and protect it from trauma. The caregiver is instructed to wash the wound, reapply the dressing, and return the child to the office or clinic as directed for wound observation. The frequency of dressing changes may vary from every other day to once a day.

Some practitioners prefer an occlusive dressing, such as a hydrocolloid, which is placed over the wound after cleansing. Hydrogel dressings, which are soothing and nonadherent, may also be used. The dressing is changed when leakage occurs—at regular intervals or at least weekly. This method eliminates the discomfort associated with frequent dressing changes but impairs visualization of the wound surface.

If there is a high probability of infection or other complications or if there is doubt about the ability to carry out instructions, the caregiver may be directed to bring the patient in daily for dressing changes and inspection. Another option is have a nurse make a home visit to inspect the wound and perform the dressing change. Frequent removal of the dressing is an effective mode of débridement. Soaking the dressing in tepid water or normal saline before removal helps to loosen the dressing and debris and reduce discomfort. Burns of the face are usually treated by an open method. The wound is washed and débrided in the same manner, and a thin film of antimicrobial ointment is applied.

A tetanus history is obtained on admission. If there is no history of immunization, or if more than 5 years have passed since the last immunization, tetanus prophylaxis is administered. There is no evidence that systemic antibiotic prophylaxis decreases the incidence of infection in small burn wounds (Herndon and others, 2002). Therefore, antibiotics should only be used when there is evidence of infection. A mild analgesic such as acetaminophen is usually sufficient to relieve discomfort; the antipyretic effect of the drug also alleviates the sensation of heat.

Most minor burns heal without difficulty, but if the wound margin becomes erythematous, gross purulence is noted, or the child develops evidence of systemic reaction, such as fever or tachycardia, hospitalization is indicated. The child should also be evaluated for functional impairment, and the caregiver should be instructed in the exercise and ambulation program. Following wound healing, an evaluation of scar maturation and range of motion will indicate any need for further therapy.

Major Burns. The first priority is airway maintenance. The inhalation of noxious agents or respiratory burns is suggested when there is a history of injury in an enclosed space; edema of the oral and nasal membranes; thermal injury to the face, nares, and upper torso; hyperemia; and blisters or evidence of trauma to the upper respiratory passages. When respiratory involvement is suspected or evident, 100% oxygen is administered and blood gas values, including carbon monoxide levels, are determined.

If the child exhibits changes in sensorium, air hunger, or other signs of respiratory distress, an endotracheal tube is inserted to maintain the airway. When severe edema of the face and neck is anticipated, intubation is performed before swelling makes intubation difficult or impossible. Controlled intubation is preferred to an emergency procedure. Intubation allows for the delivery of humidified oxygen, the removal of secretions from respiratory passages, and the provision of ventilatory support.

When full-thickness burns encircle the chest, constricting eschar may limit chest wall excursion, and ventilation of the child becomes more difficult. Escharotomy of the chest relieves this constriction and improves ventilation.

Fluid replacement therapy. The objectives of fluid therapy are to (1) compensate for water and sodium lost to traumatized areas and interstitial spaces, (2) reestablish sodium balance, (3) restore circulating volume, (4) provide adequate perfusion, (5) correct acidosis, and (6) improve renal function.

Fluid replacement is required during the first 24 hours because of fluid shifts that occur after the injury. Various formulas are used to calculate fluid needs, and the one adopted depends on practitioner preference. Crystalloid solutions are used during this initial phase of therapy. Parameters such as vital signs (especially heart rate), urine output volume, adequacy of capillary filling, and state of sensorium determine adequacy of fluid resuscitation.

After the initial 24-hour period, theoretically there is a capillary seal, and capillary permeability is restored. Colloid solutions such as albumin, plasmalyte, or fresh frozen plasma are useful in maintaining plasma volume. However, children with burn injuries usually require fluids in excess of their calculated maintenance and replacement volume. Reasons for this may include underestimation of burn size (particularly in pediatric patients), pulmonary injury that sequesters resuscitation fluid in the lung, electrical injury with greater tissue destruction than that which is visible, and a delay in the initiation of fluid resuscitation. Irreversible burn shock that persists despite aggressive fluid resuscitation remains a significant cause of death in the immediate postburn period. Fluid balance may continue to be a problem throughout the course of treatment, especially during periods in which there may be considerable evaporative loss from the wound.

Nutrition. The enhanced metabolic requirements and catabolism in severe burns make nutritional needs of paramount importance and often difficult to satisfy. The diet must provide sufficient calories to meet the increased metabolic needs and enough protein to avoid protein breakdown. Hypoglycemia can result from the stress of the burn injury because the liver glycogen stores are rapidly depleted.

A high-protein, high-calorie diet is encouraged after resolution of paralytic ileus. However, many children have poor appetites and are unable to meet energy requirements solely by oral feeding. Most children with burns in excess of 25% of the TBSA require supplementation with tube feeding. Early and continued nutritional support is an important part of therapy for seriously burned patients. Enteral feeding provides direct nourishment to the gastrointestinal tract and helps to reverse the defective gut barrier that accompanies burn shock (Hansbrough, 1998).

If nutritional requirements cannot be met entirely by the enteral route, parenteral hyperalimentation is used to supplement intake. However, enteral feeding increases blood flow in the intestinal tract, preserves gastrointestinal function, and minimizes bacterial translocation by decreasing mucosal atrophy of the intestines. These factors make enteral feeding the preferred route of nutritional support (Herndon and others, 2002).

To facilitate growth and proliferation of epithelial cells, administration of vitamins A and C is begun early in the postburn period. Zinc is also supplemented because of its important role in wound healing and epithelialization.

Medication. Antibiotics are usually not administered prophylactically. The administration of systemic antibiotics to control wound colonization is not indicated, because decreased circulation to the injured area prevents delivery of the medication to areas of deepest injury. Surveillance cultures and monitoring of the clinical course provide the most reliable indicators of developing infection. Appropriate antibiotics are instituted to treat the specific identified organism. Otitis media should not be overlooked as a source of fever in the pediatric population.

Some form of sedation and analgesia is required in the care of burned children. Morphine sulfate is the drug of choice for severe burn injuries. Morphine has extensive distribution but is metabolized rapidly; continuous infusion or frequent administration is needed for pain management in burns. Morphine is administered intravenously and titrated to individual need. The unstable circulatory status and edema formation preclude intramuscular or subcutaneous administration. When combined, midazolam (Versed) and fentanyl (Sublimaze) also provide excellent IV sedation and analgesia to control procedural pain in children with burns (Herndon and others, 2002). The oral form of fentanyl, Fentanyl Oralet, provides effective analgesia in a convenient form that the child can suck. Dosage monitoring is important because tolerance to opioids may develop. IV analgesics are most effective when they are administered just before the onset of procedural pain.

The use of short-acting anesthetic agents, such as propofol and nitrous oxide, has proved beneficial in eliminating procedural pain. Pharyngeal reflexes remain intact, thus ensuring a patent airway. Propofol (Diprivan) is an IV sedative hypnotic agent that produces sedation in less than 1 minute and lasts only a few minutes.

Nitrous oxide is a useful short-term analgesic when given in a mixture of gases on a fixed ratio of 50% nitrous oxide and 50% oxygen (Annequin and others, 2000). Initiation of action is approximately 1 minute, with peak effect reached in 3 to 5 minutes. Nitrous oxide is useful to alleviate anxiety and raise the threshold of pain during procedures. The child may self-administer the nitrous oxide mixture with assistance. For any conscious or unconscious sedation, the child must be monitored continuously during the procedure. (See Preoperative Care, Chapter 22, and Pain Assessment and Pain Management, Chapter 21.)

Management of the burn wound.   After the initial period of shock and the restoration of fluid balance, the primary concern is the burn wound. The objectives of wound management include prevention of infection, removal of devitalized tissue, and closure of the wound. The application of dressings and topical antimicrobial therapy reduce pain by minimizing the exposure to air.

Primary excision.   In children with large, full-thickness burn wounds, excision is performed as soon as the patient is hemodynamically stable after initial resuscitation. Because the burn wound precipitates an exaggerated physiologic response, many complications do not resolve until the eschar is excised and the wound is closed. Early excision of deep partial-thickness and full-thickness burns reduces the incidence of infection and the threat of sepsis.

Débridement.   Partial-thickness wounds require débridement of devitalized tissue to promote healing. Débridement is very painful and requires analgesia and a sedative before the procedure. Medications given for pain need to be readily available during this procedure and may need to be titrated up during the procedure. Atarax and Benadryl are often needed for itching that occurs after whirlpool and débridement. The itching becomes particularly bothersome as the burns heal.

Hydrotherapy is employed to cleanse the wound and involves soaking in a tub or showering once or twice a day for no more than 20 minutes. The water acts to loosen and remove sloughing tissue, exudate, and topical medications.

Hydrotherapy helps to cleanse not only the wound but the entire body and aids in maintenance of range of motion. Mesh gauze serves to entrap the exudative slough and is readily removed during hydrotherapy. Any loose tissue is carefully trimmed away before the wound is redressed.

Topical antimicrobial agents.   Methods used for managing the burn wound include:

Exposure—Wounds are left open to air; crust forms on partial-thickness wounds, and eschar forms on full-thickness burns.
Open—Topical antimicrobial agent is applied directly to the wound surface and the wound is left uncovered.
Modified—Antimicrobial is applied directly or impregnated into thin gauze and applied to the wound; gauze or net secures the area.
Occlusive—Antimicrobial is impregnated in gauze or applied directly to the wound; multiple layers of bulky gauze are placed over the primary layer and secured with gauze or net.

All of these methods provide wound coverage and employ some type of topical agent.

Topical agents do not eliminate organisms from the wound but can effectively inhibit bacterial growth. To be effective, a topical application must be nontoxic, capable of diffusing through eschar, harmless to viable tissue, inexpensive, and easy to apply. A topical ointment should not encourage the development of resistant strains of bacteria and should produce minimal electrolyte derangement. A comparison of commonly used agents is summarized in Table 30-11.

Biologic skin coverings.   Permanent coverage of extensive burns is a prolonged process that requires repeated operations for débridement and grafting. Early closure

TABLE 30-11 ■ Comparison of Common Topical Preparations

AGENT	DRESSINGS	ADVANTAGES	DISADVANTAGES
Silver nitrate 0.5% (AgNO$_3$)	Open, modified or occlusive; impedes joint movement; dressings changed twice daily; keep dressing moist, rewet at least every 2 hours	Greatly reduces evaporative losses; does not interfere with wound healing; bacteriostatic action against major burn flora, including *Pseudomonas* and *Staphylococcus*; inexpensive	Does not penetrate eschar; ineffective on established burn wound infections; little effect on *Klebsiella* and *Aerobacter* groups; stains skin, clothing, linens; makes assessment of the wound difficult because of staining; hypotonicity pulls electrolytes from the wound, depleting sodium, potassium, chloride, and magnesium; stings on application
Silver sulfadiazine 1% (AgSD)	Occlusive; motion of joints maintained; applied twice daily; do not use with a history of allergy to sulfa	Little pain on application; bactericidal by altering DNA and cell metabolism; effective against gram-positive and gram-negative bacteria; easy to apply; nontoxic	Transient neutropenia; does not penetrate eschar; forms proteinaceous gel on wound surface that is painful to remove; occasional rashes and pruritus; decreases granulocyte formation
Mafenide acetate 10% (Sulfamylon)	*Cream:* Usually open; do not apply to face; apply twice daily *Solution:* Occlusive; keep dressing moist (rewet at least every 2 hours); protect solution from light	Penetrates eschar and diffuses rapidly into burn wound and underlying tissues; effective in deep flame, electrical, and infected wounds; biostatic against many gram-positive and gram-negative organisms, including *Pseudomonas* and *Clostridium*	Difficult and painful to remove cream; pain on application; metabolic acidosis, hypercapnia, and carbonic anhydrase inhibition; inhibits wound healing; hypersensitivity in some patients
Bacitracin	Open, modified; motion of joints maintained; change dressing twice daily	Bactericidal and bacteriostatic against gram-positive organisms; low toxicity; painless application; ease of application	Limited activity against gram-negative organisms; allergic reaction in sensitive individuals

shortens the period of metabolic stress and decreases the likelihood of burn wound sepsis. In the acute phase, biologic dressings cover and protect the wound from contamination, reduce fluid and protein loss, increase the rate of epithelialization, reduce pain, and facilitate movement of joints to retain range of motion.

Allograft (homograft) skin is obtained from human cadavers that are screened for communicable diseases. Homograft is particularly useful in the coverage of surgically excised deep partial-thickness and full-thickness wounds in extensive burns when available donor sites are limited. Severe immunosuppression occurs in massively burned children, and the allograft becomes adherent. The homograft can remain in place until suitable donor sites become available. Typically, rejection is seen approximately 14 days after application. The availability of tissue banks and a supply of suitable donors limit the use of homographs.

Xenograft from a variety of species, most notably pigs, is commercially available. In large burns, the porcine xenograft is commonly applied when extensive early débridement is indicated to cover a partial-thickness burn; this provides a temporary covering for the wound until an available autograft can be applied to the full-thickness areas (Herndon and others, 2002). Pigskin dressings are replaced daily or every 2 to 3 days. Pigskin dressings are particularly effective in children with partial-thickness scald burns of the hands and face, because they allow relatively pain-free movement, which reduces contracture formation and has the added benefit of improving appetite and morale.

When applied early to a superficial partial-thickness injury, biologic dressings stimulate epithelial growth and faster wound healing. However, biologic dressings must be applied to clean wounds. If the dressing covers areas of heavy microbial contamination, infection occurs beneath the dressing. In the case of partial-thickness burns, such infection may convert the wound to a full-thickness injury.

Synthetic skin coverings are available for the management of partial-thickness burn wounds. Ideally, the dressing should provide the properties of human skin: adherence, elasticity, durability, and hemostasis. Synthetic skin substitutes are readily available, have an indefinite shelf life, and are relatively inexpensive.

Synthetic dressings are composed of a variety of materials and can be used successfully in the management of superficial partial-thickness burns and donor sites. Examples include adherent elastic films, hydroactive materials, or colloidal suspensions that are usually permeable to air, vapor, and fluids. BCG Matrix* consists of a film-backed mesh-reinforced hydrocolloid dressing.

Biobrane† is a flexible silicone-nylon membrane bonded to collagenous peptides of porcine skin. Calcium alginate is another treatment for donor sites. As with biologic dressings, it is important that the wound be free of debris before the dressing is applied. Body temperature elevation or evidence of purulence, erythema, or cellulitis around the wound edges

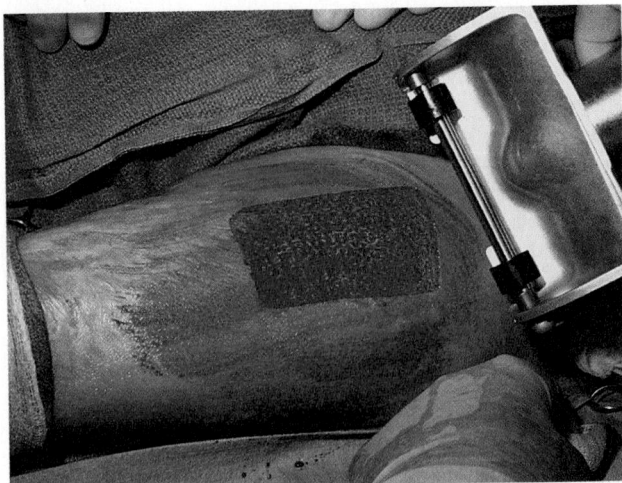

FIG. 30-20 ■ Removal of split-thickness skin graft with a dermatome.

may indicate that the wound has become infected beneath the dressing. If this occurs, prompt discontinuance of the synthetic dressing is indicated. All synthetic dressings are reputed to hasten wound healing and reduce discomfort.

Permanent skin coverings. Permanent coverage of deep partial-thickness and full-thickness burns is usually accomplished with a split-thickness skin graft. This graft consists of the epidermis and a portion of the dermis removed from an intact area of skin by a special instrument, the *dermatome* (Fig. 30-20). *The removal of skin with a dermatome is a very painful procedure that should always be done in an atraumatic fashion with the help of conscious sedation.*

With extensive burns it is often difficult to find enough viable skin to cover the wounds; therefore, available donor sites and special techniques are used. Split-thickness skin grafts may be sheet graft or mesh graft.

Sheet Graft. A sheet of skin, removed from the donor site, is placed intact over the recipient site and sutured in place; used in areas where cosmetic results are most visible (Fig. 30-21).

Mesh Graft. A sheet of skin is removed from the donor site and passed through a mesher, which produces tiny slits in the skin that allow the skin to cover 1.5 to 9 times the area of the sheet graft; results in a less desirable cosmetic and functional outcome (Fig. 30-22).

The donor site is dressed with synthetic wound coverings or fine-mesh gauze until the dressing separates at 10 to 14 days when the wound is healed. Dressings are not changed on donor sites to avoid damage to newly healed, delicate epithelium. Healed donor sites are available for reharvesting in patients with extensive burns and limited undamaged skin, but the quality of skin is decreased when multiple grafts are taken.

Artificial Skin. The development of Integra,* a product that allows the dermis to regenerate, has produced significant improvement in burn wound healing and decreased scar formation. It is applied to partial-thickness and full-

*Brennen Medical, Inc., 1290 Hammond Road, St. Paul, MN 55110; (651) 429-7413 or (800)-943-4522; website: www.brennenmedical.com.
†Bertek Pharmaceuticals, Inc., PO Box 14149, Research Triangle Park, NC 27709-4149; (888) 823-7835; website: www.bertek.com.

*Integra Life Sciences Corporation, 311 Enterprise Drive, Plainsboro, NJ 08536; (800) 654-2873; fax: (609) 275-5363; website: www.integra-ls.com.

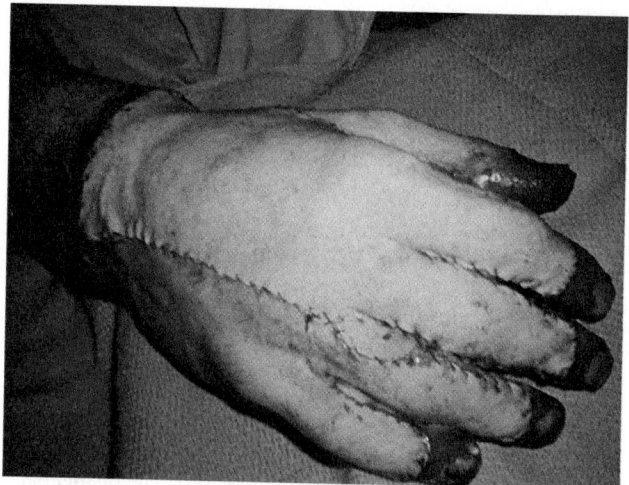

FIG. 30-21 ■ Sheet graft.

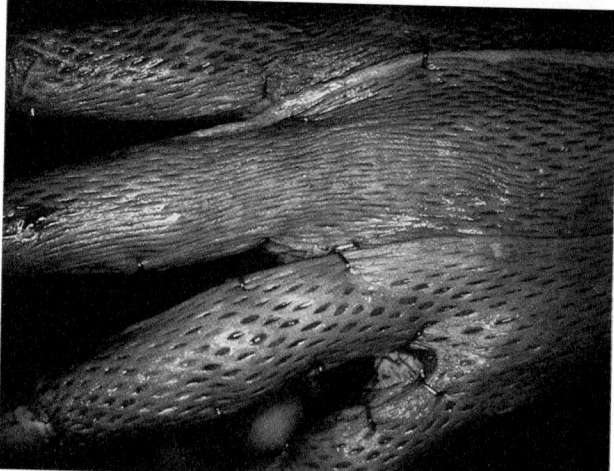

FIG. 30-22 ■ Mesh graft.

thickness burns. The two-layer membrane is made of collagen (a fibrous protein from animal tendons and cartilage) and silicone rubber (i.e., Silastic). The Silastic layer is peeled off after the dermis is formed. The application of artificial skin does not replace the grafting procedure, but it prepares the burn wound to accept an ultrathin autograft. Advantages include faster healing of the burn wound when integrity of the dermis is restored, faster healing of donor sites with the use of ultrathin grafts, and restoration of sweat glands and hair follicles. A disadvantage is its high cost.

Cultured Epithelium. When burns are extensive and donor sites for split-thickness skin grafting are limited, it is possible to culture cells from a full-thickness skin biopsy and produce coherent sheets that can be applied to clean, excised full-thickness wounds. Epithelial cell culture grafts offer the possibility of an unlimited source of autografts in patients with extensive burns. Cultured epithelial autografts are effective in early wound closure. The child's own skin is fractionated and cultured in a porcine media to form a thin epithelial layer that is applied to the burn wound. This technique offers an improved rate of survival in patients with extensive burns and limited donor sites.

Prognosis. Children differ from adults in their responses to thermal injury, and the mortality rates in young children are significantly higher than those in older children and adults. Mortality is greatest for children younger than 48 months of age. Many children who do survive have long-term functional and cosmetic impairments.

Nursing Considerations

Because the care of burned children encompasses a broad range of skills, nursing care has been divided into segments that correspond with the major phases of burn treatment. The *acute phase,* also referred to as the emergent or resuscitative phase, involves the first 24 to 48 hours. The *management phase* extends from the completion of adequate resuscitation through wound coverage. The *rehabilitative phase* begins once the majority of the wounds have healed and rehabilitation has become the predominant focus of the plan of care. This phase continues until all reconstructive

procedures and corrective measures are accomplished (often a period of months or years).

Acute Phase. The primary emphasis during the emergent phase is the treatment of burn shock and the management of pulmonary status. Monitoring vital signs, output, fluid infusion, and respiratory parameters are ongoing activities in the hours immediately after injury. IV infusion is begun immediately and is regulated to maintain a urine output of at least 1 to 2 mL/kg in children weighing less than 30 kg; an output of 30 to 50 mL/hr is expected in children weighing more than 30 kg. Urine output and specific gravity, vital signs, laboratory data, and objective signs of adequate hydration guide the rate of fluid administration.

Children who are hospitalized with burns require constant observation and assessment for complications. Alterations in electrolyte balance produce clinical symptoms of confusion, weakness, cardiac irregularities, and seizures. Changes in respiratory function and gas exchange are reflected clinically by restlessness, irritability, increased work of breathing, and alterations in blood gas values. The loss of protective function of the skin exposes burned children to increased risk of hypothermia. Edema formation and circulatory impairment result in the loss of sensation, and deep throbbing pain.

✸ NURSING ALERT

Evaluate the extremity and check the pulse every hour. If unable to palpate, use Doppler to ascertain loss of circulation and pulse. If the pulse is lost, escharotomy may be necessary to relieve the edema causing pressure on blood vessels, to restore adequate circulation.

Burn units maintain a pictorial record of the wound to record progress and for legal purposes (if child abuse is suspected). The burn wound is treated according to the protocol of the specific burn facility. The burn team monitors infection control procedures and ensures that staff and visitors comply with established protocols to prevent cross-contamination in the burn unit.

Throughout the acute phase of care, the psychosocial needs of the children and their families should not be overlooked. The child is frightened, uncomfortable, and often confused. Children may be isolated from familiar persons and surroundings; the overwhelming physical needs at this time are the primary focus of the staff and parents. In addition to feeling concern for their child, the family experiences guilt, which may be related to the fact that the parents did not or could not protect their child from injury. Consistency in the information presented and in the attitude of the staff creates a sense of familiarity and stability during the acute phase of care. Consistent caregivers can also help to decrease the patient and family's anxiety and provide coordination of care. For example, when many teams of consultants and specialists are involved in the care of the child, appointing one "spokesperson" decreases the confusion and enhances communication regarding the child's care.

Management and Rehabilitative Phases.

After the patient's condition is stabilized, the management phase begins. The multidisciplinary team concentrates on preventing wound infections, closing the wound as quickly as possible, and managing the numerous complications. Although the rehabilitative phase begins when permanent wound closure has been achieved, rehabilitation issues are identified on admission and are included in the plan of care throughout the hospital course.

● Assessment

Wound assessment and comprehensive assessment of the child's general condition and behaviors are of major importance. The nurse must assess signs of complications, infection, and the need for and effectiveness of pain management.

✎ NURSING ALERT

Disorientation in the burned patient is one of the first signs of overwhelming sepsis and may indicate inadequate hydration. Assessment of the sensorium is another important indicator of the adequacy of hydration. A spiking fever and diminished bowel sounds accompanied by paralytic ileus are noted and progressively increase over 48 to 72 hours, after which the temperature falls to subnormal limits. At this time the wound deteriorates, the white blood cell count is depressed, and septic shock becomes manifest.

● Nursing Diagnoses

Nursing diagnoses identified for the child with severe or extensive burns are included in the Nursing Care Plan on pp. 1142-1144. Additional diagnoses may be ascertained for individual children.

● Planning

The goals for the child with a burn injury and the family are as follows:

1 Child will experience reduction of pain.
2 Child will exhibit evidence of wound healing.
3 Child will receive adequate nutrition and will achieve reduction in metabolic losses.
4 Child will not experience complications during acute care.
5 Child will not experience complications during long-term care.
6 Child and family will receive emotional support.

● Implementation

Comfort Management.   The severe pain of the wound and resultant therapies, the anxiety generated by these experiences, sleep deprivation, itching related to wound healing, and the conscious and unconscious interpretations of traumatic events contribute to the psychologic behaviors commonly observed in children with burns. It is always difficult to deal with a child in pain, and inflicting pain on a helpless child is contrary to the empathic nature of nursing. Interventions to promote comfort may include medications (including IV morphine or midazolam and short-term anesthetics such as propofol), relaxation techniques, distraction therapy, behavioral techniques, operant conditioning (e.g., tokens, star chart), and family participation.

Children need age-appropriate explanations before all procedures. When children appear to accept pain with little or no response, psychologic consultation may be needed. Consistency in caregivers is important. If this is not possible, a carefully developed, multidisciplinary plan of care is necessary to provide consistency.

Care of the Burn Wound.   The nurse has a major responsibility for cleansing, debriding, and applying topical medications and dressings to the burn wound. Pain medication should be administered so that the peak effect of the drug coincides with the procedure. Children who have an understanding of the procedure to be performed and some perceived control demonstrate less maladaptive behavior. Children also respond well to participating in decisions (see Guidelines box).

Outer dressings are removed. Any dressings that have adhered to the wound can be more easily removed by applying tepid water or normal saline. Loose or easily detached tissue is débrided during the cleansing process. In dressing the wound, it is important that all areas be clean, that medication be amply applied, and that no two burned surfaces touch each other (e.g., fingers or toes; ears touching the side of the head). If they are touching, the burned surfaces will heal together, causing deformity or dysfunction.

Topical medications may be applied directly to the wound with a tongue blade or gloved hand or impregnated into fine-mesh gauze before application. Dressings are then

---

⎨ GUIDELINES

Reducing the Stress of Burn Care Procedures

Have all materials ready before beginning.
Administer appropriate analgesics and anxiolytics.
Remind the child of the impending procedure to allow sufficient time to prepare.
Allow the child to test and approve the temperature of the water.
Allow the child to select the area of the body on which to begin.
Allow the child to request a short rest period during the procedure.
Allow the child to remove the dressings if desired.
Provide something constructive for the child to do during the procedure (e.g., holding a package of dressings or a roll of gauze).
Inform the child when the procedure is near completion.
Praise the child for cooperation.

applied to assist in exudate absorption, wound débridement, and increased patient comfort. All dressings applied circumferentially should be wrapped in a distal-to-proximal manner. The dressing is applied with sufficient tension to remain in place but not so tightly as to impair circulation or limit motion. Elastic bandages are applied over dressings to prevent epithelial breakdown, decrease edema formation, stimulate circulation, and improve mobility. A stable dressing is especially important when the child is ambulatory.

Standard precautions, including the use of protective garb and barrier techniques, should be followed when caring for patients with thermal injuries. Frequent hand and forearm washing is the single most important element of the infection control program. Strict policies for cleaning the environment and patient care equipment should be implemented to minimize the risk of cross-contamination. All visitors and members of other departments should be oriented to the infection control policies, including the importance of hand and forearm washing and use of protective garb. Visitors should be screened for infection and contagious diseases before patient contact.

Nutrition.   Oral feedings are encouraged unless the child is intubated or paralytic ileus persists. Because children often lack an appetite, the child needs encouragement, help, and patience. Consultation between the caregiver and the dietitian helps to determine food preferences. Children who are old enough to participate should be included in meal planning. In addition, many children prefer an atmosphere more nearly like that provided at home. Therefore, when possible, many children enjoy sitting at a table and interacting with other children at mealtimes. Painful procedures should not be scheduled near mealtimes, because most children will be too physically exhausted and emotionally upset to eat.

Children who require enteral supplementation must be monitored for feeding intolerance and tube malposition. The nurse should also monitor and report any abdominal distention, diarrhea, or electrolyte and metabolic deviations.

Prevention of Complications

Acute Care.   The maintenance of body temperature is important to the child with burns. Core body temperature is supported when energy is conserved with an environmental temperature of 28° to 33° C (82° to 91° F). Large areas of the body should not be exposed simultaneously during dressing changes. Warmed solutions, linens, occlusive dressings, heat shields, a radiant warmer, and warming blankets assist in preventing hypothermia.

The chief danger during acute care is infection—wound infection, generalized sepsis, or bacterial pneumonia. Accurate and ongoing assessments of all parameters that provide clues to the early diagnosis and treatment of infection are essential. Symptoms of sepsis include a change in the level of consciousness, a rising or falling white blood cell count, hypothermia or hyperthermia, a loss of the progression of wound healing, increasing fluid requirements, hypoactive or absent bowel sounds, a rising or falling blood glucose level, tachycardia, tachypnea, and thrombocytopenia.

Children are reluctant to move if movement causes pain, and they are likely to assume a position of comfort. Unfortunately, the most comfortable position often encourages the formation of contractures and loss of function. Ongoing efforts to prevent contractures include maintaining proper body alignment, positioning and splinting involved extremities in extension, active and passive physical therapy, and encouraging spontaneous movement when feasible. Frequent position changes are important to promote adequate bronchopulmonary hygiene and capillary perfusion to common pressure areas. Low–air loss beds are beneficial for the morbidly obese or children with posterior grafts. Special attention should be given to areas at risk for increased pressure, such as the posterior scalp, heels, sacrum, and areas exposed to mechanical irritation from splints and dressings.

Long-Term Care.   The rehabilitative phase of care begins once wound coverage is achieved. Scar formation becomes a major problem as burn wounds heal (Fig. 30-23). Contractile properties of the scar tissue can result in disabling contractures, deformity, and disfigurement.

Uniform pressure applied to the scar decreases the blood supply. When pressure is removed, blood supply to the scar is immediately increased; therefore, periods without pressure should be brief to avoid nourishment of the hypertrophic tissue. Continuous pressure to areas of scarring can be achieved by elastic bandages or commercially available pressure garments. Because these custom-made garments are often worn for months, revisions may be required as the child grows. It is much easier to prevent scarring and contracture of the wound than to resolve an existing problem. Splints and appliances may also be needed until wound maturation is achieved (Fig. 30-24).

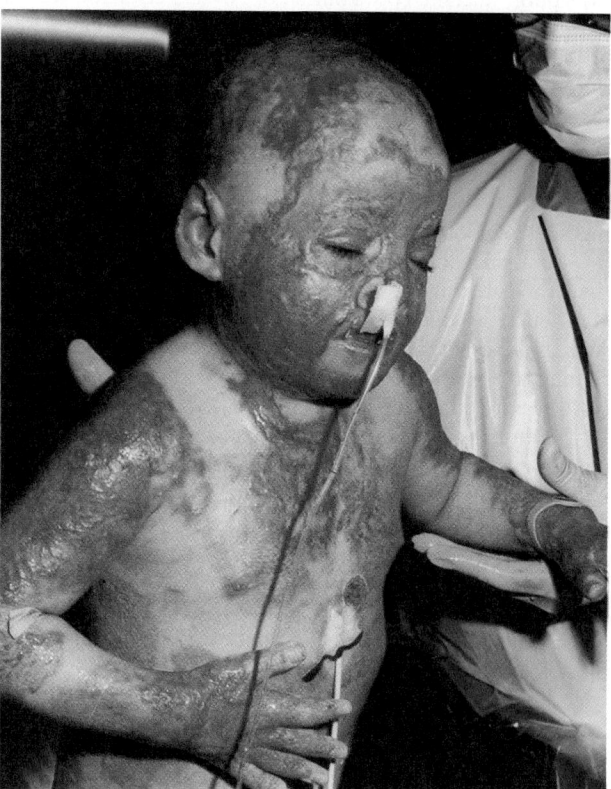

FIG. 30-23 ■ Extensive scars from flame burn. (Courtesy C.R. Boeckman, MD, Regional Burn Center, Akron, Oh.)

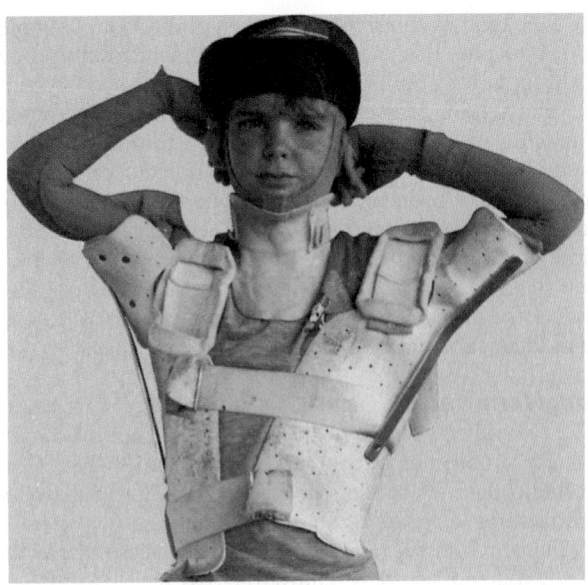

FIG. 30-24 ■ Child in elasticized (Jobst) garment and "airplane" splints.

Scar tissue has certain significant properties, particularly for growing children. Intense itching occurs in healing burn wounds and scar tissue until the scar is no longer active. Itching is usually treated with a combination of H_1 and H_2 antagonists such as cetirizine (Zyrtec) and cimetidine (Tagamet) (Baker and others, 2001), an H_1 antagonist alone, and frequent applications of a moisturizer, such as Vaseline, Cetaphil, Aquaphor, Eucerin, cocoa butter, or Nivea. Petrolatum-based ointments (Vaseline, Aquaphor) seem to spread more easily on friable skin than thick creams do. Massage therapy during the application of moisturizers is also beneficial to stretch scar tissue and aid in contracture prevention. Scar tissue has no sweat glands, and children with extensive scarring may experience difficulty during hot weather. Caregivers should be alerted to this possibility and be prepared to institute alternate methods of cooling when necessary.

Scar tissue does not grow and expand, as does normal tissue, which may create difficulties, especially in functional areas such as on the hands and over joints. Additional surgery is sometimes required to allow independent functioning in daily activities, to improve cosmetic appearance, or to restore anatomic integrity.

The nursing activities in the rehabilitative phase of treatment focus on the child and family's adaptation to the burn injury and their ability to reintegrate into the community. The psychologic pain and sequelae of severe burn injury are as intensive as the physical trauma. The impact of severe burns taxes the coping mechanisms at all ages. Very young children, who suffer acutely from separation anxiety, and adolescents, who are developing an identity, are probably the most affected psychologically. Toddlers cannot understand why the parents they love and who have protected them can leave them in such a frightening and unfamiliar place. Adolescents, in the process of achieving independence from the family, find themselves in a dependent role with a damaged body. Being different from others at a time when conformity with peers is so important is difficult to accept.

Anticipation of the return to school can be overwhelming and frightening. It is essential that health care professionals recognize the importance of preparing teachers and classmates for the child's return. Teachers need to be provided with information to assist the child and family and to promote the child's optimal adjustment. Hospital-sponsored school reentry programs use a variety of methods to provide education and information about the implications of the injury, the garments and appliances, and the need for support and acceptance. Telephone calls, videotapes, information packets, and visits by members of the health care team offer opportunities to help with reintegration into the school environment—a focal point of the child's life.

Psychosocial Support of the Child.　Children should begin early to do as much for themselves as possible and to be active participants in their care. Loss of control and perceived helplessness may result in acting-out behaviors. During illness, children regress to a previous developmental level that allows them to deal with stress. As children begin to participate in their care, they gain confidence and self-esteem. Fears and anxieties diminish with accomplishment and self-confidence. If the child demonstrates nonadherence in the rehabilitative phase, a behavior modification program can be initiated to promote or reward the child's accomplishment in care.

Children need to know that their injury and the treatments are not punishment for real or imagined transgressions and that the nurse understands their fear, anger, and discomfort. They also need body contact. This is often difficult to arrange for the child with massive burns. Stroking areas of unburned skin is comforting. Even older children enjoy sitting on the parent's lap and being cuddled and hugged. This can be a reward or a comfort in times of stress, but most of all it should be kept in mind that it is a natural part of childhood.

Psychosocial Support of the Family.　Recognizing and respecting each family's strengths, differences, and methods of coping allows the nurse to respond to their unique needs by implementing a family-centered approach to care. In the acute phase, all attention is focused on the child, and the parents feel powerless and ineffectual. Most parents feel overwhelming guilt, whether or not the guilt is justified. They feel responsible for the injury. These feelings may impede the child's rehabilitation. Parents may indulge the child and allow nonadherent behaviors that affect physical and emotional recovery. Parents need to be informed of the child's progress and helped to cope with their feelings while providing support to their child. The nurse can help them understand that it is not selfish to look after themselves and their own needs to meet the needs of their child. It is important to recognize the parents' need to grieve the change in the normal appearance of their child as a part of the grieving process. Definitive professional help may be needed for parents whose response to the injury is severe or whose response to stress is manifested in destructive behavior.

The parents are members of the multidisciplinary team and participate in the development of the plan of care. It is important to facilitate their input; to consider all aspects of the physical, emotional, social, and cultural factors affecting the child and family; and to establish a realistic home therapy program. The family's willingness to assume responsibility for care and their ability to implement the therapeutic regimen are assessed. Home, school, and other environmental factors are explored; financial concerns and available community resources are discussed; and a specific plan of care for the child, with an anticipated follow-up program, is developed.

Prevention of Burn Injury.   The best intervention is to prevent burns from occurring. Hot liquids in the kitchen and bathroom most commonly injure infants and toddlers. Hot liquids should be kept out of reach; tablecloths and dangling appliance cords are often pulled by toddlers, who spill hot grease and liquids on themselves. Electrical cords and outlets represent a potential risk to small children, who may chew on accessible cords and insert objects into outlets.

The Consumer Product Safety Commission recommends a reduction of water heater thermostats to a maximum of 48.9° C (120° F). The "dial-down" recommendation has been suggested by utility companies, burn treatment centers, medical personnel, and others interested in public safety. However, many water heaters continue to remain set at levels well above the safe level. Small children are especially at risk for scald injuries from hot tap water because of their decreased reaction time and agility, their curiosity, and the thermal sensitivity of their skin. Caregivers should never leave a child unattended in a bath and without adult supervision. Water should always be tested before a child is placed in the tub or shower.

The increased use of microwave ovens has resulted in burn injuries from the extremely hot internal temperatures generated in heated items. Baby formula, jelly-filled pastries, and hot liquids and dishes may result in cutaneous scalds or the ingestion of overheated liquids. Parents should use caution when removing items from the microwave oven and should always test the food before giving it to children.

As children mature, risk-taking behaviors increase. Matches and lighters are very dangerous in the hands of the young. Adults must remember to keep potentially hazardous items out of the reach of children; a lighter, like a match, is a tool for adult use.

Education related to fire safety and survival should begin with the very young. "Stop, drop, and roll" to extinguish a fire can be practiced. The fire escape route, including a safe meeting place away from the home in case of fire, also should be practiced.

Community activities are also very helpful in supporting burn survivors and preventing burns. The **Aluminum Cans for Burned Children (ACBC)** is an exemplary effort based in the Clifford R. Boeckman, MD, Regional Burn Center, Akron, Ohio.* Activities funded by ACBC include Burn Survivors Support Group, Burn Camp, and meetings of Juvenile Firestoppers (for children with fire-setting behavior). Adult weekend retreats and school and family education sessions are a part of this program. Burn center staff and fire department staff provide the personnel to present programs.

Additional information on burn care and prevention can be obtained from the **American Burn Association*** and the **National Safety Council.**† The **Alisa Ann Ruch Burn Foundation**‡ provides assistance to burn victims and burn centers. The **Shriners Burn Institutes** are staffed to treat pediatric patients following acute burn injuries and those requiring rehabilitative and reconstructive services as a result of scarring and functional impairment. Information can be obtained from local Shrine Temples and Shrine Clubs, from Shriners Hospitals, or by contacting the **International Shrine Headquarters.**§ The Alisa Ann Ruch Foundation and Shriners Hospitals for Crippled Children support research to improve burn care and treatment and promote public education in burn prevention.

Evaluation

The effectiveness of nursing interventions is determined by continual reassessment and evaluation of care based on the following observational guidelines:

1 Observe child's behavior during all aspects of care; listen to verbal cues; use a pain assessment record to evaluate the effectiveness of analgesia.
2 Observe the burn wound and child's general condition.
3 Observe child's eating behavior and the amount of food consumed; weigh daily or as indicated.
4 Inspect the burn wound for signs of infection; measure vital signs; observe for evidence of respiratory complications, gastric bleeding, altered hemoglobin level, and neurologic signs.
5 Observe for evidence of healing, scar formation, and contracture; assess effectiveness of physical therapy and appliances (splints, pressure garments).
6 Observe child's and family's behaviors; interview child and family regarding their feelings and concerns.

The *expected outcomes* are described in the Nursing Care Plan on pp. 1142-1144.

SUNBURN

Sunburn is a very common skin injury caused by overexposure to ultraviolet (UV) light waves. The sun emits a continuous spectrum of visible and nonvisible light rays that range in length from very short to very long. The shorter, higher-frequency waves are more damaging than longer wavelengths, but much of the light is filtered out as it travels through the atmosphere. Of the light that does filter through, *ultraviolet A (UVA) waves* are the longest and cause only minimum burning, but play a significant role in photosensitive and photoallergic reactions. They are also responsible for premature aging of the skin and potentiate the effects of *ultraviolet B (UVB)* waves. UVB waves are shorter and are responsible for

---

*Children's Hospital Medical Center of Akron, 1 Perkins Square, Akron, OH 44308-1062; (330) 543-8224; fax: (330) 379-8152; website: www.akronchildrens.org.

*625 North Michigan Avenue, Suite 1530, Chicago, IL 60611; (312) 642-9260 or (800) 548-2876; fax: (312) 642-9130; e-mail: aba@ameriburn.org.
†1121 Spring Lake Drive, Itasca, IL 60143-3201; (800) 621-7615; website: www.nsc.org.
‡20944 Sherman Way, Suite 115, Canoga Park, CA 91303; (818) 883-7700; website: www.aarbf.org.
§2900 Rocky Point Drive, Tampa, FL 33607; (800) 237-5055 (in Florida: [800] 282-9161); International Shrine Headquarters website: www.shrinershq.org; Shriners Burn Institutes website: www.shrinershq.org/Hospitals/BurnInst/.

Text continued on p. 1145.

NURSING DIAGNOSIS ■ Impaired skin integrity related to thermal injury

PATIENT GOAL 1: Will exhibit evidence of wound healing

NURSING INTERVENTIONS/*RATIONALES*

Shave hair to a 2-inch margin from the wound and area immediately surrounding the burn *to remove a reservoir for infection*

Thoroughly cleanse the wound and surrounding skin with normal saline *to decrease the risk of infection;* débride devitalized tissue *to promote healing*

Keep child from scratching and picking at the wound
  Keep fingernails clean and clipped short
  Apply socks to hands if necessary *to prevent scratching*
  Administer antipruritic medications
  Provide distraction appropriate to child's age
  Older child: explain reasons *to encourage cooperation*
  Young child: supervise activity as needed

Maintain care in handling the wound *to avoid damaging epithelializing and granulating tissues*

Offer high-calorie, high-protein meals and snacks *to meet augmented protein and calorie requirements caused by increased metabolism and catabolism*

Prevent infection, which can delay healing and convert partial-thickness wounds to full-thickness wounds by maintaining sterile technique with dressing changes

Administer supplementary vitamins and minerals—vitamins A, B, C; iron; and zinc—*to facilitate wound healing and epithelialization*

Pad burned ears *to prevent tissue necrosis caused by minimal blood flow to cartilage*

Monitor for signs/symptoms of wound infection *to ensure prompt recognition and treatment*

Wrap fingers and toes separately *to avoid tissue adherence from prolonged contact*

EXPECTED OUTCOME

Wounds heal without evidence of damage or inflammation

PATIENT GOAL 2: Will maintain integrity of skin graft

NURSING INTERVENTIONS/*RATIONALES*

Position for minimal mechanical disturbance of graft site

Place patient on low–air loss bed; turn every 2 hours

Restrain, if necessary, *to prevent graft from being dislodged*

Maintain splints or dressings *if needed for protection of the graft*

Observe grafts for evidence of hematoma/fluid accumulation; aspirate or express fluids *to ensure contact of the graft with the base*

EXPECTED OUTCOME

Skin graft remains intact

NURSING DIAGNOSIS ■ Risk for altered tissue perfusion related to circumferential burns

PATIENT GOAL 1: Will retain optimal circulation to distal regions of the affected extremity

NURSING INTERVENTIONS/*RATIONALES*

Monitor closely for signs/symptoms of circulation compression related to edema *to ensure adequate circulation perfusion* (assess numbness, tingling, color or temperature changes every 1 to 2 hours × 72 hours)

Assess diminished Doppler pulses and prolonged capillary refill *to indicate diminished distal perfusion* (Doppler checks every 1 to 2 hours × 72 hours)

Turn every 2 hours

Position extremity to elevate above the level of the heart *to prevent decreased circulation to the extremity*

Avoid restrictive dressings over the injured extremity *to prevent decreased circulation to the extremity*

EXPECTED OUTCOME

Adequate distal perfusion to the affected extremity is maintained

NURSING DIAGNOSIS ■ Pain related to skin trauma, therapies

PATIENT GOAL 1: Will experience reduction of pain to a level acceptable to child

NURSING INTERVENTIONS/*RATIONALES*

Assess need for medication (see Pain Assessment, Chapter 21)

Recognize that burn pain is often overwhelming, engulfing, and irrepressible

Position in extension *to minimize pain resulting from exercising to regain extension*

Implement passive and active exercising *to minimize contracture formation*

Reduce irritation *to prevent increased pain*

Administer medication for itching after therapy and treatments

Touch/stroke unburned areas *to provide physical contact and comfort*

Employ appropriate nonpharmacologic pain reduction techniques (see Pain Management, Chapter 21)

Promote control and predictability during painful procedures (see Guidelines Box, p. 1138)

Anticipate need for pain medication and administer before onset of severe pain and at regular intervals *to prevent recurrence* (see Pain Management, Chapter 21)

EXPECTED OUTCOME

Child exhibits reduction of pain to level acceptable to child

NURSING DIAGNOSIS ■ Risk for infection related to denuded skin, presence of pathogenic organisms, altered immune response

PATIENT GOAL 1: Will exhibit no evidence of wound infection

NURSING INTERVENTIONS/*RATIONALES*

Implement and maintain infection control precautions

Maintain careful handwashing by members of staff and visitors *to minimize exposure to infectious agents*

Wear clean or sterile gown, cap, mask, and gloves when caring for open wound areas *to minimize exposure to infectious agents*

Débride eschar, crust, and blisters *to eliminate the reservoir for organisms*

Avoid patient contact with persons who have upper respiratory or skin infection

Cover the wound or patient according to unit protocol *to provide a barrier to organisms*

Administer good oral hygiene

*Apply prescribed topical antimicrobial preparation and dressings to the wound *to control bacterial proliferation*

Obtain baseline and serial wound cultures *to ascertain any increase or changes in wound flora*

Monitor closely for signs of sepsis and infection (disorientation, tachypnea, temperature above 39.5° C [103° F], hypothermia, distention of the abdomen or intestinal ileus, change in wound appearance)

EXPECTED OUTCOMES

Possible sources of infection are eliminated

Wound displays minimal or no evidence of infection

*Dependent nursing action.

NURSING DIAGNOSIS ■ **Risk for ineffective thermoregulation related to heat loss and disruption of skin's defense mechanism to maintain body temperature**

PATIENT GOAL 1: Will maintain normal thermal regulation as evidenced by normal body temperatures ranging from 37° to 38.1° C (98.6° to 100.5° F)

NURSING INTERVENTIONS/RATIONALES

Assess patient skin for coolness, color changes, and capillary refill (acrocyanosis, nail bed color, and mottling) *to identify vascular accommodation of heat loss*

Monitor vital signs, especially temperature, *to identify significant trends*

Observe for chilling and shivering *to identify signs of heat loss*

Avoid exposure to cold stress procedures *to maintain body temperature* (limit time in tub to 20 minutes, bundling child, covering the head of a child younger than 6 months of age, using artificial heat)

EXPECTED OUTCOME

Child's temperature remains within normal limits for age

NURSING DIAGNOSIS ■ **Risk for fluid volume deficit related to normal fluid loss from tissues secondary to burn insult**

PATIENT GOAL 1: Will maintain adequate fluid hydration status during the acute postburn period

NURSING INTERVENTIONS/RATIONALES

*Administer crystalloid or colloid fluid per protocol, monitoring effect and maintaining intravenous (IV) line *to replace fluid loss related to burn injury*

Assess fluid replacement status: inadequate (skin turgor, increased pulse, decreased urine output, decreased circulation status, or change in mental status [restlessness, disorientation]) or excessive (pulmonary congestion or pulmonary edema) *to recognize appropriate fluid balance*

Monitor daily weights *to evaluate status of fluid retention or diuresis*

Observe and monitor hemodynamic parameters for changes in stability related to hypovolemia or overload *because change in blood pressure is a late sign*

Monitor laboratory results (hemoglobin, hematocrit, glucose, serum potassium, serum sodium, serum protein, phosphorus, and magnesium) *to identify fluid and electrolyte imbalance*

Administer potassium-rich or potassium-restricted fluids or foods if child is hypokalemic or hyperkalemic, respectively, *to supplement IV therapy*

EXPECTED OUTCOME

Adequate fluid resuscitation is maintained as evidenced by adequate tissue perfusion and maintenance of urine output

NURSING DIAGNOSIS ■ **Altered nutrition: less than body requirements related to increased catabolism and metabolism, loss of appetite**

PATIENT GOAL 1: Will receive optimal nourishment

NURSING INTERVENTIONS/RATIONALES

Encourage oral feeding (see Feeding the Sick Child, Chapter 22)

Provide high-calorie, high-protein meals and snacks *to avoid protein breakdown and meet augmented calorie requirements*

Provide foods child likes *to stimulate appetite*

Provide attractive meals and surroundings *to encourage eating*

Provide companionship at meals *to create a more homelike environment*

Use "contract" with older children *to encourage adherence*

Administer supplemental enteral feedings as prescribed *to meet calculated needs*

Obtain weekly weight *to monitor nutritional status*

Record accurate intake and output *to evaluate sufficiency of intake*

Monitor for diarrhea/constipation and institute prompt treatment *to avoid feeding intolerance*

EXPECTED OUTCOME

Child consumes a sufficient amount of nutrients (specify) and maintains preburn weight

NURSING DIAGNOSIS ■ **Risk for constipation and risk for diarrhea related to opioid administration, inadequate intake of nutrients, need for tube feedings**

PATIENT GOAL 1: Will have routine bowel patterns

NURSING INTERVENTIONS/RATIONALES

Monitor for diarrhea/constipation and institute prompt treatment

Record amount and consistency of stool daily

Administer antidiarrheal agents

Administer bulk laxative, stool softener, or cathartic *to avoid feeding intolerance*

Assess hydration status to correlate dehydration with development of constipation

Monitor electrolyte panel, replacing lost electrolytes via IV or tube feeding

Increase activity and ambulation *to increase peristalsis and motility*

EXPECTED OUTCOME

Normal bowel elimination pattern returns as evidenced by soft, formed stools every 1 to 2 days

NURSING DIAGNOSIS ■ **Impaired physical mobility (specify level) related to pain, impaired joint movement, scar formation**

PATIENT GOAL 1: Will achieve optimal physical functioning

NURSING INTERVENTIONS/RATIONALES

Carry out range-of-motion exercises *to maintain optimal joint and muscle function*

Encourage mobility if child is able to move extremities

Ambulate as soon as feasible

Splint involved joints in extension at night and during rest periods *to minimize contracture formation*

Encourage and promote self-help activities *to increase mobility*

Administer analgesia before painful activity (e.g., physical therapy) *so that child is more likely to cooperate and be mobile*

Encourage participation in activities of daily living and play activities *to incorporate exercise into enjoyable events*

EXPECTED OUTCOME

Child achieves functioning to level of ability

*Dependent nursing action.

Continued

PATIENT GOAL 2: Will exhibit minimal scarring

NURSING INTERVENTIONS/RATIONALES

Position in a functional attitude *for minimal deformity and optimal functioning*

Apply splints as ordered and designed *to minimize contracture*

Wrap healing tissue with elastic bandage or dress in elastic garments as ordered *to help reduce scar hypertrophy by compressing collagen and decreasing vascularity*

Provide moist wound healing

Carry out physical therapy *to minimize deformity related to scar contracture formation*

Provide treatment for pruritus *to minimize scratching and irritation of newly healed tissue*

EXPECTED OUTCOME

Wound heals with minimal scar formation; joints remain flexible and functional

---

NURSING DIAGNOSIS ■ **Disturbed body image related to perception of appearance and mobility**

PATIENT GOAL 1: Will receive adequate emotional support

NURSING INTERVENTIONS/*RATIONALES*

Convey positive attitude toward child *to demonstrate acceptance and so that child expects to get better*

Encourage parents to participate in care *to prevent the stress of separation*

Encourage as much independence as condition allows *to give child a sense of control*

Arrange for continued schooling *to encourage optimal development and sense of normalcy*

Promote peer contact where possible *to decrease isolation*

Be honest with child and family *to create a trusting nurse-client relationship*

Encourage activities appropriate to age and capabilities *to promote normalcy and increase self-esteem*

Prepare peers for child's appearance *to encourage acceptance and support*

Provide opportunities for child and family to discuss the impact of the change in appearance and lifestyle *to increase coping*

Support behaviors suggesting adaptation *to build on strengths*

EXPECTED OUTCOME

Child accepts efforts of family and caregivers

Child engages in activities with others according to age and capabilities

PATIENT GOAL 2: Will demonstrate improved body image

NURSING INTERVENTIONS/*RATIONALES*

Explore feelings concerning physical appearance *to facilitate coping with body-image changes*

Discuss feelings about returning to home, family, school, and friends *to build coping mechanisms*

Provide reinforcement of positive aspects of appearance and capabilities *to recognize and build on strengths*

Point out evidence of healing *to encourage a sense of hope*

Discuss aids that camouflage disfigurement *to facilitate coping*
Wigs
Clothing
Makeup

Provide recreational and diversional activities *to promote a sense of normalcy*

Promote constructive thinking in child *to encourage positive coping*

Help child devise a plan to address and cope with reactions of others *to increase the sense of control*

EXPECTED OUTCOME

Child discusses feelings and concerns regarding appearance and the perceived reactions of others

Child verbalizes positive suggestions for adjusting to appearance and community/peer response

PATIENT GOAL 3: Will engage in self-care activities

NURSING INTERVENTIONS/*RATIONALES*

Assist with self-care activities as needed

Encourage self-care according to capabilities

Begin to discuss "hospital discharge" early in hospitalization *so that child expects to get better*

Help child develop independence and self-help capabilities *to increase self-esteem*

EXPECTED OUTCOME

Child verbalizes and otherwise demonstrates interest in going home

Child engages in self-help activities

NURSING DIAGNOSIS ■ **Interrupted family processes related to situational crisis (child with a serious injury)**

PATIENT GOAL 1: Will be prepared for discharge and home care

NURSING INTERVENTIONS/*RATIONALES*

Teach wound care to caregiver *to achieve proficiency and increase confidence*

Discuss diet, rest, and activity *to assist in planning for a home care regimen*

Explore attitudes toward child's reentry into the family *to facilitate coping and identify a possible need for intervention*

Explore family's concept regarding child's capabilities and the possible restrictions and freedom they will allow *to assist them in planning realistically for an altered lifestyle*

Help family set realistic goals for themselves, child, and other family members *to clarify and validate the plan of home care*

Help family acquire needed equipment and supplies *to reduce anxiety*

EXPECTED OUTCOME

Family demonstrates an understanding of child's needs and the impact child's condition will have on them

Family sets realistic goals for themselves, child, and others

PATIENT FAMILY/GOAL 2: Will participate in follow-up care

NURSING INTERVENTIONS/*RATIONALES*

Coordinate team management of child and family for ongoing care *to provide continuity*

Arrange for return visits

Assess needs of the family *to determine appropriate plan of care*

Arrange for referral agencies based on needs assessment

Collaborate with school nurse *to help with child's reintegration into school and the world of peers*

Visit the school, if possible, to prepare teacher and peers *to encourage acceptance of child*

EXPECTED OUTCOME

Family maintains contact with health providers

Child attends school regularly and interacts with age-mates

See also:
Nursing Care Plan: The Child in the Hospital, Chapter 21
Nursing Care Plan: The Family of the Ill or Hospitalized Child, Chapter 21
Nursing Care Plan: The Child Who Is Terminally Ill or Dying, Chapter 18

tanning, burning, and most of the harmful effects attributed to sunlight, especially skin cancer.

Numerous factors influence the amount of UVB exposure. Maximum exposure occurs at midday (10 AM to 3 PM), when the distance from the sun to a given spot on the earth is shortest. There is more exposure at higher altitudes and near the equator, and less when the sky is hazy (although the amount of UV radiation that does penetrate is easily underestimated). Window glass effectively screens out UVB but not UVA rays. Fresh snow, water, and sand reflect UV rays, especially when the sun is directly overhead.

Sunburn is usually an epidermal burn, although severe sunburn can be a partial-thickness burn with blister formation. Treatment of sunburn involves stopping the burning process, decreasing the inflammatory response, and rehydrating the skin. Local application of cool tap water soaks, or immersion in a tepid-water bath (temperature slightly below 36.7° C [98° F]) for 20 minutes or until the skin is cool limits tissue destruction and relieves the discomfort. After the cool applications, a bland oil-in-water moisturizing lotion can be applied. Partial-thickness burns are treated the same as those from any heat source (see earlier discussion on burns).

Nursing Considerations

Protection from sunburn is the major goal of management, and the harmful effects of the sun on the delicate skin of infants and children are currently receiving increased attention. To protect skin exposed to the sun for extended periods, skin should be covered with clothing, and FDA-approved sun protection agents should be applied.

Two types of products are available for sun protection: *topical sunscreens,* which partially absorb UV light, and *sun blockers,* which block out UV rays by reflecting sunlight. The most frequently recommended sun blockers are zinc oxide and titanium dioxide ointments. Sunscreens are products containing an *SPF* based on evaluation of effectiveness against UV rays. The SPF is a number, such as 15, which indicates that if individuals normally burn in 10 minutes without a sunscreen, use of a sunscreen with SPF 15 allows them to remain in the sun 15 times 10, or 150 minutes (2½ hours) before acquiring the same degree of burns. The most effective sunscreens against UVB are *p-aminobenzoic acid (PABA)* and *PABA-esters.*

Sunscreens are applied evenly to all exposed areas, with special attention to skinfolds and areas that might become exposed as clothing shifts. Parents are directed to read labels of sunscreen products carefully for the SPF and follow the manufacturer's directions for application.

NURSING ALERT

Sunscreens are not recommended for infants younger than 6 months of age. However, infants younger than 6 months of age may have sunscreen applied over small areas of skin such as the back of hands that may not be adequately covered by clothing when they are in the sun (American Academy of Pediatrics, 1999). Infants should be kept out of the sun or physically shaded from it. Fabric with a tight weave, such as cotton, offers good protection.

Individuals who work in the community, such as teachers, day care workers, coaches, and youth-group leaders,

and relatives should all be made aware of sun safety for children. Sunscreens must be applied *liberally.*

COLD INJURY

Cold injuries are most commonly seen in very cold regions. The nature of the heat-regulating mechanisms of the body are such that the inner portion of the body, or core, produces heat and the periphery, or outer area, conserves or dissipates heat. When the body attempts to conserve heat, the outer tissues are subjected to low temperatures, and local trauma may result.

Chilblain, redness and swelling of the skin, occurs when extremities, usually the hands, are exposed intermittently to temperatures of −1.1° to 15.5° C (30° to 60° F). The response may vary but is characterized by intense vasodilation that increases the temperature of involved tissues above that of unaffected tissue and produces edematous, reddish blue patches that itch and burn. As warming takes place, the sensations become more intense, but ordinarily they subside in a few days.

Frostbite is the term used to describe tissue damage caused when excessive heat loss to local tissues allows ice crystals to form in tissues. The frostbitten part appears white or blanched, feels solid, and is without sensation. Rapid rewarming is associated with less tissue necrosis than slow thawing. It restores blood flow and shortens the period of cellular damage. Rewarming produces a flush (sometimes deep purple) and a return of sensation, which is extremely painful. Large blisters may appear in 24 to 48 hours after rewarming and begin to reabsorb within 5 to 10 days, followed by the formation of a hard black eschar. Superficial injury often heals without incident. Rewarming is accomplished by immersing the part in well-agitated water at 37.8° to 42.2° C (100° to 108° F). Discomfort is managed with analgesics and sedatives. Care of blistered skin is similar to that described for burns. It is seldom possible to estimate the extent of tissue loss until new skin layers are revealed after the eschar layer separates.

KEY POINTS

- A variety of factors can produce lesions of the skin.
- It is important for nurses to be able to describe skin lesions accurately.
- The process of wound healing consists of hemostasis, inflammation, proliferation, and remodeling.
- A moist environment promotes wound healing.
- Bacterial, viral, and fungal infections are common in childhood.
- Some skin diseases are transmitted by arthropod vectors, especially ticks.
- The most common skin infestations of childhood—scabies and pediculosis capitis—affect children of any age and from any social class.
- Contact dermatitis may involve a primary irritant or a sensitizing agent.
- Adverse reactions to drugs are manifested more often in the skin than in any other body organ.
- The most common skin disorders of infancy are diaper dermatitis, seborrheic dermatitis, and atopic dermatitis.

- Acne, a disorder affecting many adolescents, is related to excessive sebum production, the formation of comedones, and the overgrowth of the *Propionibacterium acnes* organism.

- Medication and gentle facial cleansing are the treatments of choice for acne.

- Burns are caused by thermal, chemical, electric, or radioactive agents.

- Burns are assessed on the extent, depth, and severity of the wound.

- Essentials of emergency care of burn injury include stopping the burning process, covering the burn, transporting the injured child to medical aid, and providing reassurance to the child and family.

- Management of minor burns consists of facilitating wound healing, relieving discomfort, and preventing complications.

- Management of major burns consists of facilitating wound healing, relieving discomfort, replacing destroyed skin, preventing or treating complications, and providing rehabilitation.

- Sunscreen is recommended for use when the skin is exposed to the damaging effects of the sun's rays.

- Thermal injuries to the skin can result from exposure to extreme cold.

References

American Academy of Pediatrics, Committee on Environmental Health: Ultraviolet light: a hazard to children, *Pediatrics* 104(2):328-333, 1999.

American Academy of Pediatrics, Committee on Infectious Diseases (Pickering L, editor): *2003 Red book: report of the Committee on Infectious Diseases,* ed 26, Elk Grove Village, Il, 2003, The Academy.

Annequin D and others: Fixed 50% nitrous oxide oxygen mixture for painful procedures: a French survey, *Pediatrics* 105(4):e47, 2000, available at www.pediatrics.org/cgi/content/full/105/4/e47.

Baker RAU and others: Burn wound itch control using H_1 and H_2 antagonists, *J Burn Care Rehabil* 22(4):263-268, 2001.

Bernardo LM and others: Dog bites in children treated in a pediatric emergency department, *J Spec Pediatr Nurs* 5(2):87-95, 2000.

Burkhart CN, Specht K, Nechers D: Synergistic activity of benzoyl peroxide and erythromycin, *Skin Pharmacol Appl Skin Physiol* 13(5): 292-296, 2000.

Centers for Disease Control and Prevention: Cat-scratch disease in children–Texas, September 2000-August 2001, *MMWR* 51(10): 212-214, 2002.

Food and Drug Administration: FDA issues health advisory regarding labeling changes for lindane products, *HealthInfo Tx Rep* April 2003, available at www.fda.gov/bbs/topics/ANSWERS/2003/ANS01205.html.

Frankowski BL, Weiner LB: Head lice, *Pediatrics* 110(3):638-643, 2002.

Hansbrough JF: Enteral nutritional support in burn patients, *Gastrointest Endosc Clin North Am* 8(3):645-647, 1998.

Herndon DN and others: *Total burn care,* ed 2, London, 2002, WB Saunders.

Jacobs DG, Deutsch NL, Brewer M: Suicide, depression, and isotretinoin: is there a causal link? *J Am Acad Dermatol* 45(5):S168-175, 2001.

Krasner DL, Rodeheaver GT, Sibbald RG: *Chronic wound care: a clinical source book for healthcare professionals,* ed 3, Wayne, Pa, 2001, HMP Communications.

Kronemyer B: Scratching the surface of atopic and contact dermatitis, *Infect Dis Child* 16(3):40, 2003.

Laude TA: Acne in childhood and adolescence: update on treatment choices, *Consultant* 3:457-465, 2000.

Leyden JJ: Therapy for acne vulgaris, *N Engl J Med* 336:1156-1162, 1997.

Mancini AJ: Acne vulgaris: a treatment update, *Contemp Pediatr* 17(12):122-133, 2000.

Offidani A and others: Treatment of scabies with ivermectin, *Eur J Dermatol* 9(2):100-101, 1999.

Osmond MH, Klassen TP, Quinn JV: Economic comparison of a tissue adhesive and suturing in the repair of pediatric facial lacerations, *J Pediatr* 126(6):892-895, 1995.

Russell JJ: Topical therapy for acne, *Am Fam Physician* 61(2):357-366, 2000.

Smith GA and others: Comparison of topical anesthetics without cocaine to tetracaine-adrenaline-cocaine and lidocaine infiltration during repair of lacerations: bupivacaine-norepinephrine is an effective new topical anesthetic agent, *Pediatrics* 97(3):301-307, 1996.

Wade CF: Keeping Lyme disease at bay, an integrated approach to prevention, *Am J Nurs* 100(7):26-31, 2000.

Yetman RJ, Parks D: Diagnosis and management of atopic dermatitis, *J Pediatr Health Care* 16(3):143-145, 2002.

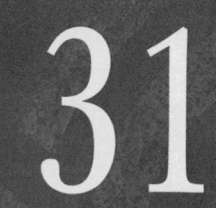

The Child With Musculoskeletal or Articular Dysfunction

DAVID WILSON

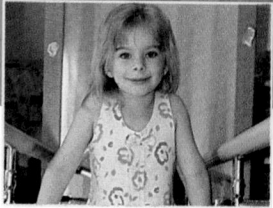

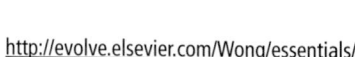

Remember to check out your companion CD-ROM

http://evolve.elsevier.com/Wong/essentials/

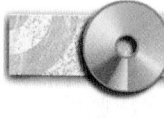
RELATED TOPICS and ADDITIONAL RESOURCES

 IN TEXT

Childhood Morbidity, *Ch. 1*
Compliance, *Ch. 22*
Family-Centered Care of the Child During
  Illness and Hospitalization, *Ch. 21*
Injury Prevention: Infant, *Ch. 10;* Toddler,
  Ch. 12; Preschooler, *Ch. 13;* School-Age
  Child, *Ch. 15;* Adolescent, *Ch. 16*
Pain Assessment; Pain Management, *Ch. 21*
Physical Examination: Back and
  Extremities, *Ch. 7*
Preparation for Procedures, *Ch. 22*
Surgical Procedures, *Ch. 22*

 CD COMPANION

Critical Thinking Exercise—Osteogenic
  Sarcoma
Case Studies—Fractures; Osteomyelitis;
  Developmental Dysplasia of the Hip
Guidelines—Assessing Trauma;
  Assessment of Traction; Traction Care
Clinical Manifestations—Developmental
  Dysplasia of the Hip; Systemic Lupus
  Erythematosus
Nursing Care Plans
NCLEX-Style Review Questions

evolve WEBSITE

WebLinks
NCLEX-Style Review Questions

 WONG'S CLINICAL MANUAL
OF PEDIATRIC NURSING, 6/E

Community and Home Care
  Instructions—Giving Nasogastric
  Tube Feedings; Gastrostomy Tube
  Feedings; Care of Child in a Cast;
  Caring for an Intermittent Infusion
  Device
Nursing Care Plans—The Child With
  Cancer; The Child With a Bone Tumor

LEARNING OBJECTIVES
On completion of this chapter the reader will be able to:

- Outline a plan for the care of a child immobilized with an injury or a degenerative disease.
- Develop a teaching plan for the parents of a child in a cast.
- Explain the functions of the various types of traction.
- Devise a nursing plan of care for the child in traction.

- Differentiate among the various congenital skeletal defects.
- Design a teaching plan for the parents of a child with a congenital skeletal deformity.
- Describe the therapies and nursing care of a child with scoliosis.
- Outline a plan of care for a child with osteomyelitis.

- Differentiate between osteosarcoma and Ewing sarcoma.
- Describe the nursing care of a child with juvenile rheumatoid arthritis.
- Demonstrate an understanding of the management of a child with systemic lupus erythematosus.

THE IMMOBILIZED CHILD

IMMOBILIZATION

One of the most difficult aspects of illness in children is the immobility it imposes. Children by nature are usually quite active, and immobility, however temporary, may have lasting consequences on the child's developmental progress. The most frequent reasons for immobility are congenital defects (e.g., spina bifida, arthrogryposis), degenerative disorders (e.g., muscular dystrophy), and infections or injuries that impair the integumentary system (severe burns), the musculoskeletal system (e.g., multiple fractures, osteomyelitis), or the neurologic system (e.g., spinal cord injury, polyneuritis, head injury). At times therapies such as traction and spinal fusion are responsible for prolonged immobilization, although the increasing trends in health care are early mobilization and discharge and outpatient treatment.

Physiologic Effects of Immobilization

Many clinical studies, including space program research, have documented predictable consequences that occur after immobilization and the absence of gravitational force. Functional and metabolic responses to restricted movement can be noted in most of the body systems. Each has a direct influence on the child's growth and development because homeostatic mechanisms thrive on normal use and need feedback to maintain dynamic equilibrium. Inactivity leads to a decrease in the functional capabilities of the whole body as dramatically as the lack of physical exercise leads to muscle weakness.

Disuse from illness, injury, or a sedentary lifestyle can limit function and potentially delay age-appropriate milestones. Most of the pathologic changes that occur during immobilization arise from decreased muscle strength and mass, decreased metabolism, and bone demineralization, which are closely interrelated, with one change leading to or affecting the other. Some results of immobilization are primary and produce a direct effect; other pathophysiologic consequences occur frequently but seem to be more indirect and are therefore secondary effects. Many pathophysiologic changes affect more than one body system, with the primary or secondary affect being demonstrated in both systems.

The major effects of immobilization are outlined briefly in Table 31-1 and are related directly or indirectly to de-creased muscle activity, which produces numerous primary changes in the musculoskeletal system with secondary alterations in the cardiovascular, respiratory, metabolic, and renal systems. The musculoskeletal changes that occur during disuse are a result of alterations in gravity and stress on the muscles, joints, and bones. Muscle disuse leads to tissue breakdown and loss of muscle mass *(atrophy)*. Muscle atrophy causes decreased strength and endurance, which may take weeks or months to restore.

During immobilization a joint contracture begins when the arrangement of collagen, the main structural protein of connective tissues, is altered, resulting in a denser tissue that does not glide as easily. Eventually muscles, tendons, and ligaments can shorten and reduce joint movement, ultimately producing contractures that restrict function. The daily stresses on bone created by motion and weight bearing maintain the balance between bone formation (osteoblastic activity) and bone reabsorption (osteoclastic activity). During immobilization, increased calcium leaves the bone, causing osteopenia (demineralization of the bones), which may predispose bone to pathologic fractures. The major musculoskeletal consequences of immobilization are (1) significant decrease in muscle size, strength, and endurance; (2) bone demineralization leading to osteoporosis; and (3) contractures and decreased joint mobility. The larger the portion of the body immobilized and the longer the immobilization, the greater the hazards of immobility.

Psychologic Effects of Immobilization

For children, one of the most difficult aspects of illness is immobilization. Throughout childhood, physical activity is an integral part of daily life and is essential for physical growth and development. It also serves children as an instrument for communication and expression and as a means for learning about and understanding their world. Activity helps them deal with a variety of feelings and impulses and provides a mechanism by which they can exert control over inner tensions. Children respond to anxiety with increased activity. Removal of this power deprives them of necessary input and a natural outlet for their feelings and fantasies. Through movement children also gain sensory input, which provides an essential element for developing and maintaining body image.

When children are immobilized by disease or as part of a treatment regimen, they experience diminished environ-

TABLE 31-1 ■ **Summary of Physical Effects of Immobilization***

PRIMARY EFFECTS	SECONDARY EFFECTS	PRIMARY EFFECTS	SECONDARY EFFECTS
MUSCULAR SYSTEM		**RESPIRATORY SYSTEM**	
Decreased muscle strength, tone, and endurance	Decreased venous return and decreased cardiac output	Decreased need for oxygen	Altered oxygen—carbon dioxide exchange and metabolism
	Decreased metabolism and need for oxygen	Decreased chest expansion and diminished vital capacity	Diminished oxygen intake
	Decreased exercise tolerance		Dyspnea and inadequate arterial oxygen saturation; acidosis
	Bone demineralization	Poor abdominal tone and distention	Interference with diaphragmatic excursion
Disuse atrophy and loss of muscle mass	Catabolism	Mechanical or biochemical secretion retention	Hypostatic pneumonia
Loss of joint mobility	Loss of strength		Bacterial and viral pneumonia
	Contractures, ankylosis of joints		Atelectasis
Weak back muscles	Secondary spinal deformities	Loss of respiratory muscle strength	Poor cough
Weak abdominal muscles	Impaired respiration		Upper respiratory infection
SKELETAL SYSTEM		**GASTROINTESTINAL SYSTEM**	
Bone demineralization—osteoporosis, hypercalcemia	Negative calcium balance	Distention caused by poor abdominal muscle tone	Interference with respiratory movements
	Pathologic fractures	No specific primary effect	Difficulty in feeding in prone position; gravitation effect on feces through ascending colon, or weakened smooth muscle tone may cause constipation
	Calcium deposits		
	Extraosseous bone formation, especially at hip, knee, elbow, and shoulder		
	Renal calculi		
Negative calcium balance	Life-threatening electrolyte imbalance		Anorexia
METABOLISM		**URINARY SYSTEM**	
Decreased metabolic rate	Slowing of all systems	Alteration of gravitational force	Difficulty in voiding in prone position
	Decreased food intake		
Negative nitrogen balance	Decline in nutritional state	Impaired ureteral peristalsis	Urinary retention in calyces and bladder
	Impaired healing		Infection
Hypercalcemia	Electrolyte imbalance		Renal calculi
Decreased production of stress hormones	Decreased physical and emotional coping capacity	**INTEGUMENTARY SYSTEM**	
		No specific primary effect	Decreased circulation and pressure leading to tissue injury and decreased healing capacity
CARDIOVASCULAR SYSTEM			Difficulty with personal hygiene
Decreased efficiency of orthostatic neurovascular reflexes	Inability to adapt readily to upright position		
	Pooling of blood in extremities in upright posture		
Diminished vasopressor mechanism	Orthostatic hypotension (intolerance) with syncope—hypotension, decreased cerebral blood flow, tachycardia		
Altered distribution of blood volume	Decreased cardiac workload		
Venous stasis	Decreased exercise tolerance		
Dependent edema	Pulmonary emboli or thrombi		
	Tissue breakdown and susceptibility to infection		

*Not all problems will apply in every situation.

mental stimuli with a loss of tactile input and an altered perception of themselves and their environment. Sudden or gradual immobilization narrows the amount and variety of environmental stimuli children receive by means of all of their senses: touch, sight, hearing, taste, smell, and proprioception—a feeling of where they are in their environment. This sensory deprivation frequently leads to feelings of isolation and boredom, and of being forgotten, especially by peers (see Family Focus box).

Physical interference with the activity of infants and young children gives them a feeling of helplessness. Even speech and language skills require sensorimotor activity and experience. Children who are restrained by casts, splints, or straps during the first 3 years of life may have more difficulty with language than children whose activities are unrestricted.

For the toddler, exploration and imitative behaviors are essential to developing a sense of autonomy; the preschooler's expression of initiative is evidenced by the need for vigorous

FAMILY FOCUS

Immobilization and Self-Esteem

Immobilization, as with any illness or disorder that is debilitating in some way, may restrict children from participating in age-appropriate activities. Children who must remain immobilized for lengthy periods may be labeled as "different," and, over time, this may result in a child feeling unaccepted. In young children, acceptance by peers is an important component in the formation of individual self-esteem. The assessment of self-esteem in young children is a critical attribute to their well-being. It is important to educate children about their illness and encourage them to engage in self-care activities. Children who have a strong sense of self-worth and confidence are able to initiate activities and explore their environment. They approach tasks and relationships with the expectation that they will be well-received and successful.

physical activity; the school-age child's development is strongly influenced by physical achievement and competition; and the adolescent relies on mobility to achieve independence. The quest for mastery at every stage of development is related to mobility.

The monotony of immobilization can lead to sluggish intellectual and psychomotor responses, decreased communication skills, increased fantasizing, and even hallucinations and disorientation. Children are likely to become depressed over loss of ability to function or the marked changes in body image. They may seek the attention of others by reverting to earlier developmental behaviors, such as wanting to be fed, bed-wetting, and baby talk.

Limbs in casts or traction transmit less than normal sensory data. Children who have limited ability to feel others touching them not only experience less tactile stimuli in a physical sense, but are also deprived of warm, loving feelings that arise from being touched. The loss of feeling derived from touch can further add to their sense of being isolated and unwanted.

Children may react to immobility by active protest, anger, and aggressive behavior, or they may become quiet, passive, and submissive. They may believe the immobilization is a justified punishment for misbehavior. Children should be allowed to discharge their anger, but it should be within the limits of safety to their self-esteem and not damaging to the integrity of others. For example, providing an object to attack rather than a person or a valued possession is safe and therapeutic. When children are unable to express anger, aggression is often displayed inappropriately through regressive behavior and outbursts of crying or temper tantrums.

Effect on Families

Even brief periods of immobilization may disrupt family function, and catastrophic illness or disability may severely tax their resources and coping abilities.

The family's needs often must be met by the services of a multidisciplinary team, and nurses play a key role in anticipating the services they will need and in coordinating conferences to plan care. In preparation for discharge, home visits are advisable, and home management is frequently planned weeks in advance of the actual discharge, including

special considerations for cultural, economic, physical, and psychologic needs. A child with a severe disability is very dependent, and caregivers need rest periods to revitalize themselves. Individual and group counseling is beneficial for pre–problem-solving situations and provides an emotional support system. Parent groups are also helpful and often allow nonthreatening social contact. The families of children with permanent disabilities need long-term resources, since some of the most difficult problems arise as they try to sustain high-quality care for many years (see Chapter 20).

Nursing Considerations

Physical assessment of the child who is immobilized for any number of reasons (illness, treatment, protection) includes a focus not only on the injured part (e.g., fracture, surgical repair), but also on the functioning of other systems that may be affected secondarily—the circulatory, renal, respiratory, muscular, and gastrointestinal systems. With long-term immobilization there may also be neurologic impairment and changes in electrolytes (especially calcium), nitrogen balance, and the general metabolic rate. The psychologic impact of immobilization should also be assessed.

Children who require prolonged total immobility and are unable to move themselves in bed should be placed on a special mattress to prevent skin breakdown. Frequent position changes also help prevent dependent edema and stimulate circulation, respiratory function, gastrointestinal motility, and neurologic sensation. Children at greater risk for skin breakdown include those with prolonged immobilization and orthotic and prosthetic devices, including wheelchairs, and plaster casts (Samaniego, 2003). Additional risk factors include poor nutrition, friction (from bed linen with traction), and moist skin (from urine or perspiration). Nursing care of children at risk includes proactive strategies for preventing skin breakdown when such conditions are present. The Modified Braden Q Scale is a reliable, objective tool that may be used in the assessment for pressure ulcer development in children who are acutely ill or who are at risk for skin breakdown from neurologic conditions and immobilization (Curley and others, 2003).

The use of antiembolism stockings may minimize or prevent dependent edema in the lower extremities. The child should be allowed as much activity as allowed within the limitations of the illness or treatment because any functional mobility, however minimal, is preferred to total immobility. High-protein, high-calorie foods are encouraged to prevent negative nitrogen balance, which may be difficult to correct by diet, especially if there is anorexia as a result of immobility and decreased gastrointestinal function (decreased motility and possibly constipation). Stimulating the appetite with small servings of attractively arranged, preferred foods may be sufficient. Sometimes, supplementary nasogastric feedings or intravenous fluids may be needed, but these are reserved for serious disability in which oral intake is impossible.

NURSING ALERT

Lying in a supine position during feeding increases the risk of aspiration. Therefore suction should be available at the bedside.

Adequate hydration and, when possible, an upright position and remobilization promote bowel and kidney function and help prevent complications in these systems. A discussion of elimination needs and toileting may help reduce embarrassment and complications of stool holding.

Children are encouraged to be as active as their condition and restrictive devices allow. This poses few problems for children, whose innate ingenuity and natural inclination toward mobility provide them with the impetus for physical activity. They need the opportunity, the materials or objects to stimulate activity, and the encouragement and participation of others. Those who are unable to move benefit from passive exercise and movement, in consultation with a physical therapist (PT).

Whenever possible, transporting the child by stretcher, wheelchair, stroller, or wagon outside the confines of the room increases environmental stimuli and provides social contact with others. Those confined to wheelchairs have specially designed chairs for increased mobility and independence. While hospitalized, children benefit from same-age visitors, computers, books, video games, and other items brought from their own room at home, all of which help them to function in a more normal way. A play therapist or child-life specialist should be consulted for recreational planning. An activity center or tray that slants can be particularly helpful for the child with limited mobility to use for drawing, coloring, writing, and playing with small toys such as trucks and cars. Children are able to express frustration, displeasure, and anger through play activities (see Chapter 21), which is helpful in the child's recovery. As soon as possible, hospitalized children should be allowed to wear their own clothes (street clothes, especially in preadolescent and adolescent girls) and resume school and preinjury activities. A parent or siblings should be allowed to stay overnight and room in with the hospitalized child to prevent the effects of family disruption from hospitalization. All efforts should be made to minimize family disruption resulting from the hospitalization. Although most of the suggestions discussed relate to hospital care, the same consultations (PT/occupational therapist/child-life/speech therapy) and environment may be considered in the home as well to help the child and family achieve independence and normalization (see Chapter 20).

Using dolls, stuffed animals, or puppets to illustrate and explain the restraining (traction, cast) method is a valuable tool for small children. Placing a cast, tubing, or other restraining equipment on the doll offers the child a nonthreatening opportunity to express, through the doll, feelings concerning the restrictions and feelings toward the nurse and other health care providers. The doll or puppet may also be used for teaching procedures such as intravenous therapy, conscious sedation, and general anesthesia to the child and family.

Children typically dislike hospital food, which is usually not tailored to their age. Parents and friends should be allowed to bring in meals from home or other sources, provided they meet necessary requirements for the illness; this enables children to have more control of their environment and will decrease resistance to treatments and schedules, which is usually common behavior evidenced when adults and children are not given any choices in an acute care setting.

One of the most useful interventions to help children cope with immobility is participation in their own care. Self-care to the maximum extent is usually well-received by children. They can help plan their daily routine, select their diet (when possible), and choose "street clothes," including innovative adornment, such as a baseball cap or brightly colored stockings, that expresses their autonomy and individuality. They are encouraged to do as much for themselves as they are able to keep muscles active and their interest alive.

Visits from significant persons, such as family members and friends, offer occasions for emotional support and also provide opportunities for learning how to care for the child. Some privacy is needed, particularly by the adolescent.

For a child with greatly restricted movement (e.g., paraplegic or quadriplegic child, child with a large bilateral hip spica cast), nursing care is often a challenge. These situations require long-term care either in the hospital or at home, but wherever the care occurs, consistent planning and coordination of activities with other health care workers and significant others are vital nursing functions.

With the increased trend in early mobilization, early discharge, and home health care, many children are discharged home within a few days of hospitalization. Follow-up treatment may take place in the home setting or an outpatient ambulatory facility.

Family Support and Home Care.   The needs of a child with severe disabilities can be very complex, and family members require time to assimilate the teachings and demonstrations needed to understand the child's situation and care. Even the child who is confined on a short-term basis can be a challenge for the family, which is usually unprepared for the problems imposed by the child's special needs. Home modification is usually needed for facilitating care, especially when it involves traction, large casts, or extended confinement. Suitable child care may be needed for times when all family members work.

Just as in the hospital, the child at home is encouraged to be as independent as possible and to follow a schedule that approximates his or her normal lifestyle as nearly as possible, such as continuing school lessons, regular bedtime, and suitable recreational activities.

TRAUMATIC INJURY

SOFT-TISSUE INJURY

Injuries to the muscles, ligaments, and tendons are common in children (Fig. 31-1). In young children, soft-tissue injury usually results from mishaps during play. In older children and adolescents, participation in sports is a common cause of such injuries.

Contusions

A contusion is damage to the soft tissue, subcutaneous structures, and muscle. The tearing of these tissues and small blood vessels and the inflammatory response lead to hemorrhage, edema, and associated pain when the child attempts to move the injured part. The escape of blood into the tissues is observed as *ecchymosis,* a black-and-blue discoloration.

Large contusions cause gross swelling, pain, and disability; those sustained while the child is participating in sports

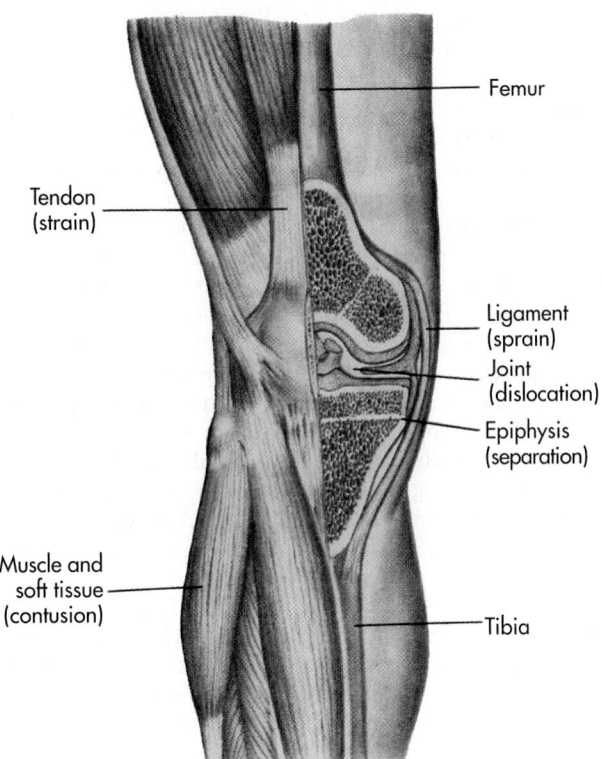

Femur

Tendon (strain)

Ligament (sprain)

Joint (dislocation)

Epiphysis (separation)

Muscle and soft tissue (contusion)

Tibia

FIG. 31-1 ■ Sites of injuries to bones, joints, and soft tissues.

usually receive immediate attention from health personnel. The less spectacular, smaller injuries may go unnoticed, allowing continued participation. However, they can become disabling after rest because of pain and muscle spasm. The young athlete is frequently instructed to "work it out" or disregard the pain. Instead of this approach, an assessment of the affected area should be first carried out by a qualified health care worker or certified athletic trainer because further damage to the site may result if the area is severely traumatized. Immediate treatment consists of cold application, as in the treatment of sprains described in the following section. Return to participation is allowed when the strength and range of motion of the affected extremity are equal to those of the opposite extremity or is demonstrated under conditions such as sport-specific tests. *Myositis ossificans* may occur from deep contusions to the biceps or quadriceps muscles; this condition may result in a restriction of flexibility of the affected limb.

Related to contusions are crush injuries that occur in children when they slam their fingers (in doors, folding chairs, or equipment) or hit their fingers (as when hammering a nail). A severe crush injury involves the bone, with swelling and bleeding beneath the nail (subungual) and sometimes laceration of the pulp of the distal phalanx. The *subungual hematoma* can be released by creating a hole at the proximal end of the nail with a battery-operated microcautery device or a heated 18-gauge needle.

Dislocations

Long bones are held in approximation to one another at the joint by ligaments. A dislocation occurs when the force of stress on the ligament is so great as to displace the normal

position of the opposing bone ends or the bone end to its socket. The predominant symptom is pain that increases with attempted passive or active movement of the extremity. In dislocations there may be an obvious deformity and inability to move the joint. Children with naturally lax joints are more prone to dislocation of joints. Dislocation of the phalanges is the most common type seen in children, followed by elbow dislocation.

The most common injury in young children is subluxation or partial dislocation of the radial head, also called "pulled elbow" or *"nursemaid's elbow."* In the majority of cases the injury occurs in a child younger than 5 years of age who receives a sudden longitudinal pull or traction at the wrist while the arm is fully extended and the forearm pronated. It usually occurs when an adult or older sibling who is holding the child by the hand or wrist gives a sudden pull or jerk to prevent a fall or attempts to lift the child by pulling the wrist, or when the child pulls away by dropping to the floor or ground. The child often cries, appears anxious, and refuses to use the affected limb. The practitioner manipulates the arm by applying firm finger pressure to the head of the radius, then supinates and flexes the forearm to return the bone structure to normal alignment. A click may be heard or felt, and functional use of the arm returns within minutes (Greene, 2001). However, the longer the subluxation is present, the longer it takes for the child to recover mobility after treatment. No anesthetic is usually required but a mild pain reliever such as acetaminophen may be given. In an older child, severe elbow injury or dislocation should be carefully evaluated by a practitioner immediately; likewise, a traumatic elbow injury in the younger child that is not a subluxation should be carefully evaluated.

In children younger than 5 years of age, the hip can be dislocated by a fall. The greatest risk after this injury is the potential loss of blood supply to the head of the femur. Relocation of the hip within 60 minutes after the injury provides the best chance for prevention of damage to the femoral head.

Shoulder dislocations occur most often in older adolescents and are often sports-related. Temporary restriction of the joint, with a sling or bandage that secures the arm to the chest in a shoulder dislocation, can provide sufficient comfort and immobilization until medical attention is received.

Simple dislocations should be reduced as soon as possible with the child under conscious sedation and often local anesthesia. Also, the use of anesthetics, such as intravenous ketamine (Ketalar) and midazolam (Versed), IV propofol (Diprivan), or fentanyl (Sublimaze), can be used to produce partial or complete analgesia. An unreduced dislocation will be complicated by increased swelling, making reduction difficult and increasing the risk of neurovascular problems. Treatment depends on the severity of the injury.

Sprains

A sprain occurs when trauma to a joint is so severe that a ligament is partially or completely torn or stretched by the force created as a joint is twisted or wrenched, often accompanied by damage to associated blood vessels, muscles, tendons, and nerves.

The presence of joint laxity is the most valid indicator of the severity of a sprain. In a severe injury the child complains of the joint "feeling loose" or as if "something is coming apart" and may describe hearing a "snap," "pop," or "tearing." Pain may or may not be the principal subjective symptom, and in some children it may prevent optimal examination of ligamentous instability. There is a rapid onset with swelling, often diffuse, accompanied by immediate disability and appreciable reluctance to use the injured joint.

Strains

A strain is a microscopic tear to the musculotendinous unit and has features in common with sprains. The area is painful to touch and swollen. Most strains are incurred over time rather than suddenly, and the rapidity of the appearance provides clues regarding severity. In general, the more rapidly the strain occurs, the more severe the injury. When the strain involves the muscular portion, there is more bleeding, often palpable soon after injury and before edema obscures the hematoma.

Therapeutic Management

The first minutes to 12 hours is the most critical period for virtually all soft-tissue injuries. Basic principles of managing sprains and other soft-tissue injuries are summarized in the acronyms *RICE* and *ICES:*

Rest	Ice
Ice	Compression
Compression	Elevation
Elevation	Support

Soft-tissue injuries should be iced immediately. This is best accomplished with crushed ice wrapped in a towel, a screwtop ice bag, or a resealable plastic storage bag. Chemical-activated ice packs are also effective for immediate treatment but are not reusable and must be closely monitored for leakage. A wet elastic wrap, which transfers cold better than dry wrap, is applied to provide compression and to keep the ice pack in place. A cloth barrier should be used between the ice container and the skin to prevent trauma to the tissues. Ice has a rapid cooling effect on tissues and reduces the pain threshold. However, ice should never be applied for more than 30 minutes at a time because of the body's homeostatic response to cold, which may trigger a decrease in vascularization at the injury site.

NURSING TIP

A plastic bag of frozen vegetables, such as peas, serves as a convenient ice pack for soft-tissue injuries. It is clean, watertight, and easily molded to the injured part. When available, snow placed in a plastic bag may serve as an ice bag.

Elevating the extremity uses gravity to facilitate venous return and reduce edema formation in the damaged area. The point of injury should be kept several inches above the level of the heart for therapy to be effective. Several pillows can be used effectively for elevation. Allowing the extremity to be dependent causes excessive fluid accumulation in the area of injury, delaying healing and causing painful swelling.

Torn ligaments, especially those in the knee, are usually treated by immobilization with a knee immobilizer or range-of-motion brace until the child is able to walk without a limp. Crutches are used for mobility to rest the affected extremity. Passive leg exercises, gradually increased to active ones, are begun as soon as sufficient healing has taken place. Parents and children are cautioned against using any form of liniment or other heat-producing preparation before examination. If the injury requires casting or splinting, the heat generated in the enclosed space can cause extreme discomfort and may even cause tissue damage. In some cases torn knee ligaments are managed with arthroscopy and ligament repair or reconstruction as necessary depending on the extent of the tear, ligaments involved, and age of the child. Surgical reconstruction of the anterior cruciate ligament (ACL) may be performed in young athletes who wish to continue in active sports (Greene, 2001).

FRACTURES

Bone fractures occur when the resistance of bone against the stress being exerted yields to the stress force. Fractures are a common injury at any age but are more likely to occur in children and older adults. Because childhood is a time of rapid bone growth, the pattern of fractures, problems of diagnosis, and methods of treatment differ in the child and the adult. In children fractures heal much faster than in adults. Consequently, children may not require as long a period of immobilization of the affected extremity as an adult with a fracture.

Fracture injuries in children are most often a result of traumatic incidents at home, at school, in a motor vehicle, or in association with recreational activities. Children's everyday activities include vigorous play that predisposes them to injury—climbing, falling down, running into immovable objects, skateboarding, and receiving blows to any part of their bodies.

Aside from automobile accidents or falls from heights, true injuries that cause fractures rarely occur in infancy; therefore, bone injury in children of that age-group warrants further investigation. In any small child, radiographic evidence of fractures at various stages of healing are, with few exceptions, a result of physical abuse. Any investigation of fractures in infants, particularly multiple fractures, should include consideration of *osteogenesis imperfecta.*

The clavicle is probably the bone most frequently broken in childhood, with approximately half of clavicle fractures occurring in children younger than 10 years of age. Common mechanisms of injury include a fall with an outstretched hand or direct trauma to the bone. In neonates, a fractured clavicle may occur with a large newborn and a small maternal pelvis.

Fractures in school-age children are often a result of bicycle-automobile or skateboard injuries. Adolescents are vulnerable to multiple and severe trauma because they are mobile on bicycles, all-terrain vehicles, skateboards, skis, snowboards, and motorcycles and are active in sports.

Epiphyseal (or Physeal) Injuries

The weakest point of long bones is the cartilage growth plate or epiphyseal plate. Consequently, this is a frequent site of damage during trauma. Detection of epiphyseal injuries is sometimes difficult, but critical. Fractures involving the epiphysis or epiphyseal plate present special problems in determining whether or not bone growth will be affected. Treatment of these fractures may include open reduction and internal fixation to prevent or reduce growth disturbances.

Types of Fractures

A fractured bone consists of fragments—the fragment closer to the midline, or the proximal fragment, and the fragment farther from the midline, or the distal fragment. When fracture fragments are separated, the fracture is **complete;** when fragments remain attached, the fracture is **incomplete.** The fracture line can be any of the following:

> **Transverse**—Crosswise, at right angles to the long axis of the bone
> **Oblique**—Slanting but straight, between a horizontal and a perpendicular direction
> **Spiral**—Slanting and circular, twisting around the bone shaft

The twisting of an extremity while the bone is breaking results in a spiral break. If the fracture does not produce a break in the skin, it is a **simple, or closed, fracture. Open,** or **compound, fractures** are those with an open wound through which the bone protrudes. If the bone fragments cause damage to other organs or tissues (e.g., the lung, bladder), the injury is said to be a **complicated** fracture. When small fragments of bone are broken from the fractured shaft and lie in the surrounding tissue, the injury is a **comminuted fracture.** This type of fracture is rare in children. The types of fractures that are seen most often in children are described in Box 31-1 and in Fig. 31-2.

> **!NURSING ALERT**
>
> A spiral fracture in children may indicate child abuse, and further assessment of the family situation should involve a multidisciplinary team.

Immediately after a fracture occurs, the muscles contract and physiologically splint the injured area. This phenomenon accounts for the muscle tightness observed over a fracture site and the deformity that is produced as the muscles pull the bone ends out of alignment. This muscle response must be overcome by traction or complete muscle relaxation (i.e., anesthesia) to realign the distal bone fragment to the proximal bone fragment.

BOX 31-1 ■ Types of Fractures in Children

Bend—Occurs when the bone is bent but not broken. A child's flexible bone can be bent 45 degrees or more before breaking. However, if bent, the bone will straighten slowly, but not completely, to produce some deformity but without the angulation seen when the bone breaks. Bends occur most commonly in the ulna and fibula, often in association with fractures of the radius and tibia.

Buckle, or torus, fracture—Produced by compression of the porous bone; appears as a raised or bulging projection at the fracture site. These fractures occur in the most porous portion of the bone near the metaphysis (the portion of the bone shaft adjacent to the epiphysis) and are more common in young children.

Greenstick fracture—Occurs when a bone is angulated beyond the limits of bending. The compressed side bends, and the tension side fails, causing an incomplete fracture similar to the break observed when a green stick is broken.

Complete fracture—Divides the bone fragments. These fragments often remain attached by a periosteal hinge, which can aid or hinder reduction.

Bone Healing and Remodeling

Bone healing is characteristically rapid in children because of the thickened periosteum and generous blood supply. When there is a break in the continuity of bone, the osteoblasts are stimulated to maximal activity. New bone cells are formed in immense numbers almost immediately after the injury and, in time, are evidenced by a bulging growth of new bone tissue between the fractured bone fragments. This is followed by deposition of calcium salts to form a **callus.**

Fractures heal in less time in children than in adults. The approximate healing times for a femoral shaft are as follows:

- Neonatal period—2 to 3 weeks
- Early childhood—4 weeks
- Later childhood—6 to 8 weeks
- Adolescence—8 to 12 weeks

Diagnostic Evaluation

A history is often lacking in childhood injuries. Infants are unable to communicate, and older children seldom volunteer information (even under direct questioning) when the injury occurred during forbidden activities. Unless they are witnesses to the injury, parents may misinterpret what the child is trying to say. In cases of child abuse, parents may give false information to protect themselves.

The child may exhibit the same manifestations seen in adults (Box 31-2). However, often a fracture is remarkably stable because of intact periosteum. The child may even be able to use an affected arm or walk on a fractured leg. Because bones are highly vascular, a soft, pliable hematoma may be felt around the fracture site.

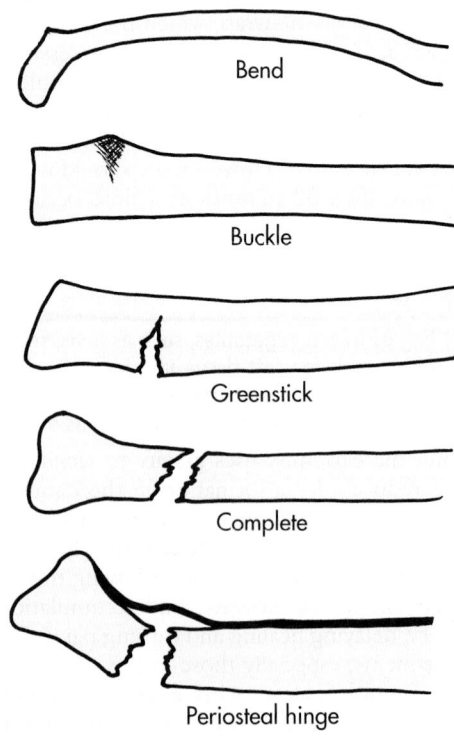

FIG. 31-2 ■ Types of fractures in children.

Radiographic examination is the most useful diagnostic tool for assessing skeletal trauma. The calcium deposits in bone make the entire structure radiopaque. Radiographic films are taken after fracture reduction and, in some cases, may be taken during the healing process to determine satisfactory progress.

Therapeutic Management

The majority of children's fractures heal well, and nonunion is rare. Most fractures are readily reduced by simple traction and immobilization until healing takes place. However, the position of the bone fragments in relation to one another influences the rapidity of healing and the residual deformity. Healing is prompt and complete with end-to-end apposition, but a gap between fragments delays (or prevents) healing. The goals of fracture management are the following:

1 To regain alignment and length of the bony fragments (reduction)
2 To retain alignment and length (immobilization)
3 To restore function to the injured parts
4 To prevent further injury

In children the bone fragments are usually realigned and immobilized by traction or by closed manipulation and casting until adequate callus is formed. Weight bearing on lower extremity fractures and active movement for the purpose of regaining function can begin after the fracture site is stable. The child's natural tendency to be active is usually sufficient to restore normal mobility, and physical therapy is rarely needed. In most cases children's fractures can be managed by closed reduction and cast immobilization, which is most often provided on an outpatient basis with reevaluation in 7 to 10 days.

Children are most frequently hospitalized for fractures of the femur and the supracondylar area of the distal humerus, which may require internal fixation and pinning; displaced supracondylar fractures in children should be treated surgically (Do and Herrera-Soto, 2003). If simple reductions cannot be achieved or if a neurovascular problem is detected after injury, observation in a hospital is indicated. Severe contusions with profound swelling cannot be treated with a cast, which would act as a tourniquet on the extrem-

BOX 31-2 ■ Clinical Manifestations of a Fracture

Signs of injury:
  Generalized swelling
  Pain or tenderness
  Deformity
  Diminished functional use of affected part
May also demonstrate:
  Bruising
  Severe muscular rigidity
  Crepitus (grating sensation at fracture site)

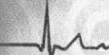

EMERGENCY TREATMENT

Fracture

Assess the extent of injury—5 Ps:
  Pain and point of tenderness
  Pulse—distal to the fracture site
  Pallor
  Paresthesia—sensation distal to the fracture site
  Paralysis—movement distal to the fracture site
Determine the mechanism of injury.
Move the injured part as little as possible.
Cover open wounds with a sterile or clean dressing.
Immobilize the limb, including joints above and below the fracture site; do not attempt to reduce the fracture or push protruding bone under the skin.
Soft splint (pillow or folded towel)
Rigid splint (rolled newspaper or magazine)
Uninjured leg can serve as a splint for a leg fracture if no splint available
Reassess neurovascular status.
Apply traction if circulatory compromise is present.
Elevate the injured limb if possible.
Apply cold to the injured area.
Call emergency medical service or transport to medical facility.

ity. A badly malaligned fracture requires traction for a period before a cast is applied.

The major methods for immobilizing a fracture, casting and traction, are described in the following sections on casting and traction.

Nursing Considerations

Nurses are frequently the persons who make the initial assessment of a child with a suspected fracture (see Emergency Treatment box). The child and parents may be frightened and upset, and the child is often in pain. Therefore, if the child is alert and there is no evidence of hemorrhage, the initial nursing interventions are directed toward calming and reassuring the child and parents so that a more extensive assessment can be more easily accomplished.

While remaining calm and speaking in a quiet voice, the nurse can ask the parents and older child to describe what happened. The child may arrive with the limb supported in some manner; if not, careful support or immobilization may be provided to the affected site. In the event that the limb is supported or immobilized, it may be best not to touch the child but to ask him or her to point to the painful area and to wiggle the fingers or toes. By this time the child may feel relatively safe and will allow someone to gently touch the area just enough to feel the pulses and test for sensation. A child's anxiety is greatly influenced by previous experiences with injury and with health personnel. However, he or she needs to be told what will happen and what to do to help. The affected limb need not be palpated, and it should not be moved unless properly splinted. If the child is at home or if the practitioner is not present to examine the child, some type of splint is applied carefully for transport to the medical facility. Parental anxiety may be heightened by the child's pain reaction and fear, and possibly by other events surrounding the accident; thus it is important to communicate to the parent that the child will receive the necessary care, including pain management.

> **! NURSING ALERT**
>
> The five "Ps" of ischemia from a vascular injury should be included in an assessment of the injury:
> 1. Pain
> 2. Pallor
> 3. Pulselessness
> 4. Paresthesia
> 5. Paralysis

THE CHILD IN A CAST

The completeness of the fracture, the type of bone involved, and the amount of weight bearing influence how much of the extremity must be included in the cast to immobilize the fracture site completely. In most cases the joints above and below the fracture are immobilized to eliminate the possibility of movement that might cause displacement at the fracture site. Four major categories of casts are used for fractures: *upper extremity* to immobilize the wrist or elbow, *lower extremity* to immobilize the ankle or knee, *spinal* and *cervical* for immobilization of the spine, and *spica casts* to immobilize the hip and knee.

The Cast

Casts are constructed from gauze strips and bandages impregnated with plaster of paris or, more commonly, from synthetic lighter weight and water-resistant materials (e.g., fiberglass and polyurethane resin).

Both types of casting produce heat from chemical reaction activated by water immediately after application. Plaster casts mold closely to the body part, take 10 to 72 hours to dry, have a smooth exterior, and are inexpensive. The newer synthetic casting material is lighter, dries in 5 to 30 minutes, permits earlier weight bearing, and is water-resistant. The disadvantage of synthetic casting is its inability to mold closely to body parts; its rough exterior, which may scratch surfaces; and increased cost.

> **FYI**
>
> Synthetic casts have special advantages for children. They come in different colors and with designs (e.g., cartoons, stripes); and they are lightweight, durable, easy to clean, and relatively water-resistant, depending on the type of inner lining used; only those with a Gore-Tex inner lining may be immersed in water without affecting the cast integrity. Bathing with a synthetic cast may be accomplished by covering the cast with a plastic bag; if the synthetic cast gets wet, it should be dried thoroughly. One drawback to immersion is the time necessary to completely dry the cast. Synthetic casts are difficult to write on. A waterproof marker or color markers may be used for writing on the cast.

Cast Application. The developmental age of the child should be considered before the cast is applied. For preschoolers who fear bodily harm and fantasize loss of an extremity, instead of immobilization, it may be helpful to use a plastic doll or stuffed animal to explain the procedure beforehand. It is also helpful to explain that the cast material will become warm but will not burn. During the application of the cast various distraction methods may be used, including a discussion of favorite pets, activities at school, blowing bubbles, and so forth. In this age-group explanations such as "This will help your arm get better" are futile because the child has no concept of causality.

Before the cast is applied, the extremities are checked for any abrasions, cuts, or other alterations in the skin surface and for the presence of rings or other items that might cause constriction from swelling; such objects are removed. A tube of cloth stockinette is stretched over the area to be casted, and bony prominences are padded with soft cotton sheeting. Some practitioners use a Gore-Tex liner under a hip spica cast to prevent continuous exposure to moisture and possible skin breakdown. Dry rolls of casting material are immersed in a pail of water. The wet rolls are put on in a bandage fashion and molded to the extremity. During application of the plaster cast, the underlying stockinette is pulled over the rough edges of the cast and secured with a layer of wet plaster 0.5 to 1 inch below the rim to form a smooth, padded edge to protect the skin.

If the practitioner does not form such a protective edge with stockinette, the rough edges of the plaster cast can be protected by a "petaled" edge. Small pieces approximately 2 to 3 inches long are cut from 1- or 1.5-inch-wide adhesive tape or moleskin. The edges are rounded with scissors, and these "petals" are placed over the edge of the cast, with each petal slightly overlapping the previous petal to form a smooth, neat edge. It is easier to apply the petal to the underside of the cast first and then bring the loose edge to the front, pressing firmly so that the edges remain securely attached. Synthetic casts usually do not require additional padding on the edges as they do not crack like plaster material might.

Nursing Considerations

The complete evaporation of the water from a hip spica cast can take 24 to 48 hours when older types of plaster materials are used. Drying occurs within minutes with fiberglass cast material. The cast must remain uncovered to allow it to dry from the inside out. Turning the child in a plaster cast at least every 2 hours will help to dry a body cast evenly and prevent complications related to immobility. A regular fan or cool-air hair dryer to circulate air may be helpful when the humidity is high.

> **! NURSING ALERT**
>
> Heated fans or dryers are not used, because they cause the cast to dry on the outside and remain wet beneath or cause burns from heat conduction by way of the cast to the underlying tissue.

A wet plaster cast should be supported by a pillow that is covered with plastic and handled by the palms of the hands to prevent indenting the cast, which can create pressure areas. A dry plaster-of-paris cast produces a hollow sound when it is tapped with the finger. If "hot spots" are felt on the cast surface (usually indicating infection beneath the area), this should be reported so that a window can be made in the cast to observe the site.

During the first few hours after a cast is applied, the chief concern is that the extremity may continue to swell to the extent that the cast becomes a tourniquet, shutting off circulation and producing neurovascular complications. To reduce the likelihood of this potential problem, the body part can be elevated, thereby increasing venous return. If edema is excessive, casts are bivalved (i.e., cut to make anterior and posterior halves that are held together with an elastic bandage). The cast and the involved extremity are observed frequently for neurovascular integrity and any signs of compromise. Permanent muscle and tissue damage can occur within 6 to 8 hours.

! NURSING ALERT

Observations such as pain (unrelieved by pain medication 1 hour after administration), swelling, discoloration (pallor or cyanosis) of the exposed portions, decreased pulses, decreased temperature, or the inability to move the distal exposed part(s) should be reported immediately.

When an extremity that has sustained an open fracture is casted, a window is often left over the wound area to allow for observation and dressing of the wound. A surgical reduction is usually casted as a closed fracture. For the first few hours after surgery, there may be substantial bleeding that will soak through the cast. Periodically the circumscribed bloodstained area should be outlined with a waterproof marker, and the time indicated to provide a guide for assessing the amount of bleeding.

Usually the child is discharged to home care after a cast is applied in the emergency department or clinic. Parents need instructions on drying and caring for the cast and checking for signs and symptoms that indicate the cast is too tight (see Family Home Care box). They should also be told to take the child to the health professional for attention if the cast becomes too loose, because a loose cast no longer serves its purpose.

Nurses can help families adapt the child's home environment to meet the temporary encumbrance of a cast. Home care creates problems of varying magnitudes, especially for children in large casts (e.g., a hip spica). Commonplace situations become problematic (e.g., transporting a child safely and comfortably in a car). Standard seat belts and car seats may not be readily adapted for use by children in some casts. There are specially designed car seats and restraints available that meet safety requirements (Fig. 31-3).* Alterations to standard car seats to accommodate the cast are not recommended, because the structure may be adversely altered.

Parents are taught the proper care of the cast (or orthotic device) and are helped to devise means for maintaining cleanliness. A superabsorbent disposable diaper is tucked beneath the entire perineal opening of the cast. A larger diaper can be applied and fastened over the small diaper and cast.

---

*For additional information contact the **Automotive Safety for Children Program,** James Whitcomb Riley Hospital for Children, Indiana University School of Medicine, 575 West Drive, Room 004, Indianapolis, IN 46202; (317) 274-2977 (in Indianapolis) or (800) 543-6227; website: www.preventinjury.org.

⌂ FAMILY HOME CARE

Cast Care

Keep the casted extremity elevated on pillows or similar support for the first day, or as directed by the health professional.

Avoid denting the plaster cast with fingertips (use palms of hand to handle) while it is still wet to avoid creating pressure points.

Observe the extremities (fingers or toes) for any evidence of swelling or discoloration (darker or lighter than a comparable extremity) and contact the health professional if noted.

Check movement and sensation of the visible extremities frequently.

Follow health professional's orders regarding any restriction of activities.

Restrict strenuous activities for the first few days.

   Engage in quiet activities but encourage use of muscles.

   Move the joints above and below the cast on the affected extremity.

Encourage frequent rest for a few days, keeping the injured extremity elevated while resting.

Avoid allowing the affected limb to hang down for any length of time.

   Keep an injured upper extremity elevated (e.g., in a sling) while upright.

   Elevate a lower limb when sitting and avoid standing for too long.

Do not allow the child to put anything inside the cast.

   Keep small items that might be placed inside the cast away from small children.

Keep a clear path for ambulation.

   Remove toys, hazardous floor rugs, pets, or other items over which the child might stumble.

Use crutches appropriately if lower limb fracture.

The crutches should fit properly, have a soft rubber tip to prevent slipping, and be well padded at the axilla.

For tightly fitting casts, transparent film dressings can be cut into strips as for petaling, and one edge applied to the cast edge and the other directly to the perineum; this forms a continuous, waterproof bridge between the perineum and the cast to prevent leakage. An additional advantage to the use of this transparent dressing is that it keeps both the skin and the cast dry while allowing for observation of skin beneath the dressing.

Older infants and small children may stuff bits of food, small toys, or other items under the cast; parents should be alerted to this possibility so that suitable preventive measures can be initiated.

Feeding the infant in a hip spica cast offers problems in positioning. Very young infants can be fed in the supine position with the head elevated, and with the infant's hips and legs supported on a pillow at the side, the parent can cuddle the infant in his or her arms during feeding. A somewhat similar position can be used for breast-feeding (i.e., with the infant supported on pillows or held in a "football" hold facing the mother with the legs behind her). An alternate position is to hold the infant upright on the caregiver's lap with the legs of the infant astride the adult's leg.

Children in spica casts usually find the prone position easier for self-feeding from a small table placed next to the dining table. The use of a conventional toilet is almost im-

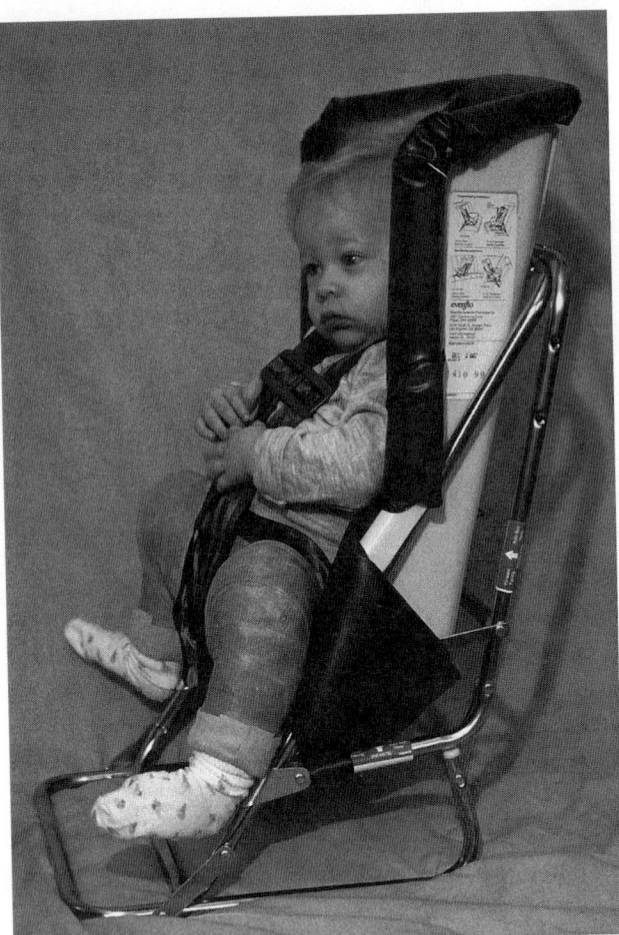

FIG. 31-3 ■ Child in a specially designed car restraint (Spelcast).

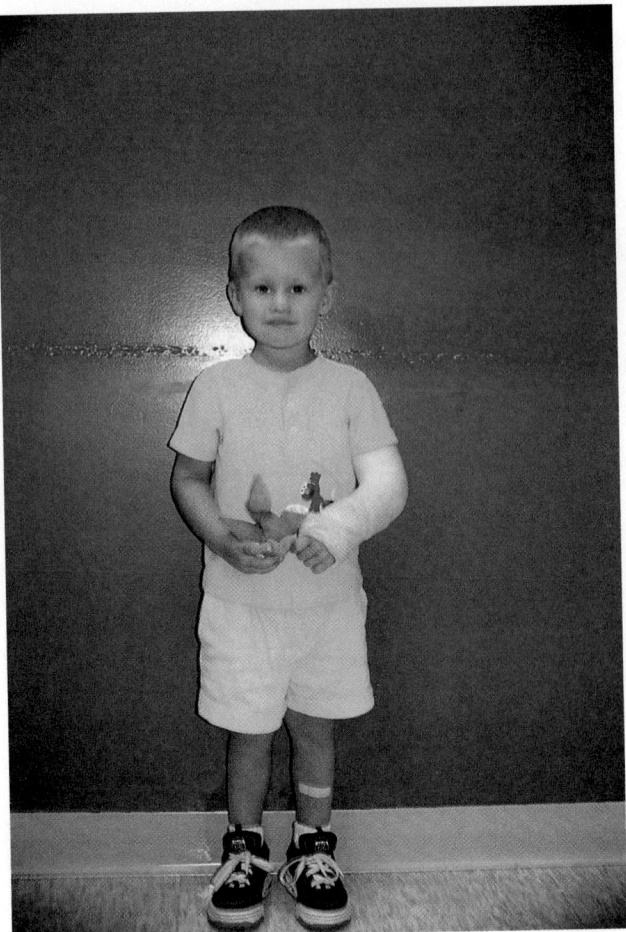

FIG. 31-4 ■ Young children usually adapt well to a cast but often fear the removal.

possible. Small bedpans or other containers offer alternatives for elimination. The nurse may suggest waterproofing methods, by devising plastic wraps, for elimination and showers. Baths are possible only if the plaster cast is kept out of the water and covered to prevent it from becoming wet from splashes.

Cast Removal.   Cutting the cast to remove it or to relieve tightness is frequently a frightening experience for children. They fear the sound of the cast cutter and are terrified that their flesh, as well as the cast, will be cut. The oscillating blade vibrates very rapidly back and forth and will not cut when placed *lightly* on the skin. Children have described it as producing a "tickly" sensation. The vibration also generates heat that may be felt by the child. Both of these feelings should be explained.

Preparation for the procedure will help reduce anxiety, especially if a trusting relationship has been established between the child and the nurse. Many young children come to regard the cast as part of themselves, which intensifies their fear of removal (Fig. 31-4). They need continual reassurance that all is going well and that their behavior is accepted. After the cast is removed, the parents and child should be given the option of keeping the cast; it may be placed in a plastic bag because of the usual odor. If the cast has been in place

for a lengthy period, decreased muscle mass will be noted. The child should be reassured that resuming exercise and routine activities will return function and appearance (provided there was no significant trauma beforehand). One concern with fiberglass casts during removal is the potential for inhalation of fiberglass particles; this may be avoided by only using a cast saw with a built-in vacuum or placing a mask on the child as age permits (Adkins, 1997).

After the cast is removed, the skin surface will be caked with desquamated skin and sebaceous secretions. Simple soaking in a bathtub is usually sufficient for their removal, but a period of several days may be required to eliminate the accumulation completely. Application of oil or lotion may provide comfort. The parents and child should be instructed not to pull or forcibly remove this material with vigorous scrubbing, because it may cause excoriation and bleeding.

THE CHILD IN TRACTION

The ever-changing health care arena has witnessed the demise of many long-term treatments involving lengthy hospitalization; one such change is in the area of traction. Most balanced skeletal traction is applied in children after a severe or complex injury to allow physiologic stability, align bone fragments, and permit closer evaluation of the injured site. Newer technology has produced orthopedic fixation

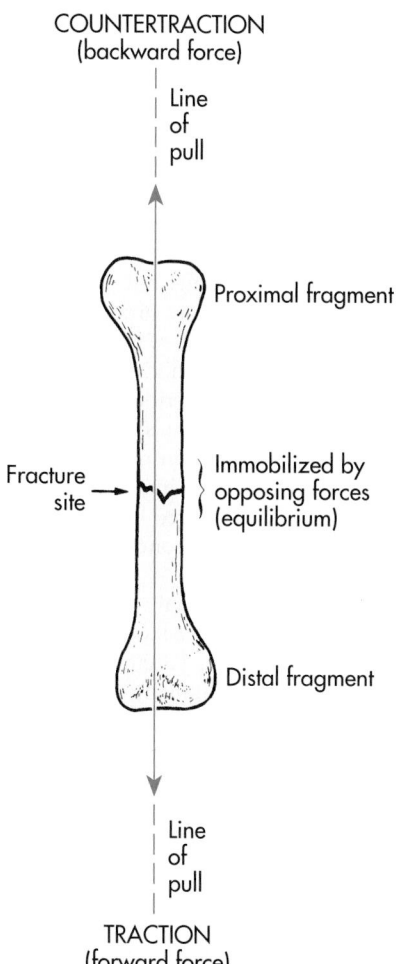

COUNTERTRACTION
(backward force)

Line
of
pull

Proximal fragment

Fracture
site →

} Immobilized by
opposing forces
(equilibrium)

Distal fragment

Line
of
pull

TRACTION
(forward force)

FIG. 31-5 ■ Application of traction to maintain bone alignment.

devices that allow partial or full mobility, thus preventing long-term immobilization and its consequences. In many situations, surgical intervention may be carried out within a matter of days; therefore, skeletal traction devices described herein may be used infrequently in many cases.

Bone fragments that cannot be aligned initially by simple traction and stabilization with a cast may require the extended pulling force supplied by continuous traction. Traction may be used for other purposes also:

■ To provide rest for an extremity
■ To help prevent or improve contracture deformity
■ To correct a deformity
■ To treat a dislocation
■ To allow preoperative or postoperative positioning and alignment
■ To provide immobilization of specific areas of the body
■ To reduce muscle spasms (rare in children)

Purposes of Traction

The three essential components of traction management are traction, countertraction, and friction (Fig. 31-5). To reduce or realign a fracture site, *traction* (forward force) is produced by attaching weight to the distal bone fragment; body weight provides *countertraction* (backward force); and the patient's contact with the bed constitutes the *frictional*

force. These forces are used to align the distal and proximal bone fragments by adjusting the line of pull upward or downward and adducting or abducting the extremity.

To attain equilibrium, the amount of forward force is adjusted by adding weight to or subtracting weight from the traction, or countertraction can be increased by elevating the foot of the bed to create a greater gravitational pull to the backward force.

The three primary purposes of traction for reduction of fractures are:

1 To fatigue the involved muscles and reduce muscle spasm so that bones can be realigned
2 To position the distal and proximal bone ends in desired realignment to promote satisfactory bone healing
3 To immobilize the fracture site until realignment has been achieved and sufficient healing has taken place to permit casting or splinting

The *all-or-none law*, characteristic of muscle contractibility, influences the complete relaxation. When muscles are stretched, muscle spasm ceases and permits the realignment of the bone ends. The continuous maintenance of traction is important during this phase because releasing the traction allows the normal contracting ability of the muscle to again cause a malpositioning of the bone ends.

The realignment of the fragments is a gradual process that is achieved more rapidly in infants, who have limited muscle tone, than in muscular teenagers. The desired line of pull and callus formation are checked periodically by radiographic examination. The traction pull to some degree immobilizes the fracture site; however, adjunctive immobilizing devices such as splints or casts are sometimes used with skeletal traction. In injuries in which there is severe soft-tissue swelling or vascular and nerve damage, it is customary to use traction until these complications have been resolved and it is safe to apply a cast. Immobilization with traction will be maintained until the bone ends are in satisfactory realignment, after which a less confining type of immobilization—a cast, pins, or external stabilization device—will be applied.

Types of Traction (General)

The pull needed for traction can be applied to the distal bone fragment in several ways (Box 31-3). The type of traction applied is determined primarily by the age of the child, the condition of the soft tissues, and the type and degree of displacement of the fracture. Fractures most commonly treated by application of traction are those involving the humerus, femur, and vertebrae. The major types of traction for specific fractures are discussed in the following sections.

Upper Extremity Traction

Treatment of fractures of the humerus by traction is accomplished by (1) *overhead suspension,* in which the arm, bent at the elbow, is suspended vertically by skin or skeletal attachment and traction is applied to the distal end of the humerus, or (2) Dunlop traction. With *Dunlop traction* (Fig. 31-6), the arm is suspended horizontally, using either skin or skeletal attachment. A skeletal wire placed in the upper arm to allow additional weight may be applied in certain instances, such as a supracondylar fracture. When skin traction is used, straps are placed on the lower and upper arm with the arm flexed to accomplish pull in two directions: one along the longitudinal direction of the upper arm and one to maintain vertical alignment of the lower arm.

Fractures of the humerus, which usually result from a fall with the arm in extension, frequently involve the supracondylar portion. These fractures especially place the patient at risk for nerve damage and angulation deformities; therefore, the fractures must be reduced carefully, sometimes with the patient under anesthesia. Because of the danger of complications, children with closed reduction of supracondylar fractures require close observation for neurovascular status and may need hospitalization. In severely malaligned fractures, closed reduction and pinning with the patient under anesthesia is followed by application of skeletal traction for a given period and then casting.

Lower Extremity Traction

The frequent site for a femoral fracture is in the middle third of the shaft. With this fracture there may be significant overriding but minimal displacement. In a fracture in the lower one third of the shaft, the pull of the gastrocnemius muscle causes the distal fragment to become downwardly displaced.

Fractures of the femur can often be reduced with immediate application of a hip spica cast in young children. When traction is required, several types may be used, based on the initial assessment.

Bryant traction is a type of running traction in which the pull is only in one direction. Skin traction is applied to the legs, which are flexed at a 90-degree angle at the hips. The child's trunk (buttocks are raised slightly off the bed) provides countertraction.

BOX 31-3 ■ Types of Traction

Manual traction—Applied to the body part by the hand placed distally to the fracture site. Manual traction may be provided during application of a cast but more commonly when a closed reduction is performed.

Skin traction—Applied directly to the skin surface and indirectly to the skeletal structures. The pulling mechanism is attached to the skin with adhesive material or an elastic bandage. Both types are applied over soft, foam-backed traction straps to distribute the traction pull.

Skeletal traction—Applied directly to the skeletal structure by a pin, wire, or tongs inserted into or through the diameter of the bone distal to the fracture.

Buck extension (Fig. 31-7) is a type of skin traction with the legs in an extended position. Except for fracture cases, turning from side to side with care is permitted, to maintain the involved leg alignment. Buck extension is used primarily for short-term immobilization, preoperatively with dislocated hips, for correcting contractures, or for bone deformities such as Legg-Calvé-Perthes disease.

Russell traction (Fig. 31-8) uses skin traction on the lower leg and a padded sling under the knee. Two lines of pull, one along the longitudinal line of the lower leg and one perpendicular to the leg, are produced. This combination of pulls allows realignment of the lower extremity and immobilizes the hip and knee in a flexed position. The hip flexion must be kept at the prescribed angle to prevent fracture malalignment, because there is no direct support under the fracture and the skin traction may slip. Special nursing measures include carefully checking the position of the traction so that the amount of desired hip flexion is maintained and damage to the common peroneal nerve under the knee does not produce footdrop.

The most common skeletal traction is *90-degree-traction* (Fig. 31-9). The lower leg is supported by a boot cast or a calf sling, and a skeletal Steinmann pin or Kirschner wire is placed in the distal fragment of the femur, resulting in a 90-degree angle at both the hip and the knee. From a nursing standpoint, this traction facilitates position changes, toileting, and prevention of complications related to traction (Houston, 1996).

Balance suspension traction (Fig. 31-10) may be used with or without skin or skeletal traction. Unless used with another traction, the balanced suspension merely suspends the leg in a desired flexed position to relax the hip and hamstring muscles and does not exert any traction directly on a body part. A *Thomas splint* extends from the groin to midair above the foot, and a *Pearson attachment* supports the lower leg. Towels or pieces of felt covered with stockinette are clipped or pinned to the splints for leg support. When the child is lifted off the bed, the traction lifts with the child without loss of alignment. This traction requires very careful checking of splints and ropes to make certain that no slippage or fraying has occurred. The traction is of great value in an older and heavier child when it is essential to lift the patient for care.

Cervical Traction

The cervical area is a vulnerable site for flexion or extension injuries to muscle, vertebrae, or the spinal cord. Cervical muscle trauma without other complications is treated with a cer-

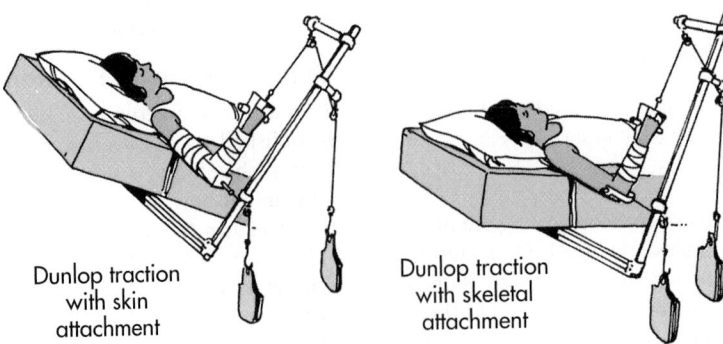

Dunlop traction
with skin
attachment

Dunlop traction
with skeletal
attachment

FIG. 31-6 ■ Dunlop traction. (Redrawn from Hilt NE, Schmitt EW: *Pediatric orthopedic nursing,* St Louis, 1975, Mosby.)

vical hard collar to relieve the weight of the head from the fracture site. When a child displaces or fractures a cervical vertebra, it may be necessary to reduce and immobilize the site with cervical skeletal traction. The spinal cord runs through the intravertebral canal, and dislocation or fracture of the vertebrae can also cause spinal cord injury. Nursing assessment of neurologic function is essential to prevent further injury during the application and use of cervical skeletal traction.

Most cervical traction is accomplished with the use of a *halo brace or halo vest.* This device consists of a steel halo attached to the head by four screws inserted into the outer skull; several rigid bars connect the halo to a vest that is worn around the chest, thus providing greater mobility of the rest of the body while avoiding cervical spinal motion altogether. If the injury has been limited to a vertebral fracture without neurologic deficit, a halo brace can be applied to permit earlier ambulation.

Cervical traction may also be accomplished by the insertion of *Crutchfield, Barton, or Gardner-Wells tongs* through

burr holes in the skull and weights attached to the hyperextended head (Fig. 31-11). As the neck muscles fatigue with constant traction pull, the vertebral bodies gradually separate so that the cord is no longer pinched between the vertebrae. Immobilization until fracture healing or surgical fixation can occur is an essential goal of cervical traction.

Nursing Considerations

To assess the child in traction, it is essential to know the purpose for which the traction is applied and to understand the basic principles of traction. Regular assessment of both the child and the traction apparatus is required (see Guidelines box). Many of the nursing problems associated with a child in traction are related to immobility.

When indicated by the attending practitioner, the nurse may remove nonadhesive skin traction. In these cases inter-

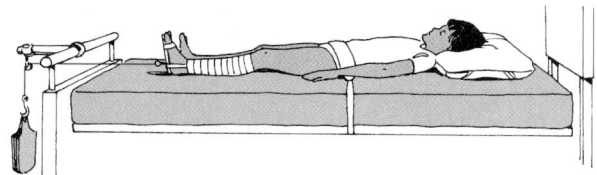

FIG. 31-7 ■ Buck extension traction. (Redrawn from Hilt NE, Schmitt EW: *Pediatric orthopedic nursing,* St Louis, 1975, Mosby.)

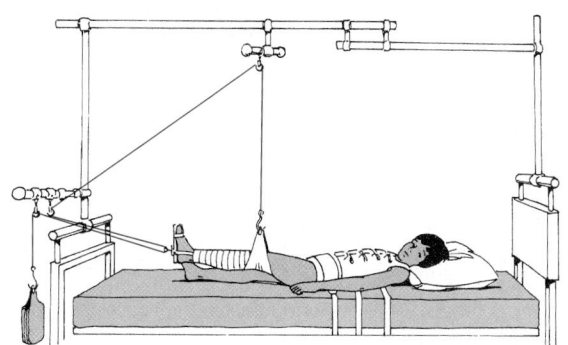

FIG. 31-8 ■ Russell traction. (Redrawn from Hilt NE, Schmitt EW: *Pediatric orthopedic nursing,* St Louis, 1975, Mosby.)

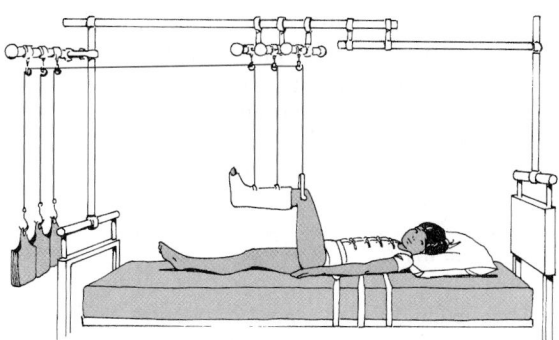

FIG. 31-9 ■ Ninety-ninety traction. (Redrawn from Hilt NE, Schmitt EW: *Pediatric orthopedic nursing,* St Louis, 1975, Mosby.)

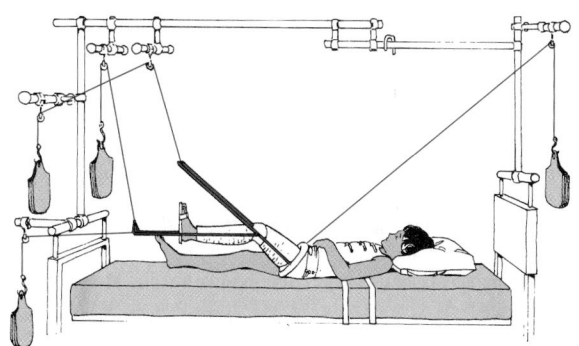

FIG. 31-10 ■ Balanced suspension with Thomas ring splint and Pearson attachment. (Redrawn from Hilt NE, Schmitt EW: *Pediatric orthopedic nursing,* St Louis, 1975, Mosby.)

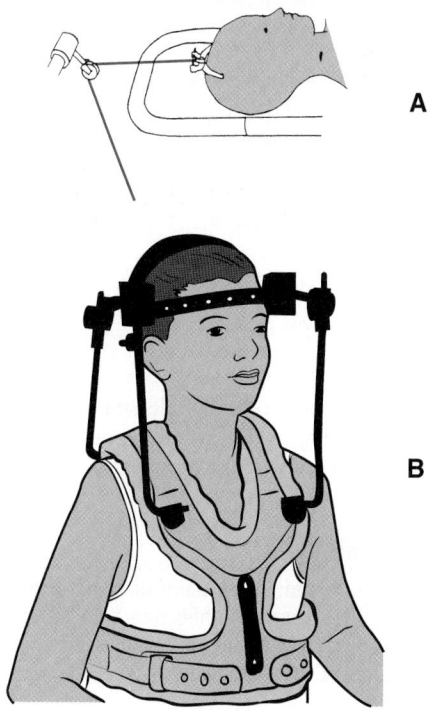

FIG. 31-11 ■ **A,** Crutchfield tong traction. **B,** Halo vest. (**A,** Redrawn from Hilt NE, Schmitt EW: *Pediatric orthopedic nursing,* St Louis, 1975, Mosby.)

GUIDELINES

Traction Care

UNDERSTAND THERAPY
Understand purpose of traction.
Understand function of traction in each specific situation.

MAINTAIN TRACTION
Check desired line of pull and relationship of distal fragment to proximal fragment.
  Check whether fragment is being directed upward, adducted, or abducted.
Check function of each component.
  Position of bandages, frames, splints
  Ropes:
    In center tract of pulley, taut, no fraying, knots tied securely
  Pulleys:
    In original position on attachment bar; have not slid from original site
    Wheels freely movable
  Weights:
    Correct amount of weight
    Hanging freely
    In safe location
Check bed position—head or foot elevated as directed for desired amount of pull and countertraction.
Do not remove skeletal traction or adhesive traction straps on skin traction.

MAINTAIN ALIGNMENT
Observe for correct body alignment with emphasis on alignment of shoulder, hip, and leg.
Check after child has moved.
Maintain correct angles at joints.

SKIN TRACTION
Replace nonadhesive straps or elastic bandage on skin traction *when permitted* or absolutely necessary, but make certain that traction on limb is maintained by someone during procedure.
Assess bandages to ascertain if they are correctly applied (diagonal or spiral), not too loose or too tight, which could cause slippage and malalignment of traction.

SKELETAL TRACTION
Check pin sites frequently for signs of bleeding, inflammation, or infection.
Cleanse and dress pin sites per institution protocol or as ordered.
Apply topical antiseptic or antibiotic daily as ordered.
Cover ends of pins with protective cord or padding to prevent child's being scratched by pin.
Note pull of traction on pin; pull should be even.
Check pin screws to be certain that screws are tight in metal clamp that attaches traction apparatus to pin.

PREVENT SKIN BREAKDOWN
Provide alternating-pressure mattress underneath hips and back.
Make total-body skin checks for redness or breakdown, especially over areas that receive greatest pressure.
Wash and dry skin at least daily.
Inspect pressure points daily or more often if risk for breakdown is observed.
Use a skin breakdown assessment scale such as Modified Braden Q.
Stimulate circulation with gentle massage over pressure areas.
Change position at least every 2 hours to relieve pressure.

PREVENT COMPLICATIONS
Check pulses in affected area and compare with pulses in contralateral site.
Assess circular dressings for excessive tightness.
Assess restrictive bandages or devices used to maintain traction on affected limb.
  Make certain that they are not too loose or too tight.
  Remove periodically and check for skin breakdown or pressure areas.
Encourage deep breathing or use of incentive spirometer.
Note any neurovascular changes, such as:
  Color in skin and nail beds
  Alterations in sensation, increased pain
  Alterations in motor ability
Take immediate action to correct problem or report to practitioner if neurovascular changes are found.
Record findings of neurovascular changes.
Carry out passive, active, or active-with-resistance exercises of uninvolved joints.
Note if any tightness, weakness, or contractures are developing in uninvolved joints and muscles.
Take measures to correct or prevent further development of weakness, such as applying footboard to prevent footdrop.

---

mittent traction is periodically released and reapplied as ordered. A child may have several types of traction at one time, and each traction must be assessed separately to avoid problems.

NURSING ALERT

Skeletal traction should be maintained as originally set by the orthopedist. When the child needs to be moved in the bed or if the traction needs to be adjusted or released for any other reason, an orthopedist is consulted.

In addition to routine skin observation and care, the child in skeletal traction will need special skin care at the pin site according to hospital policy or practitioner preference.

Frequent pin care and assessment of the insertion and exit sites is important to prevent infection. The best choice for pin cleansing agent, frequency, crust removal, and dressing application has yet to be determined by research (Bernardo, 2001). A pressure reduction device, such as a special air mattress, reduces the chance of skin breakdown.

NURSING TIP

A small hand mirror facilitates visualization of inaccessible skin areas.

When the child is first placed in traction, an increase in discomfort is common as a result of the traction pull fatiguing the muscle. It has been determined that orthopedic conditions are associated with a higher-than-average number of painful events and a higher percentage of bodily symptoms than other common conditions. Intravenous opioids, including analgesics and muscle relaxants, help during this phase of care and should be administered liberally.

> **NURSING ALERT**
>
> For skeletal traction to be effective, ensure that the weights are hanging freely at all times.

The specific nursing responsibilities for the patient in traction are outlined in the Guidelines box.

DISTRACTION

Unlike traction, which helps bones realign and fuse properly, *distraction* is the process of separating opposing bone to encourage regeneration of new bone in the created space. Distraction can also be used when limbs are of unequal lengths and new bone is needed to elongate the shorter limb.

External Fixation

The *Ilizarov external fixator (IEF)* is a common external fixation device. The IEF uses a system of wires, rings, and telescoping rods that permits limb lengthening to occur by manual distraction. In addition to lengthening bones, the device can be used to correct angular or rotational defects or to immobilize fractures (Gugenheim, 2000). The device is attached surgically by securing a series of external full or half rings to the bone with wires. External telescoping rods connect the rings to each other. Manual distraction is accomplished by manipulating the rods to increase the distance between the rings. A percutaneous ostomy is performed when the device is applied to create a "false" growth plate. A special osteotomy or corticotomy involves cutting only the cortex of the bone while preserving its blood supply, bone marrow, endosteum, and periosteum. Capillary blood flow to the transected area is essential for proper bone growth. Cut bone ends typically grow at a rate of 1 cm/month. The IEF can result in up to a 15-cm gain in length.

Nursing Considerations

Success of the IEF depends on the child's and family's cooperation; therefore, before surgery they must be fully informed of the appearance of the device, how it accomplishes bone growth and limits bone mobility, alterations in activities, and home and follow-up care. Children are involved in learning to adjust the device to accomplish distraction. Children, as well as parents, should be instructed in pin care, including observation for infection and loosening of the pins. Cleaning routines for the pin sites vary among practitioners but should not traumatize the skin.

Children who participate actively in their care report less discomfort. Because the device is external, the child and family need to be prepared for the reactions of others and assisted in camouflaging the device with appropriate apparel, such as wide-legged pants that close with self-adhering fasteners around the device (Fig. 31-12). A loose sock or stockinette may also be used over the device to decrease public awareness. Partial weight bearing is allowed, and the child learns to walk with crutches. Alterations in activity in-

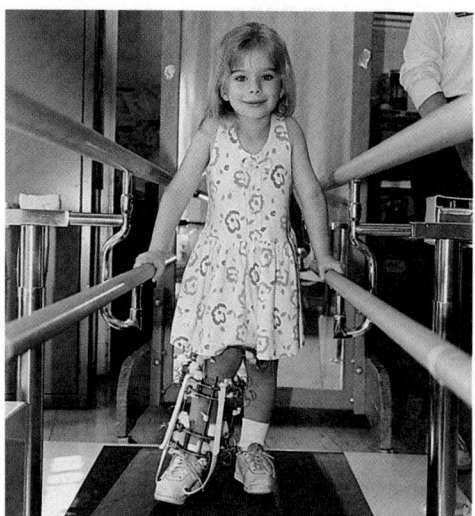

FIG. 31-12 ■ Child with Ilizarov external fixator (on right leg) during physical therapy on parallel bars

clude modifications at school and in physical education. Full weight bearing is not allowed until the distraction is completed and bone consolidation has occurred. Follow-up care is essential to maintaining appropriate distraction until the desired limb length is achieved. The device is removed surgically after the bone has consolidated, and the child may need to use crutches or have a cast for 4 to 6 weeks following removal.

AMPUTATION

A child may be born with the congenital absence of a body part, have a traumatic loss of an extremity, or need a surgical amputation for a pathologic condition such as *osteosarcoma* (see p. 1179). With today's surgical technology and the quick thinking of bystanders who save a traumatically amputated body part, some children have had fingers and arms sewn back on with variable degrees of functional use regained.

> **NURSING ALERT**
>
> For an amputated limb or body part that may be reattached, do the following:
>   Rinse limb gently with normal saline
>   Loosely wrap limb in sterile gauze
>   Place wrapped limb in a watertight bag
>   Cool (without freezing) bag in ice water (do not pack in ice because this may harm tissue)
>   Label with child's name, date and time, and transport with the child to the hospital

Surgical amputation or the surgical repair of a permanently severed limb focuses on constructing an adequately nourished stump. A smooth, healthy, padded stump, free of nerve endings, is important in prosthesis fitting and subsequent ambulation. In some situations in which there is no vascular or neurologic deficit, a cast is applied to the stump immediately after the procedure, and a pylon, metal extension, and artificial foot are attached so that the patient can walk on the temporary prosthesis within a few hours.

Nursing Considerations

Stump shaping is done postoperatively with special elastic bandaging using a figure-eight bandage, which applies pressure in a cone-shaped fashion. This technique decreases stump edema, controls hemorrhage, and aids in developing desired contours so that the child will bear weight on the posterior aspect of the skin flap rather than on the end of the stump. Stump elevation may be used during the first 24 hours, but after this time the extremity should not be left in this position, because contractures in the proximal joint will develop and seriously hamper ambulation. Monitoring proper body alignment will further decrease the risk of flexion contractures.

For older children and adolescents, arm exercises and bed pushups, as well as using parallel bars for prosthesis-training programs, help build up the arm muscles necessary for walking with crutches. Full range-of-motion exercises of joints above the amputation must be performed several times daily, using active and isotonic exercises. Young children are spontaneously active and require little encouragement.

Depending on the age of the child, children or their parents will need to learn stump hygiene, including careful soap and water washing every day and checking for skin irritation, breakdown, or infection. A tube of stockinette or powder is used to slide the prosthesis on more easily. Skin must be checked carefully every time the prosthesis is removed, and prosthesis tolerance time must be adjusted to prevent skin breakdown.

For children who have had an amputation, *phantom limb sensation* is an expected experience because the nerve-brain connections are still present. Gradually these sensations fade, although in many amputees they persist for years. Preoperative discussion of this phenomenon will aid a child in understanding these "unusual feelings" and not hiding the experiences from others. Limb pain, especially pain that increases with ambulation, should be evaluated for the possibility of a neuroma at the free nerve endings in the stump, or other problems such as a poorly fitting prosthesis or joint instability.

CONGENITAL DEFECTS

Some skeletal defects may be diagnosed at birth or within days, weeks, or months after birth. In other cases the deviation may be difficult to detect without careful inspection. Therefore it is imperative that nurses become acquainted with signs of these defects and understand the principles of therapy in order to direct others in the care and management of these children.

DEVELOPMENTAL DYSPLASIA OF THE HIP

The broad term *developmental dysplasia of the hip (DDH)* describes a spectrum of disorders related to abnormal development of the hip that may develop at any time during fetal life, infancy, or childhood. A change in terminology from congenital hip dysplasia (CHD) and congenital dislocation of the hip (CDH) to DDH more properly reflects a variety of hip abnormalities in which there is a shallow acetabulum, subluxation, or dislocation.

The incidence of hip instability of some kind is approximately 10 per 1000 live births. The incidence of frank dislocation or a dislocatable hip is 1 per 1000 live births (Wall, 2000), and approximately 30% to 50% of infants with DDH are born breech (Thompson, 2004a). The left hip is involved in 60% of cases, the right hip in 20%, and both hips in 20%. Sixty percent of the patients are girls. Caucasian children have a higher incidence of developmental dysplasia than other groups (Maher, Salmond, and Pellino, 2002).

Pathophysiology

The cause of DDH is unknown, but certain factors such as gender, birth order, family history, intrauterine position, delivery type, joint laxity, and postnatal positioning are believed to affect the risk of DDH. Predisposing factors associated with DDH may be divided into three broad categories: (1) physiologic factors, which include maternal hormone secretion and intrauterine positioning; (2) mechanical factors, which involve breech presentation, multiple fetus, oligohydramnios, and large infant size (other mechanical factors may include continued maintenance of the hips in adduction and extension that will in time cause a dislocation) and (3) genetic factors, which entail a higher incidence (6%) of DDH in siblings of affected infants and an even greater incidence (36%) of recurrence if a sibling and one parent were affected.

Some experts categorize DDH into two major groups: (1) *typical,* in which the infant is neurologically intact, and (2) *teratologic,* which involves a neuromuscular defect such as arthrogryposis or myelodysplasia (Thompson, 2004a). The teratologic forms usually occur in utero and are much less common.

Three degrees of DDH are illustrated in Fig. 31-13:

1 **Acetabular dysplasia** (or **preluxation**)—Mildest form of DDH in which there is neither subluxation nor dislocation. There is a delay in acetabular development evidenced by osseous hypoplasia of the acetabular roof that is oblique and shallow, although the cartilaginous roof is comparatively intact. The femoral head remains in the acetabulum.
2 **Subluxation**—The largest percentage of DDH, subluxation, implies incomplete dislocation of the hip and is sometimes regarded as an intermediate state in the development from primary dysplasia to complete dislocation. The femoral head remains in contact with the acetabulum, but a stretched capsule and ligamentum teres cause the head of the femur to be partially displaced. Pressure on the cartilaginous roof inhibits ossification and produces a flattening of the socket.
3 **Dislocation**—The femoral head loses contact with the acetabulum and is displaced posteriorly and superiorly over the fibrocartilaginous rim. The ligamentum teres is elongated and taut.

Factors related to infant handling are indicated in the Cultural Awareness box.

Diagnostic Evaluation

DDH is often not detected at the initial examination after birth; thus, all infants should be carefully monitored for hip dysplasia at follow-up visits throughout the first year of life. In the newborn period dysplasia usually appears as hip joint laxity rather than as outright dislocation (Fig. 31-14). Subluxation and the tendency to dislocate can be demonstrated by the Ortolani or Barlow tests (Fig. 31-14, *B, C,* and *D*).

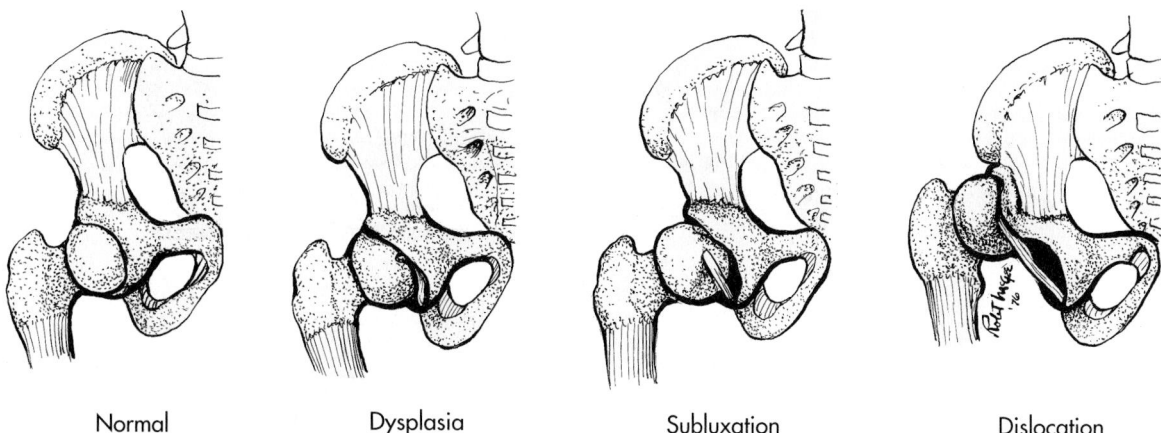

| Normal | Dysplasia | Subluxation | Dislocation |

FIG. 31-13 ■ Configuration and relationship of structures in developmental dysplasia of the hip

CULTURAL AWARENESS

Developmental Dysplasia of the Hip

A striking relationship exists between the development of the dislocation and methods of handling infants. Among the cultures with the highest incidence of dislocation, newly born infants are tightly wrapped in blankets or other swaddling material or are strapped to cradle boards. In cultures such as the Far East, where mothers traditionally carry infants on their backs or hips in the widely abducted straddle position, the disorder is virtually unknown.

The Ortolani and Barlow tests are most reliable from birth to 2 or 3 months of age. Other signs of DDH are shortening of the limb on the affected side (Galeazzi sign, Allis sign) (Fig. 31-14, *C*), asymmetric thigh and gluteal folds (Fig 31-14, *A*), and broadening of the perineum (in bilateral dislocation) (Box 31-4).

! NURSING ALERT

These tests must be performed by an experienced clinician to prevent fracture or other damage to the hip. If these tests are performed too vigorously in the first 2 days of life, when the hip subluxates freely, persistent dislocation may occur.

Radiographic examination in early infancy is not reliable, because ossification of the femoral head does not normally take place until the third to sixth month of life. However, the cartilaginous head can be visualized directly by ultrasonography. There has been debate regarding the role of ultrasound technology in diagnosing DDH in early infancy, and widespread newborn screening has been suggested; however, numerous studies reveal this approach has a high rate of false positives and subsequent overtreatment. Some experts suggest that ultrasound be used to screen hips at 2 weeks after birth in infants with clinical signs of DDH and infants with a higher risk of DDH, and to monitor the efficacy of treatment in infants with DDH (Roberts and others, 2002). In infants older than age 4 months and in children, radiographic examination is useful in confirming the diagnosis. An upward slope in the roof of the acetabulum (the acetabular angle) greater than 40 degrees

with upward and outward displacement of the femoral head is a frequent finding in older children. Computed tomography (CT) scan may be useful to assess the position of the femoral head relative to the acetabulum after closed reduction and casting.

Therapeutic Management

Treatment is begun as soon as the condition is recognized, because early intervention is more favorable to the restoration of normal bony architecture and function. The longer treatment is delayed, the more severe the deformity, the more difficult the treatment, and the less favorable the prognosis. The treatment varies with the age of the child and the extent of the dysplasia. The goal of treatment is to obtain and maintain a safe, congruent position of the hip joint to promote normal hip joint development.

Newborn to Age 6 Months. The hip joint is maintained by dynamic splinting in a safe position with the proximal femur centered in the acetabulum in an attitude of flexion. Of the numerous devices available, the *Pavlik harness* is the most widely used, and with time, motion, and gravity, the hip works into a more abducted, reduced position (Fig. 31-15). The harness is worn continuously until the hip is proved stable on clinical and radiographic examination, usually in about 3 to 5 months.

When adduction contracture is present, other devices (such as skin traction) are used to slowly and gently stretch the hip to full abduction, after which wide abduction is maintained until stability is attained. When there is difficulty in maintaining stable reduction, a hip spica cast is applied and changed periodically to accommodate the child's growth. After 3 to 6 months, sufficient stability is acquired to allow transfer to a removable protective abduction brace. The duration of treatment depends on development of the acetabulum but is usually accomplished within the first year.

Ages 6 to 18 Months. In this age-group the dislocation is not recognized until the child begins to stand and walk, when attendant shortening of the limb and contractures of hip adductor and flexor muscles become apparent. Gradual reduction by traction is used for approximately 3 weeks. An individualized home traction program may be developed

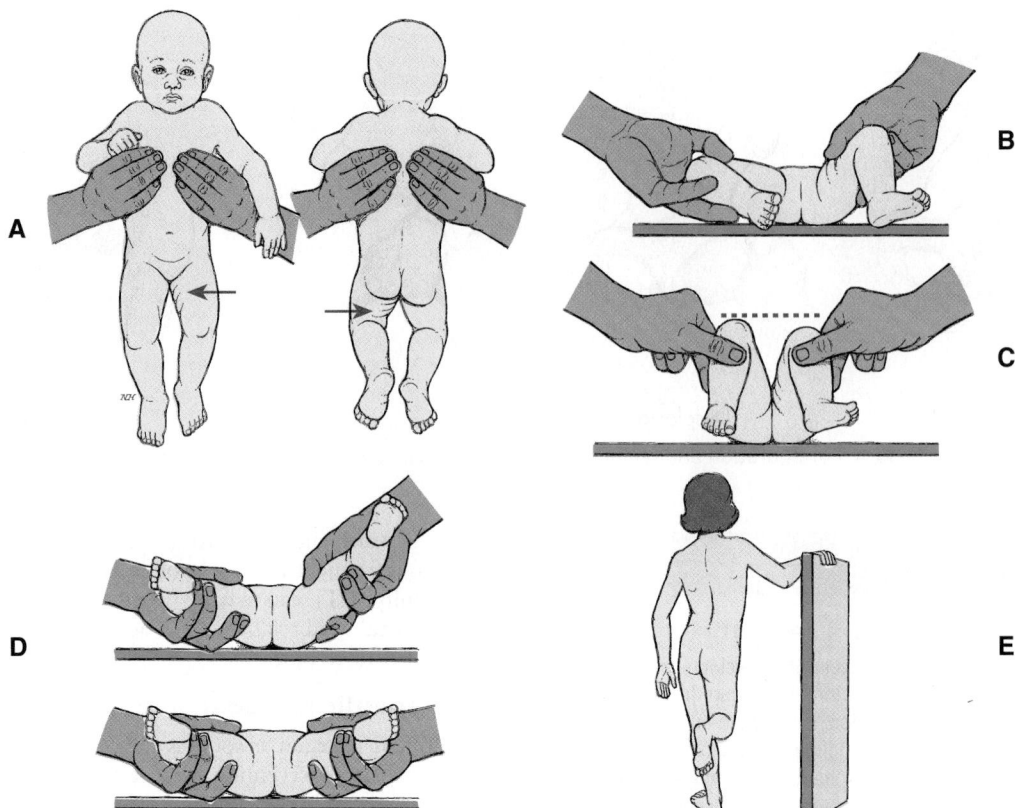

FIG. 31-14 ■ Signs of developmental dysplasia of the hip. **A,** Asymmetry of gluteal and thigh folds (Galeazzi sign). **B,** Limited hip abduction, as seen in flexion. **C,** Apparent shortening of the femur, as indicated by the level of the knees in flexion. **D,** Ortolani test clunk (in infants 1 to 2 months old). **E,** Positive Trendelenburg sign or gait (if child is weight bearing)

BOX 31-4 ■ Clinical Manifestations of Developmental Dysplasia of the Hip

INFANT
Shortening of limb on affected side (Galeazzi sign, Allis sign)
Restricted abduction of hip on affected side
Unequal gluteal folds (infant prone)
Positive Ortolani test
Positive Barlow test

OLDER INFANT AND CHILD
Affected leg shorter than the other
Telescoping or piston mobility of joint
    Head of femur can be felt to move up and down in buttock
      when extended thigh is pushed first toward child's head and
      then pulled distally
Trendelenburg sign
    When child stands first on one foot and then on the other
      (holding onto a chair, rail, or someone's hands) bearing
      weight on affected hip, pelvis tilts downward on normal side
      instead of upward, as it would with normal stability
Greater trochanter is prominent and appears above a line from
    anterior superior iliac spine to tuberosity of ischium
Marked lordosis (bilateral dislocations)
Waddling gait (bilateral dislocations)

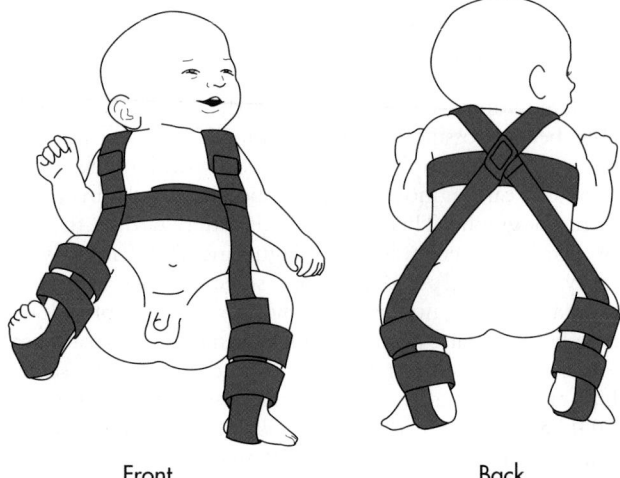

Front   Back

FIG. 31-15 ■ Child in Pavlik harness. (From Ball JW: *Mosby's pediatric patient teaching guides,* St Louis, 1998, Mosby.)

for the child preoperatively to decrease the length of hospitalization and maintain the home environment. The child then undergoes an attempted closed reduction of the hip using general anesthesia; if the hip is not reducible, an open reduction is performed. After reduction, the child is placed in a hip spica cast for 2 to 4 months until the hip is stable, at which time a flexion-abduction brace is applied.

Older Child.   Correction of the hip deformity in older children is inherently more difficult than in the preceding age-groups, because secondary adaptive changes and other etiologic factors (such as juvenile rheumatoid arthritis or nonambulatory cerebral palsy) complicate the condition. Operative reduction, which may involve preoperative traction, tenotomy of contracted muscles, and any one of several innominate osteotomy procedures designed to construct an acetabular roof, is usually required. After cast removal and before weight bearing is permitted, range-of-motion exercises help restore movement. Successful reduction and reconstruction become increasingly difficult after the age of 4 years and are usually impossible or inadvisable in children older than 6 years of age because of severe shortening and contracture of muscles and deformity of the femoral and acetabular structures.

Nursing Considerations

Nurses are in a unique position to detect DDH in early infancy. During the infant assessment process and routine nurturing activities the hips and extremities are inspected for any deviations from normal. These observations are reported to the attending practitioner, and the ambulatory child who displays a limp or an unusual gait should be referred for evaluation. This may indicate an orthopedic or neurologic problem. Nonambulatory children with cerebral palsy should also be assessed for evidence of dislocation.

The major nursing problems in the care of an infant or child in a cast or other device are related to maintenance of the device and adaptation of nurturing activities to meet the needs of the infant or child. Generally, treatment and follow-up care of these children are carried out in a clinic, practitioner's office, or outpatient unit. Hospitalization may be necessary for cast application or brace fitting but seldom exceeds 24 to 48 hours. Longer hospitalization is required for open reduction.

> **⚠ NURSING ALERT**
>
> The former practice of double- or triple-diapering for DDH is not recommended because it promotes hip extension, thus worsening proper hip development.

The primary nursing goal is teaching parents to apply and maintain the reduction device. The Pavlik harness allows for easy handling of the infant and usually produces less apprehension in the parent than heavy braces and casts. Because of the infant's rapid growth, the straps should be checked every 1 to 2 weeks for possible adjustments. It is important that parents understand the correct use of the appliance, which may or may not allow for its removal during bathing. Unbuckling or removal of the harness is determined individually on the basis of the family's level of understanding and the degree of deformity in the hip. In general, parents should not adjust the harness without supervision. The child should be examined by the practitioner before any adjustment is attempted to make certain the hips are in correct placement before the harness is resecured.

Casts and orthotic devices (braces) offer more challenging nursing and caregiver problems, because they cannot be removed for routine care, although sometimes a brace may be removed for bathing. Care of an infant or small child with a cast requires nursing innovation to reduce irritation and to maintain cleanliness of both the child and the cast, particularly in the diaper area. (See p. 1156 for care of the child in a cast.)

It is important for nurses, parents, and other caregivers to understand that children in corrective devices need to be involved in all the activities of any child in the same age-group. Confinement in a cast or appliance should not exclude children from family (or unit) activities. They can be held astride the lap for comfort and transported to areas of activity. The child may be allowed to walk in a cast or orthotic device. An adapted wheelchair, stroller, or scooter can offer mobility to the older infant or child.

CONGENITAL CLUBFOOT

Congenital *clubfoot* is a complex deformity of the ankle and foot that includes forefoot adduction, midfoot supination, hindfoot varus, and ankle equinus. Deformities of the foot and ankle are described according to the position of the ankle and foot. The more common positions involve the following variations:

- **Talipes varus**—An inversion or a bending inward
- **Talipes valgus**—An eversion or bending outward
- **Talipes equinus**—Plantar flexion in which the toes are lower than the heel
- **Talipes calcaneus**—Dorsiflexion, in which the toes are higher than the heel

Most cases of clubfoot are a combination of these positions, and the most frequently occurring type of clubfoot (approximately 95% of cases) is the composite deformity *talipes equinovarus (TEV),* in which the foot is pointed downward and inward in varying degrees of severity (Fig. 31-16). Unilateral clubfoot is somewhat more common than bilateral clubfoot and may occur as an isolated defect or in association with other disorders or syndromes, such as chromosomal aberrations, arthrogryposis (a generalized immobility of the joints), cerebral palsy, or spina bifida.

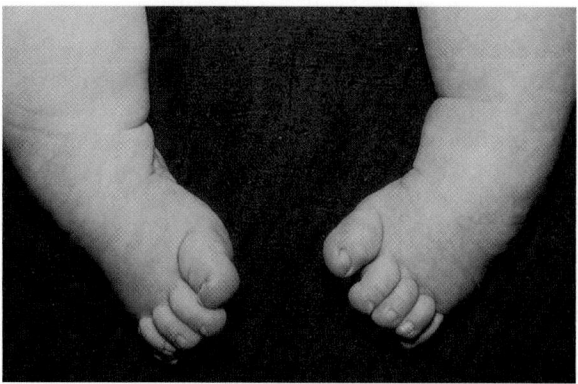

FIG. 31-16 ■ Bilateral congenital talipes equinovarus (congenital clubfoot) in 2-month-old infant. (From Zitelli BJ, Davis HW: *Atlas of pediatric physical diagnosis,* ed 4, St Louis, 2002, Mosby.)

The incidence of clubfoot in the general population is 1 to 2 per 1000 live births, with boys affected twice as often as girls. Bilateral clubfeet occur in 50% of the cases (Gilmore and Thompson, 2003). The precise cause of clubfoot is unknown. Some authorities attribute the defect to abnormal positioning and restricted movement in utero, although the evidence is not conclusive. Other experts implicate arrested or abnormal embryonic development. Arrested development during this early stage tends to result in a rigid deformity, whereas mechanical pressures from intrauterine positioning are likely causes of more flexible deformities.

Classification

The literature describes three major categories of clubfoot: (1) positional clubfoot (also called transitional, mild, or postural clubfoot), which is believed to occur primarily from intrauterine crowding and responds to simple stretching and casting; (2) syndromic (or teratologic) clubfoot, which is associated with other congenital anomalies such as myelomeningocele or arthrogryposis and is a more severe form of clubfoot that is often resistant to treatment; and (3) congenital clubfoot, also referred to as idiopathic, which may occur in an otherwise normal child and has a wide range of rigidity and prognosis.

The mild, or postural, clubfoot may correct spontaneously or may require passive exercise or serial casting. There is no bony abnormality, but there may be tightness and shortening of the soft tissues medially and posteriorly. The teratologic clubfoot is associated with other congenital anomalies such as myelodysplasia or arthrogryposis. These feet usually require surgical correction and have a high incidence of recurrence. The congenital idiopathic clubfoot, or "true clubfoot," almost always requires surgical intervention because there is bony abnormality.

Diagnostic Evaluation

The deformity is readily apparent and easily detected prenatally through ultrasonography or at birth. However, it must be differentiated from some positional deformities that can be passively corrected or overcorrected. Paralytic changes in the lower extremity of children with neuromuscular involvement often produce equinovarus deformity. An increased risk of hip dysplasia is associated with clubfoot deformities.

Therapeutic Management

The goal of treatment for clubfoot is to achieve a painless, plantigrade, and stable foot. Treatment of clubfoot involves three stages: (1) correction of the deformity, (2) maintenance of the correction until normal muscle balance is regained, and (3) follow-up observation to avert possible recurrence of the deformity. Some feet respond to treatment readily; some respond only to prolonged, vigorous, and sustained efforts; and the improvement in others remains disappointing even with maximal effort on the part of all concerned.

Serial casting is begun shortly after birth, before discharge from the nursery. Successive casts allow for gradual stretching of skin and tight structures on the medial side of the foot (Fig. 31-17). Manipulation and casting are repeated frequently (every week) to accommodate the rapid growth of early infancy. The extremity or extremities are casted until maximum correction is achieved, usually within 8 to 12 weeks. A Denis Brown splint may be used to manage feet that correct with casting and manipulation. A radiograph or ultrasound is then evaluated to see the relationship of the bones to each other. Failure to achieve normal alignment by 3 months indicates the need for surgical intervention, which may take place between 6 and 12 months of age. The foot (or feet) is immobilized postoperatively for approximately 6 to 12 weeks, and the child is allowed to walk after the cast is removed (Gilmore and Thompson, 2003).

Nursing Considerations

Nursing care of the child with clubfoot is the same as for any child who has a cast (see p. 1156). Because the child will spend considerable time in a corrective device, nursing care plans include both long-term and short-term goals. Conscientious observation of the skin and circulation is particularly important in young infants because of their rapid growth rate. Because treatment and follow-up care are handled in the orthopedist's office, clinic, or outpatient department, parent education and support are important in nursing care of these children.

Parents need to understand the overall treatment program, the importance of regular cast changes, and the role they play in the long-term effectiveness of the therapy. Reinforcing and clarifying the orthopedist's explanations and instructions, teaching parents about care of the cast or appliance (including vigilant observation for potential problems), and encouraging parents to facilitate normal development within the limitations imposed by the deformity or therapy are all part of nursing responsibilities.

METATARSUS ADDUCTUS (VARUS)

Metatarsus adductus, or metatarsus varus, is probably the most common congenital foot deformity. In most instances it is a result of abnormal intrauterine positioning, particularly in the firstborn child, and is usually detected at birth. The deformity is characterized by medial adduction of the toes and forefoot, frequently in association with inversion, and by convexity of the lateral border of the foot. Metatarsus adductus may be divided into three categories: type I, in

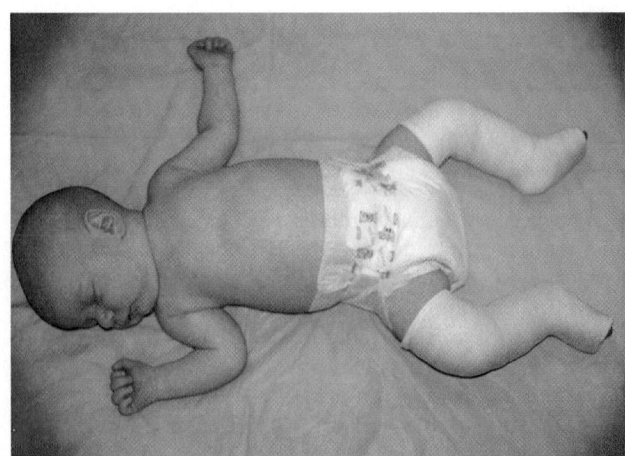

FIG. 31-17 ■ Feet casted for correction of bilateral talipes equinovarus.

which the forefoot is flexible and corrects easily with manipulation; type II, in which there is only partial flexibility in the forefoot and it corrects passively past neutral position but only to neutral position with active manipulation; and type III, in which the forefoot is rigid and will not stretch to neutral position with manipulation (Gilmore and Thompson, 2003). Unlike TEV, with which it is often confused, the angulation occurs at the tarsometatarsal joint, whereas the heel and ankle remain in a neutral position. Ankle range of motion is normal. This deformity often causes a pigeon-toed gait in the child.

Management depends on the rigidity and type of the deformity. Correction can usually be accomplished by gentle manipulation and passive stretching of the foot with types I and II, which the parent is taught to perform. Repeated and consistent stretching is continued for the first 6 weeks, after which the treatment is based on the flexibility of the foot. With type III, the child will usually require serial manipulation and casting to correct the defect. Casting is performed every 1 to 2 weeks for 6 to 8 weeks, after which a corrective shoe or orthosis may be used. Surgical correction is rarely required for the condition (Gilmore and Thompson, 2003).

Nursing Considerations

The nursing role primarily involves identifying the defect, so that early therapy and instruction of the parents can be initiated. The nurse teaches the parents how to hold the heel firmly and to stretch only the forefoot; otherwise, undue force on the heel may produce a valgus deformity. If casting or orthosis is required, the nurse instructs the parents in cast care and observation of the corrective device (see p. 1156).

SKELETAL LIMB DEFICIENCY

Congenital limb deficiencies, or reduction malformations, are manifested by a variety of degrees of loss of functional capacity. They are characterized by underdevelopment of skeletal elements of the extremities. The range of malformation can extend from minor defects of the digits to serious abnormalities, such as *amelia,* absence of an entire extremity, or *meromelia,* partial absence of an extremity, which includes *phocomelia* (seal limbs), the interposed deficiency of long bones with relatively good development of hands and feet attached at or near the shoulder or the hips. Most reduction defects are primary defects of development of the limb, but prenatal destruction of the limb can occur, such as full or partial amputation of a limb in utero from constriction of an amniotic band *(amniotic band syndrome).*

Pathophysiology

Limb deficiencies can be attributed to both heredity and environment and can originate at any stage of limb development. Formation of limbs may be suppressed at the time of limb bud formation, or there may be interference in later stages of differentiation and growth. Heredity appears to play a prominent role, and prenatal environmental insults have been implicated in a number of cases, such as the well-publicized *thalidomide* tragedy of the 1950s and early 1960s, which demonstrated a clear relationship between the time of exposure of the pregnant woman to the antiemetic

drug and the presence and type of limb deformity in the newborn. There still are many drugs that may have similar *teratogenic* effects in the first trimester of pregnancy; therefore, medication administration during this period should be carefully evaluated by the practitioner. Unfortunately, during this period, the woman may not realize her pregnant condition unless the event is highly anticipated, and inadvertent consumption of harmful medications may occur. Deletion or shortening of digits or limbs may also be associated with *chorionic villus sampling,* especially before 10 to 12 weeks of gestation; however, the incidence and relationship remain uncertain.

Therapeutic Management

Children with congenital limb deficiencies should be fitted with prosthetic devices whenever possible, and the devices should be applied at the earliest possible stage of development in an attempt to match the motor readiness of the infant. This favors natural progression of prosthetic use. For example, an infant with an upper extremity deficiency is fitted with a simple passive device, such as a mitten prosthesis, to encourage limb exploration, sitting (with the extremities needed for support), and bilateral hand activities.

Lower limb prostheses are applied when the infant begins sitting up and can maintain balance. In preparation for prosthetic devices, surgical modification may be necessary to ensure the most favorable use of the device, because severe deformity can interfere with its effective use. Phocomelic digits are preserved for controlling switches of externally powered appliances in upper extremities. Digits (in both upper and lower extremities) provide the child with surfaces for tactile exploration and stimulation. Prostheses are replaced to accommodate growth and increasing capabilities of the child.

Nursing Considerations

Prosthetic application training and habilitation are most successfully carried out in a center that specializes in meeting the special needs of these children, especially very young children and those with amputations or missing limbs. It involves a *prosthetist,* who specializes in the development, fitting, and maintenance of prosthetic limbs, and other health care workers such as PTs and occupational therapists. Parents need special attention and support and are encouraged to assist the child in making age-commensurate adjustments to the environment. Although these children need assistance, excessive overprotection may produce overdependence, with later maladjustment to school and other situations.

OSTEOGENESIS IMPERFECTA

Osteogenesis imperfecta (OI) is the most common osteoporosis syndrome in children. OI is a heterogeneous, group-inherited syndrome characterized by excessive fractures and bone deformity. There are at least five types of OI, accounting for significant disease variability. Clinical features may include the following: varying degrees of bone fragility, deformity, and fracture; blue sclerae; hearing loss; and dentinogenesis imperfecta (hypoplastic discolored teeth). The inheritance pattern is autosomal dominant in the majority of cases, although the most severe form demonstrates autosomal-recessive inheritance (Box 31-5).

BOX 31-5 ■ Classification of Osteogenesis Imperfecta

TYPE		CHARACTERISTICS
I*	A	Mild bone fragility; blue sclerae; normal teeth; hearing loss (occurs between ages 20 and 30 years); autosomal-dominant inheritance
	B	Same as A except dentinogenesis imperfecta instead of normal teeth
	C	Same as B; no bone fragility
II		Lethal; stillborn or die in early infancy; severe bone fragility, multiple fractures at birth; 10% of cases of osteogenesis imperfecta (OI); autosomal recessive inheritance
III		Severe bone fragility leads to severe progressive deformities; normal sclerae; marked growth failure; most autosomal-recessive inheritance; few autosomal-dominant inheritance
IV	A	Mild to moderate bone fragility; normal sclerae; short stature; variable deformity; autosomal-dominant inheritance
	B	Same as A except dentinogenesis imperfecta instead of normal teeth; approximately 6% of cases of OI
V		Clinically similar to IV; hyperplastic callus; collagen mutation is negative

*Two thirds of cases are type I.

Most types of OI have defects in the COL1A1 or COL1A2 genes, which code for polypeptide chains in type 1 procollagen, a precursor of type 1 collagen, a major structural component of bone. The error results in faulty bone mineralization, abnormal bone architecture, and increased susceptibility to fracture.

There are several classifications for OI based on clinical features and patterns of inheritance (see Box 31-5). Clinically, type I is the most common, with wide variability of bone fragility; some affected family members have significant deformity and disability, whereas others lead agile active lives. Type II variants are the most severe and are considered lethal in infancy. Type III OI is characterized by multiple fractures, bone deformity, and severe disability; affected individuals rarely live to 30 years of age. Type IV is similar to type I with blue or white sclerae. A new variant, or type V, has been described in which those affected have a hyperplastic callus; no collagen mutations are noted in this group (Marini, 2004).

Therapeutic Management

The treatment for OI is primarily supportive, although patients and families are optimistic about new research advances. Bone marrow transplant for severe OI was first reported in 1999 with positive results; however, this is still considered an experimental treatment (Horwitz and others, 2001). The use of bisphosphonate therapy to promote increased bone density and prevent fractures is also being evaluated. Several studies report increased bone density and decreased bone pain and fractures with intravenous pamidronate, a potent inhibitor of bone resorption (Falk and others, 2003; Zeitlin, Fassier, and Glorieux, 2003).

The goals of a rehabilitative approach to management are directed to preventing (1) positional contractures and deformities, (2) muscle weakness and osteoporosis, and (3) malalignment of lower extremity joints prohibiting weight bearing.

Several medications have been tried but appear to be of limited benefit. Lightweight braces and splints help support limbs, prevent fractures, and aid in ambulation. Physical therapy helps prevent disuse osteoporosis and strengthens muscles, which in turn improves bone density.

Surgery is sometimes used to help treat the manifestations of the disease. Surgical techniques are used to correct deformities that interfere with bracing, standing, or walking. For the child with recurrent fractures, inserting an intramedullary rod provides stability to bones.

Nursing Considerations

Infants and children with this disorder require careful handling to prevent fractures. They must be supported when they are being turned, positioned, moved, and held. Even changing a diaper may cause a fracture in severely affected infants. These children should never be held by the ankles when being diapered but should be gently lifted by the buttocks or supported with pillows.

Both parents and the affected child need education regarding the child's limitations and guidelines in planning suitable activities that promote optimal development and protect the child from harm. Realistic occupational planning and genetic counseling are part of the long-term goals of care. Educational materials and information can be obtained from the **Osteogenesis Imperfecta Foundation, Inc.,*** which also has a network that can put a family in contact with other families with a similar problem.

OI is a differential diagnosis that must be ruled out in the event of multiple fractures that may be attributed to nonaccidental injury. A detailed history, no evidence of associated soft-tissue injury, and the presence of other symptoms related to OI help to determine the diagnosis.

> **NURSING ALERT**
>
> Children with current fractures or healing fractures should be screened for osteogenesis imperfecta—the assumption that abuse or neglect is the cause of fractures in children must be carefully evaluated by a multidisciplinary team.

ACQUIRED DEFECTS

LEGG-CALVÉ-PERTHES DISEASE

Legg-Calvé-Perthes disease (LCPD) is a self-limited juvenile idiopathic avascular necrosis of the femoral head. The disease affects children ages 2 to 12 but most commonly boys between 4 and 8 years of age. Unilateral hip involvement is present in 90% of cases, it rarely occurs in African Americans, and it has a worse prognosis when detected in older children and those with severe involvement (Greene, 2001).

Pathophysiology

The cause of the disease is unknown, but there is a disturbance of circulation to the femoral capital epiphysis that produces an ischemic aseptic necrosis of the femoral head.

---

*804 West Diamond Avenue, Suite 210, Gaithersburg, MD 20878; (800) 981-2663; website: www.oif.org.

BOX 31-6 ■ Stages of Legg-Calvé-Perthes Disease

Stage I: Aseptic necrosis or infarction of the femoral capital epiphysis with degenerative changes producing flattening of the upper surface of the femoral head—***the avascular stage***

Stage II: Capital bone absorption and revascularization with fragmentation (vascular resorption of the epiphysis) that gives a mottled appearance on radiographs—***the fragmentation, or revascularization, stage***

Stage III: New bone formation, which is represented on radiographs as calcification and ossification or increased density in the areas of radiolucency; this filling-in process appears to take place from the periphery of the head centrally—***the reparative stage***

Stage IV: Gradual reformation of the head of the femur without radiolucency and, it is hoped, to a spherical form—***the regenerative stage***

During middle childhood, circulation to the femoral epiphysis is more tenuous than at other ages and can become obstructed by trauma, inflammation, coagulation defects, and a variety of other causes. The pathologic events seem to take place in four stages (Box 31-6). The entire process may encompass as little as 18 months or continue for several years. The reformed femoral head may be severely altered or appear entirely normal.

Clinical Manifestations and Diagnostic Evaluation

The onset of LCPD is usually insidious, and the history may reveal only intermittent appearance of a limp on the affected side or a symptom complex including hip soreness, ache, or stiffness that can be constant or intermittent. The parents may report seeing the child limping, and the limp becomes more pronounced with increased activity. The pain may be experienced in the hip, along the entire thigh, or in the vicinity of the knee joint. The pain and limp are usually most evident on arising and at the end of a long day of activities. The pain is usually accompanied by joint dysfunction and limited range of motion. There may be a vague history of trauma. The diagnosis is established by radiographic examination, with the definitive diagnosis being magnetic resonance imaging (MRI), which demonstrates osteonecrosis.

Therapeutic Management

Because deformity occurs early in the disease process, the aim of treatment is to keep the head of the femur contained in the acetabulum, which serves as a mold to preserve the spherical shape of the head and to maintain a full range of motion. Because LCPD is a biologic process involving revascularization of the femoral head, removal of necrotic bone, and replacement with viable bone (Greene, 2001), mechanical intervention may not produce optimal results (Roy, 1999). However, there is no agreement regarding the best treatment in terms of conservative versus surgical approaches. There has reportedly been no particular treatment that has yielded good outcomes on a consistent basis (Greene, 2001). Often, treatment approaches vary with the severity of presentation. Activity causes microfractures of the soft, ischemic epiphysis, which tend to induce synovitis,

stiffness, and adductor contractures. The initial therapy is rest and non–weight bearing, which helps reduce inflammation and restore motion. Later, active motion is encouraged. In some cases traction is applied to stretch tight adductor muscles.

Containment can be accomplished in several ways. One is the use of non–weight-bearing devices, such as an abduction brace, leg casts, or a leather harness sling, which prevent weight bearing on the affected limb. Another includes the use of various weight-bearing appliances, such as abduction-ambulation braces or casts after a period of bed rest and traction. A third consists of surgical reconstruction and containment procedures. Conservative therapy must be continued for 2 to 4 years, although braces constructed from lightweight materials allow the child to maintain a nearly normal activity level. Surgical correction, although subjecting the child to additional risks (e.g., from anesthesia, infection, blood transfusion), returns the child to normal activities in 3 to 4 months. The use of home traction has also been explored.

Prognosis. The disease is self-limited, but the ultimate outcome of therapy depends on early and efficient treatment and the age of the child at onset of the disorder. Younger children, whose epiphyses are more cartilaginous, have the best prognosis for complete recovery; however, a recent report suggests that patients younger than 5 years of age do not always have the optimal outcomes previously predicted (Fabry, Fabry, and Moens, 2003). The later the diagnosis is made, the more femoral damage has occurred before treatment is implemented. In many cases, with good patient compliance, the prognosis is excellent.

Nursing Considerations

Nurses may be the first health professionals to identify affected children and to refer them for medical evaluation. They are also persons on whom the child and the family can rely to help them understand and adjust to the therapeutic measures. Because most of the child's care is conducted on an outpatient basis, the major emphasis of nursing care is teaching the family the care and management of the corrective appliance selected for therapy. The family needs to learn the purpose, function, application, and care of the corrective device and the importance of compliance to achieve the desired outcome (see Family Focus box).

One of the most difficult aspects associated with the disorder is coping with a normally active child who feels well but must remain relatively inactive. Suitable activities must be devised to meet the needs of the child in the process of developing a sense of initiative or industry. Activities that meet the creative urges are well received.

SLIPPED FEMORAL CAPITAL EPIPHYSIS

Slipped femoral capital epiphysis (SFCE), or coxa vara, refers to the spontaneous displacement of the proximal femoral epiphysis in a posterior and inferior direction. It develops most frequently shortly before or during accelerated growth and the onset of puberty (children between the ages of 10 and 16 years: median age, 13 for boys, 12 for girls) and is most frequently observed in males and obese children. Bilateral involvement occurs in up to 40% to 50% of cases (Greene, 2001).

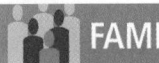

FAMILY FOCUS

Legg-Calvé-Perthes Disease

A family with five healthy children was one day startled to learn that their 2-year-old son could no longer walk. He was diagnosed with Legg-Calvé-Perthes disease. Through several years of prosthetic devices and numerous physician visits, hospitalizations, and surgeries, this family turned a potentially devastating experience into one with cherished memories.

Today, the parents reflect upon how their family coped with the reality of a debilitating disease. It was difficult for the parents to observe an eager, energetic child watch other children riding bicycles, running, or playing outdoor games. Also, they are warmed by memories of watching their other children make the difference for their sibling. They all developed a strong bond through caring and sharing with one another. Coping as a family was an easy adjustment and, most of all, therapeutic. Today, over 20 years later, the parents feel that each family member has grown with feelings of faith and trust. The experience proved to them that life will go on, and that life is what you make it!

Shona Swenson Lenss, MS, RN, FNP
Cheyenne, Wyoming

Pathophysiology

Most cases of SFCE are idiopathic, although it can be associated with endocrine disorders, renal osteodystrophy, and radiation therapy. The cause of idiopathic SFCE is multifactorial and includes obesity, physeal architecture and orientation, and pubertal hormone changes that affect physeal strength. Although obesity stresses the physeal plate, SFCE can also occur in children who are not obese. Radiographs show medial displacement of the epiphysis and uncovered upper portion of the femoral neck adjacent to the physis. There is a widened growth plate and irregular metaphysis. The capital femoral epiphysis remains in the acetabulum, but the femoral neck slips, deforming the femoral head and stretching blood vessels to the epiphysis.

Diagnostic Evaluation

The disorder is suspected when an adolescent or preadolescent youngster displays clinical signs or complains of thigh pain (Box 31-7). The diagnosis is confirmed by radiographic examination.

Therapeutic Management

Treatment goals include avoiding further slipping of the femoral head, avoiding chondrolysis and osteonecrosis, and correcting the deformity. Surgical treatment varies with the degree of displacement; methods include presurgery bed rest/traction followed by a single pin, multiple pins and screws, or osteotomy for deformity correction if needed. Postsurgery care includes non–weight bearing with crutch ambulation until acceptable, painless range of motion is achieved. SFCE with severe displacement is an emergency and requires surgical reduction and stabilization.

Nursing Considerations

Nursing care is the same as that for a child in a cast or in traction, as discussed earlier in this chapter. Postoperative care involves hemodynamic stabilization and assessment for complications.

BOX 31-7 ■ **Clinical Manifestations of Slipped Femoral Capital Epiphysis**

May be obese
Limp on affected side
Pain in hip
   Continuous or intermittent
   Frequently referred to groin, anteromedial aspect of thigh, or
     knee
Restricted internal rotation on adduction with external rotation
   deformity
Loss of abduction and internal rotation as severity increases
Shortening of lower extremity

KYPHOSIS AND LORDOSIS

The spine, consisting of numerous segments, can acquire deformity curves of three types: kyphosis, lordosis, and scoliosis (Fig. 31-18). *Kyphosis* is an abnormally increased convex angulation in the curvature of the thoracic spine (Fig. 31-18, *B*). It can occur secondary to disease processes such as tuberculosis, chronic arthritis, osteodystrophy, or compression fractures of the thoracic spine. The most common form of kyphosis is "postural." Children, especially during the time when skeletal growth outpaces growth of muscle, are prone to exaggeration of a normal kyphosis. They assume abnormal sitting and standing positions. This is particularly common in self-conscious adolescent girls who assume a round-shouldered slouching posture in an attempt to hide their developing breasts. *Scheuermann kyphosis* is a thoracic curve greater than 45 degrees with wedging greater than 5 degrees of at least three adjacent vertebral bodies and vertebral irregularity.

Postural kyphosis is almost always accompanied by a compensatory postural lordosis, an abnormally exaggerated concave lumbar curvature. Treatment of kyphosis consists of exercises to strengthen shoulder and abdominal muscles and bracing for more marked deformity. With adolescents who are significantly self-conscious in relation to their appearance the best approach is to emphasize the cosmetic value of corrective therapy and to place the responsibility on the adolescent for carrying out an exercise program at home with regular visits to and assessments by a therapist. Most adolescents respond well to selected sports as a supplement to regular exercise. Boys prefer weight lifting and other upper-body-strength–building sports. Girls may prefer swimming, ballet, or dancing. Swimming is excellent and has the added advantages of exercising all muscles, eliminating gravity, and teaching breath control. Treatment with a brace may be indicated until skeletal maturity, and surgical fusion may be considered for severe, painful, or progressive thoracic curves such as Scheuermann kyphosis.

Lordosis is an accentuation of the cervical or lumbar curvature beyond physiologic limits (Fig. 31-18, *C*). It may be a secondary complication of a disease process, a result of trauma, or idiopathic. It is often seen in association with flexion contractures of the hip, scoliosis, obesity, developmental dislocation of the hip, and slipped femoral capital epiphysis. During the pubertal growth spurt, lordosis of varying degrees is observed in teenagers, especially girls. In obese children the weight of the abdominal fat alters the center of gravity, causing a compensatory lordosis. Unlike kyphosis, severe lordosis is usually accompanied by pain.

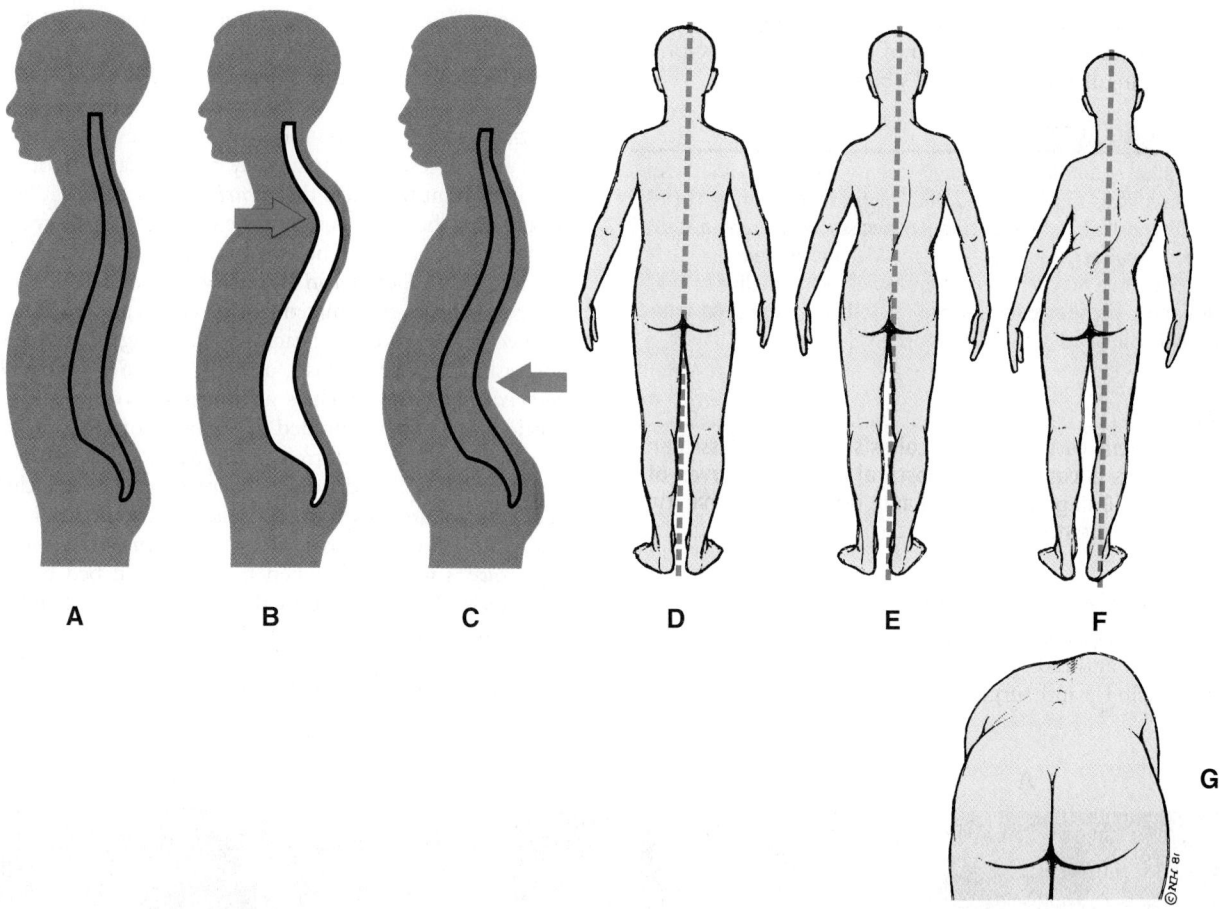

FIG. 31-18 ■ Defects of spinal column. **A,** Normal spine. **B,** Kyphosis. **C,** Lordosis. **D,** Normal spine in balance. **E,** Mild scoliosis in balance. **F,** Severe scoliosis not in balance. **G,** Rib hump and flank asymmetry seen in flexion caused by rotary component. (Redrawn from Hilt NE, Schmitt EW: *Pediatric orthopedic nursing,* St Louis, 1975, Mosby.)

Treatment involves management of the predisposing cause when possible, such as weight loss and correction of deformities. Postural exercises or support garments are helpful in relieving symptoms in some cases; however, these do not usually effect a permanent cure.

IDIOPATHIC SCOLIOSIS

Idiopathic scoliosis is a complex spinal deformity in three planes, usually involving lateral curvature, spinal rotation causing rib asymmetry, and thoracic hypokyphosis. It is the most common spinal deformity and can be further classified according to age of onset: *infantile,* at birth or up to 3 years of age, or it can develop during childhood *(juvenile),* but it is most common during the growth spurt of early adolescence *(adolescent).* Idiopathic scoliosis can be caused by a number of conditions and may occur alone or in association with other diseases, particularly neuromuscular conditions. In most cases, however, there is no apparent cause, and thus the name idiopathic scoliosis. There appears to be a genetic component to the etiology of idiopathic scoliosis; however, the exact relationship has yet to be established. The following section is limited to a discussion of adolescent idiopathic scoliosis.

Idiopathic scoliosis is most noticeable during the preadolescent growth spurt. Parents frequently bring a child for follow-up on an abnormal school scoliosis screening or because of "ill-fitting" clothes, such as poorly fitting slacks. School screening is somewhat controversial, because there are no controlled studies to demonstrate improved outcomes; however, many experts suggest that school screening has increased public and professional awareness of scoliosis and has decreased the number of significant cases of serious deformity (Newton and Wenger, 2001). The American Academy of Pediatrics recommends scoliosis screening at the time of primary practitioner visits in all preadolescent and adolescent children.

Diagnostic Evaluation

Observation is performed behind an undressed (in underpants and bra, if female) standing child, noting asymmetry of shoulder height, scapular or flank shape, or hip height and alignment. When the child bends forward at the waist (the Adams test) with hanging arms, asymmetry of the ribs and flanks may be noted. A scoliometer is also used in the initial screening to measure truncal rotation (also measured by the Adams test). Often a primary curve and a compensatory curve will place the head in alignment with the gluteal cleft. However, in the uncompensated curve the head and hips are not aligned (Fig. 31-18, *E* and *F*). (See Spine, Chapter 7, for additional information.) Definitive diagnosis is made by radiographs of the child in the standing position and use of the Cobb technique (standard measurement of angle curvature), which establishes the degree of curvature. The Risser scale is used to evaluate skeletal maturity on the radiographs; the scale assists in making a determination of the likely progression of the spinal angulature as the child's bones mature.

> **! NURSING ALERT**
>
> Intraspinal conditions or other disease processes that can cause scoliosis must be ruled out. The presence of pain, sacral dimpling or hairy patches, cutaneous vascular changes, absent or abnormal reflexes, bowel or bladder incontinence, or left thoracic curve may indicate an intraspinal abnormality such as syringomyelia, diastematomyelia, or tethered cord syndrome. An MRI scan should be obtained for evaluation.

> **FYI**
>
> Not all spinal curvatures are scoliosis. A curve of less than 10 degrees is considered a postural variation. Curves of less than 20 degrees are mild and, if nonprogressive, do not require treatment.

Therapeutic Management

Current management options include observation with regular clinical and radiographic evaluation, orthotic intervention (bracing), and surgical spinal fusion. Treatment decisions are based on the magnitude, location, and type of curve; the age and skeletal maturity of the child; and any underlying or contributing disease process.

Bracing and Exercise. For many curves in the growing child and adolescent, bracing may be the treatment of choice. It is important to realize that *bracing is not curative,* but that it may slow the progression of the curvature to allow skeletal growth and maturity. The two most common types of bracing are (1) the *Boston and Wilmington braces,* which are underarm orthoses customized from prefabricated plastic shells, with corrective forces for each patient using lateral pads and decreasing lumbar lordosis, and (2) a *TLSO (thoracolumbosacral orthosis),* which is an underarm orthosis made of plastic that is custom molded to the body and then shaped to correct or hold the deformity (Fig. 31-19). The *Milwaukee brace,* which is an individually adapted brace that includes a neck ring, is rarely used in scoliosis but is sometimes used in the treatment of kyphosis. The *Charleston nighttime bending brace* is worn only when the child is in bed because it prevents walking because of the severity of the trunk bend (Newton and Wenger, 2001). Bracing, although used as the gold standard treatment for mild to moderate curvatures, has not proved to be entirely effective in the treatment of scolio-

A   **B**   **C**

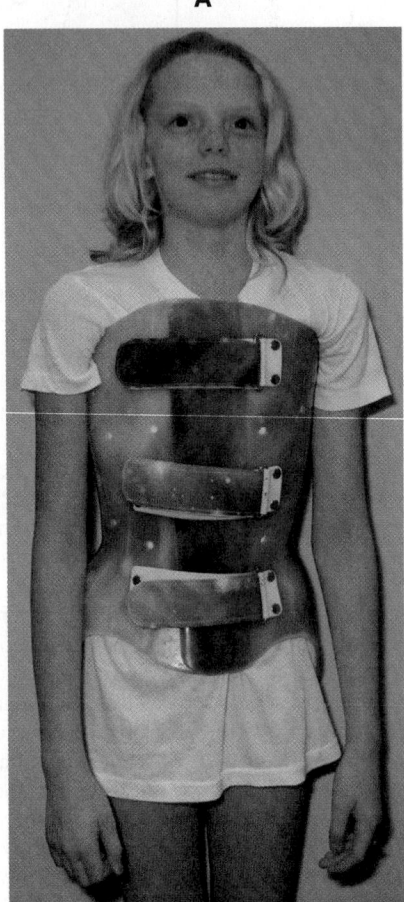 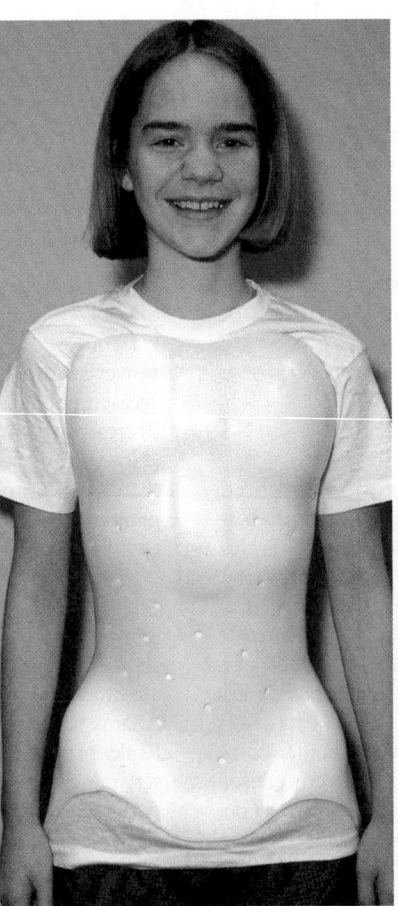 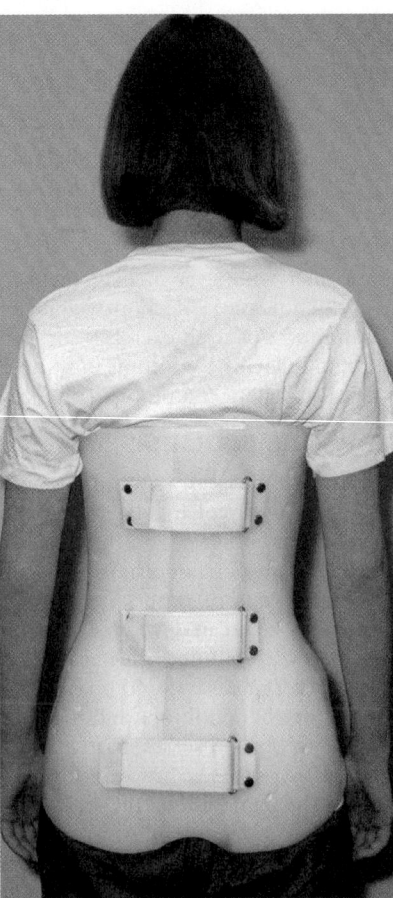

FIG. 31-19 ■ **A,** Standard thoracolumbosacral orthotic (TLSO) brace for idiopathic scoliosis. Brace may be decorated to make it more acceptable to adolescents. **B,** Variation of a standard TLSO brace that fastens in the back to provide needed support. **C,** Posterior view of same brace.

sis (Newton and Wenger, 2001), and retrospective studies show only slight variation in outcomes in regard to the type of brace used (Thompson, 2004b). Compliance in wearing the brace is difficult because of the age of the child and preoccupation with body image and appearance.

Exercises alone and chiropractic treatment are rarely of value for managing scoliosis (Thompson, 2004b); transcutaneous electrical stimulation has also proved to be an ineffective treatment for this condition. Exercises are of benefit when used in conjunction with bracing to maintain and strengthen spinal and abdominal muscles during treatment.

Surgical Management.   Surgical intervention may be required for correction of severe curves (usually 40 degrees or more). The degree of curvature and the cause determine the decision for surgery. Bracing and exercise have been universally disappointing in curves greater than 40 degrees, and paralytic and congenital curves, which will eventually progress, are best treated with early surgical stabilization if the health status of the child will allow major surgery. The age of the child and location of the curvature influence the decision for surgery, and any progressive or severe curve that does not respond to more conservative orthotic measures requires surgical correction. Difficulties with balance or seating, respiratory excursion, or pain are also considered.

The surgical technique consists of realignment and straightening with internal fixation and instrumentation combined with bony fusion *(arthrodesis)* of the realigned spine. The goals of surgical intervention are to correct the curvatures on the sagittal and coronal planes and to have a solid, pain-free fusion in a well-balanced torso, with maximum mobility of the remaining spinal segments.

There are many instrumentation systems available, including Harrington, Dwyer, Zielke, Luque, Cotrel-Dubousset, Isola, TSRH (Texas Scottish Rite Hospital), and Moss-Miami. Selection of the system is individualized according to the needs of the patient and the preference of the surgeon. Posterior or anterior approaches can be used.

The Harrington system, the first internal spinal instrumentation device, consists of distraction and compression rods, hooks, and nuts. The posterior elements are decorticated, and bone from the iliac crest or donor bone is placed across the vertebrae to provide fusion. Postoperatively the child is logrolled to prevent spinal motion and a molded plastic jacket is used to stabilize the spine until the fusion is solid.

The Luque-rod segmental spinal instrumentation provides segmental stability by the use of wires and L-shaped rods. By way of a posterior approach, the wires are threaded beneath the lamina of each vertebra and tightened around the rods resting along the transverse processes to stabilize the spine. Bone from the iliac crest or donor bone is used to fuse the spine. The advantage of this method is that the patient can be mobile within a few days and no postoperative immobilization is required. The disadvantage is the risk of nerve damage.

The Cotrel-Dubousset (CD) instrumentation combines the Harrington and L-rod approaches by using bilateral rods and hooks at many sites. Anterior approaches using the Dwyer or Zielke instrumentation involve screws into the vertebral bodies connected by a cable or rod. These systems require postoperative immobilization with a custom-fitted plastic jacket.

Nursing Considerations

Treatment for scoliosis extends over a significant portion of the affected child's period of growth. In adolescents this period is the one in which their identity, physical and psychologic, is formed. The identification of scoliosis as a "deformity," in combination with unattractive appliances and a significant surgical procedure, can have a negative effect on the already fragile adolescent body image (Noonan and others, 1997). The adolescent and family require excellent nursing care not only for physical needs to be met, but also for psychologic needs associated with the diagnosis, surgery, postoperative recovery, and eventual rehabilitation (Slote, 2002). Although these adolescents are encouraged to participate in most peer activities, necessary therapeutic modifications are likely to make them feel different and apart.

When a child first faces the prospect of a prolonged period in a brace, jacket, or other device, the therapy program and the nature of the device must be explained thoroughly to both the child and the parents so that they will have an understanding of the anticipated results, how the appliance corrects the defect, the freedoms and constraints imposed by the device, and what they can do to help achieve the desired goal. The management involves the skills and services of a team of specialists, including the orthopedist, physical therapist, orthotist (a specialist in fitting orthopedic braces), nurse, social worker, and sometimes a thoracic or pulmonary specialist.

It is difficult for a child to be restricted at any phase of development, but the adolescent needs continual positive reinforcement, encouragement, and as much independence as can be safely assumed during this time. Guidance and assistance regarding anticipated problems, such as selection of clothing and participation in social activities, are appreciated by adolescents. Socialization with peers is strongly encouraged, and every effort is expended to help the adolescent feel attractive and worthwhile.

Preoperative Care.   The preoperative workup usually involves a radiographic series, including bending and traction films, pulmonary function studies, and a number of routine laboratory studies. Because spinal surgery usually involves considerable blood loss, several options are considered preoperatively to maintain or replace blood volume. Autologous blood donations may be obtained from the patient before the surgery to replace blood loss during the operation. Other options include intraoperative blood salvage, intraoperative hemodilution, erythropoietin administration, or controlled induced hypotension, which must be carefully monitored at all times to prevent physiologic instability (Newton and Wenger, 2001).

Surgery for spinal fusion is quite complex, and often adolescents who require the procedure because of idiopathic scoliosis are not familiar with medical terms, procedures, or experiences. Preoperative teaching is critical for the adolescent to be able to cooperate and participate in his or her treatment and recovery. Extensive preoperative teaching is essential to prepare the adolescent for the postoperative and recovery course; because the surgery is quite extensive, the patient is taught how to manage his or her own patient-controlled analgesia (PCA) pump, how to log-roll, and the use and function of other equipment that will be used, such as chest tube (for anterior repair), Foley catheter, and so on. It is recommended that the child or adolescent bring a favorite toy (age-dependent) or personal items such as a favorite stuffed animal or portable compact disc player for postoperative use. Meeting with a peer who has undergone a similar surgery is also valuable (Slote, 2002).

Postoperative Care. After surgery, patients are monitored in an acute care setting and log-rolled when changing position to prevent damage to the fusion and instrumentation. Skin care is very important, and pressure-relieving mattresses or beds may be needed to prevent pressure wounds (see Maintaining Healthy Skin, Chapter 22).

In addition to the usual postoperative assessments—of wound, circulation, and vital signs—the neurologic status of the patient's extremities requires special attention. Prompt recognition of any neurologic impairment is imperative because delayed paralysis may develop that requires surgical intervention. The most common postoperative problems after spinal fusion include neurologic injury or spinal cord injury, hypotension from acute blood loss, wound infection, delayed neurologic injury, and implanted hardware complications (Newton and Wenger, 2001). The child usually has considerable pain for the first few days after surgery and requires frequent administration of pain medication, preferably the use of opioids administered on a regular schedule administered intravenously. For children able to understand the concept, PCA is recommended (see Pain Assessment; Pain Management, Chapter 21). In most cases the patient is ambulated as soon as possible; depending on the instrumentation used, most patients are ambulated by the second or third postoperative day and discharged by 1 week, depending on the surgical approach. In addition to pain management, the patient is evaluated for skin integrity, adequate urinary output, fluid and electrolyte balance, and ileus (Slote, 2002). The latter may be particularly distressful for the adolescent who is self-conscious. Discharge planning should include a timetable for follow-up with the practitioner and resumption of regular activities.

All patients are started on physical therapy as soon as they are able, beginning with range-of-motion exercises on the first postoperative day and many of the activities of daily living in the following days. Self-care, such as washing and eating, is always encouraged. Throughout the hospitalization age-appropriate activities and contact with family and friends are important parts of nursing care and planning (see Immobilization).

The family is encouraged to become involved with the patient's care to facilitate the transition from hospital to home management. An organization that provides education and services to both families and professionals is the **National Scoliosis Foundation, Inc.*** The **American Academy of Orthopaedic Surgeons†** and **Scoliosis Research Society,‡** an organization of physicians and scientists, have published an excellent book, *Scoliosis,* and the SRS has educational information available on its website.

INFECTIONS OF BONES AND JOINTS

OSTEOMYELITIS*

Osteomyelitis is an infection in the bone. *Acute osteomyelitis* is a bone infection present less than 2 weeks, *subacute osteomyelitis* is a bone infection lasting 2 to 6 weeks, and in *chronic osteomyelitis* the infection lasts more than 6 weeks. Osteomyelitis can occur at any age but is more frequent in young children and older adults. It occurs more often in boys than in girls with a 2-3:1 ratio. Other than sickle cell anemia, most children with osteomyelitis do not have significant risk factors.

Pathophysiology

Osteomyelitis can be acquired exogenously by direct inoculation of bone during trauma, puncture, or surgery—the hand and foot are commons sites. Hematogenous osteomyelitis is seeded by organisms from a preexisting infection such as tonsillitis or impetigo or from a contiguous source such as an adjacent infected bone or joint. Hematogenous osteomyelitis usually occurs in the metaphyses of long bones, the femur, or tibia. The infecting organism travels from the site of infection to the small end-artery capillary loops in the bone metaphyses, causing obstruction and initiating infection, with complications of bone destruction and abscess formation.

Any bacteria can cause osteomyelitis, but *Staphylococcus aureus* is the most common pathogen. *Haemophilus influenzae* used to be a common pathogen in the younger child; however, the incidence has decreased since the advent of *H. influenzae* vaccine. Children with sickle cell anemia are at increased risk for *Salmonella* as a causative organism.

Most cases involve the femur or tibia. In infants the diagnosis is challenging because of difficulty localizing symptoms and the increased likelihood of multiple bone involvement.

Diagnostic Evaluation

Typically children with acute hematogenous osteomyelitis present with a 2- to 7-day history of pain, warmth, tenderness, and decreased range of motion in the affected limb, and systemic symptoms of fever, irritability, and lethargy (Box 31-8). Symptoms often resemble those observed in other diseases involving bones such as arthritis or leukemia. There may be nonspecific elevation of the white blood cell count, erythrocyte sedimentation rate, and C-reactive protein. Blood cultures may be positive but can be negative in children already receiving antibiotics. Direct bone aspirates are more likely to yield a causative organism. Early plain radiographs are often normal but help rule out other diseases. Technetium-labeled bone scans are more sensitive in early disease (Karwowska and others, 1998). Ultrasound, CT, and MRI can also be useful in making the diagnosis of osteomyelitis.

---

*5 Cabot Place, Stoughton, MA 02072; (781) 341-6333 or (800) 673-6922; website: www.scoliosis.org.
†6300 North River Road, Rosemont, IL 60018-4262; (847) 698-1627.
‡611 East Wells Street, Milwaukee, WI 53202; (414) 289-9107; website: www.srs.org.

*Martha Curry, MSN, RN, CPNP, revised this section.

BOX 31-8 ■ Clinical Manifestations of Acute Osteomyelitis

GENERAL MANIFESTATIONS
History of trauma to affected bone (frequent)
Child appears very ill
Irritability
Restlessness
Elevated temperature
Rapid pulse
Dehydration

LOCAL MANIFESTATIONS
Tenderness
Increased warmth
Diffuse swelling over involved bone
Involved extremity painful, especially on movement
Involved extremity held in semiflexion
Surrounding muscles tense and resist passive movement

Therapeutic Management

As soon as blood and bone aspirate cultures are obtained, empiric parenteral antibiotics are administered pending culture results. Because *S. aureus* is the most prevalent causative organism, the empiric antibiotics are typically penicillinase-resistant penicillin and a third-generation cephalosporin. When cultures are received, the appropriate antibiotic is continued for 4 to 6 weeks. In select cases oral antibiotics may follow a shorter, intensive IV course with good results (Karwowska and others, 1998). Because of prolonged high-dose therapy, it is important to monitor hematologic, renal, hepatic, and other organ systems that might be adversely affected by the drugs (e.g., ototoxic).

Opinions differ regarding surgical intervention, but typically chronic osteomyelitis will not respond without débridement and the removal of dead bone. Débridement and amputation are frequently required in osteomyelitis in the diabetic foot and in other conditions with impaired blood flow. Antibiotic-impregnated seed implants and direct antibiotic solution instillation and drainage may be used to improve local antibiotic delivery.

Nursing Considerations

During the acute phase of illness any movement of the affected limb will cause discomfort; therefore, the child is positioned comfortably with the affected limb supported. Moving and turning are carried out carefully and gently to minimize pain. Pain medication is administered to provide comfort. Vital signs are taken and recorded frequently, and measures are implemented to reduce a significant temperature elevation.

Antibiotic therapy requires careful observation and monitoring of the IV equipment and site. Because more than one antibiotic is usually administered, the compatibility of the drugs is determined and care is taken to avoid mixing noncompatible drugs. For long-term antibiotic therapy, an intermittent infusion device or peripherally inserted central catheter (PICC) is used (see Peripheral Venous Access Devices, Chapter 22). Antibiotic therapy is often continued at home.

The child with an open wound may be placed on contact isolation. The wound is managed as prescribed. Antibiotic solution administered directly into the wound is most efficiently accomplished with a regular IV infusion setup that is prepared and regulated in the same manner as any other. The drainage tubes are connected to low Gomco or wall suction devices for continuous removal. Intake and output are measured and recorded, and the character of the wound drainage is noted. The amount and character of drainage on the wound dressing are also noted.

Casts are sometimes used for immobilization, and if so, routine cast care is carried out. The extremity is examined for sensation, circulation, and pain, and the area over the inflammation is usually left open for observation. The affected area, casted or uncasted, is assessed for color, swelling, heat, and tenderness.

The child usually has a poor appetite at first. Nourishment in the form of high-calorie liquids, such as fruit juices, gelatin, and flavored ice pops, is encouraged until the child begins to feel better. The appetite returns as the acute symptoms subside. During convalescence adequate nutrition must be maintained to aid healing and formation of new bone.

When the acute stage subsides, the child begins to feel better, the appetite improves, and the child becomes interested in the surroundings and relationships and may move about in bed. However, weight bearing on the affected limb is not permitted until healing is well under way to avoid pathologic fractures. Diversional and constructive activities become important nursing interventions. The child is usually confined to bed for some time after the acute phase but may be allowed to move about in a wheelchair when isolation and bed rest are no longer necessary. As the infection subsides, physical therapy is instituted to ensure restoration of optimum function. If amputation is required, evaluation of emotional and social support is essential for successful adaptation.

SEPTIC (SUPPURATIVE, PYOGENIC) ARTHRITIS

Infection of the joints, as with infection of bone, usually develops through hematogenous dissemination from another focus; occasionally, it may result from direct extension of a soft-tissue infection or respiratory infection. Joint infections occur predominantly in males, especially in the adolescent age-group. In infancy, however, the incidence in boys and girls is nearly equal. Any joint may be involved, but the hip, knee, shoulder, and other large joints are more commonly affected. Usually only one joint is involved.

The signs and symptoms of suppurative arthritis, unlike osteomyelitis, are usually characteristic. The presence of a warm and tender joint, painful on even gentle pressure, helps to differentiate it from osteomyelitis, in which gentle passive motion is usually tolerated. When superficial joints are involved, they are exquisitely painful and swollen; deep-seated joints show little superficial evidence. Frequently, there is a history of a traumatic injury to the affected joint. Fever, edema, erythema, and joint stiffness are present in older children but may not be demonstrated in affected infants; limited spontaneous joint mobility may be the only clinical presentation in infants. The most common pathogens are *S. aureus*, group A streptococci, and *H. influenzae*. Studies show a reduction in *H. influenzae* septic arthritis since the *H. influenzae* vaccine (Hib vaccine) (Peltola, Kallio, and Unkila-Kallio, 1998). *Neisseria gonorrhoeae* is a frequent cause of septic arthritis in sexually active adolescents. The diagnosis is made from a blood culture, joint fluid aspirate, radiographs, or MRI. Ultrasound is more helpful in determining joint effusion, especially if the hip is involved.

Therapeutic Management and Nursing Considerations

The affected joint is aspirated and evaluated for type of organism and subsequent fluid accumulation. An infection involving the hip, however, is considered a surgical emergency to prevent compromised blood supply to the head of the femur (Lampe, 2004). Antibiotic therapy is initiated after fluid aspiration and cultures. Follow-up serial aspirations may be necessary, and antibiotic regimen is maintained according to the isolated organism and the response to antibiotic therapy. Surgical intervention may also be required if there was a penetrating wound or possibly a foreign object involved. Physical therapy may be used for the child who is immobilized in a cast or traction to prevent flexion contractures. Pain management is an important aspect of nursing care, particularly for large joint involvement such as the hip. Additional nursing care is the same as for osteomyelitis.

SKELETAL TUBERCULOSIS

In children infection of bones and joints is acquired by lymphohematogenous spread at the time of primary infection. Occasionally, infection is from chronic pulmonary tuberculosis. Skeletal tubercular infection is not common in the United States but must be considered in communities with high tuberculosis case rates. The infection most likely involves the vertebrae, causing a tubercular spondylitis. If the infection is progressive, it causes Pott disease with destruction of the vertebral bodies and resultant kyphosis.

Symptoms and onset are usually insidious; the child may report persistent or intermittent pain. Other findings include joint swelling and stiffness; fever and weight loss are not common. Tubercular arthritis can also affect single joints such as a knee or hip and tends to cause severe destruction of adjacent bone. Diagnosis requires isolation of *Mycobacterium tuberculosis* from the site (bone biopsy) and patients with positive cultures are started on treatment of combined antituberculosis chemotherapy, isoniazid, rifampin, and pyrazinamide; streptomycin or other antituberculosis drugs may be required if drug resistance is encountered. Reliance on a positive purified protein derivative (PPD) skin test alone is not considered diagnostic for tuberculous arthritis. Supervised drug therapy is recommended to ensure treatment compliance. In some cases surgical débridement may be required. Tuberculous spondylitis and hip infection may involve immobilization, casting and spinal fusion.

Nursing Considerations

The nursing responsibilities are similar to those for other types of osteomyelitis and septic arthritis, in addition to monitoring tuberculosis chemotherapy and identifying positive family or environmental active disease contacts.

BONE AND SOFT-TISSUE TUMORS*

GENERAL CONCEPTS: BONE TUMORS

Neoplastic disease can arise from any tissues involved in bone growth. In children the two types that account for 85% of all primary malignant bone tumors are osteogenic sarcoma (osteosarcoma) and Ewing sarcoma.

The peak ages for occurrence during childhood are 15 to 19 years. The sexes are affected equally until puberty, at which time the ratio approaches 2:1 in favor of males. This propensity for males, with a peak incidence during adolescence, is thought to be related to the accelerated growth rate of osseous tissue. These two bone tumors have several characteristics in common, which are discussed. Specific information related to each tumor is also presented.

Diagnostic Evaluation

A primary objective in diagnosis of bone neoplasm is to rule out causes such as trauma or infection. A history and careful questioning regarding pain help determine the duration and rate of tumor growth (Box 31-9). Physical assessment focuses on the functional status of the affected area, signs of inflammation, size of the mass, involvement of regional lymph nodes, and any systemic indication of generalized malignancy.

Definitive diagnosis is based on radiologic studies such as chest radiograph, MRI, CT scans, and radioisotope bone scans that determine the extent of the disease. A needle or surgical bone biopsy is performed to determine the histologic type. Radiologic findings are characteristic for each type of tumor. In osteogenic sarcoma the needlelike bone projections present a "sunburst" appearance, whereas the layers of new bone in Ewing sarcoma have an "onionskin" or "hair-on-end" appearance (Ginsberg and others, 2002; Link, Gebhardt, and Meyers, 2002). MRI provides information regarding neurovascular structures, intramedullary bone involvement, and soft-tissue extension (Rednek, 2000).

There is no reliable biochemical test for bone cancers, although elevated alkaline phosphatase levels may occur in osteoid tumors. Several tests may be performed to rule out metastatic disease from other neoplasms. Chest CT is usually a standard procedure, because pulmonary metastasis is the most common complication of primary bone tumors. Bone marrow aspiration is helpful in diagnosing Ewing sarcoma in the rare event that the child has bone marrow metastasis.

---

*Rosalind Bryant, MSN, RN-CS, PNP, revised this section.

BOX 31-9 ■ Clinical Manifestations of Bone Tumors

Pain localized at affected site
    May be severe or dull
    Often relieved by position of flexion
Frequently brought to attention when child:
    Limps
    Curtails own physical activity
    Is unable to hold heavy objects

OSTEOSARCOMA

Osteosarcoma is the most frequently encountered malignant bone cancer in children, with a peak incidence between 10 and 25 years of age (Kline and Sevier, 2003; Link, Gebhardt, and Meyers, 2002; Meyers and Gorlick, 1997). Most primary tumor sites are in the metaphysis of long bones (wider part of the shaft, next to epiphyseal growth plate), especially in the lower extremities. More than half occur in the femur, particularly the distal portion, with the rest involving the humerus, tibia, pelvis, jaw, and phalanges.

Therapeutic Management

Optimal treatment of osteosarcoma is surgery and chemotherapy. The surgical approach consists of radical surgical resection or amputation. Depending on the tumor site, preoperative response to chemotherapy, and location of the tumor, the goal of surgery is to remove the diseased bone surrounded by a large margin of healthy bone. With tumors of the distal femur, preservation of the hip joint may be possible. Other surgical procedures include an above-the-knee amputation for tumors of the tibia or fibula, a hemipelvectomy for tumors of the innominate (hip) bone, and a forequarter amputation (removal of the arm, the scapula, and a portion of the clavicle on the affected side) for tumors of the upper humerus. *Limb-salvage procedures* entail en bloc resection of tumor-bearing bone with prosthetic replacement of the involved bone. Partial limb salvage by a *rotationplasty procedure* involves resection of the tumor, including the knee joint, with the lower part of the leg rotated 180 degrees and retransplanted to the thigh, creating a shortened leg with the ankle joint at the position of the former knee joint (Link and others, 2002).

All children with osteosarcoma receive chemotherapy to treat microscopic disease (Kline and Sevier, 2003). Antineoplastic drugs, such as high-dose methotrexate with citrovorum rescue, Adriamycin, actinomycin D, cyclophosphamide, ifosfamide, etoposide, and cisplatin, may be administered in combination or singly both before and after surgery.

Prognosis.   Surgical procedures (limb-salvage procedures, amputation, thoracotomy) accompanied by multiagent chemotherapy have significantly improved survival rates in patients with osteosarcoma. Approximately 65% to 85% of patients with nonmetastatic osteosarcoma can expect long-term survival (Redner, 2000). The patient with metastatic osteosarcoma has a survival prognosis rate of less than 50%. To improve long-term survival, a compound known as muramyl tripeptide phosphatidylethanolamine (MTP-PE) is being studied. MTP-PE is designed to stimulate macrophages to kill tumor cells, consequently reducing the risk of recurrence in patients with osteosarcoma (Dzierzbicka and others, 2003; Link and others, 2002).

Nursing Considerations

Nursing care depends on the type of surgical approach, and in either instance preparation of the child and family is crucial. Obviously, the family may have more difficulty adjusting to an amputation than a limb-salvage procedure. Honesty is essential to gain the cooperation and trust of the child. The diagnosis of cancer should not be disguised with falsehoods such as "infection." To accept the need for radical surgery, the child must be aware of the lack of alternatives for treatment. Although the task of informing the child is the responsibility of the physician, the nurse should be present for the discussion or be aware of exactly what is said to the child. The child should be told a few days before surgery, so that he or she has time to think about the diagnosis and consequent treatment and to ask questions.

Sometimes children have many questions about the prosthesis, limitations on physical ability, and prognosis in terms of cure. At other times they react with silence or with a calm manner that masks their concern and fear. Either response is part of the grieving process that accompanies a loss and must be accepted. Children should not be overwhelmed with information. A supportive approach is to answer their questions without offering additional information and to express a willingness to talk. The nurse should not push the topic unless the child initiates the discussion. Silence does not always mean nonacceptance.

The child is also informed of the need for chemotherapy and its side effects before surgery. Caution must be exercised in offering too much information at one time. It is wise to discuss hair loss with emphasis on positive aspects, such as wearing a wig or baseball cap. Because bone tumors affect adolescents and young adults, it is not unusual for them to become angry about the radical body alterations.

If an amputation is performed, the child may be fitted with a temporary prosthesis immediately after surgery, which permits early functioning and fosters psychologic adjustment. If this is not done, the child requires stump care, which is the same as for any amputee. A permanent prosthesis is usually fitted within 6 to 8 weeks. During hospitalization the child begins physical therapy to become proficient in the use and care of the device.

In rotationplasty, a prosthesis is fitted over the newly created knee joint. However, the appearance of a foot placed backward on the leg to create a substitute knee is a major change in body image. Children often need help in dealing with their own feelings and other people's reactions to the leg.

Phantom limb pain may develop after amputation. This symptom is characterized by pain, tingling, itching, burning, or cramping in the area of the amputated leg (Olsson, 1999). The child and family need to know that the sensations are real, not imagined. Amitriptyline (Elavil) has been used successfully in children to decrease the pain (Berde and others, 2002).

Discharge planning must begin early during the postoperative period. Every effort is made to promote normality and gradual resumption of realistic preamputation activities.* Role-playing in anticipation of such experiences is

---

*Information about special programs for children with amputations is available from the **Candlelighters Childhood Cancer Foundation,** PO Box 498, Kensington, MD 20895; (800) 366-2223; website: www.candlelighters.org. Information about prostheses can be obtained from the **National Amputation Foundation, Inc.,** 40 Church Street, Malverne, NY 11565; (516) 887-3600; website: http://www. nationalamputation.org/. In Canada: **War Amputations of Canada,** 1 Maybrook Drive, Scarborough, ON M1V 5K9; 1-800-250-3030 (US and Canada); (416) 297-2660; website: www.waramps.ca.

very beneficial in preparing the child for the inevitable confrontation by others. Environmental barriers, such as stairs, are assessed in terms of the accessibility of the school or home, especially because the child may need to use crutches or a wheelchair before complete healing and prosthetic competency are achieved.

The family and child need a great deal of support in adjusting not only to a life-threatening diagnosis, but also to alteration in body image and function. Because loss of a limb involves a grieving process, those caring for the child need to recognize that anger and depression are normal and necessary reactions. Often parents view the anger as a direct affront to them for allowing the amputation, or they view the depression as rejection. These are not personal attacks but the child's attempts to cope with the loss.

EWING SARCOMA (PRIMITIVE NEUROECTODERMAL TUMOR)

Ewing sarcoma, a primitive neuroectodermal tumor, is the second most common malignant bone tumor (after osteogenic sarcoma) in children and adolescents (Ginsberg and others, 2002). It arises in the marrow spaces of the bones such as the femur, tibia, fibula, ulna, humerus, vertebrae, pelvis, scapula, ribs, and skull. The disease occurs almost exclusively in individuals younger than age 30, with most occurrences in individuals between 4 and 20 years of age (Grier, 1997).

Therapeutic Management

Surgical amputation is not routinely recommended but may be considered when the results of radiotherapy render the extremity useless or deformed (such as from retarded growth in young children) or the tumor appears resectable. The treatment of choice is intensive irradiation of the involved bone combined with chemotherapy. A widely used drug regimen includes vincristine, actinomycin D, and cyclophosphamide; or ifosfamide, VP-16, and Adriamycin.

Prognosis. The prognosis is best for children who do not have metastasis at the time of diagnosis. Children with massive tumors or lung and bone marrow metastasis have a much poorer prognosis. Children with distal lesions have the best chance for cure.

Nursing Considerations

The psychologic adjustment to Ewing sarcoma is typically less traumatic than the adjustment to osteogenic sarcoma because of the preservation of the affected limb. Many families accept the diagnosis with a sense of relief in knowing that this type of bone cancer does not necessitate amputation, and initially they may not be aware of the deleterious effects on the irradiated site, especially severely affected growth, function, and appearance. Consequently, they need preparation for the various diagnostic tests, including bone marrow aspiration and surgical biopsy, and adequate explanation of the treatment regimen.

High-dose radiotherapy often causes a skin reaction of dry or moist desquamation followed by hyperpigmentation. The nurse advises the child to wear loose-fitting clothes over the irradiated area to minimize additional skin irritation. Because of increased sensitivity, the irradiated skin is protected from sunlight and sudden changes in temperature, such as avoiding use of heating pads or ice packs. The child is encouraged to use the extremity as tolerated. Occasionally, an active exercise program may be planned by the physical therapist to preserve maximum function.

The child needs the same considerations as any other patient with cancer in adjusting to the effects of chemotherapy, such as hair loss, severe nausea and vomiting, peripheral neuropathy, and possibly cardiotoxicity. Every effort should be made to outline a treatment plan that allows the child maximal resumption of a normal lifestyle and activities. See also Nursing Care Plan: The Child With Cancer (Chapter 26).

RHABDOMYOSARCOMA

The most common soft-tissue sarcoma in children is rhabdomyosarcoma. These malignant neoplasms originate from undifferentiated mesenchymal cells in muscles, tendons, bursae, and fascia or from such cells in fibrous, connective, lymphatic, or vascular tissue. These disorders derive their name from the specific tissue(s) of origin, such as *myosarcoma* (*myo*, muscle) or *rhabdomyosarcoma* (*rhabdo*, striated). Because striated (skeletal) muscle is found almost anywhere in the body, these tumors occur in many sites, the most common of which are the head and neck, especially the orbit. Sixty-five percent of the tumors occur in children younger than age 6 years, with most of the remaining cases between 10 to 18 years of age.

Diagnostic Evaluation

The initial signs and symptoms are related to the site of the tumor and compression of adjacent organs (Box 31-10). Some tumor locations, particularly the orbit, produce symptoms early in the course of the illness and contribute to rapid diagnosis and improved prognosis. Other tumors, such as those of the retroperitoneal area, produce no symptoms until they are large, invasive, and widely metastasized. Unfortunately, many of the signs and symptoms attributable to rhabdomyosarcoma are vague and frequently suggest a common childhood illness, such as "earache" or "runny nose." In some instances, a primary tumor site is never identified.

Diagnosis begins with a careful examination of the head and neck area, particularly palpation of a nontender, firm, hard mass. The nasopharynx and oropharynx are inspected for any evidence of a visible mass. Radiographic studies are performed to isolate a tumor site, accompanied by chest radiographic examinations, chest CT, bone surveys, and bone marrow aspiration to rule out metastasis. A lumbar puncture is indicated for head and neck tumors. An excisional biopsy is performed to confirm the histologic type.

Therapeutic Management

Because this tumor is highly malignant, with metastasis frequently occurring at the time of diagnosis, aggressive multimodal therapy (i.e., surgery, chemotherapy, and radiation) is recommended. Complete removal of the primary tumor is advocated whenever possible. The intergroup rhabdomyosarcoma staging system incorporates the size, invasiveness, lymph node involvement, and primary tumor site in the determina-

BOX 31-10 ■ Clinical Manifestations of Rhabdomyosarcoma According to Tumor Site

CENTRAL NERVOUS SYSTEM (CNS)
Headaches
Morning vomiting
Diplopia

ORBIT
Rapidly developing unilateral proptosis/exophthalmos
Ecchymosis of conjunctiva
Loss of extraocular movements (strabismus)
Orbital cellulitis

NASOPHARYNX
Stuffy nose (earliest sign)
Nasal obstruction—dysphagia, nasal voice (obstruction of posterior nasal conchae)
Pain (sore throat and ear)
Epistaxis
Palpable neck nodes
Visible mass in oropharynx (late sign)

PARANASAL SINUSES
Nasal obstruction
Local pain/swelling
Discharge (may be unilateral)
Sinusitis

MIDDLE EAR
Signs of chronic serous otitis media
Pain/swelling
Mass in external canal
Sanguinopurulent drainage
Facial nerve palsy
Conductive hearing loss

RETROPERITONEAL AREA (USUALLY A "SILENT" TUMOR)
Abdominal mass
Pain
Signs of intestinal or genitourinary obstruction

PERINEUM
Visible superficial mass (scrotum, vaginal or cervical areas)
Bowel or bladder dysfunction (from tumor compression)
Vaginal bleeding or mucosanguineous discharge
Extremity
Pain
Palpable fixed mass
Regional lymph node enlargement

tion of treatment and prognosis (Shamberger and others, 2002).

High-dose irradiation to the primary tumor is recommended for most tumors. Radiation usually begins after several chemotherapy courses have been given to shrink the tumor. Drugs that are cytotoxic for rhabdomyosarcoma are vincristine, actinomycin D, and cyclophosphamide, with or without Adriamycin; as well as ifosfamide, cisplatin, etoposide, and carboplatin. These may be given for 1 to 2 years.

Prognosis. With current treatment protocols, survival rates for children with tumors detected at all clinical stages have increased considerably. Tumors of the orbit, superficial

head, neck, testes, vagina, and uterus all have a 4-year survival rate of 90%. Tumors of the parameningeal area, bladder, prostate, and limbs have an approximately 65% survival rate (Shamberger and others, 2002).

Nursing Considerations

The nursing responsibilities are similar to those for other types of cancer, especially the solid tumors when surgery is used. Specific objectives include (1) careful assessment for signs of the tumor, especially during well-child examinations; (2) preparation of the child and family for the multiple diagnostic tests; and (3) supportive care during each stage of multimodal therapy. The reader is urged to review Nursing Considerations under Leukemias in Chapter 26 for physical care of the child, and Chapter 18 for emotional support of the family in the event of a poor prognosis.

DISORDERS OF JOINTS*

JUVENILE RHEUMATOID ARTHRITIS (JUVENILE IDIOPATHIC ARTHRITIS)

Juvenile idiopathic arthritis (JIA) is a new name replacing juvenile rheumatoid arthritis (JRA) in the research literature and more slowly in clinical practice. The JRA nomenclature revision to JIA was due in part to the minimally applicable reference to "rheumatoid" in JRA—in which only a small percent of children have a positive rheumatoid factor, yet the name burdens the family with images of adult disfiguring rheumatoid arthritis. Furthermore, the JRA classification system focused more on disease at onset versus disease progression, which is more important (Warren and others, 2001).

Semantics aside, JIA is an autoimmune inflammatory disease causing inflammation of joints and other tissue with an unknown cause. JIA has two peak ages of onset: between 1 and 3 years of age and between 8 and 10 years of age. Twice as many girls as boys are affected. The exact incidence is unknown, but studies suggest a minimum incidence of 4.08 per 100,000 children (Malleson, Fung, and Rosenberg, 1996). A popular theory is an infectious or environmental agent triggers an abnormal inflammatory response in a genetically predisposed child, resulting in chronic arthritis, but there is no substantiating evidence.

Pathophysiology

The disease process is characterized by chronic inflammation of the synovium with joint effusion and eventual erosion, destruction, and fibrosis of the articular cartilage. Adhesions between joint surfaces and ankylosis of joints occur if the inflammatory process persists.

Clinical Manifestations

The outcome of JIA is variable and unpredictable. The disease, even in severe forms, is rarely life-threatening but can cause significant disability. The arthritis tends to wax and wane and eventually becomes inactive in approximately 70% of the cases; however, these children may have severe or minimal joint damage remaining when active arthritis

---

*Martha Curry, MSN, RN, CPNP, revised this section.

abates. Approximately 30% of the children will have progressive arthritis into adulthood. Their arthritis can cause significant joint deformity and functional disability requiring medication, physical therapy, and perhaps future joint replacement. Chronic and acute uveitis can cause permanent vision loss if undiagnosed and not aggressively treated.

Classification of Juvenile Rheumatoid Arthritis and Juvenile Idiopathic Arthritis

JIA is not a single disease, but a heterogenous group of diseases. The three subtypes include pauciarticular onset, polyarticular onset, and systemic onset. Pauciarticular onset, which involves arthritis in four or fewer joints, accounts for 50% of all cases. Polyarticular onset, which involves more than four joints, accounts for 40% of all cases. Systemic onset has variable arthritis with systemic features of high fevers with late-evening spikes, transient maculopapular rash, hepatosplenomegaly, pericarditis, pleuritis, and lymphadenopathy. Systemic onset represents 10% of all cases. Although JIA and adult disease both involve arthritis, the diseases are distinct. In contrast to adult disease, JIA occurs in children younger than 16 years of age; children have negative rheumatoid factor in 90% of the cases, systemic features in 10% of the cases, and the associated complication of uveitis (inflammation of the iris and ciliary body) in 8% to 20% of the cases. A large portion of JIA cases—60% to 70%—tend to "burn out" and become inactive.

The universal Durban classification of JIA revised and published in 1998 lists seven disease categories, each with its own set of criteria and exclusions: systemic arthritis, oligoarthritis, rheumatoid factor–negative polyarthritis, rheumatoid factor–positive arthritis, psoriatic arthritis, enthesitis-related arthritis, and other arthritis (Petty and others, 1998).

Diagnostic Evaluation

JIA is a diagnosis of exclusion; there are no definitive tests. Both classifications are based on the clinical criteria of age of onset before 16 years, arthritis in one or more joints for 6 weeks or longer, and exclusion of other etiologies (Petty and others, 1998; Brewer and others, 1977). Laboratory tests may provide supporting evidence of disease. An elevated sedimentation rate may or may not be present. Leukocytosis is frequently present during exacerbations of systemic JIA. Antinuclear antibodies are common in JIA but are not specific for arthritis; however, they help identify children with pauciarticular disease, who are at greater risk for uveitis. Plain radiographs are the best initial imaging studies and may show soft-tissue swelling and joint space widening from increased synovial fluid in the joint. Later films can reveal osteoporosis, narrow joint space, erosions, subluxation, and ankylosis.

Therapeutic Management

There is no cure for JIA. The major goals of therapy are to control pain, preserve joint range of motion and function, minimize effects of inflammation such as joint deformity, and promote normal growth and development. Outpatient care is the mainstay of therapy; lengthy hospitalizations are infrequent in this era of managed care. The treatment plan can be exhaustive and intrusive for the child and family, including medications, physical and occupational therapy, ophthalmologic slit lamp examinations, splints, comfort measures, dietary management, school modifications, and psychosocial support.

Medications.   Many arthritis medications are available, and most are effective in suppressing the inflammatory process and relieving pain. These drugs may be given alone or in combination and are prescribed in a stepwise manner dependent on disease response to each level.

Nonsteroidal anti-inflammatory drugs (NSAIDs) are the first drugs used. Naproxen, ibuprofen, and tolmetin are approved for use in children. They are effective with few common side effects other than gastrointestinal irritation and bruising; with naproxen, skin fragility is a possible side effect. NSAIDs must be taken with food. There is unofficial use of other NSAIDs approved for arthritis in adults but not yet in children. The newer Cox-2 inhibitors, celecoxib and rofecoxib, do not affect platelet function and are presumed to cause less gastritis (Cryer and Feldman, 1998). Aspirin, once the drug of choice, has been replaced by NSAIDs because they have fewer side effects and easier administration schedules.

Methotrexate is the second-line medication used in children who have failed with NSAIDS alone (Wallace, 1998). It is started in combination with an NSAID. It is effective, with acceptable toxicity, which requires monitoring of complete blood cell counts and liver functions. Patient education about possible side effects, including discussions with teens about birth defects and avoiding alcohol, is essential.

Corticosteroids are potent immunosuppressives used for life-threatening complications, incapacitating arthritis, and uveitis. They are administered at the lowest effective dose for the briefest period and discontinued on a tapering schedule. They may be administered orally, as intraarticular joint injections, as intravenous pushes, or in eye drop form for uveitis. A single intraarticular injection may provide effective relief for children with pauciarticular disease unresponsive to NSAIDS (Padeh and Passwell, 1998). Prolonged used of systemic steroids is associated with significant side effects, including Cushing syndrome, osteoporosis, increased infection risk, glucose intolerance, cataracts, and growth suppression.

Tumor Necrosis Factor Inhibition.   *Etanercept* is a tumor necrosis factor alpha receptor blocker and an effective drug for children with JIA unresponsive to methotrexate (Lovell and others, 2003). It is given twice per week via subcutaneous injections. Possible side effects include transient allergic reaction at the injection site, increased infection risk, and rare reports of demyelinating disease and pancytopenia.

Slow-acting antirheumatic drugs (SAARDs) may require months to be effective and typically work in combination with NSAIDs. SAARDs include sulfasalazine, hydroxychloroquine, gold, and D-penicillamine. SAARDs are used less often because methotrexate has been recognized as second-line therapy.

Physical and Occupational Therapy.   Programs of physical management are individualized for each child and designed to reach the ultimate goal—preserving function or preventing deformity. Physical therapy is directed toward specific joints, focusing on strengthening muscles, mobilizing restricted joint motion, and preventing or correcting deformities. Occupational therapy assumes responsibility for generalized mobility and performance of activities of daily living.

General treatment or maintenance programs vary; physiotherapists may be involved several times weekly to monthly in management of a home program, or their visits may be limited to infrequent review of the home program for compliance, effectiveness, and need. Normal activities of daily living and the child's natural tendency to be active are usually sufficient to maintain muscle strength and joint mobility.

Exercising in a pool is excellent therapy, because it allows freedom of movement with support and minimal gravitational pull. If there is pain on motion, a hot pack or warm bath before therapy may help.

Practitioners may recommend nighttime splinting to help minimize pain and reduce flexion deformity. Joints most frequently splinted are the knees, wrists, and hands. Positioning during rest is also important. The child rests on a firm mattress with no pillow or a very low one and has no support under the knee. Loss of extension in the knee, hip, and wrist causes special problems and requires vigilance to detect the earliest signs of involvement and vigorous attention to prevent deformity with specialized passive stretching, positioning, and resting splints.

Nursing Considerations

Nursing the child with JIA involves assessment of the child's general health, the status of involved joints, and the child's emotional response to all ramifications of the disease—discomfort, physical restrictions, therapies, and self-concept.

The effects of JIA are manifest in every aspect of the child's life, including physical activities, social experiences, and personality development. Although children with severe disease may have more physical barriers to overcome, studies show that emotional and behavioral functioning is most closely linked with maternal depression and parental distress, not with physical disability (Frank and others, 1998). Nursing interventions to support the parents may foster a successful adaptation for the entire family. Parental concerns about the disease prognosis, financial and insurance issues, spouse/sibling relationships, and job and schedule conflicts must all be addressed. Referral to social workers, counselors, or support groups may be needed.

Relieve Pain. The pain of JIA is related to several aspects of the disease—disease severity, functional status, individual pain threshold, family variables, and psychologic adjustment. The aim is to provide as much relief as possible with medication and other therapies to help children tolerate the pain and cope as effectively as possible. Opioid administration is not a routine therapy for the chronic pain of JIA. Nonpharmacologic modalities have proved effective in modifying pain perception (see Pain Management, Chapter 21) and activities that aggravate pain. Behavioral and cognitive therapy, such as relaxation techniques, may be useful tools in treating arthritis pain in children (Schanberg and others, 1997).

Promote General Health. The general health of the child must be considered. A well-balanced diet with sufficient calories to maintain growth is essential. If the child is relatively inactive, caloric intake needs to match energy needs to avoid excessive weight gain, which places additional stress on affected joints. Sleep and rest are essential for children with JIA. Some children will require rest during the day; however, daytime napping that interferes with nighttime sleepiness should be avoided. A bedtime routine that involves comfort measures can help induce sleep. A firm mattress, heated water bed, electric blanket, or sleeping bag helps provide warmth, comfort, and rest. Nighttime splints needed to maintain range of motion might initially be a source of bedtime conflict. The family needs to be instructed on how to use the splint appropriately; the splint should not be painful or impede sleep. Behavior modification programs that reward splint and exercise compliance may be helpful in reducing compliance barriers. Well-child care to assess growth and development, as well as immunization requirements, needs to be coordinated between the primary care provider and the rheumatologist. Common childhood illnesses, such as upper respiratory infections, may cause arthritis to worsen; consequently, medical attention must be sought quickly for relatively minor illness to prevent arthritis flares. Effective communication between the family, the primary care provider, and the rheumatology team is essential for care coordination.

Children are encouraged to attend school, even on days when there may be some pain or discomfort. The aid of the school nurse is enlisted so that a child is permitted to take the prescribed medication at school and to arrange for rest in the nurse's office during the day. Split days or half days may help a child remain involved in school. Permitting the child to come to school late allows time to gain joint movement and reduces the time at school to avoid exhaustion. It is important that the child attend school to learn skills and engage in social interaction, especially if the JIA continues to limit physical skills. Arranging for two sets of textbooks eliminates the need to carry heavy or numerous books to and from school, thus reducing discomfort and difficulty ambulating. A formal school hearing may be necessary to obtain an individualized education plan, ensured by public law, which includes intensive school modifications.

Facilitate Compliance. The child and family are involved in the therapeutic plan. They need to know the purpose and correct use of any splints and appliances and the medication regimen. The family is instructed regarding administration of medications and the value of a regular schedule of administration to maintain a satisfactory drug level in the body. They need to know that NSAIDs should not be given on an empty stomach and to be alert for signs of medication toxicity. If evidence of drug toxicity is noted, the family is instructed to notify the health professional and follow that person's instructions.

Encourage Heat and Exercise. Heat has been shown to be beneficial to children with arthritis. Moist heat is best for relieving pain and stiffness, and the most efficient and practical method is in the bathtub with warm water. Sometimes a daily whirlpool bath, paraffin bath, or hot packs may be used as needed for temporary relief of acute swelling and pain. Hot packs are easily applied using a bath towel wrung out after being immersed in hot water or heated in a microwave oven, applied to the area, and covered with plastic for 20 minutes. Commercial pads that warm in only a few minutes in the microwave are also available. Painful hands or feet can be immersed in a pan of warm water for 10 minutes two or three times daily in addition to tub baths.

Pool therapy is the easiest method for exercising a large number of joints. Swimming activities strengthen muscles and maintain mobility in larger joints. Very small children who are frightened of the water can carry out their exercises in the bathtub. Small children love to splash, kick, and throw things in the water. Remember, adult supervision is necessary for all water activities.

Activities of daily living provide satisfactory exercise for older children to maintain maximal mobility with minimal pain. These children are encouraged in their efforts to be independent and patiently allowed to dress and groom themselves, to assume daily tasks, and to care for their belongings. It is often difficult for children to manipulate buttons, comb or brush hair, and turn faucets, but unless there is an acute flare, parents and other caregivers should not offer assistance to them. In addition, children should learn and understand why others do not help them. Many helpful devices, such as self-adhering fasteners, tongs for manipulating difficult items, and grab bars installed in bathrooms for safety, can be used to facilitate tasks. A raised toilet seat often makes the difference between dependent and independent toileting, because weak quadriceps muscles and sore knees inhibit the ability to raise the body from a low sitting position.

A child's natural affinity for play offers many opportunities for incorporating therapeutic exercises. Throwing or kicking a ball and riding a tricycle (with the seat raised to achieve maximum leg extension) are excellent moving and stretching exercises for a very young child whose daily living activities are physically limited.

An effective approach to beginning the day's activities is to awaken children early to give them their medication and then to allow them to sleep for an hour. On arising, children take a hot bath (or shower) and perform a simple ritual of limbering-up exercises, after which they commence the activities of the day, such as going to school. Exercise, heat, and rest are spaced throughout the remainder of the day according to the child's individual needs and schedules. Parents are instructed in exercises that meet the needs of the child.

> **NURSING TIP**
>
> Another method of supplying warmth before the child arises is to plug an electric blanket into an appliance timer. Set the blanket to medium or high and adjust the timer to turn on the blanket 1 hour before the child awakens (McIlvain-Simpson and Singsen, 1997).

The **Arthritis Foundation*** and the **American Juvenile Arthritis Organization*** provide services for both parents and professionals, and nurses should refer families to these agencies as an added resource.

---

*PO Box 7669, Atlanta, GA 30357-0669; (800) 283-7800; website: www.arthritis.org. In Canada, **The Arthritis Society** may be accessed for location of all local Canadian province offices; website: www.arthritis.ca.

Support Child and Family.   JIA affects every aspect of life for the child and family. Physical limitations may interfere with self-care, school participation, and recreational activities. The intensive treatment plan, including multiple medications, physical therapy, comfort measures, and medical appointments, is intrusive and very disruptive to the parents' work schedule and the family routine. To prevent isolation and encourage independence, the family is encouraged to pursue their normal activities. Unfortunately, the adaptations necessary to make that occur take resourcefulness and commitment from all family members. At diagnosis and throughout the span of JIA, it is essential to recognize signs of stress and counterproductive coping and provide the necessary support to maximize adaptation. The problems and needs of these families are discussed in Chapter 18, and the reader is directed to that chapter for guidance in planning care.

SYSTEMIC LUPUS ERYTHEMATOSUS

Systemic lupus erythematosus (SLE) is a chronic, multisystem, autoimmune disease of the connective tissues and blood vessels characterized by inflammation in potentially any body tissue. Its course and symptoms are variable and unpredictable, with mild to life-threatening complications. In addition to SLE, there are other forms of lupus, such as neonatal lupus, which occurs when maternal autoantibodies cross the placenta and cause transient lupus-like symptoms in the newborn with the potential serious complication of heart block. The remaining discussion focuses on SLE.

The estimated minimum incidence of SLE is 0.28 per 100,000 children younger than 16 years of age (Malleson, Fung, and Rosenberg, 1996). SLE is more common in girls, with an approximate 5:1 female-to-male ratio, and typically occurs between the ages of 10 and 19 years. There is a familial tendency, although many newly diagnosed patients are unaware of other affected family members. SLE has been reported in all cultures, but within the United States there has been a disproportionately higher report in African-American, Asian, and Hispanic children.

The cause of SLE is unknown. Potential triggers include hormonal imbalance, immune abnormalities, and environmental exposures, including drugs, infection, sun exposure, stress, and chemical agents.

Clinical Manifestations and Diagnostic Evaluation

The child with SLE may have any clinical manifestation (Box 31-11) with mild to life-threatening severity. The diagnosis is established when 4 of the 11 diagnostic criteria are met (Box 31-12). Kidney involvement heralds progressive disease and the need for rigorous therapeutic management.

Therapeutic Management

The goal of treatment is to ensure the health of the child by balancing the medications necessary to avoid exacerbation and complications while preventing or minimizing treatment-associated morbidity. Therapy involves the use of specific medications and general supportive care. The drugs used to control inflammation are corticosteroids administered in doses sufficient to control inflammation, then tapered to the lowest suppressive dose. Other drugs include antimalarial preparations, which are useful for rash and arthritis; NSAIDs,

BOX 31-11 ■ Clinical Manifestations of Systemic Lupus Erythematosus Related to Tissues Involved

Cutaneous lesions include the classic photosensitive erythematous malar butterfly rash extending across the nose and cheeks and sparing the nasolabial folds. Other skin findings include maculopapular rashes on any surface, discoid lesions, periungual erythema, livedo reticularis, infarcts, and alopecia.

Musculoskeletal findings include arthritis, arthralgia, myositis, and myalgia.

Central nervous system symptoms vary from headache, memory loss, and depression to seizures, psychosis, and paralysis.

Heart and lung findings may include pericarditis, myocarditis, myocardial infarction, and valvulitis. Pleural effusions, pleuritis, and pneumonitis are possible pulmonary complications.

Renal involvement, glomerulonephritis, is a serious and common complication in childhood systemic lupus erythematosus.

Lymphatic tissue involvement may include splenomegaly and generalized lymphadenopathy.

Blood abnormalities may include anemia, leukopenia, and thrombocytopenia.

Gastrointestinal symptoms include abdominal pain, nausea, vomiting, elevated lipase and amylase, and hepatomegaly.

Constitutional symptoms include weight loss, overwhelming fatigue, and low-grade fever.

BOX 31-12 ■ Classification Criteria of Systemic Lupus Erythematosus

(Requires four criteria for classification.)
1. Malar rash: fixed malar erythema
2. Discoid rash: patchy erythematous lesions
3. Photosensitivity: rash with sun exposure
4. Oral ulcers: painless ulcers in mouth/nose
5. Arthritis: swelling, tenderness, or effusion in two or more peripheral joints (nonerosive)
6. Serositis: pleuritis/pericarditis
7. Renal disorder: proteinuria/casts
8. Neurologic disorder: psychosis/seizures
9. Hematologic disorder: hemolytic anemia, thrombocytopenia, leukopenia, lymphopenia
10. Immunologic disorder: anti-dsDNA, anti-SM, antiphospholipid antibodies; lupus anticoagulant; false-positive syphilis test (RPR)
11. Antinuclear antibody

ensure compliance while minimizing the associated feeling of being different from peers (see Sunburn, Chapter 30). Patients need to be instructed to maintain regular medical supervision and seek attention quickly during illness or before elective surgical procedures, such as dental extraction, because of potential needs for increased steroids or prophylactic antibiotics. People with SLE should carry medical identification for their disease and steroid dependence.

KEY POINTS

- Immobility has a profound effect on all aspects of growth and development.
- The major physical consequences of immobilization are loss of muscle strength, endurance, and muscle mass; bone demineralization; loss of joint mobility; and contractures.
- Features of children's fractures not observed in the adult include presence of growth plate, thicker and stronger periosteum, bone porosity, more rapid healing, and less joint stiffness.
- The goals of fracture management are to regain alignment and length of bony fragments, retain alignment and length, and restore function to injured parts.
- The method of fracture reduction is determined by the age of the child, degree of displacement, amount of overriding, amount of edema, condition of the skin and soft tissues, sensation, and circulation distal to the fracture.
- The primary purposes of traction are to fatigue involved muscles and reduce muscle spasm, position bone ends in desired realignment, and immobilize the fracture site until realignment has been achieved to permit casting or splinting.
- The development of developmental dysplasia of the hip appears to be related to intrauterine, genetic, and postnatal factors.
- Treatment of clubfoot consists of manipulation and casting to correct the deformity, maintenance of the correction, and prevention of possible recurrence of the deformity.
- Acquired hip deformities are managed with non–weight-bearing devices (Legg-Calvé-Perthes disease) or surgical stabilization (slipped femoral capital epiphysis).
- Observation for scoliosis is an important part of a routine physical assessment.
- Scoliosis is managed by bracing or surgical correction.

which relieve muscle and joint inflammation; and immunosuppressive agents, such as cyclophosphamide, for renal and central nervous system disease. Antihypertensives, aspirin, and antibiotics are just a few of the additional drugs that may be necessary to treat or avoid complications.

General supportive care includes sufficient nutrition, sleep and rest, and exercise. Exposure to the sun and ultraviolet B (UVB) light is limited because of its association with SLE exacerbation.

Nursing Considerations

The principal nursing goal is to help the child and family positively adjust to the disease and therapy. The child and family must learn to recognize subtle signs of disease exacerbation and potential complications of medication therapy and to communicate these concerns to their care provider. Consequently, patient/family education is an ongoing process initiated at diagnosis and tailored to the patient's individual needs. Referral to a social worker, psychologist, or support group may help the child and family make a successful adjustment. Support groups are associated with the **Lupus Foundation of America, Inc.,*** and the **Arthritis Foundation** (see footnote on facing page).

Key issues include therapy compliance; body-image problems associated with rash, hair loss, and steroid therapy; school attendance; vocational activities; social relationships; sexual activity; and pregnancy. (See Chapter 18 for a discussion on adjusting to a chronic illness.) Specific instructions for avoiding exposure to the sun and UVB light, such as sunscreens, sun-resistant clothing, and altering outdoor activities, must be provided with great sensitivity to

* 2000 L Street NW, Suite 710, Washington, DC 20036; (202) 349-1155 or (800) 558-0121; website: www.lupus.org.

■ Bone infections are managed with vigorous antibiotic therapy, immobilization of the affected part, and (sometimes) surgical drainage.

■ Osteosarcoma is a neoplasm of bone-forming tissues; Ewing sarcoma is a neoplasm that arises from bone marrow spaces.

■ Rhabdomyosarcoma may occur almost anywhere in the body, but the most common sites are the head and neck.

■ Nursing care of the child with arthritis consists of promoting general health, relieving discomfort, preventing deformity, and preserving function.

■ Systemic lupus erythematosus is a chronic autoimmune disorder that affects the collagen tissues of the body.

References

Akins LM: Cast changes: synthetic versus plaster, *Pediatr Nurs* 23(4): 422-426,1997.

Berde CB, Billett AL, Collins JJ: Symptom management in supportive care. In Pizzo PA, Poplack DG, editors: *Principles and practice of pediatric oncology,* ed 4, Philadelphia, 2002, JB Lippincott.

Bernardo LM: Evidence-based practice for pin site care in injured children, *Orthop Nurs* 20(5):29-34, 2001.

Brewer EJ and others: Current proposed revision of JRA criteria, *Arthritis Rheum* 29(suppl 2):195-199, 1977.

Cryer B, Feldman M: Cyclooxygenase-1 and cyclooxygenase-2 selectivity of widely used nonsteroidal anti-inflammatory drugs, *Am J Med* 104:413-421, 1998.

Curley MA and others: Predicting pressure ulcer risk in pediatric patients: the Braden Q Scale, *Nurs Res* 52(1):22-33, 2003.

Do T, Herrera-Soto J: Elbow injuries in children, *Curr Opin Pediatr* 15(1):68-73, 2003.

Dzierzbicka K and others: Synthesis and cytotoxic activity of conjugates of muramyl and normuramyl dipeptides with batracylin derivatives, *J Med Chem* 46(6):978-86, 2003.

Fabry K, Fabry G, Moens P: Legg-Calvé-Perthes disease in patients under 5 years of age does not always result in a good outcome; personal experience and meta-analysis of the literature, *J Pediatr Orthop B* 12(3):222-227, 2003.

Falk MJ and others: Intravenous biphosphonate therapy in children with osteogenesis imperfecta, *Pediatrics* 111(3):573-578, 2003.

Frank RG and others: Disease and family contributors to adaptation in juvenile rheumatoid arthritis and juvenile diabetes, *Arthritis Care Res* 11(3):166-176, 1998.

Gilmore A, Thompson GH: Common childhood foot deformities, *Consult Pediatricians* 2(2):63-71, 2003.

Ginsberg JP and others: Ewing's sarcoma family of tumors: Ewing's sarcoma of bone and soft tissue and the peripheral primitive neuroectodermal tumors. In Pizzo PA, Poplack DG, editors: *Principles and practice of pediatric oncology,* ed 4, Philadelphia, 2002, JB Lippincott.

Greene WB, editor: *Essentials of musculoskeletal care,* ed 2, Rosemont, Il, 2001, American Academy of Orthopaedic Surgeons.

Gugenheim JJ Jr.: The Ilizarov fixator for pediatric and adolescent supracondylar fracture variants, *J Pediatr Orthop* 20(2):177-182, 2000.

Horwitz EM and others: Clinical responses to bone marrow transplantation in children with severe osteogenesis imperfecta, *Blood* 97(5): 1227-1331, 2001.

Houston MS: Care of the school-aged child in 90/90 traction, *Orthop Nurs* 15(2):57-64, 1996.

Karwowska A and others: Epidemiology and outcomes of osteomyelitis in the era of sequential intravenous-oral therapy, *Pediatr Infect Dis J* 17:1021-1026, 1998.

Kline NE, Sevier N: Solid tumors in children, *J Pediatr Nurs* 18(2): 96-102, 2003.

Lampe RM: Osteomyelitis and suppurative arthritis. In Behrman RE, Kliegman RM, Jenson HB, editors: *Nelson textbook of pediatrics,* ed 17, Philadelphia, 2004, WB Saunders.

Link M, Gebhardt MC, Meyers PA: Osteosarcoma. In Pizzo PA, Poplack DG, editors: *Principles and practice of pediatric oncology,* ed 4, Philadelphia, 2002, JB Lippincott.

Lovell DJ and others: Long-term efficacy and safety of etanercept in children with polyarticular-course juvenile rheumatoid arthritis: interim results from an ongoing multicenter, open-label, extended-treatment trial, *Arthritis Rheum* 48(1):218-226,2003.

Maher AB, Salmond SW, Pellino TA: *Orthopaedic nursing,* ed 3, Philadelphia, 2002, WB Saunders.

Malleson P, Fung M, Rosenberg A: The incidence of pediatric rheumatic diseases: results from the Canadian Pediatric Rheumatology Association Disease Registry, *J Rheumatol* 23(11):1981-1987, 1996.

Marini JC: Osteogenesis imperfecta. In Behrman RE, Kliegman RM, Jenson HB, editors: *Nelson textbook of pediatrics,* ed 17, Philadelphia, 2004, WB Saunders.

McIlvain-Simpson G, Singsen B: Decreasing morning stiffness, *Small Talk* 3(6):8, 1997.

Meyers PA, Gorlick R: Osteosarcoma, *Pediatr Clin North Am* 44(4): 973-989, 1997.

Newton PO, Wenger DR: Idiopathic and congenital scoliosis. In Morrissy RT, Weinstein SL, editors: *Lovell and Winter's pediatric orthopaedics,* Philadelphia, 2001, Williams & Wilkins.

Noonan KJ and others: Long term psychosocial characteristics of patients treated for idiopathic scoliosis, *J Pediatr Orthop* 17:712-717, 1997.

Olsson GL: Neuropathic pain in children. In McGrath PJ, Finley GA, editors: *Chronic and recurrent pain in children and adolescents,* Seattle, 1999, IASP Press.

Padeh S, Passwell P: Intraarticular corticosteroid injection in the management of children with chronic arthritis, *Arthritis Rheum* 41(7):1210-1214, 1998.

Peltola H, Kallio M, Unkila-Kallio L: Reduced incidence of septic arthritis in children by *Haemophilus influenzae* type b vaccination, *J Bone Joint Surg* 80B:471-473, 1998.

Petty RE and others: Revision of the proposed classification criteria for juvenile idiopathic arthritis: Durban, 1997, *J Rheumatol* 25(10): 1991-1994, 1998.

Redner A: Malignant bone tumors. In Lanzkowsky P, editor: *Pediatric hematology and oncology,* ed 3, New York, 2000, Academic Press.

Roberts CS and others: Review article: diagnostic ultrasonography: applications in orthopaedic surgery, *Clin Orthop Rel Res* 401:248-264, 2002.

Roy D: Current concepts in Legg-Calvé-Perthes disease, *Pediatr Ann* 28(12):748-751, 1999.

Samaniego IA: A sore spot in pediatrics: risk factors for pressure ulcers, *Pediatr Nurs* 29(4):278-283, 2003.

Shamberger RC, Jaksic T, Ziegler MM: General principles of surgery. In Pizzo PA, Poplack DG, editors: *Principles and practice of pediatric oncology,* ed 4, Philadelphia, 2002, JB Lippincott.

Schanberg LE and others: Pain coping and the pain experience in children with juvenile chronic arthritis, *Pain* 73(2):181-189, 1997.

Slote RJ: Psychological effects of caring for the adolescent undergoing spinal fusion for scoliosis, *Orthop Nurs* 21(6):19-28, 2002.

Thompson GH: The hip. In Behrman RE, Kliegman RM, Jenson HB, editors: *Nelson textbook of pediatrics,* ed 17, Philadelphia, 2004a, WB Saunders.

Thompson GH: The spine. In Behrman RE, Kliegman RM, Jenson HB, editors: *Nelson textbook of pediatrics,* ed 17, Philadelphia, 2004b, WB Saunders.

Wall EJ: Practical primary pediatric orthopaedics, *Nurs Clin North Am* 35(1):95-113, 2000.

Wallace CA: The use of methotrexate in childhood rheumatic disease, *Arthritis Rheum* 41:381-391, 1998.

Warren RW and others: Juvenile idiopathic arthritis (juvenile rheumatoid arthritis). In Koopman WJ, editor: *Arthritis and allied conditions,* Philadelphia, 2001, Lippincott Williams & Wilkins.

Zeitlin L, Fassier F, Glorieux FH: Modern approach to children with osteogenesis imperfecta, *J Pediatr Orthop B* 12(2):77-87, 2003.

The Child With Neuromuscular or Muscular Dysfunction

32

DAVID WILSON

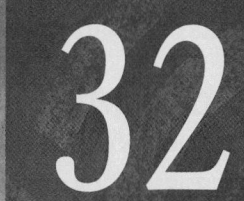

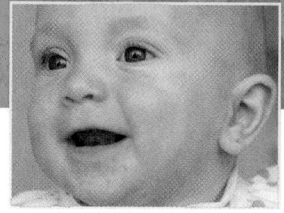

Remember to check out your companion CD-ROM

http://evolve.elsevier.com/Wong/essentials/

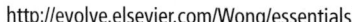

CHAPTER OUTLINE

RELATED TOPICS and ADDITIONAL RESOURCES

 IN TEXT

The Child With Cerebral Dysfunction, *Ch. 28*
Genetic Counseling, *Ch. 9*
The Immobilized Child, *Ch. 31*
Impact of Chronic Illness, Disability, or Death on the Child and Family, *Ch. 18*
Neurologic Assessment, *Ch. 7*
Nursing Care of the High-Risk Newborn and Family, *Ch. 9*
Recommendations for Routine Immunizations: Tetanus, *Ch. 10*

 CD COMPANION

Critical Thinking Exercises—Myelomeningocele; Guillain-Barré Syndrome
Clinical Manifestations—Cerebral Palsy; Spinal Muscular Atrophy; Differences Between Upper and Lower Motor Neuron Syndromes; Duchenne Muscular Dystrophy; Tetanus
Nursing Care Plans
NCLEX-Style Review Questions

evolve **WEBSITE**

WebLinks
NCLEX-Style Review Questions
 WONG'S CLINICAL MANUAL OF PEDIATRIC NURSING, 6/E
Community and Home Care Instructions—Performing Clean Intermittent Self-Catheterization
Nursing Care Plan

LEARNING OBJECTIVES
On completion of this chapter the reader will be able to:

- Discuss the nursing role in helping parents cope with a child with cerebral palsy.
- Formulate a nursing care plan for the preoperative and postoperative care of a child with myelomeningocele.
- Outline a plan of care for a child with Duchenne muscular dystrophy.
- Discuss the prevention and treatment of tetanus.
- Identify the causes of botulism in infants and children.
- List three causes of spinal cord injury in children.

CONGENITAL NEUROMUSCULAR OR MUSCULAR DISORDERS

CEREBRAL PALSY

Cerebral palsy (CP) is a nonspecific term applied to disorders characterized by early onset of impaired movement and posture. It is nonprogressive and may be accompanied by perceptual problems, language deficits, and intellectual impairment. The etiology, clinical features, and course are variable and are characterized by abnormal muscle tone and coordination as the primary disturbances. CP is the most common permanent physical disability of childhood, and the incidence is reported to be between 1.5 and 3 in every 1000 live births in the United States (Winter and others, 2002; Dabney, Lipton, and Miller, 1997). In population-based surveys the incidence of CP has risen slightly in term infants (Winter and others, 2002).

A variety of prenatal, perinatal, and postnatal factors contribute to the etiology of CP singly or multifactorially. Although the prevalent hypothesis has been that CP results from perinatal problems, especially birth asphyxia, it is now known that CP results more often from existing *prenatal* brain abnormalities—the exact cause of these abnormalities remains elusive. Intrauterine exposure to maternal infection is associated with an increased risk of CP in infants of normal birth weight and preterm infants (Gibson and others, 2003; Volpe, 2001); however, not all term infants exposed to chorioamnionitis develop CP (Grether and others, 2003). The prevalence of CP in infants born before 36 weeks' gestation and weighing less than 2000 g has been reported to be 12%; the strongest independent risk factor for development of CP was periventricular leukomalacia (Han and others, 2002). Preterm birth of extremely low birth weight (ELBW) and very low birth weight (VLBW) infants continues to be the single most important risk factor for CP, yet, in many cases, no identifiable cause is determined. Kernicterus, caused by high levels of unbound bilirubin in the neonatal period in full-term infants has also been implicated as a causative factor of CP (*MMWR*, 2001). Damage occurring as a result of shaken baby syndrome (SBS) may also result in CP in survivors (Smith, 2003).

Pathophysiology

It is difficult to establish a precise location of neurologic lesions based on etiology or clinical signs because no characteristic pathologic pattern exists. Some patients have gross malformations of the brain; others may have evidence of vascular occlusion, atrophy, loss of neurons, and degeneration. *Anoxia* plays the most significant role in the pathologic state of brain damage, which is often secondary to other causative mechanisms. A few exceptions occur and are related to anatomic areas such as spastic diplegia (associated with prematurity), caused by hypoxic infarction or hemorrhage in the area adjacent to the lateral ventricles. Ataxic CP may occur in relation to cerebral hypoplasia and, in some cases, severe hypoglycemia (Volpe, 2001). The American College of Obstetricians and Gynecologists (2003), in conjunction with the American Academy of Pediatrics, has recently published a report in which neonatal encephalopathy is defined. The report affirms that approximately 70% of cases of neonatal encephalopathy occur as a result of events occurring before the onset of labor; criteria are established to define events suffi-

BOX 32-1 ■ Clinical Classification of Cerebral Palsy

SPASTIC
May involve one or both sides
Hypertonicity with poor control of posture, balance, and coordinated motion
Impairment of fine and gross motor skills
Active attempts at motion increase abnormal postures and overflow of movement to other parts of the body

DYSKINETIC/ATHETOID
Abnormal involuntary movement
Athetosis, characterized by slow, wormlike, writhing movements that usually involve the extremities, trunk, neck, facial muscles, and tongue
Involvement of the pharyngeal, laryngeal, and oral muscles causes drooling and dysarthria (imperfect speech articulation)
Involuntary movements may take on choreoid (involuntary, irregular, jerking movements) and dystonic (disordered muscle tone) manifestations that increase in intensity with emotional stress and around adolescence

ATAXIC
Wide-based gait
Rapid, repetitive movements performed poorly
Disintegration of movements of the upper extremities when the child reaches for objects

MIXED TYPE/DYSTONIC
Combination of spasticity and athetosis

ciently capable of causing intrapartum asphyxia and cerebral palsy. Evidence indicates that events that cause the majority of CP cases occur not as a result of intrapartum asphyxia, but as a result of other causes that have been discussed previously (American Academy of Pediatrics and American College of Obstetricians and Gynecologists, 2003).

CP has been classified in several ways, but the most useful classification is based on the nature and distribution of neuromuscular dysfunction (Box 32-1).

Diagnostic Evaluation

The neurologic examination and history are the primary modalities for diagnosis of CP. A thorough knowledge of normal variations of motor development is required for detecting abnormal progress, and a careful history is elicited to detect possible etiologic factors. Early recognition is made more difficult by the lack of reliable neonatal neurologic signs; however, infants with known etiologic risk factors should be followed and evaluated closely in the first several months of life. The alert observer may be suspicious when a child demonstrates some of the manifestations outlined in Box 32-2. The child's spontaneous movements, particularly gait analysis in ambulatory children, and behavior are observed, including posture, attitude, and muscle size, function, and tone. The persistence of primitive reflexes may be of value, and two of these aid in the diagnosis: the asymmetric tonic neck reflex, or persistent Moro reflex (beyond 4 months of age), and the crossed extensor reflex (Nehring and Steele, 1996). Magnetic

BOX 32-2 ■ Clinical Signs and Symptoms of Cerebral Palsy

SPASTIC TYPE

Increased muscle tone

Increased deep tendon reflexes and clonus (sudden dorsiflexion of the ankle or rapid distal movement of the patella results in alternating spasm and relaxation of the muscles being stretched)

Flexor, adductor, and internal rotator muscles more involved than extensor, abductor, and external rotator muscles

Difficulty with fine and gross motor skills

Most common contracture is that of the heelcord

Hip adductor contractures lead to progressive subluxation and dislocation

Knee contractures

Scoliosis common

Typical gait is crouched, intoeing, scissoring

Elbow, wrist, and fingers in flexed position with thumb adducted

Motor weakness of antagonist muscle groups

ATHETOID TYPE

Purposeless, involuntary, uncontrollable movements of face and extremities

Increased movements with stress and voluntary movements, absent during sleep

Contractures rare

Normal deep tendon reflexes

ATAXIC TYPE

Disturbed coordination

Lack of equilibrium

Unsteady gait

Few orthopedic problems

Hyporeflexia

Loss of ability to gauge distance, speed, power of movement

Muscles hypotonic

Speech slurred, jerky, explosive

Nystagmus common

OTHER MANIFESTATIONS

Visual deficits (most common in spastic type)

Hearing impairment (most common in athetoid type)

Oral motor involvement resulting in drooling and feeding problems

Developmental delay (40% to 60%; most common in atonic and rigid types and spastic quadriparesis)

Sensory impairment

Seizures (approximately 40% of those with spastic hemiplegia affected)

From Maher AB, Salmond SW, Pellino TA: *Orthopaedic nursing*, ed 3, Philadelphia, 2002, WB Saunders.

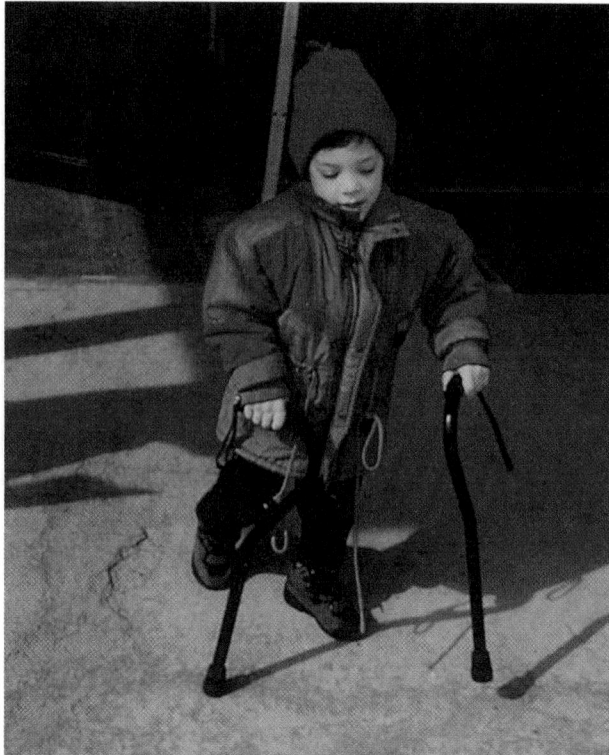

FIG. 32-1 ■ Mobilization device for child.

resonance imaging (MRI) is useful in identifying the location and extent of structural lesions and any associated pathology or anomaly; an MRI of the spine is also helpful in excluding spinal cord pathology (Johnston, 2004). Supplemental diagnostic tests may be employed, such as hearing and vision function, electroencephalography, and a genetic evaluation.

Therapeutic Management

The goals of therapy for children with CP are early recognition and promotion of optimal development to enable affected children to attain normalization and their potential within the limits of their existing health problems. The disorder is permanent, and therapy is primarily preventive and symptomatic.

There are five broad aims of therapy:

1 To establish locomotion, communication, and self-help
2 To gain optimal appearance and integration of motor functions
3 To correct associated defects as effectively as possible
4 To provide educational opportunities adapted to the individual child's needs and capabilities
5 To promote socialization experiences with other affected and unaffected children.

Each child is evaluated and managed on an individual basis. The plan of therapy may involve a variety of settings, facilities, and specially trained persons, including the parents.

Ankle-foot orthoses (AFOs, braces) are worn by many of these children and are used to help prevent or reduce deformity, increase the energy efficiency of gait, and control alignment. Other mobilization devices include wheeled scooter boards that allow children to propel themselves while on the abdomen, wheeled go-carts that provide sitting balance and serve as early "wheelchair" experience for young children, and special devices that leave the upper extremities free (Figs. 32-1 and 32-2).

Orthopedic surgery may be required to correct contracture or spastic deformities, to provide stability for an uncontrollable joint, and to provide balanced muscle power. This includes tendon-lengthening procedures (especially heelcord lengthening), release of spastic wrist flexor muscles, and correction of hip and adductor muscle spasticity or contracture to improve locomotion. A neurosurgical intervention,

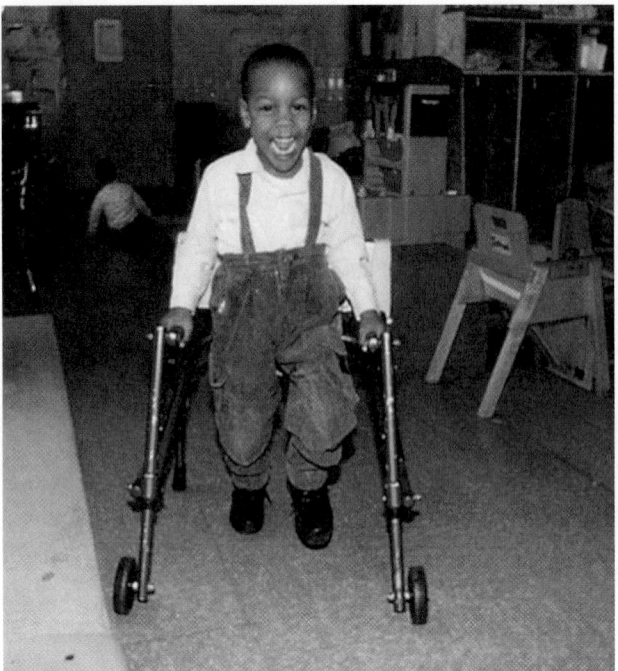

FIG. 32-2 ■ Child ambulating with use of assistive device.

selective dorsal rhizotomy, is used selectively in some children with CP. The procedure involves selectively cutting dorsal column sensory rootlets that have an abnormal response to electrical stimulation. Achieving the benefits from the surgery requires intensive physical therapy and family commitment. Because the procedure results in flaccid muscles, the child must be retaught to sit, stand, and walk.

Surgical intervention is usually reserved for the child who does not respond to the more conservative measures, but it is also indicated for the child whose spasticity causes progressive deformities. Surgery is primarily used to improve function rather than for cosmetic purposes and is followed by physical therapy.

Intense pain may occur with muscle spasms in patients with CP. Pharmacologic agents given orally (dantrolene sodium, Baclofen, and diazepam) have had little effectiveness in improving muscle coordination in children with CP; however, they are effective in decreasing overall spasticity (Jacobs, 2001). The most common side effects of these agents include hepatotoxicity (Dantrolene), drowsiness, fatigue, muscle weakness, and, less commonly, diaphoresis and constipation may be seen with Baclofen (Lioresol). Diazepam (Valium) is used frequently but should be restricted to older children and adolescents. Botulinum toxin (Botox) has become an important drug in the treatment of spasticity for CP (Jacobs, 2001). Botox is injected into the muscle, where it acts to inhibit the release of acetylcholine into a specific muscle group, thereby preventing muscle movement. When administered early in the course of the disease, contractures may be prevented, particularly in lower extremities, and surgical procedures with possible adverse effects may be avoided. The goal is to allow stretching of the muscle as it relaxes and permit ambulation with an AFO (Jacobs, 2001). The major reported adverse effect of Botox injection is pain at the injection site (Roscigno, 2002).

Neurosurgical and pharmacologic approach to managing the spasticity associated with CP involves the implantation of a pump to infuse baclofen directly into the intrathecal space surrounding the spinal cord to provide relief of spasticity. Intrathecal baclofen therapy is best suited for children with severe spasticity that interferes with activities of daily living and ambulation (Jacobs, 2001). Patients are screened before pump placement by the infusion of a "test dose" of intrathecal baclofen delivered via a lumbar puncture. Close monitoring for side effects (hypotonia, somnolence, seizures, nausea, vomiting, headache, and catheter- or pump-related problems [Albright and others, 2003]) and relief of spasticity occurs for several hours after the infusion. If a positive effect is noted, the patient is considered a candidate for pump placement. The implantation procedure is done in the operating room by a neurosurgeon. The pump, which is approximately the size of a hockey puck, is placed in the subcutaneous space of the mid-abdomen. An intrathecal catheter is tunneled from the lumbar area to the abdomen and connected to the pump. The pump is filled with baclofen and programmed to provide a set dose using a telemetry wand and a computer. Benefits of intrathecal baclofen include fewer systemic side effects, dosage titration for maximizing effects, and reversibility of therapy with removal of the pump if so desired (Jacobs, 2001). The patient may remain hospitalized for 3 to 7 days to adjust the dose and ensure proper healing. Outpatient visits to refill the pump and make dosage adjustments occur about every 4 to 6 weeks, depending on the patient's response to the treatment. This procedure is most suited for a multidisciplinary setting where rehabilitation specialists are readily available and consistently involved in the patient's ongoing care.

Antiepileptic drugs (AEDs), such as carbamazepine (Tegretol) and valproic acid (Depakote), are prescribed routinely for children who have seizures. Care of visual and auditory deficits requires the attention of appropriate specialists, and speech therapy involves the services of a speech therapist. Dental care is especially important. Regular visits to the dentist and prophylaxis, including brushing, fluoride, and flossing, should be instituted as soon as the teeth erupt. Dental care is especially important for children being given phenytoin, because they often develop gum hyperplasia.

A wide variety of technical aids is available to improve the functioning of children with CP. These include electromechanical toys that employ the concept of biofeedback and operate from a head unit. The toy is manipulated only when the head and trunk are in correct alignment. Eye-hand coordination can also be enhanced by computerized toys and games. Microcomputers combined with voice synthesizers aid children with speech difficulties to "speak." These and others print messages onto screen monitors and paper. These devices have made it apparent that some children have been erroneously considered to be mentally retarded.

Many other electronic devices allow independent functioning. Sensors can be activated and deactivated by using a head-stick, tongue, or other voluntary muscle movement over which the child has control. Voice-activated computer technology may also allow increased mobility and ambulation with specially designed devices such as wheelchairs. The application of this technology makes it possible for persons with CP to function eventually in their own residences and can be extended into the workplace.

Physical therapy is one of the most frequently used conservative treatment modalities. It requires the specialized skills of a qualified therapist with an extensive repertoire of exercise methods who can design a program to stimulate each child to achieve his or her functional goals.

An active therapy program involves the family, the physical therapist, and often other members of the health team, especially the nurse. The major approach employs traditional types of therapeutic exercises that consist of stretching, passive, active, and resistive movements applied to specific muscle groups or joints to maintain or increase range of motion, strength, or endurance.

Prognosis. Approximately 30% to 50% of individuals with CP are mentally retarded, and an even higher percentage have mild cognitive and learning deficits (Green, Greenberg, and Hurwitz, 2003); however, many children with severe spastic quadriplegic CP have normal intelligence. Growth is affected in children with spastic quadriplegia, and many children remain below the 5th percentile for age and sex. As children with CP transition to adulthood, about 30% remain in the home and are cared for by a parent or caregiver; 50% of individuals with spastic quadriplegia live in independent settings and function at appropriate social levels considering their disability (Green, Greenberg, and Hurwitz, 2003). Vocational rehabilitation and higher education is possible for adults with CP, and one study found that 53% of all persons with CP were able to work outside the home in regular jobs; one third of the severely disabled adults with CP worked outside the home (Murphy, Molnar, and Lankasky, 2000).

Nursing Considerations

Assessment

Early recognition of CP is often a result of alert observation by the nurse. Although the diagnosis may not be established until later in infancy, the nurse should be especially observant for signs in an infant who has a history that includes any of the prenatal or perinatal conditions that predispose to neonatal encephalopathy. Children who have single or multiple risk factors for CP should be carefully evaluated and followed from birth to identify abnormal signs of development. In addition, factors in the postnatal period that may contribute to hypoxic events should be monitored and prevented. Delayed attainment of developmental milestones is one of the most valuable clues to recognizing CP; therefore, developmental delays in a child offers one of the earliest indications of neurologic impairment (Box 32-3).

NURSING ALERT

The use of mobile infant walkers is discouraged. They pose a risk of injury to normal children and are especially hazardous for children with CP. Also, jumping seats, such as those that hang in doorways, should not be used.

Nursing Diagnoses

Based on a thorough assessment, several nursing diagnoses identified for the child with CP are primarily related to self-help and to facilitating mobility (see Nursing Care Plan, pp. 1193-1194). Other diagnoses may apply in specific cases.

BOX 32-3 ■ Warning Signs of Cerebral Palsy

PHYSICAL SIGNS
Poor head control after 3 months of age
Stiff or rigid arms or legs
Pushing away or arching back
Floppy or limp body posture
Cannot sit up without support by 8 months
Uses only one side of the body, or only the arms to crawl

BEHAVIORAL SIGNS
Extreme irritability or crying
Failure to smile by 3 months
Feeding difficulties
   Persistent gagging or choking when fed
   After 6 months of age, tongue pushes soft food out of the mouth

Data from Pathways Awareness Foundation: *Parents . . . if you see any of these warning signs . . . don't delay,* Chicago, 1991, The Foundation.

Planning

The goals of nursing care for the child with CP and the family are as follows:

1 Child will acquire mobility within personal capabilities.
2 Child will acquire communication skills or use appropriate assistive devices.
3 Child will engage in self-help activities.
4 Child will receive appropriate education.
5 Child will develop a positive self-image.
6 Family will receive appropriate education and support in their efforts to meet the child's needs.
7 Child will receive appropriate care if hospitalized.

Implementation

Because children with CP are being identified and treated at an earlier age, parents are participating earlier in treatment programs for their disabled child. They are taught the proper handling and home care of young children with CP and need a carefully planned program so that their change of role from parent to caregiver can be melded into the already established relationship. Nurses reinforce the therapeutic plan and assist the family in devising and modifying equipment and activities to continue the therapy program in the home.

Therapeutic interventions are those that are most appropriate for the specific problem and that best suit the needs of the individual child at any given time. CP is a complex disorder that often requires complex management of the child as well as ongoing prevention of complications. Passive range of motion exercises, stretching, and elongation exercises are valuable at any age, even at early ages when the child is unable to cooperate. They are of particular value for postural abnormalities around various joints.

Training in manual skills and activities of daily living proceeds along developmental lines and according to the child's functional level. Sitting, balancing, crawling, and walking are encouraged at appropriate ages, accompanied by stimulation of protective extension and equilibrium reactions. Hand activities are begun early to improve motor function and provide the child with sensory experiences and information about the environment. As the child progresses from simple feeding and self-care activities, training is extended to include other tasks, such as cooking or typing, that are within the child's developmental and functional capabilities.

Incorporating play into the therapeutic program often requires great ingenuity and inventiveness from those involved in the child's care. Objects and toys are chosen to provide needed sensory input, using a variety of shapes, forms, and textures. Nurses can help parents integrate therapy into play activities in natural ways.

The child may need considerable help (and patience) in learning to feed, dress, and care for personal hygiene needs. Children should be fed in the normal eating position. When they have difficulty with sucking and swallowing, it is a temptation to hold them in a semireclining posture to make use of gravity flow. This method does not promote active swallowing, however, and the neck hyperextension may even interfere with swallowing. A more flexed sitting position with arms brought forward to decrease the tendency toward back and neck extension is more natural during bottle- or spoon-feeding and encourages active swallowing (Suresh-Babu and others, 1998).

Because jaw control is compromised, more normal control can be achieved if the feeder provides stability of the oral mechanism from the side or front of the face. When directed from the front, the middle finger of the nonfeeding hand is placed posterior to the body portion of the chin, the thumb is placed below the bottom lip, and the index finger is placed parallel to the child's mandible (Fig. 32-3). Manual jaw control from the side assists with head control, correction of neck and trunk hyperextension, and jaw stabilization. The middle finger of the nonfeeding hand is placed posterior to the bony portion of the chin, the index finger is placed on the chin below the lower lip, and the thumb is placed obliquely across the cheek to provide lateral jaw stability (Fig. 32-4).

Speech training under the supervision of a speech therapist is begun early, before the child learns poor habits of communication. Parents and others can help by following the directions of the speech therapist and by talking to the child slowly and using pictures or handling objects about which the adult is speaking. Feeding techniques such as forcing the child to use the lips and tongue in eating help to facilitate speech (e.g., placing food at the side of the tongue, first one side and then the other; making the child use the lips to take food from a spoon rather than placing it directly on the tongue; and avoiding using the teeth to remove the food from the utensil). If severe dysarthria prevents articulate speech and the child has reasonable intelligence, nonverbal communication, such as sign language or voice-activated microcomputer, is used to foster communication.

As in all aspects of care, educational requirements are determined by the child's needs and potential. Children with mild to moderate involvement are generally able to participate, for varying amounts of time, in regular classes. Resource rooms are available in most schools to provide more individualized attention to a child's particular needs. Integration of these children into regular classrooms should be the initial goal. For those who are unable to benefit from formal education, a vocational training program may be ap-

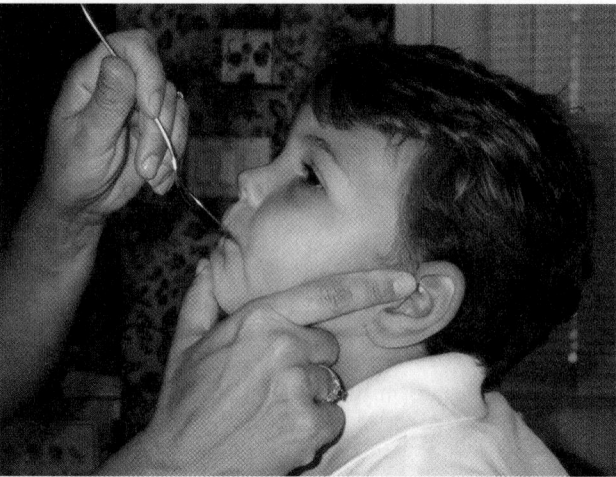

FIG. 32-3 ■ Manual jaw control provided anteriorly.

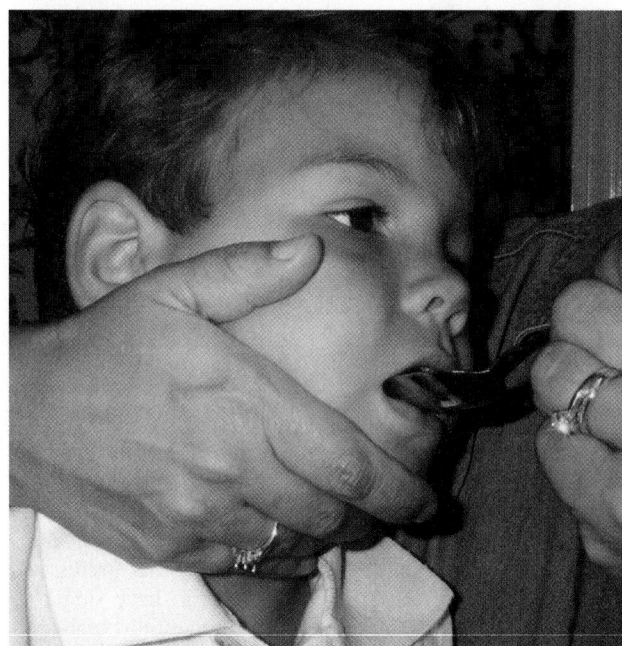

FIG. 32-4 ■ Manual jaw control provided from the side.

propriate. At adolescence, prevocational and vocational counseling and guidance are arranged. At any phase or in any setting, education is geared toward the child's assets.

Recreational outlets and after-school activities should be considered for the child who is unable to participate in the regular athletic programs and other peer activities. Some children can compete in athletic and artistic endeavors, and many games and pastimes are suited to their capabilities. Competitive sports are also becoming increasingly available to children with disabilities and offer an added dimension to physical activities. Information on training programs and competition on local, state, regional, and national levels can be obtained from the **National Disability Sports Alliance.***

---

*25 West Independence Way, Kingston, RI 02881; (401) 792-7130; website: www.ndsaonline.org.

NURSING CARE PLAN   The Child With Cerebral Palsy

NURSING DIAGNOSIS ▪ Impaired physical mobility related to neuromuscular impairment

PATIENT GOAL 1: Will acquire locomotion within capabilities (per care plan of physical therapy/occupational therapy)

NURSING INTERVENTIONS/RATIONALES

Encourage sitting, crawling, and walking as prescribed
Carry out therapies that strengthen and improve control *to facilitate optimal development*
Assist child in using reciprocal leg motion when learning to walk, if indicated in plan of care
Provide incentives to move (e.g., place toy out of child's reach)
Ensure adequate rest before attempting locomotion activities *to encourage success*
Incorporate play that encourages desired behavior *to encourage cooperation*
Employ aids such as parallel bars and crutches as prescribed *to facilitate locomotion*
Prepare child and family for surgical procedures if indicated

EXPECTED OUTCOME

Child acquires locomotion within capabilities (specify)

PATIENT GOAL 2: Will experience no or minimal deformity

NURSING INTERVENTIONS/RATIONALES

Apply and correctly use orthoses *for maximal benefit*
Carry out and teach family to perform stretching exercises as prescribed *to prevent deformities*
Employ appropriate range-of-motion exercises as prescribed *to facilitate muscle development and flexibility of joints*
Perform preoperative and postoperative care for child who requires corrective surgery

EXPECTED OUTCOME

Alignment and flexibility are maintained within child's limits

NURSING DIAGNOSIS ▪ Bathing/hygiene, dressing/grooming, feeding, toileting self-care deficits related to physical disability

PATIENT GOAL 1: Will engage in self-help activities of daily living

NURSING INTERVENTIONS/RATIONALES

Encourage child to assist with care as age and capabilities permit *to facilitate optimal development*
Select toys and activities that allow maximum participation by child and that improve motor function and sensory input *to promote self-care*
Avoid undue persistence *because child may be unable or not ready to accomplish a goal*
Encourage activities that require both unimanual and bimanual actions *to encourage optimal development*
Assist with jaw control during feeding *to facilitate eating*
Encourage use of adapted utensils, food, and clothing *to facilitate self-help* (e.g., large-bowled spoon with padded handle; finger foods and foods that adhere to, rather than slip from, utensil; clothing that opens from front with self-adhering closings rather than buttons)

Assist parents in toilet training child, *because methods may need to be individualized according to child's abilities*

EXPECTED OUTCOME

Child engages in self-help activities commensurate with capabilities

NURSING DIAGNOSIS ▪ Risk for injury, related to physical disability, neuromuscular impairment, perceptual and cognitive impairment

PATIENT GOAL 1: Will experience no physical injury

NURSING INTERVENTIONS/RATIONALES

Educate family to provide safe physical environment
    Use padded furniture *for protection*
    Use side rails on bed *to prevent falls*
    Use sturdy furniture that does not slip *to prevent falls*
    Avoid throw rugs and polished floors *to prevent falls*
Educate family to select toys appropriate to age and physical limitations *to prevent injuries*
Encourage sufficient rest *to reduce fatigue and decrease risk of injuries*
Use safety restraints when child is in chair or vehicle
Provide child who is prone to falls with protective helmet and enforce its use *to prevent head injuries*
Institute seizure precautions for susceptible child
*Administer antiepileptic drugs as prescribed *to prevent seizures*

EXPECTED OUTCOMES

Family provides a safe environment for child (specify)
Child is free of injury

NURSING DIAGNOSIS ▪ Impaired verbal communication related to hearing loss, neuromuscular impairment, cognitive impairment

PATIENT GOAL 1: Will engage in communication process within limits of impairment

NURSING INTERVENTIONS/RATIONALES

Enlist the services of a speech therapist early *to promote good habits of communication*
Talk to child slowly *to give child time to understand speech*
Use articles and pictures *to reinforce speech and encourage understanding*
Use feeding techniques *that help facilitate speech,* such as using lips, teeth, and various tongue movements
Teach and use nonverbal communication methods (e.g., sign language) for children with severe dysarthria
Help family acquire electronic equipment *to facilitate nonverbal communication* (e.g., computer with voice synthesizer)

EXPECTED OUTCOME

Child is able to communicate needs to caregivers (specify desired communication and means of accomplishment)

*Dependent nursing action.

Continued

NURSING CARE PLAN The Child With Cerebral Palsy—*cont'd*

NURSING DIAGNOSIS ■ **Imbalanced nutrition: less than body requirements related to feeding and motor problems**

PATIENT GOAL 1: Will receive optimal nutrition

NURSING INTERVENTIONS/*RATIONALES*

Provide extra calories in diet *to meet energy demands of increased muscle activity*

Monitor weight gain *to evaluate adequacy of nutritional intake*

Provide vitamin, mineral, and protein supplements if unable to meet caloric requirements with common food sources

Consult dietitian for planning adequate caloric intake based on child's individual needs

Devise aids and techniques with input from occupational/speech therapists to facilitate feeding *so that child receives adequate nourishment*

EXPECTED OUTCOMES

Child eats a balanced diet

Weight remains within acceptable limits (specify)

NURSING DIAGNOSIS ■ **Fatigue related to increased energy expenditure**

PATIENT GOAL 1: Will receive optimal rest

NURSING INTERVENTIONS/*RATIONALES*

Maintain a well-regulated schedule that allows for adequate rest and sleep periods *to prevent fatigue*

Be alert for evidence of fatigue, which tends to aggravate symptoms

EXPECTED OUTCOME

Child is sufficiently rested

PATIENT GOAL 2: Will maintain good general health

NURSING INTERVENTIONS/*RATIONALES*

Ensure regular routine health maintenance *to promote general health*
Physical assessment
Dental care
Immunizations

EXPECTED OUTCOMES

Child receives regular health assessments (specify schedule)

Child receives appropriate immunizations (specify) and dental care (specify)

NURSING DIAGNOSIS ■ **Disturbed body image related to perception of disability**

PATIENT GOAL 1: Will verbalize positive self-image

NURSING INTERVENTIONS/*RATIONALES*

Demonstrate acceptance of child through own behavior, *because children are sensitive to affective attitude of the professional*

Capitalize on child's assets and provide compensation for liabilities *to encourage positive self-image*

Praise child for accomplishments and "near" accomplishments, such as partial completion of a task

Plan activities and goals *with* the child that provide opportunities for success *to encourage cooperation and positive self-image*

Encourage grooming and age-appropriate dress *to promote acceptance by others and positive body image*

EXPECTED OUTCOME

Child exhibits behaviors that indicate positive body image (specify)

NURSING DIAGNOSIS ■ **Interrupted family processes related to a child with a lifelong disability**

PATIENT (FAMILY) GOAL 1: Will receive adequate support

NURSING INTERVENTIONS/*RATIONALES*

Refer to special support group(s) and agencies *to provide social support*

EXPECTED OUTCOMES

Family needs for support are met

See also: Nursing Care Plan: The Child With Mental Retardation, Chapter 19

Recreational activities serve to stimulate children's interest and curiosity, help them adjust to their disability, improve their functional abilities, and build self-esteem. Any accomplishment that helps children approach a "normal" way of life enhances their self-concept.

Support Family. Probably the nursing interventions most valuable to the family are support and help in coping with the emotional aspects of the disorder, many of which are discussed in relation to the child with a disability (see Chapter 18). Initially the parents need supportive counseling directed toward understanding the implications of the diagnosis and all of the feelings that it engenders. Later they need clarification regarding what they can expect from the child and from health professionals. Having a child with CP implies numerous problems of daily management and changes in family life.

The nurse needs to support the parents in their frustration, problem solving, concerns, approaches to helping the child, and lack of gratification, as well as the positive approaches they use. All of these aspects must be explored and discussed. Parents, as well as other members of the family, require much support and counseling. Siblings of a child with a disability are affected and may respond to the presence of the child with overt or less evident behavioral prob-

FAMILY FOCUS

The Reality of Acceptance of Cerebral Palsy

Acceptance is rarely achieved in the length of time implied in the literature.

In the first place, what is it? To me, it is the end of comparing my son with every other child I see. I focus on *his* gains, not society's expectations.

It is also being able to laugh periodically *at* his "clumsiness." It is "gallows humor" as he achieves adulthood; jokes about CP can be funny now.

The bitterness is gone; I am now happy for people who have children without CP.

I no longer feel sorry for my son, but rather for the people who cannot see him for the great person he is; the CP does *not* come first.

He is now a young man of 25 years and I am learning to accept his independence.

It is a "never-ending story."

Elaine A. Dunham, RN
Shriner's Hospital
Springfield, Massachusetts

lems. The family needs a relationship with nurses who can provide continued contact, support, and encouragement through the long process of habilitation.

Parents can also find help and solace from parent groups, with whom they can share problems and concerns and from whom they can derive comfort and practical information. Parent support groups are most helpful through sharing experiences and accomplishments. For example, parents can understand from others what it is like to have a child with CP, which is generally not possible from professionals (see Family Focus box). The national organization, **United Cerebral Palsy Association,*** has branches in most communities. The association provides a variety of services for children and families. A number of excellent books also are available to serve as guides for parents and nurses who work with the child with CP.

Support Hospitalized Child.

CP is not a disorder that requires hospitalization; therefore, when children with CP are hospitalized, they are usually admitted for another reason or for corrective surgery. Nursing care of the child with CP is the same as with any other child with a disability. Children with CP should be approached the same as any child in the hospital. The nurse's actions should convey acceptance, affection, and friendliness and promote a feeling of trust and dependability in the child. This is especially true with older children who have normal intelligence but who may have communication problems. Speech impairment is common in children with CP. To facilitate the care and management of these children, the therapy program should be continued, insofar as their condition allows, during the time they are hospitalized. This should be incorporated into the nursing care plan with every effort expended to make

*1660 L Street NW, Suite 700, Washington, DC 20036; (800) 872-5827; website: www.ucpa.org (also provides a listing of each state's UCP organization).

certain that the ground that has been so laboriously gained is not lost. Encouraging the parent to room-in and actively participate in the child's care facilitates a continuation of the home therapy program and helps the child adjust to an unfamiliar environment. However, it is equally important to remember that a hospitalization may be the first time a parent can defer care to a nurse and not be the primary caregiver. This respite may be crucial to the parent's well-being.

● Evaluation

The effectiveness of nursing interventions is determined by continual reassessment and evaluation of care based on the following observational guidelines:

1. Observe child's movements and use of mobilization devices.
2. Observe child's speech and ability to use communication devices.
3. Observe child's activities, especially those related to self-care.
4. Discuss with family child's activities and school attendance.
5. Observe child's interactions with others and choice of activities; interview child regarding feelings and concerns.
6. Encourage family discussion regarding their feelings and concerns and observe family members' interaction with the child.
7. Observe child's behavior and responses during hospitalization.

The *expected outcomes* are described in the Nursing Care Plan on pp. 1193-1194.

SPINA BIFIDA (MYELOMENINGOCELE)*

Abnormalities that are derived from the embryonic neural tube *(neural tube defects [NTDs])* constitute the largest group of congenital anomalies that is consistent with multifactorial inheritance. Normally the spinal cord and cauda equina are encased in a protective sheath of bone and meninges (Fig. 32-5, *A*). Failure of neural tube closure produces defects of varying degrees (Box 32-4). They may involve the entire length of the neural tube or may be restricted to a small area.

In the United States, rates of NTDs have declined from 1.3 per 1000 births (1970) to 0.3 per 1000 births after the introduction of mandatory food fortification with folic acid in 1998 (Honein, 2001). Increased use of prenatal diagnostic techniques and termination of pregnancies have also impacted the overall incidence of NTDs. (See also Prevention, p. 1199.)

Myelodysplasia refers broadly to any malformation of the spinal canal and cord. Midline defects involving failure of the osseous (bony) spine to close are called *spina bifida (SB),* the most common defect of the central nervous system. SB is categorized into two types: spina bifida occulta and spina bifida cystica.

Spina bifida occulta refers to a defect that is not visible externally. It occurs most frequently in the lumbosacral area (L5 and S1) (Fig. 32-5, *B*). SB occulta may not be apparent unless there are associated cutaneous manifestations or neuromuscular disturbances.

Spina bifida cystica refers to a visible defect with an external saclike protrusion. The two major forms of SB cystica are *meningocele,* which encases meninges and spinal fluid

*Amy Nadel Romanczuk, MSN, RN,CNS, revised this section.

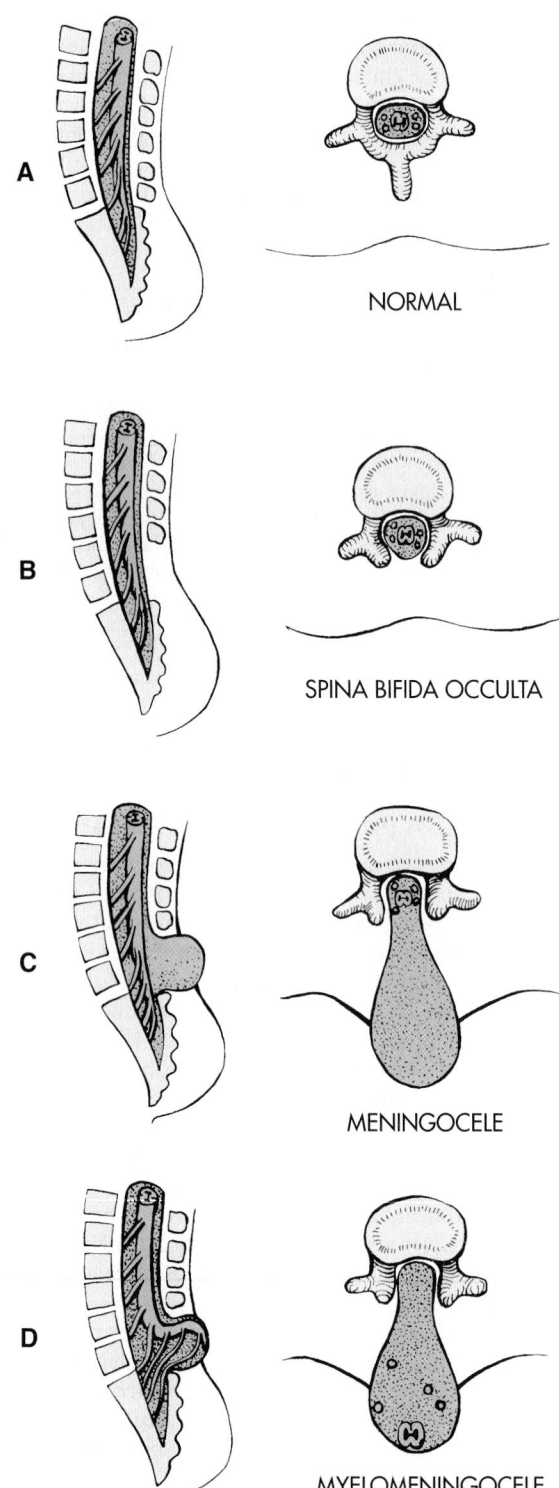

A

NORMAL

B

SPINA BIFIDA OCCULTA

C

MENINGOCELE

D

MYELOMENINGOCELE

FIG. 32-5 ■ Midline defects of osseous spine with varying degrees of neural herniations.

but no neural elements (Fig. 32-5, *C*), and ***myelomeningocele*** (or ***meningomyelocele***), which contains meninges, spinal fluid, and nerves (Fig. 32-5, *D*). Meningocele is not associated with neurologic deficit, which occurs in varying, often serious, degrees in myelomeningocele. Clinically the term *spina bifida* is used to refer to myelomeningocele.

BOX 32-4 ■ Significant Neural Tube Defects

Cranioschisis—A skull defect through which various tissues protrude

Exencephaly—Brain totally exposed or extruded through an associated skull defect; fetus usually aborted

Anencephaly—If fetus with exencephaly survives, degeneration of the brain to a spongiform mass with no bony covering; incompatible with life usually beyond a few days

Encephalocele—Herniation of brain and meninges through a defect in the skull producing a fluid-filled sac

Rachischisis or **spina bifida**—Fissure in the spinal column that leaves the meninges and spinal cord exposed

Meningocele—Hernial protrusion of a saclike cyst of meninges filled with spinal fluid (Fig. 32-5, *C*)

Myelomeningocele (meningomyelocele)—Hernial protrusion of a saclike cyst containing meninges, spinal fluid, and a portion of the spinal cord with its nerves (Fig. 32-5, *D*)

Pathophysiology

Most authorities believe that the primary defect in NTDs is a failure of neural tube closure during early development (the first 3 to 5 weeks) of the embryo. However, there is also evidence implicating a multifactorial etiology including drugs, radiation, maternal malnutrition, chemicals, and possibly a genetic mutation in folate pathways in some cases, which may result in abnormal development (Johnston and Kinsman, 2004). Additional factors predisposing to an increased risk of NTDs include prepregnancy maternal obesity, previous NTD pregnancy, and the use of AED drugs in pregnancy (Watkins and others, 2003; Frey and Hauser, 2003; Finnell, Gould, and Spiegelstein, 2003). The degree of neurologic dysfunction depends on where the sac protrudes through the vertebrae, the anatomic level of the defect, and the amount of nerve tissue involved (Rintoul and others, 2002). Most myelomeningoceles involve the lumbar or lumbosacral area (Fig. 32-6). Hydrocephalus is a frequently associated anomaly in 80% to 90% of the children.

Diagnostic Evaluation

The diagnosis of SB is made on the basis of clinical manifestations (Box 32-5) and examination of the meningeal sac. Diagnostic measures used to evaluate the brain and spinal cord include MRI, ultrasound, computed tomography (CT), and myelography.

Laboratory examinations are used primarily to determine causative organisms for the major complications of myelomeningocele—meningitis and urinary tract infections.

Prenatal Detection.   It is possible to determine the presence of some major open NTDs prenatally. Fetal ultrasound and elevated concentrations of alpha-fetoprotein (AFP), a fetal-specific gamma$_1$-globulin, in amniotic fluid may indicate the presence of anencephaly or myelomeningocele. The optimum time for performing these diagnostic tests is between 16 and 18 weeks of gestation, before AFP concentrations normally diminish and in sufficient time to permit a therapeutic abortion. Chorionic villus sampling (CVS) is also a measure for prenatal diagnosis of NTDs; however, it carries certain risks (skeletal limb depletion) and is not recommended before 10 weeks' gestation. It is recommended

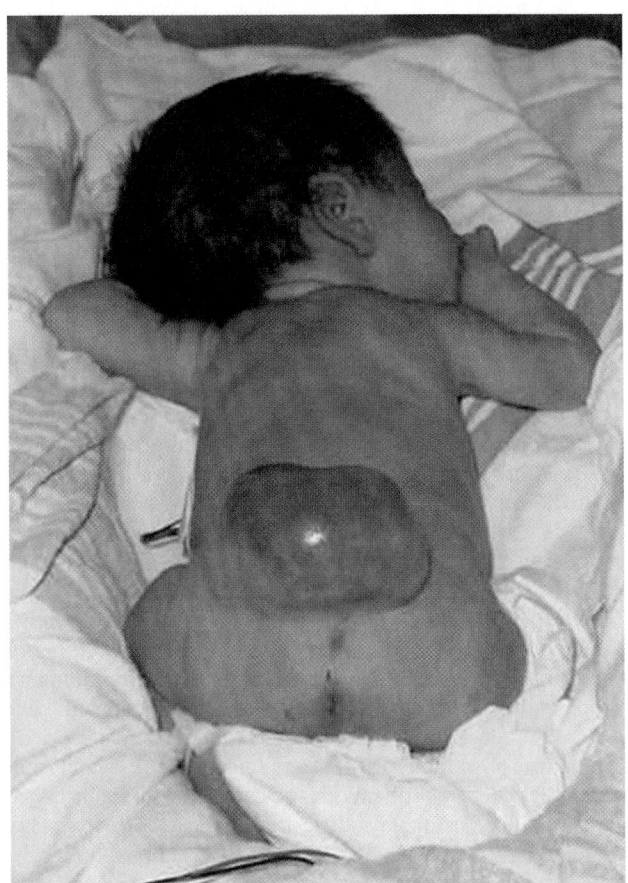

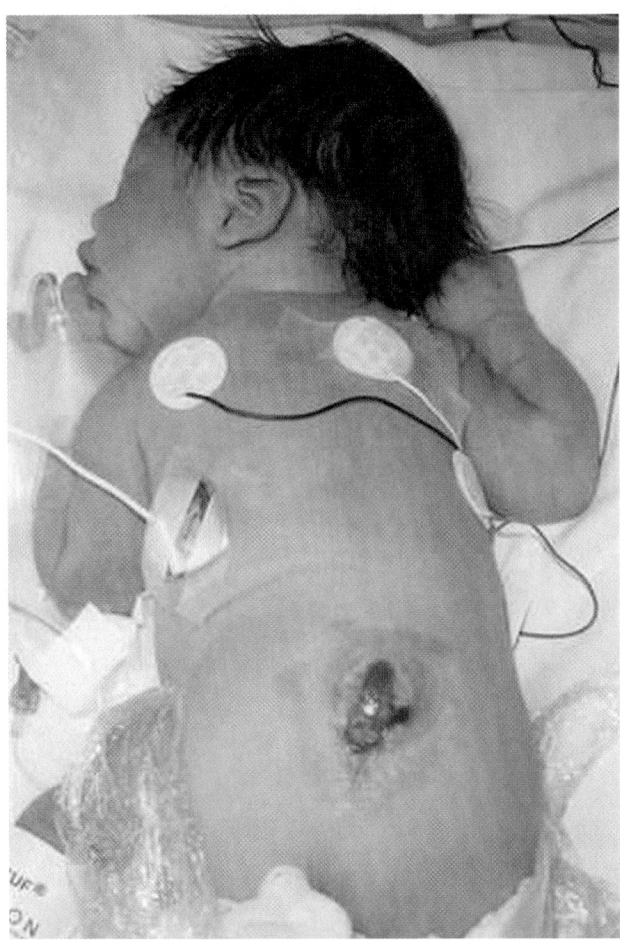

A

B

FIG. 32-6 ■ **A,** Myelomeningocele with intact sac. **B,** Myelomeningocele with ruptured sac. (Photos courtesy Dr. Robert C. Dauser, Neurosurgery, Baylor College of Medicine, Houston, Texas.)

that such diagnostic procedures be considered for all mothers who have borne an affected child, and testing is offered to all pregnant women. In addition, elective prelabor cesarean birth may result in less motor dysfunction.

Therapeutic Management

Early surgical closure of the myelomeningocele sac through fetal surgery is being evaluated in relation to prevention of injury to the exposed spinal cord tissue and the improvement of neurologic and urologic outcomes in the affected child (Hirose and others, 2001; Holmes and others, 2001; Olutoye and Adzick, 1999; Tulipan and Bruner, 1998). Initial fetal surgical success and survival rates appear to be positive; however, reports vary in relation to the success of fetal surgery in the actual reduction of urologic problems, improvement of lower leg function, and prevention of hydrocephalus in the postnatal period (Tubbs and others, 2003; Holmes and others, 2001). Some have suggested that the ethical issues surrounding fetal surgery, outcomes, and the risks involved have yet to be satisfactorily discussed and settled (Lyerly and Mahowald, 2003). Management of the child who has a myelomeningocele requires a multidisciplinary approach involving the specialties of neurology, neurosurgery, pediatrics, urology, orthopedics, rehabilitation, physical therapy, and social services as well as intensive

nursing care in a variety of specialty areas. The collaborative efforts of these specialists are focused on (1) the myelomeningocele and the problems associated with the defect—hydrocephalus, paralysis, orthopedic deformities, and genitourinary abnormalities; (2) possible acquired problems that may or may not be associated, such as meningitis, hypoxia, and hemorrhage; and (3) other abnormalities, such as cardiac or gastrointestinal malformations.

Infancy.   Initial care of the newborn involves prevention of infection; neurologic assessment, including observation for associated anomalies; and dealing with the impact of the anomaly on the family. Although meningoceles are repaired early, especially if there is danger of rupture of the sac, the philosophy regarding skin closure of myelomeningocele varies. Most authorities believe that early closure, within the first 24 to 72 hours, offers the most favorable outcome. Early closure, preferably in the first 12 to 18 hours, not only prevents local infection and trauma to the exposed tissues, but also avoids stretching of other nerve roots, which may occur as the meningeal sac expands during the first hours after birth, thus preventing further motor impairment.

Associated problems are assessed and managed by appropriate surgical and supportive measures. Shunt procedures provide relief from imminent or progressive hydrocephalus

BOX 32-5 ■ Clinical Manifestations of Spina Bifida

SPINA BIFIDA CYSTICA
Sensory disturbances usually parallel motor dysfunction
 Below second lumbar vertebra:
  Flaccid, partial paralysis of lower extremities
  Varying degrees of sensory deficit
  Overflow incontinence with constant dribbling of urine
  Lack of bowel control
  Rectal prolapse (sometimes)
 Below third sacral vertebra:
  No motor impairment
  May be saddle anesthesia with bladder and anal sphincter paralysis
Joint deformities (sometimes produced in utero):
 Talipes valgus or varus contractures
 Kyphosis
 Lumbosacral scoliosis
 Hip dislocations

SPINA BIFIDA OCCULTA
Frequently no observable manifestations
May be associated with one or more cutaneous manifestations:
 Skin depression or dimple
 Port-wine angiomatous nevi
 Dark tufts of hair
 Soft, subcutaneous lipomas
May be neuromuscular disturbances:
 Progressive disturbance of gait with foot weakness
 Bowel and bladder sphincter disturbances

(see Chapter 28). Meningitis, urinary tract infection, and ventriculitis are treated with vigorous antibiotic therapy and supportive measures. Surgical intervention for Chiari malformation (a downward herniation of the brain into the brainstem) or for tethered cord (scar tissue binding the spinal cord) is indicated only when the child is symptomatic.

Improved surgical techniques do not alter the major physical disability, spinal defect, or chronic urinary tract infections that affect the quality of life for these children. Superimposed on the physical problems are the effects that the disorder has on family life and finances, including the need for long-term specialized school and health care services.

Orthopedic Considerations. According to most orthopedists, musculoskeletal problems that will affect later locomotion should be evaluated early, and treatment, where indicated, should be instituted without delay. Neurologic assessment will determine the neurosegmental level of the lesion, recognition of spasticity and progressive paralysis, potential for deformity, and functional expectations. Orthopedic management includes prevention of joint contractures, correction of the existing deformity, prevention or minimization of the effects of motor and sensory deficits, prevention of skin breakdown, and obtaining the best possible function of affected lower extremities. Common orthopedic problems requiring attention in SB include deformities of the knees, hips, feet, and spine; fractures and insensate skin further complicate orthopedic care (Brown, 2001). Other problems that may occur later include kyphosis and scoliosis (Brown,

2001). Because children with this condition often have decreased sensitivity in lower extremities, preventive skin care is very important. A high percentage (60%) of children seen in a wound clinic for skin breakdown had myelomeningocele (Samaniego, 2003). The status of the neurologic deficit remains the most important factor in determining the child's ultimate functional abilities.

With technologic advances, a variety of lightweight orthoses are available to provide mobility to children with spinal cord lesions, including braces, special "walking" devices, and custom-built wheelchairs (see also Chapter 19). Early in infancy, intervention with passive range-of-motion exercises, positioning, and stretching exercises may help decrease the incidence of muscle contractures (Brown, 2001). Corrective surgical procedures, when indicated, are best initiated at an early age so that the child will not lag significantly behind age-mates in developmental progress. Where there is little hope for lower extremity functioning, surgery is seldom recommended unless it will improve sitting position in a wheel chair and function for activities of daily living (ADLs) and mobility.

Management of Genitourinary Function. Myelomeningocele is one of the most common causes of ***neuropathic (neurogenic) bladder dysfunction*** among children. In infants the goal of treatment is to preserve renal function. In older children the goal is to preserve renal function and achieve optimal urinary continence. Urinary incontinence is a chronic, often debilitating problem for the child. In addition, the neuropathic bladder may produce ***urinary system distress,*** characterized by symptomatic urinary tract infections, ureterohydronephrosis, and vesicoureteral reflux or renal insufficiency. The characteristics of bladder dysfunction in children vary according to the level of the neurologic lesion and the influence of bony growth and development on the spine. Therefore ongoing urologic monitoring is essential, and there is growing evidence that early intervention, based on evaluation during the neonatal period and before complications occur, serve to improve bladder function, reduce the risk of subsequent urinary system distress, and decrease the need for reconstructive surgery of the lower urinary tract (Holzbierlein and others, 2000; Kaefer and others, 1999).

Treatment of renal problems includes (1) regular urologic care with prompt and vigorous treatment of infections; (2) some type of regular emptying of the bladder, such as ***clean intermittent catheterization (CIC)*** taught to and performed by parents and self-catheterization taught to children; (3) medications to improve bladder storage and continence, such as oxybutynin chloride (Ditropan), and tolterodine (Detrol); and (4) surgical procedures such as ***vesicostomy*** (stoma created on the abdominal wall for urinary drainage) and ***augmentation enterocystoplasty*** (increases bladder capacity and reduces high bladder pressures).

Infrequently, children with myelodysplasia may develop severe dysfunction of the bladder that compromises renal function or produces debilitating urinary incontinence that is intractable to other treatments. ***Urinary diversion,*** typically using a continent neobladder constructed from bowel or stomach, may be required. Whenever feasible, the neobladder is constructed in a way that allows continence, and CIC is used to regularly evacuate urine. The appendix may also be used to create a stoma from the bladder to the abdominal wall or, in older children, the umbilicus, whereby intermittent catheterization may be done on a less conspicuous basis for normalization of daily activities (also referred to as the Mitrofanoff route).

Bowel Control.   Some degree of fecal continence can usually be achieved in most children with myelomeningocele with diet modification, regular toilet habits, and prevention of constipation and impaction. It is frequently a lengthy process. Fiber supplements, laxatives, suppositories, or enemas aid in producing regular evacuation. Older children and adolescents seeking more independence may attain bowel continence and higher quality of life after undergoing the Malone antegrade continence enema (MACE) procedure (Yerkes and others, 2003). In this procedure, the appendix or ileum is used to create a catheterizable channel with attachment of the proximal end to the colon. The distal end of the channel exits through a small abdominal stoma. Every 1 to 2 days, a catheter is passed through the stoma, allowing enema solution to be instilled directly into the colon. After administration of the enema solution, the child sits on the toilet for 30 to 60 minutes as stool is flushed out through the rectum. Frequency of enemas and volume of solution used to completely evacuate the bowel vary among individuals.

Prognosis.   The early prognosis for the child with myelomeningocele depends on the neurologic deficit present at birth, including motor ability and bladder innervation and the presence of associated neurologic anomalies. Early surgical repair of the spinal defect, antibiotic therapy to reduce the incidence of meningitis and ventriculitis, prevention of urinary system dysfunction, and early detection and correction of hydrocephalus have significantly increased the survival rate and quality of life in such children. Based on current medical knowledge and ethical considerations, aggressive management is favored for the child with myelomeningocele.

Prevention.   The widespread use of folic acid among women of childbearing age is expected to significantly decrease the incidence of SB. It has been estimated that a daily intake of 0.4 mg of folic acid in women of childbearing age will prevent 50% to 70% of all cases of neural tube defects (Centers for Disease Control and Prevention [CDC], 2001). Preliminary data show a 24% decrease in cases of spina bifida between 1996 and 2001 (Matthews, Honein, and Erickson, 2002). For women who have had a previous pregnancy affected by NTDs, folic acid intake is increased to 4 mg under supervision of a practitioner beginning 1 month before a planned pregnancy and continuing during the first trimester. Supplementation of 4 mg of folate should not be given in multivitamin preparations because of the risk of overdose of other vitamins. However, despite the recommendations of several health care and public agencies for the daily intake of 0.4 mg folic acid in the periconceptual period, a recent survey revealed that only a small percentage (42%) of women of childbearing age actually follow these guidelines (CDC, 2001). Awareness of the benefits of folic acid for the prevention of birth defects was highest in women ages 25 to 29 years of age, college-educated, married, Caucasian, and not consid-

ered overweight. These results indicate that nurses and other health care workers have an important task in disseminating information that may decrease the incidence of birth defects in children by promoting maternal consumption of folic acid.* To ensure adequate daily intake of the recommended amount of folic acid, women must take a folic acid supplement, eat a fortified breakfast cereal containing 100% of the recommended dietary allowance (RDA) of folic acid (e.g., Kellogg's Product 19, General Mills Total, Multigrain Cheerios Plus), or increase their consumption of fortified foods (cereal, bread, rice, grits, pasta) and foods naturally rich in folate (green leafy vegetables and citrus fruits). The only population in which folic acid has not proved to be effective in decreasing the incidence of NTDs is epileptic women taking antiepileptic medications during pregnancy (Finnell, Gould, and Spiegelstein, 2003).

> ⚠️ **NURSING ALERT**
>
> Because approximately half of all pregnancies in the United States are unplanned (Henshaw, 1998), adolescent girls and women of childbearing age need to be educated about the necessity of folic acid to prevent neural tube defects. The daily dose of 0.4 mg (400 μg) is most easily obtained from a multivitamin supplement.

Nursing Considerations

At birth an examination is performed to assess the intactness of the membranous cyst. During transport to the nursery, every effort is made to prevent trauma to this protective covering. In addition to the routine assessment of the newborn (see Chapter 8), the infant is assessed for the level of neurologic involvement. Movement of extremities or skin response, especially an anal reflex, that might provide clues to the degree of motor or sensory impairment is noted. It is important to observe the infant's behavior in conjunction with the stimulus, because limb movements can be induced in response to spinal cord reflex activity that has no connection with the higher centers. Observation of urine output, especially if a diaper remains dry, may indicate urinary retention. Abdominal assessment revealing bladder distention, even with a wet diaper, may indicate urinary overflow in a retentive bladder. The head circumference is measured daily (see Chapter 7), and the fontanels are examined for signs of tension or bulging.

Care of the Myelomeningocele Sac.   The infant is usually placed in an incubator or warmer so that temperature can be maintained without clothing or covers that might irritate the delicate lesion. When an overhead warmer is used, the dressings over the defect require more frequent moistening because of the dehydrating effect of the radiant heat.

Before surgical closure the myelomeningocele is prevented from drying by the application of a sterile, moist,

---

*Information is available from the Centers for Disease Control and Prevention, **Division of Birth Defects and Pediatric Genetics,** NCBDDD, CDC, 4770 Buford Highway NE, MS F-45, Atlanta, GA 30341; (888) 232-6789; website: www.cdc.gov/ncbddd/folicacid; **March of Dimes Resource Center,** 1275 Mamaroneck Avenue, White Plains, NY 10605; (888) MODIMES; website: www.modimes.org.

nonadherent dressing over the defect. The moistening solution is usually sterile normal saline. Dressings are changed frequently (every 2 to 4 hours), and the sac is closely inspected for leaks, abrasions, irritation, or any signs of infection. The sac must be carefully cleansed if it becomes soiled or contaminated. Sometimes the sac ruptures during delivery or transport, and any opening in the sac greatly increases the risk of infection to the central nervous system.

> **NURSING TIP**
>
> To prevent stool contamination of the SB defect preoperatively, obtain a surgical drape (e.g., Steri Drape*). Cut a portion of the drape to fit the infant's sacrum using nonlatex tape to secure the plastic drape to the sacrum. The rest of the drape is placed loosely over the dressing covering the defect, thus preventing exposure to stool.

> **!NURSING ALERT**
>
> Observe for early signs of infection, such as elevated temperature (axillary), irritability, and lethargy, and for signs of increased intracranial pressure (ICP), which might indicate developing hydrocephalus.

> **!NURSING ALERT**
>
> Avoid measuring rectal temperatures in infants with SB. Because bowel sphincter function is frequently affected, the thermometer can cause irritation and rectal prolapse.

One of the most difficult, important, and challenging aspects in the early care of the infant with myelomeningocele is positioning. Before surgery the infant is kept in the prone position to minimize tension on the sac and the risk of trauma. The prone position allows for optimal positioning of the legs, especially in cases of associated hip dysplasia. The infant is placed flat with the hips only slightly flexed to reduce tension on the defect. The legs are maintained in abduction with a pad between the knees to counteract hip subluxation, and a small roll is placed under the ankles to maintain a neutral foot position. A variety of aids, including diaper rolls, pads, small foam pads, or specially designed frames and appliances, can be used to maintain the desired position.

Prevent Complications. The prone position affects other aspects of the infant's care. For example, in this position the infant is more difficult to keep clean, pressure areas are a constant threat, and feeding becomes a problem. The infant's head is turned to one side for feeding. Fortunately, most defects are repaired early, and the infant can be held for feeding soon after surgery. Special care must be taken to avoid pressure on the operative site.

Diapering the infant may be contraindicated until the defect has been repaired and healing is well advanced or epithelialization has taken place. The padding beneath the diaper area is changed as needed to keep the skin dry and free of irritation. When urinary retention is detected, CIC is employed. Because the bowel sphincter is frequently affected, there is continual passage of stool, often misinterpreted as

---

*3M, St Paul, MN.

diarrhea, which is a constant irritant to the skin and a source of infection to the spinal lesion.

Areas of sensory and motor impairment are subject to skin breakdown and therefore require meticulous care. Placing the infant on a special mattress or mattress overlay reduces pressure on the knees and ankles. Periodic cleansing, application of lotion, and gentle massage aid circulation.

Gentle range-of-motion exercises are carried out to prevent contractures, and stretching of contractures is performed when indicated. However, these exercises may be restricted to the foot, ankle, and knee joint. When the hip joints are unstable, stretching against tight hip flexors or adductor muscles, which act much like bowstrings, may aggravate a tendency toward subluxation. Consultation with a physical therapist is an important aspect of the short- and long-term management of infants with myelomeningocele.

Infants with unrepaired myelomeningocele should be held in the arms and cuddled as unaffected infants are, so their need for tactile stimulation is met by caressing, stroking, and other comfort measures. To facilitate handling and to reduce parental anxiety, the infant can recline on a pillow placed in the parent's lap. Individualized developmental care with age-appropriate stimulation is provided (see Developmental Intervention and Care, Chapter 9).

Provide Postoperative Care. Postoperative care of the infant with myelomeningocele involves the same basic care as that of any postsurgical infant: monitoring vital signs, monitoring intake and output, providing nourishment, observing for signs of infection, and managing pain as needed. Care of the operative site is carried out under the direction of the surgeon and includes close observation for signs of leakage of cerebrospinal fluid. General care is continued as preoperatively.

The prone position is maintained after surgical closure, although many neurosurgeons allow a side-lying or partial side-lying position unless it aggravates a coexisting hip dysplasia or permits undesirable hip flexion. This offers an opportunity for position changes, which reduces the risk of pressure sores and facilitates feeding. If permitted, the infant can be held upright against the body, with care taken to avoid pressure on the operative site. After the effects of anesthesia have subsided and the infant is alert, feedings may be resumed unless there are other anomalies or associated complications.

Support Family and Educate About Home Care. As soon as the parents are able to cope with the infant's condition, they are encouraged to become involved in care. They need to learn how to continue at home the care that has been initiated in the hospital—positioning, feeding, skin care, and range-of-motion exercises when appropriate. They are taught CIC technique when it is prescribed. Parents also need to know the signs of complications and how to obtain assistance when needed.

The long-range planning with and support of the parents and child begin in the hospital and extend throughout childhood and even beyond. Long-term care of these children is of uncertain length, although the life expectancy is of average length, well into adulthood. Nurses assume an important role as a central member of the health team. As case manager, the nurse reviews information with the family, takes responsibility for family teaching, and acts as a liaison between inpatient and outpatient services. The child may need numerous hospitalizations over the years, and each one will be a source of stress, to which the younger child is especially vulnerable. (See Chapter 18 for a discussion of care of the child with a disability.)

Habilitation involves not only solving problems of self-help and locomotion, but also solving the most distressing problem of urinary or bowel incontinence, which threatens the child's social acceptability. Assistance with preparing the child and the school regarding the special needs of the child helps provide a better initial adjustment to this broader social experience. The **Spina Bifida Association of America*** is organized to provide services and support for families of children with spinal lesions.

Latex Allergy

Latex allergy was identified as being a serious health hazard when a report linked intraoperative anaphylaxis with latex in children with SB. The high prevalence of latex allergy (up to 80%) in children with SB has been attributed to the repeated exposure to latex products during surgery and from numerous bladder catheterizations as well as possible disease-associated factors (Mazon and others, 2000; Szepfalusi and others, 1999). Allergic reactions range from urticaria, wheezing, watery eyes, and rashes to anaphylactic shock. More severe reactions tend to occur when latex comes in contact with mucous membranes, wet skin, the bloodstream, or an airway. There also can be cross-reactions to a number of foods (e.g., banana, avocado, kiwi, chestnut). In addition to patients with SB, high-risk populations include patients with urogenital anomalies or multiple surgeries, as well as health care workers. (See Box 32-6 for medical conditions associated with SB.)

The most important goals are prevention of latex allergy and identification of children with a known hypersensitivity (see Guidelines box). High-risk and latex-allergic individuals must be managed in a *latex-safe* environment. Care must be taken so that they do not come in direct or sec-

*4590 MacArthur Boulevard NW, Suite 250, Washington, DC 20007-4226; (202) 944-3285 or (800) 621-3141; website: www.sbaa.org.

BOX 32-6 ■ Medical Conditions Associated With Risk of Latex Allergy

Spina bifida
Urogenital anomalies
Imperforate anus
Tracheoesophageal fistula
VATER association (Vertebral defects, imperforate Anus, TracheoEsophageal fistula, and Radial and renal dysplasia)
Preterm infants
Ventriculoperitoneal shunt
Mental retardation
Cerebral palsy
Quadriplegia
Multiple surgeries
Atopy

ondary contact with products or equipment containing latex *at any time* during medical treatment. Allergy testing has been used to identify latex allergy with varying success. Skin prick testing and provocation testing carry the risk of allergic reaction or anaphylaxis. The radioallergosorbent test (RAST) has been used to measure the serum level of latex-specific immunoglobulin E. The RAST has been shown to be 90% to 95% sensitive (Kellett, 1997). Pretreatment with an antihistamine and steroids (dexamethasone) before and after surgery to reduce the possibility of a serious reaction remains controversial, because it may interfere with healing.

Because children who have SB are prone to develop an allergy to latex, reducing exposure to latex, from birth on, is hoped to decrease the chance of allergy development. Latex, a natural product derived from the rubber tree, is used in combination with other chemicals to give elasticity, strength, and durability to many products.

Avoiding contact with latex is the most important intervention. The establishment of a latex-safe environment is being accomplished in many health care facilities where patients and health care workers are at high risk. In addition, there are published lists of products, such as vinyl gloves, that may be substituted for latex (see footnote to Box 32-7). Allergic reactions to latex protein can also occur when the substance is transferred to food by food-handlers wearing latex gloves, prompting several states to pass legislation that prohibits the use of latex gloves in food service (Liddle, 2001; Beezhold and others, 2000). In the health care arena it is important to use products with the lowest potential risk of sensitizing patients and staff members. User labeling for latex-containing devices that come into contact directly or indirectly with live human tissue has been proposed by the Food and Drug Administration (FDA) in 1996.

The American Nurses Association (ANA) (1997), National Institute for Occupational Safety and Health (NIOSH)

GUIDELINES

Identifying Latex Allergy

Does your child have any symptoms, such as sneezing, coughing, rashes, or wheezing, when handling rubber products (e.g., balloons, tennis or Koosh balls, adhesive bandage strips), or when in contact with rubber hospital products (e.g., gloves, catheters)?

Has your child ever had an allergic reaction during surgery?

Does your child have a history of rashes, asthma, or allergic reactions to medication or foods, especially milk, kiwi, bananas, or chestnuts?

How would you identify or recognize an allergic reaction in your child?

What would you do if an allergic reaction occurred?

Has anyone ever discussed latex or rubber allergy or sensitivity with you?

Has your child had any allergy testing?

When did your child last come in contact with any type of rubber product? Were you present?

Modified from Romanczuk A: Latex use with infants and children: it can cause problems, *MCN* 18(4):208-212, 1993.

(1997), Occupational Safety and Health Administration (OSHA) (1999), National Association of Neonatal Nurses (NANN) (2000), and other state, school, and health care organizations have issued statements on latex allergies emphasizing that all health care institutions abandon the unnecessary use of powdered latex gloves and provide latex-free equipment and latex-safe environments for patients and staff known to have or who are at high risk for developing an allergy to latex. Procedures for the identification and treatment of latex-sensitive patients, provision of latex-free medical products, and reporting of allergic events related to latex medical devices to the FDA MedWatch Program are also strongly advocated by the ANA.* In addition, the ANA recommends that each health care facility have a multidisciplinary task force to develop occupational health guidelines to ensure a safe environment for health care workers to minimize latex exposure, identify those at risk for reaction to latex, and accommodate the needs of latex-sensitive employees.

> ⚠️ **NURSING ALERT**
>
> Ask *all* patients about allergic reactions to latex, not only those at risk, during the health interview with the parent or child. Be sure that this is a routine part of all preoperative and preprocedural histories. Stress the importance of the allergy history to *all* personnel (e.g., phlebotomists).

The identification of those sensitive to latex is best accomplished through careful screening of *all* patients. (See Guidelines box for questions related to latex allergy.)

Children with latex allergy should carry or wear some form of medical identification. Education programs regarding latex hypersensitivity are aimed at those who care for high-risk groups, such as children with SB, and may include relatives, school nurses, teachers, childcare workers, and baby-sitters. In addition to educating caregivers about the child's exposure to medical products that contain latex, nurses need to inform them of common nonmedical latex objects (Box 32-7). Items brought to the hospital, such as floral bouquets, are also screened for latex balloons, which have been banned in many hospitals, and latex toys. Parents should also be given literature explaining signs and symptoms of latex hypersensitivity and appropriate emergency treatment (see Anaphylaxis, Chapter 25).

PROGRESSIVE INFANTILE SPINAL MUSCULAR ATROPHY (WERDNIG-HOFFMANN DISEASE)

Progressive infantile spinal muscular atrophy (SMA) (Werdnig-Hoffmann disease), or SMA type 1, is a disorder characterized by progressive weakness and wasting of skeletal muscles caused by degeneration of anterior horn cells. It is inherited as an autosomal-recessive trait and is the most common paralytic form of the *floppy infant syndrome (congenital hypotonia)*. The sites of the pathologic condition are the anterior

---

*The **FDA Medical Products Reporting Program,** Food and Drug Administration, 5600 Fishers Lane, Rockville, MD 20852-9787; (800) FDA-1088; fax: (800) FDA-0178; website: www.fda.gov/medwatch. Additional information regarding latex allergy may be found at the following websites: www.latexallergyhelp.com; www.latexallergyresources.org (**American Latex Allergy Association**); http://latexallergylinks.tripod.com; www.sbaa.org.

horn cells of the spinal cord and the motor nuclei of the brainstem, but the primary effect is atrophy of skeletal muscles. The age of onset is variable, but the earlier the onset, the more disseminated and severe the motor weakness. The disorder may be manifested early—often at birth—and almost always before 2 years of age. The manifestations (Box 32-8) and prognosis are categorized according to the age of onset, severity of weakness, and clinical course; some children may fluctuate between exhibiting symptoms of types 1 and 2, or types 2 and 3, in regard to clinical function (Sarnat, 2004).

Diagnostic Evaluation and Therapeutic Management

The diagnosis is based on the molecular genetic marker for the SMN (survival motor neuron) gene, which is located on chromosome 5q13. Prenatal diagnosis may be made by genetic analysis of circulating fetal cells in maternal blood (Beroud and others, 2003) or circulating fetal cells in amniotic fluid. The risk of subsequent affected offspring in carriers of the mutant gene or in families with known cases of SMA may also be evaluated genetically. Further diagnostic studies include muscle electromyography (EMG), which demonstrates a denervation pattern, and muscle biopsy; however, the genetic analysis has become the gold standard for diagnosis of the condition. There is no cure for the disease, and treatment is symptomatic and preventive, primarily preventing joint contractures and treating orthopedic problems, the most serious of which is scoliosis; hip subluxation and dislocation may also occur. Many children benefit from powered chairs, lifts, special pressure-adjustable mattresses, and accessible environmental controls. Muscle and joint contractures require careful attention and care to prevent further complications. The use of lower extremity orthoses may assist with ambulation, but eventually the child may be confined to a wheelchair as muscle atrophy progresses. Upper respiratory infections may occur and are treated with antibiotic therapy.

Prognosis. Prognosis varies according to age of onset or group as described in Box 32-8. Individuals with SMA type 1 commonly succumb to respiratory infections or failure between 1 and 24 months of age (Iannaccone and Burghes, 2002; Thompson and Berenson, 2001); however, some may live into their third or fourth decade of life. Some affected persons did not demonstrate progressive loss of strength and function (Russman, 1996).

Nursing Considerations

The infant or small child with progressive muscle weakness requires nursing care similar to that of the immobilized patient (see Chapter 31). However, the underlying goal of treatment should be to assist the child and family in dealing with the illness while progressing toward a life of normalization within the child's capabilities. Special attention to preventing muscle and joint contractures, promoting independence in performance of ADLs, and becoming incorporated into the mainstream of school when possible should be the focal point of care. In addition, parents need support and resources to be able to provide for the child and remain an intact family. Because children with neuromuscular disease have abnormal breathing patterns that often contribute to early death, it is

BOX 32-7 ■ Selected Items Possibly Containing Latex*

MEDICAL ITEMS

Adhesive bandage strips
Airways, masks (oxygen)
Anesthesia vent circuits, bags
Blood pressure cuffs and tubing
Bulb syringe
Catheters (indwelling, condom)
Chux (washable rubber pads)
Crutches (axillary, hand pads)
Dressings and wraps (various)
Elastic bandages
Electrode pads, bulbs
Endotracheal tubes
Finger cots
Gloves (sterile and examining, surgical and medical)
Heparin lock adapter
Intravenous tubing, injection ports, bags, burets
Medication vials
Nasogastric tubes
Ostomy supplies
Penrose drains
Pulse oximeters
Spacer (metered dose inhaler)
Stethoscope tubing
Suction tubing
Syringes (disposable)
Tape (cloth adhesive, paper)
Tourniquet
Urodynamics rectal pressure catheters
Vascular/compression stockings
Wheelchair cushions, tires

HOME AND COMMUNITY ITEMS

Art supplies (paint, markers, glue)
Balloons (not Mylar)
Balls (Koosh, tennis, bowling)
Cardiopulmonary resuscitation (CPR) manikins
Carpet backing, gym floor, gym mats (broadloom carpets contain no natural rubber latex. For other products, provide barrier cloth or mat)
Chewing gum
Cleaning/kitchen gloves
Condoms, contraceptive sponges, diaphragms
Dental dams and equipment
Diapers, rubber pants
Elastic exercisers
Elastic on legs, waist of clothing, rubber pants, some disposable diapers
Feeding nipples
Foam rubber lining on splints, braces
Infant toothbrush-massager
Latex paints, sealants, stains (there is no natural rubber in latex paint, although it may be present in some waterproof paints and sealants)
Pacifier
Playpits, playground surfaces with natural rubber latex
Racquet handles
Rubber bands
Water toys, swim, scuba equipment
Wheelchair cushions, tires
Zippered plastic storage bags

Modified from the Spina Bifida Association of America Fact Sheet: *Latex in the hospital environment items and home & community items,* Washington, DC, 2003, The Association.
*It is very difficult to obtain full and accurate information on the latex content of certain products, which may vary among companies and product series. Double-checking with suppliers before use with latex-allergic individuals is strongly recommended. For an updated list of latex-free items and alternative items, contact the **Spina Bifida Association of America,** 4590 MacArthur Boulevard NW, Suite 250, Washington, DC 20007-4226; Resource Center (800) 621-3141; website: www.sbaa.org.

Online Resources for Latex Allergies
Latex Allergy Links: http://latexallergylinks.tripod.com/
American Latex Allergy Association/ALERT: www.latexallergyresources.org/
Occupational Safety and Health Administration (OSHA): www.osha.gov/SLTC/latexallergy/
American Academy of Allergy, Asthma and Immunology: www.aaaai.org
Decent Exposures (latex-free undergarments) www.decentexposures.com; 1-800-524-4949

important to assess adequate oxygenation, especially during the sleep phase when shallow breathing occurs and hypoxemia may develop; home pulse oximetry may be used to assess the child during sleep and provide supplemental oxygenation treatment as necessary (Birnkrant, 2002) (see Duchenne Muscular Dystrophy for respiratory management). Supportive care also includes management of orthoses and other orthopedic equipment as required. Because children with SMA are intellectually normal, verbal, tactile, and auditory stimulation are important aspects of developmental care. Supporting them so that they can see the activities around them and transporting them in appropriate conveyances (e.g., wagon, power wheelchair) for a change of environment provide stimulation and a broader scope of contacts.

Children who are able to sit require proper support and attention to alignment to prevent deformities and other complications. Children who survive beyond infancy will need attention to educational needs and opportunities for social interaction with other children. In a recent survey parents of children with SMA type 1 expressed the belief that although care for the child was difficult, they perceived their child as having a positive quality of life (Bach and others, 2003). The parents of a child who is chronically ill require much support and encouragement (see Chapter 18). Parents who have not sought genetic counseling should be encouraged to do so to evaluate further risk potential.

JUVENILE SPINAL MUSCULAR ATROPHY (KUGELBERG-WELANDER DISEASE)

Juvenile spinal muscular atrophy (Kugelberg-Welander disease, juvenile proximal hereditary muscular atrophy) is also a result of anterior horn cell and motor nerve degeneration. The disease is characterized by a pattern of muscular weakness similar to that of infantile spinal muscular atrophy (see

BOX 32-8 ■ Clinical Manifestations of Spinal Muscular Atrophy*

GROUP 1 (WERDNIG-HOFFMANN DISEASE)
Disease acquired in utero
Hypotonia and inactivity are most prominent features
Infant lies in the frog position with legs externally rotated, abducted, and flexed at knees
Weakness
Absent deep tendon reflexes
Limited movements of shoulder and arm muscles
Active movement is usually limited to fingers and toes
Diaphragmatic breathing with intercostal retractions (diaphragmatic paralysis may occur)
Abnormal tongue movements (at rest)
Weak cry and cough
Secretions tend to pool in oropharynx
Alert facies
Normal sensation and intellect
Tire quickly during feedings (if breast-fed, may lose weight before noticeable)
Affected infants do not progress to sit alone, roll over, or walk
Early death (usually by 2 years of age) from respiratory failure or infection

GROUP 2 (INTERMEDIATE SPINAL MUSCULAR ATROPHY)
Symptoms manifest between 2 and 12 months of age
Early—weakness confined to arms and legs
Later—becomes generalized
Legs usually involved to greater extent than arms
Prominent pectus excavatum
Movements absent during complete relaxation or sleep
Some infants able to sit if placed in position
Failure to walk is common presentation
Lifespan varies from 7 months to 7 years or even longer in some cases

GROUP 3 (KUGELBERG-WELANDER SYNDROME)
Onset of symptoms in late childhood or adolescence (may be initially misdiagnosed as muscular dystrophy [limb girdle])
Normal head control and can sit unassisted by 6 to 8 months of age
Thigh and hip muscles weak
In those who manage to walk:
 Lumbar lordosis
 Waddling gait
 Genu recurvatum
 Protuberant abdomen
 Ambulation becomes increasingly difficult
 Age of onset influences ambulatory difficulty –the later (after age 2 years) the onset, the better the prognosis
 Confined to a wheelchair by second decade (may vary)
 Scoliosis is common
Deep tendon reflexes may be present early but disappear

*These classifications are general and experts suggest there may be variations in lifespan and other characteristics (Iannaccone and Burghes, 2002; Russman and others, 1992; Russman, 1996).

Box 32-8). Several modes of inheritance have been reported for the disease: autosomal-recessive, autosomal-dominant, and X-linked recessive.

The onset occurs from younger than 1 year of age into adulthood, with symptoms resembling group 3 infantile spinal muscular atrophy; proximal muscle weakness (especially of the lower limbs) and muscular atrophy are the predominant features. The disease runs a slowly progressive course. Some children lose the ability to walk 8 to 9 years after the onset of symptoms, but many can still walk after 30 years or more. Many affected persons have a normal life expectancy (Iannaccone, 1998).

Therapeutic Management and Nursing Considerations

The management is primarily symptomatic and supportive and is related to maintaining mobility as long as possible, preventing complications, and providing support to the child and family.

MUSCULAR DYSTROPHIES

Muscular dystrophies (MDs) constitute the largest and most important single group of muscle diseases of childhood. The MDs have a genetic origin in which there is gradual degeneration of muscle fibers, and they are characterized by progressive weakness and wasting of symmetric groups of skeletal muscles, with increasing disability and deformity. In all forms of MD there is insidious loss of strength, but each type differs in regard to muscle groups affected (Fig. 32-7), age of onset, rate of progression, and inheritance pattern. The most common form, *Duchenne muscular dystrophy*, is considered separately in the next section.

Facioscapulohumeral (Landouzy-Déjérine) muscular dystrophy is inherited as an autosomal-dominant disorder with onset in early adolescence. It is characterized by difficulty in raising the arms over the head, lack of facial mobility, and a forward slope of the shoulders. The progression is slow, and the lifespan is usually unaffected.

Limb-girdle muscular dystrophy is an autosomal recessive disease of later childhood or adolescence with variable but usually slow progression; it is characterized by weakness of proximal muscles of the pelvic and shoulder girdles.

Treatment of the MDs consists mainly of supportive measures, including physical therapy, orthopedic procedures to minimize deformity, and assistance for the affected child in meeting the demands of daily living.

PSEUDOHYPERTROPHIC (DUCHENNE) MUSCULAR DYSTROPHY

Duchenne muscular dystrophy (DMD) is the most severe and the most common muscular dystrophy of childhood. It is inherited as an X-linked recessive trait, and the single gene defect is located on the short arm of the X chromosome. DMD has a reportedly high mutation rate, with a positive family history in 65% of all cases (Thompson and Berenson, 2001); therefore, genetic counseling is an important aspect of the care of the family. As in all X-linked disorders, males are affected almost exclusively. At the genetic level, DMD results from mutation of the gene that encodes *dystrophin*, a protein found in skeletal muscle. The incidence is approximately 1 per 3600 male births (Sarnat, 2004). Box 32-9 describes the characteristics of DMD.

Most children with DMD reach the appropriate developmental milestones early in life, although there may be mild subtle delays. Evidence of muscle weakness usually appears

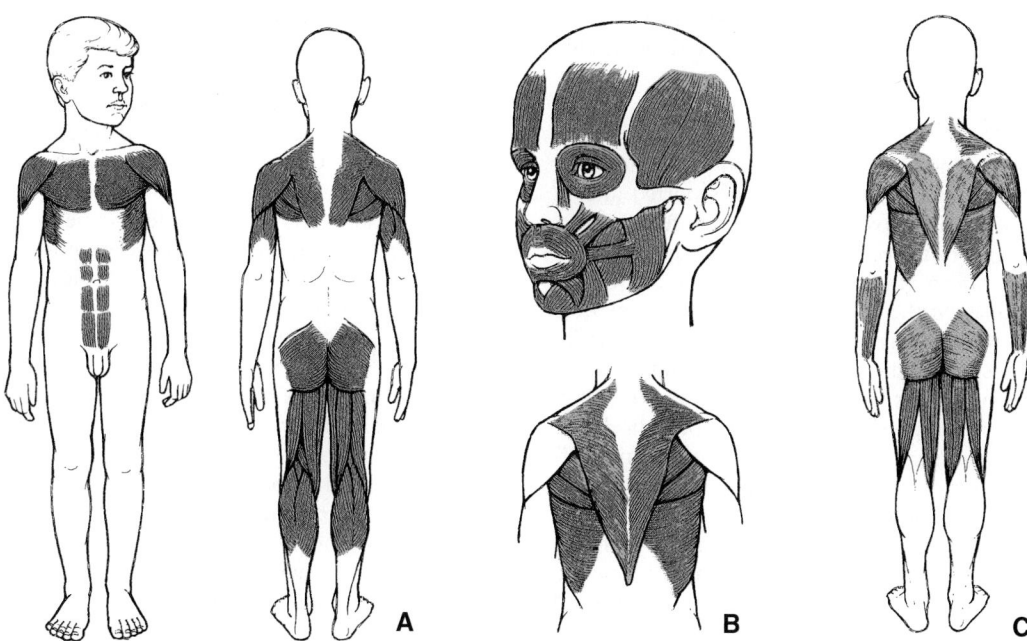

FIG. 31-7 ■ Initial muscle groups involved in muscular dystrophies. **A,** Pseudohypertrophic. **B,** Fascioscapulohumeral. **C,** Limb girdle.

BOX 32-9 ■ Characteristics of Duchenne Muscular Dystrophy

Early onset, usually between 3 and 5 years of age
Progressive muscular weakness, wasting, and contractures
Calf muscle hypertrophy in most patients
Loss of independent ambulation by 9 to 11 years of age
Slowly progressive, generalized weakness during teenage years

BOX 32-10 ■ Clinical Manifestations of Duchenne Muscular Dystrophy

Relentless progression until death from respiratory or cardiac failure
Waddling gait
Lordosis
Frequent falls
Gower sign (child turns onto side or abdomen, flexes knees to assume a kneeling position, then with knees extended gradually pushes torso to an upright position by "walking" the hands up the legs)
Enlarged muscles (especially thighs and upper arms)
    Feel unusually firm or woody on palpation
Later stages: profound muscular atrophy
Mental deficiency (common)
    Mild (about 20 IQ points below normal)
    Mental deficit present in 25% to 30% of patients
Complications:
    Contracture deformities of hips, knees, and ankles
    Disuse atrophy
    Obesity

during the third year, although there may have been a history of delay in motor development, particularly walking. Difficulties in running, riding a bicycle, and climbing stairs are usually the first symptoms noted. Later, abnormal gait on a level surface becomes apparent. In the early years, rapid developmental gains may mask the progression of the disease. Questioning the parents may reveal that the child has difficulty in rising from a sitting or supine position. Parents may also notice the child has enlarged calves (see Box 32-10).

The term *pseudohypertrophy* is derived from muscular enlargement caused by fatty infiltration. Profound muscular atrophy occurs in later stages, and as the disease progresses, contractures and deformities involving large and small joints are common complications. Ambulation usually becomes impossible by 12 years of age. Facial, oropharyngeal, and respiratory muscles are often spared until the terminal stages of the disease. Ultimately the disease process involves the diaphragm and auxiliary muscles of respiration, and cardiovascular involvement (cardiomyopathy, dysrhythmias, and heart failure) is common. Mild mental delay is common in roughly 30% of all individuals with MD, and many will have permanent learning disabilities; however, children with DMD should be transitioned into early learning programs and eventually into regular classrooms as much as possible. The eventual cause of

death is usually respiratory tract infection or cardiac failure; however, much progress has been made in providing ventilatory methods to prolong and maintain quality of life.

Diagnostic Evaluation

The diagnosis of DMD is established by DNA analysis (molecular genetic diagnosis) of peripheral blood or tissue cells obtained by muscle biopsy. Prenatal diagnosis is also possible as early as 12 weeks' gestation. Additional diagnostic evaluation may include electromyography (EMG) and muscle biopsy. If the child demonstrates the usual characteristics, has a positive family history for DMD, and the

DNA analysis is positive, the muscle biopsy may be deferred. The serum creatine phosphokinase (CK) is usually extremely elevated in children with DMD.

Therapeutic Management

No effective treatment exists for childhood MD. Increased muscle bulk and muscle power have been reported after a course of corticosteroids; however, this therapy requires further evaluation before it becomes routine management because of the side effects, particularly weight gain and osteoporosis, which may further complicate the disease process (Sarnat, 2004). Maintaining optimal function in all muscles for as long as possible is the primary goal; secondary is the prevention of contractures. It has been found that children who remain as active as possible are able to avoid wheelchair confinement for a longer time. Maintenance of function often includes stretching exercises, strength and muscle training, breathing exercises and use of incentive spirometry to increase and maintain vital lung capacity, range-of-motion exercises, surgery to release contracture deformities, bracing, and performance of activities of daily living. Parents should always be involved in making decisions about the child's care, and teaching regarding home safety and prevention of falls is important as well (Metules, 2002). Parents should also be encouraged to have the child keep follow-up appointments for medical care and physical and occupational therapy. Because respiratory infections are most troublesome in these children, flu and pneumococcal vaccines are encouraged and contact with persons with respiratory infections should be avoided. Baseline pulmonary function testing, electrocardiograms, and echocardiograms are recommended (Metules, 2002).

Eventually respiratory and cardiac problems become the central focus of the debilitating illness. Children with neuromuscular disease have abnormal breathing patterns, particularly during REM sleep, and hypoxia may occur as a result of inadequate oxygenation (Birnkrant, 2002). The child and parents should be involved in a discussion of long-term ventilation options. Cardiac and respiratory assessment during awake and asleep cycles is imperative. The use of incentive spirometry helps maintain vital capacity and breathing exercises should be taught early. Respiratory care later in life may involve the use of noninvasive IPPV (intermittent positive pressure ventilation) on a temporary or full time basis, mechanically assisted coughing (MAC), or tracheotomy and relieving airway obstruction with coughing and suctioning devices; the tracheotomy, however, is associated with more complications. Home pulse oximetry may be used to monitor oxygenation during sleep or as an adjunct to decision making regarding the use of mechanically assisted coughing to clear the airways. Several devices are available to children with neuromuscular disease to assist in clearing the airway when the cough reflex is ineffective or diminished (Birnkrant, 2002). Survival in individuals with DMD may be prolonged several years with the use of noninvasive IPPV and mechanically assisted coughing as alternatives to tracheotomy and airway suctioning (Gomez-Merino and Bach, 2002).

Genetic counseling is also recommended for parents, female siblings, and maternal aunts and their female offspring.

Research evaluating a number of treatments for DMD is in progress. These include clinical trials with glutamine and creatine monohydrate to preserve muscle strength; utrophin, a protein that is similar to dystrophin and in large quantities may counteract the effects of the deficiency of dystrophin; and the enzyme CT GalNac transferase, which blocks muscle wasting in mice (Metules, 2002). Myoblast transfer therapy (from the unaffected father) offers some hope for replacement of defective dystrophin; however, immunosuppression to prevent rejection of the foreign cells is a major drawback (Sarnat, 2004).

Nursing Considerations

The major emphasis of nursing care is to help the child and family cope with a chronic, progressive, incapacitating disease; to help design a program that will afford maximal independence and reduce the predictable and preventable disabilities associated with the disorder; and to help the child and family deal constructively with the limitations the disease imposes on their daily lives. Because of newer advances in technology, children with MD may live into early adulthood; therefore, the goals of care should also involve decisions regarding quality of life, achieving independence, and transition to adulthood.

Working closely with other team members, nurses assist the family in developing the child's self-help skills to give the child the satisfaction of being as independent as possible for as long as possible. This requires continual evaluation of the child's capabilities, which are often difficult to assess. It is not always possible to know when children seek parental assistance because they want a little extra attention, when parents are being overprotective, or when the muscles are overtired. Fortunately, most children with MD instinctively recognize the need to become as independent as possible and strive to become so.

Practical difficulties faced by families are physical limitations of housing and mobility. Parents also need assistance in buying and modifying clothing for their child. It is difficult to find clothing and footwear to wear comfortably in a wheelchair and to fit hypertrophied muscles. The parent's social activities are also restricted, and the family's activities must be continually modified to the needs of the affected child.

When the child becomes increasingly incapacitated, the family may consider home-based care, a skilled nursing facility, or respite care to provide the care needed. Unless the child is severely incapacitated, he should also be involved in the decisions regarding such care. Nurses can assist with decision making by exploring all available options and resources and support the child and family in the decision. Older boys with MD may also need psychiatric or psychologic counseling to deal with issues such as depression, anger, and quality of life (Bothwell and others, 2002). Parents also need to be encouraged to become involved in support groups because there is evidence that adequate social support from family, community, and other parents is crucial to appropriate coping in families with children with chronic illness (Bothwell and others, 2002).

Regardless of how successful the program or how well the family adapts to the disorder, superimposed on the physical and emotional problems associated with a child with a long-term disability is the constant presence of the ultimate outcome of the disease. All of the manifestations seen in the child with a chronic fatal illness are encountered in these families (see Chapter 18). The guilt feelings of the mother may be particularly pronounced in this disorder because of the mother-to-son transmission of the defective gene.

Nurses are especially valuable health professionals as they come to know the family and the family's problems. Nurses can be alert to the problems and needs of the families and make necessary referrals when supplementary services are indicated. The **Muscular Dystrophy Association of America, Inc.,*** has branches in most communities to provide assistance to families in which there is a member with muscular dystrophy.

ACQUIRED NEUROMUSCULAR DISORDERS

GUILLAIN-BARRÉ SYNDROME (INFECTIOUS POLYNEURITIS)

Guillain-Barré syndrome (GBS), also known as postinfectious polyneuritis, is an uncommon acute demyelinating polyneuropathy with a progressive, usually ascending flaccid paralysis. Children are less often affected than adults, with children between ages 4 and 10 years having higher susceptibility. *Congenital GBS* is rare yet may be seen in the neonatal period and consists of hypotonia, weakness, and decreased or absent reflexes; maternal neuromuscular disease may or may not be present. Diagnosis is established by the same criteria as in older children, yet the symptoms gradually subside over the first few months of life and there is no presence of disease by age 12 months (Sarnat, 2004).

Pathophysiology

GBS is an immune-mediated disease often associated with a number of viral or bacterial infections or the administration of certain vaccines. It has been associated with infectious mononucleosis, measles, mumps, *Campylobacter jejuni* (gastroenteritis), *Borrelia burgdorferi* (Lyme disease), *Helicobacter pylori*, and *Mycoplasma* and *Pneumocystis* infections. Onset of GBS symptoms usually occurs within 10 days of the primary infection. Pathologic changes in spinal and cranial nerves consist of inflammation and edema with rapid, segmented demyelination and compression of nerve roots within the dural sheath. Nerve conduction is impaired, producing ascending partial or complete paralysis of muscles innervated by the involved nerves. GBS has three phases:

1 **Acute**—Begins with onset of symptoms and continues until new symptoms stop appearing or deterioration ceases and may last as long as 4 weeks
2 **Plateau**—Symptoms remain constant without further deterioration and may last from days to weeks
3 **Recovery**—Patient begins to improve and progress to complete recovery and usually lasts a few days to a few weeks (Sulton, 2002).

---

*3300 East Sunrise Drive, Tucson, AZ 85718; (800) 572-1717; website: www.mdausa.org. In Canada, 2345 Yonge Street, Suite 900, Toronto, Ontario M4P 2E5; (416) 488-0030 or (800) 567-2873; website: www.mdac.ca.

BOX 32-11 ■ Clinical Manifestations of Guillain-Barré Syndrome

INITIAL SYMPTOMS
Muscle tenderness
Paresthesia and cramps (sometimes)
Proximal symmetric muscle weakness
Ascending paralysis from lower extremities
Frequently involves muscles of trunk, upper extremities, and those supplied by cranial nerves (especially facial)
Flaccid paralysis with loss of reflexes
May involve facial, extraocular, labial, lingual, pharyngeal, and laryngeal muscles
Intercostal and phrenic nerves:
  Breathlessness in vocalizations
  Shallow, irregular respirations

OTHER MANIFESTATIONS
Tendon reflexes depressed or absent
Variable degrees of sensory impairment
Muscle tenderness or sensitivity to slight pressure
Urinary incontinence or retention and constipation

Diagnostic Evaluation

Diagnosis of GBS is based on clinical manifestations (Box 32-11), cerebrospinal fluid analysis, and EMG findings. CSF analysis reveals an increased protein concentration, and EMG shows evidence of acute muscle denervation; other laboratory studies are usually noncontributory. The symmetric nature of the paralysis helps differentiate this disorder from spinal paralytic poliomyelitis, which usually affects sporadic muscles.

Therapeutic Management

Treatment of GBS is primarily supportive. In the acute phase patients are hospitalized because respiratory and pharyngeal involvement may require assisted ventilation, sometimes with a temporary tracheotomy. Treatment modalities include aggressive ventilatory support, intravenous administration of immunoglobulin (IVIG) and steroids; plasmapheresis and immunosuppressive drugs may also be used. Plasmapheresis has been shown to decrease the length of recovery in patients with severe GBS yet is expensive, and side effects include hypotension, fever, chills, urticaria, and bradycardia (Sulton, 2002). Further evidence reports equal benefits to treatment of GBS with intravenous immunoglobulin administration or plasmapheresis; both sped up recovery time in studies reviewed (Hughes and others, 2003).

Course and Prognosis. Better outcomes are associated with younger age, no requirement for mechanical respiratory assistance, slower progression of disease, normal peripheral nerve function on EMG, and treatment by plasmapheresis (Graf and others, 1999). Recovery usually begins within 2 to 3 weeks, and most patients regain full muscle strength; the recovery of muscle strength progresses in the reverse order of onset of paralysis, with lower extremity strength being the last to recover. Poor prognosis with subsequent residual effects in children is reportedly associated with the following: cranial nerve involvement, extensive disability at time of presentation, and intubation (Sarnat, 2004).

Almost all deaths are caused by respiratory failure; therefore, early diagnosis and access to respiratory support are especially important. The rate of recovery is usually related to the degree of involvement, which may extend from a few weeks to months. The greater the degree of paralysis, the longer the recovery phase.

Nursing Considerations

Nursing care is essentially supportive and is the same as that required for the child with immobilization and respiratory depression. The emphasis of care is on close observation to assess the extent of paralysis and on prevention of complications, including autonomic dysfunction (hypertension, orthostatic hypotension, syndrome of inappropriate antidiuretic hormone secretion, life-threatening dysrhythmias), respiratory dysfunction, fear and anxiety, and pain management (Sulton, 2002).

During the acute phase of GBS the child's condition should be carefully observed for possible difficulty in swallowing and respiratory involvement. The child's respiratory function is closely monitored, and oxygen source, appropriate-sized insufflation bag and mask, endotracheal intubation and suctioning equipment, tracheotomy tray, and vasoconstrictor drugs are kept available. Vital signs, including neurologic signs and level of consciousness, are monitored frequently. For the child who develops respiratory impairment, the care is the same as that for any child with respiratory distress requiring mechanical ventilation.

Throughout the recovery phase, special emphasis is placed on prevention of complications, including proper postural alignment, frequent change of position, assessment of skin at pressure points, and passive range-of-motion exercises. Respiratory care, should intubation be required, requires close monitoring of oxygenation status, usually by pulse oximetry and sometimes arterial blood gases, maintenance of an open airway with suctioning, and postural changes to prevent pneumonia. Children with oral and pharyngeal involvement may be fed via a nasogastric tube to ensure adequate feeding. Immobilization, which occurs with GBS, decreases gastrointestinal function; therefore, attention to problems such as decreased gastric emptying, constipation, and feeding residuals requires nursing assessment and appropriate collaborative interventions. Temporary urinary catheterization may be required; urinary retention is not uncommon and appropriate assessment of urinary output is vital. Sensory impairment and paralysis in the lower extremities makes the child susceptible to skin breakdown; therefore, attention should be given to meticulous skin care. A key to recovery in the child with GBS is the prevention of muscle and joint contractures, so passive range-of-motion exercises must be carried out routinely to maintain vital function. Although the child may have a generalized paralysis, cognitive function remains intact; therefore, it is important for nursing care to involve communication with the child regarding procedures and treatments that may be frightening, especially if mechanical ventilation is required. Nurses are often quite adept at devising communication tools for effective communication with patients who have compromised expressive abilities. Parents are encouraged to talk to the child and make eye and physical contact as much a possible to reassure the child during the illness.

Physical therapy is limited to passive range-of-motion exercises during the evolving phase of the disease. Later, as the disease stabilizes and recovery begins, an active physical therapy program is implemented to prevent contracture deformities and facilitate muscle recovery. This may include active exercise, gait training, and bracing.

Throughout the course of the illness, support of the child and parents is paramount. The usual rapidity of the paralysis and the long period of recovery greatly tax the emotional reserves of all family members. The parents and child benefit from repeated reassurance that recovery is occurring and from realistic information regarding the possibility of permanent disability. In the event of a residual disability, the family needs assistance in accepting and adjusting to the loss of function (see Chapter 18). The **Guillain-Barré Syndrome Foundation International*** is a nonprofit organization devoted to support, education, and research. It provides support to families from recovered persons, publishes informational literature and a newsletter, and maintains a list of practitioners experienced with the disease.

TETANUS

Tetanus, or *lockjaw,* is an acute, preventable, but often fatal disease caused by an exotoxin produced by the anaerobic spore-forming, gram-positive bacillus *Clostridium tetani.* The disorder is characterized by painful muscular rigidity primarily involving the masseter and neck muscles. There are four requirements for the development of tetanus:

1 Presence of tetanus spores or vegetative forms of the bacillus
2 Injury to the tissues
3 Wound conditions that encourage multiplication of the organism
4 A susceptible host

Tetanus spores are found in soil, dust, and the intestinal tracts of humans and animals, especially herbivorous animals. The organisms are more prevalent in rural areas but are readily carried to urban areas by the wind. The organisms are not invasive but enter the body by way of wounds, particularly a puncture wound, burn, or crushed area. They may enter through a very minor, unnoticed break in the skin, such as a thorn or needle prick, bee sting, or scratch. In the newborn, infection may occur through the umbilical cord, usually in situations in which infants are delivered in severely contaminated surroundings. The disease has the greatest incidence in months when persons are more involved in outdoor activities. Substance abusers are especially susceptible from poor injection technique and the use of street heroin, which is often mixed with quinine, a protoplasmic poison that favors the growth of the organism (American Academy of Pediatrics, 2003).

Pathophysiology

When prevention efforts are not effective and conditions are favorable, the organisms proliferate and form potent exotoxins, one of which is tetanospasmin. Tetanospasmin

---

*PO Box 262, Wynnewood, PA 19096; (610) 667-0131; website: www.guillain-barre.com.

affects the central nervous system to produce the clinical manifestations of the disease. The ideal conditions for growth of the organisms are devitalized tissues without access to air, such as wounds that have not been washed or kept clean and those that have crusted over, trapping pus beneath. The exotoxin appears to reach the central nervous system by way of either the neuron axons or the vascular system. The toxin becomes fixed on nerve cells of the anterior horn of the spinal cord and the brainstem. The toxin acts at the myoneural junction to produce muscular stiffness and lower the threshold for reflex excitability.

The incubation period for tetanus varies from 3 days to 3 weeks and averages 8 days; most cases occur within 14 days. In neonates it is usually 3 to 14 days. Shorter incubation periods have been associated with more heavily contaminated wounds, more severe disease, and a worse prognosis (American Academy of Pediatrics, 2003).

The manner of onset varies, but the initial symptoms are usually a progressive stiffness and tenderness of the muscles in the neck and jaw. Eventually all voluntary muscles are affected (Box 32-12). As the child recovers from the disease, the paroxysms become less frequent and gradually subside. Survival beyond 4 days usually indicates recovery, but complete recovery may require weeks.

The mortality rate is about 30%, but the disease is almost invariably fatal in the newborn. The incubation period is short, with the appearance of symptoms 3 to 10 days after

exposure. The first symptom is difficulty sucking, which progresses to total inability to suck, excessive crying, irritability, and nuchal rigidity (American Academy of Pediatrics, 2003).

Therapeutic Management

Preventive measures are based on the immune status of the affected child and the nature of the injury. Specific prophylactic therapy after trauma is administration of *tetanus toxoid* (tetanus antitoxin [TAT] is no longer available in the United States) (see Immunizations, Chapter 10 for age-specific recommendations).

The unprotected or inadequately immunized child who sustains a "tetanus-prone" wound (such as, but not limited to, wounds contaminated with dirt, feces, soil, and saliva; puncture wounds; avulsions; and wounds resulting from missiles, crushing, burns, and frostbite) should receive *tetanus immune globulin (TIG)*. Concurrent administration of both TIG and tetanus toxoid at separate sites is recommended both to provide protection and to initiate the active immune process. Completion of active immunization is carried out according to the usual pattern (American Academy of Pediatrics, 2003). Antibiotic treatment with penicillin G (alternatively erythromycin or tetracycline in older children with allergy to penicillin) is important in the management of tetanus as an adjunct against *Clostridia* (Arnon, 2004).

Aggressive supportive care is necessary to treat tetanus in the acute phase. The acutely ill child is best treated in an intensive care facility where close and constant observation and equipment for monitoring and respiratory support are readily available. A quiet environment is preferred to reduce external stimuli.

General supportive care, including maintenance of adequate fluid and electrolyte balance and caloric intake, is indicated. Indwelling oral or nasogastric feedings are used when necessary, but severe laryngospasm may require intravenous (IV) parenteral nutrition or gastrostomy feeding. Recurrent laryngospasm or excessive accumulation of secretions may require endotracheal intubation. TIG therapy to neutralize toxins is the most specific therapy for tetanus. Antibiotics are administered to control the proliferation of the vegetative forms of the organism at the site of infection. Local care of the wound by surgical débridement and cleansing helps reduce the numbers of proliferating organisms at the site of injury. The cleansing should be repeated several times during the first 48 hours, and deep, infected lacerations are usually exposed and débrided.

Sedatives or muscle relaxants are administered to help reduce tetanic muscle spasm and prevent seizures. Diazepam (Valium) is the drug of choice for seizure control and muscle relaxation (Arnon, 2004), but lorazepam (Ativan) may be used in some cases. Other AEDs may be administered as well. Intrathecal baclofen, magnesium sulfate, dantrolene sodium, and midazolam may also be used in the management of tetanus (Arnon, 2004). Patients with severe tetanus and those who do not respond to other muscle relaxants may require the administration of a neuromuscular blocking agent, such as rocuronium or vecuronium. Because of their paralytic effect on respiratory muscles, use of these drugs requires mechanical ventilation with endotracheal intuba-

BOX 32-12 ■ Clinical Manifestations of Tetanus

INITIAL SYMPTOMS
Progressive stiffness and tenderness of muscles in neck and jaw
Characteristic difficulty in opening the mouth *(trismus)*
Risus sardonicus (sardonic smile) caused by facial muscle spasm

PROGRESSIVE INVOLVEMENT
Opisthotonic positioning
Boardlike rigidity of abdominal and limb muscles
Difficulty swallowing
Extreme sensitivity to external stimuli (slight noise, gentle touch, or bright light):
  Trigger paroxysmal muscular contractions that last seconds to minutes
  Contractions recur with increased frequency until almost continuous (sustained, tetanic)
Laryngospasm and tetany of respiratory muscles:
  Accumulated secretions
  Respiratory arrest
  Atelectasis
  Pneumonia

OTHER ASPECTS
Mentation unaffected; patient alert
Pain, anxiety, and distress are reflected in:
  Rapid pulse
  Sweating
  Anxious facial expression
Fever usually absent or only mild

tion or tracheotomy and constant cardiopulmonary monitoring. Endotracheal tube insertion or tracheostomy is often indicated and should be performed before severe respiratory distress develops.

Nursing Considerations

In caring for the child with tetanus during the acute phase, every effort is made to control or eliminate stimulation from sound, light, and touch. Although a darkened room is ideal, sufficient light is essential so that the child can be carefully observed; light appears to be less irritating than vibratory or auditory stimuli. The infant or child is handled as little as possible, and extra effort is expended to avoid any sudden or loud noise to prevent seizures.

Medications are administered as prescribed, and vital signs, including neurologic signs, are observed and recorded at frequent intervals. The location and extent of muscle spasms and assessment of their severity are important nursing observations. Respiratory status is carefully evaluated for any signs of distress, and appropriate emergency equipment is kept available at all times. Muscle relaxants, opioids, and sedatives that may be prescribed can also cause respiratory depression; therefore, the child must be assessed for excessive central nervous system depression. Oxygen saturation is monitored, and when needed, blood gases are obtained frequently to evaluate respiratory status. Attention to hydration and nutrition may involve monitoring an IV infusion, monitoring nasogastric or gastrostomy feedings, and suctioning oropharyngeal secretions when indicated.

If a potent muscle relaxant such as vecuronium is used, the total paralysis makes oral communication impossible. The drug is not a sedative, however, and anxiety should be considered in children who are intubated. Therefore all the child's needs must be anticipated and procedures carefully explained beforehand.

Because their mental status is clear, children with tetanus are aware of what is happening to them and are often in a state of terror. They should not be left alone, and all efforts should be made to reduce anxiety, which can contribute to muscular spasms. A calm and reassuring manner and sympathetic understanding can assist immeasurably in helping a child through this crisis situation. Parents are encouraged to stay with the child to offer security and support.

BOTULISM

Botulism is an acute flaccid paralysis caused by the preformed toxin produced by the anaerobic bacillus *Clostridium botulinum*. In classic or food-borne botulism the most common source of the toxin is a contaminated food source; it was previously believed that home-canned foods were the most common source; however, this has been disproved in outbreaks associated with restaurant food. Other forms of botulism include wound botulism, infant botulism, and man-made botulism, usually a result of bioterrorism (Schechter and Arnon, 2004). In food-borne illness central nervous system symptoms appear abruptly within a few hours or gradually over several days after ingestion of contaminated food and may not be preceded by acute digestive disturbance (Box 32-13).

Treatment consists of IV administration of botulism antitoxin and general supportive measures, primarily respira-

BOX 32-13 ■ Clinical Manifestations of Botulism

GENERAL SIGNS
Weakness
Dizziness
Headache
Difficulty talking and speaking
Diplopia
Vomiting
Progressive, life-threatening respiratory paralysis

INFANT BOTULISM*
Constipation (a common symptom)
Generalized weakness
Decrease in spontaneous movements
Diminished or absent deep tendon reflexes
Loss of head control
Poor feeding
Weak cry
Reduced gag reflex
Progressive respiratory paralysis

* Most commonly diagnosed as "rule out sepsis" in the acute phase because of clinical presentation.

tory and nutritional. Toxins vary in protein-binding capacity. Some have a relatively short half-life and do not bind to tissues firmly; therefore, therapy is continued until paralysis abates. Other toxins appear to bind irreversibly to nerve endings and are therefore not amenable to neutralization.

Infant Botulism

Infant botulism, unlike the disease in older persons, is caused by ingestion of spores or vegetative cells of *C. botulinum* and the subsequent release of the toxin from organisms colonizing the gastrointestinal tract. *C. botulinum,* types A and B, are the most common causative strains of infant botulism. This form of botulism has become more prevalent than any other form. There appears to be no common food or drug source of the organisms; however, the *C. botulinum* organisms have been found in honey and light or dark corn syrup fed to affected infants (American Academy of Pediatrics, 2003). Botulism may occur in infants as young as 3 weeks of age or up to 6 months of age with peak incidence between 2 and 4 months of age (Aneja, Thomas, and Elberger, 2000).

There is wide variation in the severity of the disease, from mild constipation to progressive sequential loss of neurologic function and respiratory failure (Box 32-13). The affected infant is usually well before the onset of symptoms. Constipation is a common presenting symptom, and almost all infants exhibit generalized weakness and a decrease in spontaneous movements. Deep tendon reflexes are usually diminished or absent; cranial nerve deficits are common, as evidenced by loss of head control, difficulty in feeding, weak cry, and reduced gag reflex. The most frequently recognized form of the disease is consistent with the hypotonic infant. Presenting clinical signs often mimic those of sepsis in young infants. Botulism toxin exerts its effect by inhibiting the release of acetylcholine at the myoneural junction, thereby impairing motor activity of muscles innervated by affected nerves.

Diagnosis is made on the basis of the clinical history, physical examination, and laboratory detection of the organism in the patient's blood or stool; however, isolation of the organism may take several days; therefore suspicion of botulism by clinical presentation should involve emergent treatment (Schechter and Arnon, 2004). EMG may be helpful in establishing the diagnosis; however, results may be normal early in the course of the illness. Treatment consists of immediate administration of botulism immune globulin intravenously (BIGIV) (American Academy of Pediatrics, 2003) after the diagnosis is confirmed and supportive measures, primarily respiratory and nutritional management. Approximately 50% of affected infants will require intubation and mechanical ventilation. Trivalent equine botulinum antitoxin and bivalent antitoxin, used in adults and older children, is not administered to infants. A human-derived botulism antitoxin (BIGIV) has been recently evaluated and is now available for use in infants by the California Department of Health Services ([510] 540-2646, 24-hour telephone availability); initial clinical trials are promising, and there was a decreased need for mechanical ventilation, decreased length of stay, and decreased requirement for tube feeding (Schechter and Arnon, 2004). Antibiotic therapy is not part of the management because the botulinum toxin is an intracellular molecule and antibiotics would not be effective; aminoglycosides in particular should not be administered because they may potentiate the blocking effects of the neurotoxin (Schechter and Arnon, 2004).

The prognosis is generally good if the patient is adequately treated, although recovery may be very slow, requiring a few weeks after severe illness; the average length of stay for infant botulism is 44 days, and the fatality rate is reported to be less than 2% (Cox and Hinkle, 2002). Untreated patients may require a longer hospitalization.

> **! NURSING ALERT**
>
> Honey should not be given to infants younger than 12 months old because *Clostridia botulinum* spores, which cause infant botulism, have been isolated in the natural sweetener (CDC, 2002)

Nursing Considerations

Nursing responsibilities include observing for and reporting signs of neuromuscular weakness or impairment and providing intensive nursing care when the infant is hospitalized (see Nursing Care of the High-Risk Newborn and Family, Chapter 9). Parental support and reassurance are important (see Community Focus box). Most infants recover when the disorder is recognized and therapy is implemented. Parents should be aware that during recovery, patients tire easily when muscular action is sustained. This has important implications for timing the resumption of feedings, because of the risk of aspiration. Parents should also be advised that normal bowel action may not return for several weeks; therefore a stool softener can be beneficial. Cathartics and enemas are not advised.

SPINAL CORD INJURIES

Spinal cord injuries (SCIs) with major neurologic involvement are not a common cause of physical disability in children. However, a sufficient number of children with these

COMMUNITY FOCUS

Preventing Botulism

Home supervision and education regarding possible modes of infection (such as the use of honey as formula sweetener or to coat a pacifier nipple) are nursing responsibilities. Because the prime sources of botulism toxin are often inadequately cooked or improperly canned food, families are advised about the danger of home-canned foods, especially vegetables, fruits, fish, and condiments. Improperly cooked seafood is a common source of botulism as well. Boiling is not always adequate, particularly at high altitudes, where water boils at a lower temperature, which does not destroy the organisms.

injuries are admitted to major medical centers, and because of the increased survival rate as a result of improved management, nurses are more likely to be involved in the care of children with SCI.

Mechanisms of Injury

The most common cause of serious spinal cord damage in children is trauma involving motor vehicle crashes (MVCs) (including automobile-bicycle, all-terrain vehicles, and snowmobiles), sports injuries (especially from diving, trampoline activities, gymnastics, and football), birth trauma, and child abuse. The increased use of recreational activities involving motorized vehicles such as jet water skis and motorcycles has also increased the incidence of SCIs in children. Congenital defects of the spine such as myelomeningocele also may in some cases produce the effects of SCI.

Transverse myelitis (inflammation of the spinal cord) has also been reported to develop from inadvertent intraarterial administration of long-acting penicillin injected into the buttocks. Damage can be extensive enough to result in paraplegia or even lower limb amputation.

In motor vehicle crashes (MVCs) most SCIs in children are a result of indirect trauma caused by sudden hyperflexion or hyperextension of the neck, often combined with a rotational force. Trauma to the spinal cord without evidence of vertebral fracture or dislocation (SCIWORA) is particularly likely to occur in an MVC when proper safety restraints are not used. An unrestrained child becomes a projectile during sudden deceleration and is subject to injury from contact with a variety of objects inside and outside the vehicle. Individuals who use only a lap seat belt restraint are at greater risk of spinal cord injury than those who use a combination lap and shoulder restraint. High cervical spine injuries have been reported in children younger than 2 years of age who are restrained in forward-facing car seats. Infants who are improperly restrained in an infant car seat may experience cervical trauma in a car crash. Small children may also be severely injured by deploying front seat air bags.

Falling from heights occurs less often in children than in adults, but vertebral compression from blows to the head or buttocks can occur in water sports (diving and surfing), falls from horses, or other athletic activities. Birth injuries may occur in breech deliveries from traction force on the spinal cord during delivery of the head and shoulders. An increasing number of adolescents receive spinal cord injuries secondary to gunshot wounds, stabbings, or other violently inflicted injury.

The injury sustained can affect any of the spinal nerves, and the higher the injury, the more extensive the damage. The child can be left with complete or partial paralysis of the lower extremities *(paraplegia)* or with damage at a higher level and without functional use of any of the four extremities *(quadriplegia)*. A high cervical cord injury that affects the phrenic nerve paralyzes the diaphragm and leaves the child dependent on mechanical ventilation.

A mild but equally frightening form of cord trauma is *spinal cord compression,* a temporary neural dysfunction without visible damage to the cord. Complete quadriplegia can result but initially may not be differentiated from serious cord injury.

Therapeutic Management

The management of the child with SCI has changed dramatically in the last two decades as a result of improved technology, surgical procedures, and research into the complexity of the spinal cord and its neurologic components. Initial care begins at the scene of the accident; therefore, education and training of first responder personnel in spinal immobilization, stabilization, and transfer techniques to prevent or reduce the severity of injury is critically important. Evidence indicates that as many as one fourth of SCIs occur *after* the initial traumatic injury during transit or as a result of management during the early stages of the injury. Because of the complexity of these injuries, it is usually recommended that these persons be transported to a spinal injury center for care by specially trained health care personnel as soon as possible after the injury for appropriate diagnostic evaluation and intervention.

SCI management guidelines and standards of care have recently been published for adult and pediatric patients with spinal injuries by the American Association of Neurological Surgeons and The Congress of Neurological Surgeons. For information regarding these guidelines and a more in-depth review of SCI care, the reader is referred to the Barker and Saulino (2002) reference for a synopsis of the guidelines or the March 2002 supplement issue of *Neurosurgery* (vol 50, no 3) for the complete text.

Nursing Considerations

The nursing care of the paraplegic or quadriplegic child is complex and challenging. A multidisciplinary SCI team is equipped to manage the acute phase of the injury and some members, including the nurse, may follow the patient to eventual recovery. Nursing management is concerned with ensuring adequate initial stabilization of the entire spinal column with a rigid cervical collar with supportive blocks on a rigid backboard (Barker and Saulino, 2002). During the acute phase of the injury it is imperative that airway patency be maintained and respiratory function monitored. It is important to evaluate the extent of the neurologic damage early to establish a baseline for neurologic functioning; continual assessment of function should occur to prevent further deterioration of neurologic status as a result of spinal cord edema. The American Spinal Injury Association (ASIA) Impairment Scale may be used to assess neurologic function on a routine basis during the patient's recovery (Barker and Saulino, 2002). After the patient is admitted, further evaluation of the

patient's abilities to perform ADLs can be made with the Functional Independence Measure (FIM) scale; this scale measures the patient's abilities during recovery and need for assistance (Barker and Saulino, 2002).

NURSING ALERT

In any situation in which spinal cord injury is suspected or a possibility, the child should be calmed, reassured, and told not to move; no one should be allowed to move the child unless he or she is able to stabilize the entire spine. A rigid cervical collar is used to immobilize the cervical spine, and the child is placed supine on a rigid immobilization board. Infants and small children are removed in their car seats; no attempt should be made to take them out of the seat.

Additional nursing care is aimed at monitoring and maintenance of adequate systemic blood pressure, administration of pharmacologic agents such as methylprednisolone, and assessment for concomitant injuries or complications such as hemorrhage, which might hinder adequate recovery. Because SCI patients are particularly labile during the first few weeks after the injury, it is also important to monitor for cardiovascular complications and respiratory failure. When surgery is required, the nursing care for the child is the same as with any other major surgery involving prolonged anesthesia and major organ or skeletal trauma; preoperative teaching using age-appropriate props is essential to helping the child understand postoperative equipment, monitoring procedures, and pain management. Patients with SCI and subsequent immobilization have the same needs as those mentioned in Chapter 31. During the recovery and rehabilitation phase patients with SCI must be carefully monitored for complications of immobility such as deep vein thrombosis (DVT) and pulmonary embolus (PE).

The nurse is a crucial member of the health care team in relation to helping the family cope with the magnitude of the injury and disability, understand the extent of the disability, verbalize expected outcomes, and move the child and family toward eventual rehabilitation and normalization within the child's capabilities. The goals of rehabilitation include preparing the child and family to live at home and function as independently as possible.

Recently treatment with *functional electrical stimulation (FES)* (an implantable electrical stimulator with leads attached to the paralyzed muscles or nerves) has allowed children with certain SCIs greater mobility and functional use of paralyzed muscles to sit, stand, and walk with the aid of crutches, a walker, or other orthoses. Administration of pharmacologic agents such as clonidine hydrochloride may improve ambulation in patients with partial SCI, and exercise therapy through interactive locomotor training has been beneficial in helping some individuals with SCI regain ambulatory function (Kalb, 2003).

KEY POINTS

■ Clinical manifestations of cerebral palsy include delayed gross motor development, altered motor performance, alterations of muscle tone and subsequent muscle contractures, abnormal posture, and associated disabilities such as seizures and sensory impairment.

■ Therapy for cerebral palsy takes into account the nature of the physical disability, defects associated with the disorder, and interpersonal and social influences encountered by the affected child.

■ Care of the infant and child with myelomeningocele is directed toward protecting the meningeal sac, preventing infection and skin breakdown, observing for signs of urologic and bowel complications, and planning appropriate interventions to optimize the child's development.

■ Spinal muscular atrophy type 1 disease (Werdnig-Hoffmann disease) is characterized by progressive weakness and wasting of skeletal muscles caused by degeneration of anterior horn cells of the spinal cord.

■ Muscular dystrophies are the greatest and most important cause of neuromuscular dysfunction of childhood.

■ Children with neuromuscular disease require careful monitoring of respiratory function and prompt interventions to prevent hypoxia and further respiratory compromise.

■ Major complications of Duchenne muscular dystrophy include joint contractures, disuse atrophy, obesity, and respiratory and cardiac problems.

■ Nursing care of the child with Guillain-Barré syndrome consists of maintaining a patent airway, monitoring vital signs and neurologic signs, ensuring proper body alignment and positioning, and providing physical therapy, reassurance, and support to the child and family.

■ Tetanus occurs when tetanus spores or vegetative bacilli enter a wound and multiply in a susceptible host.

■ Infant botulism results from the release of toxins from *Clostridium botulinum* colonizing the gastrointestinal tract.

■ Therapeutic management of spinal cord injury is directed toward immobilizing the entire spinal column at the scene of the traumatic event, transporting safely by health care personnel trained to transport possible spinal trauma victims, evaluating neurologic damage, preventing further neurologic damage, and implementing an aggressive rehabilitation program designed to help achieve independence and movement.

References

Albright AL and others: Long-term intrathecal baclofen therapy for severe spasticity of cerebral origin, *J Neurosurg* 98(2):291-295, 2003.

American Academy of Pediatrics, Committee on Infectious Diseases, Pickering L, editor: *2003 Red book: report of the Committee on Infectious Diseases,* ed 26, Elk Grove Village, Il, 2003, The Academy.

American Academy of Pediatrics and American College of Obstetricians and Gynecologists: *Neonatal encephalopathy and cerebral palsy: defining the pathogenesis and pathophysiology,* Washington, DC, 2003, American College of Obstetricians and Gynecologists.

American Nurses Association: Position statement on latex allergy, *Okla Nurse* 42(4):32-33, 1997.

Aneja R, Thomas C, Elberger S: Early infantile botulism, *Emerg Med* 32(6):36-41, 2000.

Arnon SS: Tetanus *(Clostridium tetani).* In Behrman RE, Kliegman RM, Jenson HB, editors: *Nelson textbook of pediatrics,* ed 17, Philadelphia, 2004, WB Saunders.

Bach JR and others: Spinal muscular atrophy type 1 quality of life, *Am J Phys Med Rehabil* 82(2):137-142, 2003.

Barker E, Saulino MF: Special report: first-ever guidelines for spinal cord injuries, *RN* 65(10):32-37, 2002.

Beezhold DH and others: Latex protein: a hidden "food" allergen? *Allergy Asthma Proc* 21(5):301-306, 2000.

Beroud C and others: Prenatal diagnosis of spinal muscular atrophy by genetic analysis of circulating fetal cells, *Lancet* 361(9362):1013-1014, 2003.

Birnkrant DJ: The assessment and management of the respiratory complications of pediatric neuromuscular diseases, *Clin Pediatr* 41(5): 301-308, 2002.

Bothwell JE and others: Duchenne muscular dystrophy—parental perceptions, *Clin Pediatr* 41(2):105-109, 2002.

Brown JP: Orthopaedic care of children with spina bifida: you've come a long way, baby! *Orthop Nurs* 20(4):51-58, 2001.

Centers for Disease Control and Prevention: Knowledge and use of folic acid among women of reproductive age—Michigan, 1998, *MMWR* 50(10):185-189, 2001.

Centers for Disease Control and Prevention: *Botulism in the United States, 1899-1996;* available at: www.cdc.gov/ncidod/dbmd/diseaseinfo/botulism.pdf; accessed July 1, 2003; 2002.

Cox N, Hinkle R: Radiologic decision-making: infant botulism, *Am Fam Physician* 65(7):1388-1392, 2002.

Dabney KW, Lipton GE, Miller F: Cerebral palsy, *Curr Opin Pediatr* 9(1):81-88, 1997.

Finnell RH, Gould A, Spiegelstein O: Pathobiology and genetics of neural tube defects, *Epilepsia* 44(suppl 3):14-23, 2003.

Frey L, Hauser WA: Epidemiology of neural tube defects, *Epilepsia* 44(suppl 3):4-13, 2003.

Gibson CS and others: Antenatal causes of cerebral palsy: associations between inherited thrombophilias, viral and bacterial infection, and inherited susceptibility to infection, *Obstet Gynecol Surv* 58(3):209-220, 2003.

Gomez-Merino E, Bach JR: Duchenne muscular dystrophy: prolongation of life by noninvasive ventilation and mechanically assisted coughing, *Am J Phys Med Rehabil* 81(6):411-415, 2002.

Graf WD and others: Outcome in severe pediatric Guillain-Barré syndrome after immunotherapy or supportive care, *Neurology* 52(7):1494-1497, 1999.

Green L, Greenberg GM, Hurwitz E: Primary care of children with cerebral palsy, *Clin Fam Pract* 5(2):1-21, 2003.

Grether JK and others: Intrauterine exposure to infection and risk of cerebral palsy in very preterm infants, *Arch Pediatr Adolesc Med* 157(1):26-32, 2003.

Han TR and others: Risk factors of cerebral palsy in preterm infants, *Am J Phys Med Rehabil* 81(4):297-303, 2002.

Henshaw SK: Unintended pregnancy in the United States, *Fam Plan Perspect* 30:24-29, 1998.

Hirose F, Farmer DL, Albanese CT: Fetal surgery for myelomeningocele, *Curr Opin Obstet Gynecol* 13(2):215-222, 2001.

Holmes NM and others: Fetal intervention for myelomeningocele: effect on postnatal bladder function, *J Urol* 166(6):2383-2386, 2001.

Holzbierlein J and others: The urodynamic profile of myelodysplasia childhood with spinal closure during gestation, *J Urol* 164(4):1336-1339, 2000.

Honein MA: Impact of folic acid fortification of the US food supply and occurrence of neural tube defects, *JAMA* 285(23):2981-2986, 2001.

Hughes RAC and others: Intravenous immunoglobulin for Guillain-Barré syndrome, Cochrane Library (2):CD002063, 2003.

Iannaccone ST: Spinal muscular atrophy, *Semin Neurol* 18(1):19-26, 1998.

Iannaccone ST, Burghes A: Spinal muscular atrophies, *Adv Neurol* 88:83-98, 2002.

Jacobs JM: Management options for the child with spastic cerebral palsy, *Orthop Nurs* 20(3):53-59, 2001.

Johnston MV, Kinsman S: Congenital anomalies of the central nervous system. In Behrman RE, Kliegman RM, Jenson HB, editors: *Nelson textbook of pediatrics,* ed 17, Philadelphia, 2004, WB Saunders.

Johnston MV: Encephalopathies. In Behrman RE, Kliegman RM, Jenson HB, editors: *Nelson textbook of pediatrics,* ed 17, Philadelphia, 2004, WB Saunders.

Kaefer M and others: Improved bladder function after prophylactic treatment of the high risk neurogenic bladder in newborns with myelomeningocele, *J Urol* 162(3 part 2):1068-1071, 1999.

Kalb RG: Getting the spinal cord to think for itself, *Arch Neurol* 60(6):805-808, 2003.

Kellett PB: Latex allergy: a review, *J Emerg Nurs* 23(1):27-36, 1997.

Kernicterus in full-term infants—United States, 1994-1998, *MMWR* 50(23):491-494, 2001.

Liddle A: Arizona announces updates to state food-safety health codes, *Nation's Restaurant News* Oct 8, 2001.

Lyerly AD, Mahowald MB: Maternal-fetal surgery for treatment of myelomeningocele, *Clin Perinatol* 30(1):155-165, 2003.

Matthews TJ, Honein MA, Erickson JD: Spina bifida and anencephaly prevalence—United States, 1991-2001, *MMWR Recomm Rep* 51(RR-13):9-11, 2002.

Mazon A and others: Latex sensitization in children with spina bifida: follow-up comparative study after two years, *Ann Allergy Asthma Immunol* 84:207-210, 2000.

Metules T: Duchenne muscular dystrophy, *RN* 65(10):39-47, 2002.

Murphy KP, Molnar GE, Lankasky K: Employment and social issues in adults with cerebral palsy, *Arch Phys Med Rehabil* 81:807-811, 2000.

National Association of Neonatal Nurses: Position statement on latex allergy, *Central Lines* Jan 2000; available online: www.nann.org.

National Institute for Occupational Safety and Health: *NIOSH alert: preventing allergic reactions to natural rubber latex in the workplace*, 1997, DHHS pub no 97-135.

Nehring WM, Steele S: Cerebral palsy. In Jackson PL, Vessey JA, editors: *Primary care of the child with a chronic illness*, ed 2, St Louis, 1996, Mosby.

Occupational Safety and Health Administration: *Technical information bulletin—potential for allergy to natural rubber latex gloves and other natural rubber products*, April 12, 1999, US Department of Labor.

Olutoye OO, Adzick NS: Fetal surgery for myelomeningocele, *Semin Perinatol* 23(6):462-473, 1999.

Rintoul NE and others: A new look at myelomeningoceles: functional level, vertebral level, shunting, and the implications for fetal intervention, *Pediatrics* 109(3):409-413, 2002.

Roscigno CI: Addressing spasticity-related pain in children with spastic cerebral palsy, *J Neurosci Nurs* 34(3):123-131, 2002.

Russman BS: Function changes in spinal muscular atrophy II and III: the DCN/SMA group, *Neurology* 47(4):973-976, 1996.

Russman BS and others: Spinal muscular atrophy: new thoughts on the pathogenesis and classification schema, *J Child Neurol* 7(4):347-353, 1992.

Samaniego IA: A sore spot in pediatrics: risk factors for pressure ulcers, *Pediatr Nurs* 29(4):278-232, 2003.

Sarnat HB: Neuromuscular disorders. In Behrman RE, Kliegman RM, Jenson HB, editors: *Nelson textbook of pediatrics,* ed 17, Philadelphia, 2004, WB Saunders.

Schechter R, Arnon SS: Anaerobic bacterial infections: botulism (*Clostridium botulinum*). In Behrman RE, Kliegman RM, Jenson HB, editors: *Nelson textbook of pediatrics,* ed 17, Philadelphia, 2004, WB Saunders.

Smith J: Shaken baby syndrome, *Orthop Nurs* 22(3):196-203, 2003.

Sulton LL: Meeting the challenge of Guillain-Barré syndrome, *Nurs Manage* 33(7):25-30, 2002.

Suresh-Babu MV and others: Nutrition in children with cerebral palsy, *J Pediatr Gastroenterol Nutr* 26(4):484-485, 1998.

Szepfalusi Z and others: Latex sensitization in spina bifida appears disease-associated, *J Pediatr* 134(3):344-348, 1999.

Thompson GH, Berenson FR: Other neuromuscular disorders. In Morrissy RT, Weinstein SL, editors: *Lovell and Winter's pediatric orthopaedics,* ed 5, Philadelphia, 2001, Lippincott Williams & Wilkins.

Tubbs RS and others: Late gestational intrauterine myelomeningocele repair does not improve lower extremity function, *Pediatr Neurosurg* 38(3):128-132, 2003.

Tulipan N, Bruner JP: Myelomeningocele repair in utero: a report of three cases, *Pediatr Neurosurg* 28(4):177-180, 1998.

Volpe JJ: *Neurology of the newborn*, ed 4, Philadelphia, 2001, WB Saunders.

Watkins ML and others: Maternal obesity and risk for birth defects, *Pediatrics* 111(5 part 2):1152-1158, 2003.

Winter S and others: Trends in the prevalence of cerebral palsy in a population-based study, *Pediatrics* 110(6):1220-1225, 2002.

Yerkes EB and others: The Malone antegrade continence enema procedure: quality of life and family perspective, *J Urol* 169(1):320-323, 2003.

Family Assessment

Family APGAR Questionnaire

PART I

The following questions have been designed to help us better understand you and your family. You should feel free to ask questions about any item in the questionnaire.

The space for comments should be used when you wish to give additional information or if you wish to discuss the way the question is applied to your family. Please try to answer all questions.

Family is defined as the individual(s) with whom you usually live. If you live alone, your "family" consists of persons with whom you now have the strongest emotional ties.*

For each question, check only one box

	Almost always	Some of the time	Hardly ever
I am satisfied that I can turn to my family for help when something is troubling me. Comments: _____	☐	☐	☐
I am satisfied with the way my family talks over things with me and shares problems with me. Comments: _____	☐	☐	☐
I am satisfied that my family accepts and supports my wishes to take on new activities or directions. Comments: _____	☐	☐	☐
I am satisfied with the way my family expresses affection and responds to my emotions, such as anger, sorrow, and love. Comments: _____	☐	☐	☐
I am satisfied with the way my family and I share time together. Comments: _____	☐	☐	☐

*According to which member of the family is being interviewed the interviewer may substitute for the word "family" either spouse, significant other, parents, or children.

FIG. A-1 ■ Family APGAR questionnaire; may be photocopied for clinical use. **A,** Part I. (Modified from Smilkstein G, Ashworth C, Montano D: Validity and reliability of the family APGAR as a test of family function, *J Fam Pract* 15[2]:303-311, 1982.)

Continued

Family APGAR Questionnaire

PART II

Who lives in your home?* List by relationship (e.g., spouse, significant other,†child, or friend).

Please check below the column that best describes how you now get along with each member of the family listed.

Relationship	Age	Sex	Well	Fairly	Poorly
_____	__	__	☐	☐	☐
_____	__	__	☐	☐	☐
_____	__	__	☐	☐	☐
_____	__	__	☐	☐	☐
_____	__	__	☐	☐	☐
_____	__	__	☐	☐	☐

If you don't live with your own family, please list below the individuals to whom you turn for help most frequently. List by relationship, (e.g., family member, friend, associate at work, or neighbor).

Please check below the column that best describes how you now get along with each person listed.

Relationship	Age	Sex	Well	Fairly	Poorly
_____	__	__	☐	☐	☐
_____	__	__	☐	☐	☐
_____	__	__	☐	☐	☐
_____	__	__	☐	☐	☐
_____	__	__	☐	☐	☐
_____	__	__	☐	☐	☐

*If you have established your own family, consider home to be the place where you live with your spouse, children, or significant other; otherwise, consider home as your place of origin, e.g., the place where your parents or those who raised you live.

†"Significant other" is the partner you live with in a physically and emotionally nurturing relationship, but to whom you are not married.

FIG. A-1, cont'd ■ B, Part II.

Patterns of Inheritance

GLOSSARY

congenital Condition that is present at birth. The disorder may be brought about by genetic causes, nongenetic causes, or a combination of these.

familial Disorder that "runs in families" or is present in more members of a family than would be expected by chance.

genetic Disorder caused by a single harmful gene, by several genes, or by a deviation in chromosome number or structure. May or may not be apparent at birth.

genotype The genetic constitution that determines the physical and chemical characteristics of an individual.

heterozygous Having dissimilar genes at a given position (locus) on a pair of chromosomes.

homozygous Having the same genes at a given position (locus) on a pair of chromosomes.

inherited (heritable, hereditary) Synonymous with genetic, although in the past often used to describe a disorder that appeared in parent and offspring over several generations.

mutation Structural or chemical alteration in genetic material that, when changed, remains changed and is transmitted to future generations. Mutations usually occur naturally *(spontaneous)*, or can be *induced* by a variety of external agents, or *mutagens,* including temperature, certain chemicals, and radiation.

phenotype The physical or chemical characteristics of an individual, produced by the interaction of the environment with the genotype.

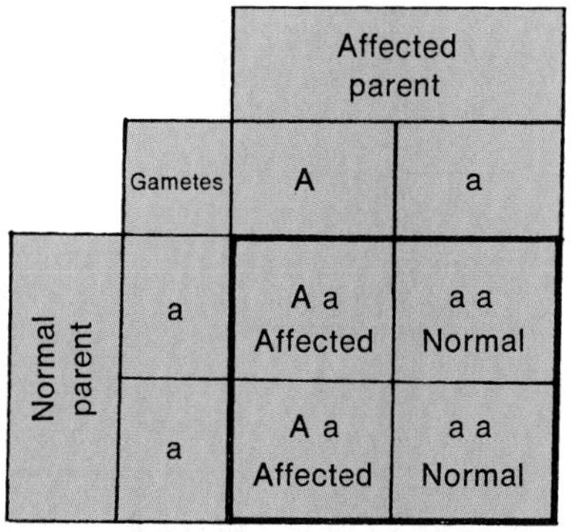

Modifications of Basic Inheritance Patterns

heterogeneity The same or similar manifestations that result from (1) different mutant genes at the same location on a chromosome or (2) mutant genes at different locations on a chromosome (such as the hemophilias, which produce defects in coagulation, and muscular dystrophies, which produce muscular weakness), but that exhibit different inheritance patterns.

linkage Phenomenon caused when genes that are located too close together on a chromosome segregate and migrate together during cell division. The characteristics the genes produce always appear together in the phenotype.

penetrance The regularity with which an inherited trait is manifested in the person who carries the gene. When a gene produces its effect on the phenotype each time it is present in the genotype, it is said to be *fully penetrant* or to exhibit *complete penetrance.* For example, achondroplasia (a form of dwarfism) is always evident whenever the gene is present. If a trait is not recognized in a person who carries the responsible gene, it is said to be *nonpenetrant* in that individual. This phenomenon accounts for what appears to be skipped generations.

pleiotropy The multiple, different, and seemingly unrelated effects associated with a particular disorder; the varied clinical features that constitute a syndrome. For example, Marfan syndrome, a disorder of the elastic fibers of connective tissue, may be manifested in an individual by any or all of the symptoms associated with it—aortic aneurysm, dislocation of the optic lens, or any of a number of skeletal deformities.

variable expressivity The degree of severity of, or the variability in, the manifestations seen in persons of a particular genotype. For instance, polydactyly can be expressed as any number of extra digits, or the extra digits may be fingers in one generation and toes in another. The severity of a disorder may be so mild as to be almost undetected or so severe that the affected individual is totally incapacitated.

Autosomal Dominant Inheritance

Characteristics of a condition caused by a dominant gene on an autosome include the following (Fig. B-1):

1 Males and females are affected with equal frequency.
2 Affected individuals have an affected parent (unless the condition is caused by a fresh mutation).
3 Half the children of a heterozygous affected parent will possess the defective gene, although it may be nonpenetrant.
4 Unaffected children of affected parents will have unaffected children (unless the gene is nonpenetrant).

FIG. B-1 ■ Possible offspring of mating between normal parent, aa, and parent with an autosomal-dominant trait, Aa.

Autosomal Recessive Inheritance

Characteristics of a condition caused by a recessive gene on an autosome include the following (Fig. B-2):

1 Males and females are affected with equal frequency.
2 Affected individuals have unaffected parents who are heterozygous for the trait.
3 There is a one in four chance that any child of two unaffected heterozygous parents will be affected.
4 Two affected parents will have affected children exclusively.
5 Affected individuals married to unaffected individuals will have normal children, all of whom will be carriers.
6 There is usually no evidence of the trait in previous generations—a negative family history.

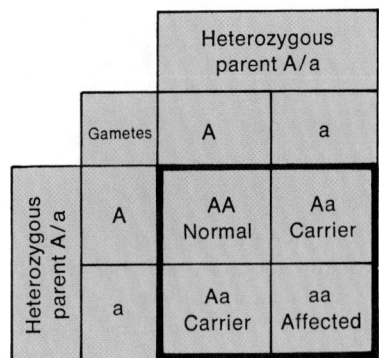

FIG. B-2 ■ Possible offspring of mating between two parents with a recessive gene, a, on an autosome.

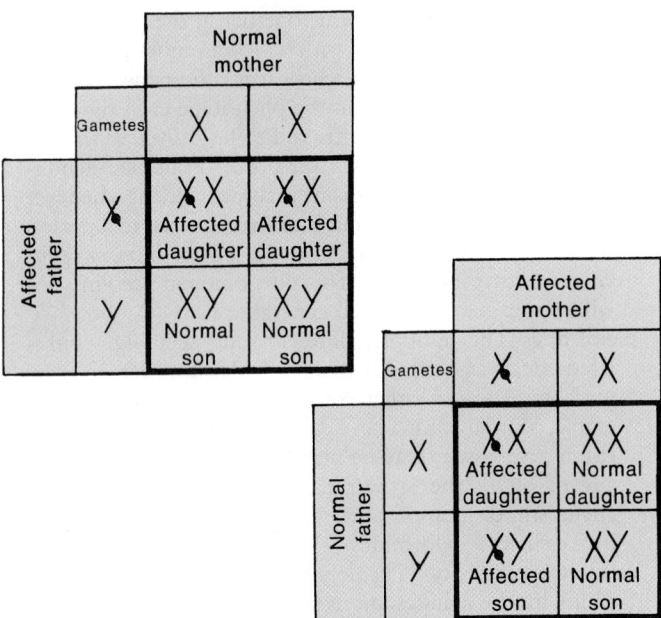

FIG. B-3 ■ Sex differences in offspring ratios in X-linked dominant inheritance. ●, Dominant allele on X chromosome.

X-Linked Dominant Inheritance

Characteristics of a condition caused by a dominant gene on an X chromosome include the following (Fig. B-3):

1 Affected individuals have an affected parent.
2 All the daughters but none of the sons of an affected male will be affected.
3 Half the sons and half the daughters of an affected female will be affected.
4 Normal children of an affected parent will have normal offspring.
5 There are no carriers.
6 The inheritance pattern shows a positive family history.

X-Linked Recessive Inheritance

Characteristics of a disorder caused by a recessive gene on the X chromosome include the following (Fig. B-4):

1 Affected individuals are principally males.
2 Affected individuals have unaffected parents (except in the rare possibility that the father is affected and the mother is a carrier).
3 Half of the female siblings of an affected male will be carriers of the trait.
4 Unaffected male siblings of an affected male cannot transmit the disorder.
5 Sons of an affected male are unaffected.
6 Daughters of an affected male are carriers.
7 The unaffected male children of a carrier female do not transmit the disorder.

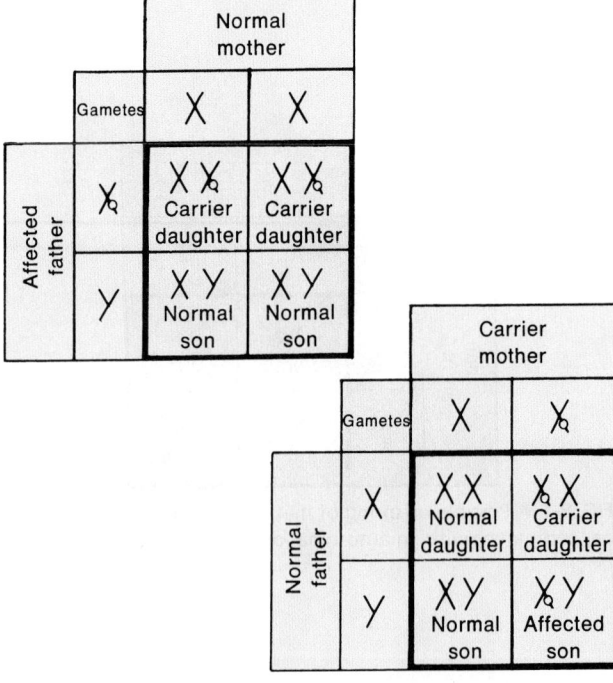

FIG. B-4 ■ Differences in offspring ratios in X-linked recessive inheritance. ○, Recessive allele on X chromosome.

Developmental/Sensory Assessment

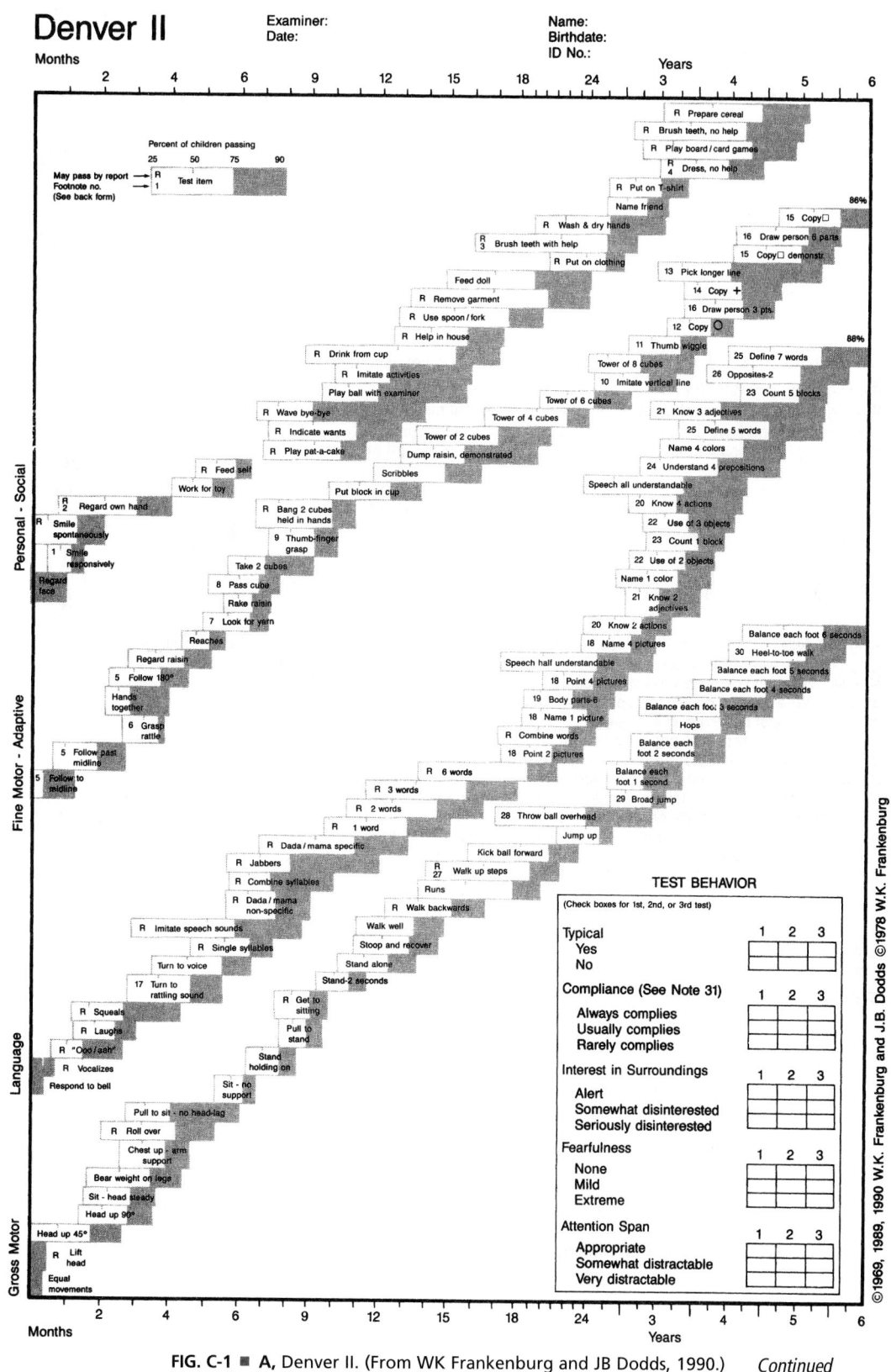

FIG. C-1 ■ A, Denver II. (From WK Frankenburg and JB Dodds, 1990.)   *Continued*

DIRECTIONS FOR ADMINISTRATION

1. Try to get child to smile by smiling, talking or waving. Do not touch him/her.
2. Child must stare at hand several seconds.
3. Parent may help guide toothbrush and put toothpaste on brush.
4. Child does not have to be able to tie shoes or button/zip in the back.
5. Move yarn slowly in an arc from one side to the other, about 8" above child's face.
6. Pass if child grasps rattle when it is touched to the backs or tips of fingers.
7. Pass if child tries to see where yarn went. Yarn should be dropped quickly from sight from tester's hand without arm movement.
8. Child must transfer cube from hand to hand without help of body, mouth, or table.
9. Pass if child picks up raisin with any part of thumb and finger.
10. Line can vary only 30 degrees or less from tester's line. /
11. Make a fist with thumb pointing upward and wiggle only the thumb. Pass if child imitates and does not move any fingers other than the thumb.

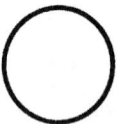 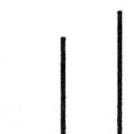 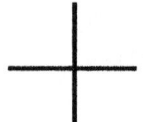 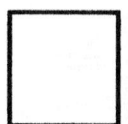

12. Pass any enclosed form. Fail continuous round motions.
13. Which line is longer? (Not bigger.) Turn paper upside down and repeat. (pass 3 of 3 or 5 of 6)
14. Pass any lines crossing near midpoint.
15. Have child copy first. If failed, demonstrate.

When giving items 12, 14, and 15, do not name the forms. Do not demonstrate 12 and 14.

16. When scoring, each pair (2 arms, 2 legs, etc.) counts as one part.
17. Place one cube in cup and shake gently near child's ear, but out of sight. Repeat for other ear.
18. Point to picture and have child name it. (No credit is given for sounds only.)
    If less than 4 pictures are named correctly, have child point to picture as each is named by tester.

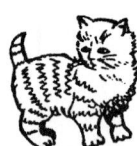 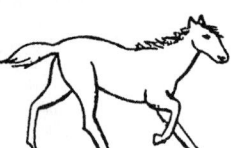 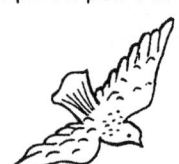 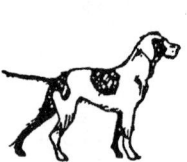 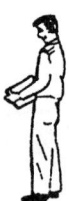

19. Using doll, tell child: Show me the nose, eyes, ears, mouth, hands, feet, tummy, hair. Pass 6 of 8.
20. Using pictures, ask child: Which one flies?... says meow?... talks?... barks?... gallops? Pass 2 of 5, 4 of 5.
21. Ask child: What do you do when you are cold?... tired?... hungry? Pass 2 of 3, 3 of 3.
22. Ask child: What do you do with a cup? What is a chair used for? What is a pencil used for?
    Action words must be included in answers.
23. Pass if child correctly places <u>and</u> says how many blocks are on paper. (1, 5).
24. Tell child: Put block **on** table; **under** table; **in front of** me, **behind** me. Pass 4 of 4.
    (Do not help child by pointing, moving head or eyes.)
25. Ask child: What is a ball?... lake?... desk?... house?... banana?... curtain?... fence?... ceiling? Pass if defined in terms of use, shape, what it is made of, or general category (such as banana is fruit, not just yellow). Pass 5 of 8, 7 of 8.
26. Ask child: If a horse is big, a mouse is __? If fire is hot, ice is __? If the sun shines during the day, the moon shines during the __? Pass 2 of 3.
27. Child may use wall or rail only, not person. May not crawl.
28. Child must throw ball overhand 3 feet to within arm's reach of tester.
29. Child must perform standing broad jump over width of test sheet (8 1/2 inches).
30. Tell child to walk forward, ⌒⌒⌒⌒➤ heel within 1 inch of toe. Tester may demonstrate.
    Child must walk 4 consecutive steps.
31. In the second year, half of normal children are non-compliant.

OBSERVATIONS:

FIG. C-1, cont'd ■ B, Directions for administration of numbered items on Denver II.

DENVER ARTICULATION SCREENING EXAM
for children 2½ to 6 years of age

Instructions: Have child repeat each word after
you. Circle the underlined sounds that he pro-
nounces correctly. Total correct sounds is the
Raw Score. Use charts on reverse side to score
results.

Name:

Hosp. No.:

Address:_____

_____

Date: _____   Child's age: _____   Examiner: _____   Raw score: ____

Percentile: _____   Intelligibility: _____   Result: _____

1. table	6. zipper	11. sock	16. wagon	21. leaf
2. shirt	7. grapes	12. vacuum	17. gum	22. carrot
3. door	8. flag	13. yarn	18. house	
4. trunk	9. thumb	14. mother	19. pencil	
5. jumping	10. toothbrush	15. twinkle	20. fish	

Intelligibility: (circle one)
   1. Easy to understand
   2. Understandable ½ the time

   3. Not understandable
   4. Can't evaluate

Comments:

Date: _____   Child's age: _____   Examiner: _____   Raw score: ____

Percentile: _____   Intelligibility: _____   Result: _____

1. table	6. zipper	11. sock	16. wagon	21. leaf
2. shirt	7. grapes	12. vacuum	17. gum	22. carrot
3. door	8. flag	13. yarn	18. house	
4. trunk	9. thumb	14. mother	19. pencil	
5. jumping	10. toothbrush	15. twinkle	20. fish	

Intelligibility: (circle one)
   1. Easy to understand
   2. Understandable ½ the time

   3. Not understandable
   4. Can't evaluate

Comments:

A

Date: _____   Child's age: _____   Examiner: _____   Raw score ____

Percentile: _____   Intelligibility: _____   Result: _____

1. table	6. zipper	11. sock	16. wagon	21. leaf
2. shirt	7. grapes	12. vacuum	17. gum	22. carrot
3. door	8. flag	13. yarn	18. house	
4. trunk	9. thumb	14. mother	19. pencil	
5. jumping	10. toothbrush	15. twinkle	20. fish	

Intelligibility: (circle one)
   1. Easy to understand
   2. Understandable ½ the time

   3. Not understandable
   4. Can't evaluate

FIG. C-2 ■ A, Denver Articulation Screening Examination (DASE) for children 2½ to 6 years of
age. (From AF Drumwright, University of Colorado Medical Center, 1971.)   *Continued*

To score DASE words: Note raw score for child's performance. Match raw score line (extreme left of chart) with column representing child's age (to the closest previous age group). Where raw score line and age column meet number in that square denotes percentile rank of child's performance when compared to other children that age. Percentiles above heavy line are ABNORMAL percentiles, below heavy line are NORMAL.

PERCENTILE RANK

Raw Score	2.5 yr.	3.0	3.5	4.0	4.5	5.0	5.5	6 years
2	1							
3	2							
4	5							
5	9							
6	16							
7	23							
8	31	2						
9	37	4	1					
10	42	6	2					
11	48	7	4					
12	54	9	6	1	1			
13	58	12	9	2	3	1	1	
14	62	17	11	5	4	2	2	
15	68	23	15	9	5	3	2	
16	75	31	19	12	5	4	3	
17	79	38	25	15	6	6	4	
18	83	46	31	19	8	7	4	
19	86	51	38	24	10	9	5	1
20	89	58	45	30	12	11	7	3
21	92	65	52	36	15	15	9	4
22	94	72	58	43	18	19	12	5
23	96	77	63	50	22	24	15	7
24	97	82	70	58	29	29	20	15
25	99	87	78	66	36	34	26	17
26	99	91	84	75	46	43	34	24
27		94	89	82	57	54	44	34
28		96	94	88	70	68	59	47
29		98	98	94	84	84	77	68
30		100	100	100	100	100	100	100

B

To score intelligibility:

	NORMAL	ABNORMAL
2½ years	Understandable ½ the time, or, "easy"	Not understandable
3 years and older	Easy to understand	Understandable ½ time Not understandable

Test result: 1. NORMAL on DASE and Intelligibility = NORMAL

2. ABNORMAL on DASE and/or Intelligibility = ABNORMAL

*If abnormal on initial screening, rescreen within 2 weeks.
If abnormal again, child should be referred for complete speech evaluation.

FIG. C-2, cont'd ■ B, Percentile rank.

DENVER EYE SCREENING TEST

Name:
Hospital No.:
Ward:
Address:

	RESCREENING: DATE:															
		Left Eye					Right Eye									
	Untestable	Abnormal	Normal	Untestable	Abnormal	Normal										
	U	3F	3P	U	3F	3P			U				Normal			
	U	3F	3P	U	3F	3P	Untestable		U							
	U	F	P	U	F	P	Abnormal		U	YES	NO		Abnormal			
		yes			yes		Normal			F	P					
										F	P		Untestable			
														Date:		

	1ST SCREENING: DATE:															
		Left Eye					Right Eye									
	Untestable	Abnormal	Normal	Untestable	Abnormal	Normal										
	U	3F	3P	U	3F	3P										
	U	3F	3P	U	3F	3P	Untestable		U							
	U	F	P	U	F	P	Abnormal		U	YES	NO		Normal			
		yes			yes		Normal			F	P		Abnormal			
										F	P		Untestable			
														Date:		

Vision Tests

1. "E" (3 years and above—3 to 5 trials) . . . . .
2. Picture card (2 1/2 – 2 11/12 yrs.—3 to 5 trials)
3. Fixation (6 months – 2 5/12 years) . . . . . .
4. Squinting . . . .

Tests for Non-Straight Eyes

1. Do your child's eyes turn in or out, or are they ever not straight? . . . .
2. Cover Test . . . .
3. Pupillary Light Reflex . . . .

Total Test Rating (Both Eyes)

Normal (passed vision test plus no squint, plus passed 2/3 tests for non-straight eyes)

Abnormal (abnormal on any vision test, squinting or 2 of 3 procedures for non-straight eyes)

Untestable (untestable on any vision test or untestable on 2/3 tests for non-straight eyes)

Future Rescreening Appointment for Total Test Rating (Abnormal or Untestable)

FIG. C-3 ■ Denver Eye Screening Test. (From WK Frankenburg and JB Dodds, University of Colorado Medical Center, 1969.)

SNELLEN SCREENING*
Preparation

1 Hang the Snellen chart on a light-colored wall so that the 20- to 30-foot lines are at eye level when children 6 to 12 years old are tested in the standing position (Fig. C-4).
2 Secure the chart to the wall with double-stick tape on the back side of all four corners. If the chart must be reversed for use of letter or E chart, secure it at the top and bottom with tacks. Make sure that the chart does not swing when in place.
3 The illumination intensity on the chart should be 10 to 30 footcandles, without any glare from windows or light fixtures. The illumination should be checked with a light meter.
4 Mark an exact 20-foot distance from the chart. Mark the floor with a piece of tape or "footprints" positioned so that the heels touch the 20-foot line.

Procedure

1 Place the child at the 20-foot mark, with the heel edging the line if the child is standing or with the back of the chair placed at the marker if the child is seated.
2 If the E chart is used, accustom the child to identifying which direction the "legs of the E" are pointing. Use a demonstration E card for this purpose.
3 Teach the child to use the occluder to cover one eye. Instruct the child to keep both eyes open during the test. Provide a clean cover card for each child and then discard after use.
4 If the child wears glasses, test only with glasses on.
5 Test both eyes together, then the right eye, then the left eye.
6 Begin with the 40- or 30-foot line and proceed with the test to include the 20-foot line.
7 With a child suspected of low vision, begin with the 200-foot line, and proceed until child can no longer correctly read three out of four or four out of six symbols on a line.

*Modified from recommendations of the National Society to Prevent Blindness: *Guide to testing distance visual acuity*, Schaumburg, Il, 1988, The Society.

8 Use covers on the Snellen chart to expose only one symbol or one line at a time. When screening kindergarten or older children, expose one line but use a pointer to point to one symbol at a time.

Recording and Referral

1 Record the last line the child read correctly (three out of four or four out of six symbols).
2 Record visual acuity as a fraction. The numerator represents the distance from the chart, and the denominator represents the last line read correctly. For example, 20/30 means that the child read the 30-foot line at a 20-foot distance.
3 Observe the child's eyes during testing and record any evidence of squinting, head tilting, thrusting the head forward, excessive blinking, tearing, or redness.
4 Only make referrals after a second screening has been made on children who are potential candidates for referral.
5 The following children should be referred for a complete eye examination:
   a Three-year-old children with vision in either eye of 20/50 or less (inability to correctly identify one more than half the symbols on the 40-foot line) *or* a two-line difference in visual acuity between the eyes in the passing range (e.g., 20/20 in one eye and 20/40 in the other)
   b All other ages and grades with vision in either eye of 20/40 or less (inability to correctly identify one or more than half the symbols on the 30-foot line)
   c All children who consistently show any of the signs of possible visual disturbances, regardless of visual acuity

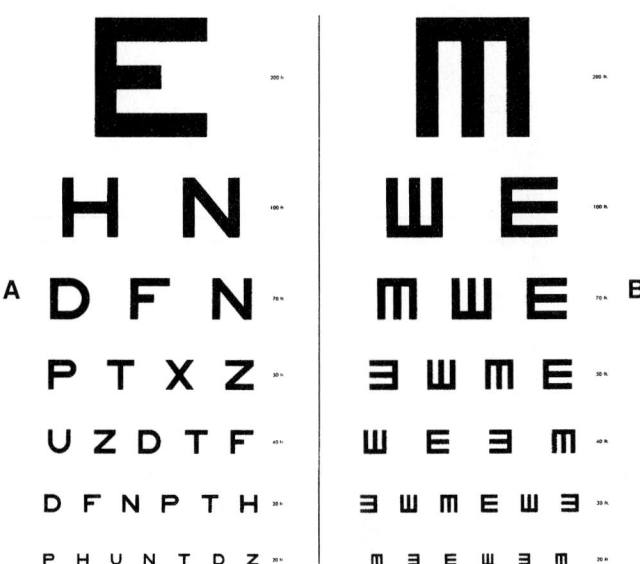

FIG. C-4 ■ Snellen chart. **A,** Letter (alphabet) chart. **B,** Symbol E chart. (From National Society to Prevent Blindness, Inc., Schaumburg, Il.)

Growth Measurements

■ Height and Weight Measurements for Boys

| AGE* | HEIGHT BY PERCENTILES | | | | | | WEIGHT BY PERCENTILES | | | | | |
| | 5 | | 50 | | 95 | | 5 | | 50 | | 95 | |
	CM	INCHES	CM	INCHES	CM	INCHES	KG	LB	KG	LB	KG	LB
Birth	46.4	18¼	50.5	20	54.4	21½	2.54	5½	3.27	7¼	4.15	9¼
3 months	56.7	22¼	61.1	24	65.4	25¾	4.43	9¾	5.98	13¼	7.37	16¼
6 months	63.4	25	67.8	26¾	72.3	28½	6.20	13¾	7.85	17¼	9.46	20¾
9 months	68.0	26¾	72.3	28½	77.1	30¼	7.52	16½	9.18	20¼	10.93	24
1	71.7	28¼	76.1	30	81.2	32	8.43	18½	10.15	22½	11.99	26½
1½	77.5	30½	82.4	32½	88.1	34¾	9.59	21¼	11.47	25¼	13.44	29½
2†	82.5	32½	86.8	34¼	94.4	37¼	10.49	23¼	12.34	27¼	15.50	34¼
2½†	85.4	33½	90.4	35½	97.8	38½	11.27	24¾	13.52	29¾	16.61	36½
3	89.0	35	94.9	37¼	102.0	40¼	12.05	26½	14.62	32¼	17.77	39¼
3½	92.5	36½	99.1	39	106.1	41¾	12.84	28¼	15.68	34½	18.98	41¾
4	95.8	37¾	102.9	40½	109.9	43¼	13.64	30	16.69	36¾	20.27	44¾
4½	98.9	39	106.6	42	113.5	44¾	14.45	31¾	17.69	39	21.63	47¾
5	102.0	40¼	109.9	43¼	117.0	46	15.27	33¾	18.67	41¼	23.09	51
6	107.7	42½	116.1	45¾	123.5	48½	16.93	37¼	20.69	45½	26.34	58
7	113.0	44½	121.7	48	129.7	51	18.64	41	22.85	50¼	30.12	66½
8	118.1	46½	127.0	50	135.7	53½	20.40	45	25.30	55¾	34.51	76
9	122.9	48½	132.2	52	141.8	55¾	22.25	49	28.13	62	39.58	87¼
10	127.7	50¼	137.5	54¼	148.1	58¼	24.33	53¾	31.44	69¼	45.27	99¾
11	132.6	52¼	143.3	56½	154.9	61	26.80	59	35.30	77¾	51.47	113½
12	137.6	54¼	149.7	59	162.3	64	29.85	65¾	39.78	87¾	58.09	128
13	142.9	56¼	156.5	61½	169.8	66¾	33.64	74¼	44.95	99	65.02	143¼
14	148.8	58½	163.1	64¼	176.7	69½	38.22	84¼	50.77	112	72.13	159
15	155.2	61	169.0	66½	181.9	71½	43.11	95	56.71	125	79.12	174½
16	161.1	63½	173.5	68¼	185.4	73	47.74	105¼	62.10	137	85.62	188¾
17	164.9	65	176.2	69¼	187.3	73¾	51.50	113½	66.31	146¼	91.31	201¼
18	165.7	65¼	176.8	69½	187.6	73¾	53.97	119	68.88	151¾	95.76	211

Modified from National Center for Health Statistics (NCHS), Health Resources Administration, Department of Health, Education and Welfare, Hyattsville, Md.
Conversion of metric data to approximate inches and pounds by Ross Laboratories.
*Years unless otherwise indicated.
†Height data include some recumbent length measurements, which make values slightly higher than if all measurements had been of stature (standing height).

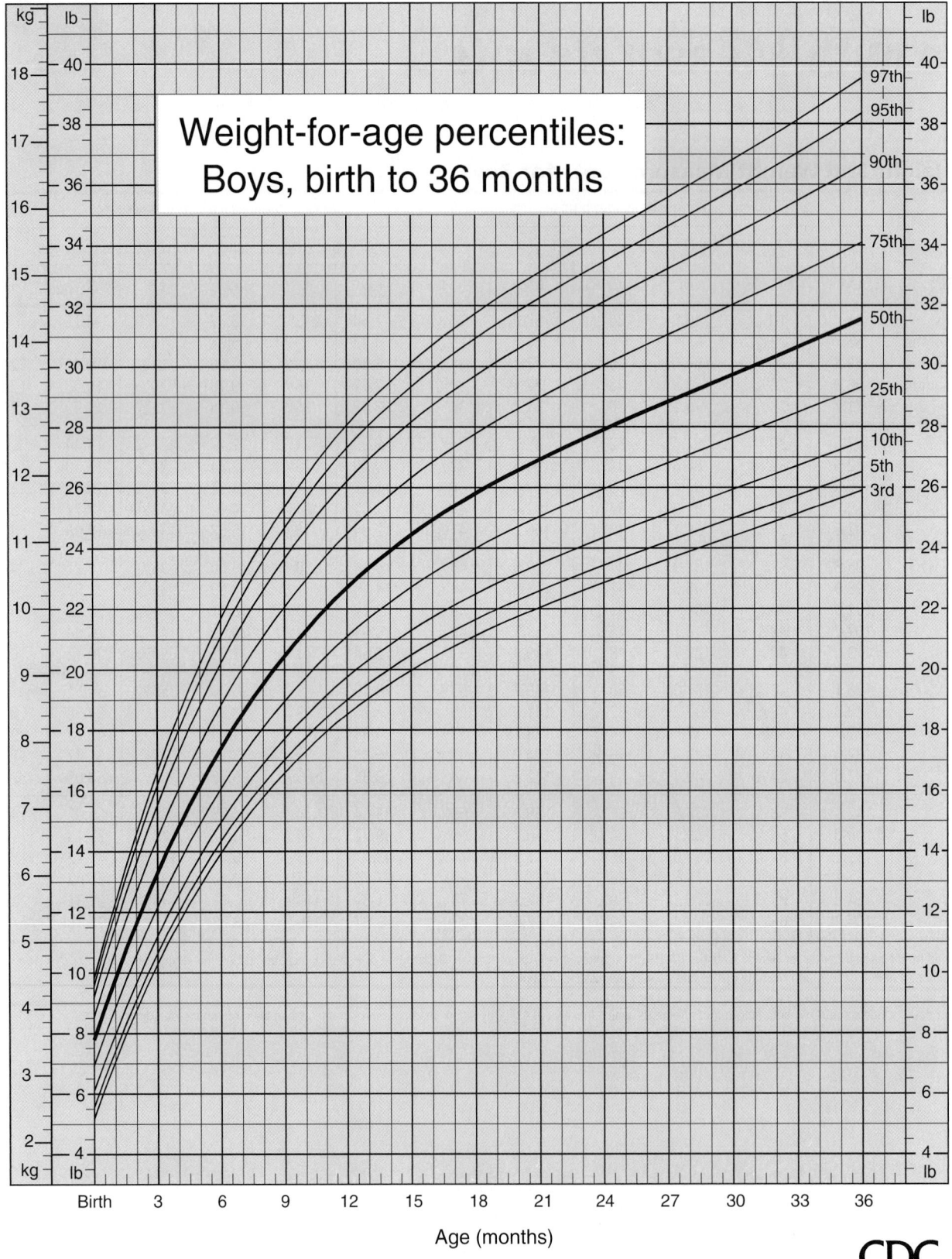

FIG. D-1 ■ Weight-for-age percentiles, boys, birth to 36 months, CDC growth charts: United States. (Developed by the National Center for Health Statistics in collaboration with the National Center for Chronic Disease Prevention and Health Promotion, 2000.)

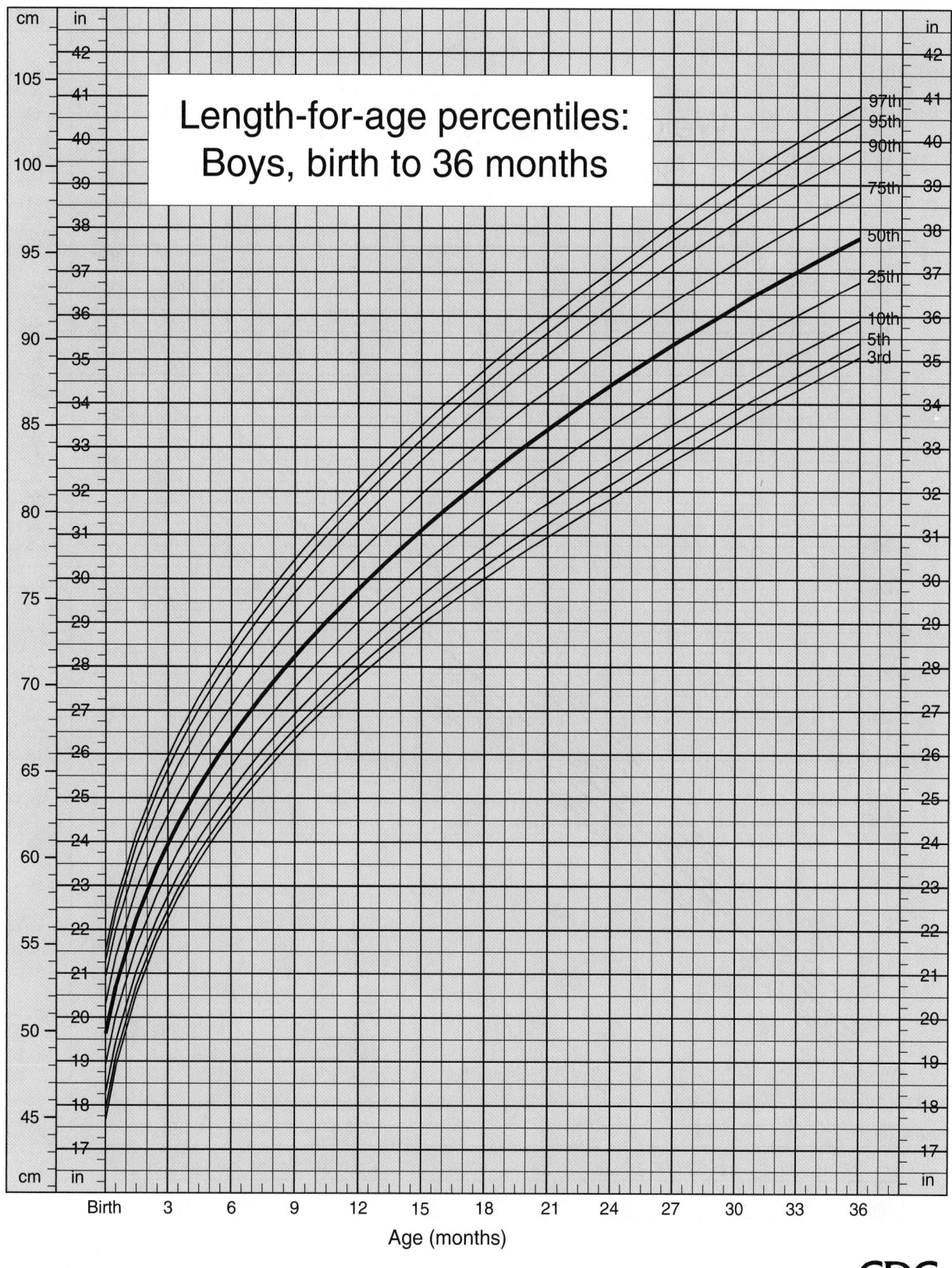

FIG. D-2 ■ Length-for-age percentiles, boys, birth to 36 months, CDC growth charts: United States. (Developed by the National Center for Health Statistics in collaboration with the National Center for Chronic Disease Prevention and Health Promotion, 2000.)

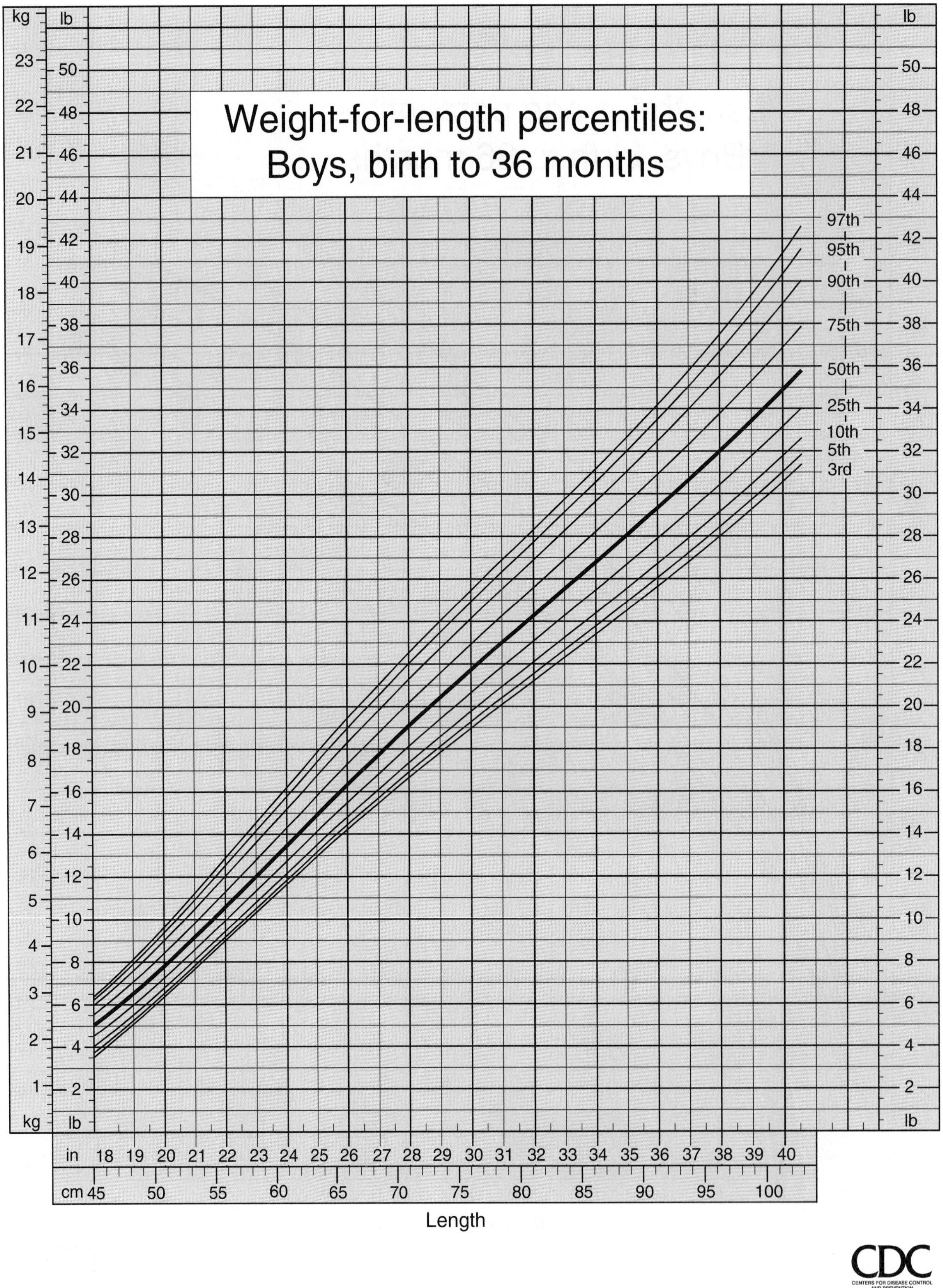

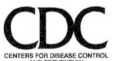

FIG. D-3 ■ Weight-for-length percentiles, boys, birth to 36 months, CDC growth charts: United States. (Developed by the National Center for Health Statistics in collaboration with the National Center for Chronic Disease Prevention and Health Promotion, 2000.)

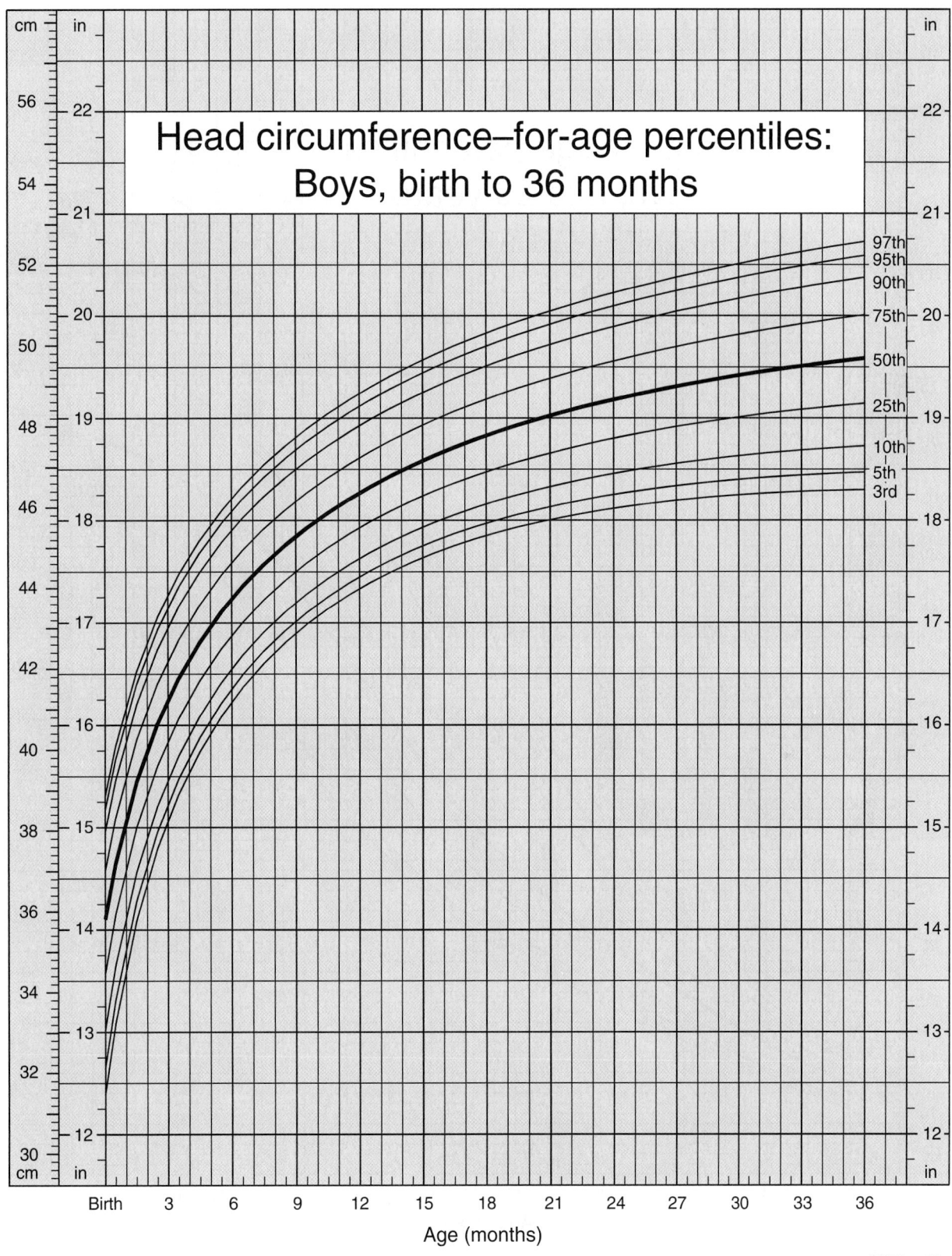

FIG. D-4 ■ Head circumference–for-age percentiles, boys, birth to 36 months, CDC growth charts: United States. (Developed by the National Center for Health Statistics in collaboration with the National Center for Chronic Disease Prevention and Health Promotion, 2000.)

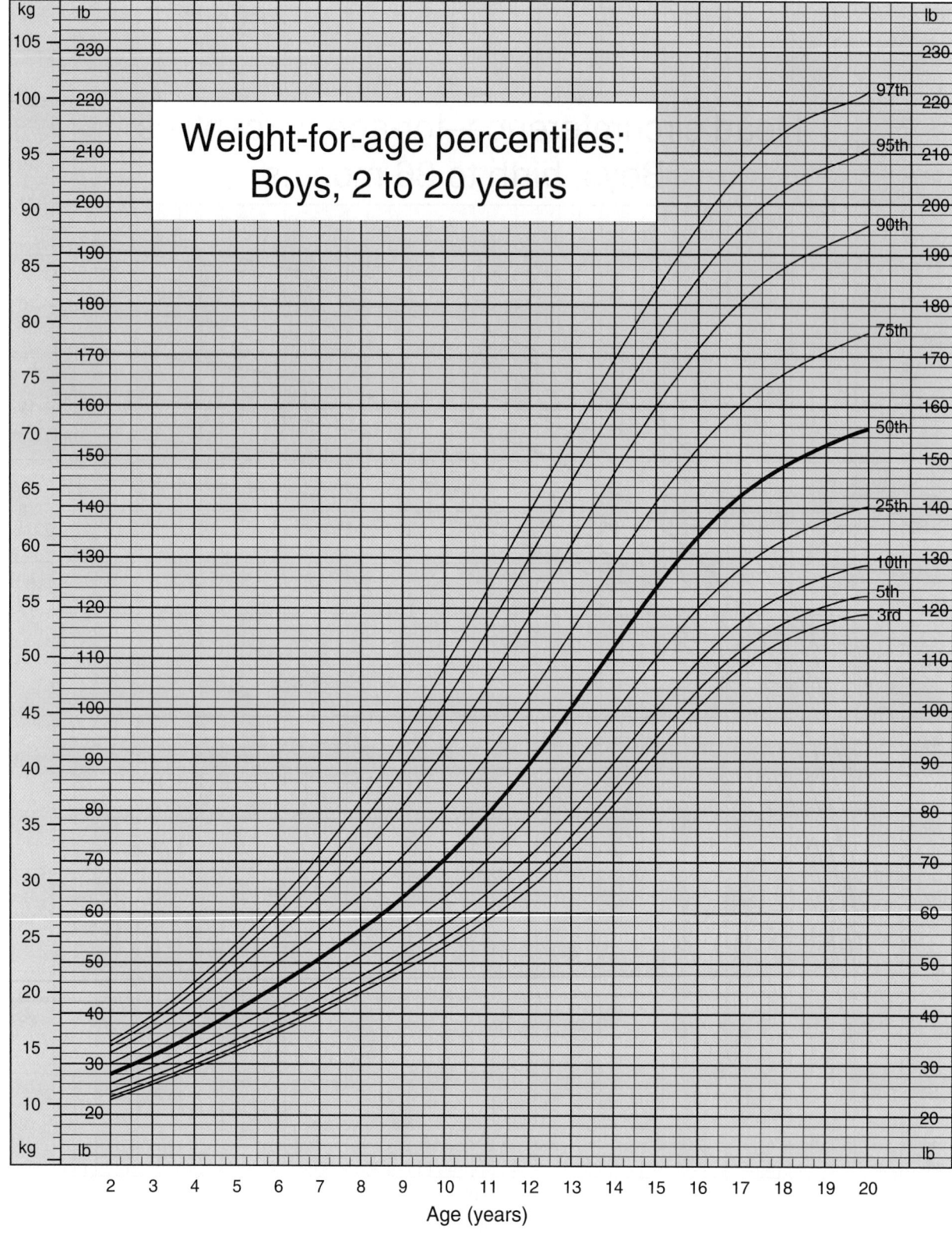

FIG. D-5 ■ Weight-for-age percentiles, boys, 2 to 20 years, CDC growth charts: United States. (Developed by the National Center for Health Statistics in collaboration with the National Center for Chronic Disease Prevention and Health Promotion, 2000.)

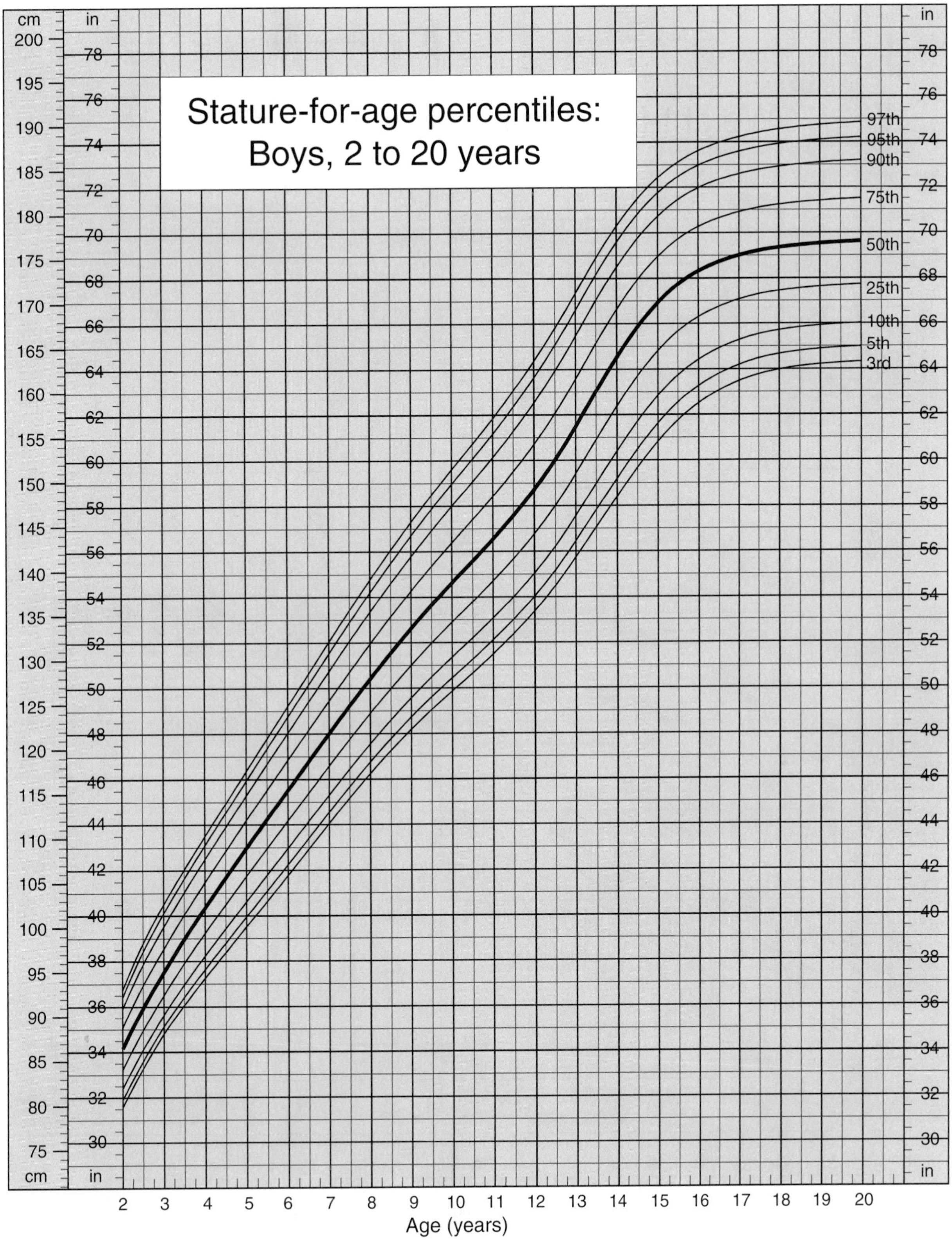

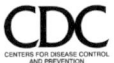

FIG. D-6 ■ Stature-for-age percentiles, boys, 2 to 20 years, CDC growth charts: United States. (Developed by the National Center for Health Statistics in collaboration with the National Center for Chronic Disease Prevention and Health Promotion, 2000.)

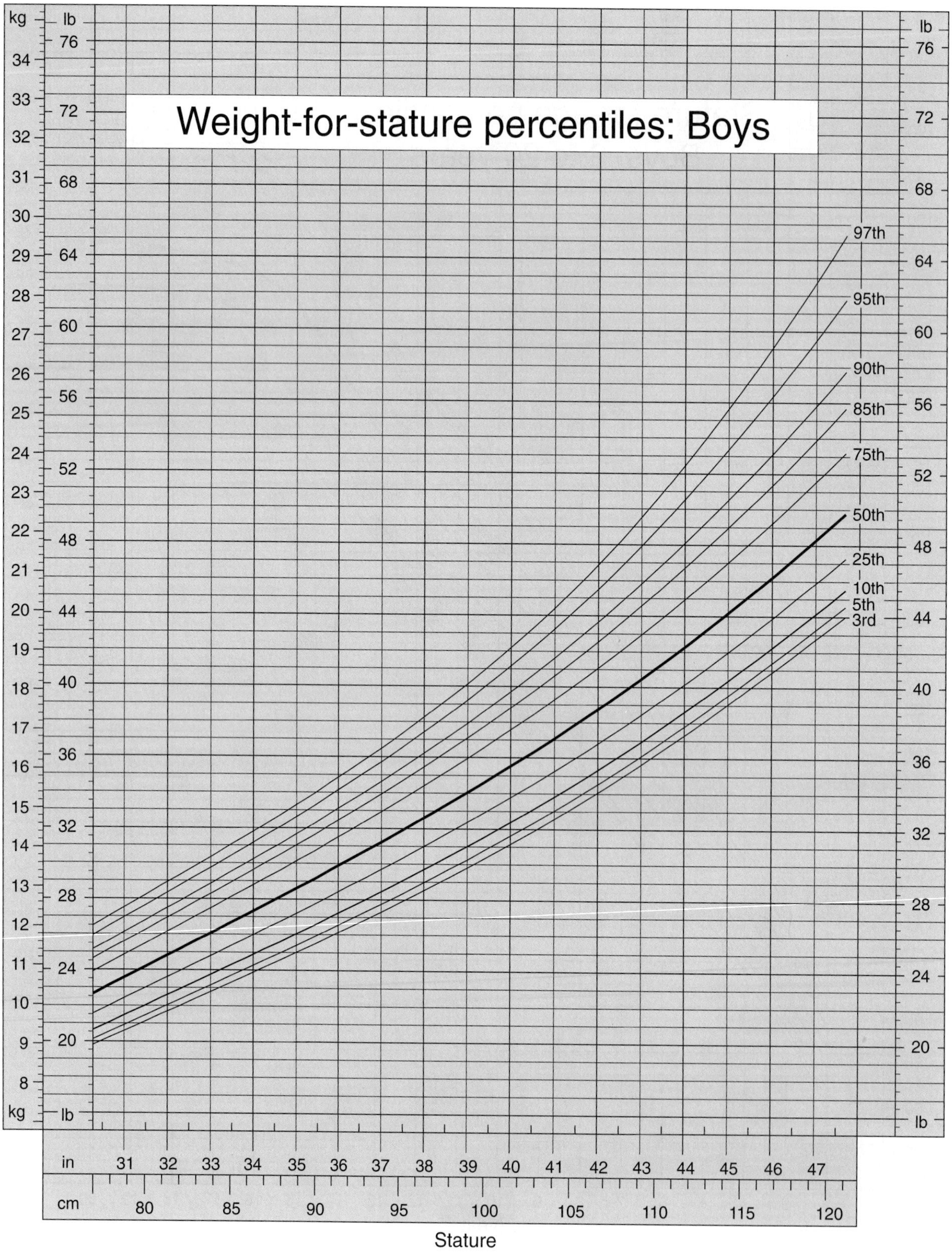

Weight-for-stature percentiles: Boys

Stature

FIG. D-7 ■ Weight-for-stature percentiles, boys, CDC growth charts: United States. (Developed by the National Center for Health Statistics in collaboration with the National Center for Chronic Disease Prevention and Health Promotion, 2000.)

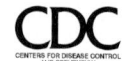

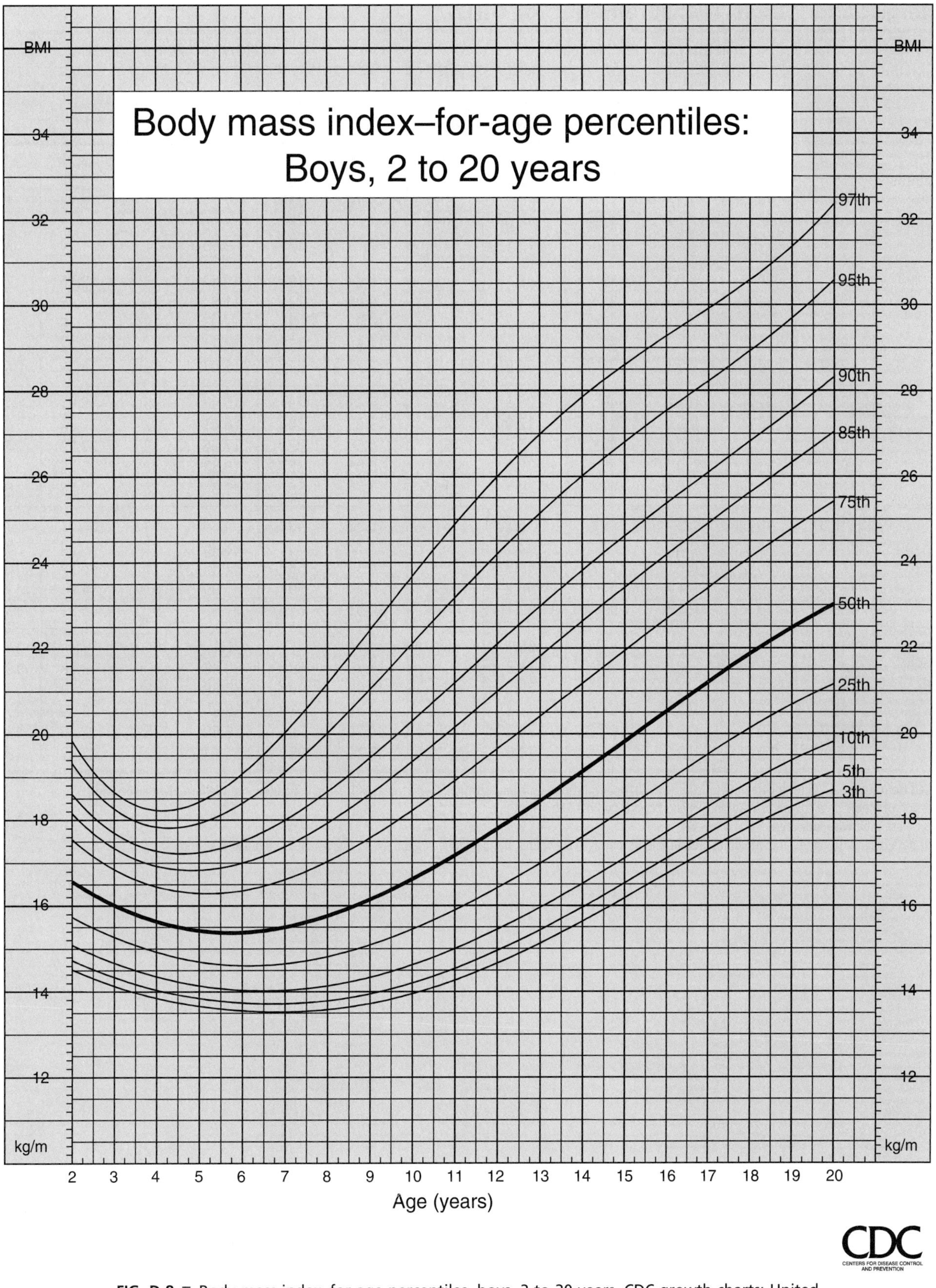
Body mass index–for-age percentiles:
Boys, 2 to 20 years
BMI
34
32
30
28
26
24
22
20
18
16
14
12
kg/m
97th
95th
90th
85th
75th
50th
25th
10th
5th
3th
2 3 4 5 6 7 8 9 10 11 12 13 14 15 16 17 18 19 20
Age (years)
CDC
CENTERS FOR DISEASE CONTROL AND PREVENTION

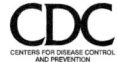

FIG. D-8 ■ Body mass index–for-age percentiles, boys, 2 to 20 years, CDC growth charts: United States. (Developed by the National Center for Health Statistics in collaboration with the National Center for Chronic Disease Prevention and Health Promotion, 2000.)

■ Height and Weight Measurements for Girls

AGE*	HEIGHT BY PERCENTILES						WEIGHT BY PERCENTILES					
	5		50		95		5		50		95	
	CM	INCHES	CM	INCHES	CM	INCHES	KG	LB	KG	LB	KG	LB
Birth	45.4	17¾	49.9	19¾	52.9	20¾	2.36	5¼	3.23	7	3.81	8½
3 months	55.4	21¾	59.5	23½	63.4	25	4.18	9¼	5.4	12	6.74	14¾
6 months	61.8	24¼	65.9	26	70.2	27¾	5.79	12¾	7.21	16	8.73	19¼
9 months	66.1	26	70.4	27¾	75.0	29½	7.0	15½	8.56	18¾	10.17	22½
1	69.8	27½	74.3	29¼	79.1	31¼	7.84	17¼	9.53	21	11.24	24¾
1½	76.0	30	80.9	31¾	86.1	34	8.92	19¾	10.82	23¾	12.76	28¼
2†	81.6	32¼	86.8	34¼	93.6	36¾	9.95	22	11.8	26	14.15	31¼
2½†	84.6	33¼	90.0	35½	96.6	38	10.8	23¾	13.03	28¾	15.76	34¾
3	88.3	34¾	94.1	37	100.6	39½	11.61	25½	14.1	31	17.22	38
3½	91.7	36	97.9	38½	104.5	41¼	12.37	27¼	15.07	33¼	18.59	41
4	95.0	37½	101.6	40	108.3	42¾	13.11	29	15.96	35¼	19.91	44
4½	98.1	38½	105.0	41¼	112.0	44	13.83	30½	16.81	37	21.24	46¾
5	101.1	39¾	108.4	42¾	115.6	45½	14.55	32	17.66	39	22.62	49¾
6	106.6	42	114.6	45	122.7	48¼	16.05	35½	19.52	43	25.75	56¾
7	111.8	44	120.6	47½	129.5	51	17.71	39	21.84	48¼	29.68	65½
8	116.9	46	126.4	49¾	136.2	53½	19.62	43¼	24.84	54¾	34.71	76½
9	122.1	48	132.2	52	142.9	56¼	21.82	48	28.46	62¾	40.64	89½
10	127.5	50¼	138.3	54½	149.5	58¾	24.36	53¾	32.55	71¾	47.17	104
11	133.5	52½	144.8	57	156.2	61½	27.24	60	36.95	81½	54.0	119
12	139.8	55	151.5	59¾	162.7	64	30.52	67¼	41.53	91½	60.81	134
13	145.2	57¼	157.1	61¾	168.1	66¼	34.14	75¼	46.1	101¾	67.3	148¼
14	148.7	58½	160.4	63¼	171.3	67½	37.76	83¼	50.28	110¾	73.08	161
15	150.5	59¼	161.8	63¾	172.8	68	40.99	90¼	53.68	118¼	77.78	171½
16	151.6	59¾	162.4	64	173.3	68¼	43.41	95¾	55.89	123¼	80.99	178½
17	152.7	60	163.1	64¼	173.5	68¼	44.74	98¾	56.69	125	82.46	181¾
18	153.6	60½	163.7	64½	173.6	68¼	45.26	99¾	56.62	124¾	82.47	181¾

Modified from National Center for Health Statistics (NCHS), Health Resources Administration, Department of Health, Education and Welfare, Hyattsville, Md.
Conversion of metric data to approximate inches and pounds by Ross Laboratories.
*Years unless otherwise indicated.
†Height data include some recumbent length measurements, which make values slightly higher than if all measurements had been of stature.

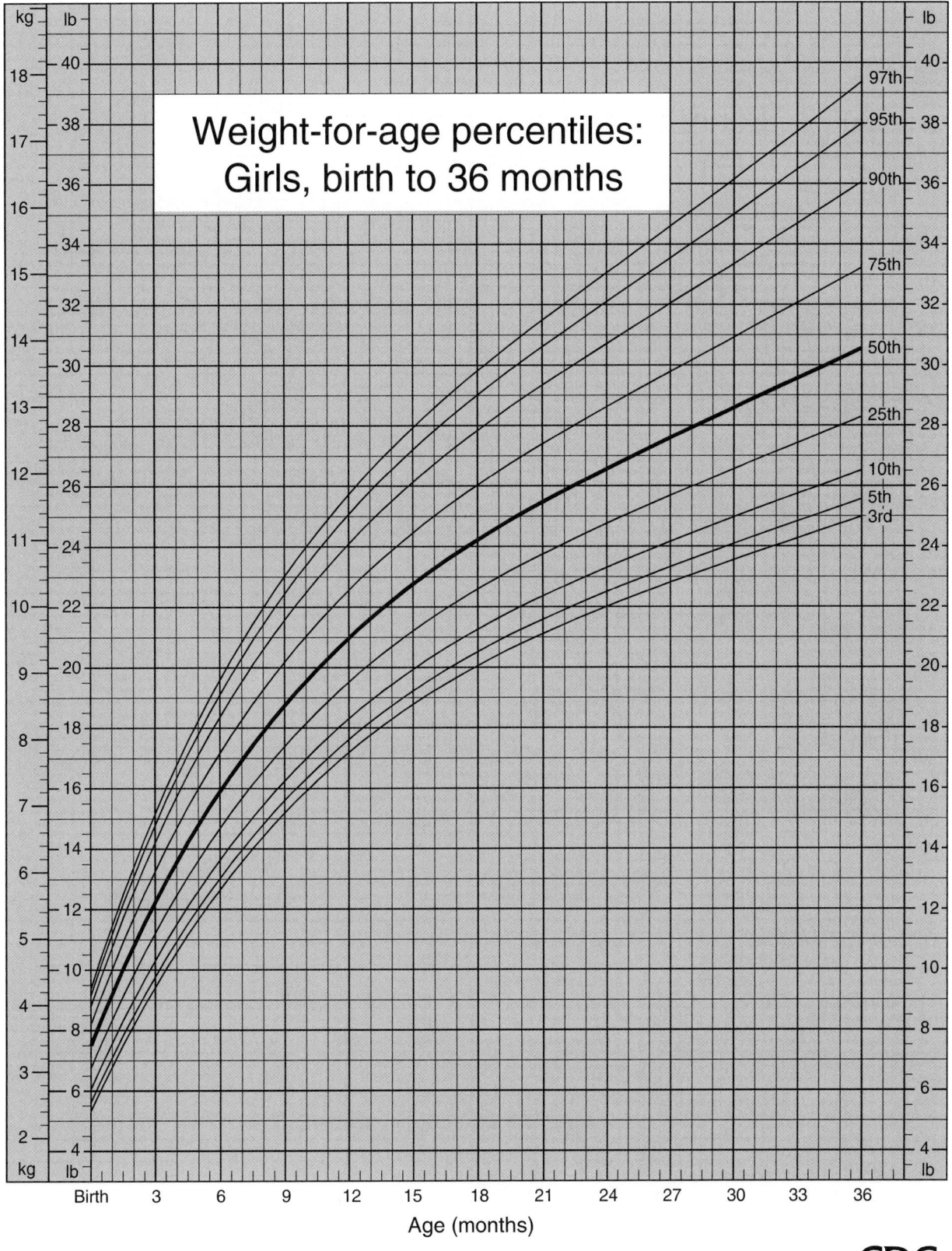

FIG. D-9 ■ Weight-for-age percentiles, girls, birth to 36 months, CDC growth charts: United States. (Developed by the National Center for Health Statistics in collaboration with the National Center for Chronic Disease Prevention and Health Promotion, 2000.)

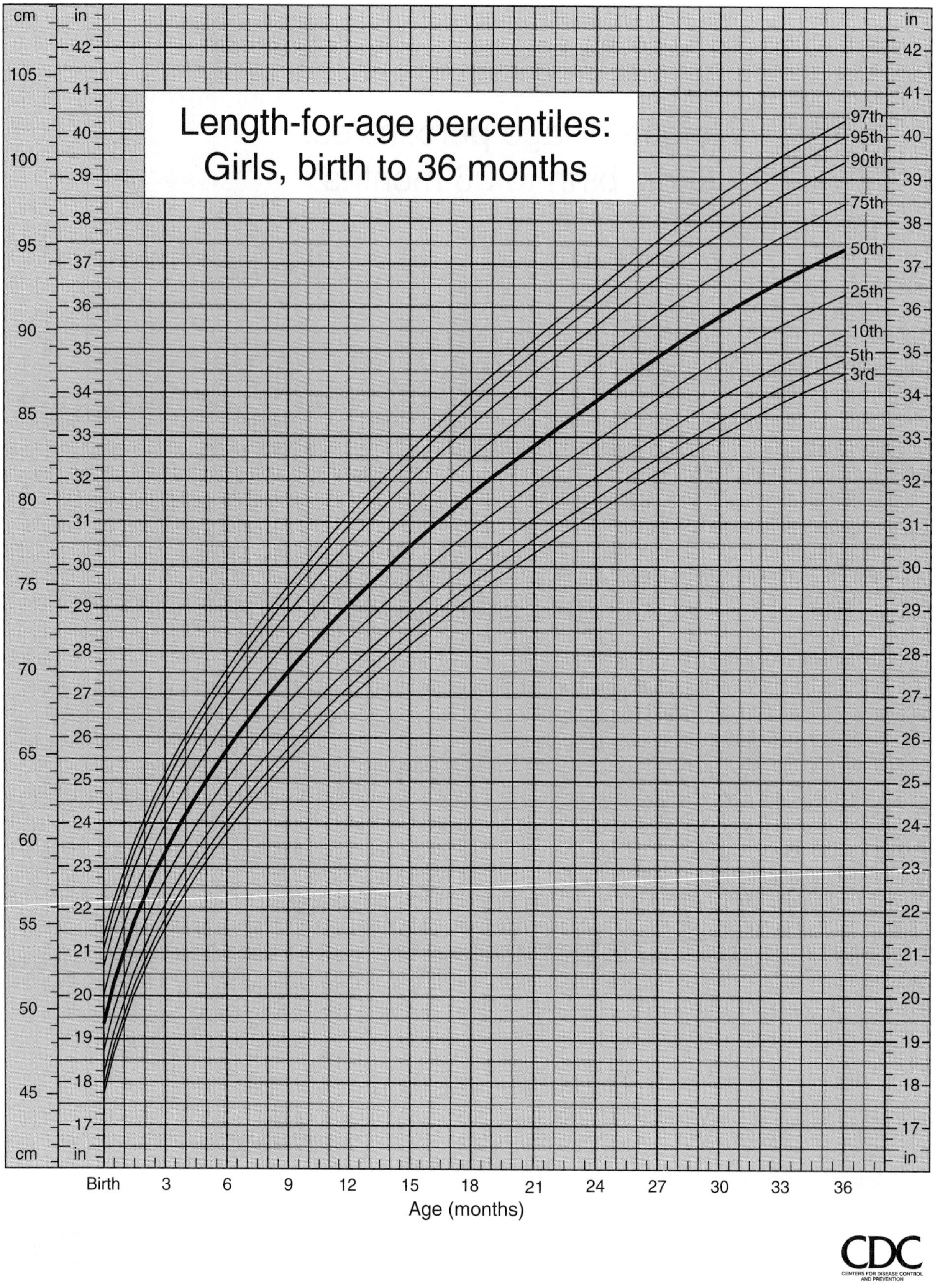

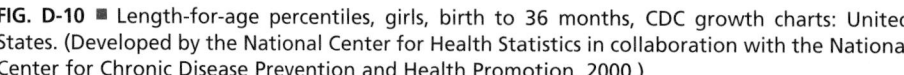

FIG. D-10 ■ Length-for-age percentiles, girls, birth to 36 months, CDC growth charts: United States. (Developed by the National Center for Health Statistics in collaboration with the National Center for Chronic Disease Prevention and Health Promotion, 2000.)

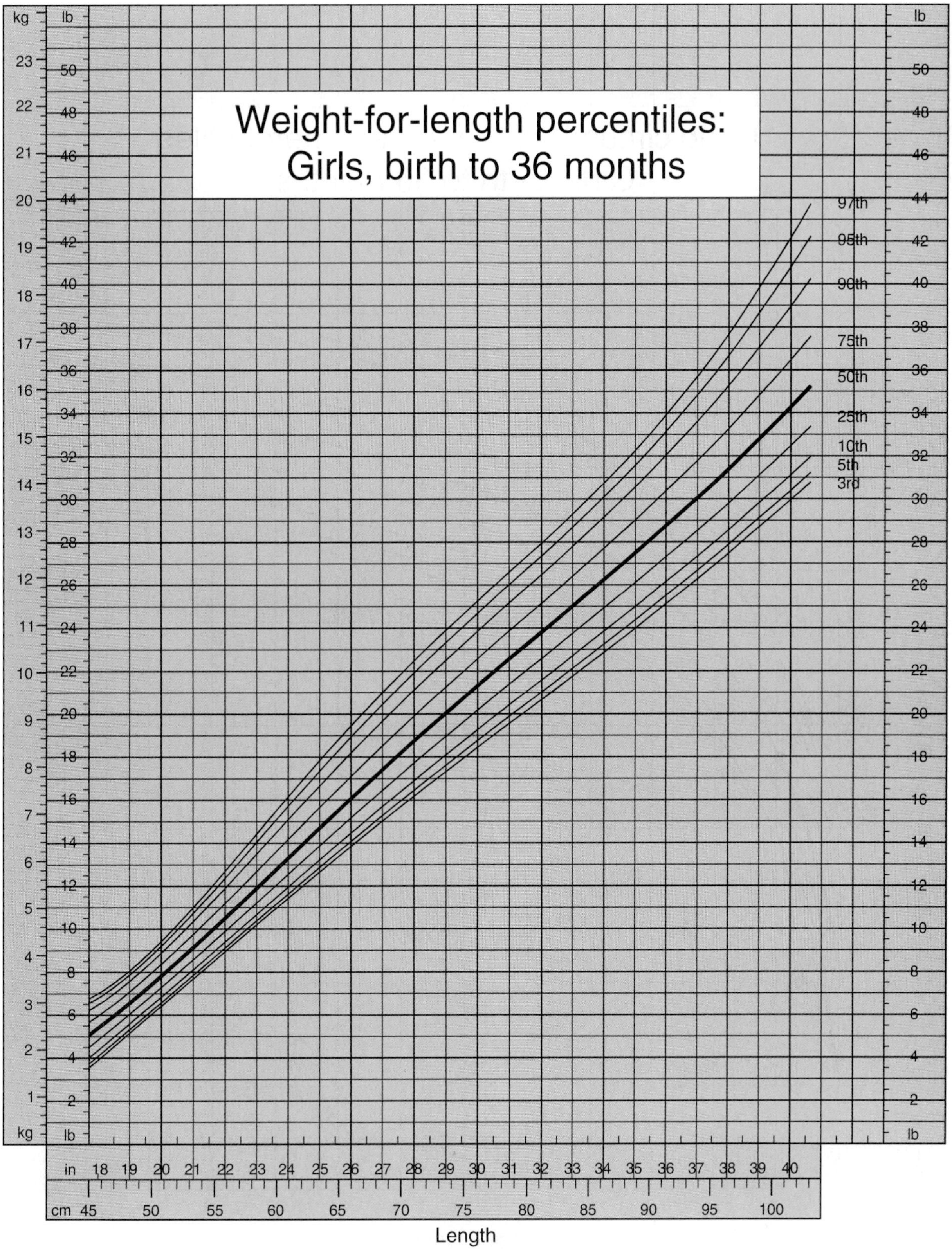

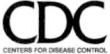

FIG. D-11 ■ Weight-for-length percentiles, girls, birth to 36 months, CDC growth charts: United States. (Developed by the National Center for Health Statistics in collaboration with the National Center for Chronic Disease Prevention and Health Promotion, 2000.)

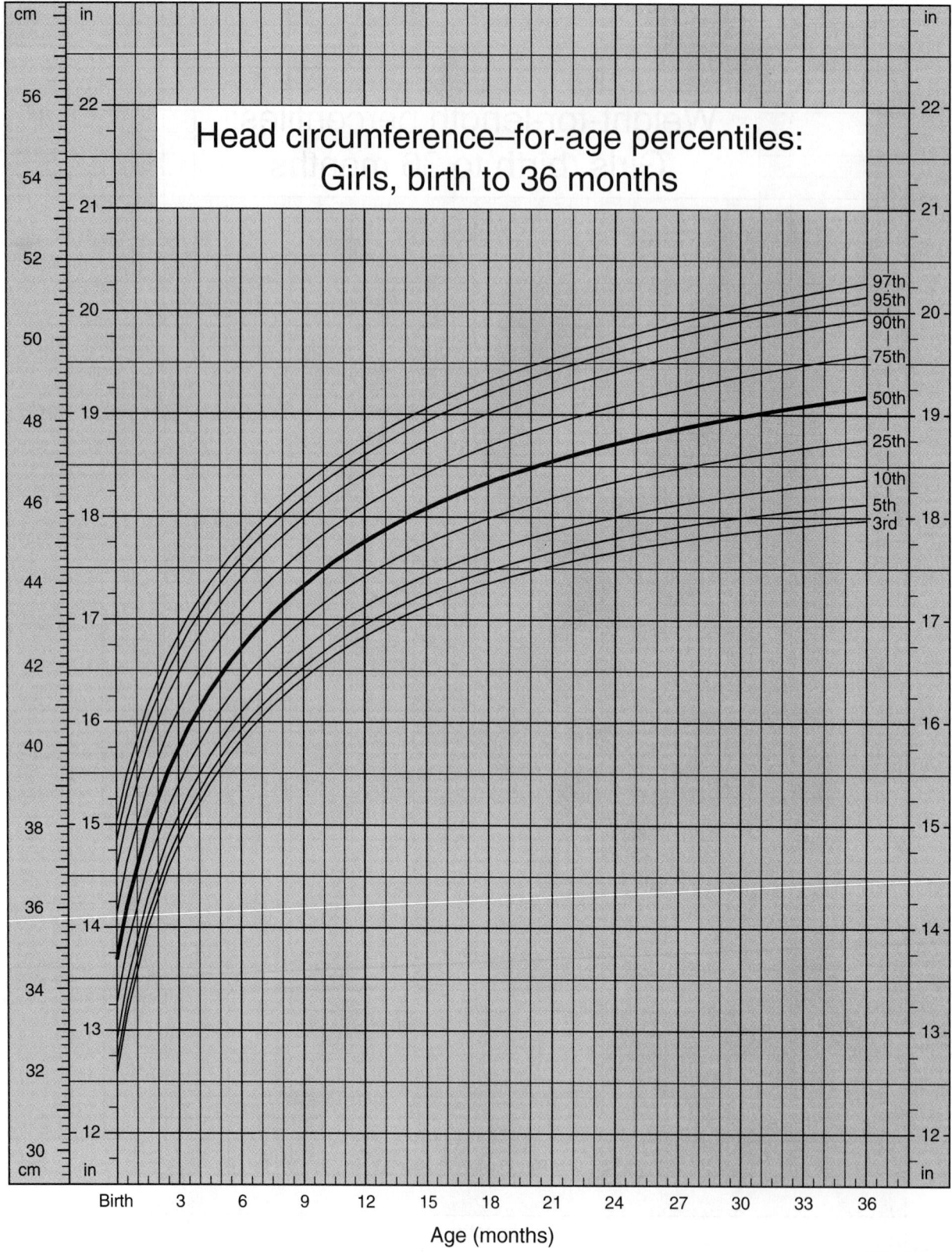

FIG. D-12 ■ Head circumference–for-age percentiles, girls, birth to 36 months, CDC growth charts: United States. (Developed by the National Center for Health Statistics in collaboration with the National Center for Chronic Disease Prevention and Health Promotion, 2000.)

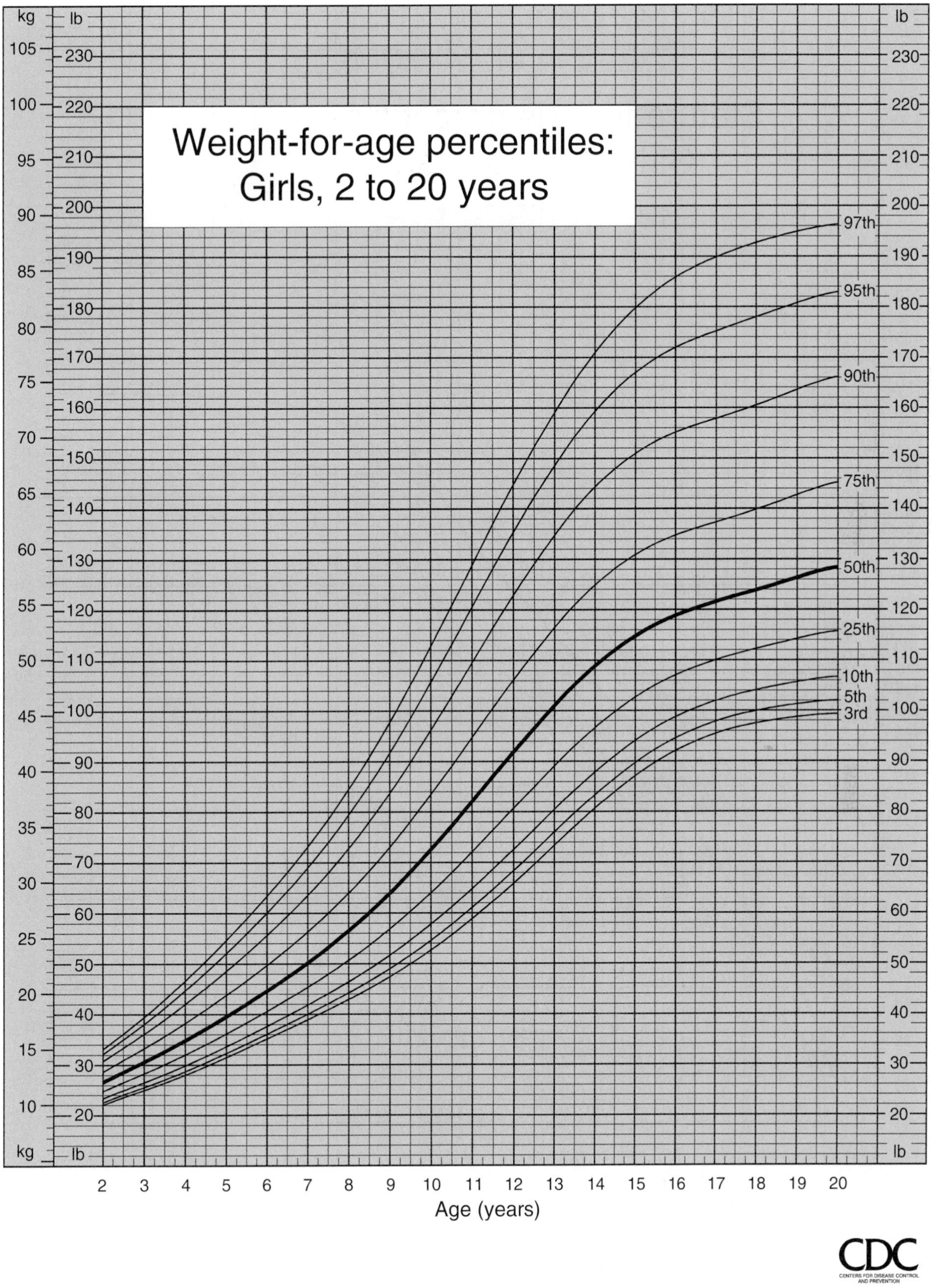

Weight-for-age percentiles: Girls, 2 to 20 years

97th
95th
90th
75th
50th
25th
10th
5th
3rd

Age (years)

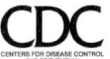

FIG. D-13 ■ Weight-for-age percentiles, girls, 2 to 20 years, CDC growth charts: United States. (Developed by the National Center for Health Statistics in collaboration with the National Center for Chronic Disease Prevention and Health Promotion, 2000.)

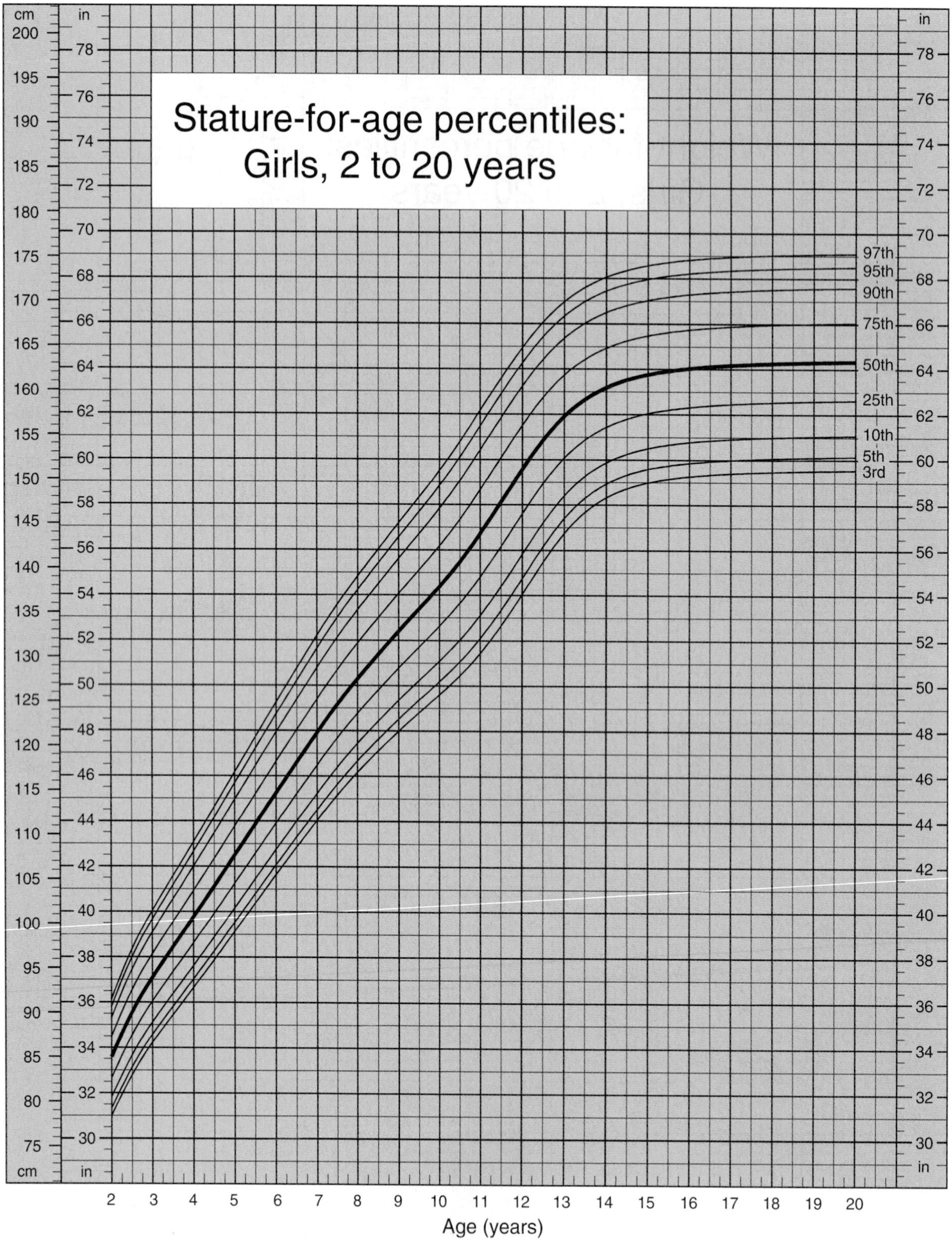

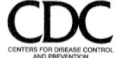

**Stature-for-age percentiles:
Girls, 2 to 20 years**

Age (years)

FIG. D-14 ■ Stature-for-age percentiles, girls, 2 to 20 years, CDC growth charts: United States. (Developed by the National Center for Health Statistics in collaboration with the National Center for Chronic Disease Prevention and Health Promotion, 2000.)

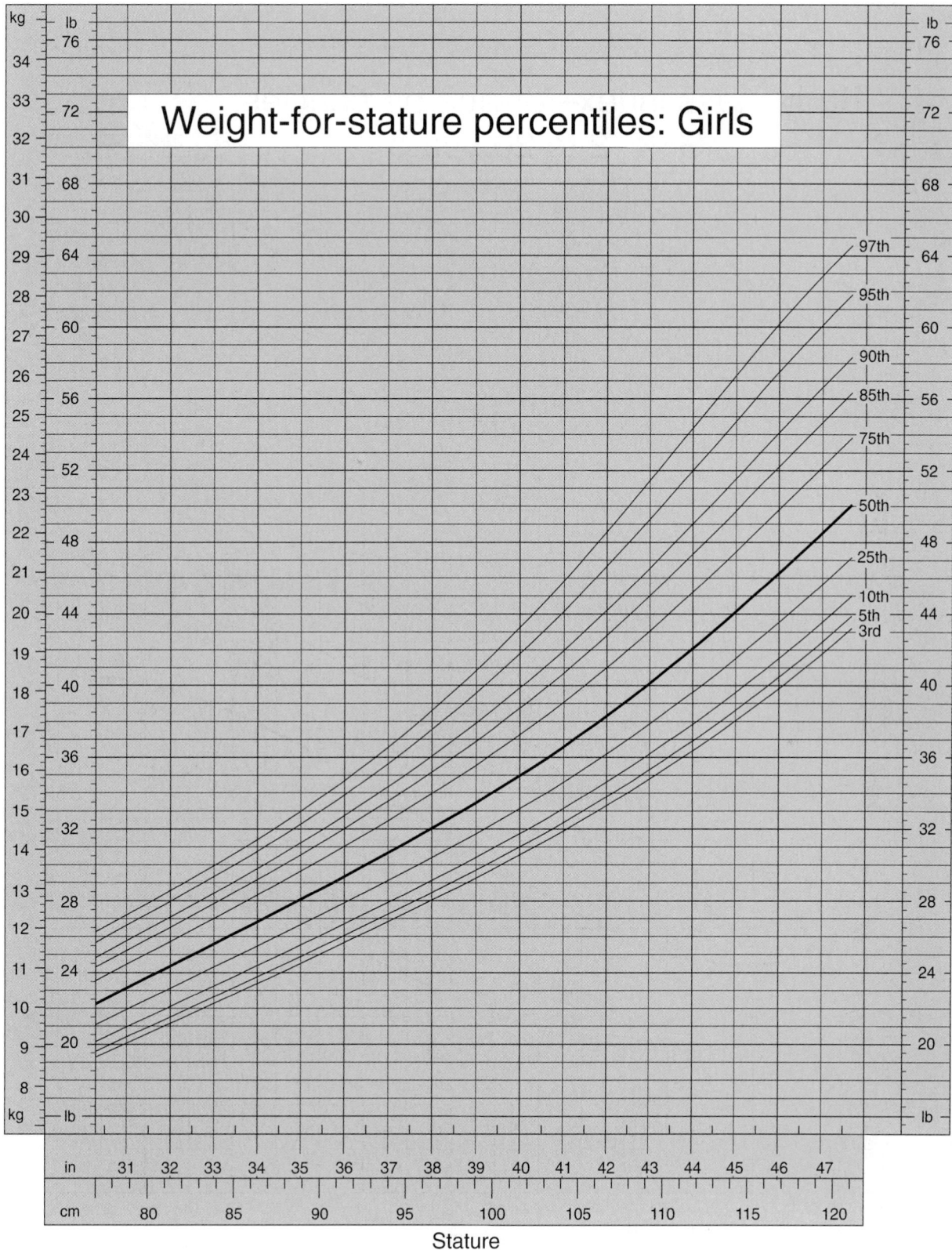

FIG. D-15 ■ Weight-for-stature percentiles, girls, CDC growth charts: United States. (Developed by the National Center for Health Statistics in collaboration with the National Center for Chronic Disease Prevention and Health Promotion, 2000.)

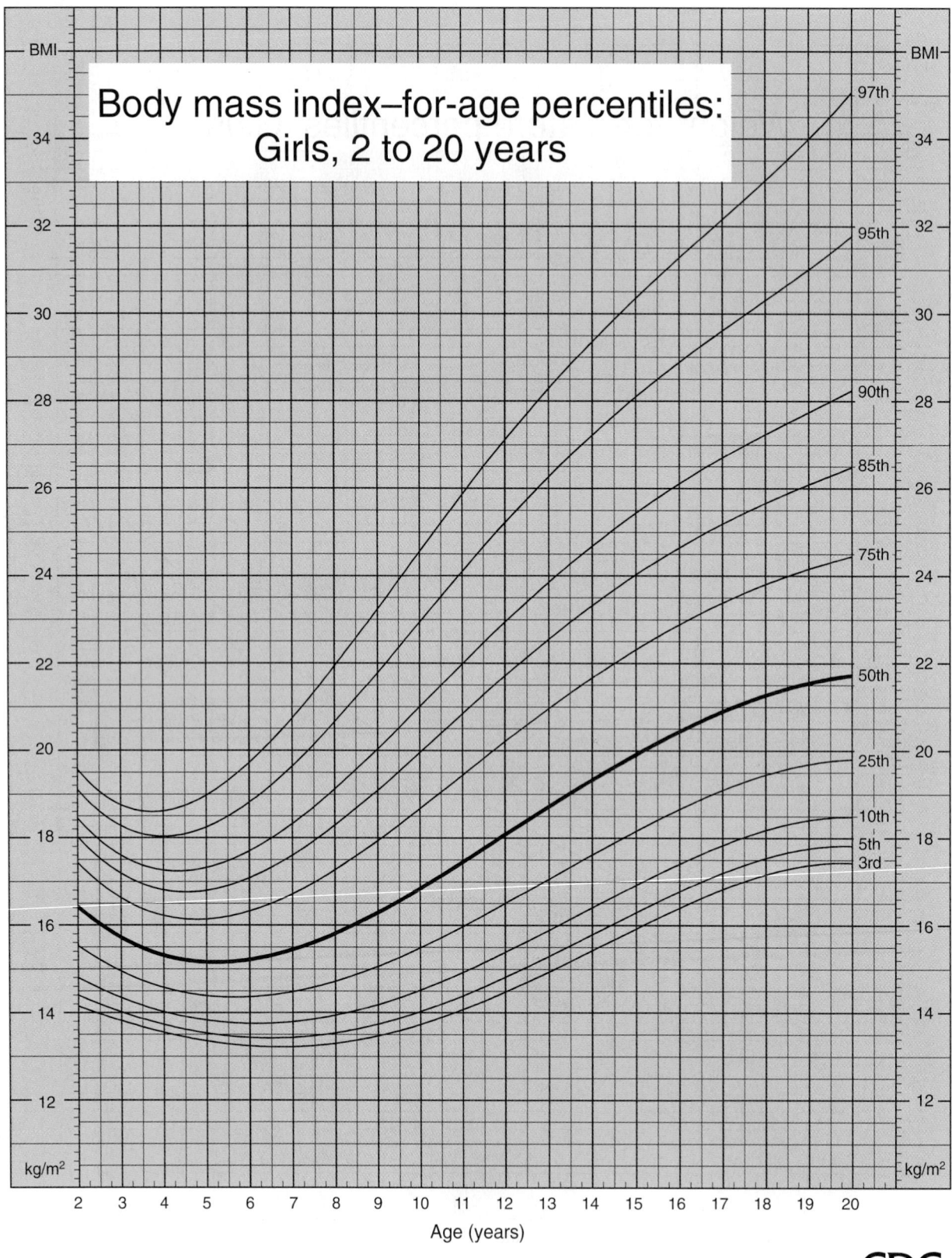

FIG. D-16 ■ Body mass index–for-age percentiles, girls, 2 to 20 years, CDC growth charts: United States. (Developed by the National Center for Health Statistics in collaboration with the National Center for Chronic Disease Prevention and Health Promotion, 2000.)

Growth Standards of Healthy Chinese Children

AGE (MONTHS OR YEARS)	WEIGHT (kg)		HEIGHT (cm)		HEAD CIRCUMFERENCE	
	BOYS	GIRLS	BOYS	GIRLS	BOYS	GIRLS
Birth	3.27	3.17	50.6	50.0	34.3	33.7
1 month	4.97	4.64	56.5	55.5	38.1	37.3
2 months	5.95	5.49	59.6	58.4	39.7	38.7
3 months	6.73	6.23	62.3	60.9	41.0	40.0
4 months	7.32	6.69	64.4	62.9	42.0	41.0
5 months	7.70	7.19	65.9	64.5	42.9	41.9
6 months	8.22	7.62	68.1	66.7	43.9	42.8
8 months	8.71	8.14	70.6	69.0	44.9	43.7
10 months	9.14	8.57	72.9	71.4	45.7	44.5
12 months	9.56	9.04	75.6	74.1	46.3	45.2
15 months	10.15	9.54	78.3	76.9	46.8	45.6
18 months	10.67	10.08	80.7	79.4	47.3	46.2
21 months	11.18	10.56	83.0	81.7	47.8	46.7
24 months	11.95	11.37	86.5	85.3	48.2	47.1
2.5 years	12.84	12.28	90.4	89.3	48.8	47.7
3 years	13.63	13.16	93.8	92.8	49.1	48.1
3.5 years	14.45	14.00	97.2	96.3	49.4	48.5
4 years	15.26	14.89	100.8	100.1	49.7	48.9
4.5 years	16.07	15.63	103.9	103.1	50.0	49.1
5 years	16.88	16.46	107.2	106.5	50.2	49.4
5.5 years	17.65	17.18	110.1	109.2	50.5	49.6
6 years	19.25	18.67	114.7	113.9	50.8	50.0
7 years	21.01	20.35	120.6	119.3	51.1	50.2
8 years	23.08	22.43	125.3	124.6	51.4	50.6
9 years	25.33	24.57	130.6	129.5	51.7	50.9
10 years	27.15	27.05	134.4	134.8	51.9	51.3
11 years	30.13	30.51	139.2	140.6	52.3	51.7
12 years	33.05	34.74	144.2	146.6	52.7	52.3
13 years	36.90	38.52	149.8	150.7	53.0	52.8

Data from Bejing Children's Hospital, 1987, China.

■ Percentiles for Triceps Skinfold

	TRICEPS SKINFOLD PERCENTILES (mm)									
	MALES					FEMALES				
AGE-GROUP (YEARS)	5	25	50	75	95	5	25	50	75	95
1-1.9	6	8	10	12	16	6	8	10	12	16
2-2.9	6	8	10	12	15	6	9	10	12	16
3-3.9	6	8	10	11	15	7	9	11	12	15
4-4.9	6	8	9	11	14	7	8	10	12	16
5-5.9	6	8	9	11	15	6	8	10	12	18
6-6.9	5	7	8	10	16	6	8	10	12	16
7-7.9	5	7	9	12	17	6	9	11	13	18
8-8.9	5	7	8	10	16	6	9	12	15	24
9-9.9	6	7	10	13	18	8	10	13	16	22
10-10.9	6	8	10	14	21	7	10	12	17	27
11-11.9	6	8	11	16	24	7	10	13	18	28
12-12.9	6	8	11	14	28	8	11	14	18	27
13-13.9	5	7	10	14	26	8	12	15	21	30
14-14.9	4	7	9	14	24	9	13	16	21	28
15-15.9	4	6	8	11	24	8	12	17	21	32
16-16.9	4	6	8	12	22	10	15	18	22	31
17-17.9	5	6	8	12	19	10	13	19	24	37
18-18.9	4	6	9	13	24	10	15	18	22	30
19-24.9	4	7	10	15	22	10	14	18	24	34

From Frisancho A: New norms of upper limb fat and muscle areas for assessment of nutritional status, *Am J Clin Nutr* 34:2540-2545, 1981.

■ Percentiles of Upper Arm Circumference

	ARM CIRCUMFERENCE PERCENTILES (mm)									
	MALES					FEMALES				
AGE-GROUP (YEARS)	5	25	50	75	95	5	25	50	75	95
1-1.9	142	150	159	170	183	138	148	156	164	177
2-2.9	141	153	162	170	185	142	152	160	167	184
3-3.9	150	160	167	175	190	143	158	167	175	189
4-4.9	149	162	171	180	192	149	160	169	177	191
5-5.9	153	167	175	185	204	153	165	175	185	211
6-6.9	155	167	179	188	228	156	170	176	187	211
7-7.9	162	177	187	201	230	164	174	183	199	231
8-8.9	162	177	190	202	245	168	183	195	214	261
9-9.9	175	187	200	217	257	178	194	211	224	260
10-10.9	181	196	210	231	274	174	193	210	228	265
11-11.9	186	202	223	244	280	185	208	224	248	303
12-12.9	193	214	232	254	303	194	216	237	256	294
13-13.9	194	228	247	263	301	202	223	243	271	338
14-14.9	220	237	253	283	322	214	237	252	272	322
15-15.9	222	244	264	284	320	208	239	254	279	322
16-16.9	244	262	278	303	343	218	241	258	283	334
17-17.9	246	267	285	308	347	220	241	264	295	350
18-18.9	245	276	297	321	379	222	241	258	281	325
19-24.9	262	288	308	331	372	221	247	265	290	345

From Frisancho A: New norms of upper limb fat and muscle areas for assessment of nutritional status, *Am J Clin Nutr* 34:2540-2545, 1981.

Common Laboratory Tests

Common Laboratory Tests and Test Results

TEST/SPECIMEN	AGE/GENDER/REFERENCE	NORMAL RANGES			
		CONVENTIONAL UNITS		INTERNATIONAL UNITS (SI)	
Acetaminophen					
Serum or plasma	Therap. conc.	10-30 μg/mL		66-200 μmol/L	
	Toxic conc.	>200 μg/mL		>1300 μmol/L	
Ammonia nitrogen					
Plasma or serum	Newborn	90-150 μg/dL		64-107 μmol/L	
	0-2 wk	79-129 μg/dL		56-92 μmol/L	
	>1 mo	29-70 μg/dL		21-50 μmol/L	
	Thereafter	0-50 μg/dL		0-35.7 μmol/L	
Antistreptolysin O titer (ASO)					
Serum	2-4 yr	<160 Todd units			
	School-age children	170-330 Todd units			
Base excess					
Whole blood	Newborn	(−10)-(−2) mEq/L		(−10)-(−2) mmol/L	
	Infant	(−7)-(−1) mEq/L		(−7)-(−1) mmol/L	
	Child	(−4)-(+2) mEq/L		(−4)-(+2) mmol/L	
	Thereafter	(−3)-(+3) mEq/L		(−3)-(+3) mmol/L	
Bicarbonate (HOC₃)					
Serum	Arterial	21-28 mEq/L		21-28 mmol/L	
	Venous	22-29 mEq/L		22-29 mmol/L	
		Premature (mg/dL)	**Full Term (mg/dL)**	**Premature (μmol/L)**	**Full Term (μmol/L)**
Bilirubin, total					
Serum	Cord	<2.0	<2.0	<34	<34
	0-1 d	<8.0	<6.0	<137	<103
	1-2 d	<12.0	<8.0	<205	<137
	2-5 d	<16.0	<12.0	<274	<205
	Thereafter	<20.0	<10.0	<340	<171
Bilirubin, direct (conjugated)					
Serum		0.0-0.2 mg/dL		0-3.4 μmol/L	
Bleeding time					
Blood from skin puncture					
Ivy	Normal	2-7 min		2-7 min	
	Borderline	7-11 min		7-11 min	
Simplate (G-D)		2.75-8 min		2.75-8 min	
Blood volume					
Whole blood	Male	52-83 mL/kg		0.052-0.083 L/kg	
	Female	50-75 mL/kg		0.050-0.075 L/kg	
C-reactive protein (CRP)					
Serum	Cord	52-1330 ng/mL		52-1330 μg/L	
	2-12 yr	67-1800 ng/mL		67-1800 μg/L	
Calcium, ionized					
Serum, plasma, or whole blood	Cord	5.0-6.0 mg/dL		1.25-1.50 mmol/L	
	Newborn, 3-24 hr	4.3-5.1 mg/dL		1.07-1.27 mmol/L	
	24-48 hr	4.0-4.7 mg/dL		1.00-1.17 mmol/L	
	Thereafter	4.8-4.92 mg/dL or 2.24-2.46 mEq/L		1.12-1.23 mmol/L	
Calcium, total					
Serum	Cord	9.0-11.5 mg/dL		2.25-2.88 mmol/L	
	Newborn, 3-24 yr	9.0-10.6 mg/dL		2.3-2.65 mmol/L	
	24-48 hr	7.0-12.0 mg/dL		1.75-3.0 mmol/L	
	4-7 d	9.0-10.9 mg/dL		2.25-2.73 mmol/L	
	Child	8.8-10.8 mg/dL		2.2-2.70 mmol/L	
	Thereafter	8.4-10.2 mg/dL		2.1-2.55 mmol/L	

Continued

■ Common Laboratory Tests and Test Results—*cont'd*

TEST/SPECIMEN	AGE/GENDER/REFERENCE	NORMAL RANGES CONVENTIONAL UNITS	NORMAL RANGES INTERNATIONAL UNITS (SI)
Carbon dioxide, partial pressure (P_{CO_2})			
Whole blood, arterial	Newborn	27-40 mm Hg	3.6-5.3 kPa
	Infant	27-41 mm Hg	3.6-5.5 kPa
	Thereafter: Male	35-48 mm Hg	4.7-6.4 kPa
	Female	32-45 mm Hg	4.3-6.0 kPa
Carbon dioxide, total (tCO_2)			
Serum or plasma	Cord	14-22 mEq/L	14-22 mmol/L
	Premature (1 wk)	14-27 mEq/L	14-27 mmol/L
	Newborn	13-22 mEq/L	13-22 mmol/L
	Infant, child	20-28 mEq/L	20-28 mmol/L
	Thereafter	23-30 mEq/L	23-30 mmol/L
Cerebrospinal fluid (CSF)			
Pressure		70-180 mm water	70-180 mm water
Volume	Child	60-100 mL	0.06-0.10 L
	Adult	100-160 mL	0.10-0.16 L
Chloride			
Serum or plasma	Cord	96-104 mEq/L	96-104 mmol/L
	Newborn	97-110 mEq/L	97-110 mmol/L
	Thereafter	98-106 mEq/L	98-106 mmol/L
Sweat	Normal (homozygote)	<40 mEq/L	<40 mmol/L
	Marginal (e.g., asthma, Addison disease, malnutrition)	45-60 mEq/L	45-60 mmol/L
	Cystic fibrosis	>60 mEq/L	>60 mmol/L
Cholesterol, total			
Serum or plasma*	Acceptable	<170 mg/dL	<4.4 mmol/L
	Borderline	170-199 mg/dL	4.4-5.1 mmol/L
	High	≥200 mg/dL	≥5.2 mmol/L
Clotting time (Lee-White)			
White blood		5-8 min (glass tubes)	5-8 min
		5-15 min (room temp)	5-15 min
		30 min (silicone tube)	30 min
Creatine kinase (CK, CPK)			
Serum	Cord blood	70-380 U/L	70-380 U/L
	5-8 hr	214-1175 U/L	214-1175 U/L
	24-33 hr	130-1200 U/L	130-1200 U/L
	72-100 hr	87-725 U/L	87-725 U/L
	Adult	5-130 U/L	5-130 U/L
Creatinine			
Serum	Cord	0.6-1.2 mg/dL	53-106 μmol/L
	Newborn	0.3-1.0 mg/dL	27-88 μmol/L
	Infant	0.2-0.4 mg/dL	18-35 μmol/L
	Child	0.3-0.7 mg/dL	27-62 μmol/L
	Adolescent	0.5-1.0 mg/dL	44-88 μmol/L
	Adult: Male	0.6-1.2 mg/dL	53-106 μmol/L
	Female	0.5-1.1 mg/dL	44-97 μmol/L
Urine, 24 hr	Premature	8.1-15.0 mg/kg/24 hr	72-133 μmol/kg/24 hr
	Full term	10.4-19.7 mg/kg/24 hr	92-174 μmol/kg/24 hr
	1.5-7 yr	10-15 mg/kg/24 hr	88-133 μmol/kg/24 hr
	7-15 yr	5.2-41 mg/kg/24 hr	46-362 μmol/kg/24 hr
Creatinine clearance (endogenous)			
Serum or plasma and urine	Newborn	40-65 mL/min/1.73 m^2	
	<40 yr: Male	97-137 mL/min/1.73 m^2	
	Female	88-128 mL/min/1.73 m^2	
Digoxin			
Serum, plasma; collect at least 12 hr after dose	Therap. conc.		
	CHF	0.8-1.5 ng/mL	1.0-1.9 nmol/L
	Arrhythmias	1.5-2.0 ng/mL	1.9-2.6 nmol/L

TEST/SPECIMEN	AGE/GENDER/REFERENCE	NORMAL RANGES	
		CONVENTIONAL UNITS	INTERNATIONAL UNITS (SI)
Serum, plasma; collect at least 12 hr after dose	Toxic conc.		
	Child	>2.5 ng/mL	>3.2 nmol/L
	Adult	>3.0 ng/mL	>3.8 nmol/L
Eosinophil count			
Whole blood, capillary blood		50-250 cells/mm³ (μL)	50-250 × 10⁶ cells/L
Erythrocyte (RBC) count			
Whole blood	Cord	3.9-5.5 million/mm³	3.9-5.5 × 10¹² cells/L
	1-3 d	4.0-6.6 million/mm³	4.0-6.6 × 10¹² cells/L
	1 wk	3.9-6.3 million/mm³	3.9-6.3 × 10¹² cells/L
	2 wk	3.6-6.2 million/mm³	3.6-6.2 × 10¹² cells/L
	1 mo	3.0-5.4 million/mm³	3.0-5.4 × 10¹² cells/L
	2 mo	2.7-4.9 million/mm³	2.7-4.9 × 10¹² cells/L
	3-6 mo	3.1-4.5 million/mm³	3.1-4.5 × 10¹² cells/L
	0.5-2 yr	3.7-5.3 million/mm³	3.7-5.3 × 10¹² cells/L
	2-6 yr	3.9-5.3 million/mm³	3.9-5.3 × 10¹² cells/L
	6-12 yr	4.0-5.2 million/mm³	4.0-5.2 × 10¹² cells/L
	12-18 yr: Male	4.5-5.3 million/mm³	4.5-5.3 × 10¹² cells/L
	Female	4.1-5.1 million/mm³	4.1-5.1 × 10¹² cells/L
Erythrocyte sedimentation rate (ESR)			
Whole blood			
Westergren (modified)	Child	0-10 mm/hr	0-10 mm/hr
	<50 yr: Male	0-15 mm/hr	0-15 mm/hr
	Female	0-20 mm/hr	0-20 mm/hr
Wintrobe	Child	0-13 mm/hr	0-13 mm/hr
	Adult: Male	0-9 mm/hr	0-9 mm/hr
	Female	0-20 mm/hr	0-20 mm/hr
Fibrinogen			
Plasma	Newborn	125-300 mg/dL	1.25-3.00 g/L
	Thereafter	200-400 mg/dL	2.00-4.00 g/L
Galactose			
Serum	Newborn	0-20 mg/dL	0-1.11 mmol/L
	Thereafter	<5 mg/dL	<0.28 mmol/L
Urine	Newborn	≤60 mg/dL	≤3.33 mmol/L
	Thereafter	≤14 mg/24 hr	<0.08 mmol/d
Glucose			
Serum	Cord	45-96 mg/dL	2.5-5.3 mmol/L
	Newborn, 1 d	40-60 mg/dL	2.2-3.3 mmol/L
	Newborn, >1 d	50-90 mg/dL	2.8-5.0 mmol/L
	Child	60-100 mg/dL	3.3-5.5 mmol/L
	Thereafter	70-105 mg/dL	3.9-5.8 mmol/L
Whole blood	Adult	65-95 mg/dL	3.6-5.3 mmol/L
CSF	Adult	40-70 mg/dL	2.2-3.9 mmol/L
Urine (quantitative)		<0.5 g/d	<2.8 mmol/d
(qualitative)		Negative	Negative
Glucose tolerance test (GTT), oral			
Serum			

Dosages	AGE/GENDER/REFERENCE	Normal	Diabetic	Normal	Diabetic
Adult: 75 g	Fasting	70-105 mg/dL	≥126 mg/dL	3.9-5.8 mmol/L	≥7.0 mmol/L
Child: 1.75 g/kg of ideal	60 min	120-170 mg/dL	≥200 mg/dL	6.7-9.4 mmol/L	≥11 mmol/L
weight up to maximum of	90 min	100-140 mg/dL	≥200 mg/dL	5.6-7.8 mmol/L	≥11 mmol/L
75 g	120 min	70-120 mg/dL	≥200 mg/dL	3.9-6.7 mmol/L	≥11 mmol/L

TEST/SPECIMEN	AGE/GENDER/REFERENCE	CONVENTIONAL UNITS	INTERNATIONAL UNITS (SI)
Growth hormone (hGH, somatotropin)			
Plasma	1 d	5-53 ng/mL	5-53 μg/L
	1 wk	5-27 ng/mL	5-27 μg/L
	1-12 mo	2-10 ng/mL	2-10 μg/L
	Fasting child/adult	<0.7-6.0 ng/mL	<0.7-6.0 μg/L

Continued

■ Common Laboratory Tests and Test Results—*cont'd*

TEST/SPECIMEN	AGE/GENDER/REFERENCE	NORMAL RANGES	
		CONVENTIONAL UNITS	INTERNATIONAL UNITS (SI)
Hematocrit (HCT, Hct)			
Whole blood	1 d (cap)	48%-69%	0.48-0.69 vol. fraction
	2 d	48%-75%	0.48-0.75 vol. fraction
	3 d	44%-72%	0.44-0.72 vol. fraction
	2 mo	28%-42%	0.28-0.42 vol. fraction
	6-12 yr	35%-45%	0.35-0.45 vol. fraction
	12-18 yr: Male	37%-49%	0.37-0.49 vol. fraction
	Female	36%-46%	0.36-0.46 vol. fraction
Hemoglobin (Hb)			
Whole blood	1-3 d (cap)	14.5-22.5 g/dL	2.25-3.49 mmol/L
	2 mo	9.0-14.0 g/dL	1.40-2.17 mmol/L
	6-12 yr	11.5-15.5 g/dL	1.78-2.40 mmol/L
	12-18 yr: Male	13.0-16.0 g/dL	2.02-2.48 mmol/L
	Female	12.0-16.0 g/dL	1.860-2.48 mmol/L
Hemoglobin A			
Whole blood		>95% of total	>0.95 fraction of Hb
Hemoglobin F			
Whole blood	1 d	63%-92% HbF	0.63-0.92 mass fraction HbF
	5 d	65%-88% HbF	0.65-0.88 mass fraction HbF
	3 wk	55%-85% HbF	0.55-0.85 mass fraction HbF
	6-9 wk	31%-75% HbF	0.31-0.75 mass fraction HbF
	3-4 mo	<2%-59% HbF	<0.02-0.59 mass fraction HbF
	6 mo	<2%-9% HbF	<0.02-0.09 mass fraction HbF
	Adult	<2.0% HbF	<0.02 mass fraction HbF
Immunoglobulin A (IgA)			
Serum	Cord blood	1.4-3.6 mg/dL	14-36 mg/L
	1-3 mo	1.3-53 mg/dL	13-530 mg/L
	4-6 mo	4.4-84 mg/dL	44-840 mg/L
	7 mo-1 yr	11-106 mg/dL	110-1060 mg/L
	2-5 yr	14-159 mg/dL	140-1590 mg/L
	6-10 yr	33-236 mg/dL	330-2360 mg/L
	Adult	70-312 mg/dL	700-3120 mg/L
Immunoglobulin D (IgD)			
Serum	Newborn	None detected	None detected
	Thereafter	0-8 mg/dL	0-80 mg/L
Immunoglobulin E (IgE)			
Serum	Male	0-230 IU/mL	0-230 kIU/L
	Female	0-170 IU/mL	0-170 kIU/L
Immunoglobulin G (IgG)			
Serum	Cord blood	636-1606 mg/dL	6.36-16.06 g/L
	1 mo	251-906 mg/dL	2.51-9.06 g/L
	2-4 mo	176-601 mg/dL	1.76-6.01 g/L
	5-12 mo	172-1069 mg/dL	1.72-10.69 g/L
	1-5 yr	345-1236 mg/dL	3.45-12.36 g/L
	6-10 yr	608-1572 mg/dL	6.08-15.72 g/L
	Adult	639-1349 mg/dL	6.39-13.49 g/L
Immunoglobulin M (IgM)			
Serum	Cord blood	6.3-25 mg/dL	63-250 mg/L
	1-4 mo	17-105 mg/dL	170-1050 mg/L
	5-9 mo	33-126 mg/dL	330-1260 mg/L
	10 mo-1 yr	41-173 mg/dL	410-1730 mg/L
	2-8 yr	43-207 mg/dL	430-2070 mg/L
	9-10 yr	52-242 mg/dL	520-2420 mg/L
	Adult	56-352 mg/dL	560-3520 mg/L
Iron			
Serum	Newborn	100-250 μg/dL	18-45 μmol/L
	Infant	40-100 μg/dL	7-18 μmol/L
	Child	50-120 μg/dL	9-22 μmol/L
	Thereafter: Male	65-170 μg/dL	12-30 μmol/L
	Female	50-170 μg/dL	9-30 μmol/L
	Intoxicated child	280-2550 μg/dL	50.12-456.5 μmol/L
	Fatally poisoned child	>1800 μg/dL	>322.2 μmol/L

TEST/SPECIMEN	AGE/GENDER/REFERENCE	NORMAL RANGES	
		CONVENTIONAL UNITS	INTERNATIONAL UNITS (SI)
Iron-binding capacity, total (TIBC)			
Serum	Infant	100-400 μg/dL	17.90-71.60 μmol/L
	Thereafter	250-400 μg/dL	44.75-71.60 μmol/L
Lead			
Whole blood	Child	<10 μg/dL	<0.48 μmol/L
Urine, 24 hr		<80 μg/dL	<0.39 μmol/L
Leukocyte count (WBC count)		× 1000 cells/mm³ (μl)	× 10⁹ cells/L
Whole blood	Birth	9.0-30.0	9.0-30.0
	24 hr	9.4-34.0	9.4-34.0
	1 mo	5.0-19.5	5.0-19.5
	1-3 yr	6.0-17.5	6.0-17.5
	4-7 yr	5.5-15.5	5.5-15.5
	8-13 yr	4.5-13.5	4.5-13.5
	Adult	4.5-11.0	4.5-11.0
		× 1000 cells/mm³ (μl)	× 10⁶ cells/L
CSF	Premature	0-25 mononuclear	0-25
		0-10 polymorphonuclear	0-10
		0-1000 RBC	0-1000
	Newborn	0-20 mononuclear	0-20
		0-10 polymorphonuclear	0-10
		0-800 RBC	0-800
	Neonate	0-5 mononuclear	0-5
		0-10 polymorphonuclear	0-10
		0-50 RBC	0-50
	Thereafter	0-5 mononuclear	0-5
Leukocyte differential count			
Whole blood	Myelocytes	0% 0 cells/mm³ (μL)	Number fraction 0
	Neutrophils ("bands")	3%-5% 150-400 cells/mm³ (μL)	Number fraction 0.03-0.05
	Neutrophils ("segs")	54%-62% 3000-5800 cells/mm³ (μL)	Number fraction 0.54-0.62
	Lymphocytes	25%-33% 1500-3000 cells/mm³ (μL)	Number fraction 0.25-0.33
	Monocytes	3%-7% 285-500 cells/mm³ (μL)	Number fraction 0.03-0.07
	Eosinophils	1%-3% 50-250 cells/mm³ (μL)	Number fraction 0.01-0.03
	Basophils	0%-0.75% 15-50 cells/mm³ (μL)	Number fraction 0-0.0075
Mean Corpuscular hemoglobin (MCH)			
Whole blood	Birth	31-37 pg/cell	0.48-0.57 fmol/cell
	1-3 d (cap)	31-37 pg/cell	0.48-0.57 fmol/cell
	1 wk-1 mo	28-40 pg/cell	0.43-0.62 fmol/cell
	2 mo	26-34 pg/cell	0.40-0.53 fmol/cell
	3-6 mo	25-35 pg/cell	0.39-0.54 fmol/cell
	0.5-2 yr	23-31 pg/cell	0.36-0.48 fmol/cell
	2-6 yr	24-30 pg/cell	0.37-0.47 fmol/cell
	6-12 yr	25-33 pg/cell	0.39-0.51 fmol/cell
	12-18 yr	25-35 pg/cell	0.39-0.54 fmol/cell
	18-49 yr	26-34 pg/cell	0.40-0.53 fmol/cell
Mean corpuscular hemoglobin concentration (MCHC)			
Whole blood	Birth	30%-36% Hb/cell or g Hb/dL RBC	4.65-5.58 mmol Hb/L RBC
	1-3 d (cap)	29%-37% Hb/cell or g Hb/dL RBC	4.50-5.74 mmol Hb/L RBC
	1-2 wk	28%-38% Hb/cell or g Hb/dL RBC	4.34-5.89 mmol Hb/L RBC
	1-2 mo	29%-37% Hb/cell or g Hb/dL RBC	4.50-5.74 mmol Hb/L RBC
	3 mo-2 yr	30%-36% Hb/cell or g Hb/dL RBC	4.65-5.58 mmol Hb/L RBC
	2-18 yr	31%-37% Hb/cell or g Hb/dL RBC	4.81-5.74 mmol Hb/L RBC
	>18 yr	31%-37% Hb/cell or g Hb/dL RBC	4.81-5.74 mmol Hb/L RBC

Continued

TEST/SPECIMEN	AGE/GENDER/REFERENCE	NORMAL RANGES	
		CONVENTIONAL UNITS	INTERNATIONAL UNITS (SI)
Mean corpuscular volume (MCV)			
Whole blood	1-3 d (cap)	95-121 μm^3	95-121 fL
	0.5-2 yr	70-86 μm^3	70-86 fL
	6-12 yr	77-95 μm^3	77-95 fL
	12-18 yr: Male	78-98 μm^3	78-98 fL
	Female	78-102 μm^3	78-102 fL
Osmolality			
Serum	Child, adult	275-295 mOsm/kg H_2O	
Urine, random		50-1400 mOsm/kg H_2O, depending on fluid intake; after 12-hr fluid restriction: >850 mOsm/kg H_2O	
Urine, 24 hr		≈300-900 mOsm/kg H_2O	
Oxygen, partial pressure (Po_2)			
Whole blood, arterial	Birth	8-24 mm Hg	1.1-3.2 kPa
	5-10 min	33-75 mm Hg	4.4-10.0 kPa
	30 min	31-85 mm Hg	4.1-11.3 kPa
	>1 hr	55-80 mm Hg	7.3-10.6 kPa
	1 d	54-95 mm Hg	7.2-12.6 kPa
	Thereafter (decreased with age)	83-108 mm Hg	11-14.4 kPa
Oxygen saturation (Sao_2)			
Whole blood, arterial	Newborn	85%-90%	Fraction saturated 0.85-9.90
	Thereafter	95%-99%	Fraction saturated 0.95-0.99
Partial thromboplastin time (PTT)			
Whole blood (Na citrate)			
Nonactivated		60-85 sec (Platelin)	60-85 sec
Activated		25-35 sec (differs with method)	25-35 sec
pH			H^+ concentration
Whole blood, arterial	Premature	7.35-7.50	31-44 nmol/L
	Birth, full term	7.11-7.36	43-77 nmol/L
	5-10 min	7.09-7.30	50-81 nmol/L
	30 min	7.21-7.38	41-61 nmol/L
	>1 hr	7.26-7.49	32-54 nmol/L
	1 d	7.29-7.45	35-51 nmol/L
	Thereafter	7.35-7.45	35-44 nmol/L
	Must be corrected for body temperature		0.1-10 $\mu mol/L$
Urine, random	Newborn/neonate	5-7	0.01-32 $\mu mol/L$ (average ≈1.0 $\mu mol/L$)
	Thereafter	4.5-8	31-100 nmol/L
Stool		7.0-7.5	
Phenylalanine			120-450 $\mu mol/L$
Serum	Premature	2.0-7.5 mg/dL	70-120 $\mu mol/L$
	Newborn	1.2-3.4 mg/dL	50-110 $\mu mol/L$
	Thereafter	0.8-1.8 mg/dL	6-12 $\mu mol/day$
Urine, 24 hr	10 d-2 wk	1-2 mg/day	24-110 $\mu mol/day$
	3-12 yr	4-18 mg/day	Trace-103 $\mu mol/day$
	Thereafter	Trace-17 mg/day	
Plasma volume			0.025-0.043 L/kg
Plasma	Male	25-43 mL/kg	0.028-0.045 L/kg
	Female	28-45 mL/kg	
Platelet count (thrombocyte count)			84-478 × $10^9/L$
Whole blood (EDTA)	Newborn (after 1 wk, same as adult)	84-478 × $10^3/mm^3$ (μl)	
	Adult	150-400 × $10^3/mm^3$ (μl)	150-400 × $10^9/L$
Potassium			3.0-6.0 mmol/L
Serum	Newborn	3.0-6.0 mEq/L	3.5-5.0 mmol/L
	Thereafter	3.5-5.0 mEq/L	3.4-4.5 mmol/L
Plasma (heparin)		3.4-4.5 mEq/L	2.5-125 mmol/L
Urine, 24 hr		2.5-125 mEq/day; varies with diet	

■ **Common Laboratory Tests and Test Results**—*cont'd*

TEST/SPECIMEN	AGE/GENDER/REFERENCE	NORMAL RANGES	
		CONVENTIONAL UNITS	INTERNATIONAL UNITS (SI)
Protein			
Serum, total	Premature	4.3-7.6 g/dL	43-76 g/L
	Newborn	4.6-7.4 g/dL	46-74 g/L
	1-7 yr	6.1-7.9 g/dL	61-79 g/L
	8-12 yr	6.4-8.1 g/dL	64-81 g/L
	13-19 yr	6.6-8.2 g/dL	66-82 g/L
Total			
Urine, 24 hr		1-14 mg/dL	10-140 mg/L
		50-80 mg/day (at rest)	50-80 mg/day
		<250 mg/day after intense exercise	<250 mg/day after intense exercise
CSF		Lumbar: 8-32 mg/dL	80-320 mg/L
Prothrombin time (PT)			
One-stage (Quick)	In general	11-15 sec (varies with type of thromboplastin)	11-15 sec
Whole blood (Na citrate)	Newborn	Prolonged by 2-3 sec	Prolonged by 2-3 sec
Two-stage modified (Ware and Seegers)			
Whole blood (Na citrate)		18-22 sec	18-22 sec
RBC count: see Erythrocyte count			
Red blood cell volume			
Whole blood	Male	20-36 mL/kg	0.020-0.036 L/kg
	Female	19-31 mL/kg	0.019-0.031 L/kg
Reticulocyte count			
Whole blood	Adults	0.5%-1.5% of erythrocytes or 25,000-75,000.mm³ (μl)	0.005-0.015 (number fraction) or 25,000-75,000 × 10⁶/L
Capillary	1 d	0.4%-6.0%	0.004-0.060 (number fraction)
	7 d	<0.1%-1.3%	<0.001-0.013 (number fraction)
	1-4 wk	<0.1%-1.2%	<0.001-0.012 (number fraction)
	5-6 wk	<0.1%-2.4%	<0.001-0.024 (number fraction)
	7-8 wk	<0.1%-2.9%	<0.001-0.029 (number fraction)
	9-10 wk	<0.1%-2.6%	<0.001-0.026 (number fraction)
	11-12 wk	0.1%-1.3%	0.001-0.013 (number fraction)
Salicylates			
Serum, plasma	Therap. conc.	15-30 mg/dL	1.1-2.2 mmol/L
	Toxic conc.	>30 mg/dL	>18.5 mmol/L
Sedimentation rate: see Erythrocyte sedimentation rate			
Sodium			
Serum or plasma	Newborn	134-146 mEq/L	134-146 mmol/L
	Infant	139-146 mEq/L	139-146 mmol/L
	Child	138-145 mEq/L	138-145 mmol/L
	Thereafter	136-146 mEq/L	40-220 mmol/L
Urine, 24 hr		40-220 mEq/L (diet dependent)	40-220 mmol/L
Sweat	Normal	<40 mEq/L	<40 mmol/L
	Indeterminate	45-60 mEq/L	45-60 mmol/L
	Cystic fibrosis	>60 mEq/L	>60 mmol/L
Specific gravity			
Urine, random	Adult	1.002-1.030	1.002-1.030
	After 12-hr fluid restriction	>1.025	>1.025
Theophylline			
Serum, plasma	Therap. conc.		
	Bronchodilator	10-20 μg/mL	56-110 μmol/L
	Premature apnea	5-10 μg/mL	28-56 μmol/L
	Toxic conc.	>20 μg/mL	>110 μmol/L
Thrombin time			
Whole blood (Na citrate)		Control time ±2 sec when control is 9-13 sec	Control time ±2 sec when control is 9-13 sec

Continued

■ Common Laboratory Tests and Test Results—*cont'd*

TEST/SPECIMEN	AGE/GENDER/REFERENCE	NORMAL RANGES CONVENTIONAL UNITS	NORMAL RANGES INTERNATIONAL UNITS (SI)
Thyroxine, total (T_3)			
Serum	Cord	8-13 μg/dL	103-168 nmol/L
	Newborn	11.5-24 (lower in low-birth-weight infants)	148-310 nmol/L
	Neonate	9-18 μg/dL	116-232 nmol/L
	Infant	7-15 μg/dL	90-194 nmol/L
	1-5 yr	7.3-15 μg/dL	94-194 nmol/L
	5-10 yr	6.4-13.3 μg/dL	83-172 nmol/L
	Thereafter	5-12 μg/dL	65-155 nmol/L
	Newborn screen (filter paper)	6.2-22 μg/dL	80-284 nmol/L

TEST/SPECIMEN	AGE/GENDER/REFERENCE	mg/dl Male	mg/dl Female	g/L Male	g/L Female
Triglycerides (TG)					
Serum, after ≥12-hr fast					
	Cord blood	10-98	10-98	0.10-0.98	0.10-0.98
	0-5 yr	30-86	32-99	0.30-0.86	0.32-0.99
	6-11 yr	31-108	35-114	0.31-1.08	0.35-1.14
	12-15 yr	36-138	41-138	0.36-1.38	0.41-1.38
	16-19 yr	40-163	40-128	0.40-1.63	0.40-1.28

TEST/SPECIMEN	AGE/GENDER/REFERENCE	CONVENTIONAL UNITS	INTERNATIONAL UNITS (SI)
Triiodothyronine, free			
Serum	Cord	20-240 pg/dL	0.3-3.7 pmol/L
	1-3 d	200-610 pg/dL	3.1-9.4 pmol/L
	6 wk	240-560 pg/dL	3.7-8.6 pmol/L
	Adults (20-50 yr)	230-660 pg/dL	3.5-10.0 pmol/L
Triiodothyronine, total (T_3-RIA)			
Serum	Cord	30-70 ng/dL	0.46-1.08 nmol/L
	Newborn	72-260 ng/dL	1.16-4 nmol/L
	1-5 yr	100-260 ng/dL	1.54-4 nmol/L
	5-10 yr	90-240 ng/dL	1.39-3.70 nmol/L
	10-15 yr	80-210 ng/dL	1.23-3.23 nmol/L
	Thereafter	115-190 ng/dL	1.77-2.93 nmol/L
Urea nitrogen			
Serum or plasma	Cord	21-40 mg/dL	7.5-14.3 mmol/L
	Premature (1 wk)	3-25 mg/dL	1.1-9 mmol/L
	Newborn	3-12 mg/dL	1.1-4.3 mmol/L
	Infant/child	5-18 mg/dL	1.8-6.4 mmol/L
	Thereafter	7-18 mg/dL	2.5-6.4 mmol/L
Urine volume			
Urine, 24 hr	Newborn	50-300 mL/d	0.050-0.3 L/day
	Infant	350-550 mL/d	0.350-0.5 L/day
	Child	500-1000 mL/d	0.500-1 L/day
	Adolescent	700-1400 mL/d	0.700-1.4 L/day
	Thereafter: Male	800-1800 mL/d	0.800-1.8 L/day
	Female	600-1600 mL/d (varies with intake and other factors)	0.600-1.6 L/day

WBC: see Leukocyte count

■ Abbreviations Used in Laboratory Tests

ABBREVIATION	TERM
cap	capillary
CHF	congestive heart failure
conc.	concentration
CSF	cerebrospinal fluid
d	day; diem
EDTA	ethylenediaminetetraacetate
g	gram
m	meter
hr	hour
L, l	liter
mEq	milliequivalent
min	minute
mm	millimeter
mm^3	cubic millimeter
mo	month
mol	mole
mOsmol	milliosmole
sec	second
SI	International system of units
Therap.	therapeutic
U	International unit of enzyme activity
vol	volume
wk	week
yr	year
>	greater than
≥	greater than or equal to
<	less than
≤	less than or equal to
±	plus/minus
≈	approximately equal to

■ Prefixes Denoting Decimal Factors

PREFIX	SYMBOL	AMOUNT
deci	d	one tenth (10^{-1})
centi	c	one hundredth (10^{-2})
milli	m	one thousandth (10^{-3})
micro	μ	one millionth (10^{-6})
nano	n	one billionth (10^{-9})
pico	p	one trillionth (10^{-12})
femto	f	one quadrillionth (10^{-15})

Dietary Reference Intakes: Recommended Dietary Allowances (RDA) and Adequate Intake (AI)*

CATEGORY	AGE (YEARS) OR CONDITION	WEIGHT (kg)	WEIGHT (lb)	HEIGHT (cm)	HEIGHT (in)	PROTEIN RDA (g/kg)	FAT-SOLUBLE VITAMINS VITAMIN A RDA (μg/d)[a]	VITAMIN D AI (μg/d)[b]	VITAMIN E RDA (mg/d)[c]	VITAMIN K AI (μg/d)
Infants	0.0-0.5	6	13	62	24		400	5	4	2
	0.5-1.0	9	20	71	28		500	5	5	2.5
Children	1-3	12	27	86	34	1.10	300	5	6	30
	4-8	20	44	115	45	0.95	400	5	7	55
Males	9-13	36	79	144	57	0.95	600	5	11	60
	14-18	61	134	174	68	0.85	900	5	15	75
	19-30	70	154	177	70	0.80	900	5	15	120
Females	9-13	37	81	144	57	0.95	600	5	11	60
	14-18	54	119	163	64	0.85	700	5	15	75
	19-30	57	126	163	64	0.80	700	5	15	90
Pregnant	≤18					+25 g/d	750	5	15	75
Lactating	≤18					+25 g/d	1200	5	19	75

*NOTE: For all nutrients, values for infants are AI

Modified from the *Dietary Reference Intake* series, National Academy of Sciences, National Academies Press, 1997, 1998, 2000, 2001; and American Academy of Pediatrics: *Pediatric nutrition handbook* ed 5, Washington, DC, 2004, National Academies Press.

[a]Retinol equivalent (RAE). 1 RAE = 1 μg retinol.

[b]Cholecalciferol. 1 μg cholecalciferol = 40 IU vitamin D. Assumes an absence of adequate exposure to sunlight.

[c]Expressed as α-tocopherol

[d]Expressed as niacin equivalents (NE); except for infants <6 months of age, expressed as preformed niacin. 1 mg niacin = 60 mg tryptophan.

[e]Expressed as dietary folate equivalents (DFE); 1 DFE = 1 μg food folate = 0.6 μg folic acid from fortified food or as a supplement consumed with food = 5 μg of a supplement taken on an empty stomach.

[f]In view of evidence linking folate intake with neural tube defects in the fetus, it is recommended that all women capable of becoming pregnant consume 400 μg from supplements or fortified foods in addition to intake of food folate from the diet.

[g]It is assumed all women will continue consuming 400 μg from supplements or fortified food until their pregnancy is confirmed and they enter prenatal care, which ordinarily occurs after the end of the preconceptional period—the critical time for formation of the neural tube.

	WATER-SOLUBLE VITAMINS							MINERALS					
VITA-MIN C RDA (mg/d)	THIAMIN RDA (mg/d)	RIBO-FLAVIN RDA (mg/d)	NIACIN RDA (mg/d)d	VITA-MIN B6 RDA (mg/d)	FOLATE RDA (μg/d)e	VITA-MIN B12 RDA (μg/d)	CALCIUM AI (mg/d)	PHOS-PHORUS RDA (mg/d)	MAGNE-SIUM RDA (mg/d)	IRON RDA (mg/d)	ZINC RDA (mg/d)	IODINE RDA (μg/d)	SELE-NIUM RDA (μg/d)
40	0.2	0.3	2	0.1	65	0.4	210	100	30	0.27	2	110	15
50	0.3	0.4	4	0.3	80	0.5	270	275	75	11	3	130	20
15	0.5	0.5	6	0.5	150	0.9	500	460	80	7	3	90	20
25	0.6	0.6	8	0.6	200	1.2	800	500	130	10	5	90	30
45	0.9	0.9	12	1	300	1.8	1300	1250	240	8	8	120	40
75	1.2	1.3	16	1.3	400	2.4	1300	1250	410	11	11	150	55
90	1.2	1.3	16	1.3	400	2.4	1000	700	400	8	11	150	55
45	0.9	0.9	12	1	300	1.8	1300	1250	240	8	8	120	40
65	1	1	14	1.2	400	2.4	1300	1250	360	15	9	150	55
75	1.1	1.1	14	1.3	400f	2.4	1000	700	310	18	8	150	55
80	1.4	1.4	18	1.9	600g	2.6	1300	1250	400	27	13	220	60
115	1.4	1.6	17	2	500	2.8	1300	1250	360	10	14	290	70

■ Estimated Safe and Adequate Daily Dietary Intakes of Selected Vitamins and Minerals[a]

CATEGORY	AGE (YEARS)	VITAMINS		TRACE ELEMENTS[b]				
		BIOTIN (μg)	PANTOTHENIC ACID (mg)	COPPER (mg)	MANGANESE (mg)	FLUORIDE (mg)	CHROMIUM (μg)	MOLYBDENUM (μg)
Infants	0-0.5	10	2	0.4-0.6	0.3-0.6	0.1-0.5	10-40	15-30
	0.5-1	15	3	0.6-0.7	0.6-1.0	0.2-1.0	20-60	20-40
Children and adolescents	1-3	20	3	0.7-1.0	1.0-1.5	0.5-1.5	20-80	25-50
	4-6	25	3-4	1.0-1.5	1.5-2.0	1.0-2.5	30-120	30-75
	7-10	30	4-5	1.0-2.0	2.0-3.0	1.5-2.5	50-200	50-150
	11+	30-100	4-7	1.5-2.5	2.0-5.0	1.5-2.5	50-200	75-250
Adults		30-100	4-7	1.5-3.0	2.0-5.0	1.5-4.0	50-200	75-250

From Food and Nutrition Board, National Research Council: *Recommended dietary allowances,* ed 10, Washington, DC, 1989, National Academy of Sciences.

[a]Because there is less information on which to base allowances, these figures are not given in the main table of RDAs and are provided here in the form of ranges of recommended intakes.

[b]Since the toxic levels for many trace elements may be only several times usual intakes, the upper levels for the trace elements given in this table should not be habitually exceeded.

■ Estimated Sodium, Chloride, and Potassium Minimum Requirements of Healthy Persons[a]

AGE	WEIGHT (kg)[a]	SODIUM (mg)[a,b]	CHLORIDE (mg)[a,b]	POTASSIUM (mg)[c]
MONTHS				
0-5	4.5	120	180	500
6-11	8.9	200	300	700
YEARS				
1	11.0	225	350	1000
2-5	16.0	300	500	1400
6-9	25.0	400	600	1600
10-18	50.0	500	750	2000
>18[d]	70.0	500	750	2000

From Food and Nutrition Board, National Research Council: *Recommended dietary allowances,* ed 10, Washington, DC, 1989, National Academy of Sciences.

[a]No allowance has been included for large, prolonged losses from the skin through sweat.

[b]There is no evidence that higher intakes confer any health benefit.

[c]Desirable intakes of potassium may considerably exceed these values (~3500 mg for adults).

[d]No allowance included for growth. Values for those younger than 18 years of age assume a growth rate at the 50th percentile reported by the National Center for Health Statistics and averaged for males and females.

■ Median Heights and Weights and Estimated Energy Requirements (EER)*

CATEGORY	AGE (YEARS) OR CONDITION	WEIGHT		HEIGHT		Energy EER (kcal/d) (male/female)
		(kg)	(lb)	(cm)	(in)	
Infants	0.0-0.5	6	13	62	24	570/520
	0.5-1.0	9	20	71	28	743/676
Children	1-3	12	27	86	34	1046/992
	4-8	20	44	115	45	1742/1642
Males	9-13	36	79	144	57	2279
	14-18	61	134	174	68	3152
	19-30	70	154	177	70	3067
Females	9-13	37	81	144	57	2071
	14-18	54	119	163	64	2368
	19-30	57	126	163	64	2403
Pregnant	1st trimester					2368
	2nd trimester					2708
	3rd trimester					2820
Lactating	1st 6 months					2698
	2nd 6 months					2768

Modified from the *Dietary Reference Intake* series, National Academy of Sciences, National Academies Press, 1997, 1998, 2000, 2001; and American Academy of Pediatrics: *Pediatric Nutrition Handbook,* ed 5, Washington, DC, 2004, National Academies Press.

*The Estimated Energy Requirement (EER) represents an average dietary energy intake that will maintain energy balance in a healthy individual based upon gender, age,

Activity intolerance
Activity intolerance, risk for
Adjustment, impaired
Airway clearance, ineffective
Allergy response, latex
Allergy response, risk for latex
Anxiety
Anxiety, death
Aspiration, risk for
Attachment, risk for impaired parent/infant/child
Autonomic dysreflexia
Body image, disturbed
Body temperature, imbalanced, risk for
Bowel incontinence
Breast-feeding, effective
Breast-feeding, ineffective
Breast-feeding, interrupted
Breathing pattern, ineffective
Cardiac output, decreased
Caregiver role strain
Caregiver role strain, risk for
Comfort, impaired
Communication, impaired verbal
Communication, readiness for enhanced
Conflict, decisional
Conflict, parental role
Confusion, acute
Confusion, chronic
Constipation
Constipation, perceived
Constipation, risk for
Coping, compromised family
Coping, defensive
Coping, disabled family
Coping, ineffective
Coping, ineffective community
Coping, readiness for enhanced
Coping, readiness for enhanced family
Denial, ineffective
Dentition, impaired
Development, risk for delayed
Diarrhea
Disuse syndrome, risk for
Diversional activity, deficient
Energy field, disturbed
Environmental interpretation syndrome, impaired
Failure to thrive, adult
Falls, risk for
Family processes, alcoholism dysfunctional
Family processes, interrupted
Family processes, readiness for enhanced
Fatigue
Fear
Fluid balance, readiness for enhanced
Fluid volume, deficient
Fluid volume excess
Fluid volume, risk for deficient

Fluid volume, risk for imbalanced
Gas exchange, impaired
Grieving
Grieving, anticipatory
Grieving, dysfunctional
Growth, risk for disproportionate
Growth and development, delayed
Health maintenance, ineffective
Health-seeking behaviors
Home maintenance, impaired
Hopelessness
Hyperthermia
Hypothermia
Identity, disturbed personal
Incontinence, functional urinary
Incontinence, reflex urinary
Incontinence, stress urinary
Incontinence, total urinary
Incontinence, urge urinary
Incontinence, risk for urge urinary
Infant behavior, disorganized
Infant behavior, readiness for enhanced organized
Infant behavior, risk for disorganized
Infant feeding pattern, ineffective
Infection, risk for
Injury, risk for
Injury, risk for perioperative-positioning
Intracranial adaptive capacity, decreased
Knowledge, deficient
Knowledge of, readiness for enhanced
Loneliness, risk for
Memory, impaired
Mobility, impaired bed
Mobility, impaired physical
Mobility, impaired wheelchair
Nausea
Neglect, unilateral
Noncompliance
Nutrition, readiness for enhanced
Nutrition, less than body requirements imbalanced
Nutrition, more than body requirements imbalanced
Nutrition, more than body requirements, risk for imbalanced
Oral mucous membrane, impaired
Pain, acute
Pain, chronic
Parenting, impaired
Parenting, readiness for enhanced
Parenting, risk for impaired
Peripheral neurovascular dysfunction, risk for
Poisoning, risk for
Posttrauma syndrome
Posttrauma syndrome, risk for
Powerlessness
Powerlessness, risk for
Protection, ineffective

Rape-trauma syndrome
Rape-trauma syndrome: compound reaction
Rape-trauma syndrome: silent reaction
Relocation stress syndrome
Relocation stress syndrome, risk for
Role performance, ineffective
Self-care deficit, bathing/hygiene
Self-care deficit, feeding
Self-care deficit, toileting
Self-concept, readiness for enhanced
Self-esteem, chronic low
Self-esteem, situational low
Self-esteem, risk for situational low
Self-mutilation
Self-mutilation, risk for
Sensory perception, disturbed
Sexual dysfunction
Sexuality patterns, ineffective
Skin integrity, impaired
Skin integrity, risk for impaired
Sleep, readiness for enhanced
Sleep deprivation
Sleep pattern, disturbed
Social interaction, impaired
Social isolation
Sorrow, chronic
Spiritual distress
Spiritual distress, risk for
Spiritual well-being, readiness for enhanced
Sudden Infant Death Syndrome, risk for
Suffocation, risk for
Suicide, risk for
Surgical recovery, delayed
Swallowing, impaired
Therapeutic regimen management, effective
Therapeutic regimen management, ineffective
Therapeutic regimen management, ineffective community
Therapeutic regimen management, ineffective family
Therapeutic regimen management, readiness for enhanced
Thermoregulation, ineffective
Thought processes, disturbed
Tissue integrity, impaired
Tissue perfusion, ineffective
Transfer ability, impaired
Trauma, risk for
Urinary elimination, impaired
Urinary elimination, readiness for enhanced
Urinary retention
Ventilation, impaired spontaneous
Ventilatory weaning response, dysfunction
Violence, risk for other-directed
Violence, risk for self-directed
Walking, impaired
Wandering

North American Nursing Diagnosis Association International: *Nursing diagnoses: definitions and classification 2003-2004,* Philadelphia, 2003, NANDA International.

Translations of Wong-Baker FACES Pain Rating Scale*

TRANSLATIONS OF WONG-BAKER FACES PAIN RATING SCALE*

0–5 coding	0	1	2	3	4	5
0-10 coding	0	2	4	6	8	10
ENGLISH	No hurt	Hurts little bit	Hurts little more	Hurts even more	Hurts whole lot	Hurts worst
SPANISH	No duele	Duele un poco	Duele un poco más	Duele mucho	Duele mucho más	Duele el máximo
FRENCH	Pas mal	Un petit peu mal	Un peu plus mal	Encore plus mal	Très mal	Très très mal
ITALIAN	Non fa male	Fa male un poco	Fa male un po di piu	Fa male ancora di piu	Fa molto male	Fa maggiormente male
PORTUGUESE	Não doi	Doi um pouco	Doi um pouco mais	Doi muito	Doi muito mais	Doi o máximo
BOSNIAN	Ne boli	Boli samo malo	Boli malo više	Boli još više	Boli puno	Boli najviše
VIETNAMESE	Không dau	Hỏi dau	Dau hỏn chút	Dau nhiêu hỏn	Dau thât nhiêu	Dau qúa dô
CHINESE†	無痛	微痛	較痛	更痛	很痛	劇痛
GREEK	Δεν Πονάϊ	Πονάϊ Λιγο	Πονάϊ Λιγο Πιο Πολν	Πονάϊ Πολν	Πονάϊ Πιο Πολν	Πονάϊ Παρα Πολν
ROMANIAN	No doare	Doare puţin	Doare un pic mai mult	Doare şi mai mult	Doare foarte tare	Doare cel mai mult

Brief Word Instructions (Above)

Point to each face using the words to describe the pain intensity. Ask person to choose face that best describes own pain and record the appropriate number. NOTE: Rating scale can be used with people 3 years and older.

NOTE: In a study of 148 children ages 4 to 5 years, there were no differences in pain scores when children used the original or brief word instructions. (In Wong D, Baker C: *Reference manual for the Wong-Baker FACES Pain Rating Scale,* Duarte, Calif, 1998, City of Hope Mayday Pain Resource Center; also available on website: http://evolve.elsevier.com/Wong/essentials/).

---

*Wong-Baker FACES Pain Rating Scale: Available at no charge from The Purdue Frederick Company, 100 Connecticut Avenue, Norwalk, CT 06850-3590; (203) 853-0123, ext. 7378 or 7314. Spanish and Portuguese translations by Ellen Johnsen; French translation from Wong DL: *Soins infirmiers pediatrie,* Quebec, 2002, Editions Etudes Vivantes, Groupe Educalivres, Inc.; Italian translation by Madeline Mitchko; Romanian translation by Bogdan R. Dinu; Bosnian translation by Barbara Bogomolov; German translation from Wong DL: *Pediatric quick reference,* Berlin, Wiesbaden, 1997, Ullstein Mosby; Vietnamese translation by Yen B. Isle; Japanese translation from *After the announcement of cancer,* Tokyo, 1993, Iwanami Shoten, Pub; Chinese translation by Hung-Shen Lin.
†Chinese translation can be read by Japanese.

Original instructions:

English

Explain to the person that each face is for a person who feels happy because he has no pain (hurt) or sad because he has some or a lot of pain. **Face 0** is very happy because he doesn't hurt at all. **Face 1** hurts just a little bit. **Face 2** hurts a little more. **Face 3** hurts even more. **Face 4** hurts a whole lot. **Face 5** hurts as much as you can imagine, although you don't have to be crying to feel this bad. Ask the person to choose the face that best describes how he or she is feeling.

Rating scale is recommended for persons age 3 years and older.

Spanish

Expliquele a la persona que cada cara representa una persona que se siente feliz porque no tiene dolor o triste porque siente un poco o mucho dolor. **Cara 0** se siente muy feliz porque no tiene dolor. **Cara 1** tiene un poco de dolor. **Cara 2** tiene un poquito más de dolor. **Cara 3** tiene más dolor. **Cara 4** tiene mucho dolor. **Cara 5** tiene el dolor más fuerte que usted pueda imaginar, aunque usted no tiene que estar llorando para sentirse asi de mal. Pidale a la persona que escoja la cara que mejor describe su proprio dolor.

Esta escala se puede usar con personas de tres años de edad o más.

French

Expliquez à la personne que chaque visage représent un personne qui est heureux parce qu'elle n'a pas point du mal ou triste parce qu'il a un peu ou beaucoup du mal. **Visage 0** est trés heureux parce qu'elle n'a pas point du mal. **Visage 1** a un petit peu de mal. **Visage 2** a plus du mal. **Visage 3** a encore plus du mal. **Visage 4** a beaucoup du mal. **Visage 5** a autant mal que vous pouvez imaginer, bien que ces mauvais sentiments ne finissent pas nécessairement a vous faire pleurer. Demandez à la personne de choisir le visage qui convient le mieux avec ses sentiments.

Ces evaluations sont recommendés pour des personnes de trois ans et davantage.

Italian

Spiegare a la persona che ogni facien è per una persona che si sente felice perchè non tiene dolore oppure triste perchè ha poco o molto dolore. **Faccia O** è molto felice perchè non tiene dolore. **Faccia 1** tiene poco dolore. **Faccia 2** tiene un po più di dolore. **Faccia 3** tiene più dolore. **Faccia 4** tiene molto dolore. **Faccia 5** tiene molto dolore che non puoi immaginare però non devi piangere per tenere dolore. Domandi ala persona di scegliere quale faccia meglio descrive come si sente.

Grado scale è raccomandata a la persona di tre anni in sù.

Portuguese

Explique a pessoa que cada face representa uma pessoa que está feliz porque não têm dor, ou triste por ter um pouco ou muita dor. **Face 0** está muito feliz porque não têm nenhuma dor. **Face 1** tem apenas um pouco de dor. **Face 2** têm um pouco mais de dor. **Face 3** têm ainda mais dor. **Face 4** têm muita dor. **Face 5** têm uma dor máxima, apesar de que nem sempre provoca o choro. Peça a pessoa que escolhe a face que melhor descreve como ele se sente.

Esta escala é aplicável a pessoas de tres anos de idade ou mais.

Romanian

Explicati copilului că fiecare desen (figură) corespunde unei persoane care este veselă, pentru că nu are nici o durere, sau unei persoane care este tristă, pentru că are dureri. **Figura 0** este foarte fericită pentru că nu are nici o durere. **Figura 1** arată că doare doar un pic. **Figura 2** arată că doare ceva mai mult. **Figura 3** arată că doare şi mai mult. **Figura 4** arată că doare foarte tare. **Figura 5** arată că doare atât de tare cât se poate imagina, chiar dacă nu este însoţita neapărat de lacrimi. Cereţi copilului (persoanei) să indice figura care exprimă cel mai bine cum se simte el.

Scala de evaluare a durerii este recomandată pentru copiii în vârstă de 3 ani şi peste.

Bosnian

Objasnite osobi da je svako lice namjenjeno za osobu koja se osjeća sretnom jer ne osjeća bol ili tužnom jer osjeća malo ili puno boli. **Lice 0** je sretno jer ne osjeća nikakvu bol. **Lice 1** osjeća samo malu bol. **Lice 2** osjeća malo više boli. **Lice 3** osjeća još veću bol. **Lice 4** osjeća puno boli. **Lice 5** osjeća onoliku bol koju je moguće zamisliti, što ne znači da osoba koja osjeća tu bol mora plakati. Upitajte osobu da izabere lice koje najbolje opisuju kako se osjeća. Skala procijene bola se preporučuje za osobe starosti 3 godine ili više.

Upirati prstom na svako lice objašnjavajući riječima intensitet boli. Pitajte dijete da izabere lice koje najbolje opisuje njihovu bol i zabilježite odgovarajući broj.

German

Erläutern Sie dem Kind, daß jedes Gesicht zu einer Person gehört, die froh darüber ist, keine Schmerzen zu haben, oder die sehr traurig ist, weil sie mäßige bis starke Schmerzen hat. **Gesicht 0** ist sehr froh, weil es keine Schmerzen hat. **Gesicht 1** sagt, es tut ein bißchen weh. **Gesicht 2** hat ein bißchen mehr Schmerzen. **Gesicht 3** sagt, es tut noch mehr weh, und **Gesicht 4,** es tut ziemlich weh. **Gesicht 5** leidet unter so starken Schmerzen, wie Du Dir nur vorstellen kannst, auch wenn dabei nicht unbedingt Tränen fließen müssen. Bitten Sie das Kind, das Gesicht auszuwählen, das seinem Empfinden am besten entspricht. Empfohlen für Kinder ab 3 Jahren.

Vietnamese

Xin cắt nghĩa cho mỗi người, từng khuôn mặt của một người căm thấy vui vẻ tại vì không có sự đau đớn hoặc, buồn vì có chút ít hay rất nhiều sự đau đớn.

Cái **mặt** với **số** 0 thì rất là vui tại vì mặt ấy không có sự đau đớn. **Mặt số** 1 chỉ đau một chút thôi. **Mặt số** 2 hơi đau hơn một chút nữa. **Mặt số** 3 đau hơn chút nữa. **Mặt số** 4 đau thật nhiều. **Mặt số** 5 đau không thể tưởng tượng, mặc dù người ta không cần phải khóc mới cảm thấy được sự buồn khổ như thế.

Bạn hỏi từng người tự chọn khuôn mặt nào diễn tả được sự đau đớn của chính mình.

Japanese

　3歳以上の患者に望ましい。それぞれの顔は、患者の痛み (pain, hurt) がないのでご機嫌な感じ、または、ある程度の痛み・沢山の痛みがあるので悲しい感じを表現していることを説明して下さい。0＝痛みがまったくないから、とても幸せな顔をしている、1＝ほんの少し痛い、2＝もう少し痛い、3＝もっと痛い、4＝とっても痛い、5＝痛くて涙を流す必要はないけれども、これ以上の痛みは考えられないほど痛い。今、どのように感じているか最もよく表わしている顔を選ぶよう、患者に求めて下さい。

Chinese

　解釋給人聽用每張臉譜來代表著一個人的感覺是因爲沒有疼痛〔傷痛〕而感快樂或是因爲些許疼痛或者是許多疼痛而感傷心。第零張臉是很快樂的因爲他一點也不覺得疼痛。第一張臉只痛一丁點兒。第二張臉又痛多了一些。第三張臉痛得更多了。第四張臉是非常痛了。第五張臉是爲人們所能想像到的劇痛既使感到這樣難過，卻不一定哭出來。請這人選擇出最能代表他現在感覺的一張臉譜。此量表適用於三歲以上的人。

Spanish-English Translations

PHYSICAL EXAMINATION:

Open your mouth	Abre la boca
Breathe deeply	Respira profundo
Turn over	Voltéate
Hoarse	Ronco
Rash or skin lesion produced by insect bite	Rozadura o una lesión en la piel producida por una picadura de insecto
Rash	Roncha, salpullido, rozadura
Ringworm	Tiña
To tighten (grip)	Apretar
To loosen	Relajar, aflojar
Bruise	Moretón
Skin "spot" (like a blanching)	Mancha
Snore, stertor	Roncar
Snoring sound	Ronquido
Swollen	Hinchado

SYMPTOMS:

I would like to know if you have . . .	Quisiera saber si tienes . . .
. . . or have had	. . . o has tenido
cough	tos
runny nose	moquera
fever	fiebre o calentura
vomiting or nausea	vómito o náusea
diarrhea	diarrea
constipation	estreñimiento
pain	dolor
Allergic reaction	Reacción alérgica
Seizure	Convulsión
Sore throat	Dolor de garganta
Diaper dermatitis	Dermatitis por el pañal
Dizzy	Mareado(a)

HISTORY:

Are you sleeping well?	¿Estás durmiendo bien?
Have you had any trauma?	¿Has tenido algún trastorno o algún trauma?
Have you had any hemorrhage or loss of blood?	¿Has tenido una hemorragia o pérdida de sangre?
Problems during pregnancy or delivery?	¿Problemas en el embarazo o parto?
Born at term or premature?	¿Nació a tiempo o fue prematuro?
Did he get better after the treatment or the medicine given?	¿Mejoró después del tratamiento o después de haberle dado la medicina?
How many times did (he/she) urinate today?	¿Cuántas veces orinó hoy?
How many wet diapers has (he/she) had?	¿Cuántos pañales ha mojado?
How many dirty diapers?	¿Cuántos pañales sucios?
Where does it hurt?	¿Dónde te duele?
When did it start?	¿Cuándo empezó?

Does (he/she) have any allergies to medicine or food?	¿ El (ella) tiene alergia a alguna medicina o comida?
Up-to-date	Al día
Contagious	Contagioso
Stool (various terms)	Excremento, heces, popo
Has (she/he) had any chronic illnesses?	¿Él (ella) ha tenido alguna enfermedad crónica?
How many times did he/she vomit today?	¿Cuántas veces vomitó hoy?
Wheezing or adventitious sounds (in lungs)	Pillido o ruidos en los pulmones
Nasal secretions	Secreción nasal
Stuffy nose	Bloqueo nasal
Breathing problems	Dificultad para respirar
Thick discharge	Flujo grueso
Wound	Herida
Blood pressure	Presión arterial
Temperature	Temperatura
Fever	Calentura, fiebre
Pulse	Pulso
Heartbeat	Latido del corazón
Airway	Vía respiratoria
Vital signs	Signos vitals

SPECIFIC CONDITIONS:

Flu	Gripa
Croup	Crup
Bronchitis	Bronquitis
Burn	Quemadura
Rash or dermatitis	Erupción o rozadura
Pneumonia	Neumonía
Pertussis	Tos ferina
Measles	Sarampión
Mumps	Paperas
Chicken pox	Varicela
Rubella	Rubéola
Polio	Polio
Tetanus	Tétano
Vomiting	Vómito
Diarrhea	Diarrea
Asthma	Asma
Mucus	Moco
Seizures	Convulsions
Drainage	Drenaje
Immunization	Vacuna
Poison ivy	Hiedra venenosa
Bacterial infection	Infección bacterial
Viral infection	Infección viral
Diaper dermatitis	Dermatitis por causa del pañal
Rash or skin lesion produced by insect bite	Rozadura o lesión de la piel hecha por una picadura de insecto
Ulcer (as in mouth ulcers or chancre sores)	Úlceras o llagas en la boca

Gastritis	Gastritis, agruras		
Constipation	Estreñimiento		
Home remedies	Tratamientos caseros		
Fracture	Fractura		
Intensive care	Cuidado intensivo		
Immunizations	Vacunas		
Animal bite	Mordida de animal		
Menstrual period	Menstruación/período		
Birth control	Anticonceptivo		

EQUIPMENT:

Can mean NG tube or urinary catheter, can be any tube that has to be inserted into body (MicKey button; gastrostomy)	Sonda, catéter urinario, tubo que se introduce en el cuerpo
Gown	Bata
Suction	Succión
Sheet	Sábana
Diaper	Pañal
Bulb syringe	Saca mocos
Clothes, clothing	Ropa
Splint or cast	Férula o yeso
Dressing, bandage	Bendaje, gaza
Infusion pump	Máquina para infusion
Tape	Cinta
Teaspoon	Cucharadita
Cup (as in small medicine cup or drinking cup)	Taza
Syringe	Jeringa
Pill	Pastilla/Píldora
Needle	Aguja
Antibiotic	Antibiótico
Cotton swab	Algodón
Pacifier	Chupón
Bottle, as in baby bottle or medicine bottle	Biberón
Juice	Jugo
Milk	Leche

BODY PARTS:

Bone	Hueso
Blood	Sangre
Tongue	Lengua
Head	Cabeza
Arm	Brazo
Finger	Dedo
Leg	Pierna
Neck	Cuello
Elbow	Codo
Foot	Pie
Ear	Oreja
Nose	Nariz
Mouth	Boca
Bladder	Vejiga
Back	Espalda
Chest	Pecho
Spleen	Bazo
Gallbladder	Vesícula

PAIN MANAGEMENT:

Do you have any pain in the . . . ?	¿Tienes dolor . . . ?
headache	de cabeza
stomachache	de estómago
backache	de espalda
chest pain	en el pecho
in the arm	en el brazo
in the legs	en las piernas
in the mouth	en la boca
in the eyes	en los ojos
in the bladder	en la vejiga
How many hours, days, months, years have you had pain in the . . .	¿Por cuántos (cuántas) horas, días, meses, años has tenido dolor en . . . ?
Please show me where it hurts.	Muéstreme dónde te duele, por favor.
What medicine are you taking for pain?	¿Qué medicina estás tomando para el dolor?
What medicine have you taken for pain?	¿Qué medicina has tomado para el dolor?
Calm down	Cálmate
This won't hurt	Esto no te va a doler

PROCEDURES:

Injection	Inyección
Lumbar puncture	Punción lumbar
Oral hydration solution (such as Pedialyte)	Suero oral o por la boca
IV fluids	Suero intravenoso o por la vena
Start an IV	Vamos a ponerle suero intra-venoso o por la vena
Normal saline drops	Gotas de solución salina
Humidity	Humedad
Vaporizer	Vaporizador de aire
Breathing treatment	Tratamiento para la respiración
Humidity in the bathroom with a hot shower running	El vapor en el baño de la re-gadera o ducha de agua caliente
Stool sample	Muestra de heces (popo) excre-mento
We need to take some blood to see what exactly (illness) (he, she) has . . .	Tenemos que tomar una mues-tra de sangre para saber con seguridad lo que el o ella tiene o padece . . .
The results of your blood test show . . .	Los resultados de la sangre muestran
The most important thing is to decrease the fever with Tylenol or Motrin	Lo más importante es reducir la fiebre con Tylenol o Motrin
We will have to catheterize (him/her)	Tendremos que ponerle una sonda en la vejiga
Topical treatment	Tratamiento tópico
To suture	Suturar
A suture	Sutura
To swab (as in "swab the mouth" or "to place a cream on . . .")	Untar

He/she should take lots of clear liquids	Debe tomar bastantes líquidos claros	
To nurse, breast-feed	Amamantar	
To burp	Eructar	
X ray	Radiografía	
CT scan	Tomografía	
Nasal drops	Gotas nasales	
Put ice on it	Póngale hielo	

MISCELLANEOUS PHRASES:

He/she will need to be hospitalized for treatment . . . observation	Tendrá que ser hospitalizado(a) para darle tratamiento . . . ser observado(a)
We need a urine specimen in this cup	Necesitamos su muestra de orina en esta taza
Take him/her to the primary doctor tomorrow	Llévelo mañana a su doctor principal o de cabecera
He/she's very sick	Está muy enfermo(a)

Index